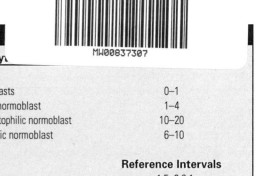

Bone Marrow Aspirate Reference Intervals (Adult)

WBC Differential	Reference Intervals (%)
Blasts	0–3
Promyelocytes	1–5
N. myelocytes	6–17
N. metamyelocytes	3–20
N. bands	9–32
N. segmented (polymorphonuclear)	7–30
Eosinophils	0–3
Basophils	0–1
Lymphocytes	5–18
Plasma cells	0–1
Monocytes	0–1
Histiocytes (macrophages)	0–1

Erythrocyte	Reference Intervals
Pronormoblasts	0–1
Basophilic normoblast	1–4
Polychromatophilic normoblast	10–20
Orthochromic normoblast	6–10

Other	Reference Intervals
M:E ratio	1.5–3.3:1
Megakaryocytes	2–10/lpf

Complete Blood Count Reference Intervals (Pediatric)

Assay	Units	0–1 d	2–4 d	5–7 d	8–14 d	15–30 d	1–2 mo	3–5 mo	6–11 mo	1–3 y	4–7 y	8–13 y
RBC	×10⁶/µL (×10¹²/L)	4.10–6.10	4.36–5.96	4.20–5.80	4.00–5.60	3.20–5.00	3.40–5.00	3.65–5.05	3.60–5.20	3.40–5.20	4.00–5.20	4.00–5.40
HGB	g/dL (g/L)	16.5–21.5 (165–215)	16.4–20.8 (164–208)	15.2–20.4 (152–204)	15.0–19.6 (150–196)	12.2–18.0 (122–180)	10.6–16.4 (106–164)	10.4–16.0 (104–160)	10.4–15.6 (104–156)	9.6–15.6 (96–156)	10.2–15.2 (102–152)	12.0–15.0 (120–150)
HCT	%	48–68	48–68	50–64	46–62	38–53	32–50	35–51	35–51	34–48	36–46	35–49
MCV	fL	95–125	98–118	100–120	95–115	93–113	83–107	83–107	78–102	76–92	78–94	80–94
MCH	pg	30–42	30–42	30–42	30–42	28–40	27–37	25–35	23–31	23–31	23–31	26–32
MCHC	g/dL	30–34	30–34	30–34	30–34	30–34	31–37	32–36	32–36	32–36	32–36	32–36
RDW	%	*	*	*	*	*	*	*	11.5–14.5	11.5–14.5	11.5–14.5	11.5–14.5
RETIC	%	1.8–5.8	1.3–4.7	0.2–1.4	0–1.0	0.2–1.0	0.8–2.8	0.5–1.5	0.5–1.5	0.5–1.5	0.5–1.5	0.5–1.5
RETIC	×10³/µL (×10⁹/L)	73.8–353.8	56.7–280.1	8.4–81.2	0.0–56.0	6.4–50.0	27.2–140.0	18.3–75.8	18.0–78.0	17.0–78.8	20–78.0	20–124.2
NRBC	/100 WBC	2–24	5–9	0–1	0	0	0	0	0	0	0	0
WBC	×10³/µL (×10⁹/L)	9.0–37.0	8.0–24.0	5.0–21.0	5.0–21.0	5.0–21.0	6.0–18.0	6.0–18.0	6.0–18.0	5.5–17.5	5.0–17.0	4.5–13.5
NEUT (ANC)	×10³/µL (×10⁹/L)	3.7–30.0	2.6–17.0	1.5–12.6	1.2–11.6	1.0–9.5	1.2–8.1	1.1–7.7	1.2–8.1	1.2–8.9	1.5–11.0	1.6–9.5
LYMPH	×10³/µL (×10⁹/L)	1.6–14.1	1.3–11.0	1.2–11.3	1.5–13.0	2.1–12.8	2.5–13.0	2.7–13.5	2.9–14.0	2.0–12.8	1.5–11.1	1.0–7.2
MONO	×10³/µL (×10⁹/L)	0.1–4.4	0.2–3.4	0.2–3.6	0.2–3.6	0.1–3.2	0.2–2.5	0.1–2.0	0.1–2.0	0.1–1.9	0.1–1.9	0.1–1.5
EO	×10³/µL (×10⁹/L)	0.0–1.5	0.0–1.2	0.0–1.3	0.0–1.1	0.0–1.1	0.0–0.7	0.0–0.7	0.0–0.7	0.0–0.7	0.0–0.7	0.0–0.5
BASO	×10³/µL (×10⁹/L)	0.0–0.7	0.0–0.5	0.0–0.4	0.0–0.4	0.0–0.4	0.0–0.4	0.0–0.4	0.0–0.4	0.0–0.4	0.0–0.3	0.0–0.3
PLT	×10³/µL (×10⁹/L)	150–450	150–450	150–450	150–450	150–450	150–450	150–450	150–450	150–450	150–450	150–450

*The RDW is markedly elevated in newborns, with a range of 14.2% to 19.9% in the first few days of life, gradually decreasing until it reaches adult levels by 6 months of age.

Pediatric reference intervals are from Riley Hospital for Children, Indiana University Health, Indianapolis, IN.

Some reference intervals are listed in common units and in international system of units (SI units) in parentheses.

ANC, Absolute neutrophil count (includes segmented neutrophils and bands); *BAND,* neutrophil bands; *BASO,* basophils; *d,* days; *EO,* eosinophils; *ESR,* erythrocyte sedimentation rate; *Hb,* hemoglobin fraction; *HCT,* hematocrit; *HGB,* hemoglobin; *lpf,* low power field; *LYMPH,* lymphocytes; *MCH,* mean cell hemoglobin; *MCHC,* mean cell hemoglobin concentration; *MCV,* mean cell volume; *M:E,* myeloid:erythroid; *mo,* month; *MONO,* monocytes; *MPV,* mean platelet volume; *N,* neutrophilic; *NEUT,* neutrophils; *NRBC,* nucleated red blood cells; *PLT,* platelets; *RBC,* red blood cell; *RDW,* red blood cell distribution width; *RETIC,* reticulocytes; *WBC,* white blood cell; *y,* year.

Please see inside back cover for additional reference interval tables.

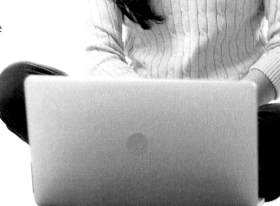

Rodak's
Hematology

Clinical Principles and Applications

Sixth Edition

Rodak's
Hematology
Clinical Principles and Applications

Elaine M. Keohane, PhD, MLS(ASCP)SH^{CM}
Professor Emeritus
Clinical Laboratory and Medical Imaging Sciences
School of Health Professions
Rutgers, The State University of New Jersey
Newark, New Jersey

Catherine N. Otto, PhD, MBA, MLS(ASCP)^{CM}, SH, DLM
Associate Professor
Clinical Laboratory and Medical Imaging Sciences
School of Health Professions
Rutgers, The State University of New Jersey
Newark, New Jersey

Jeanine M. Walenga, PhD, MLS(ASCP)H^{CM}
Professor, Thoracic-Cardiovascular Surgery, Pathology, and Physiology
Co-Director, Hemostasis and Thrombosis Research Unit
Health Sciences Division
Stritch School of Medicine
Loyola University Chicago
Maywood, Illinois
Laboratory Director, Clinical Coagulation
Laboratory Director, Urinalysis and Medical Microscopy
Associate Director, Point of Care & Referred Testing
Pathology and Laboratory Medicine
Loyola University Health System
Maywood, Illinois

ELSEVIER

RODAK'S HEMATOLOGY: CLINICAL PRINCIPLES AND APPLICATIONS, SIXTH EDITION

ISBN: 978-0-323-53045-3

Notice

Copyright 2016, 2012, 2007, 2002, 1995 by Saunders, an imprint of Elsevier, Inc.

International Standard Book Number: 978-0-323-53045-3

Executive Content Strategist: Kellie White
Senior Content Development Manager: Ellen Wurm-Cutter
Senior Content Development Specialist: Sarah Vora
Publishing Services Manager: Julie Eddy
Senior Project Manager: Richard Barber
Designer: Patrick Ferguson

Printed in the United States of America

Last digit is the print number: 9 8 7 6 5 4 3

3251 Riverport Lane
St. Louis, Missouri 63043

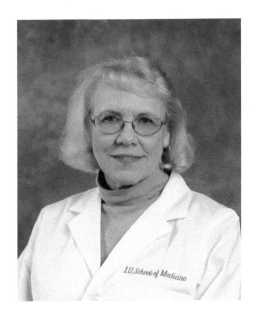

Bernadette "Bunny" F. Rodak, MS, MT(ASCP)SH, the founding author and editor of *Hematology: Clinical Principles and Applications* first published in 1995, passed away on March 22, 2016. It took courage and a love of hematology for Bunny to take on the project. For more than 20 years, and through five editions, she dedicated countless hours to publishing the highest-quality text, while mentoring and guiding five co-editors and more than 50 authors. Bunny considered it one of her greatest professional achievements, along with co-authoring five editions of the *Clinical Hematology Atlas* with her friend and colleague, Jacqueline Carr. With her great enthusiasm for hematology and life-long learning, Bunny inspired a generation of students and faculty in this country and around the world.

Bunny was a Professor of Pathology and Laboratory Medicine, and later Professor Emeritus in the Clinical Laboratory Science Program at Indiana University School of Medicine. She authored many professional publications and conducted many professional lectures and workshops throughout the United States. She used her expertise and dedication to others to lead a team of professionals to answer consumers' questions on clinical laboratory testing on the www.labtestsonline.org website. Bunny chaired the Hematology Committee of the National Credentialing Agency for Laboratory Personnel (NCA), preparing examinations to qualify clinical laboratory technicians, clinical laboratory scientists, and specialists in hematology. She was an active member of the American Society of Clinical Laboratory Science (ASCLS) for more than 40 years, including serving as editor of the journal, *Clinical Laboratory Science*. In 2013, ASCLS recognized her with their highest honor, the Robin H. Mendelson Award for her outstanding service and contributions to ASCLS, the ASCLS Education and Research Fund, and to the CLS profession.

Bunny was a pioneer and trailblazer who advanced her profession and served as a role model for her colleagues and students. She was always available to help a colleague and had a long history of community service. She lived her life with a spirit of helpfulness and kindness. We miss her smile and grace. Bunny's spirit lives on in this textbook and her colleagues are honored to continue her work.

The Current and Former Editors

To my students for being great teachers, and to Camryn, Riley, Harper, Stella, Jackie, Alana, Ken, and Jake for reminding me about the important things in life.

EMK

To the memories of Betsy Baptist, who introduced me to the Clinical Laboratory Science profession and Patricia M. Buckley, who encouraged me to chase my dreams.

CNO

To my teachers, both formal and informal, for all this fascinating knowledge in the clinical laboratory sciences, which made possible my interesting career.

JMW

Demetra Castillo, MAdEd, MLS(ASCP)^{CM}
Assistant Professor
Medical Laboratory Science
Rush University
Chicago, Illinois

Kathy W. Jones, MS, MLS(ASCP)^{CM}
Assistant Professor
College of Nursing and Health Sciences
Department of Medical and Clinical Laboratory Sciences
Auburn University, Montgomery
Montgomery, Alabama

Thomas Charles King, MD, PhD
Medical Director
Immunovia, Inc.
Marlborough, Massachusetts

Bernardino D. Madsen, MS, MLS(ASCP)
Program Director
MLT Program
Casper College
School of Health Sciences
Casper, Wyoming

Theresa McCreary, MS, MT(ASCP)SH
Research Coordinator
Office of Research Administration
DLP-Conemaugh Memorial Medical Center, LLC
Johnstown, Pennsylvania

Michelle Moy, EdD, MT(ASCP)SC
Program Director
Assistant Professor
Biological and Health Sciences
Madonna University
Livonia, Michigan

Christine M. Nebocat, MS, MLS(ASCP)^{CM}
Assistant Professor
Medical Laboratory Technology
Farmingdale State College
Farmingdale, New York
Medical Laboratory Technologist
Veterans' Affairs Center at Northport
Northport, New York

Pamela B. Primose PhD, MLS(ASCP)
Program Chair
Medical Laboratory Technology Program
Health Sciences
Ivy Tech Community College
South Bend, Indiana

Bentley H. Ried, MBA, MT(ASCP)
Program Director and Clinical Coordinator
Clinical Laboratory Clinical Laboratory Science
Howard University
Washington, District of Columbia

Linda Sykora, MSE, MLS(ASCP)SH^{CM}
Hematology Coordinator
Instructor
Division of Laboratory Science
University of Nebraska Medical Center
College of Allied Health Professions
Omaha, Nebraska

Catherine Thorp, BSC, MLT
Professor
Health Sciences
St. Lawrence College
Kingston, Ontario
Canada

CONTRIBUTORS

Nicholas C. Brehl, MEd, MLS(ASCP)^{CM}
Assistant Clinical Professor
Department of Pathology and Laboratory Medicine
Indiana University School of Medicine
Indianapolis, Indiana

Michelle Butina, PhD, MLS(ASCP)^{CM}
Program Director
Medical Laboratory Science
West Virginia University
Morgantown, West Virginia

Karen S. Clark, BS, MT(ASCP)SH
POC Supervisor
Pathology
Baptist Memorial Hospital Memphis
Memphis, Tennessee

Magdalena Czader, MD, PhD
Professor
Department of Pathology and Laboratory Medicine
Indiana University
Indianapolis, Indiana

Phillip J. DeChristopher, MD, PhD
Medical Director
Transfusion Medicine, Blood Bank, Apheresis
Professor of Pathology and Medicine
Loyola University Health System
Maywood, Illinois

Heather DeVries, BS, MT(ASCP)
Technical Specialist
Thrombosis and Hemostasis
Indiana University Health Pathology Laboratory
Indianapolis, Indiana

Kathryn Doig, PhD, MLS(ASCP)^{CM}SH^{CM}
Professor Emeritus
Biomedical Laboratory Diagnostics
Michigan State University
East Lansing, Michigan

George A. Fritsma, MS
Proprietor
The Fritsma Factor, Your Interactive Hemostasis Resource
Consultant
Laboratory Medicine
University of Alabama at Birmingham
Birmingham, Alabama
Adjunct Associate Professor
Clinical Laboratory and Medical Imaging Sciences
School of Health Professions
Rutgers, The State University of New Jersey
Newark, New Jersey
Associate Professor
Clinical Laboratory Sciences
Michigan State University
East Lansing, Michigan

Bertil Glader, MD, PhD
Professor
Pediatrics (Hematology/Oncology)
Stanford University
Stanford, California
Professor
Pathology (by courtesy)
Stanford University
Stanford, California

Linda H. Goossen, PhD, MT(ASCP)
Professor Emeritus
Diagnostic and Treatment Sciences
Grand Valley State University
Rockford, Michigan

Teresa G. Hippel, BS, MT(ASCP)SH
Quality Reviewer
Diagnostic Laboratories
Vanderbilt University Medical Center
Nashville, Tennessee

S. Renee Hodgkins, PhD, MT(ASCP)
Clinical Assistant Professor
Clinical Laboratory Science
University of Kansas Medical Center
Kansas City, Kansas

Debra A. Hoppensteadt, PhD, MT(ASCP)SH
Professor
Pathology and Pharmacology
Loyola University Chicago
Maywood, Illinois

Cynthia L. Jackson, PhD
Director of the Clinical Molecular Biology Laboratory
Department of Pathology
Lifespan Academic Medical Center
Providence, Rhode Island
Associate Professor
Pathology
Warren Alpert School of Medicine at Brown University
Providence, Rhode Island

Walter P. Jeske, PhD
Professor
Cardiovascular Research Institute
Health Sciences Division
Loyola University Chicago
Maywood, Illinois

Elaine M. Keohane, PhD, MLS(ASCP)SH^CM
Professor Emeritus
Clinical Laboratory and Medical Imaging Sciences
School of Health Professions
Rutgers, The State University of New Jersey
Newark, New Jersey

Ameet R. Kini, MD, PhD
Professor
Medical Director, Hematopathology
Pathology and Laboratory Medicine
Loyola University Health System and
Stritch School of Medicine
Loyola University Chicago
Maywood, Illinois

Clara Lo, MD
Clinical Associate Professor
Pediatric Hematology-Oncology
Stanford University
Palo Alto, California

Naveen Manchanda, MD
Associate Professor of Medicine
Department of Internal Medicine
Indiana University School of Medicine
Indianapolis, Indiana

Steven Marionneaux, MS, MT(ASCP)
Medical and Scientific Adviser
Cellavision AB
Lund, Sweden
Adjunct Assistant Professor
Clinical Laboratory and Medical Imaging Sciences
School of Health Professions
Rutgers, The State University of New Jersey
Newark, New Jersey

Peter Maslak, MD
Chief, Immunology Laboratory Service
Laboratory Medicine
Attending Physician, Leukemia Service
Internal Medicine
Memorial Sloan Kettering Cancer Center
New York, New York
Professor of Clinical Medicine
Internal Medicine
Weill Cornell Medical College
New York, New York

Shashi Mehta, PhD
Associate Professor
Clinical Laboratory and Medical Imaging Sciences
School of Health Professions
Rutgers, The State University of New Jersey
Newark, New Jersey

Kamran M. Mirza, MD, PhD, MLS(ASCP)
Assistant Professor
Medical Director, Molecular Pathology
Pathology and Laboratory Medicine
Loyola University Health System
Maywood, Illinois
Graduate Program Director, MS Program in Medical
    Laboratory Science
Medical Education
Stritch School of Medicine
Loyola University Chicago
Maywood, Illinois

Jo Ann Molnar, BS, MLS(ASCP)
Technical Specialist
Pathology and Laboratory Medicine
Loyola University Medical Center
Maywood, Illinois

Reeba A. Omman, MD
Assistant Professor
Pathology
University of Florida, Jacksonville
Jacksonville, Florida

Catherine N. Otto, PhD, MBA, MLS(ASCP)^{CM}, SH, DLM
Associate Professor
Clinical Laboratory and Medical Imaging Sciences
School of Health Professions
Rutgers, The State University of New Jersey
Newark, New Jersey

Ruth Perez, MS, MLS(ASCP)^{CM}
Clinical Coordinator, Lecturer
Clinical Laboratory and Medical Imaging Sciences
School of Health Professions
Rutgers, The State University of New Jersey
Newark, New Jersey

Tim R. Randolph, PhD, MT(ASCP)
Associate Professor
Clinical Health Sciences
Saint Louis University
St. Louis, Missouri

Kathleen M. Sakamoto, MD, PhD
Professor
Pediatrics
Stanford University
Stanford, California

Gail H. Vance, MD
Sutphin Professor of Cancer Genetics
Medical and Molecular Genetics
Indiana University School of Medicine
Indianapolis, Indiana
Professor
Pathology and Laboratory Medicine
Indiana University School of Medicine
Indianapolis, Indiana

Carolina Vilchez, MS, MLS(ASCP)H^{CM}
Clinical Educator
Medical Laboratory Science Program
The Valley Hospital
Ridgewood, New Jersey
Adjunct Assistant Professor
Clinical Laboratory and Medical Imaging Sciences
School of Health Professions
Rutgers, The State University of New Jersey
Newark, New Jersey

Jeanine M. Walenga, PhD, MLS(ASCP)H^{CM}
Professor
Thoracic-Cardiovascular Surgery, Pathology,
    and Physiology
Loyola University Chicago
Maywood, Illinois
Laboratory Director, Coagulation
Pathology and Laboratory Medicine
Loyola University Health System
Maywood, Illinois

Destiny D. Whitfield, MS, MLS(ASCP)
Medical Laboratory Scientist
Core Laboratory - Hematology
Vanderbilt University Medical Center
Nashville, Tennessee

The science of *clinical laboratory hematology* provides for the analysis of normal and pathologic peripheral blood cells, hematopoietic (blood-producing) tissue, and the cells in non-vascular body cavities such as cerebrospinal and serous fluids. Laboratory hematology also includes the analysis of the cells and coagulation proteins essential to clinical hemostasis. Hematology laboratory assay results are critical for the diagnosis, prognosis, and monitoring treatment for primary and secondary hematologic and hemostatic disorders. Similarly, hematology and hemostasis test results are used to establish safety in the perioperative period, monitor treatments during surgical procedures, and monitor transfusion needs in trauma patients.

Rodak's Hematology: Clinical Principles and Applications systematically presents basic to advanced concepts to provide a solid foundation of normal and pathologic states upon which readers can build their skills in interpreting and correlating laboratory findings in anemias, leukocyte disorders, and hemorrhagic and thrombotic conditions. It provides key features for accurate identification of normal and pathologic cells in blood, bone marrow, and body fluids. The focus, level, and detail of hematology and hemostasis testing, along with the related clinical applications, interpretation, and testing algorithms, make this text a valuable resource for all healthcare professionals managing these disorders.

The current practice of clinical laboratory hematology has been enhanced by profound changes as reflected in the numerous updates in the sixth edition of *Rodak's Hematology: Clinical Principles and Applications*. The value of the sixth edition comes from many improvements in the illustrations, tables, and layout of the chapter content, inclusion of state-of-the-art information, the addition of Catherine N. Otto as a new co-editor, joining continuing editors, Elaine M. Keohane and Jeanine M. Walenga, and fresh perspectives from new authorship of 20 chapters. Meticulous editing and attention to overall presentation of the material in the book add to the value of the sixth edition. Chapter highlights and new content are described below.

ORGANIZATION

Rodak's Hematology: Clinical Principles and Applications, sixth edition is organized into 7 parts and 43 chapters with an expanded appendix containing easy access to resource material and quick lookup reference intervals of all hematology and hemostasis parameters on the inside front and back covers to facilitate the learning process.

PART I: INTRODUCTION TO HEMATOLOGY

Chapter 1 previews the science of clinical laboratory hematology. Chapter 2 provides a comprehensive, updated coverage of quality assurance for laboratory testing with enhanced sections on method evaluation, assay validation, and a new section on multi-site validation and system-wide comparability.

PART II: BLOOD CELL PRODUCTION, STRUCTURE, AND FUNCTION

Chapters 3 and 4 include photomicrographs and figures to describe general cellular structure and function along with the morphologic and molecular details of hematopoiesis. Chapters 5, 9, and 10 discuss erythropoiesis, leukopoiesis, and megakaryopoiesis using numerous photomicrographs demonstrating ultrastructure and microscopic morphology. Chapter 6, updated with new detailed figures, and Chapter 7 examine mature red blood cell metabolism, hemoglobin structure and function, and red blood cell senescence and destruction. Iron kinetics and laboratory assessment in Chapter 8 was updated with new figures and coverage of systemic and cellular regulation of iron. Chapter 10 also includes a description of the function of platelets, detailing the primary hemostatic mechanisms of platelet adhesion, aggregation, and activation with updated figures, tables, and a new section on the platelet proteome.

PART III: LABORATORY EVALUATION OF BLOOD CELLS

Chapter 11 describes traditional (manual) clinical hematology laboratory procedures such as microscopy-based cell counts, hemoglobin and hematocrit determinations, as well as point-of-care technology. Chapter 12 includes descriptions and figures of the latest automated blood cell analyzers. New instrument parameters, capabilities, and digital data management have revolutionized the way blood specimens for the complete blood count, differential count, and morphology assessment are processed and analyzed, and how test results are reported and interpreted. Chapter 13 describes peripheral blood film examination and the differential cell count correlation to the complete blood count. Chapter 14 follows up with bone marrow aspirate and biopsy collection, preparation, examination, and reporting. Chapter 15 describes methods for analyzing normal and pathologic cells of cerebrospinal fluid, joint fluid, transudates, and exudates, illustrated with many excellent photomicrographs.

PART IV: ERYTHROCYTE DISORDERS

Chapter 16 provides an overview of the anemias and describes cost-effective diagnostic approaches that integrate patient history, physical examination, and symptoms with laboratory results for hemoglobin, red blood cell indices, reticulocyte count, and abnormal red blood cell morphology. Chapters 17 to 19 describe disorders of iron and DNA metabolism and bone marrow failure. Algorithms help the reader to distinguish types of microcytic and macrocytic anemias. Chapters 20 to 23 discuss hemolytic anemias due to intrinsic or extrinsic defects. Chapter 20 also has detailed figures that explain extravascular and intravascular hemolysis and hemoglobin catabolism. Chapters 24 and 25 provide updates in pathophysiology, diagnosis, and treatment of the hemoglobinopathies and thalassemias.

PART V: LEUKOCYTE DISORDERS

The chapters of this section were reordered beginning with non-malignant disorders, followed by an introduction to hematologic neoplasms, three chapters discussing diagnostic methodologies, followed by chapters discussing the major categories of hematologic neoplasms.

Chapter 26 is updated with many excellent photomicrographs and summary boxes of nonmalignant systemic disorders manifested by the abnormal distribution or morphology of leukocytes. These include bacterial and viral infections, various systemic disorders, and benign lymphoproliferative disorders. Chapter 27 is new to the sixth edition and provides an introduction to hematologic neoplasms, including sections on classification, molecular pathogenesis, and general categories of treatment options. Chapter 28 describes flow cytometry and its diagnostic applications, including numerous scatterplots of normal and leukemic conditions. Chapter 29 covers molecular diagnostics with many figures on basic molecular biology, end-point and real-time polymerase chain reaction, microarrays, and DNA sequencing, including next-generation sequencing. Molecular diagnosis has augmented and, in many instances, replaced long-indispensable laboratory assays. Chapter 30 provides details on traditional cytogenetic procedures for detection of quantitative and qualitative chromosome abnormalities and more sensitive methods such as fluorescence in situ hybridization (FISH) and genomic hybridization arrays. Chapters 31 to 34, with significant updating, provide the latest pathophysiologic models for acute lymphoblastic and myeloid leukemias, myeloproliferative neoplasms, myelodysplastic syndromes, and mature lymphoid neoplasms with numerous full-color photomicrographs and illustrations. Hematologic neoplasms are now classified on the basis of phenotypic, cytogenetic, and molecular genetic analyses, and diagnoses that once depended on the analysis of cell morphology and cytochemical stains now rely on flow cytometry, cytogenetic testing, FISH, end-point and real-time polymerase chain reaction assays, gene sequencing, and microarrays. The chapters cover traditional monitoring of leukemias and lymphomas at the cellular level; detection of minimal residual disease at the molecular level; and new targeted molecular, immunologic, and cellular therapies, which have dramatically improved survival.

PART VI: HEMOSTASIS AND THROMBOSIS

The chapters of this section were reordered to begin with the mechanisms of normal hemostasis followed by the hemorrhagic disorders, the thrombotic disorders, and the anticoagulant therapies. Disorder specific laboratory testing accompanies the clinical discussion of the disorder. Routine coagulation tests and instrumentation are discussed in the chapters at the end of this section. Improvements were made to most of the diagrams and figures. Chapter 35 describes in detail the plasma-based and cell-based coagulation models including the interactions between primary hemostasis, secondary hemostasis, and fibrinolysis. Chapters 36, 37, and 38 detail the hemorrhagic disorders, including the diagnosis, management, and current therapies of the acute coagulopathy of trauma and shock, von Willebrand disease, the classical hemophilias, along with the quantitative and qualitative platelet disorders. Under new authorship the chapters on platelet disorders were revamped to facilitate pedagogy. An update on thrombotic thrombocytopenic purpura (TTP) was provided, and new and revised tables and figures were incorporated. Chapters 39 and 40 update the mechanisms associated with venous and arterial thrombosis, the laboratory testing that aids in diagnosis, and management of these disorders with anticoagulant or antiplatelet drugs. In these chapters, updates to current recommendations specifically focus on deep venous thrombosis, pulmonary embolism, antiphospholipid antibodies/lupus anticoagulant, disseminated intravascular coagulation, and heparin-induced thrombocytopenia. Therapy updates in Chapter 40 cover all thrombin and factor Xa inhibitor anticoagulants, all heparin-related anticoagulants, monitoring methods for each anticoagulant in all clinical settings, as well as methods for monitoring the different classes of antiplatelet drugs. Chapter 41 details coagulation specimen collection and handling, and it covers the traditional coagulation laboratory assays that assess platelet function, the coagulation factors, and fibrinolytic parameters including the shift from clot-based to chromogenic assays. Chapter 42 reviews the latest coagulation analyzers and point-of-care instrumentation for coagulation testing.

PART VII: HEMATOLOGY AND HEMOSTASIS IN SELECTED POPULATIONS

Chapter 43 provides valuable information on the hematology and hemostasis laboratory findings in the pediatric and geriatric populations as well as a new section on pregnant populations, all correlated with information from previous chapters.

READERS

Rodak's Hematology: Clinical Principles and Applications is designed for medical laboratory scientists, medical laboratory technicians, and faculty of undergraduate and graduate educational programs in the clinical laboratory sciences. This text is also a helpful study guide for pathology and hematology-oncology residents and fellows and a valuable shelf reference for hematologists, pathologists, and hematology and hemostasis laboratory managers.

TEXTBOOK FEATURES

The outstanding value and quality of *Rodak's Hematology: Clinical Principles and Applications* reflect the educational and clinical expertise of its current and previous editors and authors who are each well-known nationally, experienced, and respected in their field of expertise. The text is enhanced by nearly 700 full-color digital photomicrographs, figures, and line art. Detailed text boxes and tables clearly summarize important information.

Each chapter contains the following for enhanced pedagogical features:

- **Learning objectives** at all taxonomy levels in the cognitive domain.
- One or two **case studies** with open-ended discussion questions at the beginning of the chapter that stimulate interest and provide opportunities for application of chapter content in real-life scenarios.
- A bulleted **summary** at the end of each chapter that provides a comprehensive review of essential material.
- **Review questions** at the end of each chapter that correlate to chapter objectives and are in the multiple-choice format used by certification examinations.

Appendices in the sixth edition were expanded and include:
- New list of major **abbreviations** in hematology and hemostasis
- New list of commonly used **formulas**
- **Answers** to case studies and review questions
- Updated **glossary**
- **Reference intervals** are provided on the inside front and back covers

The Evolve website has multiple features **for the instructor:**
- An **ExamView test bank** contains multiple-choice questions with rationales and cognitive levels.
- **Instructor's manuals** for every chapter contain key terms, objectives, outlines, and study questions.
- **Learning Objectives with taxonomy levels** are provided to supplement lesson plans.
- **Case studies** have been updated and feature discussion questions and photomicrographs when applicable.
- **PowerPoint presentations** for every chapter can be used "as is" or as a template to prepare lectures.
- The **image collection** provides electronic files of all the chapter figures that can be downloaded into PowerPoint presentations.

The Evolve website has important features for **the student and instructor:**
- **Updated information** on safety in the hematology laboratory, blood specimen collection, and care and use of the microscope is included as basic supplemental material.
- **Animations**

ACKNOWLEDGMENTS

The editors express their immense gratitude to Bernadette F. (Bunny) Rodak, who laid the foundation for *Rodak's Hematology: Clinical Principles and Applications* with her expert writing, editing, detailed figures, and especially her contribution of almost 300 outstanding digital photomicrographs. Now in its sixth edition, we are honored to continue her work on this exceptional textbook. We sincerely thank George A. Fritsma for his significant contribution to this text as a co-editor and author of 10 chapters in previous editions, for authoring five chapters in the sixth edition, for sharing his immense expertise in hemostasis, and for his constant support and encouragement. We thank Kathryn Doig for her contributions as co-editor for the third edition, author of seven chapters in previous editions, and for her tenaciousness, creativity, and care in updating three chapters authored in the sixth edition. We thank Larry J. Smith for his expertise and diligence as co-editor of the fifth edition, and for authoring a chapter in previous editions. The editors also thank the many authors who have made and continue to make significant contributions to this work. All of these outstanding professionals have generously shared their time and expertise to make *Rodak's Hematology: Clinical Principles and Applications* into a worldwide educational resource and premier reference textbook for medical laboratory scientists and technicians, as well as pathology and hematology practitioners, residents, and fellows.

We also express our appreciation to Elsevier, especially Sarah Vora, Richard Barber, and Kellie White, whose professional support and reminders kept the project on track, and to Jeanne Robertson for her superb artwork on many new figures.

Finally, and with the utmost gratitude, we acknowledge our families, friends, and professional colleagues who have supported and encouraged us through this project.

Elaine M. Keohane
Catherine N. Otto
Jeanine M. Walenga

CONTENTS

PART 7 Hematology and Hemostasis in Selected Populations

APPENDICES

1

An Overview of Clinical Laboratory Hematology

*Elaine M. Keohane**

OUTLINE

The average human possesses 5 liters of blood. Blood transports oxygen from lungs to tissues; clears tissues of carbon dioxide; transports glucose, proteins, and lipids; and moves wastes to the liver and kidneys. The liquid portion is plasma, which, among many components, provides coagulation enzymes that protect vessels from trauma and maintain the circulation.

Plasma transports and nourishes blood cells. There are three categories of blood cells: red blood cells (RBCs), or *erythrocytes*; white blood cells (WBCs), or *leukocytes*; and platelets (PLTs), or *thrombocytes*.[1] Hematology is the study of these blood cells. By expertly staining, counting, analyzing, and recording the appearance, phenotype, and genotype of all three types of cells, the medical laboratory professional is able to predict, detect, and diagnose blood diseases and many systemic diseases that affect blood cells. Physicians rely on hematology laboratory test results to select and monitor therapy for these disorders; consequently, a complete blood count (CBC) is ordered on nearly everyone who visits a physician or is admitted to a hospital.

HISTORY

The first scientists, such as Athanasius Kircher in 1657, described "worms" in the blood, and Anton van Leeuwenhoek in 1674 gave an account of RBCs,[2] but it was not until the late 1800s that Giulio Bizzozero described platelets as "petites

plaques."[3] The development of the Wright stain by James Homer Wright in 1902 opened a new world of visual blood film examination through the microscope. Although automated analyzers now differentiate and enumerate blood cells, Wright's Romanowsky-type stain (polychromatic, a mixture of acidic and basic dyes), and refinements thereof, remains the foundation of blood cell identification.[4]

In the present-day hematology laboratory, RBC, WBC, and platelet appearance is analyzed through automation or visually using $500\times$ to $1000\times$ light microscopy examination of cells fixed to a glass microscope slide and stained with *Wright* or *Wright-Giemsa stain* (Chapters 3, 12, and 13). The scientific term for cell appearance is *morphology,* which encompasses cell color, size, shape, cytoplasmic inclusions, and nuclear condensation.

RED BLOOD CELLS

RBCs are anucleate, biconcave, discoid cells filled with a reddish protein, hemoglobin, which transports oxygen and carbon dioxide (Chapters 7 and 8). RBCs appear salmon pink and measure 7 to 8 μm in diameter with a zone of pallor that occupies one third of their center (Figure 1.1A), reflecting their biconcavity (Chapters 5 and 6).

Since before 1900, physicians and medical laboratory professionals counted RBCs in measured volumes to detect anemia or

*The author extends appreciation to George A. Fritsma, whose work in prior editions provided the foundation for this chapter.

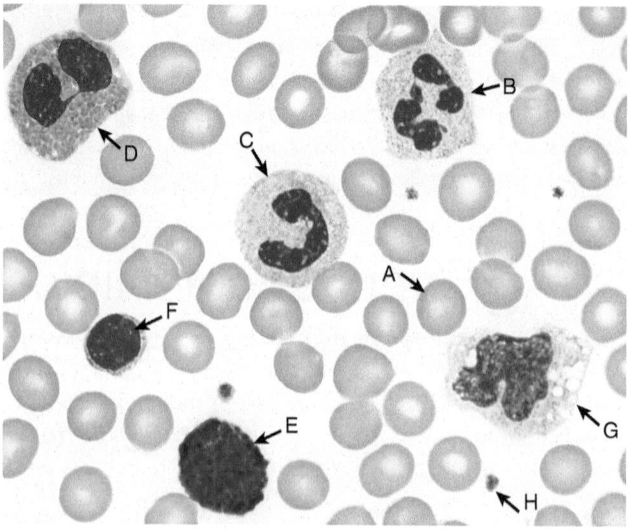

Figure 1.1 Composite of Cells Found in Peripheral Blood of Healthy Individuals. (A), Erythrocyte (red blood cell, RBC); **(B),** neutrophil (segmented neutrophil, NEUT, SEG, polymorphonuclear neutrophil, PMN); **(C),** band (band neutrophil, BAND); **(D),** eosinophil (EO); **(E),** basophil (BASO); **(F),** lymphocyte (LYMPH); **(G),** monocyte (MONO); **(H),** platelet (PLT). (Wright-Giemsa stain, ×1000.)

polycythemia. *Anemia* means loss of oxygen-carrying capacity and is often reflected in a reduced RBC count or decreased RBC hemoglobin concentration (Chapters 16 to 25). *Polycythemia* means an increased RBC count reflecting increased circulating RBC mass, a condition that leads to hyperviscosity (Chapter 32). Historically, microscopists counted RBCs by carefully pipetting a tiny alic [illegible] mal) salin [illegible] consequen [illegible] phology, [illegible] typical for [illegible] this diluti [illegible] advent of [illegible]

The dil [illegible] ber called [illegible] observed [illegible] tometer, a [illegible] and on th [illegible] and report [illegible] also called [illegible] *cubic centi* [illegible]

vocab: anemia, polycythemia
hemacytometer, µL, cc = mL,
Coulter counters, HCT, HGB,
Drabkin reagent, buffy coat, MCV,
MCH, MCHC, RDW, anisocytosis
chem vs heme vs coag

Visual [illegible] though ina [illegible] when auto [illegible] clinical laboratory. The first electronic counter, patented in 1953 by Joseph and Wallace Coulter of Chicago, Illinois, was used so widely that today automated cell counters are often called *Coulter counters,* although many high-quality competitors exist (Chapter 12).[5] The Coulter principle of direct current electrical impedance is still used to count RBCs in many automated blood cell analyzers. Fortunately, the widespread availability of automated cell counters has replaced visual RBC counting, although visual counting skills remain useful where automated counters are unavailable.

Hemoglobin, Hematocrit, and Red Blood Cell Indices

RBCs also are assayed for hemoglobin (HGB) concentration and hematocrit (HCT) (Chapter 11). Hemoglobin measurement relies on a weak solution of potassium cyanide and potassium ferricyanide, called *Drabkin reagent.* An aliquot of whole blood is mixed with a measured volume of Drabkin reagent, hemoglobin is converted to stable *cyanmethemoglobin* (hemiglobincyanide), and the absorbance or color intensity of the solution is measured in a spectrophotometer at 540 nm wavelength.[6] The color intensity is compared with that of a known standard and is mathematically converted to hemoglobin concentration. Modifications of the cyanmethemoglobin method are used in most automated applications, although some automated blood cell analyzers replace it with a formulation of the ionic surfactant (detergent) *sodium lauryl sulfate* to reduce environmental cyanide.

Hematocrit is the ratio of the volume of packed RBCs to the volume of whole blood and is manually determined by transferring blood to a plastic tube with a uniform bore, centrifuging, measuring the column of RBCs, and dividing by the total length of the column of RBCs plus plasma.[7] The normal ratio approaches 50%. Hematocrit is also called *packed cell volume* (PCV), the packed cells referring to RBCs. Often one can see a light-colored layer between the RBCs and plasma. This is the *buffy coat* and contains WBCs and platelets, and it is excluded from the hematocrit determination. The medical laboratory professional may use the three numerical results, RBC count, HGB, and HCT, to compute the RBC indices *mean cell volume* (MCV), *mean cell hemoglobin* (MCH), and *mean cell hemoglobin concentration* (MCHC) (Chapter 11). The MCV, although a volume measurement recorded in femtoliters (fL), reflects RBC diameter on a Wright-stained blood film. The MCHC, expressed in grams per deciliter (g/dL), reflects RBC staining intensity and amount of central pallor. The MCH in picograms (pg) expresses the mass of hemoglobin per cell and parallels the MCHC. A fourth RBC index, *RBC distribution width* (RDW), expresses the degree of *variation* in RBC volume. Extreme RBC volume variability is visible on the Wright-stained blood film as variation in diameter and is called *anisocytosis.* The RDW is based on the standard deviation of RBC volume and is routinely reported by automated blood cell analyzers (Chapter 12). In addition to aiding in diagnosis of anemia, RBC indices provide stable measurements for internal quality control of automated blood cell analyzers (Chapter 2). Sample reference intervals for RBC parameters are included on the inside front cover; these vary by age and gender (Chapter 43).

Medical laboratory professionals routinely use light microscopy at 500× or 1000× magnification to visually review RBC morphology, commenting on RBC diameter, color or hemoglobinization, and shape and the presence of cytoplasmic inclusions (Chapters 13 and 16). All these parameters, RBC count, HGB, HCT, indices, and RBC morphology, are employed to detect, diagnose, assess the severity of, and monitor the treatment of anemia, polycythemia, and the numerous systemic conditions that affect RBCs (Chapters 17 to 25 and Chapter 32). Automated blood cell analyzers are used in nearly all clinical laboratories to generate these data, although visual examination of the Wright-stained blood film is still essential to verify abnormal results.[8]

Reticulocytes

In the Wright-stained blood film, 0.5% to 2.5% of RBCs exceed the 7-

[handwritten note obscuring text:]
vocab
reticulocytes, WBC: neutrophils,
bands, eosinophils, basophils,
lymphocytes, monocytes,

-penia vs -cytosis

1000 (10³) more RBCs
than WBCs

These
newly
(Chapt
observe
to incr
excessi

Met
used to
vital")
ribonuc
is visual
visually
procedu
ing by t
fully au
percenta
cially se

cyte fraction (Chapter 12). However, it is still necessary to confirm automated analyzer counts visually from time to time, so medical laboratory professionals must retain this skill.

WHITE BLOOD CELLS

WBCs, or leukocytes, are a loosely related category of cell types dedicated to protecting their host from infection and injury (Chapters 4 and 9). WBCs are transported in the blood from their source, usually bone marrow or lymphoid tissue, to their tissue or body cavity destination. WBCs are so named because they are nearly colorless in an unstained cell suspension.

WBCs may be counted visually using a microscope and hemacytometer (Chapter 11). The technique is the same as RBC counting, but the typical dilution is 1:20, and the diluent is a dilute acid solution. The acid causes RBCs to *lyse* or rupture; without it, RBCs, which are 500 to 1000 times more numerous than WBCs, would obscure the WBCs. The WBC count reference intervals are included on the inside front cover. Visual WBC counting has been largely replaced by automated blood cell analyzers, but it is accurate and useful in situations in which no automation is available. Medical laboratory professionals who analyze body fluids such as cerebrospinal fluid or pleural fluid may employ visual WBC counting (Chapter 15).

A decreased WBC count is called *leukopenia,* and an increased WBC count is called *leukocytosis,* but the WBC count alone has modest clinical value. The microscopist must differentiate the categories of WBCs in the blood by using a Wright-stained blood film and light microscopy (Chapters 3, 9, and 13). The types of WBCs found in peripheral blood in healthy individuals are as follows:

- Neutrophils (NEUTs, segmented neutrophils [SEGs], polymorphonuclear neutrophils [PMNs]; Figure 1.1B). Neutrophils are

phagocytic cells whose major purpose is to engulf and destroy microorganisms and foreign material, either directly or after they have been labeled for destruction by the immune system. The term *segmented* refers to their multilobed nuclei. The cytoplasm of neutrophils contains pink- or lavender-staining granules filled with bactericidal substances. An increase in neutrophils is called *neutrophilia* and often signals bacterial infection. A decrease is called *neutropenia* and has many causes, but it is often caused by certain medications or viral infections.

- Bands (band neutrophils, BANDs; Figure 1.1C). Bands are slightly less mature neutrophils with a nonsegmented nucleus in a U or S shape. An increase in bands also signals bacterial infection and is customarily called a *left shift.*
- Eosinophils (EOs; Figure 1.1D). Eosinophils are cells with round, bright orange-red cytoplasmic granules filled with proteins involved in immune system regulation. An elevated eosinophil count is called *eosinophilia* and often signals a response to allergy or parasitic infection.
- Basophils (BASOs; Figure 1.1E). Basophils are cells with dark purple, irregular cytoplasmic granules that obscure the nucleus. The basophil granules contain histamines and various other proteins. An elevated basophil count is called *basophilia.* Basophilia is rare and often signals a hematologic disease.

The distribution of basophils and eosinophils in blood is so small compared with that of neutrophils that the terms *eosinopenia* and *basopenia* are theoretical and not used. Neutrophils, bands, eosinophils, and basophils are collectively called *granulocytes* because of their prominent cytoplasmic granules, although their functions differ.

- Lymphocytes (LYMPHs; Figure 1.1F). Lymphocytes comprise a complex system of cells that provide for host immunity. Lymphocytes recognize foreign antigens and mount *humoral* (antibodies) and *cell-mediated* antagonistic responses. On a Wright-stained blood film, most lymphocytes are nearly round, are slightly larger than RBCs, and have round featureless nuclei and a thin rim of nongranular cytoplasm. An increase in the lymphocyte count is called *lymphocytosis* and often is associated with viral infections. Accompanying lymphocytosis are often reactive lymphocytes with characteristic morphology (Chapter 26). An abnormally low lymphocyte count is called *lymphopenia* or *lymphocytopenia* and is often associated with drug therapy or immunodeficiency.
- Monocytes (MONOs; Figure 1.1G). The monocyte is an immature *macrophage* passing through the blood from its point of origin, usually the bone marrow, to a targeted tissue location. Macrophages are the most abundant cell type in the body although monocytes comprise a minor component of peripheral blood WBCs. Macrophages occupy every body cavity; some are motile and some are immobilized. Their tasks are to identify and *phagocytize* (engulf and consume) foreign particles and assist the lymphocytes in mounting an immune response through the assembly and presentation of antigen *epitopes.* On a Wright-stained blood film, monocytes have a slightly larger diameter than other WBCs, blue-gray

cytoplasm with fine azure granules, and a nucleus that is usually indented or folded. An increase in the number of monocytes is called *monocytosis.* Benign monocytosis may be found in certain infections or in inflammation (Chapter 26). Medical laboratory professionals seldom document a decreased monocyte count, so the theoretical term *monocytopenia* is seldom used.

Leukemia is an uncontrolled proliferation of a clone of malignant WBCs. Leukemia may be chronic, for example, chronic myeloid leukemia or chronic lymphocytic leukemia, or acute, for example, acute myeloid leukemia or acute lymphoblastic leukemia (Chapter 27 and Chapters 31 to 34). Leukemias may involve any of the cell lines and are categorized by their respective immunophenotypes and genetic aberrations (Chapters 28 to 30). Some leukemias are more common in a specific age group; chronic lymphocytic leukemia is more prevalent in people older than 65 years, whereas acute lymphoblastic leukemia is the most common form of childhood leukemia (Chapters 31 and 34). Medical laboratory professionals participate in characterization of leukemias using Wright-stained blood films, flow cytometric immunophenotyping, molecular diagnostic technology, cytogenetics, and molecular testing (Chapter 14 and Chapters 28 to 30).

PLATELETS

Platelets, or thrombocytes, maintain blood vessel integrity by initiating vessel wall repair. Platelets rapidly adhere to the surfaces of damaged blood vessels, form aggregates with neighboring platelets to plug the vessels, and secrete proteins and small molecules that trigger *thrombosis,* or clot formation. Platelets are the major cells that control *hemostasis,* a series of cellular and plasma-based mechanisms that seal wounds, repair vessel walls, and maintain vascular patency (unimpeded blood flow). Platelets are only 2 to 4 μm in diameter, round or oval, anucleate (for this reason some hematologists prefer to call platelets "cell fragments"), and slightly granular (Figure 1.1H). Their small size makes them appear insignificant, but they are essential to life and are extensively studied for their complex physiology. Uncontrolled platelet and hemostatic activation is responsible for deep vein thrombosis, pulmonary emboli, acute myocardial infarctions (heart attacks), cerebrovascular accidents (strokes), peripheral artery disease, and repeated spontaneous abortions (miscarriages) (Chapter 39).

The microscopist counts platelets using the same technique used in counting WBCs on a hemacytometer, although a different counting area, diluent, and dilution is usually used (Chapter 11). Owing to their small volume, platelets are hard to distinguish visually in a hemacytometer, and phase microscopy provides for easier identification. Automated blood cell analyzers have largely replaced visual platelet counting and provide greater accuracy (Chapter 12). The reference interval for the platelet count is on the inside front cover.

One advantage of automated blood cell analyzers is their ability to generate a mean platelet volume (MPV), which is unavailable through visual methods. The presence of predominantly larger platelets generates an elevated MPV value, which sometimes signals a regenerative bone marrow response to platelet consumption (Chapters 10 and 38).

Elevated platelet counts, called *thrombocytosis,* signal inflammation or trauma but convey modest intrinsic significance. *Essential thrombocythemia* is a rare malignant condition characterized by extremely high platelet counts and uncontrolled platelet production. Essential thrombocythemia is a life-threatening hematologic disorder (Chapters 32 and 38).

A low platelet count, called *thrombocytopenia,* is a common consequence of drug treatment and may be life threatening. Because the platelet is responsible for normal blood vessel maintenance and repair, thrombocytopenia is usually accompanied by easy bruising and uncontrolled hemorrhage (Chapter 38). Thrombocytopenia accounts for many hemorrhage-related emergency department visits. Accurate platelet counting contributes to patient safety because it provides for diagnosis of thrombocytopenia in many disorders or therapeutic regimens.

COMPLETE BLOOD COUNT

A complete blood count (CBC) is performed on automated blood cell analyzers and includes the RBC, WBC, and platelet counts as indicated in Box 1.1. The medical laboratory scientist may collect a blood specimen for the CBC, but a phlebotomist, nurse, physician assistant, physician, or patient care technician may also collect the specimen (Chapters 1, 3, and 42). No matter who collects, the medical laboratory professional is responsible for the integrity of the specimen and ensures that it is submitted in the appropriate anticoagulant (Chapter 42) and is free of clots and hemolysis (red-tinted plasma indicating RBC damage). The specimen must be of sufficient volume, because "short draws" result in incorrect

---

Handwritten note:

vocab

thrombocytes, CBC, vascular patency, MPV, hemolysis, short draws

-penia, -cytosis

> ### BOX 1.1   Basic Complete Blood Count Measurements Generated by Automated Blood Cell Analyzers
>
> | RBC Parameters | WBC Parameters |
> |---|---|
> | RBC count | WBC count |
> | HGB | NEUT count: % and absolute |
> | HCT | LYMPH count: % and absolute |
> | MCV | MONO count: % and absolute |
> | MCH | EO and BASO counts: % and absolute |
> | MCHC | **Platelet Parameters** |
> | RDW | PLT count |
> | RETIC | MPV |

BASO, Basophil; *EO,* eosinophil; *HGB,* hemoglobin; *HCT,* hematocrit; *LYMPH,* lymphocyte; *MCH,* mean cell hemoglobin; *MCHC,* mean cell hemoglobin concentration; *MCV,* mean cell volume; *MONO,* monocyte; *MPV,* mean platelet volume; *NEUT,* segmented neutrophil; *PLT,* platelet; *RBC,* red blood cell; *RDW,* RBC distribution width; *RETIC,* reticulocyte; *WBC,* white blood cell.

anticoagulant-to-blood ratios. The specimen must be tested or prepared for storage within the appropriate time frame to ensure accurate analysis (Chapter 2) and must be accurately registered in the work list, a process known as specimen *accession.* Accession may be automated, relying on bar code or radiofrequency identification technology, thus reducing instances of identification error.

Although all laboratory scientists and technicians are equipped to perform visual RBC, WBC, and platelet counts using dilution pipettes, hemacytometers, and microscopes, most laboratories employ automated blood cell analyzers to generate the CBC. Many blood cell analyzers also provide comments on RBC, WBC, and platelet morphology (Chapter 12). When one of the results from the blood cell analyzer is abnormal, the instrument provides an indication of this, sometimes called a *flag.* In this case a "reflex" *blood film examination* is performed (Chapter 13).

The blood film examination (described next) is a specialized, demanding, and fundamental CBC activity. Nevertheless, if all blood cell analyzer results are within reference intervals, the blood film examination is usually omitted from the CBC. However, physicians may request a blood film examination on the basis of clinical suspicion even [...] within their respective reference [...]

BLOOD FILM EXAMINATION

To accomplish a blood film ex[...] prepares a "wedge-prep" blood [...] slide, allows it to dry, and fixes [...] Wright-Giemsa stain (Chapter [...] performs an estimate of the W [...] 50× objective at 400× or 500× [...] count (with the 100× oil immer[...] nification) for comparison w [...] counts, and investigates discrep[...] systematically reviews, identifie[...] WBCs to determine their percen[...] referred to as determining the [...] WBC differential relies on th[...] acuity, and integrity, and it provides extensive diagnostic information. Finally the microscopist examines the morphology of WBCs, RBCs, and platelets by light microscopy for abnormalities of shape, diameter, color, or inclusions using 1000× magnification. Medical laboratory professionals pride themselves on their technical and analytical skills in performing the blood film examination and differential count. Visual recognition systems such as the Cellavision DM96 (Chapter 13) automate the WBC, RBC and platelet morphology assessment and WBC differential processes, but the medical laboratory professional or the hematopathologist is the final arbiter for all cell identification. Results of the CBC, including all automated blood cell analysis and blood film examination parameters and interpretive comments, are provided in paper or digital formats for physician review with abnormal results highlighted.

ENDOTHELIAL CELLS

Because they are structural and do not flow in the bloodstream, endothelial cells, the endodermal cells that form the inner surface of the blood vessel, are seldom studied in the hematology laboratory. Nevertheless, endothelial cells are important in maintaining normal blood flow, in tethering (decelerating) platelets during times of injury, and in enabling WBCs to escape from the vessel to the surrounding tissue when needed (Chapter 35). Increasingly refined laboratory methods are becoming available to assay and characterize the secretions of these important cells.

COAGULATION

Most hematology laboratories include a blood coagulation-testing department (Chapters 41 and 42). Platelets are a key component of hemostasis, as previously described; plasma coagulation is the second component (Chapter 35). The coagulation system employs a complex sequence of plasma proteins, some enzymes, and some enzyme cofactors to produce clot formation after blood vessel injury. Another six to eight enzymes exert control over the coagulation mechanism, and a third [...] and cofactors digests clots to restore vessel [...] called *fibrinolysis.* Bleeding (Chapters 36 to 38) [...] er 39) disorders are numerous and complex, [...] section of the hematology laboratory pro[...] ma-based and whole blood laboratory assays [...] lasma proteins and their interactions with [...] oratory professional focuses especially on [...] egrity for the coagulation laboratory, because [...] men defects, including clots, hemolysis, lipe[...] bin, and short draws, render the specimen [...]. High-volume coagulation tests suited to the [...] include the platelet count and MPV as de[...] *hrombin time* and *partial thromboplastin time* [...] al thromboplastin time), *thrombin time* (or [...] time), *fibrinogen assay,* and *D-dimer* assay [...] rothrombin time and partial thromboplastin [...] ly high-volume assays used in screening profiles. These tests assess each portion of the coagulation pathway for deficiencies and are used to monitor anticoagulant therapy (Chapter 40). Another 30 to 40 moderate-volume assays, mostly clot-based, are available in specialized or tertiary care facilities. The specialized or tertiary care coagulation laboratory with its interpretive complexities attracts advanced medical laboratory scientists with specialized knowledge and communication skills.

ADVANCED HEMATOLOGY PROCEDURES

Besides performing the CBC, the hematology laboratory provides *bone marrow examinations, flow cytometry immunophenotyping, cytogenetic analysis,* and *molecular diagnosis assays.* Performing these tests may require advanced preparation or particular dedication by medical laboratory scientists with a desire to specialize.

[Handwritten note: vocab: flag, reflex, specimen accession — endo levels — plasma vs buffy coat vs RBC vs serum + clot — EDTA = CBC = purple ←anti coag stuff — sodium cit. = coag = blue]

Medical laboratory scientists assist physicians with bedside *bone marrow* collection, then prepare, stain, and microscopically review bone marrow smears (Chapter 14). Bone marrow *aspirates* and *biopsy specimens* are collected and stained to analyze nucleated cells that are the immature precursors to blood cells (Chapter 4). Cells of the *erythroid* series are precursors to RBCs (Chapter 5); *myeloid* series cells mature to form bands and neutrophils, eosinophils, and basophils (Chapter 9); and *megakaryocytes* produce platelets (Chapter 10). Medical laboratory scientists, clinical pathologists, and hematologists review Wright-stained aspirate smears for morphologic abnormalities, high or low bone marrow cell concentration, and inappropriate cell line distributions. For instance, an increase in the erythroid cell line may indicate bone marrow compensation for excessive RBC destruction or blood loss (Chapter 16 and Chapters 20 to 24). The biopsy specimen, enhanced by *hematoxylin and eosin* (H&E) staining, may reveal abnormalities in bone marrow architecture indicating leukemia, bone marrow failure, or one of a host of additional hematologic disorders. Results of examination of bone marrow aspirates and biopsy specimens are compared with CBC results generated from the peripheral blood to correlate findings and develop pattern-based diagnoses.

In the bone marrow laboratory, cytochemical stains may occasionally be employed to differentiate erythroid, myeloid, and lymphoid cells. These stains include *myeloperoxidase, Sudan black B, nonspecific and specific esterases, periodic acid-Schiff, tartrate-resistant acid phosphatase, and acid phosphatase* (Chapters 31 and 32). The cytochemical stains are time-honored tests that in most laboratories have been replaced by flow cytometry immunophenotyping, molecular diagnostics, and cytogenetic techniques (Chapters 28 to 30). Since 1980, however, *immunostaining* methods have enabled identification of cell lines by detecting lineage-specific antigens on the surface or in the cytoplasm of leukemia and lymphoma cells. An example of immunostaining is a visible dye that is bound to antibodies to CD42b, a membrane protein that is present in the megakaryocytic lineage and may be diagnostic for megakaryoblastic leukemia (Chapter 31).

Flow cytometers may be *quantitative,* such as clinical flow cytometers that have grown from the original Coulter principle, or *qualitative,* including laser-based instruments that have migrated from research applications to the clinical laboratory (Chapters 12 and 28). The former devices are automated clinical blood cell analyzers that generate the quantitative parameters of the CBC through application of electrical impedance and laser or light beam interruption. Qualitative laser-based flow cytometers are mechanically simpler but technically more demanding. Both qualitative and quantitative flow cytometers are employed to analyze cell populations by measuring the effects of individual cells on laser light, such as *forward-angle fluorescent light scatter* and *right-angle fluorescent light scatter,* and by *immunophenotyping* for cell membrane epitopes using monoclonal antibodies labeled with fluorescent dyes. The qualitative flow cytometry laboratory is indispensable to leukemia and lymphoma diagnosis.

Cytogenetics (Chapter 30), a time-honored form of chromosome analysis, is employed in bone marrow aspirate examination to find gross genetic errors such as the Philadelphia chromosome, a reciprocal translocation between chromosomes 9 and 22 that is diagnostic in chronic myeloid leukemia, and t(15;17), a translocation between chromosomes 15 and 17 diagnostic in acute promyelocytic leukemia. Cytogenetic analysis remains essential to the diagnosis and treatment of leukemia.

Molecular diagnostic techniques (Chapter 29), the fastest-growing area of laboratory medicine, enhance and even replace some of the advanced hematologic methods. Real-time polymerase chain reaction, microarray analysis, fluorescence in situ hybridization, and DNA sequencing systems are sensitive and specific methods that enable medical laboratory scientists to detect various chromosome translocations and gene mutations that confirm specific types of leukemia and lymphoma, establish their therapeutic profile and prognosis, and monitor the effectiveness of treatment.

ADDITIONAL HEMATOLOGY PROCEDURES

Medical laboratory professionals provide several time-honored whole-blood methods to support hematologic diagnosis. The *glucose-6-phosphate dehydrogenase assay* phenotypically detects inherited RBC enzyme deficiency causing episodic hemolytic anemia (Chapter 24). The sickle cell solubility screening test, and confirmatory tests, hemoglobin electrophoresis and high-performance liquid chromatography, are used to detect sickle cell anemia and other inherited qualitative hemoglobin abnormalities and thalassemias (Chapters 24 and 25). One of the oldest hematology tests, the *erythrocyte sedimentation rate*, detects inflammation and roughly estimates its intensity (Chapter 31).

Finally, the medical laboratory professional reviews the cellular count, distribution, and morphology in body fluids other than blood (Chapter 15). These include cerebrospinal fluid, synovial (joint) fluid, pericardial fluid, pleural fluid, and peritoneal fluid, in which RBCs and WBCs may be present in disease and in which malignant cells may be present that require specialized detection skills. Analysis of nonblood body fluids is always performed with a rapid turnaround, because cells in these environments rapidly lose their integrity. The conditions leading to a need for body fluid analysis are invariably acute.

HEMATOLOGY QUALITY ASSURANCE AND QUALITY CONTROL

Medical laboratory professionals employ particularly complex quality control systems in the hematology laboratory (Chapter 2). Because of the unavailability of weighed standards, the measurement of cells and biological systems defies chemical standardization and requires elaborate calibration, validation, matrix effect examination, linearity, and reference interval determinations. An internal standard methodology known as the *moving average* also supports hematology laboratory applications.[10] Medical laboratory professionals in all disciplines compare methods through clinical efficacy calculations that produce clinical sensitivity, specificity, and positive and negative predictive values for each assay. They must monitor specimen integrity and test ordering patterns and ensure the integrity and delivery of reports, including numerical and narrative statements and reference interval comparisons. As in most branches of laboratory science, the hematology laboratory places an enormous responsibility for accuracy, integrity, judgment, and timeliness on the medical laboratory professional.

REFERENCES

1. Smock, K. J., & Perkins, S. L. (2014). Examination of the blood and bone marrow. In Greer, J. P., Arber, D. A., Glader, B., et al. (Eds.), *Wintrobe's Clinical Hematology*. (13th ed., pp. 1–18). Philadelphia: Lippincott Williams and Wilkins.

2. Wintrobe, M. M. (1985). *Hematology, the Blossoming of a Science: A Story of Inspiration and Effort*. Philadelphia: Lea & Febiger.

3. Bizzozero, J. (1882). Über einem neuen formbestandtheil des blutes und dessen rolle bei der Thrombose und der Blutgerinnung. *Virchows Arch Pathol Anat Physiol Klin Med, 90,* 261–332.

4. Woronzoff-Dashkoff, K. K. (2002). The Wright-Giemsa stain. Secrets revealed. *Clin Lab Med, 22,* 15–23.

5. Blades, A. N., & Flavell, H. C. (1963). Observations on the use of the Coulter model D electronic cell counter in clinical haematology. *J Clin Pathol, 16,* 158–163.

6. Klungsöyr, L., & Stöa, K. F. (1954). Spectrophotometric determination of hemoglobin oxygen saturation: the method of Drabkin & Schmidt as modified for its use in clinical routine analysis. *Scand J Clin Lab Invest, 6,* 270–276.

7. Mann, L. S. (1948). A rapid method of filling and cleaning Wintrobe hematocrit tubes. *Am J Clin Pathol, 18,* 916.

8. Barth, D. (2012). Approach to peripheral blood film assessment for pathologists. *Semin Diagn Pathol, 29,* 31–48.

9. Biggs, R. (1948). Error in counting reticulocytes. *Nature, 162,* 457.

10. Gulati, G. L., & Hyun, B. H. (1986). Quality control in hematology. *Clin Lab Med, 6,* 675–688.

Quality Assurance in Hematology and Hemostasis Testing

Heather DeVries, George A. Fritsma*

OBJECTIVES

After completion of this chapter, the reader will be able to:

1. Describe the procedures to validate and document a new or modified laboratory assay.
2. Compare a new or modified assay to a reference using statistical tests to establish accuracy.
3. Select appropriate statistical tests for a given application and interpret the results.
4. Define and compute precision using standard deviation and coefficient of variation.
5. Determine assay linearity using graphical representations and transformations.
6. Discuss analytical limits and analytical sensitivity and specificity.
7. Prepare multi-site validation protocols.
8. Explain Food and Drug Administration clearance levels for laboratory assays.
9. Compute a reference interval and a therapeutic range for a new or modified assay.
10. Interpret internal quality control using controls and moving averages.
11. Explain the benefits of participation in periodic external quality assessment.
12. Measure and describe assay clinical efficacy.
13. Interpret relative and absolute risk ratios.
14. Interpret receiver operating characteristic curves.
15. Describe methods to enhance and assess laboratory staff competence.
16. Describe a quality assurance plan to control for preanalytical and postanalytical variables.
17. List the agencies that regulate hematology and hemostasis quality.

OUTLINE

*The authors extend appreciation to David McGlasson for sharing his expertise in the preparation of this chapter.

CASE STUDY

After studying the material in this chapter, the reader should be able to respond to the following case study:

On an 8:00 a.m. assay run, the results for three levels of a preserved hemoglobin control specimen are 2 g/dL higher than the upper limit of the target interval. The medical laboratory professional reviews delta check data on the hemoglobin results for the last 10 patients in sequence and notices that the day's results are consistently 1.8 to 2.2 g/dL higher than results generated the previous day.

1. What do you call the type of error detected in this case?
2. Can you continue to analyze specimens as long as you subtract 2 g/dL from the results?
3. What aspect of the assay should you first investigate in troubleshooting this problem?

In medical laboratory science, *quality* implies the ability to provide *accurate, reproducible* assay results that offer clinically useful information.[1] Because physicians base clinical decision making on laboratory results, assay results must be *reliable*.[2] Reliability requires vigilance and effort on the part of all laboratory professionals.[3] An experienced medical laboratory scientist who is a quality assurance (QA) and quality control (QC) specialist often directs this effort.

Of the terms *quality control* and *quality assurance*, quality assurance is the broader concept, encompassing *preanalytical, analytical,* and *postanalytical* variables (Box 2.1). Quality control processes are employed to document assay validity, accuracy, and precision, including external quality assessment, publication of reference intervals (RIs) and therapeutic ranges (when applicable), and lot-to-lot validation.

Preanalytical variables (Table 2.1) are addressed in blood specimen collection texts, and in Chapter 41, which includes a section on coagulation specimen management.[4,5] Postanalytical variables are discussed briefly at the end of this chapter and are listed in Table 2.2. Quality assurance further encompasses laboratory assay utilization and physician test ordering patterns, nicknamed "pre-pre" analytical variables, and the appropriate application of laboratory assay results, sometimes called "post-post" analytical variables. There exists a combined 17% medical error rate associated with the pre-pre and post-post analytical phases of laboratory test utilization and application, prompting

BOX 2.1 Examples of Components of Quality Assurance

1. *Preanalytical* variables: assay selection based on patient indication; implementation of assay selection; patient identification and preparation; specimen collection equipment and technique; specimen transport, preparation, and storage; monitoring of specimen condition
2. *Analytical* variables: laboratory staff competence; assay and instrument selection; assay and instrument validation, including linearity, accuracy, precision, analytical measurement range (AMR), and specificity; internal quality control; external quality assessment
3. *Postanalytical* variables: accurate transcription and filing of results; content and format of laboratory report, narrative report; reference interval (RI) and therapeutic range; timeliness in communicating critical values; patient and physician satisfaction; turnaround time; cost analysis; physician application of laboratory results; patient outcome

TABLE 2.1 Preanalytical Quality Assurance Components and Laboratory Staff Responsibility

Preanalytical Component	Laboratory Staff Responsibility
Test orders	Conduct continuous utilization reviews to ensure that physician-generated orders are comprehensive and appropriate to patient indications. Inform physician about laboratory test availability and ways to avoid unnecessary orders. Reduce unnecessary repeat testing.
Test request forms	Are requisition forms legible? Can the phlebotomist confirm patient identity? Are physician orders promptly and correctly interpreted and transcribed? Is adequate diagnostic, treatment, and patient preparation information provided to assist the laboratory staff to appropriately test and interpret results?
Stat orders and timeliness	Do turnaround time expectations match clinical necessity and ensure that stat orders are reserved for medical emergencies? Does laboratory management meet established turnaround time requirements?
Specimen collection	Is the patient correctly identified, prepared, and available for specimen collection? Is fasting and therapy status appropriate for the assay? Is the tourniquet correctly applied and released at the right time? Are venipuncture sites appropriately cleansed? Are timed specimens collected at the specified intervals? Are specimen tubes collected in the specified order? Are additive tubes properly mixed? Are specimen tubes labeled correctly?
Specimen transport	Are specimens delivered intact, sealed, and within specified time limits? Are specimens maintained at the correct temperature?
Specimen management	Are specimens centrifuged correctly? Are tests begun within specified times? Are specimens and aliquots stored properly? Are coagulation specimens consistently platelet-poor?

TABLE 2.2 Postanalytical Quality Assurance and Laboratory Staff Responsibility

Postanalytical Component	Laboratory Staff Responsibility
Publication of reports	Are results accurately transcribed into the information system? Are they reviewed for errors by additional laboratory staff? If autoverification is in effect, are the correct parameters employed? Do reports provide reference intervals (RIs)? Do they flag abnormal results? Are result narratives appended when necessary? Does the laboratory staff conduct in-service education to support test result interpretation? Are critical values provided to nursing and physician staff? Are verbal reports confirmed with feedback? Are anomalous findings resolved?
Timeliness	Are turnaround times recorded and analyzed? Are laboratory reports being posted to patient charts in a timely fashion?
Patient satisfaction	Does the institution include laboratory care in patient surveys? Was specimen collection explained to the patient?

laboratory directors and scientists to develop *clinical query systems* that guide clinicians in laboratory assay selection.[6] Clinical query systems are enhanced by *reflex assay algorithms* developed in collaboration with the affiliated medical and surgical staff.[7] Equally important, a system of narrative reports that accompany and augment numerical laboratory assay output, authored by medical laboratory professionals and directors, is designed to assist physicians with case management.[7] A discussion of pre-pre and post-post analytical variables extends beyond the scope of this textbook but may be found in the references listed at the end of this chapter.[8,9] Quality control relies on the initial computation of central tendency and dispersion.

STATISTICAL SIGNIFICANCE AND EXPRESSIONS OF CENTRAL TENDENCY AND DISPERSION

Statistical Significance

When applying a statistical test such as the *Student* t-*test* of means or the *analysis of variance* (ANOVA), the statistician begins with a *null hypothesis*. The null hypothesis states that there is no difference between or among the means or variances of the populations being compared.[10] The *alternative (research) hypothesis* is the logical opposite of the null hypothesis.[11] For example, the null hypothesis may state there is no difference between the means of two data sets using the *t*-test, but the alternative hypothesis states that the null hypothesis is rejected and a statistical difference between the means does indeed exist (Table 2.3). In medical research, the null and alternative hypotheses may go unstated but are always implied.[12]

The power of a statistical test is defined as its ability to reject the null hypothesis when the null hypothesis is false. Power is expressed as *P*, which stands for the *probability* that the test is able to detect an effect. The *P* scale ranges from 0 to 1. Power is determined by the sample size (number of data points, *n*), the design of the research study, and the study's ability to control for extraneous variables.

The conventional levels for significance, or for rejecting the null hypothesis, are $P \leq 0.05$ (5%) or $P \leq 0.01$ (1%). In the former instance, there exists a 5% chance that the effect has occurred by chance alone; in the latter instance, there exists a more stringent 1% chance. Often researchers combine the statistical results, and thus the powers of several studies, to compute a common, more robust *P*-value, a process called *meta-analysis*.

The term *significant* has a specific meaning based on the *P*-value, and it should not be generalized to imply *practical* or *clinical* significance.[13] A statistical test result may indicate a statistically significant difference that is based on a selected study condition and power, but the difference may not possess practical importance because the clinical difference may be inconsequential. Experience and clinical judgment help when analyzing data, as does asking the question "Will this result generate a change in the prognosis, diagnosis, or treatment plan?"

Computing the Mean

The arithmetic mean ($\bar{X}$), or average, of a data set is the sum (Σ) of the individual data values divided by the number (*n*)

TABLE 2.3	Typical Student *t*-Test Results	
Example 1	**Reference Method**	**New or Modified Method**
n	10	10
$\bar{X}$	0.45	0.46
SD	0.01	0.02
Null hypothesis	$\bar{X}$ of control $= \bar{X}$ of test	
Selected *P*-value	0.01	
Computed *P*-value	0.085	
Computed two-tailed *t*-value	0.99	
Critical two-tailed *t*-value	2.88	
Null hypothesis is supported, means are not unequal		
Example 2	**Reference Method**	**New or Modified Method**
n	10	10
$\bar{X}$	0.40	0.44
SD	0.07	0.07
Null hypothesis	$\bar{X}$ of control $= \bar{X}$ of test	
Selected *P*-value	0.01	
Computed *P*-value	0.008	
Computed two-tailed *t*-value	3.89	
Critical two-tailed *t*-value	2.88	
Null hypothesis is rejected, means are unequal		

$\bar{X}$, Mean; *n*, number of data points; *SD*, standard deviation. In the first example of a two-tailed Student *t*-test, the difference in the means does not rise to statistical significance; the computed *P*-value exceeds the selected *P*-value, the computed *t*-value is smaller than the critical *t*-value, and the means are "not unequal." In the second example, the computed *P*-value is smaller than the selected *P*-value, the computed *t*-value exceeds the critical *t*-value, the means are unequal, and the result is statistically significant.

of data points. A data set that represents a single population, such as a series of prothrombin time results from a population, is called a *sample*. Often clinical laboratory professionals apply the terms *sample* and *specimen* interchangeably. A specimen may be defined as a single data point within a data set (sample). In the clinical laboratory, of course, a specimen often means a tube of blood or a fragment of tissue collected from a patient, which provides a single data point. The sum of sample data values above the mean is equal to the sum of the data values below the mean; however, the actual numbers of points above and below the mean are not necessarily equal.[14] The mean is a standard expression of central tendency employed in most scientific applications; however, it is profoundly affected by outliers and is unreliable in a skewed population. This is the formula for computing the arithmetic mean:

$$\text{Mean} \left(\bar{X} \right) = \frac{\left(\Sigma x \right)}{n};$$

where $\bar{X}$ = mean; Σx = sum of data point values; and *n* = number of data points.

The *geometric* mean is the *n* root of the product of *n* individual data points and is used to compute means of unlike data sets. The geometric mean of the prothrombin time RI is used to compute the prothrombin time international normalized ratio (INR) (Chapter 41). This is the formula for computing the geometric mean:

Geometric mean of n instances of $a = \sqrt[n]{a_1 a_2 \ldots a_n}$.

Determining the Median

The median is the data point that separates the upper half from the lower half of a data set (sample). To find the median, arrange the data set in numerical order and select the central data point. If the data set has an even number of data points, the median is the mean of the two central points. The median is a robust expression of central tendency in a skewed distribution because it minimizes the effects of outliers.

Determining the Mode

The mode of a data set (sample) is the data point that appears most often in the sample. The mode is not a true measure of central tendency because there is often more than one mode in a data set. For instance, a typical white blood cell histogram may be trimodal, with three modes, one each for lymphocytes, monocytes, and neutrophils. Conversely, in a Gaussian "normal"

sample, in which the data points are distributed symmetrically, the mean, median, and mode coincide at a single data point.

Computing the Variance

Variance (σ^2) expresses the deviation of each data point from its expected value, usually the mean of the data set (sample) from which the data point is drawn. The difference between each data point from the mean is squared, the squared differences are summed, and the sum of squares is divided by $n - 1$. Variance is expressed in the units of the variable squared as follows:

$$\sigma^2 = \frac{\sum \left(x_i - \bar{X} \right)^2}{\left(n - 1 \right)},$$

where σ^2 = sample variance; x_i = value of each data point; $\bar{X}$ = mean; and n = number of data points.

Computing the Standard Deviation

Standard deviation (SD), a commonly used measure of dispersion, is the square root of the variance and is the mean distance of all the data points in a sample from the sample mean (Figure 2.1). The larger the SD of a sample, the greater the

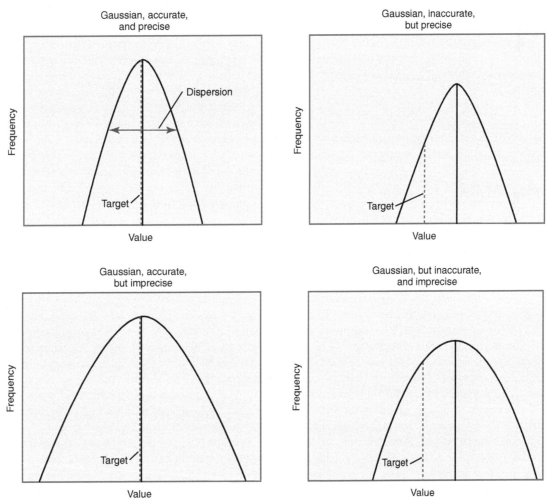

Figure 2.1 Frequency Distribution Graphs (Histograms) Generated from Repeated Assays of an Analyte. Incremental values are plotted on the horizontal *(x)* scale and number of times each value was obtained (frequency) on the vertical *(y)* scale. In this example, the values are normally distributed about their mean (symmetric, Gaussian distribution). Results from an accurate assay generate a mean that closely duplicates the reference target value. Results from a precise assay generate small dispersion about the mean, whereas imprecision is reflected in a broad curve. The ideal assay is both accurate and precise.

deviation from the mean. In clinical analyses, the SD of an assay is an expression of its quality based on its inherent dispersion or variability. The formula for SD is:

$$SD = \sqrt{\left[\frac{\sum\left(x_i - \bar{X}\right)^2}{(n-1)}\right]},$$

where SD = standard deviation; x_i = each data point value; $\bar{X}$ = mean; and n = number of data points.

SD states the confidence, or degree of *random error*, for statistical conclusions. Dispersion is typically expressed as $\bar{X} \pm 2$ SD or the 95.5% *confidence interval* (CI). Data points that are more than 2 SD from the mean are outside the 95.5% CI and may be considered abnormal. The dispersion of data points within $\bar{X} \pm 2$ SD is considered the expression of random or chance variation. Typically, $\bar{X} \pm 2$ SD is used to establish biological reference intervals (RIs or normal ranges) provided the frequency of the data points is Gaussian, or normally distributed, meaning symmetrically distributed about the mean.

Computing the Coefficient of Variation

The coefficient of variation (CV) is the *normalized expression* of the SD, ordinarily articulated as a percentage (CV%). CV% is the most commonly used measure of dispersion in laboratory medicine. CV% is expressed without units (except percentage), thus making it possible to compare data sets that use different units. The computation formula is:

$$CV\% = 100\frac{SD}{\bar{X}}$$

where $CV\%$ = coefficient of variation expressed as a percentage; SD = standard deviation; and $\bar{X}$ = mean.

METHOD VALIDATION

Before patient testing can begin, each new instrument, new assay, assay modification, or instrument-assay combination must be validated, confirming the intended results. This includes multiple instruments of the same make and model, and loaner instruments. Method validation includes proof of accuracy; precision; reportable ranges, including the analytical measurement range (AMR); and detection of interfering substances. Modifications to Food and Drug Administration (FDA)-approved assays and laboratory-developed tests (LDTs) have additional requirements, including, but not limited to, analytical sensitivity and specificity, specimen and reagent stability, and carryover. The results of these validation procedures are faithfully recorded and summarized in an evaluation that is signed by the laboratory director or designee before implementation. Multiple identical instruments and test systems require individual evaluation and approval. Documentation must be made available to laboratory assessors during periodic laboratory inspections required to maintain laboratory accreditation and licensure.[15]

Accuracy

Accuracy is the measure of agreement between an assay value and the theoretical "true value" of its analyte (Figure 2.1). Some statisticians prefer to define accuracy as the magnitude of error separating the assay result from the true value. In hematology testing, the concept of a true value is often not applicable. *Comparability* may take the place of accuracy in these situations. To test for comparability, the laboratory professional employs the laboratory's current reagent-instrument system as the reference assay for comparison to a new reagent-instrument system. Alternatively, the operator compares a reagent-instrument system to a previously validated, external reference method.

By comparison, *precision* is the expression of reproducibility or dispersion about the mean, often expressed as SD or CV%, as discussed in a subsequent section. Accuracy is easy to define but difficult to establish and maintain; precision is relatively easy to measure and maintain.

For many analytes, laboratory professionals employ *primary standards* to establish accuracy. A primary standard is a material of known, fixed composition that is prepared in pure form, often by determining its dry mass on an analytical balance. The laboratory professional dissolves the weighed standard in an aqueous solution, prepares suitable dilutions, calculates the anticipated concentration for each dilution, and assigns the calculated concentrations to assay outcomes. For example, he or she may obtain pure glucose, weigh 100 mg, dilute it in 100 mL of buffer, and assay an aliquot of the solution using photometry. The resulting absorbance would then be assigned the value of 100 mg/dL. The laboratory professional may repeat this procedure using a series of four additional glucose solutions at 20, 60, 120, and 160 mg/dL to produce a five-point *standard curve*. The curve may be reassayed several times to generate means for each concentration. Standard curve generation is automated; however, laboratory professionals retain the option of generating curves manually when necessary. The assay is then employed on human serum or plasma, with absorbance compared with the standard curve to generate a result. The matrix of a primary standard need not match the matrix of the patient specimen; the standard may be dissolved in an aqueous buffer, whereas the test specimen may be human serum or plasma.

To save time and resources, the laboratory professional may employ a secondary standard, perhaps purchased, that the vendor has previously calibrated to a primary standard. The secondary standard may be a preserved plasma preparation at a certified known concentration. The laboratory professional merely thaws or reconstitutes the secondary standard and incorporates it into the test series during validation or revalidation. Manufacturers often match secondary standards as closely as possible to the test specimen's matrix, for instance, serum to serum, plasma to plasma, and whole blood to whole blood. Primary and secondary standards are seldom assayed during routine patient specimen testing, only during calibration or when the assay tends to be unstable.

Regrettably, in hematology and hemostasis, where the analytes are often cell suspensions or enzymes, there are just a handful of primary standards: cyanmethemoglobin, fibrinogen, factor VIII, protein C, antithrombin, and von Willebrand factor.[16] For scores of analytes, the hematology and hemostasis professional relies on *calibrators*. Calibrators for hematology may be preserved human blood cell suspensions, sometimes supplemented with microlatex particles or nucleated avian red blood cells (RBCs) as surrogates for hard-to-preserve human white blood cells (WBCs). In hemostasis, calibrators may be frozen or lyophilized plasma from a pool of healthy human donors. For most of these analytes, it is impossible to prepare "weighed-in" standards; instead, calibrators are assayed using *reference methods* ("gold standards") at selected independent expert laboratories. For instance, a vendor may prepare a 1000-L lot of preserved human blood cell suspension, assay for the desired analytes within their laboratory ("in-house"), and send aliquots to five laboratories that employ well-controlled reference instrumentation and methods. The vendor obtains blood count results from all five, averages the results, compares them to their in-house values, and publishes the averages as the reference calibrator values. The vendor then distributes sealed aliquots to customer laboratories with the calibrator values published in the accompanying package inserts. Vendors may market calibrators in sets of three or five, spanning the range of assay linearity (analytical measurement range, AMR) or the range of potential clinical results; alternately, one calibrator can be diluted into multiple concentrations.

As with secondary standards, vendors attempt to match their calibrators as closely as possible to the physical properties of the test specimen. For instance, human preserved blood used to calibrate complete blood count (CBC) analytes generated by an automated blood cell analyzer is prepared to closely match the matrix of fresh anticoagulated patient blood specimens, despite the need for preservatives, refrigeration, and sealed packaging. Vendors submit themselves to rigorous certification by governmental or voluntary standards agencies in an effort to verify and maintain the validity of their products.[17]

The laboratory professional assays the calibration material using the new or modified assay and compares results with the vendor's published results. When new results parallel published results within a selected range, for example ±10%, the results are recorded and the assay is validated for accuracy. If they fail to match, the new assay is modified or a new RI, and therapeutic range when applicable, is prepared.

Medical laboratory professionals may employ locally collected fresh blood from a healthy subject as a calibrator; however, the process for validation and certification is laborious, so few attempt it. The selected specimens are assayed using reference instrumentation and methods, calibration values are assigned, and the new or modified assay is calibrated (adjusted) from these values. Routine quality control materials and the original calibrators are not suitable for accuracy evaluation.

New or modified assays may also be compared with reference methods. A reference method may be a previously employed, well-controlled assay, or an assay currently being used by an alternate laboratory. Several statistics are available to compare results of the new or modified assay to a reference method, including the Student *t*-test, analysis of variance (ANOVA), linear regression, Pearson correlation coefficient, and the Bland-Altman plot.

Statistical Tests

Comparing the Means of Two Data Sets Using the Student *t*-Test

The Student *t*-test compares the mean of a data set (sample) of a new or modified assay to the sample mean of a reference assay. In the *unpaired* t-*test* the operator assumes that population distributions are normal (Gaussian), the SDs are equal, and the

assays are independent. Often laboratory professionals use the more robust *paired* t-*test* in which the new and reference assays are performed using specimens (aliquots) from the same subjects. Laboratory professionals also choose between the *one-tailed* and *two-tailed* t-*test*, depending on whether the population being sampled has one (high *or* low) versus two (high *and* low) critical values. For instance, when assaying plasma for glucose, clinicians are concerned about both elevated and reduced glucose values, so the laboratory professional would use the two-tailed *t*-test; however, when assaying for bilirubin, clinical concern focuses only on elevated bilirubin concentrations, so the laboratory professional would apply the more robust one-tailed *t*-test in method comparison studies.

The laboratory professional generates *t*-test data by entering the paired data sets side by side into columns of a spreadsheet and applying an automated *t*-test formula. The program generates the number, mean, and variance for each data set (sample; $n_1, n_2; \bar{X}_1, \bar{X}_2; \sigma^2_1, \sigma^2_2$), and the "degrees of freedom" *(df)* for the test: $df = n_1 + n_2 - 2$. The operator selects the appropriate critical value (P), often $P \leq 0.05$. The program uses *df* and P to compare the computed *t*-value to the *standard table of critical t-values* (Table 2.4) and reports a computed *P*-value. For instance, if the two assays are performed on aliquots from each of 10 subjects, the *df* is 18. If the computed *t*-value is higher than 2.10 (critical *t*-value at $P \leq 0.05$), the means of the two data sets are unequal. Applying a stricter critical *t*-value at $P \leq 0.01$, the computed *t*-value would have to be 2.88 or higher for the means to be considered unequal.[18] To provide a more precise indication of significance, the program reports the actual computed *P*-value. If the computed *P*-value is smaller than a selected *P*-value (e.g., 0.05 or 0.01, depending on desired stringency), the means of the two data sets are unequal and the difference is "statistically significant." If the computed *P*-value is larger than the selected *P*-value, the means of the two data sets are not unequal. Table 2.3 illustrates a typical *t*-test result.

When the *t*-test indicates that two sample means are *not unequal,* the operator may choose to implement the new or modified assay. However, statistically, if two means are adjudged "not unequal," that is not the same as "equal." To increase the power of the validation, the laboratory professional often chooses to compute the *Pearson correlation coefficient* and to apply *linear regression* and the *Bland-Altman plot.*[19]

TABLE 2.4 Excerpt From the Standard Table of Critical *t*-Values for a Two-Tailed Test

df	P ≤ 0.05	P ≤ 0.01	df	P ≤ 0.05	P ≤ 0.01	df	P ≤ 0.05	P ≤ 0.01
2	4.30	9.93	12	2.18	3.06	22	2.07	2.82
4	2.78	4.60	14	2.15	2.98	24	2.06	2.80
6	2.45	3.71	16	2.12	2.92	26	2.06	2.78
8	2.31	3.36	18	2.10	2.88	28	2.05	2.76
10	2.23	3.17	20	2.09	2.85	30	2.04	2.75

The operator matches the degrees of freedom *(df)* with the test and looks up the critical *t*-value at the selected level of significance, often $P \leq 0.05$ or $P \leq 0.01$. If the computed *t*-value exceeds the critical *t*-value from the table, the null hypothesis is rejected, the means of the data sets are unequal, and the difference between the means is statistically significant.

Using Analysis of Variance to Compare Variances of More Than Two Data Sets

ANOVA accomplishes the same outcomes as the Student t-test; however, ANOVA may be applied to more than two sets of data. A laboratory professional may choose to compare two, three, or four new methods with a reference method. The ANOVA computes variance (σ^2) within each group (within-group σ^2), an overall σ^2 (between-group σ^2), and an F-statistic (similar to the t-statistic) based on dividing the between-group σ^2 by the within-group σ^2. The F-statistic is compared with a table of critical F-statistic values to determine significance analogous to the t-statistic as shown in Table 2.4.

Like the Student t-test, ANOVA is available on computer spreadsheets. The operator enters the data in one column per data set (group or sample) and applies the ANOVA formula. The test reports *between-groups* df (the number of groups − 1) and the *within-group* df (total of data points − 1 per group). The test also computes and reports the sum of squares within and between groups, the total sum of squares, the mean squares within and between groups, and the F-statistic. Spreadsheet programs compare the F-statistic to the table of critical F-values and report the P-value, which the operator then compares with the selected P-value limit to determine significance. Table 2.5 illustrates typical ANOVA results.

Comparing Data Sets Using the Pearson Correlation Coefficient

In addition to comparing means by Student t-test or variances by ANOVA, the laboratory professional compares a set of paired data to learn if the data points agree with adequate precision throughout the AMR. For instance, to validate a new prothrombin time reagent, the laboratory professional assembles 100 plasma aliquots, assays them in sequence using first the new and then the current reagents, and records the paired data points in two spreadsheet columns, x and y. He or she then applies the spreadsheet's *Pearson correlation coefficient* formula to generate a Pearson r, or *correlation coefficient*, which may range from −1.0 to +1.0. The spreadsheet uses this formula:

$$r = \frac{\left(\sum xy/n - \overline{XY}\right)}{SD_X SD_Y},$$

where r = Pearson correlation coefficient; $\sum xy$ = sum of the products of each pair of scores; n = number of values; $\overline{X}$ = mean of the x distribution; $\overline{Y}$ = mean of the y distribution; SD_X = standard deviation of the x distribution; and SD_Y = standard deviation of the y distribution.

Pearson r-values from 0 to +1.0 represent positive correlation; 1.0 equals perfect correlation. Laboratory professionals employ the Pearson formula to assess the range of values from two like assays or to compare assay results to previously assigned standard or calibrator results. Most operators set an r-value of 0.975 (or r^2-value of 0.95) as the lower limit of correlation; any Pearson r-value less than 0.975 is considered invalid because it indicates unacceptable variability from the reference method.

When the Pearson r-value result indicates the adequacy of the range of values, the linear regression r-value equation described in the next section is applied. Linear regression finds the line that best predicts x from y, but its equation does not account for dispersion. The Pearson correlation coefficient formula quantifies how x and y vary together while documenting dispersion.

Comparing Data Sets Using Linear Regression

If a set of five calibrator dilutions is tested by both a new and a reference assay, results may be analyzed by the following regression equation:

$$y = a + bx$$

$$\text{Slope}(b) = \left[n\sum XY - \left(\sum X\right)\left(\sum Y\right)\right] \Big/ \left[n\sum X^2 - \left(\sum X\right)^2\right]$$

$$\text{Intercept}(a) = \left[\sum Y - b\left(\sum X\right)\right]\Big/ n$$

where x and y are the variables; a = the intercept of the regression line and the y-axis; b = the slope of the regression line; n = number of values or data points; X = first calibrator value; Y = second calibrator value; $\sum XY$ = sum of the product of first and second calibrator values; $\sum X$ = sum of first calibrator values; $\sum Y$ = sum of second calibrator values; and $\sum X^2$ = sum of squared first calibrator values.

Perfect correlation generates a *slope* of 1 and a *y intercept* of 0 and is illustrated as a *line of identity* on a graph when plotting the values (data points) of the assay under consideration versus the reference assay (Figure 2.2). Local policy based on total error calculation establishes limits for slope and y intercept; for example, many laboratory directors reject a slope of <0.9 or >1.10 or an intercept of more than 10% above or below zero.

Slope measures *proportional systematic error*; the higher the analyte value, the greater the deviation from the line of identity. Proportional errors are caused by malfunctioning instrument components or a failure of some part of the testing process. The magnitude of the error increases with the concentration or activity of the analyte. An assay with proportional error may be invalid.

TABLE 2.5 Typical ANOVA Results

Summary of Descriptive Statistics Provided With Automated ANOVA

Group	n	Σ	$\overline{X}$	σ^2
Reference	25	63.74	2.55	1.07
Test 1	25	61.17	2.45	0.60
Test 2	25	65.08	2.60	0.68

ANOVA Example

Variation source	df	SS	MS	F	Critical F-value, $P \le 0.05$	P-Value
Between groups	2	0.32	0.17	0.20	3.12	0.82
Within groups	72	56.37	0.78			
Total	74	56.69				

ANOVA, Analysis of variance; *df*, degrees of freedom; *MS*, mean squares; *SS*, sum of squares.

The computed *F*-value does not exceed the critical *F*-value from the table of critical values. The computed *P*-value exceeds the selected *P*-value of 0.05. This test fails statistical significance at $P \le 0.05$; the null hypothesis is supported and there is no significant difference among the groups.

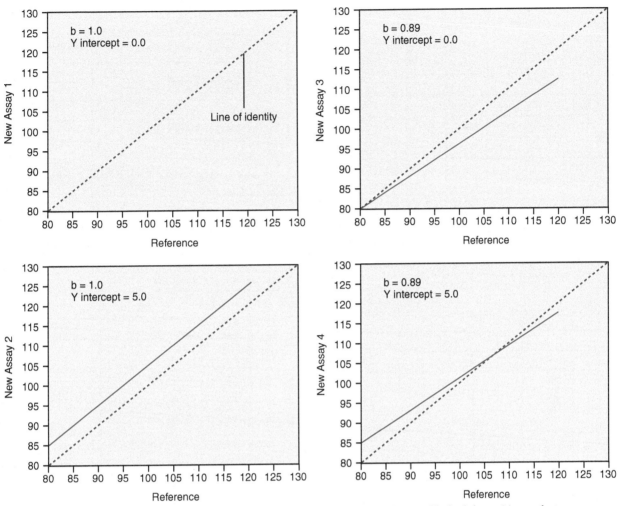

Figure 2.2   Linear Regression Comparing Four New Assays with a Reference Method. Assay 1 is a perfect correlation with the reference method and generates a line of identity in which the slope *(b)* is 1.0 and the *y* intercept is 0.0. The *y* intercept of assay 2 is 5.0, which illustrates a constant systematic error, or bias. The slope *(b)* value for assay 3 is 0.89, which illustrates a proportional systematic error. Assay 4 has both bias and proportional error. Regression analysis gains sufficient power when 40 or more specimens (calibrators and/or patients) are tested using both the new and reference assay.

Intercept measures *constant systematic error* (or *bias*, in laboratory vernacular), a constant difference between the new and reference assay regardless of assay result magnitude. A laboratory director may choose to adopt a new assay with constant systematic error but must modify the published RI.

Regression analysis gains sufficient power when 40 or more patient specimens are tested using both the new and reference assay in place of or in addition to calibrators. Data may be entered into a spreadsheet program that offers an automatic regression equation.

Comparing Data Sets Using the Bland-Altman Difference Plot

Linear regression and the Pearson correlation coefficient are essential tests of accuracy and performance; however, both are influenced by dispersion. The Bland-Altman difference plot, also known as the Tukey mean-difference plot, provides a graphical representation of agreement between two assays.[20] Similar to the *t*-test, Pearson correlation, and linear regression,

paired assay results are tabled in automated spreadsheet columns. This formula is applied:

$$S\,(x,y) = (S_1 + S_2)\,/\,2, \text{ and } S_1 - S_2$$

where S = individual coordinates

The operator computes the mean value of each specimen by the two assays and the signed difference between the values. A chart is prepared with the means plotted on the *x*-axis and the numerical or percentage differences on the *y*-axis. Difference limits are provided, characteristically at $\overline{X} \pm 2$ SD (Figure 2.3). The plot visually illustrates the magnitude of the differences. In a normal (Gaussian) distribution, 95.5% of the values are expected to fall within the limits; when more than 5% of the data points fall outside the limits, the assay is rejected.

Precision

Unlike the determination of accuracy, assessment of precision (dispersion, reproducibility, variation, random error) is a simple validation effort, because it merely requires performing a

Specimen	PTT 1	PTT 2	(S1+S2)/2	S1-S2	Difference, %
1	31.5	31.1	31.3	−0.4	−1.3
2	30.0	29.9	30.0	−0.1	−0.3
3	34.3	33.5	33.9	−0.8	−2.4
4	35.6	34.7	35.2	−0.9	−2.6
5	28.6	28.2	28.4	−0.4	−1.4
6	30.8	30.3	30.6	−0.5	−1.6
7	28.1	28.4	28.3	0.3	1.1
8	28.0	28.0	28.0	0.0	0.0
9	28.6	28.1	28.4	−0.5	−1.8
10	29.4	29.2	29.3	−0.2	−0.7

There was a total of 31 data points, 10 of which are shown.

A

Parameter	Value
n	31 (see table A for 10 of the data points)
r^2	0.999 (target ≥ 0.95)
Slope	1.05 (target = 0.9–1.1)
Intercept	1.08
$\overline{X}$ PTT 1 (reference assay)	48.09
$\overline{X}$ PTT 2	47.73
$\overline{X}$ of means (used for Bland-Altman correlation)	47.91
$\overline{X}$ difference	0.36
$\overline{X}$ difference, %	0.98
$\overline{X}$ difference, %/A versus B	0.8 (target = ±8%)
Minimum difference, %	3.92
Maximum difference, %	3.95
Maximum PTT result in seconds	110.02

B

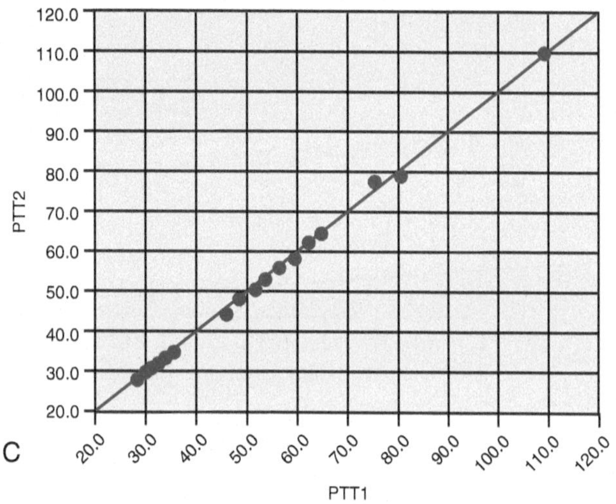

C

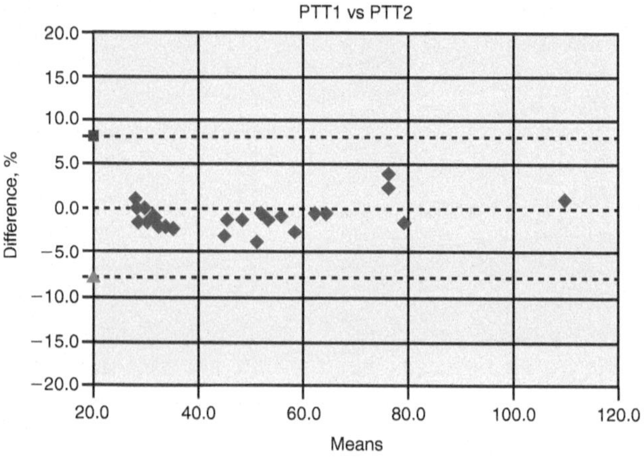

D

Figure 2.3 Bland-Altman Data and Plot. (A), Excerpt illustrating 10 of the 31 PTT result data points from a current and new reagent; (B), preliminary correlation data; (C), identity line; and (D), Bland-Altman plot based on the 31 PTT result data points. The differences between the results from each assay are within the acceptance limits; the new PTT assay is validated. *PTT,* Partial thromboplastin time.

series of assays on a single specimen or lot of reference material (Figure 2.1).[21] Precision studies always assess both *within-day* and *day-to-day* variation (random error) about the mean.[22] Precision studies are usually performed on three to five calibration specimens or QC material (unlike accuracy studies), although they may also be performed using a set of patient specimens. Managers of smaller laboratories may choose to test only two specimens or more typically QC material. To calculate within-day precision, the laboratory professional assays a single specimen at least 20 consecutive times using one reagent batch and one instrument test run. For day-to-day precision, 20 assays are required on at least 10 runs on 10 consecutive days. The day-to-day precision study employs the same source specimen and instrument but separate aliquots. If patient specimens are used in coagulation precision studies, aliquots should be prepared and frozen until ready for each run. Day-to-day precision accounts for the effects of different operators,

reagents, and environmental conditions such as temperature and barometric pressure. No matter which material is used in precision studies, their levels should be close to clinically significant decision points.

The collected data from within-day and day-to-day sequences are reduced by formula to the mean and a measure of dispersion such as SD or, most often, coefficient of variation in percent (CV%), as described in "Statistical Significance and Expressions of Central Tendency and Dispersion." The CV% documents the degree of dispersion or random error generated by an assay, a function of assay stability.

The CV% limits are established locally. For analytes based on primary standards, the within-run CV% limit may be 5% or less, and for hematology and hemostasis assays, 10% or less; however, the day-to-day run CV% limits may be as high as 30%, depending on the stability and complexity of the assay. Although accuracy, linearity, AMR, and interferences are just as important, laboratory professionals often equate the quality of an assay with its CV%. The best assay, of course, is one that combines the smallest CV% with the greatest accuracy.

Precision for visual light microscopy leukocyte differential counts on stained blood films is immeasurably broad, particularly for low-frequency eosinophils and basophils.[23] Most visual differential counts are performed by reviewing 100 to 200 leukocytes. Although impractical, it would take differential counts of 800 or more leukocytes to improve precision to measurable though inadequate levels. Automated differential counts generated by automated blood cell analyzers, however, provide CV% levels of 5% or less because these instruments count thousands of cells.

Linearity and the Analytical Measurement Range

Linearity is the ability to generate results proportional to the calculated concentration or activity of the analyte.[24] The laboratory professional dilutes a high-level calibrator to produce at least five dilutions spanning the full range of the assay. Many current analyzers are programmed to make these dilutions as part of the calibration process. For precision, these instruments assay each dilution at least twice, sometimes in triplicate. The computed values and assayed results for each dilution are paired and plotted on a linear graph on the x-scale and y-scale, respectively. The line is inspected visually for nonlinearity at the highest and lowest dilutions (Figure 2.4). The acceptable range of linearity is established just above the low value and below the high value at which linearity loss is evident. Although formulas exist for computing the limits of linearity, visual inspection is an accepted practice. Nonlinear results may be transformed using semilog or log-log graphs when necessary.

During assay runs, patient specimens with results above the linear range must be diluted and reassayed. Results from diluted specimens that fall within the linear range are valid; however, they must be multiplied by the dilution factor (reciprocal of the dilution) to produce the final concentration. Lower limits are especially important when counting platelets or assaying coagulation factors. For example, the difference between <1% and 3% coagulation factor VIII activity affects treatment options and the potential for predicting coagulation factor inhibitor formation. Likewise, the difference between a platelet count of 10,000/μL and 5000/μL affects the decision to treat with platelet concentrate.

Whereas linearity is the ability to generate a result that is proportional to the expected value, the AMR defines the upper and lower limits of those values. Verification of the AMR proves a linear relationship between measured and expected concentrations or activities of an analyte, and should include at least four concentrations, including low, mid, and high values. Laboratory professionals never report results that fall below or above the AMR because accuracy is compromised in the nonlinear regions of the assay.

Analytical Sensitivity (Lower Limit of Detection)

Analytical sensitivity (lower limit of detection, LLD) assays are coupled with linearity and AMR studies, and are required of local laboratory professionals when modifying an FDA-approved assay or developing an LDT.[25] A "zero calibrator," or blank, is assayed 10 to 20 times, and the mean and SD are computed from the results. The LLD is computed as 3 SDs above the mean of blank assay results. This limit prevents false-positive results generated by low-end assay interference, commonly called *noise*. The manufacturer or distributor typically performs limit assays in compliance with the FDA and provides the results on the package insert; however, local policies may require that results of the manufacturer's limit studies be confirmed.

Analytical Specificity

Analytical specificity is the ability of an assay to distinguish the analyte of interest from anticipated interfering substances within the specimen matrix. The laboratory professional employs subject specimens known to contain potential interferences (provided the subject consents) or "spikes" specimens with potential interfering substances and measures the effects of each upon the assay results. Except for LDTs or modifications of FDA-approved assays, analytical specificity is determined by the manufacturer and need not be confirmed at the local laboratory unless there is suspicion of interference from a particular substance not assayed by the manufacturer. Common interferences include hemolysis, lipemia, and icterus. Manufacturer specificity data are transferred from the package insert to the laboratory validation report. QC managers publish procedures on how to address the results of a specimen known to contain an interfering substance. Interference studies allow the laboratory director to intervene when a form of interference may compromise a laboratory result, for instance, when hemolysis affects the results of a chromogenic assay.

Levels of Laboratory Assay Approval

The FDA categorizes assays as *approved, cleared, modified-cleared, analyte-specific reagent* (ASR), *research use only* (RUO),

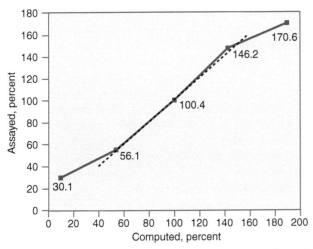

Figure 2.4 Linearity Determination. At least five dilutions of standard or calibrator material are prepared. Dilutions must span the AMR. The concentration of the analyte for each of the five dilutions is calculated and expressed as a percentage. The assayed values are plotted on the y scale and the computed values on the x scale. The linear range is selected by visual inspection, containing the dilutions for which assayed values vary in a linear manner. In this example, the limits of linearity are 56.1% to 146.2%. Assay results that fall outside these limits are inaccurate. *AMR,* Analytical measurement range.

and *laboratory-developed tests* ("home-brew").[26] When a local laboratory professional modifies an approved or cleared assay, the assay becomes categorized as modified-cleared. For instance, some facilities employ chromogenic anti-Xa heparin assays for rivaroxaban and apixaban using ASR calibrators and controls. FDA-approved or cleared assays are approved to detect or measure specific analytes and should not be used for noncleared (off-label) applications.

ASRs refer to individual reagents, and ASRs that are bundled with other ASRs or other general reagents and labeled with an intentional use are subject to premarket review requirements. RUO kits may be used on a trial basis, but the patient, facility, or a clinical trial agency bears their expense, not the third-party payer. In this case the local facility prepares an advance beneficiary notice (ABN) notifying the patient of the possibility they will be invoiced. The FDA monitors LDTs by regulating the main components, which include, but are not limited to, ASRs, locally prepared reagents, and laboratory instrumentation. Details are given in Table 2.6.

Documentation and Reliability

Validation is recorded on standard forms available from commercial sources, such as Data Innovations LLC EP Evaluator. Requirements established in the Clinical Laboratory Improvement Amendments of 1988 (CLIA) include that validation records are stored for at least 2 years in readily accessible databases and made available to laboratory assessors on request.[27,28]

Precision and accuracy records document assay reliability over specified periods. The recalibration interval may be once every 6 months or in accordance with operators' manual recommendations. Recalibration is necessary whenever reagent lots are updated unless the laboratory professional can demonstrate that

the reportable range is unchanged using lot-to-lot comparison. When control results demonstrate a shift or consistently fall outside action limits, or when an instrument is repaired, the laboratory professional repeats the validation procedure and maintains the records.

Regularly scheduled validity rechecks, lot-to-lot comparisons, instrument preventive maintenance, staff competence, and scheduled performance of internal QC and external quality assessment procedures ensure continued reliability and enhance the value of a laboratory assay to the patient and physician.

MULTI-SITE VALIDATION

Many US health care systems have multiple laboratories operating under a single CLIA license. These systems combine high-volume and low-volume laboratories, ranging from reference and hospital laboratories to acute care facilities, "satellite" clinics, and physicians' group offices. One facility, presumably the busiest, and staffed with a QC manager, serves as a central laboratory. Patients inevitably choose to have their work done at a variety of facilities, depending on physician availability or convenience.[29]

Although the QC manager tries for uniformity, the various sites may be equipped with instruments with different technologies from competing suppliers. Ideally, reagent manufacturers sequester single reagent lots to be shared among the laboratories; however, in many systems individual facilities may employ variant sole-source reagents and kits. Nevertheless, clinicians at satellite sites prefer to rely on system-wide RIs that are uniformly interpretable at their individual locations.

System-Wide Comparability

Each site validates its instrument-reagent systems, perhaps relying on central laboratory support. Subsequently, the system is validated as a whole. The QC manager verifies performance across the system with comparability studies, which resemble proficiency surveys. These are required at least twice a year, reflecting proficiency survey agency schedules.[30] Typically, the central laboratory QC manager prepares subject specimens to distribute to satellite facility personnel. For coagulation, although fresh plasma would be ideal, volume requirements may necessitate the use of frozen or preserved pooled plasma, preserved aliquots from proficiency agencies, or QC materials. QC material is only acceptable if all the sites' reagents and QC materials share the same lot number, which may not apply if the coagulometers are different. For hematology, patient anticoagulated whole blood specimens or preserved QC materials may be used. System-wide comparison efforts are most effective when all facilities are using the same reagent lots and identical or at least similar equipment. In any event, the QC manager compares satellite facility specimen results to analyze each location's accuracy. Outliers trigger troubleshooting and remedial instruction.

Multi-Site Reference Interval and Therapeutic Range

Once an assay is validated, each facility develops an RI and, when applicable, a therapeutic range, using the principles

TABLE 2.6   Categories of Assay Approval by the US Food and Drug Administration

Laboratory Assay Category	Comment
FDA-approved or cleared assay	The local facility may use package insert data for linearity, interferences, and specificity but must establish clinical accuracy and precision.
Modified approved assay	Local facility modifies an FDA-approved or cleared assay.
Analyte-specific reagent	Manufacturer may provide individual reagents, but not in kit form, and may not provide package insert validation data. Reagents are not promoted for use on specific instruments or in specific assays. Local facility performs all validation steps.
Research use only	Local facility performs all validation steps. Research use only assays are intended for clinical trials, and carriers are not required to pay. Local facility prepares an advance beneficiary notice to indicate patient may be required to pay.
Laboratory-developed assay	Assays devised locally ("home-brew"); FDA evaluates using criteria developed for FDA-approved or cleared assay kits.

FDA, Food and Drug Administration.

described in "Reference Interval and Therapeutic Range Development." Specimen collection from 20 healthy subjects is a challenge for low-volume facilities, so laboratory professionals enlist the help of larger satellites, provided both institutions serve similar population demographics. Practice guidelines discourage central laboratories from supplying healthy subject specimen aliquots to the entire system on the principle that their aliquots may not match local demographics. To reduce the inevitable confusion generated from multiple RIs, the central laboratory may develop and publish a system-wide RI from individual facility intervals, presuming the individual RIs are similar. For this purpose, the QC manager employs a statistical program such as Data Innovations LLC EP Evaluator, which the manager may choose to make available throughout the system for data collection. The computed "central" RI is distributed throughout the system and replaces individual RIs.

LOT-TO-LOT COMPARISONS

Laboratory managers reach agreements with vendors to sequester kit and reagent lots, thereby ensuring infrequent lot changes, optimistically no more than once a year.[31] The new reagent lot must arrive approximately a month before the laboratory runs out of the old lot so that *lot-to-lot comparisons* may be completed and differences resolved, if necessary. The QC manager uses control or patient specimens and prepares a range of analyte dilutions, typically five, spanning the limits of linearity. If the reagent kits provide controls, these are also included, and all are assayed using the old and new reagent lots. Results are charted as illustrated in Table 2.7.

Action limits vary by laboratory, but many managers reject the new lot when more than one specimen data point pair generates a variance greater than 10% or when all variances are positive or negative. In the latter case, the new lot may be rejected or it may be necessary to use the new lot but develop a new RI and therapeutic range.

For several analytes, lot-to-lot comparisons include revalidation of the AMR.

REFERENCE INTERVAL AND THERAPEUTIC RANGE DEVELOPMENT

Once an assay is validated, the laboratory professional develops the *RI* (also called reference range). Some laboratory professionals use the vernacular phrase *normal range*; however, statisticians prefer the term *RI*. Using strict mathematical definitions, *range* encompasses all assay results from largest to smallest, whereas *interval* is a statistic that trims outliers. The therapeutic range is correctly named, because therapeutic ranges may not be computed with the same statistical rigor as the RI.

To develop an RI, the laboratory professional carefully defines the desired healthy population and recruits representative subjects who meet the criteria to provide blood specimens. The definition may, for example, exclude smokers, women taking oral contraceptives, and people using specified over-the-counter or prescription medications. Subjects may be paid. There should be an equal number of males and females, and the chosen healthy subjects should match the institution's population *demographics* in terms of age and race. When practical, large-volume blood specimens are collected, aliquotted, and placed in long-term storage. For instance, plasma aliquots for coagulation RI development are stored indefinitely at −70° C. Laboratory directors may choose to purchase healthy subject specimen sets from plasma distributors, such as the frozen CRYO*check* Normal Donor Set (Precision BioLogic), which provides 25 carefully selected healthy subject plasmas for use in the hemostasis laboratory. These sets may be particularly useful for specialty coagulation testing when validated prior to implementation. For routine (prothrombin time [PT] and partial thromboplastin time [PTT]) assays, healthy subject sets may generate narrow RIs that are impractical for daily application. It may also be impractical to develop local RIs for infants, children, or geriatric populations (Chapter 43). In these cases the laboratory director may choose to use published (textbook) intervals.[32] In general, although published RIs are available for educational and general discussion purposes, local laboratories must generate their own RIs for adults to most closely match the demographics of the area served by their institution.

The minimum number of healthy subject specimens (data points) required to develop an RI may be determined using statistical power computations; however, practical limitations prevail.[33] For a new assay with no currently established RI, a minimum of 120 data points is necessary. In most cases, however, the assay manufacturer provides an RI in the package insert, and the local laboratory professionals need only assay 30 specimens, approximately 15 male and 15 female, to validate the manufacturer's RI, a process called *transference*. Likewise, the laboratory professional may refer to published RIs and, once they are locally validated, transfer them to the institution's report form.

QC managers assume that the population specimens employed to generate RIs will produce frequency distributions (in laboratory vernacular, *histograms*) that are normal, bell-shaped (Gaussian) curves (Figure 2.5). In a Gaussian frequency distribution the mean is at the center; the mean, median, and mode coincide; and the dispersion about the mean is identical in both directions. In many instances, however, biologic frequency

Specimen	Old Lot Value	New Lot Value	% Difference
Low value	7	6	−14.3%
Low middle value	12	12	0
Middle value	20.5	19.4	−5.4%
High middle value	31	27	−12.9%
High value	48	48	0
Old kit control 1	9	11	22.2%
Old kit control 2	22	24	9.1%
New kit control 1	10	10	0
New kit control 2	24	24	0

TABLE 2.7 Example of a Reagent Lot-to-Lot Comparison

Negative % difference indicates the new lot value is below the old lot (reference) value. The new lot is rejected because the low and high middle value results differ by more than 10%.

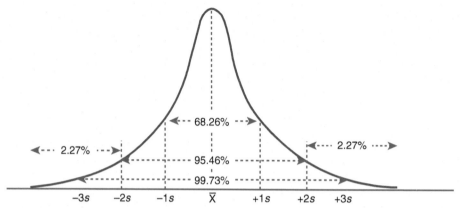

Figure 2.5 Normal (Symmetric, Gaussian) Distribution. When the test values obtained for a given subject population are normally distributed, the mean locates at the peak and the mean, mode, and median coincide. Segments of the population distribution representing ±1, ±2, and ±3 standard deviations are illustrated. In developing the reference interval (RI), laboratory directors often use ±2 standard deviations to establish the 95.5% confidence interval, or, when the precision is especially constricted, ±3 standard deviations. The ±2 standard deviations selection means that 95.46% of the test values from the healthy population are included within the limits. Consequently, 4.54%, or approximately 1 in 20 test results from theoretically healthy subjects, fall outside the interval, half (2.27%) above and half below. *s,* Standard deviation.

distributions are "log-normal" with a "tail" on the high end. For example, laboratory professionals assumed for years that the visual reticulocyte percentage RI in adults is 0.5% to 1.5%; however, repeated analysis of healthy populations in several locations has established the interval to be 0.5% to 2% because of a subset of healthy subjects whose reticulocyte counts fall at the high end of the interval.[34] QC managers may employ a log-normal distribution, or they may transform the data by replotting the curve using a semilog or log-log graphic display. The decision to transform may arise locally but eventually may become adopted as a national practice standard.

In a normal (Gaussian) distribution, the mean ($\bar{X}$) is computed by dividing the sum of the observed values by the number of data points, *n,* as shown in the equation in "Statistical Significance and Expressions of Central Tendency and Dispersion." The SD is calculated using the formula provided in the same section. A typical RI is computed as mean ±2 SDs and assumes that the distribution is normal (Gaussian). Some laboratory directors prefer ±3 SDs when the precision is especially narrow. The limits at mean ±2 SDs encompass 95.46% of results from healthy individuals, known as the *95.5% confidence interval.* This implies that 4.54% of results from theoretically healthy individuals fall outside the interval by chance alone. An SD computed from a non-Gaussian distribution may turn out to be too narrow to reflect the true RI and may thus encompass fewer than 95.5% of results from presumed healthy subjects and generate an excess of false positives. Assays with high CV% values have high levels of random error reflected in a broad curve; low CV% assays with "tight" dispersion have smaller random error and generate a narrow curve, as illustrated in Figure 2.1. The breadth of the curve may also reflect biologic variation in values of the analyte.

A few hematology and hemostasis assays are used to monitor drug therapy. For instance, the INR for prothrombin time is used to monitor the effects of oral warfarin (Coumadin) therapy, and the therapeutic range is universally established at an INR of 2 to 3. On the other hand, the therapeutic range for monitoring treatment with unfractionated heparin using the PTT assay must be established locally by graphically comparing a regression of the PTT results in seconds against the results of the *chromogenic anti-Xa heparin assay,* whose therapeutic range is established empirically as 0.3 to 0.7 international heparin units. The PTT therapeutic range is called the ex vivo *Brill-Edwards curve* and is described in Chapter 40.

If assay revalidation or lot-to-lot comparison reveals a systematic change caused by reagent or kit modifications, a new RI (and therapeutic range, when applicable) is established. The laboratory director must advise the hospital staff of RI and therapeutic range changes because failure to observe new intervals and ranges may result in diagnosis and treatment errors.

INTERNAL QUALITY CONTROL

Controls

Laboratory QC managers prepare, or more often purchase, assay *controls.* Although it may appear similar, a control is wholly distinct from a calibrator. Indeed, cautious laboratory directors may insist that controls be purchased from distributors different from those who supply their calibrators. As discussed in "Method Validation," calibrators are used to adjust or revalidate instrumentation or to develop a calibration curve. Calibrators are assayed by a reference method in expert laboratories, and their assigned value is certified. Controls are used independently of the calibration process so that systematic errors caused by deterioration of the calibrator or a change in the analytical process can be detected through internal QC. This process is continuous and is called *calibration verification.* Compared with calibrators, control materials are inexpensive and are prepared from the same matrix as patient specimens except for preservatives, lyophilization, or freezing necessary to prolong shelf life. Controls provide known values and are sampled alongside patient specimens to accomplish within-run assay validation. In nearly all instances, two controls are required per test run: one within the RI and one above or below the RI. For some assays there is reason to select controls whose values are just outside the upper or lower limit of the RI, or "slightly" abnormal. In institutions that perform continuous runs, the controls should be run at least once per shift, for instance, at 7 a.m., 3 p.m., and 11 p.m. In laboratories where assay runs are discrete events, two controls are assayed with each run.

Control results must fall within predetermined dispersion limits, typically ±2 SD. Control manufacturers provide limits; however, local laboratory professionals must validate and transfer manufacturer limits or establish their own, usually by computing SD from the first 20 control assays, during which time the previous control lot remains in service. Whenever the result for a control is outside the established limits, the run is rejected and the cause is found and corrected. The steps for correction are listed in Table 2.8.

Control results are plotted on a Levey-Jennings chart that displays each data point compared with the mean and limits (Figure 2.6).[35] The Levey-Jennings chart assumes that the control results distribute in a Gaussian manner and imprints limits

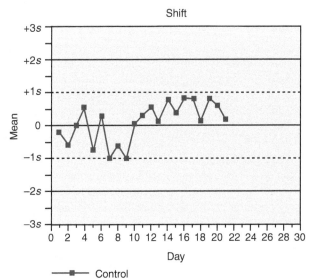

Figure 2.7 **Levey-Jennings Chart Illustrating a Systematic Error.** Control results from 21 runs in 22 days all fall within the action limits established as ±2 standard deviations; however, the final 11 control results locate above the mean. When 10 consecutive control results fall on one side of the mean, the assay has been affected by a systematic error, in this case a *Westgard 10ₓ* condition, also called a "shift" (Table 2.9). The operator troubleshoots and recalibrates the assay. *s*, Standard deviation.

at 1, 2, and 3 SD above and below the mean. In addition to being analyzed for single-run errors, the data points are examined for sequential errors over time (Figure 2.7). Both single-run and long-term control variation are a function of assay dispersion or random error and reflect the CV% of an assay.

Dr. James Westgard has established a series of internal QC rules that are routinely applied to long-term deviations, called the *Westgard rules*.[36] The rules were developed for assays that employ primary standards, but a few Westgard rules that are the most useful in hematology and hemostasis laboratories are provided in Table 2.9, along with the appropriate actions to be taken.

TABLE 2.8 Steps Used to Correct an Out-of-Control Assay Run

Step	Description
1. Reassay	When a limit of ±2 SDs is used, 5% of expected assay results fall above or below the limit.
2. Prepare new control and reassay	Controls may deteriorate over time when exposed to adverse temperatures or subjected to conditions causing evaporation.
3. Prepare fresh reagents and reassay	Reagents may have evaporated or become contaminated.
4. Recalibrate instrument	Instrument may require repair.

SD, Standard deviation.

TABLE 2.9 Westgard Rules Employed in Hematology and Hemostasis

1_{3s}	A single control value is outside the ±3 SD limit.
2_{2s}	Two control values are outside the ±2 SD limit.
R_{4s}	Two consecutive control values within a run are more than 4 SD apart.
4_{1s}	Four consecutive control values within a run exceed the mean by ±1 SD.
10_X	Also called a "shift." A series of 10 consecutive control values remain within the dispersion limits but are consistently above or below the mean.
7_T	Also called a "trend." A series of at least seven control values trend in a consistent direction.

10_X or 7_T may indicate an instrument calibration issue that has introduced a constant systematic error (bias). Shifts or trends may be caused by deterioration of reagents, pump fittings, or light sources. Abrupt shifts may reflect a reagent or instrument fitting change.

SD, Standard deviation.
In all cases, assay results are rejected and the error is identified using the steps in Table 2.8.

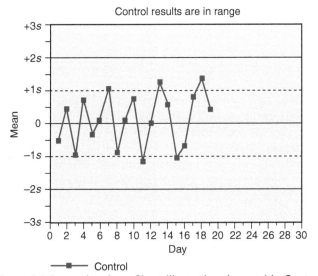

Figure 2.6 **Levey-Jennings Chart Illustrating Acceptable Control Results.** Control results from 19 runs in 20 days all fall within the action limits established as ±2 standard deviations. Results distribute evenly about the mean. *s*, Standard deviation.

Moving Average ($\overline{X}_B$) of the Red Blood Cell Indices

In 1974, Dr. Brian Bull proposed a method of employing *patient* RBC indices to monitor the stability of automated blood cell analyzers, recognizing that the RBC indices, mean cell volume (MCV), mean cell hemoglobin (MCH), and mean cell hemoglobin concentration (MCHC) remain constant on average despite individual patient variations.[37] Each consecutive sequence of 20 patient RBC index assay results is collected and treated by the moving average formula (see reference), which accumulates, "smooths," and "trims" data to reduce the effects of outliers. Each trimmed 20-specimen mean, $\overline{X}_B$, is plotted on a Levey-Jennings chart and tracked for trends and shifts using Westgard rules. The formula has been automated and embedded in the circuitry of all automated blood cell analyzers, which provide Levey-Jennings charts for MCV, MCH, and MCHC. The moving average concept has been generalized to WBC and platelet counts and to some clinical chemistry analytes, albeit with moderate success.

To begin, 500 consecutive specimens are analyzed for the mean MCV, MCH, and MCHC. A Levey-Jennings chart is prepared using ±3% of the mean or 1 SD as the action limits, and subsequent data accumulation commences in groups of 20.

The moving average method requires a computer to calculate the averages, does not detect within-run errors, and is less sensitive than the use of commercial controls in detecting systematic shifts and trends. It works well in institutions that assay specimens from generalized populations that contain minimal numbers of sickle cell or oncology patients. A population that has a high percentage of abnormal hematologic results, as may be seen in a tertiary care facility, may generate a preponderance of moving average outliers.[38] Moving average systems do not replace the use of control specimens but provide additional means to detect shifts and trends.

Delta Checks

The δ-check system compares a current analyte result with the result from the most recent previous analysis for the same patient.[39] Certain patient values remain relatively consistent over time unless there is an intervention. A result that fails a δ-check, often defined as a 20% deviation, is investigated for an intervention such as a transfusion or surgery, or for a profound change in the patient's condition subsequent to the previous analysis. If there is no ready explanation, the failed δ-check may indicate an analytical error or mislabeled specimen. In hemostasis, failed δ-checks should also encompass a review of specimen collection errors. Results that fail a δ-check are sequestered until the cause is found. Laboratory directors may require δ-checks on MCV, red cell distribution width (RDW), hemoglobin (HGB), platelet count (PLT), PT, INR, and PTT. Action limits for δ-checks are based on clinical impression and are assigned by hematology and hemostasis laboratory directors in collaboration with clinicians and laboratory staff. Computerization is essential, and δ-checks are designed only to identify gross errors, not changes in random error, or shifts or trends. There is no regulatory requirement for δ-checks.

EXTERNAL QUALITY ASSESSMENT

External quality assessment further validates the accuracy of hematology and hemostasis assays by comparing results from identical aliquots of specimens distributed at regular intervals among laboratories nationwide or worldwide. The aliquots are often called *survey* or *proficiency testing* specimens and include preserved human subject plasma and whole blood, stained peripheral blood films and bone marrow smears, and photomicrographs of cells or tissues.

In most proficiency testing systems, target (true or reference) values for the test specimens are established in-house by their manufacturer or distributor and are then further validated by preliminary distribution to a handful of "expert" laboratories. Separate target values may be assigned for various assay methods and instruments, as feasible.

Laboratories that participate in external quality assessment are directed to manage the survey specimens using the same procedures as those employed for patient specimens, that is, survey specimens should not receive special attention. Turnaround is swift, and results are sent electronically to the provider.

In addition to establishing a target value, agencies that administer surveys reduce the returned data to statistics, including the mean, median, and SD of all participant results. Provided the survey is large enough, the statistics may also be computed individually for the various instruments and assay methods. The statistics collected from participants should match the predetermined targets. If they do not, the agency troubleshoots the assay and assigns the most reliable statistics, usually the group mean and SDs.

The agency provides a report to each laboratory, illustrating its results in comparison with the target values and appending a comment if the laboratory result exceeds the established limits, usually ±2 SDs from the mean. If the specimen is a blood film or bone marrow smear, a photomicrograph, or a problem that requires a binary (positive/negative, yes/no) response, the local laboratory comment is compared with expert opinion and consensus.

Although a certain level of error is tolerated, error rates that exceed established limits result in corrective recommendations or, in extreme circumstances, loss of laboratory accreditation or licensure.

There are a number of external quality assessment agencies; however, in the United States the College of American Pathologists (CAP, cap.org) and the American Proficiency Institute (API, api-pt.com) provide the largest survey systems. Survey packages are provided for laboratories offering all levels of service. API and CAP are nongovernmental agencies; however, survey participation is necessary to meet the accreditation requirements of The Joint Commission (jointcommission.org) and to qualify for Medicare reimbursement. The North American Specialized Coagulation Laboratory Association (nascola.org) provides survey systems for specialty coagulation laboratories in the United States and Canada and is affiliated with the ECAT (External Quality Control of Diagnostic Assays and Tests, ecat.nl) Foundation External Quality Assessment Program of the Netherlands, which provides survey materials throughout Europe. Many state health agencies provide proficiency testing surveys, requiring laboratories to participate as a condition of licensure.

ASSESSING DIAGNOSTIC EFFICACY

Since the 1930s, surgeons have required the *bleeding time* test to predict the risk of intraoperative hemorrhage. The laboratory professional activates an automated lancet to make a 5-mm long, 1-mm deep incision in the volar surface of the forearm and uses a clean piece of filter paper to meticulously absorb drops of blood in 30-second intervals. The time interval from initial incision to bleeding cessation is recorded, typically 2 to 9 minutes. The test is simple and logical, and experts claimed for more than 50 years that if the incision bleeds for longer than 9 minutes, there is a risk of surgical bleeding. In the 1990s clinical researchers compared within-range and prolonged bleeding times with instances of intraoperative bleeding and found to their surprise that prolonged bleeding time results predicted fewer than 50% of intraoperative bleeds.[40,41] Many bleeds occurred despite a bleeding time shorter than 9 minutes. Thus the positive predictive value of the bleeding time for intraoperative bleeding was less than 50%, which is the probability of turning up heads in a coin toss. Today the bleeding time test is widely agreed to have no clinical efficacy and is obsolete, though still available.

Like the bleeding time test, many time-honored hematology and hemostasis assays gain credibility on the basis of logic and expert opinion. Now, however, besides being valid, accurate, linear, and precise, a new or modified assay must be diagnostically effective.[42] To compute diagnostic efficacy, the laboratory professional obtains a series of specimens from healthy subjects, volunteers who do not have the particular disease or condition being measured, called *controls;* and from patients who *conclusively possess a disease or condition.* The patients' diagnosis is based on downstream clinical outcomes, discharge notes, or the results of valid existing laboratory tests, excluding the new assay. The new assay is then applied to specimens from both the healthy control and disease patient groups to assess its efficacy.

In a perfect world, the laboratory scientist sets the *discrimination threshold* at the 95.5% CI limit (± 2 SD) of the mean. When this threshold, also called the limit or "cut point," is used, the test hopefully yields a positive result, meaning a level elevated beyond the upper limit or reduced to less than the lower limit, in every instance of disease and a negative result, within the RI, in all subjects (controls) without the disease. In reality, there is always some overlap: a "gray area" in which some positive test results are generated from nondisease specimens *(false positives)* and some negative results are generated from specimens taken from patients with proven disease *(false negatives).* False positives cause unnecessary anxiety, follow-up expense, and erroneous diagnostic leads, which are worrisome, expensive, and time consuming, but seldom fatal. False negatives fail to detect the disease and may delay treatment, a circumstance that can be potentially life threatening. The laboratory scientist employs diagnostic efficacy computations to establish the effectiveness of laboratory assays and to minimize both false-positive and false-negative results (Table 2.10). Diagnostic efficacy testing

TABLE 2.10 Diagnostic Efficacy Definitions and Binary Display

True positive	Assay correctly identifies a disease or condition in those who have it.
False positive	Assay incorrectly identifies disease or condition when none is present.
True negative	Assay correctly excludes a disease or condition in those without it.
False negative	Assay incorrectly excludes disease or condition when it is present.

	Individuals Unaffected by the Disease or Condition	Individuals Affected by the Disease or Condition
Assay is negative	True negative	False negative
Assay is positive	False positive	True positive

TABLE 2.11 Diagnostic Efficacy Study

	Individuals Unaffected by the Disease or Condition	Individuals Affected by the Disease or Condition
Assay is negative	True negative: 40	False negative: 5
Assay is positive	False positive: 10	True positive: 45

These are data on specimens from 50 individuals who are unaffected by the disease or condition and 50 individuals who are affected by the disease or condition. These data are used in the calculations in Table 2.12.

includes determination of diagnostic sensitivity and specificity, positive and negative predictive value, and receiver operating characteristic (ROC) analysis.

To start a diagnostic efficacy study, the scientist selects control specimens from healthy subjects and specimens from patients proven to have the disease or condition addressed by the assay. To make this discussion simple, assume that 50 specimens of each are chosen. All are assayed, and the results are shown in Table 2.11.

The laboratory professional next computes diagnostic sensitivity and specificity and positive and negative predictive value as shown in Table 2.12. These values are then used to consider the conditions in which the assay may be effectively employed.

Effects of Population Incidence and Odds Ratios on Diagnostic Efficacy

Epidemiologists describe population events using the terms *prevalence* and *incidence. Prevalence* describes the total number of events or conditions in a broadly defined population; for instance, the total number of patients with chronic heart disease in the United States. *Prevalence* quantitates the burden of a disease on society but is not qualified by time intervals and does not predict disease risk.

Incidence describes the number of events occurring within a randomly selected number of subjects representing a population, over a defined time; for instance, the number of new cases of heart disease per 100,000 US residents per year. Incidence

TABLE 2.12   Diagnostic Efficacy Computations*

Statistic	Definition	Formula	Example
Diagnostic sensitivity	Proportion with the disease who have a positive test result	Sensitivity (%) = TP/(TP + FN) × 100	45/(45 + 5) × 100 = 90%
Distinguish diagnostic sensitivity from analytical sensitivity. Analytical sensitivity is a measure of the smallest increment of the analyte that can be distinguished by the assay.			
Diagnostic specificity	Proportion without the disease who have a negative test result	Specificity (%) = TN/(TN + FP) × 100	40/(40 + 10) × 100 = 80%
Distinguish diagnostic specificity from analytical specificity. Analytical specificity is the ability of the assay to distinguish the analyte from interfering substances.			
Positive predictive value (PPV)	Proportion with a disease who have a positive test result compared with all individuals who have a positive test result	PPV (%) = TP/(TP + FP) × 100	45/(45 + 10) × 100 = 82%
The positive predictive value predicts the probability that an individual with a positive assay result has the disease or condition.			
Negative predictive value (NPV)	Proportion without a disease who have a negative test result compared with all individuals who have a negative test result	NPV (%) = TN/(TN + FN) × 100	40/(40 + 5) × 100 = 89%
The negative predictive value predicts the probability that an individual with a negative assay result does not have the disease or condition.			

FN, False negative; *FP*, false positive; *TN*, true negative; *TP*, true positive.
*Using data from Table 2.11.

numbers are non-cumulative. *Incidence* can be further defined, for instance, by the number of heart disease cases per 100,000 nonsmokers, 100,000 women, or 100,000 people ages 40 to 50. Scientists use incidence, not prevalence, to select laboratory assays for specific applications such as screening or confirmation.

For all assays, as diagnostic sensitivity rises, specificity declines. A *screening test* is an assay that is applied to a large number of subjects within a convenience sample where the participant's condition is unknown; for example, lipid profiles offered in a shopping mall. Assays that possess high sensitivity and low specificity make effective screening tests, although they produce a number of false positives. For instance, if the condition being studied has an incidence of 0.0001 (1 in 10,000 per year) and the false-positive rate is a modest 1%, the assay will produce 99 false-positive results for every true-positive result. Clearly such a test is useful only when the consequence of a false-positive result is minimal and follow-up confirmation is readily available.

Conversely, as specificity rises, sensitivity declines. Assays with high specificity provide effective confirmation when used in follow-up to positive results on screening assays. High-specificity assays produce a number of false negatives and should not be used as initial screening assays. A positive result on both a screening assay and a confirmatory assay provides a definitive conclusion. A positive screening result followed by a negative confirmatory test result generates a search for alternative diagnoses.

Laboratory assays are most effective when chosen to assess patients with high clinical pretest probability. In such instances, the incidence of the condition is high enough to mitigate the effects of false positives and false negatives. For instance, when a physician orders hemostasis testing for patients who are experiencing easy bruising, there is a high pretest probability, which raises the assays' diagnostic efficacy. Conversely, ordering hemostasis assays as screens of healthy individuals before elective surgery introduces a low pretest probability and reduces the efficacy of the test profile, raising the relative rate of false positives.

Epidemiologists further assist laboratory professionals by designing prospective randomized control trials to predict the relative odds ratio (or relative risk ratio, RRR) and the absolute odds ratio (or absolute risk ratio, ARR) of an intervention that is designed to modify the incidence of an event within a selected population, as illustrated in the following example.[43]

You design a 5-year study in which you select 2000 obese smokers ages 40 to 60 who have no heart disease. You randomly select 1000 for intervention: periodic laboratory assays for inflammatory markers, with follow-up aspirin for those who have positive assay results. The 1000 controls are tested with the same laboratory assays but are given a placebo that resembles aspirin. The primary endpoint is acute myocardial infarction (AMI). No one dies or drops out, and at the end of 5 years 100 of the 1000 controls and 50 of the 1000 members of the intervention arm have suffered AMIs. The control arm ratio is 100/1000 = 0.1; the intervention arm ratio is 50/1000 = 0.05; and the RRR is 0.05/0.1 = 0.5 (50%). You predict from your study that the odds (RRR) of having a heart attack are cut in half by the intervention. You repeat the study using 2000 slim nonsmokers ages 20 to 40. In this sample, 10 of the 1000 controls and 5 in the intervention group suffer AMIs; the computation is 0.005/0.01 = 0.5, same as in the obese smoker group, thus enabling you to generalize your obese smoker results to slim nonsmokers. RRR has been used extensively to support widespread medical interventions, often without regard to control arm incidence or the risks associated with generalizing to non-studied populations.

You go on to compute the ARR, which is the absolute value of the arithmetic *difference* in the event rates of the control and intervention arms. In our example using the obese smokers group, the ARR = 0.1 − 0.05 = 0.05, or 5% (not 50%, as reported in the example using RRR above). The ARR is often expressed as the number necessary to treat (NNT), the inverse of ARR. In our example, for everyone whose AMI is prevented by the laboratory test and subsequent treatment, you would have to treat 20 total subjects over a 5-year period. Further, if you reduce the ARR to an annual rate, 0.05/5 years = 0.01, or a 1% annual reduction. You conclude from your study that 100 interventions per year are required to prevent one AMI.

Finally, your RRR and ARR are not discrete integers but means computed from samples of 1000, so they must include an expression of dispersion, usually ±2 SD or a 95.5% confidence interval. Suppose the 95.5% CI for the RRR turns out to be relatively broad: −0.1 to +1.1. A ratio of 1 implies no effect from the intervention; that is, the rate of change in the intervention arm is equal to the rate of change in the control arm. Given that the 95.5% CI embraces the number 1, the intervention has failed to provide any benefit.

In summary, once a laboratory assay is verified to be accurate and precise, it must then be determined to possess diagnostic efficacy and to provide for effective intervention as determined by favorable RRR and ARR or NNT values. Application of the ROC curve may help achieve these goals.

RECEIVER OPERATING CHARACTERISTIC CURVE

A ROC curve is a further refinement of diagnostic efficacy testing that may be employed to determine the decision limit (cutoff, threshold) for an assay when the assay generates a *continuous variable.*[44] In diagnostic efficacy testing as described in the previous section, the ±2 SD limits of the RI are used as the thresholds for discriminating a positive from a negative test result. Often the "true" threshold varies from the ±2 SD limit. Using ROC analysis, the limit is adjusted by increments of 1 (or other increments depending on the analytical range), and the true-positive and false-positive rates are recomputed for each new threshold level using the same formulas provided in "Assessing Diagnostic Efficacy." The limit that is finally selected is the one that provides the largest true-positive and smallest false-positive rate (Figure 2.8). The operator generates a line graph plotting true positives on the *y*-axis and false positives on the *x*-axis. Measuring the *area under the curve* (a computer-based calculus function) assesses the overall efficacy of the assay. If the area under the curve is 0.5, the curve is at the line of identity between false and true positives and provides no discrimination. Most agree that a clinically useful assay should have an area under the curve of 0.85 or higher.[44]

ASSAY FEASIBILITY

Most laboratory managers and directors review assay feasibility before launching complex validation, efficacy, RI, and QC initiatives. Feasibility studies include a review of assay throughput (number of assays per unit time), dwell time (length of assay interval from specimen sampling to report), cost per test, cost/benefit ratio, turnaround time, and the technical skill required to perform the assay. To select a new instrument, the manager reviews issues of operator safety, footprint, overhead, compatibility with laboratory utilities and information system, the need for middleware, frequency and duration of breakdowns, and distributor support and service.

LABORATORY STAFF COMPETENCE

Staff integrity and professional staff competence are the keys to assay reliability. In the United States, California, Florida, Georgia, Hawaii, Louisiana, Montana, Nevada, New York, North Dakota, Rhode Island, Tennessee, West Virginia, and Puerto Rico enforce laboratory personnel licensure laws.[45] In these states, only licensed laboratory professionals may be employed in medical center or reference laboratories. Legislatures in Alaska, Illinois, Massachusetts, Minnesota, Missouri, Vermont, and Virginia have considered and rejected licensure bills, the bills having been opposed by competing health care specialty associations and for-profit entities. In nonlicensure states, conscientious laboratory directors employ only nationally certified professionals. Certification is available from the Board of Certification of the American Society for Clinical Pathology. Studies of laboratory errors and outcomes demonstrate that laboratories that employ only licensed or certified professionals produce the most reliable assay results.[46]

Competent laboratory staff members continuously watch for and document errors by inspecting the results of internal validation and QC programs and external quality assessment. Error is inevitable, and incidents should be documented and highlighted for quality improvement and remedial instruction. When error is associated with reprimand, the opportunity for improvement may be lost to cover-up. Except in cases of negligence, the analysis of error without blame is consistently practiced in an effort to improve the quality of laboratory services.

Proficiency Systems

Laboratory managers and directors assess and document professional staff skills using proficiency systems. The hematology laboratory manager may, for instance, maintain and secure a collection of normal and abnormal blood films, case studies, or laboratory assay reports that medical laboratory technicians and scientists are required to examine at regular intervals. Personnel who fail to reproduce the target values on examination of the blood film are provided remedial instruction. The proficiency set may also be used to assess applicants for laboratory positions. Proficiency testing systems are available from external quality assessment agencies, and proficiency reports are made accessible to laboratory assessors.

Continuing Education

The Board of Certification of the American Society for Clinical Pathology and state medical laboratory personnel licensure boards require medical laboratory technicians and scientists to participate in and document continuing education for *periodic recertification* or *relicensure.* Educators and experts deliver continuing education in the form of journal articles, case studies, online seminars (webinars), and seminars and workshops at professional meetings. Medical centers offer periodic internal continuing education opportunities (in-service education) in the form of grand rounds, lectures, seminars, and participative educational events. Presentation and discussion of current cases are particularly effective. Continuing education maintains the critical skills of laboratory personnel and provides opportunities to learn about new clinical and technical approaches. The

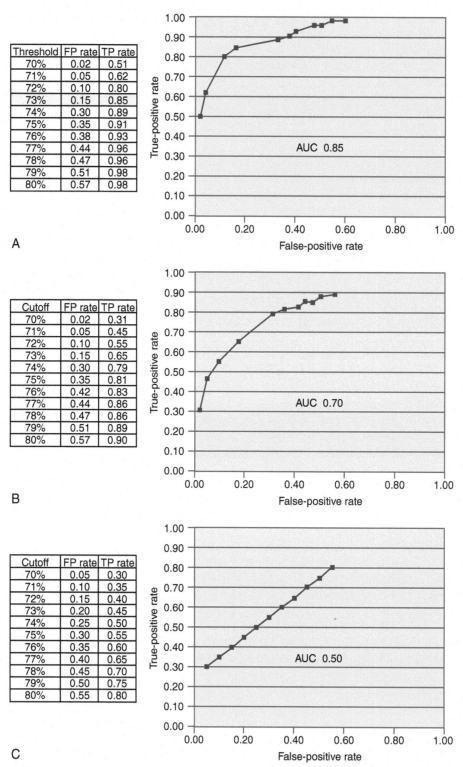

Threshold	FP rate	TP rate
70%	0.02	0.51
71%	0.05	0.62
72%	0.10	0.80
73%	0.15	0.85
74%	0.30	0.89
75%	0.35	0.91
76%	0.38	0.93
77%	0.44	0.96
78%	0.47	0.96
79%	0.51	0.98
80%	0.57	0.98

A

Cutoff	FP rate	TP rate
70%	0.02	0.31
71%	0.05	0.45
72%	0.10	0.55
73%	0.15	0.65
74%	0.30	0.79
75%	0.35	0.81
76%	0.42	0.83
77%	0.44	0.86
78%	0.47	0.86
79%	0.51	0.89
80%	0.57	0.90

B

Cutoff	FP rate	TP rate
70%	0.05	0.30
71%	0.10	0.35
72%	0.15	0.40
73%	0.20	0.45
74%	0.25	0.50
75%	0.30	0.55
76%	0.35	0.60
77%	0.40	0.65
78%	0.45	0.70
79%	0.50	0.75
80%	0.55	0.80

C

Figure 2.8 Receiver Operating Characteristic Curves. (A), The false-positive and true-positive rates for each discrimination threshold (decision point, limit) from 70% to 80% are computed and graphed as paired variables on a linear scale, false-positive rate on the horizontal *(x)* scale and true-positive rate on the vertical *(y)* scale. The assay provides acceptable discrimination between individuals affected by the disease or condition and nonaffected individuals; with an area under the curve (AUC) of 0.85, and 73% is the threshold that produces the most desirable false-positive and true-positive rates. **(B),** This assay has unacceptable discrimination between individuals affected by the disease or condition and unaffected individuals, with an AUC of 0.70. No threshold produces a desirable false-positive and true-positive rates. **(C),** This assay, with an AUC of 0.50, has no ability to discriminate. *FP,* False positive; *TP,* true positive.

American Society for Clinical Laboratory Science (ascls.org), the American Society for Clinical Pathology (ascp.org), the American Society of Hematology (hematology.org), the National Hemophilia Foundation (hemophilia.org), and the Fritsma Factor (fritsmafactor.com) are examples of the scores of organizations that direct their activities toward quality continuing education in hematology and hemostasis. Consumer Reports and the American Board of Internal Medicine (ABIM) Foundation collaborate on the Choosing Wisely program, which seeks to advance a national dialogue on avoiding wasteful or unnecessary procedures (choosingwisely.org).

The medical laboratory science profession stratifies professional staff responsibilities by educational preparation. In the United States professional levels are defined as the associate (2-year) degree level, or *medical laboratory technician*; bachelor (4-year) degree level, or *medical laboratory scientist*; and the levels of advanced degrees: master's degree, professional Doctorate in Clinical Laboratory Science (DCLS), and PhD in clinical laboratory and related sciences. Many colleges and universities offer articulation programs that enable professional personnel to advance their education and responsibility levels. Several of these institutions provide undergraduate and graduate distance-learning opportunities. A current list is maintained by the National Accrediting Agency for Clinical Laboratory Sciences (naacls.org), and the American Society for Clinical Laboratory Science publishes the *Directory of Graduate Programs for Clinical Laboratory Practitioners*. Enlightened employers encourage personnel to participate in advanced educational programs, and many provide resources for this purpose. Education contributes to quality laboratory services.

QUALITY ASSURANCE PLAN: PREANALYTICAL AND POSTANALYTICAL

In addition to keeping analytical QC records, US regulatory agencies such as the Centers for Medicare and Medicaid Services (cms.gov) require laboratory directors to maintain records of preanalytical and postanalytical QA and quality improvement efforts.[47] Although not exhaustive, Table 2.1 lists and characterizes a number of examples of preanalytical quality efforts, and Table 2.2 provides a review of postanalytical components. All QA plans provide objectives, sources of authority, scope of services, an activity calendar, corrective action, periodic evaluation,

standard protocol, personnel involvement, and methods of communication.[48]

API Paperless Proficiency Testing and CAP Q-PROBES are subscription services that provide model QA programs. Experts in QA continuously refine the consensus of appropriate indicators of laboratory medicine quality. QA programs search for events that provide improvement opportunities.

AGENCIES THAT ADDRESS HEMATOLOGY AND HEMOSTASIS QUALITY

These are representative agencies that are concerned with QA in hematology and hemostasis laboratory testing:
- Data Innovations North America (datainnovations.com). QA management software: instrument management middleware, laboratory production management software, EP Evaluator, RI tables, allowable total error tables.
- Clinical and Laboratory Standards Institute (CLSI, clsi.org). International guidelines and standards for laboratory practice. Hematology and hemostasis guidelines and standards include CLSI H02-A4, H07-A3, and H21–H48, method evaluation and assessment of diagnostic accuracy, mostly EP-prefix standards; QA and quality management systems, mostly QMS-prefix standards are available.
- Centers for Medicare and Medicaid Services (CMS, cms.gov). Administers the laws and rules developed from the *Clinical Laboratory Improvement Amendments of 1988*. Establishes *Current Procedural Terminology* (CPT) codes, reimbursement rules, and classifies assay complexity.
- American Proficiency Institute (API, api-pt.com). Laboratory proficiency testing and QA programs, continuing education programs and summaries, tutorials, and special topics library.
- College of American Pathologists (CAP, cap.org). Laboratory accreditation, proficiency testing, and QA programs; laboratory education, reference resources, and e-lab solutions.
- The Joint Commission (jointcommission.org). Medical center-wide accreditation and certification programs.
- Laboratory Medicine Quality Improvement (cdc.gov/osels/lspppo/Laboratory_Medicine_Quality_Improvement/index.html), an initiative of the US Centers for Disease Control and Prevention.

SUMMARY

- Hematology and hemostasis laboratory quality control (QC) relies on descriptive statistics that provide measures of central tendency, measures of dispersion, and significance.
- Each new assay or assay modification must be validated for accuracy, precision, linearity, analytical measurement range (AMR), specificity, and lower limit of detection (LLD) ability.
- In the hematology and hemostasis laboratory, accuracy validation usually requires a series of calibrators. Accuracy is established using the Student *t*-test, analysis of variance (ANOVA), Pearson correlation, linear regression, and the Bland-Altman distribution.

- Precision is established by using repeated within-day, and day-to-day assays, then computing the mean, standard deviation (SD), and coefficient of variation (CV) of the results.
- Vendors usually provide assay linearity, specificity, and LLD; however, laboratory managers may require that these parameters be revalidated locally. These parameters must be validated when a Food and Drug Administration (FDA)-approved assay is modified or when the laboratory professional develops a local, "laboratory-developed test."
- Internal QC is accomplished by assaying controls with each test run. Control results are compared with action limits, usually the

mean of the control assay ±2 SD. When a specified number of control values are outside the limits, the use of the assay is suspended and the laboratory professional begins troubleshooting. Control results are plotted on Levey-Jennings charts and examined for shifts and trends. Internal QC is enhanced through the use of the moving average algorithm and δ-checks.

- All conscientious laboratory directors subscribe to an external quality assessment system, also known as *proficiency testing* or *proficiency surveys.* External quality assessment enables the director to compare selected assay results with other laboratory results, nationally and internationally, as a further check of accuracy. Maintaining a good external quality assessment record is essential to laboratory accreditation. Most US states require external quality assessment for laboratory licensure.

- All laboratory assays are analyzed for diagnostic efficacy, including diagnostic sensitivity and specificity, their true-positive and true-negative rates, and positive and negative predictive values. Highly sensitive assays may be used for population screening but may poorly discriminate between the healthy and diseased population. Specific assays may be used to confirm a condition but generate a number of false negatives. Assays are chosen on the basis of the value of their intervention, based on relative or absolute risk ratios. Diagnostic efficacy computations expand to include receiver operating characteristic (ROC) curve analysis.

- Meticulous laboratory managers hire only certified or licensed medical laboratory scientists and technicians and provide regular individual proficiency tests that are correlated with in-service education. They encourage staff members to participate in continuing education activities and in-house discussion of cases. Quality laboratories provide resources for staff to pursue higher education.

- The laboratory director maintains a protocol for assessing and improving on preanalytical and postanalytical variables and finds means to communicate enhancements to other members of the health care team.

Now that you have completed this chapter, go back and read again the case study at the beginning and respond to the questions presented.

REVIEW QUESTIONS

Answers can be found in the Appendix.

1. What procedure is NOT employed to validate a new assay?
   a. Comparison of assay results to a reference method
   b. Test for assay precision
   c. Test for assay linearity
   d. Moving average algorithm

2. You validate a new assay using linear regression to compare assay calibrator results with the distributor's published calibrator results. The slope is 0.99 and the *y* intercept is +10%. What type of error is present?
   a. No error
   b. Random error
   c. Constant systematic error
   d. Proportional systematic error

3. Which is a statistical test that compares means?
   a. Bland-Altman
   b. Student *t*-test
   c. ANOVA
   d. Pearson

4. The acceptable hemoglobin control value range is 13 ± 0.4 g/dL. The control is assayed five times and produces the following five results: 12.0 g/dL 12.3 g/dL 12.0 g/dL 12.2 g/dL 12.1 g/dL
   These results are:
   a. Accurate but not precise
   b. Precise but not accurate
   c. Both accurate and precise
   d. Neither accurate nor precise

5. A WBC count control has a mean value of 6000/μL and an SD of 300/μL. What is the 95.5% confidence interval?
   a. 3000 to 9000/μL
   b. 5400 to 6600/μL
   c. 5500 to 6500/μL
   d. 5700 to 6300/μL

6. The ability of an assay to distinguish the targeted analyte from interfering substances within the specimen matrix is called:
   a. Analytical specificity
   b. Analytical sensitivity
   c. Clinical specificity
   d. Clinical sensitivity

7. The laboratory purchases reagents from a manufacturer and develops an assay using a protocol published in a volume of the *Methods in Molecular Biology* series. How would the FDA classify this assay?
   a. Cleared
   b. Research use only
   c. Analyte-specific reagent
   d. Laboratory-developed test

8. What process ensures comparability in multi-site validation?
   a. Distribution of proficiency materials to all sites
   b. Publication of individual site reference intervals
   c. Clinical sensitivity and specificity computations
   d. ROC analysis

9. A laboratory scientist measures prothrombin time for plasma aliquots from 15 healthy men and 15 healthy women. She computes the mean and 95.5% confidence interval and notes that they duplicate the manufacturer's statistics within 5%. This procedure is known as:
   a. Setting the RI
   b. Confirming linearity
   c. Determining the therapeutic range
   d. Establishing the RI by transference

10. You purchase a preserved whole blood specimen from a distributor who provides the mean values for several complete blood count analytes. What is this specimen called?
    a. Normal specimen
    b. Calibrator
    c. Control
    d. Blank

11. You perform a clinical efficacy test and get the following results:

	Unaffected by Disease or Condition	Affected by Disease or Condition
Assay is negative	40	5
Assay is positive	10	45

What is the number of false-negative results?
   a. 45
   b. 40
   c. 10
   d. 5

12. What agency provides external quality assurance (proficiency) surveys and laboratory accreditation?
   a. Clinical Laboratory Improvement Advisory Committee (CLIAC)
   b. Centers for Medicare and Medicaid Services (CMS)
   c. College of American Pathologists (CAP)
   d. The Joint Commission

13. What agency provides continuing medical laboratory education?
   a. Clinical Laboratory Improvement Advisory Committee (CLIAC)
   b. American Society for Clinical Laboratory Science (ASCLS)
   c. Centers for Medicare and Medicaid Services (CMS)
   d. College of American Pathologists (CAP)

14. Regular review of blood specimen collection quality is an example of:
   a. Postanalytical quality assurance
   b. Preanalytical quality assurance
   c. Analytical quality control
   d. External quality assurance

15. Review of laboratory report integrity is an example of:
   a. Postanalytical quality assurance
   b. Preanalytical quality assurance
   c. Analytical quality control
   d. External quality assurance

16. When performing a receiver operating curve analysis, what parameter assesses the overall efficacy of an assay?
   a. Area under the curve
   b. Performance limit (threshold)
   c. Positive predictive value
   d. Negative predictive value

17. You require your laboratory staff to annually perform manual lupus anticoagulant profiles on a set of plasmas with known values. This exercise is known as:
   a. Assay validation
   b. Proficiency testing
   c. External quality assessment
   d. Pre-pre analytical variable assay

REFERENCES

1. Westgard, J. O. (2007). *Assuring the Right Quality Right: Good Laboratory Practices for Verifying the Attainment of the Intended Quality of Test Results.* Madison, WI: Westgard QC.
2. Becich, M. J. (2000). Information management: moving from test results to clinical information. *Clin Leadersh Manag Rev, 14,* 296–300.
3. CLSI. (2011). *Quality Management System: Continual Improvement.* (3rd ed., CLSI guideline QMS06-A3). Wayne, PA: Clinical and Laboratory Standards Institute.
4. Ernst, D. J., & Ernst, C. (2017). *The Lab Draw Answer Book.* Corydon, IN: Center for Phlebotomy Education.
5. CLSI. (2017). *Collection of Diagnostic Venous Blood Specimens.* (7th ed., CLSI standard GP41). Wayne, PA: Clinical and Laboratory Standards Institute.
6. Stroobants, A. K., Goldschmidt, H. M., & Piebani, M. (2003). Error budget calculations in laboratory medicine: linking the concepts of biological variation and allowable medical errors. *Clin Chim Acta, 333,* 169–176.
7. Laposata, M. E., Laposata, M., Van Cott, E. M., et al. (2004). Physician survey of a laboratory medicine interpretive service and evaluation of the influence of interpretations on laboratory test ordering. *Arch Pathol Lab Med, 128,* 1424–1427.
8. Hickner, J., Graham, D. G., Elder, N. C., et al. (2008). Testing practices: a study of the American Academy of Family Physicians National Research Network. *Qual Saf Health Care, 17,* 194–200.
9. Laposata, M., & Dighe, A. (2007). "Pre-pre" and "post-post" analytical error: high-incidence patient safety hazards involving the clinical laboratory. *Clin Chem Lab Med, 45,* 712–719.
10. Isaac, S., & Michael, W. B. (1995). *Handbook in Research and Evaluation: A Collection of Principles, Methods, and Strategies Useful in the Planning, Design, and Evaluation of Studies in Education and the Behavioral Sciences.* (3rd ed.). San Diego: EdITS Publishers.
11. Huck, S. W. (2011). *Reading Statistics and Research.* (6th ed.). New York: Pearson.
12. Fritsma, G. A., & McGlasson, D. L. (2012). *Quick Guide to Laboratory Statistics and Quality Control.* Washington DC: AACC Press.
13. McGlasson, D. L., Plaut, D., & Shearer, C. (2006). *Statistics for the Hemostasis Laboratory, CD-ROM.* McLean, VA: ASCLS Press.
14. Westgard, J. O. (2008). *Basic Method Validation.* (3rd ed.). Madison, WI: Westgard QC.
15. Paxton, A. (August 2016). *New tests, technologies at center of 2016 CAP checklist revamp. CAP Today.* http://captodayonline.com/new-tests-technologies-center-2016-cap-checklist-revamp/. Accessed August 22, 2018.
16. CLSI. (2018). *Measurement Procedure Comparison and Bias Estimation Using Patient Samples.* (3rd ed., CLSI guideline EP09c). Wayne, PA: Clinical and Laboratory Standards Institute.
17. Clinical Laboratory Improvement Amendments. (2003). *Calibration and Calibration Verification. Brochure Number 3.* http://www.cms.gov/Regulations-and-Guidance/Legislation/CLIA/CLIA_Brochures.html. Accessed August 16, 2017.
18. CLSI. (2009). *Laboratory Instrument Implementation, Verification, and Maintenance.* (CLSI guideline GP31-A). Wayne, PA: Clinical and Laboratory Standards Institute.
19. Bartz, A. E. (1988). *Basic Statistical Concepts.* (3rd ed.). New York: Macmillan Publishing.
20. Bland, J. M., & Altman, D. G. (1986). Statistical methods for assessing agreement between two methods of clinical measurement. *Lancet, 327,* 307–310.

21. Westgard, J. O., Quam, E. F., Barry, P. L., et al. (2010). *Basic QC Practices.* (3rd ed.). Madison, WI: Westgard QC.

22. CLSI. (2008). *Protocol for the Evaluation, Validation, and Implementation of Coagulometers.* (CLSI guideline H57-A). Wayne, PA: Clinical and Laboratory Standards Institute.

23. Koepke, J. A., Dotson, M. A., & Shifman, M. A. (1985). A critical evaluation of the manual/visual differential leukocyte counting method. *Blood Cells, 11,* 173–186.

24. Rogers, M. W., Letsos, C. B., Henderson, M. P. A., et al. (2018). Method evaluation and quality control. In Bishop, M. L., Fody, E. P., & Schoeff, L. E. (Eds.), *Clinical Chemistry: Principles, Techniques, and Correlations.* (8th ed., pp. 49–86). Philadelphia: Wolters Kluwer.

25. Schork, M. A., & Remington, R. D. (2000). *Statistics with Applications to the Biological and Health Sciences.* (3rd ed.). Upper Saddle River, NJ: Prentice Hall.

26. *Commercially Distributed Analyte Specific Reagents (ASRs): Frequently Asked Questions - Guidance for Industry and FDA Staff.* https://www.fda.gov/medicaldevices/deviceregulationandguidance/guidancedocuments/ucm078423.htm. Accessed August 11, 2017.

27. *Data Innovations EP Evaluator.* http://www.datainnovations.com/products/ep-evaluator. Accessed August 17, 2017.

28. Clinical and Laboratory Improvement Amendments of 1988 Public Law 100-578, October 31, 1988.

29. CLSI. (2012). *Verification of Comparability of Patient Results Within One Health Care System.* (CLSI guideline, interim revision EP31-A-IR) Wayne, PA: Clinical and Laboratory Standards Institute.

30. Paxton, A. (September 2016). *Laboratory accreditation program 2016 checklists: Less legwork, more clarity seen in personnel changes. CAP Today.* http://captodayonline.com/less-legwork-clarity-seen-personnel-changes/. Accessed August 22, 2018.

31. CLSI. (2010). *Defining, Establishing and Verifying Reference Intervals in the Clinical Laboratory.* (3rd ed., CLSI guideline EP28-A3c). Wayne, PA: Clinical and Laboratory Standards Institute.

32. Malone, B. (2012). The quest for pediatric reference ranges: why the national children's study promises answers. *Clin Lab News, 38,* 3–4.

33. Krejcie, R. V., & Morgan, D. W. (1970). Determining sample size for research activities. *Educ Psychol Meas, 30,* 607–610.

34. Bachner, P. (1987). Quality assurance in hematology. In Howanitz, P. J., & Howanitz, J. H. (Eds.), *Laboratory Quality Assurance.* New York: McGraw-Hill.

35. Levey, S., & Jennings, E. R. (1950). The use of control charts in the clinical laboratory. *Am J Clin Pathol, 20,* 1059–1066.

36. Westgard, J. O., Barry, P. L., Hunt, M. R., et al. (1981). A multirule Shewhart chart for quality control in clinical chemistry. *Clin Chem, 27,* 493–501.

37. Bull, B. S., Elashoff, R. M., Heilbron, D. C., et al. (1974). A study of various estimators for the derivation of quality control procedures from patient erythrocyte indices. *Am J Clin Pathol, 61,* 473–481.

38. Cembrowski, G. S., Smith, B., & Tung, D. (2010). Rationale for using insensitive quality control rules for today's hematology analyzers. *Int J Lab Hematol, 32,* 606–615.

39. Ovens, K., & Naugler, C. (2012). How useful are delta checks in the 21st century? A stochastic-dynamic model of specimen mix-up and detection. *J Pathol Inform, 3,* 5.

40. Lind, S. E. (1991). The bleeding time does not predict surgical bleeding. *Blood, 77,* 2547–2552.

41. Gewirtz, A. S., Miller, M. L., & Keys, T. F. (1996). The clinical usefulness of the preoperative bleeding time. *Arch Pathol Lab Med, 120,* 353–356.

42. Tripepi, G., Jager, K. J., Dekker, F. W., et al. (2010). Measures of effect in epidemiological research. *Clin Practice, 115,* 91–93.

43. Replogle, W. H., & Johnson, W. D. (2007). Interpretation of absolute measures of disease risk in comparative research. *Fam Med, 39,* 432–435.

44. Søreide, K. (2009). Receiver-operating characteristic curve analysis in diagnostic, prognostic and predictive biomarker research. *J Clin Pathol, 62,* 1–5.

45. Rohde, R. E., Falleur, D. M., & Ellis, J. R. (March 10, 2015). Almost anyone can perform your medical laboratory tests – wait, what? *Elsevier Connect.* https://www.elsevier.com/connect/almost-anyone-can-perform-your-medical-laboratory-tests-wait-what. Accessed August 21, 2018.

46. Novis, D. A. (2004). Detecting and preventing the occurrence of errors in the practices of laboratory medicine and anatomic pathology: 15 years' experience with the College of American Pathologists' Q-PROBES and Q-TRACKS programs. *Clin Lab Med, 24,* 965–978.

47. Westgard, J. O., Ehrmeyer, S. S., & Darcy, T. P. (2004). *CLIA Final Rule for Quality Systems, Quality Assessment Issues and Answers.* Madison, WI: Westgard QC.

48. Howanitz, P. J., Hoffman, G. G., Schifman, R. B., et al. (1992). A nationwide quality assurance program can describe standards for the practice of pathology and laboratory medicine. *Qual Assur Health Care, 3,* 245–256.

3

Cellular Structure and Function

*Elaine M. Keohane**

OBJECTIVES

After completion of this chapter, the reader will be able to:

1. Describe the structure, composition, and general function of cell membranes.
2. Describe the structure, composition, and function of components of the nucleus, including staining qualities visible by light microscopy.
3. Describe the structure, composition, and general function of cytoplasmic organelles, including staining qualities visible by light microscopy, if applicable.
4. Describe the general structure and function of the hematopoietic microenvironment and the effect of growth factors.
5. Describe general types of receptor signaling mechanisms that induce specific biologic responses in cells.
6. Associate the stages of the cell cycle with activities of the cell.
7. Describe the role of cyclins and cyclin-dependent kinases in cell cycle regulation.
8. Discuss the function of checkpoints in the cell cycle and where in the cycle they occur.
9. Differentiate between apoptosis and necrosis.

OUTLINE

Knowledge of the normal structure, composition, and function of cells is fundamental to the understanding of blood cell pathophysiology covered in later chapters. From the invention of the microscope and the discovery of cells in the 1600s to the present-day highly sophisticated analysis of cell ultrastructure with electron microscopy and other technologies, a remarkable body of knowledge is available about the structure of cells and their varied organelles. Complementing these discoveries were other advances in technology that enabled detailed understanding of the biochemistry, metabolism, and genetics of cells at the molecular level. Today, highly sophisticated analysis of cells using flow cytometry, cytogenetics, and molecular genetic testing (Chapters 28, 29, and 30) has become the standard of care in diagnosis and

---

*The author extends appreciation to Keila B. Poulsen, whose work in prior editions provided the foundation for this chapter.

management of many malignant and nonmalignant blood cell diseases. This new and ever-expanding knowledge has revolutionized the diagnosis and treatment of hematologic diseases, resulting in a dramatic improvement in patient survival for many conditions that previously had a dismal prognosis. With all these advances, however, the visual examination of blood cells on a peripheral blood film by light microscopy still remains the hallmark for the initial evaluation of hematologic abnormalities.

This chapter provides an overview of the structure, composition, and function of the components of the cell; the hematopoietic microenvironment; the cell cycle and its regulation; and the process of cell death by apoptosis and necrosis.

CELL ORGANIZATION

Cells are the structural units that constitute living organisms. Cells have specialized functions and contain the components necessary to perform and perpetuate these functions (Figures 3.1 and 3.2). Regardless of shape, size, or function, human cells contain:

- A *plasma membrane* that separates the *cytoplasm* and cellular components from the extracellular environment;
- A membrane-bound *nucleus* (with the exception of mature red blood cells and platelets); and
- Other unique subcellular structures and organelles that support various cellular functions.[1,2]

Table 3.1 summarizes the cellular components and their functions, which are explained in more detail within the chapter.

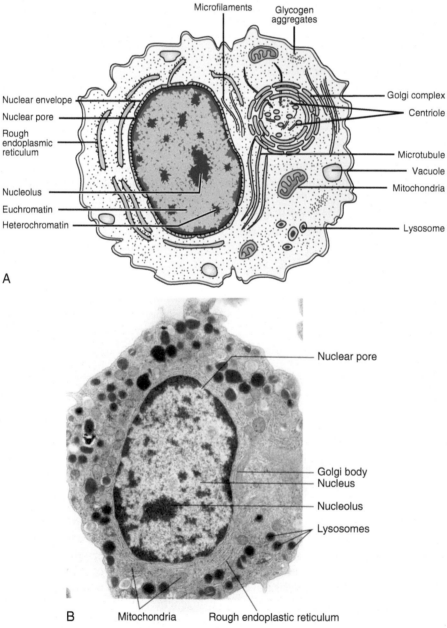

Figure 3.1 Cell Structure. (A), Schematic of an electron micrograph of cell organization and components. **(B),** Electron micrograph of a cell with labeled organelles. (B from Rodak, B. F., & Carr, J. H. [2017]. *Clinical Hematology Atlas.* [5th ed., Figure 2.3B]. St. Louis: Elsevier.)

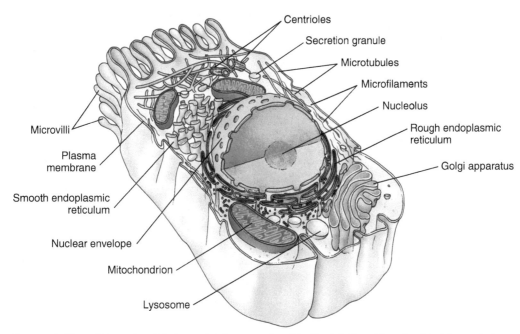

Figure 3.2 Three-Dimensional Schematic Diagram of an Idealized Cell, as Visualized by Transmission Electron Microscopy. Various organelles and cytoskeletal elements are displayed. (From Gartner L. P. [2017]. Cytoplasm. In *Textbook of Histology*. [4th ed., Figure 2.5]. Philadelphia: Elsevier.)

TABLE 3.1 Summary of Cellular Components and Functions

Organelle	Location	Appearance and Size	Function
Plasma membrane	Outer boundary of cell	Lipid bilayer consisting of phospholipids, cholesterol, proteins; glycolipids and glycoproteins form a glycocalyx	Provides physical barrier for cell; facilitates and restricts interchange of substances with environment; maintains electrochemical gradient; has receptors for signal transduction
Nucleus	Within cell	Round or oval; varies in diameter; composed of DNA and proteins; surrounded by inner and outer membranes	Controls cell division and functions; contains genetic code
Nucleolus	Within nucleus	Usually round or irregular in shape; composed of ribosomal RNA and the genes coding it, and accessory proteins; may have one to several within the nucleus	Synthesizes ribosomal RNA and assembles ribosome subunits
Ribosomes	Free in cytoplasm and on outer surface of rough endoplasmic reticulum	Macromolecular complex composed of protein and ribosomal RNA; composed of large and small subunits	Synthesizes proteins
Rough endoplasmic reticulum	Membranous network throughout cytoplasm	Branching, membrane-lined tubules and sacs; studded with ribosomes on outer surface; membrane continuous with the nuclear membrane	Synthesizes membrane-bound and secreted proteins
Smooth endoplasmic reticulum	Membranous network throughout cytoplasm	Membrane-lined tubules lacking ribosomes; continuous with rough endoplasmic reticulum	Synthesizes phospholipids and steroids; detoxifies drugs; stores calcium
Golgi apparatus	Next to nucleus and rough endoplasmic reticulum	System of stacked, membrane-bound, flattened sacs	Modifies and packages macromolecules for other organelles and for secretion
Mitochondria	Randomly distributed in cytoplasm	Elliptical or oval structures surrounded by inner and outer membranes; inner membrane has infoldings called *cristae*	Produces most of the ATP for the cell by aerobic respiration/oxidative phosphorylation

Continued

TABLE 3.1   Summary of Cellular Components and Functions—cont'd

Organelle	Location	Appearance and Size	Function
Lysosomes	Randomly distributed in cytoplasm	Membrane-bound sacs; diameter varies	Contains hydrolytic enzymes that degrade unwanted material in the cell
Microfilaments	Near nuclear envelope, plasma membrane, and mitotic processes	Double-stranded, intertwined solid structures of actin; 5–7 nm in diameter	Supports cytoskeleton and motility
Intermediate filaments	Cytoskeleton	Solid structures 8–10 nm in diameter; self-assemble into larger bundles	Provides strong structural support
Microtubules	Cytoskeleton and centrioles near nucleus	Hollow cylinder 25 nm in diameter; consists of 13 protofilaments formed from α- and β-tubulin	Maintains cell shape; involved in cell and organelle motility and the mitotic process
Centrosome	Near nucleus	Composed of two cylinder-shaped centrioles, each with nine sets of triplet microtubules; centrioles oriented at right angles to each other	Contains centrioles that serve as insertion points for mitotic spindle fibers

ATP, Adenosine triphosphate.

PLASMA MEMBRANE

The plasma membrane serves as a semipermeable outer boundary separating the cellular components from their surrounding environment. The cell membrane serves four basic functions: (1) provides a physical but flexible barrier to contain and protect cell components from the extracellular environment; (2) regulates and facilitates the interchange of substances with the environment by endocytosis, exocytosis, and selective permeability (using various membrane channels and transporters); (3) establishes electrochemical gradients between the interior and exterior of the cell; and (4) has receptors that allow the cell to respond to a multitude of signaling molecules through signal transduction pathways.[2,3]

Relevant to hematology, the membrane is also the location of cell surface glycoprotein and glycolipid molecules (surface markers or antigens) used for blood cell identity. Each type of blood cell expresses a unique repertoire of surface antigens at different stages of differentiation.[4] Antigen-specific monoclonal antibodies enable identification of these antigens using flow cytometry (Chapter 28). An international nomenclature was developed, called the *cluster of differentiation,* or *CD,* system, in which a CD number was assigned to each identified blood cell antigen.[4] More than 400 CD antigens have been identified on blood cells.[4] The CD nomenclature allows scientists, clinicians, and laboratory practitioners to communicate in a universal language for hematology research and diagnostic and therapeutic practice.

In addition to the plasma membrane, many components found within the cell (e.g., mitochondria, Golgi apparatus, nucleus, and endoplasmic reticulum) have similarly constructed membrane systems. The red blood cell membrane has been the most widely studied, and its structure and function is described in detail in Chapter 6.

To accomplish its many requirements, the cell membrane must be resilient and elastic. It achieves these qualities by being a fluid structure of proteins floating in lipids. The lipids are phospholipids and cholesterol arranged in two layers. The phosphate end of the phospholipid and the hydroxyl radical of cholesterol are polar-charged hydrophilic (water-soluble) structures that orient toward the extracellular and cytoplasmic surfaces of the cell membrane. Fatty acid chains of the phospholipids and the steroid nucleus of cholesterol are nonpolar-charged hydrophobic (water-insoluble) structures and are directed toward each other in the center of the bilayer (Figure 6.2).[3] Phospholipids are distributed asymmetrically in the membrane with mostly phosphatidylserine and phosphatidylethanolamine in the inner layer and sphingomyelin and phosphatidylcholine in the outer layer (Chapters 6 and 10). In the outer layer, carbohydrates (oligosaccharides) are covalently linked to some membrane proteins and phospholipids (forming glycoproteins and glycolipids, respectively).[3] These also contribute to the membrane structure and function.

Membrane Proteins

Cell membranes contain two types of proteins: transmembrane and cytoskeletal. Transmembrane proteins traverse the entirety of the lipid bilayer in one or more passes and penetrate the plasma and cytoplasmic layers of the membrane. The transmembrane proteins serve as channels and transporters of water, ions, and other molecules between the cytoplasm and the external environment. They also function as receptors and adhesion molecules. Cytoskeletal proteins are found only on the cytoplasmic side of the membrane and form the lattice of the cytoskeleton. The cytoplasmic ends of transmembrane proteins attach to the cytoskeletal proteins at junctional complexes to provide structural integrity to the cell and vertical support in linking the membrane to the cytoskeleton (Figure 6.3).[5] Inherited mutations in genes coding for transmembrane or cytoskeletal proteins can disrupt membrane integrity, decrease the life span of red blood cells, and lead to a hemolytic anemia. An example is hereditary spherocytosis (Chapter 21).

Membrane Carbohydrates

The carbohydrate chains of glycoproteins and glycolipids extend beyond the outer cell surface, providing an external protective carbohydrate coating called the *glycocalyx*. Substances adsorbed from the extracellular matrix also contribute to this coating. The carbohydrate moieties function in cell-to-cell recognition and adhesion and provide a negative surface charge to repel adjacent cells in circulation.

NUCLEUS

The nucleus is composed of three components: chromatin, nuclear envelope, and nucleoli. It is the control center of the cell and the largest organelle within the cell. The nucleus is composed largely of deoxyribonucleic acid (DNA) and is the site of DNA replication and transcription (Chapter 29). It controls the chemical reactions within the cell and directs its reproductive process. The nucleus has an affinity for basic dyes because of the nucleic acids contained within it; it stains deep purple with Wright stain (Chapters 5 and 9).

Chromatin

The chromatin consists of one long molecule of double-stranded DNA in each chromosome that is tightly folded with histone and nonhistone proteins. The first level of folding is the formation of *nucleosomes* along the length of the DNA molecule. Each nucleosome is 11 nm in length and consists of approximately 150 base pairs of DNA wrapped around a histone protein core.[6] The positive charge of the histones facilitates binding with the negatively charged phosphate groups of DNA. The nucleosomes are folded into 30 nm chromatin fibers, and these fibers are further folded into loops, then supercoiled chromatin fibers that greatly condense the DNA (Figure 30.3). This highly structured folding allows the long strands of DNA to be tightly condensed in the nucleus when inactive and enables segments of the DNA to be rapidly unfolded for active transcription when needed. This complex process of gene expression is controlled by transcription factors and other regulatory proteins and processes. Inappropriate silencing of genes needed for blood cell maturation contributes to the molecular pathophysiology of acute leukemias and myelodysplastic syndromes (Chapters 31 and 33).

Morphologically, chromatin is divided into two types: (1) *heterochromatin,* which has a more darkly stained, condensed clumping pattern and is the transcriptionally inactive area of the nucleus, and (2) *euchromatin,* which has a diffuse, uncondensed, open chromatin pattern and is the genetically active area of the nucleus where DNA transcription into messenger RNA (mRNA) occurs. The euchromatin is loosely coiled and turns a pale blue when stained with Wright stain. More mature cells have more heterochromatin because they are less transcriptionally active.

Nuclear Envelope

Surrounding the nucleus is a nuclear envelope consisting of two phospholipid bilayer membranes. The inner membrane surrounds the nucleus, and the outer membrane is continuous with the membrane of the endoplasmic reticulum.[1] Between the two nuclear membranes is a 30- to 50-nm perinuclear space that is continuous with the lumen of the endoplasmic reticulum.[6] Nuclear pore complexes penetrate the nuclear envelope, which allows passage of molecules between the nucleus and the cytoplasm.

Nucleoli

The nucleus contains one to several nucleoli. The nucleolus is the site of ribosomal RNA (rRNA) production and assembly into ribosome subunits. Because ribosomes synthesize proteins, the number of nucleoli in the nucleus is proportional to the amount of protein synthesis that occurs in the cell. As blood cells mature, protein synthesis decreases, and the nucleoli eventually disassemble.

Nucleoli contain a large amount of rRNA, the genes that code for rRNA (or rDNA), and ribosomal proteins. In ribosome biogenesis, rDNA is first transcribed to rRNA precursors. The rRNA precursors are processed into smaller RNA molecules and subsequently complexed with proteins forming the small and large ribosome subunits.[6] Ribosomal proteins enter the nucleus through the nuclear pores after being synthesized in the cytoplasm. After the ribosome subunits are synthesized and assembled, they are transported out of the nucleus through the nuclear pores. Once in the cytoplasm, large and small ribosome subunits self-assemble into a functional ribosome during protein synthesis (Chapter 29).[6]

CYTOPLASM

The cytoplasmic matrix is a homogeneous, continuous, aqueous solution called the *cytosol.* It is the environment in which the organelles exist and function. These organelles are discussed individually next.

Ribosomes

Ribosomes are macromolecular complexes composed of a small and large subunit of rRNA and many accessory ribosomal proteins. Ribosomes are found free in the cytoplasm or on the surface of rough endoplasmic reticulum. They may exist singly or form chains (polyribosomes). Ribosomes serve as the site of protein synthesis. This is accomplished with transfer RNA (tRNA) for amino acid transport to the ribosome, and specific mRNA molecules. The mRNA provides the genetic code for the sequence of amino acids for the protein being synthesized (Chapter 29). Cells that actively produce proteins have many ribosomes in the cytoplasm, which give it a dark blue color (basophilia) when stained with Wright stain. Cytoplasmic basophilia is particularly prominent in erythroid precursor cells when hemoglobin and other cell components are actively synthesized (Chapter 5).

Endoplasmic Reticulum

The endoplasmic reticulum (Figure 3.2) is a membrane-bound, interconnected network of flattened sacs and tubes located adjacent to the nucleus and extending throughout the cytoplasm. Its membrane is continuous with the outer membrane of the nucleus and its lumen is continuous with the perinuclear space between the outer and inner nuclear membranes. This arrangement provides a pathway for the flow of molecules between the nucleus and the cytoplasm.

Rough endoplasmic reticulum (RER) has a studded look on its outer surface because of the presence of ribosomes. RER synthesizes and processes membrane-bound proteins and proteins that will be secreted from the cell.[2] Smooth endoplasmic reticulum (SER) is continuous with the RER but does not have ribosomes. SER is involved in synthesis of phospholipids and steroids, detoxification or inactivation of harmful compounds or drugs, and calcium storage and release.[2]

Golgi Apparatus

The Golgi apparatus (Figure 3.2) is a system of membrane-bound, stacked, flattened sacs called *cisternae* that are involved in modifying, sorting, and packaging macromolecules for secretion or delivery to other organelles. It contains numerous enzymes for these activities. The Golgi apparatus locates in close proximity to the RER and the nucleus. In Wright-stained bone marrow smears of developing white blood cell precursors, the Golgi area may be observed as an unstained region next to the nucleus (Chapter 9).

Vesicles containing membrane-bound and soluble proteins from the RER enter the Golgi network on the "cis face" and are directed through the stacks where the proteins are modified, as needed, by enzymes for glycosylation, sulfation, or phosphorylation.[1,3] Vesicles with processed proteins exit the Golgi on the "trans face" to form lysosomes or secretory vesicles bound for the plasma membrane.[1,3]

Mitochondria

Mitochondria (Figure 3.3) have an outer and inner membrane separated by an intermembrane space. The inner membrane is highly convoluted forming many infoldings called *cristae*. The interior of the mitochondrion, called *mitochondrial matrix*, is surrounded by the inner membrane and contains mitochondrial DNA, ribosomes, and various enzymes and proteins.

Mitochondria generate most of the adenosine triphosphate (ATP) for the cell by aerobic respiration. In the matrix, mitochondrial enzymes oxidize pyruvate and fatty acids to acetyl coenzyme A (CoA), which is then oxidized in the citric acid cycle producing nicotinamide adenine dinucleotide (NADH) and flavin adenine dinucleotide ($FADH_2$) for the electron-transport pathway. This pathway efficiently generates ATP through oxidative phosphorylation using proteins embedded in the inner membrane.[2] The convoluted structure of the inner membrane dramatically increases its surface area and thus increases the ATP-producing capability of the cell. A component of heme biosynthesis also occurs in the mitochondrial matrix (Chapter 7).

The mitochondria are capable of self-replication. This organelle has its own circular DNA for the mitochondrial division cycle and RNA for protein synthesis. There may be fewer than 100 or up to several thousand mitochondria per cell. The number is directly related to the amount of energy required by the cell.

Lysosomes

Lysosomes contain hydrolytic enzymes bound within a membrane and are involved in the intracellular digestive process. The membrane prevents enzymes from digesting cellular components and macromolecules. Lysosomal enzymes are activated at the acidic pH of the lysosome and inactivated at the higher pH of the cytosol.[2] This protects the cell in case lysosomal enzymes are released into the cytoplasm. Lysosomes fuse with endosomes and phagosomes (Chapter 9); this allows the lysosome hydrolytic enzymes to safely digest their contents.[1] With Wright stain, lysosomes are visualized as granules in white blood cells and platelets (Chapters 9 and 10). Lysosomal lipid storage diseases result from inherited mutations in genes for enzymes that catabolize lipids. Gaucher and Neimann-Pick diseases are examples of these disorders (Chapter 26).

Microfilaments and Intermediate Filaments

Actin microfilaments are double-stranded, intertwined solid structures approximately 5 to 7 nm in diameter. They associate with myosin to enable cell motility, contraction, and intracellular transport. They locate near the nucleus and assist in cell division. They also locate near the plasma membrane and provide cytoskeletal support.

Intermediate filaments, with a diameter of approximately 8 to 10 nm, self-assemble into larger bundles.[2] They are the most durable element of the cytoskeleton and provide structural stability for the cells, especially those subjected to more physical stress, such as the epidermal layer of skin.[1] Examples include the keratins and lamins.

Microtubules

Microtubules are hollow cylindrical structures that are approximately 25 nm in diameter and vary in length. They consist of α- and β-tubulin heterodimers that self-assemble into protofilaments; 13 parallel protofilaments form each microtubule.[1,2] This arrangement gives the microtubules structural strength.

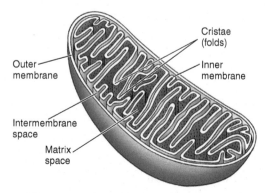

Figure 3.3 Mitochondrion Sectioned Longitudinally to Demonstrate its Outer Membrane and Folded Inner Membrane Forming Cristae. (Modified from Gartner, L. P. [2017]. Cytoplasm. In *Textbook of Histology.* [4th ed., Figure 2.28A]. Philadelphia: Elsevier.)

Tubulins can rapidly polymerize forming microtubules and then rapidly depolymerize when no longer needed by the cell.

Microtubules help support the cytoskeleton to maintain cell shape and are involved in cell motility (e.g., cilia and flagella) and the intracellular movement of some organelles.[2] Microtubules also form the mitotic spindle fibers during mitosis and are the major component of centrioles.

Centrosomes

The centrosome consists of two cylinder-shaped centrioles that are typically oriented at right angles to each other (Figure 3.2). A centriole consists of nine bundles of three microtubules each. They serve as insertion points for the mitotic spindle fibers during mitosis.

HEMATOPOIETIC MICROENVIRONMENT

Hematopoiesis occurs predominantly in the bone marrow from the third trimester of fetal life through adulthood (Chapter 4). The bone marrow microenvironment must provide for hematopoietic stem cell self-renewal, proliferation, differentiation, and apoptosis and support the developing progenitor and precursor blood cells. This protective environment is provided by stromal cells, which is a broad term for specialized endothelial cells; reticular adventitial cells (fibroblasts); adipocytes (fat cells); lymphocytes and macrophages; osteoblasts; and osteoclasts.[7] Stromal cells secrete substances that form an extracellular matrix, including collagen, fibronectin, thrombospondin, laminin, and proteoglycans (such as hyaluronate, chondroitin sulfate, and heparan sulfate).[7,8] The extracellular matrix is critical for cell growth and for anchoring developing blood cells in the bone marrow. Hematopoietic cells have various receptors for growth factors and adhesion molecules. Adhesion receptors provide a mechanism for attachment to extracellular matrix in bone marrow. Receptors also provide a means of cell-cell interaction, which is essential for regulated hematopoiesis.

Stromal cells secrete various growth factors that participate in complex processes to regulate the proliferation and differentiation of progenitor and precursor blood cells (Chapter 4). Growth factors must bind to specific receptors on their target cells to exert their effect. Most growth factors are produced by cells in the hematopoietic microenvironment and exert their effects in local cell-cell interactions. One growth factor, erythropoietin, has a hormone-type stimulation in that it is produced in another location (kidney) and exerts its effect on erythroid progenitors in the bone marrow (Chapter 5). An important feature of growth factors is their use of synergism to stimulate a cell to proliferate or differentiate. In other words, several different growth factors work together to generate a more effective response.[9] Growth factors are specific for their corresponding receptors on target cells.

Growth factor receptors are transmembrane proteins.[9] When the growth factor (or ligand) binds the extracellular domain of the receptor, a signal is transmitted to the nucleus in the cell through the cytoplasmic domain. For example, when erythropoietin binds with its receptor, it causes a conformational change in the receptor, which activates a kinase (Janus kinase 2 or JAK2) associated with its cytoplasmic domain.[9] The activated kinase in turn activates other intracellular signal transduction molecules that ultimately interact with the DNA in the nucleus to promote expression of genes required for cell growth and proliferation (Chapter 32).

Figure 3.4 provides general examples of receptor signaling mechanisms that induce specific biologic responses in hematopoietic cells.

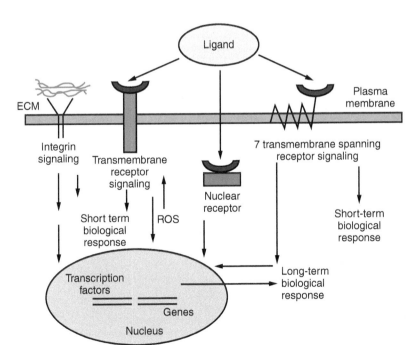

Figure 3.4 Examples of Ligands and Receptors that Transduce Biologic Responses. Signals can originate from fixed ligands (e.g., the extracellular matrix, *ECM)* or soluble ligands that are not membrane permeable and bind to extracellular regions of transmembrane receptors. Membrane-permeable ligands bind to intracellular receptors, such as the nuclear receptor family. Signals can also originate from within the cell, such as increases in levels of reactive oxygen species, *ROS.* These signals cause short-term biologic outputs without changes in gene expression or transduce medium- and long-term biologic outputs with changes in gene expression. (From Puigserver, P. [2018]. Signaling transduction and metabolomics. In Hoffman, R., Benz, E. J., Jr., Silberstein, L. E., et al. (Eds.), *Hematology: Basic Principles and Practice.* [7th ed., Figure 7.1]. Philadelphia: Elsevier.)

CELL CYCLE

Stages

The purpose of the cell cycle is to replicate DNA once and distribute identical chromosome copies equally to two daughter cells during mitosis.[10] The cell cycle is a biochemical and morphologic four-stage process through which a cell passes when it is stimulated to divide (Figure 3.5). These stages are G_1 (gap 1), S (DNA synthesis), G_2 (gap 2), and M (mitosis). G_1 is a period of cell growth and synthesis of components necessary for replication.[10] In the S stage, DNA replication takes place (Chapter 29). An exact copy of each chromosome is produced, and they pair together as *sister chromatids.* The centrosome is also duplicated during the S stage.[10] In G_2, the tetraploid DNA is checked for proper replication and damage (discussed later). The time spent in each stage can be variable, but mitosis takes approximately 1 hour.[10] During G_0 (quiescence) the cell is not actively in the cell cycle.

Mitosis or M stage involves the division of chromosomes and cytoplasm into two daughter cells. It is divided into six phases (Figure 3.5)[10]:

1. *Prophase:* the chromosomes condense, the duplicated centrosomes begin to separate, and mitotic spindle fibers appear.
2. *Prometaphase:* the nuclear envelope disassembles, the centrosomes move to opposite poles of the cell and serve as a point of origin of the mitotic spindle fibers; the sister chromatids (chromosome pairs) attach to the mitotic spindle fibers.
3. *Metaphase:* the sister chromatids align on the mitotic spindle fibers at a location equidistant from the centrosome poles.

4. *Anaphase:* the sister chromatids separate and move on the mitotic spindles toward the centrosomes on opposite poles.
5. *Telophase:* the nuclear membrane reassembles around each set of chromosomes, and the mitotic spindle fibers disappear.
6. *Cytokinesis:* the cell divides into two identical daughter cells.

Interphase is a term used for the nonmitosis stages of the cell cycle, that is, G_1, S, and G_2.

Regulation of the Cell Cycle

The cell cycle is a highly complex process that can malfunction. To prevent abnormal or mutated cells from going through the cell cycle and producing an abnormal clone, checkpoints occur in the cycle to detect abnormalities (Figure 3.5).[1,10] A restriction point in late G_1 checks for adequate nutrients and appropriate cell volume. The *G1 checkpoint* at the end of G1 checks the DNA for damage and makes the cell either wait for DNA repair or initiates apoptosis. The *S-phase checkpoint* checks DNA for damage and completion of replication. The *G2 checkpoint* takes place after DNA synthesis at the end of G_2, and it verifies that replication took place without error or damage. If damaged or unduplicated DNA is detected, then mitosis is blocked. The last checkpoint, the *metaphase checkpoint*, takes place during mitosis at the time of metaphase. The attachment and alignment of chromosomes on the mitotic spindle and the integrity of the spindle apparatus are checked.[1,10] Anaphase will be blocked if any defects are detected.

Progression through the cell cycle is regulated by cyclin and cyclin-dependent kinases (CDKs). A cyclin activates a specific

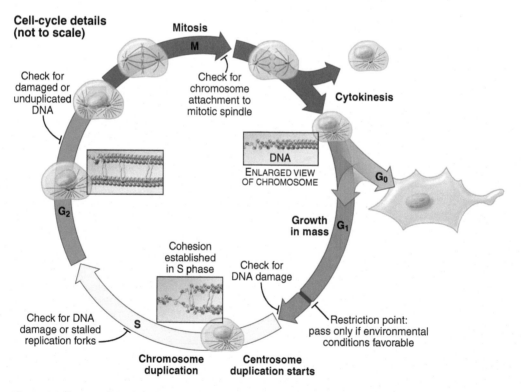

Figure 3.5 **Stages of the Cell Cycle.** Diagrams of cellular morphology and chromosome structure across the cell cycle. (Modified from Pollard, T. D., Earnshaw, W. C., Lippincott-Schwartz, J., et al. [2017]. Introduction to the cell cycle. In *Cell Biology.* [3rd ed., Figure 40.2]. Philadelphia: Elsevier.)

CDK, forms a cyclin/CDK complex, and directs the CDK to phosphorylate key substrates that drive the cell through a specific transition in the cell cycle. Cyclin is named appropriately because the concentration of specific cyclins increase and decrease at designated times in the cell cycle, and cyclin/CDK complexes drive the cycle through its successive, orderly stages. G_1 begins when external stimuli, such as growth factors, cause an increase in one or more of the D cyclins (D1, D2, D3) which then complex with CDK4 or CDK6.[10] To transition the cell from G_1 to S, cyclin E increases and binds to CDK2, forming the cyclin E/CDK2 complex. In the S stage, cyclin E degrades and cyclin A increases and complexes with CDK2, forming cyclin A/CDK2. This complex is required for progression through the S stage. Cyclin A also partners with CDK1 forming the cyclin A/CDK1 complex, which is needed for completion of S stage and the G_2 to M transition. For mitosis to occur, cyclin B must replace cyclin A and bind to CDK1, forming the cyclin B/CDK1 complex. This complex takes the cell through the intricate process of mitosis.[10,11] Degradation of cyclin B triggers the end of mitosis and initiates cytokinesis. Inhibitors of the cyclin/CDK complexes also play a primary role in cell cycle regulation.[11] Table 3.2 summarizes the actions of the major cyclins and CDKs in the cell cycle.

Tumor suppressor proteins are needed for the proper function of the checkpoints (Chapter 27). One of the first tumor suppressor genes recognized was *TP53*. It codes for the TP53 protein that detects DNA damage during G_1. It can also assist in triggering apoptosis. Many tumor suppressor genes have been described.[11] When these genes are mutated or deleted, cells with abnormal or deleted DNA/chromosomes are allowed to go through the cell cycle and replicate. Some of these cells simply malfunction, but others form malignant neoplasms, often with aggressive characteristics. For example, patients with chronic lymphocytic leukemia have a more aggressive disease with a shorter survival time when their leukemic cells lose TP53 activity either through gene mutation or deletion (Chapter 34).

TABLE 3.2 Cyclins and Cyclin-Dependent Kinases in Cell Cycle Progression

Stage	Major Activities and Complexes Required
G_1	External stimuli (e.g., growth factor) and ↑ D cyclins (D1, D2, D3) *Complex*: Cyclin D/CDK4, 6
G_1/ S	↑ Cyclin E *Complex*: Cyclin E/CDK2 required for G_1 to S transition
S	↓ Cyclin E ↑ Cyclin A *Complex*: Cyclin A/CDK2 required for progression through S stage
G_2/M	CDK1 signals end of S stage *Complex*: Cyclin A/CDK1 required for completion of S stage and G_2 to M transition
M	↓ Cyclin A ↑ Cyclin B *Complex*: Cyclin B/CDK1 required for mitosis ↓ Cyclin B signals end of mitosis

CELL DEATH BY NECROSIS AND APOPTOSIS

Cell death occurs as a normal physiologic process in the body or as a response to injury. Events that injure cells include ischemia (oxygen deprivation), mechanical trauma, toxins, drugs, infectious agents, autoimmune reactions, genetic defects including acquired and inherited mutations, and improper nutrition.[12] There are two major mechanisms for cell death: necrosis and apoptosis.[13] *Necrosis* is a pathologic process caused by direct external injury to cells such as, from burns, radiation, or toxins.[12] *Apoptosis* is a self-inflicted cell death originating from the activation signals within the cell itself.[13] Most apoptosis occurs as a normal physiologic process to eliminate potentially harmful cells (e.g., self-reacting lymphocytes [Chapter 4]), cells that are no longer needed (e.g., excess erythroid progenitors in oxygen-replete states [Chapter 5] or neutrophils after phagocytosis), and aging cells.[12] Apoptosis of older terminally differentiated cells balances with new cell growth to maintain needed numbers of functional cells in organs, hematopoietic tissue, and epithelial cell barriers, particularly in skin and the intestines. On the other hand, apoptosis also initiates in response to internal or external pathologic injury to a cell. For example, if DNA damage occurred during the replication phase of the cell cycle and the damage is beyond the capability of the DNA repair mechanisms, the cell will activate apoptosis to prevent its further progression through the cell cycle. Apoptosis can also be triggered in virally infected cells by the virus itself or by the body's immune response.[12] This is one of the mechanisms to remove virally infected cells from the body.

The first morphologic manifestation of necrosis is a swelling of the cell.[13] The cell may be able to recover from minor injury at that point. More severe damage, however, disrupts organelles and membranes; enzymes leak out of lysosomes that denature and digest DNA, RNA, and intracellular proteins; and ultimately the cell lyses.[12] An inflammatory response usually accompanies necrosis because of the release of cell contents into the extracellular space.

The morphologic manifestation of apoptosis is shrinkage of the cell.[13] The nucleus condenses and undergoes systematic fragmentation as a result of cleavage of the DNA between nucleosome subunits (multiples of 180 to 200 base pairs). The plasma membrane remains intact, but the phospholipids lose their asymmetric distribution and "flip" phosphatidylserine (PS) from the inner to the outer leaflet.[14] The cytoplasm and nuclear fragments bud off in membrane-bound vesicles. Macrophages, recognizing the PS and other signals on the membranes, rapidly phagocytize the vesicles. Thus cellular products are not released into the extracellular space and an inflammatory response is not elicited.[12] Figure 3.6 and Table 3.3 summarize the differences between necrosis and apoptosis.

Activation of apoptosis occurs through extrinsic and intrinsic pathways. Both pathways involve the activation of proteins called *caspases*. The extrinsic pathway, also called the *death receptor pathway*, initiates with the binding of ligand to a death receptor on the cell membrane. Examples of death receptors and their ligands include Fas and Fas ligand and tumor necrosis factor receptor 1 (TNFR1) and tumor necrosis factor.[15] The

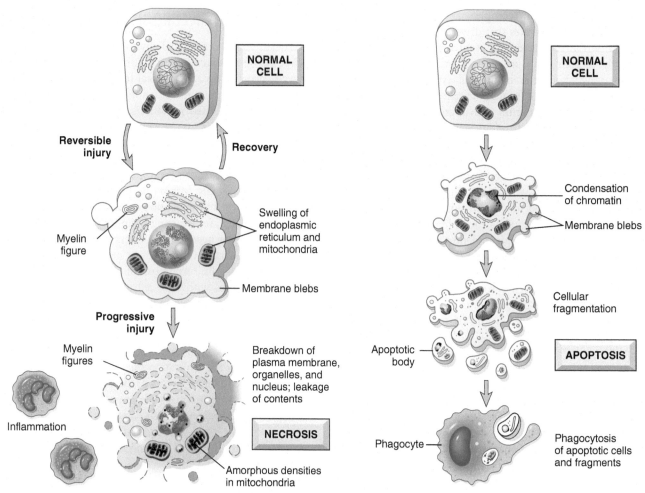

Figure 3.6 Schematic Illustration of the Morphologic Changes in Cell Injury Culminating in Necrosis or Apoptosis. (From Kumar, V., Abbas, A. K., & Aster, J. C. [2015]. Cellular responses to stress and toxic insults: adaptation, injury, and death. In *Robbins and Cotran Pathologic Basis of Disease.* [9th ed., Figure 2.8]. Philadelphia: Elsevier, Saunders.)

TABLE 3.3   Comparison of Necrosis and Apoptosis

	Necrosis	Apoptosis
Cell size	Enlarged as a result of swelling	Reduced as a result of shrinkage
Nucleus	Random breaks and lysis (karyolysis)	Condensation and fragmentation between nucleosomes
Plasma membrane	Disrupted with loss of integrity	Intact with loss of phospholipid asymmetry
Inflammation	Enzyme digestion and leakage of cell contents; inflammatory response occurs	Release of cell contents in membrane-bound apoptotic bodies, which are phagocytized by macrophages; no inflammation occurs
Physiologic or pathologic function	Pathologic; results from cell injury	Mostly physiologic to remove unwanted cells; pathologic in response to cell injury

binding recruits various adapter proteins that bind and activate caspase-8 (or sometimes caspase-10).[13,14] The intrinsic pathway is initiated by intracellular stressors (such as hypoxia, DNA damage, or membrane disruption) that stimulate the release of cytochrome c from mitochondria.[15] Cytochrome c binds to apoptotic protease-activating factor-1 (APAF-1) and caspase-9, forming an *apoptosome*, which activates caspase-9. Both pathways converge when the "initiator" caspases (8, 9, or 10) activate "executioner" caspases 3, 6, and 7, which leads to apoptosis.[13,15]

Various cellular proapoptotic and antiapoptotic proteins tightly regulate apoptosis. Examples of antiapoptotic proteins include some members of the Bcl-2 family of proteins (such as Bcl-2, Bcl-XL) as well as various growth factors (such as erythropoietin, granulocyte colony-stimulating factor, granulocyte-macrophage colony-stimulating factor, interleukin-3, and FLT3 ligand).[14] Bax, Bak, and Bid are examples of proapoptotic proteins.[14] The ratio of these intracellular proteins plays a primary role in regulating apoptosis. Any dysregulation, mutation, or translocation can cause inhibition or overexpression of apoptotic proteins, which can lead to hematologic malignancies or malfunctions.[12,14]

SUMMARY

- The cell contains cytoplasm that is separated from the extracellular environment by a plasma membrane; a membrane-bound nucleus (with the exception of mature red blood cells and platelets); and other unique subcellular structures and organelles.
- The plasma membrane is a bilayer of phospholipids, cholesterol, and proteins. Glycolipids and glycoproteins on the outer surface form the glycocalyx.
- The cytoplasm contains ribosomes for protein synthesis, which can be free in the cytoplasm or located on rough endoplasmic reticulum (RER). The RER makes most of the membrane proteins and proteins for secretion from the cell. Smooth endoplasmic reticulum (SER) lacks ribosomes; SER is involved in synthesis of phospholipids and steroids, detoxification or inactivation of harmful compounds or drugs, and calcium storage and release.
- The Golgi apparatus modifies and packages macromolecules for secretion and for transport to other cell organelles. Mitochondria make adenosine triphosphate (ATP) to supply energy for the cell. Lysosomes contain hydrolytic enzymes involved in the cell's intracellular digestive process.
- The bone marrow provides a suitable microenvironment for hematopoietic stem cell self-renewal, proliferation, differentiation, and apoptosis. Stromal cells secrete substances that form an extracellular matrix to support hematopoietic cell growth and function and help to anchor developing cells in the bone marrow. Growth factors participate in complex processes to regulate the proliferation and differentiation of hematopoietic stem and progenitor cells. Receptors and their ligands transduce signals intracellularly from the external environment to effect specific biologic responses in cells, including changes in gene expression.
- The cell cycle involves four active stages: G_1 (gap 1), S (DNA synthesis), G_2 (gap 2), and M (mitosis). Cell cycle progression is regulated by cyclins and cyclin-dependent kinases. Checkpoints in the cell cycle recognize abnormalities and initiate apoptosis.
- Two major mechanisms for cell death are necrosis and apoptosis. Necrosis is a pathologic process caused by direct external injury to cells, whereas apoptosis is a self-inflicted cell death originating from the activation signals within the cell itself. Most apoptosis occurs as a normal physiologic process to eliminate unwanted cells, but it can also be initiated in response to internal or external pathologic injury to a cell.

REVIEW QUESTIONS

Answers can be found in the Appendix.

1. The organelle involved in packaging and trafficking of cellular products is the:
   a. Nucleus
   b. Golgi apparatus
   c. Mitochondria
   d. Rough endoplasmic reticulum
2. The glycocalyx is composed of membrane:
   a. Phospholipids and cholesterol
   b. Glycoproteins and glycolipids
   c. Transmembrane and cytoskeletal proteins
   d. Rough and smooth endoplasmic reticulum
3. The "control center" of the cell is the:
   a. Nucleus
   b. Cytoplasm
   c. Membrane
   d. Microtubular system
4. The nucleus is composed largely of:
   a. RNA
   b. DNA
   c. Ribosomes
   d. Glycoproteins
5. The site of protein synthesis is the:
   a. Nucleus
   b. Mitochondria
   c. Ribosomes
   d. Golgi apparatus

6. The shape of a cell is maintained by which of the following?
   a. Microtubules
   b. Spindle fibers
   c. Ribosomes
   d. Centrioles
7. Functions of the cell membrane include all of the following *except*:
   a. Regulation of molecules entering or leaving the cell
   b. Receptor recognition of extracellular signals
   c. Maintenance of electrochemical gradients
   d. Lipid production and oxidation
8. The energy source for cells is the:
   a. Golgi apparatus
   b. Endoplasmic reticulum
   c. Nucleolus
   d. Mitochondrion
9. Ribosomes are synthesized by the:
   a. Endoplasmic reticulum
   b. Mitochondrion
   c. Nucleolus
   d. Golgi apparatus
10. Euchromatin functions as the:
    a. Site of microtubule production
    b. Transcriptionally active DNA
    c. Support structure for nucleoli
    d. Attachment site for centrioles

11. The cell cycle is regulated by:
    a. Cyclins and cyclin-dependent kinases
    b. Protooncogenes
    c. Apoptosis
    d. Growth factors

12. The transition from the G_1 to S stage of the cell cycle is regulated by:
    a. Cyclin B/CDK1 complex
    b. Cyclin A/CDK2 complex
    c. Cyclin D1
    d. Cyclin E/CDK2 complex

13. Apoptosis is morphologically identified by:
    a. Cellular swelling
    b. Nuclear condensation
    c. Rupture of the cytoplasm
    d. Rupture of the nucleus

14. Regulation of the hematopoietic microenvironment is provided by the:
    a. Stromal cells and growth factors
    b. Hematopoietic stem cells
    c. Liver and spleen
    d. Cyclins and caspases

15. Which one of the following statements is FALSE concerning cellular signal transduction?
    a. Membrane-permeable ligands can directly bind to intracellular receptors.
    b. A transmembrane receptor can transmit a signal into the cell through its intracellular domain when ligand binds its extracellular domain.
    c. The binding of membrane receptors to fixed ligands such as extracellular matrix can transmit intracellular signals.
    d. The binding of soluble ligands to membrane receptors is not able to induce changes in gene expression.

REFERENCES

1. Pollard, T. D., Earnshaw, W. C., Lippincott-Schwartz, J., et al. (2017). Introduction to cells. In *Cell Biology*. (3rd ed., pp. 3–14). Philadelphia: Elsevier.
2. Gartner, L. P. (2017). Cytoplasm. In *Textbook of Histology*. (4th ed., pp. 13–54). Philadelphia: Elsevier.
3. Mescher, A. L. (2016). The cytoplasm. In *Junqueira's Basic Histology*. (14th ed., pp. 17–52). New York: McGraw-Hill.
4. Engel, P., Boumsell L., Balderas, R., et al. (2015). CD nomenclature 2015: human leukocyte differentiation antigen workshops as a driving force in immunology. *J Immunol*, 195, 4555–4563.
5. Mohandas, N., & Gallagher, P. G. (2008). Red cell membrane: past, present, and future. *Blood*, 112, 3939–3948.
6. Mescher, A. L. (2016). The nucleus. In *Junqueira's Basic Histology*. (14th ed., pp. 53–70). New York: McGraw-Hill.
7. Dave, U. P., & Koury, M. J. (2016). Structure of the marrow and the hematopoietic microenvironment. In Kaushansky, K., Lichtman, M. A., Prchal, J. T., et al. (Eds.), *Williams Hematology*. (9th ed., pp. 53–84). New York: McGraw-Hill.
8. Kaushansky, K. (2016). Hematopoietic stem cells, progenitors, and cytokines. In Kaushansky, K., Lichtman, M. A., Prchal, J. T., et al. (Eds.), *Williams Hematology*. (9th ed., pp. 257–278). New York: McGraw-Hill.
9. Kaushansky, K. (2016). Signal transduction pathways. In Kaushansky, K., Lichtman, M. A., Prchal, J. T., et al. (Eds.), *Williams Hematology*. (9th ed., pp. 247–256). New York: McGraw-Hill.
10. Pollard, T. D., Earnshaw, W. C., Lippincott-Schwartz, J., et al. (2017). Introduction to the cell cycle. In *Cell Biology*. (3rd ed., pp. 697–712). Philadelphia: Elsevier.
11. Dai, Y., Bose, P., & Grant, S. (2016). Cell-cycle regulation and hematologic disorders. In Kaushansky, K., Lichtman, M. A., Prchal, J. T., et al. (Eds.), *Williams Hematology*. (9th ed., pp. 213–246). New York: McGraw-Hill.
12. Kumar, V., Abbas, A. K., & Aster, J. C. (2015). Cellular responses to stress and toxic insults: adaptation, injury, and death. In *Robbins and Cotran Pathologic Basis of Disease*. (9th ed., pp. 31–68). Philadelphia: Elsevier, Saunders.
13. Danial, N. N., & Hockenbery, D. M. (2018). Cell death. In Hoffman, R., Benz, E. J., Jr., Silberstein, L. E., et al. (Eds.), *Hematology: Basic Principles and Practice*. (7th ed., pp. 186–196). Philadelphia: Elsevier.
14. Reed, J. C. (2016). Apoptosis mechanisms: relevance to the hematopoietic system. In Kaushansky, K., Lichtman, M. A., Prchal, J. T., et al. (Eds.), *Williams Hematology*. (9th ed., pp. 203–212). New York: McGraw-Hill.
15. McIlwain, D. R., Berger, T., & Mak, T. W. (2013). Caspase functions in cell death and disease. *Cold Spring Harb Perspect Biol*, 5, 1–28.

Hematopoiesis

*Kamran M. Mirza**

OBJECTIVES

After completion of this chapter, the reader will be able to:

1. Define *hematopoiesis*.
2. Describe the evolution and formation of blood cells from embryo to fetus to adult, including anatomic sites and cells produced.
3. Predict the likelihood of encountering active marrow from biopsy sites when given the patient's age.
4. Relate normal and abnormal hematopoiesis to the various organs involved in the hematopoietic process.
5. Explain the stem cell theory of hematopoiesis, including the characteristics of hematopoietic stem cells, the names of various progenitor cells, and their lineage associations.

6. Discuss the roles of various cytokines and hematopoietic growth factors in differentiation and maturation of hematopoietic progenitor cells, including nonspecific and lineage-specific factors.
7. Describe general morphologic changes that occur during blood cell maturation.
8. Define *apoptosis* and discuss the relationships among apoptosis, growth factors, and hematopoietic stem cell differentiation.
9. Discuss therapeutic applications of cytokines and hematopoietic growth factors.

OUTLINE

Hematopoietic Development
    Mesoblastic Phase
    Hepatic Phase
    Medullary (Myeloid) Phase
Adult Hematopoietic Tissue
    Bone Marrow
    Liver
    Spleen
    Lymph Nodes
    Thymus

Hematopoietic Stem Cells and Cytokines
    Stem Cell Theory
    Stem Cell Cycle Kinetics
    Stem Cell Phenotypic and Functional Characterization
    Cytokines and Growth Factors
Lineage-Specific Hematopoiesis
    Erythropoiesis
    Leukopoiesis
    Megakaryopoiesis
Therapeutic Applications

CASE STUDY

After studying the material in this chapter, the reader should be able to respond to the following case study:

A 22-year-old woman visited her physician with a complaint of fatigue, fever, and frequent bruising. Specimens collected for testing included peripheral blood and bone marrow specimens. Results of the CBC: WBC = 2.5×10^9/L; HGB = 8.3 g/dL;

PLT = 50×10^9/L. Bone marrow testing confirmed the unexplained decrease in WBC, RBC, and platelets.

1. Identify the best site for collection of the bone marrow specimen. Explain.
2. Compare and contrast sites for hematopoiesis for fetus, infant, and adult.
3. What do you expect this woman's bone marrow to look like in this situation?

HEMATOPOIETIC DEVELOPMENT

Hematopoiesis is the continuous, regulated process of renewal, proliferation, differentiation, and maturation of all blood cell lines. These processes result in the formation, development, and specialization of all functional blood cells that are released from the bone marrow into the circulation. Mature blood cells have a limited lifespan (e.g., 120 days for red blood cells [RBCs]) and a cell population capable of self-renewal that sustains the system. A hematopoietic stem cell (HSC) is capable of

---

*The author extends appreciation to Larry Smith and Richard C. Meagher, whose work in previous editions provided the foundation for this chapter.

self-renewal (i.e., replenishment) and directed differentiation into all required cell lineages.[1] Thus the hematopoietic system serves as a functional model to study stem cell biology, proliferation, and maturation and their contribution to disease and tissue repair.

Hematopoiesis in the developing human can be characterized as a select distribution of embryonic cells in specific sites that rapidly changes during development.[2] In contrast, hematopoiesis in healthy adults is restricted primarily to the bone marrow. During fetal development, the restricted, sequential distribution of cells is initiated in the yolk sac and then progresses in the aorta-gonad-mesonephros (AGM) region (*mesoblastic phase*), then to the fetal liver (*hepatic phase*), and finally resides in the bone marrow (*medullary phase*). Because of the different locations and resulting microenvironmental conditions (i.e., niches) encountered, each of these locations has distinct but related populations of cells.

Mesoblastic Phase

Hematopoiesis is considered to begin around the nineteenth day of embryonic development after fertilization.[3] Early in embryonic development, cells from the mesoderm migrate to the yolk sac. Some of these cells form primitive erythroblasts in the central cavity of the yolk sac, and others (*angioblasts*) surround the cavity of the yolk sac and eventually form blood vessels.[4-7] These primitive but transient yolk sac erythroblasts are important in early embryogenesis to produce hemoglobin (Gower-1, Gower-2, and Portland) needed for delivery of oxygen to rapidly developing embryonic tissues (Chapter 7).[8] Yolk sac hematopoiesis differs from hematopoiesis that occurs later in the fetus and adult in that it occurs intravascularly (or within developing blood vessels).[8]

Cells of mesodermal origin migrate to the AGM region and give rise to HSCs for definitive or permanent adult hematopoiesis.[4,7] The AGM region was previously considered to be the only site of definitive hematopoiesis during embryonic development. However, subsequent studies clearly demonstrated that the yolk sac was the major site of adult blood formation in the embryo.[9] There is evidence to support this view via transplant experiments demonstrating T cell recovery after transplantation of yolk sac into fetuses.[10] However, other studies have theorized that de novo production of HSCs could occur at different times or locations.[11] Reports indicate that Flk1[+] HSCs separated from human umbilical cord blood could generate hematopoietic as well as endothelial cells in vitro.[12] Some reports indicate that purified murine HSCs generate endothelial cells after in vivo transplantation.[13] More recently, researchers have challenged the AGM origin of HSCs based on transgenic mouse data demonstrating that yolk sac hematopoietic cells in 7.5-day embryos express *RUNX1* regulatory elements needed for definitive hematopoiesis.[14] Overall these findings suggest that the yolk sac contains either definitive HSCs or cells that can give rise to HSCs.[14] The precise origin of the adult HSC remains unresolved.

Hepatic Phase

The hepatic phase of hematopoiesis begins at 5 to 7 gestational weeks and is characterized by recognizable clusters of developing erythroblasts, granulocytes, and monocytes colonizing the fetal liver, thymus, spleen, placenta, and ultimately the bone marrow space in the final medullary phase.[8] These varied niches support development of HSCs that migrate to them. However, the contribution of each site to the final composition of the adult HSC pool remains unknown.[15,16] Developing erythroblasts signal the beginning of definitive hematopoiesis with a decline in primitive hematopoiesis of the yolk sac. In addition, lymphoid cells begin to appear.[17,18] Hematopoiesis during this phase occurs extravascularly, with the liver remaining the major site of hematopoiesis during the second trimester of fetal life.[8] Hematopoiesis in the AGM region and the yolk sac disappear during this stage. Hematopoiesis in the fetal liver reaches its peak by the third month of fetal development, then gradually declines after the sixth month, retaining minimal activity until 1 to 2 weeks after birth[8] (Figure 4.1). The developing spleen, kidney, thymus, and lymph nodes contribute to the hematopoietic process during this phase. The thymus, the first fully developed organ in the fetus, becomes the major site of T cell production, whereas the kidney and spleen produce B cells.

Production of megakaryocytes begins during the hepatic phase. The spleen gradually decreases granulocytic production and subsequently contributes solely to lymphopoiesis. During the hepatic phase, fetal hemoglobin (Hb F) is the predominant hemoglobin, but detectable levels of adult hemoglobin (Hb A) may be present (Chapter 7).[8]

Medullary (Myeloid) Phase

Hematopoiesis in the bone marrow (termed *medullary hematopoiesis* because it occurs in the medulla or inner part of the bone cavity) begins between the fourth and fifth month of fetal development.[3] During the myeloid phase, HSCs and mesenchymal cells migrate into the core of the bone.[8] Mesenchymal cells, a type of embryonic tissue, differentiate into structural elements (e.g., stromal cells such as endothelial cells and reticular adventitial cells) that support developing hematopoietic elements.[19,20] Hematopoietic activity, especially myeloid activity, is apparent during this stage of development, and the myeloid-to-erythroid ratio gradually approaches 3:1 to 4:1 (normal adult levels).[8] By the end of 24 weeks' gestation, the bone marrow becomes the *primary* site of hematopoiesis.[8] Measurable levels of erythropoietin (EPO), granulocyte colony-stimulating factor (G-CSF), granulocyte-macrophage colony-stimulating factor (GM-CSF), and hemoglobins F and A can be detected.[8] In addition, cells at various stages of maturation can be seen in all blood cell lineages.

ADULT HEMATOPOIETIC TISSUE

In adults, hematopoietic tissue is located in the bone marrow, lymph nodes, spleen, liver, and thymus. The bone marrow contains developing erythroid, myeloid, megakaryocytic, and lymphoid cells. Lymphoid development occurs in both primary and secondary lymphoid tissue. Primary lymphoid tissue consists of the bone marrow and thymus and is where T and B lymphocytes are derived. Secondary lymphoid tissue, where lymphoid cells respond to foreign antigens, consists of the spleen, lymph nodes, and mucosa-associated lymphoid tissue.

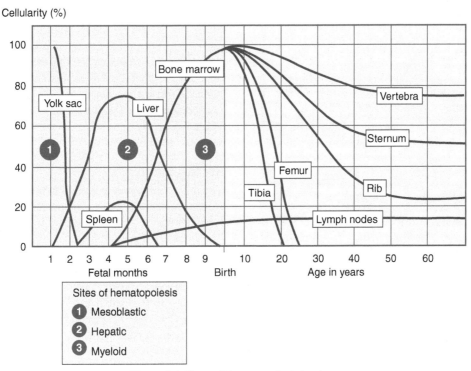

Figure 4.1 Sites of Hematopoiesis by Age.

Bone Marrow

Bone marrow, one of the largest organs in the body, is located within the cavities of the cortical bones. Resorption of cartilage and endosteal bone creates a central space within the bone. Projections of calcified bone, called *trabeculae,* radiate out from the bone cortex into the central space, forming a three-dimensional matrix resembling a honeycomb. The trabeculae provide structural support for the developing blood cells that mature within a sea of interposed mature adipocytes.

Normal bone marrow contains two major components: *red marrow,* hematopoietically active marrow that is composed of developing blood cells and their progenitors, and *yellow marrow,* hematopoietically inactive marrow composed primarily of adipocytes (fat cells), with undifferentiated mesenchymal cells and macrophages. During infancy and early childhood, all the bones in the body contain primarily red (active) marrow. Between 5 and 7 years of age, adipocytes become more abundant and begin to occupy the spaces in the long bones previously dominated by active marrow. The process of replacing the active marrow by adipocytes (yellow marrow) during development is called *retrogression* and eventually results in restriction of the active marrow in the adult to the sternum, vertebrae, scapulae, pelvis, ribs, skull, and proximal portion of the long bones (Figure 4.2). Hematopoietically inactive yellow marrow is scattered throughout the red marrow so that, in adults, there is approximately equal amounts of red and yellow marrow in these areas (Figure 4.3). The ratio of the red marrow to the yellow marrow (i.e., the hematopoietic cells to the adipocytes), often termed *marrow cellularity,* typically decreases with age. Yellow marrow is capable of reverting back to active marrow in cases of increased demand on the bone marrow, such as in excessive blood loss or hemolysis.[3]

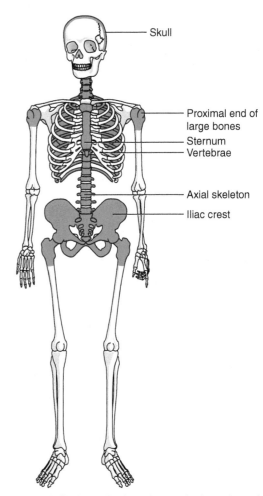

Figure 4.2 Adult Skeleton. Darkened areas depict active red marrow hematopoiesis.

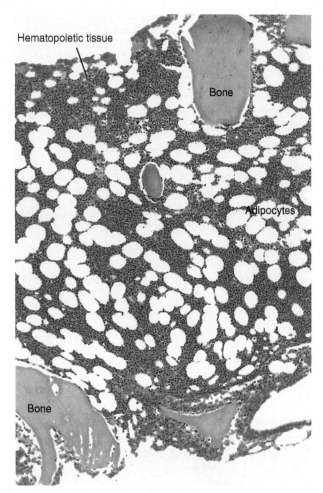

Figure 4.3 Fixed and Stained Bone Marrow Biopsy Specimen. The extravascular tissue consists of blood cell precursors and various tissue cells with scattered fat tissue. A normal adult bone marrow displays 50% hematopoietic cells and 50% fat. (Hematoxylin and eosin stain, ×100.)

The bone marrow contains hematopoietic cells, stromal cells, and blood vessels (arteries, veins, and vascular sinuses). Stromal cells originate from mesenchymal cells that migrate into the central cavity of the bone. *Stromal cells* include endothelial cells, adipocytes (fat cells), macrophages and lymphocytes, osteoblasts, osteoclasts, and reticular adventitial cells (fibroblasts).[3] *Endothelial cells* are broad, flat cells that form a single continuous layer along the inner surface of the arteries, veins, and vascular sinuses.[21] Endothelial cells regulate the flow of particles entering and leaving hematopoietic spaces in the vascular sinuses. *Adipocytes* are large cells with a single fat vacuole; they play a role in regulating the volume of the marrow in which active hematopoiesis occurs. They also secrete cytokines or growth factors that positively stimulate HSC numbers and bone homeostasis.[22,23] Macrophages function in phagocytosis, and both macrophages and lymphocytes secrete various cytokines that regulate hematopoiesis; they are located throughout the marrow space.[3,24] Other cells involved in cytokine production include endothelial cells and reticular adventitial cells. *Osteoblasts* are bone-forming cells, and *osteoclasts* are bone-resorbing cells. *Reticular adventitial cells* form an incomplete layer of cells on the abluminal surface of the vascular sinuses.[3] They extend

long, reticular fibers into the perivascular space that form a supporting lattice for the developing hematopoietic cells.[3] Stromal cells secrete a semifluid extracellular matrix that serves to anchor developing hematopoietic cells in the bone cavity. The extracellular matrix contains substances such as *fibronectin, collagen, laminin, thrombospondin, tenascin,* and *proteoglycans* (such as *hyaluronate, heparan sulfate, chondroitin sulfate,* and *dermatan*).[3,25] Stromal cells play a critical role in the regulation of hematopoietic stem and progenitor cell survival and differentiation.[21]

Red Marrow

The red marrow is composed of hematopoietic cells arranged in *extravascular cords.* Cords are located in spaces between vascular sinuses and are supported by trabeculae of spongy bone.[3] The cords are separated from the lumen of the vascular sinuses by endothelial and reticular adventitial cells (Figure 4.4). Hematopoietic cells develop in specific *niches* within the cords. *Erythroid precursors* or *erythroblasts* develop in small clusters, and the more mature forms are located adjacent to the outer surfaces of the vascular sinuses[3] (Figures 4.4 and 4.5); in addition, erythroblasts are found surrounding iron-laden

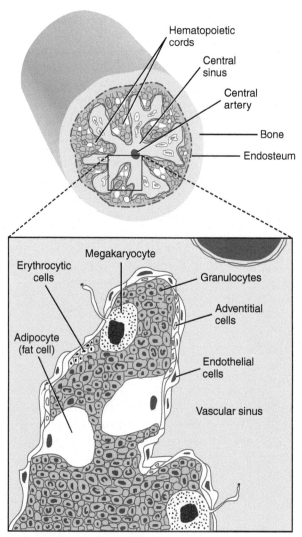

Figure 4.4 Graphic Illustration of the Arrangement of a Hematopoietic Cord and Vascular Sinus in Bone Marrow.

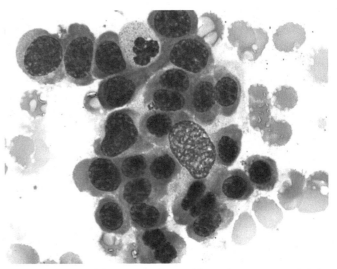

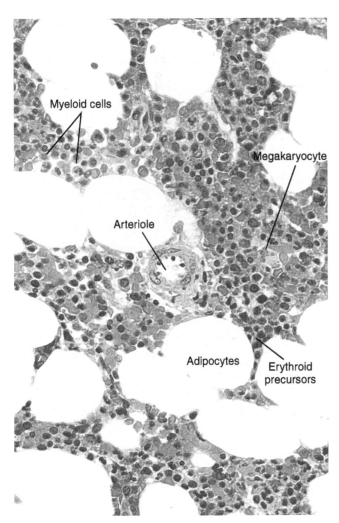

Figure 4.5 Fixed and Stained Bone Marrow Biopsy. Hematopoietic tissue reveals areas of granulopoiesis (lighter-staining cells), erythropoiesis (with darker-staining nuclei), and adipocytes (unstained areas). (Hematoxylin and eosin stain, ×400.)

Figure 4.6 Bone Marrow Aspirate. Macrophage surrounded by developing erythroid precursors. (Wright-Giemsa stain, ×1000.) (Courtesy of Peter Maslak, Memorial Sloan Kettering Cancer Center, New York, NY.)

macrophages (Figure 4.6). *Megakaryocytes* are located adjacent to the walls of the vascular sinuses, which facilitates the release of platelets into the lumen of the sinus.[3] Immature *myeloid (granulocytic) cells* through the metamyelocyte stage are located deep within the cords. As these maturing granulocytes proceed along differentiation, they move closer to the vascular sinuses.[19]

The mature blood cells of the bone marrow eventually enter the peripheral circulation by a process that is not completely understood. Through a highly complex interaction between the maturing blood cells and the vascular sinus wall, blood cells pass between layers of adventitial cells that form a discontinuous layer along the abluminal side of the sinus. Under the layer of adventitial cells is a *basement membrane* followed by a continuous layer of *endothelial cells* on the luminal side of the vascular sinus. The adventitial cells are capable of contracting, which allows mature blood cells to pass through the basement membrane and interact with the endothelial layer.

As blood cells come in contact with endothelial cells, they bind to the surface through a receptor-mediated process. Cells pass through pores in the endothelial cytoplasm, are released into the vascular sinus, and then move into the peripheral circulation.[3,26]

Marrow Circulation

The nutrient and oxygen requirements of the marrow are fulfilled by the *nutrient* and *periosteal arteries*, which enter via the bone *foramina*. The nutrient artery supplies blood only to the marrow.[20] It coils around the central longitudinal vein, which passes along the bone canal. In the marrow cavity the nutrient artery divides into ascending and descending branches that also coil around the central longitudinal vein. The arteriole branches that enter the inner lining of the cortical bone *(endosteum)* form *sinusoids* (endosteal beds), which connect to periosteal capillaries that extend from the periosteal artery.[3] The *periosteal arteries* provide nutrients for the osseous bone and the marrow. Their capillaries connect to the venous sinuses located in the endosteal bed, which empty into a larger collecting sinus that opens into the central longitudinal vein.[3] Blood exits the marrow via the central longitudinal vein, which runs the length of the marrow. The central longitudinal vein exits the marrow through the same foramen where the nutrient artery enters. Hematopoietic cells located in the endosteal bed receive their nutrients from the nutrient artery.[3]

Hematopoietic Microenvironment

The *hematopoietic inductive microenvironment,* or *niche,* plays an important role in nurturing and protecting HSCs and regulating their quiescence, self-renewal, and differentiation.[21,27] As the site of hematopoiesis transitions from yolk sac to liver to bone marrow, so must the microenvironmental niche for HSCs. The adult bone marrow HSC niche has received the most attention, although its complex nature makes studying it difficult. Stromal cells form an extracellular matrix in the niche to promote cell adhesion and regulate HSCs through complex signaling networks involving cytokines, adhesion molecules, and maintenance proteins. Key stromal cells thought to support HSCs in bone marrow niches include osteoblasts, endothelial cells, mesenchymal stem cells, CXCL12-abundant reticular cells, perivascular stromal cells, glial cells, and macrophages.[28,29]

Recent findings suggest that HSCs are predominantly quiescent, maintained in a nondividing state by intimate interactions with thrombopoietin-producing osteoblasts.[30] Opposing studies suggest that vascular cells are critical to HSC maintenance through CXCL12, which regulates migration of HSCs to the vascular niche.[31] These studies suggest a heterogeneous microenvironment that may affect the HSC differently, depending on location and cell type encountered.[32] Given the close proximity of cells within the bone marrow cavity, it is likely that niches may overlap, providing multiple signals simultaneously and thus ensuring tight regulation of HSCs.[32] Although the cell-cell interactions are complex and multifactorial, understanding these relationships is critical to the advancement of cell therapies based on HSCs such as clinical marrow transplantation.

Recent reviews, which are beyond the scope of this chapter, discuss and help to delineate between transcription factors required for HSC proliferation or function and those that regulate HSC differentiation pathways.[33,34] The importance of transcription factors and their regulatory role in HSC maturation and redeployment in hematopoietic cell lineage production are demonstrated by their intimate involvement in disease evolution, such as in leukemia. Ongoing study of hematopoietic disease continues to demonstrate the complex and delicate nature of normal hematopoiesis.

Liver

The liver consists of two lobes situated beneath the diaphragm in the abdominal cavity. The position of the liver with regard to the circulatory system is optimal for gathering, transferring, and eliminating substances through the bile duct.[35,36] The liver serves as the major site of blood cell production during the second trimester of fetal development. In adults, hepatocytes have many functions, including protein synthesis and degradation, coagulation factor synthesis, carbohydrate and lipid metabolism, drug and toxin clearance, iron recycling and storage, and hemoglobin degradation, in which bilirubin is conjugated and transported to the small intestine for eventual excretion.

Anatomically, hepatocytes are arranged in radiating plates emanating from a central vein (Figure 4.7). Adjacent to the longitudinal plates of hepatocytes are vascular sinusoids lined with endothelial cells. A small noncellular space separates the endothelial cells of the sinusoids from the plates of hepatocytes. This spatial arrangement allows plasma to have direct access to the hepatocytes for two-directional flow of solutes and fluids.

The lumen of the sinusoids contains *Kupffer cells* that maintain contact with the endothelial cell lining. Kupffer cells are macrophages that remove senescent cells and foreign debris from the blood that circulates through the liver; they also secrete mediators that regulate protein synthesis in the hepatocytes.[37] The particular anatomy, cellular components, and location in the body enables the liver to carry out many varied functions.

Liver Pathophysiology

The liver can maintain hematopoietic stem and progenitor cells to produce various blood cells (called *extramedullary hematopoiesis*) as a response to infectious agents or in pathologic

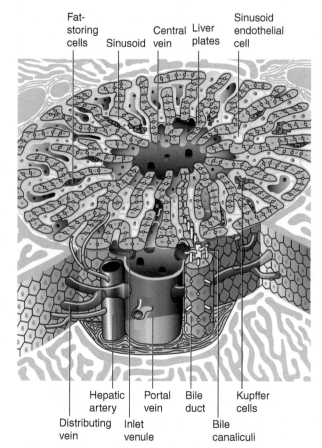

Figure 4.7 Three-dimensional Schematic of the Normal Liver.

myelofibrosis of the bone marrow.[38] It is directly affected by storage diseases of the monocyte/macrophage (Kupffer) cells as a result of enzyme deficiencies that cause hepatomegaly with ultimate dysfunction of the liver (Gaucher disease, Niemann-Pick disease; Chapter 26). In severe hemolytic anemias the liver increases the conjugation of *bilirubin* and the storage of iron. The liver sequesters membrane-damaged RBCs and removes them from the circulation. In *porphyrias,* hereditary or acquired defects in the enzymes involved in heme biosynthesis result in the accumulation of the various intermediary *porphyrins* that damage hepatocytes, erythrocyte precursors, and other tissues.

Spleen

The spleen, the largest lymphoid organ in the body, lies beneath the diaphragm behind the fundus of the stomach in the upper left quadrant of the abdomen. It is vital but not essential for life and functions as an indiscriminate filter of the circulating blood. In a healthy individual the spleen contains about 350 mL of blood.[35] The exterior surface of the spleen is surrounded by a layer of *peritoneum* covering a connective tissue capsule. The capsule projects inwardly, forming trabeculae that divide the spleen into discrete regions. Located within these regions are three types of splenic tissue: *white pulp, red pulp,* and a *marginal zone.* The white pulp consists of scattered follicles with germinal centers containing lymphocytes, macrophages, and dendritic cells. Aggregates of T lymphocytes surround arteries that pass through these germinal centers, forming a region called the *periarteriolar lymphatic sheath,* or *PALS.* Interspersed along the periphery of the PALS are lymphoid nodules containing primarily B lymphocytes. Activated B lymphocytes are found in the germinal centers.[37]

The marginal zone surrounds the white pulp and forms a reticular meshwork containing blood vessels, macrophages, memory B cells, and CD4[+] T cells.[39] The red pulp is composed primarily of vascular sinuses separated by cords of reticular cell meshwork *(cords of Billroth)* containing loosely connected specialized macrophages. This creates a sponge-like matrix that functions as a filter for blood passing through the region.[37] As RBCs pass through the cords of Billroth, there is a decrease in the flow of blood, which leads to stagnation and depletion of the RBCs' glucose supply. These cells are subject to increased damage and stress that may lead to their removal from the spleen. The spleen uses two methods for removing senescent or abnormal RBCs from the circulation: *culling,* in which the cells are phagocytized with subsequent degradation of cell organelles, and *pitting,* in which splenic macrophages remove inclusions or damaged surface membrane from the circulating RBCs.[40] The spleen also serves as a storage site for platelets. In a healthy individual, approximately 30% of the total platelet count is sequestered in the spleen.[41]

The spleen has a rich blood supply receiving approximately 350 mL/min. Blood enters the spleen through the *central splenic artery* located at the *hilum* and branches outward through the trabeculae. The branches enter all three regions of the spleen: the white pulp, with its dense accumulation of lymphocytes; the marginal zone; and the red pulp. The venous sinuses, which are located in the red pulp, unite and leave the spleen as splenic veins (Figure 4.8).[42]

Spleen Pathophysiology

As blood enters the spleen, it may follow one of two routes. The first is a slow-transit pathway through the red pulp in which the RBCs pass circuitously through the macrophage-lined cords before reaching the sinuses. Plasma freely enters the sinuses, but the RBCs have a more difficult time passing through the tiny openings created by the *interendothelial junctions* of adjacent endothelial cells (Figure 4.9). The combination of the slow passage and the continued RBC metabolism creates an environment that is acidic, hypoglycemic, and hypoxic. The increased

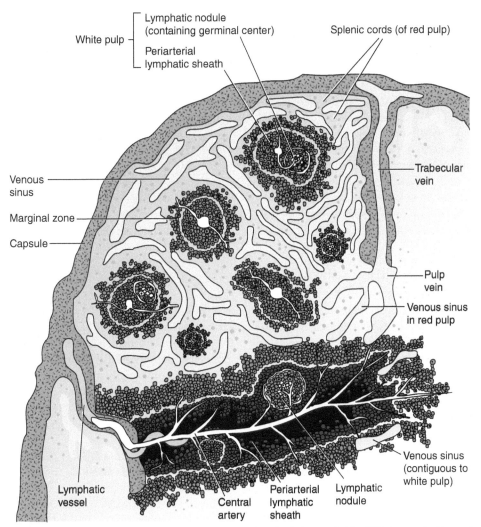

Figure 4.8 Schematic of the Normal Spleen. (From Weiss, L., & Tavossoli, M. 1970. Anatomical hazards to the passage of erythrocytes through the spleen. *Semin Hematol, 7,* 372–380.)

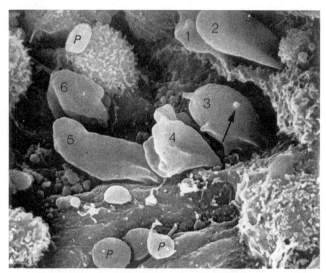

Figure 4.9 Scanning Electron Micrograph of the Spleen. Note erythrocytes (numbered 1 to 6) squeezing through the fenestrated wall in transit from the splenic cord to the sinus. The view shows the endothelial lining of the sinus wall, to which platelets (P) adhere, along with white blood cells, probably macrophages. The arrow shows a protrusion on a red blood cell (×5000). (From Weiss, L. 1974. A scanning electron microscopic study of the spleen. *Blood, 43,* 665.)

environmental stress on the RBCs circulating through the spleen leads to possible hemolysis.

In the rapid-transit pathway, blood cells enter the splenic artery and pass directly to the sinuses in the red pulp and continue to the venous system to exit the spleen. When *splenomegaly* occurs, the spleen becomes enlarged and often palpable. This occurs as a result of many conditions, including, but not limited to, chronic leukemias, inherited membrane or enzyme defects in RBCs, hemoglobinopathies, Hodgkin disease, thalassemia, malaria, and myeloproliferative neoplasms. *Splenectomy* may be beneficial in cases of excessive destruction of RBCs, such as autoimmune hemolytic anemia when treatment with corticosteroids does not effectively suppress hemolysis or in severe hereditary spherocytosis.[40,43] Splenectomy may also be indicated in severe refractory immune thrombocytopenic purpura or in storage disorders with portal hypertension and splenomegaly resulting in peripheral cytopenias.[40] After splenectomy, platelet and leukocyte counts increase transiently.[40] In sickle cell anemia, repeated splenic infarcts caused by sickled RBCs trapped in the small-vessel circulation of the spleen cause tissue damage and necrosis, which often results in *autosplenectomy* (Chapter 24).

Hypersplenism is an enlargement of the spleen resulting in some degree of pancytopenia despite the presence of a hyperactive bone marrow. The most common cause is congestive splenomegaly secondary to cirrhosis of the liver and portal hypertension. Other causes include thrombosis, vascular stenosis, other vascular deformities such as aneurysm of the splenic artery, and cysts.[44]

Lymph Nodes

Lymph nodes are organs of the lymphatic system located along the *lymphatic capillaries* that are parallel to, but not part

of, the circulatory system. These bean-shaped structures (1 to 5 mm in diameter) are typically present in groups or chains at various intervals along lymphatic vessels. They may be superficial (inguinal, axillary, cervical, supratrochlear) or deep (mesenteric, retroperitoneal). Lymph is the fluid portion of blood that escapes into the connective tissue and is characterized by a low protein concentration and the absence of RBCs. *Afferent* lymphatic vessels carry circulating lymph *to* the lymph nodes. Lymph is filtered by the lymph nodes and exits via the *efferent* lymphatic vessels located in the hilus of the lymph node.[39]

Lymph nodes can be divided into an outer region called the *cortex* and an inner region called the *medulla*. An outer capsule forms trabeculae that radiate through the cortex and provide support for the macrophages and lymphocytes located in the node. The trabeculae divide the interior of the lymph node into follicles (Figure 4.10). After antigenic stimulation, the cortical region of some follicles develop foci of activated B cell proliferation called *germinal centers.*[19,35] Follicles with germinal centers are called *secondary follicles,* whereas those without are called *primary follicles.*[39] Located between the cortex and the medulla is a region called the *paracortex,* which contains predominantly T cells and numerous macrophages. The *medullary cords* lie toward the interior of the lymph node. These cords consist primarily of plasma cells and B cells.[43] Lymph nodes have three main functions: They are a site of lymphocyte proliferation, they are involved in the initiation of the specific immune response to foreign antigens, and they filter particulate matter, debris, and bacteria entering the lymph node via the lymph.

Lymph Node Pathophysiology

Lymph nodes, by their nature, are vulnerable to the same organisms that circulate through the tissue. Sometimes increased numbers of microorganisms enter the nodes, overwhelming the macrophages and causing *adenitis* (infection or inflammation of the lymph node). More serious is the common entry into the lymph nodes of malignant cells that have broken loose from malignant tumors. These malignant cells may grow and metastasize to other lymph nodes in the same group.

Thymus

To understand the role of the thymus in adults, certain formative intrauterine processes that affect function must be considered. First, the thymus tissue originates from endodermal and mesenchymal tissue. Second, the thymus is populated initially by primitive lymphoid cells from the yolk sac and the liver. This increased population of lymphoid cells physically pushes the epithelial cells of the thymus apart; however, their long processes remain attached to one another by desmosomes. In adults, T cell progenitors migrate to the thymus from the bone marrow for further maturation.

At birth, the thymus is an efficient, well-developed organ. It consists of two lobes, each measuring 0.5 to 2 cm in diameter, and is further divided into lobules. The thymus is located in the upper part of the anterior mediastinum at about the level of the great vessels of the heart. It resembles other

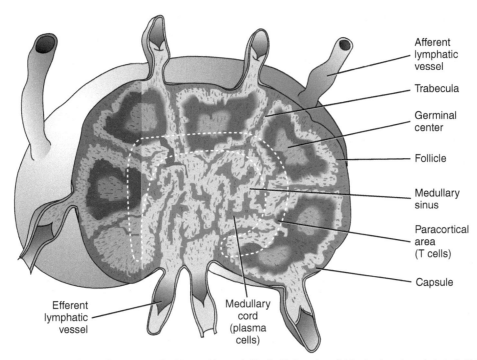

Figure 4.10 Histologic Structure of a Normal Lymph Node. Trabeculae divide the lymph node into follicles with an outer cortex (predominantly B cells) and a deeper paracortical zone (predominantly T cells). A central medulla is rich in plasma cells. After antigenic stimulation, secondary follicles develop germinal centers consisting of activated B cells. Primary follicles (not shown) lack germinal centers.

lymphoid tissue in that the lobules are subdivided into two areas: the cortex (a peripheral zone) and the medulla (a central zone) (Figure 4.11). Both areas are populated with the same cellular components—lymphoid cells, mesenchymal cells, reticular cells, epithelial cells, dendritic cells, and many macrophages—although in different proportions.[45] The cortex is characterized by a blood supply system that is unique in that it consists only of capillaries. Its function seems to be that of a "waiting zone" densely populated with progenitor T cells. When these progenitor T cells migrate from the bone marrow and first enter the thymus, they have no identifiable CD4 and CD8 surface markers *(double negative T cells)*, and they locate to the corticomedullary junction.[45] Under the influence of chemokines, cytokines, and receptors, these cells move to the cortex and express both CD4 and CD8 *(double positive T cells)*.[45] Subsequently they give rise to mature T cells that express either CD4 or CD8 surface antigen as they move toward the medulla.[45] Eventually, the mature T cells leave the thymus to populate specific regions of other lymphoid tissue, such as the T cell–dependent areas of the spleen, lymph nodes, and other lymphoid tissues. The lymphoid cells that do not express the appropriate antigens and receptors, or are self-reactive, die in the cortex or medulla as a result of apoptosis and are phagocytized by macrophages.[45] The medulla contains only 15% mature T cells and seems to be a holding zone for mature T cells until they are needed by the peripheral lymphoid tissues.[45] The thymus also contains other cell types, including B cells, eosinophils, neutrophils, and other myeloid cells.[37]

Gross examination indicates that the size of the thymus is related to age. The thymus weighs 12 to 15 g at birth, increases

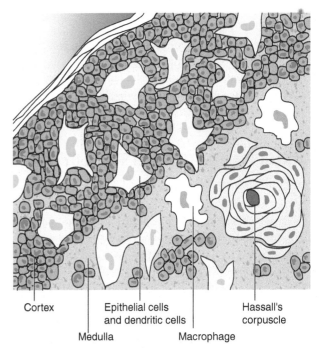

Cortex   Epithelial cells   Hassall's
          and dendritic cells   corpuscle

Medulla   Macrophage

Figure 4.11 Schematic of the Edge of a Lobule of the Thymus. Note cells of the cortex and medulla. (From Abbas, A. K., Lichtman, A. H., & Pober, J. S. 1991. *Cellular and Molecular Immunology.* Philadelphia: Saunders.)

to 30 to 40 g at puberty, and decreases to 10 to 15 g at later ages. It is hardly recognizable in old age because of atrophy (Figure 4.12). The thymus retains the ability to produce new T cells, however, as has been shown after irradiation treatment that may accompany bone marrow transplantation.

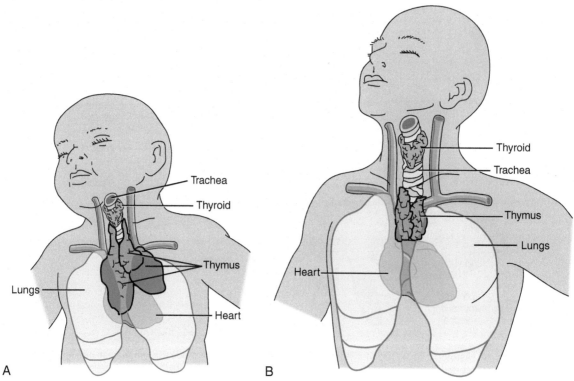

Figure 4.12 Differences in the Size of the Thymus. **(A)**, Infant. **(B)**, Adult.

Thymus Pathophysiology

Nondevelopment of the thymus during gestation results in the lack of formation of T lymphocytes. Related manifestations seen in patients with this condition are failure to thrive, uncontrollable infections, and death in infancy. Adults with thymic disturbance are not affected because they have developed and maintained a pool of T lymphocytes for life.

HEMATOPOIETIC STEM CELLS AND CYTOKINES

Stem Cell Theory

In 1961, Till and McCulloch[46] conducted a series of experiments in which they irradiated spleens and bone marrow of mice, creating a state of aplasia. These aplastic mice were given an intravenous injection of marrow cells. Colonies of HSCs were seen 7 to 8 days later in the spleens of the irradiated (recipient) mice. These colonies were called *colony-forming units–spleen* (CFU-S). These investigators later found that these colonies were capable of self-renewal and the production of differentiated progeny. The CFU-S represents what we now refer to as *committed myeloid progenitors* or *colony-forming unit–granulocyte, erythrocyte, monocyte, and megakaryocyte* (CFU-GEMM).[46,47] These cells are capable of giving rise to multiple lineages of blood cells.

Morphologically unrecognizable hematopoietic progenitor cells can be divided into two major types: noncommitted or undifferentiated HSCs and committed progenitor cells. These two groups give rise to all of the mature blood cells. Originally there were two theories describing the origin of hematopoietic progenitor cells. The *monophyletic theory* suggests that all blood

cells are derived from a single progenitor stem cell called a *pluripotent hematopoietic stem cell.* The *polyphyletic theory* suggests that each of the blood cell lineages is derived from its own unique stem cell. The monophyletic theory is the most widely accepted theory among experimental hematologists.

HSCs by definition are capable of self-renewal, are pluripotent and give rise to differentiated progeny, and are able to reconstitute the hematopoietic system of a lethally irradiated host. The undifferentiated HSCs can differentiate into progenitor cells committed to either lymphoid or myeloid lineages. These lineage-specific progenitor cells are the *common lymphoid progenitor,* which proliferates and differentiates into T, B, and natural killer lymphocyte and dendritic lineages; and the *common myeloid progenitor,* which proliferates and differentiates into individual granulocytic, erythrocytic, monocytic, and megakaryocytic lineages. The resulting limited lineage-specific progenitors give rise to morphologically recognizable, lineage-specific precursor cells (Figure 4.13 and Table 4.1). Despite the limited numbers of HSCs in the bone marrow, 6 billion blood cells per kilogram of body weight are produced each day for the entire life span of an individual.[3] Most of the cells in normal bone marrow are precursor cells at various stages of maturation.

HSCs are directed to one of three possible fates: self-renewal, differentiation, or apoptosis.[48] When the HSC divides, it gives rise to two identical daughter cells. Both daughter cells may follow the path of differentiation, leaving the stem cell pool *(symmetric division),* or one daughter cell may return to the stem cell pool and the other daughter cell may follow the path of differentiation *(asymmetric division)* or undergo apoptosis. Many

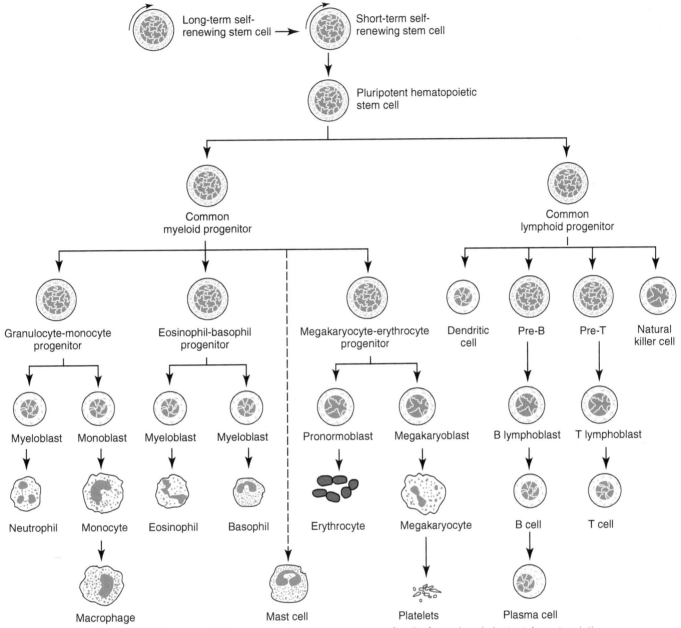

Figure 4.13 Diagram of Hematopoiesis. Note derivation of cells from the pluripotent hematopoietic stem cell.

TABLE 4.1	Culture-Derived Colony-Forming Units (CFUs)
Abbreviation	**Cell Line**
CFU-GEMM	Granulocyte, erythrocyte, megakaryocyte, monocyte
CFU-E	Erythrocyte
CFU-Meg	Megakaryocyte
CFU-M	Monocyte
CFU-GM	Granulocyte, monocyte
CFU-BASO	Myeloid to basophil
CFU-EO	Myeloid to eosinophil
CFU-G	Myeloid to neutrophil
CFU-pre-T	T lymphocyte
CFU-pre-B	B lymphocyte

theories have been proposed to describe the mechanisms that determine the fate of the stem cell. Till and McCulloch proposed that hematopoiesis is a random process whereby the HSC randomly commits to self-renewal or differentiation.[46] This model is also called the *stochastic* model of hematopoiesis. Later studies suggested that the microenvironment in the bone marrow determines whether the HSC will self-renew or differentiate (*instructive* model of hematopoiesis).[48] Researchers believe that the ultimate decision made by the HSC can be described by both the stochastic and instructive models of hematopoiesis. The initial decision to self-renew or differentiate is probably stochastic, whereas lineage differentiation that occurs later is determined by various signals from the hematopoietic inductive microenvironment in response to specific requirements of the body.

The multilineage priming model suggests that HSCs receive low-level signals from the *hematopoietic inductive microenvironment* to amplify or repress genes associated with commitment to multiple lineages. The implication is that the cell's fate is determined by intrinsic and extrinsic factors. Extrinsic regulation involves proliferation and differentiation signals from specialized niches located in the hematopoietic inductive microenvironment via direct cell-to-cell or cellular-extracellular signaling molecules.[48] Some of the cytokines released from the hematopoietic inductive microenvironment include factors that regulate proliferation and differentiation, such as KIT ligand, thrombopoietin (TPO), and FLT3 ligand. Intrinsic regulation involves genes such as *TAL1*, which is expressed in cells in the *hemangioblast*, a bipotential progenitor cell of mesodermal origin that gives rise to hematopoietic and endothelial lineages; and *GATA2*, which is expressed in later-appearing HSCs. Both these genes are essential for primitive and definitive hematopoiesis.[48] In addition to factors involved in differentiation and regulation, there are regulatory signaling factors, such as Notch-1 and Notch-2, that allow HSCs to respond to hematopoietic inductive microenvironment factors, altering cell fate.[49]

As hematopoietic cells differentiate, they take on various morphologic features associated with maturation. These include an overall decrease in cell volume and a decrease in the nucleus to cytoplasmic (N to C) ratio. Additional changes that take place during maturation occur in the cytoplasm and nucleus. Changes in the nucleus include loss of nucleoli, decrease in the diameter of the nucleus, condensation of nuclear chromatin, possible change in the shape of the nucleus, and possible loss of the nucleus. Changes occurring in the cytoplasm include decrease in basophilia, increase in the proportion of cytoplasm, and possible appearance of granules in the cytoplasm. Specific changes in each lineage are discussed in subsequent chapters.

Stem Cell Cycle Kinetics

The bone marrow is estimated to be capable of producing approximately 2.5 billion erythrocytes, 2.5 billion platelets, and 1 billion granulocytes per kilogram of body weight daily.[3] The determining factor controlling the rate of production is physiologic need. HSCs exist in the marrow in the ratio of 1 per 1000 nucleated blood cells.[4] They are capable of many mitotic divisions when stimulated by appropriate cytokines. When mitosis has occurred, the cell may reenter the cycle or go into a resting phase, termed G_0. Some cells in the resting phase reenter the active cell cycle and divide, whereas other cells are directed to terminal differentiation (Figure 4.14).

From these data, a mitotic index can be calculated to establish the percentage of cells in mitosis in relation to the total number of cells. Factors affecting the mitotic index include the duration of mitosis and the length of the resting state. Normally the mitotic index is approximately 1% to 2%. An increased mitotic index implies increased proliferation. An exception to this rule is in the case of megaloblastic anemia, in which mitosis is prolonged.[50] An understanding of the mechanism of the generative cycle aids in understanding the mode of action of specific drugs used in the treatment and management of proliferative disorders.

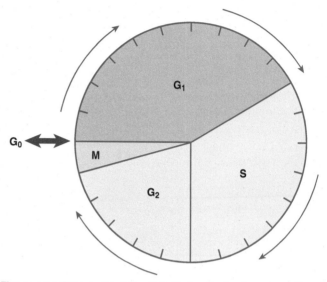

Figure 4.14 Schematic of the Cell Cycle. G_0, Resting stage; G_1, cell growth and synthesis of components necessary for cell division; S, DNA replication; G_2, premitotic phase; M, mitosis.

Stem Cell Phenotypic and Functional Characterization

The identification and origin of HSCs can be determined by immunophenotypic analysis using flow cytometry. The earliest identifiable human HSCs capable of initiating long-term cultures are $CD34^+$, $CD38^-$, HLA-DR^{low}, Thy$_1^{low}$, and Lin$^-$.[49] This population of marrow cells is enriched in primitive progenitors. The expression of CD38 and HLA-DR is associated with a loss of "stemness." The acquisition of CD33 and CD38 is seen on committed myeloid progenitors, and the expression of CD10 and CD38 is seen on committed lymphoid progenitors.[49] The expression of CD7 is seen on T-lymphoid progenitor cells and natural killer cells, and the expression of CD19 is seen on B-lymphoid progenitors (Chapter 28).[45]

Functional characterization of HSCs can be accomplished through in vitro techniques using long-term culture assays. These involve the enumeration of colony-forming units (e.g., CFU-GEMM) on semisolid media, such as methylcellulose. Primitive progenitor cells, such as the *high proliferative potential colony-forming cell* and the *long-term colony initiating cell*, also have been identified. These hematopoietic precursor cells give rise to colonies that can survive for 5 to 8 weeks and be replated.[49] In vivo functional assays also are available and require transplantation of cells into syngeneic, lethally irradiated animals, followed by transference of the engrafted bone marrow cells into a secondary recipient.[49] These systems promote the proliferation and differentiation of HSCs, thus allowing them to be characterized; they may serve as models for developing clinically applicable techniques for gene therapy and HSC transplantation.

From our rudimentary knowledge of stem cell biology, it has been possible to move from the bench to the bedside with amazing speed and success. Hematopoietic stem cell transplantation (HSCT) is more than a half-century old, and we have witnessed tremendous growth in the field as a result of the reproducibility of clinical procedures to produce similar outcomes. However, caution must be exercised because the cells capable of these remarkable clinical events are still not well defined, the niche that they inhabit is still not completely understood, and the signals that they potentially respond to are plentiful and diverse in action. Treatment of hematologic disorders is based on fundamental understanding of the biologic principles of HSC proliferation and maturation. The control mechanisms that regulate HSCs, and the requisite processes necessary to manipulate them to generate sufficient numbers for clinical use, remain largely unknown.

Cytokines and Growth Factors

A group of specific glycoproteins called *hematopoietic growth factors* or *cytokines* regulate the proliferation, differentiation, and maturation of hematopoietic precursor cells.[51] Figure 4.15

illustrates the hematopoietic system and the sites of action of some of the cytokines. These factors are discussed in more detail in subsequent chapters.

Cytokines are a diverse group of soluble proteins that have direct and indirect effects on hematopoietic cells. Classification of cytokines has been difficult because of their overlapping and redundant properties. The terms *cytokine* and *growth factor* are often used synonymously; cytokines include *interleukins (ILs), lymphokines, monokines, interferons, chemokines,* and *colony-stimulating factors (CSFs).*[51] Cytokines are responsible for stimulation or inhibition of production, differentiation, and trafficking of mature blood cells and their precursors.[52] Many of these cytokines exert a positive influence on HSCs and progenitor cells with multilineage potential (e.g., KIT ligand, FLT3 ligand, GM-CSF, IL-1, IL-3, IL-6, and IL-11).[52] Cytokines that

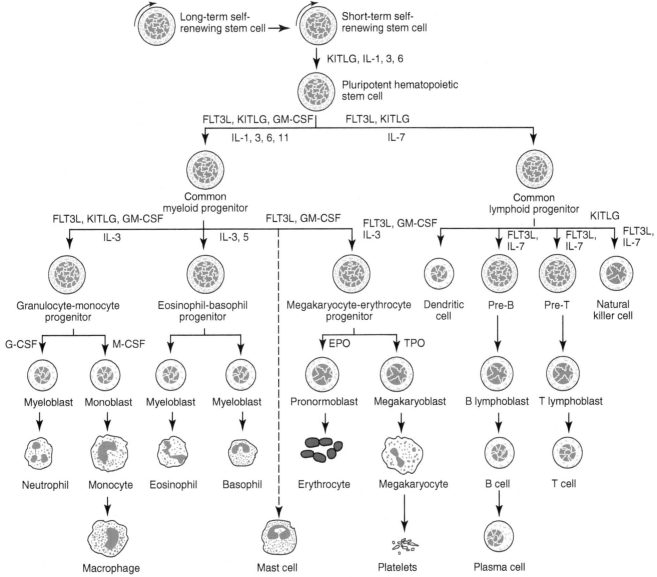

Figure 4.15 Diagram of Derivation of Hematopoietic Cells. Note sites of action of cytokines. *EPO,* Erythropoietin; *FLT3L,* FLT3 ligand; *G-CSF,* granulocyte colony-stimulating factor; *GM-CSF,* granulocyte-macrophage colony-stimulating factor; *IL-1,* interleukin-1; *IL-3,* interleukin-3; *IL-5,* interleukin-5; *IL-6,* interleukin-6; *IL-7,* interleukin-7; *IL-11,* interleukin-11; *KITLG,* KIT ligand; *M-CSF,* macrophage colony-stimulating factor; *TPO,* thrombopoietin.

exert a negative influence on hematopoiesis include transforming growth factor-β, tumor necrosis factor-α, and the interferons.[49]

Hematopoietic progenitor cells require cytokines on a continual basis for their growth and survival. Cytokines prevent hematopoietic precursor cells from dying by inhibiting apoptosis; they stimulate them to divide by decreasing the transit time from G_0 to G_1 of the cell cycle; and they regulate cell differentiation into the various cell lineages.

Apoptosis refers to programmed cell death, a normal physiologic process that eliminates unwanted, abnormal, or harmful cells. Apoptosis differs from necrosis, which is accidental death from trauma (Chapter 3). When cells do not receive the appropriate cytokines necessary to prevent cell death, apoptosis is initiated. In some disease states apoptosis is "turned on," which results in early cell death, whereas in other states apoptosis is inhibited, which allows uncontrolled proliferation of cells.[52,53]

Research techniques have accomplished the purification of many of these cytokines and the cloning of pure recombinant growth factors, some of which are discussed in detail later in this chapter. The number of cytokines identified has expanded greatly in recent years and will further increase as research continues. This chapter focuses primarily on CSFs, KIT ligand, FLT3 ligand, and IL-3. A detailed discussion is beyond the scope of this text, and the reader is encouraged to consult current literature for further details.

Colony-Stimulating Factors

CSFs are produced by many different cells. They have a high specificity for their target cells and are active at low concentrations.[51] The names of the individual factors indicate the predominant cell lines that respond to their presence. The primary target of G-CSF is the granulocytic cell line, and GM-CSF targets the granulocytic-monocytic cell line. The biologic activity of CSFs was first identified by their ability to induce hematopoietic colony formation in semisolid media. In addition, it was found in cell culture experiments that although a particular CSF may have specificity for one cell lineage, it is often capable of influencing other cell lineages as well. This is particularly true when multiple growth factors are combined.[54] Although GM-CSF stimulates the proliferation of granulocyte and monocyte progenitors, it also works synergistically with IL-3 to enhance megakaryocyte colony formation.[54]

Early-Acting Multilineage Growth Factors

Ogawa[55] described early-acting growth factors (multilineage), intermediate-acting growth factors (multilineage), and late-acting growth factors (lineage restricted). KIT ligand, also known as *stem cell factor* (SCF), is an early-acting growth factor; its receptor is the transmembrane protein, KIT. KIT is a receptor-type tyrosine-protein kinase that is expressed on HSCs and is downregulated with differentiation. The binding of KIT ligand to the extracellular domain of the KIT receptor triggers its cytoplasmic domain to induce a series of signals that are sent via signal transduction pathways to the nucleus of the HSC, stimulating the cell to proliferate. As HSCs differentiate and mature, the expression of KIT receptor decreases. Activation of the KIT receptor by KIT ligand is essential in the early stages of hematopoiesis.[52,56]

FLT3 is also a receptor-type tyrosine-protein kinase. KIT ligand and FLT3 ligand work synergistically with IL-3, GM-CSF, and other cytokines to promote early HSC proliferation and differentiation. In addition, IL-3 regulates blood cell production by controlling the production, differentiation, and function of granulocytes and macrophages.[57] GM-CSF induces expression of specific genes that stimulate HSC differentiation to the common myeloid progenitor.[58]

Interleukins

Cytokines originally were named according to their specific function, such as lymphocyte-activating factor (now called IL-1), but continued research found that a particular cytokine may have multiple actions. A group of scientists began calling some of the cytokines *interleukins*, numbering them in the order in which they were identified (e.g., IL-1, IL-2). Characteristics shared by interleukins include the following:

1. They are proteins that exhibit multiple biologic activities, such as the regulation of autoimmune and inflammatory reactions and hematopoiesis.
2. They have synergistic interactions with other cytokines.
3. They are part of interacting systems with amplification potential.
4. They are effective at very low concentrations.

LINEAGE-SPECIFIC HEMATOPOIESIS

Erythropoiesis

Erythropoiesis occurs in the bone marrow and is a complex, regulated process for maintaining adequate numbers of erythrocytes in the peripheral blood. The CFU-GEMM gives rise to the earliest identifiable colony of RBCs, called the *burst-forming unit-erythroid* (BFU-E). The BFU-E produces a large multiclustered colony that resembles a cluster of grapes containing brightly colored hemoglobin. These colonies range from a single large cluster to 16 or more clusters. BFU-Es contain only a few receptors for EPO, and their cell cycle activity is not influenced significantly by the presence of exogenous EPO. BFU-Es under the influence of IL-3, GM-CSF, TPO, and KIT ligand develop into *colony-forming unit-erythroid* (CFU-E) colonies.[47] The CFU-E has many EPO receptors and has an absolute requirement for EPO. Some CFU-Es are responsive to low levels of EPO and do not have the proliferative capacity of the BFU-E.[25] EPO serves as a differentiation factor that causes the CFU-E to differentiate into pronormoblasts, the earliest visually recognized erythrocyte precursors in the bone marrow.[59]

EPO is a lineage-specific glycoprotein produced in the *renal peritubular interstitial cells*.[25] In addition, a small amount of EPO is produced by the liver.[56] Oxygen availability in the kidney is the stimulus that activates production and secretion of EPO.[60] EPO exerts its effects by binding to transmembrane receptors expressed by erythroid progenitors and precursors.[60] EPO serves to recruit CFU-E from the more primitive BFU-E compartment, prevents apoptosis of erythroid progenitors, and induces hemoglobin synthesis[59,61] Erythropoiesis and EPO's actions are discussed in detail in Chapter 5.

Leukopoiesis

Leukopoiesis can be divided into two major categories: *myelopoiesis* and *lymphopoiesis*. Factors that promote differentiation of the CFU-GEMM into neutrophils, monocytes, eosinophils, and basophils include GM-CSF, G-CSF, macrophage colony-stimulating factor (M-CSF), IL-3, IL-5, IL-11, and KIT ligand. GM-CSF stimulates the proliferation and differentiation of neutrophil and macrophage colonies from the colony-forming unit–granulocyte-monocyte. G-CSF and M-CSF stimulate neutrophil differentiation and monocyte differentiation from the colony-forming unit–granulocyte and colony-forming unit–monocyte.[25] IL-3 is a multilineage stimulating factor that stimulates the growth of granulocytes, monocytes, megakaryocytes, and erythroid cells. Eosinophils require GM-CSF, IL-5, and IL-3 for differentiation. The requirements for basophil differentiation are less clear, but it seems to depend on the presence of IL-3 and KIT ligand. Growth factors promoting lymphoid differentiation include IL-2, IL-7, IL-12, and IL-15 and to some extent IL-4, IL-10, IL-13, IL-14, and IL-16.[53] Leukopoiesis is discussed further in Chapter 9.

Megakaryopoiesis

Earlier influences on megakaryopoiesis include GM-CSF, IL-3, IL-6, IL-11, KIT ligand, and TPO.[53] The stimulating hormonal factor TPO (also known as MPL ligand), along with IL-11, controls the production and release of platelets. The liver is the main site of production of TPO.[62,63] Megakaryopoiesis is discussed in Chapter 10.

THERAPEUTIC APPLICATIONS

Clinical use of growth factors approved by the US Food and Drug Administration has contributed numerous options in the treatment of hematologic malignancies and solid tumors. In addition, growth factors can be used as priming agents to increase the yield of HSCs during apheresis for transplantation protocols. Advances in molecular biology have resulted in cloning of the genes that are responsible for the synthesis of various growth factors and the recombinant production of large quantities of these proteins. Table 4.2 is an overview of selected

TABLE 4.2 Selected Cytokines, Characteristics, and Current and Potential Therapeutic Applications

Cytokine	Primary Cell Source	Primary Target Cell	Biologic Activity	Current/Potential Therapeutic Applications
EPO	Kidney (peritubular interstitial cell)	Bone marrow erythroid progenitors (BFU-E and CFU-E)	Simulates proliferation of erythroid progenitors and prevents apoptosis of CFU-E	Anemia of chronic renal disease (in predialysis, dialysis dependent, and chronic anemia patients) Treatment of anemia in cancer patients on chemotherapy Autologous predonation blood collection Anemia in HIV infection to permit use of zidovudine (AZT) Post autologous hematopoietic stem cell transplant
G-CSF	Endothelial cells Placenta Monocytes Macrophages	Neutrophil precursors Fibroblasts Leukemic myeloblasts	Stimulates granulocyte colonies Differentiation of progenitors toward neutrophil lineage Stimulation of neutrophil maturation	Chemotherapy-induced neutropenia Stem cell mobilization Peripheral blood/bone marrow transplantation Congenital neutropenia Idiopathic neutropenia Cyclic neutropenia
GM-CSF	T cells Macrophages Endothelial cells Fibroblasts Mast cells	Bone marrow progenitor cells Dendritic cells Macrophages NKT cells	Promotes antigen presentation T cell homeostasis Hematopoietic cell growth factor	Chemotherapy-induced neutropenia Stem cell mobilization Peripheral blood/bone marrow transplantation Leukemia treatment
IL-2	CD4$^+$ T cells NK cells B cells	T cells NK cells B cells Monocytes	Cell growth/activation of CD4$^+$ and CD8$^+$ T cells Suppress T$_{reg}$ responses Mediator of immune tolerance	Metastatic melanoma Renal cell carcinoma Non-Hodgkin lymphoma Asthma
IL-3	Activated T cells NK cells	Hematopoietic stem cells and progenitors	Proliferation of hematopoietic progenitors	Stem cell mobilization Postchemotherapy/transplantation Bone marrow failure states
IL-6	T cells Macrophages Fibroblasts	T cells B cells Liver	Costimulation with other cytokines Cell growth/activation of T cells and B cells Megakaryocyte maturation Neural differentiation Acute phase reactant	Stimulation of platelet production, but not at tolerable doses Melanoma Renal cell carcinoma IL-6 inhibitors may be promising
IL-10	CD4$^+$, Th2 T cells CD8$^+$ T cells Monocytes Macrophages	T cells Macrophages	Inhibits cytokine production Inhibits macrophages	Target lymphokines in prevention of B cell lymphoma and Epstein-Barr virus lymphomagenesis HIV infection

Continued

TABLE 4.2 **Selected Cytokines, Characteristics, and Current and Potential Therapeutic Applications—cont'd**

Cytokine	Primary Cell Source	Primary Target Cell	Biologic Activity	Current/Potential Therapeutic Applications
IL-12	Macrophages	T cells	T cell, Th1 differentiation	Allergy treatment Adjuvant for infectious disease therapy Asthma Possible role for use in vaccines
IL-15	Activated CD4$^+$ T cells	CD4$^+$ T cells CD8$^+$ T cells NK cells	CD4$^+$/CD8$^+$ T cell proliferation CD8$^+$/NK cell cytotoxicity	Melanoma Rheumatoid arthritis Adoptive cell therapy Generation of antigen-specific T cells
IFN-α	Dendritic cells NK cells T cells B cells Macrophages Fibroblasts Endothelial cells Osteoblasts	Macrophages NK cells	Antiviral Enhances MHC expression	Adjuvant treatment for stage II/III melanoma Hematologic malignancies: Kaposi sarcoma, hairy cell leukemia, and chronic myelogenous leukemia

BFU-E, Burst-forming unit-erythroid; *CFU-E,* colony-forming unit-erythroid; *EPO,* erythropoietin; *G-CSF,* granulocyte colony-stimulating factor; *GM-CSF,* granulocyte-macrophage colony-stimulating factor; *HIV,* human immunodeficiency virus; *IFN,* interferon; *IL,* interleukin; *MHC,* major histocompatibility complex; *NK,* natural killer; *NKT,* natural killer T cells; *Th1,* T helper, type 1; *Th2,* T helper, type 2; *T reg,* regulatory T cells. Adapted from Lee, S., & Margolin, K. (2011). Cytokines in cancer immunotherapy. *Cancer, 3,* 3856–3893; Kurzrock, R. (2000). Hematopoietic growth factors. In Bast, R. C., Kufe, D. W., Pollock, R. E., et al. (Eds.), *Holland-Frei Cancer Medicine.* (5th ed.) Hamilton, ON: BC Decker; Cutler, A., & Brombacher, F. (2005). Cytokine therapy. *Ann N Y Acad Sci, 1056,* 16–29; and Cazzola, M., Mercuriall, F., & Bruguara, C. (1997). Use of recombinant human erythropoietin outside the setting of uremia. *Blood, 89,* 4248–4267.

cytokines and their major functions and clinical applications. Many more examples can be found in the literature.

In addition to the cytokines previously mentioned, it is important to recognize another family of low-molecular-weight proteins known as *chemokines* (chemotactic cytokines), which complement cytokine function and help to regulate the adaptive and innate immune system. These interacting biologic mediators have amazing capabilities, such as controlling growth and differentiation, hematopoiesis, and a number of lymphocyte functions like recruitment, differentiation, and inflammation.[64-66] The chemokine field has rapidly developed and is beyond the scope of this chapter. Nevertheless, a classification system has been developed based on the positions of the first two cysteine residues in the primary structure of these molecules, and the classification system divides the chemokine family into four groups. References provide a starting point for further investigation of chemokines.[64-67]

A recent chemokine-related discovery with clinical implications has led to a successful transplantation-based HSC collection strategy targeting the HSC-microenvironment niche interaction to cause release of HSCs from the bone marrow compartment (referred to as *stem cell mobilization*) into the peripheral circulation so that they may be harvested by apheresis techniques.[68] Experimental studies conducted in the 1990s identified a critical role for CXCL12 and its receptor CXCR4 in the migration of HSCs during early development.[69] Further investigation in adult bone marrow demonstrated that CXCL12 is a key factor in the retention of HSCs within the stem cell niche. It was also found that inhibiting the CXCL12-CXCR4 interaction permitted release of HSCs into the peripheral circulation for harvesting by apheresis.[69] Plexifor (a CXCR4 antagonist) is used as a single agent and in conjunction with G-CSF in novel mobilization strategies to optimize donor stem cell collection.[68,69]

SUMMARY

- Hematopoiesis is a continuous, regulated process of blood cell production that includes cell renewal, proliferation, differentiation, and maturation. These processes result in the formation, development, and specialization of all the functional blood cells.
- During fetal development, hematopoiesis progresses through the mesoblastic, hepatic, and medullary phases.
- Organs that function at some point in hematopoiesis include the liver, spleen, lymph nodes, thymus, and bone marrow.

- The bone marrow is the primary site of hematopoiesis at birth and throughout life. In certain situations, blood cell production may occur outside the bone marrow; such production is termed *extramedullary.*
- The *hematopoietic inductive microenvironment* in the bone marrow is essential for regulating hematopoietic stem cell (HSC) maintenance, self-renewal, and differentiation.
- Monophyletic theory suggests that all blood cells arise from a single stem cell called a *pluripotent hematopoietic stem cell.*

- HSCs are capable of self-renewal. They are pluripotent and can differentiate into all the different types of blood cells. One HSC is able to reconstitute the entire hematopoietic system of a lethally irradiated host.
- As cells mature, certain morphologic characteristics of maturation allow specific lineages to be recognized. General characteristics of maturation include decreased cell diameter, decreased nuclear diameter, loss of nucleoli, condensation of nuclear chromatin, and decreased basophilia in cytoplasm. Some morphologic changes are unique to specific lineages (e.g., loss of the nucleus in red blood cells).
- Cytokines and growth factors play a major role in the maintenance, proliferation, and differentiation of HSCs and progenitor cells; they are also necessary to prevent premature apoptosis. Cytokines include interleukins, colony-stimulating factors, chemokines, interferons, and others.
- Cytokines can exert a positive or negative influence on HSCs and blood cell progenitors; some are lineage specific, and some function only in combination with other cytokines.
- Cytokines have provided new options in the treatment of hematologic malignancies and solid tumors. They are also used as priming agents to increase the yield of HSCs during apheresis for transplantation protocols.

Now that you have completed this chapter, go back and read again the case study at the beginning and respond to the questions presented.

REVIEW QUESTIONS

Answers can be found in the Appendix.

1. The process of formation and development of blood cells is termed:
   a. Hematopoiesis
   b. Hematemesis
   c. Hematocytometry
   d. Hematorrhea

2. During the second trimester of fetal development, the primary site of blood cell production is the:
   a. Bone marrow
   b. Spleen
   c. Lymph nodes
   d. Liver

3. Which one of the following organs is responsible for the maturation of T lymphocytes and regulation of their expression of CD4 and CD8?
   a. Spleen
   b. Liver
   c. Thymus
   d. Bone marrow

4. The best source of active bone marrow from a 20 year old would be:
   a. Iliac crest
   b. Femur
   c. Distal radius
   d. Tibia

5. Physiologic programmed cell death is termed:
   a. Angiogenesis
   b. Apoptosis
   c. Aneurysm
   d. Apohematics

6. Which organ is the site of sequestration of platelets?
   a. Liver
   b. Thymus
   c. Spleen
   d. Bone marrow

7. Which one of the following morphologic changes occurs during normal blood cell maturation?
   a. Increase in cell diameter
   b. Development of cytoplasm basophilia
   c. Condensation of nuclear chromatin
   d. Appearance of nucleoli

8. Which one of the following cells is a product of the common lymphoid progenitor?
   a. Megakaryocyte
   b. T lymphocyte
   c. Erythrocyte
   d. Granulocyte

9. What growth factor is produced in the kidneys and is used to treat anemia associated with kidney disease?
   a. EPO
   b. TPO
   c. G-CSF
   d. KIT ligand

10. Which one of the following cytokines is required very early in the differentiation of a hematopoietic stem cell?
    a. IL-2
    b. IL-8
    c. EPO
    d. FLT3 ligand

11. When a patient has severe anemia and the bone marrow is unable to effectively produce red blood cells to meet the increased demand, one of the body's responses is:
    a. Extramedullary hematopoiesis in the liver and spleen
    b. Decreased production of erythropoietin by the kidney
    c. Increased apoptosis of erythrocyte progenitor cells
    d. Increased proportion of yellow marrow in the long bones

12. Hematopoietic stem cells produce all lineages of blood cells in sufficient quantities over the lifetime of an individual because they:
    a. Are unipotent
    b. Have the ability of self-renewal by asymmetric division
    c. Are present in large numbers in the bone marrow niches
    d. Have a low mitotic potential in response to growth factors

REFERENCES

1. Clements, W. K., & Traver, D. (2013). Signalling pathways that control vertebrate haematopoietic stem cell specification. *Nat Rev Immunol, 13*, 336–348.

2. Tavian, M., Biasch, K., Sinka, L., et al. (2010). Embryonic origin of human hematopoiesis. *Int J Dev Biol, 54*, 1061–1065.

3. Dave, U. P., & Koury, M. J. (2016). Structure of the marrow and the hematopoietic microenvironment. In Kaushansky, K., Lichtman, M. A., Prchal, J. T., et al. (Eds.), *Williams Hematology*. (9th ed., pp. 53–84). New York: McGraw-Hill.

4. Rossmann, M. P., Orkin, S. H., & Chute, J. P. (2018). Hematopoietic stem cell biology. In Hoffman, R., Benz, E. J., Silberstein, L. E., et al. (Eds.), *Hematology Basic Principles and Practice*. (7th ed., pp. 95–110). Philadelphia: Elsevier.

5. Peault, B. (1996). Hematopoietic stem cell emergence in embryonic life: developmental hematology revisited. *J Hematother, 5*, 369–378.

6. Tavian, M., Coulombel, L., Luton, D., et al. (1996). Aorta-associated CD34+ hematopoietic cells in the early human embryo. *Blood, 87*, 67–72.

7. Ivanovs, A., Rybtsov, S., Welch, L., et al. (2011). Highly potent human hematopoietic stem cells first emerge in the intraembryonic aorta-gonad-mesonephros region. *J Exp Med, 208*, 2417–2427.

8. Palis, J., & Segal, G. B. (2016). Hematology of the fetus and newborn. In Kaushansky, K., Lichtman, M. A., Prchal, J. T., et al. (Eds.), *Williams Hematology*. (9th ed., pp. 99–118). New York: McGraw-Hill.

9. Moore, M. A., & Metcalf, D. (1970). Ontogeny of the haematopoietic system: yolk sac origin of in vivo and in vitro colony forming cells in the developing mouse embryo. *Br J Haematol, 18*, 279–296.

10. Weissman, I. L., Papaloannou, V., & Gardner, R. L. (1978). Fetal hematopoietic origins of the adult hematolymphoid system. In Clarkson, B., Marks, P. A., & Till, J. E. (Eds.), *Differentiation of Normal and Neoplastic Hematopoietic Cells*. Cold Spring Harbor, NY: Cold Spring Harbor Laboratory Press.

11. Bailey, A. S., & Fleming, W. H. (2003). Converging roads: evidence for an adult hemangioblast. *Exp Hematol, 31*, 987–993.

12. Pelosi, E., Valtieri, M., Coppola, S., et al. (2002). Identification of the hemangioblast in postnatal life. *Blood, 100*, 3203–3208.

13. Bailey, A. S., Jiang, S., Afentoulis, M., et al. (2004). Transplanted adult hematopoietic stems cells differentiate into functional endothelial cells. *Blood, 103*, 13–19.

14. Samokhvalov, I. M., Samokhvalov, N. I., & Nishikawa, S. (2007). Cell tracing shows the contribution of the yolk sac to adult haematopoiesis. *Nature, 446*, 1056–1061.

15. Delassus, S., & Cumano, A. (1996). Circulation of hematopoietic progenitors in the mouse embryo. *Immunity, 4*, 97–106.

16. DeWitt, N. (Published online 2007, June 21). Rewriting in blood: blood stem cells may have a surprising origin. *Nat Rep Stem Cells*. 10.1038/stem-cells.2007.42.

17. Dieterlen-Lievre, F., Godin, I., & Pardanaud, I. (1997). Where do hematopoietic stem cells come from? *Arch Allergy Immunol, 112*, 3–8.

18. Chang, Y., Paige, C. J., & Wu, G. E. (1992). Enumeration and characterization of DJH structures in mouse fetal liver. *EMBO J, 11*, 1891–1899.

19. Mescher, A. L. (2018). Bone. In *Junqueira's Basic Histology*. (15th ed., pp. 138–160). New York: McGraw Hill Education.

20. Ross, M. H., & Pawlina, W. (2016). Bone. In *Histology: a Text and Atlas with Correlated Cell and Molecular Biology*. (7th ed., pp. 214–253). Philadelphia: Wolters Kluwer.

21. Gupta, P., Blazar, B., Gupta, K., et al. (1998). Human CD34+ bone marrow cells regulate stromal production of interleukin-6 and granulocyte colony-stimulating factor and increase the colony-stimulating activity of stroma. *Blood, 91*, 3724–3733.

22. Rosen, C. J., Ackert-Bicknell, C., Rodriguez, J. P., et al. (2009). Marrow fat and bone marrow microenvironment: developmental, functional, and pathological implications. *Crit Rev Eukaryot Gene Expr, 19*, 109–124.

23. Scadden, D., & Silberstein, L. (2018). Hematopoietic microenvironment. In Hoffman, R., Benz, E. J., Silberstein, L. E., et al. (Eds.), *Hematology Basic Principles and Practice*. (7th ed., 119–126). Philadelphia: Elsevier.

24. Jacobsen, R. N., Perkins, A. C., & Levesque, J. P. (2015). Macrophages and regulation of erythropoiesis. *Curr Opin Hematol, 22*, 212–219.

25. Kaushansky, K. (2016). Hematopoietic stem cells, progenitors, and cytokines. In Kaushansky, K., Lichtman, M. A., Prchal, J. T., et al. (Eds.), *Williams Hematology*. (9th ed., pp. 257–278). New York: McGraw-Hill.

26. Warren, J. S., & Ward, P. A. (2016). The inflammatory response. In Kaushansky, K., Lichtman, M. A., Prchal, J. T., et al. (Eds.), *Williams Hematology*. (9th ed., pp. 279–292). New York: McGraw-Hill.

27. Klein, G. (1995). The extracellular matrix of the hematopoietic microenvironment. *Experientia, 51*, 914–926.

28. Ehninger, A., & Trumpp, A. (2011). The bone marrow stem cell niche grows up: mesenchymal stem cells and macrophages move in. *J Exp Med, 208*, 421–428.

29. Smith, J. N. P., & Calvi, L. M. (2013). Current concepts in bone marrow microenvironmental regulation of hematopoietic stem and progenitor cells. *Stem Cells, 31*, 1044–1050.

30. Yoshihara, H., Arai, F., Hosokawa, K., et al. (2007). The niche regulation of quiescent hematopoietic stem cells through thrombopoietin/Mpl signaling. *Cell Stem Cell, 1*, 685–697.

31. Morrison, S. J., & Spradling, A. C. (2008). Stem cells and niches: mechanisms that promote stem cell maintenance throughout life. *Cell, 132*, 598–611.

32. Ema, H., & Suda, T. (2012). Anatomically distinct niches regulate stem cell activity. *Blood, 120*, 2174–2181.

33. Iwasaki, H., & Akashi, K. (2007). Myeloid lineage commitment from the hematopoietic stem cell. *Immunity, 26*, 726–740.

34. Kim, S. I., & Bresnick, E. H. (2007). Transcriptional control of erythropoiesis: emerging mechanisms and principles. *Oncogene, 26*, 6777–6794.

35. Patton, K. T., & Thibodeau, G. A. (2018). Lymphatic system. In *Anatomy and Physiology*. (10th ed.). St Louis: Elsevier-Mosby.

36. Roy-Chowdhury, N., & Roy-Chowdhury, J. (2016). Liver physiology and energy metabolism. In Feldman, M., Friedman, L. S., & Brandt, L. J., (Eds.), *Sleisenger and Fordtran's Gastrointestinal and Liver Disease*. (10th ed., pp. 1223–1242). Philadelphia: Elsevier.

37. Collin, M., Hughes, D. A., & Pluddemann, A. (2014). Monocytes, macrophages, and dendritic cells. In Greer, J. P., Arber, D. A., Glader, B., et al. (Eds.), *Wintrobe's Clinical Hematology*. (13th ed., pp. 193–226). Philadelphia: Wolters Kluwer Health/Lippincott Williams & Wilkins.

38. Kim, C. H. (2010). Homeostatic and pathogenic extramedullary hematopoiesis. *J Blood Med, 1*, 13–19.

39. Freud, A. G., & Caligiuri, M. A. (2016). The organization and structure of lymphoid tissues. In Kaushansky, K., Lichtman, M. A., Prchal, J. T., et al. (Eds.), *Williams Hematology*. (9th ed., pp. 85–98). New York: McGraw-Hill.

40. Connell, N. T., Shurin, S. B., & Schiffman, F. (2018). The spleen and its disorders. In Hoffman, R., Benz, E. J., Silberstein, L. E.,

et al. (Eds.), *Hematology Basic Principles and Practice.* (7th ed., pp. 2313–2327). Philadelphia: Elsevier.

41. Warkentin, T. E. (2018). Thrombocytopenia caused by platelet destruction, hypersplenism, or hemodilution. In Hoffman, R., Benz, E. J., Silberstein, L. E., et al. (Eds.), *Hematology Basic Principles and Practice.* (7th ed., 1955–1972). Philadelphia: Elsevier.

42. VanPutte, C., Regan, J., & Russo, A. F. (2017). Lymphatic system and immunity. In *Seeley's Anatomy and Physiology.* (11th ed., pp. 779–821). New York: McGraw Hill Education.

43. Chou, S. T., & Schreiber, A. D. (2015). Autoimmune hemolytic anemia. In Orkin, S. H., Fisher, D. E., Ginsburg, D., et al. (Eds.), *Nathan and Oski's Hematology and Oncology of Infancy and Childhood.* (8th ed., pp. 411–430). Philadelphia: Elsevier.

44. Porembka, M. R., Doyl, M., & Chapman, W. C. (2014). Disorders of the spleen. In Greer, J. P., Arber, D. A., Glader, B., et al. (Eds.), *Wintrobe's Clinical Hematology.* (13th ed., pp. 1369–1383). Philadelphia: Wolters Kluwer Health/Lippincott Williams & Wilkins.

45. Paraskevas, F. (2014). T lymphocytes and natural killer cells. In Greer, J. P., Arber, D. A., Glader, B., et al. (Eds.), *Wintrobe's Clinical Hematology.* (13th ed., pp. 279–312). Philadelphia: Wolters Kluwer Health/ Lippincott Williams & Wilkins.

46. Till, T. E., & McCulloch, E. A. (1961). A direct measurement of the radiation sensitivity of normal mouse marrow cells. *Radiat Res, 14,* 213–222.

47. Quigley, J. G., Means, R. T., & Glader, B. (2014). The birth, life, and death of red blood cells: Erythropoiesis, the mature red blood cell, and cell destruction. In Greer, J. P., Arber, D. A., Glader, B., et al. (Eds.), *Wintrobe's Clinical Hematology.* (13th ed., pp. 83–124). Philadelphia: Wolters Kluwer Health/Lippincott Williams & Wilkins.

48. Metcalf, D. (2007). On hematopoietic stem cell fate. *Immunity, 26,* 669–673.

49. Verfaillie, C. (2003). Regulation of hematopoiesis. In Wickramasinghe, S. N., & McCullough, J. (Eds.), *Blood and Bone Marrow Pathology.* New York: Churchill Livingstone.

50. Antony, A. C. (2018). Megaloblastic anemias. In Hoffman, R., Benz, E. J., Silberstein, L. E., et al. (Eds.), *Hematology Basic Principles and Practice.* (7th ed., pp. 514–547). Philadelphia: Elsevier.

51. Horst Ibelfault's COPE. (2016). Cytokines Online Pathfinder Encyclopedia, version 45.1. http://www.cells-talk.com. Accessed November 21, 2017.

52. Mathur, S. C., Hutchison, R. E., & Mohi, G. (2017). Hematopoiesis. In McPherson, R. A., & Pincus, M. R. (Eds.), *Henry's Clinical Diagnosis and Management by Laboratory Methods.* (23rd ed., pp. 540–558). St. Louis: Elsevier.

53. Shaheen, M., & Broxmeyer, H. E. (2013). Cytokine/receptor families and signal transduction. In Hoffman, R., Benz, E. J., Silberstein, L. E., et al. (Eds.), *Hematology Basic Principles and Practice.* (7th ed., pp. 163–175). Philadelphia: Elsevier.

54. Sieff, C., Daley, G. Q., & Zon, L. I. (2015). Anatomy and physiology of hematopoiesis. In Orkin, S. H., Fisher, D. E., Ginsburg, D., et al. (Eds.), *Nathan and Oski's Hematology and Oncology of Infancy and Childhood.* (8th ed., pp. 3–51). Philadelphia: Elsevier.

55. Ogawa, M. (1993). Differentiation and proliferation of hematopoietic stem cells. *Blood, 81,* 2844–2853.

56. Chow, A., & Frenette, P. S. (2014). Origin and development of blood cells. In Greer, J. P., Arber, D. A., Glader, B., et al. (Eds.), *Wintrobe's Clinical Hematology.* (13th ed., pp. 65–82). Philadelphia: Wolters Kluwer Health/Lippincott Williams & Wilkins.

57. Dorssers, L., Burger, H., Bot, F., et al. (1987). Characterization of a human multilineage-colony-stimulating factor cDNA clone identified by a conserved noncoding sequence in mouse interleukin-3. *Gene, 55,* 115–124.

58. Lin, E. Y., Orlofsky, A., Berger, M. S., et al. (1993). Characterization of A1, a novel hemopoietic-specific early-response gene with sequence similarity to bcl-s. *J Immunol, 151,* 1979–1988.

59. Sawada, K., Krantz, S. B., & Dai, C. H. (1990). Purification of human burst-forming units-erythroid and demonstration of the evolution of erythropoietin receptors. *J Cell Physiol, 142,* 219–230.

60. Rizzo, J. D., Seidenfeld, J., Piper, M., et al. (2001). Erythropoietin: a paradigm for the development of practice guidelines. *Haematology, 1,* 10–30.

61. Cazzola, M., Mercuriall, F., & Bruguara, C. (1997). Use of recombinant human erythropoietin outside the setting of uremia. *Blood, 89,* 4248–4267.

62. Wolber, E. M., Ganschow, R., Burdelski, M., et al. (1999). Hepatic thrombopoietin mRNA levels in acute and chronic liver failure of childhood. *Hepatol, 29,* 1739–1742.

63. Wolber, E. M., Dame, C., Fahnenstich, H., et al. (1999). Expression of the thrombopoietin gene in human fetal and neonatal tissues. *Blood, 94,* 97–105.

64. Scales, W. E. (1992). Structure and function of interleukin-1. In Kunkel, S. L., & Remick, D. G. (Eds.), *Cytokines in Health and Disease.* New York: Marcel Dekker.

65. Zlotnik, A., & Yoshie, O. (2000). Chemokines: a new classification system and their role in immunity. *Immunity, 12,* 121–127.

66. Baggiolini, M., Dewald, B., & Moser, B. (1997). Human chemokines: an update. *Annu Rev Immunol, 15,* 675–705.

67. Murphy, P. M., Baggiolini, M., Charo, I. F., et al. (2000). International union of pharmacology. XXII. Nomenclature for chemokine receptors. *Pharmacol Rev, 52,* 145–176.

68. Luster, A. D. (1998). Chemokines—Chemotactic cytokines that mediate inflammation. *N Engl J Med, 338,* 436–445.

69. DiPersio, J. F., Uy, G. L., Yasothan, U., et al. (2009). Plerixafor. *Nat Rev Drug Discov, 8,* 105–106.

5

Erythrocyte Production and Destruction

Michelle Butina*

OBJECTIVES

After completion of this chapter, the reader will be able to:

1. List and describe erythroid precursors in order of maturity, including the morphologic characteristics, cellular activities, normal location, and length of time in the stage for each.
2. Correlate the erythroblast, normoblast, and rubriblast nomenclatures for red blood cell (RBC) stages.
3. Name the stage of erythroid development when given a written description of the morphology of a cell in a Wright-stained bone marrow preparation.
4. List and compare the cellular organelles of immature and mature erythrocytes and describe their specific functions.
5. Name the erythrocyte progenitors and distinguish them from precursors.
6. Explain the nucleus-to-cytoplasm (N:C) ratio, describe the appearance of a cell when given the N:C ratio, and estimate the N:C ratio from the appearance of a cell.
7. Explain how reticulocytes can be recognized in a Wright-stained peripheral blood film.
8. Define and differentiate the terms *polychromasia, diffuse basophilia, punctate basophilia,* and *basophilic stippling.*
9. Discuss the differences between the reticulum of reticulocytes and punctate basophilic stippling in composition and conditions for microscopic viewing.
10. Define and differentiate *erythron* and *RBC mass.*
11. Explain how hypoxia stimulates RBC production.
12. Describe the general chemical composition of erythropoietin (EPO) and name the site of production.
13. Discuss various mechanisms by which EPO contributes to erythropoiesis.
14. Define and explain apoptosis resulting from Fas/FasL interactions and how this regulatory mechanism applies to erythropoiesis.
15. Explain the effect of Bcl-XL (Bcl-2-like protein 1) and the general mechanism by which it is stimulated in erythroid progenitors.
16. Describe features of the bone marrow that contribute to establishing the microenvironment necessary for the proliferation of RBCs, including location and arrangement relative to other cells, with particular emphasis on the role of fibronectin.
17. Discuss the role of macrophages in RBC development.
18. Explain how RBCs enter the bloodstream and how premature entry is prevented and, when appropriate, promoted.
19. Describe characteristics of senescent RBCs and explain why RBCs age.
20. Explain and differentiate the two normal mechanisms of erythrocyte destruction, including location and process.

OUTLINE

Normoblastic Maturation
  Terminology
  Maturation Process
  Criteria Used in Identification of Erythroid Precursors
  Maturation Sequence
Erythrokinetics
  Hypoxia—the Stimulus to Red Blood Cell Production
  Other Stimuli to Erythropoiesis

Microenvironment of the Bone Marrow
Erythrocyte Destruction
  Macrophage-Mediated Hemolysis (Extravascular Hemolysis)
  Mechanical Hemolysis (Fragmentation or Intravascular Hemolysis)

*The author extends appreciation to Kathyrn Doig, whose work in prior editions provided the foundation for this chapter.

CASE STUDY

After studying the material in this chapter, the reader should be able to respond to the following case study:

A 42-year-old premenopausal woman has emphysema. This lung disease impairs the ability to oxygenate the blood, so patients experience significant fatigue and shortness of breath. To alleviate these symptoms, oxygen is typically prescribed, and this patient has a portable oxygen tank she carries with her at all times, breathing through a nasal cannula. Before she began using oxygen, her red blood cell (RBC) count was 5.8×10^{12}/L. After oxygen therapy for several months, her RBC count dropped to 5.0×10^{12}/L.

1. What physiologic response explains the elevation of the first RBC count?
2. What hormone is responsible? How is its production stimulated? What is the major way in which it acts?
3. What explains the decline in RBC count with oxygen therapy for this patient?

The red blood cell (RBC), or erythrocyte, provides a classic example of the biological principle that cells have specialized functions and that their structures are specific for those functions. The erythrocyte has one true function: to carry oxygen from the lung to the tissues, where the oxygen is released. This is accomplished by the attachment of the oxygen to hemoglobin, the major cytoplasmic component of mature RBCs. The role of the RBC in returning carbon dioxide to the lungs and buffering the pH of the blood is important but is quite secondary to its oxygen-carrying function. To protect this essential life function, the mechanisms controlling development, production, and normal destruction of RBCs are fine tuned to avoid interruptions in oxygen delivery, even under adverse conditions such as blood loss with hemorrhage. This chapter and subsequent chapters discussing RBC metabolism, membrane structure, hemoglobin, and iron constitute the foundation for understanding the body's response to diminished oxygen-carrying capacity of the blood, called *anemia*.

The mammalian erythrocyte is unique among animal cells in that in its mature, functional state, it does not have a nucleus. Although amphibians and birds possess RBCs, their nonmammalian RBCs retain the nuclei throughout the cells' lives. The implications of this unique mammalian adaptation are significant for cell function and life span.

NORMOBLASTIC MATURATION

Terminology

RBCs are formally called *erythrocytes*. Nucleated RBC precursors, normally restricted to the bone marrow, are called *erythroblasts*. They also may be called *normoblasts*, which refers to developing nucleated RBC precursors (i.e., blasts) with normal appearance.

Three nomenclatures are used for naming erythroid precursors (Table 5.1). The normoblastic terminology is commonly used in the United States and is descriptive of the appearance of the cells. Some prefer the rubriblast terminology because it parallels the nomenclature used for granulocyte development (Chapter 9). The erythroblast terminology is used primarily in Europe. Normoblastic terminology is used in this chapter.

Maturation Process

Erythroid Progenitors

As described in Chapter 4, the morphologically identifiable erythrocyte precursors develop from two progenitors, burst-forming unit-erythroid (BFU-E) and colony-forming unit-erythroid (CFU-E), both committed to the erythroid cell line. These erythroid progenitors are named for their ability to form colonies on semisolid media in culture experiments that enable the study of their characteristics and development.[1] The earliest committed progenitor, BFU-E, gives rise to large colonies because they are capable of multisubunit colonies (called bursts), whereas CFU-E gives rise to smaller colonies.[1]

Estimates of time spent at each stage suggest that it takes about 1 week for the BFU-E to mature to the CFU-E and another week for the CFU-E to become a pronormoblast,[2] which is the first morphologically identifiable RBC precursor. While at the CFU-E stage, the cell completes approximately three to five divisions before maturing further.[2] As seen later, it takes approximately another 6 to 7 days for the precursors to become mature enough to enter the circulation, so approximately 18 to 21 days are required to produce a mature RBC from the BFU-E.

Erythroid Precursors

Normoblastic proliferation, similar to the proliferation of other cell lines, is a process encompassing replication (i.e., division)

TABLE 5.1 Three Erythroid Precursor Nomenclature Systems

Normoblastic	Rubriblastic	Erythroblastic
Pronormoblast	Rubriblast	Proerythroblast
Basophilic normoblast	Prorubricyte	Basophilic erythroblast
Polychromatic (polychromatophilic) normoblast	Rubricyte	Polychromatic (polychromatophilic) erythroblast
Orthochromic normoblast	Metarubricyte	Orthochromic erythroblast
Polychromatic (polychromatophilic) erythrocyte*	Polychromatic (polychromatophilic) erythrocyte*	Polychromatic (polychromatophilic) erythrocyte*
Erythrocyte	Erythrocyte	Erythrocyte

*Polychromatic erythrocytes are called *reticulocytes* when observed with vital stains.

to increase cell numbers and development from immature to mature cell stages (Figure 5.1). The earliest morphologically recognizable erythrocyte precursor, the pronormoblast, is derived via the BFU-E and CFU-E from pluripotent hematopoietic stem cells, as discussed in Chapter 4. The pronormoblast is able to divide, with each daughter cell maturing to the next stage of development, the basophilic normoblast. Each of these cells can divide, with each of its daughter cells maturing to the next stage, the polychromatic normoblast. Each of these cells also can divide and mature. In the erythrocyte cell line, there are typically three and occasionally as many as five divisions[3] with subsequent nuclear and cytoplasmic maturation of the daughter cells; from a single pronormoblast, therefore, 8 to 32 mature RBCs usually result. The conditions under which the number of divisions can be increased or reduced are discussed later. The changes and cellular activities at each stage described here occur in an orderly and sequential erythroid developmental process.

Criteria Used in Identification of Erythroid Precursors

Morphologic identification of blood cells depends on a well-stained peripheral blood film or bone marrow smear (Chapters 13 and 14). In hematology, a modified Romanowsky stain, such as Wright or Wright-Giemsa, is commonly used.

The descriptions that follow are based on the use of these types of stains.

The stage of maturation of any blood cell is determined by careful examination of the nucleus and the cytoplasm. The most important features in the identification of RBCs are the nuclear chromatin pattern (texture, density, homogeneity), nuclear diameter, nucleus-to-cytoplasm (N:C) ratio (Box 5.1), presence or absence of nucleoli, and cytoplasmic color.

As erythroid precursors mature, several general trends affect their appearance. Figure 5.2 graphically represents these trends.
1. Overall diameter of the cell decreases.
2. Diameter of the nucleus decreases more rapidly than does the diameter of the cell. As a result, the N:C ratio also decreases.
3. Nuclear chromatin pattern becomes coarser, clumped, and condensed. The nuclear chromatin of erythroid precursors is inherently coarser than that of myeloid precursors. It becomes even coarser and more clumped as the cell matures, developing a raspberry-like appearance, in which the dark staining of the chromatin is distinct from the almost white appearance of the parachromatin. This chromatin/parachromatin distinction is more dramatic than in other cell lines. Ultimately the nucleus becomes quite condensed, with no parachromatin evident at all, and the nucleus is said to be *pyknotic*.

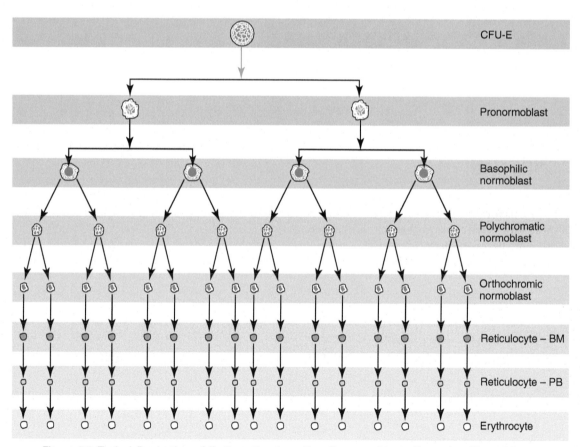

Figure 5.1 Typical Production of Erythrocytes from Two Pronormoblasts Illustrating Three Mitotic Divisions Among Precursors. *BM*, Bone marrow; *CFU*, colony-forming unit-erythroid; *PB*, peripheral blood.

The nucleus-to-cytoplasm (N:C) ratio is a morphologic feature used to identify and stage red blood cell and white blood cell precursors. The ratio is a visual estimate of the area of the cell occupied by the nucleus compared with that of the cytoplasm. If the areas of each are approximately equal, the N:C ratio is 1:1. Although not mathematically proper, it is common for ratios other than 1:1 to be referred to as if they were fractions. If the nucleus takes up less than 50% of the area of the cell, the proportion of nucleus is lower and the ratio is lower (e.g., 1:5 or less than 1). If the nucleus takes up more than 50% of the area of the cell, the ratio is higher (e.g., 3:1 or 3). In the red blood cell line, the proportion of nucleus shrinks as the cell matures and the cytoplasm increases proportionately, although the overall cell diameter grows smaller. In short, the N:C ratio decreases.

4. Nucleoli disappear. Nucleoli represent areas where the ribosomes are formed and are seen early in cell development as cells begin actively synthesizing proteins (Chapter 3). As erythroid precursors mature, nucleoli disappear, which precedes the ultimate cessation of protein synthesis.

5. Cytoplasm changes from blue to gray-blue to salmon pink. Blueness or *basophilia* is due to acidic components that attract basic stains, such as methylene blue. The degree of cytoplasmic basophilia correlates with the amount of ribosomal RNA. The ribosomes and other organelles decline over the life of the developing erythroid precursor, and the blueness fades. Pinkness, called *eosinophilia* or *acidophilia*, is due to accumulation of more basic components that attract acid stains, such as eosin. Eosinophilia of erythrocyte cytoplasm correlates with the accumulation of hemoglobin as the cell matures. Thus the cell starts out being active in protein production on the ribosomes that make the cytoplasm basophilic, transitions through a period in which the red of hemoglobin begins to mix with that blue, and ultimately ends with a thoroughly salmon pink color when the ribosomes are gone and only hemoglobin remains.

Maturation Sequence

Table 5.2 lists the stages of erythroid development in order and provides a comparison. The listing makes it appear that these stages are clearly distinct and easily identifiable. Cell maturation is a gradual process, however, with changes occurring in a generally predictable sequence but with some variation for each individual cell. The identification of a given cell's stage depends on the preponderance of characteristics, although the cell may not possess all the features of the archetypal descriptions that follow. Essential features of each stage are in italics in the

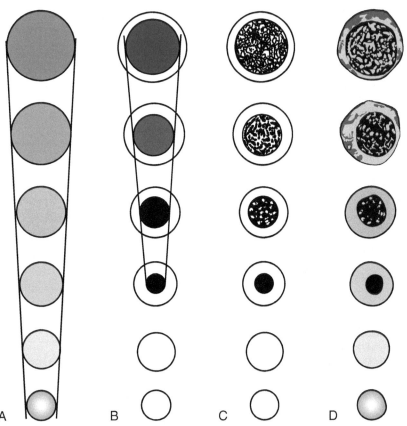

Figure 5.2 General Trends Affecting the Morphology of Erythroid Precursors During the Developmental Process. **(A),** Cell diameter decreases and cytoplasm changes from blue to salmon pink. **(B),** Nuclear diameter decreases and color changes from purplish-red to a very dark purple-blue. **(C),** Nuclear chromatin becomes coarser, clumped, and condensed. **(D),** Composite of changes during the developmental process. (Modified from Diggs, L. W., Sturm, D., & Bell, A. [1985]. *The Morphology of Human Blood Cells.* [5th ed.]. Abbott Park, Ill: Abbott Laboratories.)

TABLE 5.2   Normoblastic Series: Summary of Stage Morphology

Cell or Stage	Diameter	Nucleus-to-Cytoplasm Ratio	Nucleoli	% of Nucleated Cells in Bone Marrow	Bone Marrow Transit Time
Pronormoblast	12–20 μm	8:1	1–2	1%	24 hr
Basophilic normoblast	10–15 μm	6:1	0–1	1%–4%	24 hr
Polychromatic normoblast	10–12 μm	4:1	0	10%–20%	30 hr
Orthochromic normoblast	8–10 μm	1:2	0	5%–10%	48 hr
Bone marrow polychromatic erythrocyte*	8–10 μm	No nucleus	0	1%	24–48 hr

*Also called *reticulocyte.*

following descriptions. The cellular functions described subsequently are also summarized in Figure 5.3.

Pronormoblast (Rubriblast)

Figure 5.4 shows the pronormoblast.

Nucleus. The nucleus takes up much of the cell (N:C ratio of 8:1). The nucleus is round to oval, *containing one or two nucleoli. The purple red chromatin is open* and contains few, if any, fine clumps.

Cytoplasm. *The cytoplasm is dark blue* because of the concentration of ribosomes and RNA. The Golgi complex may be visible next to the nucleus as a pale, unstained area. Pronormoblasts may show small tufts of irregular cytoplasm along the periphery of the membrane.

Division. The pronormoblast undergoes mitosis and gives rise to two daughter pronormoblasts. More than one division is possible before maturation into basophilic normoblasts.

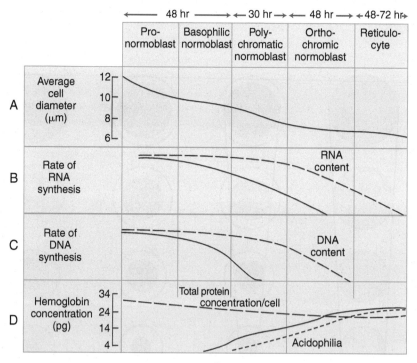

Figure 5.3 Changes in Cellular Diameter, RNA Synthesis and Content, DNA Synthesis and Content, Protein and Hemoglobin Content During Erythroid Development. **(A),** Cell diameter *(solid line)* shrinks from the pronormoblast to the reticulocyte stage. **(B),** The rate of RNA synthesis *(solid line)* for protein production is at its peak at the pronormoblast stage and ends in the orthochromic normoblast stage. RNA accumulates so that the RNA content *(dashed line)* remains relatively constant into the orthochromic normoblast stage when it begins to degrade, being eliminated by the end of the reticulocyte stage. **(C),** The rate of DNA synthesis *(solid line)* correlates to those stages of development that are able to divide: the pronormoblast, basophilic normoblast, and early polychromatic normoblast stages. DNA content *(dashed line)* of a given cell remains relatively constant until the nucleus begins to break up and is extruded during the orthochromic normoblast stage. There is no DNA (i.e., no nucleus) in reticulocytes. **(D),** The *dashed line* represents the total protein concentration, which declines slightly during maturation. Proteins other than hemoglobin predominate in early stages. The hemoglobin concentration *(solid line)* begins to rise in the basophilic normoblast stage, reaching its peak in reticulocytes and representing most of the protein in more mature cells. Hemoglobin synthesis is visible as acidophilia *(dotted line)* that parallels hemoglobin accumulation but is delayed because the earliest production of hemoglobin in basophilic normoblasts is not visible microscopically. (Modified from Granick, S., & Levere, R. D. [1964]. Heme synthesis in erythroid cells. In Moore, C. V., & Brown, E. B. [Eds.], *Progress in Hematology.* New York: Grune & Stratton.)

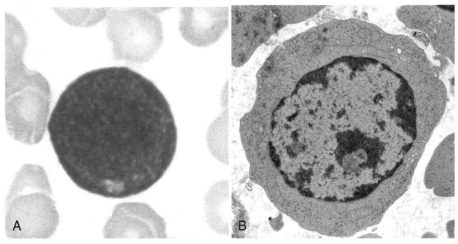

Figure 5.4 Pronormoblasts (Rubriblasts). (A), Pronormoblast. (Bone marrow, Wright-Giemsa stain, ×1000.) **(B),** Electron micrograph of a pronormoblast (×15,575). (B from Rodak, B. F., & Carr, J. H. [2017]. *Clinical Hematology Atlas.* [5th ed.]. St. Louis: Elsevier.)

Location. The pronormoblast is present only in the bone marrow in healthy states.

Cellular activity. The pronormoblast begins to accumulate the components necessary for hemoglobin production. The proteins and enzymes necessary for iron uptake and protoporphyrin synthesis are produced. Globin production begins.[4]

Length of time in this stage. This stage lasts slightly more than 24 hours.[4]

Basophilic Normoblast (Prorubricyte)

Figure 5.5 shows the basophilic normoblast.

Nucleus. *The chromatin begins to condense,* revealing clumps along the periphery of the nuclear membrane and a few in the interior. As the chromatin condenses, the parachromatin areas become larger and sharper, and the N:C ratio decreases to about 6:1. The chromatin stains deep purple-red. Nucleoli may be present early in the stage but disappear later.

Cytoplasm. When stained, *the cytoplasm may be a deeper, richer blue* than in the pronormoblast, hence the name *basophilic* for this stage.

Division. The basophilic normoblast undergoes mitosis, giving rise to two daughter cells. More than one division is possible before the daughter cells mature into polychromatic normoblasts.

Location. The basophilic normoblast is present only in the bone marrow in healthy states.

Cellular activity. Detectable hemoglobin synthesis occurs,[4] but the many cytoplasmic organelles, including ribosomes and a substantial amount of messenger ribonucleic acid (mRNA; chiefly for hemoglobin production), completely mask the minute amount of hemoglobin pigmentation.

Length of time in this stage. This stage lasts slightly more than 24 hours.[4]

Polychromatic (Polychromatophilic) Normoblast (Rubricyte)

Figure 5.6 shows the polychromatic normoblast.

Nucleus. The chromatin pattern varies during this stage of development, showing some openness early in the stage but becoming condensed by the end. *The condensation of chromatin* reduces the diameter of the nucleus considerably, so the N:C ratio

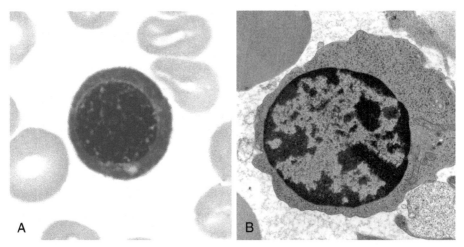

Figure 5.5 Basophilic Normoblasts (Prorubricytes). (A), Basophilic normoblast. (Bone marrow, Wright-Giemsa stain, ×1000.) **(B),** Electron micrograph of a basophilic normoblast (×15,575). (B from Rodak, B. F., & Carr, J. H. [2017]. *Clinical Hematology Atlas.* [5th ed.]. St. Louis: Elsevier.)

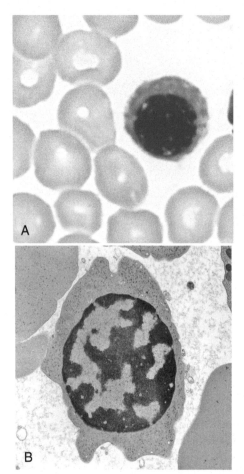

Figure 5.6 Polychromatic Normoblasts (Rubricytes). **(A),** Polychromatic normoblast. (Bone marrow, Wright-Giemsa stain, X1000.) **(B),** Electron micrograph of a polychromatic normoblast (×15,575). (B from Rodak, B. F., & Carr, J. H. [2017]. *Clinical Hematology Atlas.* [5th ed.]. St. Louis: Elsevier.)

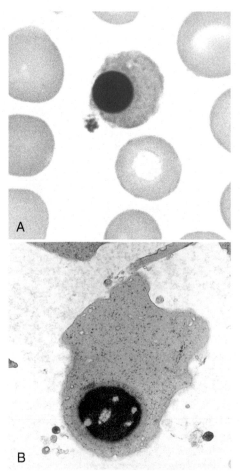

Figure 5.7 Orthochromic Normoblasts (Metarubricytes). **(A),** Orthochromic normoblast. (Bone marrow, Wright-Giemsa stain, X1000.) **(B),** Electron micrograph of an orthochromic normoblast (×20,125). (B from Rodak, B. F., & Carr, J. H. [2017]. *Clinical Hematology Atlas.* [5th ed.]. St. Louis: Elsevier.)

decreases from 4:1 to about 1:1 by the end of the stage. Notably, *no nucleoli are present.*

Cytoplasm. This is the first stage in which the pink color associated with stained hemoglobin can be seen. The stained color reflects the accumulation of hemoglobin pigmentation over time and concurrent decreasing amounts of RNA. The color produced is a mixture of pink and blue, resulting in a *murky gray-blue.* The stage's name refers to this combination of multiple colors, because *polychromatophilic* means "many color loving."

Division. This is the last stage in which the cell is capable of undergoing mitosis, although likely only early in the stage. The polychromatic normoblast goes through mitosis, producing daughter cells that mature and develop into orthochromic normoblasts.

Location. The polychromatic normoblast is present only in the bone marrow in healthy states.

Cellular activity. Hemoglobin synthesis increases, and the accumulation begins to be visible as a pinkish color in the cytoplasm. Cellular RNA and organelles are still present, particularly ribosomes, which contribute a blue color to the cytoplasm. The progressive condensation of the nucleus and disappearance of nucleoli are evidence of progressive decline in transcription of deoxyribonucleic acid (DNA).

Length of time in this stage. This stage lasts approximately 30 hours.[4]

Orthochromic Normoblast (Metarubricyte)

Figure 5.7 shows the orthochromic normoblast.

Nucleus. The nucleus is completely condensed (i.e., pyknotic) or nearly so. As a result, the N:C ratio is low or approximately 1:2.

Cytoplasm. The increase in the *salmon pink color* of the cytoplasm reflects nearly complete hemoglobin production. The residual ribosomes and RNA react with the basic component of the stain and contribute a slightly bluish hue to the cell, but that fades toward the end of the stage as the RNA and organelles are degraded.

Division. The orthochromic normoblast is not capable of division because of the condensation of the chromatin.

Location. The orthochromic normoblast is present only in the bone marrow in healthy states.

Cellular activity. Hemoglobin production continues on the remaining ribosomes using messenger RNA produced earlier. Late in this stage, the nucleus is ejected from the cell. The nucleus moves to the cell membrane and into a pseudopod-like projection. As part of the maturation process, loss of vimentin, a protein responsible for holding organelles in proper location in the cytoplasm, is probably important in the movement of the nucleus to the cell periphery.[2] Ultimately the nucleus-containing projection separates from the cell by having the membrane seal and pinch off the projection with the nucleus enveloped by cell membrane.[5] Nonmuscle myosin of the membrane is important in this pinching process.[6] The enveloped extruded nucleus, called a *pyrenocyte*,[2] is then engulfed by bone marrow *macrophages*. The macrophages recognize phosphatidylserine on the pyrenocyte surface as an "eat me" flag.[7] Other organelles are extruded and ingested in similar fashion. Often, small fragments of nucleus are left behind if the projection is pinched off before the entire nucleus is enveloped. These fragments are called *Howell-Jolly bodies* when seen in peripheral RBCs (Table 16.3 and Figure 16.1) and are typically removed from the cells by the splenic macrophage pitting process once the cell enters the circulation.

Length of time in this stage. This stage lasts approximately 48 hours.[4]

Polychromatic (Polychromatophilic) Erythrocyte or Reticulocyte

Figure 5.8 shows the polychromatic erythrocyte.

Nucleus. Beginning at the polychromatic erythrocyte stage, there is *no nucleus*. The polychromatic erythrocyte is a good example of the prior statement that a cell may not have all the classic features described but may be staged by the majority of features. In particular, when a cell loses its nucleus, regardless of cytoplasmic appearance, it is a polychromatic erythrocyte.

Cytoplasm. The cytoplasm can be compared with that of the late orthochromic normoblast in that the predominant color is that of hemoglobin yet with a bluish tinge due to some residual ribosomes and RNA. By the end of the polychromatic erythrocyte stage, *the cell is the same color as a mature RBC, salmon pink.* It remains *larger than a mature cell,* however. The shape of the cell is not the mature biconcave disc but is *irregular* in electron micrographs (Figure 5.8B).

Division. Lacking a nucleus, the polychromatic erythrocyte cannot divide.

Location. The polychromatic erythrocyte resides in the bone marrow for about 1 to 2 days and then moves into the peripheral blood for about 1 day before reaching maturity. During the first several days after exiting the marrow, the polychromatic erythrocyte is retained in the spleen for pitting of inclusions and membrane polishing by splenic macrophages, which results in the biconcave discoid mature RBC.[8]

Cellular activity. The polychromatic erythrocyte completes production of hemoglobin from a small amount of residual messenger RNA using the remaining ribosomes.[9,10] The cytoplasmic protein production machinery is simultaneously being dismantled. Endoribonuclease, in particular, digests the ribosomes. The acidic components that attract the basophilic stain decline during this stage to the point that the polychromatophilia is only slightly evident in the polychromatic erythrocytes on a peripheral blood film stained with Wright stain. A small amount of residual ribosomal RNA is present, however, and can be visualized with a vital stain such as new methylene blue, so called because the cells are stained while alive in suspension

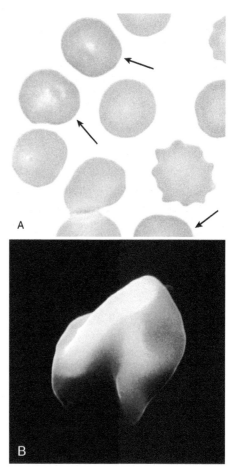

Figure 5.8 Polychromatic Erythrocytes (Shift Reticulocytes). (A), Polychromatic erythrocytes *(arrows).* (Peripheral blood, Wright-Giemsa stain, X1000) **(B),** Scanning electron micrograph of a polychromatic erythrocyte (×5000). (B from Rodak, B. F., & Carr, J. H. [2017]. *Clinical Hematology Atlas.* [5th ed.]. St. Louis: Elsevier.)

(i.e., vital), before the blood film is made (Box 5.2). The residual ribosomes appear as a mesh of small blue strands, a reticulum, or, when more fully digested, merely blue dots (Figure 5.9). When so stained, the polychromatic erythrocyte is called a *reticulocyte*. However, the name reticulocyte is often used to refer to the stage immediately preceding the mature erythrocyte,

---

BOX 5.2 Cellular Basophilia: Diffuse and Punctate

The *reticulum* of a polychromatic erythrocyte (reticulocyte) is not seen using Wright stain; however, the residual RNA imparts a bluish tinge to the cytoplasm, as seen in Figure 5.8A. Based on the Wright-stained appearance, the reticulocyte is called a *polychromatic erythrocyte* because it lacks a nucleus and is no longer an erythroblast but still has a bluish tinge. When polychromatic erythrocytes are prominent on a peripheral blood film, the examiner uses the comment *polychromasia* or *polychromatophilia*. Wright-stained polychromatic erythrocytes are also called *diffusely basophilic erythrocytes* for their regular bluish tinge. This term distinguishes polychromatic erythrocytes from red blood cells with *punctate basophilia*, in which the blue appears in distinct dots throughout the cytoplasm. More commonly known as *basophilic stippling* (Table 16.3 and Figure 16.1), punctate basophilia is associated with some anemias. Similar to the basophilia of polychromatic erythrocytes, punctate basophilia is due to residual ribosomal RNA, but the RNA is degenerate and stains deeply with Wright stain.

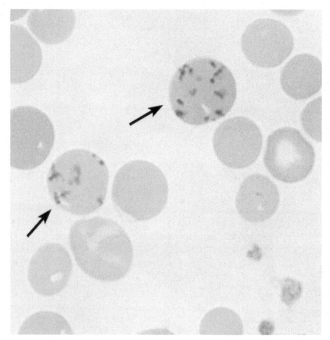

Figure 5.9 Reticulocytes *(arrows).* (Peripheral blood, new methylene blue stain, ×1000.)

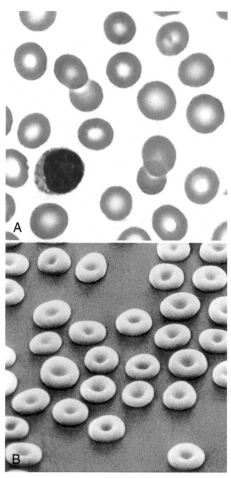

Figure 5.10 Mature Erythrocytes. (A), Mature erythrocytes and one lymphocyte. (Peripheral blood, Wright-Giemsa stain, ×1000.) **(B)**, Scanning electron micrograph of mature erythrocytes. (A from Rodak, B. F., & Carr, J. H. [2017]. *Clinical Hematology Atlas.* [5th ed.]. St. Louis: Elsevier.)

even when stained with Wright stain and without demonstrating the reticulum.

Length of time in this stage. The cell typically remains a polychromatic erythrocyte for about 3 days,[4] with the first 2 days spent in the bone marrow and the third spent in the peripheral blood, although possibly sequestered in the spleen.

Erythrocyte

Figure 5.10 shows the erythrocyte.

Nucleus. *No nucleus* is present in mature RBCs.

Cytoplasm. The mature circulating erythrocyte is a biconcave disc measuring 7 to 8 μm in diameter, with a thickness of about 1.5 to 2.5 μm. On a Wright-stained blood film, it appears as a *salmon-pink stained cell* with a *central pale area* that corresponds to the concavity. The central pallor is about one-third the diameter of the cell.

Division. The erythrocyte cannot divide.

Location and length of time in this stage. Mature RBCs remain active in the circulation for approximately 120 days.[11] Aging leads to their removal by the spleen as described subsequently.

Cellular activity. The mature erythrocyte delivers oxygen to tissues, releases it, and returns to the lung to be reoxygenated. The dynamics of this process are discussed in detail in Chapter 7. The interior of the erythrocyte contains mostly hemoglobin, the oxygen-carrying component. It has a surface area-to-volume ratio and shape that enable optimal gas exchange to occur. If the cell was spherical, it would have hemoglobin at the center of the cell that would be relatively distant from the membrane and would not be readily oxygenated and deoxygenated. With the biconcave shape, even hemoglobin molecules that are toward the center of the cell are not distant from the membrane and are able to exchange oxygen.

The cell's main function of oxygen delivery throughout the body requires a membrane that is flexible and deformable, that is, able to flex but return to its original shape. The interaction of various membrane components described in Chapter 6 creates these properties. RBCs must squeeze through small spaces such as the basement membrane of the bone marrow venous sinus. Similarly, when a cell enters the red pulp of the spleen, it must squeeze between epithelial cells to move into the venous outflow. Deformability is crucial for RBCs to enter and subsequently remain in the circulation.

ERYTHROKINETICS

Erythrokinetics is the term describing the dynamics of RBC production and destruction.[12] To understand erythrokinetics, it is helpful to appreciate the concept of the *erythron. Erythron* is the name given to the collection of all stages of erythrocytes throughout the body: the developing precursors in the bone marrow and the circulating erythrocytes in the peripheral blood and vascular spaces within organs, such as the spleen. When the term *erythron* is used, it conveys the concept of a unified functional tissue. The erythron is distinguished from the RBC *mass.* The erythron is the entirety of erythroid cells in the body, whereas the RBC mass refers only to the cells in circulation. This discussion of erythrokinetics begins by looking at erythrocytes in the bone marrow and the factors that affect their numbers, their progressive development, and their ultimate release into the peripheral blood.

Hypoxia—the Stimulus to Red Blood Cell Production

As mentioned previously, the role of RBCs is to carry oxygen. To regulate the production of RBCs for that purpose, the body requires a mechanism for sensing whether there is adequate oxygen being carried to the tissues. If tissue oxygen is inadequate, RBC production and the functional efficiency of existing cells must be enhanced. Thus a second feature of the oxygen-sensing system must be a mechanism for influencing the production of RBCs.

The primary oxygen-sensing system of the body is located in peritubular fibroblasts of the kidney.[13,14] Hypoxia, too little tissue oxygen, is detected by the peritubular fibroblasts, which then produce erythropoietin (EPO), the major stimulatory cytokine for RBCs. Under normal circumstances, the amount of EPO produced fluctuates very little, maintaining a level of RBC production that is sufficient to replace the approximately 1% of RBCs that normally die each day (discussed in section on erythrocyte destruction). When there is hemorrhage, increased RBC destruction, or other factors that diminish the oxygen-carrying capacity of the blood, the production of EPO is increased.

Increased EPO production, caused by hypoxia, is regulated by a family of transcription factor proteins, called hypoxia-inducible factors (HIFs). HIFs respond to hypoxia by binding to kidney hypoxia responsive elements located at the 5′ flanking region of the EPO gene.[15,16] This results in increased EPO gene transcription, EPO production, and ultimately increased RBC production (Box 5.3).[15,17]

Erythropoietin

Structure. EPO is a thermostable, nondialyzable, glycoprotein hormone with a molecular weight of 34 kD.[18] It consists of a *carbohydrate unit* and a *terminal sialic acid unit,* both of which play a role in the biologic activity of the hormone.[14]

Action. EPO is a true hormone, being produced at one location (kidney) and acting at a distant location (bone marrow). It is a growth factor (or cytokine) that initiates an intracellular message to the developing erythroid cells; this process is called *signal transduction.* EPO (the ligand) must bind to its receptor (EPOR) on the surface of EPO-responsive immature erythroid cells to initiate the signal or message (Figure 32.9). The interaction of EPO with its receptor initiates a cascade of intracellular events that ultimately leads to increased cell division and maturation, increased intestinal iron absorption and hemoglobin synthesis, and more RBCs entering the circulation.[14] EPO-responsive cells vary in their sensitivity to EPO as some are able to respond to low levels of EPO, whereas others require higher levels.[19,20] In healthy circumstances when RBC production needs to maintain a steady state erythropoiesis, the cells requiring only low levels of EPO respond. If EPO levels rise secondary to

---

BOX 5.3 Hypoxia and Red Blood Cell Production[2,15,17]

Steady-state hematopoiesis, occurring in healthy individuals, provides red blood cells (RBCs) at a constant rate, and erythropoiesis occurs in the linear fashion described previously. However, during times of "stress" erythropoiesis, when there is a rapid need for more RBCs such as in anemia, erythropoiesis occurs in a more adaptable manner, as described next.

The kidney is the body's hypoxia sensor and provides early detection when oxygen levels decline. Regardless of the cause of the hypoxia (e.g., decreased RBC number, defective hemoglobin, poor lung function), stimulation of RBC production is warranted because the number of RBCs present are not meeting the oxygen need. The physiologic response to hypoxia is regulated by hypoxia-inducible factors (HIFs) that result in gene expression changes, which ultimately lead to promotion of erythropoiesis. HIFs are a family of proteins that are continually produced and degraded in non-hypoxic conditions. Fundamentally, in hypoxic conditions, the proteins build up and activate the transcription of genes that will promote adaptation to the hypoxic condition. This promotion of erythropoiesis, regulated by HIFs, includes increased production of renal erythropoietin (EPO), enhanced iron uptake and intestinal absorption, and stimulation of erythroid progenitor maturation and proliferation.

Erythropoietin binds to its receptors on erythroid progenitors and early precursors, ultimately increasing the production of RBCs by (1) allowing early release of reticulocytes from the bone marrow, (2) preventing apoptotic cell death, and (3) reducing the time needed for cells to mature in the bone marrow. In severe anemia, EPO production can be increased by up to 1000-fold.

A physiologic adaptation to hypoxia occurs in the fetus and newborn as a result of the predominance of hemoglobin F, which has a higher affinity for oxygen and less readily releases oxygen to the tissues compared with adult hemoglobin A. To compensate for this hypoxia, more RBCs are produced, mediated by the action of erythropoietin. Thus a normal newborn has a relatively higher concentration of RBCs and hemoglobin compared with most adults.

---

hypoxia, however, a larger population of EPO-sensitive cells is able to respond.

The EPO receptor is a transmembrane protein homodimer with extracellular and cytoplasmic domains.[2] The binding of EPO to the extracellular domain of the EPO receptor (on erythrocyte progenitors and early precursors) results in a change in the conformation of the receptor.[2] This activates Janus-activated tyrosine kinase 2 (JAK2) signal transducers that are associated with the cytoplasmic domains of the EPO receptor.[2] JAK2 then activates downstream signal transduction pathways (such as the signal transduction and activator of transcription 5 or STAT5 pathway) that ultimately promotes transcription of specific genes in the RBC nucleus (Figure 32.9).[21] EPO has three major effects: (1) allowing early release of reticulocytes from the bone marrow, (2) preventing apoptotic cell death, and (3) reducing the time needed for cells to mature in the bone marrow. These processes are described in detail in the following sections. The essence is that EPO puts more RBCs into the circulation at a faster rate than occurs without its stimulation.

Early release of reticulocytes. EPO promotes early release of developing erythroid precursors from the bone marrow by two mechanisms. EPO induces changes in the adventitial cell layer of the bone marrow/sinus barrier that increase the width of the spaces for RBC egress into the sinus.[22] This mechanism alone, however, is insufficient for cells to leave the marrow. RBCs are held in the marrow because they express surface membrane receptors for adhesive molecules located on the bone marrow stroma, such as fibronectin (discussed later). EPO downregulates the expression of these receptors so that cells can exit the marrow earlier than they normally would.[23-25]

The result is the presence in the circulation of reticulocytes that are still very basophilic because they have not spent as much time degrading their ribosomes and RNA or making hemoglobin as they normally would before entering the bloodstream. These are called *shift reticulocytes* because they have been shifted from the bone marrow early (Figure 5.8A). Their bluish cytoplasm with Wright stain is evident, so the overall blood picture is said to have polychromasia. Even nucleated RBCs (i.e., erythroblasts or normoblasts) can be released early in cases of extreme anemia when the demand for RBCs in the peripheral circulation is great. Releasing cells from the bone marrow early is a quick fix, so to speak; it is limited in effectiveness because the available precursors in the marrow are depleted within several days and still may not be enough to meet the need in the peripheral blood for more cells. A more sustained response is required in times of increased need for RBCs in the circulation.

Inhibition of apoptosis. A second, and probably more important, mechanism by which EPO increases the number of circulating RBCs is by increasing the number of cells that will be able to mature into circulating erythrocytes. It does this by decreasing apoptosis, the programmed death of RBC progenitors.[26,27] To understand this process, an overview of apoptosis in general is helpful.

Apoptosis: programmed cell death. As noted previously, it takes about 18 to 21 days to produce an RBC from stimulation of the earliest erythroid progenitor (BFU-E) to release from the bone marrow. In times of increased need for RBCs, such as when there is loss from the circulation during hemorrhage, this time lag would be a significant problem. One way to prepare for such a need would be to maintain a store of mature RBCs in the body for emergencies. RBCs cannot be stored in the body for this sort of eventuality, however, because they have a limited life span. Therefore instead of storing mature cells for emergencies, the body produces more CFU-Es than needed at all times. When there is a steady-state demand for RBCs, the extra progenitors are allowed to die. When there is an increased demand for RBCs, however, the erythroid progenitors have about an 8- to 10-day head start in the production process. This process of intentional wastage of cells occurs by apoptosis, and it is part of the cell's genetic program.

Process of apoptosis. Apoptosis is a sequential process characterized by, among other things, the degradation of chromatin into fragments of varying size that are multiples of 180 to 185 base pairs long; protein clustering; and activation of transglutaminase. This is in contrast to necrosis, in which cell injury causes swelling and lysing with release of cytoplasmic contents that stimulate an inflammatory response (Chapter 3). Apoptosis is not associated with inflammation.[28]

During the sequential process of apoptosis, the following morphologic changes can be seen: condensation of the nucleus, causing increased basophilic staining of the chromatin; nucleolar disintegration; and shrinkage of cell volume with concomitant increase in cell density and compaction of cytoplasmic organelles, whereas mitochondria remain normal.[29] This is followed by a partition of cytoplasm and nucleus into membrane-bound apoptotic bodies that contain varying amounts of ribosomes, organelles, and nuclear material. The last stage of degradation produces nuclear DNA fragments consisting of multimers of 180 to 185 base pair segments. Characteristic blebbing of the plasma membrane is observed. The apoptotic cell contents remain membrane bound and are ingested by macrophages, which prevents an inflammatory reaction. The membrane-bound vesicles display so-called eat me signals on the membrane surface (discussed later), which promote macrophage ingestion.[30]

Evasion of apoptosis by erythroid progenitors and precursors. Thus under normal circumstances, many erythroid progenitors will undergo apoptosis. However, when increased numbers of RBCs are needed, apoptosis can be avoided. One effect of EPO is an indirect avoidance of apoptosis by removing an apoptosis induction signal. Apoptosis of erythroid precursors and progenitors is a cellular process that depends on a signal from either the inside or outside of the cell. Among the crucial molecules in the external messaging system is the death receptor Fas on the membrane of the earliest erythroid precursors, whereas its ligand, FasL, is expressed by more mature erythroid precursors.[29,31] When EPO levels are low, cell production should be at a low rate because hypoxia is not present. The excess early erythroid precursors should undergo apoptosis. This occurs when the older FasL-bearing erythroid precursors, such as polychromatic normoblasts, cross-link with Fas-marked immature erythroid precursors, such as pronormoblasts and basophilic normoblasts, which are then stimulated to undergo apoptosis.[29] As long as the more mature erythroid precursors with FasL are present in the marrow, erythropoiesis is subdued. If the FasL-bearing cells are depleted, as when EPO stimulates early bone marrow release, the younger Fas-positive precursors are allowed to develop, which increases the overall output of RBCs from the marrow. Thus early release of older precursors in response to EPO indirectly allows more of the younger precursors to mature.

A second mechanism for escaping apoptosis exists for erythroid progenitors: direct EPO rescue from apoptosis. This is the major way in which EPO is able to increase RBC production. When EPO binds to its receptor on the CFU-E, one of the effects is to reduce production of Fas ligand.[32] Thus the younger cells avoid the apoptotic signal from the older cells. Additionally, EPO is able to stimulate production of various antiapoptotic molecules, which allows the cell to survive and mature.[32,33] The cell that has the most EPO receptors and is most sensitive to EPO rescue is the CFU-E, although the late BFU-E and early pronormoblast have some receptors.[34] Without EPO, the CFU-E does not survive.[35]

As discussed previously, binding of EPO to its transmembrane receptors on erythroid progenitors and precursors activates JAK2 protein associated with its cytoplasmic domain (Figure 32.9). Activated JAK2 then phosphorylates (activates) the STAT5 pathway, leading to the production of the antiapoptotic molecule Bcl-XL (now called Bcl-2-like protein 1).[32,33] EPO-stimulated cells develop this molecule on their mitochondrial membranes, preventing release of cytochrome c, an apoptosis initiator.[36] EPO's effect is mediated by the transcription factor, GATA1, which is essential to red cell survival.[37]

Reduced marrow transit time. Apoptosis rescue is the major way in which EPO increases RBC mass, that is by increasing the number of erythroid cells that survive and mature to enter the circulation. Another effect of EPO is to increase the rate at which the surviving precursors can enter the circulation. This is accomplished by two means: increased rate of cellular processes and decreased cell cycle times.

EPO stimulates the synthesis of RNA in erythroid precursors and effectively increases the rate of the developmental process. Among the processes that are accelerated is hemoglobin production.[14] In addition, EPO induces erythroid precursors to secrete erythroferrone, which acts on hepatocytes to decrease hepcidin production.[38] This allows more iron to be absorbed from the intestines to support the increased hemoglobin synthesis (Chapter 8).[38] As mentioned earlier, another accelerated process is bone marrow egress as a result of the loss of adhesive receptors (such as the fibronectin receptor discussed later) and the acquisition of egress-promoting surface molecules.[39]

The other process that is accelerated is the cessation of division. Cell division takes time and would delay entry of cells into the circulation, so cells enter cell cycle arrest sooner. As a result, the cells spend less time maturing in the bone marrow. In the circulation, such cells are larger because of lost mitotic divisions, and they do not have time before entering the circulation to dismantle the protein production machinery that gives the bluish tinge to the cytoplasm. These cells are true shift reticulocytes similar to those in Figure 5.8A, recognizable in the Wright-stained peripheral blood film as especially large, bluish cells typically lacking central pallor. These shift reticulocytes are also called *stress reticulocytes* because they exit the marrow early during conditions of bone marrow "stress," such as in certain anemias.

EPO also can reduce the time it takes for cells to mature in the bone marrow by reducing individual cell cycle time, specifically the length of time that cells spend between mitoses.[40] This effect is only about a 20% reduction, however, so that the normal transit time in the marrow of approximately 6 days from pronormoblast to erythrocyte can be shortened by only about 1 day by this effect.

With the decreased cell cycle time and fewer mitotic divisions, the time it takes from pronormoblast to reticulocyte can be shortened by about 2 days total. If the reticulocyte leaves the marrow early, another day can be saved, and the typical 6-day transit time is reduced to fewer than 4 days under the influence of increased EPO.

Measurement of erythropoietin. Quantitative measurements of EPO are performed on plasma and other body fluids. EPO can be measured by chemiluminescence. Although the reference interval for each laboratory varies, 10 to 30 U/L is sufficient to maintain steady-state erythropoiesis in a healthy adult.[35] Increased amounts of EPO in the urine are expected in most patients with anemia, with the exception of patients with anemia caused by renal disease.

Therapeutic uses of erythropoietin. Recombinant EPO is used as therapy in certain anemias such as those associated with chronic kidney disease and chemotherapy. It is also used to stimulate RBC production before autologous blood donation and after bone marrow transplantation. The indications for EPO therapy are summarized in Table 4.2.

Unfortunately, some athletes illicitly use EPO injections to increase the oxygen-carrying capacity of their blood to enhance endurance and stamina, especially in long-distance running and cycling. The use of EPO is one of the methods of blood doping; aside from being banned in organized sports events, it increases the RBC count and blood viscosity to dangerously high levels and can lead to fatal arterial and venous thrombosis.

Other Stimuli to Erythropoiesis

In addition to tissue hypoxia, other factors influence RBC production to a modest extent. It is well documented that testosterone directly stimulates erythropoiesis, which partially explains the higher hemoglobin concentration in men than in women.[41] Also, pituitary[42] and thyroid[43] hormones have been found to affect the production of EPO and so have indirect effects on erythropoiesis.

MICROENVIRONMENT OF THE BONE MARROW

The microenvironment of the bone marrow is described in Chapter 4, and the cytokines essential to hematopoiesis are discussed there. Here the details pertinent to erythropoiesis (i.e., the erythropoietic inductive microenvironment) are emphasized, including the locale and arrangement of erythroid cells and the anchoring molecules involved.

Hematopoiesis occurs in marrow cords, essentially a loose arrangement of cells outside a dilated sinus area between the arterioles that feed the bone and the central vein that returns blood to efferent veins. Erythropoiesis typically occurs in what are called erythroid islands within the bone marrow (Figure 4.6). These islands consist of a central macrophage surrounded by erythroid precursors in various stages of development. Initial research on erythroid islands led to the theory that these central macrophages provided iron directly to the normoblasts for the synthesis of hemoglobin. However, because developing erythroid cells obtain iron via transferrin (Chapter 8), no direct contact with macrophages is needed for this. Macrophages are now known to elaborate cytokines that are vital to the maturation process of erythroid precursors and to phagocytize expelled nuclei.[44,45] Erythroid precursors would not survive without macrophage support via such stimulation.

Another role of macrophages in erythropoiesis also has been identified. Although movement of cells through the marrow cords is sluggish, developing cells would exit the marrow prematurely in the outflow were it not for an anchoring system within the marrow that holds them there until development is complete. There are three components to the anchoring system: a stable matrix of accessory and stromal

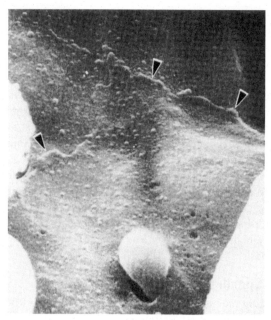

Figure 5.11 Egress of a Red Blood Cell through a Pore in an Endothelial Cell of the Bone Marrow Venous Sinus. Arrowheads indicate the endothelial cell junctions. (From De Bruyn, P. P. H. [1981]. Structural substrates of bone marrow function. *Semin Hematol, 18*, 182.)

cells to which normoblasts can attach, bridging (adhesive) molecules for that attachment, and receptors on the normoblast membrane.

The major cellular anchor for the developing normoblasts is the macrophage. Several systems of adhesive molecules and normoblast receptors tie the developing normoblasts to the macrophages.[44] At the same time, normoblasts are anchored to the extracellular matrix of the bone marrow, chiefly by fibronectin.[24]

When it comes time for RBCs to leave the marrow, they cease production of the receptors for adhesive molecules.[24] Without the receptor, cells are free to move from the marrow into the venous sinus. Entering the venous sinus requires the RBC to traverse the barrier created by the adventitial cells on the cord side, the basement membrane, and the endothelial cells lining the sinus. Egress through this barrier occurs between adventitial cells, through holes (fenestrations) in the basement membrane, and through pores in the endothelial cells[22,46,47] (Figure 5.11).

ERYTHROCYTE DESTRUCTION

All cells experience deterioration of their enzymes over time because of natural catabolism. Most cells are able to replenish needed enzymes and continue their cellular processes. As a nonnucleated cell, however, the mature erythrocyte is unable to generate new proteins, such as enzymes, so as its cellular functions decline, the cell ultimately approaches death. The average RBC has sufficient enzyme function to live 120 days. Because RBCs lack mitochondria, they rely on glycolysis for production of adenosine triphosphate (ATP). The loss of glycolytic enzymes is central to this process of cellular aging, called *senescence*, which culminates in phagocytosis by

macrophages. This is the major method by which RBCs die normally.

Macrophage-Mediated Hemolysis (Extravascular Hemolysis)

At any given time, a substantial volume of blood is in the spleen, which generates an environment that is inherently stressful on cells. Movement through the red pulp is sluggish. The available glucose in the surrounding blood is depleted quickly as cell flow stagnates, so glycolysis slows. The pH is low, which promotes iron oxidation. Maintaining reduced iron is an energy-dependent process, so factors that promote iron oxidation cause the RBC to expend more energy and accelerate the catabolism of enzymes.

In this hostile environment, aged RBCs succumb to various stresses. Their deteriorating glycolytic processes lead to reduced ATP production, which is complicated further by diminished amounts of available glucose. Membrane systems that rely on ATP begin to fail. Among these are enzymes that maintain the location and reduction of phospholipids of the membrane. Lack of ATP leads to oxidation of membrane lipids and proteins. Other ATP-dependent enzymes are responsible for maintaining the high level of intracellular potassium while pumping sodium out of the cells. As this system fails, intracellular sodium increases and potassium decreases. The effect is that the selective permeability of the membrane is lost and water enters the cell. The discoid shape is lost and the cell becomes a sphere.

RBCs must remain highly flexible to exit the spleen by squeezing through the so-called splenic sieve formed by the endothelial cells lining the venous sinuses and the basement membrane. Spherical RBCs are rigid and are not able to squeeze through the narrow spaces; they become trapped against the endothelial cells and basement membrane. In this situation, they are readily ingested by macrophages that patrol along the sinusoidal lining.

Some researchers view erythrocyte death as a nonnucleated cell version of apoptosis, termed *eryptosis*,[48] which is precipitated by oxidative stress, energy depletion, and other mechanisms that create membrane signals that stimulate phagocytosis. It is highly likely that there is no single signal but rather that macrophages recognize several. Examples of the signals that are being further investigated include binding of autologous immunoglobulin G (IgG) to band-3 membrane protein clusters, exposure of phosphatidylserine on the exterior (plasma side) of the membrane, and inability to maintain cation balance.[49] Senescent changes to leukocyte surface antigen CD47 (integrin-associated protein) may also be involved by binding thrombospondin-1, which then provides an "eat me" signal to macrophages.[50] Whatever the signal, macrophages are able to recognize senescent cells and distinguish them from younger cells; thus the older cells are targeted for ingestion and lysis.

When an RBC lyses within a macrophage, the major components are catabolized. Iron is removed from the heme. It can be stored in the macrophage as ferritin until transported out. The globin of hemoglobin is degraded and returned to the metabolic amino acid pool. The protoporphyrin component of heme is degraded through several intermediaries to bilirubin, which is released into the blood and ultimately excreted by the liver in bile. The details of bilirubin metabolism are discussed in Chapter 20.

Mechanical Hemolysis (Fragmentation or Intravascular Hemolysis)

Although most natural RBC deaths occur in the spleen, a small portion of RBCs rupture *intravascularly* (within the lumen of blood vessels). The vascular system can be traumatic to RBCs, with turbulence occurring in the chambers of the heart or at points of bifurcation of vessels. Small breaks in blood vessels and resulting clots can also trap and rupture cells.

The intravascular rupture of RBCs from purely mechanical or traumatic stress results in fragmentation and release of the cell contents into the blood; this is called *fragmentation* or *intravascular hemolysis.*

When the membrane of the RBC has been breached, regardless of where the cell is located when it happens, the cell contents enter the surrounding blood. Although mechanical lysis is a relatively small contributor to RBC demise under normal circumstances, the body still has a system of plasma proteins, including haptoglobin and hemopexin, to salvage the released hemoglobin so that its iron is not lost in the urine. Hemolysis and the functions of haptoglobin and hemopexin are discussed in Chapter 20.

SUMMARY

- Red blood cells (RBCs) develop from committed erythroid progenitor cells in the bone marrow, the burst-forming unit-erythroid (BFU-E) and colony-forming unit-erythroid (CFU-E).
- The morphologically identifiable precursors of mature RBCs, in order from youngest to oldest, are the pronormoblast, basophilic normoblast, polychromatic normoblast, orthochromic normoblast, and polychromatic erythrocyte or reticulocyte.
- As erythroid precursors age, the nucleus becomes condensed and ultimately is ejected from the cell, which produces the polychromatic erythrocyte or reticulocyte stage. The cytoplasm changes color from blue, reflecting abundant ribosomal RNA, to salmon pink as hemoglobin accumulates and the RNA is degraded. Each stage can be identified by the extent of these nuclear and cytoplasmic changes.
- It takes approximately 18 to 21 days for the BFU-E to mature to an RBC, of which about 6 days are spent as identifiable precursors in the bone marrow. The mature erythrocyte has a life span of 120 days in the circulation.
- Hypoxia of peripheral blood is detected by the peritubular fibroblasts of the kidney, which upregulates transcription of the *EPO* gene to increase the production of erythropoietin (EPO).
- EPO, the primary hormone that stimulates the production of erythrocytes, is able to rescue the CFU-E from apoptosis, shorten the time between mitoses in precursors, release reticulocytes from the marrow early, and reduce the number of mitoses of precursors.
- Apoptosis is the mechanism by which an appropriate normal production level of RBCs is controlled. Fas, the death receptor, is expressed by young erythroid precursors, and FasL, the ligand, is expressed by older erythroid precursors. As long as older cells mature slowly in the marrow, they induce the death of unneeded younger cells.

- EPO rescues CFU-E cells from apoptosis by stimulating the production of anti-apoptotic molecules that counteract the effects of Fas and FasL and simultaneously decreases Fas production by young erythroid precursors.
- Survival of erythroid precursors in the bone marrow depends on adhesive molecules, such as fibronectin, and cytokines that are secreted by macrophages and other bone marrow stromal cells. Erythroid precursors in various stages of maturation are found in erythroid islands where they surround a macrophage.
- As erythroid precursors mature, they lose adhesive molecule receptors, which allows their egress from the bone marrow. Egress occurs between adventitial cells but through pores in the endothelial cells of the venous sinus.
- Aged RBCs, or senescent cells, cannot regenerate catabolized enzymes because they lack a nucleus. The semipermeable membrane becomes more permeable to water, so the cells swell and become spherocytic and rigid. They become trapped in the splenic sieve, where they are readily phagocytized by macrophages.
- Extravascular or macrophage-mediated hemolysis accounts for most normal RBC death. The signals to macrophages that initiate RBC ingestion may include binding of autologous immunoglobulin G (IgG), expression of phosphatidylserine on the outer membrane, cation balance changes, and binding of CD47 to thrombospondin-1.
- Fragmentation or intravascular hemolysis results when mechanical factors rupture the cell membrane while the cell is in the peripheral circulation. This pathway accounts for a minor component of normal destruction of RBCs.

Now that you have completed this chapter, go back and read again the case study at the beginning and respond to the questions presented.

REVIEW QUESTIONS

Answers can be found in the Appendix.

1. Which of the following is an erythroid progenitor?
   a. Pronormoblast
   b. Reticulocyte
   c. CFU-E
   d. Orthochromic normoblast

2. Which of the following is the most mature normoblast?
   a. Orthochromic normoblast
   b. Basophilic normoblast
   c. Pronormoblast
   d. Polychromatic normoblast

3. What erythroid precursor can be described as follows: The cell is of medium size compared with other normoblasts, with an N:C ratio of nearly 1:1. The nuclear chromatin is condensed and chunky throughout the nucleus. No nucleoli are seen. The cytoplasm is gray-blue.
   a. Reticulocyte
   b. Pronormoblast
   c. Orthochromic normoblast
   d. Polychromatic normoblast

4. At which normoblastic stage does globin production begin?
   a. Orthochromic normoblast
   b. Pronormoblast
   c. Polychromatic normoblast
   d. Basophilic normoblast

5. Hypoxia stimulates RBC production by:
   a. Inducing more pluripotent stem cells into the erythroid lineage
   b. Stimulating EPO production by the kidney
   c. Increasing the number of RBC mitoses
   d. Stimulating the production of fibronectin by macrophages of the bone marrow

6. Erythropoietin can increase the production of RBCS by:
   a. Promoting apoptosis of erythroid progenitors
   b. Decreasing intravascular hemolysis
   c. Increasing EPO receptor sites
   d. Promoting early release of reticulocytes from bone marrow

7. In the bone marrow, erythroid precursors are located:
   a. Surrounding macrophages in erythroid islands
   b. Adjacent to megakaryocytes along the adventitial cell lining
   c. Surrounding fat cells in apoptotic islands
   d. In the center of the hematopoietic cords

8. Which of the following determines the timing of egress of RBCs from the bone marrow?
   a. Stromal cells decrease production of adhesive molecules over time as RBCs mature.
   b. Endothelial cells of the venous sinus form pores at specified intervals of time, allowing egress of free cells.
   c. Periodic apoptosis of pronormoblasts in the marrow cords occurs.
   d. Maturing normoblasts slowly lose receptors for adhesive molecules that bind them to stromal cells.

9. What single feature of normal RBCs is most responsible for limiting their life span?
   a. Loss of the nucleus
   b. Increased flexibility of the cell membrane
   c. Reduction of hemoglobin iron
   d. Loss of mitochondria

10. Extravascular hemolysis occurs when:
    a. RBCs are mechanically ruptured
    b. RBCs extravasate from blood vessels into the tissues
    c. Splenic macrophages ingest senescent RBCs
    d. RBCs are trapped in blood clots outside the blood vessels

REFERENCES

1. Nandakumar, S. K., Ulirsch, J. C. & Sankaran, V. G. (2016). Advances in understanding erythropoiesis: evolving perspectives. *Br J Haematol, 173,* 206–218.

2. Papayannopoulou, T., & Migliaccio, A. R. (2018). Biology of erythropoiesis, erythroid differentiation, and maturation. In Hoffman, R., Benz, E. J., Silberstein, L. E., et al. (Eds.), *Hematology: Basic Principles and Practice.* (7th ed., pp. 297–320). Philadelphia: Elsevier.

3. Shumacher, H. R., & Erslev, A. J. (1956). Bone marrow kinetics. In Szirmani, E. (Ed.), *Nuclear Hematology.* (pp. 89–132). New York: Academic Press.

4. Granick, S., & Levere, R. D. (1964). Heme synthesis in erythroid cells. In Moore, C. V., & Brown, E.B. (Eds.), *Progress in Hematology.* (vol 4., pp. 1–47). New York: Grune & Stratton.

5. Skutelsky, E., & Danon, D. (1967). An electron microscopic study of nuclear elimination from the late erythroblast. *J Cell Biol, 33,* 625–635.

6. Ubukawa, K., Guo, Y. M., Takahashi, M., et al. (2012). Enucleation of human erythroblasts involves non-muscle myosin IIB. *Blood, 119,* 1036–1044.

7. Yoshida, H., Kawane, K., Koike, M., et al. (2005). Phosphatidylserine-dependent engulfment by macrophages of nuclei from erythroid precursor cells. *Nature, 437,* 754–758.

8. Song, S. H., & Groom, A. C. (1972). Sequestration and possible maturation of reticulocytes in the normal spleen. *Can J Physiol Pharmacol, 50,* 400–406.

9. Lee, E., Choi, H. S., Hwang, J. H., et al. (2014). The RNA in reticulocytes is not just debris: it is necessary for the final stages of erythrocyte formation. *Blood Cell Mol Dis, 53,* 1–10.

10. Mills, E. W., Wangen, J., Green, R., et al. (2016). Dynamic regulation of a ribosome rescue pathway in erythroid cells and platelets. *Cell Rep, 17,* 1–10.

11. Ashby, W. (1919). The determination of the length of life of transfused blood corpuscles in man. *J Exp Med, 29,* 268–282.

12. Giblett, E. R., Coleman, D. H., Pirzio-Biroli, G., et al. (1956). Erythrokinetics: quantitative measurements of red cell production and destruction in normal subjects and patients with anemia. *Blood, 11*(4), 291–309.

13. Jacobson, L. O., Goldwasser, E., Fried, W., et al. (1957). Role of the kidney in erythropoiesis. *Nature, 179,* 633–634.

14. Kurtz, A., Wenger, R. H., & Eckardt, K. (2013). Hematopoiesis and the kidney. In Alpern, R. J., Caplan, M. J., & Moe, O. W. (Eds.), *Seldin and Giebisch's The Kidney: Physiology and Pathophysiology.* (5th ed., pp. 3087–3124). San Diego: Elsevier.

15. Haase, V. H. (2013). Regulation of erythropoiesis by hypoxia-inducible factors. *Blood Rev, 27*(1), 41–53.

16. Lee, F. S., & Percy, M. J. (2011). The HIF pathway and erythrocytosis. *Annu Rev Pathol, 6,* 165–192.

17. Liang, R., & Ghaffari, S. (2016). Advances in understanding the mechanisms of erythropoiesis in homeostasis and disease. *Br J Haematol, 174*(5), 661–673.

18. Shelton, R. N., Ichiki, A. T., & Lange, R. D. (1975). Physicochemical properties of erythropoietin: isoelectric focusing and molecular weight studies. *Biochem Med, 12,* 45–54.

19. Kaushansky, K. (2001). Hematopoietic growth factors and receptors. In Stamatoyannopoulos, G., Majerus, P. W., Perlmutter, R. M., et al. (Eds.), *The Molecular Basis of Blood Diseases.* (3rd ed., pp 25–79). Philadelphia: Saunders.

20. Broudy, V. C., Lin, N., Brice, M., et al. (1991). Erythropoietin receptor characteristics on primary human erythroid cells. *Blood, 77,* 2583–2590.

21. Parganas, E., Wang, D., Stravopodis, D., et al. (1998). Jak2 is essential for signaling through a variety of cytokine receptors. *Cell, 93*, 385–395.

22. Chamberlain, J. K., Leblond, P. F., & Weed, R. I. (1975). Reduction of adventitial cell cover: an early direct effect of erythropoietin on bone marrow ultrastructure. *Blood Cells, 1*, 655–674.

23. Patel, V. P., & Lodish, H. F. (1986). The fibronectin receptor on mammalian erythroid precursor cells: characterization and developmental regulation. *J Cell Biol, 102*, 449–456.

24. Vuillet-Gaugler, M. H., Breton-Gorius, J., Vainchenker, W., et al. (1990). Loss of attachment to fibronectin with terminal human erythroid differentiation. *Blood, 75*, 865–873.

25. Goltry, K. L., & Patel, V. P. (1997). Specific domains of fibronectin mediate adhesion and migration of early murine erythroid progenitors. *Blood, 90*, 138–147.

26. Sieff, C. A., Emerson, S. G., Mufson, A., et al. (1986). Dependence of highly enriched human bone marrow progenitors on hemopoietic growth factors and their response to recombinant erythropoietin. *J Clin Invest, 77*, 74–81.

27. Eaves, C. J., & Eaves, A. C. (1978). Erythropoietin (Ep) dose-response curves for three classes of erythroid progenitors in normal human marrow and in patients with polycythemia vera. *Blood, 52*, 1196–1210.

28. Allen, P. D., Bustin, S. A., & Newland, A. C. (1993). The role of apoptosis (programmed cell death) in haemopoiesis and the immune system. *Blood Rev, 7*, 63–73.

29. DeMaria, R., Testa, U., Luchetti, L., et al. (1999). Apoptotic role of Fas/Fas ligand system in the regulation of erythropoiesis. *Blood, 93*, 796–803.

30. Martin, S. J., Reutelingsperger, C. P., McGahon, A. J., et al. (1995). Early redistribution of plasma membrane phosphatidylserine is a general feature of apoptosis regardless of the initiating stimulus: inhibition by overexpression of Bcl-2 and Abl. *J Exp Med, 182*, 1545–1556.

31. Zamai, L., Burattini, S., Luchetti, F., et al. (2004). In vitro apoptotic cell death during erythroid differentiation. *Apoptosis, 9*, 235–246.

32. Elliott, S., Pham, E., & Mcdougall, I. C. (2008). Erythropoietins: a common mechanism of action. *Exp Hematol, 36*, 1573–1584.

33. Dolznig, H., Habermann, B., Stangl, K., et al. (2002). Apoptosis protection by the Epo target Bcl-X(L) allows factor-independent differentiation of primary erythroblasts. *Curr Biol, 12*, 1076–1085.

34. Sawada, K., Krantz, S. B., Dai, C. H., et al. (1990). Purification of human blood burst-forming units-erythroid and demonstration of the evolution of erythropoietin receptors. *J Cell Physiol, 142*, 219–230.

35. Brugnara, C., & Eckardt, K. (2016). Hematologic aspects of kidney disease. In Skorecki, K., Chertow, G. M., Marsden, P. A., et al. (Eds.), *Brenner & Rector's The Kidney.* (10th ed., pp. 1875–1911). Philadelphia: Elsevier.

36. Basanez, G., Soane, L., & Hardwick, J. M. (2012). A new view of the lethal apoptotic pore. *PLoS Biol, 10*(9), e100139.

37. Gregory, T., Yu, C., Ma, A., et al. (1999). GATA-1 and erythropoietin cooperate to promote erythroid cell survival by regulating bcl-xL expression. *Blood, 94*, 87–96.

38. Kautz, L, Jung, G., Valore, E. V., et al. (2014). Identification of erythroferrone as an erythroid regulator of iron metabolism. *Nat Genet, 46*(7), 678–684.

39. Sathyanarayana, P., Menon, M. P., Bogacheva, O., et al. (2007). Erythropoietin modulation of podocalyxin and a proposed erythroblast niche. *Blood, 110*(2), 509–518.

40. Hanna, I. R., Tarbutt, R. O., & Lamerton, L. F. (1969). Shortening of the cell-cycle time of erythroid precursors in response to anaemia. *Br J Haematol, 16*, 381–387.

41. Jacobson, W., Siegman, R. L., & Diamond, L. K. (1968). Effect of testosterone on the uptake of tritiated thymidine in bone marrow of children. *Ann N Y Acad Sci, 149*, 389–405.

42. Golde, D. W., Bersch, N., & Li, C. H. (1977). Growth hormone: species-specific stimulation of in vitro erythropoiesis. *Science, 196*, 1112–1113.

43. Popovic, W. J., Brown, J. E., & Adamson, J. W. (1977). The influence of thyroid hormones on in vitro erythropoiesis: mediation by a receptor with beta adrenergic properties. *J Clin Invest, 60*, 908–913.

44. Chasis, J. A., & Mohandas, N. (2008). Erythroblastic islands: niches for erythropoiesis. *Blood, 112*, 470–478.

45. Dzierzak, E., & Philipsen, S. (2013). Erythropoiesis: development and differentiation. *Cold Spring Harb Perspect Med, 3*(4), 1–16.

46. Chamberlain, J. K., & Lichtman, M. A. (1978). Marrow cell egress: specificity of the site of penetration into the sinus. *Blood, 52*, 959–968.

47. DeBruyn, P. P. H. (1981). Structural substrates of bone marrow function. *Semin Hematol, 18*, 179–193.

48. Lang, F., & Qadri, S. M. (2012). Mechanisms and significance of eryptosis, the suicidal death of erythrocytes. *Blood Purif, 33*(1–3), 125–130.

49. Rifkind, J. M., & Nagababu, E. (2013). Hemoglobin redox reactions and red blood cell aging. *Antiox Redox Signal, 18*(17), 2274–2283.

50. Burger, P., Hilarius-Stokman, P., de Korte, D., et al. (2012). CD47 functions as a molecular switch for erythrocyte phagocytosis. *Blood, 119*(23), 5512–5521.

6

Erythrocyte Metabolism and Membrane Structure and Function

OBJECTIVES

After completion of this chapter, the reader will be able to:

1. List the erythrocyte metabolic processes that require energy.
2. Diagram the Embden-Meyerhof anaerobic glycolytic pathway (EMP) in the red blood cell (RBC), highlighting adenosine triphosphate (ATP) consumption and generation.
3. Name the components of the hexose-monophosphate pathway (HMP) and describe the process of detoxifying peroxide.
4. Diagram the methemoglobin reductase pathway and explain its importance in maintaining functional hemoglobin.
5. Describe the RBC metabolic pathway that generates 2,3-BPG, state the effect of its formation on ATP production, and explain its importance in oxygen transport.
6. Explain the importance of the semipermeable RBC membrane.
7. Describe the arrangement and function of lipids in the RBC membrane.
8. Explain cholesterol exchange between the RBC membrane and plasma, including factors that affect the exchange.
9. Define, locate, and explain the role of RBC transmembrane proteins in maintaining membrane stability and provide examples of these proteins.
10. Discuss how ankyrin, protein 4.2, protein 4.1, actin, adducin, tropomodulin, dematin, and band 3 interact with α- and β-spectrin and the lipid bilayer of the RBC membrane.
11. Name conditions caused by mutations in transmembrane and cytoskeletal proteins that disrupt vertical and horizontal (lateral) linkages in the RBC membrane.
12. Cite the relative concentrations of RBC cytoplasmic potassium, sodium, and calcium, and name the structures that maintain those concentrations.

OUTLINE

Energy Production—Anaerobic Glycolysis
Glycolysis Diversion Pathways (Shunts)
    Hexose Monophosphate Pathway
    Methemoglobin Reductase Pathway
    Rapoport-Luebering Pathway

RBC Membrane
    RBC Deformability
    RBC Membrane Lipids
    RBC Membrane Proteins
    Osmotic Balance and Permeability

CASE STUDY

After studying the material in this chapter, the reader should be able to respond to the following case study:

Cyanosis is a blue skin coloration that occurs when the blood does not deliver enough oxygen to the tissues. It is a common sign of heart or lung disease, in which the blood fails to become oxygenated or is distributed improperly throughout the body. In the 1940s, Dr. James Deeny, an Irish physician, was experimenting with the use of vitamin C (ascorbic acid), which is a potent reducing agent, as a treatment for heart disease.[1] Unfortunately, it was ineffective for nearly all patients. However, he discovered two brothers with cyanosis and neither man was diagnosed with heart or lung disease. When he treated them with vitamin C, the skin of each brother returned to a normal, healthy pink color.[1] It was later determined that they had familial idiopathic methemoglobinemia.

1. What does it mean to say that vitamin C is a reducing agent?
2. What must be happening if vitamin C was able to reverse the cyanosis?
3. What is the significance of finding this condition in brothers?

*The author extends appreciation to Kathyrn Doig and George A. Fritsma, whose work in prior editions provided the foundation for this chapter.

There are approximately 5 million erythrocytes (red blood cells, RBCs) per microliter of circulating blood making the RBC the primary cell in the blood. The RBC lacks a nucleus, has a biconcave shape, and has an average volume of 90 fL. The biconcave shape supports deformation, enabling the circulating cell to pass smoothly through capillaries, where it readily exchanges oxygen (O_2) and carbon dioxide (CO_2) while contacting the vessel wall.[2,3] The cytoplasm of the RBC contains abundant hemoglobin (a complex of globin, protoporphyrin, and iron), which transports O_2 from the lungs to the tissues. Hemoglobin has four globin chains, and each chain contains a heme molecule with an iron in the ferrous state. This allows each hemoglobin molecule to carry four O_2 molecules (Chapter 7). The RBC also transports CO_2 and bicarbonate (HCO_3^-) from the tissues back to the lungs.

RBCs are produced through normoblastic proliferation and mature in the bone marrow (Chapter 5). The nucleus, present in maturing normoblasts, is extruded as part of the RBC maturation process, typically as the RBC moves from the bone marrow to circulation. Cytoplasmic ribosomes and mitochondria also disappear 24 to 48 hours after bone marrow release, eliminating the cells' ability to produce proteins or support oxidative metabolism.[2,3] Without mitochondria for aerobic respiration via oxidative phosphorylation, adenosine triphosphate (ATP) is produced within the cytoplasm through anaerobic glycolysis (Embden-Meyerhof pathway, EMP) for the lifetime of the cell. ATP drives mechanisms that slow the oxidation of proteins and iron by environmental peroxides and superoxide anions, maintaining hemoglobin's function and membrane integrity. Oxidation, however, eventually takes a toll, limiting the RBC circulating life span to 120 days, whereupon it is disassembled into its reusable components: globin chains and iron from hemoglobin, and phospholipids and proteins from the cell membrane. The protoporphyrin ring of hemoglobin is not reusable and is excreted as bilirubin (Chapters 5 and 20).

This chapter is one of four chapters that present the physiology of normal RBC production, structure, function, and senescence. The other chapters include Chapter 5, Erythrocyte Production and Destruction; Chapter 7, Hemoglobin Metabolism; and Chapter 8, Iron Kinetics and Laboratory Assessment. This chapter describes RBC energy production through anaerobic glycolysis, glycolysis diversion pathways that provide protective mechanisms for the RBC, and RBC membrane structure and function. Taken as a unit, these four chapters form the basis for understanding RBC disorders (anemias), as described in Chapters 16 through 25.

ENERGY PRODUCTION—ANAEROBIC GLYCOLYSIS

Lacking mitochondria, the RBC relies on anaerobic glycolysis for its energy.[4] Exchange of O_2 and CO_2 is a passive function from high partial pressure to low partial pressure; however, the cells' metabolic processes listed in Box 6.1 require energy. As energy production slows, the RBC grows senescent and is removed from the circulation (Chapter 5). Hematologists have identified hereditary deficiencies of nearly every glycolytic

---

BOX 6.1 Erythrocyte Metabolic Processes Requiring Energy

Intracellular cationic gradient maintenance
Maintenance of membrane phospholipid distribution
Maintenance of skeletal protein deformability
Maintenance of functional hemoglobin with ferrous iron
Protecting cell proteins from oxidative denaturation
Glycolysis initiation and maintenance
Glutathione synthesis
Nucleotide salvage reactions

---

enzyme, and their common result is shortened RBC survival, known collectively as *hereditary nonspherocytic hemolytic anemia* (Chapter 21).

Anaerobic glycolysis, or EMP (Figure 6.1), requires glucose to generate ATP, a high-energy phosphate source. RBCs lack internal energy stores and rely on plasma glucose to enter the cell to generate ATP. Glucose enters the RBC through facilitated diffusion via the transmembrane protein *Glut-1*.[5] Glucose is then catabolized to pyruvate (pyruvic acid) in the EMP, generating four molecules of ATP per molecule of glucose, for a net gain of two molecules of ATP. The sequential list of biochemical intermediates involved in glucose catabolism, with corresponding enzymes, is given in Figure 6.1. Glycolysis is organized into three phases in Tables 6.1 through 6.3.

The first phase of glycolysis employs glucose phosphorylation, isomerization, and diphosphorylation to yield fructose 1,6-bisphosphate (F1,6-BP). Intermediate stages employ the enzymes *hexokinase, glucose-6-phosphate isomerase,* and *6-phosphofructokinase.* The initial hexokinase and 6-phosphofructokinase steps consume a total of two ATP molecules and limit the rate of glycolysis. *Fructose-bisphosphate aldolase* then cleaves F1,6-BP to produce glyceraldehyde-3-phosphate (G3P; Figure 6.1 and Table 6.1).

The second phase of glucose catabolism converts G3P to 3-phosphoglycerate (3-PG). The substrates, enzymes, and products for this phase of glycolytic metabolism are summarized in Table 6.2. In the first step, G3P is oxidized to 1,3-bisphosphoglycerate (1,3-BPG) through the action of *glyceraldehyde-3-phosphate dehydrogenase* (G3PD) with the reduction of NAD to NADH. 1,3-BPG is dephosphorylated by *phosphoglycerate kinase,* which generates two ATP molecules and 3-PG.

The third phase of glycolysis converts 3-PG to pyruvate and generates ATP. Substrates, enzymes, and products are listed in Table 6.3. The 3-PG is isomerized by *phosphoglycerate mutase* to 2-phosphoglycerate (2-PG). *Enolase (phosphopyruvate hydratase)* then converts 2-PG to phosphoenolpyruvate (PEP). *Pyruvate kinase* (PK) splits off the phosphates, forming two ATP molecules and pyruvate. PK activity is allosterically modulated by increased concentrations of F1,6-BP, which enhances the affinity of PK for PEP.[4] Thus when the F1,6-BP is plentiful, increased activity of PK favors pyruvate production. Pyruvate may diffuse from the erythrocyte or may become a substrate for *lactate dehydrogenase (LD or LDH)* with regeneration of the oxidized form of nicotinamide adenine dinucleotide (NAD^+). The ratio of NAD^+ to the reduced form (NADH) modulates the activity of LD.

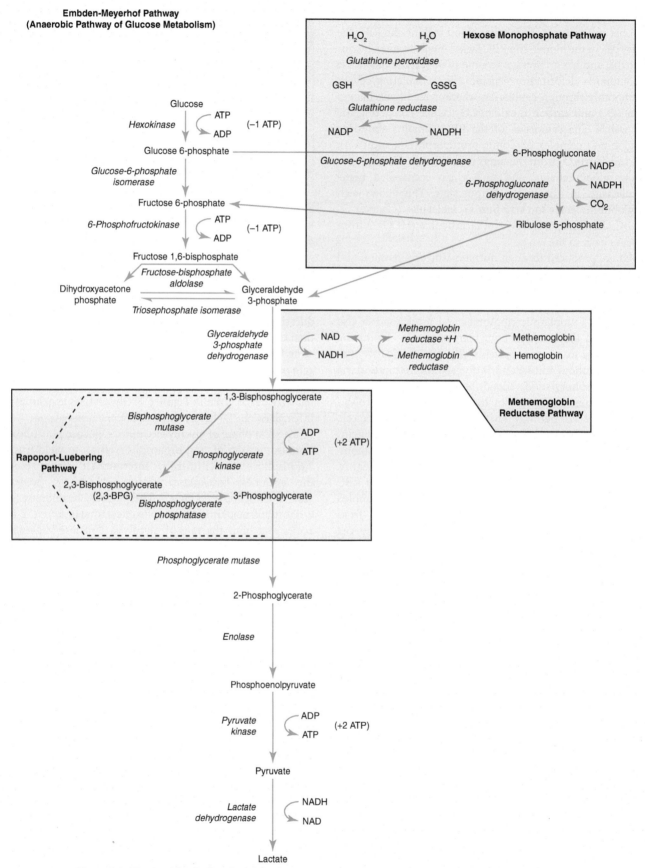

Figure 6.1 Glucose Metabolism in the Erythrocyte. Methemoglobin reductase is also called cytochrome b$_5$ reductase. *ADP,* Adenosine diphosphate; *ATP,* adenosine triphosphate; *G6PD,* glucose-6-phosphate dehydrogenase; *NAD,* nicotinamide adenine dinucleotide (oxidized form); *NADH,* nicotinamide adenine dinucleotide (reduced form); *NADP,* nicotinamide adenine dinucleotide phosphate (oxidized form); *NADPH,* nicotinamide adenine dinucleotide phosphate (reduced form).

TABLE 6.1 Glucose Catabolism: First Phase

Substrates	Enzyme	Products
Glucose, ATP	Hexokinase	G6P, ADP
G6P	Glucose-6-phosphate isomerase	F6P
F6P, ATP	6-Phosphofructokinase	F1,6-BP, ADP
F1,6-BP	Fructose-bisphosphate adolase	DHAP, G3P

ADP, Adenosine diphosphate; *ATP,* adenosine triphosphate; *DHAP,* dihydroxyacetone phosphate; *F1,6-BP,* fructose-1,6-bisphosphate; *F6P,* fructose-6-phosphate; *G3P,* glyceraldehyde-3-phosphate; *G6P,* glucose-6-phosphate.

TABLE 6.2 Glucose Catabolism: Second Phase

Substrates	Enzyme	Product
G3P, NAD	Glyceraldehyde-3-phosphate dehydrogenase	1,3-BPG, NADH
1,3-BPG, ADP	Phosphoglycerate kinase	3PG, ATP
1,3-BPG	Bisphosphoglycerate mutase	2,3-BPG
2,3-BPG	Bisphosphoglycerate phosphatase	3-PG

1,3-BPG, 1,3-Bisphosphoglycerate; *2,3-BPG,* 2,3-bisphosphoglycerate; *3-PG,* 3-phosphoglycerate; *ADP,* adenosine diphosphate; *ATP,* adenosine triphosphate; *G3P,* glyceraldehyde-3-phosphate; *NAD,* nicotinamide adenine dinucleotide (oxidized form); *NADH,* nicotinamide adenine dinucleotide (reduced form).

TABLE 6.3 Glucose Catabolism: Third Phase

Substrates	Enzyme	Product
3-PG	Phosphoglycerate mutase	2-PG
2-PG	Enolase (phosphopyruvate hydratase)	PEP
PEP, ADP	Pyruvate kinase	Pyruvate, ATP
Pyruvate, NADH	Lactate dehydrogenase*	Lactate, NAD

*The activity of lactate dehydrogenase to convert pyruvate to lactate is modulated by the ratio of NAD to NADH.
2-PG, 2-Phosphoglycerate; *3-PG,* 3-phosphoglycerate; *ADP,* adenosine diphosphate; *ATP,* adenosine triphosphate; *NAD,* nicotinamide adenine dinucleotide (oxidized form); *NADH,* nicotinamide adenine dinucleotide (reduced form); *PEP,* phosphoenolpyruvate.

GLYCOLYSIS DIVERSION PATHWAYS (SHUNTS)

Three alternate pathways, called diversions or shunts, branch from the glycolytic pathway. The three diversions are the *hexose monophosphate pathway* (HMP), the *methemoglobin reductase pathway,* and the *Rapoport-Luebering pathway.*

Hexose Monophosphate Pathway

Oxidative glycolysis occurs through a diversion of glucose catabolism into the HMP, also known as the *pentose phosphate shunt* (Figure 6.1). The HMP detoxifies peroxide (H_2O_2), which arises from O_2 reduction in the cell's aqueous environment. H_2O_2 oxidizes heme iron to the non-functional ferric state and oxidizes and denatures proteins and lipids. The HMP shunt extends the functional life span of the RBC by maintaining membrane proteins and lipids, enzymes, and hemoglobin iron in the functional, reduced, ferrous state.[4]

The HMP diverts glucose-6-phosphate (G6P) to 6-phosphogluconate (6-PG) by the action of *glucose-6-phosphate dehydrogenase* (G6PD). In the process, oxidized nicotinamide adenine dinucleotide phosphate (NADP) is converted to its reduced form (NADPH). NADPH is then available to reduce oxidized glutathione (GSSG) to reduced glutathione (GSH) in the presence of *glutathione reductase.* Glutathione is a cysteine-containing tripeptide, and the designation GSH highlights the sulfur in the cysteine moiety. Reduced glutathione becomes oxidized as it reduces peroxide to water and oxygen via *glutathione peroxidase.*

During steady-state glycolysis, 5% to 10% of G6P is diverted to the HMP. After oxidative challenge, HMP activity may increase up to thirtyfold.[6] The HMP further catabolizes 6-PG to ribulose 5-phosphate (R5P), carbon dioxide, and NADPH by the action of *6-phosphogluconate dehydrogenase.* The substrates, enzymes, and products of the HMP are listed in Table 6.4.

G6PD provides the only means of generating NADPH for glutathione reduction, and in its absence erythrocytes are particularly vulnerable to oxidative damage (Chapter 21).[7] With normal G6PD activity, the HMP detoxifies oxidative compounds and safeguards hemoglobin, sulfhydryl-containing enzymes, and membrane thiols, allowing RBCs to safely carry O_2. However, in G6PD deficiency, the most common inherited RBC enzyme deficiency worldwide, the ability to detoxify is hampered, resulting in hereditary nonspherocytic anemia.

Methemoglobin Reductase Pathway

Heme iron is constantly exposed to oxygen and peroxide.[8] Peroxide oxidizes heme iron from the ferrous (2+) to the ferric (3+) state. When the iron state is ferric, the affected hemoglobin molecule is called *methemoglobin.* Although the HMP prevents hemoglobin oxidation by reducing peroxide, it is not able to reduce methemoglobin once it forms. NADPH is able to do so, but only slowly. The reduction of methemoglobin by NADPH is rendered more efficient in the presence of *methemoglobin reductase,* also called *cytochrome b_5 reductase.* Using H^+ from NADH formed when G3P is converted to 1,3-BPG, cytochrome b_5 reductase acts as an intermediate electron carrier, returning the oxidized ferric iron to its ferrous, oxygen-carrying state (Figure 6.1). This enzyme accounts for more than 65% of the methemoglobin-reducing capacity within the RBC.[8]

Rapoport-Luebering Pathway

A third metabolic shunt generates 2,3-bisphosphoglycerate (2,3-BPG; also called 2,3-diphosphoglycerate or 2,3-DPG). 1,3-BPG

TABLE 6.4 Glucose Catabolism: Hexose Monophosphate Pathway

Substrates	Enzyme	Product
G6P, NADP	Glucose-6-phosphate dehydrogenase and 6-phosphogluconolactonase	6-PG, NADPH
6-PG, NADP	6-Phosphogluconate dehydrogenase	R5P, NADPH, CO_2

6-PG, 6-Phosphogluconate; *G6P,* glucose-6-phosphate; *NADP,* nicotinamide adenine dinucleotide phosphate (oxidized form); *NADPH,* nicotinamide adenine dinucleotide phosphate (reduced form); *R5P,* ribulose 5-phosphate.

is diverted by *bisphosphoglycerate mutase* to form 2,3-BPG (Figure 6.1). 2,3-BPG binds between the globin chains in the interior cavity of the hemoglobin tetramer to stabilize it in the deoxygenated state (tense or low oxygen affinity state). This binding shifts the hemoglobin-oxygen dissociation curve to the right, which enhances delivery of oxygen to the tissues (Chapter 7).

The 2,3-BPG forms 3-PG by the action of *bisphosphoglycerate phosphatase*. This diversion of 1,3-BPG to form 2,3-BPG sacrifices the production of two ATP molecules. There is further loss of two ATP molecules at the level of PK, because fewer molecules of PEP are formed. Because two ATP molecules were used to generate 1,3-BPG and production of 2,3-BPG eliminates the production of four ATP molecules, the cell is put into ATP deficit by this diversion. There is a delicate balance between ATP generation to support the energy requirements of cell metabolism and the need to maintain the appropriate oxygenation and deoxygenation status of hemoglobin. Acidic pH and low concentrations of 3-PG and 2-PG inhibit the activity of *bisphosphoglycerate mutase*, thus inhibiting the shunt and retaining 1,3-BPG in the EMP. These conditions and decreased ATP activate *bisphosphoglycerate phosphatase*, which returns 2,3-BPG to the glycolysis mainstream. In summary, these conditions favor generation of ATP by causing the conversion of 1,3-BPG directly to 3-PG and returning 2,3-BPG to 3-PG for ATP generation downstream by PK.

RBC MEMBRANE

RBC Membrane Deformability

RBCs are biconcave, 7 to 8 μM in diameter, with a volume range of 80 to 100 fL and a mean volume of 90 fL. Their average surface area is 140 μm^2, which is a 40% excess of surface area compared with a sphere of 7 to 8 μm in diameter.[9] This excess surface area-to-volume ratio enables RBCs to stretch undamaged up to 2.5 times their resting diameter as they pass through narrow capillaries and through splenic pores 2 μm in diameter.[10] This property is called RBC *deformability*. The RBC plasma membrane is 100 times more elastic than a comparable latex membrane, yet it has tensile (lateral) strength greater than that of steel.[9] The deformable RBC membrane provides the broad surface area and close tissue contact necessary to support the delivery of O_2 from the lungs to body tissues and to transport CO_2 from body tissues to the lungs.

RBC deformability depends not only on RBC *geometry* but also on relative cytoplasmic (hemoglobin) *viscosity*. The normal mean cell hemoglobin concentration (MCHC) ranges from 32% to 36% (Chapter 11 and inside front cover), and as MCHC rises, internal viscosity rises.[11] MCHCs greater than 36% compromise deformability and shorten the RBC life span because viscous cells become damaged as they stretch to pass through narrow capillaries or splenic pores. As RBCs age, they lose membrane surface area, while retaining hemoglobin. As the MCHC rises, the RBC, unable to pass through the splenic pores, is phagocytized and destroyed by splenic macrophages (Chapter 5).

RBC Membrane Lipids

Besides geometry and viscosity, membrane *elasticity* (pliancy) also contributes to deformability. The RBC membrane consists of approximately 8% carbohydrates, 52% proteins, and 40% lipids.[12] The *lipid* portion, equal parts of cholesterol and phospholipids, forms a bilayer universal to all animal cells (Figure 6.2). Phospholipids form an impenetrable fluid barrier as their *hydrophilic polar head groups* are arrayed on the membrane's surfaces, oriented toward both the aqueous plasma and the cytoplasm, respectively, as depicted in the fluid mosaic membrane model (FMMM).[13] Their *hydrophobic nonpolar acyl tails* arrange themselves to form a central layer sequestered (hidden) from the aqueous plasma and cytoplasm.[13] The phospholipids provide a dynamic fluidity to the membrane; if a portion of the lipid bilayer is lost, the membrane can self-seal to retain the cytoplasmic contents. The membrane also maintains extreme differences in osmotic pressure, cation concentrations, and gas concentrations between external plasma and the cytoplasm through the dynamic interaction of the lipids and proteins.[14]

Cholesterol, esterified and largely hydrophobic, resides parallel to the acyl tails of the phospholipids. It is equally distributed between the outer and inner layers of the phospholipid bilayer, and evenly dispersed within each layer, approximately one cholesterol molecule per phospholipid molecule. The β-hydroxyl group of cholesterol, the only hydrophilic domain of the molecule, anchors within the phospholipid polar heads, while the rest of the molecule becomes *intercalated* among and parallel to the acyl tails. Cholesterol confers *tensile strength* to the lipid bilayer.[15] As cholesterol concentration rises, the membrane gains strength but loses elasticity.

The ratio of cholesterol to phospholipids remains relatively constant to maintain the balance of deformability or elasticity and strength. Membrane enzymes maintain the cholesterol concentration by regularly exchanging membrane and plasma cholesterol. Deficiencies in these enzymes are associated with RBC membrane abnormalities such as *acanthocytes* and *target cells (codocytes)*[15] (Chapter 21).

The *phospholipids* are asymmetrically distributed. *Phosphatidylcholine* and *sphingomyelin* predominate in the outer layer; *phosphatidylserine (PS)* and *phosphatidylethanolamine* form most of the inner layer (Figure 6.2). Distribution of these four phospholipids is energy dependent, relying on a number of membrane-associated enzymes, termed *flippases, floppases*, and *scramblases* for their functions.[9,16] When phospholipid distribution is disrupted, as in sickle cell anemia and thalassemia (Chapters 24 and 25) or in aging RBCs, PS, the only negatively charged phospholipid, redistributes to the outer layer. Splenic macrophages possess receptors that bind to the PS displayed on *senescent* and damaged RBCs and remove them from circulation.[16] C-reactive protein and inflammatory conditions increase the PS distribution in the outer layer of the RBC membrane leading to increased RBC death (also called *eryptosis*).[17]

Membrane phospholipids and cholesterol may also *redistribute laterally* so that the RBC membrane may respond to stresses and deform within 100 milliseconds of being challenged by the

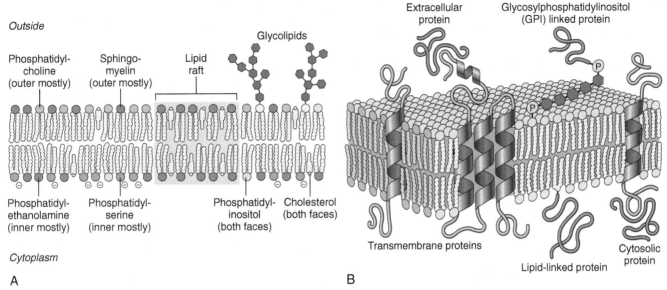

Figure 6.2 Plasma Membrane Organization and Asymmetry. (A), The plasma membrane is a bilayer of phospholipids, cholesterol, and associated proteins. The phospholipid distribution within the membrane is asymmetric; phosphatidylcholine and sphingomyelin are overrepresented in the outer leaflet, and phosphatidylserine (negative charge) and phosphatidylethanolamine are predominantly found on the inner leaflet; glycolipids occur only on the outer face where they contribute to the extracellular glycocalyx. Non-random concentration of certain membrane components such as cholesterol creates membrane domains known as lipid rafts. **(B),** Transmembrane proteins may traverse the membrane once or multiple times. Proteins may be linked to transmembrane proteins on their extracellular or intracellular domains; linked to glycosylphosphatidylinositol (GPI) anchors; or bound directly to phospholipids. Transmembrane proteins can transduce signals across the membrane. (Adapted from Mitchell, R. N. The cell as a unit of health and disease. In Kumar, V., Abbas, A. K., & Aster, J. C. [2018]. *Robbins Basic Pathology*. [10th ed., Figure 1.7]. Philadelphia: Elsevier.)

presence of a narrow passage, such as a capillary. As the proportion of cholesterol increases, however, the RBC becomes more rigid and is unable to deform as readily. In liver disease, membrane cholesterol concentration becomes increased because of an increased plasma bile salt concentration.[18] As a result, the cell membrane surface area-to-volume ratio increases giving the RBC a target cell appearance (Figure 16.1).

Glycolipids (sugar-bearing lipids) make up 5% of the external half of the RBC membrane (Figure 6.2).[19] They associate in clumps or *rafts* and support *carbohydrate side chains* that extend into the aqueous plasma to anchor the *glycocalyx*.[14] The glycocalyx is a layer of carbohydrates whose net negative charge prevents microbial attack and mechanical damage caused by adhesion to neighboring RBCs or to the endothelium. Glycolipids may bear copies of carbohydrate-based blood group antigens, such as antigens of the ABH and the Lewis blood group systems.

RBC Membrane Proteins

Although cholesterol and phospholipids constitute the principal RBC membrane structure, *transmembrane (integral)* and *cytoskeletal (skeletal, peripheral)* proteins make up 52% of the membrane structure by mass.[20] A proteomic study revealed there are at least 300 RBC membrane proteins, including 105 transmembrane proteins.[21] Some proteins have a few hundred copies per cell, and others have more than a million

copies per cell. Of the purported 300 membrane proteins, about 50 have been characterized and named.[21]

Transmembrane Proteins

The *transmembrane* proteins serve many functions including: *transport* sites, *adhesion* sites, and *signaling receptors*. Any disruption in transport protein function changes the osmotic tension of the cytoplasm, which leads to a rise in viscosity and loss of deformability. Any change affecting adhesion proteins permits RBCs to adhere to one another and to the vessel walls, promoting fragmentation (vesiculation), reducing membrane flexibility, and shortening the RBC life span. Signaling receptors bind plasma ligands and trigger activation of intracellular signaling proteins, which then initiate various energy-dependent cellular activities, a process called *signal transduction*. Through *glycosylation*, the transmembrane proteins also support *surface carbohydrates*, which join with glycolipids to make up the protective *glycocalyx*. A summary of selected transmembrane proteins and RBC functions is listed in Table 6.5.[22, 23]

Most transmembrane proteins assemble into one of two major macromolecular complexes named by their respective cytoskeletal anchorages: the *ankyrin complex* and the *actin junctional complex*, also called *protein 4.1 complex* (Figure 6.3).[23,24] The anchoring of these transmembrane complexes to cytoskeletal proteins (adjacent to the inner or cytoplasmic side of the membrane) prevents loss of the lipid bilayer. In addition, the linking

TABLE 6.5   Names and Properties of Selected Transmembrane RBC Proteins[22-32]

Transmembrane Protein	Gene	Band	MW (kD)	Copies/Cell (×10³)	% of TP	Function
Aquaporin 1	AQP1		28	120–160		Water transporter, Colton antigen
Band 3 (anion exchanger, AE1)	SLC4A1	3	90–102	1200	27%	Anion transporter, location of ABH antigens
Ca²⁺-ATPase	ATP2B1		110			Ca²⁺ transporter
Duffy	FY, DARC, ACKR1		35–43	6–13		G protein-coupled receptor, chemokine receptor, Duffy antigens, receptor for malarial parasites
Glut-1	SLC2A1	4.5	45–75	200–700	5%	Glucose transporter, location of ABH blood group antigens
Glycophorin A	GYPA	PAS-1	36	1000	85% of GP	Sialic acid transporter, location of MN blood group antigens
Glycophorin B	GYPB	PAS-4	20	250	10% of GP	Sialic acid transporter, location of Ss blood group antigens
Glycophorin C	GYPC	PAS-2	14–32	135	4% of GP	Sialic acid transporter, location of Gerbich system antigens
ICAM-4	ICAM4					Integrin adhesion
K⁺-Cl⁻ cotransporter						Transports K⁺, Cl⁻
Kell	KEL		93	3–18		Zn²⁺-binding endopeptidase, Kell antigens
Kidd	SLC14A1		43	14		Urea transporter, Kidd (Jk) antigens
Na⁺,K⁺-ATPase	ATP1A2		140	0.5		Na⁺, K⁺ transporter
Na⁺-K⁺-2Cl⁻ cotransporter						Na⁺, K⁺, Cl⁻ transporter
Rh	RHCE, RHD		30–45	200		D and CcEe antigens; stabilizes band 3 and Rh macrocomplexes[27]
RhAG	RHAG		45–100	100–200		D and CcEe antigen component; CO₂, cation, and ammonium transporter[27]

ATPase, Adenosine triphosphatase; *Duffy,* Duffy blood group system protein; *GP,* glycophorin; *ICAM,* intracellular adhesion molecule; *Kell,* Kell blood group system protein; *MW,* molecular weight; *PAS,* periodic acid-Schiff dye; *RBC,* red blood cell; *Rh,* Rh blood group system protein; *RhAG,* Rh antigen expression protein; *TP,* total protein.

of cytoskeletal proteins by the actin junctional complex provides membrane structural integrity because the cell relies on an intact cytoskeleton to maintain its biconcave shape despite deformability. Transmembrane proteins also provide vertical membrane structure.

Blood group antigens. The *blood group antigens* are located in membrane macromolecular complexes that serve as transporters, structural components, enzymes, receptors, and adhesion molecules. The carbohydrate-defined blood group antigens are supported in the RBC membrane by transmembrane proteins.[25] Half of the known transmembrane proteins (approximately 25) are involved in the macromolecular complexes that define blood antigen groups.[9] Band 3 (anion transport) and Glut-1 (glucose transport) support the majority of ABH system carbohydrate determinants.[26] Several transmembrane proteins provide peptide epitopes. For instance, glycophorin A carries the peptide-defined M and N determinants and glycophorin B carries the Ss determinants, which together comprise the MNSs system, whereas the minor glycophorins C and D carry the Gerbich system antigens.[27,28]

The Rh system employs two transmembrane lipoproteins and one *multipass* glycoprotein, each of which crosses the membrane 12 times.[29] The two lipoproteins present the D and CcEe epitopes, respectively. The expression of the D and CcEe antigens requires the separately inherited glycoprotein RhAG, which localizes near the Rh lipoproteins in the ankyrin complex. Loss of the RhAG glycoprotein prevents expression of both the D and CcEe antigens (Rh-null) and is associated with RBC morphologic abnormalities (Chapter 21). Additional blood group antigens localize to the actin junctional (4.1) complex or specialized proteins.[30-32]

The GPI anchor and paroxysmal nocturnal hemoglobinuria. A few copies of the phospholipid *phosphatidylinositol* (PI) reside in the outer, plasma-side layer of the membrane. PI serves as a base on which a glycan core of sugar molecules is synthesized, forming the glycosylphosphatidylinositol (GPI) anchor (Figure 6.2). More than 30 proteins bind to the GPI anchor and appear to float on the surface of the membrane. Two of these proteins, *decay-accelerating factor* (DAF, or CD55) and *membrane inhibitor of reactive lysis* (MIRL, or CD59), protect the RBC membrane from lysis by complement.[33]

The *phosphatidylinositol glycan anchor biosynthesis class A* (*PIGA*) gene codes for a glycosyltransferase required to add

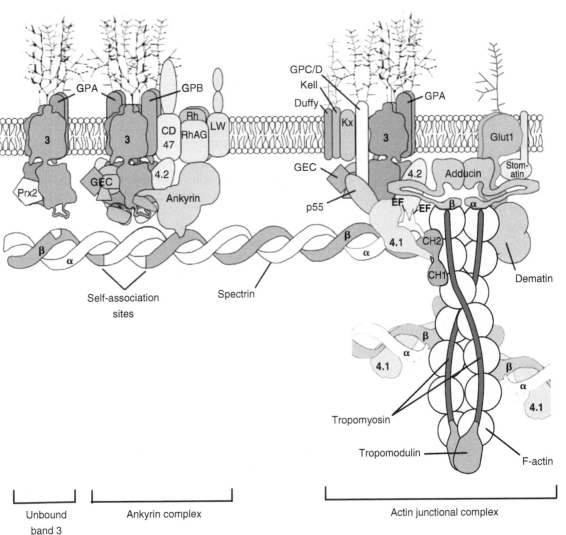

Figure 6.3 Schematic Model of the Red Cell Membrane. α- and β-Spectrins are the most abundant cytoskeletal proteins. They form antiparallel heterodimers, and two heterodimers associate head-to-head to form a tetramer. Band 3 is the most abundant transmembrane protein. The transmembrane proteins assemble into one of two complexes defined by their anchorage to either the cytoskeletal protein ankyrin or to cytoskeletal proteins actin and 4.1. The major components of the ankyrin complex are band 3 multimers and protein 4.2, which anchor the lipid bilayer to the spectrin cytoskeleton through ankyrin. Major components of the actin junctional complex (4.1 complex) are band 3 dimers, protein 4.2, and adducin, which anchor the lipid bilayer to the spectrin cytoskeleton through protein 4.1. Actin, dematin, tropomyosin, and tropomodulin are additional proteins that help link the junctional complex to the ends of the spectrin tetramers to form a hexagonal cytoskeletal lattice adjacent to the inner (cytoplasmic) lipid bilayer. The actin protofilament is drawn perpendicular to the plane of the lipid bilayer; however, it actually lies parallel to the membrane. Band 3 dimers also float untethered within the lipid bilayer. The major proteins are drawn roughly to scale. *CH1* and *CH2*, Actin-binding domains of β spectrin; *Duffy,* Duffy blood group system protein; *EF*, Ca 2^+-binding EF hand domain of α-spectrin; *GEC,* glycolytic enzyme complex (G3PD, phosphofructokinase, and aldolase); *GPA,* glycophorin A; *GPB,* glycophorin B; *GPC/D,* glycophorin C/D; *Kell,* Kell blood group system protein; *Kx,* X-linked Kell antigen expression protein; *LW,* Landsteiner-Weiner blood group system protein; *Prx2,* peroxiredoxin-2; *Rh,* Rh blood group system protein; *RhAG,* Rh-associated glycoprotein. (Adapted from Lux, S. E. [2015]. Red cell membrane. In Orkin, S. H., Fisher, D. E., Ginsburg, D., et al., [Eds.], *Nathan and Oski's Hematology and Oncology of Infancy and Childhood.* [8th ed., Figure 15.6]. Philadelphia: Saunders Elsevier, which was modified from Korsgren, C., Peters, L. L., Lux, S. E. [2010]. Protein 4.2 binds to the carboxyl-terminal EF-hands of erythroid alpha-spectrin in a calcium- and calmodulin-dependent manner. *J Biol Chem, 285,* 4757–4770.)

N-acetylglucosamine to the PI base early in the biosynthesis of the GPI anchor on the membrane. In paroxysmal nocturnal hemoglobinuria (Chapter 21), an acquired mutation in the *PIGA* gene affects the cells' ability to synthesize the GPI anchor. Without the GPI anchor, the cell membrane becomes deficient

in CD55 and CD59, and the cells are susceptible to complement-mediated hemolysis.[33]

Nomenclature. Numerical naming, for instance, band 3, protein 4.1, and protein 4.2, derives from historical (preproteomics) protein identification techniques that distinguished

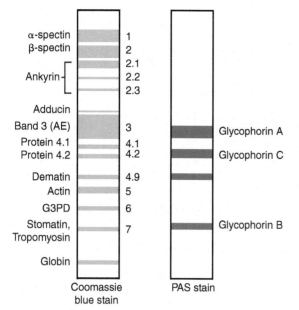

Figure 6.4 A Diagram of Sodium Dodecyl Sulfate-Polyacrylamide Gel Electrophoresis (SDS-Page) of Red Blood Cell (RBC) Membrane Proteins Stained with Coomassie Blue *(Left)* and Periodic Acid-Schiff (PAS) *(Right).* Note the positions of some of the major RBC membrane proteins. *AE,* Anion exchanger; *G3PD,* glyceraldehyde-3-phosphate dehydrogenase. (Adapted from Beck, W. S., & Tepper, R. I. [1991]. Hemolytic anemias III: Membrane disorders. In Beck, W. S. [Ed.], *Hematology* [5th ed., Figure 14.1]. Cambridge, MA: The MIT Press.)

membrane proteins using *sodium dodecyl sulfate-polyacrylamide gel electrophoresis* (SDS-PAGE), as illustrated in Figure 6.4.[34] Bands migrate through the gel, with their velocity a property of their molecular weight and net charge, and are identified using Coomassie blue dye. The glycophorins, with abundant carbohydrate side chains, are stained using periodic acid-Schiff (PAS) dye.

Band 3 and protein 4.2 are the major components of the ankyrin complex and link their associated proteins and the lipid

bilayer membrane to the spectrin cytoskeleton through ankyrin.[35,36] Likewise, band 3, protein 4.2, adducin, and actin are the major components of the actin junctional (4.1) complex and link the lipid membrane to the spectrin cytoskeleton through protein 4.1.[23-25,37] The 4.1 anchorage also includes the protein *dematin*, which links with transmembrane protein Glut-1.[38]

Cytoskeletal Proteins

The principal cytoskeletal proteins are the filamentous α-spectrin and β-spectrin (Table 6.6 and Figure 6.3), which assemble to form an *antiparallel* heterodimer held together with a series of lateral bonds.[24,39] Antiparallel means that the carboxyl (COOH) end of one strand associates with the amino (NH_3) end of the other, and the two heterodimers self-associate head-to-head to form a tetramer. The ends of the spectrin tetramers are linked in the actin junctional complex, forming a hexagonal cytoskeletal lattice adjacent to the inner (cytoplasmic) lipid bilayer. This provides *lateral or horizontal* membrane stability.[40] Because the cytoskeletal proteins do not penetrate the bilayer, they are also called *peripheral* proteins.

Spectrin stabilization. The secondary structure of both α- and β-spectrin features triple-helical repeats of 106 amino acids each; 20 such repeats make up α-spectrin, and 16 make up β-spectrin.[41] Essential to the cytoskeleton are the previously mentioned ankyrin, protein 4.1, adducin and dematin, and, in addition, *actin, tropomyosin,* and *tropomodulin* (Figure 6.3).[23,24,36] A single helix at the amino terminus of α-spectrin consistently binds a pair of helices at the carboxyl terminus of the β-spectrin chain, forming a stable triple helix that holds together the ends of the heterodimers.[24] Joining these ends are actin and protein 4.1 in the actin junctional complex. Actin forms short filaments of 14 to 16 monomers whose length is regulated by tropomyosin. Adducin and tropomodulin cap the ends of actin. Dematin appears to stabilize the actin junctional complex and helps maintain the RBC shape.[42]

TABLE 6.6   Names and Properties of Selected Cytoskeletal RBC Proteins[22-24]

Skeletal Protein	Gene	Band	MW (kD)	Copies/Cell ($\times 10^3$)	% of TP	Function
α-spectrin	SPTA1	1	240–280	242	16%	Filamentous antiparallel heterodimer, primary cytoskeletal proteins
β-spectrin	SPTB	2	220–246	242	14%	
Adducin	ADD1 ADD2	2.9	80–103	60	4%	Caps actin filament, binds Ca^{2+}/calmodulin
Ankyrin	ANK1	2.1	206–210	124	4.5%	Anchors band 3, protein 4.2, and other proteins in the ankyrin complex to spectrin
Dematin	EPB49	4.9	43–52	140	1%	Actin bundling protein
β-actin	ACTB	5	42–43	500	5.5%	Binds β-spectrin
G3PD	GAPD	6	35–37	500	3.5%	Carbohydrate metabolism, phosphorylates G3P
Protein 4.1	EPB41	4.1	66–80	200	5%	Anchors the actin junctional complex to spectrin tetramers, RBC cytoskeleton shape
Protein 4.2 (protein kinase)	EPB42	4.2	72–77	250	5%	Part of ankyrin complex, ATP binding protein
Tropomodulin	TMOD1	5	41–43	30	—	Caps actin filament
Tropomyosin	TPM3	7	27–38	70	1%	Stabilizes and regulates actin polymerization

ATP, Adenosine triphosphate; *G3PD,* glyceraldehyde-3-phosphate dehydrogenase; *MW,* molecular weight; *RBC,* red blood cell; *TP,* total protein.

Membrane deformation. Spectrin dimer bonds that appear along the length of the molecules disassociate and re-associate (open and close) during RBC deformation. Likewise, the 20 α-spectrin and 16 β-spectrin repeated helices unfold and refold.[43] These flexible interactions plus the spectrin-protein 4.1 junctions in the actin junctional complexes between the tetramers are key regulators of membrane elasticity and mechanical stability. Abnormalities in any of these proteins result in deformation-induced membrane fragmentation. For instance, *hereditary elliptocytosis* (Chapter 21) arises from one of several autosomal dominant mutations affecting the spectrin dimer-to-dimer lateral bonds or the spectrin-protein 4.1 junction.[44] These *horizontal* interaction defects inhibit the membrane's ability to rebound from deformation (Figure 6.5). Ultimately, the RBCs progressively elongate to form visible elliptocytes, which causes a mild to severe hemolytic anemia.[44-46] Conversely, autosomal dominant mutations that affect the integrity of band 3, ankyrin, protein 4.2, or α- or β-spectrin are associated with *hereditary spherocytosis* (Chapter 21).[44-46] In these cases, there are too few *vertical anchorages* to maintain membrane stability (Figure 6.5). The lipid membrane peels off in small fragments called *blebs,* or *vesicles* and immediately reseals keeping the cytoplasmic volume intact. This results in a reduced surface area-to-volume ratio and the formation of spherocytes.

Osmotic Balance and Permeability

The RBC membrane is impermeable to cations Na^+, K^+, and Ca^{2+}. It is permeable to water and the anions bicarbonate (HCO_3^-) and chloride (Cl^-), which freely exchange between plasma and RBC cytoplasm. *Aquaporin 1* (Table 6.5) is a transmembrane protein that forms pores or channels whose surface charges create inward water flow in response to internal osmotic changes. Decreases in *aquaporin 1* expression has been linked with *hereditary* spherocytosis.[47]

The ATP-dependent cation pumps *Na^+-ATPase* and *K^+-ATPase* (Table 6.5) regulate the concentrations of Na^+ and K^+, maintaining intracellular-to-extracellular ratios of 1:12 and 25:1, respectively.[48,49] *Ca^{2+}-ATPase* expels calcium from the cell, maintaining low intracellular levels of 30 to 60 nM compared with 1.8 mM in the plasma.[50] Calmodulin, a cytoplasmic Ca^{2+}-binding protein, controls the function of Ca^{2+}-ATPase. These pumps, in addition to aquaporin, maintain osmotic balance in the RBC.

The cation pumps consume a significant portion of RBC ATP production. ATP loss or pump damage permits Ca^{2+} and Na^+ influx, with water following osmotically. The cell swells, becomes spheroid, and eventually ruptures. This phenomenon is called *colloid osmotic hemolysis.* Defects in the ion channels result in red cell volume disorders, such as *overhydrated stomatocytosis* (hereditary hydrocytosis) and *dehydrated stomatocytosis* (*hereditary xerocytosis*) (Chapter 21).[51]

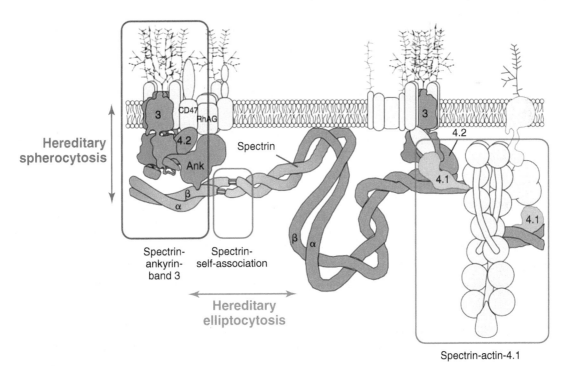

Figure 6.5 Membrane Defects in Hereditary Spherocytosis and Elliptocytosis. Hereditary spherocytosis is caused by a quantitative deficiency of spectrin, ankyrin, band 3, or protein 4.2, proteins involved in the "vertical" interactions that attach the membrane cytoskeleton to the overlying lipid bilayer with its transmembrane proteins. Hereditary elliptocytosis is caused by functional defects in the "horizontal" protein interactions that hold the cytoskeleton together. These are either defects near the head end of spectrin that impair self-association of spectrin dimers, or deficiency of protein 4.1, a protein that bolsters the attachment of spectrin to actin. (From Lux, S.E. [2015]. Disorders of the red cell membrane. In Orkin, S. H., Fisher, D. E., Ginsburg, D., et al., [Eds.], *Nathan and Oski's Hematology and Oncology of Infancy and Childhood* [8th ed., Figure 16.4]. Philadelphia: Saunders Elsevier.)

Sickle cell disease also provides an example of increased cation permeability. When hemoglobin S polymerizes on deoxygenation, the cell deforms into a sickle shape and the membrane becomes more permeable to Ca^{2+}. This causes a downstream effect of increased Na^+ and K^+, resulting in hemolysis.[50]

SUMMARY

- Glucose enters the red blood cell (RBC) by facilitated diffusion via the transmembrane protein Glut-1.
- The anaerobic Embden-Meyerhof pathway (EMP) metabolizes glucose to pyruvate, consuming two adenosine triphosphate (ATP) molecules. The EMP subsequently generates four ATP molecules per glucose molecule, a net gain of two.
- The hexose-monophosphate pathway (HMP) converts glucose to pentose and generates the reduced form of nicotinamide adenine dinucleotide phosphate (NADPH). NADPH reduces oxidized glutathione (GSSG). Reduced glutathione (GSH) reduces peroxides and protects proteins, lipids, and heme iron from oxidation.
- The methemoglobin reductase pathway converts ferric heme iron (Fe^{3+}, methemoglobin) to reduced ferrous (Fe^{2+}) form, which binds O_2.
- The Rapoport-Luebering pathway generates 2,3-BPG and enhances O_2 delivery to tissues.
- The RBC membrane is a lipid bilayer whose hydrophobic components are sequestered from aqueous plasma and cytoplasm. The membrane provides a semipermeable barrier separating plasma from cytoplasm and maintaining an osmotic differential.
- RBC membrane phospholipids are asymmetrically distributed. Phosphatidylcholine and sphingomyelin predominate in the outer layer; phosphatidylserine and phosphatidylethanolamine form most of the inner layer.
- Enzymatic plasma to membrane exchange maintains RBC membrane cholesterol.
- Acanthocytosis and target cells are associated with abnormalities in the concentration or distribution of membrane cholesterol and phospholipids.
- RBC transmembrane proteins transport ions, water, and glucose and anchor cell membrane receptors. Transmembrane proteins are critical in the ankyrin complex and the actin junctional (4.1) complex to provide the vertical membrane support and to connect the lipid bilayer to the underlying cytoskeleton to maintain membrane integrity and prevent membrane loss.
- Shape and flexibility of the RBC, which are essential to its function, depend on the cytoskeleton. The cytoskeleton is derived from cytoskeletal (peripheral) proteins on the cytoplasmic side of the lipid membrane. The major cytoskeletal proteins are α- and β-spectrin heterodimers, which associate in tetramers, and their ends connect to the actin junctional complex forming a hexagonal cytoskeletal lattice adjacent to the cytoplasmic side of the lipid bilayer. Cytoskeletal proteins provide the horizontal or lateral support for the membrane.
- Hereditary spherocytosis arises from defects in spectrin or proteins forming the ankyrin complex that provide vertical support for the membrane. Hereditary elliptocytosis is due to defects in cytoskeletal proteins that provide horizontal support for the membrane.
- RBC cytoplasmic K^+ concentration is higher than plasma K^+, whereas Na^+ and Ca^{2+} cytoplasmic concentrations are lower. Disequilibria are maintained by membrane enzymes K^+-ATPase, Na^+-ATPase, and Ca^{2+}-ATPase. Pump failure leads to cation imbalance, water influx, cell swelling, and lysis.
- Membrane proteins are extracted using sodium dodecyl sulfate, separated using polyacrylamide gel electrophoresis based on their molecular weight and net charge, and stained with Coomassie blue. Glycoproteins are stained with periodic acid-Schiff (PAS).

Now that you have completed this chapter, go back and read again the case study at the beginning and respond to the questions presented.

REVIEW QUESTIONS

Answers can be found in the Appendix.

1. Which RBC process does *not* require energy?
   a. Cytoskeletal protein deformability
   b. Maintaining cytoplasm cationic electrochemical gradients
   c. Oxygen transport
   d. Preventing the peroxidation of proteins and lipids
2. What pathway anaerobically generates energy in the form of ATP?
   a. 2,3-BPG pathway
   b. Embden-Meyerhof pathway
   c. Hexose monophosphate pathway
   d. Rapoport-Luebering pathway

3. Which is true concerning 2,3-BPG?
   a. Enhances O_2 release from hemoglobin
   b. Source of RBC ATP
   c. Source of RBC glucose
   d. The least abundant of RBC organophosphates
4. What hexose-monophosphate shunt products participate in the detoxification of peroxides?
   a. 2,3-BPG and pyruvic acid
   b. ATP and lactic acid
   c. NADPH and reduced glutathione
   d. Pyruvic and lactic acid

5. Which of the following helps maintain RBC shape?
   a. Cytoskeletal proteins
   b. Glycocalyx
   c. GPI anchor
   d. Membrane phospholipids

6. The glycolipids of the RBC membrane:
   a. Attach the cytoskeleton to the lipid layer
   b. Carry RBC antigens
   c. Constitute ion channels
   d. Provide flexibility

7. RBC membranes block passage of most large molecules, such as proteins, but allow passage of small molecules such as the cations Na^+, K^+, and Ca^{2+}. What is the term for this membrane property?
   a. Deformable
   b. Flexible
   c. Intangible
   d. Semipermeable

8. RBC membrane phospholipids are arranged:
   a. In a hexagonal lattice
   b. In chains beneath a protein cytoskeleton
   c. In two layers whose composition is asymmetric
   d. So that hydrophobic portions are facing the plasma

9. RBC membrane cholesterol is replenished from the:
   a. Cytoplasm
   b. EMB pathway
   c. Mitochondria
   d. Plasma

10. Hemoglobin iron may become oxidized to Fe^{3+} by several pathologic mechanisms. What portion of the Embden-Meyerhof pathway reduces iron to Fe^{2+}?
    a. Hexose monophosphate pathway
    b. Methemoglobin reductase pathway
    c. Rapoport-Luebering pathway
    d. 2,3-BPG shunt

11. Which of the following is an example of a transmembrane or integral membrane protein?
    a. Actin
    b. Ankyrin
    c. Glycophorin A
    d. Spectrin

12. Abnormalities in the horizontal and vertical linkages of the transmembrane and cytoskeletal RBC membrane proteins may be seen as:
    a. Enzyme pathway deficiencies
    b. Methemoglobin increase
    c. Reduced hemoglobin content
    d. Shape changes

REFERENCES

1. Percy, M. J., & Lappin, T. R. (2008). Recessive congenital methaemoglobinaemia: cytochrome b5 reductase deficiency. *Brit J Haematol, 141*, 298–308.

2. Mohandas, N. (2016). Structure and composition of the erythrocyte. In Kaushansky, K., Lichtman, M. A., Prchal, J. T., et al. (Eds.), *Williams Hematology*. (9th ed., pp. 461–478). New York: McGraw-Hill.

3. Quigley, J. G., Means, R. T., & Glader, B. (2014). The birth, life, and death of red blood cells, erythropoiesis, the mature red blood cell, and cell destruction. In Greer, J. P., Arber, D. A., Glader, B., et al. (Eds.), *Wintrobe's Clinical Hematology*. (13th ed., pp. 83–124). Philadelphia: Wolters Kluwer Health/Lippincott Williams & Wilkins.

4. van Solinge, W. W., & van Wijk, R. (2016). Erythrocyte enzyme disorders. In Kaushansky, K., Lichtman, M. A., Prchal, J. T., et al. (Eds.), *Williams Hematology*. (9th ed., pp. 689–724). New York: McGraw-Hill.

5. Zhang, J. Z., & Ismail-Beigi, F. (1998). Activation of Glut1 glucose transporter in human erythrocytes. *Arch Biochem Biophys, 356*(1), 86–92.

6. Gregg, X. T., & Prchal, J. T. (2018). Red blood cell enzymopathies. In Hoffman, R., Benz, E. J., Silberstein, L. E., et al. (Eds.), *Hematology, Basic Principles and Practice*. (7th ed., pp. 616–625). Philadelphia: Elsevier.

7. Beutler, E. (1990). Disorders of red cells resulting from enzyme abnormalities. *Semin Hematol, 27*, 137–167.

8. Agarwal, A. M., & Prchal, J. T. (2016). Methemoglobinemia and other dyshemoglobinemias. In Kaushansky, K., Lichtman, M. A., Prchal, J. T., et al. (Eds.), *Williams Hematology*. (9th ed., pp. 789–800). New York: McGraw-Hill.

9. Mohandas, N., & Gallagher, P. G. (2008). Red cell membrane: past, present, and future. *Blood, 112*, 3939–3948.

10. Kim, J., Lee, H., & Shin, S. (2015). Advances in the measurement of red blood cell deformability: a brief review. *J Cell Biotechnology, 1*, 63–79.

11. Mohandas, N., & Chasis, J. A. (1993). Red blood cell deformability, membrane material properties, and shape: regulation by transmembrane, skeletal and cytosolic proteins and lipids. *Semin Hematol, 30*, 171–192.

12. Cooper, R. A. (1970). Lipids of human red cell membrane: normal composition and variability in disease. *Semin Hematol, 7*, 296–322.

13. Singer, S. J., & Nicolson, G. L. (1972). The fluid mosaic model of the structure of cell membranes. *Science, 175*, 720–731.

14. Nicolson, G. L. (2014). The fluid mosaic model of membrane structure: still relevant to understanding the structure, function and dynamics of biological membranes after more than 40 years. *Biochim Biophys Acta, 1838*, 1451–1466.

15. Cooper, R. A. (1978). Influence of the increased membrane cholesterol on membrane fluidity and cell function in human red blood cells. *J Supramol Struct, 8*, 413–430.

16. Zhou, Q., Zhao, J., Stout, J. G., et al. (1997). Molecular cloning of human plasma membrane phospholipid scramblase. A protein mediating transbilayer movement of plasma membrane phospholipids. *J Biol Chem, 272*, 18240–18244.

17. Abed, M., Thiel, C., Towhid, S. T., et al. (2017). Simulation of erythrocyte cell membrane scrambling by C-reactive protein. *Cell Physiol Biochem, 41*, 806–818.

18. Cooper, R. A., & Jandl, J. H. (1968). Bile salts and cholesterol in the pathogenesis of target cells in obstructive jaundice. *J Clin Invest, 47*, 809–822.

19. Alberts, B., Johnson, A., Lewis, J., et al. (2015). Membrane structure. In *Molecular Biology of the Cell*. (6th ed., pp. 565–596). New York: Garland Science.

20. Steck, T. (1974). The organization of proteins in the human red blood cell membrane. *J Cell Biol, 62*, 1–19.

21. Pasini, E. M., Kirkegaard, M., Mortensen, P., et al. (2006). In-depth analysis of the membrane and cytosolic proteome of red blood cells. *Blood, 108*, 791–801.

22. Bennett, V. (1985). The membrane skeleton of human erythrocytes and its implications for more complex cells. *Annu Rev Biochem, 54*, 273–304.

23. Burton, N. M., & Bruce, L. J. (2011) Modeling the structure of the red cell membrane. *Biochem Cell Biol, 89*, 200–215.

24. Mankelow, T. J., Satchwell, T. J., & Burton, N. M. (2012). Refined views of multi-protein complexes in the erythrocyte membrane. *Blood Cells Mol Dis, 49*, 1–10.

25. Reid, M. E., & Mohandas, N. (2004). Red blood cell blood group antigens: structure and function. *Semin Hematol, 41*, 93–117.

26. Daniels, G. (2013). ABO, H, and Lewis systems. In *Human Blood Groups*. (3rd ed., pp. 11–95). West Sussex, UK: Wiley-Blackwell.

27. Daniels, G. (2013). MNS blood group system. In *Human Blood Groups*. (3rd ed., pp. 96–161). West Sussex, UK: Wiley-Blackwell.

28. Daniels, G. (2013). Gerbich blood group system. In *Human Blood Groups*. (3rd ed., pp. 410–426). West Sussex, UK: Wiley-Blackwell.

29. Daniels, G. (2013). Rh and RHAG blood group systems. In *Human Blood Groups*. (3rd ed., pp. 182–258). West Sussex, UK: Wiley-Blackwell.

30. Daniels, G. (2013). Duffy blood group system. In *Human Blood Groups*. (3rd ed., pp. 306–324). West Sussex, UK: Wiley-Blackwell.

31. Daniels, G. (2013). Kell and KX blood group systems. In *Human Blood Groups*. (3rd ed., pp. 278–305). West Sussex, UK: Wiley-Blackwell.

32. Daniels, G. (2013). Kidd blood group system. In *Human Blood Groups*. (3rd ed., pp. 325–335). West Sussex, UK: Wiley-Blackwell.

33. Parker, C. J. (2016). Paroxysmal nocturnal hemoglobinuria. In Kaushansky, K., Lichtman, M. A., Prchal, J. T., et al. (Eds.), *Williams Hematology*. (9th ed., pp. 571–582). New York: McGraw-Hill.

34. Fairbanks, G., Steck, T. L., & Wallach, D. F. (1971). Electrophoretic analysis of the major polypeptides of the human erythrocyte membrane. *Biochemistry, 10*, 2606–2617.

35. Reinhart, A. F., Casey, J. C., Kalli, A. C., et al. (2016). Band 3, the human red cell chloride/bicarbonate anion exchanger (AE1, SLC4A1), in a structural context. *Biochimica et biophysica acta, 1858*, 1507–1532.

36. Bennett, V. (1983). Proteins involved in membrane-cytoskeleton association in human erythrocytes: spectrin, ankyrin, and band 3. *Methods Enzymol, 96*, 313–324.

37. Giger, K., Habib, I. Ritchie, K., et al. (2016). Diffusion of glycophorin A in human erythrocytes. *Biochim Biophys Acta, 1858*, 2839–2845.

38. Khan, A. A., Hanada, T., Mohseni, M., et al. (2008). Dematin and adducin provide a novel link between the spectrin cytoskeleton and human erythrocyte membrane by directly interacting with glucose transporter-1. *J Biol Chem, 283*, 14600–14609.

39. Shotton, D. M., Burke, B. E., & Branton, D. (1979). The molecular structure of human erythrocyte spectrin: biophysical and electron microscope studies. *J Mol Biol, 131*, 303–329.

40. Liu, S. C., Drick, L. H., & Palek, J. (1987). Visualization of the hexagonal lattice in the erythrocyte membrane skeleton. *J Cell Biol, 104*, 527–536.

41. Speicher, D. W., & Marchesi, V. T. (1984). Erythrocyte spectrin is composed of many homologous triple helical segments. *Nature, 311*, 177–180.

42. Lu, Y., Hanada, T., Fujiwara, Y., et al. (2016). Gene disruption of dematin causes precipitous loss of erythrocyte membrane stability and severe hemolytic anemia. *Blood, 128*, 93–103.

43. An, X., Guo, X., Zhang, X., et al. (2006). Conformational stabilities of the structural repeats of erythroid spectrin and their functional implications. *J Biol Chem, 281*, 10527–10532.

44. Da Costa, L., Galimand, J., Fenneteau, O., et al. (2013). Hereditary spherocytosis, elliptocytosis, and other red cell membrane disorders. *Blood Reviews, 27*, 167–178.

45. Andolfo, I., Russo, R., Gambale, A., et al. (2016). New insights on hereditary erythrocyte membrane defects. *Haematologica, 101*, 1284–1294.

46. Gallagher, P. G. (2013). Abnormalities of the erythrocyte membrane. *Pediatr Clin North Am, 60*, 1349–1362.

47. Crisp, R. L., Maltaneri, R. E., Vittori, D. C., et al. (2016). Red blood cell aquaporin-1 expression is decreased in hereditary spherocytosis. *Ann Hematol, 95*, 1595–1601.

48. Brugnara, C. (1997). Erythrocyte membrane transport physiology. *Curr Opin Hematol, 4*, 122–127.

49. Chu, H., Puchulu-Campanella, E., Galan, J. A., et al. (2012). Identification of cytoskeletal elements enclosing the ATP pools that fuel human red blood cell membrane cation pumps. *Proc Natl Acad Sci, 109*, 12794–12799.

50. Bogdanova, A., Makhro, A., Wang, J., et al. (2013) Calcium in red blood cells – a perilous balance. *Int J Mol Sci, 14*, 9848–9872.

51. Badens, C., & Guizouarn, H. (2016). Advances in understanding the pathogenesis of the red cell volume disorders. *Br J Haematol, 174*, 674–685.

Hemoglobin Metabolism

*Catherine N. Otto**

OBJECTIVES

After completion of this chapter, the reader will be able to:

1. Describe the components and structure of hemoglobin.
2. Describe steps in heme synthesis that occur in the mitochondria and the cytoplasm.
3. Name the genes and the chromosome location and arrangement for the various polypeptide chains of hemoglobin.
4. Describe the polypeptide chains produced and the hemoglobins they form in the embryo, fetus, newborn, and adult.
5. List the three types of normal hemoglobin in adults and their reference intervals.
6. Describe mechanisms that regulate hemoglobin synthesis.
7. Describe the mechanism by which hemoglobin transports oxygen to the tissues and transports carbon dioxide to the lungs.
8. Explain the importance of maintaining hemoglobin iron in the ferrous state (Fe^{2+}).
9. Explain the significance of the sigmoid shape of the oxygen dissociation curve.
10. Correlate right and left shifts in the hemoglobin-oxygen dissociation curve with conditions that can cause shifts in the curve.
11. Differentiate T and R forms of hemoglobin and the effect of oxygen and 2,3-bisphosphoglycerate on those forms.
12. Explain the difference between adult Hb A and fetal Hb F and how that difference affects oxygen affinity.
13. Compare and contrast the composition and the effect on oxygen binding of methemoglobin, carboxyhemoglobin, and sulfhemoglobin.

OUTLINE

Hemoglobin Structure
Heme Structure
Globin Structure
Complete Hemoglobin Molecule
Hemoglobin Biosynthesis
Heme Biosynthesis
Globin Biosynthesis
Hemoglobin Assembly
Hemoglobin Ontogeny
Regulation of Hemoglobin Production
Heme Regulation

Globin Regulation
Systemic Regulation of Erythropoiesis
Hemoglobin Function
Oxygen Transport
Carbon Dioxide Transport
Nitric Oxide Transport
Dyshemoglobins
Methemoglobin
Sulfhemoglobin
Carboxyhemoglobin
Hemoglobin Measurement

CASE STUDY

After studying the material in this chapter, the reader should be able to respond to the following case study:

Hemoglobin and hemoglobin fractionation and quantification using high-performance liquid chromatography (HPLC) were performed on a mother and her newborn infant, both presumed to be healthy. The assays were part of a screening program to establish reference intervals. The mother's hemoglobin concentration was 14 g/dL, and the newborn's was 20 g/dL. The mother's hemoglobin fractions were quantified as 97% Hb A, 2% Hb A_2, and 1% Hb F by HPLC. The newborn's results were 88% Hb F and 12% Hb A.

1. Were these hemoglobin results within expected reference intervals?
2. Why were the mother's and the newborn's hemoglobin concentration so different?
3. What is the difference between the test to determine the hemoglobin concentration and the test to analyze hemoglobin by HPLC?
4. Why were the mother's and newborn's hemoglobin fractions so different?

---

*The author extends appreciation to Mary Coleman and Elaine M. Keohane, whose work in prior editions provided the foundation of this chapter.

Hemoglobin is one of the most studied proteins in the body because of the ability to easily isolate it from red blood cells (RBCs). It comprises approximately 95% of the cytoplasmic content of RBCs.[1] The body efficiently carries hemoglobin in RBCs, which provides protection from denaturation in the plasma and loss through the kidneys. Free (non-RBC) hemoglobin, generated from RBCs through hemolysis, has a short half-life outside of RBCs. When released into the plasma, it is rapidly salvaged to preserve its iron and amino acid components; when salvage capacity is exceeded, it is excreted by the kidneys (Chapter 20). The concentration of hemoglobin within RBCs is approximately 34 g/dL, and its molecular weight is approximately 64,000 Daltons.[2] Hemoglobin's main function is to transport oxygen from the lungs to tissues and transport carbon dioxide from the tissues to the lungs for exhalation. Hemoglobin also contributes to acid-base balance by binding and releasing hydrogen ions and transports nitric oxide, a regulator of vascular tone.[1,3]

This chapter covers the structure, biosynthesis, ontogeny, regulation, and function of hemoglobin. The formation, composition, and characteristics of several dyshemoglobins, namely, methemoglobin, carboxyhemoglobin, and sulfhemoglobin, are also discussed at the end of the chapter.

HEMOGLOBIN STRUCTURE

Hemoglobin is the first protein whose structure was described using x-ray crystallography.[4] The hemoglobin molecule is a globular protein consisting of two different pairs of polypeptide chains and four heme groups, with one heme group imbedded in each of the four polypeptide chains (Figure 7.1).

Heme Structure

Heme consists of a ring of carbon, hydrogen, and nitrogen atoms called *protoporphyrin IX*, with a central atom of divalent ferrous iron (Fe^{2+}) (Figure 7.2). Each of the four heme groups is positioned in a pocket of the polypeptide chain near the surface of the hemoglobin molecule. The ferrous iron in each heme molecule reversibly combines with one oxygen molecule. When the ferrous irons are oxidized to the ferric state (Fe^{3+}), they no longer can bind oxygen.

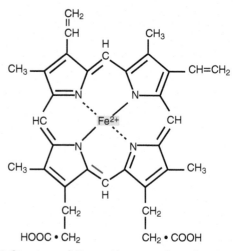

Figure 7.2 Structure of Heme. Heme consists of protoporphyrin IX with a central ferrous iron atom.

TABLE 7.1   Globin Chains

Symbol	Name	Number of Amino Acids
α	Alpha	141
β	Beta	146
γ_A	Gamma A	146 (position 136: alanine)
γ_G	Gamma G	146 (position 136: glycine)
δ	Delta	146
ϵ	Epsilon	146
ζ	Zeta	141
ϑ	Theta	Unknown

Oxidized hemoglobin is also called *methemoglobin* and is discussed later in this chapter.

Globin Structure

The four globin chains comprising each hemoglobin molecule consist of two identical pairs of unlike polypeptide chains, 141 to 146 amino acids each. Variations in amino acid sequences give rise to different types of polypeptide chains. Each chain is designated by a Greek letter (Table 7.1).[1,3]

Each globin chain is divided into eight helices separated by seven nonhelical segments (Figure 7.3).[3] The helices, designated

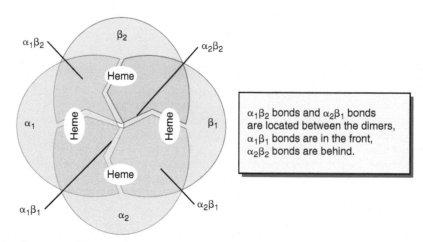

α₁β₂ bonds and α₂β₁ bonds are located between the dimers, α₁β₁ bonds are in the front, α₂β₂ bonds are behind.

Figure 7.1 Structure of Hemoglobin. Hemoglobin is a tetramer of four globin chains with a heme attached to each globin chain.

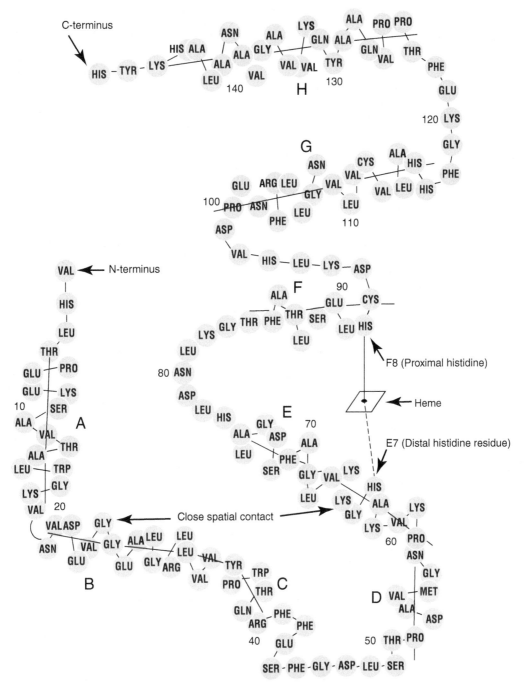

Figure 7.3 Structure of the β-globin Chain of Hemoglobin. The β-globin chain consists of helical (labeled A through H) and nonhelical segments. Heme (protoporphyrin IX with a central iron atom) is suspended in a pocket between the E and F helices. The iron atom of heme is linked to the F8 proximal histidine on one side of the heme plane (solid line). Oxygen binds to the iron atom on the other side of the plane and is close (but not linked) to the E7 distal histidine (dotted line). (Modified from Huisman, T. H., Schroder, W. A. [1971]. *New Aspects of the Structure, Function, and Synthesis of Hemoglobins.* Boca Raton: CRC Press; and modified from Stamatoyannopoulos, G. [1994]. *The Molecular Basis of Blood Diseases.* [2nd ed.]. Philadelphia: Saunders.)

A to H, contain subgroup numberings for the sequence of the amino acids in each helix and are relatively rigid and linear. Flexible nonhelical segments connect the helices, as reflected by their designations: NA for the sequence between the N-terminus and the A helix, AB between the A and B helices, and so forth, with BC, CD, DE, EF, FG, GH, and finally HC between the H helix and the C-terminus.[3]

Complete Hemoglobin Molecule

The hemoglobin molecule can be described by its primary, secondary, tertiary, and quaternary protein structures. The *primary structure* refers to the amino acid sequence of the polypeptide chains. The *secondary structure* refers to chain arrangements in helices and nonhelices. The *tertiary structure* refers to the arrangement of the helices into a pretzel-like configuration.

Globin chains loop to form a cleft pocket for heme. Each chain contains a heme group that is suspended between the E and F helices of the polypeptide chain (Figure 7.3).[2,3] The iron atom at the center of the protoporphyrin IX ring of heme is positioned between two histidine radicals, forming a proximal histidine bond within F8 and, through the linked oxygen, a close association with the distal histidine residue in E7.[3] Globin chain amino acids in the cleft are hydrophobic, whereas amino acids on the outside are hydrophilic, which renders the molecule water soluble. This arrangement also helps iron remain in its divalent ferrous form regardless of whether it is oxygenated (carrying an oxygen molecule) or deoxygenated (not carrying an oxygen molecule).

The *quaternary structure* of hemoglobin, also called a *tetramer,* describes the complete hemoglobin molecule. The complete hemoglobin molecule is spherical, has four heme groups attached to four polypeptide chains, and may carry up to four molecules of oxygen (Figure 7.4). The predominant adult hemoglobin, Hb A, is composed of two α-globin chains and two β-globin chains. Strong α_1-β_1 and α_2-β_2 bonds hold the dimers in a stable form. The α_1-β_2 and α_2-β_1 bonds are important for the stability of the quaternary structure in the oxygenated and deoxygenated forms (Figure 7.1).[1,2]

A small percentage of Hb A is *glycated.* Glycation is a posttranslational modification formed by the nonenzymatic binding of various sugars to globin chain amino groups over the life span of the RBC. The most characterized of the glycated hemoglobins is Hb A_{1c}, in which glucose attaches to the N-terminal valine of the β chain.[1] Normally, about 4% to 6% of Hb A circulates in the A_{1c} form. In uncontrolled diabetes mellitus, the amount of A_{1c} is increased proportionally to the mean blood glucose level over the preceding 2 to 3 months.

HEMOGLOBIN BIOSYNTHESIS

Heme Biosynthesis

Heme biosynthesis occurs in the mitochondria and cytoplasm of bone marrow erythroid precursors, beginning with the pronormoblast through the circulating polychromatic (also known as polychromatophilic) erythrocyte (Chapter 5). As they lose their ribosomes and mitochondria, mature erythrocytes can no longer make hemoglobin.[5]

Heme biosynthesis begins in the mitochondria with the condensation of *glycine* and *succinyl coenzyme A* (CoA) catalyzed by *aminolevulinate synthase* to form *aminolevulinic acid* (ALA) (Figure 7.5).[5] In the cytoplasm, *aminolevulinic acid dehydratase*

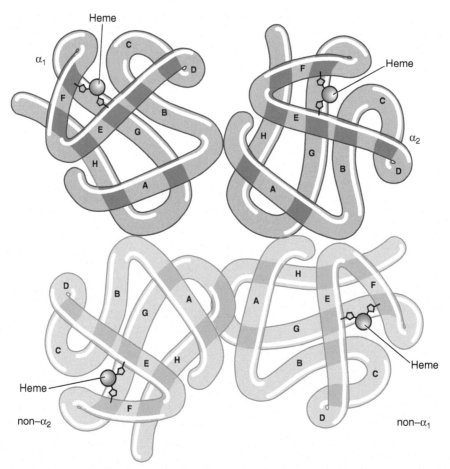

Figure 7.4 Hemoglobin Molecule Illustrating Tertiary Folding of the Four Polypeptide Chains. Heme is suspended between the E and F helices of each polypeptide chain. Pink represents α_1 *(left)* and α_2 *(right);* yellow represents non-α_2 *(left)* and non-α_1 *(right).* The polypeptide chains first form α_1-non-α_1 and α_2-non-α_2 dimers, and then assemble into a tetramer (quaternary structure) with α_1-non-α_2 and α_2-non-α_1 bonds.

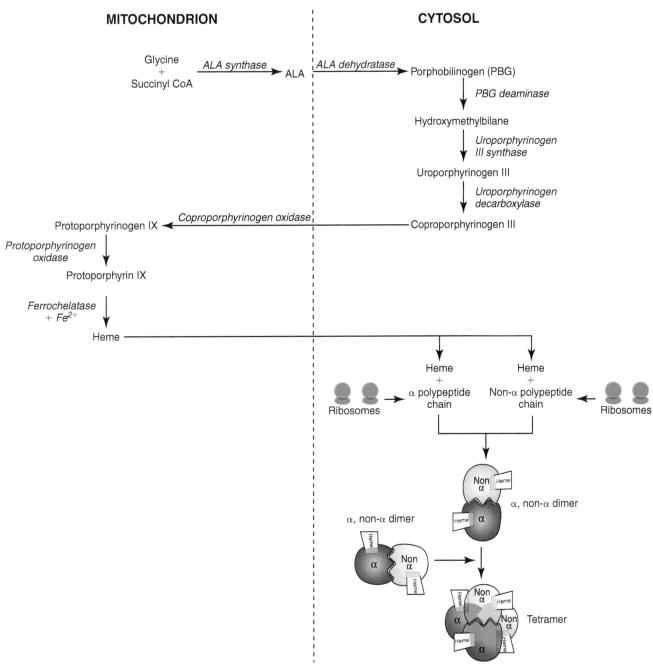

Figure 7.5 Heme Biosynthesis and Hemoglobin Assembly. Heme biosynthesis begins with the condensation of glycine and succinyl coenzyme A (CoA) forming aminolevulinic acid (ALA) in a reaction catalyzed by aminolevulinate synthase. In the cytoplasm, ALA undergoes several transformations from porphobilinogen (PBG) to coproporphyrinogen III, which, catalyzed by coproporphyrinogen oxidase, becomes protoporphyrinogen IX. In the mitochondria, protoporphyrinogen IX is converted to protoporphyrin IX by protoporphyrinogen oxidase. Ferrous (Fe^{2+}) ion is added, catalyzed by ferrochelatase to form heme. In the cytoplasm, heme assembles with an α chain and non-α chain, forming a dimer, and ultimately two dimers join to form the hemoglobin tetramer.

(also known as *porphobilinogen synthase*) converts ALA to *porphobilinogen* (PBG). PBG undergoes several transformations in the cytoplasm from *hydroxymethylbilane* to *coproporphyrinogen III*. This pathway then continues in the mitochondria until, in the final step of production of heme, Fe^{2+} combines with *protoporphyrin IX* in the presence of *ferrochelatase* (*heme synthase*) to make heme.[5]

Transferrin, a plasma protein, carries iron in the ferric (Fe^{3+}) form to developing erythroid cells (Chapter 8). Transferrin binds to transferrin receptors on erythroid precursor cell membranes and the receptors and transferrin (with bound iron) are brought into the cell in an endosome (Figure 8.5). Acidification of the endosome releases iron from transferrin. Iron is transported out of the endosome and into the mitochondria, where it is reduced to the ferrous state and is united with protoporphyrin IX to make heme. Heme leaves the mitochondria and is joined to the globin chains in the cytoplasm.

Globin Biosynthesis

Six structural genes code for six globin chains. The α- and ζ-globin genes are on the short arm of chromosome 16; the ϵ-, γ-, δ-, and β-globin gene cluster is on the short arm of chromosome 11 (Figure 25.1). In the human genome, there is one copy of each globin gene per chromatid, for a total of two genes per diploid cell, with the exception of α and γ. There are two copies of the α- and γ-globin genes per chromatid, for a total of four genes per diploid cell.

Production of globin chains takes place in erythroid precursors from the pronormoblast through the circulating polychromatic erythrocyte, but not in mature erythrocytes.[5] Transcription of the globin genes to messenger ribonucleic acid (mRNA) occurs in the nucleus, and translation of mRNA to the globin polypeptide chain occurs on ribosomes in the cytoplasm. Although transcription of α-globin genes produces more mRNA than the β-globin gene, there is less efficient translation of the α-globin mRNA.[2] Therefore, α and β chains are produced in approximately equal amounts. After translation is complete, chains are released from the ribosomes in the cytoplasm.

Hemoglobin Assembly

After their release from ribosomes, each globin chain binds to a heme molecule, then forms a heterodimer (Figure 7.5). The non-α chains have a charge difference that determines their affinity to bind to α chains. The α chain has a positive charge and has the highest affinity for a β chain because of its negative charge.[1,2] The γ-globin chain has the next highest affinity, followed by the δ-globin chain.[2] Two heterodimers then combine to form a tetramer. This completes the hemoglobin molecule.

Two α and two β chains form Hb A, the major hemoglobin present from 6 months of age through adulthood. Hb A_2 contains two α and two δ chains. Owing to a mutation in the promoter region of the δ-globin gene, production of the δ chain polypeptide is very low.[6] Consequently, Hb A_2 comprises less than 3.5% of total hemoglobin in adults. Hb F contains two α and two γ chains. In healthy adults, Hb F comprises 1% to 2% of total hemoglobin, and it is present only in a small proportion of the RBCs (uneven distribution). These RBCs with Hb F are called *F* or *A/F cells*.[1,2]

The various amino acids that comprise the globin chains affect the net charge of the hemoglobin tetramer. Electrophoresis and high-performance liquid chromatography (HPLC) are used for fractionation, presumptive identification, and quantification of normal hemoglobins and hemoglobin variants (Chapter 24). Molecular genetic testing of globin gene DNA provides definitive identification of variant hemoglobins.

HEMOGLOBIN ONTOGENY

Hemoglobin composition differs with prenatal gestation time and postnatal age. Hemoglobin changes reflect the sequential activation and inactivation (or switching) of the globin genes,

progressing from the ζ- to the α-globin gene on chromosome 16 and from the ϵ- to the γ-, δ-, and β-globin genes on chromosome 11. The ζ- and ϵ-globin chains normally appear only during the first 3 months of embryonic development. These two chains, when paired with the α and γ chains, form the embryonic hemoglobins (Figure 7.6). During the second and third trimesters of fetal life and at birth, Hb F ($\alpha_2\gamma_2$) is the predominant hemoglobin. By 6 months of age and through adulthood, Hb A ($\alpha_2\beta_2$) is the predominant hemoglobin, with small amounts of Hb A_2 ($\alpha_2\delta_2$) and Hb F.[2] Table 7.2 presents the reference intervals for the normal hemoglobin fractions at various ages.

REGULATION OF HEMOGLOBIN PRODUCTION

Heme Regulation

The key rate-limiting step in heme synthesis is the initial reaction of glycine and succinyl CoA to form ALA, catalyzed by ALA synthase (Figure 7.5). Heme inhibits the transcription of the ALA synthase gene, which leads to a decrease in heme production (a negative feedback mechanism). Heme inhibits other enzymes in the biosynthesis pathway, including ALA dehydrase and PBG deaminase. A negative feedback mechanism by heme or substrate inhibition by protoporphyrin IX is believed to inhibit the ferrochelatase enzyme.[5] Conversely, an increased demand for heme induces an increased synthesis of ALA synthase.[5]

Globin Regulation

Globin synthesis is highly regulated so that there is a balanced production of globin and heme. This is critical because an excess of globin chains, protoporphyrin IX, or iron can accumulate and damage the cell, reducing its life span.

Globin production is mainly controlled at the transcription level by a complex interaction of DNA sequences (cis-acting promoters, enhancers, and silencers) and soluble transcription factors (trans-acting factors) that bind to DNA or to one another to promote or suppress transcription.[2] Initiation of transcription of a particular globin gene requires (1) the promoter DNA sequences immediately before the 5' end or the beginning of the gene; (2) a key transcription factor called *Krüppel-like factor 1* (KLF1); (3) a number of other transcription factors (such as GATA1, Ikaros, TAL1, p45-NF-E2, and LDB1); and (4) an enhancer region of DNAse 1 hypersensitive nucleic acid sequences located more than 20 kilobases upstream (before the 5' start site of the gene) from the globin gene called the *locus control region (LCR)*.[7] For example, to activate transcription of the β-globin gene in the β-globin gene cluster on chromosome 11, the LCR, the promoter for the β-globin gene, and various transcription factors join together to form a three-dimensional active chromosome hub (ACH), with KLF1 playing a key role in connecting the complex.[7,8] Because the LCR is located a distance upstream from the β-globin gene complex, a loop of DNA is formed when the LCR and β-globin gene promoter join together in the chromosome hub.[8] The other globin genes in the cluster (ϵ-, γ-, and δ-) are maintained in the inactive state in the DNA loop, so only the β-globin gene is transcribed.[7,8]

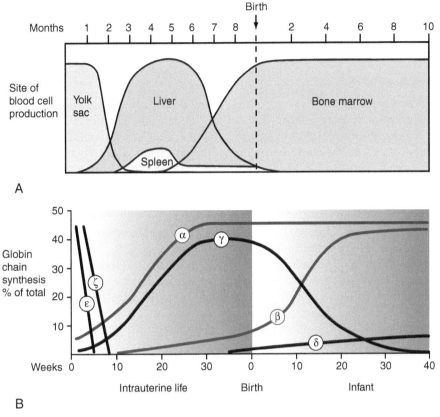

Figure 7.6 Timeline of Globin Chain Production from Intrauterine Life to Adulthood. See also Table 7.2.

TABLE 7.2	**Normal Hemoglobins**	
Stage	**Globin Chain**	**Hemoglobin**
Intrauterine		
Early embryogenesis (product of yolk sac erythroblasts)	$\zeta_2 + \epsilon_2$	Gower-1
	$\alpha_2 + \epsilon_2$	Gower-2
	$\zeta_2 + \gamma_2$	Portland
Begins in early embryogenesis; peaks during third trimester and begins to decline just before birth	$\alpha_2 + \gamma_2$	F
Birth		
	$\alpha_2 + \gamma_2$	F, 60%–90%
	$\alpha_2 + \beta_2$	A, 10%–40%
Two Years through Adulthood		
	$\alpha_2 + \gamma_2$	F, 1%–2%
	$\alpha_2 + \delta_2$	A2, <3.5%
	$\alpha_2 + \beta_2$	A, >95%

Krüppel-like factor 1 also plays a key regulatory role in the switch from γ chain to β chain production (γ-β switching) that begins in late fetal life and continues through adulthood. KLF1 is an exact match for binding to the DNA promoter sequences of the β-globin gene, whereas the γ-globin gene promoter has a slightly different sequence.[7] This results in a preferential binding to and subsequent activation of transcription of the β-globin gene.[7] KLF1 also regulates the expression of repressors of γ-globin gene transcription, such as BCL11A and MYB.[7,9]

Globin synthesis is also regulated during translation when mRNA coding for the globin chains associates with ribosomes to produce the polypeptide. Many protein factors are required to control initiation, elongation, and termination steps of translation. Heme is an important regulator of globin mRNA translation at the initiation step by promoting activation of a translation initiation factor and inactivating its repressor.[5] Conversely, when the heme level is low, the repressor accumulates and inactivates the initiation factor, thus blocking translation of the globin mRNA.[2,5]

Systemic Regulation of Erythropoiesis

When there is an insufficient quantity of hemoglobin or if the hemoglobin molecule is defective in transporting oxygen, tissue hypoxia occurs. Hypoxia is detected by the peritubular cells of the kidney, which respond by increasing production of erythropoietin (EPO). EPO increases the number of erythrocytes produced and released into the periphery; it also accelerates the rate of synthesis of erythrocyte components, including hemoglobin (Chapter 5).

Although each laboratory establishes its own reference intervals based on their instrumentation, methodology, and patient population, in general, reference intervals for hemoglobin concentration are as follows:

Men:	13.5–18.0 g/dL (135–180 g/L)
Women:	12.0–15.0 g/dL (120–150 g/L)
Newborns:	16.5–21.5 g/dL (165–215 g/L)

Reference intervals for infants and children vary according to age group. Individuals living at high altitudes have slightly higher levels of hemoglobin as a compensatory mechanism to provide more oxygen to the tissues in the oxygen-thin air. Tables on the inside front cover provide reference intervals for all age groups.

HEMOGLOBIN FUNCTION

Oxygen Transport

The function of hemoglobin is to readily bind oxygen molecules in the lung, which requires high oxygen affinity; to transport oxygen; and to efficiently unload oxygen to the tissues, which requires low oxygen affinity. During oxygenation, each of the four heme iron atoms in a hemoglobin molecule can reversibly bind one oxygen molecule. Approximately 1.34 mL of oxygen is bound by each gram of hemoglobin.[1]

The affinity of hemoglobin for oxygen relates to the partial pressure of oxygen (PO_2), often defined in terms of the amount of oxygen needed to saturate 50% of hemoglobin, called P_{50} value. The relationship is described by the oxygen dissociation curve of hemoglobin, which plots the percent oxygen saturation of hemoglobin versus the PO_2 (Figure 7.7).

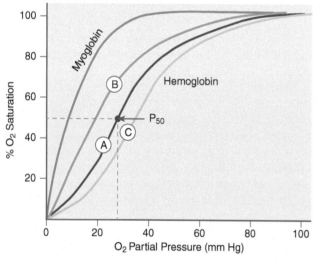

Figure 7.7 Hemoglobin-Oxygen Dissociation Curves. **(A),** Normal hemoglobin-oxygen dissociation curve. P_{50} is the partial pressure of oxygen (O_2) needed for 50% O_2 saturation of hemoglobin. **(B),** Left-shifted curve with reduced P_{50} can be caused by decreases in 2,3-bisphosphoglycerate (2,3-BPG), H^+ ions (raised pH), partial pressure of carbon dioxide (PCO_2), and/or temperature. A left-shifted curve is also seen with hemoglobin F and hemoglobin variants that have increased oxygen affinity. **(C),** Right-shifted curve with increased P_{50} can be caused by elevations in 2,3-BPG, H^+ ions (lowered pH), PCO_2, and/or temperature. A right-shifted curve is also seen with hemoglobin variants that have decreased oxygen affinity. Myoglobin, a muscle protein, produces a markedly left-shifted curve indicating a very high oxygen affinity. It is not effective in releasing oxygen at physiologic oxygen tensions.

The curve is *sigmoidal,* which indicates low hemoglobin affinity for oxygen at low oxygen tension and high affinity for oxygen at high oxygen tension.

Cooperation among hemoglobin subunits contributes to the shape of the curve. Hemoglobin that is completely deoxygenated has little affinity for oxygen. However, with each oxygen molecule that is bound, there is a change in the conformation of the tetramer that progressively increases the oxygen affinity of the other heme subunits. Once one oxygen molecule binds, the remainder of the hemoglobin molecule quickly becomes fully oxygenated.[2] Therefore, with high oxygen tension in the lungs, the affinity of hemoglobin for oxygen is high, and hemoglobin becomes rapidly saturated with oxygen. Conversely, with relatively low oxygen tension in the tissues, the affinity of hemoglobin for oxygen is low, and hemoglobin rapidly releases oxygen.

Normally, a PO_2 of approximately 27 mm Hg results in 50% oxygen saturation of the hemoglobin molecule. If there is a shift of the curve to the left, 50% oxygen saturation of hemoglobin occurs at a PO_2 of less than 27 mm Hg. If there is a shift of the curve to the right, 50% oxygen saturation of hemoglobin occurs at a PO_2 higher than 27 mm Hg.

The reference interval for arterial oxygen saturation is 96% to 100%. If the oxygen dissociation curve shifts to the left, a patient with arterial and venous PO_2 levels in the reference intervals (80 to 100 mm Hg arterial and 30 to 50 mm Hg venous) will have a higher percent oxygen saturation and a higher affinity for oxygen than a patient for whom the curve is normal. With a shift in the curve to the right, a lower oxygen affinity is seen.

In addition to the PO_2, shifts of the curve to the left or right occur if there are changes in the pH of the blood. In the tissues, a lower pH shifts the curve to the right and reduces the affinity of hemoglobin for oxygen, and the hemoglobin more readily releases oxygen. A shift in the curve because of a change in pH (or hydrogen ion concentration) is termed the *Bohr effect.* It facilitates the ability of hemoglobin to exchange oxygen and carbon dioxide (CO_2).

The concentration of 2,3-bisphosphoglycerate (2,3-BPG, formerly 2,3-diphosphoglycerate) also has an effect on oxygen affinity. In the deoxygenated state, the hemoglobin tetramer assumes a *tense* or *T* conformation that is stabilized by the binding of 2,3-BPG between the β-globin chains (Figure 7.8). The formation of salt bridges between the phosphates of 2,3-BPG and positively charged groups on the globin chains further stabilizes the tetramer in the T conformation.[1] The binding of 2,3-BPG shifts the oxygen dissociation curve to the right, favoring the release of oxygen.[1] In addition, a lower pH and higher PCO_2 in the tissues further shifts the curve to the right, favoring the release of oxygen.[1]

As hemoglobin binds oxygen molecules, a change in conformation of the hemoglobin tetramer occurs with a change in hydrophobic interactions at the $\alpha_1\beta_2$ contact point, a disruption of the salt bridges, and release of 2,3-BPG.[1] A 15-degree rotation of the $\alpha_1\beta_1$ dimer, relative to the $\alpha_2\beta_2$ dimer, occurs along the $\alpha_1\beta_2$ contact point.[2] When the hemoglobin tetramer is fully oxygenated, it assumes a *relaxed* or *R* state (Figure 7.8).

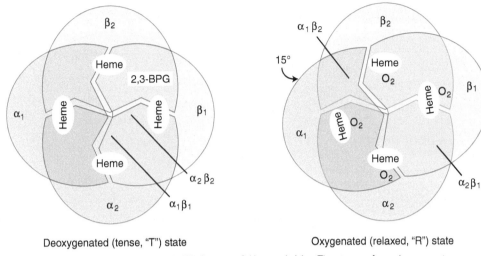

Deoxygenated (tense, "T") state   Oxygenated (relaxed, "R") state

Figure 7.8 Tense (T) and Relaxed (R) forms of Hemoglobin. The tense form incorporates one 2, 3-bisphosphoglycerate (2,3-BPG) molecule, bound between the β-globin chains with salt bridges. It is unable to transport oxygen. As hemoglobin binds oxygen molecules, the $\alpha_1\beta_1$ and $\alpha_2\beta_2$ dimers rotate 15° relative to each other as a result of the change in hydrophobic interactions at the $\alpha_1\beta_2$ contact point, salt bridges are disrupted, and 2,3-BPG is released.

Clinical conditions that produce a shift of the oxygen dissociation curve to the left include a lowered body temperature as a result of external causes; multiple transfusions of stored blood with depleted 2,3-BPG; alkalosis; and presence of hemoglobin variants with a high affinity for oxygen. Conditions producing a shift of the curve to the right include increased body temperature; acidosis; presence of hemoglobin variants with a low affinity for oxygen; and an increased 2,3-BPG concentration in response to hypoxic conditions, such as high altitude, pulmonary insufficiency, congestive heart failure, and severe anemia (Chapter 16).

The sigmoidal oxygen dissociation curve generated by normal hemoglobin contrasts with myoglobin's hyperbolic curve (Figure 7.7). Myoglobin, present in cardiac and skeletal muscle, is a 17,000-Dalton, monomeric, oxygen-binding heme protein. It binds oxygen with greater affinity than hemoglobin. Its hyperbolic curve indicates that it releases oxygen only at very low partial pressures, which means it is not as effective as hemoglobin in releasing oxygen to the tissues at physiologic oxygen tensions. Myoglobin is released into the plasma when there is damage to the muscle in myocardial infarction, trauma, or severe muscle injury, called *rhabdomyolysis.* Myoglobin is normally excreted by the kidney, but levels may become elevated in renal failure. Serum myoglobin levels aid in diagnosis of myocardial infarction in patients who have no underlying trauma, rhabdomyolysis, or renal failure. Myoglobin in the urine produces a positive result on urine biochemical analysis (by reagent test strip) for blood; this must be differentiated from a positive result caused by hemoglobin.

Hb F (fetal hemoglobin, the primary hemoglobin in newborns) has a P_{50} of 19 to 21 mm Hg, which results in a left shift of the oxygen dissociation curve and increased affinity for oxygen relative to that of Hb A. This increased affinity for oxygen is due to its weakened ability to bind 2,3-BPG.[2] There is only one amino acid difference in a critical 2,3-BPG binding site between the γ chain and the β chain that accounts for this difference in binding.[2]

In fetal life the high oxygen affinity of Hb F provides an advantage by allowing more effective oxygen withdrawal from the maternal circulation. At the same time, Hb F has a disadvantage in that it delivers oxygen less readily to tissues. The bone marrow in the fetus and newborn compensates by producing more RBCs to ensure adequate oxygenation of the tissues. This response is mediated by EPO (Chapter 5). Consequently, the RBC count, hemoglobin concentration, and hematocrit of a newborn are higher than adult values, but they gradually decrease to normal physiologic levels by 6 months of age as the γ-β switching is completed and most of the Hb F is replaced by Hb A.

Carbon Dioxide Transport

A second crucial function of hemoglobin is the transport of carbon dioxide. In venous blood, the carbon dioxide diffuses into the RBCs and combines with water to form carbonic acid (H_2CO_3). This reaction is facilitated by the RBC enzyme carbonic anhydrase. Carbonic acid then dissociates to release H^+ and bicarbonate (HCO_3^-) (Figure 7.9).

The H^+ from the second reaction binds oxygenated hemoglobin (HbO_2), and the oxygen is released from the hemoglobin because of the Bohr effect. The oxygen then diffuses out of the cell into the tissues. As the concentration of the negatively charged bicarbonate increases, it diffuses across the RBC membrane into the plasma. Chloride (Cl^-), also negatively charged, diffuses from the plasma into the cell to maintain electroneutrality across the membrane; this is called the *chloride shift* (Figure 7.9).

In the lungs, oxygen diffuses into the cell and binds to deoxygenated hemoglobin (HHb) because of the high oxygen tension. H^+ is released from hemoglobin and combines with bicarbonate to form carbonic acid. Carbonic acid is converted

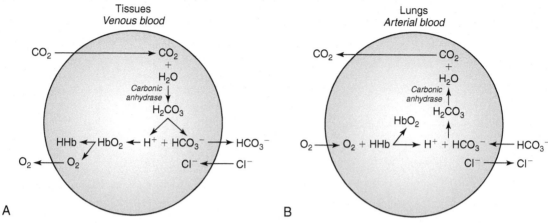

Figure 7.9 Transport and Release of Oxygen (O_2) and Carbon Dioxide (CO_2) in the Tissues and Lungs. **(A),** In the tissues, CO_2 diffuses into the red blood cell and combines with water (H_2O) to form carbonic acid (H_2CO_3). This reaction is catalyzed by carbonic anhydrase. H_2CO_3 disassociates to hydrogen (H^+) and bicarbonate (HCO_3^-) ions. H^+ binds to oxyhemoglobin (HbO_2), resulting in the release of O_2 as a result of the Bohr effect. The O_2 diffuses out of the cell into the tissues. The HCO_3^- diffuses out of the cell as its concentration increases and is replaced by chloride ($Cl-$) to maintain electroneutrality (chloride shift). Some CO_2 directly binds to the globin chains of hemoglobin. **(B),** In the lungs, O_2 binds to deoxygenated hemoglobin (HHb) because of the high oxygen tension. The H^+ dissociates from HbO_2, combines with HCO_3^- to form H_2CO_3, which then dissociates into CO_2 and H_2O. The CO_2 diffuses out of the red blood cells and is exhaled by the lungs.

to water and CO_2; the latter diffuses out of the cells and is expelled by the lungs. As more bicarbonate diffuses into the cell to produce carbonic acid, chloride diffuses back out into the plasma. Approximately 85% of the CO_2 produced in the tissues is transported by hemoglobin as H^+.[1] In this capacity, hemoglobin provides a buffering effect by binding and releasing H^+.[1] A small percentage of CO_2 remains in the cytoplasm and the remainder binds to the globin chains as a carbamino group.

Nitric Oxide Transport

A third function of hemoglobin involves the binding, inactivation, and transport of nitric oxide.[1,10] Nitric oxide is secreted by vascular endothelial cells and causes relaxation of vascular wall smooth muscle and vasodilation.[1] When released, free nitric oxide has a very short half-life, but some enters RBCs and can bind to cysteine in the β chain of hemoglobin, forming S-nitrosohemoglobin.[1,10,11] Some investigators propose that hemoglobin preserves and transports nitric oxide to hypoxic microvascular areas, which stimulates vasodilation and increases blood flow (hypoxic vasodilation).[10] In this way, hemoglobin may work with other systems in regulating local blood flow to microvascular areas by binding and inactivating nitric oxide (causing vasoconstriction and decreased blood flow) when oxygen tension is high and releasing nitric oxide (causing vasodilation and increased blood flow) when oxygen tension is low.[10] This theory is not universally accepted, and the roles of hemoglobin, endothelial cells, and nitric oxide in regulating blood flow and oxygenation of the microcirculation are still being investigated.[11]

DYSHEMOGLOBINS

Dyshemoglobins (dysfunctional hemoglobins that are unable to transport oxygen) include methemoglobin, sulfhemoglobin,

and carboxyhemoglobin. Dyshemoglobins form and may accumulate to toxic levels, after exposure to certain drugs or environmental chemicals or gasses. The offending agent modifies the structure of the hemoglobin molecule, preventing it from binding oxygen. Most cases of dyshemoglobinemia are acquired; a small fraction of methemoglobinemia cases are hereditary.

Methemoglobin

Methemoglobin (MetHb) is formed by the reversible oxidation of heme iron to the ferric state (Fe^{3+}). Normally, a small amount of methemoglobin is continuously formed by oxidation of iron during normal oxygenation and deoxygenation of hemoglobin.[11,12] However, methemoglobin reduction systems, predominantly the NADH-cytochrome b5 reductase 3 (NADH-methemoglobin reductase) pathway, normally limit its accumulation to only 1% of total hemoglobin (Chapter 6 and Figure 6.1).[11-13]

Methemoglobin cannot carry oxygen because oxidized ferric iron cannot bind it. An increase in methemoglobin level results in decreased delivery of oxygen to the tissues. Individuals with methemoglobin levels less than 25% are generally asymptomatic.[14] If the methemoglobin level increases to more than 30% of total hemoglobin, cyanosis (bluish discoloration of skin and mucous membranes) and symptoms of hypoxia (dyspnea, headache, vertigo, change in mental status) occur.[12,13] Levels of methemoglobin greater than 50% can lead to coma and death.[12,13]

An increase in methemoglobin, called *methemoglobinemia*, can be acquired or hereditary. The acquired form, also called *toxic methemoglobinemia*, occurs in normal individuals after exposure to an exogenous oxidant, such as nitrites, primaquine, dapsone, or benzocaine.[12,14] As the oxidant overwhelms the hemoglobin reduction systems, the level of methemoglobin increases, and the patient may exhibit cyanosis and symptoms of hypoxia.[11] In many cases, withdrawal of the offending oxidant is sufficient for a recovery, but if the level of methemoglobin increases to 30% or more of total hemoglobin, intravenous methylene blue is administered. Methylene blue reduces methemoglobin ferric iron to the ferrous state through NADPH-methemoglobin reductase and NADPH produced by glucose-6-phosphate dehydrogenase in the hexose monophosphate shunt (Figure 6.1).[11] In life-threatening cases, exchange transfusion may be required.[12]

Hereditary causes of methemoglobinemia are rare and include mutations in the gene for NADH-cytochrome b5 reductase 3 (CYB5R3), resulting in a diminished capacity to reduce methemoglobin, and mutations in the α-, β-, or γ-globin gene, resulting in a structurally abnormal polypeptide chain that favors the oxidized ferric form of iron and prevents its reduction.[11,12] The methemoglobin produced by the latter group is called M hemoglobin or Hb M (Chapter 24). Hb M is inherited in an autosomal dominant pattern, with methemoglobin comprising 30% to 50% of total hemoglobin.[12] There is no effective treatment for this form of methemoglobinemia.[11,12] Cytochrome b5 reductase deficiency is an autosomal recessive disorder, and methemoglobin elevations occur in individuals who are homozygous or compound heterozygous for a CYB5R3 mutation.[11,12] Most individuals with Hb M or homozygous cytochrome b5 reductase deficiency maintain methemoglobin levels less than 50%; they have cyanosis but only mild symptoms of hypoxia that do not require treatment.[11-13] Individuals heterozygous for the CYB5R3 mutation have normal levels of methemoglobin but develop methemoglobinemia, cyanosis, and hypoxia when exposed to an oxidant drug or chemical.[12,14]

Methemoglobin is assayed by spectral absorption analysis instruments such as the CO-oximeter. Methemoglobin shows an absorption peak at 630 nm.[12] With high levels of methemoglobin, the blood takes on a chocolate brown color and does not revert back to normal red color after oxygen exposure.[12,13] The methemoglobin in Hb M disease has different absorption peaks, depending on the variant.[11] Hemoglobin electrophoresis, HPLC, and DNA mutation testing are used for identification of Hb M variants. Cytochrome b5 reductase 3 deficiency is diagnosed by enzyme assays and DNA mutation testing.[11]

Sulfhemoglobin

Sulfhemoglobin is formed by irreversible oxidation of hemoglobin by drugs (such as sulfanilamides, phenacetin, nitrites, and phenylhydrazine) or exposure to sulfur chemicals in industrial or environmental settings.[11,12] It is formed by the addition of a sulfur atom to the pyrrole ring of heme and has a greenish pigment.[11] Sulfhemoglobin is ineffective for oxygen transport, and patients with elevated levels present with cyanosis. Sulfhemoglobin cannot be converted to normal Hb A; it persists for the life of the cell. Treatment consists of prevention by avoidance of the offending agent.

Sulfhemoglobin has a similar peak to methemoglobin on a spectral absorption instrument. The sulfhemoglobin spectral curve, however, does not shift when cyanide is added, a feature that distinguishes it from methemoglobin.[11]

Carboxyhemoglobin

Carboxyhemoglobin (COHb) results from the combination of carbon monoxide (CO) with heme iron. The affinity of carbon monoxide for hemoglobin is 240 times that of oxygen.[11] Once one molecule of carbon monoxide binds to hemoglobin, it shifts the hemoglobin-oxygen dissociation curve to the left, further increasing its affinity and severely impairing release of oxygen to the tissues.[11,15] Carbon monoxide has been termed the silent killer because it is an odorless and colorless gas, and victims may quickly become hypoxic.[15]

Some carboxyhemoglobin is produced endogenously, but it normally comprises less than 2% of total hemoglobin.[11] Exogenous carbon monoxide is derived from the exhaust of automobiles, tobacco smoke, and from industrial pollutants, such as coal, gas, and charcoal burning. In smokers, COHb levels may be as high as 15%.[14] As a result, smokers may have a higher hematocrit and polycythemia to compensate for the hypoxia.[11,14]

Exposure to carbon monoxide may be coincidental, accidental, or intentional (suicidal). Many deaths from house fires are the result of inhaling smoke, fumes, or carbon monoxide.[15] Even when heating systems in homes are properly maintained, accidental poisoning with carbon monoxide may occur. Toxic effects, such as headache, dizziness, and disorientation, begin to appear at blood levels of 20% to 30% COHb.[11,14] Levels of more than 40% of total hemoglobin may cause coma, seizure, hypotension, cardiac arrhythmias, pulmonary edema, and death.[11,15]

Carboxyhemoglobin may be detected by spectral absorption instruments at 540 nm.[12] It gives blood a cherry red color, which is sometimes imparted to the skin of victims.[15] A diagnosis of carbon monoxide poisoning is made if the COHb level is greater than 3% in nonsmokers and greater than 10% in smokers.[15] Treatment involves removing the carbon monoxide source and administration of 100% oxygen.[11] Use of hyperbaric oxygen therapy is controversial[15]; it is primarily used to prevent neurologic and cognitive impairment after acute carbon monoxide exposure in patients whose COHb level exceeds 25%.[15]

HEMOGLOBIN MEASUREMENT

The cyanmethemoglobin method is the reference method for hemoglobin assay.[16] A lysing agent present in the cyanmethemoglobin reagent frees hemoglobin from RBCs. Free hemoglobin combines with potassium ferricyanide contained in the cyanmethemoglobin reagent, which converts hemoglobin iron from the ferrous to the ferric state to form methemoglobin. Methemoglobin combines with potassium cyanide to form the stable pigment cyanmethemoglobin. The cyanmethemoglobin color intensity, which is proportional to hemoglobin concentration, is measured at 540 nm spectrophotometrically and compared with a standard (Chapter 11). The cyanmethemoglobin method is performed manually but has been adapted for use in automated blood cell analyzers.

Many instruments now use sodium lauryl sulfate (SLS) to convert hemoglobin to SLS-methemoglobin. This method does not generate toxic wastes (Chapter 12).

Hemoglobin electrophoresis and HPLC are used to separate the different types of hemoglobins such as Hb A, A_2, and F (Chapters 24 and 25).

SUMMARY

- The hemoglobin molecule is a tetramer composed of two pairs of unlike polypeptide chains. A heme group (protoporphyrin IX + Fe^{2+}) is bound to each of the four polypeptide chains.
- Hemoglobin, contained in red blood cells (RBCs), carries oxygen from the lungs to the tissues. Oxygen binds to ferrous iron in heme. Each hemoglobin tetramer can bind four oxygen molecules.
- Six structural genes code for the six globin chains of hemoglobin. The α- and ζ-globin genes are on chromosome 16; the ϵ-, γ-, δ-, and β-globin gene cluster is on chromosome 11. There is one copy of the δ-globin gene and one β-globin gene per chromosome, for a total of two genes per diploid cell. There are two copies of the α- and γ-globin genes per chromosome, for a total of four genes per diploid cell.
- Three hemoglobins found in normal adults are Hb A, Hb A_2, and Hb F. Hb A ($\alpha_2\beta_2$), composed of two $\alpha\beta$ heterodimers, is the predominant hemoglobin of adults. Hb F ($\alpha_2\gamma_2$) is the predominant hemoglobin in the fetus and newborn. Hb A_2 ($\alpha_2\delta_2$) is present from birth through adulthood, but at low levels.
- Hemoglobin ontogeny describes which hemoglobins are produced by the erythroid precursor cells from the fetal period through birth to adulthood.

- Complex genetic mechanisms regulate the sequential expression of the polypeptide chains in the embryo, fetus, and adult. Heme provides negative feedback regulation on protoporphyrin and globin chain production.
- The hemoglobin-oxygen dissociation curve is sigmoid because of cooperativity among the hemoglobin subunits in binding and releasing oxygen.
- 2,3-bisphosphoglycerate (2,3-BPG) produced by the glycolytic pathway facilitates the delivery of oxygen from hemoglobin to the tissues. The Bohr effect is the influence of pH on the release of oxygen from hemoglobin.
- In tissues, carbon dioxide diffuses into RBCs and combines with water to form carbonic acid (H_2CO_3). Carbonic acid is then converted to bicarbonate and hydrogen ions (HCO_3^- and H^+). Most of the carbon dioxide is carried by hemoglobin as H^+.
- Methemoglobin, sulfhemoglobin, and carboxyhemoglobin cannot transport oxygen. They can accumulate to toxic levels as a result of exposure to certain drugs, industrial or environmental chemicals, or gases. A small fraction of methemoglobinemia cases are hereditary. Cyanosis occurs in patients with increased levels of methemoglobin or sulfhemoglobin.

Now that you have completed this chapter, go back and read again the case study at the beginning and respond to the questions presented.

REVIEW QUESTIONS

Answers can be found in the Appendix.

1. A hemoglobin molecule is composed of:
   a. One heme molecule and four globin chains
   b. Ferrous iron, protoporphyrin IX, and a globin chain
   c. Protoporphyrin IX and four globin chains
   d. Four heme molecules and four globin chains
2. Normal adult Hb A contains which polypeptide chains?
   a. α and β
   b. α and δ
   c. α and γ
   d. α and ϵ
3. A key rate-limiting step in heme synthesis is suppression of:
   a. Aminolevulinate synthase
   b. Carbonic anhydrase
   c. Protoporphyrin IX reductase
   d. Glucose-6-phosphate dehydrogenase
4. Which of the following forms of hemoglobin molecule has the lowest affinity for oxygen?
   a. Tense
   b. Relaxed
5. Using the normal hemoglobin-oxygen dissociation curve in Figure 7.7 for reference, predict the position of the curve when there is a decrease in pH.
   a. Shifted to the right of normal with decreased oxygen affinity
   b. Shifted to the left of normal with increased oxygen affinity
   c. Shifted to the right of normal with increased oxygen affinity
   d. Shifted to the left of normal with decreased oxygen affinity

6. The predominant hemoglobin found in a healthy newborn is:
   a. Gower-1
   b. Gower-2
   c. A
   d. F
7. What is the normal distribution of hemoglobins in healthy adults?
   a. 80% to 90% Hb A, 5% to 10% Hb A_2, 1% to 5% Hb F
   b. 80% to 90% Hb A_2, 5% to 10% Hb A, 1% to 5% Hb F
   c. >95% Hb A, <3.5% Hb A_2, 1% to 2% Hb F
   d. >90% Hb A, 5% Hb F, <5% Hb A_2
8. Which of the following is a description of the structure of oxidized hemoglobin?
   a. Hemoglobin carrying oxygen on heme; synonymous with oxygenated hemoglobin
   b. Hemoglobin with iron in the ferric state (methemoglobin) and not able to carry oxygen
   c. Hemoglobin with iron in the ferric state so that carbon dioxide replaces oxygen in the heme structure
   d. Hemoglobin carrying carbon monoxide; hence *oxidized* refers to the single oxygen

9. In the quaternary structure of hemoglobin, the globin chains associate into:
   a. α Tetramers in some cells and β tetramers in others
   b. A mixture of α tetramers and β tetramers
   c. α Dimers and β dimers
   d. Two αβ dimers

10. How are the globin chain genes arranged?
   a. With α genes and β genes on the same chromosome, including two α genes and two β genes
   b. With α genes and β genes on separate chromosomes, including two α genes on one chromosome and one β gene on a different chromosome
   c. With α genes and β genes on the same chromosome, including four α genes and four β genes
   d. With α genes and β genes on separate chromosomes, including four α genes on one chromosome and two β genes on a different chromosome

11. The nature of the interaction between 2,3-BPG and hemoglobin is that 2,3-BPG:
   a. Binds to the heme moiety, blocking the binding of oxygen
   b. Binds simultaneously with oxygen to ensure that it stays bound until it reaches the tissues, when both molecules are released from hemoglobin
   c. Binds to amino acids of the globin chain, contributing to a conformational change that inhibits oxygen from binding to heme
   d. Oxidizes hemoglobin iron, diminishing oxygen binding and promoting oxygen delivery to the tissues

REFERENCES

1. Quigly, J. G., Means, R. T., Jr., & Glader, B. (2014). The birth, life and death of red blood cells: erythropoiesis, the mature red blood cell and cell destruction. In Greer, J. P., Arber, D. A., Glader, B., et al. (Eds.), *Wintrobe's Clinical Hematology.* (13th ed., pp. 83–124). Philadelphia: Lippincott Williams & Wilkins.

2. Steinberg, M. H., Benz, E. J., Jr, Adewoye, A. H., et al. (2018). Pathobiology of the human erythrocyte and its hemoglobins. In Hoffman, R., Benz, E. J., Silberstein, L. E., et al. (Eds.), *Hematology Basic Principles and Practice.* (7th ed., pp. 447–457). Philadelphia: Elsevier.

3. Natrajan, K., & Kutlar, A. (2016). Disorders of hemoglobin structure: sickle cell anemia and related abnormalities. In Kaushansky K., Lichtman M. A., Prchal J. T., et al. (Eds.), *Williams Hematology.* (9th ed., pp. 759–788). New York: McGraw-Hill.

4. Perutz, M. F., Rossmann, M. G., Cullis, A. F., et al. (1960). Structure of hemoglobin: a three dimensional Fourier synthesis at 5.5A resolution obtained by x-ray analysis. *Nature, 185,* 416–422.

5. Chow, A., & Frenette, P. S. (2014). Origin and development of blood cells. In Greer, J. P., Arber, D. A., Glader, B., et al. (Eds.), *Wintrobe's Clinical Hematology.* (13th ed., pp. 65–82). Philadelphia: Lippincott Williams & Wilkins.

6. Donze, D., Jeancake, P. H., & Townes, T. M. (1996). Activation of delta-globin gene expression by erythroid Krüpple-like factor: a potential approach for gene therapy of sickle cell disease. *Blood, 88,* 4051–4057.

7. Tallack, M. R., & Perkins, A. C. (2013). Three fingers on the switch: Krüppel-like factor 1 regulation of a-globin to β-globin gene switching. *Curr Opin Hematol, 20,* 193–200.

8. Tolhuis, B., Palstra, R-J., Splinter, E., et al. (2002). Looping and interaction between hypersensitive sites in the active β-globin locus. *Molecular Cell, 10,* 1453–1465.

9. Zhou, D., Liu, K., Sun, C. W., et al. (2010). KLF1 regulates BCL11A expression and gamma to beta-globin switching. *Nat Genet, 42,* 742–744.

10. Allen, B. W., Stamler, J. S., & Piantadosi, C. A. (2009). Hemoglobin, nitric oxide and molecular mechanisms of hypoxic vasodilation. *Trends Mol Med, 15,* 452–460.

11. Steinberg, M. H. (2014). Hemoglobins with altered oxygen affinity, unstable hemoglobins, M-hemoglobins, and dyshemoglobinemias. In Greer, J. P., Arber, D. A., Glader, B., et al. (Eds.), *Wintrobe's Clinical Hematology.* (13th ed., pp. 914–926). Philadelphia: Lippincott Williams & Wilkins.

12. Benz, E. J., Jr., & Ebert, B. L. (2018). Hemoglobin variants associated with hemolytic anemia altered oxygen affinity, and methemoglobinemias. In Hoffman, R., Benz, E. J., Silberstein, L. E., et al. (Eds.), *Hematology Basic Principles and Practice.* (7th ed., pp. 608–615). Philadelphia: Elsevier.

13. Skold, A., Cosco, D. I., & Klein, R. (2011). Methemoglobinemia: pathogenesis, diagnosis, and management. *South Med J, 104,* 757–761.

14. Vajpayee, N., Graham, S. S., & Bem, S. (2017). Basic examination of blood and bone marrow. In McPherson, R. A., & Pincus, M. R. (Eds.), *Henry's Clinical Diagnosis and Management by Laboratory Methods.* (23rd ed., pp. 510–539). St. Louis: Elsevier.

15. Guzman, J. A. (2012). Carbon monoxide poisoning. *Crit Care Clin, 28,* 537–548.

16. CLSI. (2000). *Reference and Selected Procedures for the Quantitative Determination of Hemoglobin in Blood.* (3rd ed., CLSI guideline H15-A3). Wayne, PA: Clinical and Laboratory Standards Institute.

Iron Kinetics and Laboratory Assessment

Kathryn Doig

OBJECTIVES

After completion of this chapter, the reader will be able to:

1. Describe the essential metabolic processes in which iron participates.
2. State whether body iron is regulated by excretion or absorption.
3. Describe the compartments in which body iron is distributed, including the relative amounts in each site.
4. Trace a molecule of iron from its absorption through the enterocyte to transport into mitochondria and then recycling via macrophages, including the names of all proteins with which it interacts and that control its kinetics.
5. Name the ionic form and number of molecules of iron that bind to one molecule of apotransferrin.
6. Explain how hepcidin regulates body iron levels.
7. Explain how individual cells acquire iron.
8. Explain how individual cells regulate the amount of iron they absorb.
9. Describe the role of each of the following in the kinetics of iron, including its location or source tissue:
   a. Divalent metal transporter 1
   b. Ferroportin
   c. Transferrin
   d. Transferrin receptor 1
   e. Transferrin receptor 2
   f. Hepcidin
   g. Erythroferrone
   h. Ferritin
10. For the proteins listed in objective 9, distinguish those that are involved in the kinetics of iron within individual cells versus those involved in systemic body iron regulation.
11. Recognize the names of proteins involved in hepatocyte iron sensing and regulation of hepcidin production, and state which contribute to upregulation or downregulation.
12. List factors that increase and decrease the bioavailability of iron.
13. Name foods high in iron, both heme containing and ionic.
14. For each of the following assays, describe the principle of the assay and the iron compartment assessed:
    a. Total serum iron
    b. Total iron-binding capacity (TIBC)
    c. Percent transferrin saturation
    d. Serum ferritin
    e. Soluble transferrin receptor (sTfR)
    f. Measures of the hemoglobin content of reticulocytes
    g. Prussian blue staining of tissues and cells
    h. Zinc protoporphyrin
15. Plot given patient values on a Thomas plot and interpret the patient's iron status.
16. Calculate the percent transferrin saturation when given total serum iron and TIBC.
17. When given reference intervals, interpret the results of each of the assays in objective 14 plus a Thomas plot and sTfR/log ferritin and recognize results consistent with decreased, normal, and increased iron status.
18. Identify instances in which sTfR, hemoglobin content of reticulocytes, sTfR/log ferritin, and Thomas plots may be needed to improve diagnosis of iron deficiency.

OUTLINE

Iron Chemistry
Iron Kinetics
   Systemic Body Iron Kinetics
   Cellular Iron Kinetics
   Iron Recycling
Dietary Iron, Bioavailability, and Demand
Laboratory Assessment of Body Iron Status
   Serum Iron
   Total Iron-Binding Capacity

Percent Transferrin Saturation
Prussian Blue Staining
Ferritin
Soluble Transferrin Receptor
Hemoglobin Content of Reticulocytes
Soluble Transferrin Receptor/Log Ferritin
Thomas Plot
Zinc Protoporphyrin

CASE STUDY

After studying the material in this chapter, the reader will be able to respond to the following case study:

In 1995, Garry, Koehler, and Simon assessed changes in stored iron in 16 female and 20 male regular blood donors aged 64 to 71.[1] They measured hemoglobin, hematocrit, serum ferritin concentration, and percent transferrin saturation in specimens from the donors, who gave an average of 15 units (approximately 485 mL/unit) of blood over 3.5 years. The investigators collected comparable data from nondonors. Of the donors, 10 women and 6 men took a dietary supplement providing approximately 20 mg of iron per day. In addition, mean dietary iron intake was 18 mg/day for the women and 20 mg/day for the men. Over the period of the study, mean iron stores in women donors decreased from 12.53 to 1.14 mg/kg of body weight. Mean iron stores in male donors declined from 12.45 to 1.92 mg/kg. Nondonors' iron stores remained unchanged. Based on hemoglobin and hematocrit results, no donors became anemic. As iron stores decreased, the calculated iron absorption rose to 3.55 mg/day for the women and 4.10 mg/day for the men—more than double the normal rate for both women and men.

1. Why did the donors' iron stores decrease?
2. Why did the donors' iron absorption rate rise? Explain using the names of all proteins involved.
3. Name the laboratory test(s) performed in the study used to evaluate directly the iron storage compartment?
4. What is the diagnostic value of the percent transferrin saturation?

Among the metals that are required for metabolic processes, none is more important than iron. It is critical to energy production in all cells, being at the center of the cytochromes of mitochondria. Oxygen needed for energy production is carried by iron in the hemoglobin molecule in red blood cells. Iron is so critical to the body that there is no mechanism for active excretion, just minimal daily loss with exfoliated skin and hair and sloughed intestinal epithelia. Iron is even recycled to conserve as much as possible in the body. To insure against times when iron may be scarce in the diet, the body stores iron as well.

The largest percentage of body iron, nearly 70% of it, is held within hemoglobin in red blood cells of various stages (Table 8.1), whereas almost 20% of body iron is in storage, mostly within hepatocytes and macrophages in the spleen and bone marrow.[2] The remaining approximately 10% is divided among the muscles, the cytochromes, various iron-containing enzymes, and the plasma.

A more functional approach to thinking about body iron distribution conceives of the iron as distributed in three compartments (Table 8.1). The *functional compartment* contains all iron that is functioning within cells including iron in hemoglobin, myoglobin (in muscles), and cytochromes (in all cells other than mature red blood cells). The *storage compartment* is the iron that is not currently functioning but is available when needed. The major repositories of this stored iron are the macrophages and hepatocytes, but every cell, except mature red blood cells, stores some iron for its own use. The third compartment is the *transport compartment* of iron that is in transit from one body site to another in the plasma.

Although the reactivity of iron ions makes them central to energy production processes, it also makes them dangerous to the stability of cells. Thus the body regulates iron carefully at the level of the whole body and also within individual cells, maintaining levels that are necessary for critical metabolic processes, while avoiding the dangers of excess iron accumulation. The conditions that develop when this balance is perturbed are described in Chapter 17. The routine tests used to assess body iron status are discussed here.

IRON CHEMISTRY

The metabolic functions of iron depend on its ability to change its valence state from reduced ferrous (Fe^{2+}) iron to the oxidized ferric (Fe^{3+}) state. Thus it is involved in oxidation and reduction reactions such as the electron transport within mitochondrial cytochromes. In cells, ferrous iron can react with peroxide via the Fenton reaction, forming highly reactive oxygen molecules.

$$Fe^{2+} + H_2O_2 = Fe^{3+} + HO^- + OH\bullet$$

The resulting hydroxyl radical ($OH\bullet$), also known as a free radical, is especially reactive as a short-lived but potent oxidizing agent, able to damage proteins, lipids, and nucleic acids. As will be described in the section on iron kinetics, there are various mechanisms within the body and individual cells to reduce the potential for this type of damage.

TABLE 8.1	Iron Compartments in Normal Humans		
Compartment	Form and Anatomic Site	Approximate Percent of Total Body Iron	Typical Iron Content (g)
Functional	Hemoglobin iron in the blood	68	2.400
	Myoglobin iron in muscles	10	0.360
	Peroxidase, catalase, cytochromes, riboflavin enzymes in all cells	3	0.120
Storage	Ferritin and hemosiderin mostly in macrophages and hepatocytes; small amounts in all cells except mature red blood cells	18	0.667
Transport	Transferrin in plasma	<1	0.001

IRON KINETICS

Systemic Body Iron Kinetics

Figure 8.1 provides an overview of systemic body iron regulation that can be a reference throughout the section on iron kinetics. The total amount of iron available to all body cells, systemic body iron, is regulated by absorption into the body because there is no mechanism for excretion.

Absorption of Iron in the Intestines

Iron can be absorbed in the intestines as heme from animal food sources or as ionic iron, mostly from vegetable sources. The means by which heme is absorbed by enterocytes is not entirely clear. Although one carrier has been identified,[3] it is actually more efficient at carrying folic acid.[4,5] So the primary heme carrier protein is still being sought.[6] Nevertheless, once the heme enters the enterocyte, likely by receptor-mediated endocytosis, the iron is freed from protoporphyrin by heme oxygenase (Figure 8.2).[7] The iron is exported from the endosome (discussed later) and enters the enterocyte cytoplasm.

Most dietary iron is nonheme ionic iron in the ferric form and must be reduced by duodenal cytochrome b (Dcytb) before it can enter the enterocyte (Figure 8.2). Once the iron is in reduced form, it is carried across the luminal side of the enterocyte by divalent metal transporter 1 (DMT1) (Figure 8.2).

Whether derived from heme or absorbed as an ion, the ferric iron can be stored as ferritin (discussed later) and used for enterocyte needs. However, most of the iron will be chaperoned through the cytoplasm to the basolaminal side of the enterocyte for transport into the plasma, though the exact nature of the chaperone remains unknown.[8]

The protein on the basolaminal side of the enterocyte that exports ferrous iron into the blood, thus truly absorbing it into the body, is ferroportin. Ferroportin is the only known protein that exports iron across cell membranes. When the body has adequate stores of iron, the hepatocytes sense that and will increase production of hepcidin, a protein able to bind to ferroportin, leading to its inactivation.[9] As a result, iron absorption into the body decreases. When the body iron begins to drop, the liver senses that change and decreases hepcidin production. As a result, ferroportin is once again active and able to transport iron into the blood. Thus homeostasis of iron is maintained by modest fluctuations in liver hepcidin production in response to body iron status. The regulation of systemic body iron is summarized in Figure 8.3.

Regulation of hepcidin production is important to understanding iron kinetics, particularly in the disease states

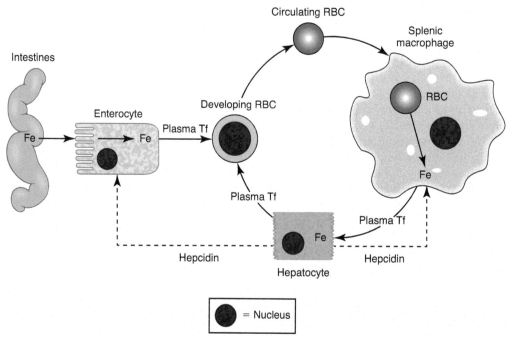

Figure 8.1 Overview of the Iron Cycle Regulating Systemic Body Iron. Iron is absorbed through the enterocyte of the duodenum and into the plasma via the portal circulation. There it binds to apotransferrin to form transferrin (Tf) for transport to cells, such as the developing red blood cells. In red blood cells the iron is used in hemoglobin that circulates with the cell until it becomes aged and is ingested by a macrophage. There the iron is removed from the hemoglobin and can be recycled into the blood for use by other cells. The level of stored and circulating body iron is detected by the hepatocyte, which is able to produce a protein, hepcidin, when iron levels get too high. Hepcidin will inactivate the absorption and recycling of iron by acting on enterocytes, macrophages, and hepatocytes. When body iron decreases, hepcidin will also decrease so that absorption and recycling are again activated. (From Doig, K. [2013]. *Iron: The Body's Most Precious Metal.* [p. 1]. McLean, VA: American Society for Clinical Laboratory Science.)

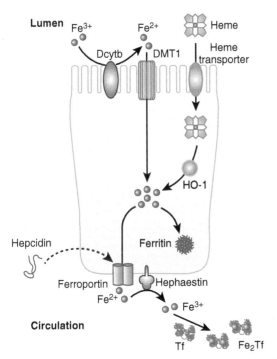

Figure 8.2 Absorption of Iron in the Small Intestine. Ferric iron (Fe^{3+}) in the intestinal lumen is reduced (Fe^{2+}) before transport across the luminal membrane of the enterocyte by the ferrireductase, duodenal cytochrome b (Dcytb). It is then able to be transported through the luminal membrane into the enterocyte cytoplasm by divalent metal transporter 1 (DMT1). Iron can also be absorbed as heme by an enterocyte membrane heme transporter. The iron is removed from heme by heme oxygenase-1 (HO-1). Some iron may be stored as ferritin. Most is chaperoned to the opposite membrane and carried into the blood by ferroportin. It is reoxidized by hephaestin as it exits for transport in the blood by transferrin (Tf). Hepcidin is a protein of hepatic origin that inhibits ferroportin from transporting iron out of the enterocyte. (Modified from Brittenham, G. M. [2018]. Pathophysiology of iron homeostasis. In: Hoffman, R., Benz, E. J., Silberstein, L. E., et al. (Eds.), *Hematology: Basic Principles and Practice.* [7th ed., p. 476, Figure 35.8]. Philadelphia: Elsevier; and Anderson, G. J., Frazer, D. M., & McLaren, G. D. [2009]. Iron absorption and metabolism. *Curr Opin Gastroenterol, 25,* p. 130, Figure 1.)

discussed in Chapter 17, but it first requires an understanding of iron transport by transferrin.

Iron Transport in the Blood

Iron exported from the enterocyte into the blood is ferrous and must be converted to the ferric form for transport in the blood. Hephaestin, a protein on the basolaminal enterocyte membrane, is able to oxidize iron as it exits the enterocyte. Once oxidized, the iron is ready for plasma transport, carried by a specific protein, apotransferrin (ApoTf) (Figure 8.2). Once iron binds, the molecule is known as transferrin (Tf). Apotransferrin binds up to two molecules of ferric iron and thus when fully loaded is often referred to as diferric transferrin or holotransferrin.

Regulation of Body Iron

The mechanism by which the hepatocytes are able to sense body iron levels and respond with hepcidin adjustments has been an area of intense research because it may hold the key to treatments for iron-related anemias (Chapter 17). Research to date has centered on two separate pathways regulating hepcidin production, with transferrin receptor 2 (TfR2) involved in both as the iron sensor.

The hepatic system for regulating hepcidin is modeled in Figure 8.4. The proteins involved include, at least, transferrin receptor 1 (TfR1), the hemochromatosis receptor (HFE), TfR2, hemojuvelin (HJV), bone morphogenic protein (BMP) and its receptor (BMPR), sons of mothers against decapentaplegic (SMAD), and matriptase-2.[10] Table 8.2 lists their functions.

When body iron is replete and transferrin is well saturated, there is more diferric transferrin available to bind to the TfR1 and TfR2 on hepatocytes. This binding contributes to a sequence of cell signaling events involving the proteins in Table 8.2 that results in the secretion of hepcidin. Hepcidin is carried in the blood to the enterocytes and macrophages, where it binds to ferroportin and leads to its inactivation, thus restricting

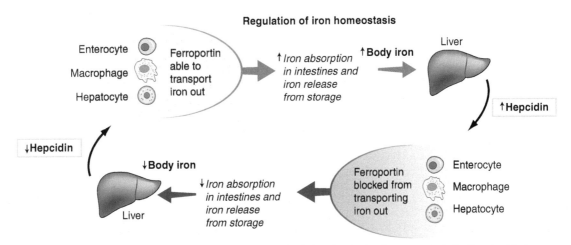

Figure 8.3 Regulation of Iron Homeostasis. When body iron levels rise (upper center), the liver is able to detect it. As a result, production of hepcidin is upregulated and secreted into the blood, where it travels to the iron-regulating cells, enterocytes, macrophages, and hepatocytes. Hepcidin will react with ferroportin in their membranes and prevent iron from exiting those cells into the blood. As a result, body iron will decline and the liver will sense it. Hepcidin production will be curtailed. As a result, ferroportin in the membranes of the iron-regulating cells will then be active and transport iron into the plasma. The cycle then repeats.

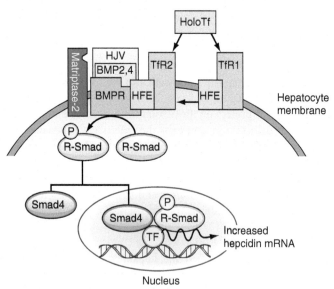

Figure 8.4 Hepatic Iron-Sensing System Leading to Hepcidin Production. One system of iron sensing by hepatocytes involves the release of the hemochromatosis receptor (HFE) from transferrin receptor 1 (TfR1) when the latter binds holotransferrin (HoloTf). The freed HFE then associates with transferrin receptor 2 (TfR2) that has bound HoloTf, bone morphogenetic protein receptor (BMPR), its ligands BMP 2 and 4, and its coreceptor, hemojuvelin (HJV). The complex is able to initiate a transcription signal by phosphorylating (P) sons of mothers against decapentaplegic (SMAD) proteins. The SMAD proteins transfer to the nucleus to activate a transcription factor (TF) that ultimately increases hepcidin production. Matriptase-2 can inactivate HJV, thus interrupting the signal transduction, and is an important mechanism to reduce hepcidin production when body iron is low. (Modified from Ganz, T. [2008]. Iron homeostasis: Fitting the puzzle pieces together. *Cell Metab, 7*, p. 290, Figure 1.)

entrance of iron into the blood. Conversely, when body iron is low, there is less diferric transferrin to trigger this pathway. In this case hepcidin production declines, ferroportin is more active, and more iron enters the blood.

The importance of the proteins in Table 8.2 to iron kinetics has been demonstrated via mutations, both natural in humans and induced in mice, that lead to either iron overload or iron deficiency. Testing for these mutations is increasing in molecular diagnostic laboratories. The diseases associated with the known human mutations are described in Chapter 17.

A second mechanism involving erythroblasts (immature red blood cells) in regulating iron kinetics has become more clear in recent years with the discovery of erythroferrone (ERFE).[11] The gene for ERFE is erythropoietin (EPO) responsive.[12] In anemias with elevated EPO levels, erythroblasts, mainly polychromatic normoblasts,[13] secrete ERFE. ERFE then acts on the liver, through mechanisms yet to be described, to reduce hepcidin production and increase iron absorption in the small intestine.[13] Thus by ERFE production, developing red blood cells control the availability of iron for their hemoglobin production. This mechanism appears to explain the excess absorption of iron in anemias, like thalassemia, in which ineffective erythropoiesis increases the number of erythroblasts that secrete ERFE.[13]

The details of the mechanism for EPO-stimulated ERFE production in erythroblasts are not yet fully elucidated. However, like hepatocytes, erythroblasts carry the TfR2, which acts as an iron sensor. TfR2 appears to enhance erythrocyte sensitivity to EPO by stabilizing the EPO receptor, thereby rescuing more cells from apoptosis, and increasing the number of cells producing ERFE.[14] Although two other products of erythroblasts, growth differentiation factor-15 (GDF-15) and twisted

TABLE 8.2   Functions and Locations of Proteins Involved in Body Iron Sensing and Hepcidin Production

Protein	Location	Function
Transferrin receptor 1 (TfR1)	Hepatocyte membrane	Binds circulating diferric transferrin and releases hemochromatosis protein (HFE) for signaling
Hemochromatosis protein (HFE)	Hepatocyte membrane	With transferrin receptor 2, associates with bone morphogenetic protein receptor (BMPR) to initiate the signal to upregulate hepcidin production
Transferrin receptor 2 (TfR2)	Hepatocyte membrane	With freed HFE, associates with BMPR to initiate the signal to upregulate hepcidin production
Bone morphogenetic protein (BMP)	Secreted product	The ligand that initiates signal transduction when it binds to its receptor in a cell membrane
Bone morphogenetic protein receptor (BMPR)	Hepatocyte (and other cells) membrane	A common membrane receptor initiating signal transduction within a cell when its ligand (BMP) binds
Hemojuvelin (HJV)	Hepatocyte membrane	A coreceptor acting with BMPR for signal transduction, leading to hepcidin production
Sons of mothers against decapentaplegic (SMAD)	Hepatocyte (and other cells) cytoplasm	A second messenger of signal transduction, phosphorylated by BMPR-HJV complex, and able to migrate to the nucleus and upregulate hepcidin gene expression
Matriptase-2	Hepatocyte membrane	Cleaves hemojuvelin to downregulate hepcidin production
Transferrin receptor 2 (TfR2)	Erythroblast membrane	Binds holotransferrin (Tf), which initiates a signal leading to secretion of erythroferrone
Erythroferrone (ERFE)	Secreted by erythroblasts	Able to downregulate hepcidin production in the liver; mechanism unknown

gastrulation protein homolog 1 (TWSG1), have been found to affect hepcidin production, their in vivo effect in humans appears to be minimal.[12]

Cellular Iron Kinetics

Cellular Iron Acquisition and Disposition

To this point the discussion has focused on absorption of iron from the diet into the body and its regulation. The focus now shifts to how individual cells are able to acquire the iron they need for their metabolic processes, and particularly to the erythroblasts that have the greatest iron demand of any body cell.

Individual cells tightly regulate the amount of iron they absorb to minimize the adverse effects of free radicals. This is accomplished by relying on a specific carrier to move iron into the cell by a process called *receptor-mediated endocytosis* (Figure 8.5). Cell membranes, including those of developing erythroblasts, possess a receptor for transferrin, TfR1. TfR1 has the highest affinity for diferric transferrin at the physiologic pH of the plasma and extracellular fluid. When TfR1 molecules bind transferrin, they move within the membrane and cluster together. Once a critical mass accumulates, the membrane begins to invaginate, progressing until the invagination pinches off a vesicle inside the cytoplasm called an *endosome*. Hydrogen

ions are pumped into the endosome. The resulting drop in pH changes the affinity of transferrin for iron, so the iron releases. Simultaneously, the affinity of TfR1 for apotransferrin at that pH increases so the apotransferrin remains bound to the receptor. The iron is exported from the endosome into the cytoplasm by DMT1.

Cytoplasmic trafficking of iron is still not fully understood despite significant research efforts. Multiple avenues are likely with some perhaps unique to erythroblasts. Some of the iron clearly finds its way to storage. There is evidence that other atoms of iron are transferred directly into the mitochondria from the endosome.[15-17] This process whereby the endosome and the mitochondria touch during iron transfer has been called "kiss and run" because the encounter is brief. In the mitochondria, iron atoms are incorporated into cytochromes, or in the case of erythroblasts, into heme for the production of hemoglobin. The direct transfer of iron into the mitochondria appears to be especially important in erythroblasts. It bypasses cytoplasmic systems that limit iron acquisition in most cells. This cytoplasmic bypass allows erythroblasts to acquire the additional iron needed for hemoglobin production.

After release of the iron to the cytoplasm, the endosome returns to the cell membrane, where its membrane fuses with the cell membrane, opening the endosome and essentially reversing

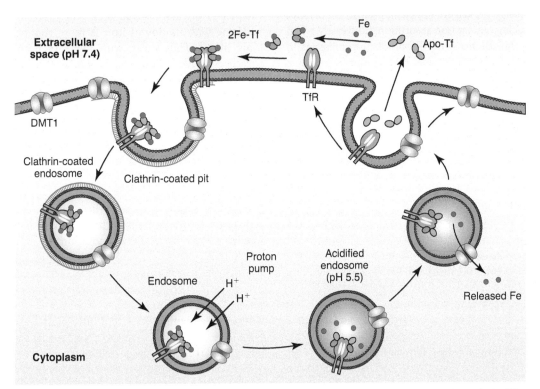

Figure 8.5 Cellular Iron Regulation. A critical mass of transferrin receptor 1 (TfR) with bound transferrin (Tf) will initiate an invagination of the membrane that ultimately fuses to form an endosome. Hydrogen ion (H⁺) inside the endosome releases the iron from Tf, and once reduced, it is transported into the cytosol by divalent mental transporter 1 (DMT1). In the cytosol, iron may be stored as ferritin or transferred to the mitochondria, where it is transported across the membrane by mitoferrin (not shown). The TfR with apotransferrin is returned to the cell membrane, where the ApoTf releases and the TfR is available to bind more Tf for iron transport into the cell. (Courtesy Thomas Walz, PhD)

its formation. At the pH of the extracellular fluid, TfR1 has a very low affinity for apotransferrin, so the apotransferrin releases into the plasma, available to bind iron once again. The TfR1 is also available again to carry new molecules of iron-carrying transferrin into the cell.

Cellular Iron Storage

Cells are able to store iron so they have a reserve if supplies of new iron decline. Although all cells, except mature erythrocytes, store iron, those cells that are central to recycling systemic body iron, macrophages and hepatocytes, contain the most (discussed later).

Ferric iron is stored in a cage-like protein called apoferritin. Once iron binds, it is known as *ferritin.* One ferritin molecule can bind more than 4000 iron ions.[18] Although ferritin is typically considered a cytoplasmic protein, it has been established that mitochondria contain ferritin as well.[19,20]

Ferritin iron can be mobilized for use during times of iron need by lysosomal degradation of the protein.[21] Partially degraded ferritin is known as hemosiderin[22] and is considered to be less metabolically available than ferritin, though greater understanding of ferritin chemistry may revise this view.

To regulate the amount of iron inside the cell and avoid free radicals, cells are able to control the amount of TfR1 on their surface. The process depends on an elegant system of iron-sensitive cytoplasmic proteins that are able to affect the posttranscriptional function of the mRNA for TfR1.[23] The result is that when iron stores inside the cell are sufficient, production of TfR1 declines, thus reducing cellular iron absorption. Conversely, when iron stores inside the cell are low, TfR1 production increases to acquire more iron. It is this process that erythroblasts must circumvent to acquire enough iron for hemoglobin production. The change in the amount of TfR1 in response to available iron is useful diagnostically to detect iron deficiency (discussed later).

Iron Recycling

When cells die, their iron is recycled. Multiple mechanisms salvage iron from dying cells. The largest percentage of recycled iron comes from red blood cells. Senescent (aging) red blood cells are ingested by macrophages in the spleen. The hemoglobin is degraded, with the iron being held by the macrophages as ferritin. Like enterocytes, macrophages possess ferroportin in their membranes.[24] This allows macrophages to be iron exporters so that the salvaged iron can be used by other cells. The exported iron is bound to plasma apotransferrin, just as if it were newly absorbed from the intestine.

Haptoglobin and hemopexin are plasma proteins that salvage plasma hemoglobin or heme, respectively, freed during fragmentation hemolysis. Because they are proteins, they do not pass readily through the glomerulus into the urine, so the bound heme iron is retained in the body. Macrophages carry a receptor for the haptoglobin-hemoglobin complex, whereas hepatocytes have a hemopexin-heme receptor, making them both important cells in iron salvage. Hepatocytes also possess ferroportin so that the salvaged iron can be exported to transferrin and ultimately to other body cells.[25] These salvage pathways are described in greater detail in Chapter 20.

DIETARY IRON, BIOAVAILABILITY, AND DEMAND

Under normal circumstances, the majority of iron for cellular processes, including hemoglobin production, derives from the recycling process described earlier. A small amount of new iron is needed daily and is acquired from the diet. Foods containing high levels of iron include red meats, legumes, and dark green leafy vegetables.[26] Although some foods may be high in iron, that iron may not be readily absorbed and thus is not bioavailable. As mentioned earlier, iron can be absorbed as either ionic iron or nonionic iron in the form of heme. Ionic iron must be in the ferrous (Fe^{2+}) form for absorption into the enterocyte via the luminal membrane carrier, DMT1. However, most dietary iron is ferric, especially from plant sources. As a result, it is not readily absorbed. Furthermore, other dietary compounds can bind iron and inhibit its absorption. These include oxalates, phytates, phosphates, and calcium.[26] Release from these binders and reduction to the ferrous form are enhanced by gastric acid, acidic foods (e.g., citrus), and an enterocyte luminal membrane ferrireductase, duodenal cytochrome b (Dcytb).[27] Nevertheless, absorption of ionic iron is limited and although the US diet contains on the order of 10 to 20 mg of iron/day, only 1 to 2 mg is absorbed.[26] This amount is adequate for most men, but menstruating women, pregnant and lactating women, and growing children usually need additional iron supplementation to meet their increased need for iron. Chapter 17 discusses this further.

Heme with its bound iron is more readily absorbed than ionic iron.[28] Thus meat, with heme in both myoglobin of muscle and hemoglobin of blood, is the most bioavailable source of dietary iron.

LABORATORY ASSESSMENT OF BODY IRON STATUS

Disease occurs when body iron levels are either too low or too high (Chapter 17). The tests used to assess body iron status are able to detect both conditions. The screening tests for iron status include serum iron, total iron-binding capacity, percent transferrin saturation, and serum ferritin. When the results of screening assays are equivocal, additional tests include Prussian blue staining of tissues, soluble transferrin receptor (sTfR), and hemoglobin content of reticulocytes. The results of measured parameters can be combined to calculate a sTfR/log ferritin ratio or graph a Thomas plot. Finally, zinc protoporphyrin is another assay with special application in sideroblastic anemia. Diagnostically the tests can be organized to assess each of the iron compartments as indicated in Table 8.3.

Serum Iron

Serum iron can be measured colorimetrically using any of several reagents such as ferrozine. The iron is first released from transferrin by acid, and then the reagent is allowed to react with the freed iron, forming a colored complex that can be detected spectrophotometrically. Reference intervals are reported separately for men, women, and children and will vary from

TABLE 8.3 Assessment of Body Iron Status

Laboratory Assay	Typical Adult Male Reference Interval	Diagnostic Use and Compartment Assessed
Serum iron level	50–160 µg/dL	Indicator of available transport iron
Total iron-binding capacity	250–400 µg/dL	Indirect indicator of transferrin level
Transferrin saturation	20%–55%	Indirect indicator of transport iron and transferrin level
Serum ferritin level	40–400 ng/mL	Indicator of iron stores
Bone marrow or liver biopsy with Prussian blue staining	Normal iron stores visualized	Visual qualitative assessment of tissue iron stores
Soluble transferrin receptor (sTfR) level	1.15–2.75 mg/L	Indicator of functional iron available in cells
sTfR/log ferritin index	0.63–1.8	Indicator of functional iron available in cells
RBC zinc protoporphyrin level	< 80 µg/dL of RBCs	Indicator of functional iron available in red blood cells
Hemoglobin content of reticulocytes	27–34 pg/cell	Indicator of functional iron available in developing red blood cells

RBC, Red blood cell.

laboratory to laboratory and from method to method. The serum iron level has limited utility on its own because of its high within-day and between-day variability; it also increases after recent ingestion of iron-containing foods and supplements. To avoid the apparent diurnal variation, the standard practice has been to collect the specimen fasting and early in the morning when levels are expected to be highest. However, this practice has recently been questioned.[29] A diurnal variation in hepcidin has been detected that may explain some of the serum iron variability and may still support the early-morning phlebotomy practice.[30,31] A typical reference interval is provided in Table 8.3.

Total Iron-Binding Capacity

The amount of iron in plasma or serum will be limited by the amount of transferrin that is available to carry it. To assess this, transferrin is maximally saturated by addition of excess ferric iron to the specimen. Any unbound iron is removed by precipitation with magnesium carbonate powder. Then the basic iron method as described in the previous section is performed on the absorbed serum, beginning with the release of the iron from transferrin. The amount of iron detected represents all the binding sites available on transferrin, that is, the total iron-binding capacity (TIBC). It is expressed as an iron value, although it is actually an indirect measure of transferrin. A typical reference interval is provided in Table 8.3.

Percent Transferrin Saturation

Because the serum iron (SI) represents the number of transferrin sites bound with iron and the TIBC represents the total number of transferrin sites for iron binding, the degree to which the available sites are occupied by iron can be calculated. The percent of transferrin saturated with iron is calculated as:

$$SI/TIBC \times 100\% = \% \text{ transferrin saturation}$$

It is important that both the SI and TIBC be expressed in the same units, but it does not matter which units are used in the calculation. A typical reference interval is provided in Table 8.3. A convenient rule of thumb evident from the table is that about one-third of transferrin is typically saturated with iron.

Prussian Blue Staining

Prussian blue is actually a chemical compound with the formula $Fe_7(CN)_{18}$.[32] The compound forms during the staining process, which uses acidic potassium ferrocyanide as the reagent/stain. The ferric iron in the tissue reacts with the reagent, forming the Prussian blue compound that is readily seen microscopically as dark blue granules or precipitate. Tissues can be graded or scored semiquantitatively by the amount of stain that is observed.

Prussian blue stain is considered the gold standard for assessment of body iron stores. Staining is conducted routinely when bone marrow or liver biopsies are collected for other purposes. Although ferric iron reacts with the reagent, ferritin is not typically detected, likely because of the intact protein cage. In high concentration, it can appear as a diffuse cytoplasmic blueness.[33] However, hemosiderin stains readily, forming distinct dark blue granules.

Ferritin

Ferritin is the iron-storage protein that functions mainly within cells, though a role for plasma ferritin as an iron transporter is under study.[34] Macrophages, including Kupffer cells, and hepatocytes have been demonstrated to secrete ferritin during in vitro studies,[35,36] yet the precise source of the plasma protein remains uncertain.[34]

Until the development of serum ferritin assays, the only way to truly assess body iron stores was to collect a bone marrow specimen and stain it with Prussian blue. Such an invasive procedure prevented regular assessment of body iron. The development of the serum immunoassay for ferritin has provided a convenient, minimally invasive, quantitative assessment of body iron stores. The level of serum ferritin has been found to correlate highly with stored iron as assessed by Prussian blue stains of bone marrow.[37] Typical reference intervals are provided in Table 8.3.

There is a significant drawback in the interpretation of serum ferritin results. Ferritin is an acute phase protein or acute phase reactant (APR).[38] The APRs are proteins that are produced, mostly by the liver, during the acute (or initial) phase of inflammation, especially during infections. They include cytokines that are nonspecific, but also other proteins with the apparent intent to suppress bacteria. Because bacteria need iron, the body's production of ferritin during an infection seems to be an attempt to sequester the iron away from the bacteria, which may be the role for plasma ferritin. Thus increases in ferritin can be induced without an increase in the amount of systemic body iron (a falsely increased result). These rises may not exceed the reference interval but may still be high enough to elevate a patient's ferritin to greater than what it would otherwise be. Ferritin values between 30 and 100 ng/mL are most equivocal, making it difficult to recognize true iron deficiency when an inflammatory condition is also present.[39] Therefore the predictive value of a ferritin result within the reference interval is weak. However, only a decreased level of stored body iron can lower ferritin levels to less than the reference interval, so the predictive value of a low ferritin result is high for iron deficiency.

Soluble Transferrin Receptor

As described previously, cells regulate the amount of TfR1 on their membrane based on the amount of intracellular iron. When the intracellular iron drops, the cell expresses more TfR1 on the membrane. A truncated form of the receptor is shed into the plasma and can be detected by immunoassay.[40] Thus increases in the soluble receptor, sTfR, reflect either increases in the amounts of TfR1 on individual cells, as in iron deficiency, or an increase in the number of cells each with a normal amount of TfR1. The latter occurs during instances of rapid erythropoiesis, such as a response to hemolytic anemia. Typical reference intervals are provided in Table 8.3.

Hemoglobin Content of Reticulocytes

Chapter 12 describes how some automated blood cell analyzers are able to report a value for the amount of hemoglobin in reticulocytes; it is analogous to the mean cell hemoglobin (MCH), but just for reticulocytes. Because, under normal conditions, the number of circulating reticulocytes represents the status of erythropoiesis in the prior 24-hour period, the amount of hemoglobin in reticulocytes provides a near real-time assessment of iron available for hemoglobin production.[41] The hemoglobin content of reticulocytes will drop when iron for erythropoiesis is restricted. A representative adult reference interval is provided in Table 8.3. Separate reference intervals may be provided for children and infants. Instrument assessment of this parameter is proprietary and each manufacturer refers to their parameter with a different name (Chapter 12).

Soluble Transferrin Receptor/Log Ferritin

Although ferritin and sTfR values alone can point to iron deficiency, the ratio of sTfR to ferritin or sTfR to log ferritin improves the identification of iron deficiency when individual assay values are equivocal.[42,43] Because the sTfR rises in iron deficiency and the ferritin (and its log) drops, these ratios are especially useful to amplify changes when one of the parameters has changed but is not outside the reference interval. A typical reference interval is provided in Table 8.3.

Thomas Plot

Thomas and Thomas[44] demonstrated that when the sTfR/log ferritin is plotted against the hemoglobin content of reticulocytes, a four-quadrant plot results that can improve the identification of iron deficiency (Figure 8.6).[45] In instances where there is *true iron deficiency*, the sTfR will rise and the ferritin will drop so that the sTfR/log ferritin will be high and the hemoglobin content of reticulocytes will be low; patient results will plot to the lower right quadrant. In instances where the ferritin may be falsely elevated by inflammation, the sTfR/log ferritin will be normal despite reduced availability of iron for hemoglobin production resulting in a low hemoglobin content in reticulocytes. In this instance patient values will plot to the lower left quadrant called *functional iron deficiency* because the systemic body stores are adequate but not available for transport and use by cells. As iron deficiency develops, other cells are starved for iron before erythrocytes; production of hemoglobin in reticulocytes remains at a normal level for as long as possible. However, the body's other iron-starved cells will increase sTfR production and systemic iron stores of ferritin will be depleted, thus elevating the sTfR/log ferritin value. These early iron-deficient patients' results will plot to the upper right quadrant called *latent iron deficiency*. By incorporating several different assessments of iron status, the use of the *Thomas plot*, as it is called, can improve the identification of iron deficiency in instances when other tests are equivocal. Chapter 17 will elucidate further the impact of various diseases on the parameters of the Thomas plot.

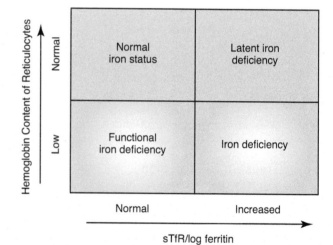

THOMAS PLOT

Figure 8.6 Thomas Plot. Plotting the ratio of soluble transferrin receptor to log ferritin (sTfR/log ferritin) against the hemoglobin content of reticulocytes produces a graph with four quadrants. Patients with values within the reference intervals for each assay will cluster in the upper left quadrant. Those with functional iron deficiency, like the anemia of chronic inflammation, will cluster at the lower left. Latent iron deficiency, before anemia develops, will cluster at the upper right with frank iron deficiency in the lower right quadrant. (Modified from Doig, K. [2013]. *Iron: The Body's Most Precious Metal.* [p. 24]. McLean, VA: American Society for Clinical Laboratory Science.)

Zinc Protoporphyrin

Zinc protoporphyrin (ZPP) accumulates in red blood cells when iron is not incorporated into heme and zinc binds instead to protoporphyrin IX. It is easily detected by fluorescence. Although ZPP will rise during iron-deficient erythropoiesis, the value of this test is greatest when the activity of the ferrochelatase is impaired, as in lead poisoning (Chapter 17).

SUMMARY

- Iron is so critical for transport and use of oxygen that the body conserves and recycles it, and it does not have a mechanism for its active excretion. Free radical production by iron ions severely damages cells and thus demands regulation. The body adjusts its iron levels by intestinal absorption, depending on need.
- Iron is absorbed into enterocytes as ferrous iron by the divalent metal transporter 1 (DMT1) on the luminal side of the cells. Heme can also be absorbed. Iron is exported into the plasma via ferroportin, a protein carrier in the enterocyte basolaminal membrane.
- Iron is carried in the plasma in ferric form attached to apo-transferrin. Each molecule of apotransferrin can bind two molecules of iron. Apotransferrin with two molecules of bound iron is called diferric transferrin or holotransferrin.
- Individual cells absorb iron when diferric transferrin binds to transferrin receptor 1 (TfR1) on their surfaces. Bound receptors cluster and invaginate the membrane to form an endosome. Iron released by acid within the endosome is exported into the cytosol, sometimes directly into mitochondria, for incorporation into cytochromes and heme. Alternatively, it can also be stored as ferritin in the cytosol. The iron-depleted endosome fuses with the cell membrane, releasing the apotransferrin and thus allowing the TfR1 on the cell membrane to bind more diferric transferrin.
- Individual cells adjust the number of transferrin receptors on their surface to regulate the amount of iron they absorb; receptor numbers rise when the cell needs additional iron but decrease when the iron in the cell is adequate. Truncated soluble transferrin receptors (sTfRs) are shed into the plasma in proportion to their number on cells.
- Cells store iron as ferritin when they have an excess. Iron can be released from ferritin when needed by degradation of the protein by lysosomes. Partially degraded ferritin can be detected in cells as stainable hemosiderin. Ferritin is secreted into the plasma in proportion to the amount of iron that is in storage. Ferritin is elevated in plasma by the acute phase response, unrelated to amounts of stored iron.
- When the hepatocyte iron-sensing system detects that body iron levels are high, the hepatocyte secretes hepcidin. Hepcidin inactivates ferroportin in enterocyte, macrophage, and hepatocyte membranes, reducing the body's absorption of new iron and the release of stored iron. When the hepatocyte senses low body iron, hepcidin secretion is reduced and ferroportin is active for intestinal iron absorption and macrophage and hepatocyte iron export and recycling.
- Hepatocytes regulate hepcidin production via two mechanisms. One involves hepatocyte transferrin receptor 2 (TfR2) sensing of transferrin saturation to initiate a transduction signal to modulate hepcidin production. The other mechanism is a response, yet uncertain, to erythroferrone secreted by developing erythroblasts that decreases hepcidin production and increases iron absorption.
- Most body iron is found in hemoglobin or stored as ferritin. Approximately 10% of all body iron is found in muscles, cytochromes and iron-containing enzymes, and plasma.
- Macrophages ingest senescent (aging) red blood cells. They salvage and store the iron derived from heme.
- Dietary iron is most bioavailable as heme from meat sources. Plant sources typically supply ferric iron that must be released from iron-binding compounds and reduced before absorption.
- Laboratory tests for assessment of iron status include total serum iron, total iron-binding capacity, percent transferrin saturation, serum ferritin, Prussian blue staining for iron in tissues, soluble transferrin receptor, the hemoglobin content of reticulocytes, and zinc protoporphyrin. Additional parameters derived from these, sTfR/log ferritin and the Thomas plot, are particularly useful for the recognition of iron deficiency when other test results are equivocal.

Now that you have completed this chapter, go back and read again the case study at the beginning and respond to the questions presented.

REVIEW QUESTIONS

Answers can be found in the Appendix.

1. Iron is transported in plasma via:
   a. Hemosiderin
   b. Ferritin
   c. Transferrin
   d. Hemoglobin

2. What is the major metabolically available storage form of iron in the body?
   a. Hemosiderin
   b. Ferritin
   c. Transferrin
   d. Hemoglobin

3. The total iron-binding capacity (TIBC) of the serum is an indirect measure of which iron-related protein?
   a. Hemosiderin
   b. Ferritin
   c. Transferrin
   d. Haptoglobin

4. For a patient with screening iron study values that are equivocal for iron deficiency, which of the following tests would be most helpful in determining whether iron deficiency is present or not?
   a. Zinc protoporphyrin
   b. Peripheral blood iron stain
   c. Soluble transferrin receptor
   d. Mean cell hemoglobin

5. What membrane-associated protein in enterocytes transports iron from the intestinal lumen into the enterocyte?
   a. DMT1
   b. Ferroportin
   c. Transferrin
   d. Hephaestin

6. Iron is transported out of macrophages, hepatocytes, and enterocytes by what membrane protein?
   a. Transferrin
   b. Ferroportin
   c. DMT1
   d. Ferrochelatase

7. Following are several of the many steps in the process from absorption and transport of iron to incorporation into heme. Place them in proper order.
   i. Transferrin picks up ferric iron.
   ii. Iron is transferred to the mitochondria.
   iii. DMT1 transports ferrous iron into the enterocyte.
   iv. Ferroportin transports iron from enterocyte to plasma.
   v. The transferrin receptor transports iron into the cell.
      a. v, iv, i, ii, iii
      b. iii, ii, iv, i, v
      c. ii, i, v, iii, iv
      d. iii, iv, i, v, ii

8. What is the fate of the transferrin receptor when it has completed its role in the delivery of iron into a cell?
   a. It is recycled to the plasma membrane and released into the plasma.
   b. It is recycled to the plasma membrane, where it can bind its ligand again.
   c. It is catabolized and the amino acids are returned to the metabolic pool.
   d. It is retained in the endosome for the life span of the cell.

9. The transfer of iron from the enterocyte into the plasma is REGULATED by:
   a. Transferrin
   b. Ferroportin
   c. Hephaestin
   d. Hepcidin

10. What is the percent transferrin saturation for a patient with total serum iron of 63 μg/dL and TIBC of 420 μg/dL?
    a. 6.7%
    b. 12%
    c. 15%
    d. 80%

11. Referring to Figure 8.6, into which quadrant of a Thomas plot would a patient's results fall with the following test results:
    Soluble transferrin receptor: increased above reference interval
    Ferritin: decreased below reference interval
    Hemoglobin content of reticulocytes: within the reference interval
    a. Normal iron status
    b. Latent iron deficiency
    c. Functional iron deficiency
    d. Iron deficiency

12. A physician is concerned that a patient is developing iron deficiency from chronic intestinal bleeding caused by aspirin use for rheumatoid arthritis. The iron studies on the patient indicate the following results:

Laboratory Assay	Adult Reference Intervals	Patient Values
Serum ferritin level	12–400 ng/mL	32 ng /mL
Serum iron level	50–160 μg/dL	45 μg/dL
Total iron-binding capacity (TIBC)	250–400 μg/dL	405 μg/dL
Transferrin saturation	20%–55%	CALCULATE IT

How would these results be interpreted?
    a. Latent iron deficiency
    b. Functional iron deficiency
    c. Iron deficiency
    d. Equivocal for iron deficiency

13. Developing erythroblasts in the bone marrow affect the supply of body iron, both absorption and recycling, by secreting which of the following hormones?
    a. Erythropoietin
    b. Erythroferrone
    c. Hepcidin
    d. Haptoglobin

14. Which of the following cells critical to iron trafficking in the body does NOT possess ferroportin?
    a. Erythroblasts
    b. Enterocytes
    c. Hepatocytes
    d. Macrophages

15. Which of the following plays a role in iron sensing so as to adjust iron absorption and recycling?
    a. Hepcidin
    b. Transferrin receptor 2
    c. Ferroportin
    d. Divalent metal transporter 1

REFERENCES

1. Garry, P. J., Koehler, K. M., & Simon, T. L. (1995). Iron stores and iron absorption: effects of repeated blood donations. *Am J Clin Nutr, 62*(3), 611–620.
2. Sharma, N., Butterworth, J., Cooper, B. T., et al. (2005). The emerging role of the liver in iron metabolism. *Am J Gastroenterol, 100*, 201–206.
3. Shayeghi, M., Latunde-Dada, G. O., Oakhill, J. S., et al. (2005). Identification of an intestinal heme transporter. *Cell, 122*(5), 789–801.
4. Le Blanc, S., Garrick, M. D., & Arredondo, M. (2012). Heme carrier protein 1 transports heme and is involved in heme-Fe metabolism. *Am J Physiol Cell Physiol, 302*, C1780–C1785.
5. Laftah, A. H., Latunde-Dada, G. O., Fakih, S., et al. (2009). Haem and folate transport by proton-coupled folate transporter/haem carrier protein 1 (SLC46A1). *Br J Nutr, 101*(8), 1150–1156.
6. Gulec, S., Anderson, G. J., & Collins, J. F. (2014). Mechanistic and regulatory aspects of intestinal iron absorption. *Am J Physiol Gastrointest Liver Physiol, 307*(4), G397–409.
7. West, A. R., & Oates, P. S. (2008). Subcellular location of heme oxygenase 1 and 2 and divalent metal transporter 1 in relation to endocytotic markers during heme iron absorption. *J Gastroenterol Hepatol, 23*(1), 150–158.
8. Philpott, C. C. (2012). Coming into view: eukaryotic iron chaperones and intracellular iron delivery. *J Biol Chem, 287*(17), 13518–13523.
9. Nemeth, E., Tuttle, M.S., Powelson, J., et al. (2004). Hepcidin regulates cellular iron efflux by binding to ferroportin and inducing its internalization. *Science, 306*(5704), 2090–2093.
10. Camaschella, C., & Silvestri, L. (2011). Molecular mechanisms regulating hepcidin revealed by hepcidin disorders. *Scientific World Journal, 11*, 1357–1366.
11. Kautz, L, Jung, G., Valore, E.V., et al. (2014). Identification of erythroferrone as an erythroid regulator of iron metabolism. *Nat Genet, 46*(7), 678–684.
12. Kim, A., & Nemeth, E. (2015). New insights into iron regulation and erythropoiesis. *Curr Opin Hematol, 22*(3), 199–205.
13. Kautz, L., Jung, G., Du, X., et al. (2015). Erythroferrone contributes to hepcidin suppression and iron overload in a mouse model of β-thalassemia. *Blood, 126*(17), 231–237.
14. Nai, A., Lindonnici, M.R., Rausa, M., et al. (2015). The second transferrin receptor regulates red blood cell production in mice. *Blood, 125*(7), 1170–1179.
15. Shaw, G. C., Cope, J. J., Li, L., et al. (2006). Mitoferrin is essential for erythroid iron assimilation. *Nature, 440*(2), 96–100.
16. Richardson, D. R., Lane, D. J. R., Becker, E. M., et al. (2010). Mitochondrial iron trafficking and the integration of iron metabolism between the mitochondrion and cytosol. *PNAS, 107*(24), 10775–10782.
17. Sheftel, A.D., Zhang, A., Brown, C., et al. (2007). Direct interorganellar transfer of iron from endosome to mitochondrion. *Blood, 110*(1), 125–132.
18. Theil, E. C. (1990). The ferritin family of iron storage proteins. *Adv Enzymol Relat Areas Mol Biol, 63*, 421–449.
19. Levi, S., Corsi, B., Bosisio, M., et al. (2001). A human mitochondrial ferritin encoded by an intronless gene. *J Biol Chem, 276*(27), 24437–24440.
20. Lane, Q. J. R., Merlot, A. M., Huang, M. L.-H., et al. (2015). Cellular iron uptake, trafficking and metabolism: key molecules and mechanisms and their roles in disease. *Biochim Biophys Acta, 1853*, 1130–1144.
21. Zhang, Y., Mikhael, M., Xu, D., et al. (2010). Lysosomal proteolysis is the primary degradation pathway for cytosolic ferritin and cytosolic ferritin degradation is necessary for iron exit. *Antioxid Redox Signal, 13*(7), 999–1009.
22. Miyazaki, E., Kato, J., Kobune, M., et al. (2002). Denatured H-ferritin subunit is a major constituent of haemosiderin in the liver of patients with iron overload. *Gut, 50*(3), 413–419.
23. Thomson, A. M., Rogers, J. T., & Leedman, P. J. (1999). Iron-regulatory proteins, iron-responsive elements and ferritin mRNA translation. *Int J Biochem Cell Biol, 31*(10), 1139–1152.
24. Abboud, S., & Haile, D. J. (2000). A novel mammalian iron-regulated protein involved in intracellular iron metabolism. *J Biolog Chem, 275*, 19906–19912.
25. Donovan, A., Lima, C. A., Pinkus, J. L., et al. (2005). The iron exporter ferroportin/Slc40a1 is essential for iron homeostasis. *Cell Metab, 1*(3), 191–200.
26. Hallberg, L. (1981). Bioavailability of dietary iron in man. *Annu Rev Nutr, 1*, 123–147.
27. McKie, A. T., Barrow, D., Latunde-Dada, G. O., et al. (2001). An iron-regulated ferric reductase associated with the absorption of dietary iron. *Science, 291*(5509), 1755–1759.
28. Layrisse, M., Cook, J. D., Martinez, C., et al. (1969). Food iron absorption: a comparison of vegetable and animal foods. *Blood, 33*, 430–443.
29. Dale, J. C., Burritt, M. F., & Zinsmeister, A. R. (2002). Diurnal variation of serum iron, iron-binding capacity, transferrin saturation, and ferritin levels. *Am J Clin Pathol, 117*, 802–808.
30. Schaap, C. C., Hendriks, J. C., Kortman, G. A., et al. (2013). Diurnal rhythm rather than dietary iron mediates daily hepcidin variations. *Clin Chem Mar, 59*(3), 527–535.
31. Kroot, J. J., Hendriks. J. C., Laarakkers, C. M., et al. (2009). (Pre) analytical imprecision, between-subject variability, and daily variations in serum and urine hepcidin: implications for clinical studies. *Anal Biochem, 389*(2), 124–129.
32. Ellis, R. *Perls Prussian Blue Staining Protocol.* http://www.ihcworld.com/_protocols/special_stains/perls_prussian_blue_ellis.htm. Accessed June 8, 2017.
33. Saito, H. (2014). Metabolism of iron stores. *Nagoya J Med Sci, 76*(3-4), 235–254.
34. Wang, W., Knovich, M. A., Coffman, L. G., et al. (2010). Serum ferritin: Past, present and future. *Biochim Biophys Acta, 1800*(8), 760–769.
35. Ghosh, S., Hevi, S., & Chuck, S. L. (2004). Regulated secretion of glycosylated human ferritin from hepatocytes. *Blood, 103*(6), 2369–2376.
36. Cohen, L. A., Gutierrez, L., Weiss, A., et al. (2010). Serum ferritin is derived primarily from macrophages through a nonclassical secretory pathway. *Blood, 116*(9), 1574–1584.
37. Lipschitz, D. A., Cook, J. D., & Finch, C. A. (1974). A clinical evaluation of serum ferritin as an index of iron stores. *N Engl J Med, 290*(22), 1213–1216.
38. Konijn, A. M., & Hershko, C. (1977). Ferritin synthesis in inflammation. I. Pathogenesis of impaired iron release. *Br J Haematol, 37*(1), 7–16.
39. Munoz, M., Garcia-Erce, J. A., & Remacha, A. F. (2011). Disorders of iron metabolism. Part II: iron deficiency and iron overload. *J Clin Pathol, 64*: 287–296.

40. Shih, Y. J., Baynes, R. D., Hudson, B. G., et al. (1990). Serum transferrin receptor is a truncated form of tissue receptor. *J Biol Chem*, *265*, 19077–19081.

41. Brugnara, C., Zurakowski, D., DiCanzio, J., et al. (1999). Reticulocyte hemoglobin content to diagnose iron deficiency in children. *JAMA*, *281*(23), 2225–2230.

42. Punnonen, K., Irjala, K., & Rajamaki, A. (1997). Serum transferrin receptor and its ratio to serum ferritin in the diagnosis of iron deficiency. *Blood*, *89*(3), 1052–1057.

43. Castel, R., Tax, M. G., Droogendijk, J., et al. (2012). The transferrin/log(ferritin) ratio: a new tool for the diagnosis of iron deficiency anemia. *Clin Chem Lab Med*, *50*(8), 1343–1349.

44. Thomas, C., & Thomas, L. (2002). Biochemical markers and hematologic indices in the diagnosis of functional iron deficiency. *Clin Chem*, *48*(7), 1066–1076.

45. Leers, M. P. G., Keuren, J. F. W., & Oosterhuis, W. P. (2010). The value of the Thomas-plot in the diagnostic work up of anemic patients referred by general practitioners. *Int J Lab Hemat*, *32*, 572–581.

Leukocyte Development, Kinetics, and Functions

Reeba A. Omman, Ameet R. Kini*

OBJECTIVES

After completion of this chapter, the reader will be able to:

1. Describe the pathways and progenitor cells involved in the derivation of leukocytes from the hematopoietic stem cell to mature forms.
2. Name the different stages of neutrophil, eosinophil, and basophil development and describe the morphology of each stage.
3. Discuss the important functions of neutrophils, eosinophils, and basophils.
4. Describe the morphology of promonocytes, monocytes, macrophages, T and B lymphocytes, and immature B cells (hematogones).
5. Discuss the functions of monocytes, macrophages, T cells, B cells, and natural killer cells in the immune response.
6. Compare the kinetics of neutrophils and monocytes.
7. Discuss in general terms how the various types of lymphocytes are produced.

OUTLINE

Granulocytes
 Neutrophils
 Eosinophils
 Basophils

 Mast Cells
Mononuclear Cells
 Monocytes
 Lymphocytes

CASE STUDY

After studying the material in this chapter, the reader should be able to respond to the following case study:

A 5-year-old girl presents with shortness of breath and wheezing. The patient gives a history of similar symptoms in the last 6 months. After the patient was given albuterol to control her acute symptoms, long-term control of her disease was achieved through the use of corticosteroids, along with monoclonal antibodies to interleukin-5 (IL-5).

1. Which leukocytes are important in mediating the clinical symptoms in this patient?
2. A complete blood count with differential was performed on this patient. What are the typical findings in such patients?
3. How did monoclonal antibodies to IL-5 help in controlling her disease?

Leukocytes (also known as *white blood cells,* or *WBCs*) are so named because they are relatively colorless compared to red blood cells. The number of different types of leukocytes varies depending on whether they are being viewed with a light microscope after staining with a Romanowsky stain (5 or 6 types) or are identified according to their surface antigens using flow cytometry (at least 10 different types). For the purposes of this chapter, the classic, light microscope classification of leukocytes will be used.

Granulocytes are a group of leukocytes whose cytoplasm is filled with granules with differing staining characteristics and whose nuclei are segmented or lobulated. Individually they include *eosinophils*, with granules containing basic proteins that stain with acid stains such as eosin; *basophils*, with granules that are acidic and stain with basic stains such as methylene blue; and *neutrophils*, with granules that react with both acid and basic stains, which gives them a pink to lavender color. Because nuclear segmentation is quite prominent in mature neutrophils, they have also been called *polymorphonuclear cells*, or *PMNs*.

Mononuclear cells are categorized into *monocytes* and *lymphocytes*. These cells have nuclei that are not segmented but

---

*The authors extend appreciation to Woodlyne Roquiz, Sameer Al Daffalha, and Anne Stiene-Martin, whose work in prior editions provided the foundation for this chapter.

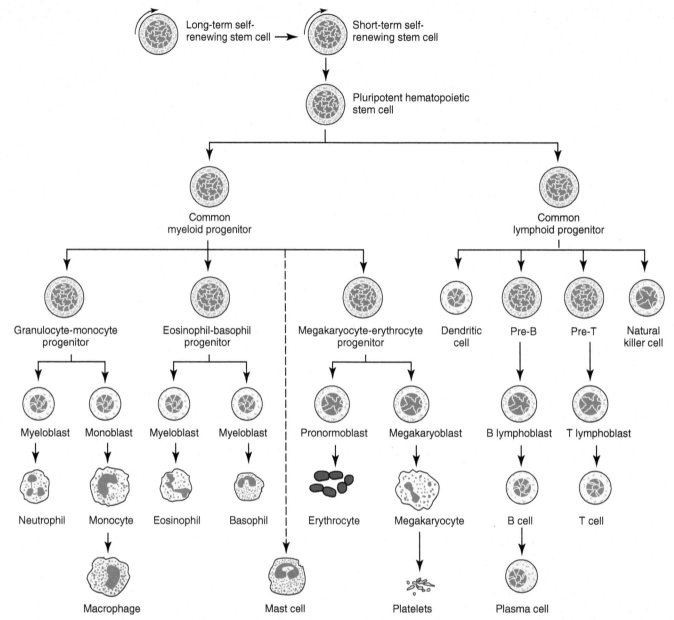

Figure 9.1 Diagram of Hematopoiesis Showing the Derivation Pathways of Each Type of Blood Cell from a Hematopoietic Stem Cell.

are round, oval, indented, or folded. Leukocytes develop from hematopoietic stem cells (HSCs) in the bone marrow, where most undergo differentiation and maturation (Figure 9.1), and then are released into the circulation. The number of circulating leukocytes varies with sex, age, activity, time of day, and ethnicity; it also differs according to whether or not the leukocytes are reacting to stress, being consumed, or being destroyed, and whether or not they are being produced by the bone marrow in sufficient numbers.[1] Reference intervals for total leukocyte counts vary among laboratories, depending on the patient population and the type of instrumentation used,

but a typical reference interval is 4.5×10^9/L to 11.5×10^9/L for adults.

The overall function of leukocytes is in mediating *immunity,* either innate (nonspecific), as in phagocytosis by neutrophils, or specific (adaptive), as in the production of antibodies by lymphocytes and plasma cells. The term *kinetics* refers to the movement of cells through developmental stages, into the circulation, and from the circulation to the tissues and includes the time spent in each phase of the cell's life. As each cell type is discussed in this chapter, developmental stages, kinetics, and specific functions will be addressed.

GRANULOCYTES

Neutrophils

Neutrophils are present in the peripheral blood in two forms according to whether the nucleus is segmented or still in a band shape. Segmented neutrophils make up the vast majority of circulating leukocytes.

Neutrophil Development

Neutrophil development occurs in the bone marrow. Neutrophils share a common progenitor with monocytes and distinct from eosinophils and basophils, known as the granulocyte-monocyte progenitor (GMP).[2] The major cytokine responsible for the stimulation of neutrophil production is granulocyte colony-stimulating factor, or G-CSF.[3,4]

There are three pools of developing neutrophils in the bone marrow (Figure 9.2): the stem cell pool, the proliferation pool, and the maturation pool.[5-8] The stem cell pool consists of HSCs that are capable of self-renewal and differentiation.[9] The proliferation (mitotic) pool consists of cells that are dividing and includes (listed in the order of maturation) common myeloid progenitors (CMPs), also known as colony-forming units–granulocyte, erythrocyte, monocyte, and megakaryocyte (CFU-GEMMs); granulocyte-monocyte progenitors (GMPs); myeloblasts; promyelocytes; and myelocytes. The third marrow pool is the maturation (storage) pool consisting of cells undergoing nuclear maturation that form the marrow reserve and are available for release: metamyelocytes, band neutrophils, and segmented neutrophils.

HSCs, CMPs, and GMPs are not distinguishable with the light microscope and Romanowsky staining and may resemble early type I myeloblasts or lymphoid cells. They can, however, be identified through surface antigen detection by flow cytometry.

Myeloblasts make up 0% to 3% of the nucleated cells in the bone marrow and measure 14 to 20 μm in diameter. They are often subdivided into type I, type II, and type III myeloblasts. The type I myeloblast has a high nucleus-to-cytoplasm (N:C) ratio of 8:1 to 4:1 (the nucleus occupies most of the cell, with very little cytoplasm), slightly basophilic cytoplasm, fine nuclear chromatin, and two to four visible nucleoli. Type I blasts have no visible granules when observed under light microscopy with Romanowsky stains. The type II myeloblast

shows the presence of dispersed *primary (azurophilic) granules* in the cytoplasm; the number of granules does not exceed 20 per cell (Figure 9.3). Type III myeloblasts have a darker chromatin and a more purple cytoplasm, and they contain more than 20 granules that do not obscure the nucleus. Type III myeloblasts are rare in normal bone marrows, but they can be seen in certain types of acute myeloid leukemias. Mufti and colleagues[10] proposed combining type II and type III blasts into a single category of "granular blasts" because of the difficulty in distinguishing type II blasts from type III blasts.

Promyelocytes comprise 1% to 5% of the nucleated cells in the bone marrow. They are relatively larger than the myeloblast cells and measure 16 to 25 μm in diameter. The nucleus is round to oval and is often eccentric. A paranuclear halo or "hof" is usually seen in normal promyelocytes but not in the malignant promyelocytes of acute promyelocytic leukemia (described in Chapter 31). The cytoplasm is evenly basophilic and full of primary (azurophilic) granules. These granules are the first in a series of granules to be produced during neutrophil maturation (Box 9.1).[11] The nucleus is similar to that described earlier for myeloblasts except that chromatin clumping (heterochromatin) may be visible, especially around the edges of the nucleus. One to three nucleoli can be seen but may be obscured by the granules (Figure 9.4).

Myelocytes make up 6% to 17% of the nucleated cells in the bone marrow and are the final stage in which cell division (mitosis) occurs. During this stage, the production of primary granules ceases and the cell begins to manufacture secondary (specific) neutrophil granules. This stage of neutrophil development is sometimes divided into early and late myelocytes. Early myelocytes may look very similar to the promyelocytes (described earlier) in size and nuclear characteristics except that patches of grainy pale pink cytoplasm representing secondary granules begin to be evident in the area of the Golgi apparatus. This has been referred to as the *dawn of neutrophilia*. Secondary neutrophilic granules slowly spread through the cell until its cytoplasm is more lavender-pink than blue. As the cell divides, the number of primary granules per cell is decreased and their membrane chemistry changes so that they are much less visible. Late myelocytes are somewhat smaller than promyelocytes (15 to 18 μm), and the nucleus

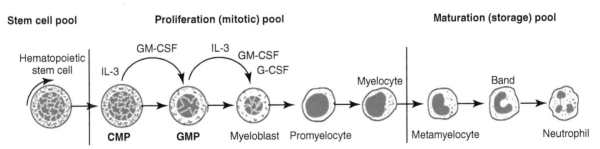

Figure 9.2 Neutrophil Development Showing Stimulating Cytokines and the Three Bone Marrow Pools.

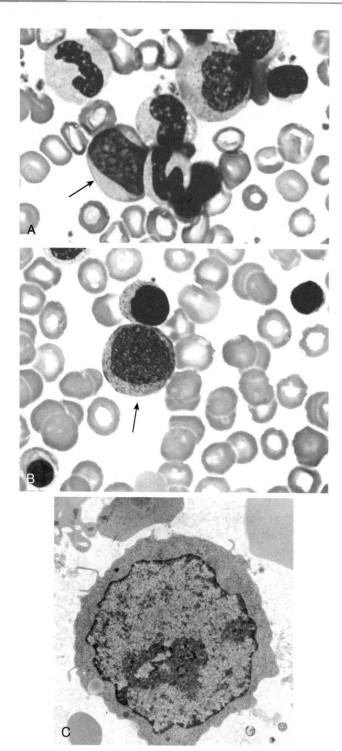

Figure 9.3 Myeloblasts. (A), Type I myeloblast *(arrow).* Note that no granules are visible in the cytoplasm. **(B),** Type II myeloblast *(arrow)* with a few azure granules in the cytoplasm. (A, B, Bone marrow, Wright-Giemsa stain, ×1000.) **(C),** Electron micrograph of a myeloblast (×16,500). (C from Rodak, B. F., & Carr, J. H. [2017]. *Clinical Hematology Atlas.* [5th ed.]. St. Louis: Elsevier.)

BOX 9.1   Neutrophil Granules

Primary (Azurophilic) Granules
Formed during the promyelocyte stage
Last to be released (exocytosis)
Contain:

- Myeloperoxidase
- Acid β-glycerophosphatase
- Cathepsins
- Defensins
- Elastase
- Proteinase-3
- Others

Secondary (Specific) Granules
Formed during myelocyte and metamyelocyte stages
Third to be released
Contain:

- β_2-Microglobulin
- Collagenase
- Gelatinase
- Lactoferrin
- Neutrophil gelatinase-associated lipocalin
- Transcobalamin I
- Others

Tertiary Granules
Formed during metamyelocyte and band stages
Second to be released
Contain:

- Gelatinase
- Collagenase
- Lysozyme
- Acetyltransferase
- β_2-Microglobulin

Secretory Granules (Secretory Vesicles)
Formed during band and segmented neutrophil stages
First to be released (fuse to plasma membrane)
Contain (attached to membrane):

- CD11b/CD18
- Alkaline phosphatase
- Vesicle-associated membrane-2
- CD10, CD13, CD14, CD16
- Cytochrome b_{558}
- Complement 1q receptor
- Complement receptor-1

---

has considerably more heterochromatin. Nucleoli are difficult to see by light microscopy (Figure 9.5).

Metamyelocytes constitute 3% to 20% of nucleated marrow cells. From this stage forward, the cells are no longer capable of division and the major morphologic change is in the shape of the nucleus. The nucleus is indented (kidney bean shaped or peanut shaped), and the chromatin is increasingly clumped. Nucleoli are absent. Synthesis of tertiary granules (also known as *gelatinase granules*) may begin during this stage. The size of the metamyelocyte is slightly smaller than that of the myelocyte (14 to 16 μm). The cytoplasm contains very little residual ribonucleic acid (RNA) and therefore little or no basophilia (Figure 9.6).

Bands make up 9% to 32% of nucleated marrow cells and 0% to 5% of the nucleated peripheral blood cells. All evidence of RNA (cytoplasmic basophilia) is absent, and tertiary granules continue to be formed during this stage. Secretory granules (also known as *secretory vesicles*) may begin to be

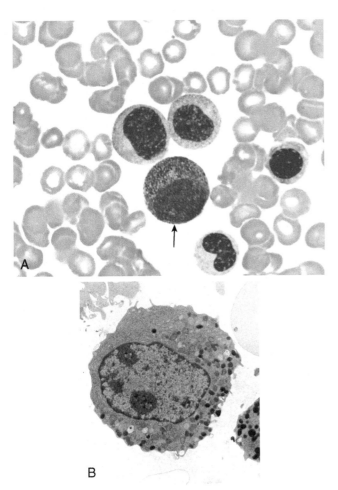

Figure 9.4 Promyelocytes. (A), Promyelocyte *(arrow)* with nucleoli and a large number of azure granules. (Bone marrow, Wright-Giemsa stain, ×1000.) **(B),** Electron micrograph of a promyelocyte (×13,000). (B from Rodak, B. F., & Carr, J. H. [2017]. *Clinical Hematology Atlas.* [5th ed.]. St. Louis: Elsevier.)

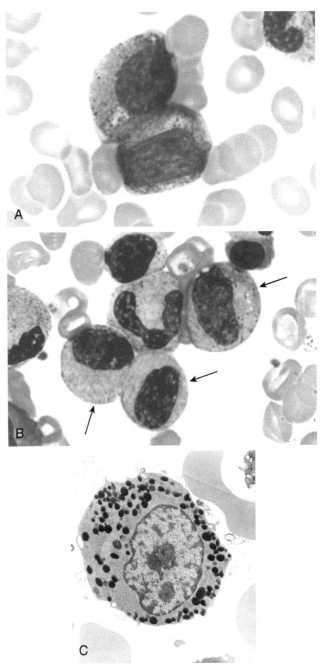

Figure 9.5 Myelocytes. (A), Two early neutrophil myelocytes. Note that they are very similar to the promyelocyte except for several light areas in their cytoplasm where specific granules are beginning to appear. **(B),** *Arrows* are pointing to three late myelocytes in the field. Their cytoplasm has few if any primary granules, and the lavender secondary granules are easily seen. (A, B, Bone marrow, Wright-Giemsa stain, ×1000.) **(C),** Electron micrograph of a late neutrophil myelocyte (×16,500). (C from Rodak, B. F., & Carr, J. H. [2017]. *Clinical Hematology Atlas.* [5th ed.]. St. Louis: Elsevier.)

formed during this stage. The nucleus is highly clumped, and the nuclear indentation that began in the metamyelocyte stage now exceeds one half the diameter of the nucleus, but actual segmentation has not yet occurred (Figure 9.7). Over the past 70 years, there has been considerable controversy over the definition of a band and the differentiation between bands and segmented forms. There have been three schools of thought concerning identification of bands, from the most conservative—holding that the nucleus in a band must have the same diameter throughout its length—to the most liberal—requiring that a filament between segments be visible before a band becomes a segmented neutrophil. The middle ground states that when doubt exists, the cell should be called a segmented neutrophil. An elevated band count was thought to be useful in the diagnosis of patients with infection. However, the clinical utility of band counts has been called into question,[12] and most laboratories no longer perform routine band counts. The Clinical and Laboratory Standards Institute (CLSI) recommends that bands should be included within the neutrophil count and not reported as a separate category because of the difficulty in reliably distinguishing bands from segmented neutrophils.[13]

Segmented neutrophils make up 7% to 30% of nucleated cells in the bone marrow. Secretory granules continue to be formed during this stage. The only morphologic difference between segmented neutrophils and bands is the presence of between two and five nuclear lobes connected by thread-like filaments (Figure 9.8). Segmented neutrophils are present in the highest

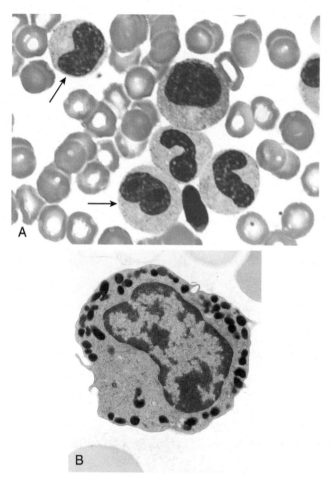

Figure 9.6 Metamyelocytes. (A), Two neutrophil metamyelocytes *(arrows)*. Note that there is no remaining basophilia in the cytoplasm, and the nucleus is indented. (Bone marrow, Wright-Giemsa stain, ×1000.) **(B),** Electron micrograph of a neutrophil metamyelocyte (×22,250). (B from Rodak, B. F., & Carr, J. H. [2017]. *Clinical Hematology Atlas.* [5th ed.]. St. Louis: Elsevier.)

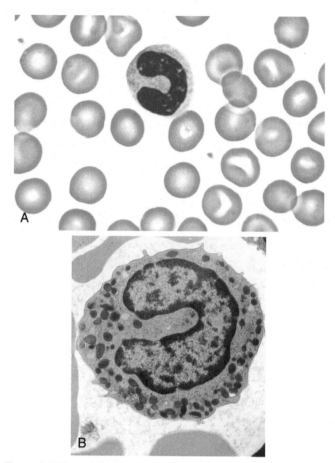

Figure 9.7 Neutrophil Bands. (A), Neutrophil band; note the nucleus is indented more than 50% of the width of the nucleus. (Peripheral blood, Wright-Giemsa stain, ×1000.) **(B),** Electron micrograph of a band neutrophil (×22,250). (B from Rodak, B. F., & Carr, J. H. [2017]. *Clinical Hematology Atlas.* [5th ed.]. St. Louis: Elsevier.)

numbers in the peripheral blood of adults (50% to 70% of leukocytes in relative numbers and 2.3 to 8.1 × 10^9/L in absolute terms). As can be seen from the table on the inside front cover, pediatric values are quite different; relative percentages can be as low as 18% of leukocytes in the first few months of life and do not begin to climb to adult values until after 4 to 7 years of age.

Neutrophil Kinetics

Neutrophil kinetics involves the movement of neutrophils and neutrophil precursors between the different pools in the bone marrow, the peripheral blood, and tissues. Neutrophil production has been calculated to be on the order of between 0.9 and 1.0 × 10^9 cells/kg per day.[14]

The proliferative pool contains approximately 2.1 × 10^9 cells/kg, whereas the maturation pool contains roughly 5.6 × 10^9 cells/kg, or a 5-day supply.[14] The transit time from the HSC to the myeloblast has not been measured. The transit time from myeloblast through myelocyte has been estimated to be roughly 6 days, and the transit time through the maturation pool is approximately 4 to 6 days.[7,14,15] Granulocyte release from the bone marrow is stimulated by G-CSF.[3,4]

Once in the peripheral blood, neutrophils are divided randomly into a circulating neutrophil pool (CNP) and a marginated neutrophil pool (MNP). The neutrophils in the MNP are loosely localized to the walls of capillaries in tissues such as the liver, spleen, and lung. There does not appear to be any functional differences between neutrophils of either the CNP or the MNP, and cells move freely between the two peripheral pools.[16] The ratio of these two pools is roughly equal overall[7,17]; however, marginated neutrophils in the capillaries of the lungs make up a considerably larger portion of peripheral neutrophils.[18] The half-life of neutrophils in the blood is relatively short at approximately 7 hours.[7,19]

Integrins and selectins are of significant importance in allowing neutrophils to marginate as well as exit the blood and enter the tissues by a process known as *diapedesis*.[20,21] Those neutrophils that do not migrate into the tissues eventually undergo programmed cell death or apoptosis and are removed by macrophages in the spleen, bone marrow, and liver.[22]

Once neutrophils are in the tissues, their life span is variable, depending on whether or not they are responding to infectious or inflammatory agents. In the absence of infectious or inflammatory agents, the neutrophil's life span is measured in hours. Spontaneous neutrophil apoptosis is regulated by pro- and antiapoptotic members of the Bcl-2 family. Some products of

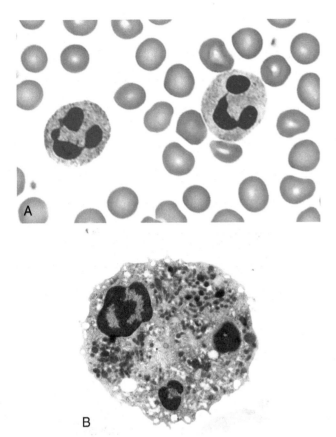

Figure 9.8 Neutrophils. (A), Segmented neutrophils, also known as a *polymorphonuclear cell* or *PMN.* (Peripheral blood, Wright-Giemsa stain, ×1000.) **(B),** Electron micrograph of a segmented neutrophil (×22,250). (B from Rodak, B. F., & Carr, J. H. [2017]. *Clinical Hematology Atlas.* [5th ed.]. St. Louis: Elsevier.)

inflammation and infection such as Mcl-1 and myeloperoxidase (MPO) tend to prolong the neutrophil's life span through antiapoptotic signals, whereas others such as MAC-1 trigger the death and phagocytosis of neutrophils.[23]

Neutrophil Functions

Neutrophils are part of the innate immune system. Characteristics of innate immunity include destruction of foreign organisms that is not antigen specific; no protection against reexposure to the same pathogen; reliance on the barriers provided by skin and mucous membranes, as well as phagocytes such as neutrophils and monocytes; and inclusion of a humoral component known as the *complement system.*

The major function of neutrophils is phagocytosis and destruction of foreign material and microorganisms. The process involves seeking (chemotaxis, motility, and diapedesis) and destruction (phagocytosis and digestion).

Neutrophil extravasation involves rolling, adhesion, crawling, and finally transmigration.[24] Neutrophil recruitment to an inflammatory site begins when chemotactic agents bind to neutrophil receptors. Chemotactic agents may be produced by microorganisms, by damaged cells, or by other leukocytes such as lymphocytes or other phagocytes. The first neutrophil response is to roll along endothelial cells of the blood vessels using stronger adhesive molecules than those used by

nonstimulated marginated neutrophils. Rolling consists of transient adhesive contacts between neutrophil selectins and adhesive molecules on the surface of endothelial cells (P selectins and E selectins). Activation is facilitated by the rolling of neutrophils on endothelium surfaces by chemokines. When integrins bind to ligands on the neutrophil surface, an outside-in signaling activates signaling pathways, stabilizes adhesion, and initiates cell motility.[20,25] Once adhesion occurs, the neutrophil scans the region while tightly attached and does not always transmigrate at the location of adhesion.[26] Active crawling depends on signaling between intercellular adhesion molecule-1 (ICAM-1) (expressed by endothelial cells) and macrophage-1 antigen (MAC-1, expressed by neutrophils).[27] Neutrophils then transmigrate in a directional manner either between endothelial cells (paracellular) or through endothelial cells (transcellular) toward the area of greatest concentration of chemotactic agents.[24]

Once at the site of infection or inflammation, neutrophils begin the process of phagocytosis (Box 9.2). They use their enormous inventory of surface receptors either to directly recognize the pathogen, apoptotic cell, or particle or to recognize opsonic molecules attached to the foreign particle such as antibodies or complement components. Surface cell receptors are primed when neutrophils are exposed to lipopolysaccharide, tumor necrosis factor-α or granulocyte-macrophage colony-stimulating factor (GM-CSF), which are recognized by Toll-like receptors.[28] With recognition comes attachment and engulfment, in which cytoplasmic pseudopodia surround the

---

BOX 9.2 Phagocytosis

Recognition and Attachment

Phagocyte receptors recognize and bind to certain foreign molecular patterns and opsonins such as antibodies and complement components.

Ingestion

Pseudopodia are extended around the foreign particle and enclose it within a "phagosome" (engulfment).

The phagosome is pulled toward the center of the cell by polymerization of actin and myosin and by microtubules.

Killing and Digestion
Oxygen Dependent

Respiratory burst through the activation of NADPH oxidase. H_2O_2 and hypochlorite are produced.

Oxygen Independent

The pH within the phagosome becomes alkaline and then neutral, the pH at which digestive enzymes work.

Primary and secondary lysosomes (granules) fuse to the phagosome and empty hydrolytic enzymes and other bactericidal molecules into the phagosome.

Formation of Neutrophil Extracellular Traps

Nuclear and organelle membranes dissolve, and activated cytoplasmic enzymes attach to DNA.

The cytoplasmic membrane ruptures, and DNA with attached enzymes is expelled so that the bacteria are digested in the external environment.

NADPH, Nicotinamide adenine dinucleotide phosphate (reduced form).

particle, forming a phagosome within the neutrophil cytoplasm.[23] Formation of the phagosome allows the reduced nicotinamide adenine dinucleotide (NADH) oxidase complex, NOX2, within the phagosome membrane to assemble; this leads to the generation of reactive oxygen species such as hydrogen peroxide, which is converted to hypochlorite by MPO.[29] Likewise, a series of metabolic changes culminate in the fusion of primary (e.g., MPO, defensins) and/or secondary (e.g., phagocytic receptors, nicotinamide adenine dinucleotide phosphate [reduced form, NADPH] oxidase) granules to the phagosome and the release of numerous bactericidal molecules into the phagosome.[30] This combination of reactive oxygen species and nonoxygen-dependent mechanisms is generally able to destroy most pathogens.

In addition to emptying their contents into phagosomes, tertiary granules degrade the extracellular matrix and act as chemotactic agents for extravasation and migration of additional neutrophils to the site of inflammation.[11,24]

A second function of neutrophils is the generation of neutrophil extracellular traps, or NETs.[31,32] NETs are extracellular thread-like structures believed to represent chains of nucleosomes from unfolded nuclear chromatin material (DNA). These structures have enzymes from neutrophil granules attached to them and have been shown to be able to trap and kill gram-positive and gram-negative bacteria as well as fungi. NETs are generated at the time that neutrophils die as a result of antibacterial activity. The term *NETosis* has been used to describe this unique form of neutrophil cell death that results in the release of NETs.

A third and final function of neutrophils is their secretory function. Neutrophils are a source of transcobalamin I or R binder protein, which is necessary for the proper absorption of vitamin B_{12}. In addition, they are a source of a variety of cytokines.

Eosinophils

Eosinophils make up 1% to 3% of nucleated cells in the bone marrow. Of these, slightly more than a third are mature, a quarter are eosinophilic metamyelocytes, and the remainder are eosinophilic promyelocytes or eosinophilic myelocytes. Eosinophils account for 1% to 3% of peripheral blood leukocytes, with an absolute number of up to 0.4×10^9/L in the peripheral blood.

Eosinophil Development

Eosinophil development is similar to that described earlier for neutrophils, and evidence indicates that eosinophils arise from the CMP.[33,34] Eosinophil lineage is established through the interaction between the cytokines interleukin-3 (IL-3), IL-5 (induced by IL-33), and GM-CSF and three transcription factors (GATA-1 (hematopoietic transcription factor), PU.1, and c/EBP). IL-5 and IL-33 are critical for eosinophil growth and survival.[35,36] Eosinophilic promyelocytes can be identified cytochemically because of the presence of Charcot-Leyden crystal protein in their primary granules. The first maturation phase that can be identified as eosinophilic using light microscopy and Romanowsky staining is the early myelocyte.

Eosinophil myelocytes are characterized by the presence of large (resolvable at the light microscope level), pale, reddish-orange secondary granules, along with azure granules in blue cytoplasm. The nucleus is similar to that described for neutrophil myelocytes. Transmission electron micrographs of eosinophils reveal that many secondary eosinophil granules contain an electron-dense crystalline core (Figure 9.9).[37]

Eosinophil metamyelocytes and bands resemble their neutrophil counterparts with respect to their nuclear shape. Secondary granules increase in number, and a third type of granule is generated called the *secretory granule* or *secretory vesicle*. The secondary granules become more distinct and refractory. Electron microscopy indicates the presence of two other organelles: lipid bodies and small granules (Box 9.3).[38]

Mature eosinophils usually display a bilobed nucleus. Their cytoplasm contains characteristic refractile, orange-red secondary granules (Figure 9.10). Electron microscopy of mature eosinophils reveals extensive secretory vesicles, and their number increases considerably when the eosinophil is stimulated or activated.[37]

Eosinophil Kinetics

The time from the last myelocyte mitotic division to the emergence of mature eosinophils from the marrow is about 3.5 days. The mean turnover of eosinophils is approximately 2.2×10^8 cells/kg per day. There is a large storage pool of eosinophils in the marrow consisting of between 9 and 14×10^8 cells/kg.[38]

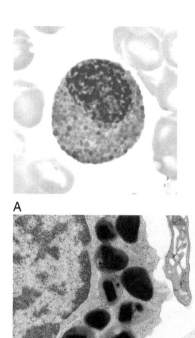

Figure 9.9 Immature Eosinophils. (A), Eosinophil myelocyte. Note the rounded nucleus and the cytoplasm in which there are numerous large, pale eosinophil granules. (Bone marrow, Wright-Giemsa stain, ×1000.) **(B),** Electron micrograph of eosinophil granules showing the central crystalline core in some of the granules. (From Rodak, B. F., & Carr, J. H. [2017]. *Clinical Hematology Atlas.* [5th ed.]. St. Louis: Elsevier).

BOX 9.3 Eosinophil Granules

Primary Granules
Formed during promyelocyte stage
Contain:
- Charcot-Leyden crystal protein

Secondary Granules
Formed throughout remaining maturation
Contain:
- Major basic protein (core)
- Eosinophil cationic protein (matrix)
- Eosinophil-derived neurotoxin (matrix)
- Eosinophil peroxidase (matrix)
- Lysozyme (matrix)
- Catalase (core and matrix)
- β-Glucuronidase (core and matrix)
- Cathepsin D (core and matrix)
- Interleukin-2, -4, and -5 (core)
- Interleukin-6 (matrix)
- Granulocyte-macrophage colony-stimulating factor (core)
- Others

Small Lysosomal Granules
Acid phosphatase
Arylsulfatase B
Catalase
Cytochrome b_{558}
Elastase
Eosinophil cationic protein

Lipid Bodies
Cyclooxygenase
5-Lipoxygenase
15-Lipoxygenase
Leukotriene C_4 synthase
Eosinophil peroxidase
Esterase

Storage Vesicles
Carry proteins from secondary granules to be released into the extracellular medium

Once in the circulation, eosinophils have a circulating half-life of roughly 18 hours[39]; however, the half-life of eosinophils is prolonged when eosinophilia occurs. The tissue destinations of eosinophils under normal circumstances appear to be underlying columnar epithelial surfaces in the respiratory, gastrointestinal, and genitourinary tracts. Survival time of eosinophils in human tissues ranges from 2 to 5 days.[40]

Eosinophil Functions

Eosinophils have multiple functions. Eosinophil granules are full of a large number of previously synthesized proteins, including cytokines, chemokines, growth factors, and cationic proteins. There is more than one way for eosinophils to degranulate in an inflammatory process. By classical exocytosis, granules move to the plasma membrane, fuse with the plasma membrane, and empty their contents into the extracellular space. Compound exocytosis is a second mechanism in which granules fuse together within the eosinophil before fusing with the plasma membrane. A third method is known as *piecemeal degranulation*, in which secretory vesicles remove specific proteins from the secondary granules. These vesicles then migrate to the plasma membrane and fuse to empty the specific proteins into the extracellular space.[37] A fourth method of degranulation is cytolysis that occurs when extracellular intact granules are deposited during cell lysis.[41]

Eosinophils play important roles in immune regulation. They transmigrate into the thymus of the newborn and are believed to be involved in the deletion of double-positive thymocytes.[42] Eosinophils are capable of acting as antigen-presenting cells and promoting the proliferation of effector T cells.[43] They are also implicated in the initiation of either type 1 or type 2 immune responses because of their ability to rapidly secrete preformed cytokines in a stimulus-specific manner. They are also important factors in acute and chronic allograft rejection.[44] Eosinophils regulate mast cell function through the release of *major basic protein* (MBP), which causes mast cell degranulation as well as cytokine production, and they also produce nerve growth factor that promotes mast cell survival and activation.

Eosinophil production is increased in infection by parasitic helminths, and in vitro studies have found that the eosinophil is capable of destroying tissue-invading helminths through the secretion of MBP and eosinophil cationic protein as well as the production of reactive oxygen species.[43] There is also a suggestion that eosinophils play a role in preventing reinfection.[45]

Finally, eosinophilia is a hallmark of allergic disorders, of which asthma has been the best studied. The number of eosinophils in blood and sputum correlates with disease severity. This has led to the suggestion that the eosinophil is one of the causes of airway inflammation and mucosal cell damage through secretion or production of a combination of basic proteins, lipid mediators, reactive oxygen species, and cytokines such as IL-5.[43] Eosinophils have also been implicated in airway remodeling (increase in thickness of the airway wall) through eosinophil-derived fibrogenic growth factors, especially in steroid-resistant asthma.[46-48] Treatment with an anti–IL-5 monoclonal antibody has been found to reduce exacerbations in certain asthmatic

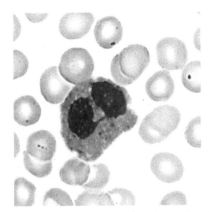

Figure 9.10 Mature Eosinophil. Note that the nucleus has only two segments, which is usual for these cells. The background cytoplasm is colorless and filled with eosinophil secondary granules. (Peripheral blood, Wright-Giemsa stain, ×1000.) (From Rodak, B. F., & Carr, J. H. [2017]. *Clinical Hematology Atlas.* [5th ed.]. St. Louis: Elsevier.)

patients.[49] Eosinophil accumulation in the gastrointestinal tract occurs in allergic disorders such as food allergy, allergic colitis, and inflammatory bowel disease such as Crohn's disease and ulcerative colitis.[50,51]

Basophils

Basophils and mast cells are two cells with morphologic and functional similarities; however, basophils are true leukocytes because they mature in the bone marrow and circulate in the blood as mature cells with granules, whereas mast cell precursors leave the bone marrow and use the blood as a transit system to gain access to the tissues where they mature. Basophils are discussed first. Basophils are the least numerous of the WBCs, making up between 0% and 2% of circulating leukocytes and less than 1% of nucleated cells in the bone marrow.

Basophil Development

Basophils are derived from progenitors in the bone marrow and spleen, where they differentiate under the influence of a number of cytokines, including IL-3 and TSLP (thymic stromal lymphopoietin).[52] Two basophil populations are identified: IL-3 elicited basophils that are immunoglobulin E (IgE) dependent and non-IgE dependent TSLP elicited basophils.[53-55] The type of mediator response is determined by the balance between these two populations.[54] Because of their very small numbers, the stages of basophil maturation are very difficult to observe and have not been well characterized. Basophils will therefore be described simply as immature basophils and mature basophils.

Immature basophils have round to somewhat lobulated nuclei with only slightly condensed chromatin. Nucleoli may or may not be apparent. The cytoplasm is blue and contains large blue-black secondary granules (Figure 9.11). Primary azure granules may or may not be seen. Basophil granules are water soluble and therefore may be dissolved if the blood film is washed too much during the staining process.

Mature basophils contain a lobulated nucleus that is often obscured by its granules. The chromatin pattern, if visible, is clumped. Actual nuclear segmentation with visible filaments occurs rarely. The cytoplasm is colorless and contains large numbers of the characteristic large blue-black granules. If any granules have been dissolved during the staining process, they often leave a reddish-purple rim surrounding what appears to be a vacuole (Figure 9.12).

Basophil Kinetics

Basophil kinetics is poorly understood because of their very small numbers.[56] This life span of basophils is relatively longer than that of the other granulocytes, 60 hours.[56] This has been attributed to the fact that when they are activated by IL-3 and IL-25, antiapoptotic pathways are initiated that prolong the basophil life span.[57]

Basophil Functions

Basophil functions are also poorly understood because of the small numbers of these cells and the lack of animal models such as basophil-deficient animals. However, the recent development of a conditional basophil-deficient mouse model promises to enhance the understanding of basophil function.[58] Previously, basophils were regarded as "poor relatives" of mast cells and minor players in allergic inflammation because, like mast cells, they have IgE receptors on their surface membranes that, when cross-linked by antigen, result in granule release.[59] Basophils functions in both innate and adaptive immunity. Basophils are capable of releasing large quantities of subtype 2 helper T cell

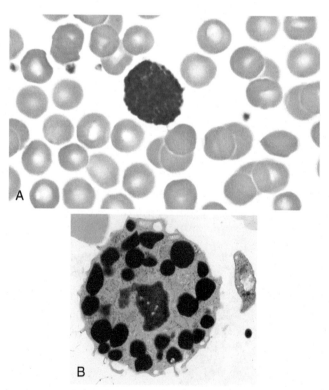

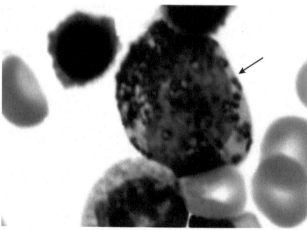

Figure 9.11 Immature Basophil *(arrow).* Note that the background cytoplasm is deeply basophilic with few large basophilic granules and there appears to be a nucleolus. (Bone marrow, Wright-Giemsa stain, ×1000.)

Figure 9.12 Basophils. (A), Mature basophil. Note that granules tend to obscure the nucleus and the background cytoplasm is only slightly basophilic. (Peripheral blood, Wright-Giemsa stain, ×1000.) **(B),** Electron micrograph of a basophil (×28,750). (B from Rodak, B. F., & Carr, J. H. [2017]. *Clinical Hematology Atlas.* [5th ed.]. St. Louis: Elsevier.)

(T_H2) cytokines such as IL-4 and IL-13 that regulate the T_H2 immune response.[60,61] Basophils also induce B cells to synthesize IgE.[62] Whereas mast cells are the effectors of IgE-mediated chronic allergic inflammation, basophils function as *initiators* of the allergic inflammation through the release of preformed cytokines.[59] Basophil activation is not restricted to antigen-specific IgE cross-linking, but it can be triggered in nonsensitized individuals by a growing list of parasitic antigens, lectins, viral superantigens, cytokines, chemokines growth factors, proteases, and components of the complement system.[62]

The contents of basophil granules are not well known. Box 9.4 provides a short list of some of the substances released by activated basophils. Moreover, mature basophils are evidently capable of synthesizing granule proteins based on activation signals. For example, basophils can be induced to produce a mediator of allergic inflammation known as *granzyme B*.[63] Mast cells can induce basophils to produce and release retinoic acid, a regulator of immune and resident cells in allergic diseases.[64] Basophils also play a role in angiogenesis through the expression of vascular endothelial growth factor (VEGF) and its receptors.[65]

Along with eosinophils, basophils are involved in the control of helminth infections by enclosing toxic egg products with granulomas and preventing tissue damage.[66] They promote eosinophilia, are associated with hindering migration of larvae to other organs, and contribute to efficient worm expulsion.[67,68] Finally, data from the basophil-deficient mouse model indicate that basophils play a nonredundant role in mediating acquired immunity against ticks.[58]

Mast Cells

Mast cells are not considered to be leukocytes. They are tissue effector cells of allergic responses and inflammatory reactions. A brief description of their development and function is included here because (1) their precursors circulate in the peripheral blood for a brief period on their way to their tissue destinations,[69] and (2) mast cells have several phenotypic and functional similarities with both basophils and eosinophils.[70]

Mast cell progenitors (MCPs) originate from the bone marrow and spleen.[69] The progenitors are then released to the blood before finally reaching tissues such as the intestine and lung, where they mediate their actions.[69] The major cytokine responsible for mast cell maturation and differentiation is KIT ligand (stem cell factor).[71] Once the MCP reaches its tissue

destination, complete maturation into mature mast cells occurs under the control of the local microenvironment (Figure 9.13).[72]

Mast cells function as effector cells in allergic reactions through the release of a wide variety of lipid mediators, proteases, proteoglycans, and cytokines as a result of cross-linking of IgE on the mast cell surface by specific allergens. Mast cells can also be activated independently of IgE, which leads to inflammatory reactions. They can function as antigen-presenting cells to induce the differentiation of T_H2 cells[73]; therefore mast cells act as mediators in both innate and adaptive immunity.[71] Mast cells can have antiinflammatory and immunosuppressive functions, and thus they can both enhance and suppress features of the immune response.[74] Finally they may act as immunologic "gatekeepers" because of their location in mucosal surfaces and their role in barrier function.[71]

MONONUCLEAR CELLS

Monocytes

Monocytes make up between 2% and 11% of circulating leukocytes, with an absolute number of up to 1.3×10^9/L.

Monocyte Development

Monocyte development is similar to neutrophil development because both cell types are derived from the GMP (Figure. 9.1). Macrophage colony-stimulating factor (M-CSF) is the major cytokine responsible for the growth and differentiation of monocytes. The morphologic stages of monocyte development are monoblasts, promonocytes, and monocytes. Monoblasts in normal bone marrow are very rare and are difficult to distinguish from myeloblasts based on morphology. Malignant monoblasts in acute monoblastic leukemia are described in

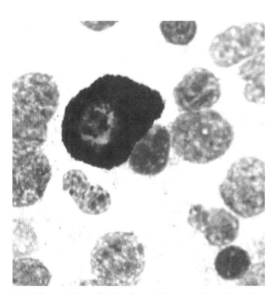

Figure 9.13 Tissue Mast Cell in Bone Marrow. Note that the nucleus is rounded and the cell is packed with large basophilic granules. Mast cells tend to be a little larger than basophils (12 to 25 μm). (Wright-Giemsa stain, ×1000.) (From Rodak, B. F., & Carr, J. H. [2017]. *Clinical Hematology Atlas.* [5th ed.]. St. Louis: Elsevier.)

BOX 9.4	**Basophil Granules**

Secondary Granules
Histamine
Platelet-activating factor
Leukotriene C_4
Interleukin-4
Interleukin-13
Vascular endothelial growth factor A
Vascular endothelial growth factor B
Heparan sulfate

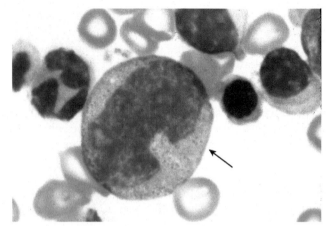

Figure 9.14 Promonocyte *(arrow).* Note that the nucleus is deeply indented and should not be confused with a neutrophil band form (compare the chromatin patterns of the two). The cytoplasm is basophilic with azure granules that are much smaller than those seen in promyelocytes. The azure granules in this cell are difficult to see and give the cytoplasm a slightly grainy appearance. (Bone marrow, Wright-Giemsa stain, ×1000.)

Chapter 31. Therefore only promonocytes and monocytes are described here.

Promonocytes are 12 to 18 μm in diameter, and their nucleus is slightly indented or folded. The chromatin pattern is delicate, and at least one nucleolus is apparent. The cytoplasm is blue and contains scattered azure granules that are fewer and smaller than those seen in promyelocytes (Figure 9.14). Electron microscopic and cytochemical studies have found that monocyte azure granules are heterogeneous with regard to their content of lysosomal enzymes, peroxidase, nonspecific esterases, and lysozyme.[75]

Monocytes appear to be larger than neutrophils (diameter of 15 to 20 μm) because they tend to stick to and spread out on glass or plastic. Monocytes are slightly immature cells whose ultimate goal is to enter the tissues and mature into macrophages, osteoclasts, or dendritic cells.

The nucleus may be round, oval, or kidney shaped but more often is deeply indented (horseshoe shaped) or folded on itself. The chromatin pattern is looser than in the other leukocytes and has sometimes been described as lace-like or stringy. Nucleoli are generally not seen with the light microscope; however, electron microscopy reveals nucleoli in roughly half of circulating monocytes. Their cytoplasm is blue-gray, with fine azure granules often referred to as *azure dust* or a ground-glass appearance. Small cytoplasmic pseudopods or blebs may be seen. Cytoplasmic and nuclear vacuoles may also be present (Figure 9.15). Based on flow cytometry immunophenotyping, three subsets of human monocytes have been described: the classical, intermediate, and nonclassical monocytes.[76] Studies have found that certain subsets of monocytes expand with infections and inflammatory and autoimmune conditions.[77] It is not clear whether the expansion is a cause or consequence of these conditions. For example, in atherosclerosis it has been found that classical monocytes advance inflammation and sift through necrotic debris, whereas nonclassical and possibly

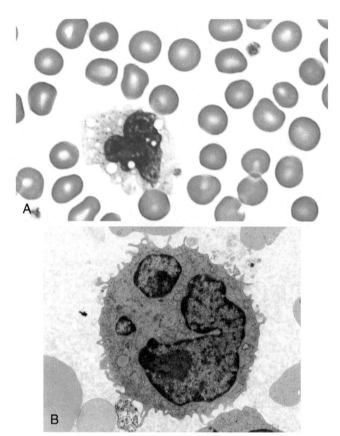

Figure 9.15 Monocytes. (A), Typical monocyte. Note the vacuolated cytoplasm, a contorted nucleus that folds on itself, the loose or lace-like chromatin pattern, and very fine azure granules. (Peripheral blood, Wright-Giemsa stain, ×1000.) **(B),** Electron micrograph of a monocyte. Note that the villi on the surface are much greater in number than is seen on neutrophils (×16,500). (B from Rodak, B. F., & Carr, J. H. [2017]. *Clinical Hematology Atlas.* [5th ed.]. St. Louis: Elsevier.)

intermediate monocyte cells reduce inflammation to support healing.[78] The exact role of monocytes in health and disease needs further exploration.

Monocyte/Macrophage Kinetics

The promonocyte pool consists of approximately 6×10^8 cells/kg, and they produce 7×10^6 monocytes/kg per hour. Under normal circumstances, promonocytes undergo two mitotic divisions in 60 hours to produce a total of four monocytes. Under conditions of increased demand for monocytes, promonocytes undergo four divisions to yield a total of 16 monocytes in 60 hours. There is no storage pool of mature monocytes in the bone marrow,[79] and unlike neutrophils, monocytes are released immediately into the circulation upon maturation. Therefore, when the bone marrow recovers from marrow failure, monocytes are seen in the peripheral blood before neutrophils and a relative monocytosis may occur. There is recent evidence, however, that a relatively large reservoir of immature monocytes resides in the subcapsular red pulp of the spleen. Monocytes in this splenic reservoir appear to respond to tissue injury such as myocardial infarction by migrating to the site of tissue injury to participate in wound healing.[80]

Like neutrophils, monocytes in the peripheral blood can be found in a marginal pool and a circulating pool. Unlike

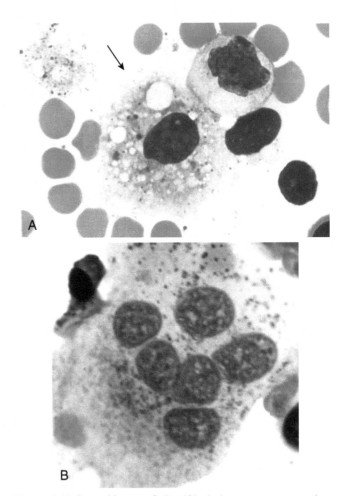

Figure 9.16 Bone Marrow Cells. (A), Active marrow macrophage *(arrow).* **(B),** Osteoclast with six nuclei. Both these cells are derived from monocytes. (A, B, Wright-Giemsa stain, ×1000.)

with neutrophils, the marginal pool of monocytes is 3.5 times the circulating pool.[81] Monocytes remain in the circulation approximately 3 days.[82] Monocytes with different patterns of chemokine receptors have different target tissues and different functions. Box 9.5 contains a list of the various tissue destinations of monocytes.[83] Once in the tissues, monocytes differentiate into macrophages, osteoclasts (Figure 9.16), or dendritic cells, depending on the microenvironment of the local tissues. Macrophages can be as large as 40 to 50 μm in diameter. They usually have an oval nucleus with a net-like (reticulated) chromatin pattern. Their cytoplasm is pale, often vacuolated, and often filled with debris of phagocytized cells or organisms.

The life span of macrophages in the tissues depends on whether they are responding to inflammation or infection, or they are "resident" macrophages such as Kupffer cells or alveolar macrophages. Resident macrophages survive far longer than tissue neutrophils. For example, Kupffer cells have a life span of approximately 21 days.[84] Inflammatory macrophages, on the other hand, have a life span measured in hours.

Monocyte/Macrophage Functions

Functions of monocytes/macrophages are numerous and varied. They can be subdivided into innate immunity, adaptive immunity, and housekeeping functions.

• *Innate immunity:* Monocytes/macrophages recognize a wide range of bacterial pathogens by means of pattern recognition receptors (Toll-like receptors) that stimulate inflammatory cytokine production and phagocytosis. Macrophages can synthesize nitric oxide, which is cytotoxic against viruses, bacteria, fungi, protozoa, helminths, and tumor cells.[30] Monocytes and macrophages also have Fc receptors and complement receptors. Hence, they can phagocytize foreign organisms or materials that have been coated with antibodies or complement components.

• *Adaptive immunity:* Both macrophages and dendritic cells degrade antigen and present antigen fragments on their surfaces (antigen-presenting cells). Because of this, they interact with and activate both T lymphocytes and B lymphocytes to initiate the adaptive immune response. Dendritic cells are the most efficient and potent of the antigen-presenting cells.

• *Housekeeping functions:* These include removal of debris and dead cells at sites of infection or tissue damage, destruction of senescent red blood cells and maintenance of a storage pool of iron for erythropoiesis, and synthesis of a wide variety of proteins, including coagulation factors, complement components, interleukins, growth factors, and enzymes.[85]

Lymphocytes

Lymphocytes are divided into three major groups: T cells, B cells, and natural killer (NK) cells. T and B cells are major players in adaptive immunity. NK cells make up a small percentage of lymphocytes and are part of innate immunity. Adaptive immunity has three characteristics: It relies on an enormous number of distinct lymphocytes, each having surface receptors for a different specific molecular structure on a foreign antigen; after an encounter with a particular antigen, memory cells are produced that will react faster and more vigorously to that same antigen on reexposure; and self-antigens are "ignored" under normal circumstances (referred to as *tolerance*).

Lymphocytes can be subdivided into two major categories: Those that participate in humoral immunity by producing antibodies and those that participate in cellular immunity by attacking foreign organisms or cells directly. Antibody-producing lymphocytes are called *B lymphocytes* or simply *B cells* because they develop in the bone marrow. Cellular immunity is accomplished by two types of lymphocytes: T cells, so named because they develop in the thymus, and NK cells, which develop in both the bone marrow and the thymus.[86-88]

Lymphocytes are different from the other leukocytes in several ways, including the following:

1. Lymphocytes are not end cells. They are resting cells, and when stimulated, they undergo mitosis to produce both memory and effector cells.
2. Unlike other leukocytes, lymphocytes recirculate from the blood to the tissues and back to the blood.
3. B and T lymphocytes are capable of rearranging antigen receptor gene segments to produce a wide variety of antibodies and surface receptors.
4. Although early lymphocyte progenitors such as the common lymphoid progenitor originate in the bone marrow, T and NK lymphocytes develop and mature outside the bone marrow.

For these reasons, lymphocyte kinetics is extremely complicated, not well understood, and beyond the scope of this chapter.

Lymphocytes make up between 18% and 42% of circulating leukocytes with an absolute number of 0.8 to 4.8 × 10⁹/L.

Lymphocyte Development

For both B and T cells, development can be subdivided into antigen-independent and antigen-dependent phases. Antigen-independent lymphocyte development occurs in the bone marrow and thymus (sometimes referred to as *central* or *primary lymphatic organs*), whereas antigen-dependent lymphocyte development occurs in the spleen, lymph nodes, tonsils, and mucosa-associated lymphoid tissue such as the Peyer's patches in the intestinal wall (sometimes referred to as *peripheral* or *secondary lymphatic organs*).

B lymphocytes develop initially in the bone marrow and go through three stages known as *pro-B, pre-B,* and *immature B cells.* It is during these stages that immunoglobulin gene rearrangement occurs so that each B cell produces a unique immunoglobulin antigen receptor. The immature B cells, which have not yet been exposed to antigen *(antigen-naive B cells),* leave the bone marrow to migrate to secondary lymphatic organs, where they take up residence in specific zones such as lymph node follicles. These immature B cells, also known as *hematogones,*[89] have a homogeneous nuclear chromatin pattern and extremely scanty cytoplasm (Figure 9.17). These cells are normally found in newborn peripheral blood and bone marrow and in regenerative bone marrows. Leukemic cells from patients with acute lymphoblastic leukemia (ALL) can sometimes resemble hematogones, but the leukemic cells can be distinguished from hematogones by flow cytometry immunophenotyping.[90]

It is in the secondary lymphatic organs or in the blood where B cells may come in contact with antigen, which results in cell division and the production of memory cells as well as effector

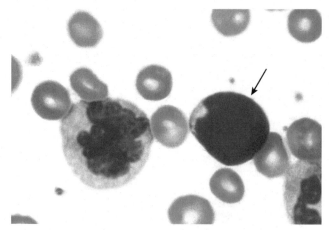

Figure 9.17 Immature B Lymphocyte or Hematogone *(arrow).* Note the extremely scanty cytoplasm. This was taken from the bone marrow of a newborn infant. (Wright-Giemsa stain, ×1000.)

cells. Effector B cells are antibody-producing cells known as *plasma cells* and *plasmacytoid lymphocytes* (Figure 9.18).

Approximately 3% to 21% of circulating lymphocytes are B cells. Resting B lymphocytes cannot be distinguished morphologically from resting T lymphocytes. Resting lymphocytes are small (around 9 μm in diameter), and the N:C ratio ranges from 5:1 to 2:1. The chromatin is arranged in

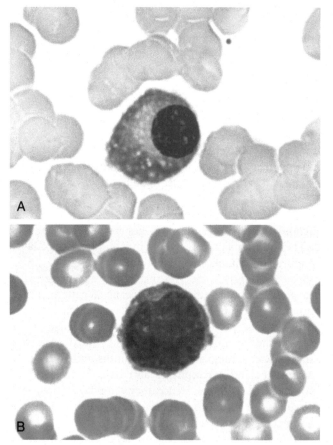

Figure 9.18 Plasma Cell vs Plasmacytoid Lymphocyte. (A), Plasma cell. **(B),** Plasmacytoid lymphocyte. These are effector cells of the B lymphocyte lineage. (A, B, Peripheral blood, Wright-Giemsa stain, ×1000.)

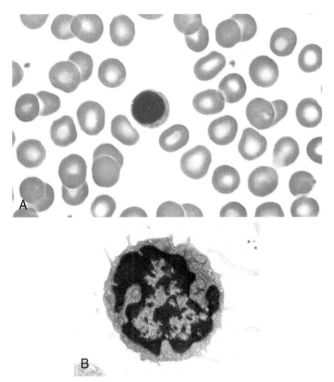

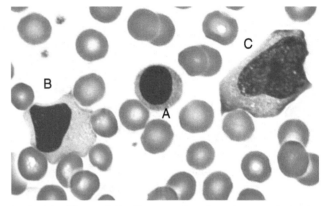

Figure 9.20 Three Cells Representing Lymphocyte Activation. A small resting lymphocyte **(A)** is stimulated by antigen and begins to enlarge to form a medium to large lymphocyte **(B)**. The nucleus reverts from a clumped to a delicate chromatin pattern with nucleoli **(C)**. The cell is capable of dividing to form effector cells or memory cells. (A-C, Peripheral blood, Wright-Giemsa stain, ×1000.)

Figure 9.19 Lymphocytes. (A), Small resting lymphocyte. (Peripheral blood, Wright-Giemsa stain, ×1000.) **(B)**, Electron micrograph of a small lymphocyte (×30,000). B from Rodak, B. F., & Carr, J. H. [2017]. *Clinical Hematology Atlas.* [5th ed.]. St. Louis: Elsevier.)

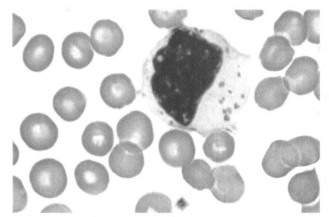

Figure 9.21 A Large Granular Lymphocyte That Could Be Either a Cytotoxic T Lymphocyte or a Natural Killer Lymphocyte. (Peripheral blood, Wright-Giemsa stain, ×1000.)

blocks, and the nucleolus is rarely seen, although it is present (Figure 9.19).

T lymphocytes develop initially in the thymus—a lymphoepithelial organ located in the upper mediastinum.[91] Lymphoid progenitor cells migrate from the bone marrow to the thymic cortex, where, under the regulation of cytokines produced by thymic epithelial cells, they progress through stages known as *pro-T, pre-T,* and *immature T cells*. During these phases they undergo antigen receptor gene rearrangement to produce T cell receptors that are unique to each T cell. T cells whose receptors react with self-antigens are allowed to undergo apoptosis.[92] In addition, T cells are subdivided into two major categories, depending on whether or not they have CD4 or CD8 antigen on their surfaces. Immature T cells then proceed to the thymic medulla, where further apoptosis of self-reactive T cells occurs. The remaining immature T cells (or *antigen-naive T cells*) then leave the thymus and migrate to secondary lymphatic organs, where they take up residence in specific zones such as the paracortical areas. T cells comprise 51% to 88% of circulating lymphocytes.

T cells in secondary lymphatic organs or in the circulating blood eventually come in contact with antigens. This results in cell activation and the production of either memory cells or effector T cells, or both (Figure 9.20). The transformation of resting lymphocytes into activated forms is the source of so-called medium and large lymphocytes that have increased amounts of cytoplasm and usually make up only about 10% of circulating lymphocytes. The morphology of effector T cells varies with the subtype of T cell involved, and they are often referred to as *reactive lymphocytes*.

NK cells are a heterogeneous group of cells with respect to their surface antigens. The majority are CD56$^+$CD16$^+$CD3$^-$CD7$^+$ large granular lymphocytes (Figure 9.21).[93] The mature NK cell is relatively large compared with other resting lymphocytes because of an increased amount of cytoplasm. Its cytoplasm contains azurophilic granules that are peroxidase negative. Approximately 4% to 29% of circulating lymphocytes are NK cells.

Lymphocyte Functions

Functions can be addressed according to the type of lymphocyte. *B lymphocytes* are essential for antibody production. In addition, they have a role in antigen presentation to T cells and may be necessary for optimal CD4 activation. B cells also produce cytokines that regulate a variety of T cell and antigen-presenting cell functions.[94]

T lymphocytes can be divided into CD4$^+$ T cells and CD8$^+$ T cells. CD4$^+$ effector lymphocytes are further subdivided into T$_H$1, T$_H$2, T$_H$17, and T$_{reg}$ (CD4$^+$CD25$^+$ regulatory T) cells. T$_H$1 cells mediate immune responses against intracellular pathogens. T$_H$2 cells mediate host defense against extracellular parasites, including helminths. They are also important in the induction of asthma and other allergic diseases. T_H17 cells are involved in the immune responses against extracellular bacteria and fungi. T_{reg} cells play a role in maintaining self-tolerance by regulating immune responses.[95,96]

CD8$^+$ effector lymphocytes are capable of killing target cells by secreting granules containing granzyme and perforin or by activating apoptotic pathways in the target cell.[97] These cells are sometimes referred to as *cytotoxic T lymphocytes.*

NK lymphocytes function as part of innate immunity and are capable of killing certain tumor cells and virus-infected cells without prior sensitization. In addition, NK cells modulate the functions of other cells, including macrophages and T cells.[98]

SUMMARY

- Granulocytes are classified according to their staining characteristics and the shape of their nuclei. Neutrophils are a major component of innate immunity as phagocytes; eosinophils are involved in allergic reactions and helminth destruction; and basophils function as initiators of allergic reactions, helminth destruction, and immunity against ticks.
- Neutrophil development can be subdivided into specific stages, with cells at each stage having specific morphologic characteristics (myeloblast, promyelocyte, myelocyte, metamyelocyte, band, and segmented neutrophil). Various granule types are produced during neutrophil development, each with specific contents.
- Eosinophil development can also be subdivided into specific stages, although eosinophilic myeloblasts are not recognizable and eosinophil promyelocytes are rare.
- Basophil development is difficult to describe, and basophils have been divided simply into immature and mature basophils.
- Mononuclear cells consist of monocytes and lymphocytes. Monocytes are precursors to tissue cells such as osteoclasts, macrophages, and dendritic cells. As a group, they perform several functions as phagocytes.

- Monocyte development can be subdivided into the promonocyte, monocyte, and macrophage stages, each with specific morphologic characteristics.
- The majority of lymphocytes are involved in adaptive immunity. B lymphocytes and plasma cells produce antibodies against foreign organisms or cells, and T lymphocytes mediate the immune response against intracellular and extracellular invaders. Both B and T lymphocytes produce memory cells for specific antigens so that the immune response is faster if the same antigen is encountered again.
- Lymphocyte development is complex, and morphologic divisions are not practical because a large number of lymphocytes develop in the thymus. Benign B-lymphocyte precursors (hematogones) as well as B-lymphocyte effector cells (plasma cells and plasmacytoid lymphocytes) have been described. Natural killer (NK) lymphocytes and cytotoxic T cells also have a distinct and similar morphology.

Now that you have completed this chapter, go back and read again the case study at the beginning and respond to the questions presented.

REVIEW QUESTIONS

Answers can be found in the Appendix.

1. Neutrophils and monocytes are direct descendants of a common progenitor known as:
   a. CLP
   b. GMP
   c. MEP
   d. HSC
2. The stage in neutrophilic development in which the nucleus is indented in a kidney bean shape and the cytoplasm has secondary granules that are lavender in color is the:
   a. Band
   b. Myelocyte
   c. Promyelocyte
   d. Metamyelocyte
3. Type II myeloblasts are characterized by:
   a. The presence of fewer than 20 primary granules per cell
   b. Basophilic cytoplasm with many secondary granules
   c. The absence of granules
   d. The presence of a folded nucleus
4. Which one of the following is a function of neutrophils?
   a. Presentation of antigen to T and B lymphocytes
   b. Protection against reexposure by same antigen
   c. Nonspecific destruction of foreign organisms
   d. Initiation of delayed hypersensitivity response

5. Which of the following cells are important in immune regulation, allergic inflammation, and destruction of tissue invading helminths?
   a. Neutrophils and monocytes
   b. Eosinophils and basophils
   c. T and B lymphocytes
   d. Macrophages and dendritic cells
6. Basophils and mast cells have high-affinity surface receptors for which immunoglobulin?
   a. A
   b. D
   c. E
   d. G
7. Which of the following cell types is capable of differentiating into osteoclasts, macrophages, or dendritic cells?
   a. Neutrophils
   b. Lymphocytes
   c. Monocytes
   d. Eosinophils
8. Macrophages aid in adaptive immunity by:
   a. Degrading antigen and presenting it to lymphocytes
   b. Ingesting and digesting organisms that neutrophils cannot
   c. Synthesizing complement components
   d. Storing iron from senescent red cells

9. Which of the following is the final stage of B cell maturation after activation by antigen?
   a. Large, granular lymphocyte
   b. Plasma cell
   c. Reactive lymphocyte
   d. Immunoblast

10. The following is unique to both B and T lymphocytes and occurs during their early development:
    a. Expression of surface antigens CD4 and CD8
    b. Maturation in the thymus
    c. Synthesis of immunoglobulins
    d. Rearrangement of antigen receptor genes

REFERENCES

1. von Vietinghoff, S., & Ley, K. (2008). Homeostatic regulation of blood neutrophil counts. *J Immunol, 181*(8), 5183–5188.
2. Gorgens, A., Radtke, S., Horn, P. A., et al. (2013). New relationships of human hematopoietic lineages facilitate detection of multipotent hematopoietic stem and progenitor cells. *Cell Cycle, 12*(22), 3478–3482.
3. Chaiworapongsa, T., Romero, R., Berry, S. M., et al. (2011). The role of granulocyte colony-stimulating factor in the neutrophilia observed in the fetal inflammatory response syndrome. *J Perinatal Med, 39*(6), 653–666.
4. Price, T. H., Chatta, G. S., & Dale, D. C. (1996). Effect of recombinant granulocyte colony-stimulating factor on neutrophil kinetics in normal young and elderly humans. *Blood, 88*(1), 335–340.
5. Iwasaki, H., & Akashi, K. (2007). Hematopoietic developmental pathways: on cellular basis. *Oncogene, 26*(47), 6687–6696.
6. Manz, M. G., Miyamoto, T., Akashi, K., et al. (2002). Prospective isolation of human clonogenic common myeloid progenitors. *Proc Natl Acad Sci U S A, 99*(18), 11872–11877.
7. Summers, C., Rankin, S. M., Condliffe, A. M., et al. (2010). Neutrophil kinetics in health and disease. *Trends Immunol, 31*(8), 318–324.
8. Terstappen, L. W., Huang, S., Safford, M., et al. (1991). Sequential generations of hematopoietic colonies derived from single nonlineage-committed CD341CD38- progenitor cells. *Blood, 77*(6), 1218–1227.
9. Adams, G. B., & Scadden, D. T. (2006). The hematopoietic stem cell in its place. *Nat Immunol, 7*(4), 333–337.
10. Mufti, G. J., Bennett, J. M., Goasguen, J., et al. (2008). Diagnosis and classification of myelodysplastic syndrome: International Working Group on Morphology of myelodysplastic syndrome (IWGM-MDS) consensus proposals for the definition and enumeration of myeloblasts and ring sideroblasts. *Haematologica, 93*(11), 1712–1717.
11. Faurschou, M., & Borregaard, N. (2003). Neutrophil granules and secretory vesicles in inflammation. *Microbes Infect, 5*(14), 1317–1327.
12. Cornbleet, P. J. (2002). Clinical utility of the band count. *Clin Lab Med, 22*(1), 101–136.
13. Clinical and Laboratory Standards Institute. (2007). *Reference Leukocyte (WBC) Differential Count (Proportional) and Evaluation of Instrumental Methods.* (2nd ed., CLSI approved standard, H20-A2). Wayne, PA: Clinical and Laboratory Standards Institute.
14. Dancey, J. T., Deubelbeiss, K. A., Harker, L. A., et al. (1976). Neutrophil kinetics in man. *J Clin Invest, 58*(3), 705–715.
15. Athens, J. W. (1963). Blood: leukocytes. *Annu Rev Physiol, 25*, 195–212.
16. Hetherington, S. V., & Quie, P. G. (1985). Human polymorphonuclear leukocytes of the bone marrow, circulation, and marginated pool: function and granule protein content. *Am J Hematol, 20*(3), 235–246.

17. Cartwright, G. E., Athens, J. W., & Wintrobe, M. M. (1964). The kinetics of granulopoiesis in normal man. *Blood, 24*, 780–803.
18. Cowburn, A. S., Condliffe, A. M., Farahi, N., et al. (2008) Advances in neutrophil biology: clinical implications. *Chest, 134*(3), 606–612.
19. Saverymuttu, S. H., Peters, A. M., Keshavarzian, A., et al. (1985). The kinetics of 111indium distribution following injection of 111 indium labelled autologous granulocytes in man. *Br J Haematol, 61*(4), 675–685.
20. Ley, K., Laudanna, C., Cybulsky, M. I., et al. (2007). Getting to the site of inflammation: the leukocyte adhesion cascade updated. *Nat Rev Immunol, 7*(9), 678–689.
21. Zarbock, A., Ley, K., McEver, R. P., et al. (2011). Leukocyte ligands for endothelial selectins: specialized glycoconjugates that mediate rolling and signaling under flow. *Blood, 118*(26), 6743–6751.
22. Furze, R. C., & Rankin, S. M. (2008). The role of the bone marrow in neutrophil clearance under homeostatic conditions in the mouse. *Faseb J, 22*(9), 3111–3119.
23. Stuart, L. M., & Ezekowitz, R. A. (2005). Phagocytosis: elegant complexity. *Immunity, 22*(5), 539–550.
24. Kolaczkowska, E., & Kubes, P. (2013). Neutrophil recruitment and function in health and inflammation. *Nat Rev Immunol, 13*(3), 159–175.
25. Cicchetti, G., Allen, P. G., & Glogauer, M. (2002). Chemotactic signaling pathways in neutrophils: from receptor to actin assembly. *Crit Rev Oral Biol Med, 13*(3), 220–228.
26. Jenne, C. N., Wong, C. H., Zemp, F. J., et al. (2013). Neutrophils recruited to sites of infection protect from virus challenge by releasing neutrophil extracellular traps. *Cell Host Microbe, 13*(2), 169–180.
27. Phillipson, M., Heit, B., Colarusso, P., et al. (2006). Intraluminal crawling of neutrophils to emigration sites: a molecularly distinct process from adhesion in the recruitment cascade. *J Exp Med, 203*(12), 2569–2575.
28. Lim, J. J., Grinstein, S., & Roth, Z. (2017). Diversity and versatility of phagocytosis: roles in innate immunity, tissue remodeling, and homeostasis. *Front Cell Infect Microbiol, 7*, 191.
29. Winterbourn, C. C., Kettle, A. J., & Hampton, M. B. (2016). Reactive oxygen species and neutrophil function. *Annu Rev Biochem, 85*, 765–792.
30. Dale, D. C., Boxer, L., & Liles, W. C. (2008). The phagocytes: neutrophils and monocytes. *Blood, 112*(4), 935–945.
31. Brinkmann, V., & Zychlinsky, A. (2007). Beneficial suicide: why neutrophils die to make NETs. *Nat Rev Microbiol, 5*(8), 577–582.
32. Brinkmann, V., & Zychlinsky, A. (2012). Neutrophil extracellular traps: is immunity the second function of chromatin? *J Cell Biol, 198*(5), 773–783.
33. Mori, Y., Iwasaki, H., Kohno, K., et al. (2009). Identification of the human eosinophil lineage-committed progenitor: revision of

phenotypic definition of the human common myeloid progenitor. *J Exp Med, 206*(1), 183–193.

34. Uhm, T. G., Kim, B. S., & Chung, I. Y. (2012). Eosinophil development, regulation of eosinophil-specific genes, and role of eosinophils in the pathogenesis of asthma. *Allergy Asthma Immunol Res, 4*(2), 68–79.

35. Johnston, L. K., & Bryce, P. J. (2017). Understanding interleukin 33 and its roles in eosinophil development. *Front Med (Lausanne), 4*, 51.

36. Johnston, L. K., Hsu, C. L., Krier-Burris, R. A., et al. (2016). IL-33 precedes IL-5 in regulating eosinophil commitment and is required for eosinophil homeostasis. *J Immunol, 197*(9), 3445–3453.

37. Melo, R. C., Spencer, L. A., Perez, S. A., et al. (2009). Vesicle-mediated secretion of human eosinophil granule-derived major basic protein. *Lab Invest, 89*(7), 769–781.

38. Giembycz, M. A., & Lindsay, M. A. (1999). Pharmacology of the eosinophil. *Pharmacol Rev, 51*(2), 213–340.

39. Steinbach, K. H., Schick, P., Trepel, F., et al. (1979). Estimation of kinetic parameters of neutrophilic, eosinophilic, and basophilic granulocytes in human blood. *Blut, 39*(1), 27–38.

40. Park, Y. M., & Bochner, B. S. (2010). Eosinophil survival and apoptosis in health and disease. *Allergy Asthma Immunol Res, 2*(2), 87–101.

41. Spencer, L. A., Bonjour, K., Melo, R. C., et al. (2014). Eosinophil secretion of granule-derived cytokines. *Front Immunol*, doi:10.3389/fimmu.2014.00496.

42. Throsby, M., Herbelin, A., Pleau, J. M., et al. (2000). CD11c1 eosinophils in the murine thymus: developmental regulation and recruitment upon MHC class I-restricted thymocyte deletion. *J Immunol, 165*(4), 1965–1975.

43. Hogan, S. P., Rosenberg, H. F., Moqbel, R., et al. (2008). Eosinophils: biological properties and role in health and disease. *Clin Exp Allergy, 38*(5), 709–750.

44. Long, H., Liao, W., Wang, L., et al. (2016). A player and coordinator: the versatile roles of eosinophils in the immune system. *Transfus Med Hemother, 43*(2), 96–108.

45. Hagan, P., Wilkins, H. A., Blumenthal, U. J., et al. (1985). Eosinophilia and resistance to Schistosoma haematobium in man. *Parasite Immunol, 7*(6), 625–632.

46. Isgro, M., Bianchetti, L., Marini, M. A., et al. (2013). The C-C motif chemokine ligands CCL5, CCL11, and CCL24 induce the migration of circulating fibrocytes from patients with severe asthma. *Mucosal Immunol, 6*(4), 718–727.

47. Mattoli, S. (2015). Involvement of fibrocytes in asthma and clinical implications. *Clin Exp Allergy, 45*(10), 1497–1509.

48. Saunders, R., Siddiqui, S., Kaur, D., et al. (2009). Fibrocyte localization to the airway smooth muscle is a feature of asthma. *J Allergy Clin Immunol, 123*(2), 376–384.

49. Robinson, D. S. (2013). Mepolizumab for severe eosinophilic asthma. *Expert Rev Respir Med, 7*(1), 13–17.

50. Hogan, S. P., Waddell, A., & Fulkerson, P. C. (2013). Eosinophils in infection and intestinal immunity. *Curr Opin Gastroenterol, 29*(1), 7–14.

51. Walsh, R. E., & Gaginella, T. S. (1991). The eosinophil in inflammatory bowel disease. *Scand J Gastroenterol, 26*(12), 1217–1224.

52. Oetjen, L. K., Noti, M., & Kim, B. S. (2016). New insights into basophil heterogeneity. *Semin Immunopathol, 38*(5), 549–561.

53. Siracusa, M. C., Saenz, S. A., Wojno, E. D., et al. (2013). Thymic stromal lymphopoietin-mediated extramedullary hematopoiesis promotes allergic inflammation. *Immunity, 39*(6), 1158–1170.

54. Siracusa, M. C., Saenz, S. A., Hill, D. A., et al. (2011). TSLP promotes interleukin-3-independent basophil haematopoiesis and type 2 inflammation. *Nature, 477*(7363), 229–233.

55. Siracusa, M. C., Kim, B. S., Spergel, J. M., et al. (2013). Basophils and allergic inflammation. *J Allergy Clin Immunol, 132*(4), 789–801; quiz 788.

56. Ohnmacht, C., & Voehringer, D. (2009). Basophil effector function and homeostasis during helminth infection. *Blood, 113*(12), 2816–2825.

57. Wang, H., Mobini, R., Fang, Y., et al. (2010). Allergen challenge of peripheral blood mononuclear cells from patients with seasonal allergic rhinitis increases IL-17RB, which regulates basophil apoptosis and degranulation. *Clin Exp Allergy, 40*(8), 1194–1202.

58. Wada, T., Ishiwata, K., Koseki, H., et al. (2010). Selective ablation of basophils in mice reveals their nonredundant role in acquired immunity against ticks. *J Clin Invest, 120*(8), 2867–2875.

59. Obata, K., Mukai, K., Tsujimura, Y., et al. (2007). Basophils are essential initiators of a novel type of chronic allergic inflammation. *Blood, 110*(3), 913–920.

60. Schroeder, J. T., MacGlashan, D. W., Jr., & Lichtenstein, L. M. (2001). Human basophils: mediator release and cytokine production. *Adv Immunol, 77*, 93–122.

61. Sullivan, B. M., & Locksley, R. M. (2009). Basophils: a nonredundant contributor to host immunity. *Immunity, 30*(1), 12–20.

62. Steiner, M., Huber, S., Harrer, A., et al. (2016). The evolution of human basophil biology from neglect towards understanding of their immune functions. *Biomed Res Int*, Article ID 8232830. doi: 10.1155/2016/8232830.

63. Tschopp, C. M., Spiegl, N., Didichenko, S., et al. (2006). Granzyme B, a novel mediator of allergic inflammation: its induction and release in blood basophils and human asthma. *Blood, 108*(7), 2290–2299.

64. Spiegl, N., Didichenko, S., McCaffery, P., et al. (2008). Human basophils activated by mast cell-derived IL-3 express retinaldehyde dehydrogenase-II and produce the immunoregulatory mediator retinoic acid. *Blood, 112*(9), 3762–3771.

65. de Paulis, A., Prevete, N., Fiorentino, I., et al. (2006). Expression and functions of the vascular endothelial growth factors and their receptors in human basophils. *J Immunol, 177*(10), 7322–7331.

66. Eberle, J. U., & Voehringer, D. (2016). Role of basophils in protective immunity to parasitic infections. *Semin Immunopathol, 38*(5), 605–613.

67. Obata-Ninomiya, K., Ishiwata, K., Tsutsui, H., et al. (2013). The skin is an important bulwark of acquired immunity against intestinal helminths. *J Exp Med, 210*(12), 2583–2595.

68. Schwartz, C., Turqueti-Neves, A., Hartmann, S., et al. (2014). Basophil-mediated protection against gastrointestinal helminths requires IgE-induced cytokine secretion. *Proc Natl Acad Sci U S A, 111*(48), E5169–E5177. doi:10.1073/pnas.1412663111.

69. Hallgren, J., & Gurish, M. F. (2011). Mast cell progenitor trafficking and maturation. *Adv Exp Med Biol, 716*, 14–28.

70. Valent, P. (1994). The phenotype of human eosinophils, basophils, and mast cells. *J Allergy Clin Immunol, 94*(6 Pt 2), 1177–1183.

71. Shea-Donohue, T., Stiltz, J., Zhao, A., et al. (2010). Mast cells. *Curr Gastroenterol Rep, 12*(5), 349–357.

72. Kambe, N., Hiramatsu, H., Shimonaka, M., et al. (2004). Development of both human connective tissue-type and mucosal-type mast cells in mice from hematopoietic stem cells with identical distribution pattern to human body. *Blood, 103*(3), 860–867.

73. Nakano, N., Nishiyama, C., Yagita, H., et al. (2009). Notch signaling confers antigen-presenting cell functions on mast cells. *J Allergy Clin Immunol, 123*(1), 74–81.e1.

74. Galli, S. J., Grimbaldeston, M., & Tsai, M. (2008). Immunomodulatory mast cells: negative, as well as positive, regulators of immunity. *Nat Rev Immunol, 8*(6), 478–486.

75. Nichols, B. A., Bainton, D. F., & Farquhar, M. G. (1971). Differentiation of monocytes. Origin, nature, and fate of their azurophil granules. *J Cell Biol, 50*(2), 498–515.

76. Ziegler-Heitbrock, L., Ancuta, P., Crowe, S., et al. (2010). Nomenclature of monocytes and dendritic cells in blood. *Blood, 116*(16), e74–80.

77. Wong, K. L., Yeap, W. H., Tai, J. J., et al. (2012). The three human monocyte subsets: implications for health and disease. *Immunol Res, 53*(1–3), 41–57.

78. Idzkowska, E., Eljaszewicz, A., Miklasz, P., et al. (2015). The role of different monocyte subsets in the pathogenesis of atherosclerosis and acute coronary syndromes. *Scand J Immunol, 82*(3), 163–173.

79. Meuret, G., Bammert, J., & Hoffmann, G. (1974). Kinetics of human monocytopoiesis. *Blood, 44*(6), 801–816.

80. Swirski, F. K., Nahrendorf, M., Etzrodt, M., et al. (2009). Identification of splenic reservoir monocytes and their deployment to inflammatory sites. *Science, 325*(5940), 612–616.

81. Meuret, G., Batara, E., & Furste, H. O. (1975). Monocytopoiesis in normal man: pool size, proliferation activity and DNA synthesis time of promonocytes. *Acta Haematol, 54*(5), 261–270.

82. Whitelaw, D. M. (1972). Observations on human monocyte kinetics after pulse labeling. *Cell Tissue Kinet, 5*(4), 311–317.

83. Kumar, S., & Jack, R. (2006). Origin of monocytes and their differentiation to macrophages and dendritic cells. *J Endotoxin Res, 12*(5), 278–284.

84. Crofton, R. W., Diesselhoff-den Dulk, M. M., & van Furth, R. (1978). The origin, kinetics, and characteristics of the Kupffer cells in the normal steady state. *J Exp Med, 148*(1), 1–17.

85. Nathan, C. F. (1987). Secretory products of macrophages. *J Clin Invest, 79*(2), 319–326.

86. Di Santo, J. P., & Vosshenrich, C. A. (2006). Bone marrow versus thymic pathways of natural killer cell development. *Immunol Rev, 214*, 35–46.

87. Lotzova, E., Savary, C. A., & Champlin, R. E. (1993). Genesis of human oncolytic natural killer cells from primitive CD34+CD33- bone marrow progenitors. *J Immunol, 150*(12), 5263–5269.

88. Res, P., Martinez-Caceres, E., Cristina Jaleco, A., et al. (1996). CD34+CD38dim cells in the human thymus can differentiate into T, natural killer, and dendritic cells but are distinct from pluripotent stem cells. *Blood, 87*(12), 5196–5206.

89. Sevilla, D. W., Colovai, A. I., Emmons, F. N., et al. (2010). Hematogones: a review and update. *Leuk Lymphoma, 51*(1), 10–19.

90. McKenna, R. W., Washington, L. T., Aquino, D. B., et al. (2001). Immunophenotypic analysis of hematogones (B-lymphocyte precursors) in 662 consecutive bone marrow specimens by 4-color flow cytometry. *Blood, 98*(8), 2498–2507.

91. Haynes, B. F. (1984). The human thymic microenvironment. *Adv Immunol, 36*, 87–142.

92. von Boehmer, H., Teh, H. S., & Kisielow, P. (1989). The thymus selects the useful, neglects the useless and destroys the harmful. *Immunol Today, 10*(2), 57–61.

93. Grossi, C. E., Cadoni, A., Zicca, A., et al. (1982). Large granular lymphocytes in human peripheral blood: ultrastructural and cytochemical characterization of the granules. *Blood, 59*(2), 277–283.

94. LeBien, T. W., & Tedder, T. F. (2008). B lymphocytes: how they develop and function. *Blood, 112*(5), 1570–1580.

95. Vignali, D. A., Collison, L. W., & Workman, C. J. (2008). How regulatory T cells work. *Nat Rev Immunol, 8*(7), 523–532.

96. Zhu, J., & Paul, W. E. (2008). CD4 T cells: fates, functions, and faults. *Blood, 112*(5), 1557–1569.

97. Rufer, N., Zippelius, A., Batard, P., et al. (2003). Ex vivo characterization of human CD8+ T subsets with distinct replicative history and partial effector functions. *Blood, 102*(5), 1779–1787.

98. Vivier, E., Tomasello, E., Baratin, M., et al. (2008). Functions of natural killer cells. *Nat Immunol, 9*(5), 503–510.

Platelet Production, Structure, and Function

Walter P. Jeske[*]

OBJECTIVES

After completion of this chapter, the reader will be able to:

1. Diagram megakaryocyte localization in bone marrow.
2. List the transcription products that trigger and control megakaryocytopoiesis and endomitosis.
3. Diagram terminal megakaryocyte differentiation, the proplatelet process, and thrombocytopoiesis.
4. Describe the ultrastructure of resting platelets in the circulation, including the plasma membrane, tubules, microfibrils, and granules.
5. List the important platelet receptors and their ligands.
6. Characterize platelet function, including adhesion, aggregation, and secretion.
7. Understand the biochemical pathways of platelet activation, including integrins, G proteins, and the eicosanoid and the inositol triphosphate-diacylglycerol pathways.

OUTLINE

CASE STUDY

After studying the material in this chapter, the reader should be able to respond to the following case study:

A 35-year-old woman noticed multiple pinpoint red spots and bruises on her arms and legs. The hematologist confirmed the presence of petechiae, purpura, and ecchymoses on her extremities and ordered a complete blood count, prothrombin time, and partial thromboplastin time. The platelet count was $35 \times 10^9/L$, the mean platelet volume was 13.2 fL, and the diameter of platelets on the Wright-stained peripheral blood film appeared to exceed 6 μm. Other complete blood count parameters and the coagulation parameters were within normal limits. A Wright-stained bone marrow aspirate smear revealed 10 to 12 small unlobulated megakaryocytes per low-power microscopic field.

1. Do these signs and symptoms indicate mucocutaneous (systemic) or anatomic bleeding?
2. What is the probable cause of the bleeding?
3. Does the patient's bleeding result from altered platelet production in the bone marrow?
4. List the growth factors involved in recruiting megakaryocyte progenitors.

*The author extends appreciation to George A. Fritsma, whose work in prior editions provided the foundation for this chapter.

MEGAKARYOCYTOPOIESIS

Platelets are nonnucleated blood cells that circulate at a concentration of 150 to 400 × 10^9/L, with average platelet counts slightly higher in women than in men and slightly lower in members of both sexes who are older than 65 years.[1] Platelets trigger primary hemostasis on exposure to subendothelial collagen or endothelial cell inflammatory proteins at the time of blood vessel injury.

Platelets arise from unique bone marrow cells called *megakaryocytes*. Megakaryocytes are the largest cells in the bone marrow and possess multiple chromosome copies (polyploid). On a Wright-stained bone marrow aspirate smear, each megakaryocyte is 30 to 50 μm in diameter with a multilobulated nucleus and abundant granular cytoplasm. Megakaryocytes account for less than 0.5% of all bone marrow cells, and on a normal Wright-stained bone marrow aspirate smear two to four megakaryocytes per 10× low-power field may be identified (Chapter 4).[2]

In healthy intact bone marrow tissue, megakaryocytes, under the influence of an array of stromal cell cytokines, cluster with hematopoietic stem cells in vascular niches adjacent to venous sinusoid endothelial cells (Figure 10.1).[3] Responding to the growth factor thrombopoietin (TPO), megakaryocyte progenitors are recruited from *common myeloid progenitors* (Chapter 4) and subsequently differentiate through several maturation stages. They extend proplatelet processes, projections that resemble strings of beads, through or between the endothelial cells and into the venous sinuses, releasing platelets from the tips of the processes into the circulation. Megakaryocytes are also found in the lungs.[4]

Megakaryocyte Differentiation and Progenitors

Megakaryocyte progenitors arise from the common myeloid progenitor under the influence of the transcription gene product, GATA-1, regulated by cofactor FOG1 (Box 10.1).[3] Megakaryocyte differentiation is suppressed by another transcription gene product, MYB, so GATA-1 and MYB act in opposition to

balance megakaryocytopoiesis with erythropoiesis, where the same progenitor cell is differentiated into the platelet cell line or the red blood cell line. Three megakaryocyte lineage-committed progenitor stages, defined by their in vitro culture colony characteristics, arise from the common myeloid progenitor (Figure 4.13). In order of differentiation, these are the least mature *burst-forming unit* (BFU-Meg), the intermediate *colony-forming unit* (CFU-Meg), and the more mature progenitor, the *light-density CFU* (LD-CFU-Meg).[5] All three progenitor stages resemble lymphocytes and cannot be distinguished by Wright-stained light microscopy. The BFU-Meg and CFU-Meg are diploid and undergo normal mitosis to maintain a viable pool of megakaryocyte progenitors. Their proliferative properties are reflected in their ability to form hundreds (BFU-Megs) or dozens (CFU-Megs) of colonies in culture (Figure 10.2).[6] The third stage, LD-CFU-Meg, undergoes *endomitosis*, a partially characterized form of mitosis unique to megakaryocytes in which DNA replication and cytoplasmic maturation are normal but cells lose their capacity to divide.

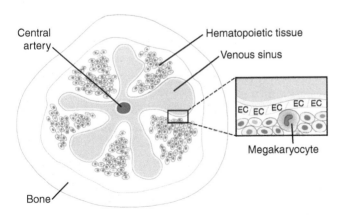

Figure 10.1 Cross Section of Bone Marrow Hematopoietic Tissue. The nerve, artery, and vein run longitudinally through the center of the marrow. Venous sinuses extend laterally from the central vein throughout the hematopoietic tissue. Differentiating and mature megakaryocytes localize to the abluminal (nonblood) surface of sinusoid-lining endothelial cells in preparation for movement into the bloodstream. *EC*, Endothelial cell.

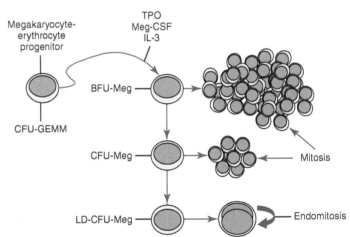

Figure 10.2 Three Stages of Megakaryocyte Progenitors. The BFU-Meg clones hundreds of daughter cells through mitosis. The CFU-Meg clones dozens of daughter cells through mitosis. The LD-CFU-Meg undergoes the first stage of endomitosis. *BFU-Meg,* Burst-forming unit megakaryocyte; *CFU-Meg,* colony-forming unit megakaryocyte; *CFU-GEMM,* colony-forming unit, granulocyte, erythrocyte, monocyte, megakaryocyte; *IL-3,* interleukin-3; *LD-CFU-Meg,* low-density CFU-Meg; *Meg-CSF,* megakaryocyte colony-stimulating factor; *TPO,* thrombopoietin.

Endomitosis

Endomitosis is a form of mitosis that lacks telophase and cyto-kinesis (separation into daughter cells). As GATA-1 and FOG1-driven transcription slows, another transcription factor, RUNX1, mediates the switch from mitosis to endomitosis by suppressing the Rho/ROCK signaling pathway. In response to the reduced Rho/ROCK signal, inadequate levels of actin and myosin (muscle fiber-like molecules) assemble in the cytoplasmic constrictions where separation would otherwise occur, preventing cytokinesis.[7] Subsequently, under the influence of transcription factor NF-E2, DNA replication proceeds to the production of 8N, 16N, or even 32N ploidy with duplicated chromosome sets.[3] Although some megakaryocytes reach 128N, this level of ploidy is unusual and may signal hematologic disease. Megakaryocytes employ their multiple DNA copies to synthesize abundant cytoplasm, which ultimately differentiates into platelets.

Terminal Megakaryocyte Differentiation

As endomitosis proceeds, megakaryocyte progenitors leave the proliferative phase and enter *terminal differentiation*, a series of stages in which microscopists become able to recognize their unique Wright-stained morphology in bone marrow aspirate films (Figure 10.3) or hematoxylin and eosin-stained bone marrow biopsy sections (Table 10.1). The morphologist, however, seldom makes the effort to distinguish MK-I, MK-II, and MK-III stages during a routine examination of a bone marrow aspirate smear.

Morphologists call the least differentiated megakaryocyte precursor the *MK-I stage* or *megakaryoblast*. Although they no longer look like lymphocytes, megakaryoblasts cannot be reliably distinguished from bone marrow myeloblasts or pronormoblasts (also named rubriblasts) using light microscopy (Figure 10.3A). The morphologist may occasionally see a vague clue: plasma membrane *blebs*, blunt projections from the

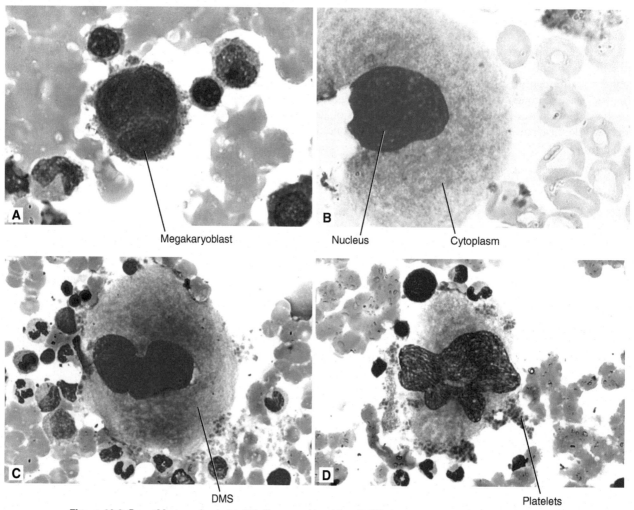

Figure 10.3 Bone Marrow Aspirate. (A), The megakaryoblast (MK-I) *(arrow)* resembles the myeloblast and pronormoblast (rubriblast); identification by morphology alone is inadvisable. This megakaryoblast has cytoplasmic "blebs" that resemble platelets. **(B),** Promegakaryocyte (MK-II). Cytoplasm is abundant, and the nucleus has minimal lobularity. **(C),** Megakaryocyte (MK-III). The nucleus is lobulated with basophilic chromatin. The cytoplasm is azurophilic and granular, with evidence of the demarcation system (DMS). **(D),** Terminal megakaryocyte shedding platelets from the proplatelet process. (A–D, Wright-Giemsa stain, ×1000.)

TABLE 10.1 Features of the Three Terminal Megakaryocyte Differentiation Stages

	MK-I	MK-II	MK-III
% of precursors	20	25	55
Diameter	14–18 μm	15–40 μm	30–50 μm
Nucleus	Round	Indented	Multilobed
Nucleoli	2–6	Variable	Not visible
Chromatin	Homogeneous	Moderately condensed	Deeply and variably condensed
Nucleus-to-cytoplasm ratio	3:1	1:2	1:4
Mitosis	Absent	Absent	Absent
Endomitosis	Present	Ends	Absent
Cytoplasm	Basophilic	Basophilic and granular	Azurophilic and granular
α-Granules	Present	Present	Present
Dense granules	Present	Present	Present
Demarcation system	Present	Present	Present

MK-I, Megakaryoblast; *MK-II*, promegakaryocyte; *MK-III*, megakaryocyte.

margin that resemble platelets. The megakaryoblast begins to develop most of its cytoplasmic ultrastructure, including procoagulant-laden α-granules, dense granules, and the demarcation system (DMS).[8]

The DMS is a series of membrane-lined channels that invade from the plasma membrane and grow inward to subdivide the entire cytoplasm. The DMS is biologically identical to the megakaryocyte plasma membrane and ultimately delineates the individual platelets during thrombocytopoiesis.

Nuclear lobularity first becomes apparent as an indentation at the 4N replication stage, rendering the cell identifiable as an *MK-II* stage, or *promegakaryocyte,* by light microscopy. The promegakaryocyte reaches its full ploidy level by the end of the MK-II stage (Figure 10.3B).

At the most abundant *MK-III* stage, the *megakaryocyte* is easily recognized at 10× magnification on the basis of its 30- to 50-μm diameter (Figure 10.3C). The nucleus is intensely indented or lobulated, and the degree of lobulation is imprecisely proportional to ploidy. When necessary, ploidy levels are measured using propidium iodide, a nucleic acid dye in megakaryocyte flow cytometry.[9] The chromatin is variably condensed with light and dark patches. The cytoplasm is azurophilic (lavender), granular, and platelet-like because of the spread of the DMS and α-granules. At full maturation, platelet shedding, or *thrombocytopoiesis,* proceeds.

Thrombocytopoiesis (Platelet Shedding)

Figure 10.3D illustrates the process of platelet shedding, termed *thrombocytopoiesis.* During thrombocytopoiesis, a single megakaryocyte may shed 2000 to 4000 platelets. In an average-size healthy human there are 10^8 megakaryocytes producing 10^{11} platelets per day. The total platelet population turns over in 8 to 9 days (the so-called platelet lifespan). In instances of high platelet consumption, such as immune thrombocytopenic purpura, platelet production may rise by as much as tenfold.

One cannot find reliable evidence for platelet budding or shedding simply by examining megakaryocytes in situ, even in well-structured bone marrow biopsy preparations. However, in megakaryocyte cultures examined by transmission electron microscopy, the DMS dilates, longitudinal bundles of tubules form, proplatelet processes develop, and transverse constrictions appear throughout the proplatelet processes. In the bone marrow environment, proplatelet processes are believed to pierce through or between sinusoid-lining endothelial cells, extend into the venous blood, and shed platelets (Figure 10.4). Thrombocytopoiesis leaves behind naked megakaryocyte nuclei to be consumed by marrow macrophages.[10]

Megakaryocyte Membrane Receptors and Markers

In specialty and tertiary care laboratories, immunostaining of fixed tissue, flow cytometry with immunologic probes, and fluorescent in situ hybridization (FISH) with genetic probes are used to identify visually indistinguishable megakaryocyte progenitors in hematologic disease. There are several megakaryocyte membrane markers that can be measured by flow cytometry, including MPL, which is the TPO receptor site present at all maturation stages, and the stem cell and common myeloid progenitor marker CD34. The CD34 marker disappears as differentiation proceeds. The platelet membrane glycoprotein (GP) IIb/IIIa (CD41/CD61) first appears on megakaryocyte progenitors and remains present throughout maturation, along with immunologic markers CD36 (platelet GP 4), CD42 (GP Ib) and CD62 (P-selectin). Cytoplasmic coagulation factor VIII, von Willebrand factor (VWF), and fibrinogen may be detected in the fully developed megakaryocyte by immunostaining (Table 10.2).[11-13]

Hormones and Cytokines of Megakaryocytopoiesis

The growth factor TPO is a 70,000 Dalton molecule that possesses 23% homology with the red blood cell-producing hormone erythropoietin.[14] Messenger ribonucleic acid (mRNA) for TPO has been found in the kidney, liver, stromal cells, and smooth muscle cells, though the liver has the most copies and is considered the primary source. TPO circulates as a hormone in plasma and is the ligand that binds the megakaryocyte and

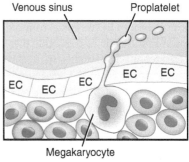

Figure 10.4 Platelet Shedding. Megakaryocyte is adjacent to the abluminal (nonblood) membrane of the sinusoid-lining endothelial cell of the bone marrow hematopoietic tissue and extends a proplatelet process through or between the endothelial cells into the vascular sinus.

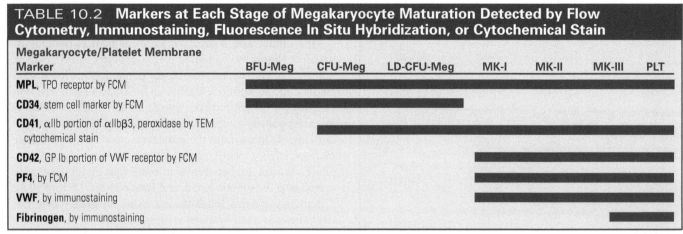

TABLE 10.2   Markers at Each Stage of Megakaryocyte Maturation Detected by Flow Cytometry, Immunostaining, Fluorescence In Situ Hybridization, or Cytochemical Stain

Megakaryocyte/Platelet Membrane Marker	BFU-Meg	CFU-Meg	LD-CFU-Meg	MK-I	MK-II	MK-III	PLT
MPL, TPO receptor by FCM	▬▬▬▬▬▬▬▬▬▬▬▬▬▬▬▬▬▬▬▬▬▬▬▬▬▬▬▬▬▬						
CD34, stem cell marker by FCM	▬▬▬▬▬▬▬▬▬▬▬▬▬						
CD41, αIIb portion of αIIbβ3, peroxidase by TEM cytochemical stain		▬▬▬▬▬▬▬▬▬▬▬▬▬▬▬▬▬▬▬▬▬▬▬▬					
CD42, GP Ib portion of VWF receptor by FCM				▬▬▬▬▬▬▬▬▬▬			
PF4, by FCM				▬▬▬▬▬▬▬▬▬▬			
VWF, by immunostaining				▬▬▬▬▬▬▬▬▬▬			
Fibrinogen, by immunostaining							▬▬▬▬

The bars indicate at which stage of differentiation the marker appears and at which stage it disappears. *BFU-Meg,* Burst-forming unit-megakaryocyte; *CFU-Meg,* colony-forming unit-megakaryocyte; *LD-CFU-Meg,* low-density colony-forming unit–megakaryocyte; *MK-I,* megakaryoblast; *MK-II,* promega-karyocyte; *MK-III,* megakaryocyte; *PLT,* platelets; *FCM,* flow cytometry; *TEM,* transmission electron microscopy; *GP,* glycoprotein; *PF4,* platelet factor 4; *TPO,* thrombopoietin; *VWF,* von Willebrand factor.

TABLE 10.3   Hormones and Cytokines That Control Megakaryocytopoiesis

Cytokine/Hormone	Differentiation to Progenitors	Differentiation to Megakaryocytes	Late Maturation	Thrombocytopoiesis	Therapeutic Agent
TPO	+	+	+	0	Available
IL-3	+	+	0	—	—
IL-6	0	0	+	+	—
IL-11	0	+	+	+	Available

IL, Interleukin; *TPO,* thrombopoietin.

platelet membrane receptor protein identified earlier, MPL, named for v-mpl, a viral oncogene associated with murine myeloproliferative leukemia. The plasma concentration of TPO is inversely proportional to platelet and megakaryocyte mass, implying that membrane binding and consequent removal of TPO by platelets is the primary platelet count control mechanism.[15] Investigators have used both in vitro and in vivo experiments to show that TPO, in synergy with other cytokines, induces stem cells to differentiate into megakaryocyte progenitors and that it further induces the differentiation of megakaryocyte progenitors into megakaryoblasts and megakaryocytes. TPO also induces the proliferation and maturation of megakaryocytes and induces thrombocytopoiesis (Table 10.3).

Synthetic TPO mimetics (analogs) elevate the platelet count in patients being treated for a variety of cancers, including acute leukemia. One commercial TPO mimetic, romiplostim (NPlate, Amgen), is a nonimmunogenic oligopeptide that is effective in raising the platelet count in patients with chronic immune thrombocytopenic purpura (ITP).[16] A second nonpeptide TPO mimetic, eltrombopag (Promacta, Novartis), binds an MPL site separate from romiplostim and is used in the treatment of chronic ITP and in patients with thrombocytopenia resulting from chronic hepatitis C or severe aplastic anemia. They may have additive effects.[17]

Other cytokines that function with TPO to stimulate megakaryocytopoiesis include interleukin-3 (IL-3), IL-6, and IL-11 (Table 10.3). IL-3 seems to act in synergy with TPO to induce the early differentiation of stem cells, whereas IL-6 and IL-11 act in the presence of TPO to enhance endomitosis, megakaryocyte maturation, and thrombocytopoiesis. An IL-11 polypeptide mimetic, oprelvekin (Neumega, Pfizer), stimulates platelet production in patients with chemotherapy-induced thrombocytopenia.[18] Other cytokines and hormones that participate synergistically with TPO and the interleukins are stem cell factor, also called kit ligand or mast cell growth factor; granulocyte-macrophage colony-stimulating factor (GM-CSF); granulocyte colony-stimulating factor (G-CSF); and acetylcholinesterase-derived megakaryocyte growth stimulating peptide.[19]

Platelet factor 4 (PF4), β-thromboglobulin, neutrophil-activating peptide 2, IL-8, and other factors inhibit in vitro megakaryocyte growth, which indicates that they may have a role in the control of megakaryocytopoiesis in vivo. Internally, reduction in the transcription factors FOG1, GATA-1, and NF-E2 diminish megakaryocytopoiesis at the progenitor, endomitotic, and terminal maturation phases.[20]

PLATELETS

The proplatelet process sheds platelets, cells consisting of granular cytoplasm with a membrane but no nucleus, into the venous sinus of the bone marrow. On a Wright-stained wedge-preparation blood film, platelets are distributed throughout the red blood cell monolayer at 7 to 21 cells per 100× field, and they average 2.5 μm in diameter[21] (Figure 1.1). The internal structure of platelets is complex but scarcely visible using light microscopy. Mean platelet volume (MPV), as measured in a buffered isotonic suspension flowing through the impedance-based detector of a clinical profiling instrument, ranges from 8 to 10 fL (Figure 12.5). A frequency distribution of platelet volume is log-normal, however, which indicates a subpopulation of large platelets (Figure 12.13). Heterogeneity in the MPV of normal healthy humans reflects random variation in platelet release volume and is not a function of platelet age or vitality, as many authors claim.[22]

Although circulating, resting platelets are biconvex, the platelets in blood collected using the anticoagulant ethylenediaminetetraacetic acid (EDTA, lavender closure tubes) tend to "round up." On a Wright-stained wedge-preparation blood film, platelets appear circular to irregular, lavender, and granular. Because of their small size, it is difficult to examine the internal structure of platelets using light microscopy.[23] In the blood, the platelet surface is even, and they flow smoothly through veins, arteries, and capillaries. In contrast to leukocytes, which tend to roll along the vascular endothelium, platelets cluster with the erythrocytes near the center of the blood vessel. Unlike erythrocytes, however, platelets move back and forth with the leukocytes from venules into the white pulp of the spleen, where both become sequestered in dynamic equilibrium.

The normal peripheral blood platelet count is 150 to 400 × 10^9/L. The platelet count decreases with increasing age, such that after 65 years of age, platelet counts of 122 to 350 × 10^9/L and 140 to 379 × 10^9/L are seen in men and women, respectively. This count represents only two thirds of total body platelets; the remaining one third is sequestered within the spleen. Sequestered platelets are immediately available in times of demand—for example, in acute inflammation or after an injury, after major surgery, or during plateletpheresis. In hypersplenism or splenomegaly, increased sequestration may cause a relative thrombocytopenia.

Reticulated platelets, sometimes known as *stress platelets,* appear in compensation for thrombocytopenia (Figure 10.5).[22] Reticulated platelets are markedly larger than ordinary mature circulating platelets; their diameter in peripheral blood films exceeds 6 μm, and their MPV reaches 12 to 14 fL.[23] Like ordinary platelets, they round up in EDTA, but in *citrated* (blue-closure tubes) whole blood, reticulated platelets are cylindrical and beaded, resembling fragments of megakaryocyte proplatelet processes. Reticulated platelets carry free ribosomes and fragments of rough endoplasmic reticulum, analogous to red blood cell reticulocytes, which triggers speculation that they arise from early and rapid proplatelet extension and release. Nucleic acid dyes such as thiazole orange bind the RNA of the endoplasmic reticulum. This property is exploited by hematology instruments to provide a quantitative evaluation of reticulated platelet production, a measurement that may be more useful than the MPV.[24] Platelet dense granule nucleotides, however, may interfere with this measurement, falsely raising the reticulated platelet count by binding nucleic acid dyes. Reticulated platelets are potentially prothrombotic and may be associated with increased risk of cardiovascular disease.[25-29]

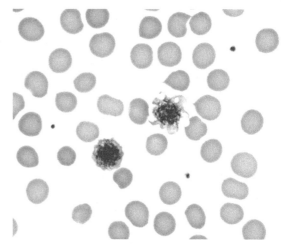

Figure 10.5 A "Stress" or "Reticulated" Platelet. The stress platelet may appear in blood circulation in compensation for thrombocytopenia. The diameter of reticulated platelets exceeds 6 μm. Reticulated platelets carry free ribosomes and fragments of rough endoplasmic reticulum, detectable in flow cytometry using nucleic acid dyes. (Peripheral blood, Wright-Giemsa stain, ×500.)

PLATELET ULTRASTRUCTURE

Platelets, although anucleate, are strikingly complex and are metabolically active. Their ultrastructure has been studied using scanning and transmission electron microscopy, flow cytometry, and molecular sequencing.

Resting Plasma Membrane

The platelet *plasma membrane* resembles any biologic membrane: a bilayer composed of proteins and lipids, as diagrammed in Figure 10.6. The predominant lipids are phospholipids, which form the basic structure, and cholesterol, which distributes

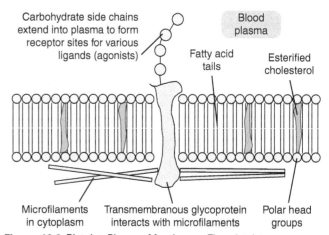

Figure 10.6 Platelet Plasma Membrane. The platelet possesses a standard biologic membrane composed of a phospholipid bilayer with polar head groups oriented toward the aqueous blood plasma (neutral phospholipids) and platelet cytoplasm (charged phospholipids) and nonpolar fatty acid tails that orient toward the center. The phospholipid backbone is interspersed with esterified cholesterol that maintains membrane integrity and function. A series of transmembranous proteins communicate with microfilaments (shown here), G-proteins, and enzymes. The transmembranous proteins support carbohydrate side chains (receptors) that extend into the plasma.

asymmetrically throughout the phospholipids. The phospholipids form a bilayer with their polar heads oriented toward aqueous environments—toward the blood plasma externally and the cytoplasm internally. Their fatty acid chains, esterified to carbons 1 and 2 of the phospholipid triglyceride backbone, orient toward each other, perpendicular to the plane of the membrane, to form a hydrophobic barrier sandwiched within the hydrophilic layers.

The neutral phospholipids phosphatidylcholine and sphingomyelin predominate in the outer blood plasma layer; the anionic or polar phospholipids phosphatidylinositol, phosphatidylethanolamine, and phosphatidylserine predominate in the inner, cytoplasmic layer. During platelet activation these phospholipids, especially phosphatidylinositol, support platelet activation by supplying arachidonic acid, an unsaturated fatty acid that becomes converted to the eicosanoids, including the potent thromboxane A_2 (detailed later in this chapter).

Esterified cholesterol moves freely throughout the hydrophobic internal layer, exchanging with unesterified cholesterol from the surrounding plasma. Cholesterol stabilizes the membrane, maintains fluidity, and helps control the transmembranous passage of materials through the selectively permeable plasma membrane.

Anchored within the membrane are glycoproteins and proteoglycans that support surface glycosaminoglycans, oligosaccharides, glycolipids, and essential plasma surface-oriented glycosylated receptors that respond to cellular and humoral stimuli, called *ligands* or *agonists*, transmitting their stimulus through the membrane to activation organelles internal to the platelet. The platelet membrane surface, called the *glycocalyx,* also absorbs albumin, fibrinogen, and other plasma proteins, in many instances transporting them to internal storage organelles using a process called *endocytosis.*

At 20 to 30 nm, the platelet glycocalyx is thicker than the analogous surface layer of leukocytes or erythrocytes. This thick layer is adhesive and responds readily to hemostatic demands. The platelet carries its functional environment with it, meanwhile maintaining a negative surface charge that repels other platelets, other blood cells, and the endothelial cells that line the blood vessels.

Surface-Connected Canalicular System

The plasma membrane invades the platelet interior, producing a unique *surface-connected canalicular system* (SCCS; Figure 10.7). The SCCS twists sponge-like throughout the platelet, enabling the platelet to store additional quantities of the same hemostatic proteins found on the glycocalyx. The SCCS also allows for enhanced interaction of the platelet with its environment, increasing access to the platelet interior as well as increasing egress of platelet release products. The glycocalyx is less developed in the SCCS and lacks some of the glycoprotein receptors present on the platelet surface. However, the SCCS is the route for endocytosis and for secretion of α-granule contents upon platelet activation.

Dense Tubular System

Parallel and closely aligned to the SCCS is the *dense tubular system* (DTS), a condensed remnant of the rough endoplasmic reticulum. The DTS sequesters Ca^{2+} and bears a number of enzymes that support platelet activation including phospholipase A_2, cyclooxygenase, and thromboxane synthetase, which support the production of thromboxane A_2, and phospholipase C, which supports production of the signaling molecules inositol triphosphate (IP_3) and diacylglycerol (DAG).

Cytoskeleton: Microfilaments and Microtubules

A thick circumferential bundle of microtubules maintains the platelet's discoid shape (Figure 10.7). The *circumferential microtubules* parallel the plane of the outer surface of the platelet and reside just within, although not touching, the plasma membrane. There are 8 to 20 tubules composed of multiple subunits of tubulin that disassemble at refrigerator temperature or when platelets are treated with colchicine. When microtubules disassemble in the cold, platelets become round, but on warming to 37° C, they recover their original disc shape. On cross section, microtubules are cylindrical, with a diameter of 25 nm. The circumferential microtubules could be a single spiral tubule.[30]

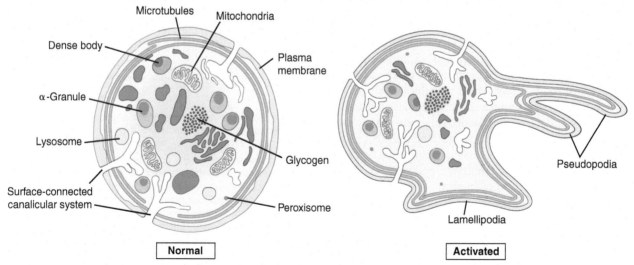

Figure 10.7 Diagram of Platelet Subcellular Organelles.

In addition to maintaining the shape of resting platelets, microtubules move inward on platelet activation to enable the expression of α-granule contents and subsequently reassemble in long parallel bundles during platelet shape change to provide rigidity to pseudopods.

In the narrow area between the microtubules and the membrane lies a thick meshwork of *microfilaments* composed of actin. *Actin* is contractile in platelets (as in muscle) and anchors the plasma membrane glycoproteins and proteoglycans. Actin also is present throughout the platelet cytoplasm, constituting 20% to 30% of platelet protein. In the resting platelet, actin is globular and amorphous, but as the cytoplasmic calcium concentration rises, actin becomes filamentous and contractile.

The cytoplasm also contains intermediate filaments, rope-like polymers 8 to 12 nm in diameter, of *desmin* and *vimentin*. The intermediate filaments connect with actin and the tubules, maintaining the platelet shape. Microtubules, actin microfilaments, and intermediate microfilaments control platelet shape change, extension of pseudopods, and secretion of granule contents.

Platelet Granules: α-Granules, Dense Granules, and Lysosomes

There are 50 to 80 *α-granules* in each platelet which stain medium gray in osmium-dye transmission electron microscopy preparations (Figure 10.7). The α-granules are filled with proteins, some endocytosed, some synthesized within the megakaryocyte and stored in platelets (Table 10.4). Several α-granule proteins are membrane bound. As the platelet becomes activated, α-granule membranes fuse with the SCCS. Their contents flow to the nearby microenvironment, where they participate in platelet adhesion and aggregation and support plasma coagulation.[31]

There are two to seven *dense granules* per platelet (Figure 10.7). These granules appear later than α-granules in megakaryocyte differentiation and stain black (opaque) when treated with osmium in transmission electron microscopy. Small molecules are probably endocytosed and are stored in the dense granules; these are listed in Table 10.5. In contrast to the α-granules, which employ the SCCS, dense granules migrate to the plasma membrane and release their contents directly into the plasma on platelet activation. Membranes of dense granules support the same integral proteins as the α-granules—P-selectin, $\alpha_{IIb}\beta_3$, and GP Ib/IX/V, for instance—which implies a common source for the membranes of both types of granules.[32]

Platelets also contain a few lysosomes that are similar to those in neutrophils (300 nm diameter granules that stain positive for arylsulfatase, β-glucuronidase, acid phosphatase, and catalase). The contents of lysosomes probably digest vessel wall matrix components during in vivo aggregation and may also digest autophagic debris.

Plasma Membrane Receptors That Provide for Adhesion

The platelet membrane contains more than 50 distinct receptors, including members of the cell adhesion molecule (CAM) *integrin* family (the CAM *leucine-rich repeat* family, the CAM

TABLE 10.4 Representative Platelet α-Granule Proteins

	Coagulation Proteins	Noncoagulation Proteins
Proteins Present in Platelet Cytoplasm and α-Granules		
Endocytosed	Fibronectin	Albumin
	Fibrinogen	Immunoglobulins
Megakaryocyte synthesized	Factor V	—
	Thrombospondin	—
	VWF	—
Proteins Present in α-Granules but not Cytoplasm		
Megakaryocyte synthesized	β-thromboglobulin	EGF
	HMWK	Multimerin
	PAI-1	PDC1
	Plasminogen	PDGF
	PF4	TGF-β
	Protein C inhibitor	VEGF/VPF
Platelet Membrane-Bound Proteins		
Restricted to α-granule membrane	P-selectin	GMP33
	—	Osteonectin
In α-granule and plasma membrane	GP IIb/IIIa	cap1
	GP IV	CD9
	GP Ib/IX/V	PECAM-1

Cap1, Adenyl cyclase-associated protein; *CD*, cluster of differentiation; *EGF*, endothelial growth factor; *GMP*, guanidine monophosphate; *GP*, glycoprotein; *HMWK*, high-molecular-weight kininogen; *PAI-1*, plasminogen activator inhibitor-1; *PDCI*, platelet-derived collagenase inhibitor; *PDGF*, platelet-derived growth factor; *PECAM-1*, platelet-endothelial cell adhesion molecule-1; *PF4*, platelet factor 4; *TGF-β*, transforming growth factor-β; *VEGF/VPF*, vascular endothelial growth factor/vascular permeability factor; *VWF*, von Willebrand factor.

TABLE 10.5 Platelet Dense Granule Contents

Small Molecule	Property
ADP	Nonmetabolic; supports neighboring platelet aggregation by binding to the $P2Y_1$ and $P2Y_{12}$ ADP receptors
ATP	Function unknown, but ATP release is detectable on platelet activation
Serotonin	Vasoconstrictor that binds endothelial cells and platelet membranes
Ca^{2+} and Mg^{2+}	Divalent cations support platelet activation and coagulation

ADP, Adenosine diphosphate; *ATP*, adenosine triphosphate; *P2Y1* and *P2Y12*, members of the purinergic receptor family (receptors that bind purines).

immunoglobulin gene family, the CAM *selectin* family), the *seven-transmembrane receptor* family, and some miscellaneous receptors (Figure 10.8).[33] Table 10.6 lists the receptors that support the initial phases of platelet adhesion and aggregation.

Several *integrins* bind collagen, enabling the platelet to adhere to the injured blood vessel lining. Integrins are heterodimeric (composed of two dissimilar proteins). CAMs integrate their ligands, which they bind on the outside of the cell, with the internal cytoskeleton, triggering activation. GP Ia/IIa, or, using integrin terminology, $\alpha_2\beta_1$, is an integrin that binds the subendothelial collagen that becomes exposed in the damaged blood vessel wall, promoting adhesion of the platelet to

the vessel wall (Table 10.6). Likewise, $\alpha_5\beta_1$ and $\alpha_6\beta_1$ bind the adhesive endothelial cell proteins *laminin* and *fibronectin*, which further promotes platelet adhesion. Another collagen-binding receptor is GP VI, a member of the *immunoglobulin gene* family, so named because the genes of its members have multiple immunoglobulin-like domains. The unclassified platelet receptor GP IV is a key collagen receptor that also binds the adhesive protein *thrombospondin*.[34]

GP Ib/IX/V is a *leucine-rich-repeat* family CAM, named for its members' multiple leucine-rich domains. GP Ib/IX/V arises from the genes *GP1BA*, *GP1BB*, *GP5*, and *GP9*. It is composed of two molecules each of GP Ibα, GP Ibβ, and GP IX, and one

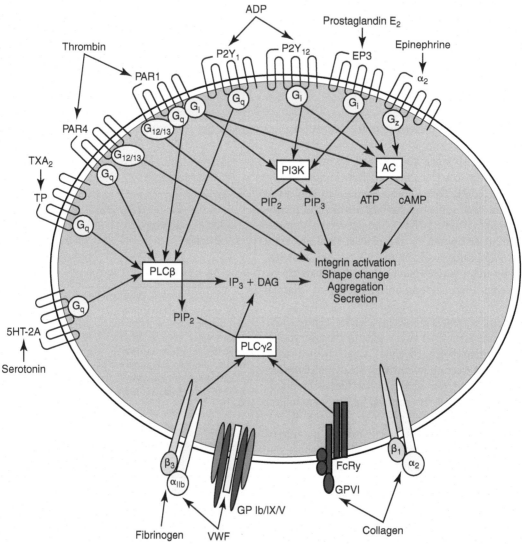

Figure 10.8 Diagram of the Platelet Membrane Receptors and Associated Activation Pathways. The seven-transmembrane repeat receptors (STRs) for serotonin, thromboxane, thrombin, adenosine diphosphate (ADP), prostaglandin E$_2$, and epinephrine are coupled to G-proteins, which become stimulated when agonists bind their respective receptors to subsequently activate phospholipase enzymes (PLCβ, PI3K), and adenyl cyclase. Integrins include collagen receptor $\alpha_2\beta_1$ and fibrinogen/VWF receptor $\alpha_{IIb}\beta_3$. The integrins and glycoproteins activate PLCγ2 that also activates the PIP$_2$ pathway. The key collagen receptor is GPVI, and the key VWF receptor is GP Ib/IX/V. *AC,* Adenyl cyclase; *DAG,* diacyl glycerol; *GP Ib/IX/V,* complex of glycoproteins Ib, IX, and V, which is the VWF receptor; *GPVI,* glycoprotein VI collagen receptor; *IP3,* inositol-1-4-5-triphosphate; *PAR1 and PAR4,* protease-activated receptors that are activated by thrombin; *PI3K,* phosphoinositide-3-kinase; *PIP2,* phosphotidylinositol-4-5 bisphosphate; *PIP3,* phosphotidylinositol-4-5 triphosphate; *PLCγ2,* phospholipase Cγ2; *PLCβ,* phospholipase Cβ; *TP,* TXA$_2$ receptor; *TXA$_2$,* thromboxane A$_2$; *VWF,* von Willebrand factor.

TABLE 10.6 Glycoprotein Platelet Membrane Receptors That Participate in Adhesion and the Initiation of Aggregation by Binding Specific Ligands

Electrophoresis Nomenclature	Current Nomenclature	Ligand	Cluster Designation	Comments
GP Ia/IIa	Integrin: $\alpha_2\beta_1$	Collagen	CD29, CD49b	Avidity is upregulated via "inside-out" activation that depends on collagen binding to GP VI.
	Integrin: $\alpha_v\beta_1$	Vitronectin		
	Integrin: $\alpha_5\beta_1$	Laminin	CD29, CD49e	
	Integrin: $\alpha_6\beta_1$	Fibronectin	CD29, CD49f	
GP VI	CAM of the immunoglobulin gene family	Collagen		Key collagen receptor, triggers activation, release of agonists that increase the avidity of integrins $\alpha_2\beta_1$ and $\alpha_{IIb}\beta_3$.
GP Ib/IX/V	CAM of the leucine-rich repeat family	VWF and thrombin bind GP Ibα; thrombin cleaves a site on GP V	CD42a, CD42b, CD42c, CD42d	GP Ib/IX/V is a 2:2:2:1 complex of GP Ibα and Ibβ, GP IX, and GP V. There are 25,000 copies on the resting platelet membrane surface, 5%–10% on the α-granule membrane, but few on the SCCS membrane. GP Ibα is the VWF-specific site. Fifty percent of GP Ibα/Ibβ is cleared from the membrane on activation. Bernard-Soulier syndrome mutations are identified for all but GP V. Bound to subsurface actin-binding protein.
GP IIb/IIIa	Integrin: $\alpha_{IIb}\beta_3$	Fibrinogen, VWF	CD41, CD61	GP IIb and GP IIIa are distributed on the surface membrane, SCCS, and α-granule membranes (30%). Heterodimer forms on activation.

CAM, Cell adhesion molecule; *GP,* glycoprotein; *SCCS,* surface-connected canalicular system; *VWF,* von Willebrand factor.

molecule of GP V which are bound noncovalently.[35] The two copies of subunit GP Ibα bind VWF and support platelet *tethering* (deceleration), necessary in capillaries and arterioles where blood flow shear rates exceed 1000 s^{-1}. The accompanying GP Ibβ molecules cross the platelet membrane and interact with actin-binding protein to provide "outside-in" signaling. Two molecules of GP IX and one of GP V help assemble the four GP Ib molecules. The subunits of the integrin GP IIb/IIIa ($\alpha_{IIb}\beta_3$), are in a low affinity conformation (α_{IIb} and β_3) as they are distributed across the plasma membrane, the SCCS, and the internal layer of α-granule membranes of resting platelets. These form their active heterodimer, $\alpha_{IIb}\beta_3$, after initiation of an "inside-out" signaling mechanism triggered by agonist binding to its receptor. Although various agonists may activate the platelet, $\alpha_{IIb}\beta_3$ is a physiologic requisite because it binds fibrinogen, generating interplatelet cohesion, called platelet aggregation. The $\alpha_{IIb}\beta_3$ integrin also binds other adhesive proteins that share the target *arginine-glycine-aspartate* (RGD) amino acid sequence with fibrinogen such as VWF, vitronectin, and fibronectin.[36]

The Seven-Transmembrane Repeat Receptors

Thrombin, thrombin receptor activation peptide (TRAP), adenosine diphosphate (ADP), epinephrine, serotonin, and thromboxane A$_2$ (TXA$_2$) (and other prostaglandins) can function individually or in combination to activate platelets (Figure 10.8). These platelet "agonists" are ligands for *seven-transmembrane repeat receptors* (STRs), so named for their unique membrane-anchoring structure. The STRs have seven hydrophobic anchoring domains supporting an external binding site and an internal

terminus that interacts with G proteins to mediate outside-in platelet signaling. The STRs expressed on the platelet surface are listed in Table 10.7.[37]

Thrombin cleaves two STRs, protease-activated receptor 1 (PAR1) and PAR4, that together have a total of 1800 membrane copies on an average platelet. Thrombin cleavage of either of these two receptors activates the platelet through G-proteins that in turn activate at least two internal physiologic pathways. Thrombin also interacts with platelets by binding or digesting two CAMs in the leucine-rich repeat family, GP Ibα and GP V, both of which are parts of the GP Ib/IX/V VWF adhesion receptor.[37]

There are about 600 copies of the high-affinity ADP receptors P2Y$_1$ and P2Y$_{12}$ per platelet.[38] These receptors are linked to different G-proteins and produce distinct intracellular signals that have complementary effects on platelet aggregation.[39] P2Y$_1$ signaling leads to an increase in intracellular calcium levels and contributes to initial platelet activation, shape change, and the formation of small reversible aggregates, whereas P2Y$_{12}$ signaling leads to a decrease in cyclic adenosine monophosphate (cAMP) levels and supports the formation of irreversible platelet aggregates.

TPα and TPβ bind TXA$_2$. This interaction produces more TXA$_2$ from the platelet, a G-protein-based autocrine (self-perpetuating) system that activates neighboring platelets. Epinephrine binds α_2-adrenergic sites that couple to G-proteins and open membrane calcium channels. The α_2-adrenergic sites function similarly to those located on heart muscle. The receptor site IP binds *prostacyclin* (prostaglandin I$_2$, PGI$_2$), a prostaglandin produced by endothelial cells. Prostacyclin binding

TABLE 10.7 **Platelet Seven Transmembrane Repeat Receptor-Ligand Interactions, G-Protein Activation, and the Effect on Platelets**

Receptor	Ligand	G-Protein	Effect
PAR1	Thrombin	G_i	Deceleration of adenylate cyclase and reduction in cAMP
		G_q	Activation of phospholipase C and increase of IP3-DAG
		G12	Activation of protein kinase C and actin microfilaments
PAR4	Thrombin	G_q	Activation of phospholipase C and increase of IP3-DAG
		G12	Activation of protein kinase C and actin microfilaments
$P2Y_1$	ADP	G_q	Activation of phospholipase C and increase of IP3-DAG
		G12	Activation of protein kinase C and actin microfilaments
$P2Y_{12}$	ADP	G_i	Deceleration of adenylate cyclase and reduction in cAMP
TPα and TPβ	TXA_2	G_q	Activation of phospholipase C and increase of IP3-DAG
		G12	Deceleration of adenylate cyclase and reduction in cAMP
α_2-adrenergic	Epinephrine	G_i	Deceleration of adenylate cyclase and reduction in cAMP
IP	PGI_2	G_S	Acceleration of adenylate cyclase and increase in cAMP (pathway is in endothelial cells not platelets, but prostacyclin affects platelet function)
$5HT_{2A}$	Serotonin	G_q	Activation of phospholipase C and increase of IP3-DAG

ADP, Adenosine diphosphate; *cAMP,* cyclic adenosine monophosphate; *DAG,* diacylglycerol; *IP,* PGI_2 receptor; *IP3,* inositol triphosphate; *PAR,* protease-activated receptor; *PGI2,* prostaglandin I_2 (prostacyclin); *STR,* seven-transmembrane repeat receptor; *TXA2,* thromboxane A_2; *P2Y1* and *P2Y12,* ADP receptors; *TPα* and *TPβ,* thromboxane receptors; *5HT,* 5-hydroxytryptamine (serotonin).

results in an increase in the internal cAMP concentration of the platelet and an inhibition of platelet activation. The platelet membrane also contains STRs for serotonin, platelet-activating factor, prostaglandin E_2, PF4, and β-thromboglobulin.[40]

Additional Membrane Receptors

About 15 clinically relevant receptors were discussed in the preceding paragraphs. The platelet contains many additional receptors. The CAM immunoglobulin family includes the intercellular adhesion molecules, or ICAMs (CD50, CD54, CD102), which play a role in inflammation and the immune reaction; platelet–endothelial cell adhesion molecule, or PECAM (CD31), which mediates platelet-to-white blood cell and platelet-to-endothelial cell adhesion; and FcγIIA (CD32), a low-affinity receptor for the immunoglobulin Fc portion that plays a role in a dangerous condition called heparin-induced thrombocytopenia (Chapter 39).[41] P-selectin (CD62) is an integrin that facilitates platelet binding to endothelial cells, leukocytes, and one another.[42] P-selectin is found on the α-granule membranes of the resting platelet but migrates via the SCCS to the surface of activated platelets. P-selectin quantification by flow cytometry is a common means for measuring in vivo platelet activation.

PLATELET ACTIVATION

Although the following discussion implies a linear and stepwise process, platelet adhesion, aggregation, and secretion often occur simultaneously.[43,44]

Adhesion: Platelets Bind Elements of the Vascular Matrix

As blood flows, vessel walls create stress, or *shear force,* measured in units labeled s^{-1}. Shear forces range from 500 s^{-1} in

venules and veins to 5000 s^{-1} in arterioles and capillaries and up to 40,000 s^{-1} in stenosed (hardened) arteries. In vessels where the shear rate is more than 1000 s^{-1}, platelet adhesion and aggregation require a defined sequence of events that involves collagen, tissue factor, phospholipid, VWF, and a number of platelet CAMs, ligands, and activators (Figure 10.9).[45]

Injury to the blood vessel wall disrupts the collagen of the extracellular matrix (ECM) (Figures 10.9A and 10.9B).[46] Damaged endothelial cells release VWF from cytoplasmic storage organelles, which then adheres to sites of injury (Figure 10.9C).[47] VWF, whose molecular weight ranges from 500,000 to 20,000,000 Daltons, circulates as a globular protein. Under shear stress, VWF becomes thread-like as it unrolls and exposes sites that weakly bind the GPIbα portion of the platelet membrane GP Ib/IX/V leucine-rich receptor. This is a reversible binding process that "tethers" thereby decelerating the forward motion of the platelet. The interaction between platelet and VWF remains localized by a liver-secreted plasma enzyme, *ADAMTS13,* also called *VWF-cleaving protease,* which digests larger VWF multimers into smaller, less biologically active forms.

At high shear rates, the VWF-GP Ibα tethering reaction is temporary and the platelet rolls along the surface unless GP VI comes in contact with the exposed ECM collagen.[48] Type I fibrillar collagen binding to platelet GP VI, which is anchored in the platelet membrane by an Fc receptor-like molecule, triggers internal platelet activation pathways, releasing TXA_2 and ADP, an "outside-in" reaction (Figure 10.8).[49] These agonists attach to their respective receptors: TPα and TPβ for TXA_2, and $P2Y_1$ and $P2Y_{12}$ for ADP, triggering an "inside-out" reaction that raises the affinity of integrin $\alpha_2\beta_1$ for collagen. The combined effect of GP Ib/IX/V, GP VI, and $\alpha_2\beta_1$ causes the platelet to become firmly affixed to the damaged surface, where it subsequently loses its discoid shape and spreads.[50]

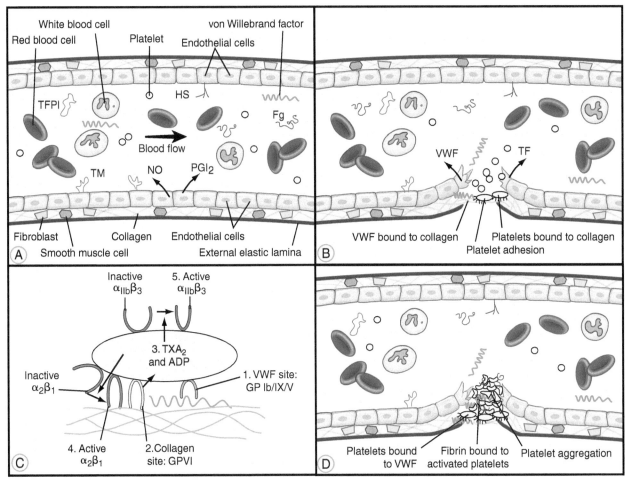

Figure 10.9 Primary Hemostasis: The Process of Platelet Response to Blood Vessel Injury. **(A),** Normal blood flow in intact vessels. RBCs and platelets flow near the center, and WBCs marginate and roll evenly along the smooth endothelium. Endothelial cells and the subendothelial matrix, which contains collagen, smooth muscle cells (in arteries) and collagen-producing fibroblasts, have several mechanisms by which they can limit blood clotting (TM, TFPI, HS) and platelet activation (NO, PGI$_2$). **(B),** Trauma to the blood vessel wall exposes subendothelial collagen and tissue factor, triggering platelet adhesion. **(C),** VWF serves as a bridge between subendothelial collagen and the platelet GP Ib/IX/V receptor. Platelet interaction with collagen via $\alpha_2\beta_1$ and GP VI receptors triggers release of TXA$_2$ and ADP and subsequent activation of the $\alpha_{IIb}\beta_3$ receptor. **(D),** Activation of $\alpha_{IIb}\beta_3$ supports platelet-platelet aggregation through binding of arginine-glycine-aspartate (RGD)–containing ligands such as fibrinogen and VWF. *ADP,* Adenosine diphosphate, *FG,* fibrinogen; *HS,* heparan sulfate; *NO,* nitric oxide; *PGI$_2$,* prostacyclin; *RBC,* red blood cells; *TF,* tissue factor; *TFPI,* tissue factor pathway inhibitor; *TM,* soluble thrombomodulin; *TXA$_2$,* thromboxane A$_2$; *VWF,* von Willebrand factor; *WBC,* white blood cells.

Aggregation: Platelets Irreversibly Cohere

In addition to collagen exposure and VWF secretion, blood vessel injury exposes *tissue factor* expressed on subendothelial smooth muscle cells and fibroblasts. Tissue factor triggers the production of thrombin, which cleaves platelet PAR1 and PAR4. This further activation generates the "collagen and thrombin activated" or *COAT* platelet, integral to the cell-based coagulation model described in Chapter 35 (Figure 10.10).

Meanwhile, the platelet activators TXA$_2$ and ADP are secreted from the platelet granules to the microenvironment, where they activate neighboring platelets through their respective receptors and trigger inside-out activation of integrin $\alpha_{IIb}\beta_3$ (GP IIb/IIIa receptor), enabling it to bind RGD sequences of fibrinogen and VWF and support platelet-to-platelet binding referred to as *platelet aggregation.* P-selectin from the α-granule

membranes moves to the surface membrane to promote binding of platelets with leukocytes.

On further activation, in conjunction with aggregation, platelets *change in shape* from discoid to round and extend pseudopods. This allows platelets to cover more surface area and it enhances platelet binding to other platelets and foreign surfaces. Membrane phospholipid asymmetry is lost, with the more polar molecules, especially phosphatidylserine, flipping to the outer layer. As platelet aggregation continues, membrane integrity is lost, and a syncytium or massive clump of platelets forms as the platelets exhaust internal energy sources.

Platelet aggregation is a key part of primary hemostasis, which in arteries may end with the formation of a "white clot," a clot composed primarily of platelets and VWF (Figure 10.9D). Although aggregation is a normal part of vessel repair, the

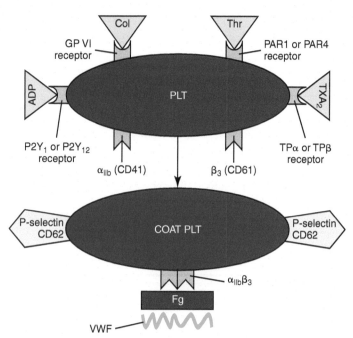

Figure 10.10 Illustration of a COAT Platelet. Further activation of the platelet yields the collagen and thrombin activated (COAT) platelet (PLT) that is able to bind other activated platelets in a process called platelet aggregation. Platelets become activated by agonists—for example, adenosine diphosphate (ADP), thromboxane A_2 (TXA_2), collagen (Col), or thrombin (Thr). P-selectin (CD62) moves from the α-granules to the platelet membrane to support platelet adhesion to foreign surfaces. The inactive α_{IIb} and β_3 units assemble to form the active arginine-glycine-aspartate (RGD) receptor $\alpha_{IIb}\beta_3$, which binds fibrinogen (Fg) and von Willebrand factor (VWF).

presence of white clots often implies inappropriate platelet activation in seemingly uninjured arterioles and arteries and is the pathologic basis for arterial thrombotic events, such as acute myocardial infarction, peripheral artery disease, and ischemic stroke. The risk of these cardiovascular events rises in proportion to the number and avidity of platelet membrane $\alpha_2\beta_1$ and GP VI receptors.[51]

The combination of polar phospholipid exposure on activated platelets, platelet fragmentation with cellular microparticle release, and secretion of the platelet's α-granule and dense granule contents triggers secondary hemostasis, called *coagulation* (Chapter 35). Fibrin and red blood cells deposit around and within the platelet syncytium to form a bulky "red clot." The red clot is essential to wound repair, but it may also be characteristic of inappropriate coagulation in venules and veins, resulting in deep vein thrombosis and pulmonary embolism.

Secretion: Activated Platelets Release Granular Contents

Outside-in activation of the platelet through STRs (such as ADP binding to $P2Y_{12}$) and the immunoglobulin gene product GP VI triggers actin microfilament contraction. Intermediate filaments also contract, moving the circumferential microtubules inward compressing the granules. Contents of α-granules and lysosomes flow through the SCCS, while dense granules migrate to the plasma membrane where their contents are secreted. The dense granule contents are small molecule vasoconstrictors and

platelet agonists that amplify primary hemostasis; most of the α-granule contents are large molecule coagulation proteins that participate in secondary hemostasis (Tables 10.4 and 10.5).

By presenting polar phospholipids on their membrane surfaces, platelets provide a localized cellular milieu that supports coagulation. *Phosphatidylserine* is the polar phospholipid on which the *factor IX/VIII (tenase)* and *factor X/V (prothrombinase)* complexes assemble. The formation of both complexes is supported by ionic calcium secreted by the dense granules.[52,53] The α-granule contents fibrinogen, factors V and VIII, and VWF (which binds and stabilizes factor VIII) are secreted and increase the localized concentrations of these essential coagulation proteins, further supporting the action of tenase and prothrombinase. Platelet secretions provide for cell-based, controlled, localized coagulation. Table 10.8 lists some additional α-granule secretion products that, although not proteins of the coagulation pathway, indirectly support hemostasis. The lists in Tables 10.4, 10.5, and 10.8 are not exhaustive because platelet granule contents continue to be identified through platelet research activities.

Generation of Platelet Microparticles

Microparticles are membrane-derived vesicles that form in response to an activating stimulus that increases the platelet intracellular concentration of calcium. Elevated levels of intracellular calcium result in an inhibition of the enzymes responsible for maintaining the asymmetric distribution of phospholipids in the plasma membrane and an activation of intracellular calpain, which cleaves the platelet cytoskeleton. Together, these effects lead to the outward blebbing of the plasma membrane and the formation of platelet microparticles. Platelet microparticles, believed to be the most abundant microparticles in the circulation, are formed after exposure of platelets to strong agonists or shear stress. These vesicles are made up of the plasma membrane and cytosolic material of the parent cell from which they are derived

TABLE 10.8 Selected Platelet α-Granule Proteins and Their Properties

α-Granule Protein	Properties
Platelet-derived growth factor	Supports mitosis of vascular fibroblasts and smooth muscle cells
Endothelial growth factor	Supports mitosis of vascular fibroblasts and smooth muscle cells
Transforming growth factor-β	Supports mitosis of vascular fibroblasts and smooth muscle cells
Fibronectin	Adhesion molecule
Thrombospondin	Adhesion molecule
Platelet factor 4	Heparin neutralization, suppresses megakaryocytopoiesis
β-thromboglobulin	Found nowhere but platelet α-granules
Plasminogen	Fibrinolysis promotion
Plasminogen activator inhibitor-1	Fibrinolysis control
α_2-Antiplasmin	Fibrinolysis control
Protein C inhibitor	Coagulation control

and retain the cell surface proteins found on the parent cell. As such, microparticles have been found to modulate inflammation, oxidative stress, angiogenesis, and thrombosis. The promotion of coagulation is the most studied platelet function and results from the expression of phosphatidylserine on the surface of the microparticles. Elevated levels of platelet microparticles in patients with hypercoagulable conditions have been shown to be predictive of adverse outcomes in some settings.[54]

PLATELET ACTIVATION PATHWAYS

G-Proteins

G-proteins control cellular activation for all cells at the inner membrane surface (Figure 10.11; Table 10.7). G-proteins are $\alpha\beta\gamma$ heterotrimers (proteins composed of three dissimilar peptides) that bind guanosine diphosphate (GDP) when inactive. Membrane receptor–ligand (agonist) binding promotes GDP release and its replacement with guanosine triphosphate (GTP). The Gα portion of the three-part G molecule briefly disassociates, exerts enzymatic guanosine triphosphatase activity, and hydrolyzes the bound GTP to GDP, releasing a phosphate radical. The G-protein resumes its resting state, but the hydrolysis step provides the necessary phosphorylation to trigger eicosanoid synthesis or the IP$_3$-DAG pathway.

Eicosanoid Synthesis

The eicosanoid synthesis pathway, alternatively called the *prostaglandin*, *cyclooxygenase*, or *thromboxane* pathway, is one of two essential platelet activation pathways triggered by G-proteins found in platelets (Figure 10.12). The platelet membrane's inner leaflet is rich in phosphatidylinositol, a phospholipid whose number 2 carbon binds numerous types of unsaturated fatty acids, but especially 5,8,11,14-eicosatetraenoic acid, commonly

called *arachidonic acid*. Membrane receptor-ligand binding and the consequent G-protein activation triggers phospholipase A$_2$, a membrane enzyme that cleaves the ester bond connecting the number 2 carbon of the triglyceride backbone with arachidonic acid. Cleavage releases arachidonic acid to the cytoplasm, where it becomes the substrate for *cyclooxygenase*, anchored in the DTS. Cyclooxygenase converts arachidonic acid to prostaglandin G$_2$ and prostaglandin H$_2$, and then *thromboxane synthetase* acts on prostaglandin H$_2$ to produce TXA$_2$. TXA$_2$ binds membrane receptors TPα or TPβ, inhibiting adenylate cyclase activity and reducing cAMP concentrations, which mobilizes ionic calcium from the DTS. The rising cytoplasmic calcium level causes contraction of actin microfilaments producing platelet shape change and further platelet activation. When reagent arachidonic acid is used as an agonist in the laboratory assay, it bypasses the membrane and directly enters the eicosanoid synthesis pathway.

The cyclooxygenase pathway in endothelial cells incorporates the enzyme *prostacyclin synthetase* in place of the thromboxane synthetase found in platelets (Figure 10.12). The eicosanoid pathway end point for the endothelial cell is prostaglandin I$_2$, or *prostacyclin*, which binds the IP receptor activating the IP$_3$-DAG pathway, leading to an acceleration of adenylate cyclase, an increase in cAMP, and a sequestration of ionic calcium to the DTS. The unavailability of ionic calcium shuts down platelet function.

Thus the endothelial cell eicosanoid pathway suppresses platelet activation in the intact blood vessel, creating a dynamic equilibrium with the eicosanoid pathway within the platelet where platelet activation occurs.

TXA$_2$ has a half-life of 30 seconds, diffuses from the platelet, and is spontaneously reduced to thromboxane B$_2$, a stable, measurable plasma metabolite. Efforts to produce a clinical

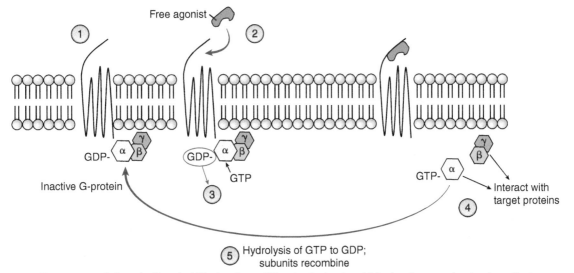

Figure 10.11 G-Protein Coupled Mechanism of Platelet Activation. (1) In the absence of a platelet activating agent (agonist), G-proteins are in a resting state bound to GDP. When an agonist binds its corresponding receptor on the platelet (2) it triggers a G-protein to swap GDP for GTP (3). The GTP-bound α-subunit of the G-protein dissociates from the $\beta\gamma$-subunit and both the α- and $\beta\gamma$-subunits interact with second messengers (Table 10.7) to mediate signal transduction within the platelet (4). Upon GTP hydrolysis (5), the α- and $\beta\gamma$-subunits reunite and the G-protein returns to a resting state bound to GDP. *GDP*, Guanosine diphosphate; *GTP*, guanosine triphosphate.

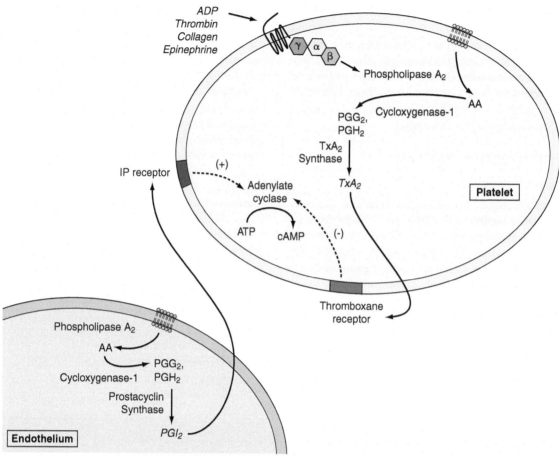

Figure 10.12 Eicosanoid Synthesis. Ligands (agonists) ADP, thrombin, collagen, or epinephrine bind their respective platelet membrane receptors. The binding activates phospholipase A₂ through the G-protein mechanism described in Figure 10.11. Phospholipase A₂ releases arachidonic acid from the platelet membrane phosphatidyl inositol. Arachidonic acid is acted on by cyclooxygenase, peroxidase, and thromboxane synthase to produce TXA₂, which activates the platelet by reducing cAMP production, thus mobilizing ionized calcium (Ca²⁺) from the dense tubules. In the endothelial cell, the eicosanoid pathway is nearly identical, except that prostacyclin synthase replaces thromboxane synthase. The resulting prostacyclin acts to reduce platelet function by increasing cAMP levels. *AA*, arachidonic acid; *ADP*, adenosine diphosphate; *ATP*, adenosine triphosphate; *cAMP*, cyclic adenosine monophosphate; *IP*, PGI₂ or prostacyclin; *PGG₂*, prostaglandin G₂; *PGH₂*, prostaglandin H₂; *PGI₂*, prostacyclin; *TXA₂*, thromboxane A₂.

assay for plasma thromboxane B₂ as a measure of platelet activity have been unsuccessful because special specimen management is required to prevent ex vivo platelet activation with unregulated release of thromboxane B₂ subsequent to collection. Thromboxane B₂ is acted on by a variety of liver enzymes to produce an array of soluble urine metabolites, including 11-dehydrothromboxane B₂, which is stable and measurable.[55,56]

Inositol Triphosphate–Diacylglycerol Activation Pathway

The *IP₃-DAG pathway* is the second G-protein-dependent platelet activation pathway. G-protein activation triggers the enzyme *phospholipase C*. Phospholipase C cleaves membrane phosphatidylinositol 4,5-bisphosphate (PIP₂) to form IP₃ and DAG, both second messengers for intracellular activation. IP₃ promotes release of ionic calcium from the DTS, which triggers actin microfilament contraction. IP₃ may also activate

phospholipase A₂. DAG triggers a multistep process: activation of phosphokinase C, which triggers phosphorylation of the protein pleckstrin, which regulates actin microfilament contraction.

PLATELET PROTEOME

Although platelets are anuclear, they contain a variety of components required for protein synthesis, including ribosomes, polyribosome complexes, and regulatory factors.[57] It has also been recently found that platelets contain microRNAs (miRNAs) and template mRNAs.[58] Proteomic analysis has indicated that platelets contain thousands of unique transcripts that can be translated in response to platelet activation and ligand binding to the GPIIb/IIIa receptor. Such mechanisms allow platelets to alter their phenotype in response to the level of activation. Additionally, it is suggested that the protein synthesis pattern of platelets can be altered by disease state.[59]

SUMMARY

- Platelets arise from bone marrow megakaryocytes, which reside adjacent to the venous sinusoid. Megakaryocyte progenitors are recruited by interleukin-3 (IL-3), IL-6, IL-11, and thrombopoietin (TPO) and mature via endomitosis.
- Platelets are released into the bone marrow through shedding from megakaryocyte proplatelet processes, a process called thrombocytopoiesis.
- Circulating platelets are complex anucleate cells with a thick surface glycocalyx bearing an assortment of coagulation factors and plasma proteins.
- The surface-connected canalicular system (SCCS) and closely aligned dense tubular system (DTS) of the platelet facilitate the storage and release of hemostatic proteins, Ca^{2+}, and enzymes.
- In platelet cytoplasm resides a system of cytoplasmic microfibrils and microtubules that accomplish platelet shape change through membrane contraction and pseudopod extension.

- Also within platelet cytoplasm are platelet α-granules and dense granules that store and secrete coagulation factors and vasoactive molecules.
- The platelet membrane supports an array of receptors that control platelet activation on binding their respective ligands.
- Platelet adhesion to VWF and exposed collagen, platelet-platelet aggregation, and platelet secretion of the substances stored within their granules are the three key functions of an activated platelet.
- Platelet activation is managed internally through G-proteins, the eicosanoid synthesis pathway, the IP_3-DAG pathway, and free ionized calcium.

Now that you have completed this chapter, go back and read again the case study at the beginning and respond to the questions presented.

REVIEW QUESTIONS

Answers can be found in the Appendix.

1. The megakaryocyte progenitor that undergoes endomitosis is:
   a. MK-I
   b. BFU-Meg
   c. CFU-Meg
   d. LD-CFU-Meg
2. The growth factor that is produced in the kidney and induces growth and differentiation of committed megakaryocyte progenitors is:
   a. IL-3
   b. IL-6
   c. IL-11
   d. Thrombopoietin
3. What platelet organelle sequesters ionic calcium and binds a series of enzymes of the eicosanoid pathway?
   a. Glycocalyx
   b. Dense granules
   c. Dense tubular system
   d. Surface connected canalicular system
4. What platelet membrane receptor binds fibrinogen and supports platelet aggregation?
   a. GP Ib/IX/V
   b. GP IIb/IIIa
   c. GP Ia/IIa
   d. $P2Y_1$
5. What platelet membrane phospholipid flips from the inner surface to the plasma surface on activation and serves as the assembly point for coagulation factors?
   a. Phosphatidylethanolamine
   b. Phosphatidylinositol
   c. Phosphatidylcholine
   d. Phosphatidylserine

6. What is the name of the eicosanoid metabolite produced from endothelial cells that suppresses platelet activity?
   a. Thromboxane A_2
   b. Arachidonic acid
   c. Cyclooxygenase
   d. Prostacyclin
7. Which of the following molecules is stored in platelet dense granules?
   a. Serotonin
   b. Fibrinogen
   c. Platelet factor 4
   d. Platelet-derived growth factor
8. What plasma protein is essential for platelet adhesion?
   a. VWF
   b. Factor VIII
   c. Fibrinogen
   d. P-selectin
9. Reticulated platelets can be enumerated in peripheral blood to detect:
   a. Impaired platelet production in disease states
   b. Abnormal organelles associated with diseases such as leukemia
   c. Increased platelet production in response to need
   d. Inadequate rates of membrane cholesterol exchange with the plasma
10. White clots:
   a. Occur primarily in the deep veins of the leg
   b. Are characteristic of the secondary hemostatic process
   c. Are largely composed of platelets and von Willebrand factor
   d. Form normally in response to vascular injury and are completely harmless

11. Upon activation, platelets secrete their α-granule contents via:
    a. The dense tubule system
    b. The surface connected canalicular system
    c. The glycocalyx
    d. Microtubules

12. Microparticles:
    a. Are stored in platelet dense granules
    b. Inhibit blood clotting
    c. Bud off of platelets after their exposure to strong agonists
    d. Exhibit no biologic activity

REFERENCES

1. Butkiewicz, A. M., Kemona, H., Dymicka-Piekarska, V., et al. (2006). Platelet count, mean platelet volume and thrombocytopoietic indices in healthy women and men. *Thromb Res, 118*, 199–204.

2. Reddy, V., Marques, M. B., & Fritsma, G. A. (2013). *Quick Guide to Hematology Testing.* (2nd Ed.). Washington, DC: AACC Press.

3. Deutsch, V. R., & Tomer, A. (2013). Advances in megakaryocytopoiesis and thrombopoiesis: from bench to bedside. *Br J Haematol, 161*, 778–793.

4. Lefrancais, E., Ortiz-Munoz, G., Caudrillier, A., et al. (2017). The lung is a site of platelet biogenesis and a reservoir for haematopoietic progenitors. *Nature, 544*, 105–109.

5. Chang, Y., Bluteau, D., Bebili, N., et al. (2007). From hematopoietic stem cells to platelets. *J Thromb Haemost, 5*(Suppl. 1), 318–327.

6. Italiano, J. E., Jr., & Hartwig, J. H. (2012). Megakaryocyte structure and platelet biogenesis. In Marder, V. J., Aird, W. C., Bennett, J. S., et al. (Eds.), *Hemostasis and Thrombosis: Basic Principles and Clinical Practice.* (6th ed., pp. 365–372). Philadelphia: Lippincott Williams & Wilkins.

7. Lordier, L., Jalil, A., Aurade, F., et al. (2008). Megakaryocyte endomitosis is a failure of late cytokinesis related to defects in the contractile ring and Rho/Rock signaling. *Blood, 112*, 3164–74.

8. Italiano, J. E., & Hartwig, J. H. (2013). Megakaryocyte and platelet structure. In Hoffman, R., Benz, E. J., Silbestein, L. E., et al. (Eds.), *Hematology: Basic Principles and Practice.* (6th ed., pp. 1797–1808). St. Louis: Elsevier.

9. Tomer, A., Harker, L. A., & Burstein, S. A. (1988). Flow cytometric analysis of normal human megakaryocytes. *Blood, 71*(5), 1244–1252.

10. Junt, T., Schulze, H., Chen, Z., et al. (2007). Dynamic visualization of thrombopoiesis within bone marrow. *Science, 317*, 1767–1770.

11. Della Porta, M. G., Lanza, F., Del Vecchio, L., & Italian Society of Cytometry (GIC). (2011). Flow cytometry immunophenotyping for the evaluation of bone marrow dysplasia. *Cytometry B Clin Cytom, 80*, 201–211.

12. Berndt, M. C., & Andrews, R. K. (2012). Major platelet glycoproteins: platelet glycoprotein Ib-IX-V. In Marder, V. J., Aird, W. C., Bennett, J. S., et al. (Eds.), *Hemostasis and Thrombosis: Basic Principles and Clinical Practice.* (6th ed., pp. 382–385). Philadelphia: Lippincott Williams & Wilkins.

13. Yee, F., & Ginsberg, M. H. (2012). Major platelet glycoproteins: integrin $a_{IIb}b_3$ (GP IIb-IIIa). In Marder, V. J., Aird, W. C., Bennett, J. S., et al. (Eds.), *Hemostasis and Thrombosis: Basic Principles and Clinical Practice.* (6th ed., pp. 386–392). Philadelphia: Lippincott Williams & Wilkins.

14. Kuter, D. J. (2010). Biology and chemistry of thrombopoietic agents. *Semin Hematol, 47*, 243–248.

15. Kaushansky, K. (2005). The molecular mechanisms that control thrombopoiesis. *J Clin Invest, 115*, 3339–3347.

16. Neunert, C., Lim, W., Crowther, M., et al. (2011). The American Society of Hematology 2011 evidence-based practice guideline for immune thrombocytopenia. *Blood, 117*, 4190–4207.

17. Bussel, J. B., & Pinheiro, M. P. (2011). Eltrombopag. *Cancer Treatment and Research, 157*, 289–303.

18. Sitaraman, S. V., & Gewirtz, A. T. (2001). Oprelvekin. Genetics Institute. *Curr Opin Investig Drugs, 2*, 1395–1400.

19. Stasi, R. (2009). Therapeutic strategies for hepatitis- and other infection-related immune thrombocytopenias. *Semin Hematol, 46*(Suppl. 2), S15–S25.

20. Yu, M., & Cantor, A. B. (2012). Megakaryopoiesis and thrombopoiesis: an update on cytokines and lineage surface markers. *Methods Mol Biol, 788*, 291–303.

21. Lance, M. D., Sloep, M., Henskens, Y. M., et al. (2012). Mean platelet volume as a diagnostic marker for cardiovascular disease: drawbacks of preanalytical conditions and measuring techniques. *Clin Appl Thromb Hemost, 18*, 561–568.

22. Leader, A., Pereg, D., & Lishner, M. (2012). Are platelet volume indices of clinical use? A multidisciplinary review. *Ann Med, 44*, 805–816.

23. Rodak, B. F., & Carr, J. H. (2013). *Clinical Hematology Atlas.* (4th ed.). St. Louis: Elsevier.

24. Michur, H., Maslanka, K., Szczepinski, A., et al. (2008). Reticulated platelets as a marker of platelet recovery after allogeneic stem cell transplantation. *Int J Lab Hematol, 30*, 519–525.

25. Tsiara, S., Elisaf, M., Jagroop, I. A., et al. (2003). Platelets as predictors of vascular risk: is there a practical index of platelet activity? *Clin Appl Thromb Hemost, 9*, 177–190.

26. Briggs, C., Harrison, P., & Machin, S. J. (2007). Continuing developments with the automated platelet count. *Int J Lab Hematol, 29*, 77–91.

27. Abe, Y., Wada, H., Sakakura, M., et al. (2005). Usefulness of fully automated measurement of reticulated platelets using whole blood. *Clin Appl Thromb Hemost, 11*, 263–270.

28. Briggs, C., Kunka, S., Hart, D., et al. (2004). Assessment of an immature platelet fraction (IPF) in peripheral thrombocytopenia. *Br J Haematol, 126*, 93–99.

29. Cesari, F., Marcucci, R., Gori, A. M., et al. (2013). Reticulated platelets predict cardiovascular death in acute coronary syndrome patients. Insights from the AMI-Florence 2 Study. *Thromb Haemost, 109*, 846–853.

30. White, J. G., & Rao, G. H. (1998). Microtubule coils versus the surface membrane cytoskeleton in maintenance and restoration of platelet discoid shape. *Am J Pathol, 152*, 597–609.

31. Blair, P., & Flaumenhaft, R. (2009). Platelet alpha-granules: basic biology and clinical correlates. *Blood Rev, 23*, 177–189.

32. Abrams, C. S., & Plow, E. F. (2013). Molecular basis for platelet function. In Hoffman, R. H., Benz, E. J., Silberstein, L. E., et al. (Eds.), *Hematology: Basic Principles and Practice.* (6th ed., pp. 1809–1820). St. Louis: Elsevier.

33. Savage, B., & Ruggeri, Z. V. (2012). The basis for platelet adhesion. In Marder, V. J., Aird, W. C., Bennett, J. S., et al. (Eds.), *Hemostasis*

and Thrombosis: Basic Principles and Clinical Practice. (6th ed., pp. 400–449), Philadelphia: Lippincott Williams & Wilkins.

34. Tandon, N. N., Kraslisz, U., & Jamieson, G. A. (1989). Identification of glycoprotein IV (CD36) as a primary receptor for platelet-collagen adhesion. *J Biol Chem, 264,* 7576–7583.

35. Li, R., & Emsley, J. (2013). The organizing principle of platelet glycoprotein Ib-IX-V complex. *J Thromb Haemost, 11*(4), 605–614.

36. Giordano, A., Musumeci, G., D'Angelillo, A., et al. (2016). Effects of glycoprotein IIb/IIIa antagonists: anti platelet aggregation and beyond. *Curr Drug Metab, 17*(2), 194–203.

37. Jackson, S. P., Nesbitt, W. S., & Kulkarni, S. (2003). Signaling events underlying thrombus formation. *J Thromb Haemost, 1,* 1602–1612.

38. Moliterno, D. J. (2008). Advances in antiplatelet therapy for ACS and PCI. *J Interven Cardiol, 21*(Suppl. 1), S18–S24.

39. Gurbel, P. A., Kuliopulos, A., & Tantry, U. S. (2015). G-protein-coupled receptor signaling pathways in new antiplatelet drug development. *Arterioscler Thromb Vasc Biol, 35,* 500–12.

40. Offermanns, S. (2006). Activation of platelet function through G protein-coupled receptors. *Circ Res, 99,* 1293–1304.

41. Greinacher, A. (2015). Heparin-induced thrombocytopenia. *New Eng J Med, 373*(3), 252–261.

42. Keating, F. K., Dauerman, H. L., Whitaker, D. A., et al. (2006). Increased expression of platelet P-selectin and formation of platelet-leukocyte aggregates in blood from patients treated with unfractionated heparin plus eptifibatide compared with bivalirudin. *Thromb Res, 118,* 361–369.

43. Ye, S., & Whiteheart, S. W. (2012). Molecular basis for platelet secretion. In Marder, V. J., Aird, W. C., Bennett, J. S., et al. (Eds.), *Hemostasis and Thrombosis: Basic Principles and Clinical Practice.* (6th ed., pp. 441–449). Philadelphia: Lippincott Williams & Wilkins.

44. Stalker, T. J., Newman, D. K., Ma, P., et al. (2012). Platelet signaling. *Handb Exp Pharmacol, 210,* 59–85.

45. Stegner, D., & Nieswandt, B. (2011). Platelet receptor signaling in thrombus formation. *J Mol Med, 89,* 109–121.

46. Tailor, A., Cooper, D., & Granger, D. N. (2005). Platelet-vessel wall interactions in the microcirculation. *Microcirculation, 12,* 275–285.

47. Zhou, Z., Nguyen, T. C., Guchhait, P., et al. (2010). Von Willebrand factor, ADAMTS-13, and thrombotic thrombocytopenic purpura. *Semin Thromb Hemost, 36,* 71–81.

48. Ruggeri, Z. M., & Mendolicchio, G. L. (2007). Adhesion mechanisms in platelet function. *Circ Res, 100,* 1673–1685.

49. Varga-Szabo, D., Pleines, I., & Nieswandt, B. (2008). Cell adhesion mechanisms in platelets. *Arterioscler Thromb Vasc Biol, 28,* 403–412.

50. Jung, S. M., Moroi, M., Soejima, K., et al. (2012). Constitutive dimerization of glycoprotein VI (GPVI) in resting platelets is essential for binding to collagen and activation in flowing blood. *J Biol Chemistry, 287,* 30000–30013.

51. Furihata, K., Nugent, D. J., & Kunicki, T. J. (2002). Influence of platelet collagen receptor polymorphisms on risk for arterial thrombosis. *Arch Pathol Lab Med, 126,* 305–309.

52. Kunicki, T. J., & Nugent, D. J. (2012). Platelet glycoprotein polymorphisms and relationship to function, immunogenicity, and disease. In Marder, V. J., Aird, W. C., Bennett, J. S., et al. (Eds.), *Hemostasis and Thrombosis: Basic Principles and Clinical Practice.* (6th ed., pp. 393–399), Philadelphia: Lippincott Williams & Wilkins.

53. Zieseniss, S., Zahler, S., Muller, I., et al. (2001). Modified phosphatidylethanolamine as the active component of oxidized low density lipoprotein promoting platelet prothrombinase activity. *J Biol Chem, 276,* 19828–19835.

54. Jeske, W. P., Walenga, J. M., Menapace, B., et al. (2016). Blood cell microparticles as biomarkers of hemostatic abnormalities in patients with implanted cardiac assist devices. *Biomarkers in Medicine, 10*(10), 1095–1104.

55. Carroll, R. C., Craft, R. M., Snider, C. C., et al. (2013). A comparison of VerifyNow with PlateletMapping – detected aspirin resistance and correlation with urinary thromboxane. *Anesth Analg, 116,* 282–286.

56. Eikelboom, J. W., & Hankey, G. J. (2004). Failure of aspirin to prevent atherothrombosis: potential mechanisms and implications for clinical practice. *Am J Cardiovasc Drugs, 4,* 57–67.

57. Zimmerman, G. A., & Weyrich, A. S. (2008). Signal-dependent protein synthesis by activated platelets. New pathways to altered phenotype and function. *Arterioscler Thromb Vasc Biol, 28,* s17–s24.

58. Rowley, J. W., Schwertz, H., Weyrich, A. S. (2012). Platelet mRNA: the meaning behind the message. *Curr Opin Hematol, 19*(5), 385–391.

59. Middleton, E. A., Campbell, R. A., Major, H. D., et al. (2016). Sepsis differentially increases protein synthesis in circulating human platelets. *Am J Respir Crit Care Med, 193,* A3670.

11

Manual, Semiautomated, and Point-of-Care Testing in Hematology

Karen S. Clark, Teresa G. Hippel, and Destiny B. Whitfield

OBJECTIVES

After completion of this chapter, the reader will be able to:

1. List the anticoagulant used for collection of blood specimens for routine hematology tests and describe general handling and processing requirements.
2. State the dimensions of the counting area of a Neubauer ruled hemacytometer.
3. Describe the performance of manual cell counts for white blood cells, red blood cells, and platelets, including types of diluting fluids, typical dilutions, and typical areas counted in the hemacytometer.
4. Calculate dilutions for cell counts when given appropriate data.
5. Calculate hemacytometer cell counts when given numbers of cells, area counted, and dilution.
6. Correct white blood cell counts for the presence of nucleated red blood cells.
7. Describe the principle of the cyanmethemoglobin assay for determination of hemoglobin.
8. Calculate the values for a standard curve for cyanmethemoglobin determination when given the appropriate data, describe how the standard curve is constructed, and use the standard curve to determine hemoglobin values.
9. Describe the procedure for performing a microhematocrit.
10. Identify sources of error in routine manual procedures discussed in this chapter and recognize written scenarios describing such errors.

11. Compare red blood cell count, hemoglobin, and hematocrit values using the rule of three.
12. Calculate red blood cell indices (mean cell volume, mean cell hemoglobin, and mean cell hemoglobin concentration) when given appropriate data, and interpret the results relative to the volume and hemoglobin content and concentration in the red blood cells.
13. Describe the principle and procedure for performing a manual reticulocyte count and the clinical value of the test.
14. Given the appropriate data, calculate the relative, absolute, and corrected reticulocyte counts and the reticulocyte production index; interpret results to determine the adequacy of the bone marrow erythropoietic response in an anemia.
15. Describe the procedure for performing the Westergren erythrocyte sedimentation rate and state its clinical utility.
16. Describe the aspects of establishing a point-of-care testing program, including quality management and selection of instrumentation.
17. Discuss the advantages and disadvantages of point-of-care testing as they apply to hematology tests.
18. Describe the principles of common instruments used for point-of-care testing for hemoglobin level, hematocrit, white blood cell counts, and platelet counts.

OUTLINE

CASE STUDIES

After studying the material in this chapter, the reader should be able to respond to the following case studies:

Case 1

The following results are obtained for a patient with normocytic, normochromic red blood cells (RBCs) on a peripheral blood film:

RBC count = 4.63×10^{12}/L

HGB = 15 g/dL

HCT = 40% (0.40 L/L)

1. Using the rule of three, given the hemoglobin concentration here, what is the expected value for the hematocrit?
2. What could cause the hemoglobin to be falsely elevated or the hematocrit to be falsely low?
3. What would you do to correct for the interferences you listed in question 2?

Case 2

For another patient, the following results are obtained:

RBC count = 3.20×10^{12}/L

HGB = 5.8 g/dL

HCT = 18.9% (0.19 L/L)

1. Calculate the red blood cell indices.
2. How would you describe the red blood cell volume and hemoglobin concentration based on these indices?
3. How should you verify this?

Case 3

The following results are obtained for a patient using a point-of-care device that employs the conductivity method to measure the hematocrit:

Sodium = 160 mmol/L (Reference interval: 135–145 mmol/L)

Potassium = 3.6 mmol/L (Reference interval: 3.5–5.5 mmol/L)

HCT = 17.0% (0.17 L/L)

HGB = 6.0 g/dL

1. Which electrolyte concentration could affect the hematocrit?
2. Would this electrolyte concentration falsely decrease or increase the hematocrit value?
3. What other factors can decrease the hematocrit value using this point-of-care device?

HCT, Hematocrit; HGB, hemoglobin.

Clinical laboratory hematology has evolved from simple observation and description of blood and its components to a highly automated, extremely technical science, including examination at the molecular level. However, some of the more basic tests have not changed significantly over the years. This chapter provides an overview of these basic tests and presents the manual and semiautomated methods that can be used in lieu of automated instrumentation. Included in this chapter is a discussion of point-of-care testing in hematology.

SPECIMEN COLLECTION

Most routine hematology tests require a whole blood specimen collected by venipuncture or skin puncture into tubes with an anticoagulant to prevent clotting. Ethylenediaminetetraacetic acid (EDTA, usually as K_2EDTA) is the most common anticoagulant for routine hematology testing, including the complete blood count (CBC) and differential count, because of its minimal effects on blood cell morphology (Chapters 12 and 13). EDTA prevents clotting in the specimen by binding (chelating) calcium required for fibrin clot formation. EDTA collection tubes are recognized by their lavender or pink stoppers. Established protocols must be followed, including accurate patient identification, proper patient preparation, and use of the appropriate body sites for venipuncture and skin puncture.

Collection tubes must be filled to the proper level to maintain an appropriate blood-to-anticoagulant ratio and mixed by inversion according to tube manufacturer requirements. Ideally specimens for CBC testing should be analyzed within 6 hours of collection if stored at room temperature, and 24 hours if stored at 4° C to minimize spurious results.[1] In addition, peripheral blood films prepared within 3 hours of collection reduce cell deterioration and morphology artifacts. Before testing, the specimen must be well mixed and inspected to ensure it is free of clots. Standard precautions and appropriate safety protocols for specimen collection and handling and discarding of contaminated equipment and supplies must be followed to prevent transmission of bloodborne pathogens.[2]

Following published protocols for specimen collection is a critically important step in providing accurate laboratory test information for patients, regardless of whether the analytical method is performed at the patient's bedside in an inpatient setting, an outpatient physician's office or a clinical laboratory. Procedures published by Clinical and Laboratory Standards Institute (CLSI) describe state of the art methods for collecting and processing blood specimens and should be followed by all health care professionals who collect blood specimens.[3,4] Important components of specimen collection that influence testing include the equipment employed to obtain the specimen, site used and technique for venipuncture or skin puncture, and handling of the specimen after collection. Further details regarding collecting blood specimens may be found on the Evolve website for this text.

MANUAL CELL COUNTS

Although most routine cell-counting procedures in the hematology laboratory are automated, it may be necessary to use manual methods when counts exceed the linearity of an instrument, when an instrument is nonfunctional and there is no backup, in remote laboratories in Third World countries, or in a disaster situation when testing is done in the field. Although the discussion in this chapter concerns whole blood, body fluid cell counts are also often performed using manual methods. Chapter 15 discusses the specific diluents and dilutions used for body fluid cell counts. Chapter 12 discusses automated cell-counting instrumentation in detail.

Manual cell counts are performed using a hemacytometer, or counting chamber, and manual dilutions made with calibrated, automated pipettes and diluents (commercially available or laboratory prepared). The principle for the performance of cell counts is essentially the same for white blood cells (WBCs), red blood cells (RBCs), and platelets; only the dilution, diluting fluid, and area counted vary. Any particle (e.g., sperm) can be counted using this system.

Equipment
Hemacytometer
The manual cell count uses a hemacytometer, or counting chamber. The most common one is the Levy chamber with improved Neubauer ruling. It is composed of two raised surfaces, each with a 3 mm × 3 mm square counting area or grid (total area 9 mm²), separated by an H-shaped moat. As shown in Figure 11.1, this grid is made up of nine 1 mm × 1 mm squares. Each of the four corner (WBC) squares is subdivided further into 16 squares, and the center square subdivided into 25 smaller squares. Each of these smallest squares is 0.2 mm × 0.2 mm, which is 1/25 of the center square or 0.04 mm². A coverslip is placed on top of the counting surfaces. The distance between each counting surface and the coverslip is 0.1 mm; thus the total *volume* of one entire grid or counting area on one side of the hemacytometer is 0.9 mm³. Hemacytometers and coverslips must meet the specifications of the National Bureau of Standards, as indicated by the initials "NBS" on the chamber. When the dimensions of the hemacytometer are thoroughly understood, the area counted can be changed to facilitate the counting of specimens with extremely low or high counts.

Calculations
The general formula for manual cell counts is as follows and can be used to calculate any type of cell count:

$$\text{Total count} = \frac{\text{cells counted} \times \text{dilution factor}}{\text{area (mm}^2) \times \text{depth (0.1)}}$$

or

$$\text{Total count} = \frac{\text{cells counted} \times \text{dilution factor} \times 10^*}{\text{area (mm}^2)}$$

*Reciprocal of depth.

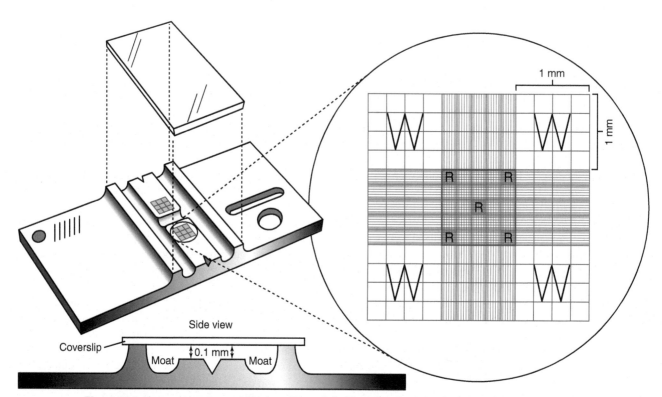

Figure 11.1 Hemacytometer and Close-up View of the Counting Areas as Seen Under the Microscope. The areas for the standard white blood cell count are labeled *W*, and the areas for the standard red blood cell count are labeled *R*. The entire center square, outlined in blue, is used for counting platelets. The side view of the hemacytometer shows a depth of 0.1 mm from the surface of the counting grid to the coverslip.

The calculation yields the number of cells per mm^3. One mm^3 is equivalent to 1 microliter (μL). The count per μL is converted to the count per liter (L) by multiplying by a factor of 10^6.

White Blood Cell Count

The WBC or leukocyte count is the number of WBCs in 1 liter (L) or 1 μL of blood. Whole blood anticoagulated with EDTA or blood from a skin puncture is diluted with 1% buffered ammonium oxalate or a weak acid solution (3% acetic acid or 1% hydrochloric acid). The diluting fluid lyses the nonnucleated RBCs in the specimen to prevent their interference in the count. The typical dilution of blood for the WBC count is 1:20. A hemacytometer is charged (filled) with the well-mixed dilution and placed under a microscope and the number of cells in the four large corner squares (4 mm^2) is counted.

PROCEDURE

1. Clean the hemacytometer and coverslip with alcohol and dry thoroughly with a lint-free tissue. Place the coverslip on the hemacytometer.
2. Make a 1:20 dilution by placing 25 μL of well-mixed blood into 475 μL of WBC diluting fluid in a small test tube.
3. Cover the tube and mix by inversion.
4. Allow the dilution to sit for 10 minutes to ensure that the RBCs have lysed. The solution will be clear once lysis has occurred. WBC counts should be performed within 3 hours of dilution.
5. Mix again by inversion and fill a plain microhematocrit tube.
6. Charge both sides of the hemacytometer by holding the microhematocrit tube at a 45-degree angle and touching the tip to the coverslip edge where it meets the chamber floor.
7. After charging the hemacytometer, place it in a moist chamber (Box 11.1) for 10 minutes before counting the cells to give them time to settle. Care should be taken not to disturb the coverslip.
8. While keeping the hemacytometer in a horizontal position, place it on the microscope stage.
9. Lower the condenser on the microscope and focus by using the low-power (10×) objective lens (100× total magnification). The cells should be distributed evenly in all of the squares.
10. For a 1:20 dilution, count all of the cells in the four corner squares, starting with the square in the upper left-hand corner (Figure 11.1). Cells that touch the top and left lines should be counted; cells that touch the bottom and right lines should be ignored (Figure 11.2). See Figure 11.3 for the appearance of WBCs in the hemacytometer using the low-power objective lens of a microscope.
11. Repeat the count on the other side of the counting chamber. The difference between the total cells counted on each side should be less than 10%. A greater variation could indicate an uneven distribution, which requires that the procedure be repeated.
12. Average the number of WBCs counted on the two sides. Using the average, calculate the WBC count using one of the equations given earlier.

BOX 11.1 How to Make a Moist Chamber

A moist chamber may be made by placing a piece of damp filter paper in the bottom of a Petri dish. An applicator stick broken in half can serve as a support for the hemacytometer.

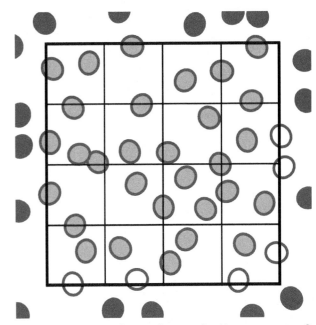

Figure 11.2 One Large Corner Square of a Hemacytometer. Cells touching the left and top lines (*solid circles*) are counted. Cells touching bottom and right (*open circles*) are not counted.

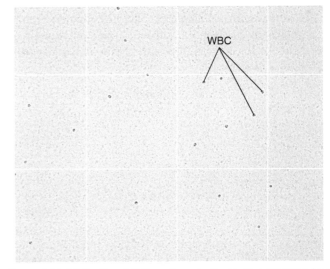

Figure 11.3 White Blood Cells as Seen in the Hemacytometer. Low power (10× objective) 100× total magnification.

Example Using the First Equation

When a 1:20 dilution is used, the four large squares on one side of the chamber yield counts of 23, 26, 22, and 21. The total count is 92. The four large squares on the other side of the chamber yield counts of 28, 24, 22, and 26. The total count is 100. The difference between sides is less than 10%.

TABLE 11.1 Manual Cell Counts with Most Common Dilutions, Counting Areas

Cells Counted	Diluting Fluid	Dilution	Objective	Area Counted
White blood cells	1% ammonium oxalate or 3% acetic acid or 1% hydrochloric acid	1:20 1:100	10× 10×	4 mm² 9 mm²
Red blood cells	Isotonic saline	1:100	40×	0.2 mm² (5 small squares of center square)
Platelets	1% ammonium oxalate	1:100	40× phase	1 mm²

The average number of cells of the two sides of the chamber is 96. Using the average in the formula:

$$\text{WBC count} = \frac{\text{cells counted} \times \text{dilution factor}}{\text{area counted (mm}^2) \times \text{depth}}$$

$$= \frac{96 \times 20}{4 \times 0.1}$$

$$= 4800/\text{mm}^3 \text{ or } 4800/\mu\text{L or}$$

$$4.8 \times 10^3/\mu\text{L or } 4.8 \times 10^9/\text{L}$$

Alternately, a 1:100 dilution may be used counting the number of cells in the entire counting area (nine large squares, 9 mm²) on both sides of the chamber (Table 11.1). As an example, if an average of 54 cells were counted in the entire counting area on both sides of the chamber:

$$\text{WBC count} = \frac{\text{cells counted} \times \text{dilution factor}}{\text{area counted (mm}^2) \times \text{depth}}$$

$$= \frac{54 \times 100}{9 \times 0.1}$$

$$= 6000/\text{mm}^3 \text{ or } 6000/\mu\text{L or}$$

$$6.0 \times 10^3/\mu\text{L or } 6.0 \times 10^9/\text{L}$$

General reference intervals for males and females in different age groups can be found on the inside front cover of this text. *Reference intervals may vary slightly according to the population tested and should be established for each laboratory.*

Sources of Error and Comments

1. The hemacytometer and coverslip should be cleaned properly before they are used. Dust and fingerprints may cause difficulty in distinguishing the cells.
2. The diluting fluid should be free of contaminants.
3. If the count is low, a greater area may be counted (e.g., 9 mm²) to improve accuracy.

4. The chamber must be charged properly to ensure an accurate count. Uneven flow of the diluted blood into the chamber results in an irregular distribution of cells. If the chamber is overfilled or underfilled, the chamber must be cleaned and recharged.
5. After the chamber is filled, allow the cells to settle for 10 minutes before counting.
6. Any nucleated red blood cells (NRBCs) present in the specimen are not lysed by the diluting fluid. The NRBCs are counted as WBCs because they are indistinguishable when seen on the hemacytometer. If five or more NRBCs per 100 WBCs are observed on the differential count on a stained peripheral blood film, the WBC count must be corrected for these cells. This is accomplished by using the following formula:

$$\frac{\text{Uncorrected WBC count} \times 100}{\text{Number of NRBCs per 100 WBCs} + 100}$$

Report the result as the "corrected" WBC count.
7. The accuracy of the manual WBC count can be assessed by performing a WBC estimate on a Wright-stained peripheral blood film made from the same specimen (Chapter 13).

Platelet Count

A platelet count is the number of platelets in 1 L or 1 μL of whole blood. Platelets adhere to foreign objects and to each other, which makes them difficult to count. They also are small and can be confused easily with dirt or debris. In this procedure, whole blood, with EDTA as the anticoagulant, is diluted 1:100 with 1% ammonium oxalate to lyse the nonnucleated RBCs. The platelets are counted in the 25 small squares in the large center square (1 mm²) of the hemacytometer using a phase-contrast microscope in the reference method described by Brecher and Cronkite.[5] A light microscope can also be used, but visualizing the platelets may be more difficult.

▌PROCEDURE

1. Make a 1:100 dilution by placing 20 μL of well-mixed blood into 1980 μL of 1% ammonium oxalate in a small test tube.
2. Mix the dilution thoroughly and charge the chamber. (Note: A special thin, flat-bottomed counting chamber is used for phase-microscopy platelet counts.)
3. Place the charged hemacytometer in a moist chamber (Box 11.1) for 15 minutes to allow the platelets to settle.
4. Platelets are counted using the 40× objective lens (400× total magnification). The platelets have a diameter of 2 to 4 μm and appear round or oval, displaying a light purple sheen when phase-contrast microscopy is used. The shape and color help distinguish the platelets from highly refractile dirt and debris. "Ghost" RBCs often are seen in the background.
5. Count the number of platelets in the 25 small squares in the center square of the grid (Figure 11.1). The area of this center square is 1 mm². Platelets should be counted on each side of the hemacytometer, and the difference between the totals should be less than 10%.

6. Calculate the platelet count by using one of the equations given earlier. Using the first equation as an example, if 200 platelets were counted in the entire center square,

$$\frac{200 \times 100}{1 \times 0.1}$$

$$= 200,000 \,/\, mm^3 \text{ or } 200,000/\mu L$$

$$\text{or } 200 \times 10^3/\mu L \text{ or } 200 \times 10^9 \,/\, L$$

7. The accuracy of the manual platelet count should be verified by performing a platelet estimate on a Wright-stained peripheral blood film made from the same specimen (Chapter 13). General reference intervals for males and females according to age groups can be found on the inside front cover of this text.

Sources of Error and Comments

1. Inadequate mixing and poor collection of the specimen can cause the platelets to clump on the hemacytometer. If the problem persists after redilution, a new specimen is needed. A skin puncture specimen is less desirable because of the tendency of the platelets to aggregate or form clumps.
2. Dirt in the pipette, hemacytometer, or diluting fluid may cause the counts to be inaccurate.
3. If fewer than 50 platelets are counted on each side, the procedure should be repeated by diluting the blood to 1:20. If more than 500 platelets are counted on each side, a 1:200 dilution should be made. The appropriate dilution factor should be used in calculating the results.
4. If the patient has a normal platelet count, the five small, RBC squares (Figure 11.1) may be counted. Then the area is 0.2 mm^2 on each side.
5. The phenomenon of "platelet satellitosis" may occur when EDTA anticoagulant is used. This refers to the adherence of platelets around neutrophils, producing a ring or satellite effect (Figure 13.1). Using sodium citrate as the anticoagulant should correct this problem. Because of the dilution in the citrate evacuated tubes, it is necessary to multiply the obtained platelet count by 1.1 for accuracy (Chapter 13).

Red Blood Cell Count

Manual RBC counts are rarely performed because of the inaccuracy of the count and questionable necessity. Use of other, more accurate manual RBC procedures, such as the microhematocrit and hemoglobin concentration, is desirable when automation is not available. Table 11.1 contains information on performing manual WBC, platelet, and RBC counts.

Disposable Blood Cell Count Dilution Systems

Capillary pipette and diluent reservoir systems are commercially available for WBC and platelet counts. One such system is Leuko Chek (Biomedical Polymers). It consists of a capillary pipette (calibrated to accept 20 μL of blood) that fits into a plastic reservoir containing 1.98 mL of 1% buffered ammonium oxalate (Figure 11.4). Blood from a well-mixed EDTA-anticoagulated specimen or from a skin puncture is allowed to enter the pipette by capillary action to the fill volume. The blood is added to the reservoir making a 1:100 dilution. After mixing the reservoir and

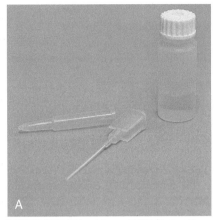

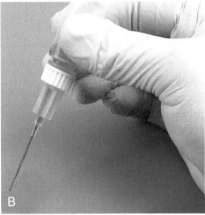

Figure 11.4 LeukoChek Blood Diluting System for Manual White Blood Cell and Platelet Counts. It consists of a 20 μL capillary pipette and plastic reservoir containing 1.98 mL of 1% buffered ammonium oxalate that makes a 1:100 dilution of whole blood. (Courtesy Biomedical Polymers, Inc., Gardner, MA.)

allowing 10 minutes for lysis of the RBCs, the reverse end of the capillary pipette is placed in the reservoir cap making a dropper. The first three or four drops of the diluted specimen are discarded, and the capillary pipette is used to charge the hemacytometer.

Both WBC and platelet counts can be done from the same diluted specimen. WBCs are counted in all nine large squares (9 mm^2) using low power (100× total magnification). Platelets are counted in the 25 small squares in the center square (1 mm^2) using high power (400× total magnification). The standard formula is used to calculate the cell counts.

Body Fluid Cell Counts

Body fluid cell counts are discussed in detail in Chapter 15.

HEMOGLOBIN DETERMINATION

The primary function of hemoglobin within the RBC is to carry oxygen to and carbon dioxide from the tissues. The cyanmethemoglobin (hemiglobincyanide) method for hemoglobin determination is the reference method approved by CLSI.[6]

Principle

In the cyanmethemoglobin method, blood is diluted in an alkaline Drabkin solution of potassium ferricyanide, potassium cyanide, sodium bicarbonate, and a surfactant. The hemoglobin is oxidized to methemoglobin (Fe^{3+}) by the potassium ferricyanide, $K_3Fe(CN)_6$. The potassium cyanide (KCN) then converts the methemoglobin to cyanmethemoglobin:

$$Hemoglobin\ (Fe^{2+}) + K_3\ Fe\ (CN)_6 \rightarrow methemoglobin\ (Fe^{3+})$$
$$+ KCN \rightarrow cyanmethemoglobin$$

The absorbance of the cyanmethemoglobin at 540 nm is directly proportional to the hemoglobin concentration. Sulfhemoglobin is not converted to cyanmethemoglobin; it cannot be measured by this method. Sulfhemoglobin fractions of more than 0.05 g/dL are seldom encountered in clinical practice, however.[7]

PROCEDURE

1. Create a standard curve, using a commercially available cyanmethemoglobin standard.
    a. When a standard containing 80 mg/dL of hemoglobin is used, the following dilutions should be made:

Hemoglobin Concentration (g/dL)	Blank	5	10	15	20
Cyanmethemoglobin standard (mL)	0	1.5	3	4.5	6
Cyanmethemoglobin reagent (mL)	6	4.5	3	1.5	0

b. Transfer the dilutions to cuvettes. Set the wavelength on the spectrophotometer to 540 nm and use the blank to set to 100% transmittance.
c. Using semilogarithmic paper, plot percent transmittance on the y-axis and the hemoglobin concentration on the x-axis. The hemoglobin concentrations of the control and patient specimens can be read from this standard curve (Figure 11.5).
d. A standard curve should be set up with each new lot of reagents. It also should be checked when alterations are made to the spectrophotometer (e.g., bulb change).
2. Controls should be analyzed with each batch of specimens. Commercial controls are available.
3. Using the patient's whole blood anticoagulated with EDTA or heparin or blood from a capillary puncture, make a 1:251 dilution by adding 0.02 mL (20 μL) of blood to 5 mL of cyanmethemoglobin reagent. The pipette should be rinsed thoroughly with the reagent to ensure that no blood remains. Follow the same procedure for the control specimens.
4. Cover and mix well by inversion or use a vortex mixer. Let stand for 10 minutes at room temperature to allow full conversion of hemoglobin to cyanmethemoglobin.
5. Transfer all the solutions to cuvettes. Set the spectrophotometer to 100% transmittance at the wavelength of 540 nm, using cyanmethemoglobin reagent as a blank.
6. Using a matched cuvette, continue reading the percent transmittance of the patient specimens and record the values.
7. Determine the hemoglobin concentration of the control specimens and the patient specimens from the standard curve.

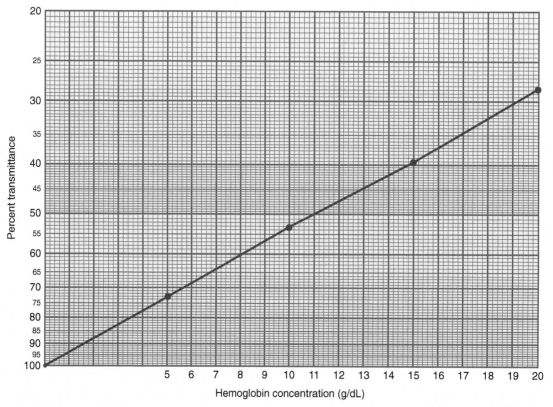

Figure 11.5 Standard Curve for Cyanmethemoglobin Standard of 80 mg/dL. A blank (100% transmittance) and four dilutions were made: 5 g/dL (72.9% transmittance), 10 g/dL (53.2% transmittance), 15 g/dL (39.1% transmittance), and 20 g/dL (28.7% transmittance).

General reference intervals can be found on the inside cover of this text.

Sources of Error and Comments

1. Cyanmethemoglobin reagent is sensitive to light. It should be stored in a brown bottle or in a dark place.
2. A high WBC count (greater than 20×10^9 /L) or a high platelet count (greater than 700×10^9 /L) can cause turbidity and a falsely high result. In this case the reagent-specimen solution can be centrifuged and the supernatant measured.
3. Lipemia also can cause turbidity and a falsely high result. It can be corrected by adding 0.01 mL of the patient's plasma to 5 mL of the cyanmethemoglobin reagent and using this solution as the reagent blank.
4. Cells containing Hemoglobin S (Hb S) S and Hemoglobin C (Hb C) may be resistant to hemolysis, causing turbidity; this can be corrected by making a 1:2 dilution with distilled water (1 part diluted specimen plus 1 part water) and multiplying the results from the standard curve by 2.
5. Abnormal globulins, such as those found in patients with plasma cell myeloma or Waldenström macroglobulinemia, may precipitate in the reagent. If this occurs, add 0.1 g of potassium carbonate to the cyanmethemoglobin reagent. Commercially available cyanmethemoglobin reagent has been modified to contain $KH_2 PO_4$ salt, so this problem is not likely to occur.
6. Carboxyhemoglobin takes 1 hour to convert to cyanmethemoglobin and theoretically could cause erroneous results in specimens from heavy smokers. The degree of error is probably not clinically significant, however.
7. Because the hemoglobin reagent contains cyanide, it is highly toxic and must be used cautiously. Consult the safety data sheet supplied by the manufacturer. Acidification of cyanide in the reagent releases highly toxic hydrogen cyanide gas. A licensed waste disposal service should be contracted to discard the reagent; reagent-specimen solutions should not be discarded into sinks.
8. Commercial absorbance standards kits are available to calibrate spectrophotometers.
9. Handheld systems are commercially available to measure the hemoglobin concentration. An example is the HemoCue[8,9] (HemoCue) (Figure 11.6) in which hemoglobin is converted to azidemethemoglobin and is read photometrically at two wavelengths (570 nm and 880 nm). This method avoids the necessity of specimen dilution and interference from turbidity. It is discussed later in the section on point-of-care testing. Another method that has been used in some automated instruments involves the use of sodium lauryl sulfate (SLS) to convert hemoglobin to SLS-methemoglobin. This method does not generate toxic wastes.[10-13]

MICROHEMATOCRIT

The hematocrit is the volume of packed RBCs that occupies a given volume of whole blood. This is often referred to as the

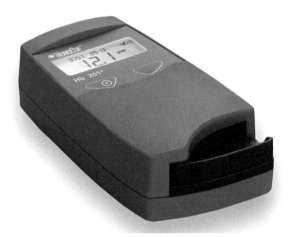

Figure 11.6 The HemoCue Hb 201 + System for Measuring Hemoglobin. (Courtesy HemoCue, Inc., Brea, CA.)

packed cell volume (PCV). It is reported either as a percentage (e.g., 36%) or in liters per liter (0.36 L/L).

PROCEDURE

1. Fill two plain capillary tubes approximately three-quarters full with blood anticoagulated with EDTA or heparin. Mylar-wrapped tubes are recommended by the National Institute for Occupational Safety and Health to reduce the risk of capillary tube injuries.[14] Alternatively, blood may be collected into heparinized capillary tubes by skin puncture. Wipe any excess blood from the outside of the tube.
2. Seal the end of the tube with the colored ring using nonabsorbent clay. Hold the filled tube horizontally and seal by placing the dry end into the tray with sealing compound at a 90-degree angle. Rotate the tube slightly and remove it from the tray. The plug should be at least 4 mm long.[14]
3. Balance the tubes in a microhematocrit centrifuge with the clay ends facing the outside away from the center, touching the rubber gasket.
4. Tighten the head cover on the centrifuge and close the top. Centrifuge the tubes at 10,000 g to 15,000 g for the time that has been determined to obtain maximum packing of RBCs, as detailed in Box 11.2. Do not use the brake to stop the centrifuge.

BOX 11.2 Determining Maximum Packing Time for Microhematocrit

The time to obtain maximum packing of red blood cells should be determined for each centrifuge. Duplicate microhematocrit determinations should be made using fresh, well-mixed blood anticoagulated with ethylenediaminetetraacetic acid (EDTA). Two specimens should be used, with one of the specimens having a known hematocrit of 50% or higher. Starting at 2 minutes, centrifuge duplicates at 30-second intervals and record results. When the hematocrit has remained at the same value for two consecutive readings, optimum packing has been achieved, and the second time interval should be used for microhematocrit determinations.[14]

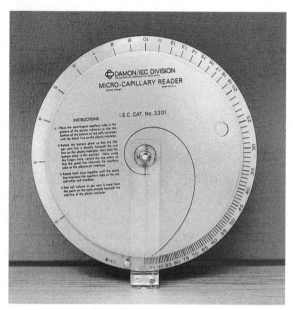

Figure 11.7 Microhematocrit Reader.

5. Determine the hematocrit by using a microhematocrit reading device (Figure 11.7). Read the level of RBC packing; do not include the buffy coat (WBCs and platelets) when taking the reading (Figure 11.8).
6. The values of the duplicate hematocrits should agree within 1% (0.01 L/L).[14]

General reference intervals according to sex and age can be found on the inside front cover of this text.

Sources of Error and Comments

1. Improper sealing of the capillary tube causes a decreased hematocrit reading as a result of leakage of blood during centrifugation. A higher number of RBCs are lost compared with plasma because of the packing of the cells in the lower part of the tube during centrifugation.
2. An increased concentration of anticoagulant (short draw in an evacuated tube) decreases the hematocrit reading as a result of RBC shrinkage.
3. A decreased or increased result may occur if the specimen was not mixed properly.
4. The time and speed of the centrifugation and the time when the results are read are important. Insufficient centrifugation or a delay in reading results after centrifugation causes hematocrit readings to increase. Time for complete packing should be determined for each centrifuge and rechecked at regular intervals. When the microhematocrit centrifuge is calibrated, one of the specimens used must have a hematocrit of 50% or higher.[14]
5. The buffy coat of the specimen should not be included in the hematocrit reading because this falsely elevates the result.
6. A decrease or increase in the readings may be seen if the microhematocrit reader is not used properly.
7. Many disorders, such as sickle cell anemia, macrocytic anemias, hypochromic anemias, spherocytosis, and thalassemia, may cause plasma to be trapped in the RBC layer even if the procedure is performed properly. The trapping of the

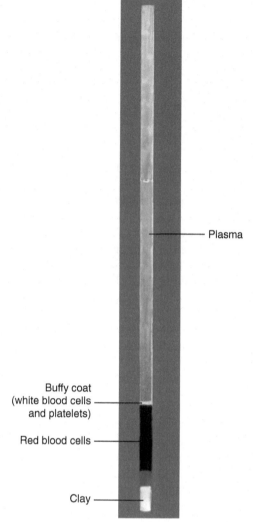

— Plasma

Buffy coat
(white blood cells
and platelets)

Red blood cells —

Clay —

Figure 11.8 Capillary Tube with Anticoagulated Whole Blood after Centrifugation. Notice the layers containing plasma, the buffy coat (white blood cells and platelets), and the red blood cells.

plasma causes the microhematocrit to be 1% to 3% (0.01 to 0.03 L/L) higher than the value obtained using automated instruments that calculate or directly measure the hematocrit and are unaffected by the trapped plasma.
8. A temporarily low hematocrit reading may result immediately after a blood loss because plasma is replaced faster than are the RBCs.
9. The fluid loss associated with dehydration causes a decrease in plasma volume and falsely increases the hematocrit reading.
10. Proper specimen collection is an important consideration. The introduction of interstitial fluid from a skin puncture or the improper flushing of an intravenous catheter causes decreased hematocrit readings.

The READACRIT centrifuge (Becton, Dickinson) uses precalibrated capillary tubes and has built-in hematocrit scales, which eliminates the need for separate reading devices (Figure 11.9). The use of SUREPREP Capillary Tubes (Becton, Dickinson) eliminates the use of sealants. They have a factory-inserted plug that seals automatically when the blood touches the plug.[15]

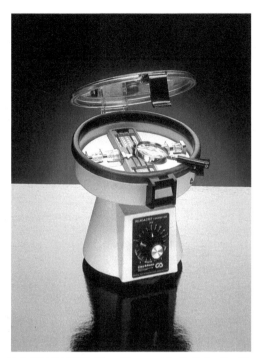

Figure 11.9 READACRIT Centrifuge with Built-in Capillary Tube Compartments and Scales to Read Hematocrit. (Courtesy and © Becton, Dickinson and Company, Franklin Lakes, NJ.)

RULE OF THREE

When specimens are analyzed by automated or manual methods, a quick visual check of the results of the hemoglobin and hematocrit can be done by applying the "rule of three." This rule applies only to specimens that have normocytic normochromic RBCs. The value of the hematocrit should be three times the value of the hemoglobin plus or minus 3: Hemoglobin (HGB) × 3 = Hematocrit (HCT) ± 3 (0.03 L/L). It should become habit for the analyst to multiply the hemoglobin by 3 mentally for every specimen; a value discrepant with this rule may indicate abnormal RBCs, or it may be the first indication of error.

For example, the following results are obtained from patients:

Case 1
HGB = 12 g/dL
HCT = 36% (0.36 L/L)
According to the rule of three,

$$HGB(12) \times 3 = HCT (36)$$

An acceptable range for the hematocrit would be 33% to 39%. These values conform to the rule of three.

Case 2
HGB = 9 g/dL
HCT = 32%
According to the rule of three,

$$HGB(9.0) \times 3 = HCT (27 \text{ versus actual value of } 32)$$

An acceptable range for hematocrit would be 24% to 30%, so these values do not conform to the rule of three.

Case 3
HGB = 15 g/dL
HCT = 36%
According to the rule of three,

$$HGB(15) \times 3 = HCT (45 \text{ versus obtained value of } 36)$$

An acceptable range for hematocrit would be 42% to 48%, so these values do not conform to the rule of three.

If values do not agree, the blood film should be examined for abnormal RBCs; causes of false increases and decreases in the hemoglobin or hematocrit values should also be investigated. In the second example the blood film reveals RBCs that are low in hemoglobin concentration (hypochromic) and are smaller in volume (microcytic), so the rule of three cannot be applied. If RBCs do appear normal, possible causes of a falsely low hemoglobin concentration or a falsely elevated hematocrit should be investigated. In the third example, the specimen is determined to have lipemic plasma causing a falsely elevated hemoglobin concentration, and a correction must be made to obtain an accurate hemoglobin value. (See Hemoglobin Determination in this chapter.)

When an unexplained discrepancy is found, the specimen analyzed before and after the specimen in question should be checked to determine whether their results conform to the rule. If they do not conform, further investigation should be done to identify the problem. A control specimen should be analyzed when such a discrepancy is found. If appropriate results are obtained for the control, random error may have occurred (Chapter 2).

RED BLOOD CELL INDICES

The mean cell volume (MCV), mean cell hemoglobin (MCH), and mean cell hemoglobin concentration (MCHC) are the RBC indices. These are calculated to determine the average volume and hemoglobin content and concentration of the RBCs in the specimen. In addition to serving as a quality control check, the indices may be used for initial classification of anemias. Table 11.2 provides a summary of the RBC indices, morphology, and correlation

TABLE 11.2 Red Blood Cell Indices, Red Blood Cell Morphology, and Disease States			
MCV (fL)	**MCHC (g/dL)**	**Red Blood Cell Morphology**	**Found In**
<80	<32	Microcytic; hypochromic	Iron deficiency anemia, anemia of inflammation, thalassemia, Hb E disease and trait, sideroblastic anemia
80–100	32–36	Normocytic; normochromic	Hemolytic anemia, myelophthisic anemia, bone marrow failure, chronic renal disease
>100	32–36	Macrocytic; normochromic	Megaloblastic anemia, chronic liver disease, bone marrow failure, myelodysplastic syndrome

Hb, Hemoglobin; *MCHC,* mean cell hemoglobin concentration; *MCV,* mean cell volume.

with various anemias. The morphologic classification of anemia on the basis of MCV is discussed in detail in Chapter 16.

Mean Cell Volume

The MCV is the average volume of the RBC, expressed in femtoliters (fL), or 10^{-15} L:

$$MCV = \frac{HCT\ (\%) \times 10}{RBC\ count\ (\times 10^{12}/L)}$$

For example, if the HCT = 45% and the RBC count = 5 × 10^{12}/L, the MCV = 90 fL.

The reference interval for MCV is 80 to 100 fL. RBCs with an MCV of less than 80 fL are microcytic; those with an MCV of more than 100 fL are macrocytic.

Mean Cell Hemoglobin

The MCH is the average weight of hemoglobin in a RBC, expressed in picograms (pg), or 10^{-12} g:

$$MCH = \frac{HGB\ (g/dL) \times 10}{RBC\ count\ (\times 10^{12}/L)}$$

For example, if the hemoglobin = 16 g/dL and the RBC count = 5 × 10^{12}/L, the MCH = 32 pg.

The reference interval for adults is 26 to 32 pg. The MCH generally is not considered in the classification of anemias.

Mean Cell Hemoglobin Concentration

The MCHC is the average concentration of hemoglobin in each individual RBC. The units used are grams per deciliter (formerly given as a percentage):

$$MCHC = \frac{HGB\ (g/dL) \times 100}{HCT\ (\%)}$$

For example, if the HGB = 16 g/dL and the HCT = 48%, the MCHC = 33.3 g/dL.

Values of normochromic RBCs range from 32 to 36 g/dL; values of hypochromic cells are less than 32 g/dL, and values of "hyperchromic" cells are greater than 36 g/dL. Hypochromic RBCs occur in thalassemias, iron deficiency, and other conditions listed in Table 11.2. The term *hyperchromic* is a misnomer: A cell does not really contain more than 36 g/dL of hemoglobin, but its shape may have become spherocytic, which makes the cell appear full. An MCHC between 36 and 38 g/dL should be checked for spherocytes. An MCHC greater than 38 g/dL should be investigated for an error in hemoglobin value (see Sources of Error and Comments in the section on hemoglobin determination). Another cause for a markedly increased MCHC could be the presence of a cold agglutinin. Incubating the specimen at 37° C for 15 minutes before analysis usually produces accurate results. Cold agglutinin disease is discussed in more detail in Chapter 23.

RETICULOCYTE COUNT

The reticulocyte is the last immature RBC stage. Normally a reticulocyte spends 2 days in the bone marrow and 1 day in the

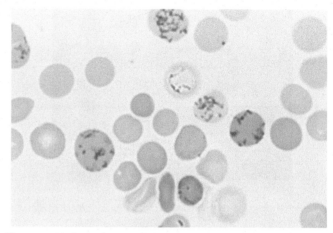

Figure 11.10 Reticulocytes. Reticulocytes are nonnucleated red blood cells with two or more blue-stained filaments or particles. (Peripheral blood, new methylene blue vital stain, ×1000.)

peripheral blood before developing into a mature RBC. The reticulocyte contains remnant cytoplasmic ribonucleic acid (RNA) and organelles such as the mitochondria and ribosomes (Chapter 5). The reticulocyte count is used to assess the erythropoietic activity of the bone marrow.

Principle

Whole blood, anticoagulated with EDTA, is stained with a supravital stain, such as new methylene blue. Any nonnucleated RBC that contains two or more particles of blue-stained granulofilamentous material after new methylene blue staining is defined as a *reticulocyte* (Figure 11.10).

PROCEDURE

1. Mix equal amounts of blood and new methylene blue stain (2 to 3 drops, or approximately 50 μL each), and allow to incubate at room temperature for 3 to 10 minutes.[16]
2. Remix the preparation.
3. Prepare two wedge films (Chapter 13).
4. In an area in which cells are close together but not touching, count 1000 RBCs under the oil immersion objective lens (1000× total magnification). Reticulocytes are included in the total RBC count (i.e., a reticulocyte counts as both an RBC and a reticulocyte).
5. To improve accuracy, have another laboratorian count the other film; counts should agree within 20%.
6. Calculate the % reticulocyte count:

$$Reticulocytes\ (\%) = \frac{number\ of\ reticulocytes \times 100}{1000\ (RBCs\ counted)}$$

For example, if 15 reticulocytes are counted,

$$Reticulocytes\ (\%) = \frac{15 \times 100}{1000} = 1.5\%$$

Or the number of reticulocytes counted can be multiplied by 0.1 (100/1000) to obtain the result.

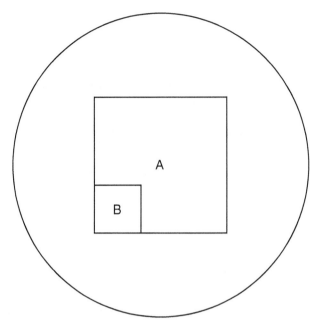

Figure 11.11 Miller Ocular Disc Counting Grid as Viewed through a Microscope. The area of square B is 1/9 the area of square A. Alternatively, square B may be in the center of square A.

Miller Disc

Because large numbers of RBCs should be counted to obtain a more precise reticulocyte count, the Miller disc was designed to reduce this labor-intensive process. The disc is composed of two squares, with the area of the smaller square measuring $\frac{1}{9}$ the area of the larger square. The disc is inserted into the eyepiece of the microscope and the grid in Figure 11.11 is seen. RBCs are counted in the smaller square, and reticulocytes are counted in the larger square. Selection of the counting area is the same as described earlier. A minimum of 112 cells should be counted in the small square, because this is equivalent to 1008 red cells in the large square and satisfies the College of American Pathologists (CAP) hematology standard for a manual reticulocyte count based on at least 1000 red cells.[17] The calculation formula for percent reticulocytes is

$$\text{Reticulocytes}\,\% = \frac{\begin{array}{c}\text{number reticulocytes in square A}\\ \text{(large square)} \times 100\end{array}}{\text{number RBCs in square B (small square)} \times 9}$$

For example, if 15 reticulocytes are counted in the large square and 112 RBCs are counted in the small square,

$$\text{Reticulocytes}\,\% = \frac{15 \times 100}{112 \times 9} = 1.5\%$$

Equation Reference Interval

General reference intervals can be found on the inside front cover of this text.

Sources of Error and Comments

1. If a patient is very anemic or polycythemic, the proportion of dye to blood should be adjusted accordingly.

2. An error may occur if the blood and stain are not mixed before the films are made. The specific gravity of the reticulocytes is lower than that of mature RBCs, and reticulocytes settle at the top of the mixture during incubation.

3. Moisture in the air, poor drying of the slide, or both may cause areas of the slide to appear refractile, and these areas could be confused with reticulocytes. The RNA remnants in a reticulocyte are not refractile.

4. Other RBC inclusions that stain supravitally include Heinz, Howell-Jolly, and Pappenheimer bodies (Table 16.3). Heinz bodies are precipitated hemoglobin, usually appear round or oval, and tend to adhere to the cell membrane (Figure 11.12). Howell-Jolly bodies are round nuclear fragments and are usually singular. Pappenheimer bodies are iron in the mitochondria whose presence can be confirmed with an iron stain, such as Prussian blue. This stain is discussed in Chapter 14.

5. If a Miller disc is used, it is important to heed the "edge rule" as described in the WBC count procedure and illustrated in Figure 11.2; significant bias is observed if the rule is ignored.[16]

Absolute Reticulocyte Count

Principle

The absolute reticulocyte count (ARC) is the actual number of reticulocytes in 1 L or 1 μL of blood.

Calculations

$$\text{ARC} = \frac{\text{reticulocytes (\%)} \times \text{RBC count } (\times 10^{12}/\,\text{L})}{100}$$

For example, if a patient's reticulocyte count is 2% and the RBC count is $2.20 \times 10^{12}/\text{L}$, the ARC is calculated as follows (note that the calculated result has to be converted from $10^{12}/\text{L}$ to $10^9/\text{L}$):

$$\text{ARC} = \frac{2 \times (2.20 \times 10^{12}/\,\text{L})}{100} = 44 \times 10^9/\,\text{L}$$

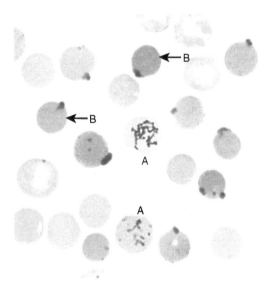

Figure 11.12 Reticulocytes and Heinz Bodies. (A), Reticulocytes. **(B),** Heinz bodies. (Peripheral blood, New methylene blue vital stain, ×1000.)

The ARC can also be reported as the number of cells per μL. Using the example just given, the RBC count in μL ($2.20 \times 10^6/\mu$L) is used in the formula, and the ARC result is $44 \times 10^3/\mu$L.

Reference Interval

Values between 20×10^9/L and 115×10^9/L are within the reference interval for most populations.[18]

Corrected Reticulocyte Count
Principle
In specimens with a low hematocrit, the percentage of reticulocytes may be falsely elevated because the whole blood contains fewer RBCs. A correction factor is used, with the average normal hematocrit considered to be 45%.

Calculation

$$\text{Corrected reticulocyte count (\%)} =$$
$$\text{reticulocyte (\%)} \times \frac{\text{patient HCT (\%)}}{45}$$

Reference Interval
Patients with a hematocrit of 35% should have an elevated corrected reticulocyte count of 2% to 3% to compensate for the mild anemia. In patients with a hematocrit of less than 25%, the count should increase to 3% to 5% to compensate for the moderate anemia. The corrected reticulocyte count depends on the degree of anemia.

Reticulocyte Production Index
Principle
Reticulocytes that are released from the marrow prematurely are called *shift reticulocytes*. These reticulocytes are "shifted" from the bone marrow to the peripheral blood earlier than usual to compensate for anemia. Instead of losing their reticulum in 1 day, as do most normal circulating reticulocytes, these cells take 2 to 3 days to lose their reticula. When erythropoiesis is evaluated, a correction should be made for the presence of shift reticulocytes if polychromasia is reported in the RBC morphology. Most normal (nonshift) reticulocytes become mature RBCs within 1 day after entering the bloodstream and thus represent 1 day's production of RBCs in the bone marrow. Cells shifted to the peripheral blood prematurely stay longer as reticulocytes and contribute to the reticulocyte count for more than 1 day. For this reason, the reticulocyte count is falsely increased when polychromasia is present, because the count no longer represents the cells maturing in just 1 day. On many automated instruments, this mathematical adjustment of the reticulocyte count has been replaced by the measurement of immature reticulocyte fraction (Chapter 12).[16]

The patient's hematocrit is used to determine the appropriate correction factor (reticulocyte maturation time in days):

Patient's Hematocrit Value (%)	Correction Factor (Maturation Time, Days)
40–45	1
35–39	1.5
25–34	2
15–24	2.5
< 15	3

Calculation
The reticulocyte production index (RPI) is calculated as follows:

$$RPI = \frac{\text{reticulocyte (\%)} \times [\text{HCT (\%)}/45\%]}{\text{maturation time}}$$

Or

$$RPI = \frac{\text{corrected reticulocyte count}}{\text{maturation time}}$$

For example, for a patient with a reticulocyte count of 7.8% and a HCT of 30%, and with polychromasia noted, the previous table indicates a maturation time of 2 days. Thus

$$RPI = \frac{7.8 \times [30/45]}{2}$$
$$RPI = 2.6$$

Reference Interval
An adequate bone marrow response usually is indicated by an RPI that is greater than 3. An inadequate erythropoietic response is seen when the RPI is less than 2.[18]

Reticulocyte Control
Several commercial controls are now available for monitoring manual and automated reticulocyte counts (e.g., Retic-Chex II, Streck Laboratories; Liquichek Reticulocyte Control [A], Bio-Rad Laboratories). Most of the controls are available at three levels. The control specimens are treated in the same manner as the patient specimens. The control can be used to verify the laboratorian's accuracy and precision when manual counts are performed.

Automated Reticulocyte Counts
The major instruments manufacturers offer are analyzers that perform automated reticulocyte counts. All the analyzers evaluate reticulocytes using optical scatter or fluorescence after the RBCs are treated with fluorescent dyes or nucleic acid stains to stain residual RNA in the reticulocytes. The percentage and the absolute count are provided. These results are statistically more valid because of the large number of cells counted. Other reticulocyte parameters that are offered on some automated instruments include a maturation index/immature reticulocyte fraction or IRF (reflecting the proportion of the more immature reticulocytes in the specimen), the reticulocyte hemoglobin concentration, and reticulocyte indices (such as the mean reticulocyte volume and distribution width). The IRF may be especially useful in detecting early erythropoietic activity after chemotherapy or hematopoietic stem cell transplantation. The reticulocyte hemoglobin is useful to detect early iron deficiency (Chapter 17). Automated reticulocyte counting is discussed in Chapter 12.

ERYTHROCYTE SEDIMENTATION RATE

The erythrocyte sedimentation rate (ESR) is ordered with other tests to detect and monitor the course of inflammatory conditions such as rheumatoid arthritis, infections, or certain malignancies. It is also useful in the diagnosis of temporal arteritis and polymyalgia rheumatica.[19] The ESR, however, is not a specific test for inflammatory diseases and is elevated in many other conditions such as plasma cell myeloma, pregnancy, anemia, and older age. It is also prone to technical errors that can falsely elevate or decrease the sedimentation rate. Because of its low specificity and sensitivity, the ESR is not recommended as a screening test to detect inflammatory conditions in asymptomatic individuals.[19] Other tests for inflammation, such as the C-reactive protein level, may be a more predictable and reliable alternative to monitor inflammation.[20]

Principle

When anticoagulated blood is allowed to stand at room temperature undisturbed for a period of time, the RBCs settle toward the bottom of the tube. The ESR is the distance in millimeters that the RBCs fall in 1 hour. The ESR is affected by RBC, plasma, and mechanical and technical factors. RBCs have a net negative surface charge and tend to repel one another. The repulsive forces are partially or totally counteracted if there are increased quantities of positively charged plasma proteins. Under these conditions the RBCs settle more rapidly as a result of the formation of rouleaux (stacking of RBCs). Examples of macromolecules that can produce this reaction are fibrinogen, β-globulins, and pathologic immunoglobulins.[21,22]

Normal RBCs have a relatively small mass and settle slowly. Certain diseases can cause rouleaux formation, in which the plasma fibrinogen and globulins are altered. This alteration changes the RBC surface, which leads to stacking of the RBCs, increased RBC mass, and a more rapid ESR. The ESR is directly proportional to the RBC mass and inversely proportional to plasma viscosity. Several methods, both manual and automated, are available for measuring the ESR. Only the most commonly used methods are discussed here.

Modified Westergren Erythrocyte Sedimentation Rate

The most commonly used method today is the modified Westergren method. One advantage of this method is that the taller column height allows the detection of highly elevated ESRs. It is the method recommended by the International Council for Standardization in Hematology and the CLSI.[19,23]

▌PROCEDURE

1. Use well-mixed blood collected in EDTA and dilute at four parts blood to one part 3.8% sodium citrate or 0.85% sodium chloride (e.g., 2 mL blood and 0.5 mL diluent). Alternatively, blood can be collected directly into special sedimentation test tubes containing sodium citrate. Standard coagulation test tubes are not acceptable because the dilution is nine parts blood to one part sodium citrate.[19]
2. Place the diluted specimen in a 200-mm column with an internal diameter of 2.55 mm or more.
3. Place the column into the rack and allow to stand undisturbed for 60 minutes at room temperature (18° to 25° C). Ensure that the rack is level.
4. Record the number of millimeters the RBCs have fallen in 1 hour. The buffy coat should not be included in the reading.

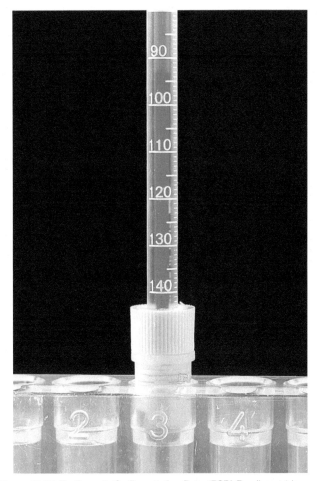

Figure 11.13 Erythrocyte Sedimentation Rate *(ESR)*. Reading at 1 hour = 93 mm, which is elevated above the reference interval.

Read the tube from the bottom of the plasma layer to the top of the sedimented RBCs (Figure 11-13). Report the result as the ESR, 1 hour = x mm.[19]

Wintrobe Erythrocyte Sedimentation Rate

When the Wintrobe method was first introduced, the specimen used was oxalate-anticoagulated whole blood. This was placed in a 100-mm column. Today, EDTA-treated or citrated whole blood is used with the shorter column. The shorter column height allows a somewhat increased sensitivity in detecting mildly elevated ESRs.

▌PROCEDURE

1. Use fresh blood collected in EDTA anticoagulant. A minimum of 2 mL of whole blood is needed.
2. After mixing the blood thoroughly, fill a Pasteur pipette using a rubber pipette bulb.
3. Place the filled pipette into the Wintrobe tube until the tip reaches the bottom of the tube.
4. Carefully squeeze the bulb and expel the blood into the Wintrobe tube while pulling the Pasteur pipette up from the bottom of the tube. There must be steady, even pressure on the bulb to expel blood into the tube as well as continuous movement of the pipette up the tube to prevent the introduction of air bubbles into the column of blood.

5. Fill the Wintrobe tube to the 0 mark.
6. Place the tube into a Wintrobe rack (tube holder) and allow to stand undisturbed for 1 hour at room temperature. The rack must be perfectly level and placed in a draft-free room.
7. Record the number of millimeters the RBCs have fallen. Read the tube from the bottom of the plasma meniscus to the top of the sedimented red cells. The result is reported in millimeters per hour.

Reference Interval

Reference intervals according to sex and age can be found on the inside front cover of this text. Table 11.3 lists some of the factors that influence the ESR.

Sources of Error and Comments

1. If the concentration of anticoagulant is increased, the ESR will be falsely low as a result of sphering of the RBCs, which inhibits rouleaux formation.
2. The anticoagulants sodium or potassium oxalate and heparin cause the RBCs to shrink and falsely elevate the ESR.
3. A significant change in the temperature of the room alters the ESR.
4. Even a slight tilt of the pipette causes the ESR to increase.
5. Blood specimens must be analyzed within 4 hours of collection if kept at room temperature (18° to 25° C).[19] If the specimen is allowed to sit at room temperature for more than 4 hours, the RBCs start to become spherical, which may

TABLE 11.3	Factors Affecting the Erythrocyte Sedimentation Rate (ESR)	
Category	**Increased ESR**	**Decreased ESR**
Blood proteins and lipids	Hypercholesterolemia Hyperfibrinogenemia Hypergammaglobulinemia Hypoalbuminemia	Hyperalbuminemia Hyperglycemia Hypofibrinogenemia Hypogammaglobulinemia Increased bile salts Increased phospholipids
Red blood cells	Anemia Macrocytosis	Acanthocytosis Anisocytosis (marked) Hemoglobin C Microcytosis Polycythemia Sickle cells Spherocytosis Thalassemia
White blood cells	Leukemia	Leukocytosis (marked)
Drugs	Dextran heparin Penicillamine Procainamide Theophylline Vitamin A	Adrenocorticotropic hormone (corticotropin) Cortisone Ethambutol Quinine Salicylates
Clinical conditions	Acute heavy metal poisoning Acute bacterial infections Collagen vascular diseases Diabetes mellitus End-stage renal failure Gout Malignancy Menstruation Multiple myeloma Myocardial infarction Pregnancy Rheumatic fever Rheumatoid arthritis Syphilis Temporal arteritis	Cachexia Congestive heart failure Newborn status
Specimen handling	Refrigerated specimen not returned to room temperature	Clotted blood specimen Delay in testing
Technique	High room temperature Tilted ESR tube Vibration	Bubbles in ESR column Low room temperature Narrow ESR column diameter

From American Society for Clinical Pathology *(ASCP)*/American Proficiency Institute *(API)*. (2006). *2nd Test Event—Educational Commentary—The Erythrocyte Sedimentation Rate and Its Clinical Utility.* http://www.api-pt.com/Reference/Commentary/2006Bcoag.pdf. Accessed April 27, 2018. API is the proficiency testing group that provides testing materials to the American Society for Clinical Pathology. The educational commentary itself is written by ASCP.

inhibit the formation of rouleaux. Blood specimens may be stored at 4° C up to 24 hours before testing, but must be rewarmed by holding the specimen at ambient room temperature for at least 15 minutes before testing.[19]

6. Bubbles in the column of blood invalidate the test results.
7. The blood must be filled properly to the zero mark at the beginning of the test.
8. A clotted specimen cannot be used.
9. The tubes must not be subjected to vibrations on the laboratory bench, which can falsely increase the ESR.
10. Hematologic disorders that prevent the formation of rouleaux (e.g., the presence of sickle cells and spherocytes) decrease the ESR.
11. The ESR of patients with severe anemia is of little diagnostic value, because it will be falsely elevated.

Disposable Kits

Disposable commercial kits are available for ESR testing (Figure 11.14). Several kits include safety caps for the columns that allow the blood to fill precisely to the zero mark. This safety cap makes the column a closed system and eliminates the error involved in manually setting the blood to the zero mark.

Automated Erythrocyte Sedimentation Rate

There are several automated ESR systems available using the traditional Westergren and Wintrobe methods, as well as alternate methods such as centrifugation and capillary photometry. These automated ESR systems usually do the following:

- Include specimen identification capability
- Require a smaller sample volume

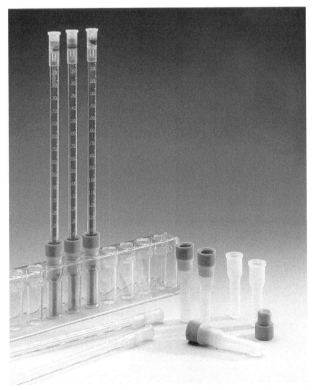

Figure 11.14 Sediplast (Polymedco) Disposable Sedimentation Rate System. (Courtesy Polymedco, Cortlandt Manor, NY.)

- Provide on-board mixing and sampling of patient's specimen
- Minimize handling of blood specimens
- Incorporate a quality control (QC) system
- Include capability of transmitting data to the laboratory information system
- Provide results within a shorter turnaround time (TAT)

Some features to consider when selecting an automated ESR system include size of the analyzer, required sample volume, specimen identification, walkaway and continuous process flow, testing time, quality control program, and interface capabilities.

ADDITIONAL TESTS

Additional manual and semiautomated methods are included in other chapters that are relevant to their clinical application. Examples include Chapter 21 for the osmotic fragility test and qualitative and quantitative assays for glucose-6-phosphate dehydrogenase and pyruvate kinase activity; Chapter 24 for the solubility test for Hb S, hemoglobin electrophoresis (alkaline and acid pH), and unstable hemoglobin test; and Chapter 25 for the vital stain for hemoglobin H and the Kleihauer-Betke acid elution test for Hb F distribution in the RBCs.

POINT-OF-CARE TESTING

Point-of-care (POC) testing offers the ability to produce rapid and accurate results that facilitate faster treatment, which can decrease hospital length of stay. This testing is rarely performed by trained laboratory personnel; most often, it is carried out by nurses. Manufacturers have created analyzers with nonlaboratory operators in mind, but results obtained using these systems are still affected by preanalytic and analytical variables. The laboratory professional's partnership with nursing is the key to success in any hospital's POC program.

Point-of-care testing is defined as diagnostic testing at or near the site of patient care. The Clinical Laboratory Improvement Amendments of 1988 (CLIA) introduced the concept of "testing site neutrality," which means that regardless of where the diagnostic testing is performed or who performs the test, all testing sites must follow the same regulatory requirements based on the "complexity" of the test. Under CLIA, POC testing (including physician-performed microscopy) is classified as "waived" or "moderately complex." Tests are classified as waived if they are determined to be "simple tests with an insignificant risk of an erroneous result." POC testing is commonly performed in hospital inpatient units, outpatient clinics, surgery centers, emergency departments, long-term care facilities, and dialysis units. For waived POC testing, facilities are required to obtain a certificate of waiver, pay the appropriate fees, and follow the manufacturers' testing instructions.[24] For any POC program to be successful, certain key elements must be present. Clear administrative responsibility, well-written procedures, a training program, quality control, proficiency testing, and equipment maintenance are essential for success. The first step is appointing a laboratory POC testing coordinator. This person not only is the "go-to" person but is also an important liaison between the laboratory and nursing staff. The second step to ensuring a successful program is to create a multidisciplinary team with authority to affect all aspects of the POC program. This committee has the authority to oversee the integrity and quality of the existing POC program and institute changes or new testing as needed. It is also important to have administrative support to help remove barriers.

A POC testing program must incorporate all of the following: A written policy that defines the program, outlines who is responsible for each part of the program. The policy indicates where testing is performed and who performs the testing. Testing procedures should clearly state how to perform the tests and address how to handle critical values and discrepant results. The program must be monitored. An ongoing evaluation of the POC testing is vital for success.

When selecting an instrument to be used in the POC testing program, it is helpful to invite vendors to demonstrate their equipment. An equipment display available for hands-on use by the operators can be very helpful in selection of the appropriate instrumentation. Patient correlation studies are useful in selecting equipment that best covers the patient population for the institution. POC operators need handheld analyzers that are lightweight, accurate, fast, and require little specimen material. The POC testing system should also address the following laboratory concerns:

- What is the range of measurement?
- How well does the test system correlate with laboratory instrumentation?
- Can it be interfaced to the laboratory information system?
- Does it provide reliable results?
- Does the company supply excellent technical support?
- Is it affordable?

Paramount to POC testing is patient safety. It is important to maintain good laboratory practices, which include use of appropriate procedures for specimen collection, identification of the patient and specimen, storage of reagents, instrument maintenance, and accurate documentation of patient test results (use of POC interfaces to the laboratory information system and electronic medical record is beneficial). Laboratory oversight is sometimes absent, and basic safety precautions necessary for waived tests can be easily overlooked, often as a result of a lack of understanding, lack of training, and high personnel turnover rates.[25]

Point-of-Care Tests

POC instruments are available to measure parameters such as hemoglobin and hematocrit; some are capable of performing a complete blood count.

Hematocrit

The most common methods for determining the hematocrit include the microhematocrit centrifuge, conductometric methods, and calculation by automated cell counters (Chapter 12).

Centrifuge-based microhematocrit systems have been available for years, and the results obtained correlate well with the results produced by standard cell counters. Nonlaboratorians

and inexperienced operators, however, may be unaware of the error that can be introduced by insufficient centrifugation time and inaccurate reading of the microhematocrit tube (see comments in the Microhematocrit section). One example of a centrifuge-based device is the Hematastat II Separation Technology. The i-STAT 1 (Abbott Laboratories)[26] (Figure 11.15 and the Epoc (Siemens Healthineers) (Figure 11.16)[27] use the conductivity method to determine the hematocrit. Plasma conducts electrical current, whereas WBCs act as insulators. In the i-STAT system, before the measured conductance is converted into the hematocrit value, corrections are applied for temperature of the specimen, size of the fluid segment being

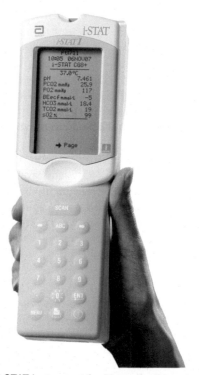

Figure 11.15 I-STAT Instrument for Measuring Hematocrit. (Courtesy Abbott Laboratories, Abbott Park, IL.)

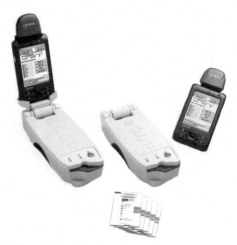

Figure 11.16 Epoc Device for Measuring Hematocrit. (Courtesy Epocal, Inc., Ottawa, Ontario, Canada.)

measured, and relative conductivity of the plasma component. The first two corrections are determined from the measured value of the calibrant conductance and the last correction from the measured concentrations of sodium and potassium in the specimen.[26]

Sources of error and comments. Conductivity of a whole blood specimen is dependent on the amount of electrolytes in the plasma portion. Conductivity does not distinguish RBCs from other nonconductive elements such as proteins, lipids, and WBCs that may be present in the specimen.

A low total protein level will falsely decrease the hematocrit. The presence of lipids can interfere with the hematocrit measurement. An increased WBC count will falsely increase the hematocrit. The presence of cold agglutinins can falsely decrease the hematocrit.[26]

Other instruments. Other instruments that measure hematocrit include the following:
- ABL 77 (Radiometer)
- IRMA (Accriva, a subsidiary of LifeHealth)
- Gem Premier (Instrumentation Laboratory Company) (Figure 11-17)

Hemoglobin Concentration

In POC testing, hemoglobin concentration is measured by modified hemoglobinometers or by oximeters integrated with a blood gas analyzer. The HemoCue hemoglobinometer (HemoCue) uses a small cuvette that contains a lysing agent and reagents to form a hemoglobin azide, which is measured by a photometer at two wavelengths (570 nm and 880 nm) (Figure 11.6).[9] This eliminates interference from turbidity in the specimen. Results obtained with the instrument compare well with those produced by reference methods, but a major source of error is mixing of blood with tissue fluid during skin puncture collection. The AVOXimeter 1000E (Instrumentation Laboratory) measures total hemoglobin by a spectrophotometric method.

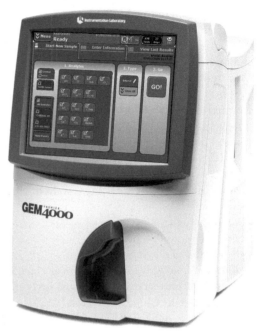

Figure 11.17 Gem Premier Instrument for Measuring Hematocrit. (Courtesy Instrumentation Laboratory Company, Lexington, MA.)

Cell and Platelet Counts

Traditional cell-counting methods can be employed at the point of care for the analysis of WBCs, RBCs, and platelets. The Ichor Hematology Analyzer (Helena Laboratories) performs a CBC along with platelet aggregation. Another option for cell quantitation and differentiation employs a buffy coat analysis method. Quantitative buffy coat analysis (QBC STAR, manufactured by QBC Diagnostics, Inc., Philipsburg, PA) involves centrifugation in specialized capillary tubes designed to expand the buffy coat layer. The components (platelets, mononuclear cells, and granulocytes) can be measured with the assistance of fluorescent dyes and a measuring device.[28]

SUMMARY

- Although most laboratories are highly automated, manual tests discussed in this chapter, such as the cyanmethemoglobin method of hemoglobin determination and centrifuge-based measurement of the microhematocrit, are used as a part of many laboratories' quality control and backup methods of analysis.
- The hemacytometer allows counts of any type of cell or particle (e.g., white blood cells [WBCs] or platelets) to be performed.
- The reference method for hemoglobin determination is based on the absorbance of cyanmethemoglobin at 540 nm. When a spectrophotometer is used, a standard curve is employed to obtain the results.
- The microhematocrit is a measure of packed red blood cell (RBC) volume.
- The rule of three specifies that the value of the hematocrit should be three times the value of the hemoglobin plus or minus 3 (%) or 0.03 (L/L). A value discrepant with this rule

may indicate abnormal RBCs or it may be the first indication of error.
- RBC indices—the mean cell volume (MCV), mean cell hemoglobin (MCH), and mean cell hemoglobin concentration (MCHC)—are calculated to determine the average volume, hemoglobin content, and hemoglobin concentration of RBCs. The indices provide an indication of possible causes of an anemia.
- The reticulocyte count, which is used to assess the erythropoietic activity of the bone marrow, is accomplished through the use of supravital stains (e.g., new methylene blue) or by flow cytometric methods.
- The erythrocyte sedimentation rate (ESR), a measure of the settling of RBCs in a 1-hour period, depends on the RBCs' ability to form rouleaux. It is used to detect and monitor conditions with inflammation such as rheumatoid arthritis, infections, and some malignancies. It is subject to many physiologic and technical errors.

- Point-of-care (POC) testing is often performed by nonlaboratory personnel. It is defined as diagnostic laboratory testing at or near the site of patient care.
- The Clinical Laboratory Improvement Amendments of 1988 (CLIA) introduced the concept of "testing site neutrality," which means that it does not matter where diagnostic testing is performed or who performs the test; all testing sites must follow the same regulatory requirements based on the "complexity" of the test.
- Tests are classified as waived if they are determined to be "simple tests with an insignificant risk of an erroneous result." Most, but not all, POC testing is waived.

- For a POC testing program to be successful, key elements such as clear administrative responsibility, well-written procedures, quality control, proficiency testing, and equipment maintenance must be present.
- Paramount to POC testing is patient safety.

Now that you have completed this chapter, read again the case studies at the beginning and respond to the questions presented.

REVIEW QUESTIONS

Answers can be found in the Appendix.

1. A 1:20 dilution of blood is made with 3% glacial acetic acid as the diluent. The four large corner squares on both sides of the hemacytometer are counted, for a total of 100 cells. What is the total WBC count ($\times 10^9$ /L)?
   a. 0.25
   b. 2.5
   c. 5
   d. 10

2. The total WBC count is 20×10^9/L. Twenty-five NRBCs per 100 WBCs are observed on the peripheral blood film. What is the corrected WBC count ($\times 10^9$/L)?
   a. 0.8
   b. 8
   c. 16
   d. 19

3. If potassium cyanide and potassium ferricyanide are used in the manual method for hemoglobin determination, the final product is:
   a. Methemoglobin
   b. Azide methemoglobin
   c. Cyanmethemoglobin
   d. Myoglobin

4. Which of the following would NOT interfere with the result when hemoglobin determination is performed by the cyanmethemoglobin method?
   a. Increased lipids
   b. Elevated WBC count
   c. Lyse-resistant RBCs
   d. Fetal hemoglobin

5. A patient has a hemoglobin level of 8.0 g/dL. According to the rule of three, what is the expected range for the hematocrit?
   a. 21% to 24%
   b. 23.7% to 24.3%
   c. 24% to 27%
   d. 21% to 27%

6. Calculate the MCV and MCHC for the following values:
   RBCs = 5.00×10^{12}/L
   HGB = 9 g/dL
   HCT = 30%

	MCV (fL)	MCHC (g/dL)
a.	30	18
b.	60	30
c.	65	33
d.	85	35

7. What does the reticulocyte count assess?
   a. Inflammation
   b. Response to infection
   c. Erythropoietic activity of the bone marrow
   d. Ability of red blood cells to form rouleaux

8. For a patient with the following test results, which measure of bone marrow red blood cell production provides the most accurate information?
   Observed reticulocyte count = 5.3%
   HCT = 35%
   Morphology—moderate polychromasia
   a. Observed reticulocyte count
   b. Corrected reticulocyte count
   c. RPI
   d. ARC

9. Given the following values, calculate the RPI:
   Observed reticulocyte count = 6%
   HCT = 30%
   a. 2
   b. 3
   c. 4
   d. 5

10. Which of the following would be associated with an elevated ESR value?
    a. Microcytosis
    b. Polycythemia
    c. Decreased globulins
    d. Inflammation

REFERENCES

1. Cornet, E., Behier, C., & Troussard, X. (2012). Guidance for storing blood samples in laboratories performing complete blood count with differential. *Int J Lab Hematol, 34,* 655–660.
2. Department of Labor OSHA. (1991). Occupational exposure to bloodborne pathogens; final rule. *Fed Reg, 56,* 64175–64182.
3. CLSI. (2007). *Procedures for the Collection of Diagnostic Blood Specimens by Venipuncture.* (6th ed., CLSI approved standard, H3-A6). Wayne, PA: Clinical and Laboratory Standards Institute.
4. CLSI. (2008). *Procedures and Devices for the Collection of Diagnostic Capillary Blood Specimens.* (6th ed., CLSI approved standard, H04-A6). Wayne, PA: Clinical and Laboratory Standards Institute.
5. Brecher, G., & Cronkite, E. P. (1950). Morphology and enumeration of human blood platelets. *J Appl Physiol, 3,* 365–377.
6. CLSI. (2000). *Reference and Selected Procedures for the Quantitative Determination of Hemoglobin in Blood.* (3rd ed., CLSI approved standard, H15-A3). Wayne, PA: Clinical and Laboratory Standards Institute.
7. Zwart, A., van Assendelft, O. W., Bull, B. S., et al. (1996). Recommendations for reference method for haemoglobinometry in human blood (ICSH Standard 1995) and specifications for international haemiglobincyanide reference preparation (4th ed.). *J Clin Pathol, 49,* 271–274.
8. von Schenck, H., Falkensson, M., & Lundberg, B. (1986). Evaluation of "HemoCue," a new device for determining hemoglobin. *Clin Chem, 32,* 526–529.
9. HemoCue. http://www.hemocue.com/. Accessed October 18, 2018.
10. MacLaren, I. A., Conn, D. M., & Wadsworth, L. D. (1991). Comparison of two automated hemoglobin methods using Sysmex SULFOLYSER and STROMATOLYSER. *Sysmex J Int, 1,* 59–61.
11. Karsan, A., MacLaren, I., Conn, D., et al. (1993). An evaluation of hemoglobin determination using sodium lauryl sulfate. *Am J Clin Pathol, 100,* 123–126.
12. Matsubara, T., & Mimura, T. (1990). Reaction mechanism of SLS-Hb Method. *Sysmex J (Japan), 13,* 206–211.
13. Fujiwara, C., Hamaguchi, Y., Toda, S., et al. (1990). The reagent SULFOLYSER for hemoglobin measurement by hematology analyzers. *Sysmex J (Japan), 13,* 212–219.
14. CLSI. (2000). *Procedure for Determining Packed Cell Volume by the Microhematocrit Method.* (3rd ed., CLSI approved standard, H07-A3). Wayne, PA: Clinical and Laboratory Standards Institute.
15. Becton Dickinson Primary Care Diagnostics. (1998). *Clay Adams brand SUREPREP capillary tubes,* Sparks, MD: Becton Dickinson Primary Care Diagnostics (product brochure).
16. CLSI. (2004). *Methods for Reticulocyte Counting (Automated Blood Cell Counters, Flow Cytometry, and Supravital Dyes).* (2nd ed., CLSI approved standard, H44-A2). Wayne, PA: Clinical and Laboratory Standards Institute.
17. College of American Pathologists. (2001). Q & A Miller disk clarification. *CAP Today, 95.* http://www.captodayonline.com/Archives/q_and_a/qa_04_04.html. Accessed October 18, 2018.
18. Koepke, J. F., & Koepke, J. A. (1986). Reticulocytes. *Clin Lab Haematol, 8,* 169–179.
19. CLSI. (2011). *Procedures for the Erythrocyte Sedimentation Rate (ESR) Test.* (5th ed., CLSI approved standard, H2-A5). Wayne, PA: Clinical and Laboratory Standards Institute.
20. Colombet, I., Pouchot, J., Kronz, V., et al. (2010). Agreement between the erythrocyte sedimentation rate and C-reactive protein in hospital practice. *Am J Med, 123,* 863.e7–863.e13.
21. Smock, K. J., & Perkins, S. L. (2014). Examination of the blood and bone marrow. In Greer, J. P., Arber, D. A., Glader, B., et al. (Eds.), *Wintrobe's Clinical Hematology.* (13th ed., pp. 1–18). Philadelphia: Lippincott Williams & Wilkins.
22. Mims, M. P. (2016). Hematology during pregnancy. In Kasushanski K., Lichtman, M. A., Prchal, J. T., et al. (Eds.), *Williams Hematology.* (9th ed., pp. 119–128). New York: McGraw-Hill.
23. Jou, J. M., Lewis, S. M., Briggs, C., et al. (2011). International Council for Standardization in Haematology: ICSH review of the measurement of the erythrocyte sedimentation rate. *Int J Lab Hematol, 33,* 125–32.
24. Centers for Medicare and Medicaid Services. Clinical Laboratory Improvement Amendments (CLIA 1988): overview. http://www.cms.hhs.gov/clia/. Accessed October 18, 2018.
25. Good Laboratory Practices. (12.17.2002). https://www.cms.gov/Regulations-and-Guidance/Legislation/CLIA/Downloads/wgoodlab.pdf. Accessed October 18, 2018.
26. Abbott Point of Care Cartridge and Hematocrit/HCT and Calculated Hemoglobin/HB information sheets, in i-STAT 1 system manual (revised June 11, 2008). Abbott Park, Ill, Abbott Laboratories.
27. Theory of operation, in Epoc System Manual, 51011600 Rev.: 00, Ottawa, Ont, Canada: Epocal, Inc., pp. 189-196. http://www.alere-epoc.com/ww/home/customer-resource-center.html. Accessed October 18, 2018.
28. QBC operator's service manual, rev B (2006) (pp. 1–2.) Philipsburg, PA: QBC Diagnostics, Inc. https://www.manualshelf.com/manual/drucker-diagnostics/qbc-star-dry-hematology-analyzer/owner-manual-english.html. Accessed October 18, 2018.

ADDITIONAL RESOURCES

College of American Pathologists, http://www.cap.org.

Howerton D, Anderson N, Bosse D, et al: Good laboratory practices for waived testing sites. Survey Findings from Testing Sites Holding a Certificate of Waiver Under the Clinical Laboratory Improvement Amendments of 1988 and Recommendations for Promoting Quality Testing. https://www.cdc.gov/mmwr/preview/mmwrhtml/rr5413a1.htm. Accessed October 18, 2018.

Centers for Disease Control and Prevention: Health disparities experienced by black or African Americans—United States. (2005). *MMWR Morb Mortal Wkly Rep, 54,* 1–32. https://www.cdc.gov/mmwr/PDF/wk/mm5401.pdf. Accessed October 18, 2018.

The Joint Commission. www.jointcommission.org

Point of Care.net. http://www.pointofcare.net.

Instrumentation Laboratory. http://us.instrumentationlaboratory.com

Abbott Point of Care. www.abbottpointofcare.com

Hemocue. www.hemocue.com

Radiometer America. www.radiometeramerica.com

Helena. www.Helena.com

Sysmex. www.sysmex.com

Automated Blood Cell Analysis

*Jo Ann Molnar**

OBJECTIVES

After completion of this chapter, the reader will be able to:

1. Explain the different principles of automated blood cell counting and analysis.
2. Describe how the general principles are implemented on different instruments.
3. Identify the parameters directly measured on the four analyzers discussed.
4. Explain the derivation of calculated or indirectly measured parameters for the same four analyzers.
5. Explain the derivation of the white blood cell differential count on the different instruments discussed.
6. Interpret and compare patient data, including white blood cell, red blood cell, and platelet histograms or cytograms or both, obtained from the four major hematology instruments.
7. Explain the general principles of automated reticulocyte counting.
8. Identify sources of error in automated cell counting and determine appropriate corrective action.

OUTLINE

General Principles of Automated Blood Cell Analysis
  Electronic Impedance
  Radiofrequency
  Optical Scatter
Principal Instruments
  Overview
  Beckman Coulter Instrumentation
  Sysmex Instrumentation

  Abbott Instrumentation
  Siemens Healthcare Diagnostics Instrumentation
Automated Reticulocyte Counting
Limitations and Interferences
  Calibration
  Instrument Limitations
  Specimen Limitations
Clinical Utility of Automated Blood Cell Analysis

CASE STUDY

After studying the material in this chapter, the reader should be able to respond to the following case study:

Review the following results from a CBC performed on an automated blood cell analyzer for a 44-year-old woman.

WBC	9.5×10^9/L
RBC	2.25×10^{12}/L
HGB	12.2 g/dL
HCT	30.4 %
MCV	135.1 fL
MCH	54.2 pg
MCHC	40.1 g/dL
RDW	26%
PLT	195×10^9/L

Refer to the reference intervals provided on the inside front cover of the book to evaluate each of the parameters.

1. Which parameter(s) do not fall within reference intervals?
2. What is the possible interference that is causing these CBC test results?
3. Explain the corrective action to be taken for this specimen.

Since the 1980s, automated blood cell analysis has virtually replaced manual hemoglobin, hematocrit, and cell counting because of its greater accuracy and precision, with the possible exception of phase platelet counting in certain circumstances. Hematology analyzers are marketed by multiple instrument manufacturers. These analyzers typically provide the eight standard hematology parameters (complete blood count [CBC]), plus a three-part, five-part, or six-part differential leukocyte count in less than 1 minute on 200 μL or less of whole blood. Automation allows more efficient workload management and more timely diagnosis and treatment of disease.

---

*The author extends appreciation to Sharral Longanbach and Martha K. Miers, whose work in prior editions provided the foundation for this chapter.

GENERAL PRINCIPLES OF AUTOMATED BLOOD CELL ANALYSIS

Despite the number of hematology analyzers available from different manufacturers and their varying levels of sophistication and complexity, most rely on only two basic principles of operation: electronic impedance (resistance) and optical scatter. *Electronic impedance,* or low-voltage direct current (DC) resistance, was developed by Coulter in the 1950s[1,2] and is the most common methodology used. *Radiofrequency* (RF), or alternating current resistance, is a modification sometimes used in conjunction with DC electronic impedance. Technicon Instruments Corporation introduced darkfield optical scanning in the 1960s, and Ortho Clinical Diagnostics followed with a laser-based optical instrument in the 1970s.[3] *Optical scatter,* using both laser and nonlaser light, is often employed in today's hematology instrumentation.

Electronic Impedance

The impedance principle of cell counting is based on the detection and measurement of changes in electrical resistance produced by cells as they traverse a small aperture. Cells suspended in an electrically conductive diluent such as saline are pulled through an aperture (orifice) in a glass tube. In the counting chamber, or transducer assembly, low-frequency electrical current is applied between an external electrode (suspended in the cell dilution) and an internal electrode (housed inside the aperture tube). Electrical resistance between the two electrodes, or impedance in the current, occurs as the cells pass through the sensing aperture, causing voltage pulses that are measurable (Figure 12.1).[4,5] Oscilloscope screens on some instruments display the pulses that are generated by the cells as they interrupt the current. The number of pulses is proportional to the number of cells counted. The height of the voltage pulse is directly proportional to the volume of the cell, which allows discrimination and counting of cells of specific volumes through the use of threshold circuits. Pulses are collected and sorted (channelized) according to their amplitude by pulse height analyzers. The data are plotted on a frequency distribution graph, or *volume distribution histogram,* with relative number on the *y*-axis and volume (channel number equivalent to a specific volume) on the *x*-axis. The histogram produced depicts the volume distribution of the cells counted. Figure 12.2 illustrates the construction of a frequency distribution graph. Volume thresholds separate the cell populations on the histogram, and the count is the cells enumerated between the lower and upper set thresholds for each population. Volume distribution histograms may be used for the evaluation of one cell population or subgroups within a population.[5] The use of proprietary lytic reagents to control shrinkage and lysis of specific cell types, as in the older Coulter S-Plus IV, STKR, and Sysmex E-5000 models, allows separation and quantitation of white blood cells (WBCs) into three populations (lymphocytes, mononuclear cells, and granulocytes) for the *three-part differential* on one volume distribution histogram.[6-8]

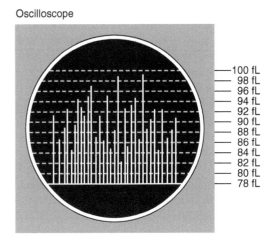

Oscilloscope

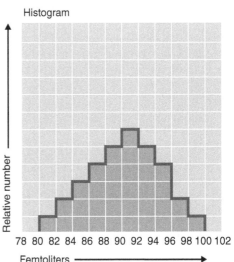

Histogram

Figure 12.2 Oscilloscope Display and Histogram. The construction of a frequency distribution graph is depicted. (Modified from Coulter Electronics. [1983]. *Significant Advances in Hematology: Hematology Education Series,* PN 4206115A. Hialeah, FL: Coulter Electronics.)

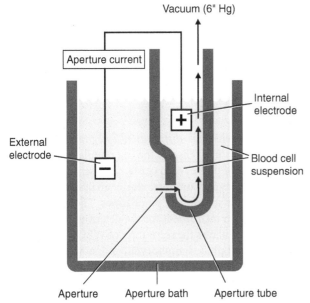

Figure 12.1 Coulter Principle of Cell Counting. (From Coulter Electronics. [1988]. *Coulter STKR Product Reference Manual, PN 4235547.* Hialeah, FL: Coulter Electronics.)

Several factors may affect volume measurements in impedance or volume displacement instruments. Aperture diameter is crucial, and the red blood cell (RBC)/platelet aperture is smaller than the WBC aperture to increase platelet counting sensitivity. On earlier systems, protein buildup occurred, decreasing the diameter of the orifice, slowing the flow of cells, and increasing their relative electrical resistance. Protein buildup results in lower cell counts, which result in falsely elevated cell volumes. Impedance instruments once required frequent manual aperture cleaning, but current instruments incorporate *burn circuits* or other internal cleaning systems to prevent or slow protein buildup.[6-9] Carryover of cells from one specimen to the next also is minimized by these internal cleaning systems. Coincident passage of more than one cell at a time through the orifice causes artificially large pulses, which results in falsely increased cell volumes and falsely decreased cell counts. This count reduction, or *coincident passage loss,* is statistically predictable (and mathematically correctable) because of its direct relationship to cell concentration and the effective volume of the aperture.[7-9] Coincidence correction typically is completed by the analyzer computer before final printout of cell counts from the instrument. Other factors affecting pulse height include orientation of the cell in the center of the aperture and deformability of the RBC, which may be altered by decreased hemoglobin content.[10,11] Recirculation of cells back into the sensing zone creates erroneous pulses and falsely elevates cell counts. A backwash or sweep-flow mechanism prevents recirculation of cells back into the sensing zone, and anomalously shaped pulses are edited out electronically.[6,7,9]

The use of hydrodynamic focusing avoids many of the potential problems inherent in a rigid aperture system. The *sample stream* is surrounded by a sheath fluid as it passes through the central axis of the aperture. Laminar flow allows the central sample stream to narrow sufficiently to separate and align the cells into single file for passage through the sensing zone.[12-14] The outer sheath fluid minimizes protein buildup and plugs, eliminates recirculation of cells back into the sensing zone with generation of spurious pulses, and reduces pulse height irregularity because off-center cell passage is prevented and better resolution of the blood cells is obtained. Coincident passage loss also is reduced because blood cells line up one after another in the direction of the flow.[15] Laminar flow and hydrodynamic focusing are discussed further in Chapter 28.

Radiofrequency

Low-voltage DC impedance, as described previously, may be used in conjunction with RF resistance, or resistance to a high-voltage electromagnetic current flowing between both electrodes simultaneously. Although the total volume of the cell is proportional to the change in DC, the cell interior density is proportional to pulse height or change in the RF signal. *Conductivity,* as measured by this high-frequency electromagnetic probe, is attenuated by nucleus-to-cytoplasm ratio, nuclear density, and cytoplasmic granulation. DC and RF voltage changes may be detected simultaneously and separated by two different pulse processing circuits.[15,16] Figure 12.3 illustrates the simultaneous use of DC and RF current.

Two different cell properties, such as low-voltage DC impedance and RF resistance, can be plotted against each other to

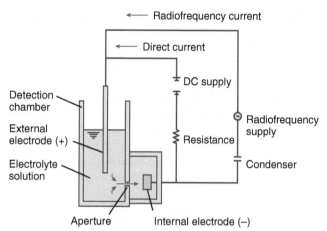

Figure 12.3 Radiofrequency/Direct Current (RF/DC) Detection Method. The simultaneous use of DC and RF in one measurement system on the Sysmex SE-9500 is depicted. (From TOA Medical Electronics Company [1997] *Sysmex SE-9500 Operator's Manual [CN 461-2464-2].* Kobe, Japan: TOA Medical Electronics Co.)

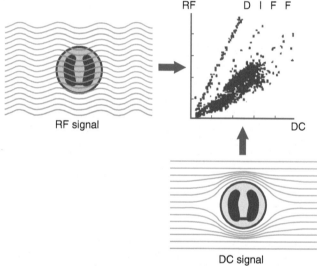

Figure 12.4 Two-Dimensional Distribution Scatterplot of Direct Current (DC) versus Radiofrequency (RF) Signals. Low-voltage DC impedance (measurement of cell volume) is plotted against RF resistance (measurement of cell interior density and nuclear volume and complexity) to form a two-dimensional distribution scatterplot. (From TOA Medical Electronics Company. [1997]. *Sysmex SE-9500 Operator's Manual* [CN 461-2464-2], Kobe, Japan: TOA Medical Electronics Co.)

create a *two-dimensional distribution cytogram* or *scatterplot* (Figure 12.4). Such plots display the cell populations as clusters, with the number of dots in each cluster representing the concentration of that cell type. Computer cluster analysis can determine absolute counts for specific cell populations. The use of multiple methods by a given instrument for the determination of at least two cell properties allows the separation of WBCs into a five-part differential (neutrophils, lymphocytes, monocytes, eosinophils, and basophils). DC and RF detection are two methods used by the Sysmex analyzers to perform WBC differentials.[15,16]

Optical Scatter

Optical scatter may be used as the primary methodology or in combination with other methods. In optical scatter systems (flow cytometers), a hydrodynamically focused sample stream is directed through a quartz flow cell past a focused light source (Figure 28.3). The light source is generally a tungsten-halogen lamp or a helium-neon *laser* (*light amplification by stimulated emission of radiation*). Laser light, termed *monochromatic light* because it is emitted at a single wavelength, differs from bright-field light in its intensity, its coherence (i.e., it travels in phase), and its low divergence or spread. These characteristics allow for the detection of interference in the laser beam and enable enumeration and differentiation of cell types.[12,17] Optical scatter may be used to study RBCs, WBCs, and platelets.

As the cells pass through the sensing zone and interrupt the beam, light is scattered in all directions. Light scatter results from the interaction between the processes of absorption, diffraction (bending around corners or the surface of a cell), refraction (bending because of a change in speed), and reflection (backward scatter of rays caused by an obstruction).[18] The detection of scattered rays and their conversion into electrical signals is accomplished by photodetectors (photodiodes and photomultiplier tubes) at specific angles. Lenses fitted with *blocker bars* to prevent nonscattered light from entering the detector are used to collect the scattered light. A series of filters and mirrors separate the varying wavelengths and present them to the photodetectors. Photodiodes convert light photons to electronic signals proportional in magnitude to the amount of light collected. Photomultiplier tubes are used to collect the weaker signals produced at a 90-degree angle and multiply the photoelectrons into stronger, useful signals. Analog-to-digital converters change the electronic pulses to digital signals for computer analysis.[12,17]

Forward-angle light scatter (0 degrees) correlates with cell volume, primarily because of diffraction of light. Orthogonal light scatter (90 degrees), or side scatter, results from refraction and reflection of light from larger structures inside the cell and correlates with degree of internal complexity. Forward low-angle scatter (2 to 3 degrees) and forward high-angle scatter (5 to 15 degrees) also correlate with cell volume and refractive index or with internal complexity.[17,19] Differential scatter is the combination of this low-angle and high-angle forward light scatter and is primarily used on Siemens systems for cellular analysis. The angles of light scatter measured by the different flow cytometers are manufacturer and method specific.

Scatter properties at different angles may be plotted against each other to generate two-dimensional cytograms or scatterplots, as on the Abbott CELL-DYN instruments.[20,21] Optical scatter may also be plotted against absorption, as on the Siemens systems,[22,23] or against volume, as on the larger Beckman Coulter systems.[9] Computer cluster analysis of the cytograms may yield quantitative and qualitative information.

PRINCIPAL INSTRUMENTS

Overview

Hematology blood cell analyzers are produced by multiple manufacturers, including, but not limited to, Abbott Laboratories[24]; HORIBA Medical[25]; Siemens Healthcare Diagnostics[26]; Beckman Coulter[27]; and Sysmex Corporation.[28] The following discussion is limited to instrumentation produced by four of these suppliers. Emphasis is not placed on sample size or

handling, speed, level of automation, or comparison of instruments or manufacturers. Likewise, technology continues to improve, and the newest (or most recent) models produced by a manufacturer may not be mentioned. Instead, a detailed description of primary methods used by these manufacturers is given to show the application of, and clarify further, the principles presented earlier and to enable the medical laboratory scientist or technician to interpret patient data, including instrument-generated histograms and cytograms. Table 12.1 summarizes methods used for the hemogram, reticulocyte, nucleated red blood cell, and WBC differential count determination on four major hematology instruments.

Hematology analyzers have some common basic components, including hydraulics, pneumatics, and electrical systems. The hydraulics system includes an aspirating unit, dispensers, diluters, mixing chambers, aperture baths or flow cells or both, and a hemoglobinometer. The pneumatics system generates the vacuums and pressures required for operating the valves and moving the sample through the hydraulics system. The electrical system controls operational sequences of the total system and includes electronic analyzers and computing circuitry for processing the data generated. Some older-model instruments have oscilloscope screens that display the electrical pulses in real time as the cells are counted. A data display unit receives information from the analyzer and prints results, histograms, or cytograms.

Specimen handling varies from instrument to instrument based on degree of automation, and systems range from discrete analyzers to walkaway systems with *front-end load* capability. Computer functions also vary, with the larger instruments having extensive microprocessor and data management capabilities. Computer software capabilities include automatic start-up and shutdown, with internal diagnostic self-checks and some maintenance; quality control, with automatic review of quality control data, calculations, graphs, moving averages, and storage of quality control files; patient data storage and retrieval, with δ checks (Chapter 2), critical value flagging, and automatic verification of patient results based on user-defined algorithms; host query with the laboratory or hospital information system to allow random access discrete testing capability; analysis of animal specimens; and even analysis of body fluids.

Beckman Coulter Instrumentation

Beckman Coulter, Inc., manufactures an extensive line of hematology analyzers, including the smaller Ac-T series that provide complete RBC, platelet, and WBC analysis with a five-part differential. The DxH800 system provides a fully automated online reticulocyte analysis, nucleated RBC (NRBC) count, and body fluid analysis.[29] Coulter instruments typically have two measurement channels in the hydraulics system for determining the hemogram data. The RBC and WBC counts and hemoglobin are considered to be measured directly. The aspirated whole-blood sample is divided into two aliquots, and each is mixed with an isotonic diluent. The first dilution is delivered to the RBC aperture chamber, and the second is delivered to the WBC aperture chamber. In the RBC chamber, RBCs and platelets are counted and discriminated by electrical impedance as the cells are pulled through each of three sensing apertures (50 μm in diameter, 60 μm in length). Particles 2 to 20 fL are

TABLE 12.1   Methods for Hemogram, Reticulocyte, Nucleated RBC, and WBC Differential Counts on Four Major Hematology Instruments

Parameter	Beckman Coulter UniCel DxH 800	Sysmex XN Series	Abbott CELL-DYN Sapphire	Siemens ADVIA 2120i
WBC	Impedance volume and conductivity and five-angle light scatter measurement	Fluorescent staining; forward light scatter and side fluorescent light detection	Light scatter (primary count), impedance (secondary count)	Light scatter and absorption
RBC	Impedance	Impedance	Impedance	Low-angle and high-angle laser light scatter
HGB	Modified cyanmethemoglobin (525 nm)	Sodium lauryl sulfate–HGB (555 nm)	Modified cyanmethemoglobin (540 nm)	Modified cyanmethemoglobin (546 nm)
HCT	(RBC × MCV)/10	Cumulative RBC pulse height detection	(RBC × MCV)/10	(RBC × MCV)/10
MCV	Mean of RBC volume distribution histogram	(HCT/RBC) × 10	Mean of RBC volume distribution histogram	Mean of RBC volume distribution histogram
MCH	(HGB/RBC) × 10	(HGB/RBC) × 10	(HGB/RBC) × 10	(HGB/RBC) × 10
MCHC	(HGB/HCT) × 100	(HGB/HCT) × 100	(HGB/HCT) × 100	(HGB/HCT) × 100
Platelet count	Impedance volume and conductivity and five-angle light scatter measurement	Impedance; light scatter; fluorescent staining, forward light scatter, and side fluorescent light detection	Dual-angle light scatter analysis; impedance count for verification; optional CD61 monoclonal antibody count	Low-angle and high-angle light scatter; refractive index
RDW	RDW as CV (%) of RBC histogram or RDW-SD (fL)	RDW-SD (fL) or RDW-CV (%)	Relative value, equivalent to CV	CV (%) of RBC histogram
Reticulocyte count	Supravital staining; impedance volume and conductivity and light scatter measurement	Fluorescent staining; forward light scatter and side fluorescent light detection	Fluorescent staining; low-angle scatter, and fluorescent light detection	Supravital staining (oxazine 750); low-angle and high-angle light scatter and absorbance
NRBC*	Impedance volume and conductivity and five-angle light scatter measurement	Fluorescent staining; forward light scatter and side fluorescent light detection	Red fluorescent dye staining; forward light scatter and fluorescent light detection	Multiangle light scatter measurements in the two WBC differential channels
WBC differential	Impedance volume and conductivity and five-angle light scatter measurement	Fluorescent staining; forward and side light scatter, and side fluorescent light detection	Multiangle polarized scatter separation (MAPSS) and three-color fluorescence detection	Peroxidase staining, light scatter and absorption; for basophils, differential lysis, low-angle and high-angle laser light scatter

CV, Coefficient of variation; *DC*, direct current; *HCT*, hematocrit; *HGB*, hemoglobin; *MCH*, mean cell hemoglobin; *MCHC*, mean cell hemoglobin concentration; *MCV*, mean cell volume; *NRBC*, nucleated red blood cell count; *RBC*, red blood cell (or count); *RDW*, RBC distribution width; *SD*, standard deviation; *VCS*, volume, conductivity, scatter; *WBC*, white blood cell (or count).
*Instruments auto-correct the WBC count for the presence of nucleated RBCs.

counted as platelets, and particles greater than 36 fL are counted as RBCs. In the WBC chamber, a reagent to lyse RBCs and release hemoglobin is added before WBCs are counted simultaneously by impedance in each of three sensing apertures (100 μm in diameter, 75 μm in length). Alternatively, some models employ consecutive counts in the same RBC or WBC aperture. After counting cycles are completed, the WBC dilution is passed to the hemoglobinometer for determination of hemoglobin concentration (light transmittance read at a wavelength of 525 nm). Electrical pulses generated in the counting cycles are sent to the analyzer for editing, coincidence correction, and digital conversion. Two of the three counts obtained in the RBC and the WBC baths must match within specified limits for the counts to be accepted by the instrument.[5,9] This multiple counting procedure prevents data errors resulting from aperture obstructions or statistical outliers and allows for excellent reproducibility on the Beckman Coulter instruments.

Pulse height is measured and categorized by pulse height analyzers; 256 channels are used for WBC and RBC analysis, and 64 channels are used for platelet analysis. Volume-distribution histograms of WBC, RBC, and platelet populations are generated. The RBC mean cell volume (MCV) is the average volume of the RBCs taken from the volume distribution data. The hematocrit (HCT), mean cell hemoglobin (MCH), and mean cell hemoglobin concentration (MCHC) are calculated from measured and derived values. The RBC distribution width (RDW) is calculated directly from the histogram as the coefficient of variation (CV) of the RBC volume distribution, with a reference interval of 11.5% to 14.5%.[5] The RDW is an index of anisocytosis, but it may be falsely skewed because it reflects the ratio of the standard deviation (SD) to MCV. That is, an RBC distribution histogram with normal divergence but a decreased MCV may imply a high RDW, falsely indicating increased anisocytosis. MCV and RDW are used by the instrument to flag possible anisocytosis, microcytosis, and macrocytosis.[9]

Platelets are counted within the range of 2 to 20 fL, and a volume-distribution histogram is constructed. If the platelet volume distribution meets specified criteria, a statistical least-squares method is applied to the raw data to fit the data to a log-normal curve. The curve is extrapolated from 0 to 70 fL, and the final count is derived from this extended curve. This fitting procedure eliminates interference from particles in the noise region, such as debris, and in the larger region, such as small RBCs. The mean platelet volume (MPV), analogous to the RBC MCV, also is derived from the platelet histogram. The reference interval for the MPV is about 6.8 to 10.2 fL. The MPV increases slightly with storage of the specimen in ethylenediaminetetraacetic acid (EDTA).[5]

Many older-model Beckman Coulter instruments, such as the STKR, and the newer, smaller models, such as the Ac-T series, provide three-part leukocyte subpopulation analysis, which differentiates WBCs into lymphocytes, mononuclear cells, and granulocytes. In the WBC channel, a special lysing reagent causes *differential shrinkage* of the leukocytes, which allows the different cells to be counted and volumetrically sized based on their impedance. A WBC histogram is constructed from the channelized data. Particles between approximately 35 and 90 fL are considered lymphocytes; particles between 90 and 160 fL are considered *mononuclears* (monocytes, blasts, immature granulocytes, and reactive lymphocytes); and particles between 160

and 450 fL are considered granulocytes. This allows the calculation of relative and absolute numbers for these three populations (Figure 12.5).[6] Proprietary computerized algorithms further allow flagging for increased eosinophils or basophils or both and interpretation of the histogram differential, including flagging for abnormal cells, such as reactive lymphocytes and blasts.[7] When cell populations overlap or a distinct separation of populations does not exist, a region alarm (R flag) may be triggered that indicates the area of interference on the volume-distribution histogram. An R1 flag represents excess signals at the lower threshold region of the WBC histogram and a questionable WBC count. This interference is visualized as a *high takeoff* of the curve and may indicate the presence of nucleated RBCs, clumped platelets, unlysed RBCs, or electronic noise.[6,7]

More recent Beckman Coulter instruments, the LH 700 Series and UniCel DxH series, generate hemogram data (including the WBC count) as before but use Coulter's proprietary *VCS (volume, conductivity, scatter) technology* in a separate channel to evaluate WBCs for the determination of a five-part differential. The VCS technology includes the volumetric sizing of cells by impedance, conductivity measurements of cells, and laser light scatter, all performed simultaneously for each cell. After RBCs are lysed and WBCs are treated with a stabilizing reagent to maintain them in a near-native state, a hydrodynamically focused sample stream is directed through the flow cell past the sensing zone. Low-frequency DC measures cell

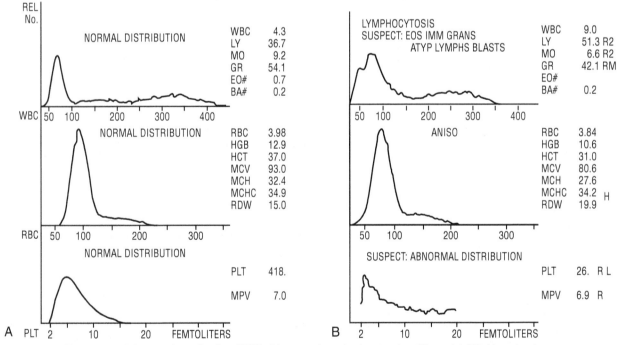

Figure 12.5 Printouts from Coulter STKR. Printouts show the interpretive differential. **(A)**, Note the three distinct white blood cell (WBC) populations, Gaussian or normal distribution of red blood cells (RBCs), and right-skewed or log-normal distribution of platelets. **(B)**, Note the left shift in the WBC histogram with possible interference at the lower threshold region. R2 flag indicates interference and loss of valley owing to overlap or insufficient separation between the lymphocyte and mononuclear populations at the 90-fL region. RM flag indicates interference at more than one region. Eosinophil data have been suppressed. Also note the abnormal platelet volume distribution with a low platelet count. Manual 200-cell differential counts on the same specimens: **(A)**, 52.5% neutrophils (47% segmented neutrophils, 5.5% bands), 41.5% lymphocytes, 4.0% monocytes, 1% basophils, 0.5% metamyelocytes, 0.5% reactive lymphocytes; **(B)**, 51% neutrophils (23% segmented neutrophils, 28% bands), 12% lymphocytes, 9.5% monocytes, 1% metamyelocytes, 1.5% myelocytes, 25% reactive lymphocytes, and 17 nucleated RBCs/100 WBCs.

volume, whereas a high-frequency electromagnetic probe measures conductivity, an indicator of cellular internal content. The conductivity signal is corrected for cellular volume, which yields a unique measurement called *opacity*. Each cell also is scanned with monochromatic laser light that reveals information about the cell surface, such as structure, shape, and reflectivity. Beckman Coulter's unique rotated light scatter detection method, which covers a 10-degree to 70-degree range, allows for separation of cells with similar volume but different scatter characteristics.[27] Beckman Coulter's newest analyzer, the UniCel DxH 800, uses volume and conductivity as well as five additional parameters: axial light loss (AL2), low-angle light scatter (LALS), median-angle light scatter (MALS), lower median–angle light scatter (LMALS), and upper median–angle light scatter (UMALS).[29, 30,] Using the data collected by the parameters listed previously, the instrument applies *data transformation,* the process by which populations of cells are separated, allowing the determination of major populations as well as the enhancement of subpopulations of cells. Once those populations are established, a technique called the *watershed concept* searches for those populations and aids in determining counts as well as flagging based on all the populations found for that specimen.[29,30]

This combination of technologies provides a three-dimensional plot or cytograph of the WBC populations, which are separated by computer cluster analysis. Two-dimensional scatterplots of the measurements represent different views of the cytograph. The scatterplot of volume (*y*-axis) versus light scatter (*x*-axis) shows clear separation of lymphocytes, monocytes, neutrophils, and eosinophils. Basophils are hidden behind the lymphocytes but are separated by conductivity because of their cytoplasmic granulation. Single-parameter histograms of volume, conductivity, and light scatter also are available.[9]

Two types of WBC flags (alarms or indicators of abnormality) are generated on all hematology analyzers that provide a WBC differential count: (1) user defined, primarily set for distributional abnormalities, such as eosinophilia or lymphocytopenia (based on absolute eosinophil or lymphocyte counts); and (2) instrument specific, primarily suspect flags for morphologic abnormalities. For *distributional flags,* the user establishes reference intervals and programs the instrument to flag each parameter as high or low. *Suspect flags* indicating the possible presence of abnormal cells are triggered when cell populations fall outside expected regions or when specific statistical limitations are exceeded. Instrument-specific *suspect* flags on the Coulter UniCel DxH 800 system and LH 700 series include immature granulocytes/bands, blasts, variant lymphocytes, nucleated RBCs, and platelet clumps. The UniCel DxH 800 also uses the International Society for Laboratory Hematology (ISLH) consensus rules in addition to the user-defined and system-defined flags for complete data analysis.[31,32] In addition to the flags listed earlier, inadequate separation of cell populations may disallow reporting of differential results by the instrument and may elicit a *review slide* message.[9,32,33]

The UniCel DxH 800 system uses VCS as well as digital signal processing from five light scatter angles for clear cellular resolution. On the LH 700 series, Coulter uses an *IntelliKinetics* application. This application is used to ensure consistency with the kinetic reactions. It provides the instrument the best signals for analysis independent of laboratory environment variations.

Compared with earlier models Coulter IntelliKinetics provides better separation of cell populations for WBCs and reticulocytes, which enables better analysis by the system algorithms.[32,33]

The UniCel DxH 800 also includes the number of nucleated RBCs as part of the standard CBC report. They are identified, counted, and subtracted from the WBC count using volume, conductivity, and the same five light scatter measurement described earlier. The AL2 measurement (which reflects the amount of light absorbed as it passes through the flow cell) initially separates the nucleated RBCs from the WBCs. Algorithms are applied using the scatter from the other angles to electronically separate and count the nucleated RBCs. Two scatterplots display the nucleated RBC data by plotting axial light loss (AL2) on the *x*-axis against low-angle light scatter (RLALS) and upper median–angle light scatter (RUMALS) on *y*-axis.

Figure 12.6 represents a standard patient printout from the Beckman Coulter UniCel DxH 800.

Sysmex Instrumentation

Sysmex Corporation, formerly TOA Medical Electronics Company, Ltd., manufactures a full line of hematology analyzers that provide complete RBC, platelet, and WBC analysis with three-part differential; the larger XT-1800i (SF-3000 and SE-9000) that performs a CBC with five-part differential; and the XE series and the newest XN series that also provide a fully automated reticulocyte count.[28,32] The newest XN series is modular. The series is scalable, and multiple modules can be combined onto one platform. Each module contains the XN-CBC and XN-DIFF with other options available, including XN-BF, the body fluid application. Included standard on the CBC and differential DIFF modules are NRBCs, RET-He (reticulocyte hemoglobin), and IRF (immature reticulocyte fraction). The platelet analysis on the XN also uses a fluorescent count, in addition to the impedance count and optical count, called the PLT-F, performed by optical measurement.[34-37] The PLT-F can be performed on each specimen or set up as a reflex based on the laboratory's PLT criteria. The method uses a fluorocell fluorescent dye (oxazine) combined with an extended PLT counting volume and time. The PLTs can be differentiated from other cells based on differences in intensity of the fluorescence combined with forward scattered light.[34] The WBC, RBC, platelet counts, hemoglobin, and HCT are considered to be measured directly. Three hydraulic subsystems are used for determining the hemogram: the WBC channel, the RBC/platelet channel, and a separate hemoglobin channel. In the WBC and RBC transducer chambers, diluted WBC and RBC samples are aspirated through the different apertures and counted using the impedance (DC detection) method for counting and volumetrically sizing cells. Two unique features enhance the impedance technology: In the RBC/platelet channel, a sheathed stream with hydrodynamic focusing is used to direct cells through the aperture, which reduces coincident passage, particle volume distortion, and recirculation of blood cells around the aperture; and in the WBC and RBC/platelet channels, *floating thresholds* are used to discriminate each cell population.[8,15,16]

As cells pass through the apertures, signals are transmitted in sequence to the analog circuit and particle volume distribution analysis circuits for conversion to cumulative cell volume

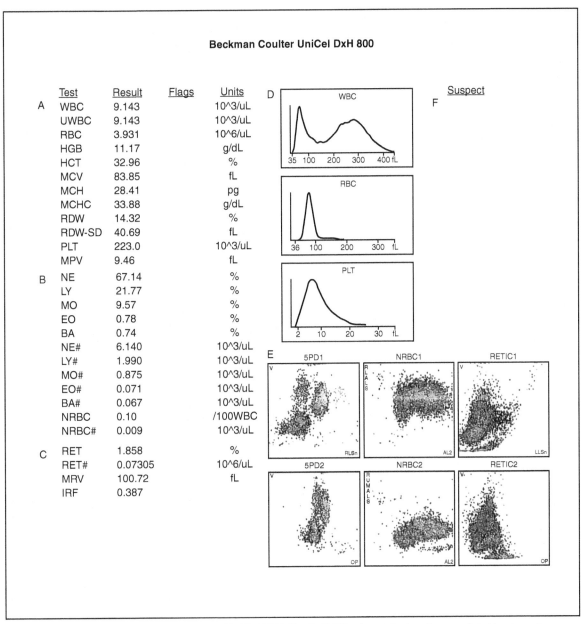

Figure 12.6 Printout from Coulter UniCel DxH 800. The DxH 800 printout displays the complete blood count (CBC), differential (DIFF), and reticulocyte data for the same patient also presented in Figures 12.7, 12.9, and 12.11 using three other hematology analyzers. **(A),** CBC data. **(B),** Differential with nucleated red blood cells (NRBCs). **(C),** Reticulocyte data, including the immature reticulocyte fraction (IRF). **(D),** Impedance histograms for white blood cells (WBC), red blood cells (RBC), and platelets (PLT). **(E),** Advanced two-dimensional optical scatterplots for WBCs, NRBCs, and reticulocytes. **(F),** Suspect area in which any specimen or system flags will display.

distribution data. Particle volume distribution curves are constructed, and optimal position of the *autodiscrimination level* (i.e., threshold) is set by the microprocessor for each cell population. The lower platelet threshold is automatically adjusted in the 2- to 6-fL volume range, and the upper threshold is adjusted in the 12- to 30-fL range, based on particle volume distribution. Likewise, the RBC lower and upper thresholds may be set in the 25- to 75-fL and 200- to 250-fL volume ranges. This floating threshold circuitry allows for discrimination of cell populations on a specimen-by-specimen basis. Cell counts are based on pulses between the lower and upper autodiscriminator levels, with dilution ratio, volume counted, and coincident passage

error accounted for in the final computer-generated numbers. In the RBC channel, the floating discriminator is particularly useful in separating platelets from small RBCs. The HCT also is determined from the RBC/platelet channel, based on the principle that the pulse height generated by the RBC is proportional to cell volume. The HCT is the RBC cumulative pulse height and is considered a true relative percentage volume of erythrocytes.[8,15] In the hemoglobin flow cell, hemoglobin is oxidized and binds to sodium lauryl sulfate (SLS), forming a stable SLS–hemoglobin complex, which is measured photometrically at 555 nm.[16]

The following indices are calculated in the microprocessor using directly measured or derived parameters: MCV, MCH,

MCHC, RDW-SD, RDW-CV, MPV, and plateletcrit. RDW-SD is the RBC arithmetic distribution width measured at 20% of the height of the RBC curve, reported in femtoliters, with a reference interval of 37 to 54 fL. RDW-CV is the RDW reported as a CV. Plateletcrit is the platelet volume ratio, analogous to the HCT. MPV is calculated from the plateletcrit and platelet count just as erythrocyte MCV is calculated from the HCT and RBC count. The proportion of platelets greater than 12 fL in the total platelet count may be an indicator of possible platelet clumping, giant platelets, or cell fragments.[8,15,16] The XE series has the capability to run the platelet counting in the optical mode, which eliminates common interferences found with impedance counting. In the optical mode, the, immature platelet fraction or IPF, can be measured to provide additional information concerning platelet kinetics in cases of thromobocytopenia.[38] Although not yet approved for reporting in the United States, subpopulations of red cells can be measured with the Sysmex XE 5000 analyzer using the upper area and lower areas of the RBC histogram to identify macrocytic cells (MacroR) and microcytic cells (MicroR).[39] Percentage of decreased and increased cellular hemoglobin content is determined from the reticulocyte channel using high-angle forward light scatter.[40] These two parameters are used in differentiation of anemias.

The SE-9000/9500 uses four detection chambers to analyze WBCs and obtain a five-part differential: the DIFF, immature myeloid information (IMI), eosinophil (EO), and basophil (BASO) chambers. The high-end instrumentation such as the XE-series and the XN series has a six-part differential: neutrophils, lymphocytes, monocytes, eosinophils, basophils, and immature granulocytes. Every differential performed generates a percentage and absolute number for immature granulocytes, thus providing valuable information about the complete differential.[28] In the DIFF detection chamber, RBCs are hemolyzed and WBCs are analyzed simultaneously by low-frequency DC and high-frequency current (*DC/RF detection method*). A scattergram of RF detection signals (*y*-axis) versus DC detection signals (*x*-axis) allows separation of the WBCs into lymphocytes, monocytes, and granulocytes. Floating discriminators determine the optimal separation between these populations. Granulocytes are analyzed further in the IMI detection chamber to determine immature myeloid information. RBCs are lysed, and WBCs other than immature granulocytes are selectively shrunk by temperature and chemically controlled reactions. Analysis of the treated sample using the DC/RF detection method allows separation of immature cells on the IMI scattergram. A similar differential shrinkage and lysis method is also used in the EO and BASO chambers. That is, eosinophils and basophils are counted by impedance (DC detection) in separate chambers in which the RBCs are lysed, and WBCs other than eosinophils or basophils are selectively shrunk by temperature and chemically controlled reactions. Eosinophils and basophils are subtracted from the granulocyte count derived from the DIFF scattergram analysis to determine the neutrophil count. User-defined distributional flags may be set, and instrument-specific suspect flags, similar to those described for the Beckman Coulter LH 700 series, are triggered for the possible presence of morphologic abnormalities.[15,16] A POSITIVE or NEGATIVE interpretive message is displayed.

In the XN-1000, fluorescent flow cytometry is used for the WBC count, WBC differential, and enumeration of nucleated RBCs. In the *WDF channel*, RBCs are lysed, WBC membranes are perforated, and the DNA and RNA in the WBCs are stained with a fluorescent dye. Plotting side scatter on the *x*-axis and side fluorescent light on the *y*-axis enables separation and enumeration of neutrophils, eosinophils, lymphocytes, monocytes, and immature granulocytes. In the *WNR channel*, the RBCs are lysed, including nucleated RBCs, and WBC membranes are perforated. A fluorescent polymethine dye stains the nucleus and organelles of the WBCs with high fluorescence intensity and stains the released nuclei of the nucleated RBCs with low intensity. Plotting side fluorescent light on the *x*-axis and forward scatter on the *y*-axis enables separation and enumeration of the total WBC count, basophils, and nucleated RBCs. The WBC count is automatically corrected when nucleated RBCs are present in the specimen. A *WPC channel* detects blasts and abnormal lymphocytes in a similar manner using a lysing agent and fluorescent dye and plotting side scatter on the *x*-axis and side fluorescent light on the *y*-axis. Figure 12.7 shows a patient report from the Sysmex XN-1000 analyzing the same patient specimen for which data are given in Figure 12.6.

Abbott Instrumentation

Instruments offered by Abbott Laboratories include the smaller CELL-DYN Emerald, which provides complete RBC, platelet, and WBC analysis with three-part differential, and the larger CELL-DYN Sapphire and the midrange CELL-DYN Ruby, both of which provide a CBC with five-part differential and random fully automated reticulocyte analysis.[32] The CELL-DYN 4000 system has three independent measurement channels for determining the hemogram and differential: an optical channel for WBC count and differential data, an impedance channel for RBC and platelet data, and a hemoglobin channel for hemoglobin determination.[20,21] The WBC, RBC, hemoglobin, and platelet parameters are considered to be measured directly. A 60- to 70-μm aperture is used in the RBC/platelet transducer assembly for counting and volumetrically sizing of RBCs and platelets by the electronic impedance method.

A unique von Behrens plate is located in the RBC/platelet counting chamber to minimize the effect of recirculating cells. Pulses are collected and sorted in 256 channels according to their amplitudes: particles between 1 and 35 fL are included in the initial platelet data, and particles greater than 35 fL are counted as RBCs. Floating thresholds are used to determine the best separation of the platelet population and to eliminate interference, such as noise, debris, or small RBCs, from the count. Coincident passage loss is corrected for in the final RBC and platelet counts. RBC pulse editing is applied before MCV derivation to compensate for aberrant pulses produced by nonaxial passage of RBCs through the aperture. The MCV is the average volume of the RBCs derived from RBC volume distribution data. Hemoglobin is measured directly using a modified hemoglobincyanide method that measures absorbance at 540 nm. HCT, MCH, and MCHC are calculated from the directly

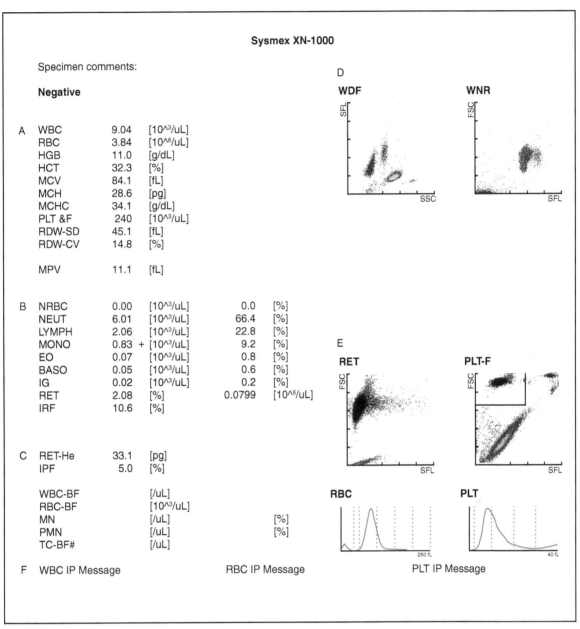

Figure 12.7 Printout from Sysmex XN-1000. The XN-1000 printout displays the complete blood count (CBC), differential (DIFF), and reticulocyte data for the same patient in Figures 12.6, 12.9, and 12.11. using three other hematology analyzers. **(A),** CBC data; note the "&F" to indicate the fluorescent platelet count result. **(B),** Nucleated red blood cells (NRBCs), six-part differential, including the immature granulocyte (IG) count, reticulocyte count (RET), and immature reticulocyte fraction (IRF). **(C),** Reticulocyte hemoglobin (RET-He), immature platelet fraction (IPF), and body fluid counts, if done. **(D),** Two scatterplots, WDF (lymphocytes, monocytes, neutrophils, eosinophils, and immature granulocytes) and WNR (white blood cell [WBC] count, basophils, and NRBCs). **(E),** RET and platelet (PLT-F) scatterplots, and RBC and PLT impedance histograms. **(F),** Specimen-related flags are listed at the bottom of the printout, if any are generated.

measured or derived parameters. The RDW, equivalent to CV, is a relative value, derived from the RBC histogram by using the 20th and 80th percentiles. The platelet analysis is based on a two-dimensional optical platelet count using fluorescent technology, the same technology used for direct nucleated RBC counting by adding a red fluorescence to the specimen to stain nucleated red cells.[41] Further analysis of platelets and platelet aggregates can be performed by using an automated CD61 monoclonal antibody to generate an immunoplatelet count.[42-44] Other indices available include MPV and plateletcrit.[20,21]

The WBC count and differential are derived from the optical channel using CELL-DYN's patented multiangle polarized scatter separation (MAPSS) technology with three-color fluorescent technology. A hydrodynamically focused sample stream is directed through a quartz flow cell past a focused light source, an argon ion laser. Scattered light is measured at multiple angles: 0-degree forward light scatter measurement is used for determination of cell volume, 90-degree orthogonal light scatter measurement is used for determination of cellular lobularity, 7-degree narrow-angle scatter measurement is used to

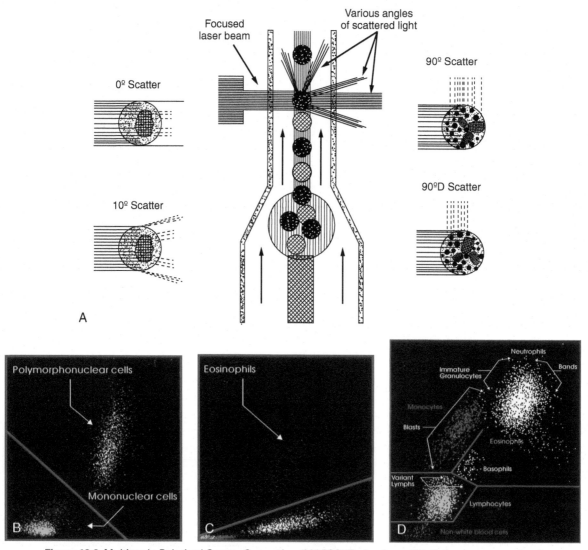

Figure 12.8 Multiangle Polarized Scatter Separation (MAPSS) Technology. (A), Cells are measured and characterized by plotting light scatter from four different angles. **(B),** Mononuclear and polymorphonuclear scatter with MAPPS technology. It plots 10-degree scatter (complexity) on the x-axis and 90-degree scatter (lobularity) on the y-axis. The system uses algorithms to further separate the two populations, displaying mononuclear on the lower left and polymorphonuclear on the upper right. **(C),** Separation and plotting of the polymorphonuclear cells into neutrophils and eosinophils based on MAPPS technology. It plots 90-degree scatter (lobularity) on the x-axis and 90-degree depolarized (90 D) scatter on the y-axis. The system uses algorithms to further separate the two populations of cells. **(D),** Scatter of all white blood cell (WBC) populations by MAPPS technology plotting 10-degree scatter (complexity) on the x-axis and 0-degree scatter (size or volume) on the y-axis. On the newer instruments, a 7-degree angle for complexity is now used instead of the 10-degree angle. The change reflects use of the midrange of the angle instead of the end range; however, it still provides the same information. (From Abbott Laboratories. [2000]. *CELL-DYN 3700 System Operator's Manual [914032C].* Abbott Park, IL: Abbott Laboratories.)

correlate with cellular complexity, and 90-degree depolarized light scatter measurement is used for evaluation of cellular granularity. Orthogonal light scatter is split, with one portion directed to a 90-degree photomultiplier tube and the other portion directed through a polarizer to the 90-degree depolarized photomultiplier tube. Light that has changed polarization (depolarized) is the only light that can be detected by the 90-degree depolarized photomultiplier tube. Various combinations of these four measurements are used to differentiate and quantify the five major WBC subpopulations: neutrophils, lymphocytes,

monocytes, eosinophils, and basophils.[20,41,45] Figure 12.8 illustrates CELL-DYN's MAPPS technology.

The light scatter signals are converted into electrical signals, sorted into 256 channels on the basis of amplitude for each angle of light measured, and graphically presented as scatterplots. Scatter information from the different angles is plotted in various combinations: 90 degrees/7 degrees, or lobularity versus complexity; 0 degrees/7 degrees, volume versus complexity; and 90 degrees depolarized/90 degrees, granularity versus lobularity. Lobularity or 90-degree scatter (*y*-axis) plotted against complexity or 7-degree scatter (*x*-axis) yields separation of mononuclear and segmented (polymorphonuclear neutrophil) subpopulations. Basophils cluster with the mononuclears in this analysis, because the basophil granules dissolve in the sheath reagent, and the degranulated basophil is a less complex cell. Each cell in the two clusters is identified as a mononuclear or segmented neutrophil for further evaluation.

The mononuclear subpopulation is plotted on a 0-degree/7-degree scatterplot, with volume on the *y*-axis and complexity on the *x*-axis. Three populations (lymphocytes, monocytes, and basophils) are seen clearly on this display. Nucleated RBCs, unlysed RBCs, giant platelets, and platelet clumps fall below the lymphocyte cluster on this scatterplot and are excluded from the WBC count and differential. Information from the WBC impedance channel also is used in discriminating these particles.[21]

The segmented neutrophil subpopulation is plotted on a 90-degree depolarized/90-degree scatterplot, with granularity or 90-degree depolarized scatter on the *y*-axis and lobularity or 90-degree scatter on the *x*-axis. Because of the unique nature of eosinophil granules, eosinophils scatter more 90-degree depolarized light, which allows clear separation of eosinophils and neutrophils on this display. Dynamic thresholds are used for best separation of the different populations in the various scatterplots. Each cell type is identified with a distinct color, so that after all classifications are made and volume (0-degree scatter) is plotted on the *y*-axis against complexity (7-degree scatter) on the *x*-axis, each cell population can be visualized easily by the operator on the data terminal screen. Other scatterplots (90 degrees/0 degrees, 90 degrees depolarized/0 degrees, 90 degrees depolarized/7 degrees) are available and may be displayed at operator request. On earlier instruments, the 7-degree angle measurement for complexity was referred to as the 10-degree angle. The change reflects use of the midrange of the angle instead of the end range; however, it still provides the same information.[46,47] As on the previously described instruments, user-defined distributional flags may be set, and instrument-specific suspect flags may alert the operator to the presence of abnormal cells.[20,46] Figure 12.9 represents a patient printout from the CELL-DYN Sapphire analyzing the same patient specimen for which data are given in Figures 12.6 and 12.7.

Siemens Healthcare Diagnostics Instrumentation

Siemens Healthcare Diagnostics Inc. manufactures the ADVIA 2120 and 2120i, the next generation of the ADVIA 120.[26,32,48] Siemens has simplified the hydraulics and operations of the analyzer by replacing multiple complex hydraulic systems with a unified fluids circuit assembly, or *Unifluidics technology.* The ADVIA 2120, 2120i, and 120 provide a complete hemogram and WBC differential, while also providing a fully automated reticulocyte count.[22,23]

Four independent measurement channels are used in determining the hemogram and differential: RBC/platelet channel, hemoglobin channel, and peroxidase (PEROX) and basophil-lobularity (BASO) channels for WBC and differential data. WBC, RBC, hemoglobin, and platelets are measured directly. Hemoglobin is determined using a modified cyanmethemoglobin method that measures absorbance in a colorimeter flow

cuvette at approximately 546 nm. The RBC/platelet method uses flow cytometric light scattering measurements determined as cells, in a sheath-stream, pass through a flow cell by a laser optical assembly (laser diode light source). RBCs and platelets are isovolumetrically sphered before entering the flow cell to eliminate optical orientation noise. Laser light scattered at two different angular intervals—low angle (2 to 3 degrees), correlating with cell volume, and high angle (5 to 15 degrees), correlating with internal complexity (i.e., refractive index or hemoglobin concentration)—is measured simultaneously (Figure 12.10). This *differential scatter technique,* in combination with isovolumetric sphering, eliminates the adverse effect of variation in cellular hemoglobin concentration on the determination of RBC volume (as seen by differences in cellular deformability affecting the pulse height generated on impedance instruments).[10,49] The Mie theory of light scatter of dielectric spheres[18] is applied to plot scatter-intensity signals from the two angles against each other for a cell-by-cell RBC volume (*y*-axis) versus hemoglobin concentration (*x*-axis) cytogram or RBC map.[19]

Independent histograms of RBC volume and hemoglobin concentration also are plotted. On the ADVIA 2120 and 120 platelets are counted and volumetrically sized using a two-dimensional (low-angle and high-angle) platelet analysis, which allows better discrimination of platelets from interfering particles, such as RBC fragments and small RBCs.[22] Larger platelets can be included in the platelet count.[23,48]

Several parameters and indices are derived from the measurements described in the previous paragraph. MCV and MPV are the mean of the RBC volume histogram and the platelet volume histogram. HCT, MCH, and MCHC are mathematically computed using RBC, hemoglobin, and MCV values. RDW is calculated as the CV of the RBC volume histogram, whereas hemoglobin distribution width (HDW), an analogous index, is calculated as the SD of the RBC hemoglobin concentration histogram. The reference interval for HDW is 2.2 to 3.2 g/dL. Cell hemoglobin concentration mean (CHCM), analogous to MCHC, is derived from cell-by-cell direct measures of hemoglobin concentration. Interferences with the hemoglobin colorimetric method, such as lipemia or icterus, affect the calculated MCHC but do not alter measured CHCM. CHCM generally is not reported as a patient result but is used by the instrument as an internal check for the MCHC and is available to the operator for calculating the cellular hemoglobin if interferences are present. Unique RBC flags derived from CHCM include hemoglobin concentration variance (HC VAR), hypochromia (HYPO), and hyperchromia (HYPER).[22,23]

Siemens hematology analyzers determine WBC count and a six-part WBC differential (neutrophils, lymphocytes, monocytes, eosinophils, basophils, and large unstained cells [LUCs]) by cytochemistry and optical flow cytometry, using the PEROX and BASO channels. LUCs include reactive or variant lymphocytes and blasts.

Peroxidase (PEROX) Channel

In the PEROX channel, RBCs are lysed, and WBCs are stained for their peroxidase activity. The following reaction is catalyzed

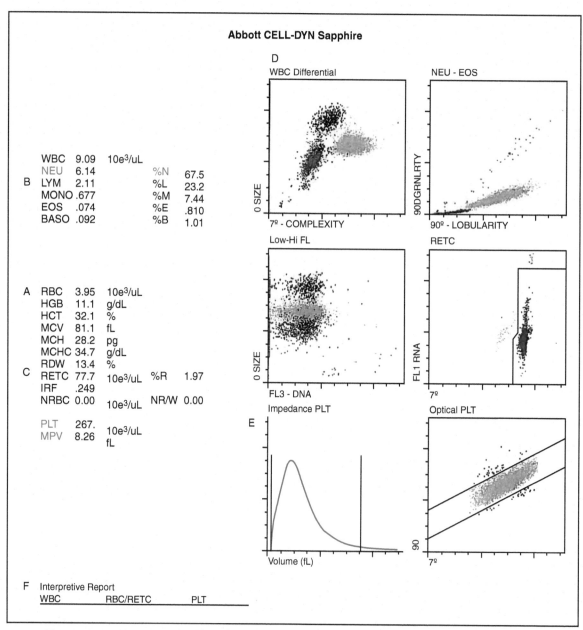

Abbott CELL-DYN Sapphire

	WBC	9.09	10e³/uL		
B	NEU	6.14		%N	67.5
	LYM	2.11		%L	23.2
	MONO	.677		%M	7.44
	EOS	.074		%E	.810
	BASO	.092		%B	1.01

	RBC	3.95	10e³/uL		
A	HGB	11.1	g/dL		
	HCT	32.1	%		
	MCV	81.1	fL		
	MCH	28.2	pg		
	MCHC	34.7	g/dL		
	RDW	13.4	%		
C	RETC	77.7	10e³/uL	%R	1.97
	IRF	.249			
	NRBC	0.00	10e³/uL	NR/W	0.00
	PLT	267.	10e³/uL		
	MPV	8.26	fL		

D WBC Differential — 0 SIZE / 7º - COMPLEXITY

NEU - EOS — 90DGRNLRTY / 90º - LOBULARITY

Low-Hi FL — 0 SIZE / FL3 - DNA

RETC — FL1 RNA / 7º

E Impedance PLT — Volume (fL)

Optical PLT — 90 / 7º

F Interpretive Report
WBC RBC/RETC PLT

Figure 12.9 Printout from CELL-DYN Sapphire. The Sapphire printout displays the complete blood count (CBC), differential (DIFF), and reticulocyte data for the same patient in Figures 12.6, 12.7, and 12.11. using three other hematology analyzers. **(A),** CBC data. **(B),** Differential count data. Note that the white blood cell (WBC) count is listed with the differential instead of the CBC data. **(C),** Reticulocyte and nucleated red blood cell (RBC) data displayed under the CBC data but before the platelet (PLT) data. **(D),** Two scattergrams for the differential; both 7-degree scatter (complexity) vs. 0-degree scatter (size or volume) and 90-degree scatter (lobularity) vs. 90-degree depolarized (90 D) scatter (granularity) are plotted for the WBCs; two histograms are also plotted for the nucleated RBC and reticulocyte data. **(E),** Impedance histogram and optical platelet scatterplot side by side. **(F),** At the bottom the interpretative report flags display if there are any for the specimen.

by cellular peroxidase, which converts the substrate to a dark precipitate in peroxidase-containing cells (neutrophils, monocytes, and eosinophils):

$$H_2O_2 + 4\text{-}chloro\text{-}1\text{-}naphthol \xrightarrow{\text{cellular peroxidase}} dark\ precipitate$$

A portion of the cell suspension is fed to a sheath-stream flow cell where a tungsten-halogen darkfield optics system is used to measure absorbance (proportional to the amount of peroxidase in each cell) and forward scatter (proportional to the volume of each cell). Absorbance is plotted on the x-axis of the cytogram, and scatter is plotted on the y-axis.[22,23] A total WBC count (WBC-PEROX) is obtained from the optical signals in this channel and is used as an internal check of the primary WBC count obtained in the basophil-lobularity channel (WBC-BASO). If significant interference occurs in the WBC-BASO count, the instrument substitutes the WBC-PEROX value.[23]

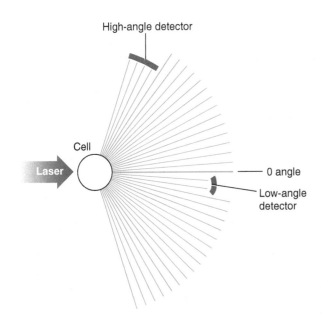

Figure 12.10 Differential Scatter Detection in the ADVIA 120. Forward high-angle scatter (5 to 15 degrees) and forward low-angle scatter (2 to 3 degrees) are detected for analysis of red and white blood cells. (From Technicon. [1993]. *Technicon H Systems Training Guide.* Tarrytown, NY: Technicon.)

Computerized cluster analysis allows classification of the different cell populations, including abnormal clusters such as nucleated RBCs and platelet clumps. Nucleated RBCs are analyzed for every specimen using four counting algorithms, which permits the system to choose the most accurate count based on internal rules and conditions. Neutrophils and eosinophils contain the most peroxidase and cluster to the right on the cytogram. Monocytes stain weakly and cluster in the midregion of the cytogram. Lymphocytes, basophils, and LUCs (including variant or reactive lymphs and blasts) contain no peroxidase and appear on the left of the cytogram, with LUCs appearing above the lymphocyte area. Basophils cluster with the small lymphocytes and require further analysis for classification.[22,23,50]

Basophil-Lobularity (BASO) Channel

In the BASO channel, cells are treated with a reagent containing a nonionic surfactant in an acidic solution. Basophils are particularly resistant to lysis in this temperature-controlled reaction, whereas RBCs and platelets lyse and other leukocytes (nonbasophils) are stripped of their cytoplasm. Laser optics, using the same two-angle (2 to 3 degrees and 5 to 15 degrees) forward scattering system of the RBC/platelet channel, is used to analyze the treated cells. High-angle scatter (proportional to nuclear complexity) is plotted on the *x*-axis, and low-angle scatter (proportional to cell volume) is plotted on the *y*-axis. Cluster analysis allows for identification and quantification of the individual cellular populations. The intact basophils are identifiable by their large low-angle scatter. The remaining nuclei are classified as mononuclear, segmented, and blast cell nuclei based on their nuclear complexity (shape and cell density) and high-angle scatter.[22,23]

Basophils fall above a horizontal threshold on the cytogram. The stripped nuclei fall below the basophils, with segmented cells to the right and mononuclear cells to the left along the *x*-axis. Blast cells uniquely cluster below the mononuclear cells. Lack of distinct separation between the segmented and mononuclear clusters indicates WBC immaturity or suspected left shift. As indicated earlier, this channel provides the primary WBC count, the WBC-BASO. Relative differential results (in percent) are computed by dividing absolute numbers of the different cell classifications by the total WBC count.[22,23]

The nucleated RBC method is based on the physical characteristics of volume and density of the nucleated RBC nuclei. These characteristics allow counting in both WBC channels on the ADVIA 2120, and algorithms are applied to determine the absolute number and percentage of nucleated RBCs. Information from the PEROX and BASO channels is used to generate differential morphology flags indicating the possible presence of reactive lymphocytes, blasts, left shift, immature granulocytes, nucleated RBCs, or large platelets or platelet clumps.[22,23,50] Figure 12.11 shows a patient printout from the ADVIA 2120i analyzing the same patient specimen for which data are given in Figures 12.6, 12.7, and 12.9.

AUTOMATED RETICULOCYTE COUNTING

Reticulocyte counting is the last of the manual cell-counting procedures to be automated and has been a primary focus of hematology analyzer advancement in recent years. The imprecision and inaccuracy in manual reticulocyte counting are due to multiple factors, including stain variability, slide distribution error, statistical sampling error, and interobserver error.[51] All these potential errors, with the possible exception of stain variability, are correctable with automated reticulocyte counting. Increasing the number of RBCs counted produces increased precision.[52] This was evidenced in the 1993 College of American Pathologists pilot reticulocyte proficiency survey (Set RT-A, Sample RT-01) on which the CV for the reported manual results was 35% compared with 8.3% for results obtained using flow cytometry.[53] Precision of automated methods has continued to improve. The manual reticulocyte results for one specimen in the 2000 Reticulocyte Survey Set RT/RT2-A showed a CV of 28.7%, whereas the CV was 2.8% for results obtained using one of the automated methods.[54] Automated reticulocyte analyzers may count 32,000 RBCs compared with 1000 cells in the routine manual procedure.[55]

Available automated reticulocyte analyzers include flow cytometry systems such as the FACS system from Becton, Dickinson or the Coulter EPICS system; the Sysmex R-3500, R-500, XE-2100, XE-5000, and XN-series systems; the CELL-DYN 3500R, 3700, and 4000 systems; the Coulter LH 750 systems and the UniCel DxH800; and the Siemens ADVIA 2120, 2120i, and 120. All these analyzers evaluate reticulocytes based on optical scatter or fluorescence after the RBCs are treated with fluorescent dyes or nucleic acid stains to stain residual RNA in the reticulocytes. Because neither the FACS nor EPICS system is generally available in the routine hematology laboratory, the discussion here is limited to the other analyzers.

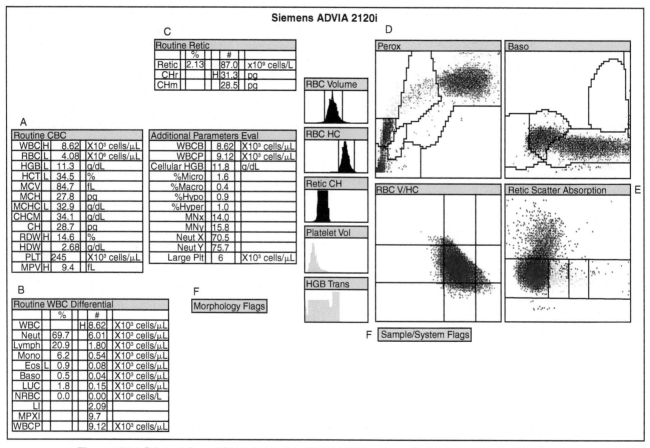

Figure 12.11 Printout from ADVIA 2120i. The ADVIA 2120i printout displays the complete blood count (CBC), differential (DIFF), and reticulocyte data for the same patient in Figures 12.6, 12.7, and 12.9. using three other hematology analyzers. **(A),** CBC data. **(B),** Six-part differential, including large unstained cells (LUCs) and nucleated red blood cells (NRBCs). **(C),** Reticulocyte information includes the cellular hemoglobin reticulocyte (CHr). **(D),** Cytograms for the differential, both the PEROX and BASO channels, on the right. **(E),** Scattergram for the reticulocyte and RBC counts; **(F),** Morphology flags and specimen/system flags where flags are displayed.

The Sysmex R-3000/3500 is a stand-alone reticulocyte analyzer that uses auramine O, a supravital fluorescent dye, and measures forward scatter and side fluorescence as the cells, in a sheath-stream, pass through a flow cell by an argon laser. The signals are plotted on a scattergram with forward scatter intensity, which correlates with volume, plotted against fluorescence intensity, which is proportional to RNA content. Automatic discrimination separates the populations into mature RBCs and reticulocytes. The reticulocytes fall into low-fluorescence, middle-fluorescence, or high-fluorescence regions, with the less mature reticulocytes showing higher fluorescence. The *immature reticulocyte fraction* (IRF) is the sum of the middle-fluorescence and high-fluorescence ratios and indicates the ratio of immature reticulocytes to total reticulocytes in a specimen. The XE-5000, the XT-2000i, and the XN series also determine the reticulocyte count and IRF by measuring forward scatter and side fluorescence. They also have a parameter called *RET-He* (reticulocyte hemoglobin equivalent) that measures the hemoglobin content of the reticulocytes.[56] It uses a proprietary polymethine dye to fluorescently stain the reticulocyte nucleic acids. This is similar to the reticulocyte hemoglobin content (CHr) parameter on the ADVIA 2120i (discussed later). Platelets, which also are counted, fall below a lower discriminator line.[57] The Sysmex SE-9500/9000 + RAM-1 module uses the same flow cytometry methodology for reticulocyte counting as the R-3500.[16] Offline specimen preparation is not required. The smaller Sysmex R-500 uses flow cytometry with a semiconductor laser as the light source and polymethine supravital fluorescent dye to provide automated reticulocyte counts.[28]

The CELL-DYN 3500R performs reticulocyte analysis by measuring 10-degree and 90-degree scatter in the optical channel (MAPSS technology) after the cells have been isovolumetrically sphered to eliminate optical orientation noise. The RBCs are stained with the thiazine dye new methylene blue N in an off-line sample preparation before the specimen is introduced to the instrument. The operator simply must change computer functions on the instrument before aspiration of the reticulocyte preparation.[46] The CELL-DYN Sapphire also uses MAPSS technology but adds fluorescence detection to allow fully automated, random access reticulocyte testing.[24,47] The RBCs are stained with a proprietary membrane-permeable fluorescent dye (CD4K530) that binds stoichiometrically to nucleic acid and emits green light as the cells, in a sheath-stream, pass through a flow cell by an argon ion laser. Platelets and reticulocytes are separated based on intensity of green fluorescence (scatter measured at 7 degrees and 90 degrees), and the reticulocyte count along with the IRF is determined.[47]

Beckman Coulter also has incorporated reticulocyte methods into its primary cell-counting instruments: LH 700 series systems and the UniCel DxH800. The Coulter method uses a new methylene blue stain and the VCS technology described earlier. Volume is plotted against light scatter (DF 5 scatterplot) and against conductivity (DF 6 scatterplot), which correlates with opacity of the RBC. Stained reticulocytes show greater optical scatter and greater opacity than mature RBCs. Relative and absolute reticulocyte counts are reported, along with mean reticulocyte volume and maturation index or IRF.[55]

The Siemens ADVIA 2120, 2120i, and 120 systems enumerate reticulocytes in the same laser optics flow cell used in the RBC/platelet and BASO channels described earlier. The reticulocyte reagent isovolumetrically spheres the RBCs and stains the reticulocytes with oxazine 750, a nucleic acid–binding dye. Three detectors measure low-angle scatter (2 to 3 degrees), high-angle scatter (5 to 15 degrees), and absorbance simultaneously as the cells pass through the flow cell. Three cytograms are generated: high-angle scatter versus absorption, low-angle scatter versus high-angle scatter (Mie cytogram or RBC map), and volume versus hemoglobin concentration. The absorption cytogram allows separation and quantitation of reticulocytes, with additional subdivision into low-absorbing, medium-absorbing, and high-absorbing cells based on amount of staining. The sum of the medium-absorbing and high-absorbing cells reflects the IRF. Volume and hemoglobin concentration for each cell are derived from the RBC map by applying Mie scattering theory.[26,58] Unique reticulocyte indices (MCVr, CHCMr, RDWr, HDWr, CHr, and CHDWr) are provided. The CHr or reticulocyte hemoglobin content of each cell is calculated as the product of the cell volume and the cell hemoglobin concentration. A single-parameter histogram of CHr is constructed, with a corresponding distribution width (CHDWr) calculated.[22,23] These reticulocyte indices are not reported on the routine patient printout but are available to the operator. Figure 12.12 is a reticulocyte printout from an ADVIA 120, showing the cytograms and reticulocyte indices.

Automation of reticulocyte counting has allowed increased precision and accuracy and has greatly expanded the analysis of immature RBCs, providing new parameters and indices that may be useful in the diagnosis and treatment of anemias. The IRF, first introduced to indicate immature reticulocytes, shows an early indication of erythropoiesis. The IRF and the absolute reticulocyte count can be used to distinguish types of anemias. Anemias with increased marrow erythropoiesis, such as hemolytic anemia, have a high total reticulocyte count and increased IRF, whereas chronic renal disease has decreased absolute count and an IRF indicating decreased marrow erythropoiesis.[58,59] An increased IRF and normal to decreased absolute reticulocyte count indicates an early response to therapy in nutritional anemias.[59] Use of both tests is a reliable indicator of changes in erythropoietic activity and may prove to be a valuable therapeutic monitoring tool in patients.[59] The reticulocyte maturity measurements also may be useful in evaluating bone marrow suppression during chemotherapy, monitoring hematopoietic regeneration after bone marrow or stem cell transplantation, monitoring renal transplant engraftment, and assessing efficacy of anemia therapy.[58-62] The reticulocyte hemoglobin content,

CHr (Advia) and Ret-He (Sysmex), provides an assessment of the availability of iron for erythropoiesis (Chapters 8 and 17). The additional reticulocyte indices derived on the ADVIA 2120 and 120 are valuable in following the response to erythropoietin therapy, and the CHr in particular has proved useful in the early detection and diagnosis of iron-deficient erythropoiesis in children.[62,63] The National Kidney Foundation Kidney Disease Outcomes Quality Initiative recommends the addition of the reticulocyte hemoglobin content to the CBC, in addition to the reticulocyte count and ferritin level, to assess the iron status in patients with chronic kidney disease.[64] Widespread use of the new parameters may be limited by the availability of instrumentation.

LIMITATIONS AND INTERFERENCES

Implementing automation in the hematology laboratory requires critical evaluation of the instrument's methods and limitations, and the performance goals for the individual laboratory. The Clinical and Laboratory Standards Institute (CLSI) has approved a standard for validation, verification, and quality assurance of automated hematology analyzers.[65] This standard provides guidelines for instrument calibration and assessment of performance criteria, including accuracy, precision, linearity, sensitivity, and specificity. The clinical accuracy (sensitivity and specificity) of the methods should be such that the instrument appropriately identifies patients who have disease and patients who do not have disease.[66] Quality control systems should reflect the laboratory's established performance goals and provide a high level of assurance that the instrument is working within its specified limits.

Calibration

Calibration is crucial in defining the accuracy of the data produced (Chapter 2). Calibration, or the process of electronically correcting an instrument for analytical bias (numerical difference from the "true" value), may be accomplished by appropriate use of reference methods, reference materials, or commercially prepared calibrators.[65] Because few instruments are precalibrated by the manufacturer, calibration must be performed at initial installation and verified at least every 6 months under the requirements of the Clinical Laboratory Improvement Act of 1988.[67] Periodic recalibration may be required after major instrument repair requiring optical alignment or part replacement.

Whole-blood calibration using fresh whole-blood specimens requires the use of reference methods, materials, and procedures to determine "true" values.[1,68,69] The International Committee for Standardization in Haematology has established guidelines for selecting a reference blood cell counter for this purpose,[1] but the cyanmethemoglobin method remains the only standard available in hematology for calibration and quality control.[70] Whole-blood calibration, which historically has been considered the preferred method for calibration of multichannel hematology analyzers, has been almost completely replaced by the use of commercial calibrators assayed using reference methods. Calibration bias is possible with the use of these calibrators because of inherent differences in stabilized

ADVIA 120

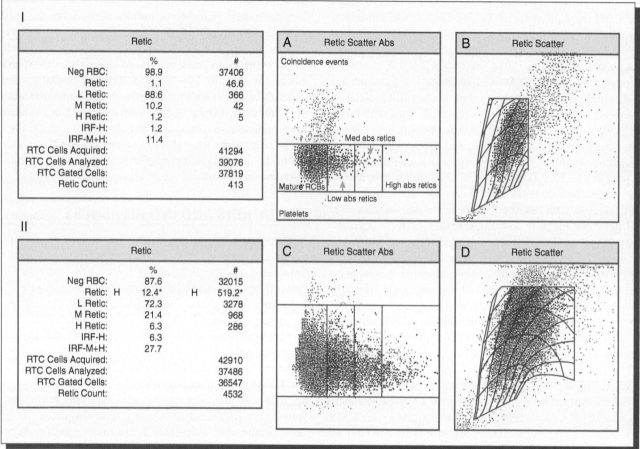

Figure 12.12 Composite Cytograms from the ADVIA 120. **(I)**, Normal reticulocyte count. **(II)**, High reticulocyte count with a large immature reticulocyte fraction (IRF). **(I-A and II-C)**, Reticulocyte scatter/absorption cytograms show high-angle (5- to 15-degree) scatter on the y-axis versus absorption on the x-axis, which allows separation of low-absorbing, medium-absorbing, and high-absorbing cells based on the amount of staining with nucleic acid-binding dye (oxazine 750). **(I-B and II-D)**, Reticulocyte scatter cytograms show low-angle (2- to 3-degree) scatter on the y-axis versus high-angle (5- to 15-degree) scatter on the x-axis (red blood cell [RBC] map). Because the RBCs are evaluated by the instrument on a cell-by-cell basis, unique reticulocyte indices can be derived.

and preserved cell suspensions.[71] It is essential that calibrations be carried out properly and verified by comparison with reference methods or review of quality control data after calibration and by external comparison studies such as proficiency testing.[1]

Instrument Limitations

The continual improvement of automated technologies has resulted in greater sensitivity and specificity of instrument flagging with detection of possible interferences in the data. The parallel improvement in instrument walk-away capabilities has increased the importance of the operator's awareness and understanding of instrument limitations, however, and of his or her ability to recognize factors that may interfere and cause erroneous laboratory results. Limitations and interferences may be related to methodology or to inherent problems in the blood specimen.

Each instrument has limitations related to methodology that are defined in instrument operation manuals and in the literature. A common limitation of impedance methods is an instrument's inability to distinguish cells reliably from other particles or cell fragments of the same volume. Cell fragments may be counted as platelets in specimens from chemotherapy-treated

patients with increased WBC fragility.[1] Likewise, schistocytes or small RBCs may interfere with the platelet count. Larger platelet clumps may be counted as WBCs, which results in a falsely decreased platelet count and potentially increases the WBC count. Micromegakaryocytes may be counted as nucleated RBCs or WBCs. RBCs containing variant hemoglobins such as Hb S or Hb C are often resistant to lysis, and the unlysed cells can be falsely counted as nucleated RBCs or WBCs and interfere in the hemoglobin reaction.[72] This phenomenon has become more apparent with the use of milder diluent and lysing reagents in the analyzers with automated WBC differential technology. Nonlysis also may be seen in specimens from patients with severe liver disease, those undergoing chemotherapy treatment, and neonates (because of increased levels of Hb F) on the older Sysmex instruments.[15] The ADVIA 2120 and 120 reports the WBC-BASO as the primary WBC count.[23] An extended lyse cycle may be used on the CELL-DYN 3500, and the newer instruments are able to provide a correct WBC impedance count when lyse-resistant RBCs are present.[21] The Sysmex SE-9000 and Sysmex SE-9500 also have an additional WBC impedance channel.[28]

Suppression of automated data, particularly WBC differential data, may occur when internal instrument checks fail or cast doubt on the validity of the data. Instruments from some manufacturers release results with specific error codes or flagging for further review. The suppression of automated differential data ensures that a manual differential count is performed, whereas the release of data with appropriate flagging mandates the need for careful review of the data and possibly a blood film examination. This suggests a difference in philosophy among the manufacturers and affects the work flow in different ways.[73] More importantly, each laboratory must establish its own criteria for directed blood film review based on established performance goals, instrument flagging, and inherent instrument limitations.

Specimen Limitations

Limitations resulting from inherent specimen problems include those related to the presence of cold agglutinins, icterus, and lipemia. Cold agglutinins manifest as a classic pattern of increased MCV (often greater than 130 fL), markedly decreased RBC count, and increased MCHC (often greater than 40 g/dL). Careful examination of the histograms or cytograms from the instruments may yield clues to this abnormality.[74] Icterus and lipemia directly affect hemoglobin measurements and related indices.[72] Table 12.2

TABLE 12.2	Conditions That Cause Interference on Most Hematology Analyzers			
Condition	Parameters Affected*	Rationale	Instrument Indicators	Corrective Action
Cold agglutinins	RBC ↓, MCV ↑, MCHC ↑, grainy appearance	Agglutination of RBCs	Dual RBC population on RBC map, or right shift on RBC histogram	Warm specimen to 37° C and rerun
Lipemia, icterus	HGB ↑, MCH ↑	↑ Turbidity affects spectrophotometric reading for HGB	HGB × 3 ≠ HCT ± 3, abnormal histogram/cytogram[†]	Plasma replacement[‡]
Hemolysis	RBC ↓, HCT↑	RBCs lysed and not counted	HGB × 3 ≠ HCT ± 3, may show lipemia pattern on histogram/cytogram	Request new specimen
Lysis-resistant RBCs with abnormal hemoglobins	WBC ↑, HGB ↑	RBCs with hemoglobin S, C, or F may fail to lyse; will be counted as WBCs	Interference at noise-WBC interface on histogram/cytogram	Perform manual dilutions, allow incubation time for lysis
Microcytes or schistocytes	RBC ↓, PLT↑	Volume of RBCs or RBC fragments less than lower RBC threshold, and/or within PLT threshold	Left shift on RBC histogram, MCV flagged if less than limits; abnormal PLT histogram may be flagged	Review blood film
Nucleated RBCs, megakaryocyte fragments, or micromegakaryoblasts	WBC ↑ (older instruments)	Nucleated RBCs or micromegakaryoblasts counted as WBCs	Nucleated RBC flag resulting from interference at noise-lymphocyte interface on histogram/cytogram	Newer instruments eliminate this error and count nucleated RBCs and correct the WBC count; count micromegakaryoblasts per 100 WBCs and correct
Platelet clumps	PLT ↓, WBC ↑	Large clumps counted as WBCs and not platelets	Platelet clumps/N flag, interference at noise-lymphocyte interface on histogram/cytogram	Redraw specimen in sodium citrate, multiply result by 1.1
WBC > 100,000/µL	HGB ↑, RBC ↑, HCT incorrect	↑ Turbidity affects spectrophotometric reading for HGB, WBCs counted with RBC count	HGB × 3 ≠ HCT ± 3, WBC count may be above linearity	Manual HCT; perform manual HGB (centrifuge/read supernatant)[‡], correct RBC count, recalculate indices; if above linearity, dilute for correct WBC count
Leukemia, especially with chemotherapy	WBC ↓, PLT ↑	Fragile WBCs, fragments counted as platelets	Platelet count inconsistent with previous results	Review film, perform phase platelet count or CD61 count
Old specimen	MCV ↑, MPV ↑, PLT ↓, automated differential may be incorrect	RBCs swell as specimen ages, platelets swell and degenerate, WBCs affected by prolonged exposure to EDTA	Abnormal clustering on WBC histogram/cytogram	Establish stability and specimen rejection criteria

↑, Increased; ↓, decreased; *EDTA,* ethylenediaminetetraacetic acid; *HGB,* hemoglobin; *HCT,* hematocrit; *MCH,* mean cell hemoglobin; *MCHC,* mean cell hemoglobin concentration; *MCV,* mean cell volume; *MPV,* mean platelet volume; *PLT,* platelet count; *RBC,* red blood cell (or count); *WBC,* white blood cell (or count).

*Manufacturer's labeling.

[†]Lipemia shows signature pattern on Siemens ADVIA 120 H cytograms.

[‡]HGB can be back-calculated from directly measured MCHC on Siemens ADVIA 120 cytograms.

summarizes conditions that cause interference on some hematology analyzers and offers suggestions for manually obtaining correct patient results. As instrumentation advances, instrumentation software can adjust or correct for some of the conditions listed. Historically a nucleated RBC flag required examination of a blood film to enumerate the nucleated RBCs and correct the WBC. All four major vendors offer online nucleated RBC enumeration and WBC correction, although the laboratory must validate the results. Lipemia interferes with the hemoglobin reading by falsely elevating the hemoglobin and associated indices. The Siemens technology uses direct measurement of the CHCM parameter, which allows back-calculation of the hemoglobin unaffected by lipemia and thus eliminates the need for the manual method of saline replacement in lipemic specimens. These two examples involving nucleated RBCs and lipemia illustrate instrument advances, and continued future improvements in technology will eliminate or decrease the need for manual intervention to obtain accurate results.

Specimen age and improper specimen handling can have profound effects on the reliability of hematology test results. These factors have even greater significance as hospitals move toward greater use of off-site testing by large reference laboratories. Specific problems with older specimens include increased WBC fragility, swelling and possible lysis of RBCs, and the deterioration of platelets.[15] Stability studies should be performed before an instrument is used, and specific guidelines should be established for specimen handling and rejection.

CLINICAL UTILITY OF AUTOMATED BLOOD CELL ANALYSIS

The use of automated hematology analyzers has directly affected the availability, accuracy, and clinical usefulness of the CBC and WBC differential count. Some parameters that are available on hematology analyzers, but cannot be derived manually, have provided further insight into various clinical conditions. The RDW, a quantitative estimate of erythrocyte anisocytosis, can be used with the MCV for initial classification of an anemia.[75,76] Although the classification scheme is not absolute, a low MCV with a high RDW suggests iron deficiency, whereas a high MCV and high RDW suggests a folate/vitamin B_{12} deficiency or myelodysplasia (Chapter 16). The immature reticulocyte fraction and the immature platelet fraction provide an early indication of engraftment success after hematopoietic stem cell transplant.[77] The reticulocyte hemoglobin content (CHr and Ret-He) provides an assessment of the iron available for hemoglobin synthesis. It is useful in the early diagnosis of iron deficiency and functional iron deficiency, as well as an early indicator of recovery after iron therapy.[62,63,78] The MPV may be useful in distinguishing thrombocytopenia caused by idiopathic thrombocytopenia purpura (high MPV), inherited macrothrombocytopenia (higher MPV), or bone marrow suppression (low MPV).[79,80] High MPV values are also associated with higher risk of acute myocardial infarction and mortality for individuals with cardiovascular disease and may have use in assessing a patient's risk of thrombosis.[80,81] However, the use of the MPV in these conditions has been hampered by the varying ability of instruments to accurately measure MPV in patients with macroplatelets (they are underestimated in impedance methods), the lack of standardization of MPV cutoff values in various conditions, and the lack of well-controlled prospective studies to prove clinical utility.[80] In addition to method variations, anticoagulation and storage time also influence the MPV, which further affects the reliability and clinical utility of MPV results.[82]

Automation of the WBC differential has had a significant impact on the laboratory work flow because of the labor-intensive nature of the manual differential count. The three-part differential available on earlier instruments generally proved suitable as a screening leukocyte differential count to identify specimens that required further workup or a manual differential count.[83-85] Partial differential counts, however, do not substitute for a complete differential count in populations with abnormalities.[86-88] The five-part or six-part automated differentials available on the larger instruments have been evaluated extensively and have acceptable clinical sensitivity and specificity for detection of distributional and morphologic abnormalities.[43,44, 89-95] Abnormal cells such as blasts and nucleated RBCs in low concentrations may not be detected by the instruments but likewise may be missed by the routine 100-cell manual/visual differential count.[94-97] The CELL-DYN Sapphire, with its added fluorescent detection technology, has been found to have high sensitivity and specificity for flagging nucleated RBCs and platelet clumps.[24,49,98] As technology continues to improve, blood film review to confirm the presence of platelet clumps or nucleated RBCs and to correct leukocyte counts for interference from platelet clumps or nucleated RBCs is becoming unnecessary, especially for nucleated RBCs, because the four major vendors now count and correct the WBC for nucleated RBCs on their high-end analyzers.[44,98,99]

Instrument evaluations based on the Clinical and Laboratory Standards Institute H20-A2 standard on reference leukocyte differential counting[100] using an 800-cell or 400-cell manual leukocyte differential count as the reference method have had acceptable correlation coefficients for all WBC types, with the possible exception of monocytes.[44,73,94,95,101-103] However, further studies using monoclonal antibodies as the reference method for counting monocytes suggest that automated analyzers yield a more accurate assessment of monocytosis than do manual methods.[104,105]

Histograms and cytograms, along with instrument flagging, provide valuable information in the diagnosis and treatment of RBC and WBC disorders. Multiple reports indicate the usefulness of histograms and cytograms in the characterization of various abnormal conditions, including RBC disorders such as cold agglutination and WBC diseases such as leukemias and myelodysplastic disorders.[32,74,94,95]

Manufacturers are developing integrated hematology workstations for the greatest automation and laboratory efficiency. The Beckman Coulter LH 1500 Automation Series is Beckman's solution to integrated hematology. The line can be customized to have two to four LH analyzers as well as SlideMakers and SlideStainers based on the laboratory's needs for efficiency and automation.[32] The Sysmex Total Hematology Automation

System (HST series) robotically links the SE-9000, R-3500 (automated reticulocyte analyzer), and SP-100 (automatic slide maker/stainer). The HST line links two XE-2100 units and one SP-100 instrument for complete automation or systemization of hematology testing. The SE-Alpha is a smaller version that links the SE-9000 and SP-100.[28] The Siemens ADVIA LabCell links the ADVIA 2120i to the track, and the Autoslide (automatic slide maker/stainer) links to the ADVIA 2120i. Finally, as a result of increasing customer needs, manufacturers have added body fluid counting to their high-end instrumentation. The Beckman Coulter UniCel DxH 800 system, the LH 780, and the Sysmex XN series and XE-5000 count WBCs and RBCs in body fluids; the ADVIA 2120i/120 counts WBCs and RBCs in body fluids and, in addition to cerebrospinal fluid WBC and RBC cell counts, performs a differential count on cerebrospinal fluid.[32,106,107] Selection of a hematology analyzer for an individual laboratory requires careful evaluation of the laboratory's needs and close scrutiny of several important instrument issues, including instrument specifications and system requirements, methods used, training requirements, maintenance needs, reagent usage, data management capabilities, staff response, and short-term and long-term expenditures.[108] All instruments claim to improve laboratory efficiency through increased automation that results in improved work flow and faster turnaround time or through the addition of new parameters that may have clinical efficacy. All four major vendors offer a slide maker/stainer that can be connected directly to their high-end analyzers. The slide makers/stainers can be programmed to make blood films for every specimen or to make films based on the laboratory's internal criteria for a film review. This reduces, but does not completely eliminate, the use of manual peripheral blood film review. Automated slide makers/stainers connect only to high-end analyzers and as such are not suitable for some laboratories. Each laboratory must assess its own efficiency needs to determine whether a slide maker and stainer is a value-added instrument to the laboratory.[109] The instrument selected should suit the workload and patient population and should have a positive effect on patient outcomes.[110] The instrument selected for a cancer center may be different from that chosen for a community hospital.[111] Ultimately, however, the instrument decision may be swayed by individual preferences.

SUMMARY

- Automated cell counting provides greater accuracy and precision compared with manual cell-counting methods.
- The primary principles of operation, electronic impedance, and optical scatter are used by most automated hematology analyzers. Radiofrequency (RF) is sometimes used in conjunction with electronic impedance.
- The electronic impedance method detects and measures changes in electrical resistance between two electrodes as cells pass through a sensing aperture. The measurable voltage changes are plotted on frequency distribution graphs, or histograms, that allow the evaluation of cell populations based on cell volume.
- RF resistance uses high-voltage electromagnetic current. Measurable changes in the RF signal are proportional to cell interior density, or conductivity. Impedance and conductivity can be plotted against each other on a two-dimensional distribution cytogram or scatterplot, which allows the evaluation of cell populations using cluster analysis.
- Optical scatter systems (flow cytometers) use detection of interference in a laser beam or light source to differentiate and enumerate cell types.
- Major manufacturers of hematology instrumentation include Beckman Coulter, Inc.; Sysmex Corporation; Abbott Diagnostics; and Siemens Healthcare Diagnostics, Inc. Table 12.1 summarizes the methods used for the hemogram, and reticulocyte, nucleated red blood cell, and white blood cell (WBC) differential counts in the newer instruments.
- Reticulocyte analysis has been incorporated into the primary cell-counting instruments of all major manufacturers. All use either fluorescent or other dyes that stain nucleic acid in reticulocytes before the cells are counted using fluorescence or absorbance and light scatter.
- Each instrument has limitations related to methodology that may result in instrument flagging of specific results or suppression of automated data. Likewise, inherent specimen problems may result in instrument flagging that indicates possible rejection of automated results.
- Automated hematology analyzers have had a significant impact on laboratory work flow, particularly automation of the WBC differential. In addition, newer parameters that can now be measured, such as the immature reticulocyte fraction (IRF) and the reticulocyte hemoglobin concentration (RET-He and CHr), have documented clinical utility.

Now that you have completed this chapter, go back and read again the case study at the beginning and respond to the questions presented.

REVIEW QUESTIONS

Answers can be found in the Appendix.

Examine the histograms/scatterplots obtained from four major instruments for the same patient specimen (Figure 12.13). Compare the results, and respond to questions 1 to 4 based on the results.

1. Which printout lets the end user know at a glance that the results are acceptable and no manual work needs to be performed?
   a. CELL-DYN Sapphire
   b. UniCel DxH 800
   c. ADVIA 2120i
   d. Sysmex XN-series

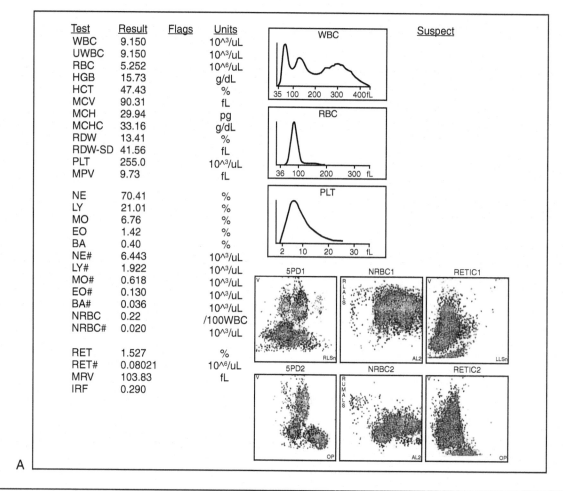

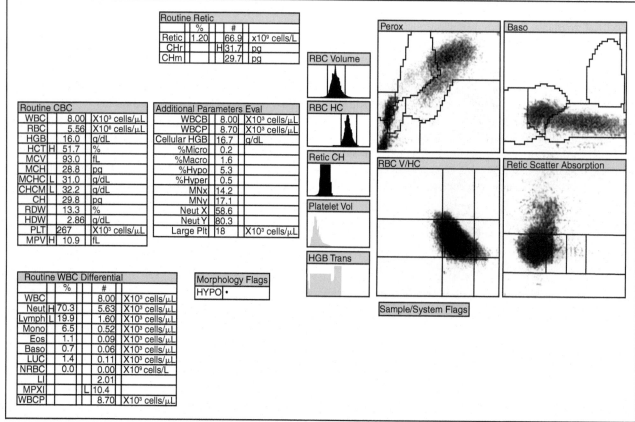

Figure 12.13 Composite Scatterplots/Histograms Obtained from Four Major Instrument Manufacturers. **(A),** Coulter UniCel DxH 800. **(B),** ADVIA 2120I.

Specimen comments:

Negative

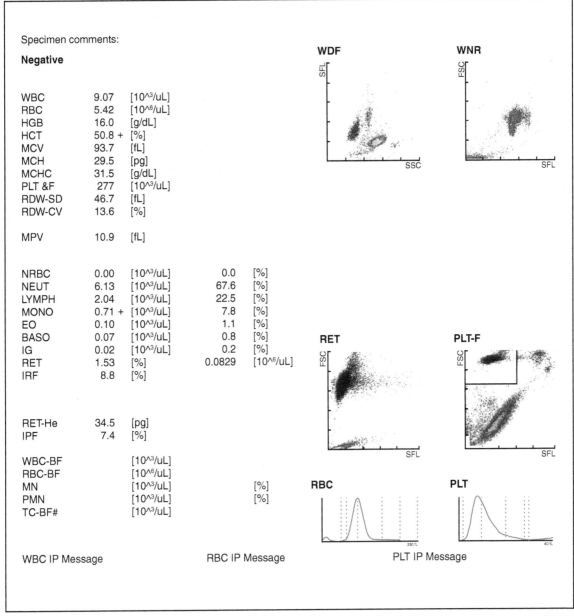

WBC	9.07	[10^3/uL]
RBC	5.42	[10^6/uL]
HGB	16.0	[g/dL]
HCT	50.8 +	[%]
MCV	93.7	[fL]
MCH	29.5	[pg]
MCHC	31.5	[g/dL]
PLT &F	277	[10^3/uL]
RDW-SD	46.7	[fL]
RDW-CV	13.6	[%]
MPV	10.9	[fL]

NRBC	0.00	[10^3/uL]	0.0	[%]
NEUT	6.13	[10^3/uL]	67.6	[%]
LYMPH	2.04	[10^3/uL]	22.5	[%]
MONO	0.71 +	[10^3/uL]	7.8	[%]
EO	0.10	[10^3/uL]	1.1	[%]
BASO	0.07	[10^3/uL]	0.8	[%]
IG	0.02	[10^3/uL]	0.2	[%]
RET	1.53	[%]	0.0829	[10^6/uL]
IRF	8.8	[%]		

RET-He	34.5	[pg]
IPF	7.4	[%]

WBC-BF		[10^3/uL]	
RBC-BF		[10^6/uL]	
MN		[10^3/uL]	[%]
PMN		[10^3/uL]	[%]
TC-BF#		[10^3/uL]	

WBC IP Message   RBC IP Message

PLT IP Message

C

Figure 12.13, cont'd (C), Sysmex XN-1000.   *Continued*

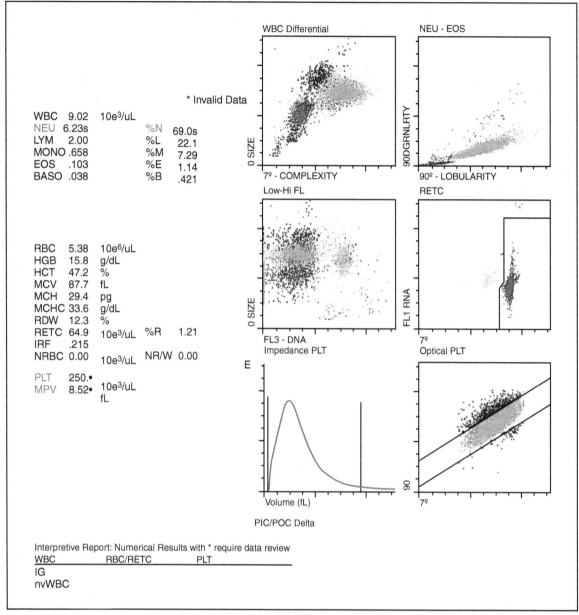

Figure 12.13, cont'd **(D)**, CELL-DYN Sapphire.

2. Which instrument printout has a system flag on the platelet count?
   a. CELL-DYN Sapphire
   b. UniCel DxH 800
   c. ADVIA 2120i
   d. XN-series

3. What do you suspect is the cause of the variation in platelet counting among the four instruments?
   a. Different instruments have different levels of sensitivity.
   b. All instruments use the same principle for counting platelets.
   c. Some instruments are susceptible to false-positive platelet flagging under certain conditions.
   d. Different instruments use different thresholds to capture and count platelets.

4. Based on the overall flagging for this specimen on each instrument, should a manual differential count be performed for this patient?
   a. Yes, because immature granulocytes are present in the specimen.
   b. Yes, because the WBC scatterplots are abnormal.
   c. No, because each differential count is complete with no system or morphology flags.

5. A patient peripheral blood film demonstrates agglutinated RBCs, and the CBC shows an elevated MCHC. What other parameters will be affected by the agglutination of the RBCs?
   a. MCV will be decreased and RBC count will be increased.
   b. MCV will be decreased and RBC count will be decreased.
   c. MCV will be increased and RBC count will be decreased.
   d. MCV will be increased and RBC count will be increased.

6. Match the cell-counting methods listed with the appropriate definition:

___ Impedance

___ RF

___ Optical scatter

a. Uses diffraction, reflection, and refraction of light waves

b. Uses high-voltage electrical waves to measure the internal complexity of cells

c. Involves detection and measurement of changes in electrical current between two electrodes

7. Low-voltage DC is used to measure:
   a. Cell nuclear volume
   b. Total cell volume
   c. Cellular complexity in the nucleus
   d. Cellular complexity in the cytoplasm

8. Orthogonal light scatter is used to measure:
   a. Cell volume
   b. Internal complexity of the cell
   c. Cellular granularity
   d. Nuclear density

9. On the Beckman Coulter instruments, hematocrit is a calculated value. Which of the following directly measured parameters is used in the calculation of this value?
   a. RDW
   b. Hemoglobin
   c. MCV
   d. MCHC

10. Match each instrument listed with the technology it uses to determine WBC differential counts.

___ Abbott CELL-DYN Sapphire

___ Siemens ADVIA 2120i

___ Sysmex XN-1000

___ Beckman Coulter UniCel DxH 800

a. Volume, conductivity, and five angles of light scatter

b. MAPSS technology and three-color fluorescence

c. Peroxidase-staining absorbance and light scatter

d. Detection of forward and side scattered light and fluorescence

REFERENCES

1. Koepke, J. A. (1991). Quantitative blood cell counting. In Koepke, J. A. (Ed.), *Practical Laboratory Hematology.* (pp. 43–60). New York: Churchill Livingstone.

2. Rappaport, E. S., Helbert, B., & Beissner, R. S. (1988). Automated hematology: where we stand. *South Med J, 81,* 365–370.

3. Dotson, M. A. (1998). Multiparameter hematology instruments. In Stiene-Martin, E. A., Lotspeich-Steininger, C. A., & Koepke, J. A. (Eds.), *Clinical Hematology: Principles, Procedures, Correlations.* (pp. 519–551). Philadelphia: Lippincott-Raven Publishers.

4. Coulter, W. H. (1956). High speed automatic blood cell counter and cell size analyzer. *Proc Natl Electron Conf, 12,* 1034.

5. Coulter Electronics. (1983). *Significant Advances in Hematology: Hematology Education Series,* PN 4206115 A. Hialeah, FL: Coulter Electronics.

6. Coulter Electronics. (1983). *Coulter Counter Model S-Plus IV with Three-Population Differential: Product Reference Manual,* PN 423560B. Hialeah, FL: Coulter Electronics.

7. Coulter Electronics. (1988). *Coulter STKR Product Reference Manual,* PN 4235547E. Hialeah, FL: Coulter Electronics.

8. TOA Medical Electronics Company. (1985). *Sysmex Model E-5000 Operator's Manual* (CN 461-2104-2). Kobe, Japan: TOA Medical Electronics Co.

9. Coulter Corporation. (1992). *Coulter STKS Operator's Guide,* PN 423592811. Hialeah, FL: Coulter Corporation.

10. Mohandas, N., Clark, M. R., Kissinger, S., et al. (1980). Inaccuracies associated with the automated measurement of mean cell hemoglobin concentration in dehydrated cells. *Blood, 56,* 125–128.

11. Arnfred, T., Kristensen, S. D., & Munck, V. (1981). Coulter counter model S and model S-plus measurements of mean erythrocyte volume (MCV) are influenced by the mean erythrocyte haemoglobin concentration (MCHC). *Scand J Clin Lab Invest, 41,* 717–721.

12. Johnson, K. L. (1992). Basics of flow cytometry. *Clin Lab Sci, 5,* 22–24.

13. Scott, R., Sethu, P., & Harnett, C. K. (2008). Three-dimensional hydrodynamic focusing in a microfluidic Coulter counter. *Rev Sci Instrum, 79,* 046104.

14. Rodriquez-Trujillo, R., Mills, C. A., Samitier, J., et al. (2007). Low cost micro-Coulter counter with hydrodynamic focusing. *Microfluid Nanofluid, 3,* 171–176.

15. TOA Medical Electronics Company. (1990). *Sysmex NE-8000 Operator's Manual* (CN 461-2326-5). Kobe, Japan: TOA Medical Electronics Co.

16. Sysmex Corporation. (1999). *Sysmex XE-2100 Operator's Manual.* Kobe, Japan: Sysmex Corp.

17. Sun, T. (2008). Principles of flow cytometry. In *Flow Cytometry and Immunohistochemistry for Hematologic Neoplasms.* (pp. 4–14). Philadelphia: Wolters Kluwer/Lippincott Williams & Wilkins.

18. Jovin, T. M., Morris, S. J., Striker, G., et al. (1976). Automatic sizing and separation of particles by ratios of light scattering intensities. *J Histochem Cytochem, 24,* 269–283.

19. Ryan, D. H. (2016). Chapter 2. Examination of blood cells. In Kaushanski, K., Lichtman, M. A., Prchal, J. T., et al. (Eds.), *Williams Hematology.* (9th ed., pp. 11–26). New York: McGraw-Hill.

20. Abbott Laboratories. (1993). *CELL-DYN 3000 System Operator's Manual* (LN 92420-92401). Abbott Park, IL: Abbott Laboratories.

21. Abbott Laboratories. (1996). *CELL-DYN 3500 System Operator's Manual* (LN 92722-92705). Abbott Park, IL: Abbott Laboratories.

22. Siemens Healthcare Diagnostics. (2009). *ADVIA 120 Operator's Guide,* V 3.01.00. Tarrytown, NY: Siemens Healthcare Diagnostics.

23. Siemens Healthcare Diagnostics. (2008). *ADVIA 2120/2120i Operator's Guide,* V4.00.00. Tarrytown, NY: Siemens Healthcare Diagnostics.

24. Abbott Diagnostics. *Diagnostic Products.* https://www.corelaboratory.abbott/us/en/offerings/category/hematology. Accessed October 26, 2018.

25. Horiba Medical. *ABX Hematology: the Product Line.* http://www.horiba.com/medical/products/hematology/. Accessed October 26, 2018.

26. Siemens Healthcare Diagnostics. *Laboratory Diagnostics.* https://usa.healthcare.siemens.com/hematology. Accessed October 26, 2018.

27. Beckman Coulter. *Hematology Systems.* https://www.beckmancoulter.com/wsrportal/wsr/diagnostics/clinical-products/hematology/index.htm. Accessed October 26, 2018.

28. Sysmex Corporation. *Hematology Products.* https://www.sysmex.com/US/en/Products/Hematology/Pages/Sysmex-Hematology-Overview.aspx. Accessed October 26, 2018.

29. Beckman Coulter. *UniCel DxH 800 Coulter Cellular Analysis System. UniCel DxH 800 wsrportal Coulter Cellular Analysis System.* https://www.beckmancoulter.com/wsrportal/wsr/diagnostics/clinical-products/hematology/unicel-dxh-800-coulter-cellular-analysis-system/index.htm. Accessed October 26, 2018.

30. Beckman Coulter. *UniCel DxH 800 Coulter Cellular Analysis System. Automated Intelligent Morphology.* https://www.beckmancoulter.com/en/learning-and-events/webinars/hematology-webinars/automated-intelligent-morphology-in-the-dxh-800-cellular-analysis-system. Accessed October 26, 2018.

31. Barnes, P. W., McFadden, S. L., Machin, S. J., et al. (2005). The international consensus group for hematology review: suggested criteria for action following automated CBC and WBC differential analysis. *Lab Hematol, 11,* 83–90.

32. CAP Today. (2017, November). *Hematology Analyzers.* Vol 31 (11), 62–73. http://www.captodayonline.com/productguides/instruments/hematology-analyzers-november-2017.html. Accessed October 26, 2018.

33. Beckman Coulter. (2003). *Coulter LH 700 Series Operator's Guide.* Fullerton, CA: Beckman Coulter.

34. Schoorl, M., Schoorl, M., Oomes, J., et al. (2013). New fluorescent method (PLT-F) on Sysmex XN 2000 Hematology Analyzers achieved higher accuracy in low platelet counting. *Am J Clin Pathol, 140,* 495–499.

35. Sysmex. *XP 300 Automated Hematology Diagnostics.* https://www.sysmex.com/US/en/Products/Hematology/Pages/Sysmex-Hematology-Overview.aspx. Accessed October 26, 2018.

36. Sysmex. *XN Series Automated Hematology Systems.* https://www.sysmex.com/us/en/Products/Hematology/XNSeries/Pages/XN-L-Automated-Hematology-Analyzer.aspx. Accessed October 26, 2018.

37. Sysmex. *Reshaping scalable automation. XN-9100 Automated Hematology Systems.* https://www.sysmex.com/us/en/Brochures/XN9100ScalableAutomationBrochure_mkt-10-1177_10252017.pdf. Accessed October 26, 2018.

38. Abe, Y., Wada, H., Tomatsu, H., et al. (2006). A simple technique to determine thrombopoiesis level using immature platelet fraction (IPF). *Thromb Res, 118,* 463–469.

39. Sysmex-Europe. *The microcytic (MICROR) and macrocytic (MACROR) red blood cell populations.* https://www.sysmex-europe.com/academy/knowledge-centre/sysmex-parameters/micrormacror.html. Accessed October 26, 2018.

40. Sysmex-Europe. *Percentage of hypo-haemoglobinsed red cells (HYPO-HE) and hyper-haemoglobinised red cells (HYPER-HE).* https://www.sysmex-europe.com/academy/knowledge-centre/sysmex-parameters/hypo-hehyper-he.html. Accessed October 26, 2018.

41. Abbott Diagnostics. *CELL-DYN Sapphire.* https://www.corelaboratory.abbott/us/en/offerings/brands/cell-dyn/cell-dyn-sapphire. Accessed October 26, 2018.

42. Matzdorff, A. C., Kühnel, G., Scott, S., et al. (1998). Comparison of flow cytometry and the automated blood analyzer system CELL-DYN 4000 for platelet analysis. *Lab Hematol, 4,* 163–168.

43. Bowden, K. L., Procopio, N., Wystepek, E., et al. (1998). Platelet clumps, nucleated red cells, and leukocyte counts: a comparison between the Abbott CELL-DYN 4000 and Coulter STKS. *Lab Hematol, 4,* 7–16.

44. Jones, R. G., Faust, A., Glazier, J., et al. (1998). CELL-DYN 4000: utility within the core laboratory structure and preliminary comparison of its expanded differential with the 400-cell manual differential count. *Lab Hematol, 4,* 34–44.

45. Abbott Diagnostics. (1992). *CELL-DYN Rainbow Classification Program,* PN 97-9427/R3-20. Abbott Park, IL: Abbott Diagnostics.

46. Abbott Laboratories. (1999). *CELL-DYN 3500 System Operator's Manual: Reticulocyte Package,* 9140293D. Abbott Park, IL: Abbott Laboratories.

47. Abbott Laboratories. (1997). *CELL-DYN 4000 Operator's Manual,* Santa Clara, CA: Abbott Laboratories.

48. Bayer Healthcare. (2005). *Bayer ADVIA 2120 Operator's Guide.* Tarrytown, NY: Bayer Healthcare.

49. Mohandas, N., Kim, Y. R., Tycko, D. H., et al. (1986). Accurate and independent measurement of volume and hemoglobin concentration of individual red cells by laser light scattering. *Blood, 68,* 506–513.

50. Harris, N., Jou, J. M., Devoto, G., et al. (2005). Performance evaluation of the ADVIA 2120 hematology analyzer: an international multicenter clinical trial. *Lab Hematol, 11,* 62–70.

51. Koepke, J. (1993). Current limitations in reticulocyte counting: implications for clinical laboratories. In Portsmann, B. (Ed.), *The Emerging Importance of Accurate Reticulocyte Counting.* (pp. 18–22). New York: Caduceus Medical.

52. Clinical and Laboratory Standards Institute. (2004). *Methods for Reticulocyte Counting (Flow Cytometry and Supravital Dyes).* (2nd ed., CLSI approved guideline, H44-A2). Wayne, PA: Clinical and Laboratory Standards Institute.

53. College of American Pathologists. (1993). *CAP Surveys: Reticulocyte (Pilot) Survey Set RT-A,* Northfield, IL: College of American Pathologists.

54. College of American Pathologists. (2000). *CAP Surveys: Reticulocyte Survey Set RT/RT2-A,* Northfield, IL: College of American Pathologists.

55. Coulter Corporation. (1993). *Introducing a New Reticulocyte Methodology using Coulter VCS Technology on Coulter STKS and MAXM Hematology Systems,* product brochure TC93003201. Miami, FL: Coulter Corp.

56. Sysmex America. (2009) *DaVita Study Demonstrates Clinical Application of Sysmex Reticulocyte Hemoglobin Equivalent (RET-He) Parameter.* https://www.sysmex.com/us/en/Company/News/Pages/DaVita-Study-Demonstrates-Clinical-Application-of-Sysmex-Reticulocyte-Hemoglobin-Equivalent-(RET-He)-Parameter.aspx. Accessed October 26, 2018.

57. TOA Medical Electronics Company. (1991). *Sysmex R-3000 Automated Reticulocyte Analyzer,* SP-9620. Los Alamitos, CA: TOA Medical Electronics Co.

58. Davis, B. H., Bigelow, N. C., van Hove, L., et al. (1998). Evaluation of automated reticulocyte analysis with immature reticulocyte fraction as a potential outcomes indicator of anemia in chronic renal failure patients. *Lab Hematol, 4,* 169–175.

59. Buttarello, M., & Plebani, M. (2008). Automated blood cell counts. *Am J Clin Pathol, 130,* 104–116.

60. Fourcade, C., Jary, L., & Belaouni, H. (1999). Reticulocyte analysis provided by the Coulter GEN-S: significance and interpretation in

regenerative and non-regenerative hematologic conditions. *Lab Hematol, 5,* 153–158.

61. Davis, B. H., & Bigelow, N. C. (1994). Automated reticulocyte analysis: clinical practice and associated new parameters. *Hematol Oncol Clin North Am, 8,* 617–630.

62. Brugnara, C., Zurakowski, D., DiCanzio, J., et al. (1999). Reticulocyte hemoglobin content to diagnose iron deficiency in children. *JAMA, 281,* 2225–2230.

63. Ullrich, C., Wu, A., Armbsy, C., et al. (2005). Screening healthy infants for iron deficiency using reticulocyte hemoglobin content. *JAMA, 294,* 924–930.

64. National Kidney Foundation. (2006). KDOQI Clinical practice guidelines and clinical practice recommendations for anemia in chronic kidney disease. *Evaluation of Anemia in CKD.* http://kdigo.org/wp-content/uploads/2016/10/KDIGO-2012-Anemia-Guideline-English.pdf. Accessed October 26, 2018.

65. CLSI. (2010). *Validation, Verificatiton, and Quality Assurance of Automated Hematology Analyzers.* (Approved standard, H26). Wayne, PA: Clinical and Laboratory Standards Institute.

66. CLSI. (2011). *Assessment of the Diagnostic Accuracy of Laboratory Tests using Receiver Operating Characteristic Curves.* (2nd ed., CLSI approved guideline, EP24). Wayne, PA: Clinical and Laboratory Standards Institute.

67. Calibration and calibration verification. *Clinical Laboratory Improvement Amendments Brochure No. 3.* https://www.cms.gov/Regulations-and-Guidance/Legislation/CLIA/Downloads/6065bk.pdf. Accessed October 26, 2018.

68. Gilmer, P. R., Williams, U., Koepke, J. A., et al. (1977). Calibration methods for automated hematology instruments. *Am J Clin Pathol, 68,* 185–190.

69. Koepke, J. A. (1977). The calibration of automated instruments for accuracy in hemoglobinometry. *Am J Clin Pathol, 68,* 180–184.

70. International Council for Standardization in Haematology. (1996). Recommendations for reference method for haemoglobinometry in human blood (ICSH Standard 1995) and specifications for international haemiglobincyanide standard. (4th ed.). *J Clin Pathol, 49,* 271–274.

71. Savage, R. A. (1985). Calibration bias and imprecision for automated hematology analyzers: an evaluation of the significance of short-term bias resulting from calibration of an analyzer with S Cal. *Am J Clin Pathol, 84,* 186–190.

72. Cornbleet, J. (1983). Spurious results from automated hematology cell counters. *Lab Med 14,* 509–514.

73. Bentley, S. A., Johnson, A., & Bishop, C. A. (1993). A parallel evaluation of four automated hematology analyzers. *Am J Clin Pathol, 100,* 626–632.

74. Strobel, S. L., Panke, T. W., & Bills, G. L. (1993). Cold erythrocyte agglutination and infectious mononucleosis. *Lab Med, 24,* 219–221.

75. Bessman, J. D., Gilmer, P. R., & Gardner, F. H. (1983). Improved classification of anemia by MCV and RDW. *Am J Clin Pathol, 80,* 322–326.

76. Marks, P. W. (2013). Approach to anemia in the adult and child. In Hoffman, R., Benz E. J. Jr, Silberstein, L. E., et al. (Eds.), *Hematology: Basic Principles and Practice.* (6th ed., pp. 418–426). Philadelphia: Elsevier, Saunders.

77. Gonçalo, A. P., Barbosa, I. L., Campilho, F., et al. (2011). Predictive value of immature reticulocyte and platelet fractions in hematopoietic recovery of allograft patients. *Transplant Proc, 43,* 241–243.

78. Brugnara, C., Schiller, B., & Moran, J. (2006). Reticulocyte hemoglobin equivalent (Ret He) and assessment of iron deficient states. *Clin Lab Haem, 29,* 303–306.

79. Noris, P., Klersy, C., & Gresele, P. (2013). Platelet size for distinguishing between inherited thrombocytopenias and immune thrombocytopenia: a multicentric, real life study. *Br J Haematol, 162,* 112–119.

80. Leader, A., Pereg, D., & Lishner, M. (2012). Are platelet volume indices of clinical use? A multidisciplinary review. *Ann Med, 44,* 805–816.

81. Chu, S. G., Becker, R. C., & Berger, P. B. (2010). Mean platelet volume as a predictor of cardiovascular risk: a systematic review and meta-analysis. *J Thromb Haemost, 8,* 148–156.

82. Reardon, D. M., Hutchinson, D., Preston, F. E., et al. (1985). The routine measurement of platelet volume: a comparison of aperture-impedance and flow cytometric systems. *Clin Lab Haematol, 7,* 251–257.

83. Allen, J. K., & Batjer, I. D. (1985). Evaluation of an automated method for leukocyte differential counts based on electronic volume analysis. *Arch Pathol Lab Med, 109,* 534–539.

84. Pierre, R. V., Payne, B. A., Lee, W. K., et al. (1987). Comparison of four leukocyte differential methods with the National Committee for Clinical Laboratory Standards (NCCLS) reference method. *Am J Clin Pathol, 87,* 201–209.

85. Payne, B. A., Pierre, R. V., & Lee, W. K. (1987). Evaluation of the TOA E-5000 automated hematology analyzer. *Am J Clin Pathol, 88,* 51–57.

86. Ross, D. W., Watson, J. S., Davis, P. H., et al. (1985). Evaluation of the Coulter three-part differential screen. *Am J Clin Pathol, 84,* 481–484.

87. Cornbleet, J., & Kessinger, S. (1985). Evaluation of Coulter S-Plus three-part differential in a population with a high prevalence of abnormalities. *Am J Clin Pathol, 84,* 620–626.

88. Miers, M. K., Fogo, A. B., Federspiel, C. F., et al. (1987). Evaluation of the Coulter S-Plus IV differential as a screening tool in a tertiary care hospital. *Am J Clin Pathol, 87,* 745–751.

89. Warner, B. A., & Reardon, D. M. (1991). A field evaluation of the Coulter STKS. *Am J Clin Pathol, 95,* 207–217.

90. Hallawell, R., O'Malley, C., Hussein, S., et al. (1991). An evaluation of the Sysmex NE-8000 hematology analyzer. *Am J Clin Pathol, 96,* 594–601.

91. Cornbleet, P. J., Myrick, D., Judkins, S., et al. (1992). Evaluation of the CELL-DYN 3000 differential. *Am J Clin Pathol, 98,* 603–614.

92. Cornbleet, P. J., Myrick, D., & Levy, R. (1993). Evaluation of the Coulter STKS five-part differential. *Am J Clin Pathol, 99,* 72–81.

93. Brigden, M. L., Page, N. E., & Graydon, C. (1993). Evaluation of the Sysmex NE-8000 automated hematology analyzer in a high-volume outpatient laboratory. *Am J Clin Pathol, 100,* 618–625.

94. Meintker, L., Ringwald, J., Rauh, M., et al. (2013). Comparison of automated differential blood cell counts from Abbott Sapphire, Siemens Advia 120, Beckman Coulter DxH 800, and Sysmex XE-2100 in normal and pathologic samples. *Am J Clin Pathol, 139,* 641–650.

95. Hotton, J., Broothaers, J., Swaelens, C., et al. (2013). Performance and abnormal cell flagging comparisons of three automated blood cell counters: Cell-Dyn Sapphire, DxH-800, and XN-2000. *Am J Clin Pathol, 140,* 845–852.

96. Rumke, C. L. (1978). The statistically expected variability in differential leukocyte counting. In Koepke, J. A. (Ed.), *Differential Leukocyte Counting,* Skokie (Ill): College of American Pathologists.

97. Koepke, J. A., Dotson, M. A., & Shifman, M. A. (1985). A critical evaluation of the manual/visual differential leukocyte counting method. *Blood Cells, 11,* 173–181.

98. Paterakis, G., Kossivas, L., Kendall, R., et al. (1998). Comparative evaluation of the erythroblast count generated by three-color fluorescence flow cytometry, the Abbott CELL-DYN 4000 hematology analyzer, and microscopy. *Lab Hematol, 4,* 64–70.

99. Bowen, K. L., Glazier, J., & Mattson, J. C. (1998). Abbott CELL-DYN 4000 automated red blood cell analysis compared with routine red blood cell morphology by smear review. *Lab Hematol, 4,* 45–47.

100. CLSI. (2007). *Reference Leukocyte (WBC) Differential Count (Proportional) and Evaluation of Instrumental Methods: Approved Standard.* (2nd ed.). CLSI document H20-A2, Wayne, PA: Clinical Laboratory and Standards Institute.

101. Warner, B. A., Reardon, D. M., & Marshall, D. P. (1990). Automated haematology analysers: a four-way comparison. *Med Lab Sci, 47,* 285–296.

102. Swaim, W. R. (1991). Laboratory and clinical evaluation of white blood cell differential counts: comparison of the Coulter VCS, Technicon H-1, and 800-cell manual method. *Am J Clin Pathol, 95,* 381–388.

103. Buttarello, M., Gadotti, M., Lorenz, C., et al. (1992). Evaluation of four automated hematology analyzers: a comparative study of differential counts (imprecision and inaccuracy). *Am J Clin Pathol, 97,* 345–352.

104. Goossens, W., Hove, L. V., & Verwilghen, R. L. (1991). Monocyte counting: discrepancies in results obtained with different automated instruments. *J Clin Pathol, 44,* 224–227.

105. Seaberg, R., & Cuomo, J. (1993). Assessment of monocyte counts derived from automated instrumentation. *Lab Med, 24,* 222–224.

106. Harris, N., Kunicka, J., & Kratz, A. (2005). The ADVIA 2120 hematology system: flow cytometry-based analysis of blood and body fluids in the routine hematology laboratory. *Lab Hematol, 11,* 47–61.

107. de Jonge, R., Brouwer, R., de Graaf, M. T., et al. (2010). Evaluation of the new body fluid mode on the Sysmex XE-5000 for counting leukocytes and erythrocytes in cerebrospinal fluid and other body fluids. *Clin Chem Lab Med, 48,* 665–675.

108. Camden, T. L. (1993). How to select the ideal hematology analyzer. *MLO Med Lab Obs, 25,* 29–33.

109. Dabkowski B. (2012, December). New fixes, configurations in automation solutions. CAP TODAY. http://www.captodayonline.com/Archives/1212/1212g_in_hematology.html. Accessed October 26, 2018.

110. van Hove, L. (1998). Guest editorial: which hematology analyzer do you need? *Lab Hematol 4,* 32–33.

111. Albitar, M., Dong, Q., Saunder, D., et al. (1999). Evaluation of automated leukocyte differential counts in a cancer center. *Lab Hematol, 5,* 10–14.

Examination of the Peripheral Blood Film and Correlation With the Complete Blood Count

Carolina Vilchez*

OBJECTIVES

After completion of this chapter, the reader will be able to:

1. List the specimen sources and collection processes that are acceptable for blood film preparation.
2. Describe the techniques for making peripheral blood films.
3. Describe the appearance of a well-prepared peripheral blood film, recognize a description of a slide that is consistent or inconsistent with that appearance, and troubleshoot problems with poorly prepared films.
4. Explain the principle, purpose, and basic method of Wright staining of blood films.
5. Identify and troubleshoot problems that cause poorly stained blood films.
6. Describe the proper examination of a peripheral blood film, including selection of the correct area, sequence of examination, and observations to be made at each magnification. Recognize deviations from this protocol.
7. Given the number of cells observed per field and the magnification of the objective, apply formulas to estimate white blood cell (WBC) and platelet counts.
8. Explain the effect that platelet satellitosis and clumping may have on automated complete blood count (CBC) results. Recognize examples of results that would be consistent with these effects.
9. Follow the appropriate course of action to recognize and correct ethylenediaminetetraacetic acid-induced pseudo-thrombocytopenia and pseudoleukocytosis.
10. Implement a systematic approach to interpretation of CBC data that results in a verbal summary of the numerical data and communicates the blood picture succinctly.
11. Calculate absolute WBC differential counts.

OUTLINE

Peripheral Blood Films
Specimen Collection
Peripheral Film Preparation
Staining of Peripheral Blood Films
Peripheral Film Examination
Summarizing Complete Blood Count Results
Organization of Complete Blood Count Results

Assessing Hematology Results Relative to Reference Intervals
Summarizing White Blood Cell Parameters
Summarizing Red Blood Cell Parameters
Summarizing Platelet Parameters

CASE STUDY

After studying the material in this chapter, the reader should be able to respond to the following case study:

A healthy-looking 56-year old man had an automated CBC performed as part of a preoperative evaluation. The results are as follows:

WBC	15.8×10^9/L
RBC	4.93×10^{12}/L
HGB	14.8 g/dL
HCT	45.1%
MCV	91.5 fL
MCH	30 pg
MCHC	32.8 g/dL
RDW	14.2%
PLT	34×10^9/L
MPV	6.6 fL

The peripheral blood film was examined and the only abnormal finding was platelet clumps.

1. Comparing the patient's results with the reference intervals on the front cover, describe the blood picture succinctly, using proper terminology for red blood cells, white blood cells, and platelets.
2. What automated results should be questioned?
3. What is the best course of action to handle this problem?

---

*The author extends appreciation to Lynn B. Maedel and Kathryn Doig, whose work in prior editions provided the foundation for this chapter.

A well-made, well-stained, and carefully examined peripheral blood film can provide valuable information regarding a patient's health. More can be learned from this test than from many other routinely performed hematologic tests. White blood cell (WBC) and platelet count estimates can be achieved, relative proportions of the different types of WBCs can be obtained, and the morphology of all three cell lines can be evaluated for abnormalities. Although routine work is now handled by the sophisticated automated instruments found in most hematology laboratories, skilled and talented laboratory professionals are essential to the reporting of reliable test results. Accurate peripheral film evaluation is quite likely to be needed for some time.

The peripheral film evaluation is the capstone of a panel of tests called the *complete blood count* (CBC) or *hemogram.* The CBC includes enumeration of cellular elements, quantitation of hemoglobin, and statistical analyses that provide a snapshot of cell appearances. These results can be derived using the manual methods and calculations described in Chapter 11 or using the automated instruments described in Chapter 12. Regardless of method, the numerical values should be consistent with the assessment derived by examining the cells microscopically. Careful examination of data in a systematic way ensures that all relevant results are noted and taken into consideration in the diagnosis.

This chapter begins with a discussion of the preparation and assessment of the blood film, followed by a systematic approach to review the CBC, including blood film evaluation. Such an evaluation can be applied in the hematology chapters that follow.

PERIPHERAL BLOOD FILMS

Specimen Collection

Sources of Specimens

Essentially all specimens received for routine testing in the hematology section of the laboratory have been collected in lavender (purple)–topped tubes. These tubes contain disodium or tripotassium ethylenediaminetetraacetic acid (EDTA), which anticoagulates the blood by chelating the calcium that is essential for coagulation. Liquid tripotassium EDTA is often preferred to the powdered form because it mixes more easily with blood. High-quality blood films can be made from the blood in the EDTA tube, provided that they are made within 4 hours of drawing the specimen.[1] Blood films from EDTA tubes that remain at room temperature for more than 5 hours often have unacceptable blood cell artifacts (echinocytic red blood cells [RBCs], spherocytes, necrobiotic leukocytes, and vacuolated neutrophils). Vacuolization of monocytes normally occurs almost immediately with EDTA but causes no evaluation problems.

The main advantages of making films from blood in the EDTA tube are that multiple slides can be made if necessary and they do not have to be prepared immediately after the blood is drawn. In addition, EDTA generally prevents platelets from clumping on the glass slide, which makes the platelet estimate more accurate during film evaluation. There are purists, however, who believe that anticoagulant-free blood is still the specimen of choice for evaluation of blood cell morphology.[2] Although some artifacts can be avoided in this way, specimens made from unanticoagulated blood pose other problems.

Under certain conditions, use of a different anticoagulant or no anticoagulant may be helpful. Some patients' blood undergoes an in vitro phenomenon called *platelet satellitosis*[3] when anticoagulated with EDTA. The platelets surround or adhere to neutrophils, which potentially causes pseudothrombocytopenia when counting is done by automated methods (Figure 13.1).[3,4] In addition, spuriously low platelet counts and falsely increased WBC counts (pseudoleukocytosis) can result from EDTA-induced platelet clumping.[5] Pseudoleukocytosis occurs when platelet agglutinates are similar in size to WBCs and automated analyzers cannot distinguish the two. The platelet clumps are counted as WBCs instead of platelets. Platelet-specific autoantibodies that react best at room temperature are one of the mechanisms known to cause this phenomenon.[6] In these circumstances the examination of a blood film becomes an important quality control strategy, identifying these phenomena so that they can be corrected before the results are reported to the patient's chart or health care provider.

Problems such as these can be eliminated by recollecting specimens in sodium citrate tubes (light blue top) and ensuring that the proper ratio of nine parts blood to one part anticoagulant is observed (a properly filled tube). These new specimens can be analyzed in the usual way by automated instruments; however, platelet counts and WBC counts from sodium citrate specimens must be corrected for the dilution of blood with the anticoagulant. In a full-draw specimen the blood is nine-tenths of the total tube volume (2.7 mL of blood and 0.3 mL of sodium citrate). The "dilution factor" is the reciprocal of the dilution (i.e., 10/9 or 1.1). The WBC and platelet counts are multiplied by 1.1 to obtain accurate counts. All other CBC parameters should be reported from the original EDTA tube specimen and slide.

Another source of blood for films is from finger and heel punctures. In general, the films are made immediately at the patient's side. There are, however, a few limitations to this procedure. First, some platelet clumping must be expected if films are made directly from a drop of finger-stick or heel-stick blood or if blood is collected in heparinized microhematocrit tubes. Generally this clumping is not enough to interfere with platelet estimates if the films are made promptly before clotting begins

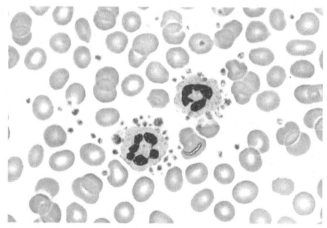

Figure 13.1 Platelet Satellitosis. (Peripheral blood, Wright-Giemsa stain, ×1000.)

in earnest. Second, only a few films can be made directly from blood from a skin puncture before the site stops bleeding. If slides are made quickly and correctly, however, cell distribution and morphology should be adequate. These problems with finger and heel sticks can be eliminated with the use of EDTA microcollection tubes, such as Microtainer tubes (Becton, Dickinson).

Peripheral Film Preparation
Types of Films

Manual wedge technique. The wedge film technique is probably the easiest to master. It is the most convenient and most commonly used method for making peripheral blood films. This technique requires at least two 3-inch × 1-inch (75-mm × 25-mm) clean glass slides. High-quality, beveled-edge microscopic slides with chamfered (beveled) corners for good lateral borders are recommended. A few more slides may be kept handy in case a good-quality film is not made immediately. One slide serves as the film slide, and the other is the pusher or spreader slide. They can then be reversed. It is also possible to make good wedge films by using a hemacytometer coverslip attached to a handle (pinch clip or tongue depressor) as the spreader.

A drop of blood (about 2 to 3 mm in diameter) from a finger, heel, or microhematocrit tube (nonheparinized for EDTA-anticoagulated blood or heparinized for capillary blood) is placed at one end of the slide. The drop also may be delivered using a Diff-Safe dispenser (Alpha Scientific). The Diff-Safe dispenser is inserted through the rubber stopper of the EDTA tube, which eliminates the need to remove it.[7] The size of the drop of blood is important; too large a drop creates a long or thick film, and too small a drop often makes a short or thin blood film. The pusher slide, held securely in the dominant hand at about a 30- to 45-degree angle (Figure 13.2A), is drawn back into the drop of blood, and the blood is allowed to spread across the width of the slide (Figure 13.2B). It is then quickly and smoothly pushed forward to the end of the slide to create a wedge film (Figure 13.2C). It is important that the entire drop be picked up and spread. Moving the pusher slide forward too slowly accentuates poor leukocyte distribution by pushing larger cells, such as monocytes and granulocytes, to the very end and sides of the film. Maintaining an even, gentle pressure on the slide is essential. It is also crucial to keep the same angle all the way to the end of the film. When the hematocrit is higher than normal (i.e., >60%), as is found in patients with polycythemia or in newborns, the angle should be lowered (i.e., 25 degrees) so the film is not too short and thick. For extremely low hematocrits, the angle may need to be raised. If two or three films are made, the best one is selected for staining and the others are disposed of properly. Some laboratories require two good films and save one unstained in case another slide is required.

The procedure just described is for a push-type wedge preparation. It is called *push* because the spreader slide is pulled into the drop of blood, and the film is made by pushing the blood along the slide. The same procedure can be modified to produce a *pulled* film. In this procedure, the spreader

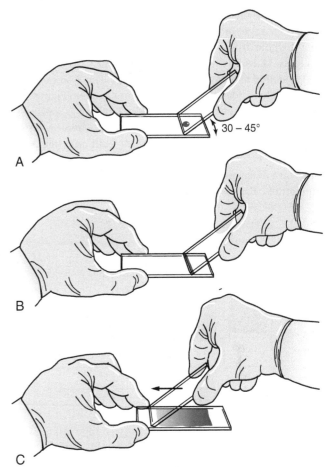

Figure 13.2 Wedge Technique of Making a Peripheral Blood Film. **(A–C.)**

slide is pushed into the drop of blood and pulled along the length of the slide to make the film. Although this method is much less commonly used, it also provides a satisfactory wedge preparation and may be easier for some individuals to perform. Other variations on the wedge technique include using the 3-inch side of the slide as the spreader slide or balancing the spreader slide on the fingers to avoid placing too much pressure on it. Learning to make consistently good blood films takes practice.

Features of a Well-Made Wedge Peripheral Blood Film

1. The film is two-thirds to three-fourths the length of the slide (Figure 13.3).
2. The film is finger shaped, very slightly rounded at the feather edge, not bullet shaped; this provides the widest area for examination.
3. The lateral edges of the film are visible.
4. The film is smooth without irregularities, holes, or streaks.

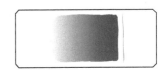

Figure 13.3 Well-made Peripheral Blood Film.

5. When the slide is held up to the light, the thin portion (feather edge) of the film has a "rainbow" appearance.
6. The whole drop of blood is picked up and spread.

Figure 13.4A-H shows unacceptable films.

Automated slide making and staining. The Sysmex SP-10 is an automated slide-making and staining system (Figure 13.5). After the instrument has performed a CBC for a specimen, a conveyor moves the racked tube to the SP-10, where its bar code is read. User-definable, onboard rules built into the system determine whether a slide is required. Criteria for a manual slide review are determined by each laboratory based on its patient population. Based on the hematocrit reading, the system adjusts the size of the drop of blood used and the angle and speed of the spreader slide in making a wedge preparation. After each blood film is prepared, the spreader slide is automatically cleaned and is ready for the next blood film to be made. Films can be produced approximately every 30 seconds. Patient identification information, such as name, number, and date for the specimen, is printed on the slide. The slide is dried, loaded into a cassette, and moved to the staining position. Based on the laboratory's desired stain protocol, stain, then buffer and rinse are added at designated times. When staining is complete, the slide is moved to a dry position, followed by a collection area where it can be picked up for microscopic evaluation. Films made offline, such as bone marrow smears and cytospin preparations, may be stained using this system as well. Other blood analyzer manufacturers, such as Beckman Coulter also have automated slide-making and staining instruments.

Drying of Films

Regardless of film preparation method, before staining, all blood films and bone marrow smears should be dried as quickly as possible to avoid drying artifact. In some laboratories a small fan is used to facilitate drying. Blowing breath on a slide is counterproductive because the moisture in breath causes RBCs to become echinocytic (crenated) or to develop water artifact (also called *drying artifact*).

Staining of Peripheral Blood Films

Pure Wright stain or a Wright-Giemsa stain (Romanowsky stain)[8] is used for staining peripheral blood films and bone marrow smears. These are considered polychrome stains because they contain both eosin and methylene blue. Giemsa stains also contain methylene blue azure. The purpose of staining blood films is simply to make the cells more visible and to allow their morphology to be evaluated. Consistent day-to-day staining quality is essential.

Methanol in the stain fixes the cells to the slide. Actual staining of cells or cellular components does not occur until the buffer is added. Oxidized methylene blue and eosin form a thiazine-eosinate complex, which stains neutral components. Because staining reactions are pH dependent, the buffer that is added to the stain should be 0.05 M sodium phosphate (pH 6.4) or aged distilled water (distilled water placed in a glass bottle for at least 24 hours; pH 6.4 to 6.8). Free methylene blue is basic and stains acidic (and basophilic) cellular components, such as ribonucleic acid (RNA). Free eosin is acidic and stains basic (and eosinophilic) components, such as hemoglobin and eosinophilic granules. Neutrophils are so named because they have cytoplasmic granules that have a neutral pH and pick up some staining characteristics from both stains. Slides must be completely dry before staining or the thick part of the blood film may come off the slide in the staining process.

Water or drying artifact has long been a nuisance to hematology laboratories. It has several appearances. It can give a moth-eaten look to the RBCs, or it may appear as a heavily demarcated central pallor. It also may appear as refractive (shiny) blotches on the RBCs. Other times, it manifests simply

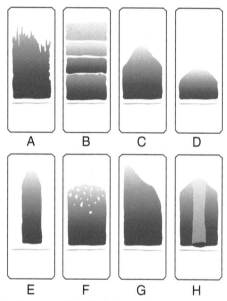

Figure 13.4 Unacceptable Peripheral Blood Films. Slide appearances associated with the most common errors are shown, but note that a combination of causes may be responsible for unacceptable films. **(A),** Chipped or rough edge on spreader slide. **(B),** Hesitation in forward motion of spreader slide. **(C),** Spreader slide pushed too quickly. **(D),** Drop of blood too small. **(E),** Drop of blood not allowed to spread across the width of the slide. **(F),** Dirt or grease on the slide; may also be due to elevated lipids in the blood specimen. **(G),** Uneven pressure on the spreader slide. **(H),** Time delay; drop of blood began to dry.

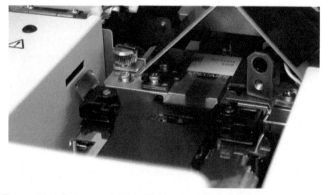

Figure 13.5 Automated Slide Making and Staining System, Sysmex SP-10. (Courtesy Sysmex America, Inc., Lincolnshire, IL.)

as echinocytes (crenation) seen in the areas of the slide that dried most slowly.

Multiple factors contribute to this problem. Humidity in the air as the slide dries may add to the punched-out, moth-eaten, or echinocytic appearance of the RBCs. It is difficult to avoid drying artifact on films from extremely anemic patients because of the very high ratio of plasma to RBCs. Water absorbed from the air into the alcohol-based stain also can contribute. Drying the slide as quickly as possible helps, and keeping a stopper tightly on the stain bottle keeps moisture out. In some laboratories, slides are fixed in pure, anhydrous methanol before staining to help reduce water artifact. More recently, stain manufacturers have used 10% volume-to-volume methanol to minimize water or drying artifact.

Wright Staining Methods

Manual technique. Traditionally, Wright staining has been performed over a sink or pan with a staining rack. Slides are placed on the rack, film side facing upward. The Wright stain may be filtered before use or poured directly from the bottle through a filter onto the slide. It is important to flood the slide completely. Stain should remain on the slide at least 1 to 3 minutes to fix the cells to the glass. Then an approximately equal amount of buffer is added to the slide. Surface tension allows very little of the buffer to run off. A metallic sheen (or green "scum") should appear on the slide if mixing is correct (Figure 13.6). More buffer can be added if necessary. The mixture is allowed to remain on the slide for 3 minutes or more (bone marrow smears take longer to stain than peripheral blood films). Timing may be adjusted to produce the best staining characteristics. When staining is complete, the slide is rinsed with a steady but gentle stream of neutral-pH water, the back of the slide is wiped to remove any stain residue, and the slide is air-dried in a vertical position.

Use of the manual Wright staining technique is desirable for staining peripheral blood films containing very high WBC counts, such as the films from leukemic patients. As with bone marrow smears, the time can be easily lengthened to enhance the staining required by the increased numbers of cells.

Understaining is common when a leukemia slide is placed on an automated slide stainer. The main disadvantages of the manual technique are the increased risk of spilling the stain and the longer time required to complete the procedure. This technique is best suited for low-volume laboratories.

Automated slide stainers. Numerous automated slide stainers are commercially available. For high-volume laboratories, these instruments are essential. Once they are set up and loaded with slides, staining proceeds without operator attention. In general, it takes 5 to 10 minutes to stain a batch of slides. The processes of fixing/staining and buffering are similar in practice to those of the manual method. The slides may be automatically dipped in stain and then in buffer and a series of rinses (Midas III, EMD Biosciences) (Figure 13.7) or propelled along a platen surface by two conveyor spirals (Hema-Tek, Siemens Healthcare Diagnostics) (Figure 13.8). In the Hema-Tek device, stain, buffer, and rinse are pumped through holes in the platen surface, flooding the slide at the appropriate time. Film quality and color consistency are usually good with any of these instruments. Some commercially prepared stain, buffer, and rinse packages do vary from lot to lot or manufacturer to manufacturer, so testing is recommended. Some disadvantages of the dip-type batch stainers are that (1) stat slides cannot be added

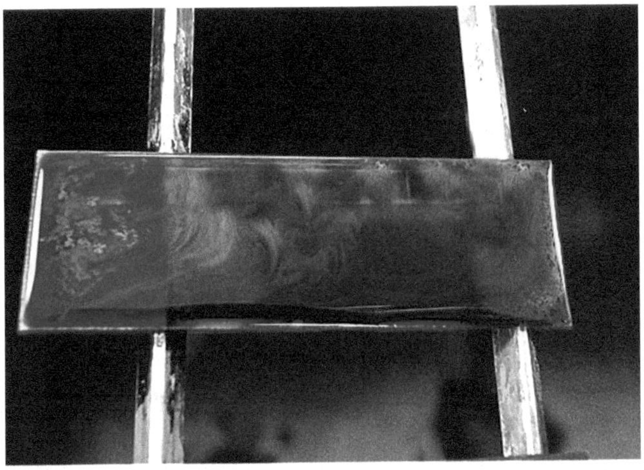

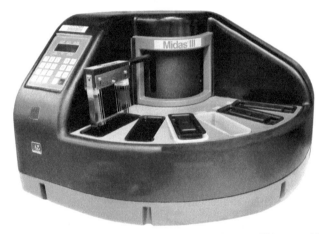

Figure 13.7 Midas III Slide Stainer. (Courtesy EM Science, Gibbstown, NJ.)

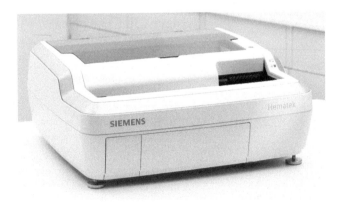

Figure 13.8 Hema-Tek 3000 Slide Stainer. (© 2014 Siemens Healthcare Diagnostics, Inc. Photo courtesy Siemens Healthcare Diagnostics.)

Figure 13.6 Manual Wright Staining of Slides. Note metallic sheen of stain indicating proper mixing.

to the batch once the staining process has begun, and (2) working or aqueous solutions of stain are stable for only 3 to 6 hours and need to be prepared often. Stat slides can be added at any time to the Hema-Tek stainer, and stain packages are stable for about 6 months.

Quick stains. Quick stains, as the name implies, are fast and easy. The whole process takes about 1 minute. Stain is purchased in a bottle as a modified Wright or Wright-Giemsa stain. The required quantity can be filtered into a Coplin jar or a staining dish, depending on the quantity of slides to be stained. Aged, distilled water is used as the buffer. Stained slides are given a final rinse under a gentle stream of tap water and allowed to air-dry. It is helpful to wipe off the back of the slide with alcohol to remove any excess stain. Quick stains are convenient and cost effective for low-volume laboratories, such as clinics and physician office laboratories, or whenever rapid turnaround time is essential. Quality is often a concern with quick stains. With a little time and patience in adjusting the staining and buffering times, however, color quality can be acceptable.

Features of a well-stained peripheral blood film. Properly staining a peripheral blood film is just as important as making a good film. Macroscopically, a well-stained blood film should be pink to purple. Microscopically, the RBCs should appear orange to salmon pink, and WBC nuclei should be purple to blue. The cytoplasm of neutrophils should be pink to tan with violet or lilac granules. Eosinophils should have bright orange refractile granules. Faulty staining can be troublesome for reading the films, causing problems ranging from minor shifts in color to the inability to identify cells and assess morphology. Trying to interpret a poorly prepared or poorly stained blood film is extremely frustrating. If possible, a newly stained film should be examined. Hints for troubleshooting poorly stained blood films are provided in Box 13.1.

The best staining results are obtained on fresh slides because the blood itself acts as a buffer in the staining process. Slides stained 1 week or longer after they are made turn out too blue. In addition, specimens that have increased levels of proteins (i.e., globulins) produce bluer-staining blood films, even when freshly stained.

BOX 13.1   Troubleshooting Poorly Stained Blood Films

First Scenario

Problems

RBCs appear gray.
WBCs are too dark.
Eosinophil granules are gray, not orange.

Causes

Stain or buffer too alkaline (most common)
Inadequate rinsing
Prolonged staining
Heparinized blood specimen

Second Scenario

Problems

RBCs are too pale or are red.
WBCs are barely visible.

Causes

Stain or buffer too acidic (most common)
Underbuffering
Overrinsing

RBC, Red blood cell; *WBC,* white blood cell.

Peripheral Film Examination

Microscopic blood film review is essential whenever instrument analysis indicates that specimen abnormalities exist. The laboratory professional evaluates the platelet and WBC count and differential, along with WBC, RBC, and platelet morphology.

Macroscopic Examination

Examining the film before placing it on the microscope stage sometimes can give the evaluator an indication of abnormalities or test results that need rechecking. For example, a film that is bluer overall than normal may indicate that the patient has increased blood proteins, as in plasma cell myeloma, and that rouleaux may be seen on the film. A grainy appearance to the film may indicate RBC agglutination, as found in cold hemagglutinin diseases. In addition, holes all over the film could mean that the patient has increased lipid levels, and some of the automated CBC parameters should be rechecked for interferences from lipemia. Markedly increased WBC counts and platelet counts can be detected from the blue specks out at the feather edge. Valuable information might be obtained before the evaluator looks through the microscope.

Microscopic Examination

The microscope should be adjusted correctly for blood film evaluation. The light from the illuminator should be properly centered, the condenser should be almost all the way up and adjusted correctly for the magnification used, and the iris diaphragm should be opened to allow a comfortable amount of light to the eye. Many individuals prefer to use a neutral density filter over the illuminator to create a whiter light from a tungsten light source. If the microscope has been adjusted for Koehler illumination, all these conditions should have been met.

10× objective examination. Blood film evaluation begins using the 10× or low-power objective lens (total magnification = 100×). Not much time needs to be spent at this magnification. However, it is a common error to omit this step altogether and go directly to the higher-power oil immersion lens. At the low-power magnification, overall film quality, color, and distribution of cells can be assessed. The feather edge and lateral edges should be checked quickly for WBC distribution. The presence of more than four times the number of cells per field at the edges or feather compared with the monolayer area of the film indicates that the film is unacceptable (i.e., a "snowplow" effect), and the film should be remade. Under the 10× objective, it is possible to check for the presence of fibrin strands; if they are present, the specimen should be rejected and another one should be collected. RBC distribution can be noted as well. Rouleaux formation or RBC agglutination is easy to recognize at this power. The film can be scanned quickly for any large abnormal cells, such as blasts, reactive lymphocytes, or even unexpected parasites. Finally, the area available for suitable examination can be assessed.

40× high-dry or 50× oil immersion objective examination. The next step is using the 40× high-dry objective (total magnification = 400×) or, as many laboratories now use, a 50× oil immersion objective (total magnification = 500×) instead. At either of these magnifications, it is easy to select the correct area of the film in which to begin the differential count and to evaluate cellular morphology. The WBC estimate also can be performed at these powers. To perform a WBC estimate, the evaluator selects an area in which the RBCs are separated from one another with minimal overlapping (where only two or three RBCs can overlap). Depending on which lens is used (40× or 50×), the procedure is the same; only the multiplication factor changes. Count the WBCs in 10 fields and determine the average number of WBCs per field. The average number of WBCs per high-power field (40×) is multiplied by 2000 (if a 50× oil lens is used, multiply by 3000) to obtain an approximation of the WBC count per microliter of blood. For example, when using a 50× oil objective, if after 10 fields are scanned it is determined that there are four to five WBCs per field, this would yield a WBC estimate of 12,000 to 15,000/μL or mm³ (12 to 15 × 10⁹/L). Box 13.2 contains a summary of the procedure for the WBC count estimate. This technique can be helpful for internal quality control, although there are inherent errors in the process. Using an area of the film that is too thick (toward the origin of the film) or too thin (toward the feather edge) affects the estimates. In addition, field diameters may vary among microscope manufacturers and models, so validation of the estimation multiplication factor should be performed first (Box 13.3). Checking for a discrepancy between the estimate and the instrument WBC count makes it easier to discover problems such as a film prepared using the wrong patient's blood specimen or a mislabeled film. In many laboratories, WBC estimates are performed on a routine basis; in others, these estimates are performed only as needed to confirm instrument values.

100× oil immersion objective examination. The 100× oil immersion objective provides the highest magnification on most standard binocular microscopes (10× eyepiece × 100× objective lens = 1000× magnification). The WBC differential count generally is performed using the 100× oil immersion

---

BOX 13.3 Validation of the White Blood Cell and Platelet Estimation Factor

1. Perform automated white blood cell (WBC) and platelet (PLT) counts on 30 consecutive fresh patient blood specimens. Make sure the results of quality control are "in control" for WBC and PLT.
2. Prepare and stain one peripheral blood film for each specimen.
3. Using the 40× high-dry or 50× oil immersion objective for the WBC estimate and the 100× oil immersion objective for the PLT estimate, select an area of the blood film in which most red blood cells (RBCs) are separated from one another with minimal overlapping of RBCs.
4. Count the number of WBCs or PLTs in 10 consecutive fields using the magnification specified in step 3, and calculate the average number of WBCs and PLTs per field.
5. For each of the 30 specimens, divide the automated WBC count by the average number of WBCs per field (40× or 50× objective); divide the automated PLT count by the average number of PLTs per field (100× objective).
6. Add the numbers obtained in step 5 for the WBCs, and divide by 30 (the number of observations in this analysis) to obtain the average ratio of the WBC count-to-WBCs per 40× or 50× field; add the numbers obtained in step 5 for the PLTs, and divide by 30 (the number of observations in this analysis) to obtain the average ratio of the PLT count–to–PLTs per 100× field.
7. Round the number calculated in step 6 to the nearest whole number to obtain an estimation factor for WBCs and PLTs at the specified magnification.

NOTE: Because of the variation in the field diameter among different microscopes, an estimation factor should be determined for each microscope in use, and that number should be used to obtain the WBC and PLT estimates when using that microscope.
Modified from Terrell, J.C. (1998).Laboratory evaluation of leukocytes. In Stiene-Martin, E.A., Lotspeich-Steininger, C.A., Koepke, J.A., (Eds.) ed, *Clinical Hematology—Principles, Procedures, Correlations*, (2nd ed., pp.337) Philadelphia: Lippincott-Raven Publishers..

BOX 13.2 Performing a White Blood Cell Estimate

1. Select an area of the blood film in which most RBCs are separated from one another with minimal overlapping of RBCs.
2. Using the 40× high-dry or 50× oil immersion objective, count the number of WBCs in 10 consecutive fields, and calculate the average number of WBCs per field.
3. To obtain the WBC estimate per microliter of blood, multiply the average number of WBCs per field by 2000* (if using the 40× high-dry objective) or 3000* (if using the 50× oil immersion objective).
4. Compare the instrument WBC count with the WBC estimate from the blood film.

Example: If an average of three WBCs were observed per field:
Using a 40× high-dry objective, the WBC estimate is 6000/μL or mm³ or 6.0 × 10⁹/L.
Using a 50× oil immersion objective, the WBC estimate is 9000/μL or mm³ or 9.0 × 10⁹/L.

RBC, Red blood cell; *WBC,* white blood cell.
*WBC estimation factors of 2000 (40× objective) and 3000 (50× objective) are provided as general guidelines. A WBC estimation factor should be determined and validated for each microscope in use (see Box 13.3).

---

objective. Performing the differential normally includes counting and classifying 100 WBCs to obtain percentages of WBC types. The RBC, WBC, and platelet morphology evaluation and the platelet estimate also are executed under the 100× oil immersion objective lens. At this magnification segmented neutrophils can be readily differentiated from bands. RBC inclusions, such as Howell-Jolly bodies, and WBC inclusions, such as Döhle bodies, can be seen easily if present. Reactive or abnormal cells are enumerated under the 100× objective as well. If present, nucleated RBCs (NRBCs) are counted and reported as NRBCs per 100 WBCs (Chapter 11).

50× oil immersion objective examination. The WBC differential and morphology examinations described for the 100× oil immersion objective also can be accomplished by experienced morphologists using a 50× oil immersion objective. The larger field of view allows more cells to be evaluated faster. Examination at this power is especially efficient for validating or verifying instrument values when a total microscopic assessment of the film is not needed. Particular cell features that may require higher magnification can be assessed by moving the parfocal 100× objective into place and then returning to the 50× objective to continue the differential. As previously mentioned, the WBC estimate also can be performed with the 50× objective, but the multiplication factor is 3000. The laboratory professional should conform to the estimation protocol of the particular laboratory.

Optimal assessment area. The tasks described, especially for the 100×, 40×, and 50× objectives, need to be performed in the best possible area of the peripheral blood film. That occurs between the thick area, or "heel," where the drop of blood was initially placed and spread, and the very thin feather edge. In the ideal area, microscopically, the RBCs are uniformly and singly distributed, with few touching or overlapping, and have their normal biconcave appearance (central pallor) (Figure 13.9A). An area that is too thin, in which there are holes in the film or the RBCs look flat, large, and distorted, is unacceptable (Figure 13.9B). A too-thick area also distorts the RBCs

by piling them on top of one another like rouleaux (Figure 13.9C). WBCs are similarly distorted, which makes morphologic evaluation more difficult and classification potentially incorrect. When the correct area of a specimen from a patient with a normal RBC count is viewed, there are generally about 200 to 250 RBCs per 100× oil immersion field.

A common problem encountered with the oil immersion objective lens is worth mentioning. If the blood film was in focus under the 10× and 40× objectives but is impossible to bring into focus under the 100× objective, the slide is probably upside down. The 100× objective does not have sufficient depth of field to focus through the slide. The oil must be completely removed before the film is put on the stage right-side up.

Performance of the white blood cell differential. Fewer manual differentials are performed today because of the superior accuracy of automated differentials and because of cost and time constraints. When indicated, however, the manual differential always should be performed in a systematic manner. When the correct area has been selected, use of a back-and-forth serpentine, or "battlement," track pattern is preferred to minimize distribution errors (Figure 13.10)[9] and ensure that each cell is counted only once. One hundred WBCs are counted and classified through the use of push-down button counters (Figure 13.11A) or newer computer-interfaced key pads (Figure 13.11B). To increase accuracy, it is advisable to count at least 200 cells when the WBC count is higher than 40×10^9/L. If the WBC count is 100×10^9/L or greater, it would be more precise and accurate to count 300 or 400 cells. Results are reported as percentages—for example, 54% segmented neutrophils, 6% bands, 28% lymphocytes, 9% monocytes, 3% eosinophils. The evaluator always should check to ensure that the sum of the percentages is 100.

Performing 100-cell differentials on extremely low WBC counts can become tedious and time consuming, even when the 50× oil immersion objective is used. In some laboratories the WBCs are concentrated by centrifugation, and buffy coat smears are made. This practice is helpful for examining the morphology of the cells; however, it is not recommended for performing differentials because of possible errors in cell distribution from centrifugation. In other laboratories evaluators may perform a 50-cell differential and multiply the results by 2 to obtain a percentage. The accuracy of this practice is questionable, and it should be avoided if possible. In some laboratories the buffy coat smear is examined for the presence of blasts, but no differential is performed. It is essential to include the side margins of the blood film in any differential so that the larger cells, such as monocytes, reactive lymphocytes, and immature cells, are not missed.

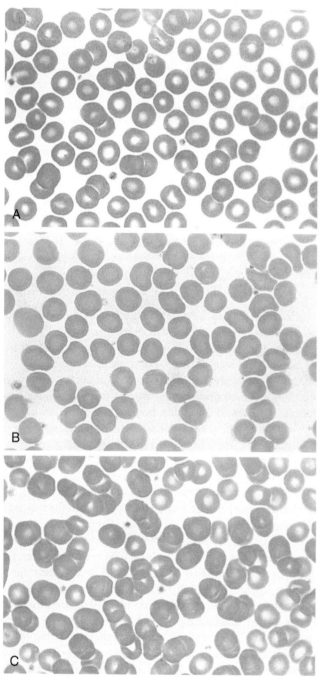

Figure 13.9 Peripheral Blood Films. (A), Photomicrograph of good area of peripheral blood film. Photomicrographs of peripheral blood film with areas too thin **(B),** and too thick **(C),** to read. (Wright-Giemsa stain, ×1000.)

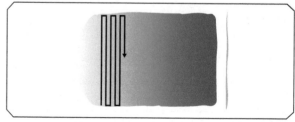

Figure 13.10 "Battlement" Pattern for Performing a Differential Count.

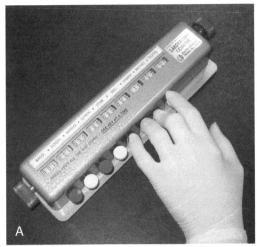

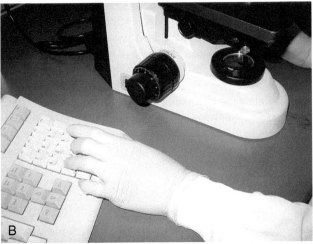

Figure 13.11 Differential Tally Counters. (A), Laboratory differential tally counter. **(B),** Computer interfaced key pad counter.

In addition to counting the cells, the evaluator assesses their appearance. If present, WBC abnormalities such as toxic granulation, Döhle bodies, reactive lymphocytes, and Auer rods (Chapters 26 and 31) are evaluated and reported. The International Council for Standardization in Haematology (ICSH) released guidelines and recommendations for the nomenclature and grading of RBCs, WBC, and platelet abnormalities.[10] Traditionally, reactive lymphocytes were reported either as a separate percentage of the 100 cells, as a percentage of the total number of lymphocytes, or semiquantitatively ("occasional" to "many"). The ICSH recommendation is to add a comment on the presence of reactive lymphocytes and to count them as a separate population of cells in the differential count if they are present in large numbers.[10] The ICSH also recommends that toxic granulation and Döhle bodies are graded as "slight" to "marked," or 1+ to 3+, and that Auer rods are reported as "present" when seen.[10] These recommendations are to be used strictly as guidelines to simplify blood film morphology reports and to help ensure better accuracy, consistency, and clinical relevance. Regardless of reporting format, each laboratory should establish criteria for reporting microscopic cell morphology.

Because the differential alone provides only partial information, reported in relative percentages, the absolute cell counts

are calculated for each cell type in some laboratories. Automated differentials already include this information.

Automation has been applied to microscopic cell identification; CellaVision is a popular digital cell morphology system.[11] It automatically identifies optimal examination areas on a slide, then locates and captures focused images of the cells. To preclassify cell images, a number of features are extracted from each individual image and are fed into a computerized visual recognition system. The digital images are presented to the operator who can review the cells on the screen, adjust any classifications, and enter comments about morphology. Images and results are stored in a local or central database enabling remote review of cell images and results for cases needing a secondary review[11] (Figure 13.12).

Red blood cell morphology. Evaluation of RBC morphology is an important part of the blood film examination and includes an assessment of cell size (microcytosis, macrocytosis), variability in size (anisocytosis), cell color (hypochromia), cell shape (poikilocytosis), and cellular inclusions (Chapter 16). Some laboratories use specific terminology for reporting the degree of abnormal morphology, such as "slight," "moderate," or "marked," or use a scale from 1+ to 3+. Other laboratories more recently have gone to a simpler report, using the term *present* for morphologic abnormalities that are clinically significant. Still other laboratories provide a summary statement regarding the overall RBC morphology that is consistent with the RBC indices and histogram. The latter methods are becoming more popular with the increased computer interfacing in most laboratories. Regardless of the reporting method used, the microscopic RBC morphology assessment should be congruent with the information given by the automated blood cell analyzer. If not, further investigation is needed.

Platelet estimate. As previously mentioned, the platelet estimate is performed under the 100× oil immersion objective lens.

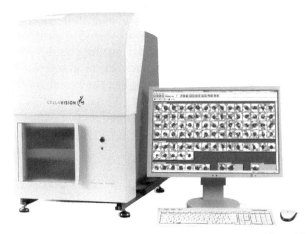

Figure 13.12 CellaVision DM9600. The CellaVision preclassifies white blood cells (WBCs) into 17 cell types, precharacterizes red blood cells (RBCs) based on 21 morphologic features, and can characterize cell morphology on body fluids cytospins such as cerebrospinal, peritoneal and pleural fluids. The operator can override the instrument's classification and identify cells that the instrument could not classify. (Courtesy Cellavision AB, Lund, Sweden.)

BOX 13.4 Performing a Platelet Estimate

1. Select an area of the blood film in which most red blood cells (RBCs) are separated from one another with minimal overlapping of RBCs.
2. Using the 100× oil immersion objective, count the number of platelets in 10 consecutive fields, and calculate the average number of platelets per field.
3. To obtain the platelet estimate per microliter of blood, multiply the average number of platelets per field by 20,000.*
4. Compare the instrument platelet count with the platelet estimate from the blood film.

Example: If an average of 20 platelets were observed per 100× oil immersion field, the platelet estimate is 400,000/μL or mm³ (400 × 10⁹/L). In instances of significant anemia or erythrocytosis, use the following formula for the platelet estimate:

$$\frac{\text{Average number of platelets/field} \times \text{total RBC count}}{200\ \text{RBCs/field}}$$

---

*A platelet estimation factor of 20,000 is provided as a general guideline. A platelet estimation factor should be determined and validated for each microscope in use (see Box 16.3).

In an area of the film where the RBCs barely touch, with minimal overlapping, the number of platelets in 10 oil immersion fields is counted. The average number of platelets per oil immersion field multiplied by 20,000 approximates the platelet count per microliter or cubic millimeter. For example, 12 to 16 platelets per oil immersion field equals about 280,000 platelets/μL or mm³ (280 × 10⁹/L) and is considered adequate. Box 13.4 contains a summary of the procedure for the platelet estimate. In situations in which the patient is anemic or has erythrocytosis, however, the relative proportion of platelets to RBCs is altered. In these instances a more involved formula for platelet estimates may be used:

$$\frac{\text{Average number of platelets/field} \times \text{total RBC count}}{200\ \text{RBCs/field}}$$

Note that 200 is the average number of RBCs per oil immersion field in the optimal assessment area.

Regardless of whether an "official" estimate is made, verification of the instrument platelet count should be included in the overall examination for internal quality control purposes. Blood film examination also includes an assessment of the morphology of the platelets, including size as well as granularity and overall appearance.

Immersion oils with different viscosities do not mix well. If slides are taken to another microscope for review, oil should be wiped off first.

SUMMARIZING COMPLETE BLOOD COUNT RESULTS

To this point, this chapter has focused on slide preparation and performance of a differential cell count. The differential is only the capstone, however, of a panel of tests collectively called the complete blood count, or *CBC*, that includes many of the routine tests described in Chapter 11. Now that the testing for the component parts has been described, interpretation of the results for the total panel can be discussed.

The CBC has evolved over time to the typical test panel reported today, including assessment of WBCs, RBCs, and platelets. The CBC provides information about the hematopoietic system, but because abnormalities of blood cells can be caused by diseases of other organ systems, the CBC also plays a role in screening those organs for disease. The CBC provides such valuable information about a patient's health status that it is among the most commonly ordered laboratory tests performed by medical laboratory scientists and laboratory technicians.

The process of interpreting the CBC test results has two phases. In phase 1 the numbers and descriptions generated by the testing are summarized using appropriate terminology. This summary provides a verbal picture of the numbers that is easy to communicate to the physician, other health care provider, or another laboratorian. It is much more convenient to be able to say, "The patient has a microcytic anemia" than to say, "The hemoglobin was low, and the mean cell volume was also low." Phase 2 of interpretation is to recognize a pattern of results consistent with various diseases and to be able to narrow the diagnosis for the given patient or perhaps even to pinpoint it so that appropriate follow-up testing or treatment can be recommended.

The following discussion focuses on phase 1 of CBC interpretation—how to collect the pertinent information and summarize it. Phase 2 of the interpretation is the essence of the remaining chapters of this book on various hematologic conditions or other metabolic conditions that have an impact on the hematologic system.

Organization of Complete Blood Count Results

Today most laboratorians perform CBCs using sophisticated automated analyzers as described in Chapter 12, but the component tests can be performed using the manual methods described in Chapter 11. The blood film assessment described in this chapter is also part of a CBC. As previously mentioned, the CBC "panel" is essentially divided into WBC, RBC, and platelet parameters.

For phase 2 interpretation, it is sometimes important to look at all three groupings of the CBC results; at other times, only one or two may be of interest. If a patient has an infection, the WBC parameters may be the only ones of interest. If the patient has anemia, all three sets—WBCs, RBCs, and platelets—may require assessment. Generally all the parameters interpreted together provide the best information, so a complete summary of the results should be generated.

Assessing Hematology Results Relative to Reference Intervals

Proper performance of the phase 1 summary of test results requires comparison of the patient values with the reference intervals. The table of reference intervals for the CBC on the inside cover of this text shows that there are different reference intervals for men and women, particularly for the RBC parameters. There also are different intervals for children of different ages, with the WBC changes the most notable. It is important to select the appropriate set of reference intervals in hematology for the gender and age of the patient.

CBC results can be reported in standard international (SI) units or in common units. For example, the following results in SI units (WBC count = 7.2 × 10^9/L, RBC count = 4.20 × 10^{12}/L, hemoglobin [HGB] = 128 g/L, hematocrit [HCT] = 0.41 L/L, and platelets [PLT] = 237 × 10^9/L) are equivalent to the following results in common units (WBC count = 7.2 × 10^3/μL, RBC count = 4.20 × 10^6/μL, HGB = 12.8 g/dL, HCT = 41%, and PLT = 237 × 10^3/μL). The older mm^3 for cell count units is equivalent to μL (Chapter 11). Because either system may be used on laboratory reports, the laboratorian should be able to easily interconvert CBC results between the systems. SI units are used for cell counts in this chapter.

Several strategies can help in determining the significance of the results. First, if the results are very far from the reference interval, it is more likely that they are truly outside the interval and represent a pathologic process. Second, if two or more diagnostically related parameters are slightly or moderately outside the interval in the same direction (both high or both low), this suggests that the results are clinically significant and associated with some pathologic process. Because some healthy individuals always have results slightly outside the reference interval, the best comparison for their results is not the reference interval but their own results from a prior time when they were known to be healthy.

Summarizing White Blood Cell Parameters

The WBC-related parameters of a routine CBC include the following:

1. Total WBC count (WBCs × 10^9/L)
2. WBC differential count values expressed as percentages, called *relative counts*
3. WBC differential count values expressed as the actual number of each type of cell (e.g., neutrophils × 10^9/L), called *absolute counts*
4. WBC morphology

Step 1

Start by ensuring that there is an accurate WBC count. Compare the WBC histogram and/or scatterplot to the respective cell counts to make sure they correlate with one another. Today's automated instruments can eliminate nucleated RBCs that falsely increase the WBC count. However, manual WBC results must be corrected mathematically to eliminate the contribution of the NRBCs (Chapter 11).

Step 2

Look at the total WBC count. When the count is elevated, it is called *leukocytosis*. When the WBC count is low, it is called *leukopenia*. As described later, increases and decreases of WBCs are associated with infections and conditions such as leukemias. Because there is more than one type of WBC, increases and decreases in the total count usually are due to changes in one of the subtypes—for example, neutrophils or lymphocytes. Determining which one is the next step.

Step 3

Examine the relative differential counts for a preliminary assessment of which cell lines are affected. The relative differential count is reported in percentages. The proportion of each cell

TABLE 13.1 Terminology for Increases and Decreases in White Blood Cells

Cell Type	Increases	Decreases
Neutrophil	Neutrophilia	Neutropenia
Eosinophil	Eosinophilia	N/A
Basophil	Basophilia	N/A
Lymphocyte	Lymphocytosis	Lymphopenia (lymphocytopenia)
Monocyte	Monocytosis	Monocytopenia

N/A, Not applicable because the reference interval begins at or near zero.

type can be described by its relative number (i.e., percent) and compared with its reference interval. Then it is described using appropriate terminology, such as a relative neutrophilia, which is an increase in neutrophils, or a relative lymphopenia, which is a decrease in lymphocytes. The terms used for increases and decreases of each cell type are provided in Table 13.1.

If the total WBC count or any of the relative values are outside the reference interval, further analysis of the WBC differential is needed. If the proportion of one of the cell types increases, then the proportion of others must decrease because the proportions are relative to one another. The second cell type may not have changed in actual number at all, however. The way to assess this accurately is with absolute differential counts.

Step 4

If not reported by the instrument, absolute counts can be calculated easily using the total WBC count and the relative differential. Multiply each relative cell count (i.e., percentage) by the total WBC count and by so doing determine the absolute count for each cell lineage.

Examine the set of WBC parameters from a CBC shown in Table 13.2. On first inspection, one may look at the WBC count and recognize that a leukocytosis is present, but it is important to determine what cell line is causing the increased count. In this case the cells are all within reference intervals relative to one another. There is no indication as to which cell line could be causing the increase in total numbers of WBCs.

When each relative number (e.g., neutrophils at 0.67 or 67%) is multiplied by the total WBC count (13.6 × 10^9/L), the absolute numbers indicate that the neutrophils are elevated (9.1 × 10^9/L compared with the reference interval provided). The acronym for absolute neutrophil count is *ANC*. The ANC is a very useful parameter for assessing neutropenia and neutrophilia. The absolute lymphocyte count (3.5 × 10^9/L) is still within the reference interval. Given this information, these results can be described as showing a leukocytosis with only an absolute neutrophilia, and the overall increase in the WBC count is due to an increase only in neutrophils. This description provides a concise summary of the WBC counts without the need to refer to every type of cell. Box 13.5 extends this concept to a convention used to describe the neutrophilic cells, and Box 13.6 addresses the clinical utility of reporting percent bands as a separate category.

TABLE 13.2   Comparison of Relative and Absolute White Blood Cell Counts

Complete Blood Count Parameter	Patient Value	Reference Interval	Interpretation Relative to Reference Interval	Description/Summary
White blood cell count	13.6	$4.3–10.8 \times 10^9/L$	Elevated	Leukocytosis
Relative Differential				
Neutrophils	67	48%–70%	WRI	
Lymphocytes	26	18%–42%	WRI	
Monocytes	3	1%–10%	WRI	
Eosinophils	3	1%–4%	WRI	
Basophils	1	0%–2%	WRI	
Absolute Differential				
Absolute neutrophils	9.1	$2.4–8.2 \times 10^9/L$	Elevated	Absolute neutrophilia
Absolute lymphocytes	3.5	$1.4–4 \times 10^9/L$	WRI	
Absolute monocytes	0.4	$0.1–1.2 \times 10^9/L$	WRI	

WRI, Within reference interval.

BOX 13.5   Summarizing Neutrophilia When Young Cells Are Present

A subtle convention in assessing the differential counts involves the presence of young cells of the neutrophilic series (e.g., bands). They typically are grouped together with the mature neutrophils in judging whether neutrophilia is present. For example, look at the following differential and the reference intervals provided in parentheses:

White blood cells	10.8	$(4.3–10.8 \times 10^9/L)$
Neutrophils	65	(48%–70%)
Bands	18	(0%–10%)
Lymphocytes	13	(18%–42%)
Monocytes	3	(1%–10%)
Eosinophils	1	(1%–4%)
Basophils	0	(0%–2%)

Although the mature neutrophils are within the reference interval, the bands exceed their reference interval. The total of the two, 83 (65% + 18%), exceeds the upper limit of neutrophilic cells even when the two intervals are combined, 80 (70% + 10%), so these results would be described as a neutrophilia even though the neutrophil value itself is within the reference interval. See steps 4 and 5 under Summarizing White Blood Cell Parameters for how to communicate the increase in bands.

BOX 13.6   Clinical Utility of Band Counts

An elevated band count was thought to be useful in the diagnosis of patients with infection. However, the clinical utility of band counts has been called into question, and most laboratories no longer perform routine band counts.[13] The Clinical and Laboratory Standards Institute (CLSI) recommends that bands and neutrophils be counted together and placed in a single category rather than in separate categories because it is difficult to reliably differentiate bands from segmented neutrophils.[14-16]

BOX 13.7   Origin of the Phrase *Left Shift*

The origin of the phrase *left shift* is a 1920s publication by Josef Arneth in which neutrophil maturity was correlated with segment count. A graphical representation was made, and the fewer the segments, the farther left was the median—hence *left shift.* This was called the *Arneth count* or *Arneth-Schilling count* and was abandoned around the time Arneth died in 1955, but the term *left shift* lived on to describe increased numbers of immature cells as an indicator of infection.

automated analyzers, which count actual numbers (i.e., produce absolute counts) and calculate relative values. Some laboratories do not report the absolute counts, so being able to calculate them is important.

As will be evident in later chapters, the findings in this example point toward a bacterial infection. Had there been an absolute lymphocytosis, a viral infection would be likely.

Step 5

Each cell line should be examined for immature cells. Young WBCs are not normally seen in the peripheral blood, and they may indicate infections or malignancies such as leukemia. For neutrophilic cells, there is a unique term that refers to the presence of increased numbers of bands or cells younger than bands in the peripheral blood: *left shift* or *shift to the left* (Box 13.7).

When young lymphocytic or monocytic cells are present, they can be reported in the differential as prolymphocytes, lymphoblasts, promonocytes, or monoblasts. When observed, young eosinophils and basophils are typically just called *immature* and are not specifically staged. For example, *eosinophilic metamyelocytes* are counted as eosinophils.

Step 6

Any abnormalities of appearance are reported in the morphology section of the report. For WBCs, abnormal morphologic features that would be noted include changes in overall

When the absolute numbers of each of the individual cell types are totaled, the sum equals the WBC count (slight differences may occur because of rounding, as in the example). This is a method for checking whether the absolute calculations are correct. Absolute counts may be obtained directly from

cellular appearance, such as cytoplasmic toxic granulation and nuclear abnormalities such as hypersegmentation. The clinical significance of these types of changes is discussed in Chapter 26.

To summarize the WBC parameters, begin with an accurate total WBC count, followed by the relative differential, or preferably the absolute counts, noting whether any abnormal young cells are present in the blood. Finally, note the presence of any abnormal morphology or inclusions.

Summarizing Red Blood Cell Parameters

RBC parameters of the CBC are as follows:
1. RBC count (RBCs $\times 10^{12}$/L)
2. HGB (g/dL)
3. HCT (% or L/L)
4. Mean cell volume (MCV, fL)
5. Mean cell hemoglobin (MCH, pg)
6. Mean cell hemoglobin concentration (MCHC, g/dL)
7. RBC distribution width (RDW, %)
8. Morphology

Step 1

Examine the hemoglobin (or hematocrit) for anemia or polycythemia. Anemia is the more common condition. If the RBC morphology is relatively normal, three times the hemoglobin approximates the hematocrit; this is called the *rule of three* (Chapter 11). If the rule of three holds, the expectation is that the following assessments will find normal RBC parameters. If the rule of three fails and all test results are reliable, further assessment should uncover some patient RBC abnormalities. Remember that the rule of three only holds true when overall RBC morphology is normocytic and normochromic.

Hemoglobin concentration (HGB) is a more reliable indicator of anemia than is the hematocrit, because the hematocrit can be influenced by the size of the RBCs. Hemoglobin concentration is a more direct indicator of the ability of the blood to carry oxygen.

Step 2

When the hemoglobin and hematocrit values have been inspected and the rule of three applied, the next RBC parameter that should be evaluated is the MCV (Chapter 11). This value provides the average RBC volume. The MCV should be correlated with the RBC histogram from the instrument and morphologic appearance of the cells using the classification first introduced by Wintrobe a century ago (Table 13.3).

The MCV is expected to be within the established reference interval (approximately 80 to 100 fL), and the RBC histogram and morphology are expected to be normal (normocytic). For a patient with anemia, classifying the anemia morphologically by the MCV narrows the range of possible causes to microcytic, normocytic, or macrocytic anemias (Chapter 16).

Step 3

Examine the MCHC to evaluate how well the cells are filled with hemoglobin. Remember that MCHC is a concentration and takes into consideration the volume of the RBCs when considering decreased or normal color. If the MCHC is within the reference interval, the cells are considered normal or *normochromic* and display typical central pallor of one-third the volume of the cell. If the MCHC is less than the reference interval, the cells are called *hypochromic*, which literally means "too little color." This correlates with a larger central pallor (hypochromia) when the cells are examined on a Wright-stained blood film.

It is possible for the MCHC to be elevated in two situations, but this does not correlate with hyperchromia. A slight elevation may be seen when cells are spherocytic (MCHC > 36 g/dL). They retain roughly normal volume but have decreased surface area. Therefore the hemoglobin is slightly more concentrated than usual, and the cells look darker with no central pallor. A more dramatic increase in MCHC (values even as high as 60) can be caused by analytical problems, often associated with patient specimen problems that falsely elevate hemoglobin measurement. Common problems of this type include interference from lipemia, icterus, or grossly elevated WBC counts. Each of these interferes with the spectrophotometric measurement of hemoglobin, thus falsely elevating the hemoglobin and affecting the calculation of the MCHC (Chapter 11). It is worth noting that the MCHC is often best used as an internal quality control parameter.

Step 4

The RDW is determined from the histogram of RBC volumes. Briefly, when the volumes of the RBCs are about the same, the histogram is narrow (Figure 13.13A). If the volumes are variable (more small cells, more large cells, or both), the histogram becomes wider. The width of the histogram, the RDW, is reflected statistically as a coefficient of variation (CV) or a standard deviation (SD). Most analyzer manufacturers provide a CV and an SD, and the operator can select which to report. Figure 13.13 depicts RBC histograms demonstrating normal, microcytosis, macrocytosis, anisocytosis, and dimorphic red cell populations.

Therefore the RDW provides information about the presence and degree of anisocytosis (variation in RBC volume). What is important is increased values only, not decreased values. If an RDW-CV reference interval is 11.5% to 14.5% and a patient has an RDW-CV of 20.6%, the patient has a more heterogeneous RBC population with more variation in cell volume (anisocytosis). If the RDW is elevated, a notation about anisocytosis is

TABLE 13.3   Interpretation of Mean Cell Volume Values Using the Wintrobe Terminology

Mean Cell Volume Value	Wintrobe Description
Within reference interval (80–100 fL)	Normocytic
Lower than reference interval (<80 fL)	Microcytic
Higher than reference interval (>100 fL)	Macrocytic

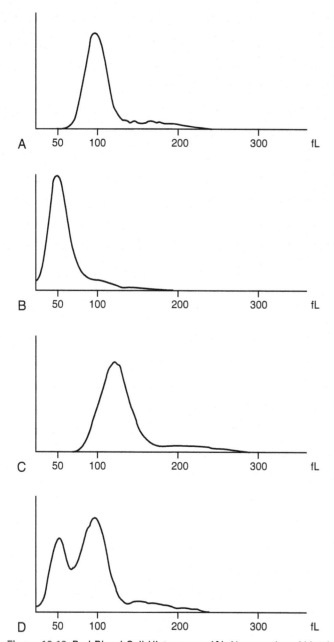

Figure 13.13 Red Blood Cell Histograms. (A), Normocytic red blood cell population with MCV of 96.8 fL and RDW-CV of 14.1%; **(B),** microcytosis with MCV of 54.6 fL and RDW-CV of 13.2%; **(C),** macrocytosis and anisocytosis with MCV of 119.2 fL and RDW-CV of 23.9%; **(D),** dimorphic red blood cells with MCV of 80.2 fL and RDW-CV of 37.2%. Note the microcytic and the normocytic red blood cell populations. Reference intervals: MCV, 80 to 100 fL; RDW-CV, 11.5% to 14.5%. *MCV,* Mean cell volume; *RDW-CV,* red blood cell distribution width, coefficient of variation.

expected in the morphologic evaluation of the blood film. Using the MCV along with the RDW provides the most helpful information (Chapter 16).

Step 5

Examine the morphology for pertinent abnormalities. Whenever anemia is indicated by the RBC parameters reported by the

analyzer, and potential abnormal RBC morphology is suggested by the indices and the rule of three, a Wright-stained peripheral blood film must be reviewed. Abnormalities include abnormal volume, abnormal shape, inclusions, immature RBCs, abnormal color, and abnormal arrangement (Chapter 16). The blood film also serves as quality control, because the morphologic characteristics seen through the microscope (e.g., microcytosis, anisocytosis) should be congruent with the results provided by the analyzer. When they do not agree, further investigation is necessary.

If everything in the morphology is normal, by convention, no notation regarding morphology is included. Therefore any notation in the morphology section requires scrutiny. All RBC-related abnormal morphologic findings should be noted, including specific poikilocytosis (abnormal shape) and the presence of RBC inclusions, such as Howell-Jolly bodies. One of the major challenges is in determining when the amount or degree of an abnormality is worth noting at all (i.e., when it should be reported). Laboratories strive for standardization of reporting. All laboratories must have good standardized morphology criteria and competent staff whose evaluations are consistent with one another and with the standardized criteria used in that facility. Generally, a semiquantitative method is used that employs terms such as *slight, moderate,* and *marked* or the numbers 1+, 2+, and 3+. Numerical ranges representing the reporting unit are defined; for example, three to six spherocytes per oil immersion field might be reported as 2+ spherocytes. Although this practice has been followed for many years, this semiquantitative method may not best serve the needs of medical staff, and many laboratories are moving toward simplifying their reports to state *present* for morphologic abnormalities. In fact, the ICSH recommends the use of qualitative grading for RBC morphology except for schistocytes; these cells will have greater clinical significance even at lower counts.[10]

The presence of immature RBCs suggests that the bone marrow is attempting to respond to an anemia. Polychromasia on the peripheral blood film indicates bone marrow response. This is manifested by the bluer color of reticulocytes that have entered the bloodstream earlier than usual in the body's attempt to improve oxygen-carrying capacity. If the anemia is severe, NRBCs also may be present. As noted earlier, it is also important to recognize NRBCs because they may falsely elevate the WBC count and may be an indication of an underlying disease process.

A better way to assess replacement erythropoiesis is with the reticulocyte count and subsequent calculation of the reticulocyte production index, if appropriate. The reticulocyte count is not normally part of the CBC, although it is now performed on the same analyzers. If the reticulocyte count is available with the CBC, its interpretation can improve the assessment of young RBCs (Chapter 11).

Step 6

Examine the RBC count and MCH. On a practical level, the RBC count is not the parameter used to judge anemia, because there are some types of anemia, such as the thalassemias (Chapter 25), in which the RBC count is normal or even elevated. Thus the assessment of anemia would be missed by relying only on the RBC count. However, this inconsistency (low hemoglobin and high RBC count) is often helpful diagnostically.

The MCH follows the MCV; that is, smaller cells necessarily hold less hemoglobin, whereas larger cells can hold more. For this reason, it is less often used than the MCV and MCHC. In the instances in which the MCH does *not* follow the MCV, the MCHC detects the discrepancy between size and hemoglobin content of the cell. The MCH is not crucial to the assessment of anemia when the other parameters are provided. In summary, when evaluating the RBC parameters of the CBC, examine the hemoglobin first, then the MCV, RDW, and MCHC. Finally, take note of any abnormal morphology.

Summarizing Platelet Parameters

The platelet parameters of the CBC are as follows:
1. Platelet count (platelets $\times 10^9$/L)
2. Mean platelet volume (MPV, fL)
3. Morphology

Step 1

The platelet count should be examined for increases (thrombocytosis) or decreases (thrombocytopenia) outside the established reference interval. A patient who has unexplained bruising or bleeding may have a decreased platelet count. The platelet count should be assessed along with the WBC count and hemoglobin to determine whether all three are decreased (pancytopenia) or increased (pancytosis). Pancytopenia is clinically significant because it can indicate a possible developing acute leukemia (Chapter 31) or aplastic anemia (Chapter 19). Pancytosis frequently is associated with a diagnosis of polycythemia vera (Chapter 32).

Step 2

Compare the instrument-generated MPV with the MPV reference interval, 6.9 to 10.2 fL, and with the platelet diameter observed on the peripheral blood film. An elevated MPV should correspond with increased platelet diameter, just as an elevated MCV reflects macrocytosis. In platelet consumption disorders such as immune thrombocytopenic purpura, an elevated MPV, accompanied by platelets 6 μm or larger in diameter (giant platelets), reflects bone marrow release of early "stress" or "reticulated" platelets, evidence for bone marrow compensation (Chapter 10 and Figure 10.5).[12,13] Comparing platelet diameter by visual inspection with MPV is a recommended quality control step; however, the MPV has a wide percent CV, which reflects interindividual variation and platelet swelling in EDTA and reduces its clinical effectiveness.[14] Some instruments identify and record a reticulated platelet count using nucleic acid dye, analogous to a reticulocyte count. Figure 13.14 demonstrates platelet histograms with a normal platelet population (A) and one with giant platelets (B).

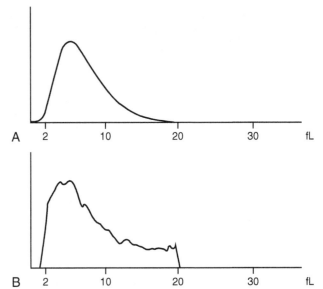

Figure 13.14 Platelet Histograms. (A), Normal with MPV of 8.0 fL; **(B),** platelet population with abnormal histogram and MPV of 9.1 fL. Although the MPV is within the reference interval, the histogram shows an increase in the number of platelets with a volume between 10 and 20 fL (curve above baseline) representing giant platelets. Reference interval for MPV: 6.8 to 10.2 fL. *MPV,* Mean platelet volume.

Step 3

Examine platelet morphology and platelet arrangement. Although the MPV can recognize abnormally large platelets, the morphologic evaluation also notes this. Some laboratories distinguish between large platelets (two times normal size) and giant platelets (more than twice as large as normal) or compare platelet size to RBC size.

Additional morphologic descriptors include terms for reporting granularity, which is most important if missing, and in this case the platelets are described as "hypogranular" or "agranular." Sometimes the abnormalities are too variable to classify, and the platelets are described simply as "bizarre" or dysplastic. In some cases, platelets can be clumped or adherent to WBCs, and these arrangements should be noted. As described previously, corrective actions can be taken to derive accurate platelet and WBC counts when these arrangements are observed on the film. Summarizing platelet parameters includes reporting total number, platelet size by either instrument MPV or morphologic evaluation, and platelet appearance.

Box 13.8 gives an example of how the entire CBC can be summarized using the steps described. When results of the CBC are properly summarized and no information has been overlooked, there is confidence that the phase 2 interpretation of the results will be reliable. Adopting a methodical approach to examining each parameter ensures that the myriad information available from the CBC can be used effectively and efficiently in patient care. Box 13.9 summarizes the systematic approach to CBC interpretation.

BOX 13.8 Applying a Systematic Approach to Complete Blood Count Summarization

A specimen from an adult male patient yields the following CBC results (refer to the reference intervals inside the front cover of this book):

WBCs	3.20×10^9/L
RBCs	2.10×10^{12}/L
HGB	8.5 g/dL
HCT	26.3%
MCV	125 fL
MCH	40.5 pg
MCHC	32.3 g/dL
RDW	20.6%
PLT	115×10^9/L

Differential:

Neutrophils	43%
Bands	2%
Lymphocytes	45%
Monocytes	10%

Morphology: hypersegmentation of neutrophils, anisocytosis, macrocytes, oval macrocytes, occasional teardrop cells, Howell-Jolly bodies, and basophilic stippling

The step-by-step assessment of the WBCs indicates that the WBC count is accurate and can be interpreted as leukopenia. Although the relative differential values are all within the reference intervals, calculation of absolute counts indicates an absolute neutropenia and lymphopenia. No unexpected young WBCs are noted, but the morphology indicates hypersegmentation of neutrophils. For the RBCs, the hemoglobin concentration (8.5) indicates that this individual is anemic. Inspection of the MCV indicates macrocytosis because the MCV is increased to more than 100 fL, the upper limit of the reference interval. Examination of the MCHC shows it to be normal, so for these results, the RBC morphology would be described as macrocytic, normochromic. The elevated RDW indicates substantial anisocytosis. There is no mention of polychromasia, so no young RBCs are seen. The morphologic description supports the interpretation of the RDW with mention of anisocytosis as a result of macrocytosis and poikilocytosis characterized by oval macrocytes and occasional teardrop cells. Howell-Jolly bodies and basophilic stippling are significant RBC inclusions. The platelet count indicates thrombocytopenia. Although MPV is not reported, the platelets are of normal size and show no morphologic abnormalities because there are no notations in the morphologic descriptions.

CBC, Complete blood count; *HCT,* hematocrit; *HGB,* hemoglobin; *MCH,* mean cell hemoglobin; *MCHC,* mean cell hemoglobin concentration; *MCV,* mean cell volume; *MPV,* mean platelet volume; *RBC,* red blood cell; *RDW,* RBC distribution width; *WBC,* white blood cell.

BOX 13.9 Systematic Approach to Complete Blood Count Interpretation

White Blood Cells

Step 1: Ensure that the WBC count is accurate. Review WBC histogram and/or scatterplot and correlate with counts. The presence of nucleated RBCs may require correction of the WBC count.

Step 2: Compare the patient's WBC count with the laboratory's established reference interval.

Steps 3 and 4: Examine the differential information (relative and absolute) on variations in the distribution of WBCs.

Step 5: Make note of immature cells in any cell line reported in the differential that should not appear in normal peripheral blood.

Step 6: Make note of any morphologic abnormalities and correlate film findings with the numerical values.

Red Blood Cells

Step 1: Examine the HGB concentration first to assess anemia.

Step 2: Examine the MCV to assess cell volume.

Step 3: Examine the MCHC to assess cell HGB concentration in RBC.

Step 4: Examine the RDW to assess anisocytosis. (Correlate both MCV and RDW with RBC histogram.)

Step 5: Examine the morphologic description and correlate with the numerical values. Look for evidence of a reticulocyte response.

Step 6: Review remaining information.

Platelets

Step 1: Examine the total platelet count.

Step 2: Examine the MPV to assess platelet volume.

Step 3: Examine platelet morphology and correlate with the numerical values.

HGB, Hemoglobin; *MCHC,* mean cell hemoglobin concentration; *MCV,* mean cell volume; *MPV,* mean platelet volume; *RBC,* red blood cell; *RDW,* RBC distribution width; *WBC,* white blood cell.

SUMMARY

- Although fewer manual peripheral blood film evaluations are performed today, much valuable information still can be obtained from a well-made and well-stained film.
- The specimen of choice for routine hematology testing is whole blood customarily collected in a lavender/purple topped tube. The tube additive is ethylenediaminetetraacetic acid (EDTA), which anticoagulates the blood by chelating plasma calcium.
- Only rarely does EDTA create problems in analyzing certain individuals' blood. EDTA-induced platelet clumping or satellitosis causes automated analyzers to report falsely decreased platelet counts (pseudothrombocytopenia) and falsely

increased white blood cell (WBC) counts (pseudoleukocytosis). This problem must be recognized through blood film examinations and the proper course of action followed to produce accurate results.

- Several methods exist for making peripheral blood films; however, the manual wedge film technique is used most often.
- Learning to make consistently good blood films takes practice. The basic technique can be modified as needed to accommodate specimens from patients with very high or very low hematocrits.
- The stain used routinely in hematology is Wright or Wright-Giemsa stain. Staining of all cellular elements occurs when

the pH-specific buffer is added to the stain already on the slide. Staining reactions depend on the pH of the cellular components.

- Wright staining is done manually, by automated techniques, or by quick stains, depending on the laboratory and the number of slides to be processed.
- Peripheral blood films and bone marrow smears always should be evaluated in a systematic manner, beginning with the 10× objective lens and finishing with the 100× oil immersion objective lens. Leukocyte differential and morphologic

evaluation, RBC and platelet morphologic evaluation, and platelet number estimate all are included.

- Use of a systematic approach to complete blood count (CBC) interpretation ensures that all valuable information is assessed and nothing is overlooked. The systematic approach to CBC interpretation is summarized in Box 13.9.

Now that you have completed this chapter, go back and read again the case study at the beginning and respond to the questions presented.

REVIEW QUESTIONS

Answers can be found in the Appendix.

1. A laboratory science student consistently makes wedge-technique blood films that are too long and thin. What change in technique would improve the films?
   a. Increasing the downward pressure on the pusher slide
   b. Decreasing the acute angle of the pusher slide
   c. Placing the drop of blood closer to the center of the slide
   d. Increasing the acute angle of the pusher slide

2. When a blood film is viewed through the microscope, the RBCs appear redder than normal, the neutrophils are barely visible, and the eosinophils are bright orange. What is the most likely cause?
   a. The slide was overstained.
   b. The stain was too alkaline.
   c. The buffer was too acidic.
   d. The slide was not rinsed adequately.

3. A stained blood film is held up to the light and observed to be bluer than normal. What microscopic abnormality might be expected on this film?
   a. Rouleaux
   b. Spherocytosis
   c. Reactive lymphocytosis
   d. Toxic granulation

4. A laboratorian using the 40× objective lens sees the following numbers of WBCs in 10 fields: 8, 4, 7, 5, 4, 7, 8, 6, 4, 6. Which of the following WBC counts most closely correlates with the estimate?
   a. 1.5×10^9/L
   b. 5.9×10^9/L
   c. 11.8×10^9/L
   d. 24×10^9/L

5. A blood film for a very anemic patient with an RBC count of 1.25×10^{12}/L shows an average of seven platelets per oil immersion field. Which of the following values most closely correlates with the estimate per microliter?
   a. 14,000
   b. 44,000
   c. 140,000
   d. 280,000

6. A blood film for a patient with a normal RBC count has an average of 10 platelets per oil immersion field. Which of the following values best correlates with the estimate per microliter?
   a. 20,000
   b. 100,000
   c. 200,000
   d. 400,000

7. What is the absolute count ($\times 10^9$/L) for the lymphocytes if the total WBC count is 9.5×10^9/L and there are 37% lymphocytes?
   a. 3.5
   b. 6.5
   c. 13
   d. 37

8. Which of the following blood film findings indicates EDTA-induced pseudothrombocytopenia?
   a. The platelets are pushed to the feathered end.
   b. The platelets are adhering to WBCs.
   c. No platelets at all are seen on the film.
   d. The slide has a bluish discoloration when examined macroscopically.

9. Which of the following is the best area to review or perform a differential on a stained blood film?
   a. Red blood cells are all overlapped in groups of three or more.
   b. Red blood cells are mostly separated, with a few overlapping.
   c. Red blood cells look flattened, with none touching.
   d. Red blood cells are separated and holes appear among the cells.

10. Use the reference intervals provided inside the front cover of this text. Given the following data, summarize the following blood picture:
    WBC: 86.3×10^9/L
    HGB: 9.7 g/dL
    HCT: 24.2%
    MCV: 87.8 fL
    MCHC: 33.5%
    PLT: 106×10^9/L
    a. Leukocytosis, normocytic-normochromic anemia, thrombocytopenia
    b. Microcytic-hypochromic anemia, thrombocytopenia
    c. Neutrophilia, macrocytic anemia, thrombocytosis
    d. Leukocytosis, thrombocytopenia

REFERENCES

1. Kennedy, J. B., Maehara, K. T., & Baker, A. M. (1981). Cell and platelet stability in disodium and tripotassium EDTA. *Am J Med Technol, 47,* 89–93.

2. Smock, K. J., & Perkins, S. L. (2014). Examination of the blood and bone marrow. In Greer, J. P., Arber, D. A., Glader, B., et al. (Eds.), *Wintrobe's Clinical Hematology.* (13th ed., pp. 1–18). Philadelphia: Wolters Kluwer Health/Lippincott Williams & Wilkins.

3. Shahab, N., & Evans, M. L. (1998). Platelet satellitism. *N Engl J Med, 338,* 591.

4. Bartels, P. C., Schoorl, M., & Lombarts, A. J. (1997). Screening for EDTA-dependent deviations in platelet counts and abnormalities in platelet distribution histograms in pseudothrombocytopenia. *Scand J Clin Lab Invest, 57,* 629–636.

5. Lombarts, A., & deKieviet, W. (1988). Recognition and prevention of pseudothrombocytopenia and concomitant pseudoleukocytosis. *Am J Clin Pathol, 89,* 634–639.

6. De Caterina, M., Fratellanza, G., Grimaldi, E., et al. (1993). Evidence of a cold immunoglobulin M autoantibody against 78 kD platelet gp in a case of EDTA-dependent pseudothrombocytopenia. *Am J Clin Pathol, 99,* 163–167.

7. Alpha Scientific Corp. *Diff-safe blood dispenser.* http://www.alpha-scientific.com/Diff-safe.html. Accessed October 28, 2018.

8. Power, K. T. (1982). The Romanowsky stains: a review. *Am J Med Technol, 48,* 519–523.

9. MacGregor, R. G., Scott, R. W., & Loh, G. L. (1940). The differential leukocyte count. *J Pathol Bacteriol, 51,* 337–368.

10. Palmer, L., Briggs, C., McFadden, S., et al. (2015). ICSH recommendation for the standardization of nomenclature and grading of peripheral blood cell morphological features. *Int J Lab Hematol, 37,* 287–303.

11. Cellavision. *Introducing CellaVision DM9600.* http://www.cellavision.com/en/our-products/products/cellavision-dm9600. Accessed October 28, 2018.

12. Briggs, C., Harrison, P., & Machin, S. J. (2007). Continuing developments with the automated platelet count. Int *J Lab Hematol, 29,* 77–91

13. Abe, Y., Wada, H., Sakakura, M., et al. (2005). Usefulness of fully automated measurement of reticulated platelets using whole blood. *Clin Appl Thromb Hemost, 11,* 263–270.

14. Ryan, D. H. (2016). Examination of the blood cells. In Kaushansky, K., Lichtman, M. A., Prchal, J. T. et al. (Eds.), *Williams Hematology.* (9th ed., pp. 11–25). New York: McGraw-Hill.

15. Cornbleet, P. J. (2002). Clinical utility of the band count. *Clin Lab Med.* Mar, 22(1), 101–136.

16. CLSI. (2007). *Reference Leukocyte (WBC) Differential Count (Proportional) and Evaluation of Instrumental Methods.* (2nd ed., approved standard, H20-A2). Wayne, PA: Clinical and Laboratory Standards Institute.

Bone Marrow Examination

*Kamran M. Mirza**

OBJECTIVES

After completion of this chapter, the reader will be able to:

1. Diagram bone marrow architecture and locate hematopoietic tissue.
2. List indications for bone marrow examinations.
3. Specify sites for bone marrow aspirate and biopsy.
4. Assemble supplies for performing and assisting in bone marrow specimen collection.
5. Assist the physician with bone marrow sample preparation subsequent to collection.
6. List the information gained from bone marrow aspirates and biopsy specimens.
7. Perform a bone marrow aspirate smear and core biopsy specimen examination.
8. List the normal hematopoietic and stromal cells of the bone marrow and their anticipated distribution.
9. Perform a bone marrow differential count and compute the myeloid-to-erythroid ratio.
10. Characterize features of hematopoietic and metastatic tumor cells.
11. Prepare specimens for and assist in performing specialized confirmatory bone marrow studies.
12. Prepare a systematic written bone marrow examination report.

OUTLINE

Bone Marrow Anatomy and Architecture
Indications for Bone Marrow Examination
Bone Marrow Specimen Collection Sites
Bone Marrow Aspiration and Biopsy
  Preparation
  Core Biopsy Procedure
  Aspiration Procedure
  Patient Care
Preparation of the Bone Marrow Specimen
  Direct Aspirate Smears
  Anticoagulated Aspirate Smears
  Crush Smears of Bone Marrow Aspirate

Concentrate (Buffy Coat) Smears
Core Biopsy Imprints (Touch Preparations)
Histologic Sections (Cell Block) of the Core Biopsy
Marrow Core Biopsy and Aspirate Smear Stains
Examining Bone Marrow Aspirate or Imprint
  Low-Power (100×) Examination
  High-Power (500×) Examination
  Prussian Blue Iron Stain Examination
Examining the Bone Marrow Core Biopsy Specimen
Definitive Bone Marrow Studies
Bone Marrow Examination Reports

CASE STUDY

After studying the material in this chapter, the reader should be able to respond to the following case study:

A patient presents with complaints of several weeks of weakness, fatigue, and malaise. Complete blood count results reveal the following:

HGB concentration: 7.5 gm/dL
HCT: 21%
RBC count: 2.5 × 10^{12}/L

Segmented neutrophils: 21 × 10^9/L (70%)
Immature neutrophils: 6 × 10^9/L (20%)
Basophils: 1.5 × 10^9/L (5%)

WBC count: 30 × 10^9/L
Platelet count: 540 × 10^9/L

Eosinophils: 0.3 × 10^9/L (1%)

Bone marrow examination reveals a hypercellular marrow with 90% myeloid precursors and 10% erythroid precursors. There are 15 megakaryocytes per 10× microscopic objective field.
1. What bone marrow finding provides information on blood cell production?
2. What is the myeloid-to-erythroid ratio in this patient, and what does it indicate?
3. What megakaryocyte distribution is normally seen in a bone marrow aspirate?

*The author extends appreciation to George A. Fritsma, whose work in prior editions provided the foundation for this chapter.

BONE MARROW ANATOMY AND ARCHITECTURE

In adults, bone marrow accounts for 3.4% to 5.9% of body weight, contributes 1600 to 3700 g or a volume of 30 to 50 mL/kg, and produces roughly 6 billion blood cells per kilogram per day in a process called hematopoiesis.[1] At birth, nearly all bones contain red hematopoietic marrow (Chapter 4). In the fifth to seventh year of life, adipocytes (fat cells) begin to replace red marrow in the long bones of the hands, feet, legs, and arms, producing yellow marrow, and by late adolescence hematopoietic marrow is limited to the lower skull, vertebrae, shoulder, pelvic girdle, ribs, and sternum (Figure 4.2). Although the percentage of bony space devoted to hematopoiesis is considerably reduced, the overall volume remains approximately constant as the individual matures.[2] Yellow marrow retains the ability to revert to active hematopoiesis by increasing red marrow volume, in conditions such as chronic blood loss or hemolytic anemia when there is increased demand.

The arrangement of red marrow and its relationship to the central venous sinus are illustrated in Figures 4.3 and 4.4. Hematopoietic tissue is enmeshed in spongy trabeculae (bony tissue) surrounding a network of sinuses that originate at the endosteum (vascular layer just within the bone) and terminate in collecting venules.[3] Adipocytes occupy approximately 50% of red hematopoietic marrow space in a 30- to 70-year-old adult, and fatty metamorphosis increases approximately 10% per decade after age 70.[4]

INDICATIONS FOR BONE MARROW EXAMINATION

Because the procedure is invasive, the decision to collect and examine a bone marrow specimen requires clinical judgment and the application of inclusion criteria. With improvements in flow cytometry phenotyping and increasing availability of 10-color laser instrumentation, immunohistochemistry, cytogenetic studies, and molecular diagnostics such as circulating tumor cell analysis, peripheral blood may often provide information historically available only from bone marrow, reducing the demand for marrow specimens. On the other hand, these advanced techniques also augment bone marrow-based diagnosis and thus potentially raise the demand for bone marrow examinations in assessment of conditions not previously diagnosed through bone marrow examination.

Table 14.1 summarizes indications for a bone marrow examination.[5] Bone marrow examination may be used to diagnose and stage hematologic and nonhematologic neoplasia, to determine the cause of cytopenias, and to confirm or exclude metabolic or infectious conditions suspected on the basis of clinical symptoms and peripheral blood findings.[6]

Each bone marrow procedure is ordered after thorough consideration of clinical and laboratory information. For instance, bone marrow examination is most likely unnecessary in anemia when the cause is apparent from red blood cell (RBC) indices, serum iron and ferritin levels, or vitamin B_{12} and folate levels. Multilineage abnormalities, circulating blasts in adults, and unexpected pancytopenia usually prompt marrow examination.

TABLE 14.1   Indications for Bone Marrow Examination

Indication	Examples
Neoplasia diagnosis	Acute leukemias
	Myeloproliferative neoplasms such as chronic leukemias, myelofibrosis
	Myelodysplastic neoplasms such as refractory anemia
	Lymphoproliferative disorders such as acute lymphoblastic leukemia
	Immunoglobulin disorders such as plasma cell myeloma, macroglobulinemia
	Metastatic tumors
Neoplasia diagnosis and staging	Hodgkin and non-Hodgkin lymphoma
Marrow failure: cytopenias	Hypoplastic or aplastic anemia
	Pure red cell aplasia
	Idiosyncratic drug-induced marrow suppression
	Myelodysplastic syndromes such as refractory anemia
	Marrow necrosis secondary to tumor
	Marrow necrosis secondary to severe infection such as parvovirus B19 infection
	Immune versus amegakaryocytic thrombocytopenia
	Sickle cell crisis
	Differentiation of megaloblastic, iron deficiency, sideroblastic, hemolytic, and blood loss anemia
	Estimation of storage iron to assess for iron deficiency
	Infiltrative processes or fibrosis
Metabolic disorders	Gaucher disease
	Mast cell disease
Infections	Granulomatous disease
	Miliary tuberculosis
	Fungal infections
	Hemophagocytic syndromes
Monitoring of treatment	After chemotherapy or radiation therapy to assess minimal residual disease
	After stem cell transplantation to assess engraftment

Bone marrow puncture is prohibited in patients with coagulopathies such as hemophilia or vitamin K deficiency, although thrombocytopenia (low platelet count) is not an absolute contraindication. Special precautions such as bridging therapy may be necessary to prevent uncontrolled bleeding when a bone marrow procedure is performed on a patient receiving anticoagulant therapy, such as Coumadin or heparin.

BONE MARROW SPECIMEN COLLECTION SITES

Bone marrow specimen collection is a collaborative effort between a medical laboratory professional and a skilled specialty physician, often a pathologist or hematologist.[7] Before bone marrow collection, a medical laboratory practitioner or phlebotomist typically collects peripheral blood for a complete blood count (CBC) with blood film examination. During bone marrow collection, the medical laboratory professional assists the physician by managing the specimens and producing initial preparations for examination.

Red marrow is gelatinous and amenable to sampling. Most bone marrow specimens consist of an *aspirate* (obtained by bone marrow aspiration) and a *core biopsy* specimen (obtained by trephine biopsy), both examined with light microscopy using varying magnification. The aspirate is examined to identify the types and proportions of hematologic cells and to look for *morphologic variance.* The core biopsy specimen demonstrates *bone marrow architecture:* the spatial relationship of hematologic cells to fat, connective tissue, and bony stroma. The core biopsy specimen is also used to estimate *cellularity.*

The core biopsy specimen is particularly important for evaluating diseases that characteristically produce focal lesions, rather than diffuse involvement of the marrow. Hodgkin lymphoma, non-Hodgkin lymphoma, multiple myeloma, metastatic tumors, amyloid, and granulomas may produce predominantly focal lesions. Granulomas, or granulomatous lesions, are cell accumulations that contain *Langerhans cells*—large, activated granular macrophages that look like epithelial cells. Granulomas signal chronic infection. The biopsy specimen also allows for morphologic evaluation of bony spicules, which may reveal changes associated with hyperparathyroidism or Paget disease.[8]

Bone marrow collection sites include the following:

- *Posterior superior iliac crest* of the pelvis (Figure 14.1). In both adults and children, this site provides adequate red marrow that is isolated from anatomic structures that are subject to injury. This site is used for both aspiration and core biopsy.
- *Anterior superior iliac crest* of the pelvis. This site has the same advantages as the posterior superior iliac crest, but the cortical bone is thicker. This site may be preferred for a patient who can only lie supine.
- *Sternum,* below the angle of Lewis at the second intercostal space. In adults, the sternum provides ample material for

aspiration but is only 1 cm thick and cannot be used for core biopsy. It is possible for the physician to accidentally pierce through the sternum and enter the pericardium, damaging the heart or great vessels.

- *Anterior medial surface of the tibia* in children younger than age 2. This site may be used only for aspiration.
- *Spinous process of the vertebrae, ribs,* or other red marrow-containing bones. These locations are available but are rarely used unless one is the site of a suspicious lesion discovered on a radiograph.

Adverse outcomes occur in less than 0.05% of marrow collections. Infections and reactions to anesthetics may occur, but the most common side effect is hemorrhage associated with platelet function disorder or thrombocytopenia.

BONE MARROW ASPIRATION AND BIOPSY

Preparation

Less than 24 hours before bone marrow collection, the medical laboratory professional or phlebotomist collects venous peripheral blood for a CBC and blood film examination using a standard collection procedure. Peripheral blood collection is often accomplished immediately before bone marrow specimen collection. The peripheral blood specimen is seldom collected after bone marrow collection to avoid stress-related white blood cell count elevation.

Most institutions purchase or assemble disposable sterile bone marrow specimen collection trays that provide the following:

- Surgical gloves
- Shaving equipment
- Antiseptic solution and alcohol pads
- Drape material
- Local anesthetic injection, usually 1% lidocaine, not to exceed 20 mL per patient
- No. 11 scalpel blade for skin incision
- Disposable Jamshidi biopsy needle (Care Fusion; Figure 14.2) or Westerman-Jensen needle (Becton, Dickinson; Figure 14.3). Both provide an obturator, core biopsy tool, and stylet.

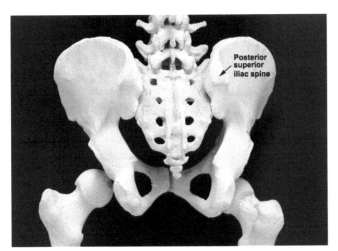

Figure 14.1 Bone Marrow Specimen Collection Site. The posterior superior iliac crest is the favored site for obtaining the bone marrow aspirate and core biopsy specimen because it provides ample marrow and is isolated from structures that could be damaged by accidental puncture. (Courtesy Indiana Pathology Images, Indianapolis, IN.)

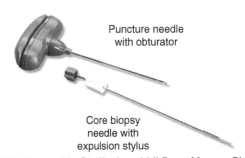

Figure 14.2 Disposable Sterile Jamshidi Bone Marrow Biopsy and Aspiration Needle. The outer puncture cannula is advanced to the medullary cavity of the bone with the obturator in place to prevent bone coring. The physician removes the obturator and slides the core biopsy needle through the cannula and into the medulla with the expulsion stylus removed. The core biopsy needle is removed from the puncture needle with the specimen in place. The specimen is expelled using the stylus. (Courtesy Care Fusion, McGaw Park, IL.)

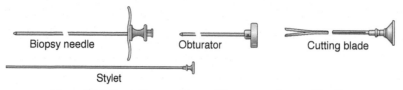

Figure 14.3 Bone Marrow Biopsy Westerman-Jensen Needle.

A Snarecoil biopsy needle also is available (Kendall Company). The Snarecoil has a coil mechanism at the needle tip that allows for capture of the bone marrow specimen without needle redirection (Figure 14.4).

- Disposable 14- to 18-gauge aspiration needle with obturator. Alternatively, the University of Illinois aspiration needle may be used for sternal puncture. The University of Illinois needle provides a flange that prevents penetration of the sternum to the pericardium.
- Microscope slides or coverslips washed in 70% ethanol
- Petri dishes or shallow circular watch glasses
- Vials or test tubes with closures
- Wintrobe hematocrit tubes
- Anticoagulant liquid tripotassium ethylenediaminetetraacetic acid (EDTA)
- Zenker fixative: potassium dichromate, mercuric chloride, sodium sulfate, and glacial acetic acid; B5 fixative: aqueous mercuric chloride and sodium acetate; or 10% neutral

formalin. Controlled disposal is required for Zenker fixative and B5 that contain toxic mercury.
- Gauze dressings

The entire procedure is depicted in Figure 14.5. After an appropriate "time out" procedure wherein the patient's name and date of birth are confirmed, the patient is asked to lie supine, prone, or in the right or left lateral decubitus position (lying on the right or left side). With attention to standard precautions, the skin is shaved if necessary, disinfected, and draped.

The physician palpates the biopsy site (Figure 14.5A), then infiltrates the skin, dermis, and subcutaneous tissue with a local anesthetic solution (Figure 14.5B) through a 25-gauge needle producing a 0.5- to 1.0-cm papule (bubble). The 25-gauge needle is replaced with a 21-gauge needle, which is inserted through the papule to the periosteum (bone surface). With the point of the needle on the periosteum, the physician injects approximately 2 mL of anesthetic over a dime-sized area while rotating the needle, and then withdraws the anesthesia needle. Next, the physician makes a 3-mm skin incision over the puncture site with a no. 11 scalpel blade to prevent skin coring during insertion of the needle.

Core Biopsy Procedure

The biopsy specimen is typically collected first, because aspiration may destroy marrow architecture; however, some health care providers prefer to take this specimen after the aspiration; there remains no gold standard. After the incision is made, the physician inserts a Jamshidi outer cannula with the obturator in place through the skin and cortex of the bone. The obturator prevents coring of skin or bone. Reciprocating rotation promotes the forward advancement of the cannula (Figure 14.5C and D). A weakening of resistance indicates penetration through the cortex to the inner medullary cavity of the bone. The physician removes the obturator, inserts the biopsy needle through the cannula, and slowly advances the needle 2 to 3 cm with continuous reciprocating rotation along the long axis (Figure 14.5E). The physician changes the needle angle slightly to separate the core cylinder specimen from its marrow cavity attachments. The biopsy needle and cannula are withdrawn from the bone, taking the core cylinder with them. The core cylinder is 1 to 1.5 cm long and 1 to 2 mm in diameter and weighs about 150 mg. The biopsy needle is placed over an ethanol-cleaned slide, and the stylus is pushed through to dislodge the core cylinder onto the slide (Figure 14.5F). Using sterile forceps, the medical laboratory professional prepares imprints (*touch preparations*) of the core biopsy onto multiple glass slides. The core cylinder is then transferred to the chosen fixative (Zenker, B5, or formalin).

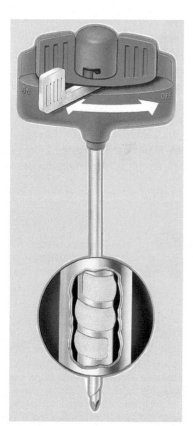

Figure 14.4 Snarecoil Bone Marrow Biopsy Needle. The coil mechanism resides within the biopsy needle as illustrated in the magnified image. The coil is turned to draw the marrow specimen into the needle. (Courtesy Tyco Healthcare/Kendall, Mansfield, MA.)

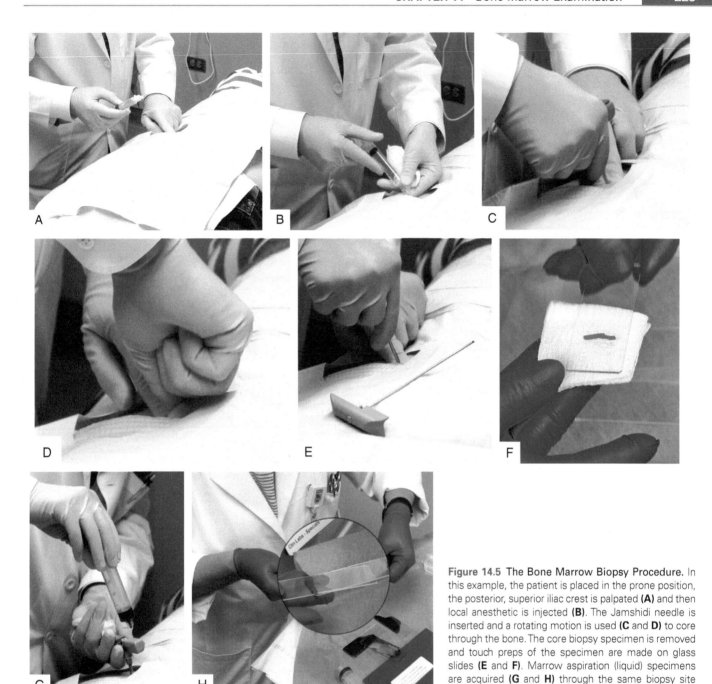

Figure 14.5 The Bone Marrow Biopsy Procedure. In this example, the patient is placed in the prone position, the posterior, superior iliac crest is palpated (**A**) and then local anesthetic is injected (**B**). The Jamshidi needle is inserted and a rotating motion is used (**C** and **D**) to core through the bone. The core biopsy specimen is removed and touch preps of the specimen are made on glass slides (**E** and **F**). Marrow aspiration (liquid) specimens are acquired (**G** and **H**) through the same biopsy site using an aspiration needle in a second quick accession.

When the Westerman-Jensen needle is used, the physician punctures through the bone cortex with the needle and the obturator in place. The obturator is then removed, the cutting blades inserted through the cannula, and the blades advanced into the medullary cavity of the bone (Figure 14.6). The cutting blades are pressed into the medullary bone, with the outer cannula held firmly in a stationary position. The physician slowly withdraws the blades so that the cannula entraps the tissue, and then withdraws the entire unit. The core cylinder is removed by inserting the probe through the cutting tip and extruding the specimen through the hub of the needle to the selected slide and fixative-containing receptacles.

Aspiration Procedure

Using the same insertion point, but in a separate location from the biopsy site, the physician inserts a 14- to 18-gauge aspiration needle such as the University of Illinois needle, with obturator, through the skin and cortex of the bone. The obturator is removed, and a 10- to 20-mL syringe is attached. The physician withdraws the plunger to create negative pressure and aspirates 1.0 to 1.5 mL of marrow into the syringe (Figure 14.5G). Collecting more than 1.5 mL dilutes the hematopoietic marrow with sinusoidal (peripheral) blood. The physician detaches the syringe and passes it *immediately* to the medical laboratory professional, who expels the material onto a series of clean and

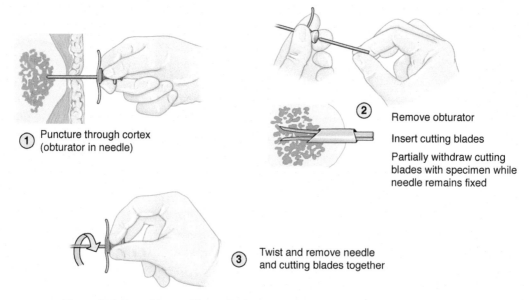

① Puncture through cortex
(obturator in needle)

② Remove obturator

Insert cutting blades

Partially withdraw cutting
blades with specimen while
needle remains fixed

③ Twist and remove needle
and cutting blades together

Figure 14.6 Bone Marrow Biopsy Technique Using the Westerman-Jensen Needle.

sterile microscopic slides or coverslips. A series of aspirate smear slides can be made (Figure 14.5H). The physician may attach a second syringe to aspirate an additional specimen for cytogenetic analysis, molecular diagnosis, or immunophenotyping using flow cytometry. The needle is then withdrawn, and pressure is applied to the wound.

If no marrow is obtained, the physician returns the obturator to the needle, advances the needle, attaches a fresh syringe, and tries again. The syringe and needle are retracted slightly and the process is repeated. If this attempt is unsuccessful, the physician removes the needle and syringe, applies pressure, and begins the procedure at a new site. If the marrow is fibrotic, acellular, or packed with leukemic cells, the first and second aspiration may be unsuccessful, known as a *dry tap*. In this case a core biopsy (described earlier) is necessary to confirm whether this is indeed a dry tap, in which case the core biopsy specimen will demonstrate a fibrotic, packed marrow (or an empty marrow in cases where the cellularity is very low), versus improper sampling (Table 14.2).

Patient Care

Subsequent to bone marrow biopsy or aspiration, the physician applies a pressure dressing and advises the patient to remain in the same position for 60 minutes to prevent bleeding.

PREPARATION OF THE BONE MARROW SPECIMEN

Direct Aspirate Smears

During the bone marrow biopsy procedure, the medical laboratory professional receives the aspirate syringe from the physician at the bedside and *immediately* transfers drops of the freshly collected marrow specimen onto six (or more) ethanol-washed microscope slides (Figure 14.5H). Marrow clots rapidly, so good organization is essential. Using spreader slides, the

TABLE 14.2 Advantages and Disadvantages of the Marrow Aspirate Smear and Marrow Core Biopsy

	Marrow Aspirate Smear	Marrow Core Biopsy
Advantages	Fast	Ability to analyze both cells and stroma
	No need for decalcification of the specimen	Represents all cells
	Quantification of cell type differential count	Explains dry taps
	Material for ancillary studies (flow, molecular)	
Disadvantages	May not represent all cells	Slow processing
	Dry tap in cases of fibrosis or hypocellularity	Decalcification precludes certain ancillary studies
	Does not represent architecture	Inability to perform quantitative differential count
	Inability to analyze the stroma	

medical laboratory professional spreads the drop into a wedge-shaped smear ½ to ¾ the length of the slide, similar to a peripheral blood film (Chapter 13). Bony spicules 0.5 to 1.0 mm in diameter and larger fat globules follow behind the spreader and become deposited on the slide. In the direct smear preparation the medical laboratory professional avoids crushing the spicules. The medical laboratory professional may lightly fan the smears (avoid blowing because the humidity in the breath distorts the morphology) to promote rapid drying in an effort to preserve cell morphology.

In the syringe the specimen consists of peripheral blood with suspended light-colored bony spicules and fat globules. The medical laboratory professional evaluates the syringe blood for spicules: More spicules are associated with a specimen with more cells to identify and categorize. If the specimen has few fat globules or spicules, the medical laboratory professional may alert the physician to collect an additional specimen.

Anticoagulated Aspirate Smears

Anticoagulated specimens are a more leisurely alternative to direct aspirate smears. The medical laboratory professional expresses the aspirate from the syringe into a vial containing EDTA and subsequently pipettes the anticoagulated aspirate to clean glass slides, spreading the aspirate using the same approach as in direct smear preparation. All anticoagulants distort cell morphology, but EDTA generates the least distortion.

Crush Smears of Bone Marrow Aspirate

To prepare crush smears, the medical laboratory professional expels a portion of the aspirate to a Petri dish or watch glass covered with a few milliliters of EDTA solution and spreads the aspirate over the surface with a sterile applicator. Individual bony spicules are transferred using applicators, forceps, or micropipettes (preferred) to several ethanol-washed glass slides. For each slide the medical laboratory professional places another glass slide directly over the specimen at a right angle and presses gently to crush the spicules. The slides are separated laterally to create two rectangular smears, which may be fanned to encourage rapid drying.

Some medical laboratory professionals prefer to transfer the aspirate directly to the slide, subsequently tilting the slide to drain off peripheral blood while retaining spicules. Once drained, the spicules are then crushed with a second slide as described earlier.

The medical laboratory professional may add one drop of 22% albumin to the EDTA solution, particularly if the specimen is suspected to contain prolymphocytes or lymphoblasts, which tend to rupture. The albumin reduces the occurrence of "smudge" or "basket" cells often seen in lymphoid marrow lesions.

The crush preparation procedure may also be performed using ethanol-washed coverslips in place of slides. The coverslip method demands adroit manipulation but may yield better morphologic information, because the smaller coverslips generate less cell rupture during separation. Use of glass slides offers the opportunity for automated staining, whereas coverslip preparations must first be affixed smear side up to slides and then stained manually (Chapter 13).

Concentrate (Buffy Coat) Smears

Buffy coat smears are useful when there are sparse nucleated cells in the direct marrow aspirate smear or when the number of nucleated cells is anticipated to be small, as in aplastic anemia. The medical laboratory professional transfers approximately 1.5 mL of EDTA-anticoagulated marrow aspirate specimen to a narrow-bore glass or plastic tube such as a Wintrobe hematocrit tube. The tube is centrifuged at 2500 g for 10 minutes and examined for four layers.

The top layer is yellowish fat and normally occupies 1% to 3% of the column. The second layer, plasma, varies in volume, depending on the amount of peripheral blood in the specimen.

The third layer consists of nucleated cells and is called the *myeloid-erythroid* (ME) layer. The ME layer is normally 5% to 8% of the total column. The bottom layer is RBCs, and its volume, like that of the plasma layer, depends on the amount of peripheral blood present. The medical laboratory professional records the ratio of the fat and ME layers using millimeter gradations on the tube.

Once the column is examined, the medical laboratory professional aspirates a portion of the ME layer with a portion of plasma and transfers the suspension to a Petri dish or watch glass. Marrow smears are subsequently prepared using the crush smear technique.

The concentrated buffy coat smear compensates for hypocellular marrow and allows for examination of large numbers of nucleated cells without interference from fat or RBCs. On the other hand, cell distribution is distorted by the procedure. Therefore the medical laboratory professional does not estimate numbers of different cell types or maturation stages on a buffy coat smear.

Core Biopsy Imprints (Touch Preparations)

Core biopsy specimens and clotted marrow may be held in forceps and repeatedly touched to a washed glass slide or coverslip so that cells attach and rapidly dry (Figure 14.5H). When touching the specimen to the glass slide, the medical laboratory professional lifts directly upward to prevent cell distortion. Imprints are valuable when the specimen has clotted or there is a dry tap (no specimen collected with the aspiration technique). The cell morphology may closely replicate aspirate morphology, although few spicules are transferred.

Histologic Sections (Cell Block) of the Core Biopsy

After the medical laboratory professional has prepared aspirate smears and has distributed aliquots of marrow for cytogenetic, molecular, and immunophenotypic studies, the remaining core biopsy specimen, spicules, or clotted specimen is submitted to histology for preparation. The specimen is suspended in 10% formalin, Zenker glacial acetic acid, or B5 fixative for approximately 2 hours.

The fixed specimen is subsequently centrifuged, and the pellet is decalcified and wrapped in an embedding bag or lens paper and placed in a paraffin-embedding cassette. A histotechnologist sections the embedded specimen, applies hematoxylin and eosin (H&E) stain, and examines the section.

Marrow Core Biopsy and Aspirate Smear Stains

Marrow aspirate smears are stained with *Wright or Wright-Giemsa stains* using the same protocols as for peripheral blood film staining (Chapter 13). Some laboratory personnel prefer to increase staining time to compensate for the relative thickness of marrow smears compared with peripheral blood films.

Marrow aspirate smears and core biopsy specimens may also be stained using an acidic potassium ferrocyanide *(Prussian blue)* solution to detect and estimate marrow storage iron or iron metabolism abnormalities (Chapter 17). Further, a number of *cytochemical* stains may be used for cell identification or differentiation (Table 14.3).

TABLE 14.3 Cytochemical Stains Used to Identify Bone Marrow Cells and Maturation Stages

Cytochemical Stain	Application
Myeloperoxidase (MPO)	Detects myeloid cells by staining cytoplasmic granular contents
Sudan black B (SBB)	Detects myeloid cells by staining cytoplasmic granular contents
Periodic acid-Schiff (PAS)	Detects lymphocytic cells and certain abnormal erythroid cells by staining of cytoplasmic glycogen
Esterases	Distinguish myeloid from monocytic maturation stages (several esterase substrates)
Tartrate-resistant acid phosphatase (TRAP)	Detects tartrate-resistant acid phosphatase granules in hairy cell leukemia

EXAMINING BONE MARROW ASPIRATE OR IMPRINT

The microscopic examination of a bone marrow specimen is critical for the diagnosis of hematologic disorders. A list of the important components of the examination, to be described in this chapter, is provided in Table 14.4. Final interpretation of the marrow should be integrated with results from the clinical history, blood film, cell counts, laboratory data, cell marker studies, and molecular or cytogenetic data.

TABLE 14.4 Components of a Bone Marrow Examination

Component	Description
Cellularity	Hypocellular, normocellular, or hypercellular classification based on ratio of hematopoietic cells to adipocytes
Megakaryocytes	Estimate using 10× objective lens (100× magnification), compare with reference interval and comment on morphology
Maturation	Narrative characterizing the maturation of the myeloid and erythroid (normoblastic, rubricytic) series
Additional hematologic cells	Narrative describing numbers and morphology of eosinophils, basophils, mast cells, lymphocytes, plasma cells, monocytes, and histiocytes if appropriate, with reference intervals
Stromal cells	Narrative describing numbers and morphology of osteoblasts, osteoclasts, bony trabeculae, fibroblasts, adipocytes, and endothelial cells; appearance of sinuses; presence of amyloid, granulomas, fibrosis, necrosis
Differential count	Numbers of all cells and cell stages observed after performing a differential count on 300–1000 cells and comparing results with reference intervals
Myeloid-to-erythroid ratio	Computed from nucleated hematologic cells excluding lymphocytes, plasma cells, monocytes, and histiocytes
Iron stores	Categorization of findings as increased, normal, or decreased iron stores

Examination of the marrow aspirate or imprint cytology begins with a low-power review of the general organization, character, and cellular quality of the whole specimen, including the presence (or absence) of bone spicules. With reference to the patient's age and clinical indication for the marrow examination, the estimation of cellularity is made as a ratio of the nucleated cells and the presence of the adipocytes. Normal, large megakaryocytes are usually easily appreciated at low power, and care should be taken in noting the presence of any cohesive clusters of nonhematopoietic cells. As a rule, hematopoietic cells are always present as discohesive cells that do not form structures. The examination then follows an algorithm of intermediate and high-power assessment that entails a detailed review of all three cell lines with the goal of assessing progressive trilineage hematopoiesis. Box 14.1 describes the uses of low- and high-power objective lenses in examining bone marrow aspirate direct smears or imprints.

Low-Power (100×) Examination

Once the bone marrow aspirate direct smear or imprint is prepared and stained, the medical laboratory professional or pathologist begins the microscopic examination using the low-power (10×) dry lens, which, when linked with 10× oculars, provides a total 100× magnification. Most bone marrow examinations are performed using a teaching format that employs projection or multiheaded microscopes to allow observation by residents, fellows, medical laboratory students, and attending staff. The microscopist locates the bony spicules, aggregations of bone, and hematopoietic cells, all of which stain dark blue (Figure 14.7). In imprints, spicules are sparse or absent; the search is for hematopoietic cells. Within these areas the microscopist selects intact and nearly contiguous nucleated cells for examination, avoiding areas of distorted morphology or areas diluted with sinusoidal blood.

Near the spicules, cellularity is estimated by observing the proportion of *hematopoietic* cells to *adipocytes* (clear fat areas).[9] For anterior or posterior iliac crest marrow, 50% cellularity is normal for patients aged 30 to 70 years. In childhood, cellularity is 80%, and after age 70, cellularity becomes

BOX 14.1 Bone Marrow Aspirate Microscopic Smear Examination: Low and High Power

Low Power: 10× Objective Lens (100× total magnification)
- Assess peripheral blood dilution
- Find bony spicules and areas of clear cell morphology
- Observe fat-to-marrow ratio, estimate cellularity
- Search for tumor cells in clusters
- Examine and estimate megakaryocytes

High Power: 50× and 100× Objective Lenses (500× and 1000× total magnification)
- Observe granulocytic and erythroid maturation
- Distinguish abnormal distribution of cells or cell maturation stages
- Perform differential count on 300–1000 cells
- Compute myeloid-to-erythroid ratio

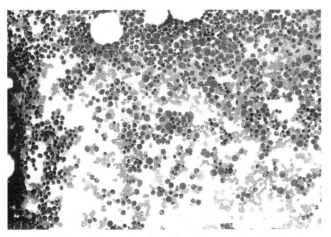

Figure 14.7 Bone Marrow Aspirate Specimen. Note the intact, contiguous cells and adipocytes. This illustrate a good site for morphologic evaluation and cell counting. (Wright-Giemsa stain, ×100.)

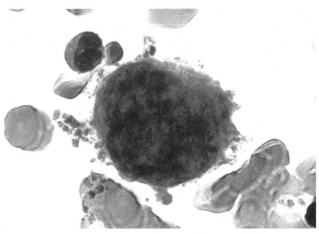

Figure 14.8 Bone Marrow Aspirate Smear Showing a Megakaryocyte. Note the platelets budding from the megakaryocyte at the plasma membrane. (Wright-Giemsa stain, ×1000.)

reduced. For those older than age 70, a rule of thumb is to subtract patient age from 100% and add ±10%. Thus for a 75-year-old, the anticipated cellularity is 15% to 35%. By comparing with the age-related normal cellularity values, the microscopist classifies the observed area as *hypocellular, normocellular,* or *hypercellular.* If a core biopsy specimen was collected, it provides a more accurate estimate of cellularity than an aspirate smear, because in aspirates there is always some dilution of hematopoietic tissue with peripheral blood. In the absence of leukemia, lymphocytes should total fewer than 30% of nucleated cells; if more are present, the marrow specimen has been substantially diluted and should not be used to estimate cellularity.[10]

Hematopoietic cells are normally discohesive (loose intercellular connections), a feature that is helpful to visualize normal cells using the 10× objective lens. At this magnification, for screening purposes, the microscopist searches for abnormal, often molded, cell clusters (syncytia) of *metastatic tumor cells* or other abnormal infiltrating cells such as *lymphoma cells or plasma cells.* Tumor cell nuclei often stain darkly (hyperchromatic), and vacuoles are seen in the cytoplasm. Tumor cell clusters are often found near the edges of the smear because of their buoyancy.

Although myeloid (granulocytic) cells and erythroid cells are best examined using 500× magnification, they may be more easily distinguished from each other using the 10× objective lens. The erythroid maturation stages stain more intensely, and their margins are more sharply defined, features more easily distinguished at lower magnification.

The microscopist evaluates *megakaryocytes* using low power (Figure 14.8). Megakaryocytes are the largest cells in the bone marrow, 30 to 50 μm in diameter, with multilobed nuclei (Chapter 10). Although in special circumstances microscopists may differentiate three megakaryocyte maturation stages-*megakaryoblast, promegakaryocyte,* and *megakaryocyte* (MK-I to MK-III)—a total megakaryocyte estimate is generally satisfactory. In a well-prepared aspirate or biopsy specimen, the microscopist observes 2 to 10 megakaryocytes per low-power field.

Deviations yield important information and are reported as decreased or increased megakaryocytes. Bone marrow megakaryocyte estimates are essential to the evaluation of peripheral blood *thrombocytopenia* and *thrombocytosis*; for instance, in immune thrombocytopenia, an increased number of marrow megakaryocytes is not uncommon.

Abnormal megakaryocytes may be small, lack granularity, or have poorly lobulated or hyperlobulated nuclei. Indications of abnormality may be visible using low power; however, conclusive descriptions require 500× or even 1000× total magnification.

High-Power (500×) Examination

Having located a suitable area on the slide for examination of the cells, the microscopist places a drop of immersion oil on the specimen and switches to the 50× objective lens, providing 500× total magnification. All of the *nucleated cells* are reviewed for morphology and normal maturation. Besides megakaryocytes, cells of the granulocytic (Figures 14.9 through 14.12) and erythroid (rubricytic, normoblastic) (Figure 14.13) series should be present, along with eosinophils, basophils, lymphocytes, plasma cells, monocytes, and histiocytes. Chapters 4, 5, and 9 provide detailed cell and cell maturation stage descriptions. Table 14.5 names all normal marrow cells and provides their expected percentages.

The microscopist searches for maturation gaps, misdistribution of maturation stages, and abnormal morphology. Although the specimen is customarily reviewed using the 50× oil immersion objective lens, the 100× oil immersion objective lens is often employed to detect small but significant morphologic abnormalities in the nuclei and cytoplasm of suspect cells.

WHO Classification of Tumors of Haematopoietic and Lymphoid Tissues (2008 and 2016) requires a 500 cell differential count of nucleated marrow cells. Many laboratory directors may mandate a different number; ranging from a differential count of 500 to 1000 nucleated cells. These seemingly large totals are rapidly reached in a well-prepared bone marrow smear at 500× magnification and compensate statistically for

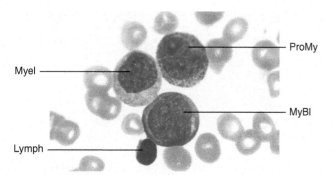

Figure 14.9 Bone Marrow Aspirate Smear. Myeloid stages include a myeloblast *(MyBl)*, promyelocyte *(ProMy)*, and myelocyte *(Myel)*. The lymphocyte *(Lymph)* diameter illustrates its size relative to the myeloid stages. The source of the lymphocyte is sinus blood. (Wright-Giemsa stain, ×1000.)

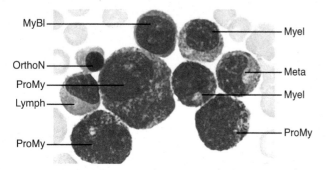

Figure 14.10 Bone Marrow Aspirate Smear. Myeloid stages include a myeloblast *(MyBl)*, promyelocytes *(ProMy)*, myelocytes *(Myel)*, and a metamyelocyte *(Meta)*. One orthochromic normoblast *(OrthoN)* and one lymphocyte *(Lymph)* are present. (Wright-Giemsa stain, ×1000.)

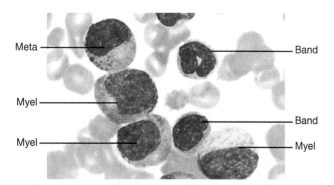

Figure 14.11 Bone Marrow Aspirate Smear. Myeloid stages include myelocytes *(Myel)*, a metamyelocyte *(Meta)*, and neutrophilic bands. (Wright-Giemsa stain, ×1000.)

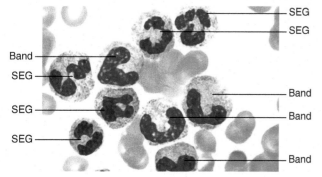

Figure 14.12 Bone Marrow Aspirate Smear. Note the neutrophilic bands and segmented neutrophils (SEGs). (Wright-Giemsa stain, ×1000.)

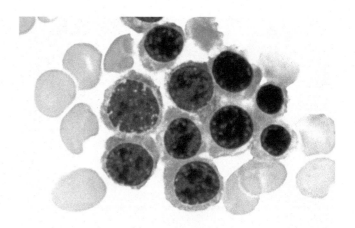

Figure 14.13 Bone Marrow Aspirate Smear. Note the island of erythroid precursors with polychromatophilic and orthochromic normoblasts. (Wright-Giemsa stain, ×1000.)

the anticipated uneven distribution of spicules and hematopoietic cells. The microscopist counts cells and maturation stages surrounding several spicules to maximize the opportunity for detecting disease-related cells. Some laboratory directors eschew the differential in favor of a thorough examination of the smear.

Many microscopists choose not to differentiate the four nucleated erythroid maturation stages, and others may combine three of the four—*basophilic, polychromatophilic,* and *orthochromic normoblasts*—in a single total, counting only *pronormoblasts* (the earliest stage) separately. In normal marrow, most erythroid precursors are either polychromatophilic or orthochromic normoblasts, and differentiation yields little additional information. On the other hand, differentiation may be helpful in megaloblastic, iron deficiency, or refractory anemia.

The microscopist may infrequently find *osteoblasts* and *osteoclasts* in the marrow aspirate specimen (Figure 14.14). Osteoblasts are responsible for bone formation and remodeling, and they derive from *endosteal* (inner lining) cells. Osteoblasts may resemble plasma cells with eccentric round to oval nuclei and abundant blue, mottled cytoplasm, but they lack the prominent Golgi apparatus characteristic of plasma cells. Additionally, they technically demonstrate tiny particles of eosinophilic "bone dust" within their cytoplasm. Osteoblasts are usually found in clusters resembling myeloma cell clusters. Their presence in marrow aspirates and core biopsy specimens is incidental; they do not signal disease, but they may create confusion.

Osteoclasts are nearly the diameter of megakaryocytes, but their multiple, evenly spaced nuclei distinguish them from multilobed megakaryocyte nuclei (Figure 14.15). Osteoclasts appear to derive from myeloid progenitor cells and are responsible for bone resorption, acting in concert with osteoblasts. Osteoclasts are recognized more often in core biopsy specimens than in aspirates.

Adipocytes, endothelial cells that line blood vessels, and fibroblast-like *reticular cells* complete the bone marrow composition (Chapter 4). *Stromal cells* and their extracellular matrix provide

TABLE 14.5   Distribution of Cells and Cell Maturation Stages in Aspirates or Imprints

Cell or Cell Maturation Stage	Normal Distribution	Cell or Cell Maturation Stage	Normal Distribution
Myeloblasts	0%–3%	Pronormoblasts/rubriblasts	0%–1%
Promyelocytes	1%–5%	Basophilic normoblasts/prorubricytes	1%–4%
Myelocytes	6%–14%	Polychromatophilic normoblasts/rubricytes	10%–20%
Metamyelocytes	3%–20%	Orthochromic normoblasts/metarubricytes	6%–10%
Neutrophilic bands	9%–32%	Lymphocytes	5%–18%
Segmented neutrophils	7%–30%	Plasma cells	0%–1%
Eosinophils and eosinophilic precursors	0%–3%	Monocytes	0%–1%
Basophils and mast cells	0%–1%	Histiocytes	0%–1%
Megakaryocytes	2–10 visible per low-power field	Myeloid-to-erythroid ratio	1.5:1–3.3:1

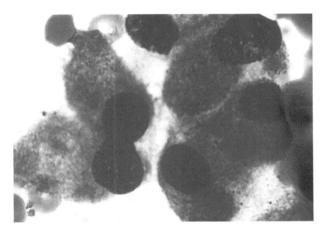

Figure 14.14 Bone Marrow Aspirate Smear Showing Osteoblasts. Note the cluster of osteoblasts that superficially resemble plasma cells. Osteoblasts have round to oval eccentric nuclei and mottled blue cytoplasm that is devoid of secretory granules. They may have a clear area within the cytoplasm but lack the well-defined central Golgi complex of the plasma cell. (A, B, C, Wright-Giemsa stain, ×1000.)

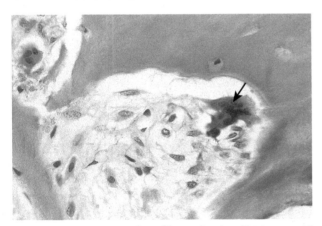

Figure 14.15 Bone Marrow Core Biopsy Section. The large multinucleated cell near the endosteal surface is an osteoclast *(arrow),* a cell that reabsorbs bone. The spindle-shaped cells are fibroblasts. (Hematoxylin and eosin stain, ×500.)

the suitable microenvironment for the maturation and proliferation of hematopoietic cells but are seldom examined for diagnosis of hematologic or systemic disease. Finally, *Langerhans cells,* giant cells with "palisade" nuclei found in granulomas, when present signal chronic inflammation.

Once the differential is completed, the *myeloid-to-erythroid* (M:E) *ratio* is computed from the total myeloid to the total nucleated erythroid cell stages. Excluded from the M:E ratio are lymphocytes, plasma cells, monocytes, histiocytes, nonnucleated erythrocytes, and nonhematopoietic stromal cells.

Prussian Blue Iron Stain Examination

A Prussian blue (acidic potassium ferrocyanide) *iron stain* is commonly used on the bone marrow aspirate smear. Figure 14.16 illustrates normal iron, absence of iron, and increased iron stores in aspirate smears. This technique is very useful for highlighting the presence of ring sideroblasts, which may be associated with both reactive and neoplastic conditions. The iron stain may be used for core biopsy specimens, but decalcifying agents used to soften the biopsy specimen during processing may leach iron, which gives a false impression of decreased or absent iron stores. For this reason, the aspirate is favored for the iron stain if sufficient spicules are present.

EXAMINING THE BONE MARROW CORE BIOPSY SPECIMEN

The standard stain for the core biopsy specimen is the *hematoxylin and eosin* (H&E) stain. Other stains and their purposes are listed in Table 14.6. Bone marrow core biopsy specimen and imprint (touch preparation) examinations are essential when the aspiration procedure yields a dry tap, which may be the result of hypoplastic or aplastic anemia, fibrosis, or tight packing of the marrow cavity with leukemic cells. The key advantage of the core biopsy specimen is preservation of bone marrow architecture so that cells, tumor clusters (Figure 14.17), and maturation stages may be examined relative to stromal elements. The disadvantage is that individual hematopoietic cell morphology is obscured.

The microscopist first examines the core biopsy specimen preparation using the 10× objective lens (100× total magnification) to assess *cellularity.* Because the sample is larger, the core biopsy specimen provides a more accurate estimate of cellularity than the aspirate. The microscopist compares cellular areas with the clear-appearing adipocytes, using a method identical to that employed in examination of aspirate smears to assess cellularity. All fields are examined because cells distribute

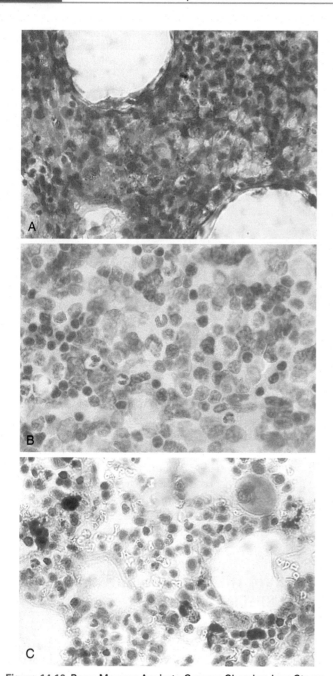

Figure 14.16 Bone Marrow Aspirate Smears Showing Iron Stores. **(A)**, Normal iron stores. **(B)**, Absence of iron stores. **(C)**, Increased iron stores. (A, B, C, Prussian blue stain, ×500.)

TABLE 14.6 Stains Used in Examination of Bone Marrow Core Biopsy Specimens

Stain	Application
Hematoxylin and eosin (H&E)	Evaluate cellularity and hematopoietic cell distribution; locate abnormal cell clusters
Prussian blue (acidic potassium ferrocyanide) iron stain	Evaluate iron stores for deficiency or excess iron; decalcification may remove iron from fixed specimens; thus EDTA chelation or the aspirate smear is preferred for iron store estimation
Reticulin and trichrome stains	Examine for marrow fibrosis
Acid-fast stains	Examine for acid-fast bacilli, fungi, or bacteria in granulomatous disease
Gram stain	Examine for acid-fast bacilli, fungi, or bacteria in granulomatous disease
Immunohistochemical stains	Establish the identity of malignant cells with stain-tagged monoclonal antibodies specific for tumor surface markers
Wright or Wright-Giemsa stain	Observe hematopoietic cell structure; cell identification is less accurate in a biopsy specimen than in an aspirate smear

EDTA, ethylenediaminetetraacetic acid.

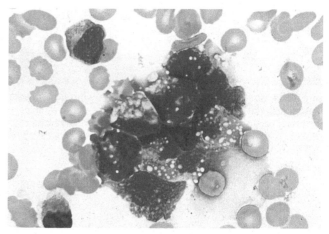

Figure 14.17 Bone Marrow Aspirate Smear Showing a Cluster or Syncytia of Tumor Cells. Nuclei are irregular and hyperchromatic, and cytoplasm is vacuolated. Cytoplasmic margins are poorly delineated. (Wright-Giemsa stain, ×500.)

unevenly. Examples of hypocellular and hypercellular core biopsy sections are provided for comparison with normocellular marrow in Figure 14.18.

Similar to what is seen on the aspirate smear, *megakaryocytes* are easily recognized by their outsized diameter and even distribution throughout the biopsy. They exhibit the characteristic lobulated nucleus, although nuclei of the more mature megakaryocytes are smaller and more darkly stained in H&E preparations than on a Wright-stained aspirate specimen. Their cytoplasm varies from light pink in younger cells to dark pink in older cells (Figure 14.19). Because of the greater sample volume, microscopists assess megakaryocyte numbers more accurately by examining a core biopsy section than an aspirate smear. Normally there are 2 to 10 megakaryocytes per 10× field, the same as in an aspirate smear or imprint. Because the core biopsy represents a 4- to 6-micron section of a paraffin block of tissue, this is a cut section and, unlike the aspirate smear, *does not* represent the entire cytologic appearance of the cells. This fact is especially important when considering larger cells such as megakaryocytes because many megakaryocytes present on a core biopsy specimen will only be partially represented because they can be cut through.

Using the 50× oil immersion objective lens, the microscopist next observes *cell distribution* relative to bone marrow stroma. For instance, in people older than age 70, normal lymphocytes may form small aggregates in nonparatrabecular regions, whereas *malignant lymphoma cell clusters* are often paratrabecular (associated with the bony region). In addition, normal lymphocytes remain as discrete cells, whereas lymphoma cells are typically pleomorphic and syncytial.

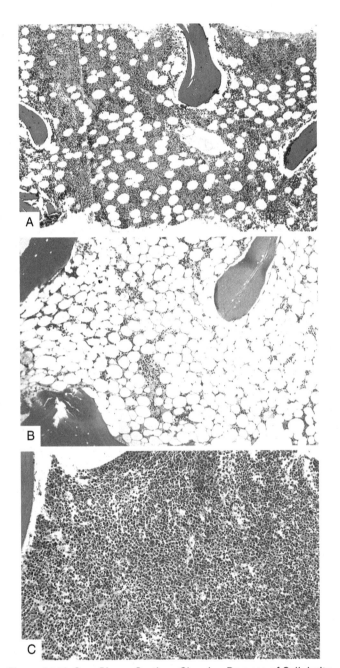

Figure 14.18 Core Biopsy Sections Showing Degrees of Cellularity.
(A), Normal cellularity, approximately 50% fat and 50% hematopoietic cells. (Hematoxylin and eosin stain, ×50.) **(B),** Hypocellularity with only fat and connective tissue cells from a patient with aplastic anemia. (Hematoxylin and eosin stain, ×100.) **(C),** Hypercellularity from a patient with chronic myelogenous leukemia with virtually 100% cellularity and no fat visible. (Hematoxylin and eosin stain, 100×.) (**B,** courtesy Dennis P. O'Malley, MD, director, Immunohistochemistry Laboratory, Indiana University School of Medicine, Indianapolis, IN.)

If no aspirate or imprint smears could be prepared, the core biopsy specimen may be stained using Wright, Giemsa, or Wright-Giemsa stains to make limited observations of cellular morphology. In Wright- or Giemsa-stained biopsy sections, myeloblasts and promyelocytes have oval or round nuclei with cytoplasm that stain blue (Figure 14.20). Neutrophilic myelocytes and metamyelocytes have light pink cytoplasm. Mature segmented neutrophils (segs) and neutrophilic bands (bands) are recognized by their smaller diameter and darkly stained C-shaped nuclei (bands) or

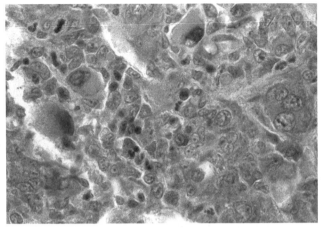

Figure 14.19 Core Biopsy Section Showing Megakaryocytes. Note the many large lobulated megakaryocytes and increased blasts. (Wright-Giemsa stain, ×400.)

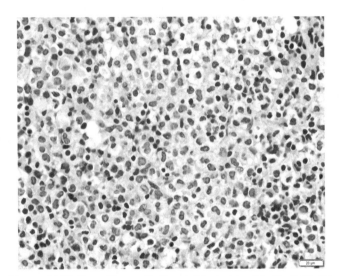

Figure 14.20 Core Biopsy Section Infiltrated by Blasts. Note the abundant cytoplasm and irregular nuclei with open chromatin of the blasts. (Hematoxylin and eosin stain, ×600.)

nuclear segments (segs). The cytoplasm of bands and segs may be light pink or may seem unstained (Figure 14.21).

The cytoplasm of *eosinophils* stains red or orange, which makes them the most brightly stained cells of the marrow (Figure 14.21). Basophils cannot be recognized on marrow biopsy specimens fixed with Zenker glacial acetic acid solution.

The following features help differentiate the most immature granulocytic cells from the most immature erythroid cells in biopsy specimens: *Early erythroid progenitor cells* typically have two or three comma-shaped nucleoli, with one nucleolus touching the nuclear envelope. These erythroid precursors tend to cluster with more mature normoblasts and often surround histiocytes. *Polychromatophilic* and *orthochromic normoblasts*, the two most common erythroid maturation stages, have centrally placed, round nuclei that stain intensely (Figure 14.22). Their cytoplasm is not appreciably stained, but the plasma membrane margin is clearly discerned, which gives the cells of these stages a "fried egg" appearance. Because erythroid cells have a tendency to cluster in small groups, they are more easily recognized using the 10× objective lens, although their individual morphology cannot be seen.

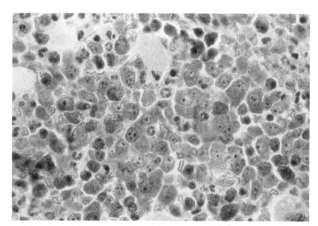

Figure 14.21 Core Biopsy Section. Note the myelocytes, metamyelocytes, bands, segmented neutrophils, and bright red-orange eosinophils. (Wright-Giemsa stain, ×400.)

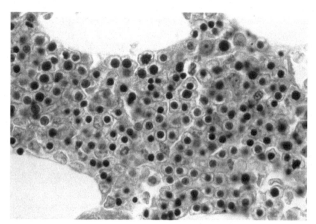

Figure 14.22 Erythroid Island in a Core Biopsy Section. Late-stage normoblasts often have a "fried egg" appearance. (Wright-Giemsa stain, ×400.)

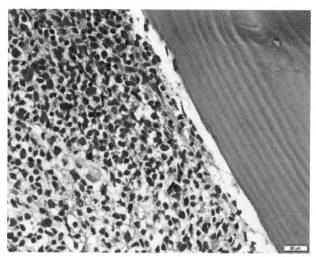

Figure 14.23 Core Biopsy with Lymphocytes. An infiltration of small mature lymphocytes is on the left (edge of bone on the right). A few are immature with larger nuclei containing a single prominent nucleolus. (Hematoxylin and eosin stain, ×600.)

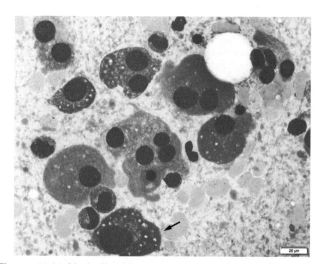

Figure 14.24 Markedly Abnormal Plasma Cells in an Aspirate Smear from a Patient with Multiple Myeloma. The plasma cell highlighted by the arrow reveals an eccentric nucleus with a perinuclear hoff (palor). Note that most other cells have lost these normal features and demonstrate voluminous vacuolated cytoplasm, multinucleation with some prominent nucleoli. (Wright-Giemsa stain, ×1000.)

Lymphocytes are among the most difficult cells to recognize in the core biopsy specimen, unless they occur in clusters. Mature lymphocytes exhibit speckled nuclear chromatin in a small, round nucleus, along with a scant amount of blue cytoplasm and slightly irregular outlines (Figure 14.23). Immature lymphocytes *(prolymphocytes)* have larger round or lobulated nuclei but still only a small rim of blue cytoplasm.

Plasma cells are difficult to distinguish from myelocytes in H&E-stained sections but are recognized using Wright-Giemsa stain as cells with eccentric dark nuclei and blue cytoplasm and a prominent pale central Golgi apparatus (Figure 14.24). The nucleus may have a "clock face" appearance to the chromatin. Characteristically, plasma cells are located in clusters of a few cells in a perivascular distribution.

DEFINITIVE BONE MARROW STUDIES

Although in many cases the aspirate smear and biopsy specimen are diagnostic, additional studies may be needed. Such studies and their applications are given in Table 14.7. These studies require additional bone marrow volume and specialized specimen collection and processing. Each study is well described in the chapter referenced in the table.

BONE MARROW EXAMINATION REPORTS

The components of a bone marrow report should be generated systematically during the microscopic review of the bone marrow specimens. In addition to the bone marrow examination components given in Table 14.4, information on patient medical history (patient identity and age, narration of symptoms, physical findings, findings in kindred, treatment) and CBC (peripheral blood CBC collected no more than 24 hours before the bone marrow puncture with hemogram and peripheral blood film examination) are included. A diagnostic narrative, which is a summary of the recorded bone marrow findings and additional laboratory chemical, microbiologic, and immunoassay tests, completes the bone marrow examination report. An example of a bone marrow examination report is provided in Figure 14.25.

Bone Marrow Pathology Report

PATIENT INFORMATION:
LAST NAME, FIRST NAME
GENDER
AGE: DOB:
Patient ID/MRN:
Account #:

PHYSICIAN INFORMATION:
LAST NAME, FIRST NAME
NAME OF HOSPITAL/MEDICAL CENTER
ADDRESS OF MEDICAL CENTER
CITY, STATE
Tel: XXX-XXX-XXXX

FINAL DIAGNOSIS:

BIOPSY SITE; BIOPSY:
- ACUTE MYELOID LEUKEMIA WITH t(8;21)(q22;q22.1); *RUNX1-RUNX1T1,* SEE COMMENT

COMMENT:
Peripheral blood film: Leukopenia, few blasts, myelocytes, neutrophils. Relative lymphocytosis. RBCs normochromic, macrocytes, mild anisocytosis. Rare teardrop cells. Normal platelet morphology.
Bone marrow aspirate: Few spicules, blasts 65% with large nuclei with fine chromatin and needle shaped Auer rods. Moderate basophilic cytoplasm with salmon-colored graules. Few mature myeloid precursors. Erythroid precursors markedly decreased, with rare binucleate rubricytes. Few eosinophil precursors noted. Dysmorphic megakaryocytes with increased nuclear lobulation.
Bone marrow imprint: Significantly increased blasts. Few mature myeloid precursors, erythroid precursors markedly decreased.
Bone marrow biopsy: Hypercellular for age; estimated at 80% cellular. Most cells are blasts, few mature myeloid precursors. Erythroid and megakaryocytic precursors markedly reduced.
Iron stain: Stainable iron in macrophages. Sideroblasts and rare ringed sideroblasts.
Flow cytometry: Analysis of the bone marrow aspirate smear demonstrates an abnormal myeloid blast population. Blasts express CD34, CD15, HLA-DR, CD33, CD19 and CD56. No phenotypic abnormalities in the lymphocytes.

Differential Counts

Date	PB	Marrow	Marrow Range (percent)		PB	Marrow	Marrow Range (percent)
Blast, unclassified	4	65	0-2	Normal lymphocytes	50	2	3-24
Myeloblasts			3-5	Reactive lymphocytes			
Promyelocytes			1-8	Lymphoblasts			
Myelocytes		14	5-21	Prolymphocytes			
Metamyelocytes			6-22	Monocytes	3		0-3
Band neutrophils			6-22	Plasma cells			0-2
Segmented neutrophils	40	4	9-27	Rubriblasts			0-4
Eosinophils	3	7		Prorubricytes			1-6
Basophils				Rubricytes			5-25
Other				Metarubricytes			1-21
Other				Erythroid		8	10-30

WBC	PLT	MPV	HGB	HCT	MCHC	
2,300	89,000	8	8.1	23	110	

Cytogenetics

ABNORMAL MALE KARYOTYPE: 45,XY,t(8;21)(q22;q22),-Y[20]

Association: This cytogenetics report renders the disease to be classified as "AML with recurrent genetic abnormalities" per the WHO classification 2016. There is also loss of the Y chromosome which is an incidental finding and of no clinical consequence in older male patients.

Prognosis: Good prognosis to chemotherapy and a high complete remission rate.

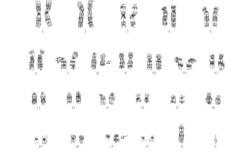

Figure 14.25 Example of a Bone Marrow Examination Report. Patient demographics, diagnosis, diagnostic comment and microscopic description, differential counts of marrow and blood with reference intervals, and cytogenetics report with karyogram can be included. *PB,* Peripheral blood; *HCT,* hematocrit; *HGB,* hemoglobin; *MCHC,* mean cell hemoglobin concentration; *MPV,* mean platelet volume; *PLT,* platelet; *WBC,* white blood cell.

TABLE 14.7 Definitive Studies Performed on Selected Bone Marrow Specimens

Bone Marrow Study	Application	Specimen	Chapter(s)
Iron stain	Identification of iron deficiency, iron overload	Fresh marrow aspirate	17
Cytochemical studies	Diagnosis of leukemias and lymphomas	Fresh marrow aspirate	26, 31, 32, 34
Cytogenetic studies	Diagnosis of acute leukemias via deletions, translocations, and polysomy; remission studies	1 mL marrow in heparin	30
Molecular studies	Polymerase chain reaction for diagnostic point mutations; minimal residual disease studies	1 mL marrow in EDTA	29
Fluorescence in situ hybridization	Staining for diagnostic mutations; minimal residual disease studies	Fresh marrow aspirate	30
Flow cytometry	Immunophenotyping, usually of malignant hematopoietic cells, clonality; minimal residual disease studies	1 mL marrow in heparin, EDTA, or ACD	28

ACD, Acid-citrate dextrose; *EDTA*, ethylenediaminetetraacetic acid.

SUMMARY

- Adult hematopoietic tissue is located in the flat bones and the ends of the long bones. Hematopoiesis occurs within the spongy trabeculae of the bone adjacent to vascular sinuses.
- Bone marrow collection is a safe but invasive procedure performed by a pathologist or hematologist in collaboration with a medical laboratory professional to obtain specimens used to diagnose hematologic and systemic disease and/or to monitor treatment.
- The necessity for a bone marrow examination should be evaluated in light of all clinical and laboratory information. In anemias for which the cause is apparent from the red blood cell indices, a bone marrow examination may not be required. Examples of indications for bone marrow examination are numerous and include (but are not limited to) unexplained cytopenias, circulating blasts, and staging of lymphomas and carcinomas.
- A peripheral blood specimen is collected for a complete blood count (CBC) no more than 24 hours before the bone marrow is collected, and the results of the CBC are reported with the bone marrow examination results.
- Bone marrow may be collected from the posterior or anterior iliac crest or sternum using sterile disposable biopsy and aspiration needles and cannulas. The site and equipment depend on how old the patient is and whether both an aspirate and a biopsy specimen are desired.

- The medical laboratory professional receives the bone marrow specimen and prepares aspirate smears, crush preparations, imprints, anticoagulated bone marrow smears, fixed biopsy sections, and specimens for confirmatory studies.
- The medical laboratory professional and pathologist collaborate with residents, fellows, attending physicians, and medical laboratory science students to stain and review bone marrow aspirate smears, biopsy sections, and confirmatory procedure results.
- Confirmatory procedures include cytochemistry, cytogenetics, immunophenotyping by flow cytometry, fluorescence in situ hybridization, and molecular diagnostics.
- The medical laboratory professional and pathologist determine cellularity and megakaryocyte distribution, then perform a differential count of 500 nucleated bone marrow cells and compute the myeloid-to-erythrocyte (M:E) ratio, comparing the results with reference intervals.
- The pathologist characterizes features of hematopoietic disease, metastatic tumor cells, and abnormalities of the bone marrow stroma and prepares a systematic written bone marrow examination report including a diagnostic narrative.

Now that you have completed this chapter, go back and read again the case study at the beginning and respond to the questions presented.

REVIEW QUESTIONS

Answers can be found in the Appendix.

1. Where is most hematopoietic tissue found in adults?
   a. Liver
   b. Lungs
   c. Spleen
   d. Long bones

2. What is the preferred bone marrow collection site in adults?
   a. Second intercostal space on the sternum
   b. Anterior or posterior iliac crest
   c. Any of the thoracic vertebrae
   d. Anterior head of the femur

3. The aspirate should be examined under low power to assess all of the following *except*:
   a. Cellularity
   b. Megakaryocyte numbers
   c. Morphology of abnormal cells
   d. Presence of tumor cell clusters

4. What is the normal myeloid to erythroid (M:E) ratio range in adults?
   a. 1.5:1 to 3.3:1
   b. 5.1:1 to 6.2:1
   c. 8.6:1 to 10.2:1
   d. 10:1 to 12:1

5. Which are the most common erythroid stages found in normal marrow?
   a. Pronormoblasts
   b. Pronormoblasts and basophilic normoblasts
   c. Basophilic and polychromatophilic normoblasts
   d. Polychromatophilic and orthochromic normoblasts

6. What cells, occasionally seen in bone marrow biopsy specimens, are responsible for the formation of bone?
   a. Macrophages
   b. Plasma cells
   c. Osteoblasts
   d. Osteoclasts

7. What is the largest hematopoietic cell found in a normal bone marrow aspirate?
   a. Osteoblast
   b. Myeloblast
   c. Pronormoblast
   d. Megakaryocyte

8. Which of the following is *not* an indication for a bone marrow examination?
   a. Pancytopenia (reduced numbers of red blood cells, white blood cells, and platelets in the peripheral blood)
   b. Anemia with RBC indices corresponding to low serum iron and low ferritin levels
   c. Detection of blasts in the peripheral blood
   d. Need for staging of Hodgkin lymphoma

9. In a bone marrow biopsy specimen, the red blood cell precursors were estimated to account for 40% of the cells in the marrow, and the other 60% were granulocyte precursors. What is the myeloid to erythroid (M:E) ratio?
   a. 4:6
   b. 1.5:1
   c. 1:1.5
   d. 3:1

10. On a bone marrow core biopsy sample, several large cells with multiple nuclei were noted. They were located close to the endosteum, and their nuclei were evenly spaced throughout the cell. What are these cells?
    a. Megakaryocytes
    b. Osteoclasts
    c. Adipocytes
    d. Fibroblasts

11. The advantage of a core biopsy bone marrow sample over an aspirate is that the core biopsy specimen:
    a. Can be acquired by a less invasive collection technique
    b. Permits assessment of the architecture and cellular arrangement
    c. Retains the staining qualities of basophils owing to the use of Zenker fixative
    d. Is better for the assessment of bone marrow iron stores with Prussian blue stain

12. Which of the following features suggests involvement of the marrow by lymphoma?
    a. Paratrabecular lymphoid aggregation
    b. Lymphoid aggregates with germinal centers
    c. Nonparatrabecular lymphoid clusters
    d. Discrete, small lymphocytes with speckled nuclear chromatin

13. Using Wright-Giemsa stain, the morphologic description of an eccentric dark nuclei with deeply basophilic (blue) cytoplasm and a prominent pale central Golgi apparatus best describes a(n):
    a. Eosinophil
    b. Basophil
    c. Lymphocyte
    d. Plasma cell

REFERENCES

1. Dave, U. P., & Koury, J. M. (2016). Structure of the marrow and the hematopoietic microenvironment. In Kaushansky, K., Lichtman, M., Prchal, J. T., et al. (Eds.), *Williams Hematology.* (9th ed., pp. 53–85). New York: McGraw Hill.

2. Farhi, D. C. (2008). *Pathology of Bone Marrow and Blood Cells.* (2nd ed.). Philadelphia: Lippincott Williams & Wilkins.

3. Foucar, K., Reichard, K., & Czuchlewski, D. (2010). *Bone Marrow Pathology.* (3rd ed.). Chicago: ASCP Press.

4. Silberstein, L., & Scadden, D. (2018). Hematopoietic microenvironment. In Hoffman, R., Benz, E. J., Silberstein, L., et al. (Eds.), *Hematology Basic Principles and Practice.* (7th ed.). St. Louis: Elsevier.

5. Reddy, V., Marques, M. B., & Fritsma, G. A. (2013). *Quick Guide to Hematology Testing.* (2nd ed.). Washington, DC: AACC Press.

6. Perkins, S. L. (2013). Examination of the blood and bone marrow. In Greer, J. P., Arber, D. A., Glader, B., et al. (Eds.), *Wintrobe's Clinical Hematology.* (13th ed.). Philadelphia: Wolters Kluwer Health/Lippincott Williams & Wilkins.

7. Ryan, D. H. (2016). Examination of the marrow. In Kaushansky, K., Lichtman, M., Prchal, J. T., et al. (Eds.), *Williams Hematology.* (9th ed., pp. 27–41). New York: McGraw Hill.

8. Krause, J. R. (1981). *Bone Marrow Biopsy,* New York: Churchill Livingstone.

9. Hartsock, R. J., Smith, E. B., & Pett, C. S. (1965). Normal variations with aging of the amount of hemopoietic tissue in bone marrow from the anterior iliac crest. *Am J Clin Pathol, 43,* 326–331.

10. Abrahamson, J. F., Lund-Johansen, F., Laerum, O. D., et al. (1995). Flow cytometric assessment of peripheral blood contamination and proliferative activity of human bone marrow cell populations. *Cytometry, 19,* 77–85.

Body Fluid Analysis in the Hematology Laboratory

*Michelle Butina**

OBJECTIVES

After completion of this chapter, the reader will be able to:

1. Describe the automated and manual methods for performing cell counts and differentials on body fluids.
2. Discuss the limitations of manual cell counts and the benefits of automated cell counts.
3. Given a description of a body fluid for cell counting, choose the appropriate diluting fluid, select a counting area, and calculate and correct (if necessary) the counts.
4. Using the proper terminology, discuss the gross appearance of body fluids, including its significance and its practical use in determining cell count dilutions.
5. Discuss the advantages and disadvantages of cytocentrifuge preparations.
6. Differentiate between traumatic spinal tap and cerebral hemorrhage on the basis of cell counts and the appearance of uncentrifuged and centrifuged specimens.
7. Identify from written descriptions normal cells found in cerebrospinal, serous, and synovial fluids.
8. Describe the characteristics of benign versus malignant cells in body fluids, and recognize written descriptions of each.
9. Differentiate exudates and transudates based on formation (cause), specific gravity, protein concentration, appearance, and cell concentration.
10. Identify crystals in synovial fluids from written descriptions, including polarization characteristics.
11. Describe the process of obtaining bronchoalveolar lavage (BAL) samples, including safety precautions for analysis; state the purpose of BAL; and recognize types of cells that normally would be found in BAL specimens.

OUTLINE

Performing Cell Counts on Body Fluids
  Automated Methods
  Manual Methods
Performing Differential Cell Counts on Body Fluids
  Manual Methods: Preparing Cytocentrifuge Slides
Cerebrospinal Fluid
  Gross Examination
  Cell Counts
  Differential Cell Counts
Serous Fluid
  Transudates Versus Exudates

Gross Examination
Differential Cell Counts
Synovial Fluid
  Gross Examination
  Differential Cell Counts
  Crystals
Bronchoalveolar Lavage Specimens
  Procedure and Precautions
  Differential Cell Counts

CASE STUDY

After studying the material in this chapter, the reader should be able to respond to the following case study:

A 33-year-old semiconscious woman was brought to the emergency department by her husband. The previous day she had complained of a headache and left work early. When she got home, she took aspirin and had a brief nap and reported she felt better that evening. Her husband stated that the next morning "she couldn't talk," so he brought her to the emergency department. A lumbar puncture was performed. The fluid that arrived in the laboratory was cloudy. The WBC count was 10.6×10^9/L. Most of the cells seen on the cytocentrifuge slide were neutrophils.

1. When multiple tubes of cerebrospinal fluid are obtained, which tube should be used for cell counts?
2. What should you look for on the cytocentrifuge slide?
3. What is the most likely diagnosis for this patient?

---

*The author extends appreciation to Bernadette F. Rodak and Leilani Collins, whose work in previous editions provided the foundation for this chapter.

The analysis of body fluids, including blood cell count and differential cell count, can provide valuable diagnostic information. This chapter is not intended to serve as a comprehensive review of all body fluids analyzed in the hematology laboratory; instead, it covers cell counting, differential cell counts, and morphology of the commonly received body fluids. The fluids discussed in this chapter include cerebrospinal fluid (CSF), serous or body cavity fluids (pleural, pericardial, and peritoneal fluids), and synovial (joint) fluids. Bronchoalveolar lavage (BAL) specimens are discussed briefly.

PERFORMING CELL COUNTS ON BODY FLUIDS

Examination of all fluids should include observation of color and turbidity, cell counts, such as total nucleated cell (TNC), white blood cell (WBC), and red blood cell (RBC), and differential cell count. Blood cell counts should be performed and cytocentrifuge slides should be prepared as quickly as possible after collection of the specimen, because WBCs begin to deteriorate within 30 minutes after collection.[1] It is important to mix the specimen gently but thoroughly before every manipulation (i.e., counting cells, preparing any dilution, and preparing cytocentrifuge slides).

Automated Methods

Historically, all body fluid (BF) cell counts were performed by manual methods using a hemacytometer for counting cells. However, this method has several limitations: It is time consuming and labor intensive, has high interobserver variability, and has poor reproducibility.[2-5] Automation of BF cell counts does overcome these difficulties, and today a large percentage of cell counts are performed on automated hematology analyzers.

The differences between whole blood and the various body fluids received in the hematology laboratory created challenges in processing cells counts until the introduction of the dedicated body fluid (BF) mode or channel that is incorporated into today's hematology analyzers. The BF mode optimizes technologies already present to account for the different cellular composition of body fluids. Manufacturers are required to provide a statement of intended use that defines which body fluids have been approved by a regulatory agency for testing on the analyzer.[2] Some features of the BF mode, dependent on analyzer and manufacturer, include extended counting for low cell counts, sample dilution not required, and flagging capabilities (e.g., possible malignant cells), all of which result in improvement of accuracy and turnaround times compared with manual methods.[2]

Manual Methods

If your laboratory does not have a hematology analyzer with a dedicated BF mode or for very low cell counts, a manual cell count may be required. Manual cell counts are performed using a hemacytometer (glass or disposable), allowing for TNC or WBC and RBC counts. In body fluid analysis the terminology *TNC* is more appropriate because nucleated cells include WBCs, tissue cells, and malignant cells. RBC counts provide clinical value for some body fluids (e.g., CSF) but not others (e.g., serous

and synovial fluids), and in these instances relevant clinical information is obtained merely from the appearance of the fluid (slightly to grossly bloody).[6]

Cell counts are performed with undiluted fluid if the fluid is clear. If the fluid is hazy or bloody, appropriate dilutions should be made to permit accurate counts of RBCs and WBC or TNC. The smallest reasonable dilution should be made. The diluting fluid for RBCs is isotonic saline. Diluting fluids for WBCs include glacial acetic acid to lyse the RBCs, or Türk solution, which contains glacial acetic acid and methylene blue to stain the nuclei of the WBCs. Acetic acid cannot be used for synovial fluids because synovial fluid contains hyaluronic acid, which coagulates in acetic acid. A small amount of hyaluronidase powder (a pinch, or what can be picked up between two wooden sticks) or one drop of 0.05% hyaluronidase in phosphate buffer per milliliter of fluid should be added to the synovial fluid sample to liquefy it before performing manual cell counts or automated cell counts (on hematology analyzer) or preparing cytocentrifuge slides.

Dilutions should be based on the turbidity of the fluid or on the number of cells seen on the hemacytometer when using an undiluted sample. If the fluid is blood tinged to slightly bloody, the RBCs can be counted using undiluted fluid, but it is advisable to use a small (1:2) dilution with Türk solution (or similar) to lyse the RBCs to provide an accurate WBC or TNC count. If the fluid is bloody, a 1:200 dilution with isotonic saline for RBCs and either a 1:2 or a 1:20 dilution with Türk solution for WBCs should be used to obtain an accurate count. The number of squares to be counted on the hemacytometer should be determined on the basis of the number of cells present. In general, all nine squares on both sides of the hemacytometer should be counted. If the number of cells is high, however, fewer squares may be counted.[5] Each square equals 1 mm². The formula for calculating the number of cells (Chapter 11) is as follows:

$$\text{Total count} = \frac{\text{cells counted} \times \text{dilution factor}}{\text{area (mm}^2) \times \text{depth (0.1)}}$$

Guidelines for manually performing cell counts and cytospin preparation are summarized in Table 15.1.

PERFORMING DIFFERENTIAL CELL COUNTS ON BODY FLUIDS

The purpose of the differential cell count is to identify the types of cells present in a fluid to provide relevant clinical information. The various cell types include WBCs, tissue cells, and malignant cells, all of which can assist in detecting infection, inflammation, hemorrhage, or malignancy.

Body fluid WBC differential counts may be performed on hematology analyzers that have a dedicated BF mode.[2] If performed on an analyzer, the WBC differential is often limited to a two-part differential consisting of polymorphonuclear cells) and mononuclear cells (additional differential results vary depending on analyzer software and technologies).[2] However, for more comprehensive differential results, including detection of

TABLE 15.1   Guidelines for Counting Fluids: Manual Methods

Test	Clear	Hazy	Blood Tinged	Cloudy	Bloody
			GROSS APPEARANCE		
WBCs	0–200/μL	>200/μL	Unknown	High	Unknown
Dilution for counting cells	None	1:2 Türk	1:2 Türk	1:20 in Türk solution	1:2 in Türk solution
No. squares to count on hemacytometer	9	9	9	9 or 4	9 or 4
RBCs	0–400/μL	Unknown	>400/μL	Unknown	>6000/μL
Dilution for counting cells	None	None	None	None	1:200 in isotonic saline
No. squares to count on hemacytometer	9 large	9 large	9 or 4 large	4 large or 5 small	5 small
Cytospin dilution (0.25 mL [5 drops] of fluid)*	Undiluted	Dilute with saline to 100–200/μL nucleated cell count	Straight or by nucleated cell count	Dilute with saline to 100–200/μL nucleated cell count	Dilute by nucleated cell count; if RBC count > 1 million/μL, make a push smear and differentiate cells that are pushed out on the end

RBC, Red blood cell; WBC, white blood cell.

*Expected cell yield (WBC count for number of cells recovered on slide): 0/μL for 0–70; 1–2/μL for 12–100; >3/μL for >100.

malignant cells, tissue cells, microorganisms, crystals, and artifacts, a manual microscopic differential must be performed. In addition, the literature maintains that a manual cell differential for CSF specimens is preferred because the differential is often crucial for diagnosis and dependent on proper identification of WBCs and malignant cells.[7,8]

Manual Methods: Preparing Cytocentrifuge Slides

The cytocentrifuge enhances the ability to identify the types of cells present in a fluid as it provides a concentration of cells for microscopic review. This centrifuge spins at a low speed, which minimizes distortion of the cellular elements and provides a "button" of cells that are concentrated into a small area on the slide. The cytocentrifuge assembly consists of a cytofunnel, filter paper to absorb excess fluid, and a glass slide. These three components are fastened together in a clip assembly, a few drops of well-mixed specimen are dispensed into the cytofunnel, and the entire assembly is centrifuged slowly. The cells are deposited onto the slide, and excess fluid is absorbed into the filter paper, which produces a monolayer of cells in a small button (Figure 15.1).

There may be some distortion of cells as a result of the centrifugation process or crowding of cells when high cell counts are present. To minimize distortion resulting from overcrowding of cells, appropriate dilutions should be made with normal saline before centrifugation. The basis for this dilution should be the WBC count or the nucleated cell count. A nucleated cell count of 200/μL or fewer provides a good basis for the differential. If a consistent amount of fluid is used when cytocentrifuge slides are prepared, a consistent yield of cells can be expected; this can be used to confirm the WBC or nucleated cell count. The area of the cell button that is used for performing the differential count is not important, but if the number of WBCs or nucleated cells present is small, use of a "systematic meander" starting at one side of the button and working toward the other side is best. In case the number of cells recovered is small, the area around the cell button should be marked on the back of the slide with a wax pencil, or premarked slides should be used to prepare cytocentrifuge slides (Figure 15.1).

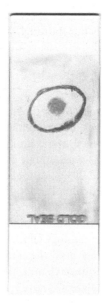

Figure 15.1 Wright-Stained Cytocentrifuge Slide. Concentrated button of cells is within a marked circle. (From Rodak, B. F., & Carr, J. H. [2017]. *Clinical Hematology Atlas.* [5th ed.]. St. Louis: Elsevier.)

CEREBROSPINAL FLUID

CSF is the only fluid that exists in quantities sufficient to sample in healthy individuals. CSF is present in volumes of 100 to 150 mL in adults, 60 to 100 mL in children, and 10 to 60 mL in newborns.[9,10] This fluid bathes the brain and spinal column and serves as a cushion to protect the brain, as a circulating nutrient medium, as an excretory channel for nervous tissue metabolism, and as lubrication for the central nervous system. CSF is collected by lumbar puncture using either the L3–4 or L4–5 interspace (Figure 15.2).[11]

Gross Examination

Normal CSF is nonviscous, clear, and colorless. A cloudy or hazy appearance may indicate the presence of WBCs (greater than 200/μL), RBCs (greater than 400/μL), or microorganisms.[9,10]

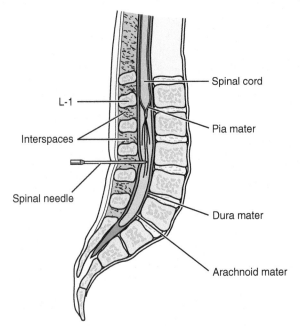

Figure 15.2 Schematic Representation of Lumbar Puncture Procedure. Spinal needle is placed between vertebrae L4–5. (From Brunzel, N. A. [2018]. *Fundamentals of Urine and Body Fluid Analysis*. [4th ed.]. St. Louis: Elsevier.)

Bloody fluid may be caused by a traumatic tap, in which blood is acquired as the puncture is performed, or by a pathologic hemorrhage within the central nervous system. If more than one tube is received, the tubes can be observed for clearing from tube to tube. If the first tube contains blood but the remaining tubes are clear or progressively clearer, the blood is the result of a traumatic puncture. If all tubes are uniformly bloody, the probable cause is an intracranial hemorrhage. When a bloody specimen is received, an aliquot should be centrifuged and the color of the supernatant should be observed and reported. A clear, colorless supernatant indicates a traumatic tap, whereas a yellowish or pinkish yellow tinge may indicate a subarachnoid hemorrhage. This yellowish color sometimes is referred to as *xanthochromia*, but because not all xanthochromia is pathologic, the Clinical and Laboratory Standards Institute recommends avoiding the term and simply reporting the actual color of the supernatant (Figure 15.3 and Table 15.2).[9]

Cell Counts

When multiple tubes of spinal fluid are collected, the cell count is generally performed on tube 3, or the tube with the lowest possibility of peripheral blood contamination. Tube 1 is used for chemistry and immunology, and tube 2 is used for microbiology. Normal cell counts in CSF are 0 to 5 WBCs/μL and 0 RBCs/μL in adults, and 0 to 30 WBCs/μL and 0 RBCs/μL in neonates. If a high RBC count is obtained, one may determine whether the source of WBCs is peripheral blood contamination by using the peripheral blood ratio of 1 WBC per 500 to 900 RBCs. If peripheral blood cell counts are known, the number of blood WBCs added to the CSF sample can be calculated using the following formula:

$$WBC_B \times \frac{RBC_{CSF}}{RBC_B} = WBCs\ added\ by\ traumatic\ puncture$$

where WBC_B is the WBC count for peripheral blood, RBC_{CSF} is the RBC count for CSF, and RBC_B is the RBC count for

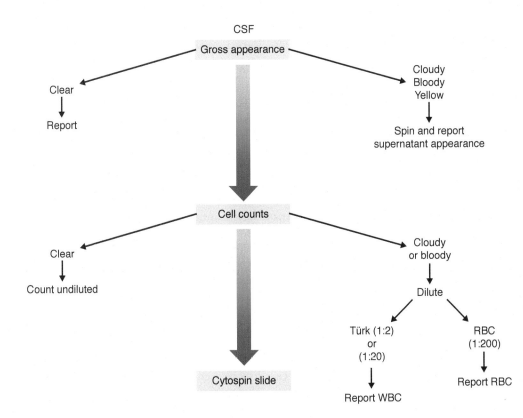

Figure 15.3 Flowchart for Examination of Cerebrospinal Fluid (CSF). *RBC,* Red blood cell; *WBC,* white blood cell. (Modified from Kjeldsberg, C., & Knight, J. [1993]. *Body Fluids.* [3rd ed.]. Chicago: ASCP Press; reprinted with permission.)

TABLE 15.2 **Characteristics of Cerebrospinal Fluid**	
Traumatic Tap	**Pathologic Hemorrhage**
Clear supernatant	Colored or hemolyzed supernatant
Clearing from tube to tube	Same appearance in all tubes
Bone marrow contamination	Erythrophages
Cartilage cells	Siderophages (may have bilirubin crystals)

peripheral blood. The corrected or true CSF WBC count (WBC$_{CSF}$) is calculated as follows[12]:

$$\text{True WBC}_{CSF} = \text{CSF WBC hemacytometer count} - \text{WBCs added}$$

Some laboratories have questioned the value of an RBC count on CSF and report only the WBC count.

A high WBC count may be found in fluid from patients with infective processes, such as meningitis. In general, WBC counts are much higher (in the thousands) in patients with bacterial meningitis than in patients with viral meningitis (in the hundreds).[13-15] The predominant cell type present on the cytocentrifuge slide (neutrophils or lymphocytes), however, is a better indicator of the type of meningitis—bacterial or viral. Elevated WBC counts also may be obtained in patients with inflammatory processes and malignancies.

Differential Cell Counts

The WBCs normally seen in CSF are lymphocytes and monocytes (Figure 15.4). In adults the predominant cells are lymphocytes, and in newborns the predominant cells are monocytes.[9,10] Neutrophils are not normal in CSF but may be seen in small numbers because of concentration techniques. When the WBC count is elevated and large numbers of neutrophils are seen, a thorough and careful search should be made for bacteria because organisms may be present in very small numbers early in bacterial meningitis (Figure 15.5). In viral meningitis the predominant cells seen are lymphocytes, including reactive or viral

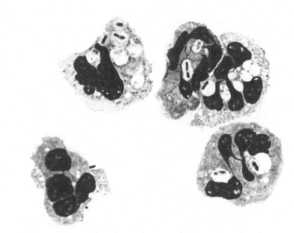

Figure 15.5 Neutrophils with Bacteria. From a patient with bacterial meningitis. (Cerebrospinal fluid, Wright-Giemsa stain, ×1000.) (From Rodak, B. F., & Carr, J. H. [2017]. *Clinical Hematology Atlas.* [5th ed.]. St. Louis: Elsevier.)

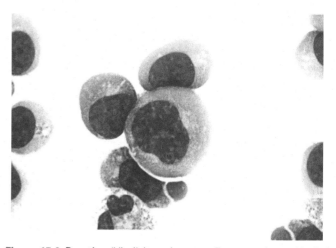

Figure 15.6 Reactive (Viral) Lymphocytes. From a patient with viral meningitis. (Cerebrospinal fluid, Wright-Giemsa stain, ×1000.)

lymphocytes and plasmacytoid lymphocytes (Figure 15.6). However, early in the course of the illness, neutrophils may predominate.[13-15] Eosinophils and basophils may be seen in response to the presence of foreign materials such as shunts, in parasitic infections, or in allergic reactions (Figure 15.7).[9,10] When nucleated RBCs are seen, bone marrow contamination resulting from accidental puncture of the vertebral body during spinal tap should be suspected and reported. In the case of bone marrow contamination, other immature neutrophils and megakaryocytes also may be seen. When there is obvious bone marrow contamination, the WBC differential is likely to be equivalent to that of the bone marrow and not that of the CSF.

Ependymal and choroid plexus cells, lining cells of the central nervous system, may be seen. These are large cells with abundant cytoplasm that stain lavender with Wright stain. They most often appear in clumps, and although they are not diagnostically significant, it is important not to confuse them with malignant cells (Figure 15.8).

Cartilage cells may be seen if the vertebral body is accidentally punctured. These cells usually occur singly, are medium to

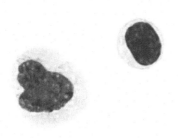

Figure 15.4 Monocye and Lymphocyte. Monocyte *(left)* and lymphocyte *(right)* seen in normal cerebrospinal fluid. (Wright-Giemsa stain, ×1000.)

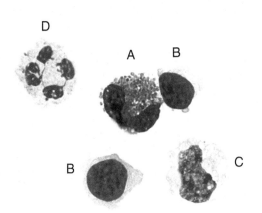

Figure 15.7 Cerbrospinal Fluid from a Patient with a Shunt. (A), Eosinophil; **(B),** lymphocytes; **(C),** monocyte; and **(D),** neutrophil. (Wright-Giemsa stain, ×1000.)

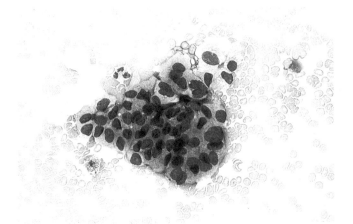

Figure 15.8 Clump of Ependymal Cells. (Cerebrospinal fluid, Wright-Giemsa stain, ×200.)

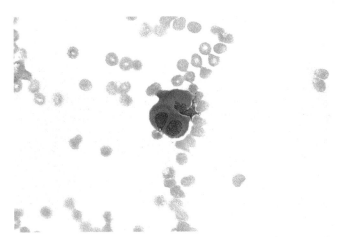

Figure 15.9 Cartilage Cells. (Cerebrospinal fluid, Wright-Giemsa stain, ×400.)

large, and have cytoplasm that stains wine red with a deep wine red nucleus with Wright stain (Figure 15.9).

Siderophages are macrophages (i.e., monocytes or histiocytes) that have ingested RBCs and, as a result of the breakdown of the RBCs, contain hemosiderin. Hemosiderin appears as large, rough-shaped, dark blue or black granules in the cytoplasm of

the macrophage. These cells also may contain bilirubin or hematoidin crystals, which are golden yellow and are a result of further breakdown of the ingested RBCs. The presence of siderophages indicates a pathologic hemorrhage. Siderophages appear approximately 48 hours after hemorrhage and may persist for 2 to 8 weeks after the hemorrhage has occurred (Figure 15.10).

A high percentage of patients with acute lymphoblastic leukemia or acute myeloid leukemia have central nervous system involvement.[9,10] It is always important to look carefully for leukemic cells (i.e., blast forms) in the CSF of patients with leukemia. Patients with lymphoma, myeloma, and chronic myeloid leukemia in blast crisis also may have blast cells in the CSF. These blast cells have the characteristics of blast forms in the peripheral blood, including a high nucleus-to-cytoplasm ratio, a fine stippled nuclear chromatin pattern, and prominent nucleoli. They are usually large cells that stain basophilic with Wright stain and have a fairly uniform appearance (Figure 15.11). If a traumatic tap has occurred and the patient has a high blast count in the peripheral blood, the blasts seen in the CSF may be the result of peripheral blood contamination and not central nervous system involvement. The possibility of peripheral blood

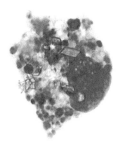

Figure 15.10 Siderophage with Bilirubin Crystals (Hematoidin). (Cerebrospinal fluid, Wright-Giemsa stain, ×400.)

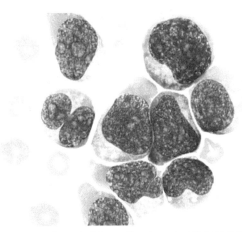

Figure 15.11 Lymphoblasts. (Cerebrospinal fluid, Wright-Giemsa stain, ×1000.) (From Rodak, B. F., & Carr, J. H. [2017]. *Clinical Hematology Atlas.* [5th ed.]. St. Louis: Elsevier.)

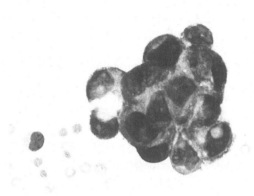

Figure 15.12 Clump of Breast Tumor Cells. (Cerebrospinal fluid, Wright-Giemsa stain, ×400.)

TABLE 15.3 Characteristics of Benign and Malignant Cells

Benign	Malignant
Have occasional large cells.	Many cells may be very large.
Are light to dark staining.	May be very basophilic.
Have rare mitotic figures.	May have several mitotic figures.
Have round to oval nucleus; nuclei are uniform in size with varying amounts of cytoplasm.	May have irregular or jagged nuclear shape.
Nuclear edge is smooth.	Edges of nucleus may be indistinct and irregular.
Nucleus is intact.	Nucleus may be disintegrated at edges.
Nucleoli are small if present.	Nucleoli may be large and prominent.
In multinuclear cells (mesothelial), all nuclei have similar appearance (size and shape).	Multinuclear cells have varying sizes and shapes of nuclei.
Have moderate to small N:C ratio.	May have high N:C ratio.
Clumps of cells have similar appearance among cells, are in the same plane of focus, and may have "windows" between cells.	Clumps of cells contain cells of varying sizes and shapes, are "three-dimensional" (require focusing up and down to see all cells), and have dark-staining borders.

N:C, Nucleus-to-cytoplasm.

contamination should be reported and the tap should be repeated in a few days.

Malignant cells resulting from metastases to the central nervous system may be found. The most common primary tumors that metastasize to the central nervous system in adults are breast, lung, and gastrointestinal tract tumors and melanoma.[9,10] In children, metastases to the central nervous system are related to Wilms tumor, Ewing sarcoma, neuroblastoma, and embryonal rhabdomyosarcoma.[10] Malignant cells are usually large with a high nucleus-to-cytoplasm ratio and are often basophilic or hyperchromic. They often occur in clumps but may occur singly. Within clumps of malignant cells, there is dissimilarity between cells, and in multinucleated cells, there may be variation in nuclear size. Clumps of malignant cells may appear three-dimensional, requiring up-and-down focusing to see the cells on different planes, and there are usually no "windows" (clear spaces) between the cells. The nuclei of these cells are usually large, often with abnormal distribution of chromatin, and they may have an indistinct or jagged border, or there may be "blebbing" at the border. Increased mitosis may be shown by the presence of several mitotic figures in the cell button. Malignant cells often have a pleomorphic appearance (Figure 15.12 and Table 15.3).

SEROUS FLUID

Serous fluids, including pleural, pericardial, and peritoneal fluids, normally exist in very small quantities and serve as lubricant between the membranes of an organ and the sac in which it is housed to reduce friction.[16] Pleural fluid is found in the space between the lungs and the pleural sac; pericardial fluid, in the space between the heart and the pericardial sac; and peritoneal fluid, between the intestine and the peritoneal sac (Figure 15.13). An accumulation of fluid in a cavity is termed an *effusion*. When an effusion is in the peritoneal cavity, it also may be referred to as *ascites* or *ascitic fluid*.[6] It would be difficult to remove these fluids from a healthy individual; the presence of these fluids in detectable amounts indicates a disease state.

Transudates Versus Exudates

As noted, the accumulation of a large amount of fluid in a cavity is called an *effusion*. There are various pathologic reasons for the formation of effusion and are due to either an increase in the production of the fluid or a decreased rate of fluid absorption.[16]

Effusions are subdivided further into *transudates* and *exudates* to distinguish whether disease is present within or outside the body cavity. In general, transudates develop as part of systemic disease processes that influence the absorption or formation of the fluid so that it accumulates, such as congestive heart failure[15,16]; whereas exudates indicate inflammatory disorders that interfere with reabsorption at the location where the fluid originates, leading to fluid accumulation associated with bacterial or viral infections, malignancy, pulmonary embolism, or systemic lupus erythematosus.[16,17] Several parameters can be measured to determine whether an effusion is a transudate or an exudate (Table 15.4). Proper determination significantly aids in identifying the diagnosis, and literature does indicate that other markers are being investigated to determine their diagnostic usefulness in differentiating the effusion.[16,18]

Gross Examination

Transudates should appear straw colored and clear, whereas the color of exudates varies (yellow, green, pink/red) and it can appear cloudy. A cloudy effusion may indicate an infectious process (leukocytes); bloody may indicate hemothorax, trauma, or malignancy; and milky often indicates the presence of chyle (fluid consisting of emulsified fats and lymph) in the pleural cavity.[19]

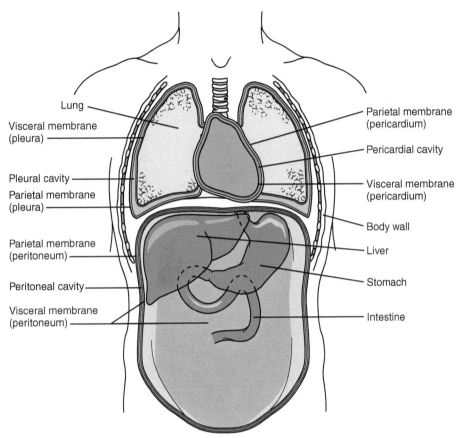

Figure 15.13 Parietal and Visceral Membranes of the Pleural, Pericardial, and Peritoneal Cavities. Parietal membranes line the body wall, whereas visceral membranes enclose organs. The two membranes are actually one continuous membrane. The space between opposing surfaces is identified as the body cavity (i.e., pleural, pericardial, and peritoneal cavities). (From Brunzel, N. A. [2018]. *Fundamentals of Urine and Body Fluid Analysis.* [4th ed.]. St. Louis: Elsevier.)

TABLE 15.4 Serous Fluid: Transudates Versus Exudates		
Characteristic	**Transudates**	**Exudates**
Specific gravity	<1.016	>1.016
Protein	<3 g/dL	>3 g/dL
Lactate dehydrogenase	<200 IU	>200 IU
White blood cells	<1000/μL (predominant cell type mononuclear)	>1000/μL
Protein: fluid-to-serum ratio	<0.5	>0.5
Lactate dehydrogenase: fluid-to-serum ratio	<0.6	>0.6
Color	Clear or straw colored	Cloudy or yellow, amber, or grossly bloody
Volume	—	Extremely large

Differential Cell Counts

The cells found in normal serous fluid are lymphocytes, histiocytes (macrophages), and mesothelial cells. Neutrophils are commonly seen in the fluid sent to the hematology laboratory for analysis but would not be present in normal fluid. When neutrophils are seen, they may have more segments and longer filaments than in peripheral blood.

Mesothelial cells are the lining cells of body cavities and are shed into these cavities constantly. These are large (12- to 30-μm) cells and have a "fried egg" appearance with basophilic cytoplasm, oval nucleus with smooth nuclear borders, stippled nuclear chromatin pattern, and one to three nucleoli.[9,10] Mesothelial cells may vary in size, may be multinucleated (including giant cells with 20 to 25 nuclei), and may have frayed cytoplasmic borders, cytoplasmic vacuoles, or both. They may occur singly, in small or large clumps, or in sheets. When they occur in clumps, there are usually "windows" between the cells. The nucleus-to-cytoplasm ratio is 1:2 to 1:3, and this is generally consistent despite the variability in cell size.[19] They tend to have a similar appearance to each other on a slide. Mesothelial cells are seen in most effusions, and their numbers are increased in sterile inflammations and decreased in tuberculous pleurisy and bacterial infections (Figure 15.14).[9]

Macrophages appear as monocytes or histiocytes in serous fluids and may contain RBCs (erythrophages) or siderotic granules (siderophages), or they may appear as signet ring cells when lipid has been ingested and the resulting large vacuole pushes the nucleus to the periphery of the cell (Figure 15.15).

Eosinophils and basophils are not normally seen. These may be present in large numbers, however, as a result of allergic reaction or sensitivity to foreign material.

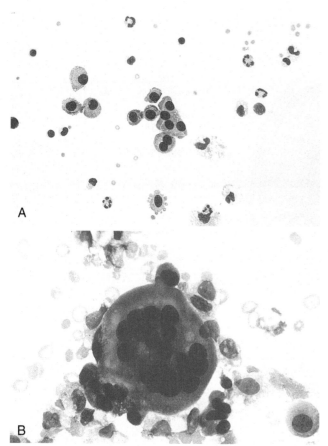

Figure 15.14 Mesothelial Cells. (A), Mesothelial cells. Note "fried egg" appearance. (Peritoneal fluid, Wright-Giemsa stain, ×200.) **(B),** Mesothelial cell with 21 nuclei. (Pleural fluid, Wright-Giemsa stain, ×400.)

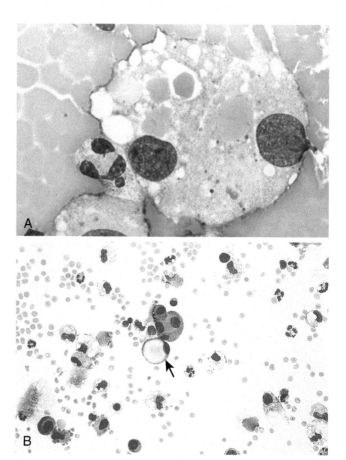

Figure 15.15 Erythrophage and Signet Ring Cell. (A), Erythrophage. (Peritoneal fluid, Wright-Giemsa stain, ×1000.) **(B),** Signet ring cell *(arrow)*. (Peritoneal fluid, Wright-Giemsa stain, ×200.)

When large numbers of neutrophils are seen, a thorough search should be made for bacteria. If possible, Gram staining should be performed on a second cytocentrifuge slide to aid in rapid identification if bacteria are found. Table 15.5 lists Gram-stained organisms most commonly seen in body fluids.

Lupus erythematosus cells may be seen in serous fluids of patients with systemic lupus erythematosus, because all the factors necessary for the formation of these cells—presence of the lupus erythematosus factor, incubation, and trauma to the cells—exist in vivo. A lupus erythematosus cell is an intact neutrophil that has engulfed a homogeneous mass of degenerated nuclear material, which displaces the normal nucleus. Lupus erythematosus cells can form in vivo and in vitro in serous and synovial fluids and should be reported (Figure 15.16).

Malignant cells are seen in serous fluids from primary or metastatic tumors. They have the characteristics of malignant cells found in CSF (Figure 15.17). Figure 15.18 presents a flow chart for examination of serous fluids.

SYNOVIAL FLUID

Gross Examination

Synovial fluid is normally present in very small amounts in the synovial cavity surrounding joints. When fluid is present in amounts large enough to aspirate, there is a disease process in

TABLE 15.5 Gram-Stained Organisms Most Commonly Seen in Body Fluids

Fluid	Organism
Cerebrospinal	Gram-negative diplococci
	Gram-positive cocci
	Gram-negative coccobacilli
	Yeast—stains gram positive
	Cryptococcus—look for capsule
Serous (peritoneal, pleural, or pericardial)	Gram-positive cocci
	Gram-negative bacilli
	Gram-positive bacilli
	Yeast—stains gram positive
Synovial (joint)	Gram-positive cocci
	Gram-negative bacilli
	Gram-negative diplococci
	Gram-negative coccobacilli

Note: If the Gram-stained organisms seen in a fluid are not listed here for that fluid, do not report Gram stain results. Save the slide for review.

the joint. Figure 15.19 demonstrates placement of the needle for synovial fluid collection from a knee. Normally this fluid is straw colored and clear. Synovial fluid contains hyaluronic acid, which makes it very viscous. A small amount (pinch) of hyaluronidase powder should be added to all joint fluids to make

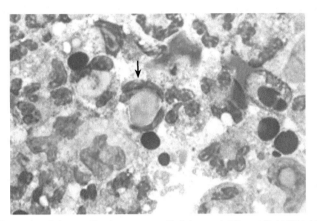

Figure 15.16 Lupus Erythematosus Cell *(arrow).* (Pleural fluid, Wright-Giemsa stain, ×1000.)

them less viscous (liquefy them) before cell counts are performed by automated methods or manual methods or cytocentrifuge slides are prepared. If a crystal analysis is to be performed, an aliquot of fluid should be removed for this purpose *before* the hyaluronidase is added.

Differential Cell Counts

Cells found in normal synovial fluid are lymphocytes, monocytes/histiocytes, and synovial cells. Synovial cells line the synovial

cavity and are shed into the cavity. They resemble mesothelial cells but are usually present in smaller numbers (Figure 15.20).

Lupus erythematosus cells may be present in synovial fluid just as in serous fluid. Malignant cells are rarely seen in synovial fluid but, when present, resemble tumor cells seen in serous fluids or CSF.

Many neutrophils are present in synovial fluid in acute inflammation of joints. As always, a careful search should be made for bacteria when many neutrophils are seen.

Crystals

Intracellular and extracellular crystals may be present in synovial fluid and are clinically significant. Crystal examination may be performed by placing a drop of fluid on a slide and adding a coverslip or by examining a cytocentrifuge preparation. However, the specimen should be fresh, without hyaluronidase added. All synovial fluids should be examined carefully for crystals using a polarizing microscope with a red compensator. The crystals most commonly seen in synovial fluids are cholesterol, calcium pyrophosphate, and monosodium urate.

Cholesterol crystals are large, flat, extracellular crystals with a notched corner.[20] They are seen in patients with chronic effusions, particularly patients with rheumatoid arthritis.

Calcium pyrophosphate crystals are seen in pseudogout. These crystals are intracellular and are small rhomboid, plate-like,

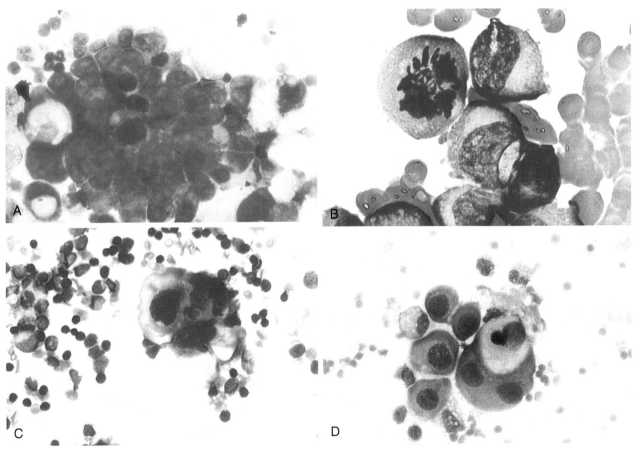

Figure 15.17 Tumor Cells. (A), Clump of tumor cells. (Pleural fluid, Wright-Giemsa stain, ×200). **(B),** Tumor cells and mitotic figure. (Pleural fluid, Wright-Giemsa stain, ×1000.) **(C),** Adenocarcinoma cells. (Pleural fluid, Wright-Giemsa stain, ×200). **(D),** Tumor cells. Note cell cannibalism. (Peritoneal fluid, Wright-Giemsa stain, ×200.)

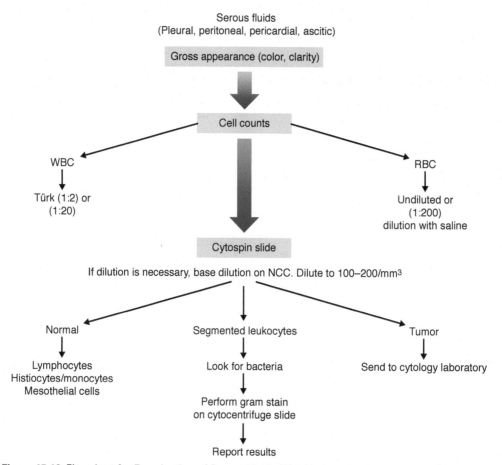

Figure 15.18 Flowchart for Examination of Serous Fluid. *NCC*, Nucleated cell count; *RBC*, red blood cell; *WBC*, white blood cell.

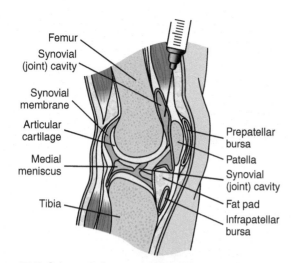

Figure 15.19 Schematic Representation of Synovial Fluid Aspiration. Note placement of the needle for synovial fluid aspiration. (From Applegate, E. [2011]. *The Anatomy and Physiology Learning System.* [4th ed.]. Philadelphia: Saunders, Elsevier.)

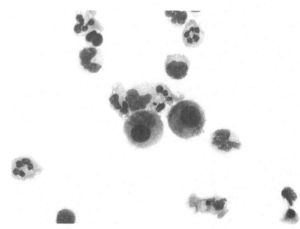

Figure 15.20 Synovial Cells. Note similarity to mesothelial cells. (Synovial fluid, Wright-Giemsa stain, ×400.)

or rod-like crystals.[20] The crystals are weakly birefringent when polarized (i.e., they do not appear bright when polarized). When the red compensator is used, calcium pyrophosphate crystals appear blue when the longitudinal axis of the crystal is parallel to the *y*-axis (Figure 15.21).[20]

Monosodium urate crystals are seen in gout. They are large needle-like crystals that may be intracellular or extracellular. These crystals are strongly birefringent when polarized. When the red compensator is used, monosodium urate crystals appear yellow when the longitudinal axis of the crystal is parallel to the *y*-axis (Figure 15.22).[20] Figure 15.23 presents a flowchart for synovial fluid analysis.

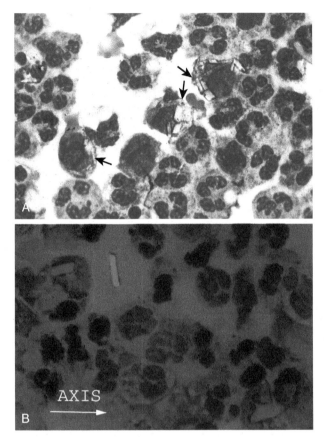

Figure 15.21 Intracellular Calcium Pyrophosphate Crystals. (Synovial fluid, **(A),** Wright-Giemsa stain, ×1000.) **(B),** Polarized with red compensator. (B Courtesy George Girgis, Indiana University Health, Indianapolis, IN.)

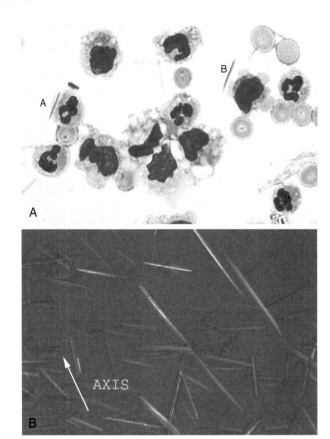

Figure 15.22 Monosodium Urate Crystals. (A), Intracellular and extracellular. (Synovial fluid, Wright-Stain, ×1000.) **(B),** Polarized with red compensator. (A from Rodak, B. F., & Carr, J. H. (2017). *Clinical Hematology Atlas.* [5th ed.]. St. Louis: Elsevier. B Courtesy George Girgis, Indiana University Health, Indianapolis, IN.)

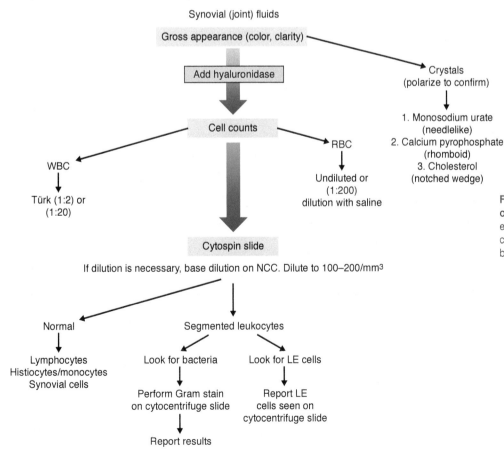

Figure 15.23 Flowchart for Examination of Synovial (Joint) Fluid. *LE,* Lupus erythematosus; *NCC,* nucleated cell count; *RBC,* red blood cell; *WBC,* white blood cell.

BRONCHOALVEOLAR LAVAGE SPECIMENS

Procedure and Precautions

Brohoalveolar lavage (BAL) specimens are not naturally occurring fluids; they are produced when the BAL procedure is performed. The procedure consists of introducing warmed saline into the lungs in 50-mL aliquots and then withdrawing it. The specimen received in the laboratory is the withdrawn fluid. The purpose of the procedure is to determine types of organisms and cells that are present in areas of the lung that are otherwise inaccessible. This procedure is performed on patients with severe lung dysfunction.

The specimen should always undergo an extensive microbiologic workup and often cytologic examination. It is common to see bacteria, yeast, or both on cytocentrifuge slides prepared from these specimens. Because samples are obtained from the interior of the lung and may contain airborne organisms, care should be taken to avoid aerosol production. Samples should be mixed and containers opened under a biologic safety hood, and a mask should be worn when performing cell counts. Because the risk of performing cell counts and preparing cytocentrifuge slides on BAL specimens outweighs the clinical relevance of the information obtained, some hematology laboratories no longer perform this procedure and defer to information reported from the microbiology laboratory.

Cell counts and cytocentrifuge preparations are performed as with any body fluid. Significant cell deterioration occurs within 30 minutes of collection, with the neutrophils disintegrating most rapidly.

Differential Cell Counts

The cell types most commonly seen in BAL specimens are neutrophils, monohistiocytes (macrophages), and lymphocytes. Mesothelial cells are not seen in BAL specimens because these cells line the body cavities and not the interior of the lung. Pneumocytes, which can resemble mesothelial cells or adenocarcinoma, may be seen in patients with acute respiratory distress syndrome.

Ciliated epithelial cells can be seen and should be reported because they indicate that the sample was obtained from the upper respiratory tract instead of deeper in the lung. These are columnar cells, with the nucleus at one end of the cell, elongated cytoplasm, and cilia at the opposite end of the cell from the nucleus. They can occur in clusters. If the sample is not aged when the cell count is performed, these cells are in motion in the hemacytometer, because they can be propelled by their cilia (Figure 15.24).

Histiocytes laden with carbonaceous material are seen in patients who use tobacco. These cells resemble siderophages in other fluids, but the carbonaceous material is black, brown, or blue-black and is more droplet-like (Figure 15.25).

Pneumocystis jirovecii (formerly *Pneumocystis carinii*) may be seen in specimens from patients infected with human immunodeficiency virus. The *P. jirovecii* organisms appear as clumps of amorphous material. Close examination of the clumps may reveal cysts (Figure 15.26).

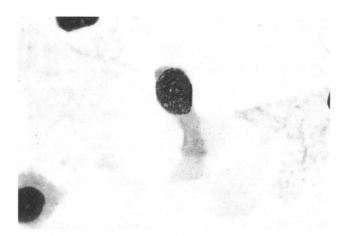

Figure 15.24 Ciliated Epithelial Cells. (Bronchoalveolar lavage fluid, Wright-Giemsa stain, ×100.)

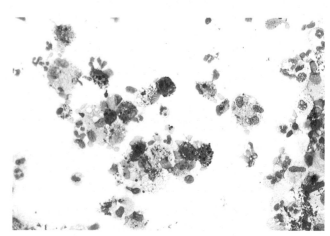

Figure 15.25 Histiocytes with Carbonaceous Material. (Bronchoalveolar lavage fluid, Wright-Giemsa stain, ×40.)

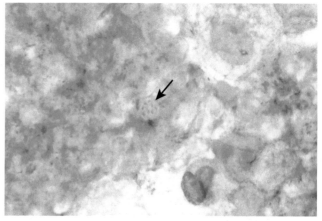

Figure 15.26 Cyst of *Pneumocystis jirovecii* (formerly *Pneumocystis carinii*). (Bronchoalveolar lavage fluid, Wright-Giemsa stain, X100.)

SUMMARY

- Cell counts and differential cell counts performed on body fluid specimens are valuable diagnostic tools.
- Cell counts are often performed on hematology analyzers that have a body fluid (BF) mode; however, they can be performed manually.
- Calibrated methods must be used when performing manual cell counts to provide accurate counts.
- Cytocentrifuge slides allow for a microscopic review of a concentrated monolayer of cells for identification of white blood cells (WBCs).
- Fluid analysis commonly performed in the hematology department include the following specimens: cerebrospinal fluid (CSF), serous (pleural, pericardial, and peritoneal) fluids, and synovial fluids.
- Normal cell types in any fluid are lymphocytes, macrophages (monocytes, histiocytes), and lining cells (ependymal cells in

CSF, mesothelial cells in serous fluids, synovial cells in joint fluids).
- Bacteria and yeast may be seen in any fluid.
- Malignant cells may be seen in any fluid but are rare in synovial fluid.
- Because of the viscosity of synovial fluid, it must be pretreated with hyaluronidase before testing to liquefy the specimen for both automated and manual test methods.
- Synovial fluid should be examined for crystals using a compensated polarizing microscope.
- Bronchoalveolar lavage (BAL) specimens are not a true body fluid, but examination of cells present may provide diagnostic information.

Now that you have completed this chapter, go back and read again the case study at the beginning and respond to the questions presented.

REVIEW QUESTIONS

Answers can be found in the Appendix.

Refer to the following scenario to answer questions 1 and 2: A spinal fluid specimen is diluted 1:2 with Türk solution to perform the TNC count. A total of six nucleated cells are counted on both sides of the hemacytometer, with all nine squares counted on both sides. Undiluted fluid is used to perform the RBC count. A total of 105 RBCs are counted on both sides of the hemacytometer, with four large squares on both sides counted.

1. The TNC count is ___/μL.
   a. 3
   b. 7
   c. 13
   d. 66
2. The RBC count is ___/μL.
   a. 131
   b. 263
   c. 1050
   d. 5830
3. Based on the cell counts, the appearance of the fluid should be:
   a. Turbid
   b. Hemolyzed
   c. Clear
   d. Cloudy
4. All of the following cells are normally seen in CSF, serous fluids, and synovial fluids *except:*
   a. Lining cells
   b. Neutrophils
   c. Lymphocytes
   d. Monocytes/histiocytes (macrophages)

5. Spinal fluid was obtained from a 56-year-old woman. On receipt in the laboratory, the fluid was noted to be slightly bloody. When a portion of the fluid was centrifuged, the supernatant was clear. The cell counts were 5200 RBCs/μL^3 and 24 WBCs/μL. On the cytocentrifuge preparation, several nucleated RBCs were seen. The differential was 52% lymphocytes, 20% neutrophils, 22% monocytes, 4% myelocytes, and 2% blasts. What is the most likely explanation for these results?
   a. Bone marrow contamination
   b. Bacterial meningitis
   c. Peripheral blood contamination
   d. Leukemic infiltration in the central nervous system
6. A 34-year-old woman with a history of breast cancer developed a pleural effusion. The fluid obtained was bloody and had a TNC count of 284/μL. On the cytocentrifuge preparation, there were several neutrophils and a few monocytes/histiocytes. There were also several clusters of large, dark-staining cells. These cell clumps appeared three-dimensional and contained some mitotic figures. What is the most likely identification of the cells in clusters?
   a. Mesothelial cells
   b. Metastatic tumor cells
   c. Cartilage cells
   d. Pneumocytes
7. A serous fluid with a clear appearance, specific gravity of 1.010, protein concentration of 1.5 g/dL, and fewer than 500 mononuclear cells/μL would be considered:
   a. Infectious
   b. An exudate
   c. A transudate
   d. Sterile

8. On the cytocentrifuge slide prepared from a peritoneal fluid sample, many large cells are seen, singly and in clumps. The cells have a "fried egg" appearance and basophilic cytoplasm, and some are multinucleated. These cells should be reported as:

a. Suspicious for malignancy
b. Macrophages
c. Large lymphocytes
d. Mesothelial cells

Refer to the following scenario to answer questions 9 and 10:
A 56-year-old man came to the physician's office with complaints of pain and swelling in his left big toe. Fluid aspirated from the toe was straw colored and cloudy. The WBC count was 2543/μL. The differential consisted mainly of neutrophils and monocytes/histiocytes. Intracellular and extracellular crystals were seen on the cytocentrifuge slide. The crystals were needle shaped and, when polarized with the use of the red compensator, appeared yellow on the *y*-axis.

9. The crystals are:

a. Cholesterol
b. Hyaluronidase
c. Monosodium urate
d. Calcium pyrophosphate

10. This patient's painful toe was caused by:

a. Gout
b. Infection
c. Inflammation
d. Pseudogout

REFERENCES

1. Glasser, L. (1981). Cells in cerebrospinal fluid. *Diagn Med, 4,* 33–50.
2. Sandhaus, L. M. (2015). Body fluid cell counts by automated methods. *Clin Lab Med, 35,* 93–103.
3. Bottini, P. V., Pompeo, D. B., Souza, M. I., et al. (2015). Comparison between automated and microscopic analysis in body fluids cytology. *Int J Lab Hematol, 37,* e16–e18.
4. Cho, Y., Chi, H., Park, S. H., et al. (2015). Body fluid cellular analysis using the Sysmex XN-2000 automatic hematology analyzer: focusing on malignant samples. *Int J Lab Hematol, 37,* 346–356.
5. Danise, P., Maconi, M., Rovetti, A., et al. (2013). Cell counting of body fluids: comparison between three automated haematology analysers and the manual microscope method. *Int J Lab Hematol, 35,* 608-613.
6. Brunzel, N. A. (2018). Physical examination of urine. In *Fundamentals of Urine and Body Fluid Analysis.* (4th ed., pp. 68–84). St. Louis: Elsevier.
7. Perné, A., Hainfellner, J. A., Womastek, I., et al. (2012). Performance evaluation of the Sysmex XE-5000 hematology analyzer for white blood cell analysis in cerebrospinal fluid. *Arch Pathol Lab Med, 136,* 194–198.
8. Tanada, H., Ikemoto, T., Masutani, R., et al. (2014). Evaluation of the automated hematology analyzer ADVIA® 120 for cerebrospinal fluid analysis and usage of unique hemolysis reagent. *Int J Lab Hematol, 36,* 83–91.
9. Kjeldsberg, C., & Knight, J. (1993). *Body fluids.* (3rd ed.). Chicago: ASCP Press.
10. Galagan, K., Blomberg, D., Cornbleet, P. J., et al. (2006). *Color Atlas of Body Fluids,* Northfield, IL: College of American Pathologists.
11. Brunzel, N.A. (2018). Cerebrospinal fluid analysis. In *Fundamentals of Urine and Body Fluid Analysis.* (4th ed., pp. 243–260). St. Louis: Elsevier.
12. CLSI. (2006). *Body Fluid Analysis for Cellular Composition.* (Approved guideline, H56-A). Wayne, PA: Clinical Laboratory and Standards Institute.
13. Bartt, R. (2012). Acute bacterial and viral meningitis. *Continuum Lifelong Learning Neurol, 18,* 1255–1270.
14. Rotbart, H. A. (2000). Viral meningitis. *Semin Neurol, 20,* 277–292.
15. Spanos, A., Harrell, F. E., & Durack, D. T. (1989). Differential diagnosis of acute meningitis. *JAMA, 262,* 2700–2707.
16. Block, D. R., & Algeciras-Schimnich, A. (2013). Body fluid analysis: clinical utility and applicability of published studies to guide interpretation of today's laboratory testing in serous fluids. *Crit Rev Cl Lab Sci, 50,* 107–124.
17. Light, R. W. (2013). The light criteria: the beginning and why they are useful 40 years later. *Clin Chest Med, 34,* 21–26.
18. Hassan, T., Al-Alawi, M., Chotirmall, S. H., et al. (2012). Pleural fluid analysis: standstill or a work in progress? *Pulm Med, 2012,* 716235. doi: 10.1155/2012/716235
19. Brunzel, N. A. (2018). Pleural, pericardial, and peritoneal analysis. In *Fundamentals of Urine and Body Fluid Analysis.* (4th ed., pp. 261–273). St. Louis: Elsevier.
20. Strasinger, S. K., & DiLorenzo, M. S. (2014). Urine sediment constituents. In *Urinalysis and Body Fluids.* (6th ed., pp. 110–146). Philadelphia: FA Davis.

16

Anemias: Red Blood Cell Morphology and Approach to Diagnosis

Naveen Manchanda*

OBJECTIVES

After completion of this chapter, the reader will be able to:

1. Define *anemia* and recognize laboratory results consistent with anemia.
2. Describe clinical findings in anemia.
3. Discuss the importance of the history and physical examination in diagnosis of anemia.
4. Explain how the body adapts to anemia and the symptoms experienced by the patient.
5. Distinguish among effective, ineffective, and insufficient erythropoiesis when given examples.
6. List laboratory procedures that are initially performed for diagnosis of anemia.
7. Discuss the importance of the reticulocyte count in the evaluation of anemia.
8. Explain the importance of examining the peripheral blood film when investigating the cause of an anemia and distinguish important findings.
9. Describe variations in red blood cell morphology such as inclusions and changes in shape, volume, or color.
10. Use an algorithm incorporating the absolute reticulocyte count to specify three groups of anemias involving decreased or ineffective red blood cell production and give one example of each.
11. Use an algorithm incorporating the mean cell volume to narrow the differential diagnosis of anemia.

OUTLINE

CASE STUDY

After studying the material in this chapter, the reader should be able to respond to the following case study:

A 45-year-old woman phoned her physician and complained of fatigue, shortness of breath on exertion, and general malaise. She requested "B$_{12}$ shots" to make her feel better. The physician asked the patient to schedule an appointment so that she could determine the cause of the symptoms before offering treatment. A point-of-care hemoglobin determination performed in the office was 9.0 g/dL. The physician then requested additional laboratory tests, including a complete blood count (CBC) with a reticulocyte count and a peripheral blood film examination.

1. Why did the physician want the patient to come to the office before she prescribed therapy?
2. How do the mean cell volume and reticulocyte count help determine the classification of the anemia?
3. Why is the examination of the peripheral blood film important in the investigation of an anemia?

*The author extends appreciation to Ann Bell and Rakesh Mehta, whose work in prior editions provided the foundation for this chapter.

Red blood cells (RBCs) perform the vital physiologic function of oxygen delivery to tissues. Hemoglobin within the RBCs has the remarkable capacity to bind oxygen in the lungs and then release it appropriately in tissues.[1] The term *anemia* is derived from the Greek word *anaimia,* meaning "without blood."[2] A decrease in hemoglobin concentration or number of RBCs results in decreased oxygen delivery to tissue, resulting in tissue hypoxia. Anemia is a common condition affecting an estimated 1.93 billion people worldwide.[3] Anemia should not be thought of as a disease but rather as a manifestation of an underlying condition or deficiency.[4,5] Therefore causes of anemia should be thoroughly investigated. This chapter provides an overview of the mechanisms, diagnosis, and classification of anemia. In the following chapters, each anemia is discussed in detail.

DEFINITION OF ANEMIA

A functional definition of *anemia* is a decrease in the oxygen-carrying capacity of the blood. It can arise if there is insufficient hemoglobin or the hemoglobin has impaired function. The former is the more frequent cause.

Anemia is defined operationally as a reduction in the hemoglobin content of blood that can be caused by a decrease in the RBC count, hemoglobin concentration, and hematocrit below the reference interval for healthy individuals of similar age, sex, and race, under similar environmental conditions.[4-8] The reference intervals are derived from large pools of "healthy" individuals; however, the definition of *healthy* is different for each of these groups. Thus these pools of "healthy" individuals may lack the heterogeneity required to be universally applied to any one of these populations of individuals.[6] This fact has led to the development of different reference intervals for individuals of different sex, age, and race.

Examples of hematologic reference intervals for the adult and pediatric populations are included on the inside cover. They are listed according to age and sex, but race, environmental, and laboratory factors can also influence the values. Each laboratory must determine its own reference intervals based on its particular instrumentation, the methods used, and the demographic characteristics and environment of its patient population. For the purpose of the discussion in this chapter, a patient is considered anemic if the hemoglobin value falls to less than those listed on the inside cover.

IMPORTANCE OF PATIENT HISTORY AND CLINICAL FINDINGS

History and physical examination are important components in making a clinical diagnosis of anemia. A decrease in oxygen delivery to tissues decreases the energy available to individuals to perform day-to-day activities. This gives rise to the classic symptoms associated with anemia, fatigue and shortness of breath. To elucidate the reason for a patient's anemia, one starts by obtaining a detailed history, which requires carefully questioning the patient, particularly with regard to diet, drug ingestion, exposure to chemicals, occupation, hobbies, travel, bleeding history, race or ethnic group, family history of disease, neurologic symptoms, previous medications, previous episodes of jaundice, and various underlying disease processes that result in anemia.[4,7-9] Therefore a thorough discussion is required to elicit any potential cause of the anemia. For example, iron deficiency can lead to an interesting symptom called *pica.*[10] Patients with pica have cravings for unusual substances such as ice (pagophagia), cornstarch, or clay. Alternatively, individuals with anemia may be asymptomatic, as can be seen in mild or slowly progressive anemias where the body is able to adapt to the slowly developing anemia.

Certain features should be evaluated closely during the physical examination to provide clues to hematologic disorders, such as skin (for petechiae), eyes (for pallor, jaundice, and hemorrhage), and mouth (for mucosal bleeding). The examination should also search for sternal tenderness, lymphadenopathy, cardiac murmurs or arrhythmias, splenomegaly, and hepatomegaly.[4,11] Jaundice is important for the assessment of anemia, because it may be due to increased RBC destruction, which suggests a hemolytic component to the anemia. Measuring vital signs is also a crucial component of the physical evaluation. Patients experiencing a rapid fall in hemoglobin concentration typically have tachycardia (fast heart rate), whereas if the anemia is long-standing, the heart rate may be normal because of the body's ability to compensate for the anemia (discussed later).

Moderate anemias (hemoglobin concentration of 7 to 10 g/dL) may cause pallor of conjunctivae and nail beds but may not produce clinical symptoms if the onset of anemia is slow.[4] However, depending on the patient's age and cardiovascular state, symptoms such as dyspnea, vertigo, headache, muscle weakness, and lethargy can occur.[4,8] Severe anemias (hemoglobin concentration of less than 7 g/dL) usually produce tachycardia, hypotension, and other symptoms of volume loss, in addition to the symptoms listed earlier. Thus severity of the anemia is gauged by the degree of reduction in hemoglobin, cardiopulmonary adaptation, and the rapidity of progression of the anemia.[4]

PHYSIOLOGIC ADAPTATIONS IN PATIENTS WITH ANEMIA

Patients who develop anemia from acute blood loss, such as with severe hemorrhage, respond with profound changes in physiologic processes to ensure adequate perfusion of vital organs and maintenance of homeostasis. In cases of severe blood loss, such as in trauma, blood volume decreases and hypotension develops, resulting in decreased blood supply to the brain and heart. As an immediate adaptation, there is sympathetic overdrive that results in increasing heart rate, respiratory rate, and cardiac output.[4,7,8] In severe anemia, blood is preferentially shunted to organs that are key to survival, including the brain, muscle, and heart.[4,7,8] This results in oxygen being preferentially supplied to vital organs even in the presence of reduced oxygen-carrying capacity. In addition, tissue hypoxia triggers an increase in RBC 2,3-bisphosphoglycerate that shifts the oxygen dissociation curve to the right (decreased oxygen affinity of hemoglobin) and results in increased oxygen delivery to tissues

---

BOX 16.1 Adaptations to Anemia

Response to Acute (Sudden) Loss of Blood
The following adaptations occur in minutes to hours:
- Increase in heart rate, respiratory rate, and cardiac output, which increases the flow of oxygenated blood
- Redistribution of blood flow from skin to essential organs (brain, heart, muscles)

Response to Slowly Developing Anemia
The following adaptations occur over days to weeks:
- Increase in erythrocyte 2,3-bisphosphoglycerate which decreases hemoglobin's affinity for oxygen and allows more oxygen release to tissues
- Increase in erythropoietin production by kidneys, which increases erythropoiesis and promotes release of more red blood cells into circulation

---

(Chapter 7).[8,12] This is also a significant mechanism in chronic anemias that enables patients with low levels of hemoglobin to remain relatively asymptomatic. Thus with slowly developing and low-grade anemia, the body develops physiologic adaptations to increase the oxygen-carrying capacity of a reduced amount of hemoglobin, which improves oxygen delivery to tissues. With persistent and severe anemia, however, the strain on the heart can ultimately lead to cardiac failure.

Reduced oxygen delivery to tissues caused by reduced hemoglobin concentration elicits an increase in erythropoietin secretion by the kidneys. Erythropoietin stimulates the erythroid precursors in the bone marrow, which leads to the release of more RBCs into the circulation[7,8] (Chapter 5).

With rapid blood loss, the hemoglobin and hematocrit may be initially unchanged because there is balanced loss of plasma and cells. However, as the drop in blood volume is compensated for by movement of fluid from the extravascular to the intravascular compartment or by administration of resuscitation fluid, there will be a dilution of RBCs and anemia. Box 16.1 summarizes the body's physiologic adaptations to anemia.

MECHANISMS OF ANEMIA

The life span of an RBC in circulation is about 120 days. In a healthy individual with no anemia, each day approximately 1% of RBCs are removed from circulation because of senescence, but the bone marrow continuously produces RBCs to replace those lost. Hematopoietic stem cells differentiate into erythroid precursor cells, and the bone marrow releases reticulocytes (immature anucleated RBCs) that mature into RBCs in the peripheral circulation. Adequate RBC production requires several nutritional factors such as iron, vitamin B_{12}, and folate. Globin (polypeptide chain) synthesis must also function normally. In conditions with excessive bleeding or hemolysis, the bone marrow must increase RBC production to compensate for the increased RBC loss. Therefore the maintenance of a stable hemoglobin concentration requires the production of functionally normal RBCs in sufficient numbers to replace the amount lost.[4]

Ineffective and Insufficient Erythropoiesis

Erythropoiesis is the term used for marrow erythroid proliferative activity. Normal erythropoiesis occurs in bone marrow and is under the control of the hormone *erythropoietin* (produced by the kidney) and other growth factors and cytokines (Chapters 4 and 5).[7,8] When erythropoiesis is effective, bone marrow is able to produce functional RBCs that replace the daily loss of RBCs.

Ineffective erythropoiesis refers to the production of erythroid precursor cells that are defective. These defective precursors often undergo apoptosis (programmed cell death) in the bone marrow before they have a chance to mature to the reticulocyte stage and be released into the peripheral circulation. Several conditions, such as megaloblastic anemia (impaired deoxyribonucleic acid [DNA] synthesis as a result of vitamin B_{12} or folate deficiency), thalassemia (deficient globin chain synthesis), and sideroblastic anemia (deficient protoporphyrin synthesis), involve ineffective erythropoiesis as a mechanism of anemia. In these anemias, peripheral blood hemoglobin concentration is low, which triggers an increase in erythropoietin production leading to increased erythropoietic activity. Although the RBC production rate is high, it is ineffective in that many of the defective erythroid precursors undergo destruction in the bone marrow. The end result is a decreased number of circulating RBCs resulting in anemia.[4,11]

Insufficient erythropoiesis refers to a decrease in the number of erythroid precursors in the bone marrow, resulting in decreased RBC production and anemia. Many factors can lead to the decreased RBC production, including a deficiency of iron (inadequate intake, malabsorption, excessive loss from chronic bleeding); a deficiency of erythropoietin (renal disease); or loss of the erythroid precursors as a result of an autoimmune reaction (aplastic anemia, acquired pure red cell aplasia) or infection (parvovirus B19). Erythropoiesis can also be suppressed by infiltration of the bone marrow space with leukemia cells or with nonhematopoietic cells (metastatic tumors, granulomas, or fibrosis), the latter called *myelophthisic anemia* with characteristic teardrop RBCs.[4,7,12]

Blood Loss and Hemolysis

Anemia can also develop as a result of acute blood loss (such as a traumatic injury) or chronic blood loss (such as an intermittently bleeding colonic polyp). Increased hemolysis results in a shortened RBC life span, thus increasing the risk for anemia. Chronic blood loss induces iron deficiency as a cause of anemia. With acute blood loss and excessive hemolysis, the bone marrow takes a few days to increase production of RBCs.[4,7,8] This response may be inadequate to compensate for a sudden excessive RBC loss as in traumatic hemorrhage or in conditions with a high rate of hemolysis and shortened RBC survival. Numerous causes of hemolysis exist, including intrinsic defects in the RBC membrane, enzyme systems, or hemoglobin, or extrinsic causes such as antibody-mediated processes, mechanical fragmentation, or infection-related destruction.[4,7,8]

LABORATORY DIAGNOSIS OF ANEMIA

Complete Blood Count With Red Blood Cell Indices

To detect the presence of anemia, the medical laboratory professional performs a complete blood count (CBC) using an automated blood cell analyzer to determine the RBC count, hemoglobin concentration, hematocrit, RBC indices, white blood cell count, and platelet count (Chapter 12). The RBC indices include the mean cell volume (MCV), mean cell hemoglobin (MCH), and mean cell hemoglobin concentration (MCHC) (Chapter 11).[13] The most important of these indices is the MCV, a measure of the average RBC volume in femtoliters (fL). Reference intervals for these determinations are listed on the inside front cover and in Table 16.1. Automated blood cell analyzers also provide the red cell distribution width (RDW), an index of variation of cell volume in an RBC population (discussed later). A reticulocyte count should be performed for every patient with anemia. As with RBCs, automated analyzers provide accurate measurements of reticulocyte counts.

The RBC histogram provided by the automated analyzer is an RBC volume frequency distribution curve with the relative number of cells plotted on the ordinate and RBC volume (fL) on the abscissa. In healthy individuals the distribution is approximately Gaussian. Abnormalities include a shift in the curve to the left (smaller cell population or microcytosis) or to the right (larger cell population or macrocytosis). A widening of the curve occurs when a population of RBCs have different volumes causing a greater variation of RBC volume about the mean. The histogram complements the peripheral blood film examination in identifying abnormal RBC populations. A discussion of histograms with examples can be found in Chapters 12 and 13.

RDW is the coefficient of variation of RBC volume expressed as a percentage.[13] It indicates the variation in RBC volume within the population measured and an increased RDW correlates with anisocytosis (variation in RBC diameter) on the peripheral blood film. Automated analyzers calculate the RDW by dividing the standard deviation of the RBC volume by the MCV and then multiplying by 100 to convert to a percentage. Clinical usefulness of the RDW is discussed later.

Reticulocyte Count

The reticulocyte count serves as an important tool to assess the bone marrow's ability to increase RBC production in response to an anemia. Reticulocytes are young RBCs that lack a nucleus but still contain residual ribonucleic acid (RNA) to complete the production of hemoglobin. Normally they circulate peripherally for only 1 day while completing their development. The adult reference interval for the reticulocyte count is 0.5% to 2.5% expressed as a percentage of the total number of RBCs.[13] The newborn reference interval is 1.5% to 6.0%, but these values change to approximately those of an adult within a few weeks after birth.[13] An absolute

reticulocyte count is determined by multiplying the percent reticulocytes by the RBC count (Table 16.1). The reference interval for the absolute reticulocyte count is 20 to 115×10^9/L, based on an adult RBC count within the reference interval (inside front cover).[4,7] A patient with a severe anemia may seem to be producing increased numbers of reticulocytes if only the percentage is considered. For example, an adult patient with 1.5×10^{12}/L RBCs and 3% reticulocytes has an absolute reticulocyte count of 45×10^9/L. The percentage of reticulocytes exceeds the reference interval, but the absolute reticulocyte count is within the reference interval. For the degree of anemia, however, both these results are inappropriately low. In other words, production of reticulocytes within the reference interval is inadequate to compensate for an RBC count that is approximately one-third of normal.

Two successive corrections are made to the reticulocyte count to obtain a better representation of RBC production. First, to obtain a corrected reticulocyte count, one corrects for the degree of anemia by multiplying the reticulocyte percentage by the patient's hematocrit and dividing the result by 45 (the average normal hematocrit). If the reticulocytes are released prematurely from the bone marrow and remain in the circulation 2 to 3 days (instead of 1 day), the corrected reticulocyte count must be divided by maturation time to determine the reticulocyte production index (RPI) (Table 16.1). The RPI is a better indication of the rate of RBC production than is the corrected reticulocyte count.[4] The reticulocyte count and derivation of RPI is discussed in Chapter 11.

In addition, state-of-the-art automated blood cell analyzers determine the fraction of immature reticulocytes among the total circulating reticulocytes, called the *immature reticulocyte fraction* (IRF). The IRF is helpful in assessing early bone marrow response after treatment for anemia and is covered in Chapter 12.

Analysis of the reticulocyte count plays a crucial role in determining whether an anemia is due to an RBC production defect or to premature hemolysis and shortened survival defect. If there is shortened RBC survival, as in the hemolytic anemias, the bone marrow tries to compensate by increasing RBC production to release more reticulocytes into the peripheral circulation. Although an increased reticulocyte count is a hallmark of the hemolytic anemias, it can also be observed after acute blood loss (Chapter 20).[4,7,8] Chronic blood loss, on the other hand, does *not* lead to an appropriate increase in the reticulocyte count, but rather leads to iron deficiency and a subsequent low reticulocyte count. Thus an inappropriately low reticulocyte count results from decreased production of normal RBCs, as a result of either insufficient or ineffective erythropoiesis.

TABLE 16.1	Formulas for Reticulocyte Counts and Red Blood Cell Indices		
Test	**Formula**	**Adult Reference Interval**
Absolute reticulocyte count ($\times 10^9$/L)	= [reticulocytes (%)/100] $\times$ RBC count ($\times 10^{12}$/L)	$20–115 \times 10^9$/L
Corrected reticulocyte count (%)	= reticulocytes (%) $\times$ patient's HCT (%)/45	—
Reticulocyte production index (RPI)	= corrected reticulocyte count/maturation time	In anemic patients, RPI should be >3
Mean cell volume (MCV) (fL)	= HCT (%) $\times$ 10/RBC count ($\times 10^{12}$/L)	80–100 fL
Mean cell hemoglobin (MCH) (pg)	= HGB (g/dL) $\times$ 10/RBC count ($\times 10^{12}$/L)	26–32 pg
Mean cell hemoglobin concentration (MCHC) (g/dL)	= HGB (g/dL) $\times$ 100/HCT (%)	32–36 g/dL

HGB, Hemoglobin; *HCT*, hematocrit; *RBC*, red blood cell.

Peripheral Blood Film Examination

An important component in the evaluation of an anemia is examination of the peripheral blood film, with particular attention to RBC diameter, shape, color, and inclusions. The peripheral blood film also serves to verify the results produced by automated analyzers. Normal RBCs on a Wright-stained blood film are nearly uniform, ranging from 7 to 8 μm in diameter. Small or microcytic cells are less than 6 μm in diameter, and large or macrocytic RBCs are greater than 8 μm in diameter. Certain shape abnormalities of diagnostic value (such as sickle cells, spherocytes, schistocytes, and oval macrocytes) and RBC inclusions (such as malarial parasites, basophilic stippling, and Howell-Jolly bodies) can be detected only by studying the RBCs on a peripheral blood film (Tables 16.2 and 16.3). Examples of abnormal shapes and inclusions are provided in Figure 16.1.

TABLE 16.2 Description of Red Blood Cell (RBC) Abnormalities and Commonly Associated Disease States

RBC Abnormality	Cell Description	Commonly Associated Disease States
Anisocytosis	Abnormal variation in RBC volume or diameter	Hemolytic, megaloblastic, iron deficiency anemias
Macrocyte	Large RBC (>8 μm in diameter), MCV > 100 fL	Megaloblastic anemia Myelodysplastic syndromes Chronic liver disease Bone marrow failure Reticulocytosis
Oval macrocyte	Large oval RBC	Megaloblastic anemia
Microcyte	Small RBC (<6 μm in diameter), MCV < 80 fL	Iron deficiency anemia Anemia of chronic inflammation Sideroblastic anemia Thalassemia/Hb E disease and trait
Poikilocytosis	Abnormal variation in RBC shape	Severe anemia; certain shapes helpful diagnostically
Spherocyte	Small, round, dense RBC with no central pallor	Hereditary spherocytosis Immune hemolytic anemia Extensive burns (along with schistocytes)
Elliptocyte, ovalocyte	Elliptical (cigar-shaped), oval (egg-shaped) RBC	Hereditary elliptocytosis or ovalocytosis Iron deficiency anemia Thalassemia major Myelophthisic anemias
Stomatocyte	RBC with slit-like area of central pallor	Hereditary stomatocytosis Rh deficiency syndrome Acquired stomatocytosis (liver disease, alcoholism) Artifact
Sickle cell	Thin, dense, elongated RBC pointed at each end; may be curved	Sickle cell anemia Sickle cell-β-thalassemia
Hb C crystal	Hexagonal crystal of dense hemoglobin formed within the RBC membrane	Hb C disease
Hb SC crystal	Finger-like or quartz-like crystal of dense hemoglobin protruding from the RBC membrane	Hb SC disease
Target cell (codocyte)	RBC with hemoglobin concentrated in the center and around the periphery resembling a target	Liver disease Hemoglobinopathies Thalassemia
Schistocyte (schizocyte)	Fragmented RBC caused by rupture in the peripheral circulation	Microangiopathic hemolytic anemia* (along with microspherocytes) Macroangiopathic hemolytic anemia[†] Extensive burns (along with microspherocytes)
Helmet cell (keratocyte)	RBC fragment in shape of a helmet	Same as schistocyte
Folded cell	RBC with membrane folded over	Hb C disease Hb SC disease
Acanthocyte (spur cell)	Small, dense RBC with few irregularly spaced projections of varying length	Severe liver disease (spur cell anemia) Neuroacanthocytosis (abetalipoproteinemia, McLeod syndrome)

Continued

TABLE 16.2　Description of Red Blood Cell (RBC) Abnormalities and Commonly Associated Disease States—cont'd

RBC Abnormality	Cell Description	Commonly Associated Disease States
Burr cell (echinocyte)	RBC with blunt or pointed, short projections that are usually evenly spaced over the surface of cell; present in all fields of blood film but in variable numbers per field[‡]	Uremia Pyruvate kinase deficiency
Teardrop cell (dacryocyte)	RBC with a single pointed extension resembling a teardrop or pear	Primary myelofibrosis Myelophthisic anemia Thalassemia Megaloblastic anemia

Hb, Hemoglobin; *MCV,* mean cell volume.

*Such as thrombotic thrombocytopenic purpura, hemolytic uremic syndrome, disseminated intravascular coagulation.

†Such as traumatic cardiac hemolysis.

‡Cells with similar morphology that are unevenly distributed in a blood film (not present in all fields) likely are due to a drying artifact in blood film preparation; these artifacts are sometimes called *crenated RBCs*.

TABLE 16.3　Erythrocyte Inclusions: Description, Composition, and Some Commonly Associated Disease States*

Inclusion	Appearance in Supravital Stain[†]	Appearance in Wright Stain	Composition of Inclusion	Associated Diseases/Conditions
Diffuse basophilia	Dark blue granules and filaments in cytoplasm (seen in reticulocytes)	Bluish tinge throughout cytoplasm; also called *polychromasia* (seen in polychromatic erythrocytes)	RNA	Hemolytic anemia After treatment for iron, vitamin B_{12}, or folate deficiency
Basophilic stippling	Dark blue-purple, fine or coarse punctate granules distributed throughout cytoplasm	Dark blue-purple, fine or coarse punctate granules distributed throughout cytoplasm	Precipitated RNA	Lead poisoning Thalassemias Hemoglobinopathies Megaloblastic anemia Myelodysplastic syndromes
Howell-Jolly body	Dark blue-purple dense, round granule; usually one per cell; occasionally multiple	Dark blue-purple dense, round granule; usually one per cell; occasionally multiple	DNA (nuclear fragment)	Hyposplenism Postsplenectomy Megaloblastic anemia Hemolytic anemia Thalassemia Myelodysplastic syndromes
Heinz body	Round, dark blue-purple granule attached to inner RBC membrane	Not visible	Denatured hemoglobin	Glucose-6-phosphate dehydrogenase deficiency Unstable hemoglobins Oxidant drugs/chemicals
Pappenheimer bodies[‡]	Irregular clusters of small, light to dark blue granules, often near periphery of cell	Irregular clusters of small, light to dark blue granules, often near periphery of cell	Iron	Sideroblastic anemia Hemoglobinopathies Thalassemias Megaloblastic anemia Myelodysplastic syndromes Hyposplenism Postsplenectomy
Cabot ring	Rings or figure-eights	Blue rings or figure-eights	Mitotic spindle remnant	Megaloblastic anemia Myelodysplastic syndromes
Hb H	Fine, evenly dispersed, dark blue granules; imparts "golf ball" appearance to RBCs	Not visible	Precipitated β-globin chains of hemoglobin	Hb H disease

Hb, Hemoglobin; *RBC,* red blood cell.

*Inclusions of hemoglobin crystals (Hb S, Hb C, Hb SC) are covered in Table 16.2.

†Such as new methylene blue.

‡Stain dark blue and are called *siderotic* granules when observed in Prussian blue stain.

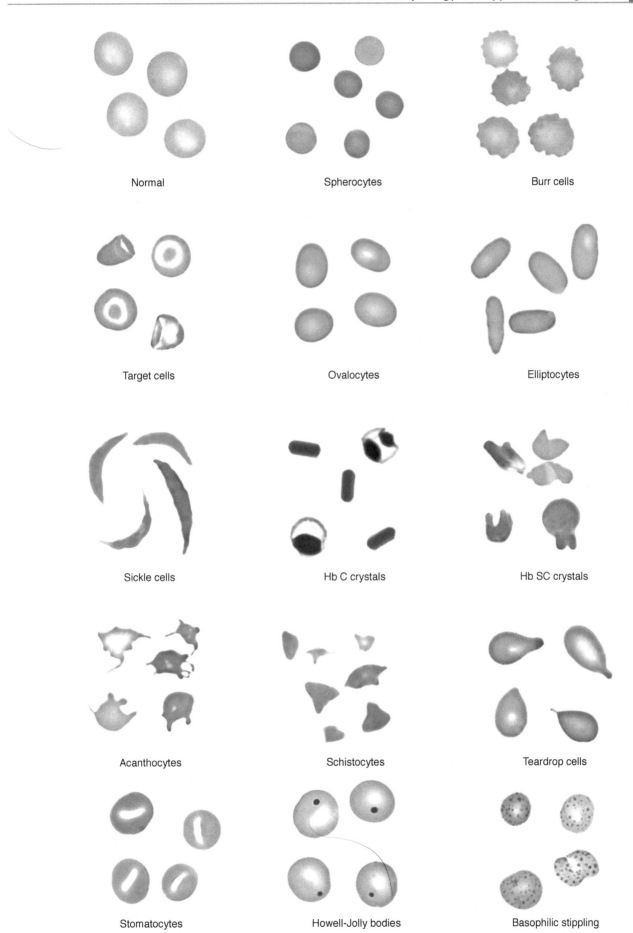

Normal

Spherocytes

Burr cells

Target cells

Ovalocytes

Elliptocytes

Sickle cells

Hb C crystals

Hb SC crystals

Acanthocytes

Schistocytes

Teardrop cells

Stomatocytes

Howell-Jolly bodies

Basophilic stippling

Figure 16.1 Red Blood Cells (RBCs): Varied RBC Shapes and Inclusions. *Hb,* Hemoglobin. (Modified from Rodak, B. F., & Carr, J. H. [2017]. *Clinical Hematology Atlas.* [5th ed.]. St. Louis: Elsevier.)

Finally, a review of the white blood cells and platelets may help show that a more generalized bone marrow problem is leading to the anemia. For example, hypersegmented neutrophils can be seen in vitamin B_{12} or folate deficiency, whereas blast cells and decreased platelets may be an indication of acute leukemia. Chapter 13 contains a complete discussion of the peripheral blood film evaluation. Information from the blood film examination always complements the data from the automated blood cell analyzer.

Bone Marrow Examination

The cause of many anemias can be determined from the history, physical examination, and results of laboratory tests on peripheral blood. When the cause cannot be determined, however, or the differential diagnosis remains broad, bone marrow aspiration and biopsy may help in establishing the cause of anemia.[4,8] Bone marrow examination is indicated for a patient with an unexplained anemia associated with or without other cytopenias, fever of unknown origin, or suspected hematologic neoplasm. Bone marrow examination evaluates hematopoiesis and can determine whether there is an infiltration of abnormal cells into the bone marrow. Important findings in bone marrow that can point to the underlying cause of the anemia include abnormal cellularity (e.g., hypocellularity in aplastic anemia); evidence of ineffective erythropoiesis and megaloblastic changes (e.g., folate/vitamin B_{12} deficiency or myelodysplastic syndromes); lack of iron on iron stains of bone marrow (the gold standard for diagnosis of iron deficiency); and the presence of granulomata, fibrosis, infectious agents, and tumor cells that may be inhibiting normal erythropoiesis. Chapter 14 discusses bone marrow procedures and bone marrow examination in detail.

Other tests that can assist in the diagnosis of anemia can be performed on a bone marrow specimen as well, including immunophenotyping of membrane antigens by flow cytometry (Chapter 28), cytogenetic studies (Chapter 30), and molecular analysis to detect specific genetic mutations and chromosome abnormalities in leukemia cells (Chapter 29).

Other Laboratory Tests

Other laboratory tests that can assist in establishing the cause of anemia include routine urinalysis (to detect hemoglobinuria or an increase in urobilinogen) with a microscopic examination (to detect hematuria or hemosiderin) and analysis of stool (to detect occult blood or intestinal parasites). Also, certain chemistry studies are very useful, such as serum haptoglobin, lactate dehydrogenase, and unconjugated bilirubin (to detect excessive hemolysis) and renal and hepatic function tests. With more patients having undergone gastric bypass surgery for obesity, certain rare deficiencies such as insufficient copper have become more common as another nutritional deficiency that can cause anemia.[14]

After the hematologic laboratory studies are completed, the anemia may be classified based on reticulocyte count, MCV, and peripheral blood film findings. Iron studies (including serum iron, total iron-binding capacity, transferrin saturation, and serum ferritin) are valuable if an inappropriately low reticulocyte count and a microcytic anemia are present. Serum vitamin B_{12} and serum folate assays are helpful in investigating a macrocytic anemia with a low reticulocyte count, whereas a direct antiglobulin test can differentiate autoimmune hemolytic anemias from other hemolytic anemias. Because of the numerous potential etiologies of anemia, the specific cause needs to be determined to initiate appropriate therapy.[11]

APPROACH TO EVALUATING ANEMIAS

The approach to the patient with anemia begins with taking a complete history and performing a physical examination.[4,7] For example, new-onset fatigue and shortness of breath suggest an acute drop in the hemoglobin concentration, whereas minimal or lack of symptoms suggests a long-standing condition where adaptive mechanisms have compensated for the drop in hemoglobin. A strict vegetarian may not be getting enough vitamin B_{12} in the diet, whereas an individual with alcoholism may not be getting enough folate. A large spleen may be an indication of hereditary spherocytosis, whereas a stool positive for occult blood may indicate iron deficiency. Thus a complete history and physical examination can yield information to narrow the possible cause or causes of the anemia and thus lead to a more rational and cost-effective approach to ordering the appropriate diagnostic tests.

The first step in the laboratory diagnosis of anemia is detecting its presence by the accurate measurement of the hemoglobin concentration, hematocrit, MCV, and RBC count and comparison of these values with the reference interval for healthy individuals of the same age, sex, race, and environment. Knowledge of previous hematologic values is valuable as a reduction of 10% or more in these values may be the first clue that an abnormal condition may be present.[4,6,15]

There are numerous causes of anemia, so a rational algorithm to initially evaluate this condition using the previously mentioned tests is required. A reticulocyte count and a peripheral blood film examination are of paramount importance in evaluating anemia.

The remainder of this chapter discusses the importance of individual RBC measurements, the MCV, reticulocyte count, and RDW and how they assist in classifying anemias so as to arrive at a specific diagnosis. Two widely used classification schemes for anemias relate to the morphology of red cells and the pathophysiologic condition responsible for the patient's anemia.

Morphologic Classification of Anemia Based on Mean Cell Volume

The MCV is an extremely important tool and is key in the *morphologic classification* of anemia. *Microcytic anemias* are characterized by an MCV of less than 80 fL with small RBCs (less than 6 μm in diameter). Microcytosis is often associated with hypochromia (increased central pallor in RBCs) and an MCHC of less than 32 g/dL. Microcytic anemias are caused by conditions that result in reduced hemoglobin synthesis. Heme synthesis is diminished in iron deficiency, iron sequestration (chronic inflammatory states), and defective protoporphyrin synthesis (sideroblastic anemia, lead poisoning). Globin chain synthesis is insufficient or defective in thalassemia and in Hb E disease. Iron deficiency is the most common cause of microcytic anemia; the low iron level is insufficient for maintaining normal erythropoiesis. Although iron deficiency anemia is characterized by abnormal iron studies, the early stages of iron deficiency do not result in microcytosis or anemia and are manifested only by reduced iron stores. The causes of iron deficiency vary in infants, children, adolescents, and adults, and it is imperative to find the cause before beginning treatment (Chapter 17).

Macrocytic anemias are characterized by an MCV greater than 100 fL with large RBCs (greater than 8 μm in diameter). Macrocytic anemias arise from conditions that result in megaloblastic or nonmegaloblastic red cell development in bone marrow. Megaloblastic anemias are caused by conditions that impair synthesis of DNA, such as vitamin B_{12} and folate deficiency or myelodysplasia. Nuclear maturation lags behind cytoplasmic development as a result of the impaired DNA synthesis. This asynchrony between nuclear and cytoplasmic development results in larger cells. All cells of the body are ultimately affected by the defective production of DNA (Chapter 18). Pernicious anemia is one cause of vitamin B_{12} deficiency, whereas pregnancy with increased requirements is a leading cause of folate deficiency. Megaloblastic anemia is characterized by oval macrocytes and hypersegmented neutrophils in the peripheral blood and by megaloblasts or large nucleated erythroid precursors in the bone marrow. The MCV in megaloblastic anemia can be markedly increased (up to 150 fL), but modest increases (100 to 115 fL) are most common.

Nonmegaloblastic forms of macrocytic anemias are also characterized by large RBCs, but in contrast to megaloblastic anemias, they are typically related to membrane changes caused by disruption of the cholesterol-to-phospholipid ratio. These macrocytic cells are mostly round, and the erythroid precursors in the bone marrow do not display megaloblastic changes. Macrocytic anemias are often seen in patients with chronic liver disease, alcohol abuse, and bone marrow failure. It is rare for the MCV to be greater than 115 fL in nonmegaloblastic anemias.

Normocytic anemias are characterized by an MCV in the range of 80 to 100 fL. The RBC morphology on the peripheral blood film must be examined to rule out a dimorphic population of microcytes and macrocytes that can yield a normal MCV. The presence of a dimorphic population can also be verified by observing a bimodal distribution on the RBC histogram produced by an automated blood cell analyzer (Chapters 12 and 13). Some normocytic anemias develop as a result of the premature destruction and shortened survival of RBCs *(hemolytic anemias),* and they are characterized by an elevated reticulocyte count. The hemolytic anemias can be further divided into those that result from intrinsic causes (membrane defects, hemoglobinopathies, and enzyme deficiencies) and those that result from extrinsic causes (immune and nonimmune RBC injury). A direct antiglobulin test helps differentiate immune-mediated RBC destruction from other causes of hemolysis. In the hemolytic anemias, reviewing the peripheral blood film provides vital information for determining the cause of the hemolysis (Tables 16.2 and 16.3 and Figure 16.1). Hemolytic anemias are discussed in Chapters 20 to 24.

Other normocytic anemias develop as a result of a decreased production of RBCs and are characterized by a decreased reticulocyte count (Chapter 19). Figure 16.2 presents an

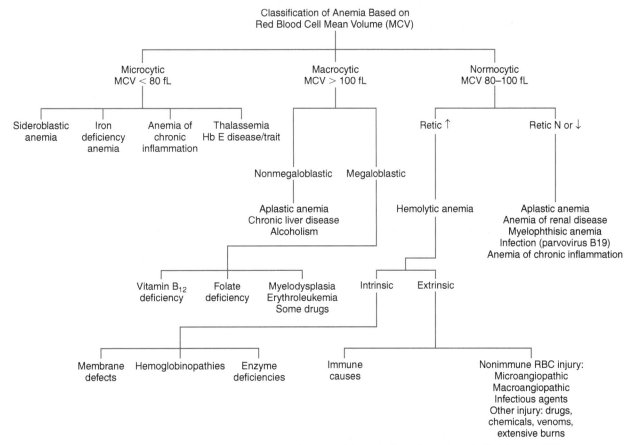

Figure 16.2 Algorithm for Morphologic Classification of Anemia Based on Mean Cell Volume (MCV). Anemia of chronic liver disease is multifactorial and can be macrocytic or normocytic; anemia of chronic inflammation can be normocytic or microcytic; and aplastic anemia can be macrocytic or normocytic. ↑, Increased; ↓, decreased; *Hb*, hemoglobin; *N*, normal; *retic*, absolute reticulocyte count.

algorithm for initial morphologic classification of anemia based on the MCV.

Morphologic Classification of Anemias and the Reticulocyte Count

The absolute reticulocyte count is useful in initially classifying anemias into the categories of decreased or ineffective RBC production (decreased reticulocyte count) and excessive RBC loss (increased reticulocyte count). Using the *morphologic classification* in the first category, when the reticulocyte count is decreased, the MCV can further classify the anemia into three subgroups: normocytic anemias, microcytic anemias, and macrocytic anemias. The excessive RBC loss category includes acute hemorrhage and the hemolytic anemias with shortened RBC survival. Figure 16.3 presents an algorithm that illustrates how anemias can be classified based on the absolute reticulocyte count and MCV.[4,7]

Morphologic Classification and the Red Blood Cell Distribution Width

The RDW can help determine the cause of an anemia when used in conjunction with the MCV. Each of the three MCV categories mentioned previously (normocytic, microcytic, macrocytic) can also be subclassified by the RDW as homogeneous (normal RDW) or heterogeneous (increased or high RDW).[7,16] For example, a decreased MCV with an increased RDW is suggestive of iron deficiency (Table 16.4). This classification is not absolute, however, because there can be an overlap of RDW values among some of the conditions in each MCV category.

Pathophysiologic Classification of Anemias and the Reticulocyte Count

In a *pathophysiologic classification* of anemia, related conditions are grouped by the mechanism causing the anemia. In this classification scheme, the anemias caused by decreased RBC production have inappropriately low reticulocyte counts (e.g., disorders of DNA synthesis and aplastic anemia) and are distinguished from other anemias caused by increased RBC destruction (intrinsic and extrinsic abnormalities of RBCs) or acute blood loss, which have increased reticulocyte counts. Some anemias have more than one pathophysiologic mechanism. Box 16.2 presents a pathophysiologic classification of anemia based on the causes of the abnormality and gives one or more examples of an anemia in each classification.

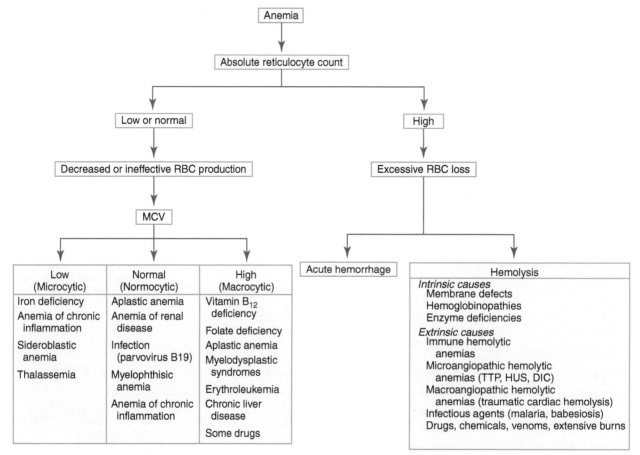

Figure 16.3 Algorithm for Evaluating Causes of Anemia Based on Absolute Reticulocyte Count and Mean Cell Volume (MCV). The list of anemias contains examples; there are numerous other causes not listed. Anemia of chronic liver disease is multifactorial and can be normocytic. *DIC,* Disseminated intravascular coagulation; *Hb,* hemoglobin; *HUS,* hemolytic uremic syndrome; *RBC,* red blood cell; *TTP,* thrombotic thrombocytopenic purpura.

TABLE 16.4 Morphologic Classification of Anemia Based on Red Blood Cell Mean Volume (MCV) and Red Blood Cell Distribution Width (RDW)*

| | MEAN CELL VOLUME | | |
	Decreased	Normal	Increased
RDW Normal	α- or β-Thalassemia trait Anemia of chronic inflammation Hb E disease/trait	Anemia of chronic inflammation Anemia of renal disease Acute hemorrhage Hereditary spherocytosis	Aplastic anemia Chronic liver disease Alcoholism Chemotherapy
RDW Increased	Iron deficiency Sickle cell-β-thalassemia	Early iron, folate, or vitamin B_{12} deficiency Mixed deficiency of iron + vitamin B_{12} or folate Sickle cell anemia Hb SC disease Myelodysplastic syndromes	Folate or vitamin B_{12} deficiency Myelodysplastic syndromes Cold agglutinin disease Chronic liver disease Chemotherapy

Hb, Hemoglobin.
*This classification scheme is not absolute because there can be overlap of RDW values among some of the conditions in each MCV category. Modified from Bessman, J. D., Gilmer, P. R., & Gardner, F. H. (1983). Improved classification of anemias by MCV and RDW. *Am J Clin Pathol, 80,* 324; and Lin, J. C. (2018). Approach to anemia in the adult and child. In Hoffman, R., Benz, E. J., Silberstein, L. E., et al. (Eds.), *Hematology: Basic Principles and Practice.* (7th ed., p. 463). Philadelphia: Elsevier.

BOX 16.2 Pathophysiologic Classification of Anemias[12]

Anemia Caused by Decreased Production of Red Blood Cells
Bone marrow failure: acquired and congenital aplastic anemia, pure red cell aplasia, anemia associated with marrow infiltration (myelophthisic)

Impairment of erythroid development:
- Disorders of DNA synthesis: megaloblastic anemia
- Disorders of hemoglobin synthesis: iron deficiency anemia, thalassemia, sideroblastic anemia, anemia of chronic inflammation
- Decreased production of erythropoietin: anemia of renal disease

Anemia Caused by Increased Red Blood Cell Destruction or Loss
Intrinsic RBC abnormality:
- Membrane defects: hereditary spherocytosis, hereditary elliptocytosis or pyropoikilocytosis, paroxysmal nocturnal hemoglobinuria

- Enzyme deficiencies: glucose-6-phosphate dehydrogenase deficiency, pyruvate kinase deficiency
- Globin abnormalities: sickle cell anemia, other hemoglobinopathies

Extrinsic RBC abnormality:
- Immune causes: warm-type autoimmune hemolytic anemia, cold agglutinin disease, paroxysmal cold hemoglobinuria, hemolytic transfusion reaction, hemolytic disease of the fetus and newborn
- Nonimmune red blood cell injuries: microangiopathic hemolytic anemia (thrombotic thrombocytopenic purpura, hemolytic uremic syndrome, HELLP syndrome, disseminated intravascular coagulation), macroangiopathic hemolytic anemia (traumatic cardiac hemolysis), infectious agents (malaria, babesiosis, bartonellosis, clostridial sepsis), other injury (chemicals, drugs, venoms, extensive burns)

Blood loss: acute blood loss anemia

HELLP, Hemolysis, elevated liver enzymes, and low platelets syndrome; *RBC*, red blood cell.
The list of anemias is not all-inclusive; numerous other conditions are not listed.

SUMMARY

- *Anemia* is defined operationally as a reduction in the hemoglobin content of blood that can be caused by a decrease in the red blood cell (RBC) count, hemoglobin concentration, and hematocrit below the reference interval for healthy individuals of the same age, sex, and race, under similar environmental conditions.
- Diagnosis of anemia is based on history, physical examination, symptoms, and laboratory test results.
- Many anemias have common manifestations. Careful questioning of the patient may reveal contributing factors, such as diet, medications, occupational hazards, and bleeding history.
- A thorough physical examination is valuable in determining the cause of anemia. Some of the areas that should be evaluated are skin, nail beds, eyes, mucosa, lymph nodes, heart, spleen, and liver.

- Moderate anemias (hemoglobin concentration between 7 and 10 g/dL) may cause pallor of conjunctivae and nail beds, but not manifest other clinical symptoms if the onset is slow. Severe anemias (hemoglobin concentration of less than 7 g/dL) usually produce pallor, dyspnea, vertigo, headache, muscle weakness, lethargy, hypotension, and tachycardia.
- Laboratory procedures helpful in the initial diagnosis of anemia include the complete blood count (CBC) with RBC indices, red blood cell distribution width (RDW), and the reticulocyte count, and examination of the peripheral blood film. Examination of a peripheral blood film is especially important in the diagnosis of hemolytic anemias.
- Bone marrow examination is usually not required for diagnosis of anemia but is indicated in cases of unexplained anemia, fever of unknown origin, or suspected hematologic neoplasm. Other tests are indicated based on the RBC

indices, history, and physical examination, such as serum iron, total iron-binding capacity, and serum ferritin (for microcytic anemias) and serum folate and vitamin B_{12} (for macrocytic anemias).

- The reticulocyte count and mean cell volume (MCV) play crucial roles in investigation of the cause of an anemia.
- Morphologic classification of anemias is based on the MCV and includes normocytic, microcytic, and macrocytic anemias. The MCV, when combined with the reticulocyte count and the RDW, also can aid in classification of anemia.

- Major subgroups of the pathophysiologic classification include anemias caused by decreased RBC production and those caused by increased RBC destruction or acute blood loss. Anemias may have more than one pathophysiologic cause.
- The cause of anemia should be determined before treatment is initiated.

Now that you have completed this chapter, go back and read again the case study at the beginning and respond to the questions presented.

REVIEW QUESTIONS

Answers can be found in the Appendix.

1. Which of the following patients would be considered anemic with a hemoglobin value of 14.5 g/dL? Refer to reference intervals inside the front cover of this text.
   a. An adult man
   b. An adult woman
   c. A newborn boy
   d. A 10-year-old girl

2. Anemia most commonly presents with which one of the following set of symptoms:
   a. Abdominal pain (from splenomegaly)
   b. Shortness of breath and fatigue
   c. Chills and fever
   d. Jaundice and enlarged lymph nodes

3. Which of the following are important to consider in the patient's history when investigating the cause of an anemia?
   a. Diet and medications
   b. Occupation, hobbies, and travel
   c. Bleeding episodes in the patient or in his or her family members
   d. All of the above

4. Which one of the following is reduced as an adaptation to long-standing anemia?
   a. Heart rate
   b. Respiratory rate
   c. Oxygen affinity of hemoglobin
   d. Volume of blood ejected from the heart with each contraction

5. An autoimmune reaction destroys the hematopoietic stem cells in the bone marrow of a young adult patient, and the amount of active bone marrow, including erythroid precursors, is diminished. Erythroid precursors that are present are normal in appearance, but there are too few to meet the demand for circulating red blood cells, and anemia develops. The reticulocyte count is low. The mechanism of the anemia would be described as:
   a. Effective erythropoiesis
   b. Ineffective erythropoiesis
   c. Insufficient erythropoiesis

6. What are the *initial* laboratory tests that are performed for the diagnosis of anemia?
   a. CBC, iron studies, and reticulocyte count
   b. CBC, reticulocyte count, and peripheral blood film examination
   c. Reticulocyte count and serum iron, vitamin B_{12}, and folate assays
   d. Bone marrow study, iron studies, and peripheral blood film examination

7. An increase in which one of the following suggests a shortened life span of RBCs and hemolytic anemia?
   a. Hemoglobin concentration
   b. Hematocrit
   c. Reticulocyte count
   d. Red cell distribution width

8. Which of the following is detectable only by examination of a peripheral blood film?
   a. Microcytosis
   b. Anisocytosis
   c. Hypochromia
   d. Poikilocytosis

9. Schistocytes, ovalocytes, and acanthocytes are examples of abnormal changes in RBC:
   a. Volume
   b. Shape
   c. Inclusions
   d. Hemoglobin concentration

10. Refer to Figure 16.3 to determine which one of the following conditions would be included in the differential diagnosis of an anemic adult patient with an absolute reticulocyte count of 20×10^9/L and an MCV of 65 fL.
    a. Aplastic anemia
    b. Sickle cell anemia
    c. Iron deficiency
    d. Folate deficiency

11. Which one of the following conditions would be included in the differential diagnosis of an anemic adult patient with an MCV of 125 fL and an RDW of 20% (reference interval 11.5% to 14.5%)? Refer to Table 16.4.
    a. Aplastic anemia
    b. Sickle cell anemia
    c. Iron deficiency
    d. Vitamin B_{12} deficiency

REFERENCES

1. Schecther, A. N. (2008). Hemoglobin research and the origins of molecular medicine. *Blood, 112,* 3927–3938.
2. *The American Heritage dictionary of the English language.* (4th ed.). (2001). Boston: Houghton Mifflin.
3. Kassebaum, N. J., & GBD 2013 Anemia Collaborators. (2016). The global burden of anemia. *Hematol Oncol Clin N Am, 30,* 247–308.
4. Means, R. T., Jr., & Glader, B. (2014). Anemia: general considerations. In Greer, J. P., Arber, D. A., Glader, B., et al. (Eds.), *Wintrobe's Clinical Hematology.* (13th ed., pp. 587–616). Philadelphia: Lippincott Williams & Wilkins, Wolters Kluwer.
5. Tefferi, A. (2003). Anemia in adults: a contemporary approach to diagnosis. *Mayo Clin Proc, 78,* 1274–1280.
6. Beutler, E., & Waalen, J. (2006). The definition of anemia: what is the lower limit of normal of the blood hemoglobin concentration? *Blood, 107,* 1747–1750.
7. Lin, J. C. (2018). Approach to anemia in the adult and child. In Hoffman, R., Benz, E. J., Silberstein, L. E., et al. (Eds.), *Hematology: Basic Principles and Practice.* (7th ed., pp. 458–467). Philadelphia: Elsevier.
8. Bunn, H. F. (2016). Approach to anemias. In Goldman, L., & Schafer, A. I. (Eds.), *Goldman-Cecil Medicine.* (25th ed., pp. 1059–1068). Philadelphia: Elsevier, Saunders.
9. Irwin, J. J., & Kirchner, J. T. (2001). Anemia in children. *Am Fam Physician, 64,* 1379–1386.
10. Kettaneh, A., Eclache, V., Fain, O., et al. (2005). Pica and food craving in patients with iron-deficiency anemia: a case-control study in France. *Am J Med, 118,* 185–188.
11. Adamson, J. W., & Longo, D. L. (2018). Anemia and polycythemia. In Kasper, D.L., Fauci, A. S., Hauser, S. L., et al. (Eds.), *Harrison's Principles of Internal Medicine.* (20th ed.). New York: McGraw-Hill.
12. Prchal, J. T. (2016). Clinical manifestations and classification of erythrocyte disorders. In Kaushansky, K., Lichtman, M. A., Prchal, J. T., et al. (Eds.), *Williams Hematology.* (9th ed., pp. 503–512). New York: McGraw-Hill.
13. Smock, K. J., & Perkins, S. L. (2014). Examination of the blood and bone marrow. In Greer, J. P., Arber, D. A., Glader, B., et al. (Eds.), *Wintrobe's Clinical Hematology.* (13th ed., pp. 1–18). Philadelphia: Lippincott Williams & Wilkins, Wolters Kluwer.
14. Halfdanarson, T. R., Kumarm, N., Li, C. Y., et al. (2008). Hematologic manifestations of copper deficiency: a retrospective review. *Eur J Haemotol, 80,* 523–531.
15. Brill, J. R., & Baumgardner, D. J. (2000). Normocytic anemia. *Am Fam Physician, 62,* 2255–2263.
16. Bessman, J. D., Gilmer, P. R., & Gardner, F. H. (1983). Improved classification of anemia by MCV and RDW. *Am J Clin Pathol, 80,* 322–326.

Disorders of Iron Kinetics and Heme Metabolism

Kathryn Doig

OBJECTIVES

After completion of this chapter, the reader will be able to:

1. Recognize complete blood count (CBC) results consistent with iron deficiency anemia, anemia of chronic inflammation, and sideroblastic anemias.
2. Given the results of classical iron studies, as well as free erythrocyte protoporphyrin (FEP), soluble transferrin receptor (sTfR), hemoglobin content of reticulocytes, sTfR/log ferritin, and Thomas plots, distinguish findings consistent with iron deficiency anemia, latent iron deficiency, anemia of chronic inflammation, sideroblastic anemias, and iron overload conditions.
3. Recognize individuals at risk for iron deficiency anemia by virtue of age, gender, diet, physiologic circumstance such as pregnancy and menstruation, or pathologic conditions such as chronic gastrointestinal bleeding.
4. Given a description of a Wright-stained bone marrow smear and the appearance of bone marrow stained with Prussian blue stain, recognize results consistent with iron deficiency anemia, anemia of chronic inflammation, or a sideroblastic anemia.
5. Recognize clinical conditions that can predispose a patient to develop anemia of chronic inflammation.
6. Recognize predisposing factors for sideroblastic anemias or conditions in which sideroblastic anemias may develop.
7. Discuss the clinical significance of increased levels of FEP.
8. Describe the pathogenesis of iron deficiency anemia, anemia of chronic inflammation, sideroblastic anemia secondary to lead poisoning, and hemochromatosis, generically.
9. Discuss the differences in disease etiology, laboratory diagnosis, and treatment between iron overload resulting from hereditary forms of hemochromatosis and transfusion-related hemosiderosis.
10. Describe the etiology of the erythropoietic porphyrias, expected CBC picture, diagnostic metabolites, and clinical presentation.

OUTLINE

General Concepts in Iron-Related Disorders
Iron-Restricted Anemias
    Iron Deficiency Anemia
    Anemia of Chronic Inflammation
Sideroblastic Anemias
    Acquired: Lead Poisoning

    Hereditary: Porphyrias
Iron Overload
    Etiology
    Pathogenesis
    Laboratory Diagnosis
    Treatment

CASE STUDY

After studying the material in this chapter, the reader should be able to respond to the following case study:

An 85-year-old slender, frail white woman was hospitalized for diagnosis and treatment of anemia suspected during a routine examination by her physician. The physician noted that she appeared pale and inquired about fatigue and tiredness. Although the patient generally felt well, she admitted to feeling slightly tired when climbing stairs. A point-of-care hemoglobin performed in the physician's office showed a dangerously low value of 3.5 g/dL, so the patient was hospitalized for further evaluation. Her hospital CBC results are as follows:

	Patient Results	Reference Intervals
WBCs ($\times 10^9$/L)	8.5	4.5–11
RBCs ($\times 10^{12}$/L)	1.66	4.3–5.9

	Patient Results	Reference Intervals
HGB (g/dL)	3.0	13.9–16.3
HCT (%)	11	39–55
MCV (fL)	66.3	80–100
MCH (pg)	18.1	26–32
MCHC (g/dL)	27.3	32–36
RDW (%)	20	11.5–14.5
Platelets ($\times 10^9$/L)	165.0	150–450
WBC differential	Unremarkable	
RBC morphology	Marked anisocytosis, marked poikilocytosis, marked hypochromia, marked microcytosis	

Continued

GENERAL CONCEPTS IN IRON-RELATED DISORDERS

Anemia may result whenever red blood cell (RBC) production is impaired, RBC life span is shortened, or there is frank loss of RBCs from the body. The anemias associated with iron and heme typically are categorized as anemias of impaired production resulting from the lack of raw materials for hemoglobin assembly. When iron is the limiting factor, the anemias are called *iron restricted*. Two important iron-restricted anemias discussed here are iron deficiency anemia and anemia of chronic inflammation. Inadequate production of protoporphyrin also leads to diminished production of heme and thus hemoglobin, but with a relative excess of iron; such anemias are described as sideroblastic and are discussed in this chapter. Blockages of protoporphyrin production at various stages in the heme synthetic pathway lead to accumulations of various porphyrins. The resulting porphyrias that are accompanied by anemia are briefly discussed. Iron metabolism can be perturbed, resulting in excess accumulations of iron, usually without anemia. These conditions, called the hemochromatoses, are included here as well. There is another group of anemias with impaired iron kinetics called *iron-loading anemias*. Often these anemias involve chronic erythroid hyperplasia as is seen in the hemoglobinopathies and thalassemias. These are diseases caused by heritable mutations affecting globin chain structure or their production. These conditions are discussed separately in Chapters 24 and 25.

An understanding of normal iron metabolism and the tests of body iron status are critical to the understanding and diagnosis of the conditions discussed in this chapter, so the reader is referred to Chapter 8, where iron kinetics and diagnostic tests are described in detail.

IRON-RESTRICTED ANEMIAS

Iron Deficiency Anemia

Etiology

Iron deficiency anemia develops when the intake of iron is inadequate to meet a standard level of demand, when the need for iron expands without compensated intake, when there is impaired absorption, or when there is chronic loss of hemoglobin from the body.

Inadequate intake. Iron deficiency anemia can develop when the erythron is slowly starved for iron. Each day,

approximately 1 mg of iron is lost from the body, mainly in the mitochondria of desquamated skin and sloughed intestinal epithelium.[1] Because the body tenaciously conserves all other iron from senescent cells, including RBCs, daily replacement of 1 mg of iron from the diet maintains iron balance and supplies the body's need for RBC production as long as there is no other source of loss. When the iron in the diet is consistently inadequate, over time the body's stores of iron become depleted. Ultimately, RBC production slows to manage the iron needs for other body cells.[2,3] With approximately 1% of cells dying naturally each day, the anemia becomes apparent when the production rate is insufficient to replace lost cells.

Increased need relative to iron supply. Iron deficiency can also develop when the level of iron intake is inadequate to meet the needs of an expanding erythron. This is the case in periods of rapid growth, such as infancy (especially in prematurity), childhood, and adolescence. For example, although both infants and adult men need about 1 mg/day of iron, that corresponds to a much higher amount per kilogram of body weight for the infant. Pregnancy and nursing place similar demands on the mother's body to provide iron for the developing fetus or nursing infant in addition to her own iron needs. In each of these instances, what had previously been an adequate intake of iron for the individual becomes inadequate as the need for iron increases.

Treatment with erythropoietin is another instance when there is rapid expansion of the erythron. The demand for iron is often so great that even individuals with adequate stores of iron will experience iron-restricted erythropoiesis because it cannot be mobilized fast enough. This is called *functional iron deficiency* because iron stores are adequate but the iron is not available to support normal erythropoiesis.

Impaired absorption. Even when the diet is adequate in iron, the inability to absorb that iron through the enterocyte into the blood will, over time, result in a deficiency of iron in the body. The impairments may be pathologic, as with malabsorption caused by celiac disease. Others may be inherited mutations of iron regulatory proteins, like the mutations of the matriptase-2 protein (Chapter 8) that lead to a persistent production of hepcidin, causing ferroportin in the enterocyte to be inactivated, thus preventing iron absorption in the intestine.[4] In addition, diseases that decrease stomach acidity impair iron absorption by decreasing the conversion of dietary ferric iron to the absorbable ferrous form. Some loss of acidity accompanies normal aging, but gastrectomy or bariatric surgeries can impair iron absorption dramatically. Medications such as stomach acid reducers can inhibit iron absorption by decreasing gastric acidity, whereas other drugs may even bind the iron in the intestine, preventing its absorption.

Chronic blood loss. A fourth way iron deficiency develops is with repeated blood donations, chronic hemorrhage, or hemolysis that results in the loss of small amounts of heme iron from the body over a prolonged period. Anemia develops when the iron loss exceeds iron intake over time and the storage iron is exhausted. Excessive heme iron can be lost through repeated blood donations; chronic gastrointestinal bleeding from ulcers, tumors, parasitosis, diverticulitis, ulcerative colitis, or hemorrhoids; and gastritis caused by alcohol or aspirin ingestion. In women, prolonged menorrhagia (heavy menstrual bleeding) or conditions such as uterine fibroid tumors or uterine malignancies can also lead to heme iron loss. Heme iron can also be lost excessively through the urinary tract with kidney stones, tumors, or chronic infections. Individuals with chronic intravascular hemolytic processes,

such as paroxysmal nocturnal hemoglobinuria, can develop iron deficiency as a result of the loss of iron in hemoglobin passed into the urine.

Pathogenesis

Iron deficiency anemia develops slowly, progressing through stages that physiologically blend into one another but are useful delineations for understanding disease progression.[5] As shown in Figure 17.1, iron is distributed among three compartments: the storage compartment, principally as ferritin in the bone marrow macrophages and liver cells; the transport compartment of serum transferrin; and the functional compartment of hemoglobin, myoglobin, and cytochromes. Hemoglobin iron and intracellular ferritin and hemosiderin constitute nearly 90% of the total distribution of iron (Table 8.1).

For a time, as an increase in demand or increased loss of iron exceeds iron intake, essentially normal iron status continues. The body strives to maintain iron balance by accelerating absorption of iron from the intestine through a decrease in the production of hepcidin in the liver. This state of declining body iron with increased absorption is not apparent in routine

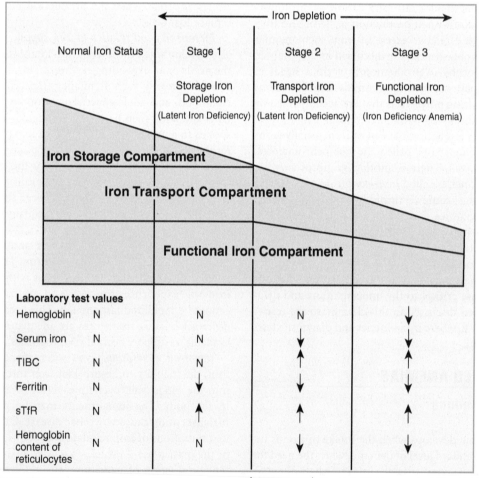

Figure 17.1 Development of Iron Deficiency Anemia. ↑, Increased; ↓, decreased; *N*, normal; *sTfR*, soluble transferrin receptor; *TIBC*, total iron-binding capacity. (Adapted from Suominen, P., Punnonen, K., Rajamaki, A., et al. [1998]. Serum transferrin receptor and transferrin receptor-ferritin index identify healthy subjects with subclinical iron deficits. *Blood, 92,* p. 2935, Figure 1; reprinted with permission.)

laboratory test results or patient symptoms. The individual appears healthy. As the negative iron balance continues, however, a stage of iron depletion develops.

Stage 1. Stage 1 of iron deficiency is characterized by a progressive loss of storage iron. RBC production and development are normal throughout this phase. However, without new iron added to storage, continuing RBC production draws down the reserve. Serum ferritin levels drop over time, which indicates the decline in stored iron, and this also could be detected in an iron stain of the bone marrow. Without evidence of anemia, though, these tests would not be performed because individuals appear healthy (latent iron deficiency). Yet stage 1 iron deficiency is common. The prevalence of stage 1 iron deficiency in the United States has been estimated in toddlers (12 to 23 months) as 15.1%, in nonpregnant women (15 to 49 years) as 10.4%, and in pregnant women (12 to 49 years) as 16.3%.[6]

Stage 2. Stage 2 of iron deficiency is defined by the exhaustion of the storage pool of iron (Figure 17.1). For a time, RBC production continues as normal, relying on the iron available in the transport compartment and that being recycled from dying cells. Quickly the hemoglobin content of reticulocytes begins to decrease, which reflects the onset of iron-restricted erythropoiesis, but because the bulk of the circulating RBCs were produced during the period of adequate iron availability, the overall hemoglobin concentration is still within the reference interval, as are the mean cell volume (MCV), mean cell hemoglobin (MCH), and mean cell hemoglobin concentration (MCHC). Thus anemia is still not evident. Although an individual's hemoglobin may begin dropping, and the RBC distribution width (RDW) may begin increasing as some smaller RBCs are released from the bone marrow, without multiple measurements over time, these changes will not be detected. Other iron-dependent tissues, such as muscles, may begin to be affected, although the symptoms may be nonspecific. The serum iron and serum ferritin levels decrease, whereas total iron-binding capacity (TIBC), an indirect measure of transferrin, increases.[7,8] Free erythrocyte protoporphyrin (FEP), the porphyrin into which iron is inserted to form heme, begins to accumulate without iron to complete heme formation. Transferrin receptors increase on the surface of iron-starved cells as they try to capture as much available iron as possible. The receptors are also shed into the blood, so the soluble transferrin receptor (sTfR) levels increase measurably. Prussian blue stain of the bone marrow in stage 2 shows essentially no stored iron, and iron-restricted erythropoiesis is evident (subsequent description). Hepcidin, though not commonly measured clinically, would be measurably decreased. Because iron deficiency in stage 2 is subclinical (latent iron deficiency) and testing is not likely to be undertaken, some authors advocate for the use of automated hypochromia measures reported with the complete blood count (CBC) to detect early iron-restricted erythropoiesis.[9,10]

Stage 3. Stage 3 of iron deficiency is frank anemia. The hemoglobin concentration and hematocrit are low relative to the reference intervals. Depletion of storage iron and diminished levels of transport iron (Figure 17.1) prevent normal development of RBC precursors. The RBCs become microcytic and

hypochromic (Figure 17.2) as their ability to produce hemoglobin is restricted. As expected, serum ferritin levels are exceedingly low. Results of other iron studies (discussed later) are also abnormal, and the FEP and sTfR levels continue to increase. The hemoglobin content of reticulocytes will continue to drop and automated hypochromia parameters will be increased. If measured, erythropoietin would be elevated but not as high as might be expected for the degree of anemia.[2,11] Hepcidin would be decreased.

In this phase the patient experiences the nonspecific symptoms of anemia, typically fatigue, weakness, and shortness of breath, especially with exertion. Pallor is evident in light-skinned individuals but also can be noted in the conjunctivae, mucous membranes, or palmar creases of dark-skinned individuals. More severe signs are not seen as often in the United States[12] but include a sore tongue (glossitis) due to iron deficiency in the rapidly proliferating epithelial cells of the alimentary tract and inflamed cracks at the corners of the mouth (angular cheilosis). Koilonychia (spooning of the fingernails) may be seen if the deficiency is long-standing. Patients also may experience cravings for nonfood items, called *pica*. The cravings may be for things such as dirt, clay, laundry starch, or, most commonly, ice (craving for the latter is called *pagophagia*).[12]

As should be evident from this discussion, numerous individuals may be iron deficient while appearing healthy. Until late in stage 2, they may experience no symptoms at all and are unlikely to come to medical attention. Even in stage 3, frankly anemic patients may not seek medical care, because the body is able to compensate remarkably for slowly developing anemia (Chapter 16), like that in the patient in the case study at the beginning of this chapter. Because results of routine screening tests included in the CBC do not become abnormal until late in stage 2 or early in stage 3, most patients are not

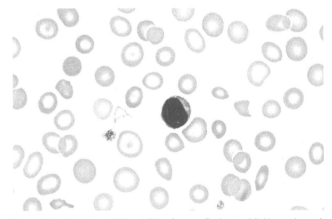

Figure 17.2 Peripheral Blood Film from a Patient with Hypochromic, Microcytic Anemia. Note the variation in red blood cell *(RBC)* diameters compared with the lymphocyte's nuclear diameter. Variation in RBC diameters is termed *anisocytosis* and corresponds to an elevated RBC distribution width *(RDW)*, a measure of variation in RBC volume. Hypochromia, microcytosis, and an elevated RDW may indicate iron deficiency anemia. Several target cells are seen. (Wright-Giemsa stain, ×1000.)

diagnosed until relatively late in the progression of the iron depletion.

Epidemiology

From the previous discussion, it is apparent that certain groups of individuals are more at risk to develop iron deficiency anemia. Menstruating women are at especially high risk. Their monthly loss of blood increases their routine need for iron, which often is not met with the standard US diet.[12] For adolescent girls, this is compounded by increased iron needs associated with growth. If women of childbearing age do not receive proper iron supplementation, pregnancy and nursing can lead to a loss of nearly 1200 mg of iron,[13] which further depletes iron stores. Succeeding pregnancies can exacerbate the problem, leading to iron-deficient fetuses.

Growing children also are at high risk. Growth requires iron for the cytochromes of all new cells, myoglobin for new muscle cells, and hemoglobin in the additional RBCs needed to supply oxygen for a larger body. The increasing need for iron as the child grows can be coupled with dietary inadequacies, especially in circumstances of poverty or neglect. Cow's milk is not a good source of iron, and infants need to be placed on iron-supplemented formula by about age 6 months, when their fetal stores of iron become depleted.[12] This assumes that the infants were able to establish adequate iron stores by drawing iron from their mothers in utero. Even though breast milk is a better source of iron than cow's milk,[14] it is not a consistent source.[15] Therefore, iron supplementation is also recommended for breastfed infants after 6 months of age.[12]

Iron deficiency is relatively rare in men and postmenopausal women because the body conserves iron so tenaciously, and these individuals lose only about 1 mg/day. Gastrointestinal disease, such as ulcers, tumors, or hemorrhoids, should be suspected in iron-deficient patients in either of these groups if the diet is known to be adequate in iron. Regular aspirin ingestion and alcohol consumption can lead to gastritis and chronic bleeding. Elderly individuals, particularly those living alone, may not eat a balanced diet, so pure dietary deficiency is seen among these individuals. In some elderly individuals, the loss of gastric acidity with age can impair iron absorption. Iron deficiency is associated with infection by hookworms, *Necator americanus* and *Ancylostoma duodenale*. The worm attaches to the intestinal wall and literally sucks blood from the gastric vessels. Iron deficiency is also associated with infection with other parasites, such as *Trichuris trichiura*, *Schistosoma mansoni*, and *Schistosoma haematobium*, in which the heme iron is lost from the body as a result of intestinal or urinary bleeding.

Soldiers subjected to prolonged maneuvers and long-distance runners also can develop iron deficiency. Exercise-induced hemoglobinuria, also called march hemoglobinuria, develops when RBCs are hemolyzed by foot-pounding trauma and iron is lost as hemoglobin in the urine.[16,17] The amount lost in the urine can be so little that it is not apparent on visual inspection of the urine. Nevertheless, in rare cases the cumulative iron loss can lead to anemia if the foot-pounding trauma is recurrent and especially severe. However, there is some evidence that well-trained professional athletes may be less subject to this effect.[18]

Laboratory Diagnosis

The early stages of iron deficiency can be detected with tests such as ferritin, but those tests are not likely to be ordered because there is virtually no physiologic evidence suggesting a declining iron state. Furthermore, those tests are not always part of comprehensive screening panels, and as a result, the progressing iron deficiency can go undetected. Nevertheless, early iron deficiency might be suspected in an individual in a high-risk group, and appropriate testing can be ordered. It is not until late in the progression that standard CBC parameters such as the hemoglobin and MCV fall to less than reference intervals and thus may prompt additional diagnostic testing. The tests for iron deficiency can be grouped into three general categories: screening, diagnostic, and specialized. The principles are discussed in more detail in Chapter 8.

Screening for iron deficiency anemia. When iron-restricted erythropoiesis is underway, the CBC results begin to show evidence of anisocytosis, microcytosis, and hypochromia (Figure 17.2). The classic picture of iron deficiency anemia in stage 3 includes a decreased hemoglobin concentration. An RDW greater than 15% is expected and may precede the decrease in hemoglobin.[19] For patients in high-risk groups, the elevated RDW can be an early and sensitive indicator of iron deficiency that is provided in a routine CBC.[20] As the hemoglobin concentration continues to fall, microcytosis and hypochromia become more prominent, with progressively declining values for the MCV, MCH, and MCHC. Automated measures of microcytosis and hypochromia may detect these changes before they are noticeable on the peripheral blood film.[10] The RBC count ultimately becomes decreased, though lagging behind the drop in indices, as does the hematocrit. Polychromasia may be apparent early, although it is not a prominent finding. Poikilocytosis, including occasional target cells and elliptocytes, may be present, although no particular shape is characteristic or predominant. Thrombocytosis may be present, particularly if the iron deficiency results from chronic bleeding, but this is not a diagnostic parameter. White blood cells are typically normal in number and appearance. Iron deficiency should be suspected when the CBC findings show a hypochromic, microcytic anemia with an elevated RDW but no consistent shape changes to the RBCs.

Diagnostic testing for iron deficiency. Biochemical iron studies remain the backbone for diagnosis of iron deficiency, though some argue that modern automated blood cell analyzers can supplant the biochemical studies.[21] The biochemical analyses include assays of serum iron, TIBC, transferrin saturation, and serum ferritin; Chapter 8 covers the principle of each assay and technical considerations affecting test performance and interpretation. Serum iron is a measure of the amount of iron bound to transferrin (transport protein) in the serum. TIBC is an indirect measure of transferrin and the available binding sites for iron. The percent of transferrin binding sites occupied by iron can be calculated from the total iron and the TIBC:

$$\text{Transferrin saturation (\%)} = \frac{\text{serum iron }(\mu g/dL) \times 100}{\text{TIBC }(\mu g/dL)}$$

Ferritin provides an intracellular storage repository for metabolically active iron. Yet ferritin is secreted into blood, and serum levels reflect the levels of iron stored within cells. Serum ferritin is an easily accessible surrogate for stainable bone marrow iron. Iron studies are used collectively to assess the iron status of an individual. Table 17.1 shows that, as expected, serum ferritin and serum iron values are decreased in iron deficiency anemia, a state called *sideropenia*. Transferrin levels increase when the hepatocytes detect low iron levels, and research shows that this is a transcriptional and posttranscriptional response to low iron levels.[7,8,22] The result is a decline in the iron saturation of transferrin that is more dramatic than might be expected simply from the decrease in serum iron level. The biochemical markers of iron deficiency are rarely assayed on non-anemic patients, though some results (such as serum ferritin) are abnormal during the latent period.

Instrument manufacturers have developed parameters that can be reported with a CBC to enhance detection of latent iron deficiency and that are even more sensitive to iron deficiency anemia. These include sensitive and quantitative detection of hypochromia and microcytosis.[10,21,23,24] Because these are early indicators of impending anemia, they can provide an early alert during the latent period. On some instruments, these newer assays remain for research use only pending approval from the Food and Drug Administration.

Reticulocyte parameters also support the diagnosis of iron deficiency. A low absolute reticulocyte count confirms a diminished rate of effective erythropoiesis because this is a nonregenerative anemia.[2] The amount of hemoglobin in reticulocytes can be assessed on some automated blood cell analyzers (Chapter 12).[21] The hemoglobin content of reticulocytes is analogous to the MCH, but for reticulocytes only. The MCH is the average weight of hemoglobin per cell across the entire RBC population. Some of the RBCs are nearly 120 days old, whereas others are just 1 to 2 days old. If iron deficiency is developing, the MCH does not change until a substantial proportion of the cells are iron deficient, and the diagnosis is effectively delayed for weeks or months after iron-restricted erythropoiesis begins. Measuring the hemoglobin content of reticulocytes enables detection of iron-restricted erythropoiesis within days as the first iron-deficient cells leave the bone marrow. It is a sensitive indicator of iron deficiency. Even in stage 2 of iron deficiency, before anemia is apparent, the hemoglobin content of reticulocytes will be low.[21] The disadvantage is that a CBC is unlikely to be ordered for non-anemic patients who demonstrate no symptoms. An order for reticulocyte parameters is even less likely.

Specialized tests of iron status. Other tests, although not commonly used for the diagnosis of iron deficiency, show abnormalities that become important in the differential diagnosis of similar conditions. Test results for the accumulated porphyrin precursors to heme are elevated (Table 17.1). FEP accumulates when iron is unavailable. In the absence of iron, FEP may be preferentially chelated with zinc to form zinc protoporphyrin (ZPP).[25] The FEP and zinc chelate can be assayed fluorometrically, although they are not particularly valuable in the diagnosis of iron deficiency. Soluble transferrin receptors (sTfR) can be assayed using immunoassay. Levels increase as the disease progresses, and individual cells seek to take in as much iron as possible.[26]

A bone marrow assessment is not indicated for suspected uncomplicated iron deficiency. A therapeutic trial of iron (discussed in Response to Treatment) provides a less invasive and less expensive diagnostic assessment. However, marrow examination for iron is routinely performed when a bone marrow specimen is collected for other reasons. With routine stains, the iron-deficient bone marrow appears hyperplastic early in the progression of the disease, with a decreased myeloid-to-erythroid ratio as a result of increased erythropoiesis.[12] As the disease progresses, hyperplasia subsides and the profound deficiency of iron leads to slowed RBC production.[3] Polychromatic normoblasts (i.e., rubricytes) show the most dramatic morphologic changes (Figure 17.3). Nuclear-cytoplasmic asynchrony is evident, with cytoplasmic maturation lagging behind nuclear

TABLE 17.1 Results of Iron Studies in Microcytic Anemias

	Iron Deficiency Anemia	β-thalassemia Minor	Anemia of Chronic Inflammation	Sideroblastic Anemia	Lead Poisoning
Serum ferritin	↓	↑/N	↑/N	↑	N
Serum iron	↓/N	↑/N	↓	↑	Variable
TIBC	↑	N	↓	↓/N	N
Transferrin saturation	↓	↑/N	↓/N	↑	↑
FEP/ZPP	↑	N	↑	↑	↑ (marked)
sTfR	↑	N	N	N	N
Hemoglobin content of reticulocytes	↓	↓	↓	N	N
BM iron (Prussian blue reaction)	No stainable iron	↑/N	↑/N	↑	N
Sideroblasts in BM	None	N	None/very few	↑ (ring)	N (ring)
Other special tests		↑ Hb A$_2$	Specific tests for inflammatory disorders or malignancy		↑ ALA in urine ↑ Blood lead levels

↑, Increased; ↓, decreased; *ALA*, aminolevulinic acid; *BM*, bone marrow; *FEP/ZPP*, free erythrocyte protoporphyrin/zinc protoporphyrin; *Hb*, hemoglobin; *N*, normal; *sTfR*, soluble transferrin receptor.

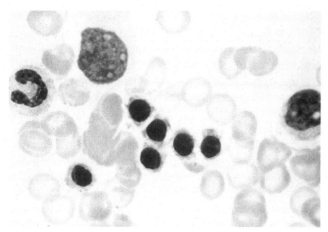

Figure 17.3 Bone Marrow Smear From a Patient with Iron Deficiency Anemia. The later-stage nucleated red blood cells show the characteristic "shaggy" cytoplasm which is also very blue because of delayed maturation relative to the nucleus (i.e., nuclear-cytoplasmic asynchrony). (Wright-Giemsa stain, ×1000.) (Courtesy Ann Bell, University of Tennessee, Memphis.)

maturation. Without the pink provided by hemoglobin, the cytoplasm remains bluish after the nucleus has begun to condense. The cell membranes appear irregular and are usually described as "shaggy."

Treatment and Its Effects

Treatment. The first therapy for iron deficiency is to treat any underlying contributing cause, such as hookworms, tumors, or ulcers. As in the treatment of simple nutritional deficiencies or increased need, dietary supplementation is necessary to replenish the body's iron stores. Oral supplements of ferrous sulfate are the standard prescription.[12] The supplements should be taken on an empty stomach to maximize absorption. Many patients experience side effects such as nausea and constipation, however, which leads to poor patient compliance. Vigilance on the part of the health care providers is important to ensure that patients complete the course of iron replacement, which usually lasts 6 months or longer.[27] Use of oral bovine lactoferrin to provide iron supplementation has been studied in developing nations.[28,29] The intestinal side effects are reduced compared with ferrous sulfate while being equally effective in correcting iron deficiency.

In rare cases in which intestinal absorption of iron is impaired (e.g., in conditions like gastric achlorhydria, celiac disease, or matriptase-2 mutations causing iron-refractory iron deficiency anemia or IRIDA), intravenous administration of iron dextrans can be used, although the side effects of this therapy are notable.[12] Because of the risks associated with RBC transfusions, they are rarely warranted for the correction of uncomplicated iron deficiency unless the patient's hemoglobin level has become dangerously low, like the patient in this chapter's case study.

Response to treatment. When optimal treatment with iron is initiated, the effects are quickly evident. The hemoglobin content of reticulocytes will correct within 2 days.[21] Reticulocyte counts (relative and absolute) begin to increase within 5 to 10 days.[27] The anticipated rise in hemoglobin appears in

2 to 3 weeks, and levels should return to normal for the individual by about 2 months after the initiation of adequate treatment.[30] The peripheral blood film and indices still reflect the microcytic RBC population for several months, with a biphasic population including the younger normocytic cells. The normocytic population eventually predominates. Iron therapy must continue for another 3 to 4 months to replenish the storage pool and prevent a relapse.

It is common and reasonable for care providers to assume that iron deficiency is due to dietary deficiency because that is the case in most instances of iron deficiency. Thus supplementation should correct it. If the patient has been adherent to the therapeutic regimen, the failure to respond to iron treatment points to the need for further investigation. The patient may be experiencing continued occult loss of blood or inadequate absorption, justifying additional diagnostics. The rare, but likely underdiagnosed, hereditary causes of iron deficiency should be considered. Alternatively, causes of hypochromic, microcytic anemia unrelated to iron deficiency, such as thalassemia, should be investigated.

Anemia of Chronic Inflammation

Anemia is commonly associated with systemic diseases, including chronic inflammatory conditions such as rheumatoid arthritis, chronic infections such as tuberculosis or human immunodeficiency virus infection, and malignancies. Cartwright[31] was the first to suggest that although the underlying diseases seem quite disparate, the associated anemia may be from a single cause, proposing the concept of anemia of chronic disease. This anemia ranks only behind iron deficiency anemia in incidence worldwide and is common among hospitalized patients.[32,33]

Etiology

Although the anemia associated with chronic systemic disorders was originally called *anemia of chronic disease,* chronic blood loss is not among the conditions leading to the anemia of chronic disease. Chronic blood loss results in quantitative iron deficiency. Anemia of chronic disease is more correctly termed *anemia of chronic inflammation,* because inflammation is the unifying factor among the three aforementioned general types of conditions in which this anemia is seen. The central feature of anemia of chronic inflammation is sideropenia in the face of abundant iron stores. The cause is now understood to be largely impaired ferrokinetics and thus iron-restricted erythropoiesis. However, impaired erythropoiesis and shortened RBC life span are also contributors.

Impaired ferrokinetics. As explained in detail in Chapter 8, hepcidin is a hormone produced by hepatocytes to regulate body iron levels, particularly absorption of iron in the intestine and release of iron from macrophages and hepatocytes. Hepcidin interacts with and causes degradation of transmembrane protein ferroportin, which exports iron from enterocytes into the blood, thus reducing the amount of iron absorbed into the blood from the intestine.[34] Macrophages and hepatocytes also use ferroportin to export and recycle iron into blood and are affected by hepcidin.[34,35] Conversely, when systemic body iron

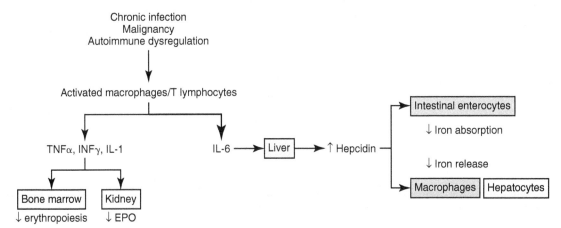

Figure 17.4 Mechanisms of Anemia in Chronic Inflammatory Conditions. Chronic infections (bacterial, viral, parasitic, or fungal), malignancy, or autoimmune dysregulation result in the release of inflammatory cytokines from activated macrophages and T lymphocytes. Interleukin-6 *(IL-6)* promotes liver production of hepcidin, an acute phase reactant that impairs iron absorption in intestinal enterocytes and iron release from macrophages and hepatocytes. Inflammatory cytokines, such as tumor necrosis factor-α *(TNF-α)*, interleukin-1 *(IL-1)*, and interferon-γ *(INF-γ)*, also inhibit erythropoiesis and decrease erythropoietin *(EPO)* production by the kidney. Although these latter mechanisms contribute to the anemia of chronic inflammation, the hepcidin-induced inhibition of intestinal iron absorption and iron release from storage sites in macrophages and hepatocytes is the more significant cause of the anemia. (Adapted from Weiss, G., & Goodnough, L. T. [2005]. Anemia of chronic disease. *N Engl J Med, 352*, p. 1013, Figure 1.)

levels decrease, hepcidin production by hepatocytes decreases,[36] and enterocytes export more iron into the blood. Macrophage and hepatocyte release of iron also increases. When systemic iron levels are high, hepcidin increases, enterocytes export less iron into the blood, and macrophages and hepatocytes retain iron.

Hepcidin is an acute phase reactant.[37] During inflammation, the liver increases the synthesis of hepcidin in response to interleukin-6 produced by activated macrophages.[33,38] This increase occurs regardless of systemic iron levels in the body. As a result, during inflammation, there is a decrease in iron absorption from the intestine and iron release from macrophages and hepatocytes (Figure 17.4). Although there is plenty of iron in the body, it is unavailable to developing RBCs because it is sequestered in the macrophages and hepatocytes.

The elevation of hepcidin during inflammation may be a nonspecific defense against invading bacteria.[39] If the body can sequester iron, it reduces the iron available to bacteria and thus contributes to their demise. Although a hepcidin rise is not harmful during disorders of short duration, chronically high levels of hepcidin sequester iron for long periods, which leads to diminished production of RBCs.

A second iron-related acute phase reactant seems to contribute to anemia of chronic inflammation, although probably to a much smaller extent than hepcidin. Lactoferrin is an iron-binding protein in the granules of neutrophils. Its avidity for iron is greater than that of transferrin. Lactoferrin is important to prevent phagocytized bacteria from using intracellular iron for their metabolic processes.[40] Lactoferrin may also provide protection for the phagocyte from oxidized iron that forms when reactive oxygen species (ROS) are produced during phagocytosis.[41]

During infection and inflammation, neutrophil lactoferrin is released into the blood and extracellular spaces with the death of neutrophils. There it scavenges iron that would otherwise induce oxidative damage. In this way, lactoferrin is anti-inflammatory. When it is carrying iron, lactoferrin binds to macrophages and liver cells that take up and salvage the iron. Because of high hepcidin, however, the macrophages and hepatocytes cannot export iron and it remains sequestered away from erythroblasts. Erythroblasts cannot acquire iron salvaged by lactoferrin directly because they do not have lactoferrin receptors.

The result of these effects during chronic inflammation is a functional iron deficiency; iron is present in abundance in storage but unavailable to developing erythroblasts. This maldistribution of iron can be seen histologically with iron stains of bone marrow that show iron in macrophages but not in erythroblasts (Figure 14.16C). The effect on the developing erythroblasts is essentially no different from a mild iron deficiency because they are effectively deprived of the iron. So, like iron deficiency anemia, this is iron-restricted erythropoiesis.

Diminished erythropoiesis. Production of inflammatory cytokines (such as tumor necrosis factor-α and interleukin-1 from activated macrophages and interferon-γ from activated T cells) also impairs proliferation of erythroid progenitor cells, diminishes their response to erythropoietin, and decreases production of erythropoietin by the kidney (Figure 17.4).[33,42]

Shortened red blood cell life span. A third factor contributing to the anemia of chronic inflammation is a shortened RBC life span. The cause appears to be an extracellular mechanism but without clear identification to date.[33] However, inflammation appears to induce increased production of hemophagocytic macrophages.[42] Although inflammatory suppression and shortened RBC life span contribute to the anemia of chronic inflammation, the impaired ferrokinetics is the most significant cause of the anemia.

Laboratory Diagnosis

The peripheral blood picture in anemia of chronic inflammation is that of a mild anemia, with hemoglobin concentration usually 8 to 10 g/dL and without reticulocytosis. The cells are usually normocytic and normochromic. Although microcytosis and hypochromia can be seen, they typically represent coexistent iron deficiency.[42] The inflammatory condition leading to the anemia also may cause leukocytosis, thrombocytosis, or both. Iron studies (Table 17.1) show low serum iron and TIBC values. Because hepatocyte production of transferrin is regulated by intracellular iron levels, the low TIBC (an indirect measure of transferrin) reflects the abundant iron stores in hepatocytes. The transferrin saturation may be normal or low. The serum ferritin level, as an acute phase reactant, is usually increased beyond the value that would be expected for the same patient in the absence of the inflammatory condition. It may not be outside the reference interval, but it is nevertheless increased. The failure to incorporate iron into heme results in elevation of FEP, although this test typically is not used diagnostically. The hemoglobin content of reticulocytes will be decreased, demonstrating the iron-restricted erythropoiesis, but the sTfR will be normal, reflecting normal intracellular iron. The bone marrow shows hypoproliferation of the RBCs, consistent with the lack of reticulocytes in the peripheral blood. Prussian blue stain of the bone marrow confirms abundant stores of iron in macrophages, although not in RBC precursors, but bone marrow examination is not usually required in the diagnostic evaluation.

Patients with iron deficiency anemia who have an inflammatory condition present a special diagnostic dilemma. The iron deficiency may be missed because of the increase in serum ferritin levels associated with the inflammation. Serum ferritin values in the 30 to 100 ng/mL range are most equivocal.[33,42] Iron deficiency anemia and anemia of chronic inflammation may be distinguished in such situations, or their coexistence can be verified, by measuring sTfRs in the serum.[43] These receptors are sloughed from cells into the blood. As noted earlier, levels increase during iron deficiency anemia but remain essentially normal during anemia of chronic inflammation.

Additional modifications to the use of the sTfR assay have been developed to better distinguish iron deficiency, latent iron deficiency, and anemia of chronic inflammation. The principles of these assays and calculations are discussed in Chapter 8 along with the measurement of the hemoglobin content of reticulocytes, also discussed in Chapter 12. It is expected that the sTfR/log ferritin will rise most dramatically in iron deficiency as the numerator rises and the denominator falls; in anemia of chronic inflammation, both remain essentially normal, and thus a normal ratio results (Figure 17.5).[44] The hemoglobin content of reticulocytes will be reduced in both iron deficiency and anemia of chronic inflammation. However, when graphed against the sTfR/log ferritin in a Thomas plot (Figure 8.6), the two conditions may be distinguished, sometimes better than with the sTfR/log ferritin alone (Chapter 8).[45,46] Additional research should help resolve this diagnostic dilemma.

Treatment

Therapeutic administration of erythropoietin can correct anemia of chronic inflammation,[47] but iron must be administered

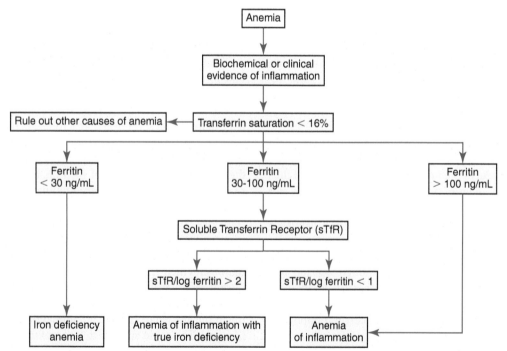

Figure 17.5 Algorithm for Diagnosis and Differentiation of Iron Deficiency Anemia and the Anemia of Chronic Inflammation. Patients with iron deficiency may exhibit normal ferritin levels in the range of 30 to 100 ng/mL when there is a rise of ferritin as a result of coexistent anemia of chronic inflammation. Use of the soluble transferrin receptor assay in conjunction with ferritin can help distinguish these conditions or establish their coexistence. *sTfR,* Soluble transferrin receptor in mg/L. (Adapted from Weiss, G., & Goodnough, L. T. [2005]. Anemia of chronic disease. *N Engl J Med, 352,* p. 1020, Figure 2.)

concurrently because stored body iron remains sequestered and unavailable (i.e., functional iron deficiency).[48] The anemia is typically not severe, however, and this costly treatment is warranted only in select patients. At present, the best course of treatment is effective control or alleviation of the underlying condition. However, various anti-hepcidin therapies are being investigated.[2]

SIDEROBLASTIC ANEMIAS

Just as anemia can result from inadequate supplies of iron for production of hemoglobin, diseases that interfere with the production of protoporphyrin also can produce anemia. (Protoporphyrin synthesis is discussed in Chapter 7.) As in iron deficiency, the anemia may be microcytic and hypochromic. In contrast to iron deficiency, however, iron is abundant in the bone marrow. A Prussian blue stain of the bone marrow shows erythroblasts with iron deposits in the mitochondria surrounding the nucleus. Its presence in the mitochondria shows that the iron is awaiting incorporation into heme. These *ring (or ringed) sideroblasts* are the hallmark of the sideroblastic anemias (Figure 17.6).

The sideroblastic anemias are a diverse group of diseases that include hereditary and acquired conditions (Box 17.1). Among the hereditary forms, X-linked and autosomal varieties of this condition are known. Some patients experience at least modest

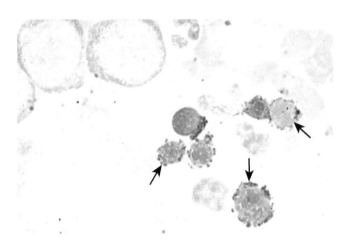

Figure 17.6 Ring Sideroblasts *(arrows)* in Bone Marrow. (Prussian blue stain, ×1000.)

BOX 17.1 Disorders Included in Sideroblastic Anemias

Hereditary
X-linked
Autosomal

Acquired
Primary sideroblastic anemia (refractory)
Secondary sideroblastic anemias caused by drugs and bone marrow toxins
   Antitubercular drugs
   Chloramphenicol
   Alcohol
   Lead
   Chemotherapeutic agents

---

improvement of anemia with pharmacologic doses of pyridoxine (vitamin B_6) to stimulate heme synthesis.[49] Pyridoxine is a cofactor in the first step of porphyrin synthesis (Figure 7.5) in which glycine is condensed with succinyl coenzyme A to form aminolevulinic acid.

Acquired: Lead Poisoning

The acquired conditions leading to sideroblastic anemia constitute a diverse group in themselves. Certain drugs, such as chloramphenicol or isoniazid, can induce sideroblastic anemia.[50] Other toxins, including heavy metals, also have been implicated. Among these, lead is a significant public health concern. Adults may be exposed to leaded compounds at work if proper safety precautions are not in place. Adults and children living in older homes can be exposed to lead from paints produced before the 1970s. They are at risk if dust is created during renovations or paint is permitted to peel. Toddlers and crawling infants are at special risk from getting dust on their hands and placing them in their mouths. Lead leached from service pipes by improperly treated drinking water can also be a source of the toxin. Several cities in the United States that have experienced this have been spotlighted in the news in recent years.[51]

Although anyone can experience lead poisoning, it is of special concern in children because the metal affects the central nervous system as well as the hematologic system, leading to impaired mental development and anemia.[52] In children and adults with lead poisoning, a peripheral neuropathy[53] can be seen with abdominal cramping and vomiting or seizures.

Lead interferes with porphyrin synthesis at several steps. The most critical are as follows (Figure 7.5):
1. The conversion of aminolevulinic acid (ALA) to porphobilinogen (PBG) by ALA dehydratase (also called *PBG synthase*); the result is the accumulation of aminolevulinic acid.
2. The incorporation of iron into protoporphyrin IX by ferrochelatase (also called *heme synthase*); the result is accumulation of iron and protoporphyrin in the mitochondria.[54]

Accumulated ALA is measurable in the urine, and protoporphyrin is measurable in an extract of RBCs as FEP or ZPP. Chapter 8 describes the principles of these assays.

Anemia, when present in lead poisoning, is most often normocytic and normochromic; however, with chronic exposure to lead, a microcytic, hypochromic blood picture may be seen. The degree of anemia in adults may not be dramatic, but in children it may be more profound. The reticulocyte count in acute poisoning may be quite elevated, which suggests that the anemia has a hemolytic component. The presence of a hemolytic component is supported by studies showing impairment of the pentose-phosphate shunt by lead,[55] which makes the cells sensitive to oxidant stress as in glucose-6-phosphate dehydrogenase deficiency (Chapter 21). Although the bone marrow may show erythroid hyperplasia, consistent with the elevated reticulocyte count, in some patients it may be hypoplastic.[56] Basophilic stippling is a classic finding associated with lead toxicity. Lead inhibits pyrimidine 5'-nucleotidase, an enzyme involved in the breakdown of ribosomal ribonucleic acid (RNA) in reticulocytes.[57] This causes undegraded ribosomes to aggregate, forming basophilic stippling. The size of the aggregates in lead poisoning is typically large, so the stippling is heavier than that seen in many anemias and thus represents truly punctate basophilia. Because basophilic stippling is also seen in other anemias, this is not a pathognomonic finding but an expected finding, and whenever punctate basophilic stippling is seen, lead poisoning should be under consideration.

Removal of the drug or toxin is usually successful for the treatment of acquired sideroblastic anemias. In the case of lead poisoning, calcium disodium edetate (CaNa$_2$EDTA) and/or dimercaprol are often used to chelate the lead present in the body so it can be excreted in the urine.[56] The other impacts of lead poisoning, such as mental impairments in children, are often more sustained.

Hereditary: Porphyrias

Lead poisoning is an example not only of an acquired sideroblastic anemia but also of an acquired porphyria. The porphyrias are diseases characterized by impaired production of the porphyrin component of heme. The impairments to heme synthesis may be acquired, as with lead poisoning, or hereditary. The term *porphyria* is most often used to refer to the hereditary conditions that impair production of protoporphyrin. Among the inherited disorders, single deficiencies of most enzymes in the synthetic pathway for heme have been identified (Figure 7.5). Although even the autosomal dominant conditions are relatively rare, the disease has been influential historically. The intermarrying European monarchies of past centuries were plagued with some variants of the porphyrias in which psychosis is a prominent clinical feature.

When an enzyme in heme synthesis is missing, the products from earlier stages in the pathway accumulate in cells that actively produce heme, such as erythrocytes and hepatocytes. The excess porphyrins leak from the cells as they age or die and may be excreted in urine or feces, which allows diagnosis. The accumulated products also deposit in body tissues. Some of the accumulated products are fluorescent. Their deposition in skin can lead to photosensitivity with severe burns on exposure to sunlight. Accumulation during childhood leads to fluorescence of developing teeth and bones. Only three of the porphyrias have hematologic manifestations; the others have a greater effect on liver cells. Even in those with hematologic effects, the hematologic impact is relatively minimal, and photosensitivity is a greater clinical problem. The fluorescence of some accumulated compounds can be used diagnostically, for example to measure FEP (Chapter 8). In a bone marrow specimen the erythroblasts will be bright red under a fluorescent microscope. Table 17.2 summarizes the deficient enzymes, affected genes, inheritance, and clinical and laboratory features that can be used in the diagnosis of the hematologically significant porphyrias.

IRON OVERLOAD

Chapter 8 describes the body's tenacity in conserving iron. For some individuals, this tenacity becomes the basis for disease related to excess iron accumulations in nearly all cells. Iron overload may be primary, as in hereditary hemochromatosis, or secondary to chronic anemias and their treatments. In both cases the toxic effects of excess iron lead to serious health problems as lipids, proteins, nucleic acids, and heme iron become oxidized.

TABLE 17.2 Erythropoietic Porphyrias

		Congenital Erythropoietic Porphyria (CEP)	Erythropoietic Protoporphyria (EPP)	X-linked Erythropoietic Protoporphyria (XLEPP)
Enzyme affected		Uroporphyrinogen III synthase deficiency	Ferrochelatase deficiency	ALA-synthase 2 (gain of function)
Affected gene		*UROS*	*FECH*	*ALAS2*
Inheritance		Autosomal recessive	Autosomal recessive	X-linked dominant
Clinical features		Photosensitivity, hemolytic anemia	Photosensitivity; anemia is mild if present	Photosensitivity; mild microcytic, hypochromic anemia with reticulocyte response is possible
Laboratory Features				
Red blood cells	Protoporphyrin	N	↑↑↑	↑
	Uroporphyrin	↑↑↑	N	N
	Coproporphyrin	↑↑	N	N
Urine	Porphobilinogen	N	N	N
	Uroporphyrin	↑↑↑	N	N
	Coproporphyrin	↑↑	N	N
Feces	Protoporphyrin	N	↑↑	N or ↑
	Coproporphyrin	↑	N	N
Confirmatory tests		↓↓↓ Uroporphyrinogen III synthase activity	↓↓ Ferrochelatase activity	↑↑ ALA-synthase activity
		Genetic testing	Genetic testing	↑↑ FEP/ZPP
				Genetic testing

↑, Minimally increased levels; ↑↑, moderately increased levels; ↑↑↑, markedly increased levels; ↓↓, moderately decreased levels; ↓↓↓, markedly decreased levels; FEP/ZPP, free erythrocyte protoporphyrin/zinc protoporphyrin.
(Adapted from Desnick, R. J., Balwani, M. [2015]. The porphyrias. In Kasper, D. L., Fauci, A., Hauser, S., et al. [Eds.], *Harrison's Principles of Internal Medicine*. [19th ed., p. 2422]. New York: McGraw Hill Education.)

Etiology

Excess accumulation of iron results from acquired or hereditary conditions in which the body's rate of iron acquisition exceeds the rate of loss, which is usually about 1 mg/day. Regardless of the source of the iron, the body's first reaction is to store excess iron in the form of ferritin and, ultimately, hemosiderin within cells. Eventually the storage system is overwhelmed, and, as described later, parenchymal cells are damaged in organs such as the liver, heart, and pancreas.

Accumulation of excess iron may be an acquired condition. It occurs when there is a need for repeated transfusions, as in the treatment of anemias such as sickle cell anemia and β-thalassemia major (Chapters 24 and 25). The iron present in the transfused RBCs exceeds the usual 1 mg/day of iron typically added to the body's stores by a healthy diet. This is sometimes called *transfusion-related hemosiderosis.*

Some chronic anemias, usually hereditary hemolytic anemias (e.g., β-thalassemia major), are innately iron loading, even without transfusion therapy. Hemolytic anemias cause the bone marrow to develop a compensatory erythroid hyperplasia. As described in Chapter 8, erythroblasts are able to downregulate hepcidin production by secreting erythroferrone. If there are more erythroblasts than usual, as in compensatory erythroid hyperplasia, then erythroferrone is increased, hepcidin is decreased, and more than the usual amount of iron is absorbed and recycled. With chronic hemolytic anemias, this leads to excessive accumulation of iron. Although this is seen most often with hereditary hemolytic anemias, the iron loading is secondary to the hereditary condition that causes the hemolysis. If the hemolysis is controlled, the iron loading subsides. Thus this is acquired iron overload in a hereditary anemia.

On the other hand, hemochromatosis may develop as a result of mutations in genes for proteins controlling iron kinetics (Table 8.2) so that feedback regulation of iron is impaired and the body continues to absorb iron, even when stores are full. This is a true hereditary iron overload. An autosomal recessive disease was recognized for many years before modern methods allowed a molecular investigation of its cause. In the mid-1990s, a mutation was identified affecting the hereditary hemochromatosis (HFE) protein,[58] and shortly after that, additional mutations of the same gene were identified.[59,60] With reliable and specific molecular tests, individuals with the phenotypic disease (i.e., excess iron deposition in tissues) were soon discovered who did not have the HFE mutations. Trying to explain their diseases led to discovery of the other proteins that are now known to be involved in iron kinetics. What has emerged is a picture of hereditary hemochromatosis as a general phenotype that can be produced by various genotypes when a gene for an iron regulatory protein is mutated (Table 17.3). The biologic default is to absorb and store iron, and the regulatory mechanisms typically dampen that process. Failure of normal regulation as a result of mutations leads to excessive absorption and storage, causing the diseases collectively known as the *hereditary hemochromatoses.* Although substantial understanding of the proteins involved in iron kinetics has emerged in the past 2 decades in large part from studying patients with various mutations, more remains to be discovered.

TABLE 17.3   Known Mutations Producing Hemochromatosis Phenotypes

Feature	Hemochromatosis, Type 1 (*HFE*-Associated Hereditary Hemochromatosis)	Hemochromatosis, Type 2A Juvenile (*HFE2*-Related Juvenile Hemochromatosis)	Hemochromatosis, Type 2B Juvenile (*HAMP*-Related Juvenile Hemochromatosis)	Hemochromatosis, Type 3 (*TFR2*-Related Hereditary Hemochromatosis)	Hemachromatosis, Type 4 (Ferroportin-Related Iron Overload)	Hemachromatosis, Type 5
Affected gene	*HFE*	*HFE2 (HJV)*	*HAMP*	*TFR2*	*SLC40A1*	*FTH1*
Mutated protein	Hereditary hemochromatosis protein	Hemojuvelin	Hepcidin	Transferrin receptor protein 2	Solute carrier family 40 member 1 (ferroportin-1)	Ferritin heavy chain
Normal function of affected protein	Participates in signaling complex for hepcidin regulation	Hepatocyte coreceptor in signaling complex for hepcidin regulation	Downregulates ferroportin-mediated iron transport in macrophages, hepatocytes and enterocytes	Hepatic iron sensor to regulate hepcidin expression	Transports iron out of enterocytes, hepatocytes, and macrophages	Iron storage
Age of onset of symptoms (yr)	30–40	Teens–20	Teens–20	20–40, mild	30–40	*
Inheritance pattern of most common alleles	Autosomal recessive	Autosomal recessive	Autosomal recessive	Autosomal recessive	Autosomal dominant	Autosomal dominant

TfR1, Transferrin receptor 1; *TfR2*, transferrin receptor 2.
*Found in three members of a Japanese family.
Names of hemochromatosis types from Online Mendelian Inheritance of Man: https://www.omim.org/entry/235200.
Approved gene symbols from The Human Genome Organization (HUGO) Gene Nomenclature Committee (HGNC): http://www.genenames.org.
Approved protein names from Uni Prot KB, 2002–2014 UniProt Consortium: http://www.uniprot.org.

Table 17.3 describes each of the known forms of hemochromatosis, its mutated protein, age of onset, inheritance pattern, and the nature of the mutation and its effect. Because mutations of the *HFE* gene remain the most common, that form of the disease will be discussed here with some references to differences seen in other forms of the disease. However, in general, the most common hereditary hemochromatoses involve mutated proteins that impair hepcidin regulation of ferroportin activity. Other iron overload conditions, such as hemochromatosis type 5 and hypotransferrinemia, involve mutations of proteins involved in iron kinetics but not the hepcidin-ferroportin axis. They are not all named hemochromatosis, likely because of a different phenotype, and some may be considered among the iron-loading anemias.

Homozygous hereditary hemochromatosis involving the *HFE* gene occurs in approximately 5 of 1000 northern Europeans.[61] Heterozygosity approaches 13%.[61] The first two mutations known to produce the hereditary hemochromatosis phenotype involve *HFE*, a gene on the short arm of chromosome 6 that encodes an HLA class I-like molecule that is closely linked to HLA-A.[58] The most common of the two mutations substitutes tyrosine for cysteine at position 282 (Cys282Tyr or C282Y), whereas the other substitutes aspartate for histidine at position 63 (His63Asp or H63D).[59] Other mutations are now known.[60] The normal HFE protein binds β_2-microglobulin intracellularly.[59] This binding is necessary for the HFE to appear on the cell surface, where it interacts with transferrin receptor 1 (TfR1). HFE is bound to TfR1 until TfR1 binds transferrin, and then the HFE is released. It subsequently associates with transferrin receptor 2 (TfR2), bone morphogenetic protein (BMP) and its receptor, and hemojuvelin (HJV). This complex initiates a signal for hepcidin production, ultimately reducing iron absorption. The mutated HFE molecule either does not bind β_2-microglobulin and thus does not reach the cell surface or, if it does reach the cell surface, does not bind TfR1 or associate properly with TfR2.[62] In any case the result is that when HFE protein is mutated, the BMP-BMPR mediated signal to produce hepcidin is diminished. Without hepcidin, ferroportin in the intestinal enterocyte membrane is continually active, transporting iron into the blood even when body stores are already replete.

Pathogenesis

The processes described previously lead to increased amounts of iron in parenchymal cells throughout the body. The first cellular reaction to excess iron is to form ferritin and ultimately hemosiderin, essentially a degenerate and non-metabolically active form of ferritin. When cells exhaust the capacity to store iron as hemosiderin, free iron (ferrous) accumulates intracellularly. In the presence of oxygen, ferrous iron initiates the generation of superoxide and other free radicals, which results in the peroxidation of membrane lipids (Chapter 8).[63] The membranes affected include not only the cell membranes but also mitochondrial, nuclear, and lysosomal membranes. Cell respiration is compromised, and lysosomal enzymes are released intracellularly. Vitamins E and C can act to moderate the effects and interrupt the chain reaction, but in iron overload,

even these protective mechanisms are overwhelmed. The ultimate result is cell death caused by irreversible membrane damage.

Because all cells except mature RBCs, require iron and have the cellular machinery for iron acquisition, most cells have the potential for iron damage. The tissues most obviously affected are the skin, where deposition of hemosiderin gives the skin a golden color; the liver, where cirrhosis-induced jaundice and subsequent cancer may develop; and the pancreas, where damage results in diabetes mellitus. Thus hemochromatosis has been characterized as "bronzed diabetes." But the heart muscle also is especially vulnerable to excessive iron deposition, which leads to congestive heart failure. Early diagnosis and treatment (discussed later) can prevent the development of these secondary effects of iron overload. Hepatocellular carcinoma occurs more often in patients with hemochromatosis. Mutations of the *p53* tumor suppressor gene seem to contribute to the pathogenesis of the carcinoma,[64,65] and there is some evidence that the free radicals produced by iron cause the mutations in the *p53* gene.[66]

The disease (i.e., hemochromatosis phenotype) is rarer than the *C282Y* gene frequency predicts, so the penetrance of the genes is not complete.[61] Other factors also affect the development of clinical disease, including the particular mutation, zygosity, presence of other physiologic conditions, diet, and other environmental influences.

In classic hereditary hemochromatosis (*HFE* mutations), individuals usually harbor 20 to 30 g of iron by the time their disease becomes clinically evident at the age of 40 to 60 years.[67] This is almost 10 times the amount of stored iron in healthy individuals and represents just 1 to 2 mg/day of excess iron absorbed over many years.[68] In the juvenile forms of the disease associated with mutations to the hepcidin or hemojuvelin genes, the process of iron accumulation is accelerated, so these effects may appear as early as the teenage years.

In the slower-developing diseases, phenotypic expression of the tissue damage in hereditary hemochromatosis is more common in men, although the gene frequency of HFE mutations is not higher in men. This is because the blood loss associated with menstruation and childbirth forestalls the effects of excess iron in affected women, and they usually develop clinical symptoms later in life than affected men. In each sex, homozygous individuals develop clinical disease faster than heterozygotes.

The amount of iron available in the diet for absorption affects the rate at which disease can develop. Substances that can promote iron absorption even in normal individuals, such as ascorbic acid and alcohol, also affect absorption in individuals with hemochromatosis. In transfusion-related hemosiderosis, the frequency of transfusions over time affects the rate of development of clinical disease.

Laboratory Diagnosis

Laboratory testing in hemochromatosis serves four purposes. It can be used to screen for the condition, diagnose the cause of organ damage, pinpoint the mutation for family genetic counseling, and monitor treatment. Elevations of transferrin saturation or serum ferritin can be used as a screening test for hereditary hemochromatosis.[69] Although screening was estimated to be performed cost effectively in populations with a disease prevalence of at least 3 per 1000,[70] large-scale screening programs remain controversial, even in Europe, where the incidence of the disease is high.[71]

Individuals with undiagnosed hereditary hemochromatosis may come to medical attention because of organ function problems leading to nonspecific physical complaints (e.g., abdominal pain), or the disease may be discovered incidentally with routine laboratory testing. Abnormal results on common tests of liver function (e.g., elevated alanine transaminase levels) may be among the first laboratory findings that lead a care provider to order further testing to identify the cause. Because inflammation is minimal, however, a finding of diminished levels of the liver's synthetic products, such as albumin, may be more helpful. If hereditary hemochromatosis is among the disorders being considered to explain organ dysfunction, serum iron, transferrin saturation, and serum ferritin testing are warranted because elevations in these values are among the earliest findings in most forms of hemochromatosis. Genetic testing for known mutations provides confirmation of the diagnosis for most patients with hereditary hemochromatosis. It is especially valuable for testing nonaffected family members who can be counseled in lifestyle changes to prevent the phenotype from developing or for whom early treatment interventions can prevent organ damage.

Whether hemochromatosis is acquired or hereditary, the serum ferritin level provides an assessment of the degree of iron overload and can be monitored after treatment is initiated to reduce iron stores. Hemoglobin concentration and hematocrit are inexpensive tests that can also be used to monitor treatment, as described later.

Determination of the actual extent of tissue damage is beyond the scope of the clinical laboratory. Liver biopsy with assessment of iron staining and degree of scarring in liver specimens is essential to determining the degree of organ damage.

Treatment

The treatment of secondary tissue damage, such as liver cirrhosis and heart failure, follows standard protocols. Treatment of the underlying condition leading to excess iron accumulation is also needed. Hereditary hemochromatosis and transfusion-related hemosiderosis require different treatment approaches. In forms of hereditary hemochromatosis, withdrawal of blood by phlebotomy provides a simple, inexpensive, and effective means of removing iron from the body. The regimen calls for weekly phlebotomy early in treatment to remove about 500 mL of blood per treatment. Maintenance phlebotomies are required about every 3 months for life.[72] Hemoglobin levels are monitored, and a mild anemia is sought and maintained. Such monitoring is an easy and inexpensive substitute for iron studies because, as explained in the discussion of iron deficiency, iron stores must be exhausted before anemia develops.

Individuals who rely on transfusions to maintain hemoglobin levels and prevent anemia cannot be treated with phlebotomy. Instead, iron-chelating drugs are used to bind excess iron in the body for excretion (Chapter 25). Deferoxamine is the classic treatment, although it is not without side effects.[73] The drug typically is administered subcutaneously with an infusion pump over 8 to 12 hours to maximize exposure time for iron binding. When absorbed into the bloodstream with its bound iron, it is readily excreted in the urine. Recently oral iron chelators have been developed.[74-76] Although they also have side effects, the convenience of oral administration with the potential for improved patient outcomes may lead to a greater reliance on this form of treatment.

▎SUMMARY

- Impaired iron kinetics or heme metabolism can result in microcytic, hypochromic anemias.
- Three conditions affecting iron kinetics can result in microcytic, hypochromic anemias: iron deficiency anemia, anemia of chronic inflammation, and sideroblastic anemias, especially lead poisoning. The red blood cells (RBCs) in thalassemias also may be microcytic and hypochromic, and this condition must be differentiated from the anemias of disordered iron metabolism.
- Iron deficiency results from inadequate iron intake, increased need, decreased absorption, or excessive loss. All four of these situations create a relative deficit of body iron that over time results in a microcytic, hypochromic anemia.
- Infants, children, and women of childbearing age are at greatest risk for iron deficiency anemia. If iron deficiency anemia is present in men and postmenopausal women, the possibility of gastrointestinal bleeding should be investigated because it is the primary, although not the only, cause of iron loss.
- Iron deficiency is suspected when the complete blood count (CBC) shows microcytic, hypochromic RBCs and elevated RBC distribution width (RDW) but no consistent morphologic abnormality. The diagnosis is confirmed with iron studies showing low levels of serum iron and serum ferritin, elevated total iron-binding capacity (TIBC), and decreased transferrin saturation.
- Inadequate dietary iron is treated by oral supplementation, and with good patient adherence, the anemia should be corrected within 3 months. Gastrointestinal distress resulting from iron supplements can make patient adherence a significant concern. Other causes of iron deficiency must be treated by eliminating the underlying cause or with intravenous iron administration.
- Anemia of chronic inflammation is associated with chronic infections such as tuberculosis, chronic inflammatory conditions such as rheumatoid arthritis, and malignancies. It may be a microcytic, hypochromic anemia, but most often it is a mild normocytic, normochromic anemia.
- In anemia of chronic inflammation, increased levels of hepcidin, an acute phase reactant, decrease iron absorption in the intestines and sequester iron in macrophages and hepatocytes. Bone marrow macrophages show abundant stainable iron, whereas developing erythroblasts show inadequate iron (iron-restricted erythropoiesis). Inflammatory cellular products also impair the production and action of erythropoietin. RBC life span is shortened.

- Iron studies in the anemia of chronic inflammation show decreased serum iron level, decreased TIBC, decreased or normal transferrin saturation, and normal or increased ferritin level.
- Sideroblastic anemias develop when the synthesis of protoporphyrin or the incorporation of iron into protoporphyrin is blocked. The result is accumulation of iron in the mitochondria of developing erythroblasts. When stained with Prussian blue, the iron appears in deposits around the nucleus of the developing erythroblasts in the bone marrow. These cells are called *ring sideroblasts.*
- Protoporphyrin synthesis and iron incorporation into protoporphyrin can be blocked when any of the enzymes of the heme synthetic pathway are deficient or impaired. Deficiencies of these enzymes may be hereditary, as in the porphyrias, or acquired, as in heavy metal poisoning. The most common of the latter conditions is lead poisoning.
- Iron studies in sideroblastic anemias show elevated levels of serum iron and serum ferritin, decreased or normal TIBC, and increased transferrin saturation. Test values for the accumulating products of the heme synthetic pathway, such as zinc protoporphyrin (ZPP) or free erythrocyte protoporphyrin (FEP), are also elevated.
- Lead interferes with several steps in heme synthesis, preventing iron incorporation into heme and resulting in a normocytic, normochromic anemia, although with long-term exposure it can be microcytic and hypochromic. Lead also impairs the pentose-phosphate shunt, which adds a hemolytic component to the anemia.
- Children are especially vulnerable to the effects of lead on the central nervous system, which may result in irreversible brain damage. Treatment consists of removing the source of lead from the patient's environment and, if necessary, chelating drug therapy to facilitate excretion of lead in the urine. Central nervous system effects are typically not reversed with treatment.
- Porphyrias are diseases in which porphyrin production is impaired. They can be acquired, such as lead poisoning, or inherited with mutations affecting enzymes in the heme synthetic pathway.
- Three hereditary porphyrias have hematologic manifestations including anemia and fluorescent erythroblasts caused by accumulated porphyrins.
- Because the body has no mechanism for iron excretion, iron overload can occur when transfusions are used to sustain patients with chronic anemias such as β-thalassemia major (called *transfusion-related hemosiderosis*).
- Iron-loading anemias are those with erythroid hyperplasia that increases levels of erythroferrone leading to decreased hepcidin, increased ferroportin activity, and increased iron absorption.
- A defective *HFE* gene can lead to hereditary hemochromatosis by decreased hepcidin production. Affected men develop symptoms earlier in life than women; homozygotes develop more severe disease than heterozygotes.
- Mutations of other genes affecting iron regulation can produce a phenotype similar to that of hereditary hemochromatosis. When the hepcidin or hemojuvelin gene is mutated, the disease develops early in life, affecting even teenagers.
- Free iron becomes available in cells when ferritin and hemosiderin become saturated. Free iron causes tissue damage by creating free radicals that lead to cell membrane damage and perhaps mutations. The liver, pancreas, skin, and heart muscle are especially vulnerable to damage by excess iron deposition.
- Elevated transferrin saturation or serum ferritin can be an indicator of hemochromatosis that can be diagnosed fully using genetic testing to identify mutated genes.
- Hereditary hemochromatosis and similar diseases are treated by lifelong periodic phlebotomy to induce a mild iron deficiency anemia and keep body iron levels low. Transfusion-related hemosiderosis must be treated with iron-chelating drugs.

Now that you have completed this chapter, go back and read again the case study at the beginning and respond to the questions presented.

REVIEW QUESTIONS

Answers can be found in the Appendix.

1. The mother of a 4-month-old infant who is being breastfed sees her physician for a routine postpartum visit. She expresses concern that she may be experiencing postpartum depression because she does not seem to have any energy. Although the physician is sympathetic to the patient's concern, she orders a CBC and iron studies seeking an organic explanation for the patient's symptoms. The results are as follows:
   CBC: all results within reference intervals except the RDW, which was 15%.
   Serum iron: decreased
   TIBC: increased
   % transferrin saturation: decreased
   Serum ferritin: decreased
   Correlate the patient's laboratory and clinical findings. What can you conclude?

   a. The results of the iron studies reveal findings consistent with a thalassemia that was apparently previously undiagnosed.
   b. The patient is in stage 2 of iron deficiency, before frank anemia develops.
   c. The results of the iron studies are inconsistent with the CBC results, and a laboratory error should be suspected.
   d. There is no evidence of a hematologic explanation for the patient's symptoms.

2. A bone marrow biopsy was performed as part of the cancer staging protocol for a patient with Hodgkin lymphoma. Although no evidence of spread of the tumor was apparent in the bone marrow, other abnormal findings were noted, including a slightly elevated myeloid-to-erythroid ratio. WBC and RBC morphology appeared normal, however. The Prussian blue stain showed abundant stainable iron in the marrow macrophages. The patient's CBC revealed a hemoglobin of 10.8 g/dL, but RBC indices were within reference intervals. RBC morphology was unremarkable. These findings are consistent with:
   a. Anemia of chronic inflammation
   b. Sideroblastic anemia
   c. Thalassemia
   d. Iron deficiency anemia

3. Predict the iron study results for the patient with Hodgkin lymphoma described in question 2.

	Serum Iron Level	TIBC	% Transferrin Saturation	Serum Ferritin Level
a.	Decreased	Increased	Decreased	Decreased
b.	Increased	Normal	Increased	Normal
c.	Increased	Increased	Normal	Increased
d.	Decreased	Decreased	Normal	Normal

4. A 35-year-old white woman went to her physician complaining of headaches, dizziness, and nausea. The headaches had been increasing in severity over the past 6 months. This was coincident with her move into an older house built about 1900. She had been renovating the house, including stripping paint from the woodwork. Her CBC results showed a mild hypochromic, microcytic anemia, with polychromasia and basophilic stippling noted. Which of the following tests would be most useful in confirming the cause of her anemia?
   a. Serum lead level
   b. Serum iron level and TIBC
   c. Absolute reticulocyte count
   d. Prussian blue staining of the bone marrow to detect iron stores in macrophages

5. In men and postmenopausal women whose diets are adequate, iron deficiency anemia most often results from:
   a. Increased need associated with aging
   b. Impaired absorption in the gastric mucosa
   c. Chronic gastrointestinal bleeding
   d. Diminished resistance to hookworm infections

6. Which one of the following individuals is at greatest risk for the development of iron deficiency anemia?
   a. A 15-year-old boy who eats mainly junk food
   b. A 37-year-old woman who has never been pregnant and has amenorrhea
   c. A 63-year-old man with reactivation of tuberculosis from his childhood
   d. A 40-year-old man who lost blood during surgery to repair a fractured leg

7. Which of the following individuals is at the greatest risk for the development of anemia of chronic inflammation?
   a. A 15-year-old girl with asthma
   b. A 40-year-old woman with type 2 diabetes mellitus
   c. A 65-year-old man with hypertension
   d. A 30-year-old man with severe rheumatoid arthritis

8. In what situation will increased levels of free erythrocyte protoporphyrin be present?
   a. Loss of function mutation to one of the enzymes in the heme synthesis pathway
   b. A mutation that prevents heme attachment to globin so that protoporphyrin remains free
   c. Any condition that prevents iron incorporation into protoporphyrin IX
   d. When red blood cells lyse, freeing their contents into the plasma

9. In the pathogenesis of the anemia of chronic inflammation, hepcidin levels:
   a. Decrease during inflammation and reduce iron absorption from enterocytes
   b. Increase during inflammation and reduce iron absorption from enterocytes
   c. Increase during inflammation and increase iron absorption from enterocytes
   d. Decrease during inflammation and increase iron absorption from enterocytes

10. Sideroblastic anemias result from:
    a. Sequestration of iron in hepatocytes
    b. Inability to incorporate heme into apohemoglobin
    c. Sequestration of iron in myeloblasts
    d. Failure to incorporate iron into protoporphyrin IX

11. In general, most instances of hereditary hemochromatoses result from mutations that impair:
    a. The manner in which developing red cells acquire and manage iron
    b. The hepcidin-ferroportin iron regulatory system
    c. The TfR-Tf endocytic iron acquisition process for body cells other than red blood cells
    d. The function of divalent metal transporter in enterocytes and macrophages

12. In the erythropoietic porphyrias, mild anemia may be accompanied by what distinctive clinical finding?
    a. Gallstones
    b. Impaired night vision
    c. Unintentional nighttime leg movements
    d. Heightened propensity for sunburn

Also review Chapter 8, questions 4, 10, 11, and 12, which are pertinent to the diagnostic value of various tests of iron status.

REFERENCES

1. Hallberg, L. (1981). Bioavailability of dietary iron in man. *Annu Rev Nutr, 1,* 123–147.
2. Kim, A., & Nemeth, E. (2015). New insights into iron regulation and erythropoiesis. *Curr Opin Hematol, 22*(3), 199–205.
3. Nai, A., Lidonnici, M. R., Rausa, M., et al. (2015). The second transferrin receptor regulates red blood cell production in mice. *Blood, 125*(7), 1170–1179.
4. Silvestri, L., Guillem, F., Pagani, A., et al. (2009). Molecular mechanisms of the defective hepcidin inhibition in TMPRSS6 mutations associated with iron-refractory iron deficiency anemia. *Blood, 113*(22), 5605–5608.
5. Suominen, P., Punnonen, K., Rajamaki, A., et al. (1998). Serum transferrin receptor and transferrin receptor-ferritin index identify healthy subjects with subclinical iron deficits. *Blood, 92,* 2934–2939.
6. Gupta, P. M., Hammer, H. C., Suchdev, P. S., et al. (2017). Iron status of toddlers, non-pregnant females, and pregnant females in the United States. *Am J Clin Nutr, 106*(Suppl 6), 1640S–1646S.
7. Rolfs, A., Kvietikova, I., Gassmann, M., et al. (1997). Oxygen-regulated transferrin expression is mediated by hypoxia-inducible factor-1. *J Biol Chem, 272*(32), 20055–20062.
8. Frise, M. C., & Robbins, P. A. (2015). Iron, oxygen, and the pulmonary circulation. *J Appl Physiol, 119*(12), 1421–1431.
9. Buttarello, M., Pajola, R., Novello, E., et al. (2016). Evaluation of the hypochromic erythrocyte and reticulocyte hemoglobin content provided by the Sysmex XE-5000 analyzer in diagnosis of iron deficiency erythropoiesis. *Clin Chem Lab Med, 54*(12), 1939–1945.
10. Urrechaga, E., Borque, L., & Escanero, J. F. (2016). Clinical value of hypochromia markers in the detection of latent iron deficiency in nonanemic premenopausal women. *J Clin Lab Anal, 30,* 623–627.
11. de Klerk, G., Rosengarten, P. C. J., Vet, R. J. M., et al. (1981). Serum erythropoietin (ESF) titers in anemia. *Blood, 58*(6), 1164–1170.
12. Goodnough, L. T., & Nemeth, E. (2014). Iron deficiency and related disorders. In Greer, J. P., Arber, D. A., Glader, D., et al. (Eds.), *Wintrobe's Clinical Hematology.* (13th ed., pp. 617–642). Philadelphia: Lippincott Williams & Wilkins.
13. McMahon, L. P. (2010). Iron deficiency in pregnancy. *Obstet Med, 3*(1), 17–24.
14. Saarinen, U. M., Siimes, M. A., & Dallman, P. R. (1977). Iron absorption in infants: high bioavailability of breast milk iron as indicated by the extrinsic tag method of iron absorption and by the concentration of serum ferritin. *J Pediatr, 91,* 36–39.
15. Siimes, M. A., Vuori, E., & Kuitunen, P. (1979). Breast milk iron: a declining concentration during the course of lactation. *Acta Paediatr Scand, 68,* 29–31.
16. Wouthuyzen-Bakker, M., & van Assen, S. (2015). Exercise-induced anaemia: a forgotten cause of iron deficiency aneaemia in young adults. *Br J Gen Pract, 65*(634), 268–269.
17. Janakiraman, K., Shenoy, S., & Sandhu, J. S. (2011). Intravascular haemolysis during prolonged running on asphalt and natural grass in long and middle distance runners. *J Sports Sci, 29*(12), 1287–1292.
18. Lippi, G., Schena, F., Salvagno, G. L., et al. (2012). Foot-strike haemolysis after a 60-km ultramarathon. *Blood Transfus, 10*(3), 377–383.
19. Thompson, W. G., Meola, T., Lipkin, M., Jr., et al. (1988). Red cell distribution width, mean corpuscular volume, and transferrin saturation in the diagnosis of iron deficiency. *Arch Intern Med, 148,* 2128–2130.
20. McClure, S., Custer, E., & Bessman, J. D. (1985). Improved detection of early iron deficiency in nonanemic subjects. *JAMA, 253,* 1021–1023.
21. Brugnara, C., Schiller, B., & Moran, J. (2006). Reticulocyte hemoglobin equivalent (Ret He) and assessment of iron deficient states. *Clin Lab Haem, 29,* 303–306.
22. Cox, L. A., & Adrian, G. S. (1993). Postranscriptional regulation of chimeric human transferrin genes by iron. *Biochemistry, 32,* 4738–4745.
23. Urrechaga, E., Borque, L., & Escanero, J.F. (2013). Biomarkers of hypochromia: the contemporary assessment of iron status and erythropoiesis. *BioMed Res Int, 2013,* 603786.
24. Hoffmann, J. J. M. L., Urrechaga, E., & Aguirre, U. (2015). Discriminant indices for distinguishing thalassemia and iron deficiency in patients with microcytic anemia: a meta-analysis. *Clin Chem Lab Med, 53*(12), 1883–1894.
25. Lamola, A. A., Joselow, M., & Yamane, T. (1975). Zinc protoporphyrin (ZPP): a simple, sensitive fluorometric screening test for lead poisoning. *Clin Chem, 21,* 93–97.
26. Huebers, H. A., Beguin, Y., Pootrakul, P., et al. (1990). Intact transferrin receptors in human plasma and their relation to erythropoiesis. *Blood, 75,* 102–107.
27. O'Sullivan, D. J., Higgins, P. G., & Wilkinson, J. F. (1955). Oral iron compounds: a therapeutic comparison. *Lancet, 2,* 482–485.
28. Rezk, M., Dawood, R., Abo-elnasr, M., et al. (2016). Lactoferrin versus ferrous sulphate for the treatment of iron deficiency anemia during pregnancy: a randomized clinical trial. *J Matern Fetal Neonatal Med, 29*(9), 1387–1390.
29. Paesano, R., Berlutti, F., Pietropaoli, M., et al. (2010). Lactoferrin efficacy versus ferrous sulfate in curing iron disorders in pregnant and non-pregnant women. *Int J Immunopathol Pharmacol, 23*(2), 577–587.
30. Swan, H. T., & Jowett, G. H. (1959). Treatment of iron deficiency with ferrous fumarate: assessment by a statistically accurate method. *BMJ, 2,* 782–787.
31. Cartwright, G. E. (1966). The anemia of chronic disorders. *Semin Hematol, 3,* 351–375.
32. Sears, D. A. (1992). Anemia of chronic disease. *Med Clin North Am, 76,* 567–579.
33. Poggiali, E., De Amicis, M. M., & Motta, I. (2014). Anemia of chronic disease: a unique defect of iron recycling for many different chronic diseases. *Euro J Int Med, 25,* 12–17.
34. Nemeth, E., Tuttle, M. S., Powelson, J., et al. (2004). Hepcidin regulates iron efflux by binding to ferroportin and inducing its internalization. *Science, 306,* 2090–2093.
35. Rivera, S., Liu, L., Nemeth, E., et al. (2005). Hepcidin excess induces the sequestration of iron and exacerbates tumor-associated anemia. *Blood, 105,* 1797–1802.
36. Nicolas, G., Bennoun, M., Devaux, I., et al. (2001). Lack of hepcidin gene expression and severe tissue iron overload in upstream stimulatory factor 2 (USF2) knockout mice. *Proc Natl Acad Sci U S A, 98,* 8780–8785.
37. Nicolas, G., Chauvet, C., Viatte, L., et al. (2002). The gene encoding the iron regulatory peptide hepcidin is regulated by anemia, hypoxia, and inflammation. *J Clin Invest, 110,* 1037–1044.
38. Wang, C. Y., & Babitt, J. L. (2016). Regulation in the anemia of inflammation. *Curr Opin Hematol, 23*(3), 189–197.
39. Ganz, T., & Nemeth, E. (2015). Iron homeostasis in host defense and inflammation. *Nat Rev Immunol, 15,* 500–510.
40. Masson, P. L., Heremans, J. F., & Schonne, E. (1969). Lactoferrin: an iron binding protein in neutrophilic leukocytes. *J Exp Med, 130,* 643–658.

41. Cutone, A., Rosa, L., Lepanto M. S., et al. (2017). Lactoferrin efficiently counteracts the inflammation-induced changes of the iron homeostasis system in macrophages. *Front Immunol, 8,* 705.

42. Akilesh, H. M., Buechler, M. B., Duggan, J. M., et al. (2019). Chronic TLR7 and TLR9 signaling drives anemia via differentiation of specialized hemophagocytes. *Science, 363*(6423), DOI:10.1126/science.aao5213.

43. Mast, A. E., Blinder, M. A., Gronowski, A. M., et al. (1998). Clinical utility of the soluble transferrin receptor and comparison with serum ferritin in several populations. *Clin Chem, 44,* 45–51.

44. Castel, R., Tax, M. G., Droogendijk, J., et al. (2012). The transferrin/log(ferritin) ratio: a new tool for the diagnosis of iron deficiency anemia. *Clin Chem Lab Med, 50,* 1343–1349.

45. Thomas, C., & Thomas, L. (2002). Biochemical markers and hematologic indices in the diagnosis of functional iron deficiency. *Clin Chem, 48,* 1066–1076.

46. Leers, M. P. G., Keuren, J. F. W., & Oosterhuis, W. P. (2010). The value of the Thomas-plot in the diagnostic work up of anemic patients referred by general practitioners. *Int J Lab Hemat, 32,* 572–581.

47. Pincus, T., Olsen, N. J., Russell, I. J., et al. (1990). Multicenter study of recombinant human erythropoietin in correction of anemia in rheumatoid arthritis. *Am J Med, 89,* 161–168.

48. Arndt, U., Kaltwasser, J. P., Gottschalk, R., et al. (2005). Correction of iron-deficient erythropoiesis in the treatment of anemia of chronic disease with recombinant human erythropoietin. *Ann Hematol, 84,* 159–166.

49. Horrigan, D. L., & Harris, J. W. (1964). Pyridoxine responsive anemia: analysis of 62 cases. *Adv Intern Med, 12,* 103–174.

50. Verwilghen, R., Reybrouck, G., Callens, L., et al. (1965). Antituberculosis drugs and sideroblastic anemia. *Br J Haematol, 11,* 92–98.

51. Sanburn J. (2016). The toxic tap. *Time, 187*(3), 32–39.

52. Benson, P. (1965). Lead poisoning in children. *Dev Med Child Neurol, 7,* 569–571.

53. Campbell, A. M., & Williams, E. R. (1968). Chronic lead intoxication mimicking motor neurone disease. *BMJ, 4,* 582.

54. Granick, S., Sassa, S., Granick, J. L., et al. (1972). Assays for porphyrins, delta-aminolevulinic acid dehydratase, and porphyrinogen synthetase in microliter samples of blood: application to metabolic defects involving the heme pathway. *Proc Natl Acad Sci U S A, 69,* 2381–2385.

55. Lachant, N. A., Tomoda, A., & Tanaka, K. R. (1984). Inhibition of the pentose phosphate shunt by lead: a potential mechanism for hemolysis in lead poisoning. *Blood, 63,* 518–524.

56. Lowry, J.A. Childhood lead poisoning: Management. *UpToDate.* https://www.uptodate.com/contents/childhood-lead-poisoning-management. Accessed November 19, 2017.

57. Valentine, W. N., Paglia, D. E., Fink, K., et al. (1976). Lead poisoning. Association with hemolytic anemia, basophilic stippling, erythrocyte pyrimidine 5'-nucleotidase deficiency, and intraerythrocytic accumulation of pyrimidines. *J Clin Invest, 58,* 926–932.

58. Feder, J. N., Gnirke, A., Thomas, W., et al. (1996). A novel MHC class I-like gene is mutated in patients with hereditary hemochromatosis. *Nat Genet, 13,* 399–408.

59. Waheed, A., Parkkila, S., Zhou, X. Y., et al. (1997). Hereditary hemochromatosis: effect of C282Y and H63D mutations on association with β$_2$-microglobulin, intracellular processing, and cell surface expression of the HFE protein in COS-7 cells. *Proc Natl Acad Sci U S A, 94,* 12384–12389.

60. Brissot, P., Bardou-Jacquet, E., Troadec, M. B., et al. (2010). Molecular diagnosis of genetic iron-overload disorders. *Expert Rev Mol Diagn, 10,* 755–763.

61. Beutler, E. (2003). The *HFE* Cys282Tyr mutation as a necessary but not sufficient cause of clinical hereditary hemochromatosis. *Blood, 101,* 3347–3350.

62. Lebron, J. A., & Bjorkman, P. J. (1999). The transferrin receptor binding site on HFE, the class I MHC-related protein mutated in hereditary hemochromatosis. *J Mol Biol, 289,* 1109–1118.

63. McCord, J. M. (1998). Iron, free radicals, and oxidative injury. *Semin Hematol, 35,* 5–12.

64. Vautier, G., Bomford, A. B., Portmann, B. C., et al. (1999). p53 mutations in British patients with hepatocellular carcinoma: clustering in genetic hemochromatosis. *Gastroenterology, 117,* 154–160.

65. Hussain, S. P., Schwank, J., Staib, F., et al. (2007). TP53 mutations and hepatocellular carcinoma: insights into the etiology and pathogenesis of liver cancer. *Oncogene, 26*(15), 166–176.

66. Hussain, S. P., Raja, K., Amstad, P. A., et al. (2000). Increased p53 mutation load in nontumorous human liver of Wilson disease and hemochromatosis: oxyradical overload diseases. *Proc Natl Acad Sci U S A, 97,* 12770–12775.

67. Niederau, C., Strohmeyer, G., & Stremmel, W. (1996). Long term survival in patients with hereditary hemochromatosis. *Gastroenterology, 110,* 1107–1119.

68. Bothwell, T. H., & MacPhail, A. P. (1998). Hereditary hemochromatosis: etiologic, pathologic, and clinical aspects. *Semin Hematol, 35,* 55–71.

69. Nadakkavukaran, I. M., Gan, E. K., & Olynyk, J. K. (2012). Screening for hereditary haemochromatosis. *Pathology, 44,* 148–152.

70. Phatak, P. D., Guzman, G., Woll, J. E., et al. (1994). Cost effectiveness of screening for hemochromatosis. *Arch Intern Med, 154,* 769–776.

71. Rogowski, W. H. (2009). The cost-effectiveness of screening for hereditary hemochromatosis in Germany: a remodeling study. *Med Decis Making, 29,* 224–238.

72. Edwards, C. Q., & Barton, J. C. (2014). Hemochromatosis. In Greer, J. P., Arber, D. A., Glader, D., et al. (Eds.), *Wintrobe's Clinical Hematology.* (13th ed., pp. 662–681). Philadelphia: Lippincott Williams & Wilkins.

73. Borgna-Pignatti, C., & Galanello, R. (2014). Thalassemias and related disorders: quantitative disorders of hemoglobin synthesis. In Greer, J. P., Arber, D. A., Glader, D., et al. (Eds.), *Wintrobe's Clinical Hematology.* (13th ed., pp. 862–913). Philadelphia: Lippincott Williams & Wilkins.

74. Cappellini, M. D., & Pattoneri, P. (2009). Oral iron chelators. *Annu Rev Med, 60,* 25–38.

75. Imran, F., & Phatak, P. (2009). Pharmacoeconomic benefits of deferasirox in the management of iron overload syndromes. *Expert Rev Pharmacoecon Outcomes Res, 9,* 297–304.

76. Elalfy, M. S., Adly, A. M., Wali, Y., et al. (2015). Efficacy and safety of a novel combination of two oral chelators deferasirox/deferiprone over deferoxamine/deferiprone in severely iron overloaded young beta thalassemia major patients. *Eur J Haematol, 95*(5), 411–420.

Anemias Caused by Defects of DNA Metabolism

Linda H. Goossen

OBJECTIVES

After completion of this chapter, the reader will be able to:

1. Discuss the relationships among macrocytic anemia, megaloblastic anemia, and pernicious anemia, and classify anemias appropriately within these categories.
2. Discuss the physiologic roles of folate and vitamin B_{12} in DNA production and the general metabolic pathways in which they act.
3. Describe the absorption and distribution of vitamin B_{12}, including carrier proteins and the biologic activity of various vitamin-carrier complexes.
4. Describe the biochemical basis for development of anemia with deficiencies of vitamin B_{12} and folate, and explain the cause of the accompanying megaloblastosis.
5. Recognize individuals at risk for megaloblastic anemia by virtue of age, dietary habits, or physiologic circumstance such as pregnancy, drug regimens, or pathologic conditions.
6. Recognize complete blood count, reticulocyte count, red and white blood cell morphologies and bone marrow findings consistent with megaloblastic anemia.
7. Given the results of tests measuring levels of serum vitamin B_{12}, serum methylmalonic acid, serum folate, plasma or serum homocysteine, and antibodies to intrinsic factor, determine the likely cause of a patient's deficiency.
8. Recognize results of bilirubin and lactate dehydrogenase tests that are consistent with megaloblastic anemia and explain why the test values are elevated in this condition.

OUTLINE

Etiology
  Physiologic Roles of Vitamin B_{12} and Folate
  Defect in Megaloblastic Anemia
    Caused By Deficiency in Folate and
    Vitamin B_{12}
  Other Causes of Megaloblastosis
Systemic Manifestations of Folate and Vitamin B_{12}
  Deficiency

Causes of Vitamin Deficiencies
  Folate Deficiency
  Vitamin B_{12} Deficiency
Laboratory Diagnosis
  Screening Tests
  Specific Diagnostic Tests
Macrocytic Nonmegaloblastic Anemias
Treatment

CASE STUDY

After studying the material in this chapter, the reader should be able to respond to the following case study:

During a holiday visit, the children of a 76-year-old man noticed that he seemed more forgetful than usual and that he had difficulty walking. Concerned about the possibility of a mild stroke, the children insisted that he see his physician. The physician diagnosed peripheral neuropathy affecting the father's ability to walk. In addition, the physician noted that he was pale and slightly jaundiced and ordered a complete blood count (CBC). The results were as follows:

	Patient Results	Reference Intervals
WBCs ($\times 10^9$/L)	3.2	4.5–11.0
RBCs ($\times 10^{12}$/L)	2.22	4.60–6.00

	Patient Results	Reference Intervals
HGB (g/dL)	8.5	14.0–18.0
HCT (%)	27.0	40–54
MCV (fL)	121.6	80–100
MCH (pg)	38.3	26–32
MCHC (g/dL)	31.5	32–36
RDW (%)	18.0	11.5–14.5
Platelets ($\times 10^9$/L)	115	150–450
Reticulocytes (%)	1.8	0.5–2.5

WBC differential: unremarkable with the exception of hypersegmentation of neutrophils

Continued

Impaired deoxyribonucleic acid (DNA) metabolism causes systemic effects by impairing production of all rapidly dividing cells of the body. These are chiefly the cells of the skin, the epithelium of the gastrointestinal tract, and the hematopoietic tissues. Because these all must be replenished throughout life, any impairment of cell production is evident in these tissues first. Patients may experience symptoms in any of these systems, but the blood provides a ready tissue for analysis. The hematologic effects, especially megaloblastic anemia, have come to be recognized as the hallmark of the diseases affecting DNA metabolism.

ETIOLOGY

The root cause of megaloblastic anemia is impaired DNA synthesis. The anemia is named for the very large cells of the bone marrow that develop a distinctive morphology (discussed in Laboratory Diagnosis) because of a reduction in the number of cell divisions. Megaloblastic anemia is one example of a macrocytic anemia. Box 18.1 shows the classification of macrocytic anemias. Understanding the cause of megaloblastic anemia requires a review of DNA synthesis with particular attention to the roles of vitamin B_{12} (cobalamin) and folic acid (folate).

Physiologic Roles of Vitamin B_{12} and Folate

Vitamin B_{12} (cobalamin) is an essential nutrient consisting of a tetrapyrrole (corrin) ring containing cobalt that is attached to 5,6-dimethylbenzimidazolyl ribonucleotide. It has various analogs, including hydroxycobalamin and cyanocobalamin (forms often found in food and supplements) and coenzyme forms, methylcobalamin and 5′-deoxyadenosylcobalamin (Figure 18.1). Vitamin B_{12} is a coenzyme in two biochemical reactions in humans. One is isomerization of methylmalonyl coenzyme A (CoA) to succinyl CoA, which requires vitamin B_{12} (in the deoxyadenosylcobalamin form) as a cofactor and is catalyzed by the enzyme methylmalonyl CoA mutase (Figure 18.2). In the absence of vitamin B_{12}, the impaired activity of methylmalonyl CoA mutase leads to a high level of serum methylmalonic acid (MMA), which is useful for the diagnosis of vitamin B_{12} deficiency (discussed in Laboratory Diagnosis). The second reaction is the transfer of a methyl group from 5-methyltetrahydrofolate (5-methyl THF) to homocysteine, which thereby generates methionine. This reaction is catalyzed by the enzyme methionine synthase and uses vitamin B_{12} (in the methylcobalamin form) as a coenzyme (discussed later in this section). Methylcobalamin is synthesized through reduction and methylation of vitamin B_{12}.

BOX 18.1 Classification of Macrocytic Anemias by Cause

Megaloblastic Anemia
Folate deficiency
  Inadequate intake
  Increased need
  Impaired absorption (e.g., inflammatory bowel disease)
  Impaired use due to drugs
  Excessive loss with renal dialysis
Vitamin B_{12} deficiency
  Inadequate intake
  Increased need
  Impaired absorption
    Failure to split from food
    Failure to split from haptocorrin
    Lack of intrinsic factor
      Pernicious anemia
      Helicobacter pylori infection
      Gastrectomy
      Hereditary intrinsic factor deficiency
  General malabsorption (e.g., inflammatory bowel disease)
  Inherited errors in absorption or transport
    Imerslund-Gräsbeck syndrome
    Transcobalamin deficiency
  Competition for the vitamin
    Diphyllobothrium latum (fish tapeworm) infection
    Blind loop syndrome
Other causes of megaloblastosis
  Myelodysplastic syndrome
  Acute erythroid leukemia
  Congenital dyserythropoietic anemia
  Reverse transcriptase inhibitors

Macrocytic, Nonmegaloblastic Anemias
Normal newborn status
Reticulocytosis
Liver disease
Chronic alcoholism
Bone marrow failure

This reaction represents the link between folate and vitamin B_{12} coenzymes and appears to account for the requirement for both vitamins in normal erythropoiesis.[1,2]

Folate is the general term used for any form of the vitamin folic acid. Folic acid is the synthetic form in supplements and fortified food. Folates consist of a pteridine ring attached to para-aminobenzoate with one or more glutamate residues (Figure 18.3).

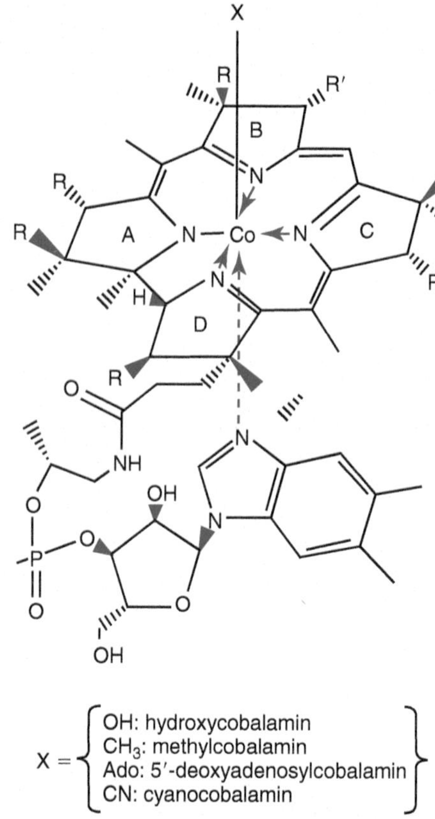

Figure 18.1 Structure of Vitamin B$_{12}$ (Cobalamin) and its Analogs.
The basic structure of cobalamin includes a tetrapyrrole (corrin) ring with
a central cobalt atom linked to 5,6-dimethylbenzimidazolyl ribonucleotide.
Hydroxycobalamin and cyanocobalamin are forms often found in food and
supplements and methylcobalamin and 5'-deoxyadenosylcobalamin are
coenzyme forms. (From Scott, J. M., & Browne, P. [2006]. Megaloblastic
anemia. In Caballero, B., Allen, L., & Prentice, A. [Eds.], *Encyclopedia of
human nutrition.* [2nd ed., p. 113]. Oxford: Academic Press.)

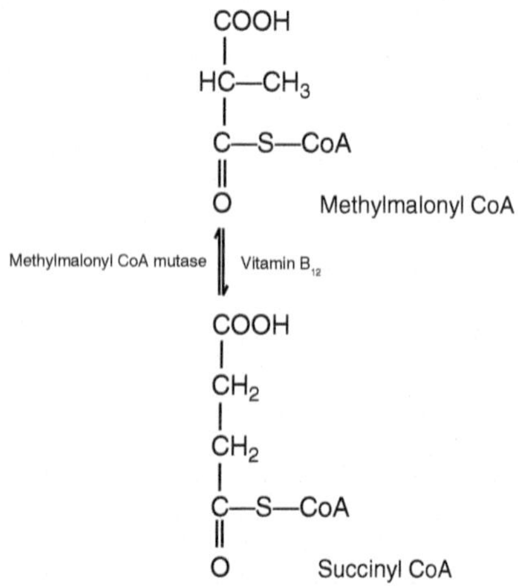

**Figure 18.2 Role of Vitamin B$_{12}$ in the Metabolism of Methylmalo-
nyl Coenzyme A (CoA).** Vitamin B$_{12}$, in the 5'-deoxyadenosylcobalamin
form, is a coenzyme in the isomerization of methylmalonyl CoA to succinyl CoA. The reaction is catalyzed by the enzyme methylmalonyl CoA
mutase.

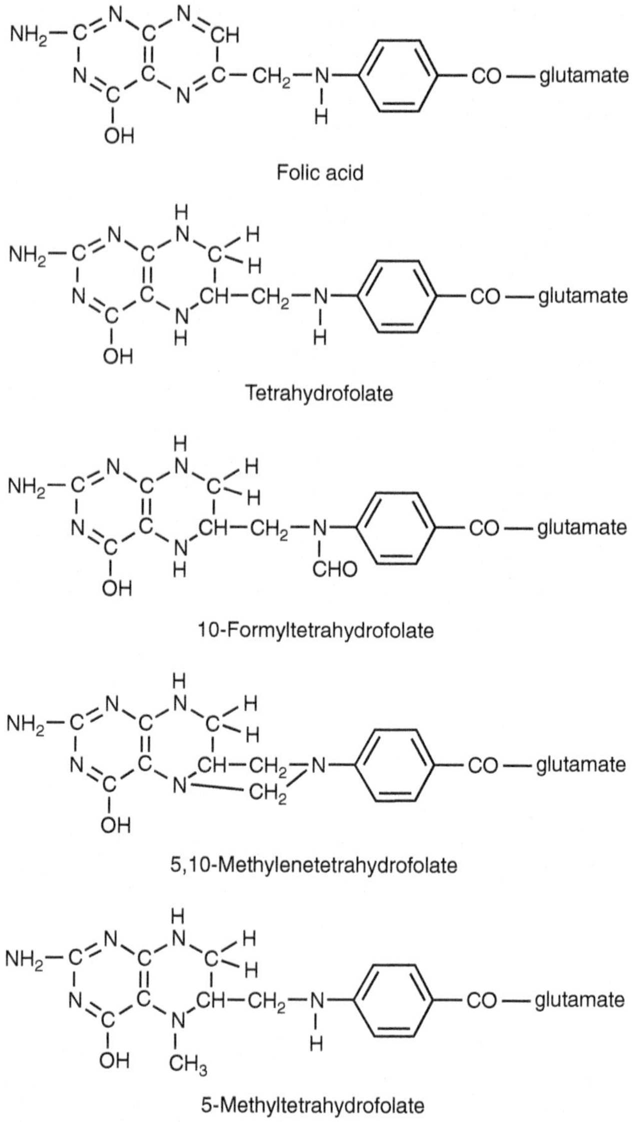

**Figure 18.3 Structure of Synthetic Folic Acid and the Naturally
Occurring Forms of the Vitamin.** (From Scott, J. M., & Browne, P. [2006].
Megaloblastic anemia. In Caballero, B., Allen, L., & Prentice, A. [Eds.],
Encyclopedia of human nutrition. [2nd ed., p. 114]. Oxford: Academic
Press.)

The function of folate is to transfer carbon units in the form of
methyl groups from donors to receptors. In this capacity folate
plays an important role in the metabolism of amino acids and
nucleotides. Deficiency of the vitamin leads to impaired cell replication and other metabolic alterations. Folate circulates in the
blood predominantly as 5-methyl THF.[3] 5-Methyl THF is metabolically inactive until it is demethylated to tetrahydrofolate
(THF), whereupon folate-dependent reactions may take place.

Folate has an important role in DNA synthesis. As seen in
Figure 18.4, within the cytoplasm of the cell, a methyl group is
transferred from 5-methyl THF to homocysteine, which converts
it to methionine and generates THF. This reaction is catalyzed
by the enzyme methionine synthase and requires vitamin B$_{12}$ in
the form of methylcobalamin as a cofactor. THF is then converted to 5,10-methylenetetrahydrofolate (5,10-methylene THF);
the methyl group for this reaction comes from serine as it is

converted to glycine. The methyl group of 5,10-methylene THF is then transferred to deoxyuridine monophosphate (dUMP), which converts it to deoxythymidine monophosphate (dTMP). This reaction is catalyzed by thymidylate synthase and results in the conversion of 5,10-methylene THF to dihydrofolate (DHF). Deoxythymidine monophosphate is a precursor to deoxythymidine triphosphate (dTTP), which, like the other nucleotide triphosphates, is a building block of the DNA molecule. THF is regenerated by the conversion of DHF to THF by the enzyme dihydrofolate reductase. Because some of the folate is catabolized during the cycle, the regeneration of THF also requires additional 5-methyl THF from the plasma. Once in the cell, folate is rapidly polyglutamated by the addition of one to six glutamic acid residues. This conjugation is required for retention of THF in the cell, and it also promotes attachment of folate to enzymes.[4]

Defect in Megaloblastic Anemia Caused By Deficiency in Folate and Vitamin B$_{12}$

When either folate or vitamin B$_{12}$ is deficient, thymidine nucleotide production for DNA synthesis is impaired. Folate deficiency has the more direct effect, ultimately preventing the methylation of dUMP. The effect of vitamin B$_{12}$ deficiency is more indirect, preventing the production of THF from 5-methyl THF. When vitamin B$_{12}$ is deficient, progressively more and more of the folate becomes metabolically trapped as 5-methyl

THF. This constitutes what has been called the *folate trap* as 5-methyl THF accumulates and is unable to supply the folate cycle with THF. Some 5-methyl THF also leaks out of the cell if it is not readily polyglutamated. This results in a decrease in intracellular folate.[5] In addition, when either folate or vitamin B$_{12}$ is deficient, homocysteine accumulates because methionine synthase is unable to convert it to methionine without vitamin B$_{12}$ as a cofactor (Figure 18.4).

In this state of diminished thymidine availability, uridine is incorporated into DNA.[6] The DNA repair process can remove the uridine, but without available thymidine to replace it, the repair process is unsuccessful. Although the DNA can unwind and replication can begin, at any point where a thymidine nucleotide is needed, there is essentially an empty space in the replicated DNA sequence, which results in many single-strand breaks. When excisions at opposing DNA strand sites coincide, double-strand breaks occur. Repeated DNA strand breaks lead to fragmentation of the DNA strand.[4] The resulting DNA is nonfunctional, and the DNA replication process is incomplete. Cell division is halted, resulting in either cell lysis or apoptosis[7] of many erythroid progenitors and precursors within the bone marrow. Cells that survive continue the abnormal maturation with a fewer number of red blood cells (RBCs) released into the circulation. This abnormal blood cell development is called *ineffective hematopoiesis*. The dependency of DNA production on folate has been used in cancer chemotherapy (Box 18.2).

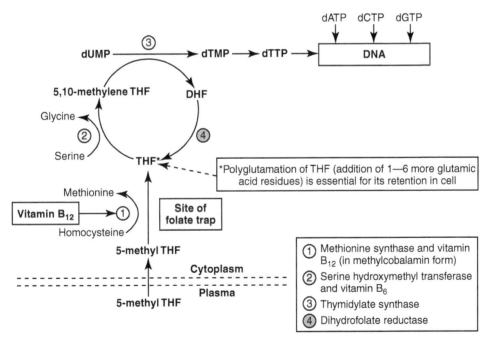

Figure 18.4 Role of Folate and Vitamin B$_{12}$ in DNA Synthesis. Folate enters the cell as 5-methyltetrahydrofolate (5-methyl THF). In the cell, a methyl group is transferred from 5-methyl THF to homocysteine, converting it to methionine and generating tetrahydrofolate (THF). This reaction is catalyzed by methionine synthase and requires vitamin B$_{12}$ as a cofactor. THF is then converted to 5,10-methylene THF by the donation of a methyl group from serine. The methyl group of 5,10-methylene THF is then transferred to deoxyuridine monophosphate (dUMP), which converts it to deoxythymidine monophosphate (dTMP) and converts 5,10-methylene THF to dihydrofolate (DHF). This reaction is catalyzed by thymidylate synthase. dTMP is a precursor of deoxythymidine triphosphate (dTTP), which is used to synthesize DNA. THF is regenerated by the conversion of DHF to THF by the enzyme dihydrofolate reductase. A deficiency of vitamin B$_{12}$ prevents the conversion of THF from 5-methyl THF; as a result, folate becomes metabolically trapped as 5-methyl THF. This constitutes the "folate trap."

BOX 18.2   Disruption of the Folate Cycle in Cancer Chemotherapy

Folate has a complex relationship with cancer. Folate deficiency leads to DNA strand breaks, which leave the DNA vulnerable to mutation. In this way, folate deficiency is a risk factor for the initiation of cancer. The central role of folate in cell division also makes it a target for chemotherapeutic drugs used to treat cancer. Folate analogs can be used to compete for folate in DNA production and result in impaired cell division. Cells in the cell cycle, such as cancer cells and other normally rapidly dividing cells such as epithelium and blood cell precursors, are most susceptible to the drug interference. Methotrexate, used in treatment of leukemia and arthritis, is an example of a folate antimetabolite drug. Methotrexate has a higher affinity for dihydrofolate reductase than does tetrahydrofolate. Thus methotrexate enters the folate cycle in preference to tetrahydrofolate, and the folate cycle is blocked by the drug. Methotrexate treatment typically is followed by what is known as *leucovorin rescue*. Leucovorin is a folic acid derivative that can be administered to counteract the effects of methotrexate or other folate antagonists.

In addition to the increased apoptosis of erythroid progenitor and precursor cells in the bone marrow discussed earlier, the remaining erythroid precursors are larger than normally seen during the final stages of erythropoiesis, and their nuclei are immature-appearing compared with the cytoplasm. In contrast to the normally dense chromatin of comparable normoblasts, the nuclei of megaloblastic erythroid precursors have an open, finely stippled, reticular pattern.[5] The nuclear changes seen in the megaloblastic erythroid precursors are related to cell cycle delay, prolonged resting phase, and arrest in nuclear maturation. Electron microscopy reveals that reduced synthesis of histones is also responsible for morphologic changes in the chromatin of megaloblastic erythroid precursors.[8] Ribonucleic acid (RNA) function is not affected by vitamin B_{12} or folate deficiency because RNA contains uracil instead of thymidine nucleotides, so cytoplasmic development progresses normally. The slower maturation rate of the nucleus compared with the cytoplasm is called *nuclear-cytoplasmic asynchrony*. Together the accumulation of cells with nuclei at earlier stages of development and cells with increased diameter and immaturity result in the appearance of erythroid precursors in the bone marrow that are pathognomonic of megaloblastic anemia.[7] Because ineffective hematopoiesis affects all three blood cell lineages, pancytopenia is also evident, with certain distinctive cellular changes (discussed in Laboratory Diagnosis).

Other Causes of Megaloblastosis

Vitamin B_{12} and folate deficiency are not the only causes of megaloblastic erythroid precursors. Dysplastic erythroid precursors in myelodysplastic syndrome (MDS) can also have megaloblastoid features (Chapter 33). In MDS, however, the macrocytic erythrocytes and their precursors characteristically show delayed cytoplasmic and nuclear maturation, including cytoplasmic vacuole formation, nuclear budding, multinucleation, and nuclear fragmentation, and thus may be distinguished from the megaloblastic erythroid precursors seen in the vitamin deficiencies. In addition, nuclear-cytoplasmic asynchrony and megaloblastic erythroid precursors may be seen in congenital dyserythropoietic anemia (CDA) types I and III

(Chapter 19). The CDAs are rare conditions that usually manifest in childhood and may be distinguished from the acquired causes of megaloblastosis by clinical history and morphologic differences. In CDA I, internuclear chromatin bridging of erythroid precursors or binucleated forms are observed, and in CDA III, giant multinucleated erythroblasts are present. Another rare condition in which erythroid precursors have a megaloblastic appearance is acute erythroid leukemia, previously classified as FAB M6 (Chapter 31). In this condition the erythroblasts are macrocytic, and the immature appearance of the nuclear chromatin is similar to the more open appearance of the chromatin in megaloblasts. There are usually other aberrant findings in erythroid leukemia, including an increase of myeloblasts in the bone marrow; however, an experienced morphologist can discern the subtle differences. Reverse transcriptase inhibitors, used to treat human immunodeficiency virus (HIV) infections, interfere with DNA production and may also lead to megaloblastic changes.[9]

Although the conditions described in this section are characterized by megaloblastic morphology, they are due to acquired or inherited mutations in progenitor cells or interference with DNA synthesis and are refractive to therapy with vitamin B_{12} or folic acid.

SYSTEMIC MANIFESTATIONS OF FOLATE AND VITAMIN B_{12} DEFICIENCY

When DNA synthesis and subsequent cell division are impaired by lack of folate or vitamin B_{12}, megaloblastic anemia and its systemic manifestations develop. With either vitamin deficiency, patients may experience general symptoms related to anemia (fatigue, weakness, and shortness of breath) and symptoms related to the alimentary tract. Loss of epithelium on the tongue results in a smooth surface and soreness (glossitis). Loss of epithelium along the gastrointestinal tract can result in gastritis, nausea, or constipation.

Although the blood pictures seen with the two vitamin deficiencies are indistinguishable, the clinical presentations vary. After dietary deficiency or malabsorption begins, it takes a few years to develop a vitamin B_{12} deficiency but only a few months to develop a folate deficiency, reflecting the storage capacity of each vitamin in the body. In vitamin B_{12} deficiency, neurologic symptoms may be pronounced and may even occur in the absence of anemia.[5] These include memory loss, numbness and tingling in toes and fingers, loss of balance, and further impairment of walking by loss of vibratory sense, especially in the lower limbs.[10] Neuropsychiatric symptoms may also be present, including personality changes and psychosis. These symptoms seem to be the result of demyelination of the spinal cord and peripheral nerves, but the relationship of this demyelination to vitamin B_{12} deficiency is unclear. The roles of increases in tumor necrosis factor-α, a neurotoxic agent, and decreases in epidermal growth factor, a neurotrophic agent, in the development of neurologic symptoms in vitamin B_{12}-deficient patients are being researched.[11,12]

At one time, folate deficiency was believed to be more benign clinically than vitamin B_{12} deficiency. Later research suggested that low levels of folate and the resulting high homocysteine levels were risk factors for cardiovascular disease.[13] More recent research has provided mixed results, with studies both refuting this association[14,15] and substantiating the association between high circulating homocysteine levels and the risk of cardiovascular disease.[16,17] Several studies suggest that high folate levels provide a cardioprotective effect in diabetic patients and certain ethnic populations.[14,18,19] The evidence at this time is unclear as to whether persistent suboptimal folate status may have a significant long-term health impact. In addition, there is evidence of depression, peripheral neuropathy, and psychosis related to folate deficiency.[20,21] Folate levels appear to influence the effectiveness of treatments for depression.[22] Folate deficiency during pregnancy can result in impaired formation of the fetal nervous system, resulting in neural tube defects such as spina bifida,[23] despite the fact that the fetus accumulates folate at the expense of the mother. Pregnancy requires a considerable increase in folate to fulfill the requirements related to rapid fetal growth, uterine expansion, placental maturation, and expanded blood volume.[3] Ensuring adequate folate levels in women of childbearing age is particularly important because many women are likely to be unaware of their pregnancy during the first crucial weeks of fetal development. Fortification of the US food supply with folic acid in grain and cereal products was mandated by the Food and Drug Administration in 1998 to lower the risk of neural tube defects in the unborn.

CAUSES OF VITAMIN DEFICIENCIES

In general, vitamin deficiencies may arise because the vitamin is in relatively short supply, because use of the vitamin is impaired, or because of excessive loss. Folate deficiency can be caused by all of these mechanisms.

Folate Deficiency
Inadequate Intake
Folate is synthesized by microorganisms and higher plants. Folate is ubiquitous in foods, but a generally poor diet can result in deficiency. Good sources of folate include leafy green vegetables, dried beans, liver, beef, fortified breakfast cereals, and some fruits, especially oranges.[3,24] Folates are heat labile, and overcooking of foods can diminish their nutritional value.[3]

Increased Need
Increased need for folate occurs during pregnancy and lactation when the mother must supply her own needs plus those of the fetus or infant. Infants and children also have increased need for folate during growth.[3]

Impaired Absorption
Food folates must be hydrolyzed in the gut before absorption in the small intestine; however, only 50% of what is ingested is available for absorption.[3] A rare autosomal recessive deficiency of a folate transporter protein (PCFT) severely decreases intestinal absorption of folate.[5,25] Once across the intestinal cell, most folate is transported in the plasma as 5-methyl THF unbound to any specific carrier.[10] Its entry into cells, however, is by both carrier systems and receptors.[26]

Folate absorption may also be impaired by intestinal disease, especially sprue and celiac disease. Sprue is characterized by weakness, weight loss, and steatorrhea (fat in the feces), which is evidence that the intestine is not absorbing food properly. It is seen in the tropics (tropical sprue), where its cause is generally considered to be overgrowth of enteric pathogens.[27] Celiac disease (nontropical sprue) has been traced to intolerance of gluten in some grains[27] (gluten-induced enteropathy) and can be controlled by eliminating wheat, barley, and rye products from the diet. Surgical resection of the small intestine and inflammatory bowel disease can also decrease folate absorption.

Impaired Use of Folate
Numerous drugs decrease absorption of folic acid or impair folate metabolism (Box 18.3).[28] Antineoplasic, antibacterial, and antiseizure agents are particularly known for this,[28] and the result is macrocytosis with frank megaloblastic anemia. Because folate deficiency results in inhibition of cell replication, several anticancer drugs, including methotrexate, are folate inhibitors.[3] In most instances, supplementation with folic acid or reduced folic acid (in the form of folinic acid) is sufficient to override the impairment and allow the patient to continue therapy.[28]

Excessive Loss of Folate
Physiologic loss of folate occurs through the kidney. The amount is small and not a cause of deficiency. Patients undergoing renal dialysis lose folate in the dialysate, however; thus supplemental folic acid is routinely provided to these individuals to prevent megaloblastic anemia.[10]

Vitamin B12 Deficiency
Inadequate Intake
Although true dietary deficiency of vitamin B_{12} is rare, this condition is possible for strict vegetarians (vegans) who do not eat meat, eggs, or dairy products. Although it is an essential vitamin for animals, plants cannot synthesize vitamin B_{12} and thus it is not available from vegetable sources. The best dietary sources are animal products such as liver, dairy products, fish,

---

BOX 18.3   Some Drugs That May Lead to Impaired Use of Folate

Impair Folate Metabolism
- Methotrexate: antiarthritic, chemotherapeutic
- 5-Fluorouracil: chemotherapeutic
- Hydroxyurea: antimetabolite
- Pyrimethamine: antimalarial
- Pentamidine: antimicrobial
- Trimethoprim: antimicrobial

Impair Folate Absorption
- Metformin: oral antidiabetic
- Cholestyramine: cholesterol lowering
- Birth-control pills: hormones
- Penicillins: antibiotics
- Phenytoin: anticonvulsant

shellfish, and eggs.[29] In contrast to the heat-labile folate, vitamin B_{12} is not destroyed by cooking.

Increased Need

Increased need for vitamin B_{12} occurs during pregnancy, lactation, and growth. Because of the vigorous cell replication, what would otherwise be a diet adequate in vitamin B_{12} can become inadequate during these periods.

Impaired Absorption

Vitamin B_{12} in food is released from food proteins primarily in the acid environment of the stomach, aided by pepsin, and is subsequently bound by a specific salivary protein, haptocorrin, also known as *R protein* or *transcobalamin I* (Figure 18.5). In the small intestine, vitamin B_{12} is released from haptocorrin by the action of pancreatic proteases, including trypsin. It is then bound by intrinsic factor, which is produced by gastric parietal

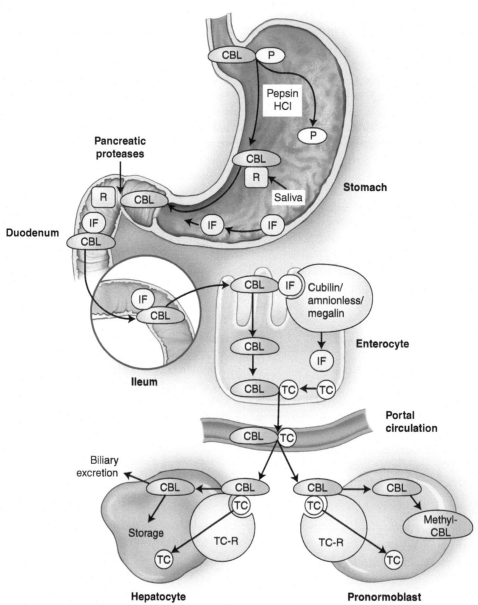

Figure 18.5 Normal Absorption of Vitamin B_{12}. Dietary vitamin B_{12} (cobalamin, CBL) is food protein (P) bound. In the stomach, pepsin and hydrochloric acid (HCl) secreted by parietal cells release CBL from P. CBL then binds haptocorrin (R protein, R), released from salivary glands, and remains bound until intestinal pancreatic proteases, including trypsin, catalyze its release. Parietal cells secrete intrinsic factor (IF), which binds CBL in the duodenum. Cubilin-amnionless (cubam) and megalin receptors in ileal enterocytes bind CBL-IF, and once inside the enterocyte, release CBL from IF. Enterocytes produce transcobalamin (TC), which binds CBL and transports it through the portal circulation. Bone marrow pronormoblast membrane TC receptors (TC-R) bind CBL-TC, and release CBL from TF inside the cell, where it is converted to methylcobalamin (methyl-CBL). Methyl-CBL is a coenzyme that supports homocysteine-methionine conversion. Hepatocyte TC-R receptors bind CBL-TC and release the CBL, which is moved to storage organelles or excreted through the biliary system.

cells. Vitamin B_{12} binding to intrinsic factor is required for absorption by ileal enterocytes that possess receptors for the complex. These receptors are cubilin-amnionless complex, collectively known as *cubam,* which binds the vitamin B_{12}-intrinsic factor complex, and megalin, a membrane transport protein.[5,26,29-32] Once in the enterocyte, the vitamin B_{12} is then freed from intrinsic factor and bound to transcobalamin (previously called *transcobalamin II*) and released into the circulation. In the plasma, only 10% to 30% of the vitamin B_{12} is bound to transcobalamin; the remaining 75% is bound to transcobalamin I and III, referred to as the *haptocorrins.*[29,33] The vitamin B_{12}-transcobalamin complex, termed *holotranscobalamin* (holoTC), is the metabolically active form of vitamin B_{12}. Holotranscobalamin binds to specific receptors on the surfaces of many different cells and enters the cells by endocytosis,[26] with subsequent release of vitamin B_{12} from the carrier.[34] The body maintains a substantial reserve of absorbed vitamin B_{12} in hepatocytes[4] and kidney cells.[26]

The absorption of vitamin B_{12} can be impaired by (1) failure to separate vitamin B_{12} from food proteins in the stomach, (2) failure to separate vitamin B_{12} from haptocorrin in the intestine, (3) lack of intrinsic factor, (4) malabsorption, and (5) competition for available vitamin B_{12}.

Failure to separate vitamin B_{12} from food proteins. A condition known as *food-cobalamin malabsorption* is characterized by hypochlorhydria and the resulting inability of the body to release vitamin B_{12} from food or intestinal transport proteins for subsequent binding to intrinsic factor. Food-cobalamin malabsorption is caused primarily by the reduced gastric acidity in atrophic gastritis or atrophy of the stomach lining that often occurs with increasing age.[35] It also occurs with gastric bypass surgery and the long-term use of histamine type 2 receptor blockers and proton pump inhibitors, which reduce gastric acidity for the treatment of ulcers and gastroesophageal reflux disease.[35]

Failure to separate vitamin B_{12} from haptocorrin. Lack of gastric acidity or lack of trypsin as a result of chronic pancreatic disease can prevent vitamin B_{12} absorption because the vitamin remains bound to haptocorrin in the intestine and unavailable to intrinsic factor.[10]

Lack of intrinsic factor. Lack of intrinsic factor constitutes a significant cause of impaired vitamin B_{12} absorption. It is most commonly a result of autoimmune disease, as in pernicious anemia, but can also result from hereditary intrinsic factor deficiency or loss of parietal cells in *Helicobacter pylori* infection or after total or partial gastrectomy.

Pernicious anemia. Pernicious anemia is an autoimmune disorder characterized by impaired absorption of vitamin B_{12} because of an intrinsic factor deficiency.[34] This condition is called *pernicious anemia* because the disease was fatal before its cause was discovered. The incidence per year is roughly 25 new cases per 100,000 persons older than 40 years of age.[5] Pernicious anemia most often manifests in the sixth decade or later but can also be found in children. Patients with pernicious anemia have an increased risk of developing gastric tumors.[4]

In pernicious anemia, autoimmune lymphocyte-mediated destruction of gastric parietal cells severely reduces the amount of intrinsic factor secreted in the stomach. Pathologic CD4 T cells inappropriately recognize and initiate an autoimmune response against the H^+/K^+-adenosine triphosphatase embedded in the membrane of parietal cells.[36] A chronic inflammatory infiltration follows, which extends into the wall of the stomach.[37] Over a period of years and even decades, there is progressive development of atrophic gastritis, resulting in the loss of the parietal cells with their secretory products, H^+ and intrinsic factor. The loss of H^+ production in the stomach constitutes achlorhydria. Low gastric acidity was previously an important diagnostic criterion for pernicious anemia. Serum gastrin levels can be markedly elevated as a result of the gastric achlorhydria.[4] The absence of intrinsic factor can also be detected using the Schilling test. However, because the test requires a 24-hour urine collection and the use of radioactive cobalt in vitamin B_{12} to trace absorption, safer diagnostic tests are currently used (discussed in Laboratory Diagnosis).

Another feature of the autoimmune response in pernicious anemia is the production of antibodies to intrinsic factor and gastric parietal cells that are detectable in serum.[38,39] The most common antibody to intrinsic factor blocks the site on intrinsic factor where vitamin B_{12} binds, which inhibits the formation of the intrinsic factor-vitamin B_{12} complex and prevents the absorption of the vitamin.[37] These blocking antibodies are present in serum or gastric fluid in 70% to 90% of patients with pernicious anemia and their presence is highly specific for the disease.[5] Parietal cell antibodies are detectable in the serum of 50% to 90% of patients with pernicious anemia.[5,37,39]

Other causes of lack of intrinsic factor. A lack of intrinsic factor may also be related to *H. pylori* infection. Left untreated, colonization of the gastric mucosa with *H. pylori* progresses until the parietal cells are entirely destroyed, a process involving both local and systemic immune mechanisms.[40,41] In addition, partial or total gastrectomy, which results in removal of intrinsic factor-producing parietal cells, invariably leads to vitamin B_{12} deficiency.

Impaired absorption of vitamin B_{12} can also be caused by hereditary intrinsic factor deficiency. This is a rare autosomal recessive disorder characterized by the absence or impaired function of intrinsic factor. In contrast to the acquired forms of pernicious anemia, histology and gastric acidity are normal.[31]

Malabsorption. General malabsorption of vitamin B_{12} can be caused by the same conditions interfering with folate absorption, such as celiac disease, tropical sprue, and inflammatory bowel disease.

Inherited errors of vitamin B_{12} absorption and transport. Imerslund-Gräsbeck syndrome is a rare autosomal recessive condition caused by mutations in the genes for either cubilin or amnionless. This defect results in decreased endocytosis of the intrinsic factor-vitamin B_{12} complex by ileal enterocytes. Transcobalamin deficiency is another rare autosomal recessive condition resulting in a deficiency of physiologically available vitamin B_{12}.[26,31,42]

Competition for vitamin B_{12}. Competition for available vitamin B_{12} in the intestine may come from intestinal organisms. The fish tapeworm *Diphyllobothrium latum* is able to split vitamin B_{12} from intrinsic factor, rendering the vitamin unavailable for host absorption.[43] Also, *blind loops,* portions of the intestines that are stenotic as a result of surgery or inflammation, can become overgrown with intestinal bacteria that compete effectively with the host for available vitamin B_{12}.[10] In both these cases, the host is unable to absorb sufficient vitamin B_{12}, and megaloblastic anemia results.

LABORATORY DIAGNOSIS

The tests used in the diagnosis of megaloblastic anemia include screening tests and specific diagnostic tests to identify the specific vitamin deficiency and perhaps its cause.

Screening Tests

Five tests used to screen for megaloblastic anemia are the complete blood count (CBC), reticulocyte count, white blood cell (WBC) manual differential, serum bilirubin, and lactate dehydrogenase.

Complete Blood Count and Reticulocyte Count

Slight macrocytosis often is the earliest sign of megaloblastic anemia. Patients with uncomplicated megaloblastic anemia are expected to have decreased hemoglobin and hematocrit values, pancytopenia, and reticulocytopenia. Megaloblastic anemia develops slowly, and the degree of anemia is often severe when first detected. Hemoglobin values of less than 7 or 8 g/dL are not unusual.[4] When the hematocrit is less than 20%, erythroblasts with megaloblastic nuclei, including an occasional promegaloblast, may appear in the peripheral blood. The mean cell volume (MCV) is usually 100 to 150 fL and commonly is greater than 120 fL, although coexisting iron deficiency, thalassemia trait, or inflammation can prevent macrocytosis. The mean cell hemoglobin (MCH) is elevated by the increased volume of the cells, but the mean cell hemoglobin concentration (MCHC) is usually within the reference interval because hemoglobin production is unaffected. The red blood cell distribution width (RDW) is also elevated.

The characteristic morphologic findings of megaloblastic anemia in the peripheral blood include oval macrocytes (enlarged oval RBCs) (Figure 18.6) and hypersegmented neutrophils with six or more lobes (Figure 18.7).[44] Impaired cell production results in a low absolute reticulocyte count, especially in light of the severity of the anemia, and polychromasia is not observed on the peripheral blood film. Additional morphologic changes may include the presence of teardrop cells (dacryocytes), RBC fragments, and microspherocytes. These smaller cells further increase the RDW. The presence of schistocytes sometimes leads to a paradoxically lower MCV than is seen in less severe cases. These erythrocyte changes reflect the severity of the dyserythropoiesis and should not be taken as evidence of microangiopathic hemolysis. Nucleated RBCs, Howell-Jolly bodies, basophilic stippling, and Cabot rings may also be observed.

White Blood Cell Manual Differential Count

Hypersegmentation of neutrophils is essentially pathognomonic for megaloblastic anemia. It appears early in the course of the disease[39] and may persist for up to 2 weeks after treatment is initiated.[5] Hypersegmented neutrophils noted in the WBC

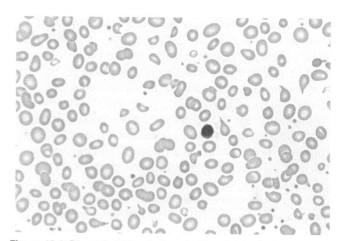

Figure 18.6 Blood Cell Morphology in Megaloblastic Anemia. Note the oval macrocytes, teardrop cells (dacryocytes), other red blood cell abnormalities, and a small lymphocyte for size comparison. (Peripheral blood, Wright-Giemsa stain, ×500.)

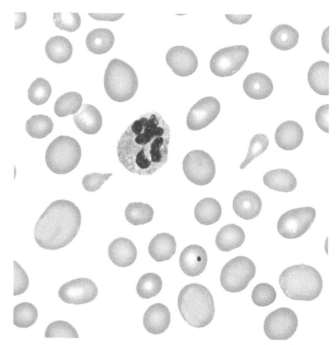

Figure 18.7 Blood Cell Morphology in Megaloblastic Anemia. Note the hypersegmented neutrophil, oval macrocytes, and a Howell-Jolly body. (Peripheral blood, Wright-Giemsa stain, ×1000.) (From Rodak, B. F., & Carr, J. H. [2017]. *Clinical Hematology Atlas.* [5th ed.]. St. Louis: Elsevier.)

differential report are a significant finding and require a reporting rule that can be applied consistently because even healthy individuals may have an occasional one. One such rule is to report hypersegmentation when there are at least 5 five-lobed neutrophils per 100 WBCs or at least 1 six-lobed neutrophil is noted.[10] Some laboratories perform a lobe count on 100 neutrophils and then calculate the mean. In megaloblastic anemia, the mean lobe count should be greater than 3.4.[10] The cause of the hypersegmentation is not understood, despite considerable investigation.[45] Recent advances in the understanding of growth factors and their impact on transcription factors may yet solve this mystery. Nevertheless, a search for neutrophil hypersegmentation on a peripheral blood film constitutes an inexpensive yet sensitive screening test for megaloblastic anemia.

Bilirubin and Lactate Dehydrogenase Levels

Although generally considered a nutritional anemia, megaloblastic anemia is in one sense a hemolytic anemia. Because many erythroid progenitors and precursors die during division in bone marrow, many RBCs never enter the circulation (ineffective hematopoiesis), so a decrease in reticulocytes occurs in the peripheral blood. The usual signs of hemolysis are evident in the serum, including an elevation in levels of total and indirect bilirubin and lactate dehydrogenase (predominantly RBC derived).

The constellation of findings, including macrocytic anemia, moderate to marked pancytopenia, reticulocytopenia, oval macrocytes, and hypersegmented neutrophils plus increased levels of total and indirect bilirubin and lactate dehydrogenase, justifies further testing to confirm a diagnosis of megaloblastic anemia and determine its cause. Occasionally the classic findings may be obscured by coexisting conditions such as iron deficiency or thalassemia, which makes the diagnosis more challenging. Most hematologic aberrations do not appear until vitamin deficiency is fairly well advanced (Box 18.4).[46]

Specific Diagnostic Tests
Bone Marrow Examination

Modern tests for vitamin deficiencies and autoimmune antibodies have made bone marrow examination an infrequently used diagnostic test for megaloblastic anemia. Nevertheless, it remains the reference confirmatory test to identify the megaloblastic appearance of the developing erythroid precursors.

Megaloblastic, in contrast to *macrocytic,* anemia refers to specific morphologic changes in the developing erythroid precursors. The cells are characterized by a nuclear-cytoplasmic asynchrony in which the cytoplasm matures as expected with increasing pinkness as hemoglobin accumulates. The nucleus lags behind, however, appearing younger than expected for the degree of maturity of the cytoplasm (Figure 18.8). This asynchrony is most striking at the stage of the polychromatic normoblast. The cytoplasm appears pinkish-blue as expected for that stage, but the nuclear chromatin remains more open than expected, similar to that in the nucleus of a basophilic normoblast. Overall the bone marrow is hypercellular, with a reduced myeloid-to-erythroid ratio of about 1:1 by virtue of the increased erythropoietic activity. Hematopoiesis is ineffective, however, and although cell production in the bone marrow is increased, the apoptosis of hematopoietic cells in the marrow results in peripheral pancytopenia.

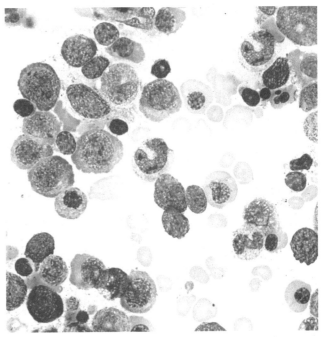

Figure 18.8 Erythroid Precursors in Megaloblastic Anemia. Note nuclear-cytoplasmic asynchrony. (Bone marrow, Wright-Giemsa stain, ×500.) (From Rodak, B. F., & Carr, J. H. [2017]. *Clinical hematology atlas.* [5th ed.]. St. Louis: Elsevier.)

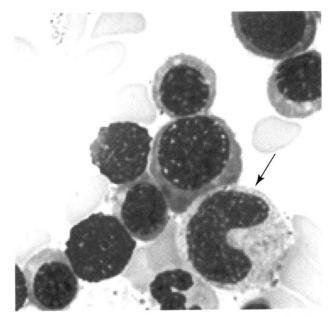

Figure 18.9 Giant Band (Early) in Megaloblastic Anemia. (Bone marrow, Wright-Giemsa stain, original magnification ×1000.)

The WBCs are also affected in megaloblastic anemia and appear larger than normal. This is most evident in metamyelocytes and bands, because in the usual development of neutrophils, the cells should be getting smaller at these stages. The effect creates "giant" metamyelocytes and bands (Figure 18.9).

Megakaryocytes do not show consistent changes in megaloblastic anemia. They may be either increased or decreased in number and may show diminished lobulation. The latter finding is not consistently seen, however, and even when present, it is difficult to assess.

BOX 18.4 Sequence of Development of Megaloblastic Anemias

1. Decrease in vitamin levels
2. Hypersegmentation of neutrophils in peripheral blood
3. Oval macrocytes in peripheral blood
4. Megaloblastosis in bone marrow
5. Anemia

Assays for Folate, Vitamin B$_{12}$, Methylmalonic Acid, and Homocysteine

Although bone marrow aspiration is confirmatory for megaloblastosis, the invasiveness of the procedure and its expense mean that other testing is performed more often than a bone marrow examination. Furthermore, the confirmation of megaloblastic morphology in the marrow does not identify its cause. Tests for serum levels of folate and vitamin B$_{12}$ are readily available using immunoassay; serum vitamin B$_{12}$ may also be assayed by competitive binding chemiluminescence.[47] However, there are a number of interferences with these assays that can cause false increased and decreased results[5,47] (Box 18.5); reflexive testing to MMA and homocysteine (discussed later) can increase diagnostic accuracy. RBC folate levels may also be measured. Unlike serum folate levels, which fluctuate with diet, RBC folate values are stable and may be a more accurate reflection of true folate status[48]; however, current RBC folate tests have less than optimal sensitivity and specificity and have not been validated in actual patients with normal and deficient folate levels. Thus the serum folate level is preferred over RBC folate level in the United States as the initial test for evaluation of folate deficiency.[5]

Some laboratories conduct a reflexive assay for MMA if vitamin B$_{12}$ levels are low. As indicated previously, in addition to playing a role in folate metabolism, vitamin B$_{12}$ is a cofactor in the conversion of methylmalonyl CoA to succinyl CoA by the enzyme methylmalonyl CoA mutase (Figure 18.2). If vitamin B$_{12}$ is deficient, methylmalonyl CoA accumulates. Some of it hydrolyzes to methylmalonic acid, and the increase can be detected in serum and urine. Because MMA is also elevated in patients with impaired renal function, the test is not specific, and thus increased levels cannot be definitively related to vitamin B$_{12}$ deficiency.[3] Methylmalonic acid is assayed by gas chromatography-tandem mass spectrometry.

Homocysteine levels are affected by deficiencies in either folate or vitamin B$_{12}$. 5-Methyl THF donates a methyl group to homocysteine in the generation of methionine. This reaction uses vitamin B$_{12}$ as a coenzyme (Figure 18.4). Thus a deficiency in either folate or vitamin B$_{12}$ results in elevated levels of homocysteine. Total homocysteine can be measured in either plasma or serum. Homocysteine may be assayed by gas chromatography-mass spectrometry, high-performance liquid chromatography, or fluorescence polarization immunoassay. Homocysteine levels are also elevated in patients with renal failure and dehydration. Figure 18.10 presents an algorithm of the analysis of these analytes in the diagnosis of vitamin B$_{12}$ and folate deficiency.

Gastric Analysis and Serum Gastrin

Gastric analysis may be used to confirm achlorhydria, an expected finding in pernicious anemia. Achlorhydria occurs in other conditions, however, including natural aging. When other causes of vitamin B$_{12}$ deficiency have been eliminated, a finding of achlorhydria is supportive, although not diagnostic, of pernicious anemia. The H^{+} concentration is determined by pH measurement.

As a result of the gastric achlorhydria, serum gastrin levels can be markedly elevated.[4] Serum gastrin is measured by immunoassay, including chemiluminescent immunometric assays.

Antibody Assays

Antibodies to intrinsic factor and parietal cells can be detected in the serum of most patients with pernicious anemia. Various immunoassays can detect intrinsic factor-blocking antibodies; parietal cell antibodies can be detected by indirect fluorescent antibody techniques or enzyme-linked immunosorbent assays. Anti-intrinsic factor antibodies are highly specific and confirmatory for pernicious anemia, but their absence does not rule out the condition. The test for parietal cell antibodies is nonspecific and not clinically useful for the diagnosis of pernicious anemia.[5]

Figure 18.11 presents an algorithm for the diagnosis of pernicious anemia using tests for serum vitamin B$_{12}$, methylmalonic acid, intrinsic factor blocking antibody, and serum gastrin levels.

Holotranscobalamin Assay

Holotranscobalamin is the metabolically active form of vitamin B$_{12}$. Until recently, methods for measuring holotranscobalamin were

---

BOX 18.5   Causes of False Increases and Decreases of Vitamin B$_{12}$ and Folate Assays[5,47]

False Increases in Vitamin B$_{12}$ Assay Results

Assay technical failure

Occult malignancy

Alcoholic liver disease

Renal disease

Increased transcobalamin I and II binders (e.g., myeloproliferative states, hepatomas, and fibrolamellar hepatic tumors)

Activated transcobalamin II-producing macrophages (e.g., autoimmune diseases, monoblastic leukemias, and lymphomas)

Release of cobalamin from hepatocytes (e.g., active liver disease)

High serum anti-intrinsic factor antibody titer

False Decreases in Vitamin B$_{12}$ Assay Results

Haptocorrin deficiency

Folate deficiency

Plasma cell myeloma

Human immunodeficiency virus

Pregnancy

Plasma cell myeloma

Transcobalamin I deficiency

Megadose vitamin C therapy

False Increases in Folate Assay Results

Recent meal

Alcoholism

False Decreases in Folate Assay Results

Severe anorexia requiring hospitalization

Acute alcohol consumption

Normal pregnancy

Anticonvulsant therapy

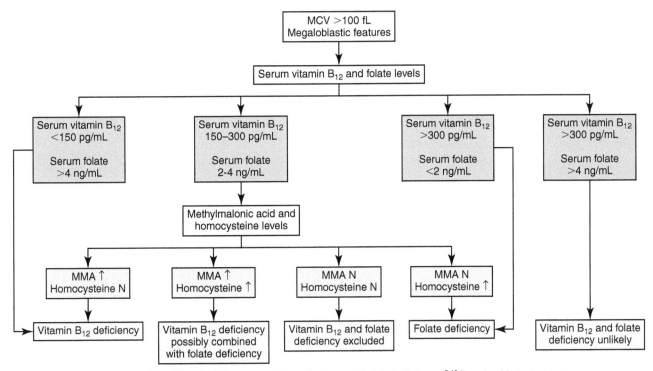

Figure 18.10 Algorithm for Diagnosis of Vitamin B_{12} and Folate Deficiency.[5,40] The algorithm uses serum assays for folate, vitamin B_{12}, methylmalonic acid, and homocysteine to differentiate the conditions. ↑, Increased; *MCV*, mean cell volume; *MMA*, methylmalonic acid; *N*, within reference interval.

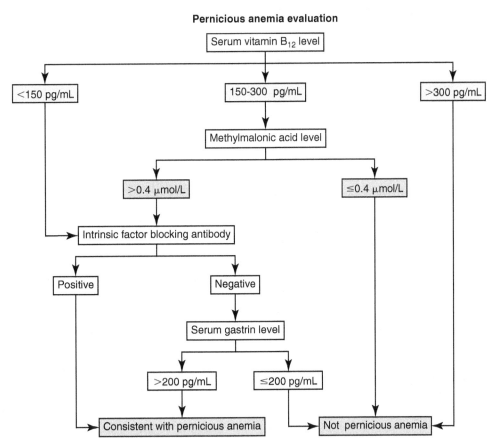

Figure 18.11 Algorithm for Diagnosis of Pernicious Anemia. (Adapted from Klee, G. G. [2000]. Cobalamin and folate evaluation: Measurement of methylmalonic acid and homocysteine vs vitamin B_{12} and folate. *Clin Chem, 46*, 1281.)

TABLE 18.1   Laboratory Tests Used to Diagnose Vitamin B₁₂ and Folate Deficiency

		Folate Deficiency	Vitamin B₁₂ Deficiency
Screening tests	Complete blood count	↓ HGB, HCT, RBCs, WBCs, PLTs ↑ MCV, MCH	Same as Folate Deficiency
	Manual differential count	Hypersegmented neutrophils, oval macrocytes, anisocytosis, poikilocytosis, RBC inclusions	Same as Folate Deficiency
	Absolute reticulocyte count	↓	↓
	Serum total and indirect bilirubin	↑	↑
	Serum lactate dehydrogenase	↑	↑
Specific diagnostic tests	Bone marrow examination*	Erythroid hyperplasia (ineffective) Presence of megaloblasts	Same as Folate Deficiency
	Serum vitamin B₁₂	N	↓
	Serum folate	↓	N or ↑†
	RBC folate	↓	N or ↓†
	Serum methylmalonic acid	N	↑
	Serum/plasma homocysteine	↑	↑
	Antibodies to intrinsic factor and gastric parietal cells	Absent	Present in pernicious anemia
	Serum gastrin	N	Can be markedly elevated in pernicious anemia
	Gastric analysis*	N	Achlorhydria in pernicious anemia
	Holotranscobalamin assay‡	N	↓
	Stool analysis for parasites	Negative	*Diphyllobothrium latum* may be the cause of deficiency

↑, Increased; ↓, decreased; *HCT,* hematocrit; *HGB,* hemoglobin; *MCH,* mean cell hemoglobin; *MCV,* mean cell volume; *N,* within reference interval; *PLT,* platelet; *RBC,* red blood cell; *WBC,* white blood cell.

*Bone marrow examination and gastric analysis are not usually required for diagnosis.

†Without vitamin B₁₂, the cell is unable to produce intracellular polyglutamated tetrahydrofolate; therefore 5-methyltetrahydrofolate leaks out of the cell, which results in a decreased level of intracellular folate.

‡Holotranscobalamin level is also decreased in transcobalamin deficiency.

manual and not suitable for use in clinical laboratories. Newer, more rapid immunoassays using monoclonal antibodies specific for holotranscobalamin have been developed in the past several years that are both sensitive and specific.[49,50] Recent studies support the use of holotranscobalamin to detect vitamin B₁₂ deficiency and recommend its use in screening for metabolic vitamin B₁₂ deficiency.[51-53]

Stool Analysis for Parasites

When vitamin B₁₂ is found to be deficient, a stool analysis for eggs or proglottids of the fish tapeworm *D. latum* may be part of the diagnostic workup.

Table 18.1 contains a summary of laboratory tests used to diagnose vitamin B₁₂ and folate deficiency.

MACROCYTIC NONMEGALOBLASTIC ANEMIAS

The macrocytic nonmegaloblastic anemias are macrocytic anemias in which DNA synthesis is unimpaired. The macrocytosis tends to be mild; the MCV usually ranges from 100 to 110 fL and rarely exceeds 120 fL. Patients with nonmegaloblastic, macrocytic anemia lack hypersegmented neutrophils and oval macrocytes in the peripheral blood and megaloblasts in the bone marrow. Macrocytosis may be physiologically normal, as in the newborn (Chapter 43), or the result of a pathologic condition, as in liver disease, chronic alcoholism, or bone marrow failure. Reticulocytosis is a common cause of macrocytosis. Figure 18.12 presents an algorithm for the preliminary investigation of macrocytic anemias.

TREATMENT

Treatment should be directed at the specific vitamin deficiency established by the diagnostic tests and should include addressing the cause of the deficiency (e.g., better nutrition, treatment for *D. latum*) if possible. Vitamin B₁₂ may be administered intramuscularly to treat pernicious anemia to bypass the need for intrinsic factor. High-dose oral vitamin B₁₂ treatment is increasingly popular in the treatment of pernicious anemia.[35,54,55] Regardless of the treatment modality, those with pernicious anemia or malabsorption must have lifelong vitamin replacement therapy. Folic acid can be administered orally. The inappropriate treatment of vitamin B₁₂ deficiency with folic acid improves the anemia but does not correct or stop the progress of the neurologic damage, which may advance to an irreversible state.[3] Thus proper diagnosis before treatment is important. Iron is often supplemented concurrently to support the rapid cell production that accompanies effective treatment.

When proper treatment is initiated, the body's response is prompt and brisk and can be used to confirm the accuracy of the diagnosis. Bone marrow morphology will begin to revert to a normoblastic appearance within a few hours of treatment. A substantial reticulocyte response is apparent at about 1 week, with hemoglobin increasing toward normal levels in about 3 weeks.[11] Hypersegmented neutrophils disappear from the peripheral blood within 2 weeks of initiation of treatment.[5] Thus with proper treatment, hematologic parameters may return to normal within 3 to 6 weeks and correction of the megaloblastic anemia may occur in 6 to 8 weeks.[56]

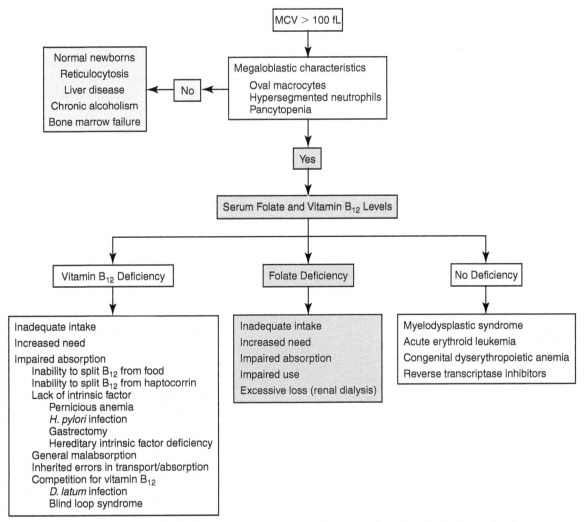

Figure 18.12 Algorithm for Preliminary Investigation of Macrocytic Anemias. *MCV,* Mean cell volume.

SUMMARY

- Impaired DNA synthesis affects all rapidly dividing cells of the body, including those in skin, gastrointestinal tract, and bone marrow. The effect on hematologic cells results in megaloblastic anemia.
- Vitamin B₁₂ and folate are needed for the production of thymidine nucleotides for DNA synthesis. Deficiencies of either vitamin impair DNA replication, halt cell division, and increase apoptosis, which results in ineffective hematopoiesis and megaloblastic morphology of erythroid precursors.
- Vitamin B₁₂ deficiency is associated with peripheral neuropathies and neuropsychiatric abnormalities as a result of demyelinization of nerves in the peripheral and central nervous system. Peripheral neuropathy and depression also may accompany folate deficiency. Folate deficiency in early pregnancy can lead to neural tube defects in the fetus.
- Lack of vitamin B₁₂ leads to the accumulation of methylmalonic acid (MMA) and homocysteine. Folate deficiency, in particular, leads to elevation of homocysteine levels and possible risk of coronary artery disease.
- Folate deficiency may result from inadequate intake, increased need with growth or pregnancy, impaired absorption,

impaired use, or excessive loss. The action of folate can be impaired by drugs such as those used to treat seizures or cancer. Renal dialysis patients experience significant folate loss to the dialysate.
- Vitamin B₁₂ deficiency arises from inadequate intake, increased need, or inadequate absorption. Inadequate intake of vitamin B₁₂, although possible, is uncommon because vitamin B₁₂ is ubiquitous in animal products. Pregnancy, lactation, and growth create increased need for vitamin B₁₂.
- Absorption of vitamin B₁₂ depends on production of intrinsic factor by parietal cells of the stomach. Vitamin B₁₂ binds to transcobalamin, forming holotranscobalamin, the metabolically active form of the vitamin.
- Impaired absorption of vitamin B₁₂ can be caused by several mechanisms. Decrease in gastric acid production or lack of trypsin in the intestine causes vitamin B₁₂ to be excreted in the stool rather than absorbed. Malabsorption can be caused by intestinal disorders, such as sprue, celiac disease, and inflammatory bowel disease. Competition for vitamin B₁₂ can develop from an intestinal parasite (*Diphyllobothrium latum*) or bacteria in intestinal blind loops. Lack of intrinsic

factor may result from loss of gastric parietal cells with pernicious anemia, *Helicobacter pylori* infection, gastrectomy, or inherited intrinsic factor deficiency.

- Pernicious anemia is vitamin B_{12} deficiency resulting from an autoimmune disease that causes destruction of gastric parietal cells. H^+ and intrinsic factor secretion is lost. Antibodies to parietal cells or intrinsic factor, or both, are detectable in the serum.

- Classic complete blood count findings in megaloblastic anemia include decreased hemoglobin, hematocrit, and red blood cell (RBC) count; leukopenia; thrombocytopenia; decreased absolute reticulocyte count; elevated mean cell volume (MCV; usually greater than 120 fL); elevated RBC distribution width (RDW) and mean cell hemoglobin (MCH); mean cell hemoglobin concentration (MCHC) within the reference interval; and oval macrocytes and hypersegmented neutrophils observed on the peripheral blood film. Additional abnormal laboratory test findings may include elevated levels of total and indirect serum bilirubin and lactate dehydrogenase as a result of the hemolysis and apoptosis of megaloblastic erythroid precursors within the bone marrow.

- The bone marrow in megaloblastic anemia is hyperplastic with increased erythropoiesis; however, it is ineffective because of increased apoptosis of developing cells. Erythroid precursors show nuclear-cytoplasmic asynchrony, with the nuclear maturation lagging behind the cytoplasmic maturation. Giant metamyelocytes and bands are evident.

- The cause of megaloblastic anemia is determined using specific immunoassays for serum folate and vitamin B_{12}. Immunoassays for holotranscobalamin and antibodies to intrinsic factor can aid in the diagnosis of pernicious anemia. Additional tests for gastrointestinal disease or parasites may be needed.

- Treatment of megaloblastic anemia is directed at correcting the cause of the deficiency and supplementing the missing vitamin.

- For pernicious anemia, lifelong supplementation with vitamin B_{12} is necessary.

Now that you have completed this chapter, go back and read again the case study at the beginning and respond to the questions presented.

REVIEW QUESTIONS

Answers can be found in the Appendix.

1. Which of the following findings is consistent with a diagnosis of megaloblastic anemia?
   a. Hyposegmentation of neutrophils
   b. Decreased serum lactate dehydrogenase level
   c. Absolute increase in reticulocytes
   d. Increased MCV

2. A patient has a clinical picture of megaloblastic anemia. The serum folate level is decreased, and the serum vitamin B_{12} level is 600 pg/mL (reference interval is 200 to 900 pg/mL). What is the expected value for the methylmalonic acid assay?
   a. Increased
   b. Decreased
   c. Within the reference interval

3. Which one of the following statements characterizes the relationships among macrocytic anemia, megaloblastic anemia, and pernicious anemia?
   a. Macrocytic anemias are megaloblastic.
   b. Macrocytic anemia is pernicious anemia.
   c. Megaloblastic anemia is macrocytic.
   d. Megaloblastic anemia is pernicious anemia.

4. Which of the following CBC findings is most suggestive of a megaloblastic anemia?
   a. MCV of 103 fL
   b. Hypersegmentation of neutrophils
   c. RDW of 16%
   d. Hemoglobin concentration of 9.1 g/dL

5. In the following description of a bone marrow smear, find the statement that is *inconsistent* with the expected picture in megaloblastic anemia.
   "The marrow appears hypercellular with a myeloid-to-erythroid ratio of 1:1 due to prominent erythroid hyperplasia. Megakaryocytes appear normal in number and appearance. WBC elements appear larger than normal, with especially large metamyelocytes, although they otherwise appear morphologically normal. Erythroid precursors also appear large. There is nuclear-cytoplasmic asynchrony, with the nucleus appearing more mature than expected for the color of the cytoplasm."
   a. Erythroid nuclei that are more mature than cytoplasm
   b. Larger than normal WBC elements
   c. Larger than normal erythroid precursors
   d. Normal appearance of megakaryocytes

6. Which one of the following findings would be *inconsistent* with elevated titers of intrinsic factor blocking antibodies?
   a. Hypersegmentation of neutrophils
   b. Low levels of methylmalonic acid
   c. Macrocytic RBCs
   d. Low levels of vitamin B_{12}

7. Which of the following is the most metabolically active form of absorbed vitamin B_{12}?
   a. Transcobalamin
   b. Intrinsic factor-vitamin B_{12} complex
   c. Holotranscobalamin
   d. Haptocorrin-vitamin B_{12} complex

8. Folate and vitamin B_{12} work together in the production of:
   a. Amino acids
   b. RNA
   c. Phospholipids
   d. DNA

9. The macrocytosis associated with megaloblastic anemia results from:
   a. Reduced numbers of cell divisions with normal cytoplasmic development
   b. Activation of a gene that is typically active only in mega-karyocytes
   c. Reduced concentration of hemoglobin in the cells so that larger cells are needed to provide the same oxygen-carrying capacity
   d. Increased production of reticulocytes in an attempt to compensate for the anemia

10. Which one of the following groups has the highest risk for pernicious anemia?
    a. Malnourished infants
    b. Children during growth periods
    c. Persons older than 60 years of age
    d. Pregnant women

REFERENCES

1. Scott, J. M. (1999). Folate and vitamin B$_{12}$. *Proc Nutr Soc, 58,* 441–448.
2. Wickramasinghe, S. N. (1999). The wide spectrum and unre-solved issues of megaloblastic anemia. *Semin Hematol, 36,* 3–18.
3. Miller, J. W. (2013). Folic acid. In Caballero, B. (Ed.), *Encyclopedia of Human Nutrition.* (3rd ed., pp. 262–269). Amsterdam: Elsevier/Academic Press.
4. Carmel, R. (2014). Megaloblastic anemias: disorders of impaired DNA synthesis. In Greer, J. P., Arber, D. A., Glader, B., et al. (Eds.), *Wintrobe's Clinical Hematology.* (13th ed., pp. 927–953). Philadelphia: Lippincott Williams & Wilkins.
5. Antony, A. C. (2018). Megaloblastic anemias. In Hoffman, R., Benz, E. J., Silberstein, L. E., et al. (Eds.), *Hematology: Basic Prin-ciples and Practice.* (7th ed., pp. 514–545). Philadelphia: Elsevier.
6. Wickramasinghe, S. N., & Fida, S. (1994). Bone marrow cells from vitamin B$_{12}$- and folate-deficient patients misincorporate uracil into DNA. *Blood, 83,* 1656–1661.
7. Koury, M. J., Horne, D. W., Brown, Z. A., et al. (1997). Apoptosis of late stage erythroblasts in megaloblastic anemia: association with DNA damage and macrocyte production. *Blood, 89,* 4617–4623.
8. Das, K. C., Das, M., Mohanty, D., et al. (2006). Megaloblastosis: from morphos to molecules. *Med Princ Pract, 14,* 2–14.
9. Geené, D., Sudre, P., Anwar, D., et al. (2000). Causes of macrocy-tosis in HIV-infected patients not treated with zidovudine. Swiss HIV Cohort Study. *J Infect, 40,* 160–163.
10. Carmel, R., & Rosenblatt, D. S. (2003). Disorders of cobalamin and folate metabolism. In Handin, R. I., Lux, S. E., & Stossel, T. P. (Eds.), *Blood: Principles and Practice of Hematology.* (2nd ed., pp. 1361–1398). Philadelphia: Lippincott Williams & Wilkins.
11. Solomon, L. R. (2007). Disorders of cobalamin (vitamin B$_{12}$) metabolism: emerging concepts in pathophysiology, diagnosis and treatment. *Blood Rev, 21,* 113–130.
12. Scalabrino, G., & Peracchi, M. (2006). New insights into the pathophysiology of cobalamin deficiency. *Trends Mol Med, 12,* 247–254.
13. Morrison, H. I., Schaubel, D., Desmeules, M., et al. (1996). Serum folate and risk of fatal coronary heart disease. *JAMA, 275,* 1893–1896.
14. Voutilainen, S., Virtanen, J. K., Rissanen, T. H., et al. (2004). Serum folate and homocysteine and the incidence of acute coronary events: the Kuopio Ischaemic Heart Disease Risk Factor Study. *Am J Clin Nutr, 80,* 317–323.
15. de Bree, A., Verschuren, W. M., Blom, H. J., et al. (2003). Coronary heart disease mortality, plasma homocysteine, and B-vitamins: a prospective study. *Atherosclerosis, 166,* 369–377.
16. Blom, H. J., & Smulders, Y. (2011). Overview of homocysteine and folate metabolism. With special references to cardiovascular disease and neural tube defects. *J Inherit Metab Dis, 346,* 75–81.
17. Humphrey, L. L., Rongwei, F., Rogers, K., et al. (2008). Homocys-teine level and coronary heart disease incidence: a systematic review and meta-analysis. *Mayo Clin Proc, 83,* 1203–1212.
18. Soinio, M., Marniemi, J., Laakso, M., et al. (2004). Elevated plasma homocysteine level is an independent predictor of coro-nary heart disease events in patients with type 2 diabetes melli-tus. *Ann Intern Med, 140,* 94–100.
19. Lindeman, R. D., Romero, L. J, Yau, C. L., et al. (2003). Serum ho-mocysteine concentrations and their relation to serum folate and vitamin B$_{12}$ concentrations and coronary artery disease preva-lence in an urban, bi-ethnic community. *Ethn Dis, 13,* 178–185.
20. Bottiglieri, T., Laundry, M., Crellin, R., et al. (2000). Homocysteine, folate, methylation, and monoamine metabolism in depression. *J Neurol Neurosurg Psychiatry, 69,* 228–232.
21. Kronenberg, G., Colla, M., & Endres, M. (2009). Folic acid, neu-rodegenerative and neuropsychiatric disease. *Curr Mol Med, 9,* 315–323.
22. Alpert, J. E., Mischoulon, D., Nierenberg, A. A., et al. (2000). Nu-trition and depression: focus on folate. *Nutrition, 16,* 544–546.
23. Blom, H. J., Shaw, G. M., den Heijer, M., et al. (2006). Neural tube defects and folate: case far from closed. *Nat Rev Neurosci, 7,* 724–731.
24. Gallagher, M. L. (2004). Vitamins. In Mahan, L. K., & Escott-Stump, S. (Eds.), *Krause's Food, Nutrition, and Diet Therapy.* (11th ed., pp. 74–119). Philadelphia: Saunders.
25. Qui, A., Jansen, M., Sakaris, A., et al. (2006). Identification of an intestinal folate transporter and the molecular basis for heredi-tary folate malabsorption. *Cell, 127,* 917–928.
26. Moestrup, S. K. (2006). New insights into carrier binding and epithelial uptake of the erythropoietic nutrients cobalamin and folate. *Curr Opin Hematol, 13,* 119–123.
27. Nath, S. K. (2005). Tropical sprue. *Curr Gastroenterol Rep, 7,* 343–349.
28. Hesdorffer, C. S., & Longo, D. L. (2015). Drug-induced megalo-blastic anemia. *N Engl J Med, 373,* 1649–1658.
29. Green, R. (2013). Vitamin B$_{12}$ physiology, dietary sources, and requirements. In Caballero, B. (Ed.), *Encyclopedia of Human Nutrition.* (3rd ed., pp. 351–356). Amsterdam: Elsevier/Academic Press.
30. He, Q., Madsen, M., Kilkenney, A., et al. (2005). Amnionless function is required for cubilin brush-border expression and in-trinsic factor-cobalamin (vitamin B$_{12}$) absorption in vivo. *Blood, 106,* 1447–1453.

31. Watkins, D., Morel, C. F., & Rosenblatt, D. S. (2017). Inborn errors of folate and cobalamin transport and metabolism. In Sarafoglou, K., Hoffman, G. F., & Roth, K. S. (Eds.), *Pediatric Endocrinology and Inborn Errors of Metabolism*. (2nd ed., pp. 287–308). New York: McGraw-Hill.

32. Fyfe, J. C., Madsen, M., Hojrup, P., et al. (2004). The functional cobalamin (vitamin B_{12})-intrinsic factor receptor is a novel complex of cubilin and amnionless. *Blood, 103*, 1573–1579.

33. Afman, L. A., Van Der Put, N. M. J., Thomas, C. M. G., et al. (2001). Reduced vitamin B_{12} binding by transcobalamin II increases the risk of neural tube defects. *QJM, 94*, 159–166.

34. Kozyraki, R., & Cases, O. (2013). Vitamin B_{12} absorption: mammalian physiology and acquired and inherited disorders. *Biochimie, 95*, 1002-1007.

35. Dali-Youcef, N., & Andres, E. (2009). An update on cobalamin deficiency in adults. *QJM, 102*, 17–28.

36. Karlsson, F. A., Burman, P., Loof, L., et al. (1988). Major parietal cell antigen in autoimmune gastritis with pernicious anemia in the acid-producing H^+,K^+-adenosine triphosphatase of the stomach. *J Clin Invest, 81*, 475–479.

37. Toh, B. H., Van Driel, I. R., & Gleeson, P. A. (1997). Pernicious anemia. *N Engl J Med, 337*, 1441–1448.

38. Fernandez-Banares, F., Monzon, H., & Forme, M. (2009). A short review of malabsorption and anemia. *World J Gastroenterol, 15*, 4644–4652.

39. Wickramasinghe, S. N. (2006). Diagnosis of megaloblastic anemia. *Blood Rev, 20*, 299–318.

40. Kaferle, J., & Strzoda, C. E. (2009). Evaluation of macrocytosis. *Am Fam Physician, 79*(3), 203–208.

41. Kaptan, K., Beyan, C., Ural, A. U., et al. (2000). *Helicobacter pylori*—is it a novel causative agent in vitamin B_{12} deficiency? *Arch Intern Med, 160*, 1349–1353.

42. Morel, C. F., Watkins, D., Scott, P., et al. (2005). Prenatal diagnosis for methylmalonic acidemia and inborn errors of vitamin B_{12} metabolism and transport. *Mol Genet Metab, 86*, 160–171.

43. Nyberg, W., Gräsbeck, R., Saarni, M., et al. (1961). Serum vitamin B_{12} levels and incidence of tape worm anemia in a population heavily infected with *Diphyllobothrium latum*. *Am J Clin Nutr, 9*, 606–612.

44. Zittoun, J., & Zittoun, R. (1999). Modern clinical testing strategies in cobalamin and folate deficiency. *Semin Hematol, 36*, 35–46.

45. Wickramasinghe, S. N. (1999). The wide spectrum and unresolved issues in megaloblastic anemia. *Semin Hematol, 36*, 3–18.

46. Carmel, R. (1999). Introduction: beyond megaloblastic anemia. *Semin Hematol, 36*, 1–2.

47. Oberley, M. J., & Yang, D. T. (2013). Laboratory testing for cobalamin deficiency in megaloblastic anemia. *Am J Hematol, 88*, 522–526.

48. Piyathilake, C. J., Robinson, C. B., & Cornwell, P. (2007). A practical approach to red blood cell folate analysis. *Anal Chem Insights, 2*, 107–110.

49. Brady, J., Wilson, L., McGregor, L., et al. (2008). Active B_{12}: a rapid, automated assay for holotranscobalamin on the Abbott AxSYM analyzer. *Clin Chem, 54*(3), 567–573.

50. Ulleland, M., Eilertsen, I., Quadros, E. V., et al. (2002). Direct assay for cobalamin bound to transcobalamin (holo-transcobalamin) in serum. *Clin Chem, 48*(3), 526–532.

51. Heil, S. G., de Jonge, R., de Rotte, M. C. F. J., et al. (2012). Screening for metabolic vitamin B_{12} deficiency by holotranscobalamin in patients suspected of vitamin B_{12} deficiency: a multicenter study. *Ann Clin Biochem, 49*, 184–189.

52. Valente, E., Scott, J. M., Ueland, P-M., et al. (2011). Diagnostic accuracy of holotranscobalamin, methylmalonic acid, serum cobalamin, and other indicators of tissue vitamin B_{12} status in the elderly. *Clin Chem, 37*(6), 856–863.

53. Nexo, E., & Hoffmann-Lucke, E. (2011). Holotranscobalamin, a marker of vitamin B-12 status: analytical aspects and clinical utility. *Am J Clin Nutr, 94*(1), 1S-7S.

54. Carmel, R. (2008). How I treat cobalamin (vitamin B_{12}) deficiency. *Blood, 112*(6), 2214–2221.

55. Butler, C. C., Vidal-Alaball, J., & Cannings-John, R., et al. (2006). Oral vitamin B_{12} versus intramuscular vitamin B_{12} for vitamin B_{12} deficiency: a systematic review of randomized controlled trials. *Fam Pract, 23*, 279–285.

56. Stabler, S. P. (2013). Vitamin B_{12} deficiency. *N Engl J Med, 368*, 149–160.

Bone Marrow Failure

Clara Lo, Bertil Glader, and Kathleen M. Sakamoto*

CASE STUDY

After studying the material in this chapter, the reader should be able to respond to the following case study:

A 16-year-old girl presented to her pediatrician with jaundice. Her pediatrician checked liver enzyme and bilirubin levels, which were elevated. Hepatitis A, B, and C serologic tests were all negative. She was referred to a gastroenterologist, who diagnosed her with autoimmune hepatitis. With immunomodulatory treatment, her hepatitis improved. However, over the next several months, she noticed increasing fatigue and bruising. She also developed heavier menses, with menstrual cycles lasting up to 2 weeks. Physical examination revealed pallor and scattered ecchymoses with petechiae on her chest and shoulders with no other abnormalities. Complete blood count results were as follows:

	Patient Results	Reference Intervals
WBCs ($\times 10^9$/L)	2.0	4.5–11.0
HGB (g/dL)	7.9	12.0–15.0

	Patient Results	Reference Intervals
MCV (fL)	104	80–100
Platelets ($\times 10^9$/L)	15	150–450
Reticulocytes (%)	0.6	0.5–2.5
Reticulocytes ($\times 10^9$/L)	16	20–115
Neutrophils ($\times 10^9$/L)	0.5	2.3–8.1
Lymphocytes ($\times 10^9$/L)	0.4	0.8–4.8

Serum vitamin B_{12} and folate levels were within reference intervals. Bone marrow aspirate revealed mild dyserythropoiesis but normal myelopoiesis and megakaryopoiesis. Iron stain revealed normal stores. A bone marrow biopsy specimen was moderately hypocellular (15%) with a reduction in all three cell lines. There was no increase in reticulin or blasts. Cytogenetic testing revealed a normal karyotype, and results of flow

Continued

*The authors extend appreciation to Elaine M. Keohane, whose work in prior editions provided the foundation for this chapter.

cytometry for paroxysmal nocturnal hemoglobinuria (PNH) cells were negative.

1. What term is used to describe a decrease in all cell lines in the peripheral blood?
2. Which anemia of bone marrow failure should be considered?

3. How would an increase in either reticulin or blasts alter the preliminary diagnosis?
4. How would the severity of this patient's condition be classified?
5. What treatment modality would be considered for this patient?

PATHOPHYSIOLOGY OF BONE MARROW FAILURE

Bone marrow failure is the reduction or cessation of blood cell production affecting one or more cell lines. Pancytopenia, or decreased numbers of circulating red blood cells (RBCs), white blood cells (WBCs), and platelets, is seen in most cases of bone marrow failure, particularly in severe or advanced stages.

The pathophysiology of bone marrow failure includes (1) destruction of hematopoietic stem cells as a result of injury by drugs, chemicals, radiation, viruses, or autoimmune mechanisms; (2) premature senescence and apoptosis of hematopoietic stem cells as a result of genetic mutations; (3) ineffective hematopoiesis caused by stem cell mutations or vitamin B_{12} or folate deficiency; (4) disruption of the bone marrow microenvironment that supports hematopoiesis; (5) decreased production of hematopoietic growth factors or related hormones; and (6) loss of normal hematopoietic tissue as a result of infiltration of the marrow space with abnormal cells.

Clinical consequences of bone marrow failure vary, depending on the extent and duration of the cytopenias. Severe pancytopenia can be rapidly fatal if untreated. Some patients may initially be asymptomatic, and their cytopenia may be detected during a routine blood examination. Thrombocytopenia can result in bleeding and increased bruising. Decreased RBCs and hemoglobin can result in fatigue, pallor, and cardiovascular complications. Sustained neutropenia increases the risk of life-threatening bacterial or fungal infections.

This chapter focuses on aplastic anemia, a bone marrow failure syndrome resulting from damaged or defective stem cells (mechanisms 1 and 2 listed earlier). Bone marrow failure resulting from other mechanisms may present similarly to aplastic anemia, and differentiation is discussed later. Because there are many mechanisms involved in the various bone marrow failure syndromes, accurate diagnosis is essential to ensure appropriate treatment.

APLASTIC ANEMIA

Aplastic anemia is a rare but potentially fatal bone marrow failure syndrome. In 1888 Ehrlich provided the first case report of aplastic anemia involving a patient with severe anemia, neutropenia, and a hypocellular marrow on postmortem examination.[1] The name *aplastic anemia* was given to the disease by Vaquez and Aubertin in 1904.[2] The characteristic features of aplastic anemia include pancytopenia, reticulocytopenia, bone marrow hypocellularity, and depletion of hematopoietic stem cells (Box 19.1). Approximately 80% to 85% of aplastic anemia

---

BOX 19.1 Characteristic Features of Aplastic Anemia

Pancytopenia
Reticulocytopenia
Bone marrow hypocellularity
Depletion of hematopoietic stem cells

---

cases are acquired, whereas 15% to 20% are inherited/congenital.[3] Box 19.2 provides an etiologic classification.[3-5]

Acquired Aplastic Anemia

Acquired aplastic anemia is classified into two major categories: idiopathic and secondary. Idiopathic acquired aplastic anemia has no known cause. Secondary acquired aplastic anemia is associated with an identified cause. Approximately 70% of all aplastic anemia cases are idiopathic, whereas 10% to 15% are secondary.[3] Idiopathic and secondary acquired aplastic anemia have similar clinical and laboratory findings. Patients may initially present with macrocytic or normocytic anemia and reticulocytopenia. Pancytopenia may develop slowly or progress at a rapid rate, with complete cessation of hematopoiesis.

Incidence

In North America and Europe the annual incidence is approximately 1 in 500,000.[6] In Asia and East Asia the incidence is two

---

BOX 19.2 Etiologic Classification of Bone Marrow Failure

Acquired Aplastic Anemia (80%–85% of Cases)
Idiopathic (70% of cases)
Secondary (10%–15% of cases)
  Dose dependent/predictable
    Cytotoxic drugs
    Benzene
    Radiation
  Idiosyncratic
    Drugs (Box 19.3)
    Chemicals
      Insecticides
      Cutting/lubricating oils
  Viruses
    Epstein-Barr virus
    Hepatitis virus (non-A, non-B, non-C, non-G)

Human immunodeficiency virus
Miscellaneous conditions
  Paroxysmal nocturnal hemoglobinuria
  Autoimmune diseases
  Pregnancy

Inherited/Congenital Bone Marrow Failure Syndromes (15%–20% of Cases)
Fanconi anemia
Dyskeratosis congenita
Shwachman-Bodian-Diamond syndrome

to three times higher than in North America or Europe, which may be due to environmental and/or genetic differences.[7] Aplastic anemia can occur at any age, with peak incidence at 15 to 25 years and the second highest frequency at older than 60 years.[4,6,8] There is no gender predisposition.[6]

Etiology

As the name indicates, the cause of idiopathic aplastic anemia is unknown. Secondary aplastic anemia is associated with exposure to certain drugs, chemicals, radiation, or infections. Cytotoxic drugs, radiation, and benzenes are responsible for 10% of secondary aplastic anemia cases and suppress the bone marrow in a predictable, dose-dependent manner.[4,5] Depending on the dose and exposure duration, the bone marrow generally recovers after withdrawal of the agent. Alternatively, approximately 70% of cases of secondary aplastic anemia occur as a result of idiosyncratic reactions to drugs or chemicals. In idiosyncratic reactions the bone marrow failure is unpredictable and unrelated to dose.[4] Documentation of a responsible factor or agent in these cases is difficult because evidence is primarily circumstantial and symptoms may occur months or years after exposure. Some drugs associated with idiosyncratic secondary aplastic anemia are listed in Box 19.3.[4,8]

Generally, idiosyncratic secondary aplastic anemia is a rare event and likely is due to a combination of genetic and environmental factors in susceptible individuals. There are no readily available tests that predict individual susceptibility to these idiosyncratic reactions. However, genetic variations in immune response pathways or metabolic enzymes may play a role.[4] There is an approximately twofold higher incidence of human leukocyte antigen-DR2 (HLA-DR2) and its major serologic split, HLA-DR15, in aplastic anemia patients compared with the general population, but the relationship of this finding to disease pathophysiology has not been elucidated.[9,10] There are also reports that genetic polymorphisms in enzymes that metabolize benzene increase susceptibility to toxicity, even at low exposure levels.[4,11] These include polymorphisms in glutathione S-transferase (GST) enzymes (GSTT1 and GSTM1), myeloperoxidase, nicotinamide adenine dinucleotide phosphate (reduced form, NADPH), quinine oxidoreductase 1, and cytochrome oxidase P450 2E1.[11] A deficiency in GST as a result of the *GSTT1* null genotype is overrepresented in Caucasians, Hispanics, and Asians with aplastic anemia, with a frequency of 30%, 28%, and 75%, respectively.[12] Caucasian patients with aplastic anemia also have a higher frequency (22%) of the *GSTM1/GSTT1* null genotype than the general population.[12] GST is important for metabolism and neutralization of chemical toxins, and deficiencies of this enzyme may increase the risk of aplastic anemia. Further study is required to assess how these genetic variations, and other yet undiscovered factors, contribute to aplastic anemia.

Acquired aplastic anemia occurs occasionally as a complication of infection with Epstein-Barr virus, human immunodeficiency virus (HIV), hepatitis virus, and human parvovirus B19.[4] In 2% to 10% of patients with acquired aplastic anemia, there is a history of acute nontypable hepatitis (non-A, non-B, etc.) occurring 1 to 3 months before the onset of pancytopenia; this is thought to represent autoimmune hepatitis.[13] The acquired aplastic anemia in these cases may be mediated by such mechanisms as interferon-γ (IFN-γ) and cytokine release.[13]

Aplastic anemia associated with pregnancy is a rare occurrence, with fewer than 100 cases reported in the literature.[14] Approximately 10% of individuals with acquired aplastic anemia have a concomitant autoimmune disease[15] and approximately 10% develop hemolytic or thrombotic manifestations of paroxysmal nocturnal hemoglobinuria (PNH).[16] The overlap between acquired aplastic anemia and PNH is discussed later.

Pathophysiology

The primary lesion in acquired aplastic anemia is a quantitative and qualitative deficiency of hematopoietic stem cells. Stem cells of patients with acquired aplastic anemia have diminished colony formation in methylcellulose cultures.[17] The hematopoietic stem and early progenitor cell compartment is identified by expression of CD34 surface antigens. The CD34$^+$ cell population in the bone marrow of patients with acquired aplastic anemia can be 10% or lower than that seen in healthy individuals.[17] In addition, these CD34$^+$ cells have increased expression of Fas receptors that mediate apoptosis and increased expression of apoptosis-related genes.[18-20]

Bone marrow stromal cells are functionally normal in acquired aplastic anemia. They produce normal or even increased quantities of growth factors and are able to support the growth of CD34$^+$ cells from healthy donors in culture and in vivo after transplantation.[4,21] Individuals with aplastic anemia also have

---

BOX 19.3 Selected Drugs Reported to Have a Rare Association With Idiosyncratic Secondary Aplastic Anemia

Antiarthritics
Gold compounds
Penicillamine

Antibiotics
Chloramphenicol
Sulfonamides

Anticonvulsants
Carbamazepine
Hydantoins
Phenacemide

Antidepressants
Dothiepin
Phenothiazine

Antidiabetic Agents
Chlorpropamide
Tolbutamide
Carbutamide

Antiinflammatories (Nonsteroidal)
Diclofenac
Fenbufen

Fenoprofen
Ibuprofen
Indomethacin
Naproxen
Phenylbutazone
Piroxicam
Sulindac

Antiprotozoals
Chloroquine
Quinacrine

Antithyroidals
Methimazole
Methylthiouracil

Carbonic Anhydrase Inhibitors
Methazolamide
Mesalazine
Acetazolamide

elevated serum levels of erythropoietin, thrombopoietin, granulocyte colony-stimulating factor (G-CSF), and granulocyte-macrophage colony-stimulating factor (GM-CSF).[22] In addition, serum levels of FLT3 ligand, a growth factor that stimulates proliferation of stem and progenitor cells, is up to 200 times higher in patients with severe aplastic anemia compared with healthy controls.[22,23] However, despite their elevated levels, growth factors are generally unsuccessful in correcting the cytopenias found in acquired aplastic anemia.

The severe depletion of hematopoietic stem and progenitor cells from the bone marrow may be due to direct damage to stem cells, immune damage to stem cells, or other unknown mechanisms. Direct damage to stem and progenitor cells results from deoxyribonucleic acid (DNA) injury after exposure to cytotoxic drugs, chemicals, radiation, or viruses.[4]

Immune damage to stem cells results from exposure to drugs, chemicals, viruses, or other agents that cause an autoimmune cytotoxic T lymphocytic destruction of stem and progenitor cells.[24] An autoimmune pathophysiology was first suggested in the 1970s when aplastic anemia patients undergoing pretransplant immunosuppressive conditioning had an improvement in cell counts.[25] Further evidence supporting an autoimmune pathophysiology include (1) elevated blood and bone marrow cytotoxic (CD8[+]) T lymphocytes with an oligoclonal expansion of specific T cell clones[26]; (2) increased T cell production of such cytokines as IFN-γ and tumor necrosis factor-α (TNF-α), which inhibit hematopoiesis and induce apoptosis[27-29]; (3) upregulation of T-bet, a transcription factor that binds to the promoter of the IFN-γ gene[30]; (4) increased TNF-α receptors on CD34[+] cells[31]; and (5) improvement in cytopenias after immunosuppressive therapy (IST).[4,24] Approximately two-thirds of patients with acquired aplastic anemia respond to IST.[32] The nonresponders may have a severely depleted stem cell compartment or other pathophysiologic factors contributing to their cytopenias.[32]

Possible autoimmune mechanisms include mutation of stem cell antigens and disruption of immune regulation. Young and colleagues showed that environmental exposures may alter self-proteins, induce expression of abnormal or novel antigens, or induce an immune response that cross-reacts with self-antigens.[24,28] Solomou and colleagues. demonstrated that CD4[+]CD25[+]FOXP3[+] regulatory T cells are decreased in aplastic anemia.[33] These regulatory T cells normally suppress autoreactive T cells, and a deficit of these cells may facilitate an autoimmune reaction. Furthermore, a number of individuals with aplastic anemia have single nucleotide polymorphisms in IFN-γ/[+]874 TT, TNF-α/−308 AA, transforming growth factor-β1/−509 TT, and interleukin-6/−174 GG.[34] These polymorphisms result in cytokine overproduction and may impart a genetic susceptibility to aplastic anemia as well as contribute to its severity.[34]

The specific antigens responsible for triggering and sustaining the autoimmune attack on stem cells are unknown. Candidate antigens have been identified from aplastic anemia patient sera, including kinectin,[35] diazepam-binding inhibitor-related protein 1,[36] and moesin.[37] These proteins are expressed in hematopoietic progenitor cells, but their role in the pathogenesis of aplastic anemia requires further investigation.

Approximately one-third of patients with acquired aplastic anemia have shortened telomeres in their peripheral blood granulocytes compared with age-matched controls.[38,39] Telomeres protect the ends of chromosomes from damage and erosion, and cells with abnormally short telomeres undergo proliferation arrest and premature apoptosis. Telomerase is an enzyme complex that repairs and maintains telomeres. Approximately 10% of patients with acquired aplastic anemia and shortened telomeres have a mutation in the telomerase complex gene for either the ribonucleic acid (RNA) template (TERC) or the reverse transcriptase (TERT).[39-41] The cause for shortened telomeres in the other 90% of patients may be due to stress hematopoiesis or other yet unidentified mutations.[39] In stress hematopoiesis there is an increase in progenitor cell turnover, and the telomeres become shorter with each cell division.

Approximately 4% of patients with acquired aplastic anemia and shortened telomeres have mutations in the Shwachman-Bodian-Diamond syndrome (SBDS) gene.[42] The SBDS gene product is involved in ribosome biogenesis, and its relationship to telomere maintenance is currently unknown.[42] TERT/TERC and SBDS mutations also occur in the inherited bone marrow failure syndromes dyskeratosis congenita (DC) and SBDS, respectively, and some patients diagnosed with acquired aplastic anemia who have these mutations may actually have DC or SBDS.[3,4] Correct differentiation between acquired aplastic anemia and inherited bone marrow failure syndromes has important implications for appropriate treatment and prognosis. Immunosuppressive therapy is not nearly as effective in inherited bone marrow failure compared with acquired aplastic anemia. Furthermore, hematopoietic stem cell transplantation, the only known curative treatment for DC and SBDS and a treatment option for acquired aplastic anemia, should not be performed with HLA-matched siblings who test positive for the same genetic mutation.[39] Shortened telomeres occur more often in patients whose pancytopenia does not respond to immunosuppressive therapy.[43] Defective telomere maintenance may be another pathophysiologic mechanism of stem cell injury, imparting susceptibility to aplastic anemia after an environmental insult.[39,41]

Clinical Findings

Symptoms vary in acquired aplastic anemia, ranging from asymptomatic to severe. Patients usually present with symptoms of insidious-onset anemia, with pallor, fatigue, and weakness. Severe and prolonged anemia can result in serious cardiovascular complications, including tachycardia, hypotension, cardiac failure, and death. Symptoms of thrombocytopenia are also varied and include petechiae, bruising, epistaxis, mucosal bleeding, menorrhagia, retinal hemorrhages, intestinal bleeding, and intracranial hemorrhage. Fever and bacterial or fungal infections are unusual at initial presentation but may occur after prolonged periods of neutropenia. Splenomegaly and hepatomegaly are typically absent.

Laboratory Findings

Pancytopenia is typical, although initially only one or two cell lines may be decreased. The absolute neutrophil count is

TABLE 19.1   Diagnostic Criteria for Aplastic Anemia

	MAA	SAA	VSAA
Bone marrow	Hypocellular bone marrow plus at least two of the following:	Bone marrow cellularity < 25%,* plus at least two of the following:	Same as SAA
Neutrophils ($\times 10^9$/L)	0.5–1.5	0.2–0.5	<0.2
Platelets ($\times 10^9$/L)	20–50	<20	Same as SAA
Other	HGB ≤ 10 g/dL plus reticulocytes < 30 × 10^9/L	Reticulocytes < 20 × 10^9/L or < 1% corrected for HCT	Same as SAA

*Or 25% to 50% cellularity with < 30% residual hematopoietic cells.
HCT, Hematocrit; *HGB,* hemoglobin; *MAA,* moderate aplastic anemia; *SAA,* severe aplastic anemia; *VSAA,* very severe aplastic anemia.

decreased, and the absolute lymphocyte count may be normal or decreased. The hemoglobin is usually less than 10 g/dL, the mean cell volume (MCV) is increased or normal, and the percent and absolute reticulocyte counts are decreased. Table 19.1 lists the diagnostic criteria for aplastic anemia by degree of severity.[6,8,44,45]

Neutrophils, monocytes, and platelets are decreased in the peripheral blood, and the RBCs are macrocytic or normocytic (Figure 19.1). Toxic granulation may be observed in the neutrophils, but the RBCs and platelets are usually normal in appearance. Leukemic blasts and other immature blood cells are characteristically absent. The serum iron level and percent transferrin saturation may be increased, which reflects decreased iron use for erythropoiesis. Liver function test results may be abnormal in cases of hepatitis-associated aplastic anemia.

Approximately two-thirds of patients have small numbers (less than 25%) of PNH clones in the peripheral blood,[46] but only 10% of patients develop a sufficient number of PNH cells to have the clinical and biochemical manifestations of PNH

disease.[16] PNH is characterized by an acquired stem cell mutation resulting in lack of the glycosylphosphatidylinositol (GPI)-linked proteins CD55 and CD59. The absence of CD55 and CD59 on the surface of the RBCs renders them more susceptible to complement-mediated cell lysis. It is important to test for PNH in acquired aplastic anemia because of the increased risk of hemolytic or thrombotic complications (Chapter 21). Historically, PNH diagnosis depended on the Ham acid hemolysis test: Patients' cells were placed in acidified serum, and a positive result demonstrated lysis of RBCs. However, this test was poorly sensitive, because complement-mediated hemolysis was detected only in the presence of large numbers of circulating PNH cells. The Ham test has been replaced by flow cytometric analysis for proteins linked to the GPI anchor; CD55 and CD59 on RBCs, and CD24 and CD14 on granulocytes and monocytes.[8,46,47] In addition, flow cytometry for the GPI anchor (FLAER assay) is the newest and most sensitive assay for detecting PNH cells among granulocytes (Chapter 21).[48]

Bone marrow aspirate and biopsy specimens have prominent fat cells with areas of patchy marrow cellularity. Biopsy specimens are required for accurate quantitative assessment of marrow cellularity, and severe hypocellularity is a characteristic feature of aplastic anemia (Figure 19.2). Erythroid, granulocytic, and megakaryocytic cells are decreased or absent.

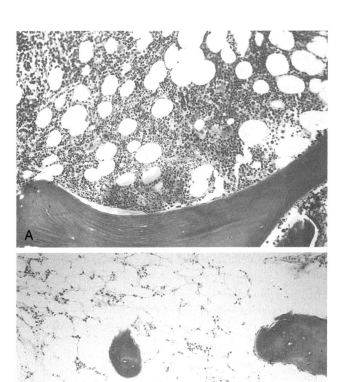

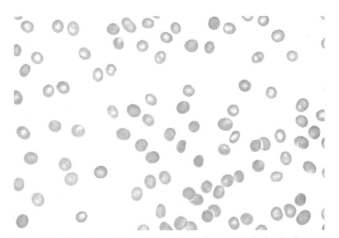

Figure 19.1 Peripheral Blood Film of a Patient with Aplastic Anemia. Note occasional macrocytes and absence of white blood cells and platelets. (Wright-Giemsa stain, ×1000.)

Figure 19.2 Biopsy of Normal and Hypoplastic Bone Marrow. (A), Normal bone marrow tissue section. **(B),** Hypoplastic bone marrow tissue section from a patient with aplastic anemia. (A, B, Hematoxylin and eosin stain, ×100.) (Courtesy Ann Bell, University of Tennessee, Memphis.)

Dyserythropoiesis may be present, but there is typically no dysplasia of the granulocyte or platelet cell lines. Blasts and other abnormal cell infiltrates are characteristically absent. Reticulin staining is usually normal.

In patients receiving immunosuppressive therapy, the risk of developing an abnormal karyotype is 14% at 5 years and 20% at 10 years.[49] Monosomy 7 and trisomy 8 are the most common cytogenetic abnormalities.[47,49] Cytogenetic analysis using conventional culture techniques often underestimates the incidence of karyotype abnormalities because of bone marrow hypocellularity and scarcity of cells in metaphase.[50] Alternatively, interphase fluorescence in situ hybridization (FISH) using DNA probes for specific chromosome abnormalities may be used. In comparison to conventional cytogenetic analysis, FISH has greater sensitivity in the detection of chromosome abnormalities and can also be performed using nondividing cells.[50] In a study performed by Kearns and colleagues, FISH detected monosomy 7 or trisomy 8 in 26% of aplastic anemia patients who had a normal karyotype by conventional cytogenetic testing.[50]

Patients with an inherited bone marrow failure syndrome may be misdiagnosed with acquired aplastic anemia if symptoms manifest in late adolescence or adulthood or if the patients lack the typical clinical and physical characteristics of an inherited marrow failure syndrome (e.g., abnormal thumbs, short stature).[3,4] Consideration of inherited bone marrow failure syndromes in the differential diagnosis of acquired aplastic anemia is essential because these conditions require a different therapeutic approach. The inherited bone marrow failure syndromes are discussed later in the chapter.

Treatment and Prognosis

Severe acquired aplastic anemia requires immediate attention to prevent serious complications. If a causative agent is identified, its use should be discontinued. Blood product replacement should be given judiciously to avoid alloimmunization.[8] Platelets should not be transfused at counts greater than 10,000/μL, unless the patient is bleeding.[8]

One of the most important early decisions is determining whether the patient is a candidate for bone marrow transplantation (BMT). BMT is the treatment of choice for patients with severe aplastic anemia who are younger than 40 years of age and have an HLA-identical sibling.[4,8] Unfortunately, only 20% to 30% of patients meet these criteria.[4] Therefore, IST, consisting of antithymocyte globulin and cyclosporine, is used for patients older than 40 years of age and for patients without an HLA-identical sibling.[8,16] Antithymocyte globulin decreases the number of activated T cells, and cyclosporine inhibits T cell function, thereby suppressing the autoimmune reaction against the stem cells. For patients with severe acquired aplastic anemia who are not responsive to IST, BMT from a high-resolution HLA-matched unrelated donor is an option.[8,51] With advances in modern transplantation protocols, overall survival rates are now only slightly lower with high-resolution HLA-matched unrelated donors compared with HLA-matched siblings.[4] The response rate for a second course of IST is approximately 65% for those who experienced relapse and only 30% for those whose disorder was initially refractive to IST.[52] Individuals with

PNH cells (CD55− CD59−) are almost twice as likely to respond to IST than are those who lack these cells.[46] In addition, the presence of both PNH cells and HLA-DR2 increases the likelihood of response by 3.5-fold.[53] G-CSF, other hematopoietic growth factors, and steroids do not increase overall survival or improve the response rate; therefore they are not recommended for routine use.[8,54,55]

There have been promising results from a phase 1/2 study evaluating the addition of eltrombopag, a thrombopoietin mimetic, to standard IST for severe aplastic anemia, with higher hematologic response in study patients compared with historical cohorts.[56] Eltrombopag's mechanism of action in aplastic anemia is unclear but may be due to stimulatory effects on stem and progenitor cells. Further studies are currently underway to evaluate the efficacy of eltrombopag in pediatric severe aplastic anemia.

Other supportive therapy includes antibiotic and antifungal prophylaxis in cases of prolonged neutropenia. Patients with mild to moderate aplastic anemia may not require treatment but must be monitored periodically for pancytopenia and abnormal cells.

The overall outcome for patients with acquired aplastic anemia has dramatically improved in the past two decades. Children have higher survival rates compared with adults with both BMT and IST as first-line treatment.[51] With BMT, the 10-year survival for those aged 1 to 20 and those older than 40 years is 86% and 56%, respectively; with IST, 10-year survival for those same age groups is 84%, and 58%, respectively.[51] Additional outcomes in the IST-treated patients include a 10-year risk of developing hemolytic or thrombotic PNH and a 10% to 20% risk of myelodysplastic syndrome (MDS) or leukemia.[16,47] Development of monosomy 7 predicts poor outcome, with a greater likelihood of unresponsiveness to IST and progression to MDS or leukemia.[49]

Inherited/Congenital Bone Marrow Failure Syndromes

Compared with acquired aplastic anemia, patients with inherited/congenital bone marrow failure syndromes present at an earlier age and may have characteristic physical stigmata. The three most common inherited/congenital bone marrow failure disorders associated with pancytopenia are Fanconi anemia, dyskeratosis congenita, and Shwachman-Bodian-Diamond syndrome.

Fanconi Anemia

Fanconi anemia (FA) is a chromosome instability disorder characterized by aplastic anemia, physical abnormalities, and cancer susceptibility. In 1927 Dr. Guido Fanconi first described this syndrome in three brothers with skin pigmentation, short stature, and hypogonadism.[57] FA has a prevalence of 1 to 5 cases per million.[58] The carrier rate is 1 in 300 in the United States and Europe, with a threefold higher prevalence in Ashkenazi Jews and South African Africaners.[59] FA is the most common of the inherited bone marrow failure syndromes.

Clinical findings. Patients with FA have variable features and symptoms. Physical malformations may be present at birth, though hematologic abnormalities may not appear until older childhood or adulthood. Furthermore, only two-thirds of patients have physical malformations.[3,58,60] These anomalies vary considerably, though there is a higher frequency of skeletal abnormalities (thumb malformations, radial hypoplasia, microcephaly, hip dislocation, and scoliosis); skin pigmentation (hyperpigmentation, hypopigmentation, café-au-lait lesions); short stature; and abnormalities of the eyes, kidneys, and genitals.[58-60] Low birth weight and developmental delay are also common.

The symptoms associated with pancytopenia usually become apparent at 5 to 10 years of age, though some patients may not present until adulthood.[3,59] Individuals with FA also have an increased cancer risk. This includes an increased incidence of leukemia in childhood and solid tumors (e.g., oral, esophageal, anogenital, cervical) in adulthood.[61] In approximately 5% of cases a malignancy is diagnosed before the FA is recognized.[61]

Genetics and pathophysiology. Patients with FA typically have biallelic mutations or deletions in one of at least 21 genes: *FANCA, FANCB, FANCC, FANCD1 (BRCA2), FANCD2, FANCE, FANCF, FANCG (XRCC9), FANCI, FANCJ (BRIP1/ BACH1), FANCL, FANCM, FANCN (PALB2), FANCO (RAD51C), FANCP (SLX4), FANCQ (ERCC4 or XPF), FANCR (RAD51), FANCS (BRCA1), FANCT (UBE2T), FANCU (XRCC2),* and *FANCV* (MAD2L2, REV7).[58,62] The mode of inheritance is autosomal recessive except for *FANCB*, which is X-linked recessive. Mutations in the *FANCA* gene occur with the highest frequency (60%); this is followed by *FANCC* (14%) and *FANCG* (10%), whereas mutations in the other *FANC* genes are much less common.[3,60,63] The relationship between mutations in the FA genes and disease pathology is not clear. Cells are highly susceptible to chromosome breakage after exposure to DNA cross-linking agents. FA cells may also have accelerated telomere shortening and apoptosis, a late S-phase cell cycle delay, hypersensitivity to oxidants, and cytokine dysregulation.[3,58,60,64]

The range of FA protein function is not completely known, but these proteins participate in a highly elaborate DNA damage response pathway. The FA pathway consists of a nuclear core complex, a protein ID complex, and effector proteins.[60,64] The FA proteins A, B, C, E, F, G, L, and M form the nuclear core complex; proteins D2 and I form the ID complex; and the effector proteins are D1, J, N, O, P, Q, R, S, T, U, and V.[60,62,64] The core complex facilitates the monoubiquitylation and activation of the ID complex. The ID complex then localizes with effector DNA repair proteins at foci of DNA damage to effect DNA repair.[60,64]

Laboratory findings. Laboratory results are similar to those in acquired aplastic anemia, with pancytopenia, reticulocytopenia, and a hypocellular bone marrow. Macrocytic RBCs are often the first detected abnormality, and thrombocytopenia usually precedes the development of the other cytopenias.[58] Fetal hemoglobin (Hb F) may be strikingly elevated, and α-fetoprotein is also increased.[58]

Chromosomal breakage analysis is the diagnostic test for Fanconi anemia.[58] Patients' peripheral blood lymphocytes are cultured with the DNA cross-linking agents diepoxybutane (DEB) or mitomycin C (MMC). Compared with normal lymphocytes, FA cells have a greater number of characteristic chromosome breaks and ring chromosomes, indicating increased fragility.[3,58] Caution must be taken in interpreting peripheral blood results because they may be negative in the 10% to 15% of FA patients who have somatic mosaicism as a result of a reversion of one abnormal allele to the normal type.[3,58] Chromosome breakage studies can be performed on cultured skin fibroblasts from a skin biopsy specimen in these cases.[58,65] Diagnosis is confirmed by genetic testing for FA gene mutations or deletions.[58]

Treatment and prognosis. More than 90% of FA patients develop bone marrow failure by 40 years of age.[61] Furthermore, one-third of patients develop MDS and/or acute myeloid leukemia (AML) by a median age of 14 years, and 25% develop solid tumors by a median age of 26 years.[61,66] Squamous cell carcinomas of the head and neck, anogenital region, and skin are the most common solid tumors, followed by tumors of the liver, brain, and kidney.[61] Patients with FA have an increased risk of developing vulvar cancer (4300-fold), esophageal cancer (2300-fold), AML (800-fold), and head/neck cancer (700-fold) compared with the general population.[67] Approximately 3% of patients develop more than one type of malignancy.[66] Left untreated, death by 20 years of age secondary to bone marrow failure or malignancy is common. Patients with mutations in the *FANCC* gene experience bone marrow failure at a particularly young age and have the poorest survival.[58,66] Increased telomere shortening in FA cells is associated with more severe pancytopenia and a higher risk of malignancy. However, the precise role of telomere shortening in the evolution of bone marrow failure and cancer is currently unclear.[68]

Supportive treatment for cytopenia includes transfusions and administration of cytokines (G-CSF and GM-CSF).[58,59] The only curative treatment is hematopoietic stem cell transplant, preferably from an HLA-identical sibling, although high-resolution (molecular) HLA-matched unrelated donors can be used with almost the same success rate.[69] It is important to screen donor siblings for FA with DNA breakage studies and gene mutation analysis before transplant. Patients should also have decreased intensity pretransplant conditioning because of their underlying chromosomal instability.[58,66] Gene therapy has been attempted in clinical trials but has not been successful.

Dyskeratosis Congenita
DC is a rare inherited bone marrow failure syndrome with an incidence of approximately 4 cases per million per year.[58,70]

Clinical findings. DC is characterized by mucocutaneous abnormalities, bone marrow failure, and pancytopenia. The typical clinical presentation involves a triad of abnormal skin pigmentation, dystrophic nails, and oral leukoplakia. Skin and nail findings usually appear before 10 years of age.[3,58] By age 30, 80% to 90% of patients have bone marrow abnormalities.[3] Patients can also manifest a wide range of multisystem abnormalities, including pulmonary fibrosis, liver disease, developmental delay, short stature, microcephaly, prematurely gray hair or hair loss, immunodeficiency, dental caries, and periodontal disease.[58,71] Patients have a 40% risk of cancer by age 50, most commonly AML, MDS, and epithelial malignancies.[70]

Genetics and pathophysiology. DC chromosomes have very short telomeres, and inherited defects in the telomerase complex are implicated in the pathophysiology.[71] The telomerase complex synthesizes telomere repeats to elongate chromosome ends, maintaining the telomere length needed for cell survival.

Patients with DC typically have mutations in one of at least 11 genes. The mode of inheritance is X-linked recessive, autosomal dominant, or autosomal recessive.[3,58,71] The best-characterized form results from one or more mutations on the long arm of the X-chromosome on the *DKC1* gene coding for dyskerin. Dyskerin is a ribonucleoprotein involved in RNA processing, and it associates with TERC (telomerase RNA component) in the telomerase complex. Autosomal dominant forms are mainly caused by mutations in the genes that encode TERC, TERT (telomerase enzyme), or TINF2 (component of the shelterin complex that regulates telomere length).[58,71] In the autosomal recessive form, mutations in *TERT, RTEL1, ACD, CTC1, NHP2, NOP10, PARN,* and *WRAP53* have been identified.[58,71] The proteins encoded by these genes are also involved in telomere maintenance. Although the exact pathophysiologic mechanisms are still unknown, the shortened telomeres in DC cause premature death in the rapidly dividing cells in the bone marrow and epithelium and likely lead to genomic instability and a predisposition to cancer.[3,58,72]

Laboratory findings. Pancytopenia and macrocytic RBCs are typical peripheral blood findings. The fetal hemoglobin level may also be increased. About 75% of patients have an identified mutation in one of the 11 telomerase complex genes and can be diagnosed by genetic testing.[58,71] A flow cytometry FISH (flow-FISH) test for detection of very short telomeres in WBC subsets is used as a diagnostic test for those with suspected DC who lack mutations in known genes.[72] Patients with FA, SBDS, and acquired aplastic anemia may also have cells with shortened telomeres, though they are not found in multiple WBC subsets.[72] In contrast, DC cells often have shortened telomeres in several WBC subsets, including naive T cells and B cells.[72]

Treatment and prognosis. Median survival for patients with DC is 42 years.[70] Approximately 60% to 70% of deaths are due to bone marrow failure complications. Approximately 10% to 15% of deaths result from severe pulmonary disease, and 10% of deaths result from malignancies.[3,58] Treatment with hematopoietic stem cell transplantation has not been optimal because of the high incidence of fatal pulmonary fibrosis and vascular complications.[3] Although androgen therapy produces a transient response in 50% to 70% of patients, it does not halt the progression of the bone marrow failure.[3]

Shwachman-Bodian-Diamond Syndrome

SBDS is a multisystem disorder characterized by pancreatic insufficiency, cytopenia, skeletal abnormalities, and a predisposition for hematologic malignancies. The incidence has been estimated to be approximately 8.5 cases per 1 million live births.[58]

Clinical findings. Patients with SBDS have peripheral blood cytopenia and decreased pancreatic enzyme secretion.[45] The pancreatic insufficiency causes gastrointestinal malabsorption, which typically presents in early infancy.[3] Patients have neutropenia and immune dysfunction and are at increased risk of severe infections and sepsis.[45,73] Nearly all SBDS patients have delayed bone maturation, and approximately 50% have failure to thrive and short stature.[45,74]

Genetics and pathophysiology. SBDS is an autosomal recessive disorder, and 90% of patients have biallelic mutations in the *SBDS* gene.[3,45,73] The *SBDS* gene is involved in ribosome biogenesis and mitotic spindle stability,[71,75] but its relationship to the disease manifestations is currently unknown. There are quantitative and qualitative deficiencies in CD34$^+$ cells, dysfunctional bone marrow stromal cells, increased apoptosis and mitotic spindle destabilization in hematopoietic cells, and short telomeres in peripheral blood granulocytes.[3,45,73,75]

Laboratory findings. Nearly all patients with SBDS have neutropenia (less than 1.5×10^9 neutrophils/L).[76] Half of patients also develop anemia or thrombocytopenia, and one fourth develop pancytopenia.[76] The RBCs are usually normocytic but can be macrocytic, and approximately two-thirds of patients have elevated Hb F.[45,76] Bone marrow is usually hypocellular but can be normal or even hypercellular. Because of pancreatic insufficiency, 72-hour fecal fat testing shows increased fat excretion, and serum trypsinogen and isoamylase levels are decreased compared with age-related reference intervals.[73] Compared with cystic fibrosis, which can have a similar malabsorption presentation, patients with SBDS have normal sweat chloride tests. Testing for the *SBDS* gene mutation is commercially available and should be done in suspected patients and their parents.

Treatment and prognosis. In some cases no treatment of hematologic features is needed. However, if needed, treatment consists of G-CSF for neutropenia, transfusion support for anemia and thrombocytopenia, and enzyme replacement for pancreatic insufficiency. The risk of AML and MDS is approximately 19% at 20 years and 36% at 30 years.[77] Allogeneic stem cell transplantation is recommended in cases of severe pancytopenia, AML, or MDS. Unfortunately, despite supportive care and attempted curative therapy, 5-year overall survival is 60% to 65%, with many deaths occurring from severe infections and malignancy.[45,73] Poor outcomes after transplant occur as a result of graft failure, transplant-related toxicities, and recurrent leukemia.[73]

Differential Diagnosis

A distinction must be made between acquired aplastic anemia, inherited/congenital bone marrow failure syndromes, and other causes of pancytopenia, including PNH, MDS, megaloblastic anemia, and leukemia. The importance of a correct diagnosis is clear because diagnostic conclusions dictate therapeutic management and prognosis. The distinguishing features of these conditions are listed in Tables 19.2 and 19.3.[3,8]

Alternative diagnoses include lymphoma, myelofibrosis, and mycobacterial infections, which also may present with pancytopenia. However, these diagnoses often can be distinguished with a careful history, physical examination, and laboratory testing. Review of a peripheral blood film by an experienced

TABLE 19.2 Differentiation of Aplastic Anemia From Other Causes of Pancytopenia

Condition	Peripheral Blood	Bone Marrow	Laboratory Test Results	Clinical Findings
Failure of Bone Marrow to Produce Blood Cells				
Aplastic anemia	No immature WBCs or RBCs; ↓ reticulocytes; MCV ↑ or normal	Hypocellular; blasts and abnormal cells absent; reticulin normal; RBC dyspoiesis may be present; WBC and platelet dyspoiesis absent	Acquired: PNH cells* may be present; chromosome abnormalities may be present Inherited/congenital: Table 19.3	Splenomegaly absent
Increased Destruction of Blood Cells				
PNH	Reticulocytes ↑; MCV ↑ or normal; nucleated RBCs present or absent	Erythroid hyperplasia; may be hypocellular	PNH cells* present; hemoglobinuria +/−; chromosome abnormalities may be present	Splenomegaly absent; thrombosis may be present
Ineffective Hematopoiesis				
Myelodysplastic syndrome	Variable pancytopenia; reticulocytes ↓; MCV ↑ or normal; blasts and abnormal WBCs, RBCs, and platelets may be present	Hypercellular; 20% of cases hypocellular; dyspoiesis in one or more cell lines present; blasts and immature cells present; reticulin ↑	Chromosome abnormalities usually present	Splenomegaly uncommon
Megaloblastic anemias	MCV ↑; oval macrocytes; hypersegmented neutrophils	Hypercellular with megaloblastic features	Serum vitamin B₁₂ or folate or both ↓	Splenomegaly absent
Bone Marrow Infiltration				
Acute leukemia	Blasts present	Hypercellular; blasts ↑; reticulin ↑	Chromosome abnormalities usually present	Splenomegaly may be present
Hairy cell leukemia	Hairy cells present; monocytes ↓	Hairy cells† and fibrosis present; reticulin ↑	Hairy cells present; TRAP +	Splenomegaly present (60%–70% of cases)

↑, Increased; ↓, decreased; +, positive result; +/−, positive or negative result; *MCV*, mean cell volume; *PNH*, paroxysmal nocturnal hemoglobinuria; *RBC*, red blood cell; *TRAP*, tartrate-resistant acid phosphatase; *WBC*, white blood cell.
*PNH erythrocytes are detected by flow cytometry by their lack of expression of CD59; PNH granulocytes and monocytes lack CD24 and CD14 (Chapter 21).
†Hairy cells are detected by flow cytometry by their expression of CD19, CD20, CD22, CD11c, CD25, CD103, and FMC7.

TABLE 19.3 Key Characteristics of Inherited/Congenital Bone Marrow Failure Anemias

Condition	Genetics*	Peripheral Blood	Bone Marrow	Laboratory Test Results	Clinical Findings
Caused by Bone Marrow Hypoplasia					
FA	AR (most), XLR; mutations identified in at least 21 genes	Pancytopenia; reticulocytes ↓; MCV ↑	Hypocellular with ↓ in all cell lines	Chromosome breakage with DEB/MMC; majority have mutations or deletions in FA genes; *FANCA* mutations occur with highest frequency (60%); Hb F may be ↑	Physical malformations may be present; risk of cancers, leukemia, MDS
DC	AR, XLR, AD; mutations identified in at least 11 genes	Pancytopenia; reticulocytes ↓; MCV ↑	Hypocellular with ↓ in all cell lines	75% have mutations or deletions in DC genes; *DKC1* mutations occur with highest frequency (30%); very short telomeres in WBC subsets by flow-FISH; Hb F may be ↑	Physical malformations may be present; pulmonary disease; risk of cancers, leukemia, MDS
SBDS	AR; mutations identified in 1 gene	Neutropenia; pancytopenia (25% of cases); reticulocytes ↓; MCV ↑ or normal	Hypocellular, normocellular, or hypercellular	90% have mutations in *SBDS* gene; serum trypsinogen and isoamylase ↓ for age; Hb F may be ↑	Pancreatic insufficiency; physical malformations may be present; risk of infections, leukemia, MDS
DBA	AD (most); XLR; mutations identified in at least 17 genes	Anemia; reticulocytes ↓; MCV ↑	Erythroid hypoplasia	70% have mutations or deletions in DBA genes; *RPS19* mutations occur with highest frequency (25%); erythrocyte adenosine deaminase ↑; Hb F may be ↑	Physical malformations may be present; risk of cancers, leukemia, MDS

Continued

TABLE 19.3 Key Characteristics of Inherited/Congenital Bone Marrow Failure Anemias—cont'd

Condition	Genetics*	Peripheral Blood	Bone Marrow	Laboratory Test Results	Clinical Findings
Caused by Ineffective Hematopoiesis					
CDA I	AR; mutations identified in at least 2 genes	Anemia; reticulocytes ↓; MCV ↑; poik, baso stipp, Cabot rings	Hypercellular; erythroid precursors megaloblastoid with internuclear chromatin bridges and < 5% binucleated forms	Mutations in *CDAN1* or *C15orf41* genes; spongy, "Swiss cheese" heterochromatin in erythroblasts by electron microscopy	Physical malformations may be present; iron overload; splenomegaly; hepatomegaly
CDA II	AR; mutations identified in at least 1 gene	Anemia; reticulocytes ↓; MCV normal; poik, baso stipp	Hypercellular; erythroid precursors normoblastic with 10%–35% binucleated forms	Mutations in *SEC23B* gene; positive Ham test (no longer done)	Physical malformations may be present; iron overload; jaundice; gallstones; splenomegaly
CDA III	AD; mutations identified in at least 1 gene	Mild anemia; reticulocytes ↓; MCV ↑; poik, baso stipp	Hypercellular; erythroid precursors megaloblastoid with giant multinucleated forms with up to 12 nuclei	Mutations in *KIF23* gene	Treatment usually not needed

↑, Increased; ↓, decreased; *AD*, autosomal dominant; *AR*, autosomal recessive; *baso stipp*, basophilic stippling; *CDA*, congenital dyserythropoietic anemia; *DBA*, Diamond-Blackfan anemia; *DC*, dyskeratosis congenita; *DEB*, diepoxybutane; *FA*, Fanconi anemia; *flow-FISH*, flow cytometry with fluorescence in situ hybridization; *Hb F*, fetal hemoglobin; *MCV*, mean cell volume; *MDS*, myelodysplastic syndrome; *MMC*, mitomycin C; *poik*, poikilocytosis; *RBC*, red blood cell; *SBDS*, Shwachman-Bodian-Diamond syndrome; *SDS-PAGE*, sodium dodecyl sulfate polyacrylamide gel electrophoresis; *XLR*, X-linked recessive.
*Gene mutations identified as of 2017; genetic discovery is ongoing.

morphologist is important. If needed, bone marrow evaluation and molecular testing for chromosome abnormalities and gene mutations can further distinguish these diagnoses. Anorexia nervosa also may present with pancytopenia. In these cases the bone marrow is hypocellular and has a decreased number of fat cells.[8] The cytopenias revert with correction of the underlying disease.

OTHER FORMS OF BONE MARROW FAILURE

Pure Red Cell Aplasia

Pure red cell aplasia (PRCA) is a rare disorder of erythropoiesis characterized by a selective and severe decrease in erythroid precursors in an otherwise normal bone marrow. Patients have severe anemia (usually normocytic), reticulocytopenia, and normal WBC and platelet counts. PRCA may be acquired or congenital. It is important to distinguish between acquired and congenital forms because they require different therapeutic approaches.

Acquired Pure Red Cell Aplasia

Acquired PRCA may occur in children or adults and can be acute or chronic. Primary PRCA may be idiopathic or autoimmune-related. Secondary PRCA may occur in association with an underlying thymoma, hematologic malignancy, solid tumor, infection, chronic hemolytic anemia, collagen vascular disease, or exposure to drugs or chemicals.[78,79] Therapy is first directed at treatment of the underlying condition, but IST may be considered if the PRCA is not responsive. Cyclosporine is associated with a higher response rate (65% to 87%) than

corticosteroids (30% to 62%) and is better suited for long-term maintenance if needed.[79]

The acquired form of PRCA in young children is also known as *transient erythroblastopenia of childhood* (TEC). A history of viral infection is found in half of patients, which is thought to trigger an immune mechanism that targets red cell production.[80] The anemia is typically normocytic, and Hb F and erythrocyte adenosine deaminase levels usually are normal.[78,80] Red cell transfusion support is the mainstay of therapy if the child is symptomatic from anemia. Normalization of erythropoiesis occurs within weeks in the vast majority patients.[80] There may be a genetic predisposition to TEC in some families.[80]

Congenital Pure Red Cell Aplasia: Diamond-Blackfan Anemia

Diamond-Blackfan anemia (DBA) is a congenital erythroid hypoplastic disorder of early infancy with an estimated incidence of 7 to 10 cases per million live births.[58] Mutations have been identified in at least 17 genes: those that encode structural ribosome proteins, *RPS7*, *RPS10*, *RPS17*, *RPS19*, *RPS24*, *RPS26*, *RPS27*, *RPS28*, and *RPS29* in the 40S subunit and *RPL5*, *RPL11*, *RPL15*, *RPL26*, *RPL27*, *RPL31*, and *RPL35A* in the 60S subunit, as well as the gene encoding *GATA1*, a transcription factor important for hematopoieisis.[58,71,81] Mutations in the *RPS19* gene occur with the highest frequency (25%), followed by *RPL11* and *RPS26* (approximately 6% each); the other known mutations are uncommon.[71,81,82] An additional 15% to 20% of cases can be accounted for by haplo-deletions of these same ribosome genes, but many mutations still remain unidentified.[58,83] Nearly 50% of DBA mutations are linked to an autosomal dominant inheritance pattern, less than 1% with an X-linked recessive pattern (*GATA1*), and sporadic mutations have also been reported.[58,71,81] Mutations in ribosomal proteins disrupt ribosome biogenesis in DBA, but the pathophysiologic mechanisms leading to the clinical manifestations are currently unknown.

More than 90% of patients show signs of the disorder during the first year of life, with a median age of 8 weeks; however, some patients with DBA are asymptomatic until adulthood.[84] Approximately half of patients have characteristic physical anomalies, including craniofacial dysmorphisms, short stature, and neck and thumb malformations.[58,84]

The characteristic peripheral blood finding is a severe macrocytic anemia with reticulocytopenia.[58] The WBC count is normal or slightly decreased, and the platelet count is normal or slightly increased. Bone marrow examination distinguishes DBA from the hypocellular marrow in aplastic anemia, because there is normal cellularity of myeloid cells and megakaryocytes and hypoplasia of erythroid cells. The karyotype in DBA is usually normal, and genetic testing can identify a DBA-related mutation in about 70% of patients.[58] In most cases, Hb F and erythrocyte adenosine deaminase are increased; these findings distinguish DBA from TEC, in which these levels are normal.[58,81] Other features distinguishing DBA from TEC are detailed in Table 19.4.

Therapy includes RBC transfusions and corticosteroids. Although 50% to 75% of patients respond to corticosteroid therapy, side effects can be severe with long-term use, including immunosuppression and growth delay.[58,81] Overall survival is 75% at 40 years.[84] Bone marrow transplantation improves outcomes, with greater than 90% overall survival in patients younger than 10 years old transplanted with an HLA-matched related donor, and 80% in those with a matched unrelated donor.[81]

Congenital Dyserythropoietic Anemia

The congenital dyserythropoietic anemias (CDAs) are a heterogeneous group of rare disorders characterized by refractory anemia, reticulocytopenia, hypercellular bone marrow with markedly ineffective erythropoiesis, and distinctive dysplastic changes in bone marrow erythroblasts. Megaloblastoid development occurs in some types, but it is not related to vitamin B_{12} or folate deficiency. Granulopoiesis and thrombopoiesis are normal. The anemia varies from mild to moderate, even among affected siblings. Secondary hemosiderosis arises from chronic intramedullary and extramedullary hemolysis, as well as increased iron absorption associated with ineffective erythropoiesis. Iron overload develops even in the absence of blood transfusions. Jaundice, cholelithiasis, and splenomegaly are also common findings. CDAs do not progress to aplastic anemia or hematologic malignancies.[85]

Symptoms of CDA usually occur in childhood or adolescence but may first appear in adulthood.[58] CDA is classified into three major types: CDA I, CDA II, and CDA III. There are rare variants that do not fall into these categories, and they have been assigned to four other groups: CDA IV through CDA VII.[58,85] Whether CDA types IV through VII actually are separate entities is a matter of some controversy. This merely may be a reflection of the insensitive tests to classify CDA disorders. Further gene mutation studies should clarify this issue.

CDA I is inherited in an autosomal recessive pattern and is characterized by a mild to severe chronic anemia. More than 150 cases have been reported.[86] CDA I is caused by mutations in the *CDAN1* or *C15orf41* genes.[58] *CDAN1* (chromosome 15) encodes codanin-1, a cell-cycle regulated nuclear protein.[87,88] The exact role of *CDAN1* and *C15orf41* mutations in the pathophysiology of CDA I is unknown. Malformations of fingers or toes, brown skin pigmentation, and neurologic defects are found more often in CDA I than in the other CDA subtypes. The hemoglobin usually ranges from 6.5 g/dL to 11.5 g/dL, with a mean of 9.5 g/dL.[85] RBCs are macrocytic and may exhibit marked poikilocytosis, basophilic stippling, and Cabot rings. The erythroblasts are megaloblastoid and characteristically have internuclear chromatin bridges or nuclear stranding (Figure 19.3). There are less than 5% binucleated erythroblasts. The characteristic feature of the CDA I erythroblast is a spongy heterochromatin with a "Swiss cheese" appearance.[85] Treatment includes IFN-α and iron chelation.[58,86]

CDA II is the most common subtype and is inherited in an autosomal recessive pattern. More than 300 cases have been

TABLE 19.4 Distinguishing Characteristics of Diamond-Blackfan Anemia (DBA) and Transient Erythroblastopenia of Childhood (TEC)

Test Result	DBA*	TEC*
Erythrocyte ADA ↑ at diagnosis	85%	5%
MCV ↑ at diagnosis	80%	5%
MCV ↑ in remission	80%	0%
Hb F ↑ at diagnosis	50%–85%	1%–2%
Hb F ↑ in remission	50%–85%	0%

↑, Increased; *ADA*, adenosine deaminase; *Hb F*, fetal hemoglobin; *MCV*, mean cell volume.
*Percent of patients displaying the test results.
Modified from D'Andrea, A. D., Dahl, N., Guinan, E. C., et al. (2002). Marrow failure. *Hematology Am Soc Hematol Educ Program*, 58–72.

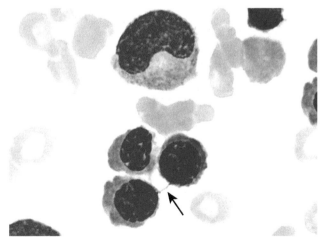

Figure 19.3 Erythroid Precursors with Nuclear Bridging (arrow) Indicating Dyserythropoiesis. (Bone marrow, Wright-Giemsa stain, ×1000.) (Modified from Rodak, B. F., & Carr, J. H. [2017]. *Clinical Hematology Atlas.* [5th ed.]. St. Louis: Elsevier.)

reported.[86] It results from mutations in the *SEC23B* gene on chromosome 20.[89] *SEC23B* encodes a component of the coat protein complex (COPII) that forms vesicles for transport of secretory proteins from the endoplasmic reticulum to the Golgi apparatus.[90] Its exact role in the pathophysiology of CDA II is unknown. The anemia in CDA II is mild to moderate, with hemoglobins ranging from 9 g/dL to 12 g/dL and a mean hemoglobin of 11 g/dL.[85] On peripheral blood film, RBCs are normocytic with anisocytosis, poikilocytosis, and basophilic stippling. The bone marrow has normoblastic erythropoiesis, with 10% to 35% binucleated forms and rare multinucleated forms.[85] Occasional pseudo-Gaucher cells are also evident.[85] Circulating RBCs hemolyze with the Ham acidified serum test but not with the sucrose hemolysis test.[58] For this reason, CDA II is also known as *HEMPAS* (*h*ereditary *e*rythroblastic *m*ultinuclearity with *p*ositive *a*cidified *s*erum).[58] The Ham test is no longer used for CDA II confirmation, given the difficulty of appropriate quality control and the relative lack of testing availability in most laboratories.[85] RBCs also show abnormal migration of band 3 using sodium dodecyl sulfate polyacrylamide gel electrophoresis.[85] Treatment includes splenectomy and iron chelation.[58,86]

CDA III is the least common of the CDA subtypes, with about 60 cases reported in the literature, the majority being from one Swedish family.[91] This familial autosomal dominant form is associated with mutations in the *KIF23* gene, which codes for a protein involved in cytokinesis.[91,92] The nonfamilial or sporadic form is extremely rare, with fewer than 20 cases reported.[86,91] The anemia is mild, and the hemoglobin is usually in the range of 8 to 14 g/dL, with a mean of 12 g/dL.[85] RBCs are macrocytic, and poikilocytosis and basophilic stippling are evident. The bone marrow has megaloblastic changes, and giant erythroblasts with up to 12 nuclei are a characteristic feature. Patients rarely require RBC transfusions, and iron overload does not occur.

Myelophthisic Anemia

Myelophthisic anemia is due to the infiltration of abnormal cells into the bone marrow and subsequent destruction and replacement of normal hematopoietic cells. Metastatic solid tumor cells (particularly from lung, breast, and prostate), fibroblasts, and inflammatory cells (such as those found in miliary tuberculosis and fungal infections) have been implicated.[93,94] Cytopenia results from the release of substances such as cytokines and growth factors that suppress hematopoiesis and destroy stem, progenitor, and stromal cells.[94] With disruption of normal bone marrow architecture by the infiltrating cells, the marrow releases immature hematopoietic cells. Furthermore, because of the unfavorable bone marrow environment, stem and progenitor cells migrate to the spleen and liver and establish extramedullary hematopoietic sites.[94] Because blood cell production in the liver and spleen is inefficient, these extramedullary sites also release immature cells into the circulation.[93]

The severity of anemia is mild to moderate, with normocytic erythrocytes and reticulocytopenia. Peripheral blood findings include teardrop erythrocytes and nucleated RBCs, as well as immature myeloid cells (*leukoerythroblastic blood picture*)

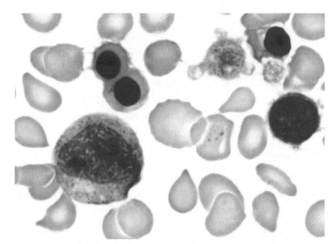

Figure 19.4 Myelophthisic Anemia Showing a Leukoerythroblastic Blood Picture. Note a myelocyte, three orthochromic normoblasts, a giant platelet with abnormal morphology, a micromegakaryocyte, and teardrop red blood cells. (Peripheral blood, Wright-Giemsa stain, ×1000.)

and megakaryocyte fragments (Figure 19.4).[93] The infiltrating abnormal cells are detected in a bone marrow aspirate or biopsy specimen.

Anemia of Chronic Kidney Disease

Anemia is a common complication of chronic kidney disease (CKD), with a positive correlation between anemia and renal disease severity.[95,96] The Centers for Disease Control and Prevention reported that in 2017 approximately 30 million adults in the United States had CKD.[97] The primary cause of anemia in CKD is inadequate renal production of erythropoietin.[95,96] Without erythropoietin, the bone marrow lacks adequate stimulation to produce RBCs. Another contributor to the anemia of CKD is chronic inflammation. Inflammatory cytokines increase production of hepcidin by the liver, which decreases the iron available for erythropoiesis (Chapter 17).[96,98] Uremia also inhibits erythropoiesis and increases RBC fragility.[98,99] Furthermore, hemodialysis and frequent blood draws result in chronic blood loss. Anemia of CKD is normocytic and normochromic with reticulocytopenia. Burr cells are a common peripheral blood film finding in cases complicated by uremia.

Anemia in CKD can lead to cardiovascular complications, cognitive impairment, and suboptimal quality of life.[96] The 2012 Kidney Disease: Improving Global Outcomes (KDIGO) Clinical Practice Guideline for Anemia recommends periodic hemoglobin testing in patients with CKD and investigation of the anemia if the hemoglobin is less than 13.0 g/dL in adult men and less than 12 g/dL in adult women.[95] In anemic adult CKD patients, a trial of oral iron (non-dialysis patients) or intravenous iron (dialysis patients) is recommended when the transferrin saturation is ≤ 30% and serum ferritin level is ≤ 500 ng/mL.[95] The Guideline also recommends consideration of therapy with an erythropoiesis-stimulating agent (ESA) if the hemoglobin falls below 10 g/dL.[95] Using ESA therapy to maintain the hemoglobin at more than 11.5 g/dL is not recommended because of the increased risk of cardiovascular complications.[95] Successful therapy requires adequate iron stores, so plasma ferritin level and percent transferrin saturation are also periodically monitored.

Patients may become hyporesponsive to ESA therapy because of functional iron deficiency (FID). In FID the bone marrow is unable to release iron rapidly enough to accommodate the accelerated erythropoiesis. The transferrin saturation remains less than 20%, but the serum ferritin level is normal or increased, indicating adequate iron stores.[100] Patients with FID may require intravenous iron therapy to reach or maintain target hemoglobin levels, even with high ESA doses.[100] Researchers have proposed diagnostic criteria for FID in CKD: decreased reticulocyte hemoglobin content and increased soluble transferrin receptor (Chapter 8), and greater than 10% hypochromic RBCs in the peripheral blood.[100,101] Other causes of ESA hyporesponsiveness include chronic inflammatory disease, infection, malignancy, aplastic anemia, antibody-mediated pure red cell aplasia, and some hemoglobin disorders.

SUMMARY

- Bone marrow failure is the reduction or cessation of blood cell production affecting one or more cell lines. Pancytopenia (decreased red blood cells, white blood cells, and platelets) is a common finding. Sequelae of pancytopenia include weakness and fatigue, infections, and bleeding.
- Aplastic anemia may be acquired or inherited/congenital. Acquired aplastic anemia may be idiopathic or secondary to drugs, chemical exposures, radiation, or viruses. Acquired aplastic anemia may also occur with conditions such as paroxysmal nocturnal hemoglobinuria, autoimmune diseases, and pregnancy.
- Bone marrow failure in acquired aplastic anemia occurs from destruction of hematopoietic stem cells by direct toxic effects of a drug, autoimmune T cell targeting of stem cells, or other unknown mechanisms. The autoimmune reactions are rare adverse events after exposure to drugs, chemicals, or viruses. They are *idiosyncratic* in that they are unpredictable, and severity is unrelated to the dose or duration of exposure.
- Aplastic anemia is classified as nonsevere, severe, or very severe, based on bone marrow hypocellularity, absolute neutrophil count, platelet count, hemoglobin level, and reticulocyte count. The severity classification helps guide treatment decisions.
- Preferred treatment for severe acquired aplastic anemia is bone marrow transplant for younger patients with an HLA-identical sibling. For those without a matched sibling donor and for older adults, immunosuppressive therapy (IST) with antithymocyte globulin and cyclosporine is recommended.
- Fanconi anemia (FA), dyskeratosis congenita (DC), and Shwachman-Bodian-Diamond syndrome (SBDS) are inherited bone marrow failure syndromes with progressive bone marrow failure, and patients may present with characteristic physical malformations. FA is inherited in an autosomal recessive or X-linked pattern, and mutations in at least 21 genes have been identified. A positive chromosome breakage study with diepoxybutane is diagnostic. DC can be X-linked, autosomal dominant, or autosomal recessive, and mutations in at least 11 genes have been identified. SBDS is autosomal recessive and is associated with mutations in the *SBDS* gene.
- Telomerase complex defects play a role in the pathophysiology of inherited bone marrow failure syndromes and some acquired aplastic anemias. The defects result in the inability of telomerase to elongate telomeres at the ends of chromosomes, which leads to premature hematopoietic stem cell senescence and apoptosis.
- Pure red cell aplasia is a disorder of erythrocyte production. Acquired transient erythroblastopenia of childhood (TEC) and Diamond-Blackfan anemia (DBA) are disparate subtypes with distinct causes, clinical features, and courses. Mutations in at least 17 genes have been identified in DBA.
- Patients with congenital dyserythropoietic anemia (CDA) exhibit refractory anemia, reticulocytopenia, secondary hemosiderosis, and distinct abnormalities of erythroid precursors. Three major subtypes are recognized: CDA I, CDA II, and CDA III.
- Myelophthisic anemia results from the replacement of normal bone marrow cells with abnormal cells, such as metastatic tumor cells, fibroblasts, and inflammatory cells. The main cause of anemia of chronic kidney disease is inadequate production of erythropoietin by the kidneys.

Now that you have completed this chapter, go back and read again the case study at the beginning and respond to the questions presented.

REVIEW QUESTIONS

Answers can be found in the Appendix.

1. The clinical consequences of pancytopenia include:
   a. Pallor and thrombosis
   b. Kidney failure and fever
   c. Fatigue, infection, and bleeding
   d. Weakness, hemolysis, and infection

2. Idiopathic acquired aplastic anemia is due to a(n):
   a. Drug reaction
   b. Benzene exposure
   c. Inherited mutation in stem cells
   d. Unknown cause

3. The pathophysiologic mechanism in acquired idiosyncratic aplastic anemia is:
   a. Replacement of bone marrow cells by abnormal cells
   b. Destruction of stem cells by autoimmune T cells
   c. Defective production of hematopoietic growth factors
   d. Inability of bone marrow stroma to support stem cells
4. Based on the criteria in Table 19.1, what is the aplastic anemia classification of a 15-year-old girl with a bone marrow cellularity of 10%, hemoglobin of 7 g/dL, absolute neutrophil count of 0.1×10^9/L, and platelet count of 10×10^9/L?
   a. Nonsevere
   b. Moderate
   c. Severe
   d. Very severe
5. The most consistent peripheral blood findings in severe aplastic anemia are:
   a. Hairy cells, monocytopenia, and neutropenia
   b. Macrocytosis, thrombocytopenia, and neutropenia
   c. Blasts, immature granulocytes, and thrombocytopenia
   d. Polychromasia, nucleated RBCs, and hypersegmented neutrophils
6. The treatment that has shown the best success rate in young patients with severe aplastic anemia is:
   a. Immunosuppressive therapy
   b. Long-term red blood cell and platelet transfusions
   c. Administration of hematopoietic growth factors and androgens
   d. Bone marrow transplant with an HLA-identical sibling
7. The test that is most useful in differentiating Fanconi anemia from other causes of pancytopenia is:
   a. Bone marrow biopsy
   b. Ham acidified serum test
   c. Diepoxybutane-induced chromosome breakage
   d. Flow cytometric analysis of CD55 and CD59 cells

8. Mutations in genes that code for the telomerase complex may induce bone marrow failure by causing which one of the following?
   a. Resistance of stem cells to normal apoptosis
   b. Autoimmune reaction against telomeres in stem cells
   c. Decreased production of hematopoietic growth factors
   d. Premature death of hematopoietic stem cells
9. Diamond-Blackfan anemia differs from Fanconi anemia in that in the former:
   a. Reticulocyte count is increased
   b. Fetal hemoglobin is decreased
   c. Only erythropoiesis is affected
   d. Congenital malformations are absent
10. Which anemia should be suspected in a patient with refractory anemia, reticulocytopenia, hemosiderosis, and binucleated erythrocyte precursors in the bone marrow?
    a. Fanconi anemia
    b. Dyskeratosis congenita
    c. Acquired aplastic anemia
    d. Congenital dyserythropoietic anemia
11. The primary pathophysiologic mechanism of anemia associated with chronic kidney disease is:
    a. Inadequate production of erythropoietin
    b. Excessive hemolysis
    c. Hematopoietic stem cell mutation
    d. Toxic destruction of stem cells
12. Which one of the following findings is *not* consistent with myelophthisic anemia?
    a. Reticulocytosis
    b. Teardrop RBCs
    c. Extramedullary hematopoiesis
    d. Leukoerythroblastic blood picture

REFERENCES

1. Ehrlich, P. (1888). Über einen Fall von Anämie mit Bemerkungen über regenerative Veränderungen des Knochenmarks. *Charite Annal, 13,* 301.
2. Vaquez, M. H., & Aubertin, C. (1904). L'anémie pernicieuse d'après les conceptions actuelles. *Bull Soc Med Hop Paris, 21,* 288–297.
3. Dokal, I., & Vulliamy, T. (2008). Inherited aplastic anaemias/bone marrow failure syndromes. *Blood Rev, 22,* 141–153.
4. Young, N. S., & Maciejewski, J. P. (2018). Aplastic anemia. In Hoffman, R., Benz, E. J., Silberstein, S. E., et al. (Eds.), *Hematology: Basic Principles and Practice.* (7th ed., pp. 394–414). Philadelphia: Elsevier.
5. Muir, K. R., Chilvers, C. E. D., Harriss, C., et al. (2003). The role of occupational and environmental exposures in the aetiology of acquired severe aplastic anaemia: a case control investigation. *Br J Haematol, 123,* 906–914.
6. International Agranulocytosis and Aplastic Anemia Study. (1987). Incidence of aplastic anemia: the relevance of diagnostic criteria. *Blood, 70,* 1718–1721.
7. Kojima, S. (2002). Aplastic anemia in the Orient. *Int J Hematol, 76*(suppl 2), 173–174.

8. Scheinberg, P., & Young, N. (2012). How I treat acquired aplastic anemia. *Blood, 102,* 1185–1196.
9. Nimer, S. D., Ireland, P., Meshkinpour, A., et al. (1994). An increased HLA DR2 frequency is seen in aplastic anemia patients. *Blood, 84,* 923–927.
10. Saunthararajah, Y., Nakamura, R., Nam, J. M., et al. (2002). HLA-DR15 (DR2) is overrepresented in myelodysplastic syndrome and aplastic anemia and predicts a response to immunosuppression in myelodysplastic syndrome. *Blood, 100,* 1570–1574.
11. Dougherty, D., Garte, S., Barchowsky, A., et al. (2008). NQO1, MPO, CYP2E1, GSTT1 and GSTM1 polymorphisms and biological effects of benzene exposure—a literature review. *Toxicol Lett, 182,* 7–17.
12. Sutton, J. F., Stacey, M., Kearns, W. G., et al. (2004). Increased risk for aplastic anemia and myelodysplastic syndrome in individuals lacking glutathione S-transferase genes. *Pediatr Blood Cancer, 42,* 122–126.
13. Gonzalez-Casas, R., Garcia-Buey, L., Jones, E. A., et al. (2009). Systematic review: hepatitis-associated aplastic anaemia—a syndrome associated with abnormal immunological function. *Aliment Pharmacol Ther, 30,* 6–43.
14. Choudhry, V. P., Gupta, S., Gupta, M., et al. (2002). Pregnancy associated aplastic anemia—a series of 10 cases with review of literature. *Hematol, 7,* 233–238.

15. Stalder, M. P., Rovó, A., Halter, J., et al. (2009). Aplastic anemia and concomitant autoimmune diseases. *Ann Hematol, 88,* 659–665.

16. Frickhofen, N., Heimpel, H., Kaltwasser, J. P., et al. (2003). Antithymocyte globulin with or without cyclosporin A: 11-year follow-up of a randomized trial comparing treatments of aplastic anemia. *Blood, 101,* 1236–1242.

17. Maciejewski, J. P., Selleri, C., Sato, T., et al. (1996). A severe and consistent deficit in marrow and circulating primitive hemato-poietic cells (long-term culture-initiating cells) in acquired aplastic anemia. *Blood, 88,* 1983–1991.

18. Philpott, N. J., Scopes, J., Marsh, J. C. W., et al. (1995). Increased apoptosis in aplastic anemia bone marrow progenitor cells: possible pathophysiologic significance. *Exp Hematol, 23,* 1642–1648.

19. Maciejewski, J. P., Selleri, C., Sato, T., et al. (1995). Increased expression of Fas antigen on bone marrow CD34 sup[+] cells of patients with aplastic anaemia. *Br J Haematol, 91,* 245–252.

20. Zeng, W., Chen, G., Kajigaya, S., et al. (2004). Gene expression profiling in CD34 cells to identify differences between aplastic anemia patients and healthy volunteers. *Blood, 103,* 325–332.

21. Novitzky, N., & Jacobs, P. (1995). Immunosuppressive therapy in bone marrow aplasia: the stroma functions normally to support hematopoiesis. *Exp Hematol, 23,* 1472–1477.

22. Koijima, S. (1998). Hematopoietic growth factors and marrow stroma in aplastic anemia. *Int J Hematol, 68,* 19–28.

23. Wodnar-Filipowicz, A., Lyman, S. D., Gratwohl, A., et al. (1996). Flt3 ligand level reflects hematopoietic progenitor cell function in aplastic anemia and chemotherapy-induced bone marrow aplasia. *Blood, 88,* 4493–4499.

24. Young, N. S., & Maciejewski, J. (1997). The pathophysiology of acquired aplastic anemia. *N Engl J Med, 336,* 1365–1372.

25. Mathe, G., Amiel, J. L., Schwarzenberg, L., et al. (1970). Bone marrow graft in man after conditioning by antilymphocytic serum. *Br Med J, 2,* 131–136.

26. Risitano, A. M., Maciejewski, J. P., Green, S., et al. (2004). In-vivo dominant immune responses in aplastic anaemia: molecular tracking of putatively pathogenic T-cell clones by TCR beta-CDR3 sequencing. *Lancet, 364,* 355–364.

27. Hara, T., Ando, K., Tsurumi, H., et al. (2004). Excessive produc-tion of tumor necrosis factor-alpha by bone marrow T lympho-cytes is essential in causing bone marrow failure in patients with aplastic anemia. *Eur J Haematol, 73,* 10–16.

28. Young, N. S. (2000). Hematopoietic cell destruction by immune mechanisms in acquired aplastic anemia. *Semin Hematol, 37,* 3–14.

29. Selleri, C., Sato, T., Anderson, S., et al. (1995). Interferon-gamma and tumor necrosis factor-alpha suppress both early and late stages of hematopoiesis and induce programmed cell death. *J Cell Physiol, 165,* 538–546.

30. Solomou, E. E., Keyvanfar, K., & Young, N. S. (2006). T-bet, a Th1 transcription factor, is up-regulated in T cells from patients with aplastic anemia. *Blood, 107,* 3983–3991.

31. Kasahara, S., Hara, T., Itoh, H., et al. (2002). Hypoplastic myelo-dysplastic syndromes can be distinguished from acquired aplastic anaemia by bone marrow stem cell expression of the tumour necrosis factor receptor. *Br J Haematol, 118,* 181–188.

32. Young, N. S., Calado, R. T., & Scheinberg, P. (2006). Current con-cepts in the pathophysiology and treatment of aplastic anemia. *Blood, 108,* 2509–2519.

33. Solomou, E. E., Rezvani, K., Mielke, S., et al. (2007). Deficient CD4+ CD25+ FOXP3+ T regulatory cells in acquired aplastic anemia. *Blood, 110,* 1603–1606.

34. Gidvani, V., Ramkissoon, S., Sloand, E. M., et al. (2007). Cytokine gene polymorphisms in acquired bone marrow failure. *Am J Hematol, 82,* 721–724.

35. Hirano, N., Butler, M. O., von Bergwelt-Baildon, M. S., et al. (2003). Autoantibodies frequently detected in patients with aplastic anemia. *Blood, 102,* 4567–4575.

36. Feng, X., Chuhjo, T., Sugimori, C., et al. (2004). Diazepam-binding inhibitor-related protein 1: a candidate autoantigen in acquired aplastic anemia patients harboring a minor population of paroxysmal nocturnal hemoglobinuria-type cells. *Blood, 104,* 2425–2431.

37. Takamatsu, H., Feng, X., Chuhjo, T., et al. (2007). Specific antibodies to moesin, a membrane-cytoskeleton linker protein, are frequently detected in patients with acquired aplastic anemia. *Blood, 109,* 2514–2520.

38. Ball, S. E., Gibson, F. M., Rizzo, S., et al. (1998). Progressive telomere shortening in aplastic anemia. *Blood, 91,* 3582–3592.

39. Calado, R. T., & Young, N. S. (2008). Telomere maintenance and human bone marrow failure. *Blood, 111,* 4446–4455.

40. Xin, Z-T., Beauchamp, A. D., Calado, R. T., et al. (2007). Func-tional characterization of natural telomerase mutations found in patients with hematologic disorders. *Blood, 109,* 524–532.

41. Yamaguchi, H., Calado, R. T., Ly, H., et al. (2005). Mutations in *TERT,* the gene for telomerase reverse transcriptase, in aplastic anemia. *N Engl J Med, 352,* 1413–1424.

42. Calado, R. T., Graf, S. A., Wilkerson, K. L., et al. (2007). Mutations in the *SBDS* gene in acquired aplastic anemia. *Blood, 110,* 1141–1146.

43. Brummendorf, T. H., Maciejewski, J. P., Mak, J., et al. (2001). Telomere length in leukocyte subpopulations of patients with aplastic anemia. *Blood, 97,* 895–900.

44. Camitta, B. M., Thomas, E. D., Nathan, D. G., et al. (1976). Severe aplastic anemia: a prospective study of the effect of early marrow transplantation on acute mortality. *Blood, 48,* 63–70.

45. Bacigalupo, A., Hows, J., Gluckman, E., et al. (1988). Bone marrow transplantation (BMT) versus immunosuppression for the treatment of severe aplastic anaemia (SAA): a report of the EMBT SAA working party. *Br J Haematol, 70,* 177–182.

46. Sugimori, C., Chuhjo, T., Feng, X., et al. (2006). Minor popula-tion of CD55[-]CD59[-] blood cells predicts response to immuno-suppressive therapy and prognosis in patients with aplastic anemia. *Blood, 107,* 1308–1314.

47. Socie, G., Rosenfeld, S., Frickhofen, N., et al. (2000). Late clonal diseases of treated aplastic anemia. *Semin Hematol, 37,* 91–101.

48. Sutherland, D. R., Kuek, N., Azcona-Olivera, J., et al. (2009). Use of FLAER-based WBC assay in the primary screening of PNH clones. *Am J Clin Pathol, 132,* 564–572.

49. Maciejewski, J. P., Risitano, A., Sloand, E., et al. (2002). Distinct clinical outcomes for cytogenetic abnormalities evolving from aplastic anemia. *Blood, 99,* 3129–3135.

50. Kearns, W. G., Sutton, J. F., Maciejewski, J. P., et al. (2004). Genomic instability in bone marrow failure syndromes. *Am J Hematol, 76,* 220–224.

51. Bacigalupo, A., Giammarco, S., & Sica, S. (2016). Bone marrow transplantation versus immunosuppressive therapy in patients with acquired severe aplastic anemia. *Int J Hematol, 104,* 168–174.

52. Scheinberg, P., Nunez, O., & Young, N. S. (2006). Retreatment with rabbit anti-thymocyte globulin and ciclosporin for patients with relapsed or refractory severe aplastic anaemia. *Br J Haematol, 133,* 622–627.

53. Maciejewski, J. P., Follmann, D., Nakamura, R., et al. (2001). Increased frequency of HLA-DR2 in patients with paroxysmal nocturnal hemoglobinuria and the PNH/aplastic anemia syndrome. *Blood, 98,* 3513–3519.

54. Socie, G., Mary, J-Y., Schrezenmeier, H., et al. (2007). Granulocyte-stimulating factor and severe aplastic anemia: a survey by the European group for blood and marrow transplant (EBMT). Blood, 109, 2794–2796.

55. Gurion, R., Gafter-Gvili, A., Paul, M., et al. (2009). Hematopoietic growth factors in aplastic anemia patients treated with immunosuppressive therapy—systematic review and meta-analysis. *Hematologica, 94,* 712–719.

56. Townsley, D. M., Scheinberg, P., Winkler, T., et al. (2017). Eltrombopag added to standard immunosuppression for aplastic anemia. *N Engl J Med, 376,* 1540–1550.

57. Fanconi, G. (1927). Familiaere infantile perniziosaartige Anaemie (pernizioeses Blutbild und Konstitution). *Jahrbuch Kinderheil, 117,* 257–280.

58. Dror, Y. (2018). Inherited bone marrow failure syndromes. In Hoffman, R., Benz, E. J., Silberstein, L. E., et al. (Eds.), *Hematology: Basic Principles and Practice.* (7th ed., pp. 350–393). Philadelphia: Elsevier.

59. Tischkowitz, M. D., & Hodgson, S. V. (2003). Fanconi anaemia. *J Med Genet, 40,* 1–10.

60. Green, A. M., & Kupfer, G. M. (2009). Fanconi anemia. *Hematol Oncol Clin North Am, 23,* 193–214.

61. Alter, B. P. (2003). Cancer in Fanconi anemia, 1927–2001. *Cancer, 97,* 425–440.

62. Gueiderikh, A., Rosselli, F., & Neto, J. B. C. (2017). A never-ending story: the steadily growing family of the FA and FA-like genes. *Genet Mol Biol, 40,* 398–407.

63. Shimamura, A., & Alter, B. P. (2010). Pathophysiology and management of inherited bone marrow failure syndromes. *Blood Rev, 24,* 101–122.

64. Levitus, M., Joenje, H., & de Winter, J. P. (2006). The Fanconi anemia pathway of genomic maintenance. *Cell Oncol, 28,* 3–19.

65. Pinto, F. O., Leblanc, T., Chamousset, D., et al. (2009). Diagnosis of Fanconi anemia patients with bone marrow failure. *Haematologica, 94,* 487–495.

66. Kutler, D. I., Singh, B., Satagopan, J., et al. (2003). A 20-year perspective on the International Fanconi Anemia Registry (IFAR). *Blood, 101,* 1249–1256.

67. Rosenberg, P. S., Greene, M. H., & Alter, B. P. (2003). Cancer incidence in persons with Fanconi anemia. *Blood, 101,* 822–826.

68. Li, X., Leteurtre, F., Rocha, V., et al. (2003). Abnormal telomere metabolism in Fanconi's anaemia correlates with genomic instability and the probability of developing severe aplastic anaemia. *Br J Haematol, 120,* 836–845.

69. MacMillan, M. L., DeFor, T. E., Young, J. A., et al. (2015). Alternative donor hematopoietic cell transplantation for Fanconi anemia. *Blood, 125,* 3798–3804.

70. Alter, B. P., Giri, N., Savage, S. A., et al. (2009). Cancer in dyskeratosis congenita. *Blood, 113,* 6549–6557.

71. Wegman-Ostrosky, T., & Savage, S. A. (2017). The genomics of inherited bone marrow failure: from mechanism to the clinic. *Br J Haematol, 177,* 526–542.

72. Alter, B. P., Baerlocher, G. M., Savage, S. A., et al. (2007). Very short telomere length by flow fluorescence in situ hybridization identifies patients with dyskeratosis congenita. *Blood, 110,* 1439–1447.

73. Burroughs, L., Woolfrey, A., & Shimamura, A. (2009). Shwachman-Diamond syndrome: a review of the clinical presentation,

molecular pathogenesis, diagnosis, and treatment. *Hematol Oncol Clin North Am, 23,* 233–248.

74. Myers, K. C., Rose, S. R., Rutter, M. M., et al. (2013). Endocrine evaluation of children with and without Shwachman-Bodian-Diamond syndrome gene mutations and Shwachman-Diamond syndrome. *J Pediatr, 162,* 1235–1240.

75. Austin, K. M., Gupta M. L. Jr., Coats, S. A., et al. (2008). Mitotic spindle destabilization and genomic instability in Shwachman-Diamond syndrome. *J Clin Invest, 118,* 1511–1518.

76. Dror, Y., & Freedman, M. H. (2002). Shwachman-Diamond syndrome. *Br J Haematol, 118,* 701–713.

77. Donadieu, J., Leblanc, T., Meunier, B. B., et al. (2005). Analysis of risk factors for myelodysplasias, leukemias and death from infection among patients with congenital neutropenia. Experience of the French Severe Chronic Neutropenia Study Group. *Hematologica, 90,* 45–53.

78. Maciejewski, J. P., & Thota, S. (2018). Acquired disorders of red cell, white cell, and platelet production. In Hoffman, R., Benz, E. J., Silberstein, L. E., et al. (Eds.), *Hematology: Basic Principles and Practice.* (7th ed., pp. 425–444). Philadelphia: Elsevier.

79. Sawada, K., Hirokawa, M., & Fujishima, N. (2009). Diagnosis and management of acquired pure red cell aplasia. *Hematol Oncol Clin North Am, 23,* 249–259.

80. Shaw, J., & Meeder, R. (2007). Transient erythroblastopenia of childhood in siblings: case report and review of the literature. *J Pediatr Hematol Oncol, 29,* 659–660.

81. Lipton, J. M., & Ellis, S. R. (2009). Diamond-Blackfan anemia: diagnosis, treatment, and molecular pathogenesis. *Hematol Oncol Clin North Am, 23,* 261–282.

82. Boria, I., Garelli, E., Gazda, H. T., et al. (2010). The ribosomal basis of Diamond-Blackfan anemia: mutation and database update. *Hum Mutat, 12,* 1269–1279.

83. Farrar, J. E., Vlachos, A., Atsidaftos, E., et al. (2011). Ribosomal protein gene deletions in Diamond-Blackfan anemia. *Blood, 118,* 6943–6951.

84. Lipton, J. M., Atsidaftos, E., Zyskind, I., et al. (2006). Improving clinical care and elucidating the pathophysiology of Diamond Blackfan anemia: an update from the Diamond Blackfan anemia registry. *Pediatr Blood Cancer, 46,* 558–564.

85. Renella, R., & Wood, W. G. (2009). The congenital dyserythropoietic anemias. *Hematol Oncol Clin North Am, 23,* 283–306.

86. Heimpel, H. (2004). Congenital dyserythropoietic anemias: epidemiology, clinical significance, and progress in understanding their pathogenesis. *Ann Hematol, 83,* 613–621.

87. Dgany, O., Avidan, N., Delaunay, J., et al. (2002). Congenital dyserythropoietic anemia type I is caused by mutations in codanin-1. *Am J Hum Genet, 71,* 1467–1474.

88. Noy-Lotan, S., Dgany, O., Lahmi, R., et al. (2009). Codanin-1, the protein encoded by the gene mutated in congenital dyserythropoietic anemia type I (*CDAN1*), is cell cycle-regulated. *Haematologica, 94,* 629–637.

89. Schwarz, K., Iolascon, A., Verissimo, F., et al. (2009). Mutations affecting secretory COPII coat component SEC23B cause congenital dyserythropoietic anemia type II. *Nat Genet 41,* 936–940.

90. Kirchhausen, T. (2007). Making COPII coats. *Cell, 129,* 1325–1336.

91. Liljeholm, M., Irvine, A. F., Vikberg, A. L., et al. (2013). Congenital dyserythropoietic anemia type III (CDA III) is caused by a mutation in kinesin family member, *KIF23. Blood, 121,* 4791–4799.

92. Iolascon, A., Heimpel, H., Wahlin, A., et al. (2013). Congenital dyserythropoietic anemias: molecular insights and diagnostic approach. *Blood, 122,* 2162–2166.

93. Reddy, V. V. B., & Prchal, J. T. (2016). Anemia associated with marrow infiltration. In Kaushansky, K., Lichtman, M. A., Prchal, J. T., et al. (Eds.), *Williams Hematology.* (9th ed., pp. 657–660). New York: McGraw-Hill.

94. Makoni, S. N., & Laber, D. A. (2004). Clinical spectrum of myelophthisis in cancer patients. *Am J Hematol, 76,* 92–93.

95. Kidney Disease: Improving Global Outcomes (KDIGO) Anemia Work Group. (2012). KDIGO Clinical Practice Guideline for Anemia in Chronic Kidney Disease. *Kidney Inter, Suppl 2,* 279–335.

96. Crowther, M. A., & Iqbal, A. (2018). Hematologic manifestations of renal disease. In Hoffman, R., Benz, E. J., Silberstein, L. E., et al. (Eds.), *Hematology: Basic Principles and Practice.* (7th ed., pp. 2244–2246). Philadelphia: Elsevier.

97. National Center for Chronic Disease Prevention and Health Promotion. (2017). National Chronic Kidney Disease Fact Sheet, 2017. Centers for Disease Control and Prevention. https://www.cdc.gov/diabetes/pubs/pdf/kidney_factsheet.pdf. Accessed March 17, 2018.

98. Ganz, T. (2016). Anemia of chronic disease. In Kaushansky, K., Lichtman, M. A., Prchal, J. T., et al. (Eds.), *Williams Hematology.* (9th ed., pp. 549–558). New York: McGraw-Hill.

99. Macdougall, I. C. (2001). Role of uremic toxins in exacerbating anemia in renal failure. *Kidney Int, 59*(Suppl. 78), S67–S72.

100. Wish, J. B. (2006). Assessing iron status: beyond serum ferritin and transferrin saturation. *Clin J Am Soc Nephrol, 1,* S4–S8.

101. Bovy, C., Gothot, A., Delanaye, P., et al. (2007). Mature erythrocyte parameters as new markers of functional iron deficiency in haemodialysis: sensitivity and specificity. *Nephrol Dial Transplant, 22,* 1156–1162.

Introduction to Increased Destruction of Erythrocytes

Kathryn Doig

OBJECTIVES

After completion of this chapter, the reader will be able to:

1. Define *hemolysis* and recognize its hallmark clinical findings.
2. Differentiate a hemolytic disorder from hemolytic anemia by definition and recognition of laboratory findings.
3. Discuss methods of classifying hemolytic anemias and apply the classification to an unfamiliar anemia.
4. Describe the processes of fragmentation (intravascular) and macrophage-mediated (extravascular) hemolysis, including sites of hemolysis, catabolic products, and time frame for the appearance of those products after hemolysis.
5. Describe protoporphyrin catabolism (bilirubin production), including metabolites and their sites of production and excretion.
6. Describe mechanisms that salvage hemoglobin and heme during fragmentation hemolysis.
7. Describe changes to bilirubin metabolism and iron salvage systems that occur when the rate of fragmentation or macrophage-mediated hemolysis increases.
8. Identify, explain the diagnostic value, and interpret the results of laboratory tests that indicate increased hemolysis and erythropoiesis.
9. Differentiate between hemolytic anemias and other causes of increased erythropoiesis given laboratory or clinical information.
10. Differentiate between hemolytic anemias and other causes of bilirubinemia given laboratory or clinical information.
11. Interchange conjugation terminology for bilirubin fractions with Van den Bergh reaction terminology.
12. Explain the principle of the Van den Bergh reaction to quantitate and fractionate bilirubin in body fluids.

OUTLINE

Classification
Hemolysis
  Normal Macrophage-Mediated Hemolysis and Bilirubin Metabolism
  Plasma Hemoglobin Salvage During Normal Fragmentation Hemolysis
Excessive Macrophage-Mediated (Extravascular) Hemolysis

Excessive Fragmentation (Intravascular) Hemolysis
Clinical Features
Laboratory Findings
  Tests of Accelerated Red Blood Cell Destruction
  Tests of Increased Erythropoiesis
  Laboratory Tests to Identify Specific Hemolytic Processes
Differential Diagnosis

CASE STUDY

After studying the material in this chapter, the reader should be able to respond to the following case study:

A 34-year-old woman was admitted to the hospital for a vaginal hysterectomy. Except for excessive menstrual bleeding, she was in otherwise good health, and all of her preoperative laboratory test results were within their respective reference intervals. There was no excessive blood loss during or after surgery, and recovery was uneventful except for some expected pain, for which

the patient received ibuprofen. Three days after surgery, the patient began to experience abdominal pain and pass "root beer"-colored urine. A CBC at that time revealed a hemoglobin level of 5.8 g/dL.

1. What process is indicated by the root beer-colored urine?
2. What laboratory tests can be used to differentiate the cause of the hemolysis?
3. Based on the patient's clinical presentation, predict the results expected for each test listed for question 2.

This chapter presents an overview of the hemolytic process and provides a foundation that is applicable in the following chapters on red blood cell (RBC) disorders. The term *hemolysis* or *hemolytic disorder* refers to increased rate of destruction (lysis) of RBCs, shortening their life span. The reduced number of cells results in reduced tissue oxygenation and increased erythropoietin production by the kidney. When the patient is otherwise healthy, the bone marrow responds by accelerating erythrocyte production, which leads to reticulocytosis. A hemolytic process is present without anemia if bone marrow is able to compensate by accelerating RBC production sufficiently to replace RBCs lost through hemolysis. Healthy bone marrow can increase its production of RBCs by four to eight times normal.[1,2] Therefore significant RBC destruction must occur before an anemia develops during hemolysis. A *hemolytic anemia* results when the rate of RBC destruction exceeds the increased rate of RBC production.

CLASSIFICATION

Many anemias have a hemolytic component, including anemia associated with vitamin B_{12} or folate deficiency and anemia of chronic inflammation, renal disease, and iron deficiency. In these conditions, hemolysis alone does not cause anemia, and so they are not typically classified as hemolytic disorders. Rather, these anemias develop as a result of the inability of bone marrow to increase production of RBCs. Because hemolysis is not the primary underlying cause, these disorders are considered anemias with a secondary hemolytic component.

When hemolysis is the primary feature, anemias can be classified as follows:
- Acute versus chronic
- Inherited versus acquired
- Intrinsic versus extrinsic
- Intravascular versus extravascular
- Fragmentation versus macrophage-mediated

Every hemolytic condition can be classified according to each of these descriptors. Table 20.1 shows this and provides a noncomprehensive list of hemolytic anemias categorized in this way. This chapter focuses on the mechanism of hemolysis, that is, the distinction between fragmentation and macrophage-mediated hemolytic conditions. Other classifying schemes are summarized here briefly for application in the chapters that follow.

Acute versus *chronic hemolysis* delineates the clinical presentation. Acute hemolysis has a rapid onset and is isolated (sudden), episodic, or paroxysmal, as in *paroxysmal cold hemoglobinuria* or *paroxysmal nocturnal hemoglobinuria*. Patients with paroxysmal cold hemoglobinuria experience hemolysis after exposure to cold, and patients with paroxysmal nocturnal hemoglobinuria may experience intermittent episodes of hemolysis. A hemolytic transfusion reaction is an example of a single acute incident. Whatever the cause, acute hemolysis either disappears or subsides between episodes, during which time the patient's condition may return to normal.

Chronic hemolysis may not be evident if the bone marrow is able to compensate, but it may be punctuated over time with hemolytic *crises* that cause anemia. Glucose-6-phosphate dehydrogenase deficiency is such a condition. RBC life span is chronically shortened, but bone marrow compensation prevents anemia. When the cells are challenged with oxidizing agents

TABLE 20.1 Classification of Selected Hemolytic Anemias by Primary Cause and Type of Hemolysis		
	Predominantly Fragmentation (Intravascular) Hemolysis	**Predominantly Macrophage-Mediated (Extravascular) Hemolysis**
Extrinsic defects	**Agents From Outside the RBC**	
	Immune hemolysis: cold antibody Microangiopathic hemolysis Infectious agents, as in malaria Thermal injury Chemicals/drugs Venoms **Prosthetic heart valve**	Immune hemolysis: warm antibody Drugs
	Membrane Abnormalities	
	Spur cell anemia of severe liver disease Paroxysmal nocturnal hemoglobinuria	**Hereditary membrane defects**
Intrinsic defects	**Abnormalities of the RBC Interior**	
	Enzyme defects such as G6PD deficiency **Globin abnormalities such as sickle cell disease, thalassemia**	

G6PD, Glucose-6-phosphate dehydrogenase; *RBC*, red blood cell.
Green text indicates acute or episodic hemolysis.
Red text indicates chronic hemolysis.
Some conditions may exhibit mixed presentations under certain circumstances. It is evident that most hereditary conditions lead to chronic hemolysis, whereas acquired conditions are more often acute. Furthermore, the intrinsic red blood cell defects typically are due to hereditary conditions, whereas extrinsic factors typically lead to acquired hemolytic disorders.

Acquired conditions (right column label, spanning Agents From Outside the RBC and upper Membrane Abnormalities rows)
Hereditary conditions (right column label, spanning lower Membrane Abnormalities and Abnormalities of the RBC Interior rows)

such as antimalarial drugs, a dramatic acute hemolytic event occurs. When the drug is withdrawn, compensation returns.

Other chronic conditions result in anemia that is so severe that the bone marrow cannot generate cells fast enough to compensate for the anemia. Thalassemia major is an example of such a condition. Although RBC production is brisk, each cell possesses an inadequate complement of one type of globin chain, and functional hemoglobin production is decreased overall. As a result, the oxygen-carrying capacity of blood is chronically low. Cells lyse in thalassemia because excess normal globin chains precipitate inside erythroid cells, which leads to hemolysis and exacerbates the chronically reduced hemoglobin production.

Inherited hemolytic conditions, such as thalassemia, are passed to offspring by mutant genes from the parents. *Acquired* hemolytic disorders develop in individuals who were previously hematologically normal but acquire an agent or condition that lyses RBCs. Infectious diseases such as malaria are an example.

Hemolytic disorders are also classified as involving *intrinsic* or *extrinsic* RBC defects, with the latter caused by the action of external agents. This is the classification scheme used for subsequent chapters in this book. Examples of *intrinsic* hemolytic disorders are abnormalities of the RBC membrane, enzymatic pathways, or the hemoglobin molecule. With intrinsic defects, if RBCs of the affected patient were to be transfused into a healthy individual, they would still have a shortened life span because the defect is in the RBC. If normal RBCs are transfused into a patient who has an intrinsic defect, the transfused cells have a normal life span because the transfused cells are normal.

Extrinsic hemolytic conditions are those that arise from outside the RBC, typically substances in plasma or conditions affecting the anatomy of the circulatory system. Even though malaria protozoa and other infectious agents are within the RBC, they are classified as extrinsic because the RBC was normal until it was invaded by an outside agent. An antibody against RBC antigens and a prosthetic heart valve are examples of noninfectious extrinsic agents that can damage RBCs. In extrinsic hemolysis, cross-transfusion studies have shown that the patient's RBCs have a normal life span in the bloodstream of a healthy individual, but normal cells are lysed more rapidly in the patient's circulation. These studies confirm that something outside the RBCs is causing the hemolysis. (Of course, in the case of intracellular parasites, cross-transfusion study is not applicable.) Most intrinsic defects are inherited; most extrinsic ones are acquired (Table 20.1). A few exceptions exist, such as paroxysmal nocturnal hemoglobinuria, an acquired disorder involving an intrinsic defect (Chapter 21).

Intrinsic disorders are subclassified as membrane defects, enzyme defects, and hemoglobinopathies. Extrinsic hemolysis may be immunohemolytic, traumatic, or microangiopathic or may be caused by infectious agents, chemical agents (drugs and venoms), or physical agents (Table 20.1).

Another classification scheme is based on the site of hemolysis and is related to the general mechanism of lysis. *Intravascular* hemolysis occurs by *fragmentation*. Although this

takes place most often within the bloodstream, RBCs can lyse by fragmentation in the spleen and bone marrow as well. *Macrophage-mediated* hemolysis occurs when RBCs are engulfed by macrophages and lysed inside the phagocyte by their digestive enzymes. The designation *extravascular,* meaning outside the vessels, can refer either to lysis within the macrophage and not in the bloodstream or to the fact that most of the macrophages are in tissues, chiefly the spleen and liver, and thus are outside the vasculature. Commonly the terms *fragmentation* and *intravascular* are used interchangeably, as are *macrophage-mediated* and *extravascular*. The mechanistic classifying scheme is useful because screening laboratory tests rely on the differences in the hemolytic processes. However, the exact cause of the hemolysis must still be determined by targeted testing in order for appropriate treatment to be implemented.

HEMOLYSIS

Normal Macrophage-Mediated Hemolysis and Bilirubin Metabolism

Detection of hemolysis depends partly on detection of RBC breakdown products. A prominent product is bilirubin. The process of normal bilirubin production is described to clarify the relationship between hemolysis and increased bilirubin levels.

RBCs live approximately 120 days. During this time, they undergo various metabolic and chemical changes that result in membrane alterations and a loss of deformability. Under normal circumstances, macrophages of the mononuclear phagocyte system (or reticuloendothelial system) recognize these changes and phagocytize the aged erythrocytes (Chapter 5), producing a macrophage-mediated hemolytic process that removes approximately 1% of the RBCs per day. The organs involved include the spleen, bone marrow, liver, lymph nodes, and circulating monocytes, but it is primarily the macrophages in spleen and liver that process senescent RBCs.

The majority of RBC degradation occurs inside macrophages as enzymes of the macrophage phagolysosome rupture phagocytized erythrocytes and salvage or metabolize the contents (Figure 20.1). Hemoglobin is hydrolyzed into heme and globin; the latter is further degraded into amino acids that return to the amino acid pool. Iron is released from heme, returned to plasma via ferroportin, bound to its protein carrier molecule (transferrin), and recycled to needy cells thus salvaging virtually all RBC iron (Chapter 8). The protoporphyrin component is catabolized and the products are processed in the liver, move to the intestines, where they facilitate dietary fat absorption, and then are excreted mostly in the stool. Bilirubin and urobilinogen are the excretory products derived from the protoporphyrin component of heme.

Figure 20.2 illustrates protoporphyrin catabolism. While protoporphyrin is inside the macrophage, heme oxygenase acts on it, breaking the protoporphyrin ring to yield a linear molecule, biliverdin. The lungs excrete a byproduct of that reaction, carbon monoxide. The green biliverdin is reduced to bilirubin, a nonpolar yellow molecule that is secreted into the blood

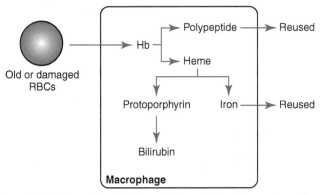

Figure 20.1 Normal Catabolism of Hemoglobin. Macrophages lyse ingested red blood cells *(RBCs)* and separate hemoglobin *(Hb)* into globin chains and heme components. Amino acids from the globin chains are reused. Heme is degraded to iron and protoporphyrin. Iron is returned to the blood to be reused. Protoporphyrin is degraded to un-conjugated bilirubin.

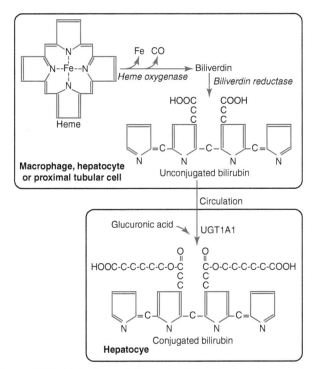

Figure 20.2 Catabolism of Heme to Bilirubin. In cells containing heme oxygenase, iron is removed from heme, and the protoporphyrin ring is opened up to form an intermediate, biliverdin. Biliverdin is converted to unconjugated bilirubin by biliverdin reductase. The unconjugated bilirubin is secreted into the blood and binds to albumin for transport to the liver. When unconjugated bilirubin enters the hepatocyte, UGT1A1 (uridine diphosphate glucuronosyltransferase family 1 member A1, formerly glucuronyl transferase) adds two molecules of glucuronic acid to form bisglucuronosyl bilirubin, also called conjugated bilirubin.

(Box 20.1). This form of bilirubin is called unconjugated for reasons that will be evident shortly. Because it is hydrophobic, this form of bilirubin must bind to albumin to be transported in blood to the liver.

An understanding of blood circulation in the liver is needed to appreciate the subtleties of hepatic bilirubin metabolism.

BOX 20.1 Visualizing the Color Changes of Hemoglobin Degradation

The degradation of heme can be seen in bruises in fair-skinned individuals or in the sclera of the eye after a vascular bleed. The same process that macrophages facilitate can occur in tissues. At first the extravasated but deoxygenated blood gives the injury the purple-red appearance of hemoglobin. As the hemoglobin is degraded, the color changes to a greenish hue due to the biliverdin, but ultimately it becomes yellow due to the bilirubin.

Blood enters the liver lobule at the periphery via a hepatic artery and also from a portal vein bringing blood from the intestines (Figure 4.7). Blood from each vessel enters the endothelial cell-lined sinusoids that run between rows of hepatocytes. The loose structure of the sinusoids leads to the characterization of the blood as percolating through the lobule and around the hepatocytes toward the central vein. Here the blood drains into progressively larger veins that leave the liver to enter the inferior vena cava.

Bilirubin formed in macrophages and secreted in blood, enters the liver sinusoid via the hepatic artery. In the liver sinusoid, bilirubin dissociates from albumin so that it can be carried into the hepatocyte by organic anion transporter (OAT) proteins, chiefly OATP1B3.[3,4] Once inside the hepatocyte, bilirubin is bound to glutathione S-transferase, known as ligandin, for transport to the endoplasmic reticulum.[5] There, unconjugated bilirubin is joined (i.e., conjugated) with one to two molecules of a sugar acid, glucuronic acid, by uridine diphosphate (UDP) glucuronosyltransferase family 1 member A1 (UGT1A1), previously known as glucuronyl transferase. The molecules formed include monoglucuronosyl bilirubin, with just a single glucuronic acid added, and bisglucuronosyl bilirubin, previously known as bilirubin diglucuronide, which has two glucuronic acid molecules added. Addition of glucuronic acids makes the bilirubin molecules polar and water soluble. They are also called *conjugated* bilirubin or *direct* bilirubin (Box 20.2). Thus the bilirubin originally released from macrophages that lacks glucuronic acids is termed *unconjugated bilirubin* or *indirect* bilirubin (Box 20.2).

In the structure of the liver lobule (Figure 4.7), small ducts called canaliculi run from the central vein outward along the lateral sides between hepatocytes. They receive the bile excreted by hepatocytes and channel it toward the exterior of the lobule where the canaliculi join into larger bile ducts that ultimately collect the bile into the common bile duct. Conjugated bilirubin is actively excreted by hepatocytes into the canaliculi by a unidirectional and adenosine triphosphate (ATP)-dependent membrane protein, multidrug resistant protein 2 (MRP2).[4,6] Once in the bile canaliculi, conjugated bilirubin continues down to the common bile duct and eventually into the intestines (Figure 20.3). There it assists with the emulsification of fats for absorption from the diet.

Under normal conditions, hepatocytes at the exterior of the lobule receive the highest concentration of unconjugated

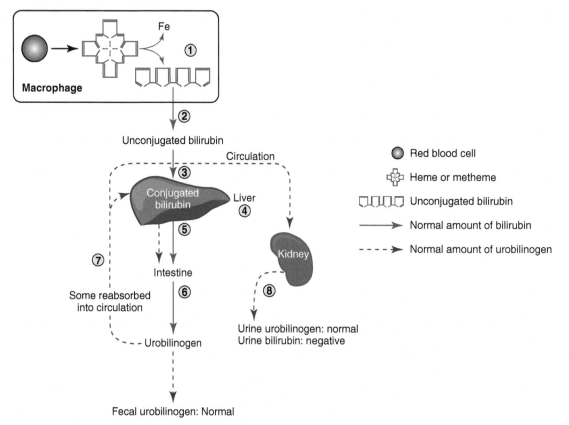

Figure 20.3 Normal Macrophage-Mediated Hemolysis. *1,* In a macrophage, hemoglobin is degraded to heme, the iron is released, and the protoporphyrin ring is converted to unconjugated bilirubin. *2,* Macrophages release unconjugated bilirubin into the blood, where it binds to albumin for transport to the liver. *3,* Unconjugated bilirubin enters the hepatocyte. *4,* The hepatocyte converts unconjugated bilirubin to conjugated bilirubin. *5,* Conjugated bilirubin leaves the liver in the bile and enters the small intestine. *6,* Bacteria in the large intestine convert conjugated bilirubin to urobilinogen, most of which is excreted in the stool. *7,* Some of the water-soluble urobilinogen is reabsorbed in the portal circulation, and most is recycled through the liver for excretion. *8,* A small component of the reabsorbed urobilinogen is filtered and excreted in the urine. (Adapted from Brunzel, N. A. [2013]. *Fundamentals of Urine and Body Fluid Analysis.* [3rd ed., p. 141, Figure 7-8]. St. Louis: Elsevier.)

bilirubin in the blood entering the sinus. Having conjugated the bilirubin, they are not always able to export all of it into the bile duct. Therefore they export conjugated bilirubin into sinusoidal blood via a second MRP (MRP3), which is localized to the sinusoidal side of hepatocytes.[4] It can then be absorbed downstream by more centrilobular hepatocytes via a second OAT protein, OATP1B1, in the sinusoidal membrane.[4] OATP1B1 has a very high affinity for conjugated bilirubin.[4] The absorbed, conjugated bilirubin can then be exported into the canaliculi by these downstream hepatocytes.

Once conjugated bilirubin enters the intestines, it is oxidized by gut bacteria into various water-soluble compounds, collectively called *urobilinogen*. Most urobilinogen is oxidized further to stercobilin and similar compounds that give the brown color to stool. This is the usual and ultimate route for excretion of most red cell-derived protoporphyrin.

Some conjugated bilirubin and urobilinogen molecules are absorbed by osmosis from the intestines into the blood of the portal circulation (Figure 20.3). The portal circulation (blood vessels that surround the intestines to absorb nutrients) collects these bile products and carries them directly to the liver in this enterohepatic circulation. These bilirubin derivatives enter the lobule via the portal veins and flow into the sinusoidal blood. Most of the intestinally absorbed and hepatocyte-secreted conjugated bilirubin in the sinusoidal blood is absorbed into hepatocytes by OATP1B1 and recycled directly into the bile.[7] Urobilinogen is similarly recycled into the bile. A miniscule amount of direct bilirubin remains in the blood entering the central vein, along with a larger amount of urobilinogen. These compounds are filtered at the renal glomerulus and excreted in the urine. So although conjugated bilirubin is virtually undetectable in urine because of efficient recycling in the liver, a measurable amount of urobilinogen can be expected normally. This is the second, but much smaller, route of excretion for protoporphyrins. The yellow color of urine is not caused by the urobilinogen, which is colorless. It is a result of urobilin, a stool derivative of urobilinogen that is also water soluble and absorbed via the portal circulation.

Plasma Hemoglobin Salvage During Normal Fragmentation Hemolysis

Fragmentation hemolysis is the result of trauma to the RBC membrane that causes a breach sufficient for the cell contents, chiefly hemoglobin, to spill directly into plasma (Box 20.3). Approximately 10% to 20% of normal RBC destruction is via fragmentation,[8] usually secondary to turbulence and anatomic restrictions in the vasculature.

Because hemoglobin is filtered through the glomerulus, some iron could be lost daily with even normal amounts of fragmentation hemolysis. In addition, free hemoglobin, and especially free heme, can scavenge nitric oxide and cause iron-induced oxidative damage to cells. These effects are magnified in conditions such as sickle cell disease, hemolytic transfusion reactions, and sepsis. Thus several mechanisms exist to salvage

hemoglobin iron and prevent oxidation reactions (Box 20.4). They are collectively called the *haptoglobin-hemopexin-methemalbumin system* (Figure 20.4).

When free in plasma, hemoglobin exists mostly as α/β dimers[9] that rapidly complex to a liver-produced plasma protein called *haptoglobin*. By binding to haptoglobin, hemoglobin avoids filtration at the glomerulus and the iron is saved from urinary loss. Haptoglobin binds a hemoglobin dimer in a conformation that is very similar to the binding of the complementary dimer in the native hemoglobin structure, so the conformation of the complex has been termed a *pseudotetramer*.[10,11] In this complex the hemes are sequestered, as they are in intact hemoglobin, so that cells are protected from their oxidative properties.[10] As the plasma is carried to various tissues, the complex is taken up by macrophages, principally those in the liver, spleen, bone marrow, and lung.[12] In these tissues, macrophages express CD163, the haptoglobin scavenger receptor, on their membranes. Once the hemoglobin-haptoglobin complex binds to CD163, the entire complex is internalized into the macrophage in a lysosome.[12,13] Inside the lysosome, iron is salvaged, globin is catabolized, and protoporphyrin is converted to unconjugated bilirubin, just as though an intact RBC had been ingested by the macrophage. Haptoglobin is also degraded within the lysosome.

The level of haptoglobin in plasma is typically adequate to salvage only the small amount of plasma hemoglobin generated each day because of normal fragmentation of RBCs. If fragmentation hemolysis is accelerated, haptoglobin is depleted because the liver's production does not increase in response to the increased consumption of haptoglobin. (discussed in Excessive Fragmentation [Intravascular] Hemolysis later in this chapter).

A second mechanism of iron salvage and oxidation prevention involves *hemopexin* (Figure 20.4). The iron in free plasma hemoglobin rapidly becomes oxidized, forming methemoglobin. The heme molecule (actually *metheme* or *hemin*) readily dissociates from the globin and binds to another liver-produced plasma protein, hemopexin.[14,15] This binding also saves the iron from urinary loss and prevents oxidant injury to cells and tissues. The latter role of hemopexin may actually be more critical, as free metheme has high redox activity. It readily diffuses across cell membranes and into extracellular spaces oxidizing proteins, lipids, and nucleic acids. In so doing, it sensitizes cells to

---

BOX 20.3 Laboratory Impact of Significant Hemoglobinemia

The results of a routine complete blood count are unreliable for patients with significant hemoglobinemia. Under normal circumstances, the measured hemoglobin represents the hemoglobin present inside the red blood cells. For individuals with hemoglobinemia, the intracellular hemoglobin and the plasma hemoglobin both are measured. The hemoglobin value therefore is falsely elevated. An unrealistically high value for mean cell hemoglobin concentration may provide a clue to this problem, which can be remedied in several ways (Chapters 11 and 12).

BOX 20.4 Therapeutic Applications of Haptoglobin and Hemopexin

During severe fragmentation hemolysis, the oxidizing capabilities of hemoglobin and heme cause serious tissue damage. Both readily transfer into extravascular spaces, damaging cells and causing organ dysfunction, such as renal failure. When hemoglobin binds to haptoglobin and heme binds to hemopexin, they are retained in the vasculature, diminishing tissue damage. As a result, the two proteins are gaining serious consideration as therapeutic agents that could be used during instances of fragmentation hemolysis to reduce organ damage. Haptoglobin has been used in Japan since 1985. Hemopexin has not yet been used clinically, but Schaer and colleagues report that both salvage proteins are under investigation by US and European pharmaceutical firms.[9]

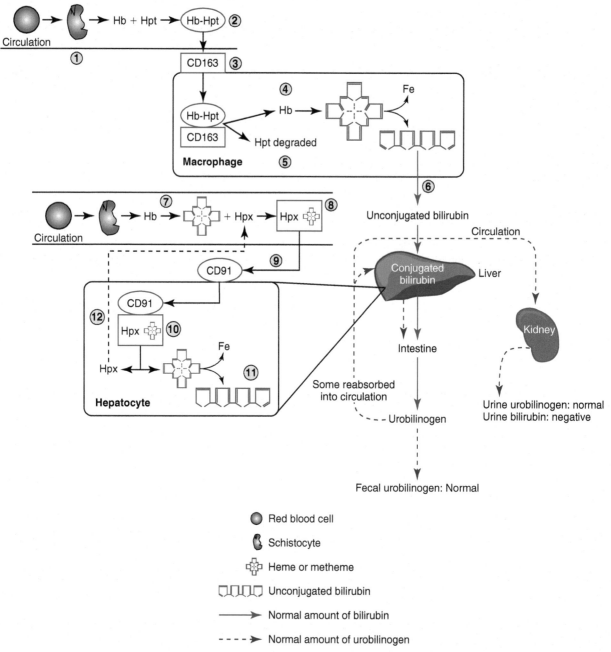

Red blood cell

Schistocyte

Heme or metheme

Unconjugated bilirubin

———▶ Normal amount of bilirubin

- - - -▶ Normal amount of urobilinogen

Figure 20.4 Normal Fragmentation Hemolysis. *1,* Normally a small number of red blood cells lyse within the circulation, forming schistocytes and releasing hemoglobin *(Hb)* into the blood, mostly as α/β dimers. *2,* The plasma protein haptoglobin *(Hpt)* binds a hemoglobin dimer in a complex. *3,* The hemoglobin-haptoglobin complex binds to CD163 on the surface of macrophages in various organs. *4,* The complex is internalized into the macrophage, where the hemoglobin dimer is released. The hemoglobin dimer is degraded to heme, the iron is released, and the protoporphyrin ring is converted to unconjugated bilirubin. *5,* The haptoglobin is degraded. *6,* The unconjugated bilirubin released into the blood is bound to albumin and processed through the liver as in Figure 20.3 (steps 2 to 8). *7,* When free hemoglobin is released into the blood with fragmentation, the iron is rapidly oxidized, forming methemoglobin, and the heme (metheme) molecule dissociates from the globin. *8,* The plasma protein hemopexin *(Hpx)* binds free metheme into a complex. *9,* The hemopexin-metheme complex binds to CD91 on the surface of hepatocytes. *10,* The complex is internalized into the hepatocyte. *11,* The iron is released from the metheme, and the protoporphyrin ring is converted to unconjugated bilirubin, ready for conjugation and further processing, as in Figure 20.3 (steps 4 to 8). *12,* Hemopexin is recycled to the blood. Note that metheme can also bind to albumin, forming metheme-albumin (not shown), but this complex is temporary because metheme is rapidly transferred to hemopexin. (Adapted from Brunzel, N. A. [2013]. *Fundamentals of Urine and Body Fluid Analysis.* [3rd ed., p. 141, Figure 7-8]. St. Louis: Elsevier.)

proinflammatory stimuli.[16] Metheme toxicity is a major factor in the lethality of systemic conditions such as sepsis or hemolytic transfusion reactions. This observation has led to experiments using hemopexin as a therapy[16] (Box 20.4).

Hemopexin-metheme binds to ligand nonspecific CD91 receptor, lipoprotein receptor-related protein (LRP1),[17] chiefly on hepatocytes. The complex is internalized by endocytosis.[18] The fate of the internalized heme remains an area of research because some studies suggest that intact heme can be incorporated into needed proteins within the hepatocyte, like cytochromes, and others suggest it is broken down to bilirubin with reuse of the iron.[18] It appears that under normal circumstances the bulk of the hemopexin is recycled to blood from the hepatocyte.[16,19]

A third mechanism of iron salvage is the metheme-albumin system. Albumin acts as a carrier for many molecules, including metheme. This is just a temporary holding state for metheme, merely by virtue of the high concentration of albumin in plasma. But metheme is rapidly transferred to hemopexin, when available, which has a higher binding affinity for metheme than does albumin.[20] The hemopexin-metheme complex then travels to the liver for processing.

The prevailing view has been that these salvage systems work somewhat sequentially. Haptoglobin binds hemoglobin until it is saturated and depleted. Then hemopexin binds metheme until it is saturated. And then albumin binds metheme. More recent theories suggest that these systems work simultaneously, particularly during accelerated hemolysis, and that hemopexin acts to prevent heme toxicity at all times.[16,21]

If the haptoglobin-hemopexin salvage systems are overloaded, the excess (met) hemoglobin and metheme will be filtered into the urine. Normally this is a negligible amount so that the kidney is not significantly involved in normal iron salvage. Yet it has been known for some time that proximal tubular cells can reabsorb iron in various forms because iron staining of tubular cells in urinary sediment during periods of excessive hemolysis demonstrates the presence of hemosiderin. The entire picture of renal handling of iron and related proteins is an area of active research yet to be fully elucidated. However, an emerging picture suggests that under normal circumstances a small amount of filtered transferrin is salvaged by transferrin receptors on the apical surface of proximal tubular cells.[22] This may be the normal source of iron for those cells' metabolic needs. Ferroportin has been identified on the basolateral membrane of proximal tubular cells, suggesting that renal cells are then able to transfer additional salvaged iron back into the blood.[23] Once again, these systems evolved to manage the amount and "form" of iron present in normal urinary filtrate. During excessive fragmentation hemolysis, other forms of iron are presented to and processed by the kidney.

EXCESSIVE MACROPHAGE-MEDIATED (EXTRAVASCULAR) HEMOLYSIS

Many hemolytic anemias are a result of increased macrophage-mediated hemolysis (Figure 20.5), during which more than the usual number of RBCs are removed from the circulation daily. Under normal circumstances, senescent RBCs display surface markers that identify them to macrophages as aged cells requiring removal (Chapter 5). Pathologic processes also lead to expression of the same markers, so cells are recognized and removed. If the number of affected cells increases beyond the quantity normally removed each day as a result of senescence, and if the bone marrow cannot compensate, then anemia develops. As an example, when excessive oxidation of hemoglobin causes increased formation of Heinz bodies, aggregates of denatured hemoglobin, they bind to the interior of the RBC membrane. That binding then leads to changes to the exterior of the membrane. Those changes are detected by macrophages and the cells are removed from circulation prematurely. A similar process occurs when intracellular parasites are present or when complement or immunoglobulins are on the surface of the RBC.

When an RBC is ingested by a macrophage, it is lysed within a phagolysosome, and the contents are processed entirely within the macrophage as described previously. The contents of the RBC are not detected in plasma because it is lysed inside the macrophage, and the contents are degraded there, hence the designation *extravascular hemolysis.* Because defective RBCs display markers like those of senescent RBCs, macrophage-mediated hemolysis of defective cells occurs most often in the spleen and liver, where macrophages possess receptors for those markers.

Sometimes the macrophage ingests a portion of the membrane, leaving the remainder to reseal. Little, if any, cytoplasmic volume is lost, but with less membrane, the cell becomes a spherocyte, the characteristic shape change associated with macrophage-mediated hemolysis. Although the spherocyte may enter the circulation, its survival is shortened because of its rigidity and inability to traverse the splenic sieve during subsequent passages through the red pulp. It may become trapped against the basement membrane of the splenic sinus and be fully ingested by a macrophage, or it may lyse mechanically because of its rigidity and in so doing contribute a fragmentation component to what is otherwise a macrophage-mediated process.

In macrophage-mediated hemolytic anemias, the total plasma bilirubin level rises as RBCs are lysed prematurely. The rise of the total bilirubin is due to the increase of the unconjugated fraction (Figure 20.5). As long as the liver is healthy, it processes the increased load of unconjugated bilirubin, producing more than the usual amount of conjugated bilirubin that enters the intestine. Increased urobilinogen forms in the intestines and is subsequently absorbed by the portal circulation and excreted by the kidney. Increased direct bilirubin is also absorbed into the portal (enterohepatic) circulation but is reprocessed through the hepatocytes and into the bile. Increased urobilinogen is detectable in the urine because it is (1) absorbed more than direct bilirubin into the portal circulation and (2) not reprocessed through the liver as completely as direct bilirubin. Although there is an increase in unconjugated bilirubin in the plasma, none of it appears in urine because it is bound to albumin and cannot pass through the glomerulus. These findings are summarized in Table 20.2.

Hemopexin may play an especially important role in macrophage-mediated hemolysis. If macrophages ingest more than one to two erythrocytes, the released heme can be toxic to them.[21,24] They possess a membrane heme exporter, feline

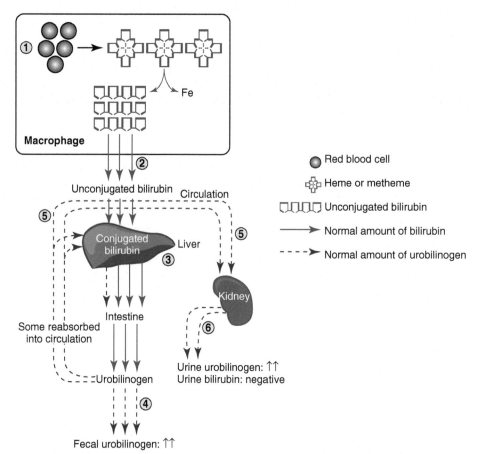

Figure 20.5 Excess Macrophage-Mediated Hemolysis. *1,* More than the usual number of red blood cells are ingested each day by macrophages. *2,* An increased amount of unconjugated bilirubin is produced, released into the blood, and binds to albumin. *3,* When increased unconjugated bilirubin is presented to the liver, an increased amount of conjugated bilirubin is made and excreted into the intestine. *4,* When an increased amount of conjugated bilirubin is present in the intestine, an increased amount of urobilinogen is formed and excreted in the stool. *5,* Increased urobilinogen in the intestine results in increased urobilinogen reabsorbed into the blood. *6,* Increased urobilinogen in the blood results in increased urobilinogen filtered and excreted in the urine. (Adapted from Brunzel, N. A. [2013]. *Fundamentals of Urine and Body Fluid Analysis.* [3rd ed., p. 141, Figure 7-8]. St. Louis: Elsevier.)

TABLE 20.2 **Comparison of Laboratory Findings Indicating Accelerated Red Blood Cell Destruction in Fragmentation Versus Macrophage-Mediated Hemolysis**

Test Specimen	Result	Fragmentation	Macrophage Mediated
Serum	Total bilirubin	↑	↑
	Indirect (unconjugated) bilirubin	↑	↑
	Direct (conjugated) bilirubin	WRI	WRI
	Lactate dehydrogenase activity (RBC fraction)	↑	sl ↑
	Haptoglobin	↓	sl ↓
	Free hemoglobin	↑	sl ↑
	Hemopexin	↓	sl ↓
Urine	Urobilinogen	↑	↑
	Free hemoglobin	Positive	Negative
	Methemoglobin	Positive	Negative
	Prussian blue staining of urine sediment	Positive	Negative
Anticoagulated whole blood	Hemoglobin, hematocrit, RBC count	↓	↓
	Schistocytes	Often present	
	Spherocytes		Often present
	Glycated hemoglobin	↓	↓
Special tests	Endogenous carbon monoxide	↑	↑
	Erythrocyte life span	↓	↓

↑, Typically increased; *sl*↑, typically only slightly increased, minor component; ↓, typically decreased; *RBC,* red blood cell; *WRI,* within the reference interval.

leukemia virus subgroup C receptor (FLVCR), that permits them to rid themselves of excess heme.[21] Hemopexin then is important to accept the exported free heme during macrophage-mediated hemolysis to prevent heme toxicity to other cells.[21]

EXCESSIVE FRAGMENTATION (INTRAVASCULAR) HEMOLYSIS

Although fragmentation hemolysis is a minor component of normal RBC destruction, it can be a major feature of pathologic processes. Dramatic examples of fragmentation hemolysis are the traumatic, physical lysis of RBCs caused by prosthetic heart valves and the exit of mature intracellular RBC parasites, such as malaria protozoa, by bursting out of cells. In these instances the fragmentation destruction of RBCs can cause profound anemias.

Excessive fragmentation hemolysis is characterized by the appearance in the plasma of the contents of RBCs, chiefly hemoglobin, and thus the development of (met)hemoglobinemia. As a result, the iron salvage proteins form complexes with their respective ligands (Figure 20.6A and B); hemoglobin-haptoglobin, metheme-hemopexin, and metheme-albumin.

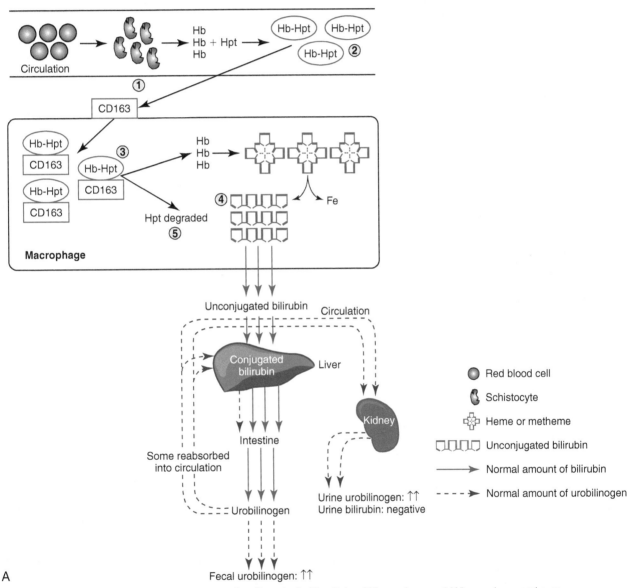

Figure 20.6 (A), Excess Fragmentation Hemolysis: The Role of Macrophages. *1,* When an increased number of red blood cells lyse by fragmentation, more than the usual amount of hemoglobin *(Hb)* is released into the blood, mostly as α/β dimers. *2,* Haptoglobin *(Hpt)* binds the increased hemoglobin dimers, forming more than usual numbers of complexes. *3,* The hemoglobin-haptoglobin complexes are taken up by macrophages bearing the CD163 receptor in various organs. *4,* An increased amount of hemoglobin dimers is released from the complexes. The hemoglobin is degraded to heme, the iron is released, and the protoporphyrin ring is converted to unconjugated bilirubin. The increased amount of unconjugated bilirubin is then transported to the liver and processed as with excess macrophage-mediated hemolysis (Figure 20.5, steps 2 to 6). *5,* Degradation of haptoglobin is accelerated compared with normal.

Continued

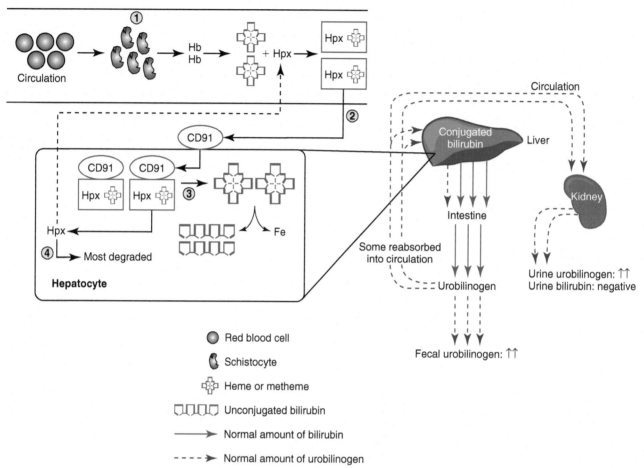

Circulation

Hb
Hb

+ Hpx →

Hpx

Hpx

CD91

CD91   CD91

Hpx   Hpx

Most degraded

Hepatocyte

Fe

Conjugated
bilirubin   Liver

Circulation

Kidney

Intestine

Some reabsorbed
into circulation

Urobilinogen

Urine urobilinogen: ↑↑
Urine bilirubin: negative

Fecal urobilinogen: ↑↑

⬤ Red blood cell

  Schistocyte

  Heme or metheme

  Unconjugated bilirubin

———➤ Normal amount of bilirubin

- - - -➤ Normal amount of urobilinogen

B

Figure 20.6, cont'd (B), Excess Fragmentation Hemolysis: The Role of the Liver. *1,* If the amount of hemoglobin released from lysing red blood cells exceeds the capacity of haptoglobin, the unbound free hemoglobin is rapidly oxidized, forming methemoglobin, and the metheme molecule dissociates from the globin. *2,* Hemopexin binds to metheme, and the complex is captured by the CD91 receptor on hepatocytes. *3,* The complex is internalized by the hepatocyte, the iron is released from the metheme, and the protoporphyrin ring is converted to unconjugated bilirubin and ultimately to conjugated bilirubin to be processed, as in Figure 20.5, steps 3 to 6. *4,* Although a small of amount of hemopexin is recycled to the blood, most is degraded. Metheme can also temporarily bind to albumin, forming metheme-albumin (not shown), but metheme is rapidly transferred to hemopexin.

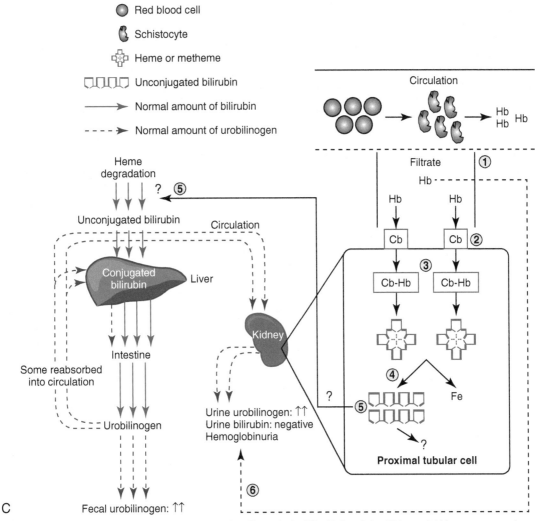

Figure 20.6, cont'd (C), Excess Fragmentation Hemolysis: The Role of the Kidney. *1,* When excess red blood cells lyse by fragmentation and other systems are saturated, free (met)hemoglobin enters the urinary filtrate. *2,* Cubilin *(Cb)* on the luminal side of the proximal tubular cells binds proteins for reabsorption, including hemoglobin. *3,* Cubilin carries hemoglobin into the proximal tubular cells. *4,* The hemoglobin is degraded to heme, the iron is released, and the protoporphyrin ring is converted to unconjugated bilirubin as in a macrophage and conjugated as in a hepatocyte. *5,* The fate of the bilirubin is uncertain, as it may be secreted to the filtrate or reabsorbed into the blood. *6,* When the amount of hemoglobin exceeds the capacity of the proximal tubular cells to absorb it from the filtrate, hemoglobinuria occurs.

Continued

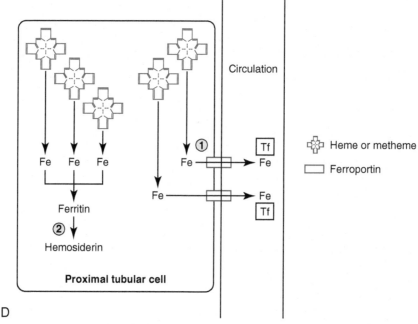

D

Figure 20.6, cont'd (D), Fate of Iron Removed from Salvaged Hemoglobin in the Kidney. *1,* Iron (Fe) salvaged from absorbed hemoglobin can be transported into the circulation by ferroportin on the basolaminal side of the tubular cell. In the blood it will be bound to transferrin (Tf) for transport. *2,* Iron in excess of what can be transported into the circulation is stored as ferritin, and some is converted to hemosiderin. If the tubular cell is sloughed into the filtrate and appears in the urine sediment, the hemosiderin can be detected using the Prussian blue stain. (A–C, Adapted from Brunzel, N. A. [2013]. *Fundamentals of Urine and Body Fluid Analysis.* [3rd ed., p. 141, Figure 7-8]. St. Louis: Elsevier.)

The complexes are then cleared within minutes from plasma by complexing with their respective receptors.[15,17,19] The levels of free haptoglobin will drop because more than the usual amounts of the complex will form and be taken up by macrophages (Table 20.2). The endocytosed protein is not recycled to the plasma and there is no compensatory increase in production, so the plasma is depleted of haptoglobin. The levels of free hemopexin can also decrease even though it is normally recycled. It appears that the hepatic recycling system can become saturated when there are high levels of metheme to be salvaged.[17] During these circumstances, hemopexin then gets degraded within the hepatocyte and plasma levels fall. Still the drop in hemopexin is not as dramatic as the decline of haptoglobin,[8] because some recycling continues.

In roughly the same time frame that hemoglobin appears in the plasma, it can also appear in the urine (hemoglobinuria) (Table 20.2) if the amount of liberated hemoglobin and heme exceeds the salvage capacity of the plasma proteins. Increased amounts of iron-containing proteins are then absorbed into the proximal tubular cells (Figure 20.6C).

Glomerular filtrate is low in protein compared with plasma. However it is not devoid of filtered proteins, including some that carry iron or iron-containing proteins, such as transferrin, albumin, and lactoferrin. As mentioned previously, transferrin receptors appear on the apical surface of proximal tubular cells, perhaps to provide for the iron needs of those cells.[25] The proximal tubular cells also possess the megalin-cubilin-amnionless receptor endocytosis system.[25,26] These receptors are not specific for heme/iron-containing proteins. Rather, they are responsible for nonspecific but very efficient reabsorption of a variety of proteins from the urinary filtrate. Megalin and cubilin have each been shown to bind hemoglobin and myoglobin.[26] Additionally, megalin can bind lactoferrin, and cubilin can bind transferrin.[26] The kinetics of such nonspecific competitive reabsorption favors the iron-containing proteins when they are present in high concentrations as during a hemolytic episode.

Proximal tubular cells are able to catabolize heme via heme-oxygenase-1,[27] thus freeing and salvaging the iron for export to the plasma by ferroportin in the basolaminal membrane.[23] Proximal tubular cells also possess UGT1A1 to conjugate bilirubin.[28] Its disposition is uncertain at this time. MRP2 on the apical membrane may allow secretion of the conjugated bilirubin into the filtrate/urine.[29,30] However, the presence of OAT proteins in the basolaminal membrane may allow reabsorption into the plasma for ultimate liver excretion.[30] Future research may clarify this.

Proximal tubular cell iron in excess of what can be transported into the circulation gets stored as ferritin, and some is converted to hemosiderin (Figure 20.6D). If the tubular cell is sloughed into the filtrate and appears in the urine sediment, the hemosiderin can be detected using the Prussian blue stain. This provides evidence that excess iron in some form, such as hemoglobin, has been salvaged from the filtrate.

Elevated levels of plasma indirect bilirubin and urinary urobilinogen are also measurable, although not immediately, because time is needed to produce these products. The time course of these findings assists with the differential diagnosis. After an acute onset, a rise in reticulocytes several days later would also be seen.

CLINICAL FEATURES

Clinical findings typical of hemolysis may be prominent if the hemolytic process is the primary cause of anemia. For patients in whom hemolysis is secondary, however, other clinical features may be more noticeable. If hemolysis is sufficient to result in anemia, patients experience the general symptoms of fatigue, dyspnea, and dizziness to a degree that is consistent with the severity and rate of development of the anemia. The associated signs of pallor and tachycardia can be expected.

Increase in plasma bilirubin gives a yellow tinge, not only to the plasma but also to body tissues. It is readily evident in the sclera of the eyes for all patients, but also the skin of fair-skinned individuals. *Jaundice* refers to the yellow color of the skin and sclera, whereas *icterus* describes yellow plasma and tissues. An increase in plasma bilirubin and subsequent jaundice can occur in other conditions besides hemolysis, such as hepatitis or gallstones. If the jaundice is the result of hemolysis, it is called *hemolytic jaundice* or *prehepatic jaundice,* which reflects the predominance of unconjugated bilirubin in plasma. The lipid solubility of unconjugated bilirubin also leads to deposition in the brain when hemolysis affects newborns (Chapter 23) because the blood-brain barrier is not fully developed. This can lead to a type of brain damage called *kernicterus*, which refers to the yellow coloring (icterus) of the brain tissue.

The frequency or constancy of jaundice provides clues to the cause. In glucose-6-phosphate dehydrogenase deficiency, for example, jaundice is periodic, appearing after an oxidative crisis. In thalassemia, jaundice is chronic. Jaundice may not be present at all if hemolysis is minimal and the liver is able to process the additional bilirubin, as is often the case in hereditary elliptocytosis.

Some signs differentiate chronic from acute hemolysis. Splenomegaly can develop, particularly with chronic macrophage-mediated hemolytic processes. Gallstones (cholelithiasis) can occur whenever hemolysis is chronic; the constantly increased amount of bilirubin in the bile leads to the formation of the stones.[31] When hemolysis is chronic in children, the persistent compensatory bone marrow hyperplasia can lead to bone deformities because the bones are still forming (Figure 25.3). For patients in whom an acquired, acute hemolytic process develops, the associated malaise, aches, vomiting, and possible fever may cause it to be confused with an acute infectious process. Profound prostration and shock may develop, particularly with acute fragmentation hemolysis. Flank pain, oliguria, or anuria develop, which leads to acute renal failure, one of the life-threatening effects of heme toxicity.

Other clinical features may offer a clue as to whether hemolysis is macrophage-mediated or caused by fragmentation. In particular, brown urine, associated with (met)hemoglobinuria, points to a fragmentation hemolytic process.

LABORATORY FINDINGS

In patients with the clinical features of hemolytic anemia, laboratory tests typically show evidence of increased erythrocyte destruction and the compensatory increase in the rate of erythropoiesis. Other tests that are specific to a particular diagnosis also may be indicated.

Tests of Accelerated Red Blood Cell Destruction
Bilirubin

In either fragmentation or macrophage-mediated hemolysis, the increased rate of hemoglobin catabolism results in increased amounts of plasma unconjugated bilirubin and carbon monoxide. The elevation of bilirubin may be evident visually in icteric serum or plasma. Bilirubin assays should reveal an increase indirect fraction resulting in an increase in total bilirubin. If liver function is normal, conjugated bilirubin is formed and excreted as urobilinogen in the stool, and the serum level of direct (conjugated) bilirubin remains within the reference interval. No bilirubin is detected in the urine because unconjugated bilirubin is bound to albumin for plasma transport and the complex is not filtered by the glomerulus. The urinary urobilinogen level may be increased, however, because there is increased urobilinogen in the stool and more than usual amounts are absorbed by the portal circulation. In some patients, serum indirect (unconjugated) bilirubin values can be misleadingly low because the amount of bilirubin in the blood depends on the rate of RBC catabolism as well as hepatic function. If the rate of hemolysis is low and liver function is normal, the total serum bilirubin level can be within the reference interval. Quantitative measurements of fecal urobilinogen, however, would demonstrate an increase.

Plasma Hemoglobin, Urine Hemoglobin, and Urine Hemosiderin

Visual examination of plasma and urine may suggest fragmentation hemolysis. The presence of methemoglobin, methemalbumin, and hemopexin-heme imparts a coffee-brown color to plasma, strongly suggestive of fragmentation hemolysis. When these compounds are present in urine, the color is more often described as root beer- or beer-colored. In a properly collected blood specimen the normal physiologic fragmentation hemolysis produces a plasma hemoglobin level of less than 1 mg/dL.[32] Plasma does not become visibly red/brown until the plasma hemoglobin level is at 50 mg/dL.[32] Typical values during hemolytic processes may be as low as 15 mg/dL, so an increase in plasma hemoglobin may not always be visible.[33] As a quick check, a urinalysis test strip for blood can be used on plasma to detect hemolysis that may not be visible.

Hemoglobin/heme from fragmentation hemolysis can be detected in urine when the capacity of the plasma salvage systems is exceeded and the hemoglobin/heme is filtered into the urine. The urinalysis test strip for blood can be positive even when the hemoglobin is not present in a high enough concentration to change the color of the urine significantly. Because the product entering the urine is free hemoglobin/heme, the sediment will be negative for red blood cells. However, renal tubular cells sloughed into the filtrate during the period after hemoglobinuria can demonstrate deposits of hemosiderin (iron) when stained with Prussian blue stain (i.e., hemosiderinuria), resulting from absorbed hemoglobin.

Complete Blood Count

For a patient with a hemolytic process, a complete blood count (CBC) may provide clues to the cause. Whether the hemolysis has been sufficient to cause anemia will be reflected by the hemoglobin, hematocrit, and number of RBCs. Spherocytes can be expected to be seen with macrophage-mediated hemolysis (Table 20.2), whereas fragmented cells, or schistocytes, are noted with fragmentation hemolysis.

Haptoglobin and Hemopexin

Haptoglobin can be quantified by methods such as immunoturbidimetry. A substantial decline in the serum haptoglobin level indicates fragmentation hemolysis. In what is mostly a macrophage-mediated hemolysis, there can still be a minor component of fragmentation lysis involving spherical cells that are fragile, so a more modest decline in haptoglobin level can be seen. In short, whenever the level of hemoglobin in the plasma increases, the haptoglobin level declines. In one study a low haptoglobin level indicated an 87% probability of hemolytic disease.[34] Haptoglobin measurement is, however, prone to both false-positive and false-negative results. Low values suggest hemolysis but may be due instead to impaired synthesis of haptoglobin caused by liver disease. Alternatively, a patient with hemolysis may have a relatively normal haptoglobin level if there is also a complicating infection or inflammation, because haptoglobin is an acute phase reactant. For diagnosis of hemolysis, quantification of hemopexin may also demonstrate a low value, yet it is not often measured, relying instead on the more dramatic haptoglobin decline to detect fragmentation hemolysis. However, some researchers recommend assay of hemopexin and plasma heme to create a more complete picture of a patient's hemolytic process.[21] Hemopexin assays may ultimately be more valuable for detection of hemopexin depletion in conditions such as sepsis.[16]

Carbon Monoxide

Tests to determine the rate of endogenous carbon monoxide production have been developed because carbon monoxide is produced in the first step of heme breakdown by heme oxygenase. Values of 2 to 10 times the normal rate have been detected in some patients with hemolytic anemia,[35] but testing for carbon monoxide production is not typically required for clinical diagnosis.

Red Blood Cell Survival

General evidence of reduced RBC survival can be gleaned by measuring glycated hemoglobin (usually by the Hb A_{1c} test).[36] Glycated hemoglobin increases over the life of a cell as it is exposed to plasma glucose. The glycated hemoglobin level usually is decreased in chronic hemolytic disease because the cells have less exposure to plasma glucose before early lysis. The magnitude of the decrease is related to the magnitude of the hemolytic process over the previous 4- to 8-week period. However, there is significant variability in RBC life span among hematologically normal individuals,[36] so use of glycated hemoglobin for detection of hemolysis is problematic without baseline values for individuals. Glycated hemoglobin levels are now widely used as an indicator of diabetes mellitus because the increased rate of glycation

with elevated plasma glucose levels leads to an increase in the glycated hemoglobin value. Coexistence of hemolysis with diabetes leads to falsely lowered glycated hemoglobin values, however, and is a recognized problem in the interpretation of glycated hemoglobin values for glucose control.

A more exact RBC survival assay uses random labeling of blood with chromium-51 radioisotope. This is the reference method for RBC survival studies published by the International Committee for Standardization in Hematology.[37] A sample of blood is collected, mixed with the isotope, and returned to the patient. The labeled cells are all ages, reflecting normal peripheral blood. This method differs from cohort labeling in which RBCs are labeled with radioactive iron or heavy nitrogen as they are produced in the bone marrow, thus the labeled cells are generally the same age. In both methods the disappearance of the label from the blood is measured over time. As measured using the random chromium labeling technique, the normal half-time of chromium is 25 to 32 days.[37] A half-time of 20 to 25 days suggests mild hemolysis; 15 to 20 days, moderate hemolysis; and less than 15 days, severe hemolysis.[37] Both cohort and random techniques have significant limitations,[38] including being time consuming, expensive, and requiring the use of radioactive isotopes. Therefore these methods are not often used clinically but are used for research, particularly in the search for improved methods of determining RBC survival.

Lactate Dehydrogenase

Serum lactate dehydrogenase activity is often increased in patients with fragmentation hemolysis because of the release of the enzyme from ruptured RBCs, but other conditions, such as myocardial infarction or liver disease, also can cause increases. Although enzyme isoform fractionation could be used to identify lactate dehydrogenase of RBC origin, this test is generally not needed. Rather, when other results point to fragmentation hemolysis, one should expect an increase in the level of serum lactate dehydrogenase and other RBC enzymes and should not be misled into assuming that there is other organ damage (Table 20.2).

Tests of Increased Erythropoiesis

If bone marrow is healthy, the hypoxia associated with hemolysis leads to increased erythropoiesis. Recognition of this increase may be a first clue to the presence of a hemolytic process, particularly if the liver is able to clear the unconjugated bilirubin and prevent jaundice. Laboratory findings indicating increased erythropoiesis include an increase in circulating reticulocytes and, in severe cases, nucleated RBCs, as well as associated changes in the CBC and bone marrow, described more fully in the next section (Table 20.3). These findings are persistently present in chronic hemolytic disease and are evident within 3 to 6 days after an acute hemolytic episode. Increased erythropoiesis is not unique to hemolytic anemias, however, and so it is not diagnostic. Similar results are expected after hemorrhage and with successful specific therapy for anemia caused by iron, folate, or vitamin B_{12} deficiency. An assessment of erythropoiesis can determine the effectiveness of the bone marrow response, however, and should be factored into the differential diagnosis (discussed in Differential Diagnosis).

TABLE 20.3 Hematologic Findings Indicating Accelerated Red Blood Cell Production

Specimen	Findings
Anticoagulated peripheral blood	Increased absolute reticulocyte count, immature reticulocyte fraction, reticulocyte production index
	Rising mean cell volume (compared with baseline)
	Polychromasia, nucleated RBCs
Bone marrow	Erythroid hyperplasia

RBC, Red blood cell.

Complete Blood Count and Red Blood Cell Morphology

Peripheral blood film evaluation is crucial. An increase in polychromatic RBCs (reticulocytes) and nucleated RBCs represents bone marrow compensation for hemolysis or blood loss. Schistocytes are expected with excessive fragmentation hemolysis, whereas spherocytes may be seen with macrophage-mediated processes. Additional morphologic changes to RBCs may point toward the cause of the hemolysis (discussed later).

An increase in the mean cell volume (MCV) is usually seen with extreme compensatory reticulocytosis resulting from the larger, prematurely released "shift" reticulocytes. The increase must be assessed by comparison with the value seen early in hemolysis, before the shift reticulocytes have emerged. The MCV may not increase to greater than the reference interval but rather may be more than the baseline value for that patient. Exceptions occur if the hemolytic condition itself involves smaller cells that counter the increased volume of the reticulocytes. In hereditary spherocytosis, microspherocytes are the cause of the anemia and the MCV may be within the reference interval even when larger shift reticulocytes are generated; hence the importance of a baseline value for comparison. In other circumstances, numerous schistocytes may outnumber the reticulocytes so that the MCV remains low or normal.

The red cell distribution width, RDW, can be expected to rise with reticulocytosis. Though the MCV may not elevate to more than the reference interval, the addition of larger reticulocytes can be expected to extend the range of cell volumes. Thus the previously mentioned situations where there are small cells with the larger reticulocytes may be reflected by a rise in the RDW. Alternatively, morphologic examination of the peripheral blood film can also reveal this anisocytosis.

Leukocytosis and thrombocytosis may accompany acute hemolytic anemia and are considered reactions to the hemolytic process. Conversely, conditions that directly cause leukocytosis, such as sepsis, might cause hemolysis. Low platelet counts in association with other signs of hemolysis may indicate a platelet-consuming microangiopathic process, such as disseminated intravascular coagulopathy.

Reticulocyte Count

The reticulocyte count is the most commonly used test to detect accelerated erythropoiesis and is expected to rise during hemolysis or hemorrhage. Assuming the bone marrow is healthy and there are adequate nutrients, all measures of reticuloycyte production should rise: absolute reticulocyte count, relative reticulocyte count, reticulocyte production index, and immature reticulocyte fraction. The association of reticulocytosis with hemolysis is so strong that if an anemic patient has an elevated reticulocyte count and hemorrhage is ruled out, a cause of hemolysis should be investigated. The reticulocyte increase usually correlates well with the severity of the hemolysis. Exceptions occur during aplastic crises of some hemolytic anemias and in some immunohemolytic anemias with hypoplastic marrow, which suggests that the autoantibodies were directed against the bone marrow erythroid precursors and circulating erythrocytes.[32] Chapters 11 and 16 describe the interpretation of reticulocyte indices in patients with anemia.

Bone Marrow Examination

Bone marrow examination is usually not necessary to diagnose hemolytic anemia. If conducted, however, bone marrow examination will reveal erythroid hyperplasia that results in peripheral blood reticulocytosis. As the erythroid component (the denominator) of the myeloid-to-erythroid ratio increases, the overall ratio decreases. (The myeloid-to-erythroid ratio is defined in Chapter 14.) As always, the cellularity of bone marrow should be determined on a core biopsy specimen, rather than an aspirated specimen, for a more accurate assessment.

Laboratory Tests to Identify Specific Hemolytic Processes

As noted earlier, the appearance of spherocytes or schistocytes on a peripheral blood film can point to a hemolytic cause for anemia. Other abnormalities found on the film, such as elliptocytes, acanthocytes, burr cells, sickle cells, target cells, agglutination, erythrophagocytosis, or parasites, may help reveal the specific disorder causing the hemolysis (Table 20.4).

Other tests for diagnosis of specific types of hemolytic anemia are discussed in subsequent chapters. They include the direct antiglobulin test, osmotic fragility test, eosin-5'-maleimide binding test, Heinz body test, RBC enzyme studies, and immunophenotyping.

TABLE 20.4 Morphologic Abnormalities Associated With Hemolytic Anemia

RBC Morphology	Hemolytic Disorders
Spherocytes	Hereditary spherocytosis, IgG-mediated immune hemolytic anemia, thermal injury to RBCs
Elliptocytes (ovalocytes)	Hereditary elliptocytosis
Acanthocytes	Abetalipoproteinemia, severe liver disease (spur cell anemia)
Burr cells	Pyruvate kinase deficiency, uremia
Schistocytes	Microangiopathic hemolytic anemia, traumatic cardiac hemolytic anemia, IgM-mediated immune hemolytic anemia
Erythrophagocytosis	Damage to RBC surface, especially due to complement-fixing antibodies
RBC agglutination	Cold agglutinins, immunohemolytic disease

Ig, Immunoglobulin; *RBC,* red blood cell.

DIFFERENTIAL DIAGNOSIS

Differential diagnosis of hemolytic anemias incorporates several intersecting lines of deduction. The first is to establish the hemolytic nature of the anemia. A rapid decrease in hemoglobin concentration (e.g., 1 g/dL per week) from levels previously within the reference interval can signal hemolysis when hemorrhage and hemodilution have been ruled out. Jaundice and reticulocytosis provide additional confirmation of a hemolytic cause for an anemia of at least several days' duration. When only the indirect (unconjugated) fraction of the total serum bilirubin is elevated, hemolytic jaundice is confirmed. An elevated urinary urobilinogen level strengthens the conclusion.

The rapid decrease in hemoglobin during an acute hemolytic episode, however, usually is apparent before reticulocytosis and bilirubinemia develop. For acute hemolysis, hemoglobinemia and hemoglobinuria are expected with fragmentation causes; therefore their absence suggests a macrophage-mediated cause. RBC morphology and haptoglobin levels can assist in differentiating fragmentation from a macrophage-mediated cause. Figure 20.7 is a graphic representation of the general timeline of the events in acute fragmentation and macrophage-mediated hemolysis. In chronic hemolysis, persistence of hemoglobinemia, hemoglobinuria, decreased serum haptoglobin level, indirect bilirubinemia, and reticulocytosis can be expected, depending on the mechanism of the hemolysis.

Hemolytic anemias must be differentiated from other anemias associated with bilirubinemia, reticulocytosis, or both. Anemia with reticulocytosis but without bilirubinemia is expected during recovery from hemorrhage not treated with transfusion or with effective treatment of deficiencies such as iron deficiency. Anemia that results from hemorrhage into a body cavity is characterized by reticulocytosis during recovery and bilirubinemia as a result of catabolism of the hemoglobin in the hemorrhaged cells. RBC morphology should remain normal throughout the event, however. Anemias associated with ineffective erythropoiesis, such as megaloblastic anemia, are essentially hemolytic, with the cell death occurring in the bone marrow. Bilirubinemia and elevated serum lactate dehydrogenase levels are to be expected, but the reticulocyte count is low. Because most of the RBCs never reach the periphery, such anemias are typically classified as anemias of diminished production rather than as hemolytic anemias. As summarized in Table 20.5, the differential diagnosis in each of these instances may rely on negative results of tests for increased cell destruction or accelerated production.

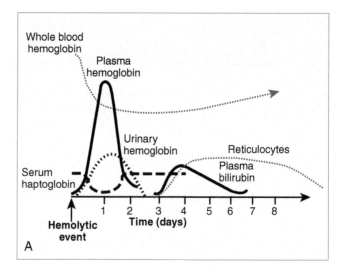

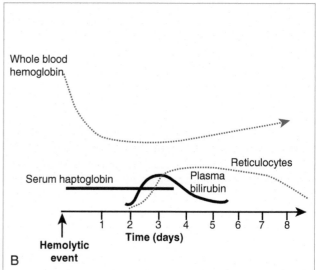

Figure 20.7 Hemolysis Timelines. (A), Example of fragmentation (intravascular) hemolysis timeline. During fragmentation hemolysis, hemoglobin is detectable in plasma and urine for a period very soon after the hemolysis occurs. Haptoglobin levels will drop as the plasma hemoglobin rises. When hemolysis ends, the hemoglobin will disappear from plasma and urine as the haptoglobin returns to normal. However, the protoporphyrin of salvaged hemoglobin will be processed to bilirubin that will rise after the hemolytic event. Assuming the hemolysis has resulted in anemia, reticulocyte indices will also rise several days after the hemolytic event. **(B),** Example of macrophage-mediated (extravascular) hemolysis timeline. With macrophage-mediated hemolysis, the contents of the red blood cells do not enter the blood, so evidence of hemolysis is delayed until bilirubin and reticulocytes rise.

TABLE 20.5	Differential Diagnosis of Hemolytic Anemias Versus Other Causes of Indirect Bilirubinemia and Reticulocytosis			
	Hemoglobin Level	Indirect Bilirubinemia	Reticulocytosis	Spherocytes or Schistocytes
Hemolytic anemia—acute, fragmentation	Rapidly dropping	Delayed	Delayed	Schistocytes
Hemolytic anemia—acute, macrophage-mediated	Rapidly dropping	Delayed	Delayed	Spherocytes
Hemolytic anemia—chronic, fragmentation	Persistently low	Persistent	Persistent	Schistocytes
Hemolytic anemia—chronic, macrophage-mediated	Persistently low	Persistent	Persistent	Spherocytes
Acute hemorrhage	Rapidly dropping	Absent	Delayed	Absent

Continued

TABLE 20.5 **Differential Diagnosis of Hemolytic Anemias Versus Other Causes of Indirect Bilirubinemia and Reticulocytosis—cont'd**

	Hemoglobin Level	Indirect Bilirubinemia	Reticulocytosis	Spherocytes or Schistocytes
Hemodilution	Rapidly dropping	Absent	Absent	Absent
Recovery from hemorrhage	Rising	Absent	Present	Absent
Treated anemia (iron, vitamin B$_{12}$, or folate deficiency)	Rising	Absent or declining	Present	Absent
Hemorrhage into a body cavity	Rapidly dropping	Delayed	Delayed	Absent
Ineffective erythropoiesis (e.g., megaloblastic anemia)	Dropping	Persistent	Absent	Absent

SUMMARY

- A hemolytic disorder is a condition in which there is increased destruction of red blood cells (RBCs) and a compensatory acceleration in RBC production by the bone marrow.
- A hemolytic anemia develops when the bone marrow is unable to compensate for the shortened survival of the RBCs.
- Hemolytic anemias can be classified as acute or chronic, intravascular or extravascular, acquired or inherited, intrinsic or extrinsic, and fragmentation or macrophage mediated.
- Most RBC death in healthy individuals occurs via macrophages of the spleen and liver. A small amount occurs by fragmentation due to mechanical trauma.
- Hemoglobin from RBCs is converted to heme and globin within macrophages. Heme is further degraded to iron, carbon monoxide, and unconjugated bilirubin. The bilirubin is secreted into the blood, where it binds to albumin and is transported to the liver. In the liver, bilirubin is conjugated with glucuronic acid and excreted as bile into the intestines, and it is converted to urobilinogen by intestinal bacteria. Some urobilinogen is reabsorbed into the portal circulation and reexcreted through the liver. A small amount of urobilinogen remains in the blood, and it is excreted by the kidney into the urine.
- In macrophage-mediated (extravascular) hemolytic anemia, there is an increase in unconjugated bilirubin in the plasma and an increase in urobilinogen in the stool and urine. Spherocytes may be seen on the peripheral blood film.
- Signs of fragmentation (intravascular) hemolysis include (met)hemoglobinemia, (met)hemoglobinuria, and hemosiderinuria.

- Serum haptoglobin is markedly decreased or absent. Schistocytes may be seen on the peripheral blood film.
- Jaundice can result from increased serum unconjugated bilirubin during any hemolytic anemia.
- Major clinical features of chronic inherited hemolytic anemia are varying degrees of anemia, jaundice, splenomegaly, and the development of cholelithiasis. In children, bone abnormalities may develop as a result of accelerated erythropoiesis.
- Laboratory studies providing evidence of hemolytic anemia include tests for increased RBC destruction and compensatory increase in the rate of erythropoiesis. Elevated serum indirect bilirubin level with a normal serum direct bilirubin level suggests accelerated RBC destruction. A moderate to marked decrease in serum haptoglobin level suggests a fragmentation cause of hemolysis. The reticulocyte count is the most commonly used laboratory test to identify accelerated erythropoiesis, including an elevation of the immature reticulocyte fraction. Other tests that are specific to a particular diagnosis also may be needed.
- Hemolytic anemias must be differentiated from other anemias with reticulocytosis, including the post-acute hemorrhage state and recovery from iron, vitamin B$_{12}$, or folate deficiency, and from those with bilirubinemia, such as with internal bleeding.

Now that you have completed this chapter, go back and read again the case study at the beginning and respond to the questions presented.

REVIEW QUESTIONS

Answers can be found in the Appendix.

1. The term *hemolytic disorder* in general refers to a disorder in which there is:
   a. Increased destruction of RBCs in the blood, bone marrow, or spleen
   b. Excessive loss of RBCs from the body
   c. Inadequate RBC production by the bone marrow
   d. Increased plasma volume with unchanged red cell mass
2. RBC destruction that occurs when macrophages ingest and destroy RBCs is termed:
   a. Extracellular
   b. Macrophage mediated
   c. Intra-organ
   d. Extrahematopoietic

3. A sign of hemolysis that is typically associated with both fragmentation and macrophage-mediated hemolysis is:
   a. Hemoglobinuria
   b. Hemosiderinuria
   c. Hemoglobinemia
   d. Elevated urinary urobilinogen level

4. An elderly white woman is evaluated for worsening anemia, with a decrease of approximately 0.5 mg/dL of hemoglobin each week. The patient is pale, and her skin and eyes are slightly yellow. She complains of extreme fatigue and is unable to complete the tasks of daily living without napping in mid-morning and midafternoon. She also tires with exertion, finding it difficult to climb even five stairs. Which of the features of this description points to a hemolytic cause for her anemia?
   a. Pallor
   b. Yellow skin and eyes
   c. Need for naps
   d. Tiredness on exertion

5. Which of the following tests provides a good indication of accelerated erythropoiesis?
   a. Urine urobilinogen level
   b. Hemosiderin level
   c. Reticulocyte count
   d. Glycated hemoglobin level

6. A 5-year-old girl was seen by her physician several days before the current visit and was diagnosed with pneumonia. She was prescribed a standard course of antibiotics. Her mother has brought her to the physician again because the girl's urine began to darken after the first visit and now is alarmingly dark. The girl has no history of anemia, and there is no family history of any hematologic disorder. The CBC shows a mild anemia, polychromasia, and a few schistocytes. This anemia could be categorized as:
   a. Acquired, fragmentation
   b. Acquired, macrophage mediated
   c. Hereditary, fragmentation
   d. Hereditary, macrophage mediated

7. A patient has a personal and family history of a mild hemolytic anemia. The patient has consistently elevated levels of total and indirect serum bilirubin and urinary urobilinogen. The serum haptoglobin level is consistently decreased, whereas the reticulocyte count is elevated. The latter can be seen as polychromasia on the patient's peripheral blood film. Spherocytes are also noted. Which one of the findings reported for this patient is *inconsistent* with a classical diagnosis of fragmentation hemolysis?
   a. Elevated total and indirect serum bilirubin
   b. Elevated urinary urobilinogen
   c. Decreased haptoglobin
   d. Spherocytes on the peripheral blood film

8. Under normal circumstances, the major fraction of bilirubin in the plasma is:
   a. Unconjugated bilirubin secreted by in the liver
   b. Urobilinogen reabsorbed from the intestines
   c. Macrophage-secreted indirect bilirubin
   d. Direct bilirubin conjugated by hepatocytes

9. A patient has anemia that has been worsening over the last several months. The hemoglobin level has been declining slowly, with a drop of 1.5 g/dL of hemoglobin over about 6 weeks. Polychromasia and anisocytosis are seen on the peripheral blood film, consistent with the elevated reticulocyte count and red cell distribution width (RDW). Serum levels of total bilirubin and indirect fractions are normal. The urinary urobilinogen level also is normal. When these findings are evaluated, the conclusion is drawn that the anemia does not have a hemolytic component. Based on the data given here, why was hemolysis ruled out as the cause of the anemia?
   a. The decline in hemoglobin is too gradual to be associated with hemolysis.
   b. The elevation of the reticulocyte count suggests a malignant cause.
   c. Evidence of increased protoporphyrin catabolism is lacking.
   d. Elevated RDW points to an anemia of decreased production.

10. Which of the following sets of test results is typically expected with chronic fragmentation hemolysis?

	Serum Haptoglobin	Urine Hemoglobin	Urine Sediment Prussian Blue Stain
a.	Increased	Positive	Positive
b.	Decreased	Negative	Negative
c.	Decreased	Positive	Positive
d.	Increased	Positive	Negative

REFERENCES

1. Crosby, W. H., & Akeroyd, J. H. (1952). The limit of hemoglobin synthesis in hereditary hemolytic anemia. *Am J Med, 13*, 273–283.
2. Hillman, R. S., & Henderson, P. A. (1969). Control of marrow production by the level of iron supply. *J Clin Invest, 48*(3), 454–460.
3. Cui, Y., Konig, J., Leier, I., et al. (2001). Hepatic uptake of bilirubin and its conjugates by the human organic anion transporter SLC21A6. *J Biol Chem, 276*, 9626–9630.
4. Keppler, D. (2014). The roles of MRP2, MRP3, OATP1B1, and OATP1B3 in conjugated hyperbilirubinemia. *Drug Metab Dispos, 42*, 561–565.
5. Sticova, E., & Jirsa, M. (2013). New insights in bilirubin metabolism and their clinical implications. *World J Gastroent, 19*(38), 6398–6407.
6. Keppler, D., & Kartenbeck, J. (1996). The canalicular conjugate export pump encoded by the cmrp/cmoat gene. *Prog Liver Dis, 14*, 55–67.
7. van de Steeg, E., Wagenaar, E., van der Kruijssen, C. M., et al. (2010). Organic anion transporting polypeptide 1a/1b-knock-out

mice provide insights into hepatic handling of bilirubin, bile acids, and drugs. *J Clin Invest, 120,* 2942–2952.

8. Quigley, J. G., Means, R. T., & Glader, B. (2014). The birth, life, and death of red blood cells: erythropoiesis, the mature red blood cell, and cell destruction. In Greer, J. P., Arber, D. A., Glader, B., et al. (Eds.), *Wintrobe's Clinical Hematology.* (13th ed., pp. 83–124). Philadelphia: Wolters Kluwer Health/Lippincott Williams & Wilkins.

9. Schaer, D. J., Buehler, P. W., Alayash, A. I., et al. (2013). Hemolysis and free hemoglobin revisited: exploring hemoglobin and hemin scavengers as a novel class of therapeutic proteins. *Blood, 121,* 1276–1284.

10. Andersen, C. B. F., Torvund-Jensen, M., Nielsen, M. J., et al. (2012). Structure of the haptoglobin-haemoglobin complex. *Nature, 489,* 456–460.

11. Ratanasopa, K., Chakane, S., Ilyas, M., et al. (2013). Trapping of human hemoglobin by haptoglobin: molecular mechanisms and clinical applications. *Antiox Redox Signal, 18,* 2364–2374.

12. Etzerodt, A., & Moestrup, S. (2013). CD163 and inflammation: biological, diagnostic and therapeutic aspects. *Antioxid Redox Signal, 18,* 2352–2363.

13. Kristiansen, M., Graversen, J. H., Jacobsen, C., et al. (2001). Identification of the haemoglobin scavenger receptor. *Nature, 409,* 198–201.

14. Tolosano, E., & Altruda, F. (2002). Hemopexin: structure, function, and regulation. *DNA Cell Biol, 21,* 297–306.

15. Delanghe, J. R., & Langlois, M. R. (2001). Hemopexin: a review of biological aspects and the role in laboratory medicine. *Clin Chim Acta, 312,* 13–23.

16. Smith, A. (2014). Protection against heme toxicity: hemopexin rules, OK? In Ferreira, G. C. (Ed.), *Handbook of Porphyrin Science: With Applications to Chemistry, Physics, Materials Science, Engineering, Biology and Medicine. 30,* 311–388.

17. Hvidberg, V., Maniecki, M. B., Jacobsen, C., et al. (2005). Identification of the receptor scavenging hemopexin-heme complexes. *Blood, 106,* 2572–2579.

18. Tolosano, E., Fagoonee, S., Morello, N., et al. (2010). Heme scavenging and the other facets of hemopexin. *Antioxid Redox Signal, 12,* 305–320.

19. Smith, A., & Morgan, W. T. (1979). Haem transport to the liver by haemopexin. *Biochem J, 182,* 47–54.

20. Morgan, W. T., Liem, H. H., Sutor, R. P., et al. (1976). Transfer of heme from heme-albumin to hemopexin. *Biochem Biophys Acta, 444,* 435–445.

21. Smith, A., & McCulloh, R. J. (2016). Hemopexin and haptoglobin: allies against heme toxicity from hemoglobin not contenders. *Frontiers in Physiol, 6*(Article 187), 1–20.

22. Zhang, D., Meyron-Holtz, E., & Rouault, T. A. (2007). Renal iron metabolism: transferrin iron delivery and the role of iron regulatory proteins. *J Am Soc Nephrol, 18,* 401–406.

23. Wolff, N., Liu, W., Fenton, R. A., et al. (2011). Ferroportin 1 is expressed basolaterally in rat kidney proximal tubule cells and iron excess increases its membrane trafficking. *J Cell Mol Med, 15,* 209–219.

24. Kondo, H., Saito, K., Grasso, J. P., et al. (1988). Iron metabolism in the erythrophagocytosing Kupffer cell. *Hepatology, 8*(1), 32–38.

25. Thevenod, F., & Wolff, N. A. (2016). Iron transport in the kidney: implications for physiology and cadmium nephrotoxicity. *Metallomics, 8,* 17–42.

26. Christiansen, E. I., Verroust, P. J., & Nielsen, R. (2009). Receptor-mediated endocytosis in renal proximal tubule. *Pfulgers Arch-Eur J Physiol, 458,* 1039–1048.

27. Ferenbach, D. A., Kluth, D. C., & Hughes, J. (2010). Hemeoxygenase-1 and renal ischaemia-reperfusion injury. *Exp Nephrol, 115,* e33–e37.

28. Gaganis, P., Miners, J. O., Brennan, J. S., et al. (2007). Human renal cortical and medullary UDP-glucuronosyltransferases (UGTs): immunohistochemical localization of UGT2B7 and UGT1A enzymes and kinetic characterization of S-naproxen glucuronidation. *J Pharmacol Exp Ther, 323*(2), 422–30.

29. Schaub, T. P., Kartenbeck, J., Konig, J., et al. (1999). Expression of the MRP2 gene-encoded conjugate export pump in human kidney proximal tubules and in renal cell carcinoma. *J Am Soc Nephrol, 10,* 1159–1169.

30. Brandoni, A., Hazelhoff, M. H., Bulacio, R. P., et al. (2012). Expression and function of renal and hepatic organic anion transporters in extrahepatic cholestasis. *World J Gastroent, 18*(44), 6387–6397.

31. Trotman, B. W. (1991). Pigment gallstone disease. *Gastroent Clin North Am, 20,* 111–126.

32. Means, R. T. Jr., & Glader, B. (2014). Anemia: general considerations. In Greer, J. P., Arber, D. A., Glader, B., et al. (Eds.), *Wintrobe's Clinical Hematology.* (13th ed., pp. 587–616). Philadelphia: Wolters Kluwer Health/Lippincott Williams & Wilkins.

33. Crosby, W. H., & Dameshek, W. (1951). The significance of hemoglobinemia and associated hemosiderinuria, with particular reference to various types of hemolytic anemia. *J Lab Clin Med, 38,* 829–841.

34. Marchand, A., Galen, R. S., & Van Lente, F. (1980). The predictive value of serum haptoglobin in hemolytic disease. *JAMA, 243,* 1909–1911.

35. Coburn, R. F. (1970). Endogenous carbon monoxide production in man. *N Engl J Med, 282,* 207–209.

36. Cohen, R. M., Franco, R. S., Khera, P. K., et al. (2008). Red cell life span heterogeneity in hematologically normal people is sufficient to alter HbA1c. *Blood, 112,* 4284–4291.

37. International Committee for Standardization in Haematology. (1980). Recommended method for radioisotope red cell survival studies. *Br J Haematol, 45,* 659–666.

38. Korell, J., Coulter, C. V., & Duffull, S. B. (2011). Evaluation of red blood cell labeling methods based on a statistical model for red blood cell survival. *J Theor Biol, 291,* 88–98.

Intrinsic Defects Leading to Increased Erythrocyte Destruction

*S. Renee Hodgkins**

OBJECTIVES

After completion of this chapter, the reader will be able to:

1. Describe the intrinsic cell properties that affect red blood cell (RBC) deformability.
2. Explain how defects in vertical and horizontal membrane protein interactions can result in a hemolytic anemia.
3. Compare and contrast hereditary spherocytosis, hereditary elliptocytosis, and hereditary ovalocytosis, including the inheritance pattern, mutated membrane proteins, mechanism of hemolysis, typical RBC morphology, and clinical and laboratory findings.
4. Compare and contrast the RBC morphology and laboratory findings of hereditary spherocytosis and immune-associated hemolytic anemias.
5. Explain the principle, interpretation, and limitations of the osmotic fragility and eosin-5′-maleimide (EMA) binding tests in the diagnosis of hereditary spherocytosis.
6. Describe the causes, pathophysiology, RBC morphology, and clinical and laboratory findings of hemolytic anemias characterized by stomatocytosis.

7. Describe the causes and pathophysiology of hereditary and acquired conditions characterized by acanthocytosis.
8. Describe the cause, pathophysiology, clinical manifestations, laboratory findings, and treatment for paroxysmal nocturnal hemoglobinuria.
9. Compare and contrast the inheritance pattern, pathophysiology, clinical symptoms, and typical laboratory findings of glucose-6-phosphate dehydrogenase deficiency and pyruvate kinase deficiency.
10. Given the history, symptoms, laboratory findings, and a representative microscopic field from a peripheral blood film for a patient with a suspected intrinsic hemolytic anemia, discuss possible causes of the anemia and indicate the data that support these conclusions.

OUTLINE

Red Blood Cell Membrane Abnormalities
   Red Blood Cell Membrane Structure and Function
   Hereditary Red Blood Cell Membrane Abnormalities
   Acquired Red Blood Cell Membrane Abnormalities

Red Blood Cell Enzymopathies
   Glucose-6-Phosphate Dehydrogenase Deficiency
   Pyruvate Kinase Deficiency
   Other Enzymopathies

CASE STUDY

After studying the material in this chapter, the reader should be able to respond to the following case study:

A 45-year-old man sought medical attention for the onset of chest pain. Physical examination revealed slight jaundice and splenomegaly. The medical history included gallstones, and there was a family history of anemia. A complete blood count (CBC) yielded the following results:

	Patient Results	Reference Intervals
WBCs (×10⁹/L)	13.4	3.6–10.6
RBCs (×10¹²/L)	4.20	4.60–6.00

	Patient Results	Reference Intervals
HGB (g/dL)	11.9	14.0–18.0
HCT (%)	32.4	40–54
MCV (fL)	77.1	80–100
MCH (pg)	28.3	26–32
MCHC (g/dL)	36.7	32–36
RDW (%)	22.9	11.5–14.5
Platelets (×10⁹/L)	290	150–450

*The author extends appreciation to Elaine M. Keohane, whose work in prior editions provided the foundation for this chapter.

The peripheral blood film revealed anisocytosis, polychromasia, and sphero-cytes (Figure 21.1).

1. From the data given, what is a likely cause of the anemia?
2. What additional laboratory tests would be of value in establishing the diagnosis, and what abnormalities in the results of these tests would be expected to confirm your impression?
3. What is the cause of this type of anemia?

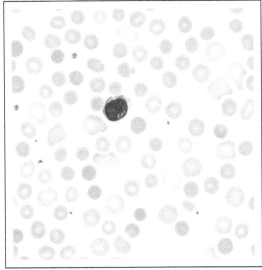

Figure 21.1 Peripheral Blood Film for the Patient in the Case Study. (Wright-Giemsa stain, ×500.) (From Rodak, B. F., & Carr, J. H. [2017]. *Clinical Hematology Atlas.* [5th ed.]. Philadelphia: Elsevier.)

Intrinsic hemolytic anemias comprise a large group of disorders in which defects in the red blood cells (RBCs) result in premature hemolysis and anemia. Intrinsic disorders can be divided into abnormalities of the RBC membrane, metabolic enzymes, or hemoglobin. Most of these defects are hereditary. This chapter covers defects in the RBC membrane and enzymes causing hemolytic anemia. Chapter 24 covers qualitative hemoglobin disorders, and Chapter 25 covers quantitative hemoglobin disorders (thalassemias).

RED BLOOD CELL MEMBRANE ABNORMALITIES

Red Blood Cell Membrane Structure and Function

The RBC maintains a biconcave discoid shape that is essential for normal function and survival for 120 days in the peripheral circulation. The key to maintaining this shape is the plasma membrane, a lipid bilayer embedded with proteins and connected to an underlying protein cytoskeleton (Figure 6.2). The insoluble lipid portion serves as a barrier to separate the vastly different ion and metabolite concentrations of the interior of the RBC from its external environment, the blood plasma. The concentration of the constituents in the cytoplasm is tightly regulated by proteins embedded in the membrane that serve as pumps and channels for movement of ions and other material between the RBC's interior and the blood plasma. Various membrane proteins also act as receptors, RBC antigens, enzymes, and support for the surface carbohydrates. The lipid bilayer remains intact because two transmembrane protein complexes embedded in the membrane anchor it to a two-dimensional protein lattice (cytoskeleton) immediately beneath its surface (Chapter 6).[1] Together the transmembrane proteins and underlying cytoskeleton provide structural integrity, cohesion, and mechanical stability to the cell.

In their life span, RBCs must repeatedly maneuver through very narrow capillaries and squeeze through the splenic sieve (narrow slits or fenestrations in the endothelial cell lining of the splenic sinuses) as they move from the splenic cords to the sinuses. To accomplish this without premature lysis, the RBCs must have *deformability,* or the ability to repeatedly bend, stretch, distort, and then return to the normal discoid, biconcave shape.[2] The cellular properties that enable RBC deformability include the RBC's biconcave, discoid geometry; the elasticity (pliancy) of its membrane; and its cytoplasmic viscosity (Chapter 6).[3,4]

The biconcave, discoid geometry of the RBC is dependent on vertical and horizontal interactions between the transmembrane and cytoskeletal proteins (listed in Tables 6.5 and 6.6).[3] Two transmembrane protein complexes, the ankyrin complex and actin (protein 4.1) junctional complex, provide *vertical* structural integrity to the cell by anchoring the lipid bilayer to the underlying spectrin cytoskeleton.[3,5,6] In the ankyrin complex, ankyrin and protein 4.2 link transmembrane proteins (band 3, RhAG, and other associated proteins) to β-spectrin in the cytoskeleton.[6-8] In the actin junctional complex, protein 4.1 and actin link transmembrane proteins (band 3, GLUT1, and other associated proteins) to β-spectrin in the cytoskeleton, with protein 4.2, adducin, dematin, tropomyosin, and tropomodulin as accessory proteins (Figure 6.3).[6,9] These interactions are called *vertical* because they are perpendicular to the plane of the cytoskeleton. Vertical interactions prevent the loss of membrane, which would result in decreased surface area-to-volume ratio of the RBC.[3,5] Two major cytoskeletal proteins, α-spectrin and β-spectrin, interact laterally with each other to form antiparallel heterodimers, which link with other spectrin heterodimers to form tetramers. The ends of spectrin tetramers are joined in the actin junctional complex with the accessory proteins mentioned earlier, thus linking the spectrin tetramers in a two-dimensional lattice.[3,10,11] These proteins provide *horizontal* mechanical stability, which prevents the membrane from fragmenting in response to mechanical stress.[3,5]

Factors that affect the elasticity of the cell are not as clear. Interactions between the spectrin dimers and their junctional complexes are flexible and allow for movement as the RBCs stretch and bend.[3,11] In addition, the ability of spectrin repeats to unfold and refold is likely to be one of the determinants of membrane elasticity.[11,12]

The cytoplasmic viscosity depends on the concentration of hemoglobin, as well as the maintenance of the proper cell volume by the normal functioning of various channels and pumps that allow the passage of ions, water, and macromolecules in and out of the cell.[3]

A defect in the RBCs that changes the membrane geometry, its elasticity, or the viscosity of the cytoplasm affects RBC deformability and can result in premature hemolysis and anemia.[3] The RBC membrane is discussed in more detail in Chapter 6; the reader is encouraged to review that chapter when studying defects in the membrane.

Hereditary Red Blood Cell Membrane Abnormalities

Most defects in the RBC membrane that can cause hemolytic anemia are hereditary; however, acquired defects also exist. Hereditary RBC membrane defects have historically been classified by morphologic features. The major disorders are hereditary spherocytosis, characterized by spherocytes, and hereditary elliptocytosis, characterized by elliptical RBCs. Hereditary pyropoikilocytosis, a variant of hereditary elliptocytosis, is characterized by marked poikilocytosis and heat sensitivity. Other less common membrane disorders include hereditary ovalocytosis, overhydrated hereditary stomatocytosis (also called hereditary hydrocytosis), and dehydrated hereditary stomatocytosis (also called hereditary xerocytosis). Hereditary membrane defects can also be classified as those that affect membrane structure (altering geometry and elasticity) and those that affect membrane transport (altering cytoplasmic viscosity) (Box 21.1).[11] The

> ### BOX 21.1 Classification of Major Hereditary Membrane Defects Causing Hemolytic Anemia
>
> **Mutations That Alter Membrane Structure**
> Hereditary spherocytosis
> Hereditary elliptocytosis/pyropoikilocytosis
> Hereditary ovalocytosis (Southeast Asian ovalocytosis)
>
> **Mutations That Alter Membrane Transport Proteins**
> Overhydrated hereditary stomatocytosis (hereditary hydrocytosis)
> Dehydrated hereditary stomatocytosis (hereditary xerocytosis)

membrane structural defects can be further divided into those that affect vertical membrane protein interactions and those that affect horizontal membrane protein interactions.[5,11] The major hereditary membrane defects are described in Table 21.1.

Mutations That Alter Membrane Structure

Hereditary spherocytosis. Hereditary spherocytosis (HS) is a heterogeneous group of hemolytic anemias caused by defects in proteins that disrupt the vertical interactions between transmembrane proteins and the underlying protein cytoskeleton. HS has worldwide distribution and affects 1 in 2000 to 3000 individuals of northern European ancestry.[6,11,13] In 75% of families, it is inherited as an autosomal dominant trait and is expressed in heterozygotes who have one affected parent.[6] Homozygotes are rare; such patients present with severe hemolytic anemia but have asymptomatic parents.[13] In approximately 25% of cases, the inheritance is nondominant, with some autosomal recessive cases.[11,13]

Pathophysiology. HS results from gene mutations in which the defective proteins disrupt the vertical linkages between the lipid bilayer and the cytoskeletal network (Figure 6.5).[5] Various mutations in five known genes can result in the HS phenotype (Table 21.1). Mutations can occur in genes for (1) cytoskeletal proteins, including *ANK1*, which codes for ankyrin (40% to 65% of cases in the United States and Europe; 5% to 10% of cases in Japan); *SPTA1*, which codes for α-spectrin (fewer than 5% of cases); *SPTB*, which codes for β-spectrin (15% to 30% of cases); and *EPB42*, which codes for protein 4.2 (fewer than 5% of cases in the United States and Europe; 45% to 50% of cases in Japan); and (2) a transmembrane protein, band 3 which is coded by *SLC4A1* (20% to 35% of cases).[6,11] Less than 10% of cases involve de novo mutations, with most affecting the ankyrin gene.[13] A mutation database for HS lists 130 different mutations (*ANK1*, 52; *SCL4A1*, 49; *SPTA1*, 2; *SPTB*, 19; and *EPB42*, 8).[14] Because of the vertical interactions of the transmembrane proteins and cytoskeletal protein lattice, a primary mutation in one gene may have a secondary effect on another protein in the membrane. For example, primary mutations in *ANK1* result in both ankyrin and spectrin deficiencies in the RBC membrane.[13,15,16] In approximately 10% of patients, no mutation is identified.[11]

The defects in vertical membrane protein interactions cause RBCs to lose unsupported lipid membrane over time because of local disconnections of the lipid bilayer and underlying cytoskeleton. Essentially, small portions of the membrane form vesicles; the vesicles are released with little loss of cell volume.[13] The RBCs acquire a decreased surface area-to-volume ratio, and the cells become spherical. These cells do not have the deformability of normal biconcave discoid RBCs, and their survival in the spleen is decreased.[4,13,15] As the spherocytes attempt to move through the narrow, elliptical fenestrations of the endothelial cells lining the splenic sinusoids (2 to 3 μm in diameter), they acquire further membrane loss or become trapped and are rapidly removed by the macrophages of the red pulp of the spleen.[4,11,13] In addition, as the RBCs are sequestered in the spleen, the membrane can acquire yet more damage, lose more

TABLE 21.1   Characteristics of Major Hemolytic Anemias Caused by Hereditary Membrane Defects

Condition	Inheritance Pattern	Deficient Protein (Mutated Gene)	Pathophysiology	Typical RBC Morphology	Clinical Findings/ Comments
Hereditary spherocytosis	75% autosomal dominant 25% nondomi- nant	Ankyrin (ANK1) Band 3 (SLC4A1) α-Spectrin (SPTA1) β-Spectrin (SPTB) Protein 4.2 (EPB42)	Mutation in protein that disrupts vertical membrane interactions between transmembrane pro- teins and underlying cytoskele- ton; loss of membrane and ↓ surface area-to-volume ratio	Spherocytes, polychromasia	Varies from asymptomatic to severe Typical features: spleno- megaly, jaundice, anemia
Hereditary elliptocytosis	Autosomal dominant	α-Spectrin (SPTA1) β-Spectrin (SPTB) Protein 4.1 (EPB41)	Mutation in protein that disrupts the horizontal linkages in the cytoskeleton; loss of mechanical stability of membrane	Few to 100% ellipto- cytes; schistocytes in severe cases	90% of cases asymptom- atic; 10% of cases show moderate to severe anemia
Hereditary pyropoi- kilocytosis (rare subtype of heredi- tary elliptocytosis)	Autosomal recessive	α-Spectrin (SPTA1) β-Spectrin (SPTB) Homozygous or compound heterozygous	Mutation in spectrin that disrupts horizontal linkages in cytoskele- ton; severe RBC fragmentation	Elliptocytes, schisto- cytes, microsphero- cytes	Severe anemia
Southeast Asian ovalocytosis	Autosomal dominant	Band 3 (SLC4A1); only one known mutation	Mutation in band 3 that causes excessive membrane rigidity; only exists in heterozygous state	30% oval cells with one or two transverse ridges	Asymptomatic or mild hemolysis; prevalent in some areas of Southeast Asia
Overhydrated hereditary stomatocytosis (hereditary hydrocytosis)	Autosomal dominant	Rh-associated glycoprotein (RHAG) Others unknown	Mutation in protein that causes ↑ membrane permeability to sodium and potassium; high intracellular sodium causes influx of water, ↑ cell volume (↑ MCV), and ↓ cytoplasmic viscosity (↓ MCHC)	Stomatocytes (5%–50%), macrocytes	Moderate to severe hemo- lytic anemia; splenec- tomy is contraindicated because of thrombotic risk
Dehydrated heredi- tary stomatocyto- sis (hereditary xerocytosis)	Autosomal dominant	Piezo-type mechanosensitive ion channel component 1 (PIEZO1) Potassium calcium-activated channel subfamily N member 4 (KCNN4)	Mutation in protein that causes ↑ membrane permeability to potas- sium; low intracellular potassium causes loss of water from cell, ↓ cell volume (↓ MCV), and ↑ cyto- plasmic viscosity (↑ MCHC)	Target cells, burr cells, stomatocytes (<10%), RBCs with "puddled" hemoglobin at periph- ery, desiccated cells with spicules	Mild to moderate anemia, splenomegaly; may lead to fetal loss, hydrops fetalis; may be accompanied by pseudohyperkalemia

↑, Increased; ↓, decreased; *MCHC*, mean cell hemoglobin concentration; *MCV*, mean cell volume; *RBC*, red blood cell.

lipid membrane, and become more spherical as a result of splenic conditioning.[4,13,15] The conditioning may be enhanced by the acidic conditions in the spleen and the prolonged contact of the RBCs with macrophages.[13,15] Low glucose and adenosine triphos- phate (ATP) levels and phagocyte-produced free radicals, which cause oxidative damage, may also play a role (Figure 21.2).[13,15]

In HS, RBC membranes also have abnormal permeability to cations, particularly sodium and potassium, which is likely a result of disruption of the integrity of the protein cytoskele- ton.[4,17] The cells become dehydrated, but the exact mechanism is not clear. Excess activity of the Na^+-K^+ ATPase may cause a reduction in intracellular cations, causing more water to diffuse out of the cell.[4,13] This results in an increase in viscosity and cellular dehydration.[13] The abnormality is not related to defects in cation transport proteins, and dehydration occurs regardless of the type of primary mutation causing the HS.[17]

Clinical and laboratory findings. Symptomatic HS has three key clinical manifestations: anemia, jaundice, and spleno- megaly. Symptoms of HS may first appear in infancy, childhood,

or adulthood, or even at an advanced age.[16] There is wide varia- tion in symptoms. Silent carriers are clinically asymptomatic with normal laboratory findings and usually are identified only if they are the parents of a child with recessively inherited HS.[4,13,16] Approximately 20% to 30% of patients have mild HS and are asymptomatic because an increase in erythropoiesis compensates for the RBC loss.[4,6] They usually have normal he- moglobin levels but may show subtle signs of HS, with a slight increase in serum bilirubin in the range of 1.0 to 2.0 mg/dL, an increased reticulocyte count of up to 6%, and a few spherocytes on the peripheral blood film.[4,6,16] Mild HS may first become evident during pregnancy, during illnesses that cause spleno- megaly (such as infectious mononucleosis), or in aging, when the rate of erythropoiesis starts to decline.[13,16] Approximately 60% of patients have moderate HS with incompletely compen- sated hemolytic anemia, hemoglobin levels greater than 8 g/dL, serum bilirubin more than 2 mg/dL, reticulocyte counts in the range of 6% to 10% (typically >8%), and spherocytes on the peripheral blood film.[4,6,11,16] Jaundice is seen at some time in

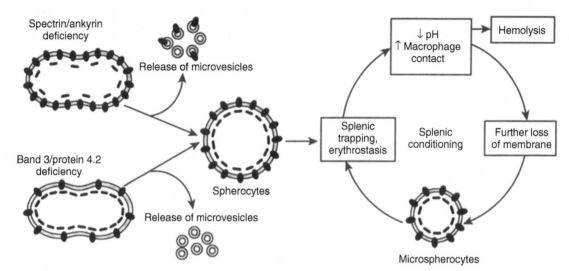

Figure 21.2 Pathophysiology of Hereditary Spherocytosis. The primary defect in hereditary spherocytosis is a loss of membrane resulting in a deficiency of membrane surface area. Decreased surface area may be produced by different mechanisms: (1) Defects of spectrin, ankyrin, or protein 4.2 lead to reduced density of the membrane skeleton, destabilizing the overlying lipid bilayer and releasing band 3-containing microvesicles. (2) Defects of band 3 lead to band 3 deficiency and loss of its lipid-stabilizing effect. This results in the loss of band 3-free microvesicles. Both pathways result in membrane loss, decreased surface area-to-volume ratio, and formation of spherocytes with decreased deformability. These deformed erythrocytes become trapped in the hostile environment of the spleen (low pH, low glucose and high oxidant levels, and contact with macrophages). Splenic conditioning results either in hemolysis or further membrane damage forming microspherocytes, thus amplifying the cycle of red cell membrane injury. (From Gallagher, P. G. [2018]. Red blood cell membrane disorders. In Hoffman, R., Benz, E. J., Silberstein, L. E., et al. (Eds.), *Hematology: Basic Principles and Practice.* [7th ed., Figure 45.2]. Philadelphia: Elsevier.)

about half these patients, usually during viral infections. About 5% to 10% of patients have moderate to severe HS, with hemoglobin levels usually in the range of 6 to 8 g/dL, serum bilirubin between 2 to 3 mg/dL, and reticulocyte counts greater than 10%.[4,6,16] About 3% to 5% of patients have severe HS, with hemoglobin levels less than 6 g/dL, serum bilirubin greater than 3 mg/dL, and reticulocyte counts greater than 10%.[4,6,15] Patients with severe HS are usually homozygous for HS mutations and require regular transfusions.[13] Splenomegaly is found in about

half of young children and in 75% to 95% of older children and adults with HS.[4,11,15]

The hallmark of HS is spherocytes on the peripheral blood film. When present in patients with childhood hemolytic anemia and a family history of similar abnormalities, the uniform spherocytes are highly suggestive of HS. Some of these are microspherocytes, appearing as small, round, dense RBCs that are filled with hemoglobin and lack a central pallor (Figure 21.3). Normal-appearing RBCs, along with polychromasia and varying

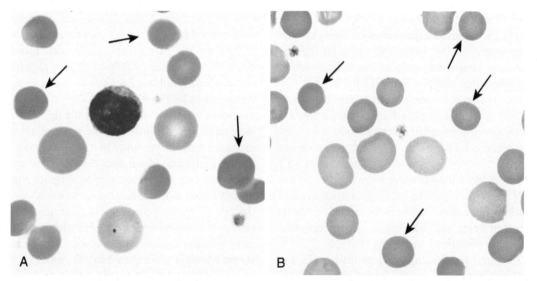

Figure 21.3 Spherocytes (*arrows*), (A and B). (Peripheral blood, Wright-Giemsa stain, ×1000.)

degrees of anisocytosis and poikilocytosis, are present. In addition to spherocytes, occasionally other RBC morphologic variants may be observed in some types of mutations: acanthocytes in some β-spectrin mutations,[18] pincered or mushroom-shaped cells in some cases of band 3 deficiency in patients without splenectomy,[19] and ovalostomatocytes in homozygous *EPB4.2* mutations.[20] Note that spherocytes are not specific for HS and can be seen in other hereditary and acquired conditions.

Because of the spherocytosis, patients with moderate to severe HS have an increase in the mean cell hemoglobin concentration (MCHC) greater than 36 mg/dL.[4,16,21] The mean cell volume (MCV) is variable, ranging from within the reference interval to slightly below.[6,13] Several blood cell analyzers have newer technology that allow for direct measurement of a cell hemoglobin concentration mean (CHCM) of intact cells and/or parameters that estimate the hyperdense cell percentage (% Hyper) through various methods.[21] A cutoff of greater than 4% hyperchromic (hyperdense) cells has been proposed to screen patients for HS when family history and RBC indices are consistent with HS.[6,21,22] Biochemical evidence of extravascular hemolysis may be present in moderate to severe forms of HS, and the extent is dependent on the severity of the hemolysis. This includes a decrease in serum haptoglobin level and an increase in levels of serum indirect bilirubin and lactate dehydrogenase (Chapter 20). Bone marrow shows erythroid hyperplasia as a result of the increased demand for RBCs to replace the circulating spherocytes that are prematurely destroyed, but bone marrow analysis is not required for diagnosis.

Additional tests. In patients with a family history of HS, splenomegaly, an increased MCHC and reticulocyte count, and spherocytes on the peripheral blood film, no further special testing is needed for the diagnosis of HS.[16] In cases in which HS is suspected but the family history and mode of inheritance are not clear or there are atypical clinical or laboratory findings, further special testing is needed to confirm a diagnosis.[16] No one method will detect all cases of HS, so a combination of methods is needed for definitive diagnosis.

Osmotic fragility. The osmotic fragility test demonstrates increased RBC fragility in blood specimens in which the RBCs have decreased surface area-to-volume ratios. Blood is added to a series of tubes with increasingly hypotonic sodium chloride (NaCl) solutions. In each tube, water enters and leaves the RBCs until equilibrium is achieved. In 0.85% NaCl, the amount of water entering the cell is equivalent to the water leaving the cell because the intracellular and extracellular osmolarity is the same. In a hypotonic solution, more water will enter the cell to dilute the intracellular contents until equilibrium is reached between the cytoplasm and the hypotonic extracellular solution. As this phenomenon occurs, the cells swell. As the RBCs are subjected to increasingly hypotonic solutions, even more water will enter the RBCs until the internal volume is too great and lysis occurs. Because spherocytes already have a decreased surface area-to-volume ratio, they lyse in less hypotonic solutions than normal-shaped, biconcave RBCs and thus have increased osmotic fragility.

In the procedure a standard volume of fresh, heparinized blood is mixed with NaCl solutions ranging from 0.85% (isotonic

saline) to 0.0% (distilled water) in 0.05% to 0.1% increments.[23] After a 30-minute incubation at room temperature, the tubes are centrifuged and the absorbance of the supernatant is measured spectrophotometrically at 540 nm.[23] The percent hemolysis is calculated for each tube as follows[23]:

$$\% \text{ hemolysis} = \frac{A_{x\%} - A_{0.85\%}}{A_{0.0\%} - A_{0.85\%}} \times 100$$

$A_{x\%}$ is the absorbance in the tube being measured, $A_{0.85\%}$ is the absorbance in the 0.85% NaCl tube (representing no hemolysis), and $A_{0.0\%}$ is the absorbance in the 0.0% NaCl tube (representing complete hemolysis). The hemolysis percentage for each NaCl concentration is plotted, and an osmotic fragility curve is drawn (Figure 21.4). Normal biconcave RBCs show initial hemolysis at 0.45% NaCl, and complete hemolysis generally occurs between 0.35% and 0.30% NaCl. If the curve is shifted to the left, the patient's RBCs have increased osmotic fragility with initial hemolysis at a NaCl concentration greater than 0.5%. Conversely, if the curve is shifted to the right, the RBCs have decreased osmotic fragility. Decreased osmotic fragility is found in conditions in which RBCs have increased surface area-to-volume ratios (such as a population of target cells in thalassemia).

Incubating the blood at 37° C for 24 hours before performing the test (called the *incubated osmotic fragility test*) allows HS cells to become more spherical and is often needed to detect mild cases. Patients who have increased osmotic fragility only when their blood is incubated tend to have mild disease and a low number of spherocytes in the total RBC population.

The osmotic fragility test is time consuming, and it requires a fresh heparinized blood specimen collected without trauma (to avoid hemolysis) and accurately made NaCl solutions. Specimens are stable for 2 hours at room temperature or 6 hours if the specimen is refrigerated.[23] Although the osmotic fragility test is the traditional screening method for HS, a major

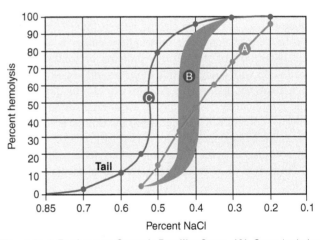

Figure 21.4 Erythrocyte Osmotic Fragility Curve. (A), Curve in thalassemia showing two cell populations: one with increased fragility *(lower left of curve)* and one with decreased fragility *(upper right of curve).* **(B),** Normal curve. **(C),** Curve indicating increased fragility, as in hereditary spherocytosis. The tail represents erythrocytes with increased osmotic fragility after conditioning in the spleen.

drawback of the test is its lack of sensitivity.[16] In a 2011 study of 150 HS patients by Bianchi and colleagues, the sensitivity for the unincubated test was 68%, with only a modest increase in sensitivity to 81% with the incubated test.[24] In nonsplenectomized HS patients with compensated anemia, those sensitivity figures dropped to only 53% and 64%, respectively.[24] Thus a normal osmotic fragility does not exclude a diagnosis of HS especially in mild cases.[21] The osmotic fragility test is also nonspecific. A result indicating increased fragility does not differentiate between HS and spherocytosis caused by other conditions, such as thermal RBC injury (burns), immune hemolytic anemias, and other acquired disorders.[13,16] These disadvantages have led some not to recommend this test for routine use.[16]

Eosin-5′-maleimide binding test. The eosin-5′-maleimide (EMA) binding test has been proposed as a more sensitive alternative for confirmation of HS.[16] EMA is a fluorescent dye that binds to transmembrane proteins band 3, Rh, RhAg, and CD47 in the RBC membrane.[25] When measured in a flow cytometer, specimens from HS patients show a lower mean fluorescence intensity (MFI) compared with normal controls and from patients with spherocytes caused by immune-mediated hemolysis.[25] The result is reported in percentage decrease in MFI when the patient specimen is compared with normal controls.[6,21] The sensitivity and specificity of the EMA-binding assay varies from 93% to 97% and 94% to 99%, respectively.[6,21,24,26] Positive tests can also occur with congenital dyserythropoietic anemia type II, Southeast Asian ovalocytosis, and hereditary pyropoikilocytosis (HPP), but these are rare conditions.[6,21,24,27] The EMA binding test offers advantages in that it is suitable for low-volume pediatric specimens, it can be performed within 3 hours, specimens are acceptable for analysis up to 7 days after collection, and gating can be used to eliminate the interference from transfused or fragmented RBCs.[6] However, there is disagreement among laboratories on the percentage MFI decrease cutoff value for HS, and standardization is needed across laboratories.[6,21,27]

Other tests. In atypical HS cases, additional tests may be required to identify the defective proteins.[16] Sodium dodecyl sulfate-polyacrylamide gel electrophoresis (SDS-PAGE) can be used to identify membrane protein deficiencies by electrophoretic separation of the various proteins in solubilized RBC membranes with quantification of the proteins by densitometry (Figure 6.4).[13,16] Membrane proteins can also be quantified by radioimmunoassay.[13] Variation in membrane surface area and cell water content can be determined by osmotic gradient ektacytometry.[28] The ektacytometer is a laser-diffraction viscometer that records the laser diffraction pattern of a suspension of RBCs exposed to constant shear stress in solutions of varying osmolality from hypotonic to hypertonic. An RBC osmotic deformability index is calculated and plotted against the osmolality of the suspending solution to generate an osmotic gradient deformability profile.[28] This method is available only in specialized laboratories; however, because of the advantages of distinguishing multiple RBC membrane disorders, this test may be included in future HS guidelines.[6,13,16,28]

Several other tests have been used for diagnosis of HS, but they are cumbersome to perform; lack sensitivity and specificity,

or both; and are not widely used in the United States.[4,13] The acidified glycerol lysis test measures the amount of hemolysis after patient RBCs are incubated with a buffered glycerol solution at an acid pH. The test has a sensitivity of 95% but is not specific in that other conditions with spherocytes will yield a positive result, including autoimmune hemolytic anemias.[24,29] In the autohemolysis test, the patient's RBCs and serum are incubated for 48 hours, with and without glucose. Normal controls generally have less than 5.0% hemolysis at the end of the 48-hour incubation period, and they have less than 1.0% hemolysis if glucose is added. Glucose catabolism (anaerobic glycolysis) provides the ATP to drive the cation pumps to help maintain the osmotic balance in the RBCs. In HS the hemolysis is 10% to 50%, which corrects considerably but not to the reference interval when glucose is added. The test has a sensitivity similar to that of the incubated osmotic fragility test.[4,13] The hypertonic cryohemolysis test is based on the fact that cells from HS patients are particularly sensitive to cooling at 0° C in hypertonic solutions.[30] The percent hemolysis is calculated after the patient's RBCs are incubated in buffered 0.7 mol/L sucrose, first at 37° C for 10 minutes and then at 0° C for 10 minutes. Normal cells show 3% to 15% hemolysis, whereas RBCs in HS have greater than 20% hemolysis.[30] Increased hemolysis can also occur in Southeast Asian ovalocytosis, some types of hereditary elliptocytosis, and congenital dyserythropoietic anemia type II.[16,30]

Molecular techniques for detection of genetic mutations are not usually required for diagnosis of HS.[13,16] Molecular studies are often performed after the identification of a deficient protein by SDS-PAGE. Because of the wide genetic diversity and shared mutations across RBC membrane defects, molecular testing often does not provide any additional information in patients whose family history confirms HS but could confirm diagnosis in a patient with no family history (recessive inheritance or de novo mutation).[22] Molecular testing may also be useful in patients who have been recently transfused because traditional methods are invalidated by the presence of donor RBCs in the patient's circulation.[31]

Complications. Although most patients with HS have a well-compensated hemolytic anemia and are rarely symptomatic, complications may occur that require medical intervention. Patients may experience various crises, classified as hemolytic, aplastic, and megaloblastic.[13] Hemolytic crises are rare and usually associated with viral syndromes. In aplastic crises there is a dramatic decrease in hemoglobin level and reticulocyte count. The crisis usually occurs in conjunction with parvovirus B19 infection, which suppresses erythropoiesis, and patients can become rapidly and severely anemic, often requiring transfusion.[16] This complication is more common in children, but it can occur in adults.[13,16] Patients with moderate and severe HS can also develop folic acid deficiency resulting from increased folate utilization to support the chronic erythroid hyperplasia in the bone marrow.[13] This phenomenon is termed *megaloblastic crisis* and is particularly acute during pregnancy and during recovery from an aplastic crisis. Providing folic acid supplementation to patients with moderate and severe HS avoids this complication.[16] About half of patients, even those with mild disease, also experience cholelithiasis (bilirubin stones in the gallbladder or bile ducts) as a result of the chronic hemolysis.[13] Chronic ulceration or dermatitis of the legs is a rare complication.[13]

Treatment. Mild HS usually requires no treatment.[16] Patients with severe HS usually require regular transfusions.[13,15,16] Splenectomy is recommended for moderate to severe cases, results in longer RBC survival in the peripheral blood, and helps prevent gallstones by decreasing the amount of hemolysis and thus the amount of bilirubin produced.[13,16] The major drawbacks of splenectomy are the lifelong risk of overwhelming sepsis and death from encapsulated bacteria and an increased risk of cardiovascular disease with age.[13,16] Because infants and young children are especially susceptible to post-splenectomy sepsis, splenectomy is usually postponed until after the age of 6 years.[16] In a nationwide sample of 1657 children (aged 5 to 12 years) with HS who underwent splenectomy, there were no cases of postoperative sepsis and no fatalities from any cause during hospitalization for the surgery.[32] Partial splenectomy has been performed in young children with severe HS, but further evaluation of the risks and benefits of this procedure is needed.[13,16]

After splenectomy, spherocytes are still apparent on the blood film, and all the changes in RBC morphology typically seen after splenectomy are also observed, including Howell-Jolly bodies, target cells, and Pappenheimer bodies (Figure 21.5). Reticulocyte counts decrease to the high-reference interval, and the anemia is usually corrected. Leukocytosis and thrombocytosis are present. Bilirubin levels decrease but may remain in the high-reference interval. Occasionally a patient does not improve because of an accessory spleen missed during surgery or the accidental autotransplantation of splenic tissue during splenectomy. In these cases, hemolysis may resume years later.[13]

Differential diagnosis. HS must be distinguished from immune-related hemolytic anemia with spherocytes. Family history and evaluation of family members, including parents, siblings, and children of the patient, help differentiate the hereditary disease from the acquired disorder. Immune disorders

with spherocytes are usually characterized by a positive result on the direct antiglobulin test (DAT) (Chapter 23), whereas the results are negative in HS. Increased osmotic fragility is not diagnostic of HS, because the spherocytosis found in acquired hemolytic anemia also results in increased osmotic fragility. The EMA binding test, however, shows decreased fluorescence in HS. The typical clinical and laboratory findings in HS are summarized in Table 21.2.

Hereditary elliptocytosis. Hereditary elliptocytosis (HE) is a heterogeneous group of hemolytic anemias caused by defects in proteins that disrupt the horizontal or lateral interactions in the protein cytoskeleton. It reportedly exists in all of its forms in 1 in 2000 to 1 in 4000 individuals in the United States, but because the majority of cases are asymptomatic, the actual prevalence is not known.[13,33] The disease is more common in Africa and Mediterranean regions, where there is a high prevalence of malaria. The prevalence in West Africa of certain spectrin mutations associated with HE is between 0.6% and 1.6%.[13] The molecular basis for the association of elliptocytosis and malaria is unknown. The inheritance pattern in HE is mainly autosomal dominant.[11,13]

Pathophysiology. HE results from gene mutations in which the defective proteins disrupt the horizontal linkages in the

TABLE 21.2 **Typical Clinical and Laboratory Findings in Hereditary Spherocytosis (HS)**	
Clinical manifestations	Splenomegaly Anemia* Jaundice (can be intermittent)
Mode of inheritance	75% autosomal dominant 25% nondominant
Complete blood count results	↓ Hemoglobin* ↑ Mean cell hemoglobin concentration ↑ Reticulocyte count ↑ Hyperchromic (hyperdense) RBCs†
Peripheral blood film findings‡	Spherocytes Polychromasia
Direct antiglobulin test result	Negative
Indicators of hemolysis	↓ Serum haptoglobin ↑ Serum lactate dehydrogenase ↑ Serum indirect bilirubin
Selected additional tests for atypical cases	Not required for diagnosis of HS with the typical features listed above ↓ Fluorescence in eosin-5'-maleimide binding test by flow cytometry ↑ Osmotic fragility and incubated osmotic fragility tests§ SDS-PAGE analysis of membrane proteins

↑, Increased; ↓, decreased; *RBC,* red blood cell; *SDS-PAGE,* sodium dodecyl sulfate-polyacrylamide gel electrophoresis.
*Varies with severity of HS and ability of the bone marrow to compensate for the hemolysis.
†As measured on some automated blood cell analyzers.
‡With some rare mutations, acanthocytes, pincered cells, stomatocytes, or ovalocytes may be seen in addition to spherocytes.
§A result within the reference interval does not rule out HS; similar results can be observed in conditions other than HS.

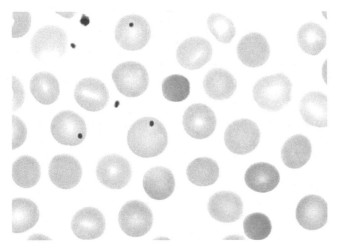

Figure 21.5 Red Blood Cell Morphology in Hereditary Spherocytosis after Splenectomy. Note the Howell-Jolly bodies and spherocytes. (Peripheral blood, Wright-Giemsa stain, ×1000.)

protein cytoskeleton and weaken the mechanical stability of the membrane (Figure 6.5).[4,5] The HE phenotype can result from various mutations in at least three genes: *SPTA1*, which codes for α-spectrin (65% of cases); *SPTB*, which codes for β-spectrin (30% of cases); and *EPB41*, which codes for protein 4.1 (5% of cases) (Table 21.1).[11,33] A mutation database for HE is available and lists 46 different mutations.[14] The spectrin mutations disrupt spectrin dimer interactions and the *EPB41* mutations result in weakened spectrin interactions with actin junctional complexes.[6,11] RBCs are biconcave and discoid at first but become elliptical over time after repeated exposure to the shear stresses in the peripheral circulation.[13] The extent of the disruption of the spectrin dimer interactions seems to be associated with the severity of the clinical manifestations.[11] In severe cases the protein cytoskeleton is weakened to such a point that cell fragmentation occurs. As a result, there is membrane loss and a decrease in surface area-to-volume ratio that reduces the deformability of the RBCs. The damaged RBCs become trapped or acquire further damage in the spleen, which results in extravascular hemolysis and anemia. In general, patients who are heterozygous for a mutation are asymptomatic, and their RBCs have a normal life span; those who are homozygous for a mutation or compound heterozygous for two mutations can have moderate to severe anemia that can be life threatening.[6,11]

Elliptocytosis can also be seen in patients with the Leach phenotype who lack Gerbich antigens and glycoprotein C (GPC).[4] The phenotype is due to a mutation in the genes for GPC and results in the absence of the glycoprotein in the RBC membrane.[34] The Gerbich antigens are normally expressed on the extracellular domains of GPC and thus are absent in this condition. Heterozygotes have normal RBC morphology, and homozygotes have mild elliptocytosis but no anemia.[4] The reason for the elliptocyte morphology may be a defect in the interaction between GPC and protein 4.1 in the actin junctional complex.[4]

The RBCs in HE patients all show some degree of decreased thermal stability. Cases in which the RBCs show marked RBC fragmentation on heating were previously classified as HPP. HPP is now considered a severe form of HE that exists in either the homozygous or compound heterozygous state.[11,13]

Clinical and laboratory findings. The vast majority of patients with HE are asymptomatic, and only about 10% have moderate to severe anemia.[11] Some may have a mild compensated hemolytic anemia, as evidenced by a slight increase in the reticulocyte count and a decrease in haptoglobin level, or develop transient hemolysis in response to other conditions such as viral infections, pregnancy, hypersplenism, or vitamin B_{12} deficiency.[13] Often an asymptomatic patient is diagnosed after a peripheral blood film is examined for another condition. Rarely, heterozygous parents with undiagnosed, asymptomatic HE have offspring who are homozygous or compound heterozygous for their mutations and have moderate to very severe hemolysis. Some of these asymptomatic parents have normal RBC morphology and laboratory tests.[13]

The characteristic finding in HE is elliptical or cigar-shaped RBCs on the peripheral blood film in numbers that can vary from a few to 100%[4] (Figure 21.6). The number of

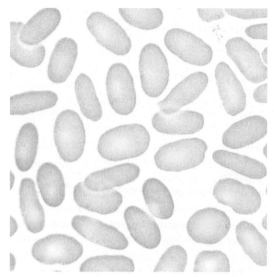

Figure 21.6 Red Blood Cell Morphology in Hereditary Elliptocytosis. (Peripheral blood, Wright-Giemsa stain, X1000.) (From Rodak, B. F., & Carr, J. H. [2017]. *Clinical Hematology Atlas.* [5th ed.]. Philadelphia: Elsevier.)

elliptocytes does not correlate with disease severity.[4] Investigation of elliptocytosis begins by taking a thorough patient and family history, performing a physical examination, and examining the peripheral blood films of the parents.[4] Other laboratory tests may be needed to rule out other conditions in which elliptocytes may be present, such as iron deficiency anemia, thalassemia, megaloblastic anemia, myelodysplastic syndrome, and primary myelofibrosis.[4] In these cases the elliptocytes usually comprise less than one-third of the RBCs.[35] An acquired defect in the gene for protein 4.1 may be found in myelodysplastic syndrome.[36] In the homozygous or compound heterozygous states the anemia is moderate to severe, the osmotic fragility is increased, and biochemical evidence of excessive hemolysis is present. The peripheral blood film in patients with the HPP phenotype shows extreme poikilocytosis with fragmentation, microspherocytosis, and elliptocytosis similar to that in patients with thermal burns (Figure 21.7A). The MCV is very low (50 to 65 fL) because of the RBC fragments.[4,35] RBCs in the HPP phenotype show marked thermal sensitivity. After incubation of a blood specimen at 41° C to 45° C, the RBCs fragment (Figure 21.7B).[13] Normal RBCs do not fragment until reaching a temperature of 49° C. Thermal sensitivity is not specific for HPP, however; it also occurs in cases of HE with spectrin mutations.[4,13] RBCs with the HPP phenotype show a lower fluorescence than RBCs in HS when incubated with eosin-5'-maleimide and analyzed by flow cytometry.[37] Mutation screening using molecular tests or quantification of membrane proteins by SDS-PAGE may be also be performed.

As in HS, patients with moderate or severe hemolytic anemia as a result of HE can develop cholelithiasis because of bilirubin gallstones, and hemolytic, aplastic, and megaloblastic crises can occur.

Treatment. Asymptomatic HE patients require no treatment. HE patients who are significantly anemic and show signs

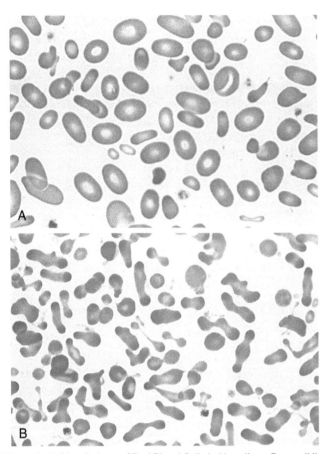

Figure 21.7 Morphology of Red Blood Cells in Hereditary Pyropoikilocytosis. **(A),** Morphology without incubation. **(B),** Morphology after 1 hour incubation at 45° C. (A, B, Peripheral blood, Wright-Giemsa stain, × 500.)

of hemolysis respond well to splenectomy.[4] Transfusions are occasionally needed for life-threatening anemia.

Hereditary ovalocytosis (Southeast Asian ovalocytosis). Hereditary ovalocytosis or Southeast Asian ovalocytosis (SAO) is a condition caused by a mutation in the gene for band 3 that results in increased rigidity of the membrane and resistance to invasion by malaria.[3,4] It is common in the malaria belt of Southeast Asia, where its prevalence can reach 30%.[13,38] The inheritance pattern is autosomal dominant, and all patients identified are heterozygous.[3,4]

Pathophysiology. SAO is the result of one mutation, a deletion of 27 base pairs in the gene, *SLC4A1*, and 9 amino acids in its encoded protein, band 3.[38,39] Deletion occurs at the interface between the transmembrane and cytoplasmic domains.[4,38,40] The mutation causes an increase in membrane rigidity that may be due to tighter binding of band 3 to ankyrin or decreased lateral mobility of band 3 in the membrane.[4,13,38] RBC membranes also have decreased elasticity as measured by ektacytometry and micropipette aspiration.[3,38] The molecular mechanism responsible for the increased membrane rigidity that results from the band 3 mutation has not yet been elucidated.[3,4]

Clinical and laboratory findings. In patients with SAO, hemolysis is mild or absent. On a peripheral blood film, typical cells of SAO are oval RBCs with one to two transverse bars or ridges and usually comprise about 30% of the RBCs.[3,13] No treatment is required for this condition.

Mutations That Alter Membrane Transport Proteins

RBC volume is regulated by various membrane proteins that serve as passive transporters, active transporters, and ion channels. When RBCs lose the ability to regulate volume, the cells are prematurely hemolyzed. Cell volume is determined by the intracellular concentration of cations, particularly sodium.[11] If the total cation content is increased, water enters the cell and increases the cell volume, forming a stomatocyte. If the total cation content is decreased, water leaves the cell, which decreases the cell volume and produces a dehydrated RBC, also called a *xerocyte.*

Hereditary stomatocytosis comprises a group of heterogeneous conditions in which the RBC membrane leaks monovalent cations. The two major categories are overhydrated hereditary stomatocytosis (hereditary hydrocytosis) and dehydrated hereditary stomatocytosis (hereditary xerocytosis). Molecular characterization of these conditions is ongoing and should provide a better means of classification and clearer understanding of their pathophysiology.

Overhydrated hereditary stomatocytosis (hereditary hydrocytosis). Overhydrated hereditary stomatocytosis (OHS) is a very rare hemolytic anemia that results from a defect in membrane cation permeability that causes the RBCs to be overhydrated.[3,6] It is inherited in an autosomal dominant pattern.[11,13]

Pathophysiology. In OHS the RBC membrane is excessively permeable to sodium and potassium at 37° C.[41] There is an influx of sodium into the cell that exceeds the loss of potassium, which results in a net increase in the intracellular cation concentration. As a result, more water enters the cell, and the cell swells and becomes stomatocytic. Because of the water influx, the cytoplasm has decreased density and viscosity. The increase in cell volume without an increase in membrane surface area causes premature hemolysis in the spleen.[3] Most patients also have a secondary deficiency of stomatin, a transmembrane protein, but its gene is not mutated.[6,41,42] Stomatin may participate in regulation of ion channels, but its role in OHS is unclear.[41] Mutations in the *RHAG* gene that codes for RhAG protein, along with a deficiency of the RhAG protein in the membrane have been found in some patients with OHS.[41,42] RhAG is a transmembrane protein involved in cation transport.[42]

Clinical and laboratory findings. OHS can cause moderate to severe hemolytic anemia. Diagnostic features include 5% to 50% stomatocytes on the peripheral blood film (Figure 21.8), macrocytes (MCV of 110 to 150 fL), decreased MCHC (24 to 30 g/dL), reticulocytosis, reduced RBC potassium concentration, elevated RBC sodium concentration, and increased net cation content in the RBCs.[3,6] Because of the increased cell volume, the RBCs have a decreased surface area-to-volume ratio and increased osmotic fragility.[11] Splenectomy is not recommended in OHS because it is associated with an increased risk of thromboembolic complications.[3]

Dehydrated hereditary stomatocytosis (hereditary xerocytosis). Dehydrated hereditary stomatocytosis (DHS) or hereditary xerocytosis (HX) is an autosomal dominant hemolytic anemia as a result of a defect in membrane cation permeability that causes the RBCs to be dehydrated.[3,4] It is the most common form of stomatocytosis.[4]

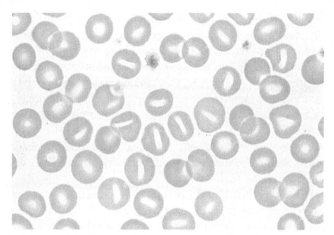

Figure 21.8 Red Blood Cell Morphology in Hereditary Stomatocytosis. (Peripheral blood, Wright-Giemsa stain, ×1000.)

Pathophysiology. In DHS/HX the RBC membrane is excessively permeable to potassium. The potassium leaks out of the cell, but this is not balanced by an increase in sodium. Because of the reduced intracellular cation concentration, water is lost from the cell.[3,4] Most cases are due to mutations in the *PIEZO1* gene that codes for the Piezo-type mechanosensitive ion channel component 1 protein in the RBC membrane.[43-45] The PIEZO1 protein combines with other proteins to form a pore in the membrane to mediate cation transport, and it is important for RBC volume regulation.[43,45] The mutations result in an increase in ion channel activity and an increase in cation transport.[45] Mutations in the *KCNN4* gene have also been reported.[45] *KCNN4* encodes the potassium calcium-activated channel subfamily N member 4 (also called Gardos channel) and, when mutated, affects the transport function of the channel.[45]

Clinical and laboratory findings. Patients with DHS/HX generally have mild to moderate anemia, reticulocytosis, jaundice, and mild to moderate splenomegaly.[4,11] Fetal loss, hydrops fetalis, and neonatal hepatitis can also be features of DHS/HX.[4] The RBCs are dehydrated with decreased MCV, increased cell viscosity and MCHC, and decreased osmotic fragility.[4,11,45] The RBC morphology includes stomatocytes (usually fewer than 10%), target cells, burr cells, desiccated cells with spicules, and RBCs in which the hemoglobin appears to be puddled in discrete areas on the cell periphery.[4,11] Most patients with DHS/HX do not require treatment. Splenectomy does not improve the anemia and is contraindicated because it increases the risk of thromboembolic complications.[3,4]

Other Hereditary Membrane Defects With Stomatocytes

Familial pseudohyperkalemia. Familial pseudohyperkalemia (FP) is a rare autosomal dominant disorder in which excessive potassium leaks out of the RBCs at room temperature in vitro but not at body temperature in vivo.[6] Complete blood count (CBC) parameters are near the reference intervals, although some patients have a mild anemia.[6,29] Occasional stomatocytes may be observed on the peripheral blood film.[6] Mutations in the *ABCB6* gene (encoding a mitochondrial porphyrin transporter) have been identified.[45]

Cryohydrocytosis. Cryohydrocytosis (CHC) is another rare disorder that manifests as a mild to moderate hemolytic anemia with stomatocytosis caused by cold-induced leakage of sodium and potassium from the RBCs.[6,45] The RBCs have marked increase in cation permeability, cell swelling, and hemolysis when stored at 4° C for 24 to 48 hours.[29] Mutations in *SLC4A1* encoding band 3 have been identified in some patients, which cause it to leak cations out of the RBCs, whereas other patients have a deficiency in membrane stomatin or, rarely, mutations in *GLUT1 (SCL2A1)* encoding a glucose transporter.[4,6,29,45]

Rh Deficiency syndrome. Rh deficiency syndrome comprises a group of rare hereditary conditions in which expression of Rh membrane proteins is absent (Rh-null) or decreased (Rh-mod).[4,13] Cases of the syndrome can be genetically divided into the amorph type (caused by mutations in Rh proteins) and the regulatory type (caused by mutations in a protein that regulates Rh gene expression).[4,13] Patients with Rh deficiency syndrome present with mild to moderate hemolytic anemia. Stomatocytes and occasional spherocytes may be observed on the peripheral blood film. Symptomatic patients may be treated by splenectomy, which improves the anemia.

Other Hereditary Membrane Defects With Acanthocytes

Acanthocytes (spur cells) are small, dense RBCs with a few irregular projections that vary in width, length, and surface distribution (Figure 21.9). These are distinct from burr cells (echinocytes), which typically have small, uniform projections evenly distributed on the surface of the RBC (Chapter 16). The differentiation is easier to make on scanning electron micrographs and on wet preparations than on dried blood films.[35] A small number of burr cells (less than 3% of RBCs) can be present on the peripheral blood films of healthy individuals, whereas increased numbers of burr cells are observed in uremia and pyruvate kinase deficiency.[13,35] Acanthocytes, however, are not present on peripheral blood films of healthy individuals but can be

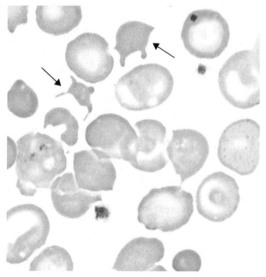

Figure 21.9 Two Acanthocytes *(arrows)*. Note that cells are dense with irregularly spaced projections of varying length. (Peripheral blood, Wright-Giemsa stain, ×1000.)

found in hereditary neuroacanthocytosis (including abetalipo-proteinemia), and acquired conditions such as spur cell anemia in severe liver disease (discussed later), myelodysplasia, malnutrition, and hypothyroidism.[13]

Neuroacanthocytosis. Neuroacanthocytosis is a term used to describe a group of rare inherited disorders characterized by neurologic impairment and acanthocytes on the peripheral blood film. Three disorders are provided as examples in this group: abetalipoproteinemia, McLeod syndrome, and chorea acanthocytosis.[46]

Abetalipoproteinemia (ABL) is a rare autosomal recessive disorder characterized by fat malabsorption, progressive ataxia, neuropathy, retinitis pigmentosa, and acanthocytosis.[46] ABL can first manifest with steatorrhea and failure to thrive in young children (because of fat malabsorption) or as ataxia and neuropathy in young adults (because of decreased absorption of fat-soluble vitamin E).[46] ABL is caused by mutations in the *MTP* (microsomal triglyceride transfer protein) gene; *MTP* is needed to transfer and assemble lipids onto apolipoprotein B.[46] The mutations result in an absence in the plasma of chylomicrons, very low density lipoproteins (which transport triglycerides), and low-density lipoproteins (which transport cholesterol).[13,46] Consequently, triglycerides and cholesterol are decreased but sphingomyelin is increased in plasma.[13] Because RBC membrane lipids are in equilibrium with plasma lipids, the RBC membrane acquires increased sphingomyelin, which decreases the fluidity of the RBC membrane and results in the shape change. The shape defect is not present in developing erythroid precursors and reticulocytes but progresses as RBCs age in the circulation.[13] Other unknown mechanisms may also contribute to the formation of acanthocytes in ABL. Usually, 50% to 90% of the RBCs are acanthocytes.[4,13] Affected individuals have a mild hemolytic anemia, normal RBC indices, and normal to slightly elevated reticulocyte counts.[13] Early treatment with high doses of vitamins A and E can reduce the neuropathy and retinopathy.[13] Patients with other related disorders, such as hypobetalipoproteinemia caused by mutations in the *APOB* gene, also may have acanthocytosis and neurologic disease.[4,46]

The *McLeod syndrome* (MLS) is an X-linked disorder caused by mutations in the *KX* gene.[47] *KX* codes for the Kx protein, a membrane precursor of Kell blood group antigens.[46] Men who lack Kx on their RBCs have reduced expression of Kell antigens, reduced RBC deformability, and shortened RBC survival.[46] Patients with MLS have variable acanthocytosis (up to 85%), mild anemia, and late-onset (aged 40 to 60 years), slowly progressive chorea (movement disorders), peripheral neuropathy, myopathy, and neuropsychiatric manifestations.[46,47] Some female heterozygote carriers may have acanthocytes, but neurologic symptoms are rare. Clinical manifestations in females depend on the proportion of RBCs with the normal X chromosome inactivated versus those with the mutant X chromosome inactivated.[13,47]

Chorea acanthocytosis (ChAc) is a rare autosomal recessive disorder characterized by chorea, hyperkinesia, cognitive impairments, and neuropsychiatric symptoms.[46] The mean age of onset of the neurologic symptoms is 35 years.[46] In patients with ChAc, 5% to 50% of RBCs on the peripheral blood film are acanthocytes.[46] ChAc is caused by mutations in *VPS13A,* a gene

that codes for chorein, a protein with uncertain cellular functions.[47] Chorein may be involved in trafficking proteins to the cell membrane; consequently, a deficiency of chorein may lead to abnormal membrane protein structure and acanthocyte formation.[46]

Acquired Red Blood Cell Membrane Abnormalities
Acquired Stomatocytosis

Stomatocytosis may occur as a drying artifact on Wright-stained peripheral blood films. A medical laboratory professional should examine many areas on several films before categorizing the result as stomatocytosis, because in true stomatocytosis such cells should be found in all areas of the blood film. In healthy individuals, 3% to 5% of RBCs may be stomatocytes.[4] In wet preparations in which RBCs are diluted in their own plasma and examined under phase microscopy, stomatocytes tend to be bowl shaped or uniconcave, rather than the normal biconcave shape. This technique can eliminate some of the artefactual stomatocytosis, but target cells also may appear bowl shaped in solution. Acute alcoholism and a wide variety of other conditions (such as malignancies and cardiovascular disease) as well as certain medications have been associated with acquired stomatocytosis.[4,13]

Spur Cell Anemia

A small percentage of patients with severe liver disease develop a hemolytic anemia with acanthocytosis called *spur cell anemia.* In severe liver disease there is excess free cholesterol because of the presence of abnormal plasma lipoproteins. The free cholesterol preferentially accumulates in the outer leaflet of the RBC membrane.[4,13] The spleen remodels the membrane into the acanthocyte shape giving the RBC long, rigid projections.[13] Because of this remodeling, they become entrapped and hemolyzed in the spleen, which results in a rapidly progressive anemia of moderate severity, splenomegaly, and jaundice.[4,13] Spur cell anemia in end-stage liver disease has a poor prognosis. The anemia may resolve, however, if the patient is able to undergo liver transplantation.[4]

Paroxysmal Nocturnal Hemoglobinuria

Paroxysmal nocturnal hemoglobinuria (PNH) is a rare chronic intravascular hemolytic anemia caused by an acquired clonal hematopoietic stem cell mutation that results in circulating blood cells that lack glycosylphosphatidylinositol (GPI)-anchored proteins on their surfaces, such as CD55 and CD59.[48] Absence of CD55 and CD59 on the surface of the RBCs renders them susceptible to spontaneous lysis by complement. Because the mutation occurs in a hematopoietic stem cell, the defect is also found in platelets, granulocytes, monocytes, and lymphocytes.[49] PNH is uncommon, with an annual incidence of two to five new cases per million persons in the United States.[50]

Pathophysiology of the hemolytic anemia. The GPI anchor consists of a phosphatidylinositol (PI) molecule and a glycan core. The phosphatidylinositol is incorporated in the outer leaflet of the lipid bilayer membrane. The glycan core consists of glucosamine, three mannose residues, and ethanolamine phosphate. At least 24 genes code for enzymes and proteins

GPI-linked protein

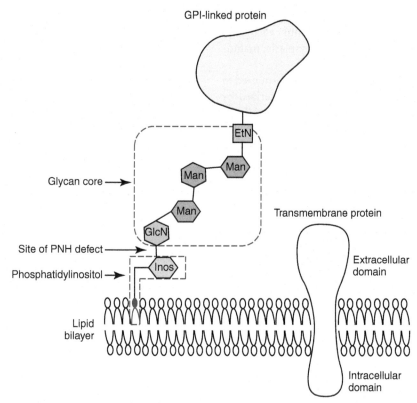

Glycan core →

EtN

Man

Man

Man

GlcN

Site of PNH defect →

Phosphatidylinositol →

Inos

Transmembrane protein

Extracellular domain

Lipid bilayer

Intracellular domain

Figure 21.10 Glycosylphosphatidylinositol (GPI) Anchor for Attachment of Surface Proteins to the Cell Membrane. *Left:* The structure of a GPI-anchored protein. The GPI anchor consists of phosphatidylinositol in the outer leaflet of the lipid bilayer, which is connected to a glycan core consisting of glucosamine *(GlcN)*, three mannose *(Man)* residues, and ethanolamine phosphate *(EtN)*. A protein is linked to the anchor at its C-terminus by an amide bond. The result is a surface protein with a fluid and mobile attachment to the cell surface. The GPI anchor and GPI-linked protein is extracellular. In paroxysmal nocturnal hemoglobinuria *(PNH)*, a mutation occurs in the PIGA gene encoding phosphatidylinositol glycan anchor biosynthesis class A (PIG-A), one of seven subunits of a glycosyl transferase enzyme needed to add N-acetylglucosamine to the inositol *(Inos)* component of the phosphatidylinositol molecule *(arrow* shows location of the PNH defect). The mutated PIG-A enzyme subunit inhibits or prevents the first step in the biosynthesis of the GPI anchor. *Right:* In contrast, a transmembrane protein has an extracellular domain, a short transmembrane domain, and an intracellular domain. (Adapted from Parker, C. J., & Ware, R. E. [2015]. Paroxysmal nocturnal hemoglobinuria. In Orkin, S. H., Fisher, D. E., Ginsburg, D., et al. (Eds.), *Nathan and Oski's Hematology and Oncology of Infancy and Childhood.* [8th ed., Figure 14.1]. Philadelphia: Elsevier.)

involved in the biosynthesis of the GPI anchor.[50] GPI-anchored proteins attach to the ethanolamine in the glycan core by an amide bond at their C-termini (Figure 21.10).

In PNH a hematopoietic stem cell acquires a mutation in the *PIGA* gene that codes for phosphatidylinositol glycan anchor biosynthesis class A (PIG-A), also known as phosphatidylinositol *N*-acetylglucosaminyltransferase subunit A.[51] It is one of seven subunits of a glycosyl transferase enzyme needed to add *N*-acetylglucosamine to phosphatidylinositol.[48-50] This is the first step in the biosynthesis of the GPI anchor in the endoplasmic reticulum membrane. The *PIGA* gene is located on the X chromosome, and more than 180 different mutations have been identified.[49] Without a fully functional glycosyl transferase enzyme, the hematopoietic stem cell is unable to effectively synthesize the glycan core on phosphatidylinositol in the membrane; therefore the cell is deficient in membrane GPI anchors. Without GPI anchors, all the progeny of the mutated stem cell are unable to express any of the approximately 20 currently

known GPI-anchored proteins found on normal blood cells.[48] The GPI-anchored proteins are complement regulators, enzymes, adhesion molecules, blood group antigens, or receptors.[49,50] Relevant to the presence of hemolysis in PNH, two GPI-anchored proteins are absent or deficient on the RBC membrane: decay accelerating factor (DAF, or CD55) and membrane inhibitor of reactive lysis (MIRL, or CD59).[50] CD55 and CD59 are complement-inhibiting proteins. CD55 inhibits the complement alternate pathway C3 and C5 convertases, and CD59 prevents the formation of the membrane attack complex.[48] When CD55 and CD59 are absent from the RBC surface, the cell is unable to prevent the activation of complement, and spontaneous and chronic intravascular hemolysis occurs. Out of all the genes needed for GPI anchor synthesis, *PIGA* is the only one located on the X chromosome. Therefore only one acquired mutation in the *PIGA* gene is needed for the PNH phenotype in a stem cell (males have only one X chromosome, and in females one of the X chromosomes is inactivated).[48]

The *PIGA* mutant clone coexists with normal hematopoietic stem cells and progenitors, which results in a population of RBCs that is GPI-deficient and a population that is normal.[48] Some patients have a greater expansion of the mutant clone, a higher percentage of circulating GPI-deficient RBCs, and a more severe chronic hemolytic anemia.[48] On the other hand, other patients have minimal expansion of the mutant clone and have a lower percentage of circulating GPI-deficient RBCs. These patients may be asymptomatic and may not require any treatment. It is unclear why there is a greater expansion of the GPI-deficient clone and chronic hemolysis in some patients and not others.

Patients with PNH also display *phenotypic mosaicism*.[48,50] The mosaicism results when a single patient is able to harbor normal clones as well as mutant clones with different *PIGA* mutations. Those different mutations result in variable expression of CD55 and CD59 on the RBCs within an individual patient, giving rise to three RBC phenotypes: type I, type II, and type III.[48,49] Type I RBCs are phenotypically normal, express normal amounts of CD55 and CD59, and undergo little or no complement-mediated hemolysis. Type II RBCs are the result of a *PIGA* mutation that causes only a partial deficiency of CD55 and CD59, and these cells are relatively resistant to complement-mediated hemolysis. Type III RBCs are the result of a *PIGA* mutation that causes a complete deficiency of the GPI anchor, and therefore no CD55 and CD59 proteins are anchored to the RBC surface. Type III RBCs are highly sensitive to spontaneous lysis by complement. The most common RBC phenotype in PNH is a combination of type I and type III cells, whereas the second most common has all three types.[48] When the severity of the hemolysis in PNH is being assessed, both the relative amount and the type of circulating RBCs are considered.

In addition to hemolysis, patients with PNH may have bone marrow dysfunction that contributes to the severity of the anemia. Many patients have a history of bone marrow failure caused by acquired aplastic anemia or myelodysplastic syndrome that precedes or coincides with the onset of PNH, resulting in a hypoplastic PNH presentation.[50-52]

Clinical manifestations. The onset of PNH most often occurs in the third or fourth decade, but it can occur in childhood and advanced age.[48-50] The major clinical manifestations and complications of PNH are those associated with hemolytic anemia, thrombosis, and bone marrow failure (Table 21.3).[50-53] Anemia is mild to severe, depending on the predominant type of RBC, the degree of hemolysis, and the presence of bone marrow failure. Dark urine (hemoglobinuria) and jaundice occur as a result of intravascular hemolysis. In addition, free hemoglobin released during intravascular hemolytic episodes rapidly scavenges and removes nitric oxide (NO). The decreased NO can manifest as smooth muscle dystonia (esophageal spasms, dysphagia, erectile dysfunction, abdominal and back pain) or platelet activation and thrombosis.[49,50] The most common thrombotic manifestation is hepatic vein thrombosis (called *Budd-Chiari syndrome*), which obstructs venous outflow from the liver, causing a serious, often fatal complication.[50] Patients also may develop chronic renal disease as a result of renal

TABLE 21.3 Clinical Manifestations in Paroxysmal Nocturnal Hemoglobinuria (PNH)[50-53]

Clinical Findings	Cause
Symptoms of anemia Fatigue Shortness of breath	Intravascular hemolysis; bone marrow failure
Thrombosis Budd-Chiari syndrome (hepatic vein thrombosis) Deep vein thrombosis Portal hypertension Pulmonary embolism Stroke	Intravascular hemolysis; platelet activation caused by depletion of nitric oxide by free hemoglobin
Smooth muscle dystonia Abdominal and/or back pain Dysphagia Erectile dysfunction Esophageal spasms Fatigue	Intravascular hemolysis; depletion of nitric oxide by free hemoglobin
Dark urine	Intravascular hemolysis; hemoglobinuria
Jaundice	Increased serum indirect bilirubin
Chronic kidney disease/renal tubule damage	Intravascular hemolysis; microvascular thrombosis due to platelet activation; accumulation of iron caused by repeated hemoglobinuria

tubule damage from microvascular thrombosis and accumulation of iron during episodes of hemoglobinuria.[50]

Classification. The International PNH Interest Group proposed three subcategories of PNH: classic PNH, hypoplastic PNH (PNH in the setting of another specified bone marrow disorder), and subclinical PNH (Table 21.4).[48,50,52] In classic PNH there is clinical and biochemical evidence of intravascular hemolysis, reticulocytosis, a cellular bone marrow with erythroid hyperplasia and normal morphology, and a normal karyotype. In addition, more than 30% to 50% of the circulating neutrophils are GPI deficient.[48,50,52] In hypoplastic PNH, patients have evidence of hemolysis and a concomitant bone marrow failure syndrome such as aplastic anemia, refractory anemia/myelodysplastic syndrome, or other myelopathy (e.g., myelofibrosis). The number of GPI-deficient neutrophils is variable but is usually less than 20% to 30% of the total neutrophils.[48,50] In subclinical PNH, patients have no clinical or biochemical evidence of hemolysis but have a small subpopulation of GPI-deficient neutrophils that comprise less than 1% of the total circulating neutrophils.[48,52] Subclinical PNH also occurs in the setting of a bone marrow failure syndrome.

Laboratory findings. Biochemical evidence of intravascular hemolysis includes decreased levels of serum haptoglobin, increased levels of plasma hemoglobin, serum indirect bilirubin and lactate dehydrogenase, hemoglobinuria, and hemosiderinuria (Chapter 20). Hemolysis can be exacerbated by conditions such as infections, strenuous exercise, and surgery.[50] The major

TABLE 21.4   **Major Laboratory Findings in Paroxysmal Nocturnal Hemoglobinuria (PNH)**[48,50-52]

	Classic PNH	Hypoplastic PNH*	Subclinical PNH*
Hemoglobin	↓	↓	↓
Reticulocytes	↑	↓	↓
Cytopenias	Mild to moderate	Moderate to severe	Moderate to severe
Bone marrow	Normocellular to hypercellular with erythroid hyperplasia Normal to near-normal morphology Decreased iron	Evidence of bone marrow failure: Hypocellular (<25%) May have dysplastic morphology, ↑ blasts, or other myelopathy	Evidence of bone marrow failure: Hypocellular (<25%) May have dysplastic morphology, ↑ blasts, or other myelopathy
Circulating PNH granulocytes (GPI deficient)[†] by flow cytometry	>30%–50%	<20%–30%	<1%
Evidence of intravascular hemolysis[‡]	Frequent, marked	Intermittent, mild to moderate	None
DAT	Negative	Negative	Negative

↑, Increased; ↓ decreased; *DAT,* direct antiglobulin test.
*PNH in the setting of a bone marrow failure syndrome such as aplastic anemia, refractory anemia/myelodysplastic syndrome, or other myelopathy (e.g., myelofibrosis).
[†]Measured by high-sensitivity flow cytometry with anti-CD24 and fluorescein-labeled proaerolysin variant (FLAER)
[‡]Evidence of intravascular hemolysis includes elevated plasma hemoglobin, serum lactate dehydrogenase, and serum indirect bilirubin; decreased serum haptoglobin; and hemoglobinuria and hemosiderinuria.

laboratory findings associated with classic, hypoplastic, and subclinical PNH are summarized in Table 21.4.[48,50-52] Hemoglobinuria is present in only 25% of patients at diagnosis, but it will occur in most patients during the course of the illness.[52] Very few patients report periodic hemoglobinuria at night, a symptom for which the condition was originally named.[50] Hemosiderinuria as a result of chronic intravascular hemolysis may be detected with Prussian blue staining of the urine sediment.

In classic PNH, reticulocyte counts are mildly to moderately increased, with less elevation than would be expected in other hemolytic anemias of comparable severity. The MCV may be slightly elevated because of the reticulocytosis. The DAT is negative. If the patient does not receive transfusions, iron deficiency develops as a result of the loss of hemoglobin iron in the urine, and the RBCs become microcytic and hypochromic. Serum iron studies (serum iron, total iron-binding capacity, and serum ferritin) are performed to detect iron deficiency (Chapter 17). Folate deficiency often occurs if there is chronic erythroid hyperplasia and a greater need for folate, which leads to secondary macrocytosis. Pancytopenia may occur if there is concomitant bone marrow failure.

Bone marrow aspirate and biopsy specimens are examined for evidence of an underlying bone marrow failure syndrome, abnormal cells, and cytogenetic abnormalities.[52] The bone marrow may be normocellular to hypercellular with erythroid hyperplasia in response to the hemolysis (classic PNH), or it may be hypocellular with concomitant bone marrow failure (hypoplastic and subclinical PNH).[50] A finding of dysplasia or certain chromosome abnormalities is helpful in diagnosis of a myelodysplastic syndrome (Chapter 33). An abnormal karyotype is found in 20% of patients with PNH.[50]

Confirmation of PNH requires demonstration of GPI-deficient cells in the peripheral blood. Flow cytometric analysis

(Chapter 28) of RBCs with fluorescence-labeled anti-CD59 determines the proportion of types I, II, and III RBCs and thus can provide an assessment of the severity of the hemolysis (Figure 21.11).[48,50] Type I cells with normal expression of CD59 show the highest intensity level of fluorescence; type II cells with a partial deficiency of CD59 show moderate fluorescence; and type III cells with no CD59 are negative for fluorescence. Patients with a greater proportion of type III cells (complete deficiency of GPI-anchored proteins) are expected to have a high-grade hemolysis.[48,52] Patients with a high percentage of type II cells (partial deficiency of GPI-anchored proteins) and a low percentage of type III cells may have only modest hemolysis.[48-52] A high-sensitivity two-parameter flow cytometry method using labeled anti-CD59 and anti-CD235a (anti-glycophorin A) was able to detect type III PNH RBCs with a sensitivity of 0.002% (1 in 50,000 normal cells).[54] However, flow cytometry methods to detect PNH RBCs have two major disadvantages. They underestimate the percentage of type III cells because RBCs lacking CD59 undergo rapid complement lysis in the circulation.[52] In addition, these methods cannot accurately determine the percentage of PNH RBCs after recent transfusion.

Because of the inherent problems with flow cytometry methods to detect PNH RBCs, diagnosis of PNH is accomplished by detection of the absence of GPI-anchored proteins on white blood cells (WBCs) using multiparameter flow cytometry. The absence of at least two GPI-anchored proteins in two WBC lineages (usually granulocytes and monocytes) is recommended for greater diagnostic accuracy.[50,54] Methods typically use fluorescent monoclonal antibodies to GPI-anchored proteins (such as CD59, CD55, CD24, CD16, CD66b, CD14), along with lineage-specific antibodies to non-GPI-anchored proteins (such as CD15 and CD64) to identify granulocytes and monocytes, respectively.[50,54,55] An alternative flow cytometric

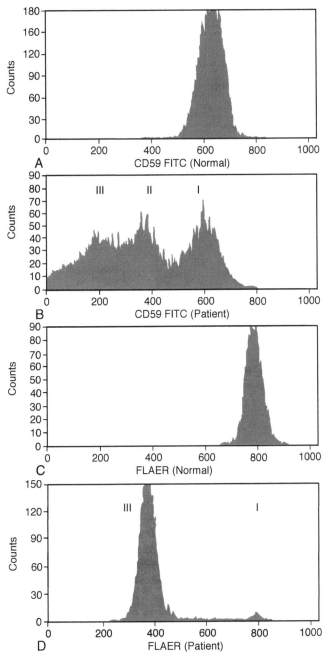

Figure 21.11 Flow Cytometric Analysis of Peripheral Blood Cells from a Patient with Paroxysmal Nocturnal Hemoglobinuria (PNH) and a Healthy (Normal) Control. **(A),** Fluorescence intensity of erythrocytes from a healthy control after staining with anti-CD59. **(B),** Fluorescence intensity of erythrocytes from an untransfused patient with PHN after staining with anti-CD59. Type II cells are "blended" between the type I (normal) and type III cells. **(C),** Fluorescence intensity of granulocytes from a healthy control stained with FLAER. **(D),** Fluorescence intensity of granulocytes from the same patient with PHN as in B after staining with FLAER. Note that the granulocytes are almost exclusively type III cells. A small population of type I granulocytes is present. *FITC,* Fluorescein isothiocyanate; *FLAER,* fluorescein-labeled proaerolysin variant.(From Brodsky, R. A. [2018]. Paroxysmal nocturnal hemoglobinuria. In Hoffman, R., Benz, E. J., Silberstein, L. E., et al. (Eds.), *Hematology: Basic Principles and Practice.* [7th ed., Figure 31.2]. Philadelphia: Elsevier.)

method uses a fluorescein-labeled proaerolysin variant (FLAER).[53-56] FLAER binds directly to the glycan core of the GPI anchor with a high signal-to-noise ratio. The absence of binding on granulocytes and/or monocytes is indicative of GPI deficiency (Figure 21.11).[54-56] Using multiparameter flow cytometry with FLAER in combination with monoclonal antibodies to GPI-anchored antigens and lineage-specific antigens increases sensitivity and specificity for detection of GPI-deficient granulocytes and monocytes.[54,55] A high-sensitivity four-color protocol using FLAER, CD24, CD15, and CD45 for granulocytes and FLAER, CD14, CD64, and CD45 for monocytes was able to detect GPI-deficient granulocytes and monocytes with a sensitivity of 0.01% (1 in 10,000) and 0.04% (1 in 2500), respectively.[54] The results are not affected by recent transfusions because neutrophils and monocytes have a short life span in stored donor blood; therefore it can reliably be used to estimate the percentage of GPI-deficient granulocytes and monocytes in recently transfused patients.[50] The high sensitivity is also important for posttherapy monitoring of PNH clones.

The sugar water test (sucrose hemolysis test) and the Ham test (acidified serum lysis test) have insufficient sensitivity for diagnosis of PNH and have been replaced by flow cytometric techniques.

Treatment. In 2007, the US Food and Drug Administration approved eculizumab for the treatment of hemolysis in PNH.[57] Eculizumab is a humanized monoclonal antibody that binds to complement C5, prevents its cleavage to C5a and C5b, and thus inhibits the formation of the membrane attack unit.[57] Eculizumab is the treatment of choice for patients with classic PNH. It results in an improvement of the anemia and a decrease in transfusion requirements.[51,53,57,58] There is also a reduction in the lactate dehydrogenase level in the serum, reflecting a reduction in hemolysis.[57,58] In a study by Hillmen and colleagues of 195 patients taking eculizumab for a duration of 30 to 66 months, 96.4% of patients did not have an episode of thrombosis, and in 93%, markers of their chronic kidney disease stabilized or even improved.[58] Because of the inhibition of the complement system, patients taking eculizumab have an increased risk for infections with *Neisseria meningitidis* and need to be vaccinated before administration of the drug.[57] Patients continue to have a mild to moderate anemia and reticulocytosis likely because of extravascular hemolysis of RBCs sensitized with C3 (eculizumab does not inhibit complement C3).[48,59] To address this issue, research is under way to identify therapies that target the early events of complement activation, including monoclonal antibodies to C3, but a universal inhibition of C3 may increase the patient's susceptibility to infections and immune complex disease.[59] A promising new therapy under investigation is a novel recombinant fusion protein (TT30) designed to prevent the formation of C3 convertase only on the membranes of GPI-deficient RBCs.[59] Because of the expense and administration (intravenous) of eculizumab, novel complement inhibitors that have a longer half-life or oral administration are in high demand. Several drugs are currently in clinical trials including C5 inhibitors, C3 inhibitors and a complement alternative pathway inhibitor.[51,53]

Eculizumab is not curative and does not address the bone marrow failure complications of PNH. Other treatments for PNH are mainly supportive. Iron therapy is given to help alleviate the iron deficiency caused by the urinary loss of hemoglobin, and folate supplementation is given to replace the folate consumed in accelerated erythropoiesis. Administration of androgens and glucocorticoids to ameliorate anemia is not universally accepted.[48] Anticoagulants are used in the treatment of thrombotic complications. In suitable patients with severe intravascular hemolysis, hematopoietic stem cell transplantation with an HLA-matched sibling donor may be an option and can be a curative therapy, but with an overall survival of only 50% to 60%.[48]

PNH is a disease with significant morbidity and mortality. Before eculizumab, thrombosis was the major cause of death, and the median survival after diagnosis was approximately 10 years.[48] Long-term studies of patients on eculizumab therapy are in progress, and early results show a decrease in the debilitating complications and an increase in survival of patients with PNH.[58]

RED BLOOD CELL ENZYMOPATHIES

The major function of RBCs is to transport oxygen to the tissues over their life span of 120 days. For RBCs to do that effectively, they need functional enzymes to maintain glycolysis, preserve the shape and deformability of the cell membrane, keep hemoglobin iron in a reduced state, protect hemoglobin and other cellular proteins from oxidative denaturation, and degrade and salvage nucleotides. Deficiencies in RBC enzymes may impair these functions to varying degrees and decrease the life span of the cell. The most important metabolic pathways are the Embden-Meyerhof pathway (anaerobic glycolysis) and the hexose monophosphate (pentose) shunt[60] (Figure 6.1). The most commonly encountered enzymopathies are deficiencies of glucose-6-phosphate dehydrogenase and pyruvate kinase. Other RBC enzymopathies are rare.[60]

Glucose-6-Phosphate Dehydrogenase Deficiency

RBCs normally produce free oxygen radicals (O_2^-) and hydrogen peroxide (H_2O_2) during metabolism and oxygen transport, but they have multiple mechanisms to detoxify these oxidants (Chapter 6). Occasionally RBCs are subjected to an increased level of oxidants (*oxidant stress*) as a result of exposure to certain oxidizing drugs, foods, chemicals, and herbal supplements and even through reactive oxygen molecules produced in the body during infections. If allowed to accumulate in RBCs, these reactive oxygen species would oxidize and denature hemoglobin, membrane proteins, and lipids and ultimately cause premature hemolysis. Therefore the capacity of RBCs to detoxify oxidants, especially during oxidant stress, is critical to maintain their normal life span.

Glucose-6-phosphate dehydrogenase (G6PD) is one of the important intracellular enzymes needed to protect hemoglobin and other cellular proteins and lipids from oxidative denaturation.

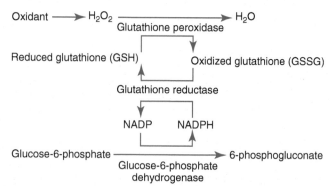

Figure 21.12 Function of Glucose-6-Phosphate Dehydrogenase (G6PD). G6PD converts glucose-6-phosphate (from the Embden-Meyerhof pathway) to 6-phosphogluconate generating the reduced form of nicotinamide adenine dinucleotide phosphate (NADPH). Glutathione reductase uses the NADPH to reduce oxidized glutathione (GSSG) to reduced glutathione (GSH). Glutathione peroxidase uses the GSH to detoxify hydrogen peroxide to water.

G6PD catalyzes the first step in a series of reactions that detoxify hydrogen peroxide formed from oxygen radicals (Figure 21.12). In the hexose monophosphate shunt (Chapter 6), G6PD generates reduced nicotinamide adenine dinucleotide phosphate (NADPH) by converting glucose-6-phosphate to 6-phosphogluconate. In the next step, glutathione reductase uses the NADPH to reduce oxidized glutathione (GSSG) to reduced glutathione (GSH) and NADP. In the final reaction, glutathione peroxidase uses the GSH generated in the previous step to detoxify hydrogen peroxide to water (H_2O).[60-62] GSSG is formed in the reaction and is rapidly transported out of the cell. During oxidant stress, RBCs with normal G6PD activity are able to readily detoxify hydrogen peroxide to prevent cellular damage and safeguard hemoglobin. G6PD is especially critical to the cell because it provides the only means of generating NADPH. Consequently, G6PD-deficient RBCs are particularly vulnerable to oxidative damage and subsequent hemolysis during oxidant stress.[60-62]

The *G6PD* gene is located on the X chromosome. It codes for the G6PD enzyme, which assembles into a dimer and tetramer in its functional configuration.[60] With the X-linked inheritance pattern, men can be normal hemizygotes (have the normal allele) or deficient hemizygotes (have a mutant allele). Women can be normal homozygotes (both alleles normal), deficient homozygotes (both alleles have same mutation), compound heterozygotes (each allele has a different mutation), or heterozygotes (have one normal allele and one mutant allele). The G6PD enzyme activity in female heterozygotes lies between normal and deficient because of the random inactivation of one of the X chromosomes in each cell (lyonization).[60-62] Therefore RBCs of female heterozygotes are a mosaic, with some cells having normal G6PD activity and some cells having deficient G6PD activity. Because X inactivation is random, the proportion of normal to G6PD-deficient RBCs varies among different heterozygous women.[62] Some heterozygous women experience acute hemolytic episodes after exposure to oxidants if they have a high proportion of G6PD-deficient RBCs.

G6PD deficiency is the most common RBC enzyme defect, with a prevalence of 5% of the global population, or approximately 400 million people worldwide.[63] The prevalence of G6PD deficiency varies by geographic location: sub-Saharan Africa (7.5%), the Middle East (6.0%), Asia (4.7%), Europe (3.9%), and the Americas (3.4%).[63] In the United States the prevalence of G6PD deficiency in African American males is approximately 10%.[60] G6PD deficiency has the highest prevalence in geographic areas in which malaria is endemic because of the selective pressure of malaria.[64] Studies in Africa show that G6PD deficiency (A⁻ variant) in hemizygous males confers protection against life-threatening *Plasmodium falciparum* malaria.[65] This protective effect is not observed in heterozygous females because of their mosaicism of normal and G6PD-deficient RBCs.[65] In a 2010 case-control study in Pakistan, G6PD deficiency (Mediterranean variant) conferred protection against *Plasmodium vivax* infection, also with a greater protective effect in hemizygous males.[66] This protective effect may be due to parasite susceptibility to excess free oxygen radicals produced in G6PD-deficient RBCs.[67] In addition, significant oxidative damage may occur to the RBCs early after parasite invasion so that these early-infected cells are more readily phagocytized with elimination of the parasite.[68] However, a meta-analysis of 28 malarial G6PD studies suggested a strong publication bias toward a negative correlation between G6PD deficiency and *P. falciparum*.[69] This meta-analysis failed to demonstrate a protective effect of G6PD deficiency in severe malarial infection (particularly female heterozygotes) except in African populations. It did show, however, a negative correlation between G6PD deficiency and hyperparasitemia, suggesting that G6PD deficiency may decrease parasite load.[69]

A mutation database published in 2016 reported 217 known mutations in the *G6PD* gene, with approximately 84% of them being single missense mutations.[70] An amino acid substitution changes the structure of the enzyme and thus affects its function, stability, or both. In addition, more than 400 variant isoenzymes have been identified.[62] The normal or wild-type G6PD variant is designated G6PD-B.[60,62] Some G6PD variants have significantly reduced enzyme activity, whereas others have mild or moderately reduced activity or normal activity. The different variants of G6PD have been divided into classes by the World Health Organization, based on clinical symptoms and amount of enzyme activity (Table 21.5).[70,71] Several recent studies have shown that the severity of G6PD deficiency is determined by the catalytic activity and the protein stability of the G6PD variant.[72,73]

Pathophysiology

G6PD-deficient RBCs cannot generate sufficient NADPH to reduce glutathione and thus cannot effectively detoxify the hydrogen peroxide produced on exposure to oxidative stress. Oxidative damage to cellular proteins and lipids occurs, particularly affecting hemoglobin and the cell membrane. Oxidation converts hemoglobin to methemoglobin and forms sulfhydryl groups and disulfide bridges in hemoglobin polypeptides. This leads to decreased hemoglobin solubility and precipitation as Heinz bodies.[60] Heinz bodies adhere to the inner RBC membrane, causing irreversible membrane damage (Figure 11.12). Because of the membrane damage and loss of deformability, RBCs with Heinz bodies are rapidly removed from the circulation by intravascular and extravascular hemolysis.[62] Reticulocytes have approximately five times more G6PD activity than older RBCs, because enzyme activity decreases as the cells age. Therefore during exposure to oxidants, the older RBCs with less G6PD are preferentially hemolyzed.[64]

Clinical Manifestations

The vast majority of individuals with G6PD deficiency are asymptomatic throughout their lives. However, some patients have clinical manifestations. The clinical syndromes are acute hemolytic anemia, neonatal jaundice (hyperbilirubinemia), and chronic hereditary nonspherocytic hemolytic anemia (HNSHA).[64]

Acute Hemolytic anemia. *Oxidative stress* can precipitate a hemolytic episode, and the main triggers are certain oxidizing drugs or chemicals, infections, and ingestion of fava beans.

TABLE 21.5 Classification of Glucose-6-Phosphate Dehydrogenase (G6PD) Variants by the World Health Organization

Class	G6PD Enzyme Activity	Clinical Manifestations	Examples of Variants
I	Severely deficient: <1% activity or not detectable	Chronic, hereditary nonspherocytic hemolytic anemia; severity is variable; rare	G6PD-Serres G6PD-Madrid
II	Severely deficient: <10% activity	Severe, episodic acute hemolytic anemia associated with infections, certain drugs, and fava beans; not self-limited and may require transfusions during hemolytic episodes	G6PD-Mediterranean G6PD-Chatham
III	Mild to moderately deficient: 10%–60% activity	Episodic, acute hemolytic anemia associated with infections and certain drugs; self-limited	G6PD-A⁻ G6PD-Canton
IV	Mildly deficient to normal: 60%–150% activity	None	G6PD-B (wildtype) G6PD-A⁺*
V	Increased: >150% activity	None	

From Beutler, E., Gaetani, G., der Kaloustian, V., et al. (1989). World Health Organization (WHO) Working Group. Glucose-6-phosphate dehydrogenase deficiency. *Bull World Health Organ, 67,* 601–611; and Minucci, A., Moradkhani, K., Hwang, M. J., et al. (2012). Glucose-6-phosphate dehydrogenase (G6PD) mutations database: Review of the "old" and update of the new mutations. *Blood Cells Mol Dis, 48,* 154–165.
*May also manifest as class III

BOX 21.2 Drugs Causing Predictable Hemolysis in Glucose-6-Phosphate Dehydrogenase (G6PD) Deficiency[74,75]

Drugs with Strong Evidence-Based Support for an Association with Drug-Induced Hemolysis

Dapsone
Methylthioninium chloride (methylene blue)
Nitrofurantoin
Phenazopyridine
Primaquine
Rasburicase
Tolonium chloride (toluidine blue)

Drugs with Well-Documented Case Reports for an Association with Drug-Induced Hemolysis

Cotrimoxazole
Quinolones
Sulfadiazine

Hemolysis secondary to drug exposure is the classic manifestation of G6PD deficiency. The actual discovery of G6PD deficiency in the 1950s was a direct consequence of investigations into the development of hemolysis in certain individuals after ingestion of the antimalarial agent primaquine.[60] Box 21.2 lists drugs that show strong evidence-based association with hemolysis in G6PD-deficient individuals or have been reported in well-documented case reports.[74,75] Primaquine and sulfa drugs are among the most commonly associated with hemolysis. The degree of hemolysis can vary, depending on the dosage, coexisting infection, concomitant use of other drugs, or type of mutation.[74] Exposure to naphthalene in mothballs and some herbal supplements have also been associated with hemolysis in some G6PD-deficient individuals.[60]

Individuals with class II and III G6PD deficiency are clinically and hematologically normal until the offending drug is taken. Clinical hemolysis can begin abruptly within hours or occur gradually 1 to 3 days after the drug is taken.[62,64] Typical symptoms include chills, fever, headache, nausea, and back pain.[60] A rapid drop in hemoglobin may occur, and the anemia can range from mild to very severe. Hemoglobinuria is a usual finding and indicates that the hemolysis is intravascular, although some extravascular hemolysis occurs. Reticulocytes increase within 4 to 6 days.[62] Generally, with class III variants such as G6PD-A⁻, the hemolytic episode is self-limiting because the newly formed reticulocytes have higher G6PD activity. With class II variants such as G6PD-Mediterranean, the RBCs are severely G6PD deficient, so the hemolytic episode may be longer and the hemolysis is not self-limiting.[62]

Infection is probably the most common cause of hemolysis in individuals with G6PD deficiency. During the episode, the hemoglobin can drop 3 to 4 g/dL if reticulocyte production is suppressed by the infection.[60] The hemolysis resolves after recovery from the infection.[62] The mechanism of hemolysis induced by acute and subacute infection is poorly understood, but the generation of hydrogen peroxide by phagocytizing leukocytes may play a role.[62] Diminished liver function may contribute further to the oxidant stress by allowing the accumulation of oxidizing metabolites. Infectious agents implicated in hemolytic episodes include bacteria, viruses, and rickettsia.

Favism is a rare, severe hemolytic episode that occurs in some G6PD-deficient individuals after ingestion of fava beans. Favism can initially manifest with a sudden onset of acute intravascular hemolysis within hours of ingesting fava beans, or hemolysis can occur gradually over a period of 24 to 48 hours.[62] Hemoglobinuria is one of the first signs. Specific patient factors may affect the severity of the hemolysis, including the type of mutation, the presence of underlying disorders, and the amount of fava beans ingested. Only a small percentage of G6PD-deficient individuals manifest favism, and most of these have the G6PD-Mediterranean variant.

Neonatal hyperbilirubinemia. Neonatal hyperbilirubinemia is associated with G6PD deficiency. Jaundice generally appears 2 to 3 days after birth without concomitant anemia.[64] The jaundice is mainly attributed to inefficient conjugation of indirect bilirubin by the liver rather than to excessive hemolysis.[76] These neonates must be closely monitored because the hyperbilirubinemia can be severe and cause bilirubin encephalopathy (kernicterus) and permanent brain damage.[62] Severe hyperbilirubinemia occurs more often in infants who, in addition to a mutated *G6PD* gene, are homozygous for a mutation in the promoter region of the uridine diphosphate (UDP) glucuronosyltransferase family 1 member A1 *(UGT1A1)* gene, which impairs their ability to conjugate and excrete indirect bilirubin.[62] In addition, the particular G6PD variant and environmental factors (such as drugs given to the mother or infant, the presence of infection, and gestational age) probably play an important role in the occurrence of neonatal hyperbilirubinemia, because a wide variation exists in frequency and severity in different populations with G6PD deficiency.

Chronic hereditary nonspherocytic hemolytic anemia. A small percentage of G6PD-deficient patients have chronic HNSHA, as evidenced by persistent hyperbilirubinemia, decreased serum haptoglobin level, and increased serum lactate dehydrogenase level. Most of these patients are diagnosed at birth as having neonatal hyperbilirubinemia, and the hemolysis continues into adulthood. They usually do not have hemoglobinuria, which suggests that the ongoing hemolysis is extravascular as opposed to intravascular. RBC morphology is unremarkable. These patients also are vulnerable to acute oxidative stress from the same agents as those affecting other G6PD-deficient individuals and may have acute episodes of hemoglobinuria. The severity of HNSHA is extremely variable, likely related to the type of mutation in the *G6PD* gene.

Laboratory Findings

General tests for hemolytic anemia. The anemia occurring during a hemolytic crisis may range from moderate to extremely severe and is usually normocytic and normochromic. The morphology of G6PD-deficient RBCs is normal except during a hemolytic episode. The degree of RBC morphology change during a hemolytic episode varies, depending on the severity of the hemolysis. In some patients, the change is not striking, but in other individuals with severe variants, marked anisocytosis, poikilocytosis, spherocytosis, and schistocytosis may occur.[62] Bite cells (RBCs in which the margin appears indented and the hemoglobin is concentrated) may be observed in rare cases of drug-induced hemolysis but should not be considered a specific feature of G6PD deficiency.[62,77] Bite cells are absent in acute and chronic hemolytic states associated with common G6PD-deficient variants, and they can also be found in other conditions.[62,77] Heinz bodies (precipitated denatured hemoglobin) can form in patients with G6PD deficiency but cannot be detected with Wright staining. They can be visualized with supravital stains, such as crystal violet, as dark purple inclusions attached to the inner RBC membrane (Figure 11.12). The reticulocyte count is increased and may reach 30% of RBCs. Consistent with intravascular hemolysis, the serum haptoglobin level is severely decreased, the serum lactate dehydrogenase activity is elevated, and there is hemoglobinemia and hemoglobinuria. The indirect bilirubin level is also elevated. The WBC count is moderately elevated, and the platelet count varies. Importantly, the DAT is negative, indicating that an immune cause of the hemolysis is unlikely (Chapter 23). Table 21.6 contains a summary of the clinical and laboratory findings in G6PD deficiency during an acute hemolytic episode.

Tests for G6PD deficiency. The two major categories of tests for G6PD deficiency are quantitative and qualitative biochemical assays for G6PD activity (phenotypic assays) and deoxyribonucleic acid (DNA) based molecular tests for mutation detection (genotypic assays). Quantitative spectrophotometric assays are the gold standard to determine G6PD activity, make a definitive diagnosis, and assess the severity of the deficiency.[60,78] The assays are based on the direct measurement of NADPH generated by the patient's G6PD in the reaction shown in Figure 21.13. The assays require venous blood collected in heparin or ethylenediaminetetraacetic acid (EDTA) anticoagulant. A hemolysate is prepared and incubated with the substrate/cofactor (glucose-6-phosphate/NADP) reagent. The rate of NADPH formation is proportional to G6PD activity and is measured as an increase in absorbance at 340 nm by spectrophotometry.[60,78] The activity is typically reported as a ratio of the units of G6PD activity per gram of hemoglobin (IU/g hemoglobin [Hb]), so a standard hemoglobin assay must be done on the same specimen used for the G6PD assay. Cutoff points to determine G6PD deficiency are usually set at less than 20% of normal activity (usually less than 4.0 IU/g Hb), but this varies by method, laboratory, and population screened.[75]

Qualitative tests are designed as rapid screening tools to distinguish normal from G6PD-deficient patients. G6PD deficiency is defined by various methods as less than 20% to 50% of normal G6PD activity.[75,78,79] Similar to quantitative assays, these tests also incubate a lysate of heparin or EDTA-anticoagulated blood with a glucose-6-phosphate/NADP reagent to generate NADPH (Figure 21.13). The endpoint in qualitative tests, however, is visually observed, and the results are reported as "G6PD-deficient" or "normal." Qualitative tests with deficient or intermediate results are reflexed to the quantitative assay for verification of the G6PD deficiency.

The fluorescent spot test is based on the principle that the NADPH generated in the reaction is fluorescent, while the NADP in the reagent is not fluorescent. Blood and glucose-6-phosphate/NADP reagent are incubated and spotted on filter paper in timed intervals. Specimens with normal G6PD activity appear as moderate to strong fluorescent spots under long-wave ultraviolet (UV) light; specimens with decreased or no

---

TABLE 21.6 Typical Clinical and Laboratory Findings in Glucose-6-Phosphate Dehydrogenase (G6PD) Deficiency During Acute Hemolytic Episode

History	Recent infection, administration of drugs associated with hemolysis, or ingestion of fava beans
Clinical manifestations	Chills, fever, headache, nausea, back pain, abdominal pain Jaundice Dark urine
Complete blood count results	↓ Hemoglobin (moderate to severe) ↓ Reticulocyte count
Peripheral blood film findings	Polychromasia RBC morphology varies from normal to marked anisocytosis, poikilocytosis, spherocytosis, or schistocytosis, depending on severity
Direct antiglobulin test result	Negative
Indicators of hemolysis	↓ Serum haptoglobin (severe) ↑ Serum lactate dehydrogenase ↑ Serum indirect bilirubin ↑ Plasma hemoglobin Hemoglobinuria
Selected additional tests	↓ G6PD activity (mild to severe); may be falsely normal as a result of reticulocytosis, leukocytosis, or thrombocytosis and in individuals with mild deficiencies DNA-based mutation detection usually needed to identify heterozygous females Heinz bodies observed on supravital stain

↑, Increased; ↓, decreased; *DNA*, deoxyribonucleic acid; *RBC*, red blood cell.

$$\text{Glucose-6-phosphate + NADP} \xrightarrow{\text{G6PD}} \text{6-Phosphogluconate + NADPH}$$

Not fluorescent   Fluorescent; ↑ absorbance at 340 nm

Figure 21.13 Principle of the Glucose-6-Phosphate Dehydrogenase (G6PD) Activity Assay. G6PD (in patient's hemolysate) converts glucose-6-phosphate to 6-phosphogluconate with the conversion of oxidized nicotinamide adenine dinucleotide phosphate (NADP) (not fluorescent) to the reduced form of nicotinamide adenine dinucleotide phosphate (NADPH) (fluorescent). In the quantitative assay the rate of production of NADPH is proportional to G6PD activity and is measured as an increase in absorbance at 340 nm by spectrophotometry. In the qualitative assay the appearance of a fluorescent spot under ultraviolet light when the reaction mixture is spotted on filter paper indicates normal G6PD activity.

activity do not fluoresce or display weak fluorescence compared with a normal control.

Dye-reduction qualitative assays use the same G6PD enzymatic reaction but have a second step in which the NADPH reduces a dye, giving a visually observed color change. An example is BinaxNOW (Alere/Abbott), which is a handheld device that uses the enzyme chromographic test (ECT) method.[80] Hemolysate is applied to one section of a lateral flow test strip in the device. The specimen migrates to the reaction pad of the strip containing the glucose-6-phosphate/NADP substrate/cofactor and a nitroblue tetrazolium dye.[80] If the specimen has normal G6PD activity, the NADPH generated reduces the dye to a formazan product that is visually observed as a brown-black color on the reaction pad.[80] This method has a sensitivity of 98% in detecting deficient specimens with G6PD activity less than 4.0 U/g Hb.[80] In another formazan-based test, the NADPH reduces a tetrazolium monosodium salt (WST-8) substrate, forming a formazan orange-colored product.[79] The dye-reduction methods have an advantage because they do not need a UV light for visualization. A disadvantage of the BinaxNOW method, however, is its higher cost compared with other assays. Rapid, point-of-care screening methods that do not require a venipuncture specimen are in development.

Biochemical qualitative screening tests are reliable to identify hemizygous males and homozygous or compound heterozygous mutant females with severe deficiency (less than 20% of normal activity) but lack the sensitivity to detect mild and moderate deficiencies found in some class III G6PD deficiency and in heterozygous females. They also have subjective endpoints that may affect test reproducibility and accuracy.

Phenotypic assays for G6PD activity have several additional limitations. As covered earlier in the chapter, reticulocytes have higher G6PD activity compared with mature RBCs. Reticulocytosis typically occurs as a response to an acute hemolytic episode and will falsely increase the patient's G6PD activity over baseline values.[60,78] G6PD deficiency should be suspected when a patient with reticulocytosis has an unexpectedly normal G6PD activity result; that is because a patient with a normal G6PD enzyme and reticulocytosis is expected to have high G6PD activity. To avoid falsely elevated or falsely normal results, biochemical assays for G6PD activity should not be performed during acute hemolysis. The testing should be performed after the reticulocyte and total RBC counts have returned to baseline, which may take 2 weeks to 2 months after the hemolytic episode.[75,78] Another limitation of phenotypic assays is that testing cannot be done after recent transfusion because the mixture of donor and patient RBCs does not reflect the patient's true G6PD activity. WBCs and platelets also contain G6PD activity, but they generally do not interfere with the assay. However, in cases of severe anemia, or in severe leukocytosis or thrombocytosis, the buffy coat should be removed from the specimen before preparing the hemolysate to avoid falsely elevating the G6PD activity.[78]

DNA-based mutation detection (genotyping) is available in larger hospital and reference laboratories. Typically the DNA is extracted from WBCs isolated from whole blood. Because the vast majority of G6PD mutations involve single nucleotide substitutions, molecular testing is straightforward. Although there are approximately 217 known mutations, rapid polymerase chain reaction-based methods can be used that target specific mutations with high prevalence in a particular geographic area, racial group, or ethnic group.[70,78] If targeted mutation testing is negative, whole-gene DNA sequencing is required.[78]

DNA-based testing is best suited for prenatal testing, family studies, and identification of heterozygous females who typically have indeterminate or normal biochemical (phenotypic) tests because of their mosaicism of normal and G6PD-deficient cells.[60,78] DNA-based methods can be done on patients who were recently transfused because donor WBCs have a short half-life in stored blood and will not interfere with the test. In addition, DNA-based tests are not affected by reticulocytosis and can be done during an acute hemolytic episode.

The disadvantage of DNA-based methods is the requirement for technical expertise and specialized equipment. In addition, knowing the genotype of heterozygous females does not predict the clinical phenotype in terms of the proportion of normal and G6PD-deficient cells.[75]

An additional application of tests for G6PD deficiency is screening asymptomatic patients before prescribing the drugs listed in Box 21.2. Screening is recommended for patients with a family history of G6PD deficiency or for those who are members of ethnic/racial groups with a high prevalence of G6PD variants.

Treatment

Treatment for G6PD-deficient patients with acute hemolysis begins with discontinuing drugs associated with hemolysis. Most hemolytic episodes, especially in individuals with G6PD-A⁻, are self-limited. In patients with more severe types, such as G6PD-Mediterranean, RBC transfusions may be required. Screening is important in populations that have a high incidence of G6PD deficiency. The prevention of acute hemolytic anemia is difficult because multiple causes exist; however, some cases of acute hemolytic anemia are easily preventable, such as by avoidance of fava bean consumption and drugs known to induce hemolysis. Neonates in high-risk populations should be screened for hyperbilirubinemia associated with G6PD deficiency and treated immediately to prevent kernicterus and permanent brain damage.

Favism is a relatively dangerous manifestation and potentially fatal in individuals who do not have access to appropriate medical facilities and a transfusion service. Prevention of drug-induced disease is possible by choosing alternate drugs when possible. In cases in which the offending drugs must be used, especially in individuals with G6PD-A⁻, the dosage can be lowered to decrease the hemolysis to a manageable level. Infection-induced hemolysis is more difficult to prevent but can be detected early in the course of the episode and treated if necessary. Most episodes resolve without treatment but may be severe enough to warrant RBC transfusion. In patients with hemoglobin levels greater than 9 g/dL with persistent hemoglobinuria, close monitoring is important. Neonates with moderate hyperbilirubinemia and jaundice secondary to G6PD deficiency can be treated with phototherapy, but those with severe hyperbilirubinemia may require exchange transfusion.[60]

Pyruvate Kinase Deficiency

Pyruvate kinase (PK) is a rate-limiting key enzyme of the glycolytic pathway of RBCs. It catalyzes the conversion of phosphoenolpyruvate to pyruvate, forming ATP (Figure 6.1). PK deficiency is an autosomal recessive disorder, with an estimated prevalence of 1 per 20,000 in the white population.[81] It is the most common form of hereditary nonspherocytic hemolytic anemia and is found worldwide.[60,62] PK deficiency is due to a mutation in the *PKLR* gene that codes for PK in RBCs and hepatocytes. A mutation database published in 2016 reported 256 mutations with 72% being single nucleotide substitutions (missense), about 9% deletions, and 3% insertions, while 13% affect the promoter region and introns.[82] Symptomatic hemolytic anemia occurs in homozygotes or compound heterozygotes. Certain mutations are more common in the United States, parts of Europe, and Asia.[60,82] There is a high prevalence of PK-deficient homozygotes with the same point mutations in two isolated, consanguineous communities in the United States: an Amish kindred in Pennsylvania (1436G > A) and children born into polygamist families in a small town in the Midwest (1529G > A).[83,84]

Pathophysiology

The mechanisms causing hemolysis and premature destruction of PK-deficient cells are not completely known. Metabolic consequences of PK deficiency is a depletion of cellular ATP and an increase in 2,3-bisphosphoglycerate (2,3-BPG).[85,86] The increase in 2,3-BPG shifts the hemoglobin-oxygen dissociation curve to the right and decreases the oxygen affinity of hemoglobin[85] (Chapter 7). This promotes greater release of oxygen to the tissues and enables affected individuals to tolerate lower levels of hemoglobin.[60,85,86] ATP depletion also affects the ability of the cell to maintain its shape and membrane integrity.

Clinical Manifestations

Individuals with PK deficiency have a wide range of clinical presentations, varying from severe neonatal anemia and hyperbilirubinemia requiring exchange or multiple transfusions to a fully compensated hemolytic process in apparently healthy adults.[85] Most patients, however, have manifestations of chronic hemolysis, including anemia, jaundice, splenomegaly, and increased incidence of gallstones (because of the production of excessive bilirubin).[60] Rarely, folate deficiency (as a result of accelerated erythropoiesis), bone marrow aplasia (usually caused by parvovirus B19 infection), and skin ulcers can occur.[77,86] Pregnancy carries the risk of fetal loss and exacerbation of the anemia in the mother.[83] There is an increased risk of iron overload and organ damage that occurs with age, even in the absence of transfusions.[83,86,87] The mechanism of dysregulation of iron homeostasis is not clear but may be related to a decrease in or lack of response to hepcidin, the major iron-regulating protein.[83]

Laboratory Findings

The hemoglobin level is variable, depending on the extent of the hemolysis. Reticulocytosis is usually present, but not in proportion to the severity of the anemia, because the reticulocytes are preferentially destroyed in the spleen.[60,86] After splenectomy, the number of circulating reticulocytes can increase fivefold.[86] In addition to showing anisocytosis, poikilocytosis, and polychromasia, the peripheral blood film reveals a variable number of burr cells, or echinocytes (in the range of 3% to 30%), which increase in number after splenectomy.[86] The post-splenectomy peripheral blood film may also show Howell-Jolly bodies, Pappenheimer bodies, and target cells. The WBC and platelet counts are normal or slightly increased. Patients usually have the characteristic laboratory findings of chronic hemolysis, including increased serum indirect bilirubin and lactate dehydrogenase levels, decreased serum haptoglobin level, and increased urinary urobilinogen. The osmotic fragility is usually normal, and the DAT is negative.

Tests for PK deficiency include quantitative and qualitative biochemical assays for PK activity (phenotypic assays) and DNA-based molecular tests for mutation detection (genotypic assays). In the quantitative PK assay, a hemolysate is prepared from patient's anticoagulated blood after careful removal of the WBCs. WBCs have a very high PK level, and contamination of the hemolysate with WBCs falsely increases the result (i.e., in a PK deficiency, the result could be falsely normal).[86] The reagents include phosphoenolpyruvate, adenosine diphosphate (ADP), lactate dehydrogenase, and the reduced form of NADH. In the first step of the reaction, the patient's PK converts phosphoenolpyruvate to pyruvic acid, and a phosphate is transferred to ADP, forming ATP. In the second step, lactate dehydrogenase converts the pyruvic acid to lactic acid, and the NADH is converted to its oxidized form, NAD (Figure 21.14). The rate of NAD formation is proportional to PK activity and is measured as a decrease in absorbance at 340 nm by spectrophotometry. The activity is typically reported as a ratio of the units of PK activity per gram of hemoglobin (IU/g Hb). More complex techniques may be necessary when some variant forms of PK are suspected.[86]

The enzyme pyruvate kinase catalyzes the following reaction:

1. ADP + Phosphoenolpyruvic acid $\xrightarrow{\text{Pyruvate kinase}}$ ATP + Pyruvic acid

The pyruvic acid formed then takes part in the following reaction:

2. Pyruvic acid + NADH (Fluorescent) $\xrightarrow{\text{Lactate dehydrogenase}}$ Lactic acid + NAD (Not fluorescent; ↓absorbance at 340 mn)

Figure 21.14 Principle of the Pyruvate Kinase (PK) Activity Assay. The reagent contains adenosine diphosphate (ADP), phosphoenolpyruvic acid, lactate dehydrogenase, and the reduced form of nicotinamide adenine dinucleotide (NADH). In the first step, PK (in patient's hemolysate) converts phosphoenolpyruvic acid to pyruvic acid, and a phosphate is transferred to ADP, forming adenosine triphosphate (ATP). In the second step, lactate dehydrogenase converts pyruvic acid to lactic acid with the conversion of NADH (fluorescent) to the oxidized form of nicotinamide adenine dinucleotide (NAD) (not fluorescent). In the quantitative assay, the rate of production of NAD is proportional to PK activity and is measured as a decrease in absorbance at 340 nm by spectrophotometry. In the qualitative assay the disappearance of fluorescence under ultraviolet light when the reaction mixture is spotted on filter paper indicates normal PK activity.

Qualitative tests for PK deficiency are used for screening and are based on the same principle as that described earlier; the hemolysate and reagents are incubated and spotted onto filter paper. The loss of fluorescence is visually evaluated to determine the oxidation of NADH to NAD.[88]

Mutation detection (genotypic testing) can be accomplished by sequencing the exons, flanking regions, and promoter region of the *PKLR* gene.[82,86] Molecular testing is superior in sensitivity and specificity, is applicable for use in prenatal testing, confirms patients with borderline enzyme deficiencies, and enables correlation of certain mutations with disease severity.[60,83,86]

Treatment

No specific therapy is available for PK deficiency except supportive treatment and RBC transfusion as necessary. Splenectomy is beneficial in severe cases, and after this procedure the hemoglobin level usually increases enough to reduce or eliminate the need for transfusion.[77] Splenectomy, however, results in a lifelong increased risk of sepsis by encapsulated bacteria. Hematopoietic stem cell transplant may be curative for children with severe hemolytic disease who have an unaffected HLA-identical sibling for a donor.[83]

Other Enzymopathies

Pyrimidine 5′-nucleotidase type 1 (P5′NT-1) is an enzyme needed for the degradation and elimination of ribosomal ribonucleic acid (RNA) in reticulocytes. P5′NT-1 removes the phosphate from pyrimidine 5′ ribonucleoside monophosphate to form ribonucleoside and inorganic phosphate. These degradation products are then able to diffuse out of the cell.[60] P5′NT-1 deficiency is inherited in an autosomal recessive manner.[60,89] It is the third most common RBC enzyme deficiency that causes hereditary nonspherocytic hemolytic anemia (after G6PD and

PK deficiencies) with only 100 cases reported worldwide.[60,89,90] The *NT5C3A* gene codes for P5′NT-1, and more than 20 different mutations have been reported.[89] A recent proteomics study revealed that P5′NT-1-deficient patients also had a decrease in transketolase, an enzyme in the pentose phosphate pathway.[90]

Patients who are homozygotes or compound heterozygotes for *NT5C3A* mutations develop chronic hemolytic anemia. The P5′NT-1-deficient RBCs accumulate pyrimidine ribonucleoside monophosphates, which precipitate and appear as very coarse *basophilic stippling* in the cell.[60,89] These RBCs ultimately undergo premature hemolysis. Most patients have a mild to moderate anemia with reticulocytosis, jaundice, and splenomegaly.[89] Diagnostic tests include measurement of P5′NT-1 activity and the concentration of intracellular pyrimidine nucleotides in RBCs and DNA-based testing for mutations.[89] Therapy consists of supportive RBC transfusions as needed.

Other RBC enzymopathies are rarely encountered. In addition to PK deficiency, deficiencies of other enzymes of the RBC Embden-Meyerhof pathway that cause hereditary nonspherocytic hemolytic anemia have been described, including hexokinase, glucose-6-phosphate isomerase, 6-phosphofructokinase, fructose-bisphosphate aldolase, triosephosphate isomerase, and phosphoglycerate kinase.[62] All these deficiencies are autosomal recessive conditions, except for phosphoglycerate kinase deficiency, which is X-linked. Mutations in enolase are rare, and their association with hemolytic anemia is uncertain.[62] Deficiencies in glyceraldehyde-3-phosphate dehydrogenase and lactate dehydrogenase are not associated with hemolytic anemia.[62] Phosphoglycerate mutase deficiency results in a depletion of 2,3-bisphosphoglycerate. This causes a shift in the hemoglobin-oxygen dissociation curve to the left and an increased affinity of hemoglobin for oxygen. The resulting tissue hypoxia manifests as a mild erythrocytosis.[62]

SUMMARY

- The red blood cell (RBC) membrane must have deformability for RBCs to maneuver through the microcirculation and the splenic sieve over its life span of 120 days. Cellular properties that enable deformability are the biconcave, discoid shape of the cell; viscoelasticity of the membrane; and cytoplasmic viscosity.
- Two transmembrane protein complexes, the ankyrin complex and actin (protein 4.1) junctional complex, provide vertical structural integrity to the cell by anchoring the lipid bilayer to the underlying spectrin skeleton. α-Spectrin, β-spectrin, and their accessory proteins form a two-dimensional lattice to provide horizontal mechanical stability to the membrane.
- Hereditary spherocytosis (HS) is caused by mutations that disrupt the vertical membrane protein interactions, which results in loss of membrane, decrease in surface area-to-volume ratio, and formation of spherocytes that undergo extravascular hemolysis in the spleen. Patients with HS have anemia, splenomegaly, jaundice, an increased mean cell hemoglobin concentration (MCHC), spherocytes and polychromasia on the peripheral blood film, a negative direct antiglobulin test (DAT), and biochemical evidence of

hemolysis. RBCs in HS show decreased fluorescence in the eosin-5′-maleimide binding test by flow cytometry, and osmotic fragility is usually increased.
- Hereditary elliptocytosis (HE) and hereditary pyropoikilocytosis (HPP) are caused by mutations that disrupt the horizontal interactions in the protein cytoskeleton, which results in loss of mechanical stability of the membrane. Elliptocytes are present on the peripheral blood film. Only 10% of HE patients have moderate or severe anemia. HPP is a severe thermal-sensitive form of HE in which extreme poikilocytosis along with schistocytes, microspherocytes, and elliptocytes are seen on the peripheral blood film.
- Hereditary ovalocytosis, also called Southeast Asian ovalocytosis (SAO), is caused by a mutation in band 3 that increases membrane rigidity. The prevalence is high in Southeast Asia, and hemolysis is mild or absent; typical cells are oval with one to two transverse bars or ridges.
- Hereditary stomatocytosis is a group of disorders characterized by an RBC membrane that leaks cations. In overhydrated hereditary stomatocytosis (OHS) or hereditary hydrocytosis, RBCs have increased mean cell volume (MCV),

decreased cytoplasmic viscosity and MCHC, and stomatocytes on the peripheral blood film. In dehydrated hereditary stomatocytosis (DHS) or hereditary xerocytosis (HX), RBCs have decreased MCV and increased cytoplasmic viscosity and MCHC, and the peripheral blood film shows burr cells, target cells, few stomatocytes, and cells with puddled hemoglobin at the periphery. Stomatocytosis may also occur in Rh deficiency syndrome and in a variety of acquired conditions.

- Neuroacanthocytosis comprises a group of inherited disorders characterized by neurologic impairment and the presence of acanthocytes on the peripheral blood film. Major disorders in this group include abetalipoproteinemia, McLeod syndrome, and chorea acanthocytosis. Acquired acanthocytosis can occur in severe liver disease (spur cell anemia).
- Paroxysmal nocturnal hemoglobinuria (PNH) is due to an acquired hematopoietic stem cell mutation that results in the lack of glycosylphosphatidylinositol (GPI)-anchored proteins on blood cell surfaces. CD55 and CD59, complement-regulating proteins, are partially or completely deficient on RBCs, which makes the RBCs susceptible to spontaneous complement lysis. Flow cytometry is a sensitive method to detect the absence of the GPI anchor and GPI-anchored proteins on cell surfaces. The rate of hemolysis in classic PNH improves after treatment with eculizumab, a complement C5 inhibitor.

- Glucose-6-phosphate dehydrogenase (G6PD) deficiency is the most common RBC enzymopathy, but the vast majority of patients are asymptomatic. Patients with class II and III G6PD variants may develop acute hemolytic anemia after infections or after ingestion of certain drugs or fava beans. A small percentage of patients have class I G6PD variant and chronic hereditary nonspherocytic hemolytic anemia (HNSHA).
- Most patients with pyruvate kinase (PK) deficiency have symptoms of hemolysis. Burr cells are commonly observed on the peripheral blood film. PK deficiency is the most common cause of HNSHA.

Now that you have completed this chapter, go back and read again the case study at the beginning and respond to the questions presented.

REVIEW QUESTIONS

Answers can be found in the Appendix.

1. In HS, a characteristic abnormality in the CBC results is:
   a. Decreased MCH
   b. Decreased platelet and WBC counts
   c. Increased MCHC
   d. Increased MCV

2. The altered shape of the spherocyte in HS is due to:
   a. Abnormal precipitation of the hemoglobin molecule
   b. A mutated RBC membrane protein affecting vertical protein interactions
   c. A mutated RBC membrane protein affecting horizontal protein interactions
   d. Defective RNA catabolism and clearance

3. Which one of the following sets of results is consistent with HS?
   a. Decreased osmotic fragility, negative DAT result
   b. Decreased osmotic fragility, positive DAT result
   c. Increased osmotic fragility, negative DAT result
   d. Increased osmotic fragility, positive DAT result

4. The RBCs in HE are abnormally shaped and have unstable cell membranes as a result of:
   a. Defects in horizontal membrane protein interactions
   b. Deficiency in cation pumps in the RBC membrane
   c. Lack of Rh antigens in the RBC membrane
   d. Mutations in the ankyrin complex

5. The peripheral blood film for patients with mild HE is characterized by:
   a. Densely stained RBCs with a few irregular projections
   b. Elliptical RBCs
   c. Oval RBCs with one or two transverse ridges
   d. Overhydrated RBCs with oval central pallor

6. Laboratory test results for patients with HPP include all of the following *except*:
   a. Increased MCV and normal RDW
   b. Low fluorescence when incubated with eosin-5′-maleimide
   c. Marked poikilocytosis with elliptocytes, RBC fragments, and microspherocytes
   d. RBCs that show marked thermal sensitivity at 41° C to 45° C

7. Acanthocytes are found in association with:
   a. Abetalipoproteinemia
   b. G6PD deficiency
   c. Rh deficiency syndrome
   d. Vitamin B_{12} deficiency

8. The most common manifestation of G6PD deficiency is:
   a. Acute hemolytic anemia caused by drug exposure or infections
   b. Chronic hemolytic anemia caused by cell shape change
   c. Chronic hemolytic anemia caused by intravascular RBC lysis
   d. Mild compensated hemolysis caused by ATP deficiency

9. A patient experiences an episode of acute intravascular hemolysis after taking primaquine for the first time. The physician suspects that the patient may have G6PD deficiency and orders an RBC G6PD assay 3 days after the hemolytic episode began. How will this affect the test result?
   a. Absence of enzyme activity
   b. False decrease in enzyme activity due to hemoglobinemia
   c. False increase in enzyme activity due to reticulocytosis
   d. No effect on enzyme activity

10. The most common defect or deficiency in the anaerobic glycolytic pathway that causes chronic HNSHA is:
    a. Glucose-6-phosphate dehydrogenase deficiency
    b. Lactate dehydrogenase deficiency
    c. Methemoglobin reductase deficiency
    d. Pyruvate kinase deficiency

11. Which of the following laboratory tests would be best to confirm PNH?
    a. Acidified serum test (Ham test)
    b. Flow cytometry for detection of eosin-5′-maleimide binding on erythrocytes
    c. Flow cytometry for FLAER binding, CD24 on granulocytes, and CD14 on monocytes
    d. Osmotic fragility test

12. A 22-year-old man with a moderate decrease in hemoglobin level and a decrease in RBC, WBC, platelet, and reticulocyte counts has a history of infrequent and mild episodes of hemolysis with hemoglobinuria. His bone marrow showed 15% cellularity with no abnormal cells, and flow cytometry revealed that 15% of his circulating granulocytes were GPI deficient. He most likely has:
    a. A hereditary RBC membrane defect
    b. Classic PNH
    c. Hypoplastic PNH
    d. Subclinical PNH

REFERENCES

1. Mohandas, N., & Evans, E. (1994). Mechanical properties of the red cell membrane in relation to molecular structure and genetic defects. *Annu Rev Biophys Biomol Struct, 23*, 787–818.
2. Mohandas, N., & Chasis, J. A. (1993). Red blood cell deformability, membrane material properties and shape: regulation by transmembrane, skeletal and cytosolic proteins and lipids. *Semin Hematol, 30*, 171–192.
3. Mohandas, N., & Gallagher, P. G. (2008). Red cell membrane: past, present, future. *Blood, 112*, 3939–3948.
4. Coetzer, T. L. (2016). Erythrocyte membrane disorders. In Kaushansky. K., Lichtman, M. A., Prchal, J. T., et al. (Eds.), *Williams Hematology.* (9th ed., pp. 661–688). New York: McGraw-Hill.
5. Palek, J., & Jarolim, P. (1993). Clinical expression and laboratory detection of red blood cell membrane protein mutations. *Semin Hematol, 30*, 249–283.
6. Da Costa, L., Galimand, J., Fenneteau O., et al. (2013). Hereditary spherocytosis, elliptocytosis, and other red cell membrane disorders. *Blood Rev, 27*, 167–178.
7. Bennett, V. (1983). Proteins involved in membrane-cytoskeleton association in human erythrocytes: spectrin, ankyrin, and band 3. *Methods Enzymol, 96*, 313–324.
8. Nicolas, V., Le Van Kim, C., Gane, P., et al. (2003). Rh-RhAG/ankyrin-R, a new interaction site between the membrane bilayer and the red cell skeleton, is impaired by Rhnull-associated mutation. *J Biol Chem, 278*, 25526–25533.
9. Salomao, M., Zhang, X., Yang, Y., et al. (2008). Protein 4.1R-dependent multiprotein complex: new insights into the structural organization of the red blood cell membrane. *Proc Natl Acad Sci U S A, 105*, 8026–8031.
10. An, X., Debnath, G., Guo, X., et al. (2005). Identification and functional characterization of protein 4.1R and actin-binding sites in erythrocyte beta-spectrin: regulation of the interactions by phosphatidylinositol-4,5-bisphosphate. *Biochemistry, 44*, 10681–10688.
11. Narla, J., & Mohandas, N. (2017). Red cell membrane disorders. *Int J Lab Hem, 39*(Suppl. 1), 47–52.
12. An, X., Guo, X., Zhang, X., et al. (2006). Conformational stabilities of the structural repeats of erythroid spectrin and their functional implications. *J Biol Chem, 281*, 10527–10532.
13. Gallagher, P. G. (2018). Red blood cell membrane disorders. In Hoffman, R., Benz, E. J., Silberstein, L. E., et al. (Eds.), *Hematology: Basic Principles and Practice.* (7th ed., pp. 626–647). Philadelphia: Elsevier.
14. National Human Genome Research Institute. *Red Cell Membrane Disorder Mutations Database.* http://research.nhgri.nih.gov/RBCmembrane/. Accessed August 10, 2017.
15. Perrotta, S., Gallagher, P. G., & Mohandas, N. (2008). Hereditary spherocytosis. *Lancet, 372*, 1411–1426.
16. Bolton-Maggs, P. H. B., Langer, J. C., Iolascon, A., et al. (2011). Guidelines for the diagnosis and management of hereditary spherocytosis—2011 update. *Br J Haematol, 156*, 37–49.
17. De Franceschi, L., Olivieri, O., Miraglia del Giudice, E., et al. (1997). Membrane cation and anion transport activities in erythrocytes of hereditary spherocytosis: effects of different membrane protein defects. *Am J Hematol, 55*, 121–128.
18. Hassoun, H., Vassiliadis, J. N., Murray, J., et al. (1997). Characterization of the underlying molecular defect in hereditary spherocytosis associated with spectrin deficiency. *Blood, 90*, 398–406.
19. Dhermy, D., Galand, C., Bournier, O., et al. (1997). Heterogenous band 3 deficiency in hereditary spherocytosis related to different band 3 gene defects. *Br J Haematol, 98*, 32–40.
20. Bouhassira, E. E., Schwartz, R. S., Yawata, Y., et al. (1992). An alanine-to-threonine substitution in protein 4.2 cDNA is associated with a Japanese form of hereditary hemolytic anemia (protein 4.2NIPPON). *Blood, 79*, 1846–1854.
21. Farias, M. G. (2017). Advances in laboratory diagnosis of hereditary spherocytosis. *Clin Chem Lab Med, 55*(7), 944–948.
22. King, M.-J., Garçon, L., Hoyer, J. D., et al and the International Council for Standardization in Haematology. (2015). ICSH guidelines for the laboratory diagnosis of nonimmune hereditary red cell membrane disorders. *Int J Lab Hematol, 37*(3), 304–325.
23. Hansen, D. M. (1998). Hereditary anemias of increased destruction. In Steine-Martin, E. A., Lotspeich-Steininger, C. A., & Koepke, J. A., (Eds.), *Clinical Hematology: Principles, Procedures, Correlations.* (2nd ed., pp. 255–256). Philadelphia: Lippincott.
24. Bianchi, P., Fermo, E., Vercellati, C., et al. (2012). Diagnostic power of laboratory tests for hereditary spherocytosis: a comparison study in 150 patients groups according to molecular and clinical characteristics. *Haematologica, 97*, 516–523.
25. King, M-J., Smythe, J., & Mushens, R. (2004). Eosin-5- maleimide binding to band 3 and Rh-related proteins forms the basis of a screening test for hereditary spherocytosis. *Br J Haematol, 124*, 106–113.
26. Kar, R., Mishra, P., & Pati, H. P. (2008). Evaluation of eosin-5-maleimide flow cytometric test in diagnosis of hereditary spherocytosis. *Int J Lab Hematol, 32*, 8–16.
27. Mackiewicz, G., Bailly, F., Favre, B., et al. (2012). Flow cytometry test for hereditary spherocytosis. *Haematologica, 97*, e47.

28. Da Costa, L., Suner, L., Galimand, J., et al. (2016). Diagnostic tool for red blood cell membrane disorders: assessment of a new generation ektacytometer. *Blood Cells Mol Dis, 56*(1), 9–22.

29. King, M. J., & Zanella, A. (2013). Hereditary red cell membrane disorders and laboratory diagnostic testing. *Int J Lab Hem, 35,* 237–243.

30. Streichman, S., & Gescheidt, Y. (1998). Cryohemolysis for the detection of hereditary spherocytosis: correlation studies with osmotic fragility and autohemolysis. *Am J Hematol, 58,* 206–212.

31. Agarwal, A. M., Nussenzveig, R. H., Reading, N. S., et al. (2016). Clinical utility of next-generation sequencing in the diagnosis of hereditary haemolytic anaemias. *Br J Haematol, 174*(5), 806–814.

32. Abdullah, F., Zhang, Y., Camp, M., et al. (2009). Splenectomy in hereditary spherocytosis: review of 1,657 patients and application of the pediatric quality indicators. *Pediatr Blood Cancer, 52,* 834–837.

33. Gallagher, P. G. (2004). Hereditary elliptocytosis: spectrin and protein 4.1R. *Semin Hematol, 41,* 142–164.

34. Winardi, R., Reid, M., Conboy, J., et al. (1993). Molecular analysis of glycophorin C deficiency in human erythrocytes. *Blood, 81,* 2799–2803.

35. Gallagher, P. G. (2013). Abnormalities of the erythrocyte membrane. *Pediatr Clin N Am, 60,* 1349–1362.

36. Ideguchi, H., Yamada, Y., Kondo, S., et al. (1993). Abnormal erythrocyte band 4.1 protein in myelodysplastic syndrome with elliptocytosis. *Br J Haematol, 85,* 387–392.

37. King, M-J., Telfer, P., MacKinnon, H., et al. (2008). Using the eosin-5-maleimide binding test in the differential diagnosis of hereditary spherocytosis and hereditary pyropoikilocytosis. *Cytometry B Clin Cytom, 74B,* 244–250.

38. Mohandas, N., Winardi, R., Knowles, D., et al. (1992). Molecular basis for membrane rigidity of hereditary ovalocytosis. A novel mechanism involving the cytoplasmic domain of band 3. *J Clin Invest, 89,* 686–692.

39. Liu, S-C., Zhai, S., Palek, J., et al. (1990). Molecular defect of the band 3 protein in Southeast Asian ovalocytosis. *N Engl J Med, 323,* 1530–1538.

40. Schofield, A. E., Tanner, M. J. A., Pinder, J. C., et al. (1992). Basis of unique red cell membrane properties in hereditary ovalocytosis. *J Mol Biol, 223,* 949–958.

41. Bruce, L. J. (2009). Hereditary stomatocytosis and cation leaky red cells—recent developments. *Blood Cells Mol Dis, 42,* 216–222.

42. Bruce, L. J., Guizouam, H., Burton, N. M., et al. (2009). The monovalent cation leak in overhydrated stomatocytic red blood cells results from amino acid substitutions in the Rh-associated glycoprotein. *Blood, 113,* 1350–1357.

43. Zarychanski, R., Schulz, V. P., Houston, B. L., et al. (2012). Mutations in the mechanotransduction protein PIEZO1 are associated with hereditary xerocytosis. *Blood, 120,* 1908–1915.

44. Bae, C., Gnanasambandam, R., Nicolai, C., et al. (2013). Xerocytosis is caused by mutations that alter the kinetics of the mechanosensitive channel PIEZO1. *Proc Natl Acad Sci U S A, 110,* E1162–E1168.

45. Gallagher, P. G. (2017). Disorders of erythrocyte hydration. *Blood, 130,* 2699–2708.

46. Rampoldi, L., Danek, A., & Monaco, A. P. (2002). Clinical features and molecular bases of neuroacanthocytosis. *J Mol Med, 80,* 475–491.

47. Walker, R. H., Jung, H. H., Dobson-Stone, C., et al. (2007). Neurologic phenotypes associated with acanthocytosis. *Neurology, 68,* 92–98.

48. Parker, C. J. (2015). Paroxysmal nocturnal hemoglobinuria. In Kaushansky, K., Lichtman, M. A., Prchal, J. T., et al. (Eds.), *Williams Hematology.* (9th ed., pp. 571–582). New York: McGraw-Hill.

49. Besslar, M., & Hiken, J. (2008). The pathophysiology of disease in patients with paroxysmal nocturnal hemoglobinuria. *Hematology Am Soc Hematol Educ Program,* 104–110.

50. Brodsky, R. A. (2018). Paroxysmal nocturnal hemoglobinuria. In Hoffman, R., Benz, E. J., Silberstein, L. E., et al. (Eds.), *Hematology: Basic Principles and Practice.* (7th ed., pp. 415–424). Philadelphia: Elsevier.

51. Hill, A., DeZern, A. E., Kinoshita, T., et al. (2017). Paroxysmal nocturnal haemoglobinuria. *Nat Rev Dis Primers, 3,* 17028.

52. Parker, C., Omine, M., Richards, S., et al. (2005). Diagnosis and management of paroxysmal nocturnal hemoglobinuria. *Blood, 106,* 3699–3709.

53. Griffin, M., & Munir, T. (2017). Management of thrombosis in paroxysmal nocturnal hemoglobinuria: a clinician's guide. *Ther Adv Hematol, 8*(3), 119–126.

54. Sutherland, R. D., Keeney, M., & Illingworth, A. (2012). Practical guidelines for the high-sensitivity detection and monitoring of paroxysmal nocturnal hemoglobinuria clones by flow cytometry. *Cytometry Part B, 82B,* 195–208.

55. Preis, M., & Lowrey, C. H. (2014). Laboratory tests for paroxysmal nocturnal hemoglobinuria. *Am J Hematol, 89,* 339–341.

56. Sutherland, D. R., Kuek, N., Azcona-Olivera, J., et al. (2009). Use of FLAER-based WBC assay in the primary screening of PNH clones. *Am J Clin Pathol, 132,* 564–572.

57. Dmytrijuk, A., Robie-Suh, K., Cohen, M. H., et al. (2008). FDA report: eculizumab (Soliris) for the treatment of patients with paroxysmal nocturnal hemoglobinuria. *Oncologist, 13,* 993–1000.

58. Hillmen, P., Muus, P., Röth, A., et al. (2013). Long-term safety and efficacy of sustained eculizumab treatment in patients with paroxysmal nocturnal hemoglobinuria. *Br J Haematol, 162,* 62–73.

59. Risitano, A. M., Notaro, R., Pascariello, C., et al. (2012). The complement receptor 2/factor H fusion protein TT30 protects paroxysmal nocturnal hemoglobinuria erythrocytes from complement-mediated hemolysis and C3 fragment opsonization. *Blood, 119,* 6307–6316.

60. Gregg, X. T., & Prchal, J. T. (2018). Red blood cell enzymopathies. In Hoffman, R., Benz, E. J., Silberstein, L. E., et al. (Eds.), *Hematology: Basic Principles and Practice.* (7th ed., pp. 616–625). Philadelphia: Elsevier.

61. Cappellini, M. D., & Fiorelli, G. (2008). Glucose-6-phosphate dehydrogenase deficiency. *Lancet, 371,* 64–74.

62. van Solinge, W. W., & van Wijk, R. (2016). Erythrocyte enzyme disorders. In Kaushansky, K., Lichtman, M. A., Prchal, J. T., et al. (Eds.), *Williams Hematology.* (9th ed., pp. 689–724). New York: McGraw-Hill.

63. Nkhoma, E. T., Poole, C., Vannappagari, V., et al. (2009). The global prevalence of glucose-6-phosphate dehydrogenase deficiency: a systematic review and meta-analysis. *Blood Cells Mol Dis, 42,* 267–278.

64. Luzzatto, L. (2006). Glucose 6-phosphate dehydrogenase deficiency: from genotype to phenotype. *Hematologica, 91,* 1303–1306.

65. Guindo, A., Fairhurst, R. M., Doumbo, O. K., et al. (2007). X-linked G6PD deficiency protects hemizygous males but not heterozygous females against severe malaria. *PLoS, 4*(3), e66.

66. Leslie, T., Briceno, M., Mayan, I., et al. (2010). The impact of phenotypic and genotypic G6PD deficiency on risk of Plasmodium vivax infection: a case-control study amongst Afghan refugees in Pakistan. *PLoS, 7*(5), e1000283.

67. Clark, I. A., & Hunt, N. H. (1983). Evidence for reactive oxygen intermediates causing hemolysis and parasite death in malaria. *Infect Immun, 39*, 1–6.

68. Cappadoro, M., Giribaldi, G., O'Brien, E., et al. (1998). Early phagocytosis of glucose-6-phosphate dehydrogenase (G6PD)-deficient erythrocytes parasitized by *Plasmodium falciparum* may explain malaria protection in G6PD deficiency. *Blood, 92*, 2527–2534.

69. Mbanefo, E. C., Ahmed, A. M., Titouna, A., et al. (2017). Association of glucose-6-phosphate dehydrogenase deficiency and malaria: a systematic review and meta-analysis. *Sci Rep, 7*, 45963.

70. Gómez-Manzo, S., Marcial-Quino, J., Vanoye-Carlo, A., et al. (2016). Glucose-6-phosphate dehydrogenase: update and analysis of new mutations around the world. *Int J Mol Sci, 17*(12), 2069.

71. Beutler, E., Gaetani, G., der Kaloustian, V., et al. (1989). Glucose-6-phosphate dehydrogenase deficiency. World Health Organization (WHO) Working Group. *Bull World Health Organ, 67*(6), 601–611.

72. Boonyuen, U., Chamchoy, K., Swangsri, T., et al. (2017). A trade off between catalytic activity and protein stability determines the clinical manifestations of glucose-6-phosphate dehydrogenase (G6PD) deficiency. *Int J Biol Macromol, 104*, 145–156.

73. Cunningham, A. D., Colavin, A., Huang, K. C., et al. (2017). Coupling between protein stability and catalytic activity determines pathogenicity of G6PD variants. *Cell Rep, 18*(11), 2592–2599.

74. Youngster, I., Arcavi, L., Schechmaster, R., et al. (2010). Medications and glucose-6-phosphate dehydrogenase deficiency: an evidence-based review. *Drug Saf, 33*, 713–726.

75. Luzzatto, L., & Seneca, E. (2014). G6PD deficiency: a classic example of pharmacogenetics with on-going clinical implications. *Br J Haematol, 164*, 469–480.

76. Kaplan, M., Muraca, M., Vreman, H. J., et al. (2005). Neonatal bilirubin production-conjugation imbalance: effect of glucose-6-phosphate dehydrogenase deficiency and borderline prematurity. *Arch Dis Child Fetal Neonatal Ed, 90*, F123–F127.

77. Prchal, J. T., & Gregg, X. T. (2005). Red cell enzymes. *Hematol Am Soc Hematol Educ Program*, pp. 19–23.

78. Minucci, A., Giardina, B., Zuppi, C., et al. (2009). Glucose-6-phosphate dehydrogenase laboratory assay: how, when, and why? *IUBMB Life, 61*, 27–34.

79. Tantular, I. S., & Kawamoto, F. (2003). An improved simple screening method for detection of glucose-6-phosphate dehydrogenase deficiency. *Trop Med Int Health, 8*, 569–574.

80. Tinley, K. E., Loughlin, A. M., Jepson, A., et al. (2010). Evaluation of a rapid qualitative enzyme chromatographic test for glucose-6-phosphate dehydrogenase deficiency. *Am J Trop Med Hyg, 82*, 210–214.

81. Beutler, E., & Gelbart, T. (2000). Estimating the prevalence of pyruvate kinase deficiency from the gene frequency in the general white population. *Blood, 95*, 3585–3588.

82. Canu, G., De Bonis, M., Minucci, A., et al. (2016). Red blood cell PK deficiency: An update of PK-LR gene mutation database. *Blood Cells Mol Dis, 57*, 100–109.

83. Rider, N. L., Strauss, K. A., Brown, K., et al. (2011). Erythrocyte pyruvate kinase deficiency in an old-order Amish cohort: longitudinal risk and disease management. *Am J Hematol, 86*, 827–834.

84. Christensen, R. D., Yaish, H. M., Johnson, C. B., et al. (2011). Six children with pyruvate kinase deficiency in one small town: molecular characterization of the PK-LR gene. *J Pediatr, 159*, 695–697.

85. Van Wijk, R., & van Solinge, W. W. (2005). The energy-less red blood cell is lost: erythrocyte enzyme abnormalities of glycolysis. *Blood, 106*, 4034–4042.

86. Zanella, A., Fermo, E., Bianchi, P., et al. (2005). Red cell pyruvate kinase deficiency: molecular and clinical aspects. *Br J Haematol, 130*, 11–25.

87. Andersen, F. D., d'Amore, F., Nielsen, F. C., et al. (2004). Unexpectedly high but still asymptomatic iron overload in a patient with pyruvate kinase deficiency. *Hematol J, 5*, 543–545.

88. Tsang, S. S., & Feng, C. S. (1993). A modified screening procedure to detect pyruvate kinase deficiency. *Am J Clin Pathol, 99*, 128–131.

89. Zanella, A., Bianchi, P., Fermo, E., et al. (2006). Hereditary pyrimidine 5'-nucleotidase deficiency: from genetics to clinical manifestations. *Br J Haematol, 133*, 113–123.

90. Barasa, B., van Oirschot, B., Bianchi, P., et al. (2016). Proteomics reveals reduced expression of transketolase in pyrimidine 5'nucleotidase deficient patients. *Proteomics Clin Appl, 10*(8), 859–869.

Extrinsic Defects Leading to Increased Erythrocyte Destruction—Nonimmune Causes

*Catherine N. Otto**

OBJECTIVES

After completion of this chapter, the reader will be able to:

1. Describe the general pathophysiology and clinical laboratory findings in microangiopathic hemolytic anemia, including the characteristic red blood cell morphology.
2. Compare and contrast the pathophysiology, clinical symptoms, and typical laboratory findings in thrombotic thrombocytopenic purpura, hemolytic uremic syndrome, HELLP (*h*emolysis, *e*levated *l*iver enzymes, and *l*ow *p*latelet count) syndrome, and disseminated intravascular coagulation.
3. Explain the pathophysiology and typical laboratory features of traumatic cardiac hemolytic anemia and exercise-induced hemoglobinuria.
4. Describe the life cycle of *Plasmodium,* including the hepatic and erythrocytic cycles, and the insect vector.
5. Explain the pathophysiologic mechanisms in *P. falciparum* infection that lead to anemia and neurologic manifestations.
6. Describe the pathophysiology, laboratory findings, and peripheral blood morphology in hemolytic anemia due to babesiosis, clostridial sepsis, bartonellosis, drugs, chemicals, venoms, and extensive burns.
7. Given the history, symptoms, laboratory findings, and a representative microscopic field from a peripheral blood film of a patient with suspected extrinsic, nonimmune hemolytic anemia, discuss possible causes of the anemia and indicate the data that support the conclusions.

OUTLINE

Microangiopathic Hemolytic Anemia
  Thrombotic Thrombocytopenic Purpura
  Hemolytic Uremic Syndrome
  HELLP Syndrome
  Disseminated Intravascular Coagulation
Macroangiopathic Hemolytic Anemia
  Traumatic Cardiac Hemolytic Anemia
  Exercise-Induced Hemoglobinuria
Hemolytic Anemia Caused by Infectious Agents
  Malaria

  Babesiosis
  Clostridial Sepsis
  Bartonellosis
Hemolytic Anemia Caused by Other Red Blood Cell Injury
  Drugs and Chemicals
  Venoms
  Extensive Burns (Thermal Injury)

CASE STUDY

After studying the material in this chapter, the reader should be able to respond to the following case study:

A 24-year-old woman was brought to the emergency department with a 2-day history of fever, chills, excessive sweating, nausea, and general malaise. Because she had recently returned from a 3-week family trip to Ghana in Western Africa, the treating physician ordered a CBC and examination of thin and thick peripheral blood films. The following are the patient's laboratory results:

	Patient Results	Reference Intervals
WBCs ($\times 10^9$/L)	11.0	4.5–11.0
HGB (g/dL)	8.7	12.0–15.0

	Patient Results	Reference Intervals
HCT (%)	22	35–49
MCV (fL)	92	80–100
Platelets ($\times 10^9$/L)	176	150–450

Inclusions were noted on the thin and thick peripheral blood films (Figures 22.1 and 22.2).

Based on the results of the CBC and peripheral blood films, the patient was treated with oral quinine sulfate and doxycycline.

Continued

aThe author extends appreciation to Elaine M. Keohane, whose work in prior editions provided the foundation for this chapter.

CASE STUDY—cont'd

1. Identify the inclusions present on the thin and thick peripheral blood films.
2. What is the likely diagnosis for this patient?
3. What clues in the history support this diagnosis?

4. What are the pathophysiologic mechanisms for the anemia in this disease?

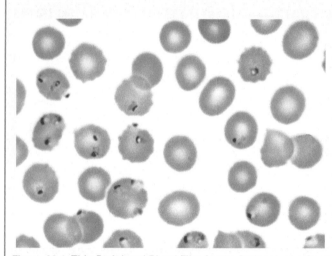

Figure 22.1 Thin Peripheral Blood Film for the Patient in the Case Study. (Wright-Giemsa stain, ×1000.)

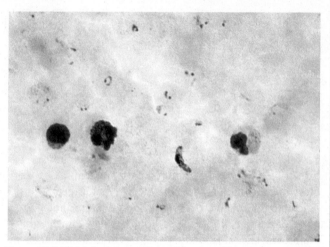

Figure 22.2 Thick Peripheral Blood Film for the Patient in the Case Study. (Wright-Giemsa stain, ×1000.) (Courtesy Linda Marler, Indiana Pathology Images, Indianapolis, IN.)

Extrinsic hemolytic anemias comprise a diverse group of disorders in which red blood cells (RBCs) are structurally and functionally normal, but a condition outside of the RBCs causes premature hemolysis. The extrinsic hemolytic anemias can be divided into conditions with nonimmune and immune causes. A common feature in the nonimmune extrinsic hemolytic anemias is the presence of a condition that causes physical or mechanical injury to the RBCs. This injury can be caused by abnormalities in the microvasculature (microangiopathic) or the heart and large blood vessels (macroangiopathic), infectious agents, chemicals, drugs, venoms, or extensive burns. The nonimmune disorders causing hemolytic anemia are discussed in this chapter and are summarized in Box 22.1. In immune hemolytic anemia, hemolysis is mediated by antibodies, complement, or both, and these conditions are covered in Chapter 23.

Examination of a peripheral blood film is important in suspected extrinsic hemolytic anemias, because observation of abnormal RBC morphology, such as schistocytes, spherocytes, or the presence of intracellular organisms, provides an important clue to the diagnosis.

MICROANGIOPATHIC HEMOLYTIC ANEMIA

Microangiopathic hemolytic anemias (MAHAs) are a group of potentially life-threatening disorders characterized by RBC fragmentation and thrombocytopenia. The RBC fragmentation occurs intravascularly by the mechanical shearing of RBC membranes as the cells rapidly pass through turbulent areas of small blood vessels that are partially blocked by microthrombi or damaged endothelium.[1,2] Upon shearing, RBC membranes

---

BOX 22.1 Extrinsic Conditions Causing Nonimmune Red Blood Cell Injury and Hemolytic Anemia

Microangiopathic Hemolytic Anemia
Thrombotic thrombocytopenic purpura
Hemolytic uremic syndrome
HELLP syndrome
Disseminated intravascular coagulation

Macroangiopathic Hemolytic Anemia
Traumatic cardiac hemolytic anemia
Exercise-induced hemoglobinuria

Infection
Malaria
Babesiosis
Clostridial sepsis
Bartonellosis

RBC Injury Due to Other Causes
Chemicals
Drugs
Venoms
Extensive Burns

HELLP, Hemolysis, elevated liver enzymes, and low platelet count; *RBC,* red blood cell.

---

quickly reseal with minimal escape of hemoglobin, but the resulting fragments (called *schistocytes*) are distorted and become rigid.[1] The spleen clears the rigid RBC fragments from the circulation through the extravascular hemolytic process (Chapter 20).[1]

Laboratory evidence of the hemolytic anemia includes a decreased hemoglobin level, increased reticulocyte count, increased serum indirect (unconjugated) bilirubin, increased serum lactate dehydrogenase (LD) activity, decreased serum haptoglobin level, and increased urine urobilinogen. In some cases the fragmentation is so severe that intravascular hemolysis occurs with varying amounts of hemoglobinemia, hemoglobin-uria, and markedly decreased levels of serum haptoglobin.[1] The presence of schistocytes on the peripheral blood film is a characteristic feature of microangiopathic hemolytic anemia. RBC shearing may also produce helmet cells and, occasionally, microspherocytes. Polychromasia and nucleated RBCs may also be present on the blood film, depending on the severity of the anemia.

Thrombocytopenia is also a feature of microangiopathic hemolytic anemia; it is due to the consumption of platelets in thrombi that form in the microvasculature.[3] Thus these disorders are sometimes called *thrombotic microangiopathies*.[4,5]

The major microangiopathic hemolytic anemias include thrombotic thrombocytopenic purpura (TTP), hemolytic uremic syndrome (HUS), HELLP (*h*emolysis, *e*levated *l*iver enzymes, *l*ow *p*latelet count) syndrome, and disseminated intravascular coagulation (DIC).[1,4,5] TTP and HUS can be difficult to differentiate because they have overlapping clinical and laboratory findings (Box 22.2). Definitive diagnosis, however, is critical because they have different etiologies and require different treatments.[3] This chapter provides an overview of these conditions. TTP, HUS, and HELLP syndrome are covered in more detail in Chapter 38. DIC is covered in more detail in Chapter 39.

Thrombotic Thrombocytopenic Purpura

Thrombotic thrombocytopenic purpura is a rare, life-threatening disorder characterized by the abrupt appearance of microangiopathic hemolytic anemia, severe thrombocytopenia, and markedly elevated serum LD activity.[2,6] Neurologic dysfunction, fever, and renal failure may also occur, but they are not consistently present.[2,6] TTP is most commonly found in adults in their fourth decade, but it can present at any age.[5,6] There is a higher incidence in females than in males.[5]

BOX 22.2 Laboratory Findings in Thrombocytopenic Purpura and Hemolytic Uremic Syndrome

Hematologic
Decreased hemoglobin
Decreased platelets
Increased reticulocyte count

Peripheral Blood Film
Schistocytes
Polychromasia
Nucleated red blood cells (severe cases)

Biochemical
Markedly increased lactate dehydrogenase activity[a]
Increased serum total and indirect bilirubin
Decreased serum haptoglobin level
Hemoglobinemia
Hemoglobinuria
Proteinuria, hematuria, casts[b]

[a]From systemic ischemia and hemolysis; more commonly found in TTP.
[b]From acute renal failure; more commonly found in HUS.

TTP is caused by a deficiency of the von Willebrand factor-cleaving protease known as *a d*isintegrin *a*nd *m*etallo-protease with a *t*hrombospondin type 1 motif, member *13* (ADAMTS13).[6–9] ADAMTS13 regulates the size of circulating von Willebrand factor (VWF) by cleaving ultralong VWF multimers (ULVWF) into shorter segments that have less hemostatic potential.[6,10] VWF multimers circulate in a folded conformation so that their cleavage sites for ADAMTS13 (in the A2 domain) and binding sites for platelets (GP Ibα receptor in the A1 domain) are hidden.[5,6,10] These sites normally become accessible only when the ULVWF multimer is "unrolled or stretched out," which occurs (1) during its release from endothelial cells, (2) during passage through small blood vessels with very high shear forces, or (3) after binding to collagen in the subendothelium after vascular injury (Chapters 36 and 38).[5,6,10] Once unrolled, ADAMTS13 binds to the cleavage sites on the ULVWFs and cuts them into smaller multimers.[6,10] Thus ADAMTS13 serves an important antithrombotic function by preventing VWF from excessively binding and activating platelets.[6]

When ADAMTS13 is deficient, however, the hyperreactive ULVWF multimers adhere to the endothelial cells of the microvasculature, where they readily unroll as a result of hydrodynamic shear forces.[5–7,10] Platelets are then able to bind to A1 domains of ULVWF multimers, and platelet aggregation is triggered.[5,6] Platelet-VWF microthrombi accumulate in and block small blood vessels, leading to severe thrombocytopenia; ischemia in the brain, kidney, and other organs; and hemolytic anemia due to RBC rupture as they pass through blood vessels partially blocked by microthrombi.[2,3,7] Intravascular hemolysis along with extensive tissue ischemia result in a striking increase in serum LD activity that is characteristic of TTP.[5]

TTP can be idiopathic, secondary, or inherited. Idiopathic TTP has no known precipitating event.[5,6] In idiopathic TTP, autoantibodies to ADAMTS13 inhibit its activity, causing a severe deficiency.[5,8,9] These autoantibodies are usually of the IgG class but can be IgM or IgA.

Secondary TTP can be triggered by infections, pregnancy, surgery, trauma, inflammation, and disseminated malignancy, possibly by depressing the synthesis of ADAMTS13.[3,5] Other conditions may induce an inhibitory reaction to ADAMTS13, including hematopoietic stem cell transplantation; autoimmune disorders; human immunodeficiency virus (HIV); and certain drugs, such as quinine, ticlopidine, and trimethoprim.[3–6,11] Secondary TTP is heterogeneous, and the mechanisms that trigger the TTP pathophysiology are not completely clear.[3]

Inherited TTP, also called Upshaw-Schülman syndrome, is a severe ADAMTS13 deficiency caused by mutations in the *ADAMTS13* gene.[5,6,12] Over 75 different mutations have been identified, and symptomatic individuals are either homozygous for one of the mutations or compound heterozygous for two different mutations.[5,12,13] Inherited TTP may present in infancy or childhood, with recurrent episodes throughout life; however, some patients may not be symptomatic until adulthood after their system is stressed by pregnancy or a severe infection.

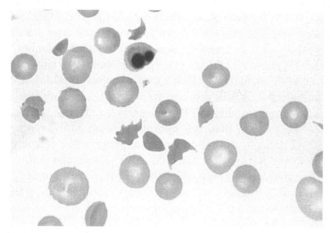

Figure 22.3 Peripheral Blood Film from a Patient with Thrombotic Thrombocytopenic Purpura. Note the schistocytes and a nucleated red blood cell. (Wright-Giemsa stain, ×1000.)

Typical initial laboratory findings in all types of TTP include a hemoglobin level of 8 to 10 g/dL, a platelet count of 10 to 30 × 10⁹/L, and schistocytes on the peripheral blood film (Figure 22.3).[6] After the bone marrow begins to respond to the anemia, polychromasia and nucleated RBCs may also be present on the blood film. The white blood cell (WBC) count is often increased, and immature granulocytes may appear. The bone marrow shows erythroid hyperplasia and a normal number of megakaryocytes. Hemoglobinuria occurs when there is extensive intravascular hemolysis. Various amounts of protein, RBCs, and urinary casts may also be present in the urine, depending on the extent of the renal damage. Results of coagulation tests are usually within the reference interval, which differentiates TTP from DIC. An elevation of serum indirect bilirubin level does not occur for several days after an acute onset of hemolysis, but serum LD activity will be markedly elevated, and the serum haptoglobin level will be reduced.

In idiopathic and inherited TTP, ADAMTS13 activity is usually severely reduced to less than 5% to 10% of normal.[4,6,7] In secondary TTP the ADAMTS13 deficiency is not as severe. ADAMTS13 autoantibodies can be detected in idiopathic TTP but are absent in inherited TTP.[6]

Approximately 80% to 90% of patients with idiopathic TTP respond favorably to plasma exchange therapy due to the removal of the offending ADAMTS13 autoantibody and infusion of replacement ADAMTS13 enzyme from donor plasma.[6,11] Therefore it is important that this type of TTP be recognized and quickly treated with plasma exchange therapy to avoid a fatal outcome. Corticosteroids are also administered to suppress the autoimmune response.[5,6] Approximately one third of patients who respond to plasma exchange experience recurrent episodes of TTP.[4] Rituximab (anti-CD20) is effective in suppressing an autoantibody response in some patients with relapsing TTP.[6] Patients with secondary TTP generally do not respond well to plasma exchange, and the prognosis in these cases is poor, except when the TTP is related to autoimmune disease, pregnancy, or ticlopidine use.[11,13] Plasma exchange is not required in inherited TTP, which is treated by infusion of fresh frozen plasma to supply the deficient ADAMTS13 enzyme.[3,4,6]

Hemolytic Uremic Syndrome

HUS is characterized by microangiopathic hemolytic anemia, thrombocytopenia, and acute renal failure from damage to endothelial cells in the glomerular microvasculature.[3,5] There are two general types: typical and atypical HUS. Typical HUS (Shiga toxin-associated HUS, or Stx-HUS) is caused by bacteria that produce Shiga toxin and is preceded by an episode of acute gastroenteritis, often with bloody diarrhea.[5] Atypical HUS (aHUS) is caused by unregulated activation of the alternative complement pathway.[3,5] Patients with HUS have the typical laboratory findings of microangiopathic hemolytic anemia. However, the platelet count is only mildly to moderately decreased, and evidence of renal failure is usually present, including an elevated level of serum creatinine, proteinuria, hematuria, and the presence of hyaline, granular, and RBC casts in the urine (Box 22.2).

The Stx-HUS type comprises 90% of cases of HUS.[5,14] The most common cause is infection with Shiga-like toxin-1-producing *Escherichia coli* (STEC), such as serotype O157:H7, but strains of toxin-producing *Shigella* have also been implicated.[4,5] Stx-HUS occurs most often in young children but can be found in patients of all ages. Patients initially have acute gastroenteritis, often with bloody diarrhea, and after approximately 5 to 13 days develop oliguria and other symptoms of renal damage.[5] About one fourth of patients also develop neurologic manifestations.[5,14]

E. coli and *Shigella* serotypes implicated in HUS release Shiga toxins (Stx-1 and Stx-2, also called *verotoxins*) that are absorbed from the intestines into the plasma. The toxins have an affinity for the Gb3 glycolipid receptors (CD77) on endothelial cells, particularly those in the glomerulus and brain.[4,5,15] The toxin is transported into the endothelial cells, where it inhibits protein synthesis and causes endothelial cell injury and eventual apoptosis.[5,15] Shiga toxin, together with many cytokines secreted as a result of the infection, also induces changes in endothelial cells that are prothrombotic, including expression of tissue factor, adhesion molecules, and secretion of increased amounts of ULVWF multimers.[4,5,15] Endothelial cell damage can cause stenosis (narrowing) of small blood vessels, which can be exacerbated by the activation of platelets and formation of platelet-fibrin thrombi.[3,5,15] The resultant blockages in the microvasculature of the glomeruli result in acute renal failure.[3,15] Endothelial damage and microthrombi can also occur in the microvasculature of the brain and other organs.[3,5] There is no specific treatment for Stx-HUS; patients are provided supportive care as needed, including hydration, dialysis, and transfusions.[14,15] Symptoms usually resolve spontaneously in 1 to 3 weeks, and the prognosis is favorable for most patients.[14]

Atypical HUS comprises about 10% of cases of HUS and can first present in infancy, childhood, or adulthood.[5,16] The characteristic feature is uncontrolled activation of the alternative complement system, which causes endothelial cell injury, activation of platelets and coagulation factors, and formation of platelet-fibrin thrombi that obstruct the microvasculature in the glomerulus and other organs.[3,5] Approximately 50% to 70% of aHUS patients have inherited mutations in genes that code for components of the alternative complement pathway or its regulatory proteins.[5,16] Inactivating mutations have been identified in genes for complement regulatory proteins, including complement factor H, complement factor I, membrane cofactor protein, and thrombomodulin.[3,5,16] Activating mutations have been identified in the genes for complement factors B and C3.[3,5,16] An acquired form of aHUS is associated with autoantibodies to complement factor H and accounts for approximately 5% to 10% of cases.[5] In the remaining cases no mutation or autoantibodies have been identified.[5] aHUS may be triggered by hematopoietic stem cell therapy, pregnancy, infection, inflammation, surgery, or trauma.[3] Plasma exchange and plasma infusion have limited efficacy in aHUS.[5,16] In recent studies therapy with eculizumab (antibody to C5) has improved platelet counts and renal function in aHUS patients and may become the therapy of choice.[16]

Differential diagnosis of aHUS and TTP is difficult due to the similarities in their clinical presentation and initial laboratory findings (Chapter 38). Both are life-threatening disorders that require rapid action to prevent a fatal outcome; plasma exchange is most beneficial for TTP, and eculizumab is more likely to benefit patients with aHUS.[5,16] Assays for ADAMTS13 activity, ADAMTS13 inhibitors, and anti-ADAMTS13 antibodies are available and typically performed in a reflex algorithm. The current assays lack optimization and standardization; they are commonly only performed in reference laboratories. DNA analysis for complement system gene mutations is available in specialized laboratories, but the results are not timely enough to be used in initial therapy decisions.[16] More sensitive, specific, and rapid tests are needed for definitive diagnosis of these two conditions.

HELLP Syndrome

HELLP syndrome, a serious complication in pregnancy, is named for its characteristic presentation of *h*emolysis, *e*levated *l*iver enzymes, and *l*ow *p*latelet count. It occurs in approximately 0.5% of all pregnancies but develops in approximately 4% to 12% of pregnancies with preeclampsia and 30% to 50% of pregnancies with eclampsia, most often in the third trimester.[17,18] In preeclampsia, abnormalities in the development of placental vasculature result in poor perfusion and hypoxia. As a result, antiangiogenic proteins, such as soluble vascular endothelial growth factor receptor-1 (sVEGFR-1), are released from the placenta which bind to and inactivate placental and endothelial growth factors.[18] Continued vascular insufficiency of the placenta results in maternal endothelial cell dysfunction, which leads to platelet activation and fibrin deposition in the microvasculature, particularly in the liver.[18]

Anemia, biochemical evidence of hemolysis, and schistocytes on the peripheral blood film are found as in other microangiopathies. A low platelet count and increased serum LD and aspartate aminotransferase (AST) activity are major diagnostic criteria for HELLP syndrome and are used to assess the severity of the disease (Chapter 38).[17,18] The platelet count in conjunction with LD and AST levels serve as a predictor of maternal morbidity and mortality with the platelet count serving as differentiation between the three risk categories.[18,19] Patients with platelet counts less than 50 × 10⁹/L have the greatest risk of bleeding and have a greater incidence of morbidity and mortality.[18,19] Patients with platelet counts between 50 and 100 × 10⁹/L have a moderate risk of bleeding, and those with a platelet count greater than 100 × 10⁹/L do not have a risk of bleeding.[18,19] Serum LD activity is elevated, which reflects hepatic necrosis and hemolysis. Serum AST can be markedly elevated due to severe hepatocyte injury. The prothrombin time and partial thromboplastin time are within reference intervals, which distinguishes HELLP syndrome from DIC. Therapy includes delivery of the fetus and placenta as soon as possible, along with supportive care to control electrolytes, fluid balance, hypertension, and prevent seizures.[18,19] The mortality rate is 3% to 5% for the mother and 9% to 24% for the fetus.[18]

Disseminated Intravascular Coagulation

DIC is characterized by the widespread activation of the hemostatic system, resulting in fibrin thrombi formation throughout the microvasculature. Major clinical manifestations are organ damage due to obstruction of the microvasculature and bleeding due to the consumption of platelets and coagulation factors and secondary activation of fibrinolysis. DIC is a complication of many disorders, such as metastatic cancers, acute leukemias, infections, obstetric complications, crush or brain injuries, acute hemolytic transfusion reactions, extensive burns, snake or spider envenomation, and chronic inflammation (Table 39.6).

Thrombocytopenia of varying degrees is a consistent finding. Approximately half of patients have schistocytes on the peripheral blood film; however, this finding is not required for a DIC diagnosis.[20] The prothrombin time and partial thromboplastin time are prolonged, the fibrinogen level is decreased, and the D-dimer level is increased in DIC, which distinguish it from the other microangiopathies. Tables 39.7 and 39.8 contain the primary and specialized tests used in the diagnosis of DIC.

MACROANGIOPATHIC HEMOLYTIC ANEMIA

Traumatic Cardiac Hemolytic Anemia

Mechanical hemolysis can occur in patients with prosthetic cardiac valves due to the turbulent blood flow through and around the implanted devices.[18,21] Hemolysis is usually mild, and anemia does not generally develop due to compensation by the bone marrow.[21] Severe hemolysis is rare and is usually due to paravalvular leaks in prosthetic cardiac valves.[21] Hemolysis can also occur in patients with cardiac valve disease prior to corrective surgery.[18] The anemia that occurs in severe cases is usually normocytic but can be microcytic if iron deficiency develops due to chronic urinary hemoglobin loss.

Depending on the severity of the hemolysis and the ability of the bone marrow to compensate for the reduced RBC life span, patients can be asymptomatic or present with pallor, fatigue, and even heart failure.[21] Schistocytes are a characteristic feature found on the blood film due to mechanical fragmentation of the RBCs (Figure 22.4). The reticulocyte count is increased, but the platelet count is within the reference interval. Serum LD activity and levels of serum indirect bilirubin and plasma hemoglobin are elevated, and the serum haptoglobin

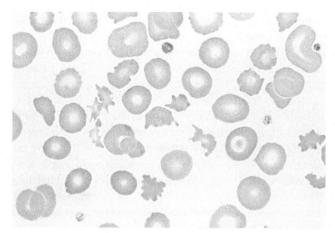

Figure 22.4 Peripheral Blood Film from a Patient with Traumatic Cardiac Hemolytic Anemia. Note the presence of schistocytes. (Wright-Giemsa stain, ×1000.)

level is decreased. Hemoglobinuria may be observed in severe hemolysis. Hemosiderinuria and a decreased level of serum ferritin occur with chronic hemoglobinuria due to the urinary loss of iron.

Surgical repair or replacement of the prosthesis may be required if the anemia is severe enough to require transfusions. For patients with hemoglobinuria, iron supplementation is provided to replace urinary iron loss. Folic acid may also be required, because deficiencies can occur due to the increased erythropoietic activity in the bone marrow.[21]

Exercise-Induced Hemoglobinuria

RBC lysis, with an increase in free plasma hemoglobin and a decrease in the serum haptoglobin level, has been demonstrated in some individuals after long-distance running and, to a lesser extent, after intensive cycling and swimming[1,22–24]; however, frank hemoglobinuria after exercise is a rare occurrence.[25] Exercise-induced hemoglobinuria has been reported mainly in endurance runners, but has also been observed after strenuous hand drumming.[22,26] Various causes have been proposed, including mechanical trauma from the forceful, repeated impact of the feet or hands on hard surfaces[22,23,26]; increased RBC susceptibility to oxidative stress[27]; and exercise-induced alterations in membrane cytoskeletal proteins.[28,29]

Exercise-induced hemoglobinuria does not usually cause anemia unless the hemoglobinuria is particularly severe and recurrent.[1,25] Laboratory findings include a decreased level of serum haptoglobin, an elevated level of free plasma hemoglobin, and hemoglobinuria observed after strenuous exercise. Patients also have a slight increase in mean cell volume (MCV) and reticulocyte count. Schistocytes are not present on the peripheral blood film except in rare cases.[25,26] Exercise-induced hemoglobinuria is a diagnosis of exclusion, and other possible causes of hemolysis and hemoglobinuria should be investigated and ruled out.[25] There is no treatment for the disorder other than minimizing the physical impact on the feet with padding in shoes, running on softer terrain or, if hemolysis is severe, discontinuing the activity.

HEMOLYTIC ANEMIA CAUSED BY INFECTIOUS AGENTS

Malaria

Malaria is a potentially fatal condition caused by infection of RBCs with protozoan parasites of the genus *Plasmodium*. Most human infections are caused by *P. falciparum* and *P. vivax*, but *P. ovale*, *P. malariae*, and a fifth species, *P. knowlesi*, also infect humans. *P. knowlesi*, a natural parasite of macaque monkeys, is easily misdiagnosed as *P. malariae* by microscopy, because the organisms are difficult to distinguish morphologically. Since 2004 hundreds of microscopically identified cases of *P. malariae* infection in Malaysia were found actually to be caused by *P. knowlesi* when polymerase chain reaction (PCR) assays were used, including tests on archival blood films from 1996.[30–32] With the use of molecular techniques, *P. knowlesi* malaria is now known to be widespread in Malaysia, and cases have been reported in other areas of Southeast Asia, although the US Centers for Disease Control and Prevention considers this to be a zoonotic malaria.[30–33]

Prevalence

Approximately 3.4 billion people live in areas in which malaria is endemic and are at risk for the disease.[34] Worldwide in 2016, there were an estimated 216 million cases of malaria, with 445,000 deaths, mostly in children younger than 5 years of age.[34] The majority of deaths were in Africa (91%), followed by Southeast Asia (6%) and the Eastern Mediterranean region (2%).[34] The World Health Organization is coordinating a major global effort to control and eliminate malaria. These efforts include implementation of indoor chemical spraying, distribution of millions of insecticide-treated sleeping nets in high-risk areas, and promotion of policies for appropriate treatment in regions of endemic disease.[34]

Approximately 1700 cases of malaria are diagnosed annually in the United States, with a majority of the cases associated with travel to a malaria-endemic country.[33] *P. falciparum* and *P. vivax* cause most of the infections seen in the United States.

Plasmodium Life Cycle

Malaria is transmitted to humans by the bite of an infected female *Anopheles* mosquito. During a blood meal, sporozoites from the salivary gland of the mosquito are injected into the skin and migrate into the bloodstream of the human host. Sporozoites rapidly leave the circulating blood and invade hepatic parenchymal cells to begin exoerythrocytic schizogony, the parasite's asexual cycle. After 5 to 16 days (depending on the species), hepatic cells rupture, and each cell releases tens of thousands of merozoites into the bloodstream to invade circulating RBCs, thus beginning erythrocytic schizogony.[35] Inside the erythrocyte the merozoite grows and metabolizes hemoglobin. The merozoite becomes a ring form, which grows into a mature trophozoite, then into an immature schizont (chromatin dividing), and finally into a mature schizont that contains merozoites. Merozoites are released from erythrocytes into the bloodstream and invade other RBCs to continue the asexual cycle. As the infection continues, cycles often recur at regular intervals as all the individual parasitic cycles become synchronous; this produces paroxysms of fever and chills at a frequency that varies by species. Resting stages of *P. vivax* and *P. ovale,* called *hypnozoites,* can remain dormant in the liver and produce a relapse months or years later.[36,37]

Some merozoites enter RBCs and form male and female gametocytes (sexual stages). Gametocytes are ingested by an *Anopheles* mosquito when it takes in a blood meal. The female gamete is fertilized by the male gamete in the mosquito gut to produce a zygote, which becomes an ookinete that migrates to the outer wall of the mosquito midgut and develops into an oocyst. The oocyst produces sporozoites that are released into the hemocele and migrate to the salivary glands of the mosquito. When the mosquito takes in a blood meal, the sporozoites are inoculated into the human host.

Other modes of transmission include congenital infection and transmission by blood transfusion, organ transplantation, or sharing of syringes and needles, but malaria acquired by these routes and local mosquito-transmitted malaria occur infrequently in the United States.[33]

Pathogenesis

If an individual is bitten by infected mosquitos, the clinical outcome may be (1) no infection, (2) *asymptomatic parasitemia* (the patient has no symptoms, but parasites are present in the blood), (3) *uncomplicated malaria* (the patient has symptoms and parasitemia but no organ dysfunction), or (4) *severe malaria* (the patient has symptoms, parasitemia, and major organ dysfunction).[34,36] The clinical outcome depends on parasite factors (species, number of sporozoites injected, multiplication rate, virulence, drug resistance), host factors (age, pregnancy status, immune status, previous exposure, genetic polymorphisms, nutrition status, coinfection with other pathogens, and duration of infection), geographic and social factors (endemicity, poverty, and availability of prompt and effective treatment), and other as yet unknown factors.[35,36,38]

In areas of high *Plasmodium* transmission, most individuals develop immunity, and major risk groups for severe malaria are children younger than 5 years of age and women in their first pregnancy.[39] Even in these risk groups, severe malaria is infrequent.[36] On the other hand, immunity is low or nonexistent in individuals living in regions with low *Plasmodium* transmission and in travelers to regions where malaria is endemic, so all age groups are at risk for severe malaria.[39] Most cases of severe malaria are due to *P. falciparum;* however, *P. vivax* and *P. knowlesi* can also cause severe disease.[31,35] Infection with *P. malariae* or *P. ovale,* however, is usually uncomplicated and benign. Hyperparasitemia, defined as greater than 2% to 5% of the total RBCs parasitized, is usually present in severe malaria.[39] Major complications of severe malaria include respiratory distress syndrome, metabolic acidosis, circulatory shock, renal failure, hepatic failure, hypoglycemia, severe anemia (defined as a hemoglobin level below 5 g/dL),[39] poor pregnancy outcome, and cerebral malaria.[35] Even with treatment the fatality rate of severe malaria is 10% to 20%.[39]

Causes of anemia in malaria include direct lysis of infected RBCs during schizogony, immune destruction of infected and noninfected RBCs in the spleen, and inhibition of erythropoiesis and ineffective erythropoiesis.[37,38] Destruction of noninfected RBCs contributes significantly to the anemia. In the invasion process parasites shed proteins that bind to infected and noninfected RBCs.[40] These proteins may change the RBC membrane in noninfected cells, allowing adherence of immunoglobulins and complement, thus enhancing their removal by the spleen.[40,41]

Malaria parasites metabolize hemoglobin, forming toxic hemozoin, or malaria pigment. When RBCs lyse in schizogony, the hemozoin and other toxic metabolites are released, which results in an inflammatory response and cytokine imbalance.[40] Abnormal levels of tumor necrosis factor-α and interferon-γ result in inhibition of erythropoiesis and ineffective erythropoiesis; increased levels of interleukin-6 stimulate hepcidin production in the liver, which decreases the iron available to developing RBCs (Chapter 17).[40] In areas where malaria is endemic poor nutrition and coinfection with hookworm or HIV contributes to the anemia, inflammation, and cytokine imbalance.[38,40]

P. falciparum is unique and particularly lethal in that infected RBCs adhere to endothelial cells in the microvasculature of internal organs, including the brain, heart, lung, liver, kidney, dermis, and placenta.[35,36] This contributes to the pathogenesis by obstructing the microvasculature and decreasing oxygen delivery to organs and by protecting the parasite from clearance by the spleen.[35,36] In the placental microvasculature, adherence of infected RBCs to endothelial cells results in local inflammation that can cause severe maternal anemia, decreased fetal growth, premature delivery, and an increased risk of fetal loss.[35,36] In the brain microvasculature, adherence of infected RBCs to endothelial cells can cause lethal cerebral malaria. Infected RBCs express a parasite protein on their membranes, called *Plasmodium falciparum* erythrocyte membrane protein 1 (*Pf*EMP1). *Pf*EMP1 mediates binding of infected RBCs to cell receptors, particularly CD36 on platelets and some endothelial cells.[35,42] Adherence of infected RBCs in the brain has been attributed to a complex formed by VWF released by cytokine-stimulated endothelial cells, platelets bound to the VWF, and infected RBCs bound to platelet CD36.[43] A recent mechanism has been proposed whereby a specific variant of *Pf*EMP1, expressed on the surface of RBCs infected with certain strains of *P. falciparum*, specifically binds to endothelial protein C receptor (EPCR) on endothelial cells lining the microvessels in the brain.[44] This binding prevents the activation of protein C (an inhibitor of activated factors V and VIII), creating a local hypercoagulable state resulting in fibrin deposition and parasite sequestration in the brain microvasculature and symptoms of severe cerebral malaria.[44]

The ability of the parasite to invade RBCs affects the extent of the parasitemia and the severity of the disease. *P. vivax* and *P. ovale* can only invade reticulocytes, and *P. malariae* can only invade older RBCs. On the other hand, *P. falciparum* and *P. knowlesi* are able to invade RBCs of all ages and thus can lead to very high levels of parasitemia.[35,37] *P. vivax* requires Duffy antigens on RBCs for invasion, so individuals lacking Duffy antigens are resistant to infection with *P. vivax.* The expansion of the Duffy-negative population in West Africa seems to be an effective genetic adaptation because *P. vivax* infection is almost nonexistent in West Africa.[35]

Clinical and Laboratory Findings

The clinical symptoms of malaria are variable and can include fever, chills, rigors, sweating, headache, muscle pain, nausea, and diarrhea. In severe malaria jaundice, splenomegaly, hepatomegaly, shock, prostration, bleeding, seizures, or coma may occur.[39] In patients with chronic malaria or with repeated malarial infections the spleen may be massively enlarged.

During fevers the WBC count is normal to slightly increased; however, neutropenia may develop during chills and rigors. In chronic malaria with anemia the reticulocyte count is decreased due to the negative effect of inflammation on erythropoiesis. In severe malaria one or more of the following laboratory features are found: metabolic acidosis, decreased serum glucose (less than 40 mg/dL), increased serum lactate, increased serum creatinine, decreased hemoglobin level (less than 5 g/dL), hemoglobinuria, and hyperparasitemia.[39]

Microscopic Examination

Often malarial parasites are discovered during a review of the peripheral blood film, as a component of the complete blood count (CBC) and manual differential. Identification of malaria and its species is customarily performed in clinical microbiology. In the hematology laboratory, however, it is important to recognize the presence of intracellular organisms (bacteria, malaria and other parasites) in order to ensure rapid diagnosis and treatment for these infections. Malarial infection can be diagnosed microscopically by demonstration of the parasites in the peripheral blood. Optimally, as for any situation in which there is an infection, blood should be collected before treatment is initiated.[37,45] At least two thick and two thin peripheral blood films should be made as soon as possible after collection of venous blood in ethylenediamine tetraacetic acid (EDTA) anticoagulant for examination by laboratory professionals.[45] Malarial parasite detection and species identification require specific expertise and experience. A platelet lying on top of an erythrocyte in a thin blood film may be confused with a malarial parasite by an inexperienced observer (Figure 22.5).

Plasmodium species. *P. vivax* is widely distributed and causes 40% of human malaria cases worldwide (Figures 22.6 and 22.7).[39] It is the predominant species in Asia and South and Central America, but it also occurs in Southeast Asia, Oceania, and the Middle East.[33] It is rare in Africa and virtually absent in West Africa.[33]

P. ovale is found mainly in West Africa and India (Figure 22.8).[33]

P. malariae is found worldwide but at low frequency (Figure 22.9). The highest prevalence is in East Africa and India.[33]

P. falciparum is the predominant species in sub-Saharan Africa, Saudi Arabia, Haiti, and the Dominican Republic (Figures 22.1 and 22.10).[33] It is also found in Asia, Southeast Asia, the Philippines, Indonesia, and South America.[33] *P. falciparum* can produce high parasitemia (greater than 50% of RBCs infected) due to its ability to invade RBCs of all ages.

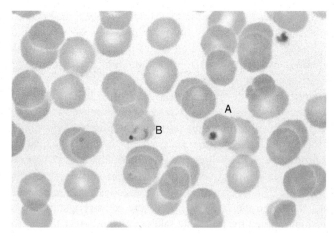

Figure 22.5 Peripheral Blood Film with a Platelet on Top of a Red Blood Cell **(A)** Compared with an Intraerythrocytic *Plasmodium vivax* Ring Form **(B)**. (Wright-Giemsa stain, ×1000.)

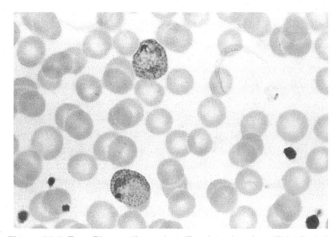

Figure 22.6 Two *Plasmodium vivax* Trophozoites in a Thin Peripheral Blood Film. Note that the infected red blood cells are enlarged and contain Schüffner stippling, and the trophozoites are large and ameboid in appearance. (Wright-Giemsa stain, ×1000.)

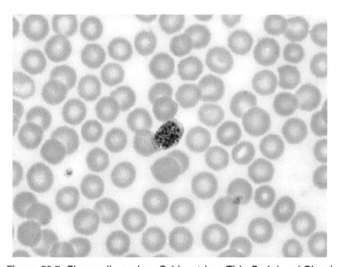

Figure 22.7 *Plasmodium vivax* Schizont in a Thin Peripheral Blood Film. Note the number of merozoites and the presence of brown hemozoin pigment. (Wright-Giemsa stain, ×1000.) (Courtesy Linda Marler, Indiana Pathology Images, Indianapolis, IN.)

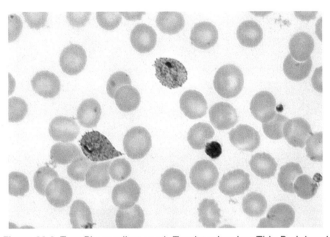

Figure 22.8 Two *Plasmodium ovale* Trophozoites in a Thin Peripheral Blood Film. Note that the infected cells are enlarged, oval, have fringed edges, and contain Schüffner stippling. (Wright-Giemsa stain, ×1000.) (Courtesy Linda Marler, Indiana Pathology Images, Indianapolis, IN.)

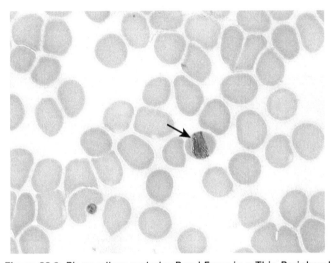

Figure 22.9 *Plasmodium malariae* Band Form in a Thin Peripheral Blood Film. (Wright-Giemsa stain, ×1000.) (Courtesy Linda Marler, Indiana Pathology Images, Indianapolis, IN.)

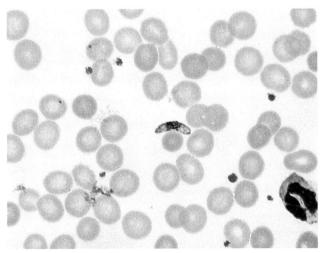

Figure 22.10 *Plasmodium falciparum* Crescent-Shaped Gametocyte in a Thin Peripheral Blood Film. (Wright-Giemsa stain, ×1000.) (Courtesy Linda Marler, Indiana Pathology Images, Indianapolis, IN.)

P. knowlesi is widespread in Malaysia, and cases have been reported in Myanmar, the Philippines, and Thailand (Figure 22.11).[33]

Other Tests for Diagnosis

Fluorescent dyes may be used to stain *Plasmodium* species; they are sensitive for parasite detection but are not useful for speciation.[37] Molecular-based tests (e.g., PCR) can be used for detection and speciation of malarial parasites and are especially helpful in cases of mixed infections, low parasitemia, and infection with *P. knowlesi*. A rapid antigen test, the BinaxNOW Malaria Test, has been approved by the US Food and Drug Administration (FDA) for use in the United States.[45] It is based on the detection of *P. falciparum* histidine-rich protein II and generic *Plasmodium* aldolase.[45] The sensitivity of the test is low when there are fewer than 100 parasites per microliter of blood.[37,45] Therefore thick and thin blood film microscopy should be performed along with the antigen test.[45]

Babesiosis

Babesiosis is a tick-transmitted disease caused by intraerythrocytic protozoan parasites of the genus *Babesia*. There are hundreds of species of *Babesia*; a few are known to cause disease in humans. *B. microti* is the most common cause of babesiosis in the United States, where it was originally called *Nantucket fever* because the first cluster of cases was found on Nantucket Island, off Massachusetts, in 1969 and the early 1970s.[46,47] The sexual cycle of *B. microti* occurs in the tick, *Ixodes scapularis*, whereas its asexual cycle primarily occurs in the white-footed mouse, the reservoir host in the United States.[48] Humans are incidental hosts and become infected after injection of sporozoites during a blood meal by infected ticks. Other *Babesia* species, such as *B. duncani* and *B. divergens*, can be found sporadically in humans.[47–49] Babesia may also be transmitted by transfusion of RBCs from asymptomatic donors.[48,49]

Geographic Distribution

The areas in which *B. microti* is endemic in the United States are southern New England, New York State, New Jersey, Wisconsin, and Minnesota.[47–49] *B. duncani* occurs along the Pacific Coast (northern California to Washington); *B. divergens*-like organisms are found in Missouri, Kentucky, and Washington state; and *B. divergens* and *B. venatorum* occur in Europe.[47,49,50] Isolated cases of babesiosis have also been reported in Asia, Africa, Australia, and South America.[47,50]

Clinical Findings

The incubation period for *B. microti* infection ranges from 1 to 9 weeks.[47] Infection is asymptomatic in perhaps a third of individuals, so the exact prevalence is unknown.[47,51] In other individuals *B. microti* causes a mild to severe hemolytic anemia.[47,48] The patient usually experiences fever and nonrespiratory flu-like symptoms, including chills, headache, sweats, nausea, arthralgias, myalgia, anorexia, and fatigue, that last from several weeks to months. Jaundice, splenomegaly, or hepatomegaly may be present. Some individuals progress to severe, life-threatening

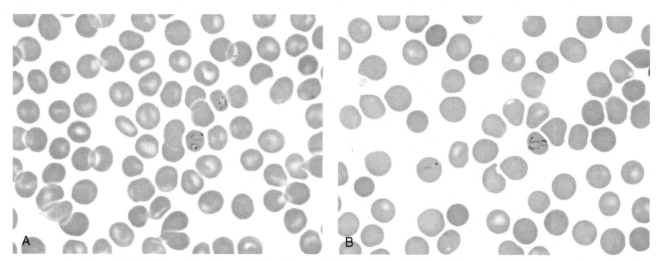

Figure 22.11 *Plasmodium knowlesi* Ring Forms **(A)** and a Ring Form and Trophozoite **(B)** in a Thin Peripheral Blood Film. (Wright-Giemsa stain, ×1000.) (Courtesy Wadsworth Center Laboratories, New York State Department of Health, New York, NY.)

disease due to acute respiratory failure, congestive heart failure, renal shutdown, liver failure, central nervous system involvement, or disseminated intravascular coagulation. Severe disease may occur at any age, but it is more common in individuals over 50 years of age.[1,47] Immune deficiency due to asplenia, malignancy, immunosuppressive drugs, or HIV infection increases the risk of severe disease.[1,47,48]

Laboratory Findings and Diagnosis

Evidence of hemolytic anemia is usually present in symptomatic infection, including a decreased hemoglobin level, an increased reticulocyte count, a decreased serum haptoglobin level, and bilirubinemia. Leukopenia, thrombocytopenia, hemoglobinuria, and proteinuria may also be present, along with abnormal results on renal and liver function tests.[47]

The diagnosis of babesiosis is made by demonstration of the parasite on Wright-Giemsa-stained thin peripheral blood films (Figures 22.12 and 22.13). Parasitemia may be low (fewer than 1% of RBCs affected) in early infections, but as many as 80% of RBCs may be infected in asplenic patients.[52] In cases of low parasitemia, babesiosis can be diagnosed by detection of IgG and IgM antibodies to *B. microti* by indirect immunofluorescent antibody assay.[48] The sensitivity of the assay ranges from 88% to 96%.[53] Definitive species identification requires PCR-based methods.[47,48]

Clostridial Sepsis

Sepsis with massive intravascular hemolysis, which is often fatal, is a rare complication of infection with *Clostridium perfringens,* an anaerobic gram-positive bacillus. *C. perfringens* grows very rapidly (7-minute doubling time) and produces an α-toxin with phospholipase C and sphingomyelinase activity that hydrolyzes RBC membrane phospholipids.[54,55] RBCs become spherical and extremely susceptible to osmotic lysis, which results in sudden, massive hemolysis and dark red plasma and urine.[1,54,56] The hematocrit may drop to below 10%.[1,56] Intravascular hemolysis can trigger DIC and renal

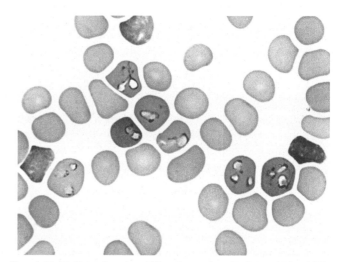

Figure 22.12 *Babesia microti* Ring Forms in a Peripheral Blood Film. Note the varying appearance of the ring forms and the presence of multiple ring forms in individual red blood cells. (Wright-Giemsa stain, ×1000.)

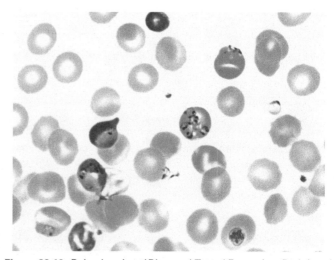

Figure 22.13 *Babesia microti* Ring and Tetrad Forms in a Peripheral Blood Film. (Wright-Giemsa stain, ×1000.)

failure. Spherocytes, microspherocytes, and toxic changes to neutrophils can be observed on a peripheral blood film.[1,54,56] Some conditions that increase the risk of clostridial sepsis and hemolytic anemia include malignancies (genitourinary, gastrointestinal, and hematologic), solid organ transplantation, postpartum or postabortion infections, biliary surgery, acute cholecystitis, and deep wounds.[1,54,57,58] Rapid therapy with transfusions, antibiotics, and fluid management is critical for patient survival.[58] The prognosis is grave, and many patients die despite intensive treatment.

Bartonellosis

Human bartonellosis (Carrión disease) is transmitted by the bite of a female sandfly and is endemic in certain regions of Peru, Ecuador, and Colombia.[59,60] It is caused by *Bartonella bacilliformis,* a small, pleomorphic, intracellular coccobacillus that adheres to RBCs and causes hemolysis.[1,61] The bacteria produce a protein called *deformin* that forms pits or invaginations in the RBC membrane.[1,61] There are two clinical stages: the first stage is characterized by acute hemolytic anemia; the second or chronic verruga stage is characterized by the eruption of skin lesions and warts on the extremities, face, and trunk. The acute phase begins with fever, malaise, headache, and chills, followed by pallor, jaundice, general lymphadenopathy, and, less commonly, hepatosplenomegaly.[59–61] Over several days, there is rapid hemolysis, with the hematocrit falling below 20% in two thirds of patients.[59,61] Polychromasia, nucleated RBCs, and mild leukocytosis with a left shift are observed on the peripheral blood film. The mortality rate is approximately 10% for hospitalized patients and 90% for those who are untreated.[59,60] Diagnosis is made by blood culture and observation of bacilli or coccobacilli on the RBCs on a Wright-Giemsa-stained peripheral blood film. During the acute phase, 80% of the RBCs can be involved.[1] Serologic diagnosis with indirect immunofluorescent antibody or immunoblotting has a sensitivity of 89%.[60]

HEMOLYTIC ANEMIA CAUSED BY OTHER RED BLOOD CELL INJURY

Drugs and Chemicals

Hemolytic anemia of varying severity may result from drugs or chemicals that cause the oxidative denaturation of hemoglobin, leading to the formation of methemoglobin and Heinz bodies.[1] Examples of agents that can cause hemolytic anemia in individuals with normal RBCs include dapsone, a drug used to treat leprosy and dermatitis herpetiformis,[1,62] and naphthalene, a chemical found in mothballs.[63] Individuals deficient in glucose-6-phosphate dehydrogenase (G6PD) are particularly sensitive to the effects of oxidative agents. For example, primaquine can cause hemolytic anemia in G6PD-deficient individuals (Chapter 21).[39]

Typical laboratory findings include a decrease in hemoglobin level, increase in the reticulocyte count, increase in serum indirect bilirubin, and decrease in serum haptoglobin level. In severe drug- or chemical-induced hemolytic anemia, Heinz

bodies (denatured hemoglobin) may be observed in RBCs. Heinz bodies, only visualized with a supravital stain, appear as round, blue granules attached to the inner RBC membrane (Figure 11.12). Exposure to high levels of arsine hydride, copper, and lead can also cause hemolysis.[1,64]

Venoms

Envenomation from contact with snakes, spiders, bees, or wasps can induce hemolytic anemia in some individuals. The hemolysis can occur acutely or be delayed 1 or more days after a bite or sting.[1,64] The severity of the hemolysis depends on the amount of venom injected, and in severe cases renal failure and death can result. Some mechanisms by which venoms can induce hemolysis are direct disruption of the RBC membrane, alteration of the RBC membrane that results in complement-mediated lysis, and initiation of DIC.[64] Hemolytic anemia has been reported after bites from poisonous snakes (e.g., some cobras and pit vipers) and the brown recluse spider (*Loxosceles reclusa* and *Loxosceles laeta*), and after multiple stings (50 or more) by bees or wasps.[1,64–68]

Extensive Burns (Thermal Injury)

Warming normal RBCs to 49° C in vitro induces RBC fragmentation and budding.[1] Patients with extensive burns manifest similar RBC injury with acute hemolytic anemia. Schistocytes, spherocytes, and microspherocytes are observed on the peripheral blood film (Figure 22.14), but the damaged RBCs are usually cleared by the spleen within 24 hours of the burn injury.[64] In addition to resulting from acute hemolysis, anemia associated with extensive burns is also caused by blood loss during surgical excision and grafting of burn wounds, nutritional deficiency, impaired metabolism, and anemia of chronic inflammation.[69] Overheating of blood in malfunctioning blood warmers prior to transfusion can also result in RBC fragmentation and hemolysis of the donor RBCs.[1]

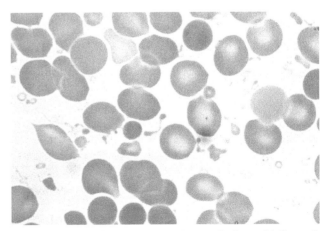

Figure 22.14 Peripheral Blood Film From a Patient with Extensive Burns. Note the presence of schistocytes, microspherocytes, and spherocytes. (Wright-Giemsa stain, ×1000.)

SUMMARY

- A common feature of the nonimmune extrinsic hemolytic anemias is the presence of a condition that causes physical or mechanical injury to RBCs. These conditions include microangiopathic hemolytic anemia; macroangiopathic hemolytic anemia; some infections; exposure to certain drugs, chemicals, or venoms; and extensive burns.
- Microangiopathic hemolytic anemia is characterized by the shearing of RBCs as they pass through small blood vessels partially blocked by microthrombi. Fragmented RBCs (called *schistocytes*) are formed, and premature RBC destruction results in hemolytic anemia. Ischemic injury to the brain, kidney, and other organs also occurs. Thrombocytopenia also occurs as a result of consumption in microthrombi. Major microangiopathic hemolytic anemias are thrombotic thrombocytopenic purpura (TTP), hemolytic uremic syndrome (HUS), HELLP (*h*emolysis, *e*levated *l*iver enzymes, *l*ow *p*latelet count) syndrome, and disseminated intravascular coagulation (DIC).
- TTP is a rare disorder found predominantly in adults and characterized by microangiopathic hemolytic anemia, severe thrombocytopenia, a markedly increased serum lactate dehydrogenase activity, and variable symptoms of fever, neurologic dysfunction, and renal failure. Idiopathic TTP is due to autoimmune antibodies to the VWF-cleaving protease ADAMTS13 causing a severe functional deficiency. Secondary TTP is associated with stem cell transplantation, disseminated cancer, pregnancy, and use of certain drugs. Inherited TTP is due to mutations in the *ADAMTS13* gene.
- HUS is characterized by microangiopathic hemolytic anemia, thrombocytopenia, and acute renal failure. Typical HUS (Stx-HUS) comprises 90% of cases, is found predominantly in young children, and is caused by toxin-producing strains of *E. coli.* Atypical HUS (aHUS) is due to inherited mutations in genes coding for complement components and regulators or autoantibodies to complement factor H. It also occurs secondary to organ transplantation, cancer, pregnancy, HIV infection, and some drugs.
- HELLP syndrome is a serious complication of pregnancy presenting with microangiopathic hemolytic anemia, thrombocytopenia, and elevated levels of liver enzymes.
- DIC is due to the widespread intravascular activation of the hemostatic system and formation of fibrin thrombi; coagulation factors and platelets are consumed in the intravascular thrombi, and secondary fibrinolysis occurs. Schistocytes are found in approximately half of the cases.
- Macroangiopathic hemolytic anemia is caused by traumatic cardiac hemolysis (RBC fragmentation from damaged or prosthetic cardiac valves) or exercise-induced hemolysis (mechanical trauma from forceful impact on feet or hands or from strenuous exercise). The platelet count is normal in both conditions; schistocytes are seen only in traumatic cardiac hemolysis.
- Infections associated with hemolytic anemia due to invasion of RBCs include malaria and babesiosis. Hemolysis in bartonellosis is due to attachment of the bacteria to red blood cells and production of a lytic protein. Hemolysis in clostridial sepsis is due to the production of α-toxin.
- Identification of parasite genus and species requires experience and expertise and is usually performed by laboratory professionals in clinical microbiology.
- In malaria, severe anemia is due to direct lysis of infected RBCs, immune destruction of infected and uninfected RBCs in the spleen, and inhibition of erythropoiesis.
- *Plasmodium* (five species) and *Babesia* organisms are identified by the morphology of their intraerythrocytic stages on a Wright-Giemsa-stained peripheral blood film. *Plasmodium* species are transmitted to humans by mosquitoes, whereas a tick is the vector for *Babesia.*
- Hemolytic anemia can also be caused by injury to RBCs by drugs, chemicals, venoms, and extensive burns (thermal injury). In patients with extensive burns, schistocytes, spherocytes, and microspherocytes are observed on the peripheral blood film.

Now that you have completed this chapter, go back and read again the case study at the beginning and respond to the questions presented.

REVIEW QUESTIONS

Answers can be found in the Appendix.

1. Which one of the following is a feature found in *all* microangiopathic hemolytic anemias?
   a. Pancytopenia
   b. Thrombocytosis
   c. Intravascular RBC fragmentation
   d. Prolonged prothrombin time and partial thromboplastin time

2. Typical laboratory findings in TTP and HUS include:
   a. Schistocytosis and thrombocytopenia
   b. Anemia and reticulocytopenia
   c. Reduced levels of lactate dehydrogenase and aspartate aminotransferase
   d. Increased levels of free plasma hemoglobin and serum haptoglobin

3. The pathophysiology of idiopathic TTP involves:
   a. Shiga toxin damage to endothelial cells and obstruction of small blood vessels in glomeruli
   b. Formation of platelet-VWF thrombi due to autoantibody inhibition of ADAMTS13
   c. Overactivation of the complement system and endothelial cell damage due to loss of regulatory function
   d. Activation of the coagulation and fibrinolytic systems with fibrin clots throughout the microvasculature

4. Which of the following tests yields results that are abnormal in DIC but are usually within the reference interval or just slightly abnormal in TTP and HUS?
   a. Indirect serum bilirubin and serum haptoglobin
   b. Prothrombin time and partial thromboplastin time
   c. Lactate dehydrogenase and aspartate aminotransferase
   d. Serum creatinine and serum total protein

5. Which of the following laboratory results may be seen in *both* traumatic cardiac hemolytic anemia and exercise-induced hemoglobinuria?
   a. Schistocytes on the peripheral blood film
   b. Thrombocytopenia
   c. Decreased serum haptoglobin
   d. Hemosiderinuria

6. Which *Plasmodium* species is widespread in Malaysia, has RBCs with multiple ring forms, has band-shaped early trophozoites, shows a 24-hour erythrocytic cycle, and can cause severe disease and high parasitemia?
   a. *P. falciparum*
   b. *P. vivax*
   c. *P. knowlesi*
   d. *P. malariae*

7. One week after returning from a vacation in Rhode Island, a 60-year-old man experienced fever, chills, nausea, muscle aches, and fatigue of 2 days' duration. A complete blood count (CBC) showed a WBC count of 4.5×10^9/L, a hemoglobin level of 10.5 g/dL, a platelet count of 134×10^9/L, and a reticulocyte count of 2.7%. The medical laboratory scientist noticed tiny ameboid ring forms in some of the RBCs and some tetrad forms in others. These findings suggest:
   a. Bartonellosis
   b. Malaria
   c. Babesiosis
   d. Clostridial sepsis

8. What RBC morphology is characteristically found within the first 24 hours following extensive burn injury?
   a. Macrocytosis and polychromasia
   b. Burr cells and crenated cells
   c. Howell-Jolly bodies and bite cells
   d. Schistocytes and microspherocytes

9. A 36-year-old woman was brought to the emergency department by her husband because she had experienced a seizure. He reported that she had been well until that morning, when she complained of a sudden headache and malaise. She was not taking any medications and had no history of previous surgery or pregnancy. Laboratory studies showed a WBC count of 15×10^9/L, a hemoglobin level of 7.8 g/dL, a platelet count of 18×10^9/L, and schistocytes and helmet cells on the peripheral blood film. Chemistry test results included markedly elevated serum lactate dehydrogenase activity and a slight increase in the level of total and indirect serum bilirubin. The urinalysis results were positive for protein and blood, but there were no RBCs in the urine sediment. Prothrombin time and partial thromboplastin time were within the reference interval. When the entire clinical and laboratory picture is considered, which of the following is the most likely diagnosis?
   a. HUS
   b. HELLP syndrome
   c. TTP
   d. Exercise-induced hemoglobinuria

10. Which of the following laboratory test results are abnormal in HELLP syndrome but not in DIC?
   a. Aspartate aminotransferase
   b. Prothrombin time
   c. Platelet count
   d. Hemoglobin

REFERENCES

1. Mentzer, W. C., & Schrier, S. S. (2018). Extrinsic nonimmune hemolytic anemias. In Hoffman, R., Benz, E. J. Jr, Silberstein, L. E., et al. (Eds.), *Hematology: Basic Principles and Practice.* (7th ed., pp. 663–672). Philadelphia: Elsevier.

2. Moake, J. L. (2002). Thrombotic microangiopathies. *N Engl J Med, 347,* 589–600.

3. Tsai H-M. (2013). Thrombotic thrombocytopenic purpura and the atypical hemolytic uremic syndrome. *Hematol Oncol Clin N Am, 27,* 565–584.

4. Moake, J. (2009). Thrombotic microangiopathies: multimers, metalloprotease, and beyond. *Clin Transl Sci, 2,* 366–373.

5. Schneidewend R., Epperla N., & Friedman K. D. (2018). Thrombotic thrombocytopenic purpura and the hemolytic uremic syndrome. In Hoffman, R., Benz, E. J. Jr, Silberstein, L. E., et al. (Eds.), *Hematology: Basic Principles and Practice.* (7th ed., pp. 1984–2000). Philadelphia: Elsevier.

6. Crawley, J. T. B., & Scully, M. A. (2013). Thrombotic thrombocytopenic purpura: basic pathophysiology and therapeutic strategies. *Hematology Am Soc Hematol Educ Program,* 292–299.

7. Moake, J. L., Rudy, C. K., Troll, J. H., et al. (1982). Unusually large plasma factor VIII: von Willebrand factor multimers in chronic relapsing thrombotic thrombocytopenic purpura. *N Engl J Med, 307,* 1432–1435.

8. Furlan, M., Robles, R., Galbusera, M., et al. (1998). von Willebrand factor-cleaving protease in thrombotic thrombocytopenic purpura and the hemolytic-uremic syndrome. *N Engl J Med, 339,* 1578–1584.

9. Tsai, H-M., & Lian, E C-Y. (1998). Antibodies to von Willebrand factor-cleaving protease in acute thrombotic thrombocytopenic purpura. *N Engl J Med, 339,* 1585–1594.

10. Zhang, Q., Zhou, Y. F., Zhang, C. Z., et al. (2009). Structural specializations of A2, a force-sensing domain in the ultralarge vascular protein von Willebrand factor. *Proc Natl Acad Sci U S A, 106,* 9226–9231.

11. Kremer Hovinga, J. A., Vesely, S. K., Terrell, D. R., et al. (2010). Survival and relapse in patients with thrombotic thrombocytopenic purpura. *Blood, 115,* 1500–1511.

12. Lotta, L. A., Garagiola, I., Palla, R., et al. (2010). ADAMTS13 mutations and polymorphisms in congenital thrombotic thrombocytopenic purpura. *Hum Mutat, 31,* 11–19.

13. Mariotte, E., & Veyradier, A. (2015). Thrombotic thrombocytopenic purpura; from diagnosis to therapy. *Curr Opin Crit Care, 21,* 593–601.

14. Scheiring, J., Rosales, A., & Zimmerhackl, L. B. (2010). Clinical practice: today's understanding of the haemolytic uraemic syndrome. *Eur J Pediatr, 169,* 7–13.

15. Petruzziello, T. N., Mawji, I. A., Khan, M., et al. (2009). Verotoxin biology: molecular events in vascular endothelial injury. *Kidney Int, 75*, S17–S19.

16. Cataland, S. R., & Wu, H. F. (2014). Diagnosis and management of complement mediated thrombotic microangiopathies. *Blood Reviews, 28*, 67–74.

17. Haram, K., Svendsen, E., & Abildgaard, U. (2009). The HELLP syndrome: clinical issues and management. *BMC Pregnancy Childbirth, 9*, 1–15.

18. Baker, K. R., & Moake, J. (2016). Fragmentation hemolytic anemia. In Kaushansky, K., Lichtman, M. A., Prchal, J. T., et al. (Eds.), *Williams Hematology*. (9th ed., pp. 801–808). New York: McGraw-Hill.

19. Martin, J. N. (2013). Milestones in the quest for best management of patients with HELLP syndrome (micorangiopathic hemolytic anemia, hepatic dysfunction, thrombocytopenia). *Int J Gynecol Obstet, 121*, 202–207.

20. Lesesve, J. F., Martin, M., Banasiak, C. et al. (2014). Schistocytes in disseminated intravascular coagulation. *Int J Lab Hematol, 36*, 439–443.

21. Shapira, Y., Vaturi, M., & Sagie, A. (2009). Hemolysis associated with prosthetic heart valves a review. *Cardiol Rev, 17*, 121–124.

22. Davidson, R. J. L. (1964). Exertional haemoglobinuria: a report on three cases with studies on the haemolytic mechanism. *J Clin Pathol, 17*, 536–540.

23. Telford, R. D., Sly, G. J., Hahn, A. G., et al. (2003). Footstrike is the major cause of hemolysis during running. *J Appl Physiol, 94*, 38–42.

24. Selby, G. B., & Eichner, E. R. (1986). Endurance swimming, intravascular hemolysis, anemia, and iron depletion. New perspective on athlete's anemia. *Am J Med, 81*, 791–794.

25. Shaskey, D. J., & Green, G. A. (2000). Sports haematology. *Sports Med, 29*, 27–38.

26. Tobal, D., Olascoaga, A., Moreira, G., et al. (2008). Rust urine after intense hand drumming is caused by extracorpuscular hemolysis. *Clin J Am Soc Nephrol, 3*, 1022–1027.

27. Smith, J. A., Kolbuch-Braddon, M., Gillam, I., et al. (1995). Changes in the susceptibility of red blood cells to oxidative and osmotic stress following submaximal exercise. *Eur J Appl Physiol, 70*, 427–436.

28. Beneke, R., Bihn, D., Hütler, M., et al. (2005). Haemolysis caused by alterations of alpha- and beta-spectrin after 10 to 35 min of severe exercise. *Eur J Appl Physiol, 95*, 307–312.

29. Yusof, A., Leithauser, R. M., Roth, H. J., et al. (2007). Exercise-induced hemolysis is caused by protein modification and most evident during the early phase of an ultraendurance race. *J Appl Physiol, 102*, 582–586.

30. Singh, B., Lee, K. S., Matusop, A., et al. (2004). A large focus of naturally acquired *Plasmodium knowlesi* infections in human beings. *Lancet, 363*, 1017–1024.

31. Cox-Singh, J., Davis, T. M. E., Lee, K. S., et al. (2008). *Plasmodium knowlesi* malaria in humans is widely distributed and potentially life-threatening. *Clin Infect Dis, 46*, 165–171.

32. Lee, K. S., Cox-Singh, J., Brooke, G., et al. (2009). *Plasmodium knowlesi* from archival blood films: further evidence that human infections are widely distributed and not newly emergent in Malaysian Borneo. *Int J Parasitol, 39*, 1122–1128.

33. Centers for Disease Control and Prevention. (2014). *Malaria Facts*. https://www.cdc.gov/malaria/about/index.html. Accessed July 9, 2018.

34. World Health Organization. (2013). *World Malaria Report 2013*. Geneva: WHO Press. http://www.who.int/malaria/publications/world-malaria-report-2017/report/en/. Accessed July 9, 2018.

35. Miller, L. H., Baruch, D. I., Marsh, K., et al. (2002). The pathogenic basis of malaria. *Nature, 415*, 673–679.

36. Wellems, T. E., Hayton, K., & Fairhurst, R. M. (2009). The impact of malaria parasitism: from corpuscles to communities. *J Clin Invest, 119*, 2496–2205.

37. Garcia, L. S. (2010). Malaria. *Clin Lab Med, 30*, 93–129.

38. Ekvall, H. (2003). Malaria and anemia. *Curr Opin Hematol, 10*, 108–114.

39. World Health Organization. (2015). *Guidelines for Treatment of Malaria*. (3rd ed.). Geneva: WHO Press.

40. Haldar, K., & Mohandas, N. (2009). Malaria, erythrocytic infection, and anemia. *Hematology Am Soc Hematol Educ Program*, 87–93.

41. Waitumbi, J. N., Opollo, M. O., Muga, R. O., et al. (2000). Red cell surface changes and erythrophagocytosis in children with severe *Plasmodium falciparum* anemia. *Blood, 95*, 1481–1486.

42. Craig, A., & Scherf, A. (2001). Molecules on the surface of the *Plasmodium falciparum* infected erythrocyte and their role in malaria pathogenesis and immune evasion. *Mol Biochem Parasitol, 115*, 129–143.

43. Bridges, D. J., Bunn, J., van Mourik, J. A., et al. (2010). Rapid activation of endothelial cells enables *Plasmodium falciparum* adhesion to platelet-decorated von Willebrand factor strings. *Blood, 115*, 1472–1474.

44. Aird, W. C., Mosnier, L. O., & Fairhurst, R. M. (2014). *Plasmodium falciparum* picks (on) EPCR. *Blood, 123*, 163–167.

45. Centers for Disease Control and Prevention. *Malaria Diagnosis (U.S.)—Microscopy*. https://www.cdc.gov/malaria/diagnosistreatment/microscopy.html. Accessed July 11, 2018.

46. Ruebush, T. K., II, Juranek, D. D., Spielman, A., et al. (1981). Epidemiology of human babesiosis on Nantucket Island. *Am J Trop Med Hyg, 30*, 937–941.

47. Vannier, E., & Krause, P. J. (2009). Update on babesiosis. *Interdiscip Perspect Infect Dis, 2009*, 984568.

48. Centers for Disease Control and Prevention. *Babesiosis*. https://www.cdc.gov/parasites/babesiosis/. Accessed July 10, 2018.

49. Sanchez, E., Vannier, E., Wormser, G. P., et al. (2016). Diagnosis, treatment, and prevention of Lyme disease, human granulocytic anaplasmosis, and babesiosis. *JAMA, 315*(16), 1767–1777.

50. Hildebrandt, A., Gray, J. S., & Hunfeld, K. P. (2013). Human babesiosis in Europe: what clinicians need to know. *Infection, 41*, 1057–1072.

51. Krause, P. J., McKay, K., Gadbaw, J., et al. (2003). Increasing health burden of human babesiosis in endemic sites. *Am J Trop Med Hyg, 68*, 431–436.

52. Blevins, S. M., Greenfield, R. A., & Bronze, M. S. (2008). Blood smear analysis in babesiosis, ehrlichiosis, relapsing fever, malaria, and Chagas disease. *Cleve Clin J Med, 75*, 521–530.

53. Krause, P. J., Telford, S. R. 3rd., Ryan, R., et al. (1994). Diagnosis of babesiosis: evaluation of a serologic test for the detection of *B. microti* antibody. *J Infect Dis, 169*, 923–926.

54. Kapoor, J. R., Montiero, B., Tanoue, L., et al. (2007). Massive intravascular hemolysis and a rapid fatal outcome. *Chest, 132*, 2016–2019.

55. Urbina, P., Flores-Díaz, M., Alape-Girón, A., et al. (2009). Phospholipase C and sphingomyelinase activities of the *Clostridium perfringens* α-toxin. *Chem Phys Lipids, 159,* 51–57.

56. Merino, A., Pereira, A., & Castro, P. (2009). Massive intravascular haemolysis during *Clostridium perfringens* sepsis of hepatic origin. *Eur J Haematol, 84,* 278–279.

57. Barrett, J. P., Whiteside, J. L., & Boardman, L. A. (2002). Fatal clostridial sepsis after spontaneous abortion. *Obstet Gynecol, 99,* 899–901.

58. Simon, T. G., Bradley, J., Jones, A., et al. (2014). Massive intravascular hemolysis from *Clostricium perfringens* septicemia: a review. *J Int Care Med, 29*(6), 327–333.

59. Maguina, C., & Gotuzzo, E. (2000). Bartonellosis new and old. *Infect Dis Clin North Am, 14,* 1–22.

60. Huarcaya, E., Maguina, C., Torres, R., et al. (2004). Bartonellosis (Carrion's disease) in the pediatric population of Peru: an overview and update. *Braz J Infect Dis, 8,* 331–339.

61. Lichtman, M. A. (2016). Hemolytic anemia resulting from infections with microorganisms. In Kaushansky, K., Lichtman, M. A., Prchal J. T., et al. (Eds.), *Williams Hematology.* (9th ed., pp. 815–822). New York: McGraw-Hill.

62. Ranawaka, R. R., Mendis, S., & Weerakoon, H. S. (2008). Dapsone-induced haemolytic anemia, hepatitis and agranulocytosis in a leprosy patient with normal glucose-6-phosphate-dehydrogenase activity. *Lepr Rev, 79,* 436–440.

63. Lim, H. C., Poulose, V., & Tan, H. H. (2009). Acute naphthalene poisoning following the non-accidental ingestion of mothballs. *Singapore Med J, 50,* e298–e301.

64. Herrmann, P. C. (2016). Erythrocyte disorders as a result of chemical and physical agents. In Kaushansky, K., Lichtman, M. A., Prchal J. T., et al. (Eds.), *Williams Hematology.* (9th ed., pp. 809–814). New York: McGraw-Hill.

65. Athappan, G., Balaji, M. V., Navaneethan, U., et al. (2008). Acute renal failure in snake envenomation: a large prospective study. *Saudi J Kidney Dis Transpl, 19,* 404–410.

66. McDade, J., Aygun, B., & Ware, R. E. (2010). Brown recluse spider (*Loxosceles reclusa*) envenomation leading to acute hemolytic anemia in six adolescents. *J Pediatr, 156,* 155–157.

67. Kolecki, P. (1999). Delayed toxic reaction following massive bee envenomation. *Ann Emerg Med, 33,* 114–116.

68. Paudel, B., & Paudel, K. (2009). A study of wasp bites in a tertiary hospital of western Nepal. *Nepal Med Coll J, 11,* 52–56.

69. Posluszny, J. A., & Gamelli, R. L. (2010). Anemia of thermal injury: combined acute blood loss anemia and anemia of critical illness. *J Burn Care Res, 31,* 229–242.

Extrinsic Defects Leading to Increased Erythrocyte Destruction—Immune Causes

*Ruth Perez**

OBJECTIVES

After completion of this chapter, the reader will be able to:

1. Define *immune hemolytic anemia* and indicate the types of antibodies involved.
2. Compare and contrast mechanisms of immune hemolysis mediated by immunoglobulin M (IgM) and IgG antibodies.
3. Describe typical laboratory findings in immune hemolytic anemia and the importance of the direct antiglobulin test (DAT).
4. Compare and contrast four types of autoimmune hemolytic anemia in terms of immunoglobulin class involved, temperature for optimal reactivity of the autoantibody, proteins detected by the DAT on the patient's red blood cells, presence or absence of complement activation, type and site of hemolysis, and specificity of the autoantibody.
5. Relate results of the DAT to the pathophysiology and clinical findings in autoimmune hemolytic anemia.
6. Describe two types of hemolytic transfusion reactions, the usual immunoglobulin class involved, typical site of hemolysis, and important laboratory findings.
7. Describe the cause, pathophysiology, and laboratory findings in Rh and ABO hemolytic disease of the fetus and newborn (HDFN).
8. Describe three mechanisms of drug-induced immune hemolysis.
9. Compare and contrast the pathophysiology of immune hemolysis caused by drug-dependent and drug-independent antibodies, including related laboratory findings.
10. Given a patient history and results of a complete blood count, peripheral blood film examination, pertinent biochemical tests on serum and urine, and the direct and indirect antiglobulin tests, determine the type of immune hemolysis.

OUTLINE

Overview of Immune Hemolytic Anemias
  Pathophysiology of Immune Hemolysis
  Laboratory Findings in Immune Hemolytic Anemia
Autoimmune Hemolytic Anemia
  Warm Autoimmune Hemolytic Anemia
  Cold Agglutinin Disease
  Paroxysmal Cold Hemoglobinuria
  Mixed-Type Autoimmune Hemolytic Anemia

Alloimmune Hemolytic Anemias
  Hemolytic Transfusion Reaction
  Hemolytic Disease of the Fetus and Newborn
Drug-Induced Immune Hemolytic Anemia
  Mechanisms of Drug-Induced Immune Hemolysis
  Antibody Characteristics
  Nonimmune Drug-Induced Hemolysis
  Treatment

CASE STUDY

After studying the material in this chapter, the reader should be able to respond to the following case study:

A 37-year-old man sought medical attention from his general practitioner for malaise, shortness of breath, and difficulty concentrating for the past 5 days. Physical examination revealed an otherwise healthy adult with tachycardia. There was no significant medical history and the patient was not taking any medications. The physician ordered a complete blood count (CBC), urinalysis,

comprehensive metabolic panel (CMP), and electrocardiogram (ECG). The following are the patient's key laboratory results:

	Patient Results	Reference Intervals
WBC ($\times 10^9$/L)	12.4 (corrected)	3.6–10.6
HGB (g/dL)	7.1	14.0–18.0
MCV (fL)	105.4	80.0–100.0

Continued

*The author extends appreciation to Elaine M. Keohane and Kim A. Przekop, whose work in prior editions provided the foundation for this chapter.

	Patient Results	Reference Intervals
MCHC (g/dL)	36.3	32.0–36.0
RDW (%)	17.3	11.5–14.5
PLT (×10⁹/L)	325	150–450
Reticulocytes (%)	18.1	0.5–2.5
Neutrophils (%)	72	50–70
Bands (%)	10	0–5

The ECG was normal. The blood cell analyzer printout flagged for nucleated red blood cells (and corrected the WBC for them), 3+ anisocytosis, and reticulocytosis. The peripheral blood film had moderate spherocytes, moderate polychromasia, few macrocytes, marked anisocytosis, and 15 nucleated red blood cells/100 WBCs (Figure 23.1). Occasional schistocytes and neutrophilia with a slight left shift were also observed on the blood film (not shown in figure). The urinalysis report included 2+ protein, 2+ blood, and increased urobilinogen, with 0 to 5 RBCs seen on microscopic examination. Patient's serum was moderately icteric, and total serum bilirubin was increased. The patient was admitted for further testing. Serum haptoglobin was decreased, serum indirect (unconjugated) bilirubin and lactate dehydrogenase (LD) were elevated, and urine hemosiderin was positive.

A type and screen was ordered. The antibody screen was negative at the immediate spin and 37° C incubation phase but showed 3+ agglutination in the antihuman globulin (AHG) phase for all panel cells and the autocontrol. The direct antiglobulin test (DAT) showed 3+ agglutination with polyspecific AHG and monospecific anti-IgG but was negative with monospecific anti-C3b/C3d (complement). An acid elution was performed on the patient's RBCs, and the eluate showed 2+ reactions with all panel cells and autocontrol at the AHG phase. The patient was diagnosed with warm autoimmune hemolytic anemia (WAIHA) and started on 1 mg/kg per day prednisone until the hemoglobin reached 10.0 g/dL (2 weeks of treatment). The patient was continued on prednisone for 4 months with slowly decreasing levels of the drug. He also received bisphosphonates, vitamin D, and calcium to prevent osteoporosis, an adverse effect of prednisone.

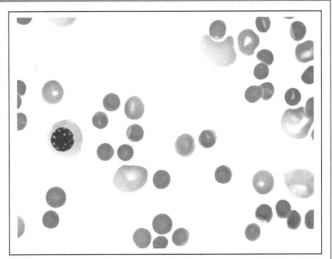

Figure 23.1 Peripheral Blood Film from the Patient in the Case Study. (Wright-Giemsa stain, ×1000.)

At 3 weeks postdiagnosis, spherocytes were no longer present on the peripheral blood film, urinalysis was normal, and the DAT was negative.

1. Explain why the WBC count, MCV, RDW, and reticulocyte count results were elevated.
2. Describe the immune mechanism that caused the spherocytosis, and explain why spherocytes have a shortened life span.
3. Relate the chemistry, urinalysis, and blood bank results with the pathophysiology of the patient's anemia.
4. Explain why the treatment was effective, and explain if the patient's WAIHA was acute or chronic.

OVERVIEW OF IMMUNE HEMOLYTIC ANEMIAS

Immune hemolytic anemia and nonimmune hemolytic anemia are two broad categories comprising the extrinsic hemolytic anemias, disorders in which red blood cells (RBCs) are structurally and functionally normal but a condition outside of the RBCs causes premature hemolysis. Nonimmune extrinsic hemolytic anemias are the result of physical or mechanical injury to RBCs and are covered in Chapter 22. Immune hemolytic anemias are conditions in which RBC survival is shortened as a result of an antibody-mediated mechanism. The antibody may be an *autoantibody* (directed against a self RBC antigen), an *alloantibody* (directed against an RBC antigen of another person), or an antibody directed against a drug (or its metabolite) taken by the patient. Some antibodies are able to activate the classical complement pathway, which results in the attachment of activated complement proteins to the RBC membrane. RBCs with bound antibody or complement are prematurely removed from the circulation extravascularly by macrophages (because of their receptors for complement and the Fc component of antibody), intravascularly by complement-mediated hemolysis, or by a combination of both mechanisms.[1] Anemia develops when the amount of hemolysis exceeds the ability of bone marrow to replace RBCs that are destroyed. The degree of anemia varies from asymptomatic and mild to severe and life threatening.

Immune hemolytic anemias may be classified into the following groups: autoimmune hemolytic anemia, alloimmune hemolytic anemia, and drug-induced immune hemolytic anemia (Box 23.1).[1,2] It is important to determine the cause of an immune hemolytic anemia so that the appropriate therapy can be administered to the patient.

Pathophysiology of Immune Hemolysis

In immune hemolysis an antibody binds to an antigen on the surface of RBCs, which signals premature removal of those cells from the circulation through extravascular or intravascular hemolysis (Chapter 20). Two classes or isotypes of antibodies involved in most immune hemolytic anemias are immunoglobulin G (IgG) and M (IgM). IgG is a monomer in a Y-like structure with two identical heavy chains (γ H chains) and two identical light chains (either κ or λ) connected by disulfide bonds.[3] At the top of the Y-like structure are two antigen-binding (Fab) domains, each formed from the N-terminus of the variable domain of one light and one heavy chain. IgG has one Fc domain (stem of the Y) consisting of the C-termini of the two heavy chains (Figure 23.2). IgM is a pentamer consisting of five monomeric units connected by disulfide linkages at

BOX 23.1 Classification of Immune Hemolytic Anemias

Autoimmune Hemolytic Anemia
Warm autoimmune hemolytic anemia (WAIHA)
  Idiopathic
  Secondary
    Lymphoproliferative disorders
    Nonlymphoid neoplasms
    Collagen-vascular disease
    Immunodeficiency disorders
    Viral infections
Cold agglutinin disease (CAD)
  Idiopathic
  Secondary
    Acute: infections (*Mycoplasma pneumoniae*, infectious mononucleosis, other viruses)
    Chronic: lymphoproliferative disorders
Paroxysmal cold hemoglobinuria (PCH)
  Idiopathic
  Secondary
    Viral infections
    Syphilis
Mixed-type autoimmune hemolytic anemia

Alloimmune Hemolytic Anemias
Hemolytic transfusion reaction (HTR)
Hemolytic disease of the fetus and newborn (HDFN)

Drug-Induced Immune Hemolytic Anemia (DIIHA)
Drug dependent
Drug independent

the C-termini of their heavy chains (μ H chains).[3,4] Because the composition, structure, and size of IgG and IgM are different, their properties and mechanisms in mediating hemolysis are also different.

The classical complement pathway is an important mediator of immune hemolysis. Major proteins of the classical complement pathway are designated C1 through C9, and their components or fragments are designated with lowercase suffixes. The first protein, C1, has three components: C1q, C1r, and C1s. After an antibody binds to its specific antigens on the RBC surface, C1q must bind to two adjacent antibody Fc domains to activate the pathway.[4] Theoretically only one IgM molecule is needed for complement activation because of its larger pentameric structure with five Fc domains; however, at least two molecules of monomeric IgG in close proximity are required for C1q attachment.[4] Therefore IgM antibodies are highly effective in activating complement, whereas IgG antibodies are unable to activate the pathway unless there is a sufficient number of IgG molecules on the RBC surface.[4,5] In addition, subclasses IgG1 and IgG3 have high binding affinity for C1q, whereas subclasses IgG2 and IgG4 have minimal ability to bind complement.[4,5]

The binding of C1q to adjacent Fc domains requires calcium and magnesium ions and activates C1r, which then activates C1s. This activated C1q-C1r-C1s complex is an enzyme that cleaves C4 and then C2, which results in the binding of a small number of C4bC2a complexes to the RBC membrane. C4bC2a complex is an active *C3 convertase* enzyme that cleaves C3 in plasma; the result is the binding of many C3b molecules to C4bC2a on the RBC surface. The last phase of the classical pathway occurs when C4bC2aC3b *(C5 convertase)* converts C5 to C5b, which combines with C6, C7, C8, and multiple C9s to form the *membrane attack complex (MAC)*. The MAC resembles a cylinder that inserts into the lipid bilayer of the membrane, forming a pore that allows water and small ions to enter the cell, causing lysis (Figure 23.3).[3] Negative regulators inhibit various complement proteins and complexes in the pathway to prevent uncontrolled activation and excessive hemolysis.[1,3,4]

Hemolysis mediated by IgM antibodies requires complement and can result in both extravascular and intravascular hemolysis.[5] When IgM molecules attach to the RBC surface in relatively low density, complement activation results in C3b binding to the membrane, but complement inhibitors prevent full activation of the pathway to the terminal membrane attack complex.[1,5] C3b-sensitized RBCs are destroyed by extravascular hemolysis, predominantly by macrophages (Kupffer cells) in the liver, which have C3b receptors. Some C3b on RBCs can be cleaved, however, which leaves the C3d fragment on the cell. RBCs sensitized with only C3d are not prematurely removed from circulation because macrophages lack a C3d receptor.[5] In severe cases of immune hemolysis involving heavy sensitization of RBCs with IgM antibody, significantly more complement is activated, which overwhelms complement inhibitors. In these cases, complement activation proceeds from C1 to C9 and results in rapid intravascular hemolysis.[5]

Hemolysis mediated by IgG antibodies occurs with or without complement and predominantly by extravascular mechanisms.[5] RBCs sensitized with IgG are removed from circulation by macrophages in the spleen, which have receptors for the Fc component of IgG1 and IgG3.[1,5] IgG antibodies are not efficient in activating complement, and intravascular hemolysis by full activation of complement from C1 to C9 is rare (except with anti-P in paroxysmal cold hemoglobinuria).[5] However, if there is a high density of IgG1 or IgG3 bound to antigens on RBCs, some complement is activated and C3b binds to the membrane. If both IgG and C3b are on the RBC membrane, there is faster clearance from the circulation by macrophages in both the spleen and the liver.[1,5] Often, IgG-sensitized RBCs are only partially phagocytized by macrophages, which results in removal of some membrane. Spherocytes are the result of this process, and they are the characteristic cell of IgG-mediated hemolysis.[5] The spherocytes are eventually removed from circulation by entrapment in the red pulp of the spleen (splenic cords), where they are rapidly phagocytized by macrophages (Chapter 5).[5] The mechanisms of immune hemolysis are summarized in Table 23.1.

Laboratory Findings in Immune Hemolytic Anemia

Laboratory findings in immune hemolytic anemia are similar to the findings in other hemolytic anemias and include

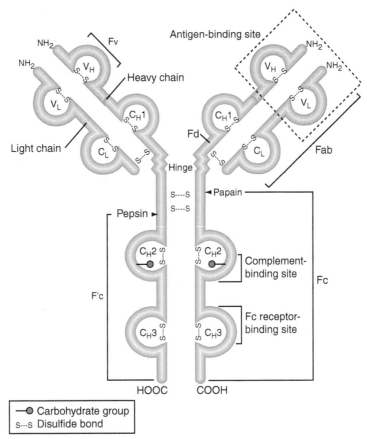

Figure 23.2 Schematic of an Immunoglobulin G (IgG) Molecule. IgG consists of two heavy chains and two light chains. Note the antigen binding sites at the amino (NH$_2$) end formed by the variable region (Fv) of one heavy chain and one light chain. Note the Fc region at the carboxyl (COOH) end of the heavy chains. The chains are held together by disulfide linkages. (From McPherson, R. A., Riley, R. S., & Massey, H. D. [2017]. Laboratory evaluation of immunoglobulin function and humoral immunity. In McPherson, R. A. & Pincus, M. R. (Eds.), *Henry's Clinical Diagnosis and Management by Laboratory Methods.* [23rd ed., Figure 46.1, p. 914]. St. Louis: Elsevier.)

decreased hemoglobin; increased reticulocyte count; increased levels of indirect serum bilirubin and lactate dehydrogenase; and decreased serum haptoglobin level. If hemolysis is predominantly intravascular, or extravascular hemolysis is severe, the haptoglobin level will be moderately to severely decreased, plasma hemoglobin will be increased, and the patient may have hemoglobinuria or even hemosiderinuria (in cases of chronic hemolysis) (Chapter 20). Mean cell volume (MCV) may be increased because of reticulocytosis and RBC agglutination (if present). Leukocytosis and thrombocytosis may occur along with increased erythroid proliferation in bone marrow.[1] Findings on the peripheral blood film include polychromasia (as a result of reticulocytosis), spherocytes (caused by IgG-mediated membrane damage by macrophages), and occasionally RBC agglutination.[5] Nucleated RBCs, fragmented RBCs or schistocytes, and erythrophagocytosis (phagocytes engulfing RBCs) may also be observed on the peripheral blood film.[1]

To determine whether the hemolysis is due to an immune mechanism, a *direct antiglobulin test* (DAT) is performed. The DAT detects in vivo sensitization of the RBC surface by IgG, C3b, or C3d.[2] In the DAT procedure, polyspecific antihuman globulin (AHG) is added to saline-washed patient RBCs. Polyspecific AHG has specificity for the Fc portion of human IgG and complement components C3b and C3d; agglutination will occur if a critical number of any of these molecules is present on the RBC surface (Figure 23.4).[2] If the DAT result is positive with polyspecific AHG, then RBCs are tested with monospecific anti-IgG and anti-C3b/C3d to identify the type of sensitization. If IgG is detected on RBCs, elution procedures are used to remove the antibody from RBCs for identification.

Specificity of the IgG antibody may be determined by assessing the reaction of the eluate with screening and panel reagent RBCs (RBCs genotyped for the major RBC antigens) using the *indirect antiglobulin test* (IAT) (Figure 23.4). Identification of any circulating alloantibodies or autoantibodies by the IAT is also important in the investigation.[2] The DAT result may be negative in patients with some immune hemolytic anemias.[2] In addition, other disorders beside immune

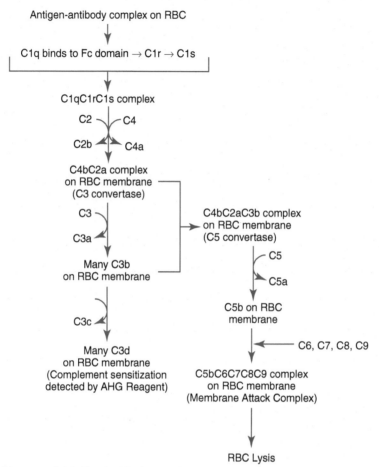

Figure 23.3 Diagram of the Classical Pathway of Complement Activation. C1q is activated by binding to adjacent Fc domains of immunoglobulin bound to RBC antigen. C1q activates C1r; C1r activates C1s which forms the complex, C1qC1rC1s. The complex activates C2 and C4 to form the C4bC2a complex (C3 convertase) on the membrane. The complex converts C3 to many C3b molecules on the membrane. If there is no further activation, C3b will degrade to C3d on the membrane, which can be detected by polyspecific antihuman globulin (AHG). C3b can also form the complex C4bC2aC3b (C5 convertase), which converts C5 to C5b on the membrane. C5b forms the membrane attack complex, C5bC6C7C8C9, which inserts into the bilipid layer, causing lysis.

TABLE 23.1	Major Mechanisms of Immune Hemolysis	
	IgM Mediated	**IgG Mediated**
Extravascular hemolysis	IgM activation of classical complement pathway from C1 to C3b only; clearance of C3b-sensitized RBCs by macrophages mainly in liver	Clearance of IgG-sensitized RBCs by macrophages mainly in spleen Formation of spherocytes by partial phagocytosis of IgG-sensitized RBCs; spherocytes cleared by macrophages after entrapment in spleen IgG* activation of classical complement pathway from C1 to C3b only; requires high-density IgG on RBC surface; clearance of IgG- and C3b-sensitized RBCs by macrophages in spleen and liver
Intravascular hemolysis	Full IgM activation of classical complement pathway from C1 to C9 and direct RBC lysis; requires high-density IgM on RBCs to overcome complement inhibitors	Full IgG activation of classical complement pathway from C1 to C9 and direct RBC lysis; requires very high-density IgG on RBCs for activation and to overcome complement inhibitors; uncommon

Ig, Immunoglobulin; *RBC,* red blood cell.
*IgG3 and IgG1 are most efficient in complement activation.

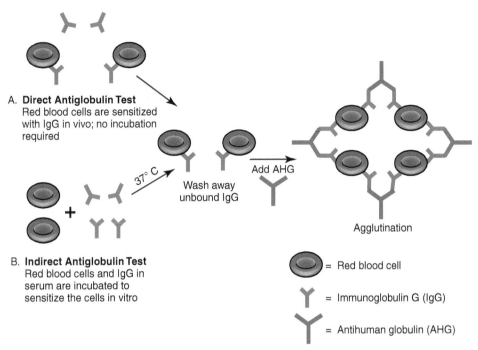

Figure 23.4 Graphic Representation of the Direct and Indirect Antihuman Globulin Reaction. **(A),** The direct antiglobulin test (DAT) detects immunoglobulin G (IgG) antibodies that are bound to corresponding antigens on the patient's red blood cells in vivo. It does not require an incubation step. **(B),** The indirect antiglobulin test (IAT) requires a 37° C incubation step to bind IgG antibodies (from patient's serum or from typing reagents) to corresponding antigens on red blood cells in vitro. Polyspecific antihuman globulin (AHG) is a mixture of antibodies to IgG and complement components C3d/C3b. The anti-IgG produces agglutination by binding to the Fc domain of immunoglobulin G (IgG) antibodies that are bound to antigens on the red blood cell membranes. Similarly, the anti-C3d/C3b produces agglutination by binding to the respective complement components if present on the red blood cell membranes (reaction not shown). Monospecific AHG has specificity for either IgG or C3b/C3d. Although AHG is depicted as an IgG antibody in this figure, in some reagents it can be an IgM isotype.

hemolytic anemia can cause a positive DAT.[2] Therefore diagnosis of immune hemolytic anemia cannot rely solely on the DAT and must take into account the patient history; symptoms; recent medications; previous transfusions; coexisting conditions, including pregnancy; and results of applicable hematologic, biochemical, and serologic tests.[2,5]

AUTOIMMUNE HEMOLYTIC ANEMIA

Autoimmune hemolytic anemia (AIHA) is a rare disorder characterized by premature RBC destruction and anemia caused by autoantibodies that bind to the RBC surface with or without complement activation. AIHA can affect both children and adults, and its annual incidence is estimated to be between 1 and 3 per 100,000 individuals.[6] In children, more males are affected, but in adults, more females are affected.[6] Autoantibodies may arise as a result of immune system dysregulation and loss of immune tolerance, exposure to an antigen similar to an autoantigen, B-lymphocyte neoplasm, or other unknown reason.[1,6] The type, amount, and duration of antigen exposure and genetic and environmental factors may also contribute to development of autoantibodies.[5] Anemia can be mild or severe, and onset can be acute or gradual. Severity of the anemia depends on autoantibody characteristics (titer, ability to react

at 37° C, ability to activate complement, and specificity and affinity for the autoantigen), antigen characteristics (density on RBCs, immunogenicity), and patient factors (age, ability of bone marrow to compensate for the hemolysis, function of macrophages, complement proteins and regulators, and underlying conditions).[1,6]

Autoimmune hemolytic anemias may be divided into four major categories based on the characteristics of the autoantibody and the mechanism of hemolysis: warm autoimmune hemolytic anemia, cold agglutinin disease, paroxysmal cold hemoglobinuria, and mixed-type AIHA (Table 23.2).[2,5,6]

Warm Autoimmune Hemolytic Anemia

Warm autoimmune hemolytic anemia (WAIHA) is the most commonly encountered autoimmune hemolytic anemia, comprising up to 70% to 80% of cases.[1,5] Autoantibodies causing WAIHA react optimally at 37° C, and the vast majority of them are IgG.[1] WAIHA may be classified as idiopathic or secondary. In patients with idiopathic WAIHA, the cause is unknown. Secondary WAIHA may occur in many conditions such as lymphoproliferative diseases (chronic lymphocytic leukemia, B-lymphocytic lymphomas, and Waldenström macroglobulinemia), nonlymphoid neoplasms (thymoma and cancers of the colon, kidney, lung, and ovary), autoimmune disorders

TABLE 23.2	**Characteristics of Autoimmune Hemolytic Anemias**			
	Warm Autoimmune Hemolytic Anemia	**Cold Agglutinin Disease**	**Paroxysmal Cold Hemoglobinuria**	**Mixed-Type Autoimmune Hemolytic Anemia**
Immunoglobulin class	IgG (rarely IgM, IgA)	IgM	IgG	IgG, IgM
Optimum reactivity temperature of autoantibody	37° C	4° C; reactivity extends to greater than 30° C	4° C	4° to 37° C
Sensitization detected by direct antiglobulin test	IgG or IgG + C3d; only C3d uncommon	C3d	C3d	IgG and C3d
Complement activation	Variable	Yes	Yes	Yes
Hemolysis	Extravascular primarily	Extravascular; some intravascular	Intravascular	Extravascular and intravascular
Autoantibody specificity	Panreactive or Rh complex; rarely specific Rh or other antigen	I (most), i (some), Pr (rare)	P	Panreactive; unclear specificity
Other laboratory findings	Polychromasia, spherocytes, occasionally decreased PLT count	RBC agglutination may be present	Polychromasia, spherocytes (common), schistocytes, NRBCs, anisocytosis, poikilocytosis, and erythrophagocytosis	Varies

Ig, Immunoglobulin; *NRBCs,* nucleated red blood cells; *PLT,* platelet; *RBC,* red blood cell.

(rheumatoid arthritis, scleroderma, polyarteritis nodosa, Sjögren syndrome, and systemic lupus erythematosus), immunodeficiency disorders, and viral infections.[1,5]

The onset of WAIHA is usually insidious, with symptoms of anemia (fatigue, dizziness, dyspnea), but some cases can be acute and life threatening with fever, jaundice, splenomegaly, and hepatomegaly, especially in children with WAIHA secondary to viral infections.[1,5] Massive splenomegaly, lymphadenopathy, fever, petechiae, ecchymosis, or renal failure in adults suggests an underlying lymphoproliferative disorder.[1,5]

Although most autoantibodies that cause WAIHA are IgG, rare cases involving IgA autoantibodies as well as cases with fatal outcomes caused by warm-reacting IgM antibodies have been reported.[1,2] Hemolysis is predominantly extravascular in WAIHA, and cases of fulminant intravascular hemolysis are rare.[5]

The DAT is positive in more than 95% of patients, with approximately 85% of patients having IgG alone or both IgG and C3d on their RBCs, and 10% to 14% having C3d only.[1,2,5] In 1% to 4% of patients, the DAT is negative because of IgA or IgM autoantibodies that are not detected by the polyspecific AHG; IgG or C3d in an amount less than the reagent detection limit; dissociation of IgG antibodies with low avidity during the washing phase of the DAT; or various technical errors.[1,2,5] Therefore a negative DAT result does not rule out autoimmune hemolytic anemia.

Warm autoantibodies are usually panreactive; that is, they will agglutinate all screening and panel cells, donor RBCs, and the patient's own RBCs, so the specificity of the autoantibody is not apparent.[2,5] In some cases Rh complex specificity can be demonstrated.[2,5] Rarely, a specific autoantibody to an antigen in the Rh blood group system is identified. Autoantibodies to other antigens (such as LW, Jk, K, Di, Ge, Lu, M, N, S, U, En[a], and Wr[b]) are occasionally identified.[2,5] For most patients

(approximately 80%) the autoantibody can be detected in the serum. Because the autoantibody is panreactive, it may mask reactions of alloantibodies with RBC panel cells. If an RBC transfusion is necessary, it is crucial to perform tests to determine whether clinically significant *allo*antibodies are also present.[5]

Anemia in WAIHA can be mild or severe, with RBC life span sometimes reduced to 5 days or less.[1] Laboratory findings for serum and urine reflect the predominantly extravascular hemolysis that occurs in IgG-mediated immune hemolysis. Polychromasia and spherocytes are typical findings on the peripheral blood film (Figure 23.1). Occasionally WAIHA is accompanied by immune thrombocytopenic purpura and a decreased platelet count, a condition known as *Evans syndrome,* which occurs primarily in children.[6,7]

In symptomatic but non-life-threatening WAIHA, a glucocorticosteroid such as prednisone is the initial treatment of choice.[1,2,8,9] Approximately 70% to 80% of patients show improvement with prednisone, but only about 20% to 40% achieve a long-term response.[1,8] Many adult patients need to be on a long-term maintenance dosage to remain asymptomatic.[1] A serious side effect of glucocorticosteroid treatment (initially and long term) is an increased risk of osteoporosis and bone fractures.[1] Guidelines from the American College of Rheumatology indicate that patients on glucocorticosteroids may benefit from vitamin D, calcium, and bisphosphonate therapy to prevent osteoporosis, but each patient's situation should be evaluated on an individual basis.[10]

In patients with chronic WAIHA who are refractive to prednisone therapy or require long-term, high-dose prednisone therapy, second-line therapy usually includes a choice of either splenectomy or rituximab.[1,8,9] Splenectomy achieves a favorable response only in about 50% of patients, both initially and long term.[1,8] Rituximab is a monoclonal anti-CD20 antibody that binds to the corresponding antigen found on B lymphocytes. In a recent meta-analysis of 21 studies (409 patients) of the efficacy and safety of rituximab in WAIHA, Reynaud and colleagues found an overall response rate of 73% with a low incidence of adverse effects; they suggested that rituximab may be a superior choice over invasive (splenectomy) or toxic (immunosuppression) therapies.[11] However, there are few studies on the long-term efficacy and safety of rituximab in WAIHA, and as of this publication, rituximab is not FDA-approved for this indication.[1,8] Immunosuppressive drugs, such as cyclophosphamide or azathioprine, are the third-line therapy for refractory WAIHA because the toxicity and side effects may be severe.[1,6,9] Hematopoietic stem cell transplantation (HSCT) has been used in the past for severe, refractory, life-threatening autoimmune syndromes, including hemolytic anemia and Evans syndrome, but is a therapy of last resort.[9] In secondary WAIHA, successful management of the underlying condition often controls the hemolysis and anemia. WAIHA with a critically low hemoglobin level requires RBC transfusion. If the autoantibody has broad specificity, all RBC units may be incompatible with the autoantibody.[1,2,5] In such cases a check for underlying alloantibodies is performed, and extended phenotype matching for Rh, Kell, Kidd, and Ss antigens may be recommended to prevent further alloimmunization.[1] In addition, a minimum volume of RBCs is given, and the patient is carefully monitored during the transfusion.

Cold Agglutinin Disease

Cold agglutinins are autoantibodies of the IgM class that react optimally at 4° C and are commonly found in healthy individuals. These nonpathologic cold agglutinins are polyclonal, occur in low titers (less than 1:64 at 4° C), and have no reactivity above 30° C.[1,5] Most pathologic cold agglutinins are monoclonal, occur at high titers (greater than 1:1000 at 4° C), and are capable of reacting at temperatures greater than 30° C.[2] Because pathologic cold agglutinins can react at body temperature, they may induce cold agglutinin disease (CAD). Cold agglutinins that are able to bind RBC antigens near or at 37° C (high thermal amplitude) cause more severe symptoms.[1,12,13] CAD is also recognized as a clonal lymphoproliferative B cell disorder.[6,12] It comprises approximately 15% to 20% of the cases of autoimmune hemolytic anemia.[6]

In CAD, IgM autoantibodies bind to RBCs when the patient is exposed to cold temperatures, particularly in peripheral circulation and vessels of the skin, where temperatures can drop to 30° C.[13] During the brief transit of RBCs through these colder areas, IgM autoantibodies activate the classical complement pathway.[12] When RBCs return to the central circulation, the IgM antibody dissociates, but C3b components remain on the cell.[2,12] Hemolysis is predominantly extravascular by hepatic macrophages, which have receptors for C3b.[1,12] However, if the autoantibody has a high thermal amplitude or there is a deficiency in complement regulatory proteins, full complement activation and intravascular hemolysis can occur.[2,14]

Acute CAD occurs secondary to *Mycoplasma pneumoniae* infection, infectious mononucleosis, and other viral infections.

These cold agglutinins are polyclonal IgM, with a normal distribution of κ and λ light chains.[2,5] Chronic CAD is a rare hemolytic anemia that typically occurs in middle-aged and elderly individuals, and the autoantibody is usually monoclonal IgM with κ light chains.[6,12,13] In a study of 86 patients with chronic CAD by Berentsen and colleagues, the median age at onset was 67 years, with the median age at death reported to be 82 years.[12] Chronic CAD can be idiopathic, but it is usually secondary as a result of an underlying lymphoproliferative neoplasms such as B-lymphocytic lymphoma, Waldenström macroglobulinemia, or chronic lymphocytic leukemia.[12]

Clinical manifestations are variable in chronic CAD. Most patients have a mild anemia with a hemoglobin result ranging from 9 to 12 g/dL, but others can develop life-threatening anemia with hemoglobin levels falling to less than 5 g/dL, especially after exposure to cold temperatures.[5,13] Individuals often experience fluctuations between mild and severe symptoms, and approximately half of those affected require transfusions over the course of the disease.[12] Symptoms include fatigue, weakness, dyspnea, pallor (caused by the anemia), and acrocyanosis.[13] *Acrocyanosis* is a bluish discoloration of the extremities (fingers, toes, feet, earlobes, nose) as a result of RBC autoagglutination, which causes local capillary stasis and decreased oxygen delivery to the affected areas.[1,2,13] Some patients also have episodes of hemoglobinuria, especially after exposure to cold temperatures.[2,13] In contrast, patients with acute CAD may have mild to severe hemolysis that appears abruptly within 2 to 3 weeks after onset of infectious mononucleosis, other viral infection, or *M. pneumoniae* infection, but it resolves spontaneously within days to a few weeks.[13]

The DAT result is positive with polyspecific AHG because of the presence of C3d on the RBC surface.[1] Specificity of the cold agglutinin is most often anti-I but can be anti-i or, very rarely, anti-Pr.[2,14] Virtually all adult RBCs are positive for I antigen, so anti-I will agglutinate all screening and panel cells, donor RBCs, and the patient's own RBCs at room temperature and at temperatures greater than 30° C, depending on the thermal amplitude of the autoantibody. Anti-I will show weaker or negative reactions with cord RBCs (cord cells are negative for I antigen but positive for i antigen).[2]

A cold agglutinin test determines the titer of the autoantibody at 4° C. Pathologic cold agglutinins can reach titers of 1:10,000 to 1:1,000,000 at 4° C.[1,5] Blood specimens for cold agglutinin testing must be maintained at 37° C after collection to prevent binding of the autoantibody to the patient's own RBCs, which can falsely decrease the antibody titer in the serum. Alternatively, a specimen anticoagulated with ethylenediaminetetraacetic acid (EDTA) can be warmed for 15 minutes at 37° C to dissociate autoabsorbed antibody before determining the titer.

When a high-titer cold agglutinin is present, an EDTA-anticoagulated blood specimen can show visible agglutinates in the tube at room temperature or cooler.[1] Agglutination can also be observed on the peripheral blood film (Figure 23.5). Blood specimens from patients with cold agglutinins must be warmed to 37° C for at least 15 minutes before complete blood count analysis by automated blood cell analyzers. RBC agglutination grossly elevates the mean cell volume, reduces the RBC

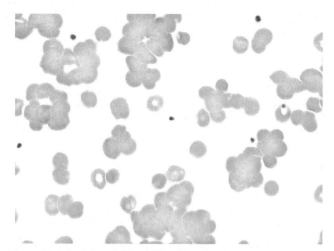

Figure 23.5 Peripheral Blood Film Showing Red Blood Cell Agglutination. (Wright-Giemsa stain, ×1000.)

count, and has unpredictable effects on other indices (Chapter 12). When the specimen is warmed to 37° C, antibody dissociates from RBCs and agglutination usually disappears. If not, a new specimen is collected and maintained at 37° C for the entire time before testing. To avoid agglutination on a peripheral blood film, the slide can also be warmed to 37° C before the application of blood. Cold agglutinins can also interfere with ABO typing.[2]

Acute CAD associated with infections is self-limiting, and cold agglutinin titers are usually less than 1:4000.[13] If hemolysis is mild, no treatment is required; however, patients with severe hemolysis require transfusion and supportive care.[13] Patients with chronic CAD and mild anemia are regularly monitored and advised to avoid cold temperatures.[1] In chronic CAD with moderate to severe symptoms, rituximab produces a partial response in about half of patients as a result of its targeting and ultimate destruction of B lymphocytes containing the CD20 antigen, but median remission is less than a year.[15] Rituximab-fludarabine and rituximab-bendamustine combination therapies have a better response rate, 76% and 71% respectively, with the later combination having fewer side effects and better tolerability.[16,17] Plasmapheresis is used in severe cases but provides only temporary benefit.[1] Corticosteroid therapy and immunosuppressive therapy with cyclophosphamide and chlorambucil are not effective for most patients.[13,14] Splenectomy is also not effective because C3b-sensitized RBCs in IgM-mediated autoimmune hemolysis are cleared primarily by the liver.[1,5,13]

RBC transfusion is reserved for patients with life-threatening anemia or cardiovascular or cerebrovascular symptoms.[1] If transfusion is needed, the presence of clinically significant *allo*antibodies must be ruled out.[2] In CAD cases involving an autoantibody with wide thermal amplitude, detection of coexisting warm-reactive alloantibodies can be time consuming and difficult. During transfusion, the patient is kept warm, small amounts of blood are given while the patient is observed for symptoms of a hemolytic transfusion reaction, and a blood warmer is used to minimize in vivo reactivity of the cold autoantibody.[1]

Paroxysmal Cold Hemoglobinuria

Paroxysmal cold hemoglobinuria (PCH) is an acute form of cold-reactive hemolytic anemia. PCH can be idiopathic or secondary. Secondary PCH was associated with late-stage syphilis, but now it is most commonly seen in young children after a viral respiratory infection.[1,2,13] PCH is rare in adults. The prevalence of PCH has been reported to be as high as 32% to 40% of children with autoimmune hemolytic anemia, with a median age at presentation of 5 years.[18,19]

Anti-P autoantibody, also called the *Donath-Landsteiner antibody,* is a complement-binding IgG hemolysin with specificity for P antigen on RBCs. Anti-P autoantibody is biphasic in that at cold temperatures it binds to the P antigen on RBCs and partially activates complement (C1 to C4), but full complement activation (C3 through C9) and hemolysis occur only upon warming to 37° C.[20] Anti-P autoantibody binds RBC antigen optimally at 4° C and has a thermal amplitude of less than 20° C. At warmer temperatures, anti-P autoantibody dissociates from RBCs; the titer is usually less than 1:64.[13]

Children typically present with acute fever, malaise, and back, leg, and/or abdominal pain 1 to 2 weeks after an upper respiratory tract infection.[13] Pallor, jaundice, and dark urine caused by hemoglobinuria are often present.[13] The abrupt onset of hemolysis causes a rapidly progressing and severe anemia, with hemoglobin levels often dropping to less than 5 g/dL.[13] Exposure to cold temperatures may precipitate hemolytic manifestations in some patients, but cold exposure is not required for the majority of patients to manifest symptoms; the reasons for this have yet to be explained.[2,19]

Reticulocytosis is typical but can be preceded by reticulocytopenia.[13] The peripheral blood film shows polychromasia and spherocytes, but schistocytes, nucleated RBCs, anisocytosis, poikilocytosis, and erythrophagocytosis can also be observed.[13] At first, leukopenia may be present; later, leukocytosis occurs.[13] In addition, laboratory findings typical for intravascular hemolysis are found. Because anti-P autoantibody is dissociated from RBCs at body temperature, the DAT result is usually positive for C3d only.[2,18]

The classic Donath-Landsteiner screening test for anti-P is done by collecting blood specimens in two tubes (without anticoagulant), one for the patient test and the other for the patient control.[19] The patient test specimen is incubated first at 4° C for 30 minutes (to allow anti-P binding to the P antigen and partial complement activation on RBCs) and then at 37° C for 30 minutes (to allow full activation of the complement pathway to lysis). The patient control tube is kept at 37° C for both incubations (a total of 60 minutes). After centrifugation serum is examined for hemolysis. A positive test result for anti-P is indicated by hemolysis in the patient test specimen incubated first at 4° C and then at 37° C and no hemolysis in the patient control specimen kept at 37° C. In the control tube, anti-P is not able to bind to antigen at 37° C, so complement is not activated and hemolysis does not occur.[19] Initial test results may be falsely negative as a result of low complement and/or anti-P levels in the patient specimen because of the brisk hemolysis in vivo.[19] Incubating patient serum with complement and papain-treated compatible group O RBCs increases the sensitivity of the test in detecting anti-P. Enzyme treatment provides greater exposure of the P antigen on the RBC surface for antibody binding.[19]

PCH is severe but self-limiting and resolves in several days to a few weeks, with an excellent prognosis.[1,13,18] In most patients, anemia is severe and can be life threatening, so transfusion is usually needed until the symptoms resolve. Because anti-P autoantibody reacts only at lower temperatures and P antigen-negative blood is very rare, P-positive blood can be transfused.[2]

Mixed-Type Autoimmune Hemolytic Anemia

Mixed-type AIHA occurs very infrequently.[21] In this condition the patient simultaneously develops an IgG autoantibody with optimum reactivity at 37° C (WAIHA) and a pathologic IgM autoantibody that reacts optimally at 0° C to 10° C but has a thermal amplitude of greater than 30° C (CAD).[21] Patients with WAIHA and a nonpathogenic cold agglutinin (i.e., an agglutinin that does not react at a temperature greater than 20° C) should not be classified as having a mixed-type AIHA because the cold agglutinin is not clinically significant.[13]

Hemolysis results from a combination of extravascular and intravascular mechanisms. The disease course appears to be chronic, with intermittent episodes of severe anemia.[5,13] The DAT is positive with IgG only, C3d only, or both IgG and C3d.[2] The warm autoantibody is typically panreactive with unclear specificity, whereas the cold-reacting antibody usually has anti-I specificity.[5] Treatment is the same as that described for WAIHA.[5]

ALLOIMMUNE HEMOLYTIC ANEMIAS

Hemolytic Transfusion Reaction

One of the most severe and potentially life-threatening complications of blood transfusion is a hemolytic transfusion reaction (HTR) caused by immune-mediated destruction of donor cells by an antibody in the recipient. The offending antibody in the recipient may be IgM or IgG, complement may be partially or fully activated or not activated at all, and hemolysis may be intravascular or extravascular, depending on the characteristics of the antibody. HTRs can have an acute or delayed onset.[2]

Acute Hemolytic Transfusion Reaction

Acute hemolytic transfusion reactions (AHTRs) occur within minutes to hours of initiation of a transfusion.[22] The most common cause of AHTR is accidental transfusion of ABO-incompatible donor RBCs into a recipient. An example is transfusion of group A RBCs into a group O recipient. The recipient has preformed, non-RBC stimulated anti-A (IgM) that is capable of fully activating complement to C9 upon binding to the A antigen on donor RBCs. There is rapid, complement-mediated intravascular hemolysis and activation of the coagulation system. ABO-incompatible RBC transfusions are usually a result of clerical error and have been estimated to occur in approximately 1 in 40,000, whereas the estimated risk of ABO HTR is 1:80,000.[2] Severity of AHTR is variable and is affected by the infusion rate and volume of blood transfused.[2,23] AHTR carries an estimated mortality rate of 2%.[22] AHTRs can occur as a result of incompatibilities involving other blood group systems, but these are rare.[22]

Symptoms of severe intravascular hemolysis found in ABO-related AHTRs begin within minutes or hours and may include chills, fever, urticaria, tachycardia, nausea and vomiting, chest and back pain, shock, anaphylaxis, pulmonary edema, congestive heart failure, and bleeding as a result of disseminated intravascular coagulation (DIC). The transfusion should be immediately terminated on first appearance of symptoms. Treatment is urgent and includes efforts to prevent or correct shock, maintain renal circulation, and control DIC.[23]

The immediate investigation of a suspected HTR includes a clerical check for errors, an examination of a posttransfusion blood specimen for hemolysis, and performance of the DAT on RBCs in a posttransfusion specimen.[22] If an AHTR occurred, hemoglobinemia and hemoglobinuria are detectable and the DAT result is positive. DAT findings may be negative, however, if all the donor cells are lysed.[22] Hemoglobin and serum haptoglobin levels decrease, but serum indirect bilirubin will not begin to rise until 2 to 3 days after the episode. ABO and Rh typing, antibody screen, and cross-matching are repeated on recipient and donor specimens to identify the blood group incompatibility. Coagulation tests such as D-dimer, fibrinogen, factors V and VIII, and platelet count can help reveal and assess the risk of DIC.[2]

Delayed Hemolytic Transfusion Reaction

Delayed hemolytic transfusion reaction (DHTR) may occur days to weeks after transfusion as the titer of alloantibodies increases.[2,23] Often the patient has been alloimmunized by pregnancy or previous transfusion, but the antibody titer was lower than the level of serologic detection at the time of transfusion. The second exposure to the antigen results in an increase in titer (anamnestic response). The antibody is usually IgG, is reactive at 37° C, and may or may not be able to partially or fully activate complement. Antibodies most often implicated in DHTRs are directed against antigens in the Duffy and Kidd blood group systems.[22,23] Patient's antibody binds to transfused RBCs, which leads to extravascular hemolysis, with or without complement activation. The principal signs are an inadequate posttransfusion hemoglobin increase, positive DAT results for IgG and/or C3d, morphologic evidence of hemolysis (spherocytes, polychromasia), and an increase in serum indirect bilirubin.[22] Management of DHTR includes monitoring of kidney function, especially in acutely ill patients.[22]

Hemolytic Disease of the Fetus and Newborn

Hemolytic disease of the fetus and newborn (HDFN) occurs when an IgG alloantibody produced by the mother crosses the placenta into the fetal circulation and binds to fetal RBCs that are positive for the corresponding antigen. IgG-sensitized fetal RBCs are cleared from the circulation by macrophages in the fetal spleen (extravascular hemolysis), and an anemia gradually develops. There is erythroid hyperplasia in the fetal bone marrow and extramedullary erythropoiesis in the fetal spleen, liver, kidneys, and adrenal glands.[24] As a result, many nucleated RBCs are released into the fetal circulation. If anemia is severe in utero, it can lead to generalized edema, ascites, and a condition called *hydrops fetalis,* which is fatal if untreated.[2,24] Anti-Kell antibodies are notable because they also cause anemia by suppressing fetal erythropoiesis.[24]

Rh Hemolytic Disease of the Fetus and Newborn

In Rh HDFN, which causes the highest number of fetal fatalities, an Rh (D)-negative mother has preformed anti-D antibodies (IgG, reactive at 37° C) from exposure to the D antigen either through immunization in a previous pregnancy with a D-positive baby or from previous transfusion of blood products with D-positive RBCs. In subsequent pregnancies the anti-D crosses the placenta, and if the fetus is D positive, the anti-D binds to D antigen sites on the fetal RBCs. These anti-D-sensitized fetal RBCs are cleared from the circulation by macrophages in the fetal spleen, and anemia and hyperbilirubinemia develop. Amniocentesis is accurate at predicting severe fetal anemia, but it is an invasive procedure and carries some risk of fetal loss.[24] If severe fetal anemia and HDFN caused by anti-D are suspected, a percutaneous umbilical fetal blood specimen can be obtained and tested for the hemoglobin level to determine the severity of the anemia; in addition, a noninvasive assessment of anemia can be done by ultrasound measurement of fetal cerebral blood flow.[2,24]

Laboratory findings. ABO, Rh typing, and an antibody screen are performed on the mother when the fetus is between 10 and 16 weeks' gestation and again at 28 weeks' gestation.[24] The antibody screen during pregnancy detects antibodies other than those caused by ABO incompatibility.[2] If the antibody screen is positive for a clinically significant antibody, an RBC panel is performed to identify the specificity of the antibody. Certain antibodies may be ignored if their corresponding antigens are poorly developed at birth, such as anti-I, anti-P1, anti-Le[a] and -Le[b]. Mothers with initial positive antibody screens are retested with an antibody screen every month until 28 weeks, then every 2 weeks thereafter; antibody titers are reported from each specimen. Titration of the antibody does not predict the severity of HDFN; rather, it helps determine when to monitor for HDFN by additional methods, such as spectrophotometric analysis of amniotic fluid bilirubin.[2,24] After the first affected pregnancy, the antibody titer is no longer useful, and other means of monitoring the fetus are used, such as amniocentesis and ultrasonography.[24]

An unimmunized D-negative mother receives antenatal Rh immune globulin (RhIG) at 28 weeks' gestation and again within 72 hours of delivery of a D-positive infant to prevent alloimmunization to the D antigen.[2] Even one antenatal dose of 200 μg RhIG will reduce by half the risk of the mother developing anti-D antibodies and having a child with HDFN in the next pregnancy.[25] Rh-negative women who experience spontaneous or induced abortion also receive Rh immune globulin.

At delivery, newborn testing is performed on umbilical cord blood. Neonates with Rh HDFN have a decreased hemoglobin level, increased reticulocyte count, and increased level of serum indirect bilirubin. The peripheral blood film shows polychromasia and many nucleated RBCs. ABO (only forward typing), Rh typing, and the DAT are also performed. The DAT result is positive for IgG, and anti-D can be demonstrated in an eluate of the infant's RBCs.[24]

Treatment for the affected infant. Treatment for a fetus affected by HDFN may include intrauterine transfusion, whereby pooled hemolyzed blood is removed via amniocentesis from the fetal abdomen and replaced with a small amount of fresh RBCs. This procedure can be used to correct fetal anemia and prevent hydrops fetalis.[26] Cordocentesis is also used, whereby fresh RBCs are injected into the umbilical vein. Survival rates of fetuses receiving transfusions are 85% to 90%; the risk of premature death from these procedures varies from 1% to 3%.[26] After delivery, the neonate may need exchange transfusions and phototherapy to reduce the level of serum indirect bilirubin and prevent kernicterus (bilirubin accumulation in the brain).[24] Prolonged postnatal anemia can be the result of a slow decrease of maternal antibody in the newborn's circulation; rare cases of prolonged anemia are documented in infants who received intrauterine transfusions.[27,28]

Hemolytic Disease of the Fetus and Newborn Caused by Other Blood Group Antibodies

ABO HDFN is more common than Rh HDFN and may occur during the first pregnancy. Unlike Rh HDFN, ABO HDFN is asymptomatic or produces mild hyperbilirubinemia and anemia. ABO HDFN is seen in some type A or B infants born to type O mothers who produce IgG anti-A and anti-B, which are capable of crossing the placenta. The disease is milder than Rh HDFN likely because A and B antigens are poorly developed on fetal and newborn RBCs, and other cells and tissues express A and B antigens, which reduces the amount of maternal antibody directed against fetal RBCs. The DAT result for the newborn with ABO HDFN is only weakly positive and may be negative. Spherocytes and polychromasia on the peripheral blood film are typical.[2] Table 23.3 presents a comparison of HDFN caused by ABO and Rh incompatibility.

HDFN can be caused by other IgG antibodies, particularly antibodies to the K, c, and Fy[a] antigens.[2] HDFN caused by other blood group antibodies is rare.[24,29-32] Antibody screening in the first trimester can assist in identifying rare antibodies that can cause HDFN.[33] Varying degrees of anemia, jaundice, and kernicterus are the adverse clinical outcomes in all forms of HDFN.

TABLE 23.3 Characteristics of Rh and ABO Hemolytic Disease of the Fetus and Newborn

	Rh	ABO
Blood groups	Mother: Rh (D) negative Child: Rh (D) positive	Mother: O Child: A or B
Severity of disease	Severe	Mild
Jaundice	Severe	Mild
Spherocytes on peripheral blood film	Rare	Usually present
Anemia	Severe	If present, mild
Direct antiglobulin test	Positive	Negative or weakly positive

DRUG-INDUCED IMMUNE HEMOLYTIC ANEMIA

Drug-induced immune hemolytic anemia (DIIHA) is very rare, with an estimated annual incidence of about 1 per million persons.[34] This condition is suspected when there is a sudden decrease in hemoglobin after administration of a drug, clinical and biochemical evidence of extravascular or intravascular hemolysis, and a positive DAT result.[35] More than 125 drugs have been reported to cause DIIHA, with the most common drug categories being antimicrobial (particularly penicillins and cephalosporins), antiinflammatory, and antineoplastic drugs.[36-38] The most common drugs implicated in DIIHA in the last 10 years are piperacillin, cefotetan, and ceftriaxone.[39] Severe, even fatal, cases have been reported.[34,37,40,41]

Mechanisms of Drug-Induced Immune Hemolysis

Various theories have been proposed to explain the mechanisms of DIIHA.[34,41] Three generally accepted mechanisms involve an antibody produced by the patient as a result of exposure to the drug and include drug adsorption, drug-RBC membrane protein immunogenic complex, and RBC autoantibody induction

(Figure 23.6). A fourth mechanism, drug-induced nonimmunologic protein adsorption (NIPA), can result in a positive DAT result, but no drug or RBC antibody is produced by the patient. This mechanism is discussed at the end of this section.

1. *Drug adsorption:* The patient produces an IgG antibody to a drug. When the drug is taken by the patient, the drug binds strongly to the patient's RBCs. The IgG drug antibody binds to the drug attached to the RBCs, usually without complement activation. Because the offending antibody is IgG and is strongly attached to the RBCs via the drug, hemolysis is extravascular by splenic macrophages, which remove the antibody- and drug-coated RBCs from the circulation.

2. *Drug-RBC membrane protein immunogenic complex:* A drug binds loosely to an RBC membrane protein to form a drug-RBC protein immunogenic complex or epitope. The patient produces an IgM and/or IgG antibody that binds to the complex on the RBCs, and complement is fully activated, which causes acute intravascular hemolysis.

3. *RBC autoantibody induction:* A drug induces the patient to produce IgG warm-reactive autoantibodies against RBC

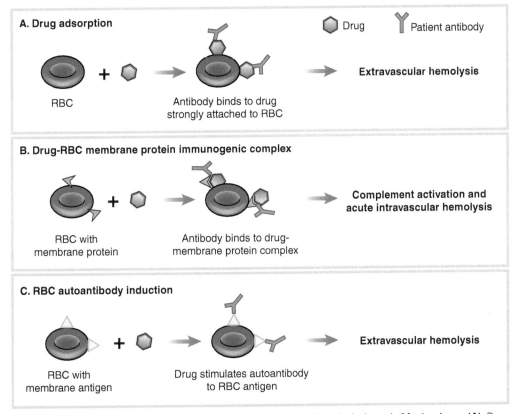

A. Drug adsorption

⬡ Drug   Y Patient antibody

RBC + ⬡ → Antibody binds to drug strongly attached to RBC → **Extravascular hemolysis**

B. Drug-RBC membrane protein immunogenic complex

RBC with membrane protein + ⬡ → Antibody binds to drug-membrane protein complex → **Complement activation and acute intravascular hemolysis**

C. RBC autoantibody induction

RBC with membrane antigen + ⬡ → Drug stimulates autoantibody to RBC antigen → **Extravascular hemolysis**

Figure 23.6 Graphic Representation of Drug-Induced Immune Hemolytic Anemia Mechanisms. (A), Drug adsorption. A drug binds (adsorbs) tightly to the red blood cell (RBC) membrane. The patient produces an antidrug immunoglobulin G (IgG) antibody that binds to the drug. RBCs coated with adsorbed drug bound with antidrug antibodies are removed from circulation by macrophages in the spleen (extravascular hemolysis). **(B),** Drug-RBC membrane protein immunogenic complex. A drug loosely binds to an RBC membrane protein forming a drug-RBC protein complex. The patient produces an IgG and/or IgM (not shown) antibody that binds to the complex, causing complement activation and acute intravascular hemolysis. **(C),** RBC autoantibody induction. A drug induces the patient to produce IgG warm-reactive autoantibodies against RBC self-antigens. The IgG autoantibodies bind to the corresponding antigens on the RBC surface. RBCs coated with IgG autoantibodies are removed from circulation by macrophages in the spleen (extravascular hemolysis).

self-antigens. These autoantibodies react at 37° C, and the laboratory findings are indistinguishable from those in WAIHA. Hemolysis is extravascular and is mediated by macrophages predominantly in the spleen.

Several authors have suggested that all drug-induced immune hemolysis is explained by a single mechanism, known as the *unifying theory*. This theory proposes that a drug interacts with the RBC membrane and generates multiple immunogenic epitopes that can elicit an immune response to the drug alone, to the drug-RBC membrane protein combination, or to an RBC membrane protein alone.[2,36,42] Diagnosis of DIIHA can only be made if the antibody screen is positive and the RBC eluate contains an antibody.[1]

Antibody Characteristics

Antibodies implicated in DIIHA can be divided into two general types: drug-dependent (most common) and drug-independent antibodies.[2,36] Some drugs are able to induce a combination of both types of antibodies.[34,41,42]

Drug-Dependent Antibodies

Drug-dependent antibodies only react in vitro when the suspected drug or its metabolite is present.[2,36] There are two types of drug-dependent antibodies:

1. *Antibodies that react only with drug-treated cells*[2]: These are IgG drug antibodies that bind to the drug when it is strongly associated with the RBC surface (drug adsorption mechanism). Because they have bound IgG, RBCs are cleared from the circulation extravascularly by macrophages in the spleen, and a hemolytic anemia gradually develops. Complement is not usually activated. If the DIIHA is not recognized, the patient may continue to take the drug to a point in which life-threatening anemia develops.[2,34] Examples of drugs that elicit antibodies in this category are penicillin, ampicillin, and many cephalosporins.[2,36,38,39] Laboratory features include a positive DAT reaction with anti-IgG, whereas the reaction with anti-C3b/C3d is usually negative. In the IAT, the patient's serum and an eluate of the patient's cells react only with drug-treated RBCs and not with untreated RBCs.[2]

2. *Antibodies that react only in the presence of the drug*[2]: These IgG and/or IgM antibodies bind to the drug or its metabolite only when it is weakly associated in a drug-RBC membrane protein complex (drug-RBC membrane protein immunogenic complex mechanism). The antibodies activate complement and trigger acute intravascular hemolysis that may progress to renal failure.[2] Hemolysis occurs abruptly after short periods of drug exposure or upon readministration of the drug.[34] Examples of drugs that elicit antibodies in this category are piperacillin and some second- and third-generation cephalosporins.[2,38,39] Laboratory features include a positive DAT reaction with anti-C3b/C3d and occasionally with anti-IgG. In the IAT, patient's serum reacts with untreated, normal RBCs only in the presence of the drug.

Drug-Independent Antibodies

Drug-independent antibodies are IgG, warm-reactive, RBC autoantibodies induced by the drug (RBC autoantibody induction mechanism). These autoantibodies have the same serologic reactivity as those causing WAIHA, and they do not require the presence of the drug for in vitro reactivity. Hemolysis is extravascular, mediated by macrophages predominantly in the spleen, usually with a gradual onset of anemia. A common example of a drug in this category is fludarabine.[2,39] Laboratory features include a positive DAT reaction with anti-IgG. In the IAT, patient's serum and an eluate of the patient's cells generally react at 37° C with all screening and panel RBCs and with the patient's own RBCs.[2]

Nonimmune Drug-Induced Hemolysis

In *drug-induced nonimmunologic protein adsorption (NIPA)*, the patient does not produce an antibody to the drug or to RBCs. The mechanism is also called the *membrane modification method,* because certain drugs such as high-dose clavulanate and cisplatin can alter the RBC membrane so that numerous proteins, including IgG and complement, adsorb onto the RBC surface.[36,41] Examples of drugs that cause NIPA and a positive DAT are cephalothin, diglycoaldehyde, cisplatin, oxaliplatin, and β-lactamase inhibitors.[2,38,39] This phenomenon is usually asymptomatic and results in a positive DAT finding, but only rarely has hemolysis been reported.[38] The IAT on patient's serum and an eluate of patient's RBCs yield negative results.[2,39]

Treatment

After a DIIHA is recognized and confirmed, the first treatment is to discontinue the drug. Most patients will gradually show improvement within a few days to several weeks.[34] In cases in which a warm-reacting autoimmune antibody is present, the positive DAT result may persist for months after a hematologic recovery. If anemia is severe, the patient may require RBC transfusion or plasma exchange.[34] Regardless of mechanism, future episodes of DIIHA are prevented by avoidance of the drug.

▌ SUMMARY

- Immune hemolytic anemias are classified into autoimmune hemolytic anemia, alloimmune hemolytic anemia, and drug-induced immune hemolytic anemia.
- Hemolysis mediated by immunoglobulin M (IgM) requires complement; hemolysis may be extravascular (mainly in the liver) if complement is partially activated to C3b, or intravascular if complement is fully activated to C9.

- Hemolysis mediated by IgG occurs with or without complement activation; IgG-sensitized red blood cells (RBCs) are removed from the circulation by macrophages in the spleen; partial phagocytosis produces spherocytes, which are prematurely trapped in the spleen and phagocytized; IgG- and C3b-sensitized RBCs are removed by macrophages in the spleen and liver.

- Laboratory findings in immune hemolytic anemia include decreased hemoglobin level, increased reticulocyte count, increased levels of serum indirect bilirubin and lactate dehydrogenase, and decreased serum haptoglobin level. The peripheral blood film may show polychromasia, spherocytes (IgG-mediated hemolysis), or RBC agglutination (cold agglutinins). The direct antiglobulin test (DAT) detects in vivo sensitization of RBCs by IgG and/or C3b/C3d.
- Classification of autoimmune hemolytic anemia (AIHA) includes warm autoimmune hemolytic anemia (WAIHA), cold agglutinin disease (CAD), paroxysmal cold hemoglobinuria (PCH), and mixed-type autoimmune hemolytic anemia.
- WAIHA is the most common form of AIHA and involves IgG autoantibodies with optimum reactivity at 37° C. Anemia varies from mild to severe, and characteristic morphologic features on the peripheral blood film are polychromasia and spherocytes.
- CAD is caused by an IgM autoantibody with optimum reactivity at 4° C and a thermal amplitude of greater than 30° C. RBC agglutination may be observed on a peripheral blood film, and agglutinates may cause interference with complete blood count analysis on automated blood cell analyzers.
- PCH is due to a biphasic IgG autoantibody with anti-P specificity. The antibody binds to P antigen on RBCs and partially activates complement at 4° C; complete complement activation and hemolysis occur upon warming the specimen to 37° C.
- Acute hemolytic transfusion reactions (AHTRs) occur within minutes to hours after the start of an RBC transfusion and most often involve transfusion of ABO-incompatible blood; the hemolysis is predominantly intravascular. Delayed hemolytic transfusion reactions (DHTRs) may occur days or weeks after the transfusion and represent an anamnestic response to a donor RBC antigen; hemolysis is usually extravascular.
- Hemolytic disease of the fetus and newborn (HDFN) occurs when an IgG alloantibody produced by the mother crosses the placenta into the fetal circulation and binds to fetal RBCs that are positive for the corresponding antigen. IgG-sensitized fetal RBCs are cleared from the circulation by macrophages in the fetal spleen, and an anemia gradually develops; the usual laboratory findings in the neonate are anemia, hyperbilirubinemia, and a positive DAT result.
- ABO HDFN is more common than Rh HDFN and produces no symptoms or mild anemia. Rh HDFN caused by anti-D results in severe anemia. Antenatal administration of Rh immune globulin to a D-negative mother when the fetus is at 28 weeks' gestation and within 72 hours after delivery of a D-positive baby prevents immunization to the D antigen.
- In drug-induced immune hemolytic anemia (DIIHA), the patient produces antibodies to (1) a drug only, (2) a complex of a drug loosely bound to an RBC membrane protein, or (3) an RBC membrane protein only. In vitro reactions of antibodies in DIIHA may be drug dependent or drug independent.

Now that you have completed this chapter, go back and read again the case study at the beginning and respond to the questions presented.

REVIEW QUESTIONS

Answers can be found in the Appendix.

1. Immune hemolytic anemia is due to a(n):
   a. Structural defect in the RBC membrane
   b. Allo- or autoantibody against an RBC antigen
   c. T cell immune response against an RBC antigen
   d. Obstruction of blood flow by intravascular thrombi

2. The pathophysiology of immune hemolysis with IgM antibodies always involves:
   a. Complement
   b. Autoantibodies
   c. Abnormal hemoglobin molecules
   d. Alloantibodies

3. In hemolysis mediated by IgG antibodies, which abnormal RBC morphology is typically observed on the peripheral blood film?
   a. Spherocytes
   b. Nucleated RBCs
   c. RBC agglutination
   d. Macrocytes

4. The most important finding in the diagnostic investigation of a suspected autoimmune hemolytic anemia is:
   a. Detection of a low hemoglobin and hematocrit
   b. Observation of hemoglobinemia in a specimen
   c. Recognition of a low reticulocyte count
   d. Demonstration of IgG and/or C3d on the RBC surface

5. In autoimmune hemolytic anemia, a positive DAT is evidence that an:
   a. IgM antibody is in the patient's serum
   b. IgG antibody is in the patient's serum
   c. IgM antibody is sensitizing the patient's red blood cells
   d. IgG antibody is sensitizing the patient's red blood cells

6. Which of the following is *not* a mechanism of drug-induced hemolytic anemia?
   a. Drug adsorption on red blood cell membrane
   b. Drug-RBC membrane protein immunogenic complex
   c. RBC autoantibody induction
   d. IgM autoantibody sensitization of RBCs after exposure to cold temperatures

7. Which of the following describes a penicillin-induced AIHA?
   a. Extravascular hemolysis, positive DAT with IgG, gradual anemia
   b. Intravascular, possible renal failure, positive DAT with C3d
   c. Extravascular hemolysis, positive DAT with C3d, acute onset
   d. Intravascular hemolysis, positive DAT with IgG

8. Which one of the following statements is *true* about DHTR?
   a. It usually is due to an ABO incompatibility
   b. Hemoglobinemia and hemoglobinuria often occur
   c. It is due to an anamnestic response after repeat exposure to a blood group antigen
   d. The DAT yields a positive result for C3d only

9. Chronic secondary CAD is most often associated with:
   a. Antibiotic therapy
   b. *M. pneumoniae* infection
   c. B cell malignancies
   d. Infectious mononucleosis

10. A 63-year-old man is being evaluated because of a decrease in hemoglobin of 5 g/dL after a second cycle of fludarabine for treatment of chronic lymphocytic leukemia. The patient's DAT result is strongly positive for IgG only, and antibody testing on his serum and an eluate of his RBCs yield positive results with all panel cells and the patient's own cells. This suggests which mechanism of immune hemolysis for this patient?
    a. Drug-RBC membrane protein complex
    b. Drug adsorption
    c. RBC autoantibody induction
    d. Drug-induced nonimmunologic protein adsorption

11. A group A Rh-negative mother gave birth to a group O Rh-positive baby. The baby is at risk for HDFN if:
    a. This was the mother's first pregnancy
    b. The mother has IgG ABO antibodies
    c. The mother was previously immunized to the D antigen
    d. The mother received Rh immune globulin before delivery

REFERENCES

1. Michel, M., & Jäger, U. (2018). Autoimmune hemolytic anemia. In Hoffman, R., Benz, E. J., Silberstein, L. E., et al. (Eds.), *Hematology: Basic Principles and Practice*. (7th ed., pp. 648–662). Philadelphia: Elsevier.

2. Leger, R. M., & Borge, P. D. (2017). The positive direct antiglobulin test and immune-mediated hemolysis. In Fung, M. K., Eder, A. F., Spitalnik, S. L., et al. (Eds.), *Technical Manual*. (19th ed., pp. 385–411). Bethesda, MD: American Association of Blood Banks.

3. Araten, D. J., Mandle, R. J., Isenman, D. E., et al. (2018). Complement and immunoglobulin biology leading to clinical translation. In Hoffman, R., Benz, E. J., Silberstein, L. E., et al. (Eds.), *Hematology: Basic Principles and Practice*. (7th ed., pp. 261–284). Philadelphia: Elsevier.

4. Morgan, B. P. (2013). Complement. In Paul, W. E. (Ed.), *Fundamental Immunology*. (7th ed., pp. 863–890). Philadelphia: Lippincott Williams & Wilkins.

5. Friedberg, R. C., & Johari, V. P. (2014). Autoimmune hemolytic anemia. In Greer, J. P., Arber, D. A., Glader, B., et al. (Eds.), *Wintrobe's Clinical Hematology*. (13th ed., 746–765). Philadelphia: Lippincott Williams & Wilkins.

6. Michel, M. (2011). Classification and therapeutic approaches in autoimmune hemolytic anemia: an update. *Expert Rev Hematol, 4*, 607–618.

7. Dhingra, K., Jain, D., Mandal, S., et al. (2008). Evans syndrome: a study of six cases with review of literature. *Hematology, 13*, 356–360.

8. Salama, A. (2015). Treatment options for primary autoimmune hemolytic anemia: a short comprehensive review. *Transfus Med Hemother, 42*, 294–301.

9. Kalfa, T. A. (2016). Warm antibody autoimmune hemolytic anemia. *Hematology Am Soc Hematol Educ Program, 2016*, 690–697.

10. Buckley, L., Guyatt, G., & Fink, H. A. (2017). 2017 American College of Rheumatology guideline for the prevention and treatment of glucocorticoid-induced osteoporosis. *Arthritis Care Res, 69*(8), 1095–1110.

11. Reynaud, Q., Durieu, I., Dutertre, M., et al. (2015). Efficacy and safety of rituximab in autoimmune hemolytic anemia: a meta-analysis of 21 studies. *Autoimmun Rev, 14*(4), 304–313.

12. Berentsen, S., Beiske, K., & Tjonnfjord, G. (2007). Primary chronic cold agglutinin disease: an update on pathogenesis, clinical features and therapy. *Hematology, 12*, 361–370.

13. Petz, L. (2008). Cold antibody autoimmune hemolytic anemias. *Blood Rev, 22*, 1–15.

14. Berentsen, S., Ulvestad, E., Langholm, R., et al. (2006). Primary chronic cold agglutinin disease: a population based clinical study of 86 patients. *Haematologica, 91*, 460–466.

15. Schöllkopf, C., Kjeldsen, L., Bjerrum, O. W., et al. (2006). Rituximab in chronic cold agglutinin disease: a prospective study of 20 patients. *Leuk Lymphoma, 47*, 253–260.

16. Berentsen, S., Randen, U., Vagan, A., et al. (2010). High response rate and durable remissions following fludarabine and rituximab combination therapy for chronic cold agglutinin disease. *Blood, 116*, 3180–3184.

17. Berensten, S., Randen, U., Oksman, M., et al. (2017). Bendamustine plus rituximab for chronic cold agglutinin disease: results of a Nordic prospective multicenter trial. *Blood, 130*(4), 537–541.

18. Karafin, M., Shirey, S., Ness, P., et al. (2012). A case study of a child with chronic hemolytic anemia due to a Donath-Landsteiner positive, IgM anti-I autoantibody. *Pediatr Blood Cancer, 59*, 953–955.

19. Gertz, M. (2007). Management of cold haemolytic syndrome. *Br J Haematol, 138*, 422–429.

20. Sokol, R., Hewitt, S., & Stamps, B. (1981). Autoimmune haemolysis: an 18 year study of 865 cases referred to a regional transfusion centre. *Br Med J, 282*, 2023–2027.

21. Mayer, B., Yurek, S., Kiesewetter, H., et al. (2008). Mixed-type autoimmune hemolytic anemia: differential diagnosis and critical review of reported cases. *Transfusion, 48*, 2229–2234.

22. McCullough, J., Refaai, M. A., & Cohn, C. S. (2016). Blood procurement and red cell transfusion. In Kaushansky, K., Lichtman, M. A., Prchal, J. T., et al. (Eds.), *Williams Hematology*. (9th ed., pp. 2365–2380). New York: McGraw-Hill.

23. Eder, A., & Chambers, L. (2007). Noninfectious complications of blood transfusion. *Arch Pathol Lab Med, 131*, 708–718.

24. Fasano, R. M., Hendrickson, J. E., & Luban, N. L. C. (2016). Alloimmune hemolytic disease of the fetus and newborn. In Kaushansky, K., Lichtman, M. A., Prchal, J. T., et al. (Eds.),

Williams Hematology. (9th ed., pp. 847–862). New York: McGraw-Hill.

25. Koelewijn, J., Haas, M., Vrijkotte, T., et al. (2008). One single dose of 200 µg of antenatal RhIG halves the risk of anti-D immunization and hemolytic disease of the fetus and newborn in the next pregnancy. *Transfusion, 48,* 1721–1729.

26. Dodd, J. M., Windrim, R. C., & van Kamp, I. L. (2012). Techniques of intrauterine fetal transfusion for women with red-cell isoimmunisation for improving health outcomes. *Cochrane Database Syst Rev,* (9), CD007096.

27. Patel, L. L., Myers, J. C., Palma, J. P., et al. (2013). Anti-Ge3 causes late-onset hemolytic disease of the newborn: the fourth case in three Hispanic families. *Transfusion, 53,* 2152–2157.

28. Dorn, I., Schlenke, P., & Hartel, C. (2010). Prolonged anemia in an intrauterine-transfused neonate with Rh-negative hemolytic disease: no evidence for anti-D-related suppression of erythropoiesis in vitro. *Transfusion, 50,* 1064–1070.

29. Michalewska, B., Wielgos, M., Zupanska, B., et al. (2008). Anti-Coᵃ implicated in severe haemolytic disease of the foetus and newborn. *Transfus Med, 18,* 71–73.

30. Dohmen, S., Muit, J., Ligthart, P., et al. (2008). Anti-e found in a case of hemolytic disease of the fetus and newborn makes use of the IGHV3 superspecies genes. *Transfusion, 48,* 194–194.

31. van Gammeren, A. J., Overbeeke, M. A., Idema, R. N., et al. (2008). Haemolytic disease of the newborn because of rare anti-Vel. *Transfus Med, 18,* 197–198.

32. Li, B. J., Jiang, Y. J., Yuan, F., et al. (2010). Exchange transfusion of least incompatible blood for severe hemolytic disease of the newborn due to anti-Rh17. *Transfus Med, 20,* 66–69.

33. Koelewijn, J. M., Vrijkotte, T. G., van der Schoot, C. E., et al. (2008). Effect of screening for red cell antibodies, other than anti-D, to detect hemolytic disease of the fetus and newborn: a population study in the Netherlands. *Transfusion, 48,* 941–952.

34. Garratty, G. (2010). Immune hemolytic anemia associated with drug therapy. *Blood Rev, 24,* 143–150.

35. Johnson, S., Fueger, J., & Gottschall, J. (2007). One center's experience: the serology and drugs associated with drug-induced hemolytic anemia—a new paradigm. *Transfusion, 47,* 697–702.

36. Garratty, G. (2009). Drug-induced immune hemolytic anemia. *Hematology Am Soc Hematol Educ Program, 2009,* 73–79.

37. Garratty, G., & Arndt, P. (2007). An update on drug-induced immune hemolytic anemia. *Immunohematology, 23,* 105–119.

38. Renard, D., & Rosselet, A. (2017). Drug-induced hemolytic anemia: pharmacological aspects. *Transfus Clin Biol, 24*(3), 110–114.

39. Garratty, G., & Arndt, P. A. (2014). Drugs that have been shown to cause drug-induced immune hemolytic anemia or positive direct antiglobulin tests: some interesting findings since 2007. *Immunohematology, 30*(2), 66–79.

40. Gupta, S., Piefer, C., Fueger, J., et al. (2010). Trimethoprim-induced immune hemolytic anemia in a pediatric oncology patient presenting as an acute hemolytic transfusion reaction. *Pediatr Blood Cancer, 55,* 1201–1203.

41. Arndt, P., Garratty, G., Isaak, E., et al. (2009). Positive direct and indirect antiglobulin tests associated with oxaliplatin can be due to drug antibody and/or drug-induced nonimmunologic protein adsorption. *Transfusion, 49,* 711–718.

42. Salama, A. (2009). Drug-induced immune hemolytic anemia. *Expert Opin Drug Saf, 8,* 73–79.

Hemoglobinopathies (Structural Defects in Hemoglobin)

Tim R. Randolph

OBJECTIVES

After completion of this chapter, the reader will be able to:

1. Explain the difference between structural hemoglobin disorders and thalassemias, and describe the types of mutations found in the structural disorders.
2. Describe globin gene structure and the development of normal human hemoglobins throughout prenatal and postnatal life.
3. Differentiate between homozygous and heterozygous states and the terms *disease* and *trait* as they relate to the hemoglobinopathies.
4. Given the hemoglobin genotypes of parents involving common β chain variants, determine the possible genotypes of their children using a Punnett square.
5. Describe the general geographic distribution of common hemoglobin variants and the relationship of that distribution with the prevalence of malaria.
6. For disorders involving hemoglobin (Hb) S and Hb C, describe the genetic mutation, effect of the mutation on the hemoglobin molecule, inheritance pattern, pathophysiology, symptoms, clinical findings, peripheral blood findings, laboratory diagnosis, and genetic counseling and treatment considerations.
7. Describe the genetic mutation, clinical findings, and laboratory diagnosis for disorders involving Hb C-Harlem, Hb E, Hb O-Arab, Hb D, and Hb G.
8. Describe the clinical and laboratory findings for the compound heterozygous disorders of Hb S with Hb C, β-thalassemia, Hb D, Hb O-Arab, Hb Korle Bu, and Hb C-Harlem.
9. Describe the electrophoretic mobility of Hb A, Hb F, Hb S, and Hb C at an alkaline pH, and explain how other methods (including the Hb S solubility test, citrate agar electrophoresis at acid pH, and high-performance liquid chromatography) are used to distinguish Hb S and Hb C from other hemoglobins with the same alkaline electrophoresis mobility.
10. Describe the genetic mutations, inheritance patterns, pathophysiology, and clinical and laboratory findings in hemoglobin variants that result in methemoglobinemia.
11. Describe the inheritance patterns, causes, and clinical and laboratory findings of unstable hemoglobin variants.
12. Discuss the pathophysiology of hemoglobin variants with increased and decreased oxygen affinities, and explain how they differ from unstable hemoglobins.
13. Given a case history and clinical and laboratory findings, interpret test results to identify the hemoglobin variants present in the patient.

OUTLINE

CASE STUDY

After studying the material in this chapter, the reader should be able to respond to the following case study:

An 18-year-old African American woman was seen in the emergency department for fever and abdominal pain. The following results were obtained on a complete blood count:

	Patient Results	Reference Intervals
WBCs ($\times 10^9$/L)	11.9	3.6–10.6
RBCs ($\times 10^{12}$/L)	3.67	4.00–5.40
HGB (g/dL)	10.9	12.0–15.0
HCT (%)	32.5	35–49
RDW (%)	19.5	11.5–14.5
Platelets ($\times 10^9$/L)	410	150–450
Segmented neutrophils (%)	75	50–70
Lymphocytes (%)	18	18–42
Monocytes (%)	3	2–11
Eosinophils (%)	3	1–3
Basophils (%)	1	0–2
Reticulocytes (%)	3.1	0.5–2.5

A typical field in the patient's peripheral blood film is shown in Figure 24.1. Alkaline hemoglobin electrophoresis showed 50.9% Hb S and 49.1% Hb C.

1. Select confirmatory tests that should be performed and describe the expected results.
2. Describe the characteristic red blood cell morphology on the peripheral blood film.

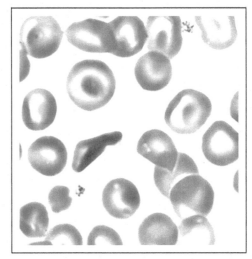

Figure 24.1 Peripheral Blood Film for the Patient in the Case Study. (Wright-Giemsa stain, ×1000.) (Courtesy Ann Bell, University of Tennessee, Memphis.)

3. Based on the electrophoresis and red blood cell morphology results, what diagnosis is suggested?
4. If this patient were to marry a person of genotype Hb AS, what would be the expected frequency of genotypes for each of four children?

Hemoglobinopathy refers to a disease state *(opathy)* involving the hemoglobin (Hb) molecule. Hemoglobinopathies are the most common genetic diseases, affecting approximately 7% of the world's population.[1] More than 300,000 children are born each year with some form of inherited hemoglobin disorder and approximately 80% occur in mid- to low-income countries.[2] All hemoglobinopathies result from a genetic mutation in one or more genes that affect hemoglobin synthesis. The genes that are mutated can code for either proteins that make up the hemoglobin molecule (globin or polypeptide chains) or proteins involved in synthesizing or regulating synthesis of the globin chains. Regardless of the mutation encountered, all hemoglobinopathies affect hemoglobin synthesis in one of two ways: qualitatively or quantitatively. In qualitative hemoglobinopathies, hemoglobin synthesis occurs at a normal or near-normal rate, but the hemoglobin molecule has an altered amino acid sequence within the globin chains. This change in amino acid sequence can alter the structure of the hemoglobin molecule (structural defect) and its function (qualitative defect). In contrast, thalassemias result in a reduced rate of hemoglobin synthesis (quantitative) but do not affect the amino acid sequence of the affected globin chains. A reduction in the amount of hemoglobin synthesized produces an anemia and stimulates the production of other hemoglobins not affected by the mutation in an attempt to compensate for the anemia. Based on this distinction, hematologists divide hemoglobinopathies into two categories: structural defects (qualitative) and thalassemias (quantitative). To add confusion to the classification scheme, many hematologists also refer to *only* the structural defects as hemoglobinopathies. This chapter describes the structural or qualitative defects that are referred to as *hemoglobinopathies*; the quantitative defects (thalassemias) are described in Chapter 25.

STRUCTURE OF GLOBIN GENES

As discussed in Chapter 7, there are six functional human globin genes located on two different chromosomes. Two of the globin genes, α and ζ, are located on chromosome 16 and are referred to as *α-like genes*. The remaining four globin genes, β, γ, δ, and ε, are located on chromosome 11 and are referred to as *β-like genes*. In the human genome there is one copy of each globin gene per chromatid, for a total of two genes per diploid nucleus, with the exception of α and γ. There are two copies of the α and γ genes per chromatid, for a total of four genes per diploid nucleus. Each globin gene codes for the corresponding globin chain: the α-globin genes *(HBA1* and *HBA2)* are used as the template to synthesize the α-globin chains, the β-globin gene *(HBB)* codes for the β-globin chain, the γ-globin genes *(HBG1* and *HBG2)* code for the γ-globin chains, and the δ-globin gene *(HBD)* codes for the δ-globin chain.

HEMOGLOBIN DEVELOPMENT

As discussed in Chapter 7, each human hemoglobin molecule is composed of four globin chains: a pair of α-like chains and a pair of β-like chains. During the first 3 months of embryonic life, only one α-like gene (ζ) and one β-like gene (ϵ) are activated, which results in the production of ζ- and ϵ-globin chains that pair to form hemoglobin Gower-1 ($\zeta_2\epsilon_2$). Shortly thereafter, α and γ chain synthesis begins, which leads to the production of Hb Gower-2 ($\alpha_2\epsilon_2$) and Hb Portland ($\zeta_2\gamma_2$). Later in fetal development, ζ and ϵ synthesis ceases; this leaves α and γ chains, which pair to produce Hb F ($\alpha_2\gamma_2$), also known as *fetal hemoglobin*. During the 6 months after birth, γ chain synthesis gradually decreases and is replaced by β chain synthesis so that Hb A ($\alpha_2\beta_2$), also known as *adult hemoglobin*, is produced. BCL11A and Krüppel-like factor 1 (KLF1), zinc-finger transcriptional repressors, are necessary to silence the γ-globin gene and are part of a complex mechanism involved in γ-β switching; mutations in the gene that codes for either factor results in elevated Hb F levels.[3] The remaining δ-globin gene, becomes activated around birth, producing δ chains at low levels that pair with α chains to produce the second adult hemoglobin, Hb A_2 ($\alpha_2\delta_2$). Normal adults produce Hb A (95%), Hb A_2 (less than 3.5%), and Hb F (less than 1% to 2%).

GENETIC MUTATIONS

More than 1200 structural hemoglobin variants (hemoglobinopathies) are known to exist throughout the world, and more are being discovered regularly (Table 24.1).[4,5] Each of these

TABLE 24.1 Genetic Abnormalities of Hemoglobin Variants

NUMBER OF VARIANTS BY GLOBIN CHAIN*				
	α	β	δ	γ	Total
Point mutations with amino acid substitution	444	564	73	97	1178
Deletions	19	37	1	1	58
Insertions	12	16	0	0	28
Duplications	1	1	0	0	2
Total	476	618	74	98	1266
Fusions	—	—	—	—	9**

*The table provides a relative distribution of mutation types and only includes structural variants. Fifty one of the variants are also categorized as thalassemias. Mutations include those identified as of 2017; genetic discovery is ongoing.

**Seven fusions involve the β and δ chains; two fusions involve the β and γ chains.

Data from Patrinos, G. P., Giardine, B., Riemer, W., et al. (2004). Improvements in the HbVar database of human hemoglobin variants and thalassemia mutations for population and sequence variation studies, *Nucl Acids Res, 32*(database issue), D537-541. http://globin.cse.psu.edu/hbvar/menu.html. Accessed August 1, 2017.

hemoglobin variants results from one or more genetic mutations that alter the amino acid sequence of a hemoglobin polypeptide chain. Some of these changes alter the molecular structure of the hemoglobin molecule, ultimately affecting hemoglobin function. The types of genetic mutations that occur in the hemoglobinopathies include point mutations, deletions, insertions, and fusions involving one or more of the adult globin genes, namely, α, β, γ, and δ.[5]

Point mutation is the most common type of genetic mutation occurring in the hemoglobinopathies. Point mutation is the replacement of one original nucleotide in the normal gene with a different nucleotide. Because one nucleotide is replaced by one nucleotide, the codon triplet remains intact, and the reading frame is unaltered. This results in the substitution of one amino acid in the globin chain product at the position corresponding to the codon containing the point mutation. As can be seen in Table 24.1, 1178 of the 1275 known hemoglobin variants result from a point mutation that causes an amino acid substitution. It also is possible to have two point mutations occurring in the same globin gene, which results in two amino acid substitutions within the same globin chain. More than 35 mutations occur by this mechanism.[5]

Deletions involve the removal of one or more nucleotides, whereas insertions result in the addition of one or more nucleotides. Usually deletions and insertions are not divisible by three and disrupt the reading frame, which leads to the nullification of synthesis of the corresponding globin chain. This is the case for the quantitative thalassemias (Chapter 25). In hemoglobinopathies, the reading frame usually remains intact, however; the result is the addition or deletion of one or more amino acids in the globin chain product, which sometimes affects the structure and function of the hemoglobin molecule. Of the 1275 variants described in Table 24.1, 58 variants result from deletions and 28 from insertions.[5]

Chain extensions occur when the stop codon is mutated so that translation continues beyond the typical last codon. Amino acids continue to be added until another stop codon is reached by chance. This process produces globin chains that are longer than normal. Significant globin chain extensions usually result in degradation of the globin chain and a quantitative defect. If the extension of the globin chain is insufficient to produce significant degradation, however, the defect is qualitative and is classified as a hemoglobinopathy. Hemoglobin molecules with extended globin chains fold inappropriately, which affects hemoglobin structure and function.

Gene fusions occur when two normal genes break between nucleotides, switch positions, and anneal to the opposite gene. For example, if a β-globin gene and a δ-globin gene break in similar locations, switch positions, and reanneal, the resultant genes would be $\beta\delta$ and $\delta\beta$ fusion genes in which the head of the fusion gene is from one original gene and the tail is from the other. If the reading frames are not disrupted and the globin chain lengths are similar, the genes are transcribed and translated into hybrid globin chains. The fusion chains fold differently, however, and affect the corresponding hemoglobin function. Nine fusion globin chains have been identified (Table 24.1).

ZYGOSITY

Zygosity refers to the association between the number of gene mutations and the level of severity of the resultant genetic defect. Generally there is a level of severity associated with each normal gene that is mutated and used to synthesize the globin chain product. For the normal adult globin genes, there are four copies of the α and γ genes and two copies of the β and δ genes. In theory, this could result in four levels of severity for α and γ gene mutations and two levels of severity for the β and δ gene mutations. Expressed another way, if all things were equal, it would require twice as many mutations within the α and γ genes to produce the same physiologic effect as mutations within the β and δ genes. Because the γ and δ genes are transcribed and translated at such low levels in adults, however, mutations of either gene have little impact on overall hemoglobin function. In addition, because the dominant hemoglobin in adults, Hb A, is composed of α and β chains, β gene mutations affect overall hemoglobin function to a greater extent than the same number of α gene mutations. This partially explains the greater number of identified β chain variants compared with α chain variants, because a single β gene mutation is more likely to create a clinical condition than a single α gene mutation.

The inheritance pattern of β chain variants is referred to as *heterozygous* when only one β gene is mutated and *homozygous* when both β genes are mutated. The terms *disease* and *trait* are also commonly used to refer to the homozygous (disease) and heterozygous (trait) states.

PATHOPHYSIOLOGY

Pathophysiology refers to the manner in which a disorder translates into clinical symptoms. The impact of point mutations on hemoglobin function depends on the chemical nature of the substituted amino acid, where it is located in the globin chain, and the number of genes mutated (zygosity). The charge and size of the substituted amino acid may alter the folding of the affected globin chain. A change in charge affects the interaction of the substituted amino acid with adjacent amino acids. In addition, the size of the substituted amino acid makes the globin chain either more (large amino acids) or less (small amino acids) bulky. Therefore the charge and the size of the substituted amino acid determine its impact on hemoglobin structure by potentially altering the tertiary structure of the globin chain and the quaternary structure of the hemoglobin molecule. Changes in hemoglobin structure may affect function. Location of the substitution within the globin chain also has an impact on the degree of structural alteration and hemoglobin function based on its positioning within the molecule and the interactions with the surrounding amino acids. In the case of the sickle cell mutation, one amino acid substitution results in hemoglobin polymerization, leading to the formation of long hemoglobin crystals that stretch the red blood cell (RBC) membrane and produce the characteristic crescent moon or sickle cell shape.

Zygosity also affects the pathophysiology of the disease. In β-hemoglobinopathies, zygosity predicts two severities of disease. In homozygous β-hemoglobinopathies, in which both β genes are mutated, the variant hemoglobin becomes the dominant hemoglobin type and normal hemoglobin (Hb A) is absent. Examples are sickle cell disease (SCD, caused by Hb SS) and Hb C disease (Hb CC). In heterozygous β-hemoglobinopathies, one β gene is mutated and the other is normal, which suggests a 50/50 distribution. In an attempt to minimize the impact of the abnormal hemoglobin, however, the variant hemoglobin is usually present in lesser amounts than Hb A. Patients with homozygous SCD (Hb SS) inherit a severe form of the disease that occurs less often but requires lifelong medical intervention, which must begin early in life, whereas heterozygotes (Hb AS) are much more common but rarely experience overt symptoms.

Fishleder and Hoffman[6] divided the structural hemoglobins into four groups: abnormal hemoglobins that result in hemolytic anemia, such as Hb S and the unstable hemoglobins; abnormal hemoglobins that result in methemoglobinemia, such as Hb M; hemoglobins with either increased or decreased oxygen affinity; and abnormal hemoglobins with no clinical or functional effect. Imbalanced chain production also may be associated in rare instances with a structurally abnormal chain, such as Hb Lepore,[4] because of reduced production of the abnormal chain. A functional classification of selected hemoglobin variants is summarized in Box 24.1.

Many of the variants are clinically insignificant because they do not produce any physiologic effect. As discussed previously, most clinical abnormalities are associated with the β chain, followed by the α chain. Involvement of the γ and δ chains does occur, but because of the small amount of hemoglobin involved, it is rarely detected and is usually of no clinical consequence. Box 24.2 lists clinically significant abnormal hemoglobins. The most commonly occurring of the abnormal hemoglobins and the most severe is Hb S.

NOMENCLATURE

As hemoglobins were reported in the literature, they were designated by letters of the alphabet. Normal adult hemoglobin and fetal hemoglobin were called *Hb A* and *Hb F*. By the time the middle of the alphabet was reached, however, it became apparent that the alphabet would be exhausted before all mutations were named. Currently some abnormal hemoglobins are assigned a common designation and a scientific designation. The common name is selected by the discoverer and usually represents the geographic area where the hemoglobin was identified. A single capital letter is used to indicate a special characteristic of the hemoglobin

BOX 24.1   Functional Classification of Selected Hemoglobin (Hb) Variants

I. Homozygous: Hemoglobin Polymorphisms: Most Common Variants

Hb S: $\alpha_2\beta_2^{6Val}$ (severe hemolytic anemia; sickling)

Hb C: $\alpha_2\beta_2^{6Lys}$ (mild hemolytic anemia)

Hb D-Punjab: $\alpha_2\beta_2^{121Gln}$ (no anemia)

Hb E: $\alpha_2\beta_2^{26Lys}$ (mild microcytic anemia)

II. Heterozygous: Hemoglobin Variants Causing Functional Aberrations or Hemolytic Anemia in the Heterozygous State

A. Hemoglobins Associated with Methemoglobinemia and Cyanosis

Hb M-Boston: $\alpha_2^{58Tyr}\beta_2$

Hb M-Iwate: $\alpha_2^{87Tyr}\beta_2$

Hb Auckland: $\alpha_2^{87Asn}\beta_2$

Hb Chile: $\alpha_2\beta_2^{28Met}$

Hb M-Saskatoon: $\alpha_2\beta_2^{63Tyr}$

Hb M-Milwaukee-1: $\alpha_2\beta_2^{67Glu}$

Hb M-Milwaukee-2: $\alpha_2\beta_2^{92Tyr}$

Hb F-M-Osaka: $\alpha_2\gamma_2^{63Tyr}$

Hb F-M-Fort Ripley: $\alpha_2\gamma_2^{92Tyr}$

B. Hemoglobins Associated with Altered Oxygen Affinity

1. Increased affinity and erythrocytosis

Hb Chesapeake: $\alpha_2^{92Leu}\beta_2$

Hb J-Capetown: $\alpha_2^{92Gln}\beta_2$

Hb Malmo: $\alpha_2\beta_2^{97Gln}$

Hb Yakima: $\alpha_2\beta_2^{99His}$

Hb Kempsey: $\alpha_2\beta_2^{99Asn}$

Hb Ypsi (Ypsilanti): $\alpha_2\beta_2^{99Tyr}$

Hb Hiroshima: $\alpha_2\beta_2^{146Asp}$

Hb Rainier: $\alpha_2\beta_2^{145Cys}$

Hb Bethesda: $\alpha_2\beta_2^{145His}$

2. Decreased affinity (may have mild anemia or cyanosis)

Hb Kansas: $\alpha_2\beta_2^{102Thr}$

Hb Titusville: $\alpha_2^{94Asn}\beta_2$

Hb Providence: $\alpha_2\beta_2^{82Asn}$

Hb Agenogi: $\alpha_2\beta_2^{90Lys}$

Hb Beth Israel: $\alpha_2\beta_2^{102Ser}$

Hb Yoshizuka: $\alpha_2\beta_2^{108Asp}$

C. Unstable Hemoglobins

1. Hemoglobin may precipitate as Heinz bodies after splenectomy

Severe hemolysis: no improvement after splenectomy

Hb Bibba: $\alpha_2^{136Pro}\beta_2$

Hb Hammersmith: $\alpha_2\beta_2^{42Ser}$

Hb Bristol-Alesha: $\alpha_2\beta_2^{67Asp\ or\ 67Met}$

Hb Olmsted: $\alpha_2\beta_2^{141Arg}$

Severe hemolysis: improvement after splenectomy

Hb Torino: $\alpha_2^{43Val}\beta_2$

Hb Ann Arbor: $\alpha_2^{80Arg}\beta_2$

Hb Genova: $\alpha_2\beta_2^{28Pro}$

Hb Shepherds Bush: $\alpha_2\beta_2^{74Asp}$

Hb Köln: $\alpha_2\beta_2^{98Met}$

Hb Wien: $\alpha_2\beta_2^{130Asp}$

Mild hemolysis: intermittent exacerbations

Hb Hasharon: $\alpha_2^{47His}\beta_2$

Hb Leiden: $\alpha_2\beta_2^{6\ or\ 7}$ (Glu deleted)

Hb Freiburg: $\alpha_2\beta_2^{23}$ (Val deleted)

Hb Seattle: $\alpha_2\beta_2^{70Asp}$

Hb Louisville: $\alpha_2\beta_2^{42Leu}$

Hb Zurich: $\alpha_2\beta_2^{63Arg}$

Hb Gun Hill: $\alpha_2\beta_2^{91-95}$ (5 amino acids deleted)

No disease

Hb Etobicoke: $\alpha_2^{84Arg}\beta_2$

Hb Sogn: $\alpha_2\beta_2^{14Arg}$

Hb Tacoma: $\alpha_2\beta_2^{30Ser}$

2. Tetramers of normal chains; appear in α-thalassemias

Hb Bart: γ_4

Hb H: β_4

Modified from Elghetany, M. T., Schexneider, K. I., & Banki, K. (2017). Erythrocytic disorders. In McPherson, R. A., & Pincus, M. R. (Eds.), *Henry's Clinical Diagnosis and Management by Laboratory Methods.* (23rd ed., p. 580). St. Louis: Elsevier. Originally modified from Winslow, R. M., Anderson, W. F. (1983). The hemoglobinopathies. In Stanbury, J. B., Wyngaarden, J. B., Fredrickson, D. S., et al. (Eds.), *The Metabolic Basis of Inherited Disease.* (5th ed., pp. 2281–2317). New York: McGraw-Hill.

Updated from Patrinos, G. P., Giardine, B., Riemer, C., et al. (2004). Improvements in the HbVar database of human hemoglobin variants and thalassemia mutations for population and sequence variation studies, *Nucl Acids Res, 32* (database issue), D537–541. http://globin.cse.psu.edu/hbvar/menu.html. Accessed August 1, 2017.

Arg, Arginine; *Asn,* asparagine; *Asp,* aspartic acid; *Cys,* cysteine; *Gln,* glutamine; *Glu,* glutamic acid; *His,* histidine; *Leu,* leucine; *Lys,* lysine; *Met,* methionine; *Pro,* proline; *Ser* serine; *Thr,* threonine; *Tyr,* tyrosine; *Val,* valine.

variants, such as hemoglobins demonstrating identical electrophoretic mobility but containing different amino acid substitutions, as in Hb G-Philadelphia, Hb G-Copenhagen, and Hb C-Harlem. The variant description also can involve scientific designations that indicate the variant chain, the sequential and the helical number of the abnormal amino acid, and the nature of the substitution. The designation [β_6 (A_3) Glu →Val] for the Hb S mutation indicates the substitution of valine for glutamic acid in the A helix in the β chain at position 6.[4]

HEMOGLOBIN S

Sickle Cell Anemia

History

Although the origin of sickle cell anemia has not been identified, symptoms of the disease have been traced in one Ghanaian family back to 1670.[7] Sickle cell anemia was first reported by a Chicago cardiologist, Herrick, in 1910 in a West Indian student with severe anemia. In 1917 Emmel recorded that sickling occurred in non-anemic patients and in patients who were severely

The term *sickle cell disease* is used to describe a group of symptomatic hemoglobinopathies that have in common sickle cell formation and the associated crises. Patients with SCD are either homozygous for Hb S (SS) or are compound heterozygotes expressing Hb S in combination with another hemoglobin β chain mutation like Hb C or β-thalassemia. SCDs are the most common form of hemoglobinopathy, with Hb SS and the variants Hb SC and Hb S-β-thalassemia (Hb S-β-thal) occurring most often.

Inheritance Pattern

As stated earlier, globin genes that have two copies per chromosome resulting in four loci are α (chromosome 16) and γ (chromosome 11). Globin genes that have one copy per chromosome resulting in two loci are β and γ (chromosome 11). β-Hemoglobin variants are inherited as autosomal codominants, with one gene inherited from each parent.[4]

Patients with SCD (Hb SS, Hb SC, or Hb S-β-thal) have inherited a sickle (S) gene from one parent and an S, C, or β-thalassemia gene from the other. Among patients with SCD, individuals who are homozygotes (Hb SS) have more severe disease than individuals who are compound heterozygotes for Hb S (Hb SC or Hb S-β-thal). Heterozygotes (Hb AS) are generally asymptomatic but may have mild symptoms and may develop adverse events when subjected to extreme exertion as in military boot camp and high-level athletics.[11] Using Hb S and Hb C as examples, Figure 24.2 illustrates the inheritance of abnormal hemoglobins involving mutations in the β gene.

Prevalence

The highest frequency of the sickle cell gene is found in sub-Saharan Africa, where each year approximately 250,000 babies are born with SCD (Hb SS), representing 0.74% of all live births occurring in this area.[2,12] In contrast, approximately 2600 babies are born annually with SCD in North America and 1300 in Europe.[12] Globally the sickle cell gene occurs at the highest frequency in five geographic areas: sub-Saharan Africa,

anemic. In 1927 Hahn and Gillespie described the pathologic basis of the disorder and its relationship to the hemoglobin molecule. These investigators showed that sickling occurred when a solution of RBCs was deficient in oxygen and that the shape of the RBCs was reversible when that solution was oxygenated again.[4,8] In 1946 Beet reported that malarial parasites were present less often in blood films from patients with SCD than in individuals without SCD.[9] It was determined that the sickle cell trait confers a resistance against infection with *Plasmodium falciparum* occurring early in childhood between the time that passively acquired immunity dissipates and active immunity develops.[10] In 1949 Pauling showed that when Hb S is subjected to electrophoresis, it migrates differently than does Hb A. This difference was found to be caused by an amino acid substitution in the globin chain. Pauling and coworkers[4] defined the genetics of the disorder and clearly distinguished heterozygous sickle trait (Hb AS) from the homozygous state (Hb SS).

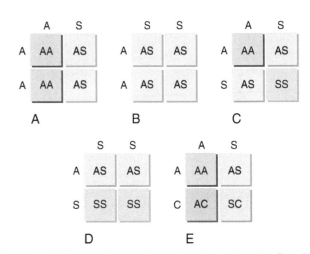

Figure 24.2 Punnett Square Examples Illustrating the Standard Method for Predicting the Inheritance of Abnormal Hemoglobins. Each parent contributes one gene.

Arab-India, the Americas, Eurasia, and Southeast Asia. In 2010 these five geographic areas accounted for 64.4%, 22.7%, 7.4%, 5.4%, and 0.1%, respectively, of all neonates born globally with sickle cell trait, and 75.5%, 16.9%, 4.6%, 3.0%, and 0% respectively, of all neonates born globally with sickle cell disease. Three countries accounted for approximately 50% of neonates with SS and AS genotypes: Nigeria, India, and DR Congo.[13] In the United States between 1 in 300 to 1 in 400 African American births (2000 annually) are diagnosed with sickle cell disease. Between 60% to 65% inherited two Hb S alleles (Hb SS), 25% to 30% have one Hb S and one Hb C allele (Hb SC), and 9% have a Hb S mutation with a β^0-thalasemia mutation.[14] Although in the United States, SCD is found mostly in individuals of African descent, it also has been found in individuals from the Middle East, India, and the Mediterranean area (Figure 24.3). SCD can also be found in individuals from the Caribbean and Central and South America. The sickle cell mutation is becoming more prominent in southern India, particularly in certain tribes.[15] Estimates indicate that 25,000 babies are born annually with sickle cell anemia in India.[2]

Etiology and Pathophysiology

Hb S is defined by the structural formula $\alpha_2\beta_2^{6Glu\rightarrow Val}$, which indicates that on the β chain at position 6, glutamic acid is replaced by valine. The mutation occurs in nucleotide 17, where thymine replaces adenine, resulting in a change in codon 6 and the substitution of valine (GTG) for glutamic acid (GAG) at amino acid position 6.[12] Glutamic acid has a net charge of (-1), whereas valine has a net charge of (0). This amino acid substitution produces a change in charge of $(+1)$, which affects the

electrophoretic mobility of the hemoglobin molecule. This amino acid substitution also affects the way the hemoglobin molecules interact with one another within the erythrocyte cytosol. Nonpolar (hydrophobic) valine is placed in the position that polar glutamic acid once held. Because glutamic acid is polar, the β chain folds in such a way that glutamic acid extends outward from the surface of the hemoglobin tetramer to bind water and contribute to hemoglobin solubility in the cytosol. In the mutated chain the hydrophobic valine is also extended outward, but instead of binding water, it seeks a hydrophobic niche with which to bind. When Hb S is fully oxygenated, the quaternary structure of the molecule does not produce a hydrophobic pocket for valine, which would allow the hemoglobin molecules to remain soluble in the erythrocyte cytosol like Hb A and maintain the normal biconcave disc shape of the RBCs. However, the natural allosteric change that occurs on deoxygenation creates a hydrophobic pocket in the area of phenylalanine 85 and leucine 88, which allows the valines from adjacent hemoglobin S molecules to bind. This hemoglobin pairing creates an orientation that facilitates other hemoglobin molecules to form electrostatic bonds between amino acids and becomes the seed for polymer formation. Other hemoglobin pairs polymerize, forming a hemoglobin core composed of four hemoglobin molecules that elongate in a helical formation. An outer layer of 10 hemoglobin molecules forms around the 4-hemoglobin-molecule core, creating the long, slender Hb S polymer.[16-19] Hb S molecules within the RBCs become less soluble, forming *tactoids* or liquid crystals of Hb S polymers that grow in length beyond the diameter of the RBC, causing sickling. In homozygotes the sickling

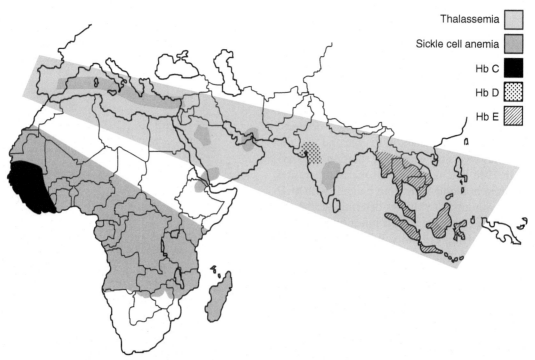

Figure 24.3 Geographic Distribution of Common Inherited Structural Hemoglobin Variants and the Thalassemias. (Modified from Hoffbrand, A. V., Pettit, J. E. [1993]. *Essential Haematology.* [3rd ed.]. Oxford: Blackwell Scientific.)

process begins when oxygen saturation decreases to less than 85%. In heterozygotes, sickling does not occur unless the oxygen saturation of hemoglobin is reduced to less than 40%. The blood becomes more viscous when polymers and sickle cells form.[20] Increased blood viscosity and sickle cell formation slow blood flow. In addition to a decrease in oxygen tension, there is a reduction in pH and an increase in 2,3-bisphosphoglycerate. Reduced blood flow prolongs the exposure of Hb S-containing RBCs to a hypoxic environment, and the lower tissue pH decreases oxygen affinity, which further promotes sickling. The end result is occlusion of capillaries and arterioles by sickled RBCs and infarction of surrounding tissue.

Sickle cells occur in two forms: reversible sickle cells and irreversible sickle cells.[21] Reversible sickle cells are Hb S-containing RBCs that change shape in response to oxygen tension. Reversible sickle cells circulate as normal biconcave discs when fully oxygenated but undergo hemoglobin polymerization, show increased viscosity, and change shape on deoxygenation. The vasoocclusive complications of SCD are thought to be due to reversible sickle cells that are able to travel into the microvasculature in the biconcave disk conformation because of their normal rheologic properties when oxygenated and then become distorted and viscous as they become deoxygenated, converting to the sickle cell configuration in the vessel.

In contrast, irreversible sickle cells do not change their shape regardless of the change in oxygen tension or degree of hemoglobin polymerization. These cells are seen on the peripheral blood film as elongated sickle cells with a point at each end. Irreversible sickle cells are likely recognized as abnormal by the spleen and removed from circulation, which prevents them from entering the microcirculation and causing vasoocclusion.

Not only the oxygen tension but also the level of intracellular hydration affects the sickling process. When RBCs containing Hb S are exposed to a low oxygen tension, hemoglobin polymerization occurs. Polymerized deoxyhemoglobin S activates a membrane channel called P_{sickle} that is otherwise inactive in normal RBCs. These membrane channels open when the blood partial pressure of oxygen decreases to less than 50 mm Hg. Open P_{sickle} channels allow the influx of Ca^{2+}, raising the intracellular calcium levels and activating a second membrane channel called the *Gardos channel*. An activated Gardos channel causes the efflux of K^+, which stimulates the efflux of Cl^- through another membrane channel to maintain charge equilibrium across the RBC membrane. The efflux of these ions leads to water efflux and intracellular dehydration, effectively increasing the intracellular concentration of Hb S and intensifying polymerization. Another contributor to K^+ and Cl^- efflux and the resultant dehydration is the K^+/Cl^- cotransporter system (Kcc1). Ironically, this system is activated by dehydration and positively charged hemoglobins such as Hb S and Hb C. The K^+/Cl^- cotransporter pathway is also activated by the low pH encountered in the spleen and kidneys. One potential explanation for the altered function of the membrane channels is oxidative damage triggered by Hb S polymerization. Injury to the RBC membrane induces adherence to endothelial surfaces, which causes RBC aggregation, produces ischemia, and exacerbates Hb S polymerization.[10]

Another important factor in the pathophysiology of SCD involves the redistribution of phospholipids in the RBC membrane, which contributes to hemolysis, vasoocclusive crisis, stroke, and acute chest syndrome. In the lipid bilayer membranes of normal RBCs choline phospholipids, like sphingomyelin and phosphatidylcholine, are located on the outer plasma layer whereas aminophospholipids, like phosphatidylserine (PS) and phosphatidylethanolamine, are primarily on the inner cytoplasmic layer. This asymmetric distribution of membrane phospholipids is accomplished by adenosine triphosphate-dependent enzymes called *translocases* or *flippases* (Chapter 6). Inhibition of flippases and activation of an enzyme called *scramblase* cause a more random distribution of membrane phospholipids, which increases the number of choline phospholipids on the interior half of the membrane and the number of aminophospholipids on the exterior membrane surface. The sickle cells of homozygotes (Hb SS) express 2.1% PS on RBC exterior surfaces compared with 0.2% for normal Hb AA controls.[22,23] Hb S polymerization may produce microparticles (discussed later) and iron complexes that adhere to the RBC membrane and generate reactive oxygen species, which, along with increased intracellular calcium and protein kinase C activation, may contribute to flippase inhibition and scramblase activation.[24,25] PS on the exterior surface of RBCs binds thrombospondin on vascular endothelial cells,[26] enhancing adherence between RBCs and the vessel wall and contributing to vasoocclusive crisis, activation of coagulation, and decreased RBC survival.[27,28] In addition, RBCs with PS on the external membrane surface are vulnerable to hydrolysis by secretory phospholipase A_2 ($sPLA_2$), which generates lysophospholipids and fatty acids like lysophosphatidic acid. This results in vascular damage that contributes to acute chest syndrome.[29,30]

Microparticles, previously known as "cellular dust," are submicron (100 to 1000 nm in diameter), unilamellar vesicles derived from parent cells that contribute to the pathophysiology of sickle cell disease. In sickle cell patients, microparticle vesicles contain a lipid bilayer with transmembrane and cytoskeletal proteins and a variety of cytoplasmic proteins, RNA, and mediators derived primarily from RBCs, platelets, endothelial cells, and monocytes. Microparticles are generated when these cells undergo stimulation, activation, or apoptosis. They form a complex biosystem that participates in cellular communication in normal and pathologic conditions after their phagocytosis by other cells, their binding to cell surface receptors, or their fusion with the cell membrane of target cells.[31]

In sickle cell disease, microparticles play a role in inflammation, coagulation, apoptosis, and angiogenesis. Inflammation and vasoocclusive crisis can induce the release of microparticles, which can, in turn, further modulate the inflammatory response. It is well established that inflammation can activate white blood cells (WBCs) and promote sickling, modulate the endothelium to increase RBC adhesion, and activate coagulation through tissue factor activation, all of which promotes vascular obstruction.[31] Chronic hypercoagulability observed in patients with SCD may be initiated by tissue factor aberrantly expressed by circulating blood cells or by microparticles derived from them. It is possible that the detection, quantification, and identification of microparticle subtypes could be used diagnostically or prognostically to predict clinical outcomes.[31]

In addition, initiation of vasoocclusion is thought to represent an interrelationship among hemolysis, inflammation, cellular adhesion, and gut flora translocated to the blood. Chronic hemolysis (intra- and extravascular) cause an increase in free heme iron and stimulates synthesis and release of erythropoietin. Increased erythropoietin and heme iron stimulate the release of placental growth factor, a vascular-endothelial growth factor that activates inflammatory pathways in the lung, producing reactive airway disease, which is common in children with SCD. Simultaneously, heme iron turnover in monocytes and macrophages stimulates a 200-fold increased expression of Toll-like receptor-4 (TLR-4) on their surface that presumably binds lipopolysaccharides on normal flora translocated from the gut to the blood.[32] This ligand binding activates the monocytes and macrophages, stimulating cytokine release and inflammation. Leukotrienes and cytokines, particularly interleukin 13 (IL-13), participate in reactive airway disease and stimulate the expression of P- and E-selectins on neutrophils, platelets, and endothelial cells, promoting vasoocclusion. Leukotrienes and IL-13 also stimulate the release of more placental growth factor to perpetuate the pathway.[32]

Clinical Features

Clinical manifestations of SCD can vary from no symptoms to a potentially lethal state. Symptoms also vary between ethnic groups with Indian patients expressing a much milder disease than their African counterparts.[15] People with SCD can develop a variety of symptoms as listed in Box 24.3. More than 1200 hemoglobin variants are known; however, only eight genotypes cause severe disease: Hb SS, Hb S-β^0-thal, severe Hb S-β^+-thal, Hb SD-Punjab, Hb SO-Arab, Hb SC-Harlem, Hb CS-Antilles, and Hb S-Quebec-CHORI. These eight clinically significant forms are listed in the order of severity and can have high morbidity and mortality rates. Three additional genotypes produce moderate disease: Hb SC, moderate Hb S-β^+-thal, and Hb AS-Oman. Three produce mild disease: mild Hb S-β^{silent}-thal, Hb SE, and Hb SA-Jamaica Plain. Two produce very mild disease: Hb S-HPFH and Hb S with a variety of mild variants.[12] Symptom variability in patients with SCD and across the genotypes listed earlier are largely caused by the intracellular ratio of Hb S to Hb F, as well as factors that affect vessel tone and cellular activation.[33] Individuals affected with SCD are characteristically symptom free until the second half of the first year of life because of the protective effect of Hb F.[34] In the first 6 months of life, mutant β chains gradually replace normal γ chains, which causes Hb S levels to increase and Hb F levels to decrease. RBCs containing Hb S become susceptible to hemolysis, and a progressive hemolytic anemia and splenomegaly may become evident.

Many individuals with SCD undergo episodes of recurring pain termed *crises*. Sickle cell crises were described by Diggs as "any new syndrome that develops rapidly in patients with SCD owing to the inherited abnormality."[35] The pathogenesis of the acute painful episode first described by Diggs is not fully understood. Various crises may occur: vasoocclusive or "painful," splenic sequestration, chronic hemolytic, megaloblastic, and aplastic. These crises and other sequellae of SCD are described next.

BOX 24.3 Clinical Features of Sickle Cell Disease

I. Vasoocclusion
  A. Causes
    Acidosis
    Hypoxia
    Dehydration
    Infection
    Fever
    Extreme cold
  B. Clinical manifestations
    1. Bones:
      Pain
      Hand-foot dactylitis
      Infection (osteomyelitis)
    2. Lungs:
      Pneumonia
      Acute chest syndrome
    3. Liver:
      Hepatomegaly
      Jaundice
    4. Spleen:
      Sequestration splenomegaly
      Autosplenectomy

  5. Penis:
    Priapism
  6. Eyes:
    Retinal hemorrhage
  7. Central nervous system
  8. Urinary tract:
    Renal papillary necrosis
  9. Leg ulcers
II. Bacterial infections
  A. Sepsis
  B. Pneumonia
  C. Osteomyelitis
III. Hematologic defects
  A. Chronic hemolytic anemia
  B. Megaloblastic episodes
  C. Aplastic episodes
IV. Cardiac defects
  A. Enlarged heart
  B. Heart murmurs
V. Other clinical features
  A. Stunted growth
  B. High-risk pregnancy

Vasoocclusive crisis. The hallmark of SCD is vasoocclusive crisis (VOC), which accounts for most hospital and emergency department visits. This acute, painful aspect of SCD occurs with great predictability and severity in many individuals and can be triggered by acidosis, hypoxia, dehydration, infection and fever, and exposure to extreme cold. Painful episodes manifest most often in bones, lungs, liver, spleen, penis, eyes, central nervous system, and urinary tract.

The pathogenesis of vasoocclusion in SCD is not fully understood, but Hb S polymerization and sickling of RBCs play a major role, with other factors also affecting this process. Most VOC events occur in capillaries and postcapillary venules.[6,36] The list of possible risk factors includes polymerization, decreased deformability, sickle cell–endothelial cell adherence, endothelial cell activation, WBC and platelet activation, hemostatic activation, and altered vascular tone.[36] Interrelationships among these risk factors is shown in Figure 24.4. Vasoocclusion can be triggered by any of these factors under various circumstances. During inflammation, increased WBCs interacting with endothelium, platelet activation causing elevation of thrombospondin level, or clinical dehydration resulting in an increase in von Willebrand factor can trigger RBC adherence to endothelium, precipitating vascular obstruction. Another mechanism of obstruction can be dense cells, which are less deformable and are at greatest risk for intracellular polymerization because of their higher Hb S concentration.[37,38] Vasoocclusive episodes gradually consume the patient organ by organ, through the destructive and debilitative effects of cumulative infarcts. Approximately 8% to 10% of SCD patients develop cutaneous manifestations in the form of ulcers or sores on the lower leg.[12]

The abnormal interaction between sickle cells and vascular endothelium seems to have a great impact on the vasoocclusive event. Endothelial adherence correlates significantly with the severity of painful episodes. In addition, sickle cell adherence to vascular endothelium results in intimal hyperplasia that can slow blood flow. Cells of patients with Hb SC disease produce less sickling with fewer adherent RBCs.[8]

The frequency of painful episodes varies from none to six per year.[8] On average, each episode persists for 4 to 5 days, although protracted episodes may last for weeks.

Splenic sequestration and infarcts. Splenic sequestration is characterized by a sudden trapping of blood in the spleen, which leads to a rapid decline in hemoglobin, often to less than 6 g/dL. This phenomenon occurs most often in infants and young children whose spleens are chronically enlarged. Children experiencing splenic sequestration episodes may have earlier onset of splenomegaly and a lower level of Hb F at 6 months of age.[8] Crises are often associated with respiratory tract infections.

Repeated splenic infarcts produce scarring resulting in diminished splenic tissue and abnormal function. Gradual loss of splenic function is referred to as *autosplenectomy* and is evidenced by the presence of Howell-Jolly and Pappenheimer bodies in RBCs on the peripheral blood film. Loss of splenic function contributes to an increased risk of bacterial infections.

Acute chest syndrome. Acute chest syndrome (ACS) is defined as an acute illness with fever and/or other respiratory symptoms (incuding cough, chest pain, and dyspnea) that displays pulmonary infiltrates on chest radiograph. ACS is the second most common cause of hospitalization and third most common cause of death among adults with SCD with more than 10% of adults dying from complications linked to chronic lung disease and pulmonary hypertension.[14,39] Pulmonary infection, fat embolism, and pulmonary infarction are the most common inciting factors, resulting in a decreased alveolar oxygen tension that induces Hb S polymerization and sickle cell formation. Sickle cells and vasoocclusion further decrease pulmonary blood flow and alveolar oxygen tension, causing further polymerization, thus exacerbating the syndrome. Hypoxia, along with fat emboli, can upregulate VCAM1, inducing RBC adhesion and increasing vasoocclusion. In children, ACS generally is precipitated by infection characterized by fever, cough, and tachypnea (rapid breathing). ACS often develops within 24 to 72 hours after hospitalization for a vasoocclusive crisis.[14] ACS is also linked with sPLA$_2$, discussed previously. An increase in sPLA$_2$ is a predictor of ACS in patients with SCD[40] and correlates with the degree of lung damage. sPLA$_2$ rises 24 to 48 hours before symptoms of ACS begin.[41] In addition to the ACS symptoms (fever, hypoxia, tachypnea, and chest pain), chest radiographs, complete blood count (CBC), creatinine, liver function tests, arterial blood gases (ABG), and blood and/or sputum cultures are helpful in making the diagnosis. The CBC will often indicate a rapid decline in hemoglobin and platelet count. Creatinine and liver function tests are used to monitor organ function and predict organ failure primarily from fat emboli. ABG testing is used to monitor lung function, and a type and screen is ordered because blood transfusions are often

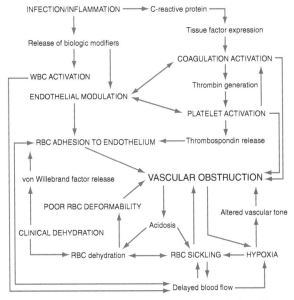

Figure 24.4 Numerous Risk Factors for Vasoocclusion Illustrating Physiological Interrelationships. *RBC,* Red blood cell; *WBC,* white blood cell. (From Embury, S. H., Hebbel, R. P., Mohandas, N., et al. [1994]. *Sickle Cell Disease: Basic Principles and Clinical Practice.* [p. 322, Figure 5]. Philadelphia: Lippincott Williams & Wilkins.)

necessary. Blood and sputum cultures are ordered to investigate the cause of ACS and to treat underlying infections. Treatment and continuous monitoring must be promptly initiated to reduce morbidity and mortality. Oxygen is administered to maintain saturation at ≥95% and intravenous fluids to prevent dehydration. Pain relief is essential but opioids can reduce respiration so overdosing is avoided. Incentive spirometry and chest physiotherapy are helpful to maintain adequate ventilation. Respiratory infection is presumed so antibiotics are prescribed to all patients and tailored to treat confirmed infections. The more severe cases of ACS benefit from blood or exchange transfusions, and many patients have rapid and dramatic improvements.[42]

Fat embolism syndrome and bone marrow necrosis. Fat embolism syndrome (FES) secondary to bone marrow necrosis (BMN) is a rare but often fatal sequalae of SCD. Often associated with long bone fractures, FES has also been observed in nontramatic conditions. It occurs more often in Hb SC (43%) and at similar frequency in Hb S-β$^+$-thal (17%) and Hb SS (19%). The cause is unknown but hypothesized to be BMN from a hypoxic event. Necrotic bone marrow material and fat particles are released into circulation and deposit in the lung, where they fragment. Small fat droplets reenter circulation via pulmonary capillaries and terminate in various organs, causing damage. It is thought that these fat emboli produce organ ischemia, stimulating the release of vasoactive amines and inflammatory mediators. Damage to the lung can cause acute respiratory distress syndrome. In addition to bone marrow and lung damage, patients often experience neurologic (brain) and renal damage. Patients generally present with back, bone, and abdomen pain and fever and fatigue associated with BMN and may rapidly progress to respiratory failure and central nervous system depression from FES. Altered mental status and respiratory distress are the most consistent findings and signal rapid deterioration within hours that is often fatal if not detected and treated swiftly.[43]

Laboratory evaluation is critical to differentiate FES/BMN from conditions with similar presentation. The CBC indicates a rapid drop in hemoglobin (>20%) and platelet count (>50%) from admission values with many nucleated RBCs and a left shift in the differential. The reticulocyte count is low because of the BMN. Chemical analysis shows elevated lactate dehydrogenase, ferritin, creatinine, alkaline phosphatase, and bilirubin, indicating end organ damage. A bone marrow evaluation is diagnostic showing myeloid necrosis, focal hypoplasia, loss of fat, and eosinophilic material in the background. However, patient demise often precedes bone marrow analysis. Fiberoptic bronchoscopy and bronchial lavage show intracellular fat in macrophages, and magnetic resonance imaging demonstrates the characteristic "star field" pattern indicating infarction. Rapid treatment with either multiple transfusions or red cell exchange (RCE) must be administered quickly and often results in complete recovery. In contrast, delayed diagnosis and treatment often results in death or permanent neurologic damage. Mortality rates in patients receiving RCE is 29% compared with simple transfusion (61%) and no transfusion (91%).[43]

Pulmonary hypertension. Pulmonary hypertension (PHT) is a serious and potentially fatal sequela of SCD. Among patients with SCD, PHT has a prevalence of about 33%, with 10% of patients manifesting a more severe type.[44] The mortality rate for sickle cell patients who develop PHT is 40% at 40 months.[44] An association has been documented between the development of PHT and the nitrous oxide (NO) pathway. NO is produced from the action of endothelial NO synthase (eNOS) on arginine, which causes vasodilation. Patients with SCD have a decrease in NO, and this leads to vasoconstriction and hypertension.[4,44] In addition, low NO levels in the blood fail to inhibit endothelin-1, a potent vasoconstrictor, which results in additional vasoconstriction and hypertension.[39] The connection between NO and SCD involves the hemolytic crisis. RBC hemolysis releases high levels of arginase, which degrades arginine; the result is less NO production from eNOS.[45,46] In addition, the free hemoglobin released from hemolyzed RBCs scavenges NO, which further reduces the levels and exacerbates the vasoconstriction and hypertension.[44] Blood arginine and NO levels drop a few days before the onset of acute chest syndrome, a finding suggesting that the NO pathway is a connection among SCD, PHT, and asthma.[39,47] Treatment with large doses of arginine reduces pulmonary artery pressure, but the effect is not sustainable and does not reduce mortality. An increased tricuspid regurgitation velocity (TRV) and blood N-terminal pro b-type natriuretic peptide (NT-ProBNP) levels greater than 160 ng/L were found to be good predictors of PHT and are associated with a higher mortality rate.[36]

Bacterial infections. Bacterial infections pose a major problem for SCD patients, who have increased susceptibility to life-threatening infections from *Staphylococcus aureus, Streptococcus pneumoniae,* and *Haemophilus influenzae.* Acute infections are common causes of hospitalization and have been the most common causes of death, especially in the first 3 years of life.[1] Bacterial infections of the blood (septicemia) are exacerbated by the autosplenectomy effect as the spleen gradually loses its ability to function as a secondary lymphoid tissue to effectively clear organisms from the blood.

Chronic hemolysis. Chronic hemolytic anemia is characterized by shortened RBC survival (between 16 and 20 days)[48] with a corresponding decrease in hemoglobin and hematocrit, an elevated reticulocyte count, and jaundice. Continuous screening and removal of sickle cells by the spleen perpetuate the chronic hemolytic anemia and autosplenectomy effect. Because other conditions (such as hepatitis and gallstones) may cause jaundice, chronic hemolysis is difficult to diagnose in sickle cell patients.[22] RBC hemolysis releases free hemoglobin, which disrupts the arginine-NO pathway, resulting in the sequestration and lowering of NO.[34,48] Decreased NO levels lead to endothelial cell activation, vasoconstriction, adherence of RBCs to the endothelium, and pulmonary hypertension, as previously discussed.[48] Another major sequelae of hemolysis is renal hyperfiltration and dysfunction, which can be detected early by an increased glomerular filtration rate of 140 mL/min per 1.73 m^3 or greater found in 71% of patients with SCD.[49] Progression of renal dysfunction can be identified by detecting microalbuminuria (>4 to 5 mg/mmol), followed by proteinuria and terminating in elevated blood urea nitrogen and creatinine levels. Angiotensin-converting enzyme inhibitors (ACEIs) have been found to lower proteinuria in SCD patients.[36]

Megaloblastic episodes. Megaloblastic episodes result from the sudden arrest of erythropoiesis caused by folate depletion. Folic acid deficiency as a cause of exaggerated anemia in SCD is extremely rare in the United States. It is common practice to prescribe prophylactic folic acid for patients with SCD, however.[8]

Aplastic episodes. Aplastic episodes (bone marrow failure) are the most common life-threatening hematologic complications and are usually associated with infection, particularly parvovirus infection.[37] Aplastic episodes present clinical problems similar to those seen with other hemolytic disorders.[50] Sickle cell patients usually can compensate for the decrease in RBC survival by increasing bone marrow output. When the bone marrow is suppressed temporarily by bacterial or viral infections, however, the hematocrit decreases substantially with no reticulocyte compensation. Most aplastic episodes are short lived, however, and require no therapy. Spontaneous recovery is characterized by the presence of nucleated RBCs and an increase in the number of reticulocytes in the peripheral blood. If anemia is severe and the bone marrow remains aplastic, transfusions are necessary. If patients are not transfused in a timely fashion, death can occur.[50]

Cardiac abnormalities. Patients also experience cardiac defects, including enlarged heart and heart murmurs. In patients with severe anemia, cardiomegaly can develop as the heart works harder to maintain adequate blood flow and tissue oxygenation. Increased cardiac workload along with increased bone marrow erythropoiesis increases calorie burning, contributing to a reduced growth rate.[51] When patients enter childbearing age, pregnancy becomes risky.[4]

Bone and skin abnormalities. Impaired blood supply to the head of the femur and humerus results in a condition called *avascular necrosis* (AVN). About 50% of patients with SCD develop AVN by age 35 years.[52] Physical therapy and surgery to relieve intramedullary pressure within the head of the long bones are effective, but hip and/or shoulder implants become necessary in most patients experiencing AVN.[52] Similarly, leg ulcers are a common complication of SCD. Ulcers tend to heal slowly, develop unstable scars, and recur at the same site, becoming a chronic problem, with associated chronic pain.[50]

Stroke. Hemorrhagic or ischemic stroke occurs in approximately 11% of children with SCD before age 20 years.[14] Screening children with transcranial Doppler is recommended annually between the ages of 2 to 16 years.[14] Silent microstrokes can lead to headaches, poor school performance, reduced intelligence quotient (IQ), and overt central nervous system dysfunction. Neurologic examination followed by magnetic resonance imaging and, if available, transcranial Doppler ultrasonography or magnetic resonance angiography is recommended to detect microstrokes.[51]

Retinopathy. Retinopathy occurs at a rate of 45% in patients with Hb SC, 11% with Hb SS, and 17% with Hb S-β-thal by early adulthood.[14] Visual acuity is lost as a result of retinopathy caused by retinal ischemia and neovascularization. Beginning at age 10 years, children with SCD should have annual dilated opthamalogic examinations and vitrectomy in severe cases to detect early retinal injury. When proliferative retinopathy is detected, laser photocoagulation is performed and vitrectomy can be done to resolve severe vitreous hemorrhage.[14]

Incidence With Malaria

The sickle gene occurs with greatest frequency in Central Africa, the Near East, the Mediterranean region, and parts of India. Sickle gene frequency parallels the incidence of *P. falciparum* and seems to offer some protection against cerebral falciparum malaria in young patients. Malarial parasites are living organisms within the RBCs that use the oxygen within the cells. This reduced oxygen tension causes the cells to sickle, which results in injury to the cells. These injured cells tend to become trapped within the blood vessels of the spleen and other organs, where they are easily phagocytized by scavenger macrophages. Selective destruction of RBCs containing parasites decreases the number of malarial organisms and increases the time for immunity to develop. One explanation for this phenomenon is that the infected cell is uniquely sickled and destroyed, probably in an area of the spleen or liver, where phagocytic cells are plentiful, and the oxygen tension is significantly decreased.[53]

Laboratory Diagnosis

SCD is a chronic hemolytic anemia, classified morphologically as normocytic, normochromic. The characteristic diagnostic cell observed on a Wright-stained peripheral blood film is a long, curved cell with a point at each end (Figure 24.5). Because of its appearance, the cell was named a *sickle cell.*[35] The peripheral blood film shows marked poikilocytosis and anisocytosis with normal RBCs, sickle cells, target cells, nucleated RBCs, along with a few spherocytes, basophilic stippling, Pappenheimer bodies, and Howell-Jolly bodies. The presence of sickle cells and target cells is the hallmark of SCD. There is moderate to marked polychromasia with a reticulocyte count between 10% and 25%, corresponding with the hemolytic state and the resultant bone marrow response. The RBC distribution width (RDW) is increased as a result of moderate anisocytosis. The mean cell volume (MCV) is not as elevated as one would expect, however, given the elevated reticulocyte count. An aplastic crisis can be heralded by a decreased reticulocyte count. Moderate leukocytosis is usually present (sometimes 40 to 50 × 10^9 WBC/L) with neutrophilia and a mild shift toward immature granulocytes. The leukocyte alkaline phosphatase score is not elevated when neutrophilia is caused by sickle cell crisis alone when no underlying infection is present. Thrombocytosis is usually present. The bone marrow shows erythroid hyperplasia, reflecting an attempt to compensate for the anemia, which results in polychromasia and an increase in reticulocytes and nucleated RBCs in the peripheral blood. Levels of immunoglobulins, particularly immunoglobulin A, are elevated in all forms of SCD. Serum ferritin levels are normal in young patients but tend to be elevated later in life. Chronic hemolysis is evidenced by elevated levels of indirect and total bilirubin with the accompanying jaundice.

The diagnosis of SCD is generally a two-step process begun by first demonstrating the insolubility of deoxygenated Hb S in solution followed by confirmation of its presence using hemoglobin electrophoresis, high-performance liquid

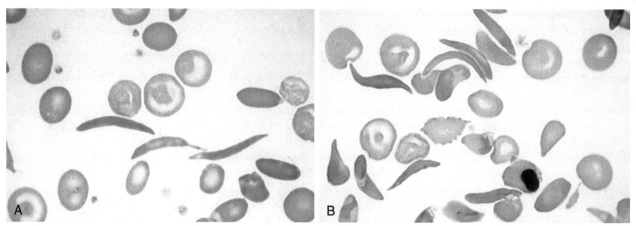

Figure 24.5 Peripheral Blood Films for a Patient with Sickle Cell Disease. (A), Note anisocytosis, polychromasia, three sickle cells, target cells, and normal platelets. **(B),** Note anisocytosis, poikilocytosis, sickle cells, target cells, and one nucleated red blood cell. Platelets are not present in this field, but their numbers were adequate in this patient. (A, B, Wright-Giemsa stain, X1000.) (Courtesy Ann Bell, University of Tennessee, Memphis.)

chromatography (HPLC), or capillary electrophoresis. For more complicated cases, isoelectric focusing, tandem mass spectrometry, or DNA analysis may be needed. An older screening test detects Hb S insolubility by inducing sickle cell formation on a glass slide. A drop of blood is mixed with a drop of 2% sodium metabisulfite (a reducing agent) on a slide, and the mixture is sealed under a coverslip. The hemoglobin inside the RBCs is reduced to the deoxygenated form; this induces polymerization and the resultant sickle cell formation, which can be identified microscopically. This method is slow and cumbersome and is rarely used.

Hemoglobin solubility test. The most common screening test for Hb S, called the hemoglobin solubility test, capitalizes on the decreased solubility of deoxygenated Hb S in solution, producing turbidity. Blood is added to a buffered salt solution containing a reducing agent, such as sodium hydrosulfite (dithionite), and a detergent-based lysing agent (saponin). Saponin dissolves membrane lipids, causing release of hemoglobin from RBCs, and dithionite reduces iron from the ferrous to the ferric oxidation state. Ferric iron is unable to bind oxygen, converting hemoglobin to the deoxygenated form. Deoxygenated Hb S polymerizes in solution, which renders it turbid, whereas solutions containing nonsickling hemoglobins remain clear (Figure 24.6). False-positive results for Hb S can occur with hyperlipidemia, in a few rare hemoglobinopathies, and when too much blood is added to the test solution; false-negative results can occur in infants younger than 6 months and in those with low hematocrits. Other hemoglobins that give a positive result on the solubility test include Hb C-Harlem (Georgetown), Hb C-Ziguinchor, Hb S-Memphis, Hb S-Travis, Hb S-Antilles, Hb S-Providence, Hb S-Oman, Hb Alexander, and Hb Porte-Alegre.[4,8] All these hemoglobins have two amino acid substitutions: the Hb S substitution ($\beta^{6Glu \rightarrow Val}$) and another unrelated substitution. Hb S-Antilles is particularly important because it can cause sickling in the heterozygous state.

Hemoglobin fractionation and quantification. Alkaline hemoglobin electrophoresis is a common first step in confirmation of

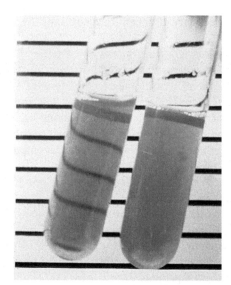

Figure 24.6 Hemoglobin Solubility Test for the Presence of Hemoglobin S. In a negative test result *(left),* the solution is clear and the lines behind the tube are visible. In a positive test result *(right),* the solution is turbid because of the polymerization of hemoglobin (Hb) S and the lines are not visible. (Courtesy Ann Bell, University of Tennessee, Memphis.)

hemoglobinopathies. Electrophoresis is based on the separation of hemoglobin molecules in an electric field primarily as a result of differences in total molecular charge. In alkaline electrophoresis, hemoglobin molecules assume a negative charge and migrate toward the anode (positive pole). Historically, alkaline hemoglobin electrophoresis was performed on cellulose acetate medium, but it is being replaced by agarose medium. Nonetheless, because some hemoglobins have the same charge and therefore the same electrophoretic mobility patterns, hemoglobins that exhibit an abnormal electrophoretic pattern at an alkaline pH may be subjected to electrophoresis at an acid pH for definitive separation. In an acid pH some hemoglobins assume a negative charge and migrate toward the anode, whereas others are positively charged and migrate toward the cathode (negative pole). For example, Hb S migrates with Hb D and Hb G on alkaline electrophoresis

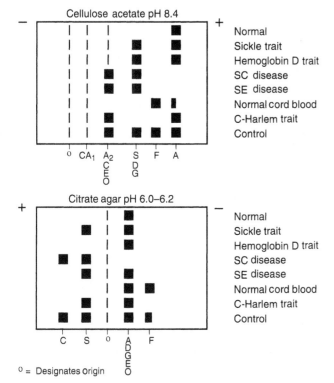

Figure 24.7 Relative Mobilities of Normal and Variant Hemoglobins in Various Conditions Measured by Electrophoresis on Cellulose Acetate at an Alkaline pH and Citrate Agar at an Acid pH. The relative amount of hemoglobin is not proportional to the size of the band; for example, in sickle cell trait (hemoglobin [Hb] AS), the bands may appear equal but the amount of Hb A exceeds that of Hb S. (From Schmidt, R. M., & Brosious, E. F. [1976]. *Basic Laboratory Methods of Hemoglobinopathy Detection.* [6th ed.]. HEW Pub. No. [CDC] 77-8266. Atlanta: Centers for Disease Control and Prevention.)

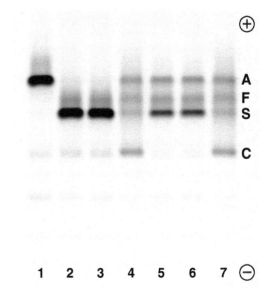

Figure 24.8 Electrophoretic Separation of Hemoglobins (Hb) at Alkaline pH. *1,* Normal adult; *2* and *3,* 17-year-old patient with sickle cell anemia (Hb SS); *5* and *6,* patient with sickle cell anemia, recently transfused (note the presence of Hb A from the transfused red blood cells); *4* and *7,* Hbs A/F/S/C standard (Hydragel 7 Hemoglobin/Hydrasys System, Sebia Electrophoresis, Norcross, GA). (Modified from Elghetany, M. T., Schexneider, K. I., & Banki, K. [2017]. Erythrocytic disorders. In McPherson, R. A., & Pincus, M. R. [Eds.], *Henry's Clinical Diagnosis and Management by Laboratory Methods.* [23rd ed., p. 580, Figure 32.17]. St. Louis: Elsevier.)

but separates from Hb D and Hb G on acid electrophoresis. Hb D and Hb G are further differentiated from Hb S in that they produce a negative result on the hemoglobin solubility test. Similarly, Hb C migrates with Hb E and Hb O on alkaline electrophoresis but separates on acid electrophoresis. Figure 24.7 shows electrophoretic patterns for normal and abnormal hemoglobins. Figure 24.8 shows the electrophoretic separation of a normal adult and a patient with SCD (Hb SS) at an alkaline pH. HPLC and capillary electrophoresis are gaining in popularity because these methods are more automated, the instruments are more user friendly, and they can be used to confirm hemoglobin variants observed with electrophoresis (Figure 24.9).

HPLC separates hemoglobin types in a cation exchange column and usually requires only one sample injection. Unlike electrophoresis, HPLC can identify and quantify low levels of Hb A_2 and Hb F, but comigration of Hb A_2 and Hb E occurs. Therefore HPLC is best used in the diagnosis of thalassemias rather than hemoglobinopathies because quantification of low levels of normal and abnormal hemoglobin levels is necessary to distinguish thalassemias.

Capillary electrophoresis, like agarose electrophoresis, separates hemoglobin types based on charge in an alkaline buffer but does so using smaller volumes and produces better separation than traditional agarose electrophoresis. Semiautomated

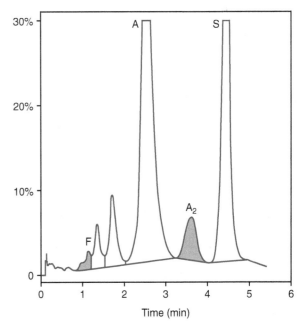

Figure 24.9 Ion-Exchange High-Performance Liquid Chromatography (HPLC) Separation of Hemoglobins (Hbs) in a Patient with Sickle Cell Trait Demonstrating Hbs F, A, A_2, and an Abnormal Hb in the S Window. (Bio-Rad Variant Classic Hb Testing System, BioRad Laboratories, Philadelphia). (Modified from Elghetany, M. T., Schexneider, K. I., & Banki, K. [2017]. Erythrocytic disorders. In McPherson, R. A., & Pincus, M. R. [Eds.], *Henry's Clinical Diagnosis and Management by Laboratory Methods.* [23rd ed., p. 580, Figure 32.16]. St. Louis: Elsevier.)

systems allow for the testing of multiple samples in parallel with computerized analysis of results. Capillary electrophoresis is also economical because each capillary can accommodate at least 3000 runs.[1]

Isoelectric focusing (IEF) is a confirmatory technique that is expensive and complex, requiring well-trained and experienced laboratory personnel. The method uses an electrical current to push the hemoglobin molecules across a pH gradient. The charge of the molecules changes as they migrate through the pH gradient until the hemoglobin species reaches its isoelectric point (net charge of zero). With a net charge of zero, migration stops and the hemoglobin molecules accumulate at their isoelectric position. Molecules with isoelectric point differences of as little as 0.02 pH units can be effectively separated.[1]

Neonatal screening requires a more sophisticated approach, often using three techniques: adapted IEF, HPLC, and reversed-phase HPLC. This multisystem approach is needed to distinguish not only the multitude of hemoglobin variants but also the numerous thalassemias. The more progressive laboratories use a combination of two or more techniques to improve identification of hemoglobin variants. Some reference laboratories may use mass spectroscopy, matrix-assisted laser desorption-ionization time-of-flight (MALDI-TOF) mass spectrometry, or IEF to separate hemoglobin types, or nucleic acid identification of the genetic mutation.[1,54]

Patients with Hb SS or Hb SC disease lack normal β-globin chains, so they have no Hb A. In Hb SS, the Hb S level is usually greater than 80%. The Hb F level is usually increased (1% to 20%), and when Hb F constitutes more than 20% of hemoglobin, it modulates the severity of the disease. This is especially true in newborns and in patients with hereditary persistence of fetal hemoglobin.[34] The Hb A_2 level is usually normal. Hb A_2 quantification is useful in differentiating Hb SS from Hb S-β-thal because Hb A_2 is increased in the latter (Chapter 25).

Assessment of inflammation. Typical sequelae of SCD may be predicted, and the effectiveness of treatment monitored, if reliable biomarkers of inflammation can be identified. Among the common indicators of inflammation, the WBC count is a good predictor of sickle cell complications and mortality, whereas the erythrocyte sedimentation rate (ESR) and C-reactive protein (CRP) level exhibit variability too great to reliably predict episodes. However, CRP and sPLA$_2$ are both elevated during VOC and acute chest syndrome. Other markers, such as IL-6, IL-10, and protein S, are showing promise as useful indicators in clinical practice.[55] Annexin A5, a protein bound to lipids in the plasma membrane of endothelial cells and platelets, has been found to elevate before and during VOC.[56] Lipid damage from oxidative stress can be predicted by plasma elevations of malondialdehyde (MDA) and depleted α-tocopherol. In addition, α-tocopherol rises with CRP during bouts of inflammation. Of all the biomarkers evaluated, IL-6, IL-10, vascular cell adhesion molecule 1 (VCAM-1), and sPLA$_2$ are the most promising at predicting impending crisis.[57]

Treatment

Supportive care has been the mainstay of therapy for SCD and includes adequate hydration, prophylactic vitamin therapy, avoidance of low-oxygen environments, analgesia for pain, and aggressive antibiotic therapy with the first signs of infection. Hydration maintains good blood flow and reduces vasoocclusive crises. Prophylactic oral penicillin V is recommended for children younger than 5 years to avoid infection and the associated morbidity and mortality.[14,58] When infections occur, prompt antibiotic treatment reduces the associated morbidity and mortality.[9,58] Avoidance of strenuous exercise, high altitudes, and unpressurized air travel maintains high oxygen tensions and reduces the sickling phenomenon. Treatment for painful episodes includes ensuring optimal hydration, rapidly treating associated infection, oxygen therapy, and effectively relieving pain. Analgesics are the foundation of pain management, with nonsteroidal antiinflammatory drugs usually given to manage mild to moderate pain.[58,59] In the acute setting, parenteral opioids are used for severe pain, whereas short- and long-acting oral opioids are prescribed and closely monitored when severe pain becomes chronic.[58,59] Blood exchange transfusion (BET) is the treatment of choice for severe VOCs and ACS.[36] Painful crises tend to increase with age, and physicians must be aware of opiate tolerance and rebound pain after opiate therapy, called central sensitization. Repeated painful crises can result in hypersensitivity to repeated pain by increasing peripheral inflammation, increased neurotransmitter release, increased calcium influx into postsynaptic junctions, and other pathways that increase pain signals to the brain.[48] This phenomenon can be misinterpreted as drug intolerance, causing inappropriate dose escalation, or as drug-seeking behavior, causing inappropriate termination of treatment. The most appropriate response to opioid tolerance and central sensitization is a gradual dose reduction to reset the pain receptors followed by switching to opioids that are less sensitive to this phenomenon.[48] The patient should be examined on a regular basis, and routine testing should be done to establish baseline pain values for the patient during nonsickling periods.

Children younger than 3 years often experience *hand-foot syndrome,* characterized by pain and swelling in the hands and feet.[36] Treatment usually consists of increasing intake of fluids and analgesics for pain.

Pneumococcal disease has been a leading cause of morbidity and mortality in children, especially children younger than 6 years. With immunization and prophylactic antibiotics, however, this is now a preventable complication.[7] Immunization with the 13-valent conjugate pneumococcal vaccine series is recommended to begin shortly after birth.[58] The 23-valent pneumococcal vaccine is recommended at 2 years, with a booster at the age of 5 years.[58] Standard immunizations should be given according to the schedule recommended by the US Preventive Services Task Force and the Advisory Committee for Immunization Practices (ACIP) including annual administration of influenza vaccine beginning at age 6 months.[14,45,58,59] The risk of invasive bacterial infection increases in older children and adults with SCD genotypes mainly because of reduced splenic function as a result of repeated infarcts.[21,58]

Transfusions can be used to prevent the complications of SCD. More specifically, chronic transfusions, given at a frequency of eight or more per year, are used to prevent stroke, symptomatic anemia, priapism, leg ulcers, pulmonary hypertension, delayed pubescence, splenomegaly, and chronic pain and to improve exercise tolerance and sense of well-being. In other circumstances, such as central nervous system infarction, hypoxia with infection, stroke, episodes of acute chest syndrome, and preparation for surgery, transfusions are used to decrease blood viscosity and the percentage of circulating sickle cells. Before all but simple surgeries, Hb SS patients are transfused with normal Hb AA blood to achieve a hemoglobin of 10 g/dL in an effort to prevent complications in surgery.[58,60] For chronically transfused children, a Hb S level of less than 30% immediately before the next transfusion is recommended.[58,59] Transfused units for all SCD patients should be matched for C, E, and K antigens.[58,59] Maintenance transfusions should be given in pregnancy if the mother experiences vasoocclusive or anemia-related problems or if there are signs of fetal distress or poor growth.[21] Nonetheless, transfusion therapy has the potential to cause transfusion reactions, transfusion-related infections, and iron overload. Of the three, iron overload is the most common.

Iron overload has been associated with endocrine dysfunction[61] and cardiac disease.[62] Iron chelators have been effective in treating iron overload by chelating and removing excess iron from the body through excretion in the urine or feces. Deferoxamine, approved by the US Food and Drug Administration (FDA) in 1982, is administered by continuous pump infusion over 8 to 12 hours, or by twice daily subcutaneous injections.[63] Oral iron chelators deferasirox (FDA approved in 2005) and deferiprone (FDA approved in 2011) are more conveniently administered through three daily doses and one daily dose, respectively.[63] All three chelators can have adverse effects and issues with patient compliance. The use of combinations of chelators or alternating days of chelators to decrease adverse effects and improve compliance is the subject of ongoing study.[63]

Allogeneic bone marrow or hematopoietic stem cell transplantation is the only curative therapy and has been performed in more than 1000 patients with SCD worldwide.[64] Unfortunately, few patients qualify because of the lack of HLA-matched, related donors. Only 14% of patients with SCD have HLA-identical sibling donors.[65] The risks of graft rejection, graft-versus-host disease, and mortality must be weighed against disease severity. The event-free survival rates for patients receiving transplants from HLA-identical related donors are between 80% and 90% for SCD.[64-66] Patients chosen for transplantation are generally children younger than age 17 with severe complications of SCD (i.e., stroke, acute chest syndrome, and refractory pain). In addition, morbidity and mortality after transplantation increase with age, which places another restriction on transplantation therapy There is evidence that transplantation restores some splenic function, but its effect on established organ damage is unknown.[67] Transplantation of cord blood stem cells from HLA-identical related and unrelated donors is associated with a disease-free survival rate of 83% to 90%.[64,68] The primary benefits of using cord blood as a source of stem cells is its lower immunogenicity as a donor source and that banking of cord blood increases the number of units available to achieve an HLA match. However, the volume of a cord blood sample often is too little for adult patients.[68] Newer transplantation protocols involve reduced intensity conditioning (RIC) and donor sample manipulations to include ex vivo CD34$^+$ cell selection and T-cell depletion.[65] Some researchers are now focusing on the use of in utero stem cell transplantation to produce engraftment while the immune system of the fetus has the capability for HLA tolerance. Others are attempting to genetically alter fetal hematopoietic stems cells to overcome HLA mismatches.[69]

Hydroxycarbamide (hydroxyurea) therapy has offered some promise in relieving the sickling disorder by increasing the proportion of Hb F in the RBCs of individuals with SCD. Hydroxyurea can be administered to children beginning at age 9 months at pediatric dose regimens to reduce symptoms and prolong life, in part by increasing Hb F levels.[14] Daily dosing produces a better HbF response compared with sequential weekly dosing.[70] Because Hb F does not copolymerize with Hb S, increasing production of Hb F can avoid some complications of SCD. The severity of the disease expression and the number of irreversible sickle cells are inversely proportional to the extent to which Hb F synthesis persists. Individuals in whom Hb F levels stabilize at 12% to 20% of total hemoglobin may have little or no anemia and few, if any, vasoocclusive attacks. Levels of 4% to 5% Hb F may modulate the disease, and levels of 5% to 12% may suppress the severity of hemolysis and lessen the frequency of severe episodes.[37] Drug compliance is best monitored by an increasing MCV, whereas a decreasing LD might be an indicator of treatment response.[36] Response to hydroxycarbamide is variable among SCD patients, but high baseline Hb F level, neutrophil level, and reticulocyte count are the best predictors of Hb F response.[71]

Prevention of intracellular RBC dehydration reduces intracellular Hb S polymerization, thus reducing VOC. The uses of senicapoc to inhibit Gardos channels and Mg^{2+} to modulate K^+/Cl^- transport systems produce increased hemoglobin levels and decreased numbers of dense RBCs, resulting in reduced hemolysis but no clear reduction in VOC.[72-75]

Recently L-glutamine has been FDA approved to reduce acute complications of SCD in patients 5 years and older.[76] L-glutamine is converted to free glutamine in the blood, which is taken up by RBCs and degraded, producing antioxidant molecules that neutralize oxidants to maintain RBC flexibility. In clinical trials, patients taking L-glutamine experienced fewer sickle cell crises, fewer hospital admissions and emergency visits for pain, and fewer episodes of acute chest syndrome.[76]

New treatment strategies are being investigated to protect against free hemoglobin and free heme to reduce or prevent organ damage. Haptoglobin supplementation has been found experimentally to reduce vasculotoxic injury.[32] Haptoglobin/hemoglobin complexes are too large to penetrate endothelial cell-cell tight junctions, allowing hemoglobin to bind CD163 receptors on monocytes, macrophages, and dendritic for elimination (Chapter 20). When hemoglobin enters the subendothelial space, its NO scavenging activity causes vasculotoxic injury.

Similarly, hemopexin binds free heme and directs it to hepatocytes for removal rather than to macrophages, where the heme stimulates macrophages toward the M1 proinflammatory phenotype. Combination therapy using both agents represents a natural strategy to ameliorate vasculotoxic effects and reduce or prevent organ injury.[32]

Another novel therapeutic approach is to test drugs that target adhesion of circulating blood cells to the endothelium. Rivipansel (GMI-1070) blocks P-selectin and E-selectin, which are highly expressed on endothelial cells and platelets of patients with SCD.[32] Phase II trials in patients with SCD experiencing VOC indicated a reduction in time of resolution and decreased opioid use. Intravenous immunoglobulin G (IVIG) is being investigated to stabilize neutrophil Mac-1 activation in VOC.[32] Lastly, AKT2 inhibitors in combination with hydroxyurea are being tested in a mouse model to reduce neutrophil adhesion, platelet-neutrophil aggregation, endothelial E-selectin, and intercellular adhesion molecule 1 to improve survival.[32]

Anti-sickling drugs bind to Hb S molecules and inhibit sickling by increasing oxygen affinity and maintaining Hb S in the oxyhemoglobin state. 5-Hydroxymethylfurfural (5-HMF), vanillin derivatives, GBT440, and trizole sulfate are currently being investigated in clinical trials.[77] 5-HMF binds the N-terminal valine of the α chains that stabilizes the R state (relaxed) to increase oxygen affinity for Hb S. 5-HMF has also been found to inhibit P_{sickle} and Gardos channels to prevent dehydration.[77] Lastly, 5-HMF also increases the RBC's ability to generate NO to promote vasodilation and blood flow.[77] The effect of 5-HMF is improved when combined with hydroxycarbamide (hydroxyurea). Derivatives of vanillin have been found to also increase oxygen affinity of Hb S and destabilize HbS polymer contacts. GBT440 also binds the N-terminal valine of the α chains similar to 5-HMF, but it also influences the intradimer interface and the heme pockets to increase oxygen affinity. Triazole sulfide binds to βCys93 and βC112 and to the central water cavity to stabilize the R state and increase oxygen affinity to a greater degree than 5-HMF. The main challenge is the concentration of anti-sickling drug needed to bind the approximately 200 to 300 million hemoglobin molecules in each RBC. Large, nontoxic doses may be difficult to achieve and maintain, especially because most of these drugs have a short half-life.[77]

In addition to transplantation, gene therapy also offers the chance of a cure. The initial approach to gene therapy performed in mice was to transfect a wild-type β-globin gene into a lentiviral vector, expose the viral vector to patient stem cells, allow for gene integration, and transplant autologous stem cells back into the patient. Although gene integration into the patient's genome was successful, controlling the genomic position of the wild-type gene was unpredictable resulting great variation in gene expression rates. Modifications in the gene regulatory elements and lentivirus characteristics reduced mutagenic integration and improved gene expression. This approach was successful in a few human trials, but the insertion stimulated growth of myeloid cells with malignant potential.[65] Further modifications were made to the lentivirus, which is currently in phase I and II clinical trials in patients with β-thalassemia and SCD, and preliminary results are promising.[65]

Course and Prognosis

Proper management of SCD has increased the life expectancy of patients from 14 years in 1973 to the current average life span of greater than 50 years.[78] For men and women who are compound heterozygotes for Hb SC, the average life span is 60 and 68 years, respectively, with a few patients living into their seventies.[33,79] Individuals with Hb SS can pursue a wide range of vocations and professions. They are discouraged, however, from jobs that require strenuous physical exertion or exposure to high altitudes or extreme environmental temperature variations.

Newborn screening for hemoglobinopathies has significantly reduced mortality in children with SCD by enabling prompt and comprehensive medical care. The most common form of screening is HPLC followed by confirmation using hemoglobin electrophoresis and genotyping methods.[80]

Sickle Cell Disease and Pregnancy

Managing pregnant patients with SCD is challenging and involves interventions before conception, prenatally, during delivery, and postpartum.

Preconception. Repeated microvascular occulusion in patients with SCD increases the risk of cardiomyopathy (four times greater risk), renal disease, proteinuria, pulmonary hypertension (six times greater risk), hypercoagulability, osteonecrosis, and hepatic necrosis, all of which greatly complicate pregnancy.[81] When present, these conditions require management by a multidiscipinary approach. The father should be tested to predict the risk of the child having SCD and genetic counseling should be recommended as appropriate. Immunizations should be current and the patient should be typed and screened for alloantibodies. Medications that affect pregnancy like ACEIs or angiotensin II receptor blockers for cardiomyopathy and hydroxyurea must be discontinued before conception or switched to a safer agent.[81]

Prenatal (Antenatal). Women with SCD have a sixfold increased risk of maternal death and a 2.2 times greater risk of fetal death.[81] Fetal ultrasound should be performed during the first trimester and at 20, 32, and 36 weeks gestation. Pregnant women should continue with folic acid at 5 mg/day or greater to prevent neural tube defects. Because pregnant patients with SCD develop blood clots five times more often, thromboembolism prophylaxis is recommended once hospitalized.[81] Although prophylactic transfusion therapy is controversial, it may ameliorate chronic organ dysfunction, acute chest syndrome, and frequent pain crises. Therapeutic transfusions are indicated if patients experience severe anemia, refractory pain crises, reticulocytopenia, septicemia, and intrapartum complications. To minimize alloimmunization, blood products should be matched for C, D, E, and Kell antigens and leukoreduced.[81]

During delivery (intrapartum). To minimize complications, delivery is recommended between 38 to 40 weeks. To reduce sickling risk, patients should be on oxygen and kept warm and well hydrated, and local anesthesia should be used rather than general anesthesia. If a cesarean section is warranted or if the fetus has late decelerations, the patient should be transfused to maintain a hemoglobin level at 10 g/dL.[81]

Postpartum. Patients should remain hospitalized for 3 days postpartum to monitor fluid status, blood cell counts, renal function, and liver function and for evidence of vasoocclusive crisis, which occurs in 25% of patients.[81] Because thromboembolism is a risk, patients should be mobilized early and thromboprophylaxis should be restarted 12 hours after delivery and continued for 6 weeks for a cesarean section. For nursing mothers, hydroxyuria should not be restarted until breastfeeding is discontinued.[81]

Sickle Cell Trait

The term *sickle cell trait* (SCT) refers to the heterozygous state (Hb AS) and describes a benign condition that generally does not affect mortality or morbidity except under conditions of extreme exertion. It occurs in approximately 8% of African Americans, but also can be found in individuals from Central America, Asia, and the Mediterranean region.[1]

Individuals with SCT are generally asymptomatic and present with no significant clinical or hematologic manifestations. Under extremely hypoxic conditions, however, systemic sickling and vascular occlusion with pooling of sickled cells in the spleen, focal necrosis in the brain, rhabdomyolysis, and even death can occur. In circumstances such as severe respiratory infection, unpressurized flight at high altitudes, and anesthesia in which pH and oxygen levels are sufficiently lowered to cause sickling, patients may develop splenic infarcts. Failure to concentrate urine is the only consistent abnormality found in SCT patients. This abnormality is caused by diminished perfusion of the kidney vasa recta, which impairs concentration of urine by renal tubules. Renal papillary necrosis with hematuria has been described in some patients.[8]

Although much controversy exists as to the potential connection between strenuous exercise and severe to fatal adverse events in patients with SCT, at least 46 cases have been documented in the literature (39 military recruits and 7 athletes).[82] These deaths largely were due to cardiac or renal failure or rhabdomyolysis. Opponents of the connection of SCT and fatal events argue that these events occur in sickle cell-negative people, many people with SCT do not develop adverse events, fatal sickle crisis cannot be adequately established in patients encountering such events, and similar events have not been clearly documented in patients with sickle cell disease. However, it has been found that military recruits with SCT have a 21 times greater risk of exercise-related death than recruits with normal hemoglobin.[82] Similar data have not been established in athletes with SCT, but evidence is mounting that SCT is associated with sudden death in competitive athletes.[11] In 2010 the National Collegiate Athletic Association mandated SCT screening with the hemoglobin solubility test for all student athletes in division I sports.[11] This mandate continued with division II sports in 2012 and division III sports in 2013.[11] Athletes experiencing an adverse event present with cramping, dyspnea, muscle pain, severe weakness, fatigue, and exhaustion that evolves into a gradual deterioration over several minutes and often terminating in rhabdomyolysis. These events occur more often after strenuous physical exertion early in the athletic season, at high temperatures, at high altitudes, and after interval training. These events constitute a medical emergency that requires immediate monitoring of vital signs, administration of oxygen

and intravenous hydration, cooling, and transport to a medical facility.[11]

The peripheral blood film in SCT has normal RBC morphology, with the exception of a few target cells. No abnormalities in the leukocytes and thrombocytes are seen. The hemoglobin solubility screening test yields positive results, and SCT is diagnosed by detecting the presence of Hb S and Hb A on hemoglobin electrophoresis or HPLC. In individuals with SCT, electrophoresis reveals approximately 40% or less Hb S and approximately 60% or more Hb A, Hb A_2 level is normal or slightly increased, and Hb F level is within the reference interval. Levels of Hb S less than 40% can be seen in patients who also have α-thalassemia or iron or folate deficiency.[21] No treatment is required for this benign condition, and the patient's life span is not affected.

HEMOGLOBIN C

Hb C was the next hemoglobinopathy after Hb S to be described and in the United States is found almost exclusively in the African American population. Spaet and Ranney reported this disease in the homozygous state (Hb CC) in 1953.[8]

Prevalence, Etiology, and Pathophysiology

Hb C is found in 17% to 28% of people of West African extraction and in 2% to 3% of African Americans.[4] It is the most common nonsickling variant encountered in the United States and the third most common in the world.[4] Hb C is defined by the structural formula $\alpha_2\beta_2^{6Glu \rightarrow Lys}$, in which lysine replaces glutamic acid in position 6 of the β chain. Lysine has a $+1$ charge and glutamic acid has a -1 charge, so the result of this substitution is a net change in charge of $+2$, which has a different structural effect on the hemoglobin molecule and electrophoresis mobility pattern compared with the Hb S substitution.

Similar to Hb S, Hb C forms polymers intracellularly. Unlike HbS the structure of Hb C polymers differ and they form under high oxygen tension. Hb S polymers are long and thin, whereas the polymers in Hb C form a short, thick crystal within the RBCs. As a result of electrostatic interactions between the positively charged B6-lysyl side chain and the negativity charged adjacent groups, Hb C is less soluble than Hb A in RBCs and crystalizes in the oxygenated state. Band 3 within the RBC membrane serves as a nucleation center for Hb C crystal formation.[83] The shorter Hb C crystal does not alter RBC shape to the extent that Hb S does, so there is less splenic sequestration and hemolysis.

Clinical Features

Homozygous hemoglobin C disease (Hb CC) manifests as a milder disease compared with SCD. Mild splenomegaly and hemolysis may be present. In addition, vasoocclusive crises do not occur. Heterozygous hemoglobin C trait (Hb AC) is asymptomatic.

Laboratory Diagnosis

A mild to moderate, normochromic, normocytic anemia occurs in homozygous Hb C disease. Occasionally, some microcytosis and mild hypochromia may be present. There is a marked

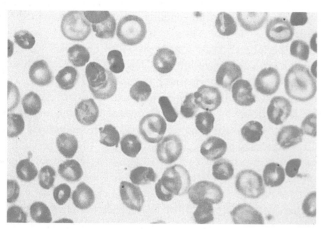

Figure 24.10 Peripheral Blood Film of a Patient with Hemoglobin C Disease. Note one hemoglobin C crystal and target and folded cells. (Wright-Giemsa stain, ×1000.) (Courtesy Ann Bell, University of Tennessee, Memphis.)

increase in the number of target cells and a slight to moderate increase in the number of reticulocytes (2% to 3%), and nucleated RBCs may be present in peripheral blood.

Hexagonal crystals of Hb C form within RBCs and may be seen on the peripheral blood film (Figure 24.10). Many crystals appear extracellularly with no evidence of a cell membrane. In some cells, hemoglobin is concentrated within the boundary of the crystal. Crystals are densely stained and vary in size and appear oblong with pyramid-shaped or pointed ends. These crystals may be seen on wet preparations by washing RBCs and resuspending them in a solution of sodium citrate or hypertonic saline.[12,83]

Hb C yields a negative result on the hemoglobin solubility test, and definitive diagnosis is made using electrophoresis, HPLC, or nucleic acid testing. No Hb A is present in Hb CC disease. In addition, Hb C is present at levels of greater than 90%, with Hb F at less than 7% and Hb A_2 at approximately 2%. In Hb AC trait, about 60% Hb A and 30% Hb C are present. On alkaline hemoglobin electrophoresis Hb C migrates in the same position as Hb A_2, Hb E, and Hb O-Arab (Figure 24.7). Hb C is separated from these other hemoglobins on citrate agar electrophoresis at an acid pH (Figure 24.7).

Treatment and Prognosis

No specific treatment is required. This disorder becomes problematic only if infection occurs, if splenomegaly becomes painful, or if mild chronic hemolysis leads to gallbladder disease. Genetic counseling is recommended because Hb C in combination with Hb S results in SCD and can have severe symptoms similar to Hb SS.

HEMOGLOBIN C-HARLEM (HEMOGLOBIN C-GEORGETOWN)

Hb C-Harlem (Hb C-Georgetown) has a double substitution on the β chain.[5,21] The substitution of valine for glutamic acid at position 6 of the β chain is identical to the Hb S substitution, and the substitution at position 73 of aspartic acid for asparagine is the same as the Hb Korle Bu mutation. The double

mutation is termed *Hb C-Harlem (Hb C-Georgetown)* because the abnormal hemoglobin migrates with Hb C on alkaline hemoglobin electrophoresis. Patients heterozygous for this anomaly are asymptomatic, but patients with compound heterozygosity for Hb S and Hb C-Harlem have crises similar to those with Hb SS disease.[84]

A positive solubility test result may occur with Hb C-Harlem, and hemoglobin electrophoresis or HPLC is necessary to confirm the diagnosis. On alkaline hemoglobin electrophoresis, Hb C-Harlem migrates in the C position (Figure 24.7). Citrate agar electrophoresis at pH 6.2, however, shows migration of Hb C-Harlem in the S position (Figure 24.7). Because so few cases have been identified, the clinical outcome for homozygous individuals affected with this abnormality is uncertain,[84] but heterozygotes appear normal.

HEMOGLOBIN E

Prevalence, Etiology, and Pathophysiology

Hb E was first described in 1954.[85] The variant has a prevalence of 30% in Southeast Asia and can reach rates of 50% in border areas of Cambodia, Laos and Thailand. Hb E has also been found in Bangladesh, India, and Madagascar.[8] As a result of the influx of immigrants from these areas, Hb E prevalence has increased in the United States. It occurs infrequently in African Americans and whites. Hb E is a β chain variant in which lysine is substituted for glutamic acid in position 26 ($\alpha_2\beta_2^{26Glu \rightarrow Lys}$). As with Hb C, this substitution results in a net change in charge of +2, but because of the position of the substitution, hemoglobin polymerization does not occur. However, the amino acid substitution at codon 26 inserts a cryptic splice site at the junction of exon 1 and intron 1 that causes abnormal alterative splicing and decreased transcription of functional mRNA for the Hb E globin chain.[86] Reduced Hb E synthesis explains Hb E levels in heterozygotes of between 25% to 30%.[8] Thus the Hb E mutation is both a qualitative defect (because of the amino acid substitution in the globin chain) and a quantitative defect with a β-thalassemia phenotype (because of decreased production of the mutated globin chain).[86] Hb E is often coinherited with either α-thalassemia, β-thalassemia, or other hemoglobin variants including Hb S forming Hb SE disease. This creates a wide range of clinical severities, with Hb E-β-thalassemia being the most severe. [8]

Clinical Features

The homozygous state (Hb EE) manifests as a mild anemia with microcytes and target cells. RBC survival time is shortened. The condition is not associated with clinically observable icterus, hemolysis, or splenomegaly. The main concern in identifying homozygous Hb EE is differentiating it from iron deficiency, β-thalassemia trait, and Hb E-β-thal (Chapter 25).[86] Because the highest incidence of the Hb E gene is in areas of Thailand where malaria is most prevalent, it is thought that *P. falciparum* multiplies more slowly in Hb EE RBCs than in Hb AE or Hb AA RBCs and that the mutation may give some protection against malaria.[1] Hb E trait is asymptomatic. However, Hb E-β[0]-thal results in symptoms more severe than Hb EE and more closely

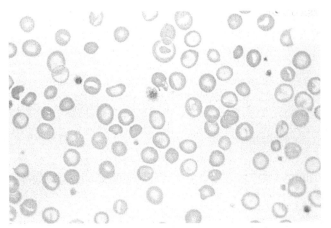

Figure 24.11 Peripheral Blood Film of a Patient with Hemoglobin E Trait. Note the microcytes and target cells. (Wright-Giemsa stain, ×1000.) (From Hematology Tech Sample H-1. [1991]. American Society of Clinical Pathologists, Chicago, IL.)

resembles the severity β-thalassemia major, requiring regular blood transfusions.[1]

Laboratory Diagnosis

Hb E does not produce a positive hemoglobin solubility test result and must be confirmed using electrophoresis or HPLC. In the homozygous state there is greater than 90% Hb E, mild anemia (hemoglobin between 11.0 to 13.0 g/dL), a very low MCV (55 to 65 fL), few to many target cells, and a normal reticulocyte count. The heterozygous state has normal hemoglobin levels, a mean MCV of 65 fL, slight erythrocytosis, target cells[1] (Figure 24.11), and approximately 25% to 30% Hb E. Patients with Hb E-β⁺-thal have an anemia that varies in severity (hemoglobin between 6.5 to 9.5 g/dL), depending on the β-thalassemia mutation, and those with Hb E-β⁰-thal have an even more severe anemia depending on the degree of Hb F compensation.[8] On alkaline hemoglobin electrophoresis, Hb E migrates with Hb C, Hb O, and Hb A$_2$ (Figure 24.7). On citrate agar electrophoresis at an acid pH, Hb E can be separated from Hb C, but it comigrates with Hb A and Hb O (Figure 24.7).

Treatment and Prognosis

No therapy is required with Hb E disease and trait. Some patients may experience splenomegaly and fatigue, however. Genetic counseling is recommended, and the Hb E gene mutation should be discussed in the same manner as a mild β-thalassemia allele.[86] Patients with Hb E-β⁰-thal are treated like β-thalassemia major with chronic transfusion therapy, iron chelation therapy, splenectomy with hypersplenism, and hydroxyurea in severe cases.[8]

HEMOGLOBIN O-ARAB

Hb O-Arab is a β chain variant caused by the substitution of lysine for glutamic acid at amino acid position 121 ($\alpha_2\beta_2{}^{121\text{Glu}\rightarrow\text{Lys}}$).[5,21] It is a rare disorder found in Kenya, Israel, Egypt, and Bulgaria and in 0.4% of African Americans.[21] No clinical symptoms are exhibited by individuals who carry this variant, except for mild splenomegaly in homozygotes.[5] When Hb O-Arab is inherited with Hb S, however, severe clinical symptoms similar to those in Hb SS result.[5]

Homozygous individuals have mild hemolytic anemia, with many target cells on the peripheral blood film and a negative result on the hemoglobin solubility test. The presence of this hemoglobin variant must be confirmed using electrophoresis or HPLC. Because Hb O-Arab migrates with Hb A$_2$, Hb C, and Hb E on alkaline hemoglobin electrophoresis, citrate agar electrophoresis at an acid pH is required to differentiate it from Hb C (Figure 24.7). Hb O-Arab is the only hemoglobin to move just slightly away from the point of application toward the cathode on citrate agar at an acid pH. No treatment is generally necessary for individuals with Hb O-Arab.

HEMOGLOBIN D AND HEMOGLOBIN G

Hb D and Hb G are a group of at least 16 β chain variants (Hb D) and 6 α chain variants (Hb G) that migrate in an alkaline pH at the same electrophoretic position as Hb S.[4,8,21] This is because their α and β subunits have one fewer negative charge at an alkaline pH than Hb A, as does Hb S. They do not sickle, however, when exposed to reduced oxygen tension.

Most variants are named for the place where they were discovered. Hb D-Punjab and Hb D-Los Angeles are identical hemoglobins in which glutamine replaces glutamic acid at position 121 in the β chain ($\alpha_2\beta_2{}^{121\text{Glu}\rightarrow\text{Gln}}$). Hb D-Punjab occurs in about 3% of the population in northwestern India, and Hb D-Los Angeles is seen in fewer than 2% of African Americans.

Hb G-Philadelphia is an α chain variant of the G hemoglobins in which lysine replaces asparagine at position 68 ($\alpha_2{}^{68\text{Asn}\rightarrow\text{Lys}}\beta_2$).[5] The Hb G-Philadelphia variant is the most common G variant encountered in African Americans and is seen with greater frequency than the Hb D variants. The Hb G variant is also found in Ghana.[4,8,21]

Hb D and Hb G do not sickle and produce a negative hemoglobin solubility test result. On alkaline electrophoresis, Hb D and Hb G have the same mobility as Hb S (Figure 24.7). Hb D and Hb G can be separated from Hb S on citrate agar at pH 6.0 (Figure 24.7). These variants should be suspected whenever a hemoglobin band is encountered that migrates in the S position on alkaline electrophoresis and has a negative result on the hemoglobin solubility test. In the homozygous state (Hb DD), there is greater than 95% Hb D, with normal amounts of Hb A$_2$ and Hb F.[33] Hb DD can be confused with the compound heterozygous state for Hb D and β⁰-thalassemia. The two disorders can be differentiated based on the MCV, levels of Hb A$_2$, and family studies. HbD-β⁰-thal produces a low MCV and an elevated Hb A$_2$, whereas both values are usually normal in Hb DD disease.[4,8,21]

Hb D and Hb G are asymptomatic in the heterozygous state. Hb D disease (Hb DD) is marked by mild hemolytic anemia and chronic nonprogressive splenomegaly. No treatment is required.[4,8,21] When Hb D is coinherited with β⁰-thalassemia, patients have mild microcytic anemia, but when inherited with Hb S it usually produces a mild form of sickle cell disease.[8]

COMPOUND HETEROZYGOSITY WITH HEMOGLOBIN S AND ANOTHER β-GLOBIN GENE MUTATION

Compound heterozygosity is the inheritance of two different mutant genes that share a common genetic locus, in this case the β-globin gene locus.[87] Because there are two β-globin genes, these compound heterozygotes have inherited Hb S from one parent and another β chain hemoglobinopathy or thalassemia from the other parent. Compound heterozygosity of Hb S with Hb C, Hb D, Hb O, or β-thalassemia may produce hemolytic anemia of variable severity. Inheritance of Hb S with other hemoglobins, such as Hb E, Hb G-Philadelphia, and Hb Korle Bu, causes disorders of no clinical consequence.[87]

Hemoglobin SC

Hb SC is the most common compound heterozygous syndrome that results in a structural defect in the hemoglobin molecule in which different amino acid substitutions are found on each of two β-globin chains. At position 6, glutamic acid is replaced by valine (Hb S) on one β-globin chain and by lysine (Hb C) on the other β-globin chain. The prevalence of Hb SC is 25% in West Africa. The incidence in the United States is approximately 1 in 833 births per year.[86,88]

Clinical Features

Hb SC disease usually results in a milder form of SCD, but it can be severe in some cases. Growth and development are delayed compared with normal children. Unlike Hb SS, Hb SC usually does not produce significant symptoms until the teenage years. Hb SC disease may cause all the vasoocclusive complications of sickle cell anemia, but episodes are less frequent and damage is less disabling. Hemolytic anemia is moderate, and many patients exhibit moderate splenomegaly. Proliferative retinopathy is more common and more severe than in sickle cell anemia.[89] Respiratory tract infections with *S. pneumoniae* are common.[8]

Patients with Hb SC disease live longer than patients with Hb SS and have fewer painful episodes, but this disorder is associated with considerable morbidity and mortality, especially after age 30.[90] In the United States the median life span for men is 60 years and for women 68 years.[33]

Laboratory Diagnosis

The CBC indicates a mild normocytic, normochromic anemia with many features associated with sickle cell anemia. The hemoglobin level is usually 11 to 13 g/dL, and the reticulocyte count is 3% to 5%. On the peripheral blood film there are a few sickle cells, target cells, and intraerythrocytic crystalline structures. Crystalline aggregates of hemoglobin (SC crystals) form in some cells, where they protrude from the membrane (Figure 24.12).[87] Hb SC crystals often appear as a hybrid of Hb S and Hb C crystals. They are longer than Hb C crystals but shorter and thicker than Hb S polymers and are often branched.

The hemoglobin solubility test is positive because of the presence of Hb S. Electrophoretically, Hb C and Hb S migrate in almost equal amounts (45%) on alkaline electrophoresis, and Hb F is normal. Hb C is confirmed on citrate agar at an acid pH, where it is separated from Hb E and Hb O. Hb A_2 migrates with Hb C, and its quantification is of no consequence in Hb SC disease. Determination of Hb A_2 becomes vital, however, if a patient is suspected of having Hb C concurrent with β-thalassemia (Chapter 25).

Treatment and Prognosis

Therapy similar to that for SCD is given to individuals with Hb SC disease.[84]

Hemoglobin S-β-Thalassemia

Compound heterozygosity for Hb S and β-thalassemia is the most common cause of sickle cell syndrome in patients of Mediterranean descent and is second to Hb SC disease among all compound heterozygous sickle disorders. Hb S-β-thal usually causes a clinical syndrome resembling that of mild or moderate sickle cell anemia. The severity of this compound heterozygous condition depends on the β chain production of the affected β-thalassemia gene. If there is no β-globin chain production from the β-thalassemia gene (Hb S-β⁰-thal), the clinical course is similar to that of Hb SS. If there is production

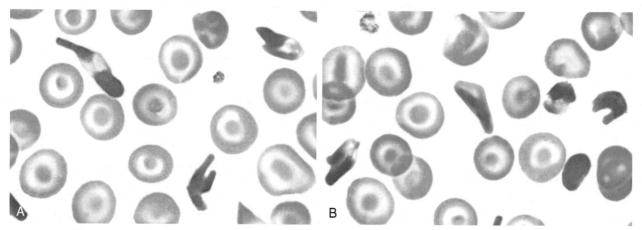

Figure 24.12 Peripheral Blood Films for a Patient with Hemoglobin SC Disease. (A) and **(B)**, Note intraerythrocytic, blunt-ended SC crystals and target cells. (A, B, Wright-Giemsa stain, ×1000.) (Courtesy Ann Bell, University of Tennessee, Memphis.)

of some level of β-globin chain (Hb S-β⁺-thal), patients tend to have a milder condition than patients with Hb SC. These patients can be distinguished from individuals with SCT because of the presence of greater amounts of Hb S than of Hb A, increased levels of Hb A_2 and Hb F, microcytosis from the thalassemia, hemolytic anemia, abnormal peripheral blood morphology, and splenomegaly (Chapter 25).[21,87]

Hemoglobin SD and Hemoglobin SG-Philadelphia

Hb SD is a compound heterozygous and Hb SG-Philadelphia a double heterozygous sickle cell syndrome.[21] Hb SG-Philadelphia is asymptomatic because Hb G is associated with an α gene mutation that still allows for sufficient Hb A to be produced. Hb SD syndrome may cause a mild to severe hemolytic anemia because both β chains are affected. Some patients with Hb SD may have severe vasoocclusive complications. The Hb SD syndrome in African Americans usually is due to the interaction of Hb S with Hb D-Los Angeles (Hb D-Punjab).

The peripheral blood film findings for Hb SD disease are comparable to those seen in less severe forms of Hb SS disease. Because Hb D and Hb G comigrate with Hb S on alkaline electrophoresis, citrate agar electrophoresis at an acid pH is necessary to separate Hb S from Hb D and Hb G. The clinical picture is valuable in differentiating Hb SD and Hb SG. The treatment for Hb SD disease is similar to treatment for patients with SCD and is administered according to the severity of the clinical condition.

Hemoglobin SO-Arab and Hb SD-Punjab

Hb SO-Arab and Hb SD-Punjab are rare compound heterozygous hemoglobinopathies that cause severe chronic hemolytic anemia with vasoocclusive episodes.[8,21] Both mutations replace glutamic acid at position 121; O-Arab substitutes lysine and D-Punjab substitutes glutamine. Glutamic acid at position 121 is located on the outer surface of the hemoglobin tetramer, which enhances the polymerization process involving Hb S. Hb SO-Arab can be mistaken for Hb SC on alkaline electrophoresis because Hb C and Hb O-Arab migrate at the same position; however, differentiation is made on citrate agar at an acid pH because these hemoglobins do not comigrate. Therapy is similar to treatment for patients with SCD. Similarly, Hb D-Punjab comigrates with Hb S on alkaline electrophoresis, making this mutation look like SCD. Hb O-Arab and Hb D-Punjab are not clinically significant in either the heterozygous or the homozygous form.[1]

Hemoglobin S-Korle Bu

Hb Korle Bu is a rare hemoglobin variant with substitution of aspartic acid for asparagine at position 73 of the β chain.[5,21] When inherited with Hb S, it interferes with lateral contact between Hb S fibers by disrupting the hydrophobic pocket for $β_6$ valine, which inhibits Hb S polymerization. The compound heterozygous condition Hb S-Korle Bu is asymptomatic.

CONCOMITANT CIS MUTATIONS WITH HEMOGLOBIN S

A concomitant cis mutation with Hb S involves a second mutation on the same gene along with Hb S. Three cis mutations will be described: Hb C-Harlem, Hb S-Antilles, and Hb S-Oman.

Hemoglobin C-Harlem

Hb C-Harlem has two substitutions on the β chain: the sickle mutation and the Korle Bu mutation. Patients heterozygous for only Hb C-Harlem are asymptomatic. The compound heterozygous Hb SC-Harlem state resembles Hb SS clinically. Hb C-Harlem yields a positive result on the hemoglobin solubility test and migrates to the Hb C position on alkaline electrophoresis and to the Hb S position on citrate agar electrophoresis at an acid pH.[5,21,84]

Hemoglobin S-Antilles and Hemoglobin S-Oman

Hb S-Antilles bears the Hb S mutation ($β^{6Glu→Val}$) along with a substitution of isoleucine for valine at position 23.[91] Hb S-Oman also has the Hb S mutation with a second substitution of lysine for glutamic acid at position 121.[92] In both these hemoglobin variants, the second mutation enhances Hb S such that significant sickling can occur even in heterozygotes.[1]

Table 24.2 summarizes common clinically significant hemoglobinopathies, including general characteristics and treatment options.

HEMOGLOBIN M

Hb M is caused by a variety of mutations in the α-, β-, and γ-globin genes, all of which result in production of methemoglobin, hence the Hb M designation.[93] These genetic mutations result in a structural abnormality in the globin portion of the molecule. Most M hemoglobins involve a substitution of a tyrosine amino acid for either the proximal (F_8) or the distal (E_7) histidine amino acid in the α, β, or γ chains. These substitutions cause heme iron to auto-oxidize, which results in methemoglobinemia. Hb M has iron in the ferric state (Fe^{3+}) and is unable to carry oxygen, which produces cyanosis. Seven hemoglobin variants affecting the α or β chains have been classified as M hemoglobins: Hb M-Boston, Hb M-Iwate, and Hb Auckland (α chain variants); and Hb Chile, Hb M-Saskatoon, Hb M-Milwaukee-1, and Hb M-Milwaukee-2 (β chain variants), all named for the locations in which they were discovered.[5] Two variants affect the γ chain, namely, Hb F-M-Osaka and Hb F-M-Fort Ripley,[5] but symptoms disappear when Hb A replaces Hb F at age 3 to 6 months.

Hb M variants have altered oxygen affinity and are inherited as autosomal dominant disorders. Affected individuals have 30% to 50% methemoglobin (healthy individuals have less than 1%) and may appear cyanotic. Ingestion of oxidant drugs, such as sulfonamides, can increase methemoglobin to life-threatening levels. Methemoglobin causes the blood specimen to appear brown. Heinz bodies may be seen sometimes on wet preparations because methemoglobin causes globin chains to precipitate (Figure 11.12). Diagnosis is made by spectral absorption of the hemolysate or by hemoglobin electrophoresis. Absorption spectrum peaks are determined at various wavelengths. The unique absorption range of each Hb M variant is identified when these are compared with the spectrum of normal blood.

Before electrophoresis, all hemoglobin types are converted to methemoglobin by adding potassium cyanide to the specimen so that any migration differences observed are only the result of an amino acid substitution, not differences in iron states. On

TABLE 24.2   Common Clinically Significant Hemoglobinopathies

Hemoglobin Disorder	Abnormal Hemoglobin	Structural Defect	Groups Primarily Affected	Hemoglobin Solubility Test Results	Hemoglobins Present	Red Blood Cell Morphology	Symptoms/Organ Defects	Treatment
Sickle cell anemia (homozygous)	Hb S	$\alpha_2\beta_2^{6Glu\to Val}$	African, African American, Middle Eastern, Indian, Mediterranean	Positive	0% Hb A, > 80% Hb S, 1%–20% Hb F, 2%–5% Hb A$_2$	Sickle cells, target cells, nucleated RBCs, polychromasia, Howell-Jolly bodies, basophilic stippling	Vasoocclusion, bacterial infections, hemolytic anemia, aplastic episodes; affects bones, lungs, liver, spleen, penis, eyes, central nervous system, urinary tract	Transfusions, antibiotics, analgesics, bone marrow transplant, hydroxyurea
Hb C disease (homozygous)	Hb C	$\alpha_2\beta_2^{6Glu\to Lys}$	African, African American	Negative	0% Hb A, >90% Hb C, <7% Hb F, 2% Hb A$_2$	Hb C crystals, target cells, nucleated RBCs, occasionally some microcytes	Mild splenomegaly, mild hemolysis	Usually none, antibiotics
Hb SC-Harlem* (Hb C-Georgetown)	Hb C-Harlem, Hb S	$\alpha_2\beta_2^{6Glu\to Val}$ and $\alpha_2\beta_2^{73Asp\to Asn}$ on same gene and $\alpha_2\beta_2^{6Glu\to Val}$	Rare, so uncertain; African, African American	Positive	Hb C-Harlem migrates with Hb C at alkaline pH; migrates with Hb S at acid pH	Target cells	Compound heterozygotes with Hb SC-Harlem have symptoms similar to Hb SS	Similar to Hb SS
Hb E disease (homozygous)	Hb E	$\alpha_2\beta_2^{26Glu\to Lys}$	Southeast Asian, African, African American	Negative	0% Hb A, 95% Hb E, 2%–4% Hb A$_2$; migrates with Hb A$_2$, Hb C, and Hb O at alkaline pH	Target cells, microcytes	Mild anemia, mild splenomegaly, no symptoms	Usually none
Hb O-Arab (homozygous)	Hb O-Arab	$\alpha_2\beta_2^{121Glu\to Lys}$	Kenyan, Israeli, Egyptian, Bulgarian, African American	Negative	0% Hb A, 95% Hb O, 2%–4% Hb A$_2$; migrates with Hb A$_2$, Hb C, and Hb E at alkaline pH	Target cells	Mild splenomegaly	Usually none
Hb D disease (rare homozygous)	Hb D-Punjab (Hb-D Los Angeles)	$\alpha_2\beta_2^{121Glu\to Gln}$	Middle Eastern, Indian	Negative	95% Hb D, normal Hb A$_2$ and Hb F; migrates with Hb S at alkaline pH	Target cells	Mild hemolytic anemia, mild splenomegaly	Usually none

Continued

TABLE 24.2 Common Clinically Significant Hemoglobinopathies—cont'd

Hemoglobin Disorder	Abnormal Hemoglobin	Structural Defect	Groups Primarily Affected	Hemoglobin Solubility Test Results	Hemoglobins Present	Red Blood Cell Morphology	Symptoms/Organ Defects	Treatment
Hb G disease (rare homozygous)	Hb G, Hb G-Philadelphia	$\alpha_2^{68Asn\rightarrow Lys}\beta_2$	African American, Ghanaian	Negative	95% Hb G, normal Hb A$_2$ and Hb F; migrates with S at alkaline pH	Target cells	Mild hemolytic anemia, mild splenomegaly	Usually none
Hb SC* disease	Hb S, Hb C	$\alpha_2\beta_2^{6Glu\rightarrow Val}$ and $\alpha_2\beta_2^{6Glu\rightarrow Lys}$	Same as Hb S	Positive	45% Hb S, 45% Hb C, 2%–4% Hb A$_2$, 1% Hb F	Sickle cells, Hb SC crystals, target cells	Same as those for Hb SS except milder	Similar to that for Hb SS but less intensive
Hb S-β-thalassemia*	Hb S + β-thalassemia mutation	$\alpha_2\beta_2^{6Glu\rightarrow Val}$ and β^0 or β^+	Same as Hb S	Positive	Hb S variable, some Hb A in β$^+$; increased Hb A$_2$ and Hb F	Sickle cells, target cells, microcytes	Hemolytic anemia, splenomegaly	Similar to that for Hb SS; varies depending on amount of Hb A present
Hb SD* disease	Hb S, Hb D	$\alpha_2\beta_2^{6Glu\rightarrow Val}$ and $\alpha_2\beta_2^{121Glu\rightarrow Gln}$	Same as Hb S	Positive	45% Hb S, 45% Hb D, 2%–4% Hb A$_2$, 1% Hb F; Hb S and D comigrate at alkaline pH	Sickle cells, target cells	Similar to those for Hb SS but milder	Similar to that for Hb SS but less intensive
Hb SG†	Hb S, Hb G	$\alpha_2\beta_2^{6Glu\rightarrow Val}$ and $\alpha_2^{68Asn\rightarrow Lys}\beta_2$	Same as Hb S	Positive	45% Hb S, 45% Hb G, 2%–4% Hb A$_2$, 1% Hb F; Hb S and G comigrate at alkaline pH	Target cells	No symptoms	Usually none
Hb SO-Arab*	Hb S, Hb O-Arab	$\alpha_2\beta_2^{6Glu\rightarrow Val}$ and $\alpha_2\beta_2^{121Glu\rightarrow Lys}$	Same as Hb S	Positive	45% Hb S, 45% Hb O, 2%–4% Hb A$_2$, 1% Hb F	Sickle cells, target cells	Similar to those for Hb SS	Similar to that for Hb SS

Asn, Asparagine; *Asp,* aspartic acid; *Gln,* glutamine; *Glu,* glutamic acid; *Hb,* hemoglobin; *Lys,* lysine; *Val,* valine.

*Compound heterozygous.

†Double heterozygous.

alkaline electrophoresis, Hb M migrates slightly more slowly than Hb A. The electrophoresis should be performed on agar gel at pH 7.1 for clear separation. Further confirmation may be obtained using HPLC or DNA-based globin gene analysis. No treatment is necessary. Diagnosis is essential to prevent inappropriate treatment for other conditions, such as cyanotic heart disease.

UNSTABLE HEMOGLOBIN VARIANTS

Unstable hemoglobin variants result from genetic mutations to globin genes creating hemoglobin products that precipitate in vivo, producing Heinz bodies and causing a hemolytic anemia.[93] More than 185 variants of unstable hemoglobin exist.[5] The majority of these are β chain variants, and most others are α chain variants. Only a few are γ and δ chain variants. Most unstable hemoglobin variants have no clinical significance, although the majority have increased oxygen affinity. About 25% of unstable hemoglobins are responsible for hemolytic anemia, which varies from compensated mild anemia to severe hemolytic episodes.[93,94]

At one time the anemia was referred to as *congenital nonspherocytic hemolytic anemia* or *congenital Heinz body anemia*. This disorder is more properly called *unstable hemoglobin disease*. The syndrome appears at or just after birth, depending on the globin chains involved. It is inherited in an autosomal dominant pattern. All patients are heterozygous; apparently the homozygous condition is incompatible with life. The instability of the hemoglobin molecule may be due to (1) substitution of a charged for an uncharged amino acid in the interior of the molecule, (2) substitution of a polar for a nonpolar amino acid in the hydrophobic heme pocket, (3) substitution of an amino acid in the α and β chains at the intersubunit contact points, (4) replacement of an amino acid with proline in the α helix section of a chain, and (5) deletion or elongation of the primary structure.[93,94]

Clinical Features

Unstable hemoglobin disorder is usually detected in early childhood in patients with hemolytic anemia accompanied by jaundice and splenomegaly. Fever or ingestion of an oxidant exacerbates the hemolysis. Severity of the anemia depends on the degree of instability of the hemoglobin molecule. Unstable hemoglobin precipitates in vivo and in vitro in response to factors that do not affect normal hemoglobins, such as drug ingestion and exposure to heat or cold. Hemoglobin precipitates in RBCs as Heinz bodies. Precipitated hemoglobin attaches to the inner cell membrane, causing clustering of band 3, attachment of autologous immunoglobulin, and macrophage activation. In addition, Heinz bodies can be trapped mechanically in the splenic sieve, which shortens RBC survival. Oxygen affinity of these cells is also abnormal.[93,94]

The most prevalent unstable hemoglobin is Hb Köln. Other unstable hemoglobins include Hb Hammersmith, Hb Zurich, and Hb Gun Hill.[5] Because of the large variability in the degree of instability in these hemoglobins, the extent of hemolysis varies greatly. For some of the variants, such as Hb Zurich, the presence of an oxidant is required for any significant hemolysis to occur.[93,94]

Laboratory Diagnosis

RBC morphology varies. It may be normal or show slight hypochromia and prominent basophilic stippling, which possibly is caused by excessive clumping of ribosomes. Before splenectomy, hemoglobin levels range from 7 to 12 g/dL, with a 4% to 20% reticulocyte count. After splenectomy, anemia is corrected, but reticulocytosis persists. Heinz bodies can be shown using a supravital stain (Figure 11.12). After splenectomy, Heinz bodies are larger and more numerous. Many patients excrete dark urine that contains dipyrrole.[93,94]

Many unstable hemoglobins migrate in the normal AA pattern and thus are not detected on electrophoresis. Other tests used to detect unstable hemoglobins include the isopropanol precipitation test, which is based on the principle that an isopropanol solution at 37° C weakens the bonding forces of the hemoglobin molecule. If unstable hemoglobins are present, rapid precipitation occurs in 5 minutes and heavy flocculation occurs after 20 minutes. Normal hemoglobin does not begin to precipitate until after approximately 40 minutes. The heat denaturation test also can be used. When incubated at 50° C for 1 hour, heat-sensitive unstable hemoglobins show a flocculent precipitation, whereas normal hemoglobin shows little or no precipitation. Significant numbers of Heinz bodies appear after splenectomy, but even in individuals with intact spleens, with longer incubation and the addition of an oxidative substance such as acetylphenylhydrazine, unstable hemoglobins form more Heinz bodies than does the blood from individuals with normal hemoglobins. Other techniques, such as isoelectric focusing, can resolve many hemoglobin variants with only a slight alteration in their isoelectric point, and globin chain analysis can be performed by HPLC or DNA-based globin gene analysis.[93,94]

Treatment and Prognosis

Patients are treated to prevent hemolytic crises. In severe cases the spleen must be removed to reduce sequestration and rate of removal of RBCs. Because unstable hemoglobin disease is rare, prognosis in the affected individuals is unclear. Patients are cautioned against the use of sulfonamides and other oxidant drugs. They also should be informed of the potential for febrile illnesses to trigger a hemolytic episode.[93,94]

HEMOGLOBINS WITH INCREASED AND DECREASED OXYGEN AFFINITY

More than 380 hemoglobin variants have been discovered to have abnormal oxygen affinity.[4,93-95] Most are high-affinity variants and have been associated with familial erythrocytosis. The remaining hemoglobin variants are characterized by low oxygen affinity. Many of these are associated with mild to moderate anemia.[2]

As described in Chapter 7, normal Hb A undergoes a series of allosteric conformational changes as it converts from a fully deoxygenated to a fully oxygenated form. These conformational changes affect hemoglobin function and its affinity for oxygen. When normal hemoglobin is fully deoxygenated (tense state), it has low affinity for oxygen and other heme ligands and high affinity for allosteric effectors, such as Bohr protons and 2,3-bisphosphoglycerate. In the oxygenated (relaxed) state, hemoglobin has a high affinity for heme ligands, such as oxygen, and a low affinity for Bohr protons and 2,3-bisphosphoglycerate. The transition from the tense to the relaxed state involves a series of structural changes that have a marked effect on hemoglobin function. If an amino acid substitution lowers the stability of the tense structure, transition to the relaxed state occurs at an earlier stage in oxygen binding, and hemoglobin has increased oxygen affinity and decreased heme-heme interaction or cooperativity (Chapter 7). One example of a β chain variant is Hb Kempsey. This unstable hemoglobin variant has amino acid substitutions at sites crucial to hemoglobin function.[93,95]

Hemoglobins With Increased Oxygen Affinity

The high-affinity variants, like other structurally abnormal hemoglobins, show an autosomal dominant pattern of inheritance. Affected individuals have equal volumes of Hb A and the abnormal variant. Exceptions to this are compound heterozygotes for Hb Abruzzo and β-thalassemia and for Hb Crete and β-thalassemia, in which the proportion of abnormal hemoglobin is greater than 85%.[93,95]

More than 200 variant hemoglobins with high oxygen affinity have been discovered.[5] Such hemoglobins fail to release oxygen on demand, and hypoxia results. Kidneys sense the hypoxia and respond by increasing the release of erythropoietin, which leads to a compensatory erythrocytosis. These variants differ from unstable hemoglobin, which also may have abnormal oxygen affinity, in that they do not precipitate in vivo to produce hemolysis and there is no abnormal RBC morphology.[93,95]

Most individuals are asymptomatic and have no physical symptoms except a ruddy complexion. Erythrocytosis is usually detected during routine examination because the patient generally has a high RBC count, hemoglobin, and hematocrit. The WBC count, platelet count, and peripheral blood film findings are generally normal. In some cases, hemoglobin electrophoresis may establish a diagnosis. An abnormal band that separates from the A band is present on alkaline electrophoresis in some variants; however, if a band is not found, the diagnosis of increased oxygen affinity cannot be ruled out. In some cases the abnormal hemoglobin can be separated using citrate agar electrophoresis (pH 6.0). Measurement of oxygen affinity is required for definitive diagnosis.[93,95]

Patients with high-oxygen-affinity hemoglobins live normal lives and require no treatment. Diagnosis should be made to avoid unnecessary treatment of the erythrocytosis as a myeloproliferative neoplasm or a secondary erythrocytosis.[93,95]

Hemoglobins With Decreased Oxygen Affinity

Hemoglobins with decreased oxygen affinity quickly release oxygen to the tissues, which results in normal to decreased hemoglobin concentration, slight anemia, and cyanosis. More than 170 variant hemoglobins with low oxygen affinity have been discovered.[5] The best known of these hemoglobins is Hb Kansas, which has an amino acid substitution of asparagine by threonine at position 102 of the β chain. These hemoglobins may be present when cyanosis and a normal arterial oxygen tension coexist, and most may be detected by starch gel electrophoresis, HPLC, or DNA-based globin gene analysis.[93,95]

GLOBAL BURDEN OF HEMOGLOBINOPATHIES

The prevalence of hemoglobinopathies has already been presented in this chapter, and the bulk of these conditions occurs in underdeveloped countries. However, as developing countries work to decrease deaths from malnutrition, infectious diseases, and other conditions, more patients with hemoglobinopathies will survive and remain consumers of the health care system. For example, in 1944 thalassemia was first identified in Cypress. However, during the post-World War II recovery period, as the death rate decreased, the prevalence of thalassemias increased.[2] In 1970 it was estimated that in the absence of systems to control the disease, within 40 years 78,000 units of blood would be needed each year, requiring that 40% of the population serve as donors.[2] If left unchecked, the cost to maintain thalassemia therapy would exceed the country's total health care budget. In contrast, efforts to develop prenatal screening and genetic counseling programs have reduced the birth rate of SCD.[2] It is clear that hemoglobinopathies are a worldwide problem requiring planning, investment, and interventions from around the globe to optimize the impact on patients with the disease without debilitating the health care systems of developing countries where the disease is prevalent.

▮ SUMMARY

- Hemoglobinopathies are genetic disorders of globin genes that produce structurally abnormal hemoglobins with altered amino acid sequences, which can affect hemoglobin function and stability.
- Hemoglobin (Hb) S is the most common hemoglobinopathy, resulting from a substitution of valine for glutamic acid at position 6 of the β-globin chain, and primarily affects people of African descent.
- Hb S polymerizes in red blood cells (RBCs) because of abnormal interaction with adjacent tetramers when it is in the deoxygenated form, producing sickle-shaped RBCs.
- In homozygous Hb SS, polymerization of hemoglobin may result in severe episodic conditions; however, factors other

than hemoglobin polymerization may account for vasoocclusive episodes in sickle cell patients.
- The most clinically significant hemoglobinopathies are Hb SS, Hb SC, and Hb S-β-thalassemia; Hb SS causes the most severe disease.
- Individuals with sickle cell trait (Hb AS) are clinically asymptomatic but can manifest symptoms under extreme exertion.
- Sickle cell anemia (Hb SS) is a normocytic, normochromic anemia, characterized by a single band in the S position on hemoglobin electrophoresis, a single Hb S peak on high-performance liquid chromatography (HPLC), and a positive hemoglobin solubility test. The median life expectancy of patients with SCD is greater than 50 years.

- Hb C and Hb E are the next most common hemoglobinopathies after Hb S and cause mild hemolysis in the homozygous state. In the heterozygous states these hemoglobinopathies are asymptomatic.
- Hb C is found primarily in people of African descent.
- On peripheral blood films from patients with Hb CC, hexagonal crystals may be seen with and without apparent RBC membrane surrounding them.
- Hb EE results in a microcytic anemia and is found primarily in people of Southeast Asian descent.
- Other variants, such as unstable hemoglobins and hemoglobins with altered oxygen affinity, can be identified, and many cause no clinical abnormality.

- Laboratory procedures employed for diagnosis of hemoglobinopathies are the complete blood count, peripheral blood film evaluation, reticulocyte count, hemoglobin solubility test, and methods to quantify normal and variant hemoglobins, including hemoglobin electrophoresis (alkaline and acid pH), HPLC, and capillary electrophoresis.
- Advanced techniques available for hemoglobin identification include isoelectric focusing and DNA-based analysis of the globin genes.

Now that you have completed this chapter, go back and read again the case study at the beginning and respond to the questions presented.

REVIEW QUESTIONS

Answers can be found in the Appendix.

1. A qualitative abnormality in hemoglobin may involve all of the following *except:*
   a. Replacement of one or more amino acids in a globin chain
   b. Addition of one or more amino acids in a globin chain
   c. Deletion of one or more amino acids in a globin chain
   d. Decreased production of a globin chain

2. The substitution of valine for glutamic acid at position 6 of the β chain of hemoglobin results in hemoglobin that:
   a. Is unstable and precipitates as Heinz bodies
   b. Polymerizes to form tactoid crystals
   c. Crystallizes in a hexagonal shape
   d. Contains iron in the ferric (Fe^{3+}) state

3. Patients with SCD usually do not exhibit symptoms until 6 months of age because:
   a. The mother's blood has a protective effect
   b. Hemoglobin levels are higher in infants at birth
   c. Higher levels of Hb F are present
   d. The immune system is not fully developed

4. Megaloblastic episodes in SCD can be prevented by prophylactic administration of:
   a. Iron
   b. Folic acid
   c. Steroids
   d. Erythropoietin

5. Which of the following is the most definitive test for Hb S?
   a. Hemoglobin solubility test
   b. Hemoglobin electrophoresis at alkaline pH
   c. Osmotic fragility test
   d. Hemoglobin electrophoresis at acid pH

6. A patient presents with mild normochromic, normocytic anemia. On the peripheral blood film, there are a few target cells, rare nucleated RBCs, and hexagonal crystals within and lying outside of the RBCs. Which abnormality in the hemoglobin molecule is most likely?
   a. Decreased production of β chains
   b. Substitution of lysine for glutamic acid at position 6 of the β chain
   c. Substitution of tyrosine for the proximal histidine in the β chain
   d. Double amino acid substitution in the β chain

7. A well-mixed specimen obtained for a CBC has a brown color. The patient is being treated with a sulfonamide for a bladder infection. Which of the following could explain the brown color?
   a. The patient has Hb M.
   b. The patient is a compound heterozygote for Hb S and thalassemia.
   c. The incorrect anticoagulant was used.
   d. Levels of Hb F are high.

8. Through routine screening, prospective parents discover that they are both heterozygous for Hb S. What percentage of their children potentially could have sickle cell anemia (Hb SS)?
   a. 0%
   b. 25%
   c. 50%
   d. 100%

9. Painful crises in patients with SCD occur as a result of:
   a. Splenic sequestration
   b. Aplasia
   c. Vasoocclusion
   d. Anemia

10. The screening test for Hb S that uses a reducing agent, such as sodium dithionite, is based on the fact that hemoglobins that sickle:
    a. Are insoluble in reduced, deoxygenated form
    b. Form methemoglobin more readily and cause a color change
    c. Are unstable and precipitate as Heinz bodies
    d. Oxidize quickly and cause turbidity

11. DNA analysis documents a patient has inherited the sickle mutation in both β-globin genes. The two terms that best describe this genotype are:
    a. Homozygous/trait
    b. Homozygous/disease
    c. Heterozygous/trait
    d. Heterozygous/disease

12. In which of the following geographic areas is Hb S most prevalent?
    a. India
    b. South Africa
    c. United States
    d. Sub-Saharan Africa

13. Which hemoglobinopathy is more common in Southeast Asian patients?
    a. Hb S
    b. Hb C
    c. Hb O
    d. Hb E

14. Which of the following Hb S compound heterozygotes exhibits the mildest symptoms?
    a. Hb S-β-thalassemia
    b. Hb SG
    c. Hb SC-Harlem
    d. Hb SC

15. A 1-year-old Indian patient presents with anemia, and both parents claim to have an "inherited anemia" but can't remember the type. The peripheral blood shows target cells, and the hemoglobin solubility is negative. Alkaline hemoglobin electrophoresis shows a single band at the "Hb C" position and a small band at the "Hb F" position. Acid hemoglobin electrophoresis shows two bands. The most likely diagnosis is:
    a. Hb CC
    b. Hb AC
    c. Hb CO
    d. Hb SC

16. Unstable hemoglobins exhibit all of the following findings *except*:
    a. Globin chains that precipitate intracellularly
    b. Heinz body formation
    c. Elevated reticulocyte count
    d. Only homozygotes are symptomatic

REFERENCES

1. Wajeman, H., & Moradkhani, K. (2011). Abnormal hemoglobins: detection and characterization. *Indian J Med Res, 134*, 538–546.
2. Weatherall, D. J. (2011). The challenges of haemoglobinopathies in resource-poor countries. *Br J Haematol, 154*, 736–744.
3. Bauer, D. E., & Orkin, S. H. (2011). Update on fetal hemoglobin gene regulation in hemoglobinopathies. *Curr Opin Pediatr, 23*, 1–8.
4. Wang, W. C. (2014). Sickle cell anemia and other sickling syndromes. In Greer, J. P., Arber, D.A., Bertil, G., et al. (Eds.), *Wintrobe's Clinical Hematology*. (Vol. 1, 13th ed., pp. 1038–1082). Philadelphia: Wolters Kluwer Health/Lippincott Williams & Wilkins.
5. Patrinos, G. P., Giardine, B., Riemer, C., et al. (2004). Improvements in the HbVar database of human hemoglobin variants and thalassemia mutations for population and sequence variation studies. *Nucl Acids Res, 32*(database issue), D537–541. http://globin.cse.psu.edu/hbvar/menu.html. Accessed July 31, 2017.
6. Fishleder, A. J., & Hoffman, G. C. (1987). A practical approach to the detection of hemoglobinopathies. Part II: the sickle cell disorders. *Lab Med, 18*, 441–443.
7. Konotey-Ahulu, F. I. (1974). The sickle cell diseases. Clinical manifestations including the "sickle crisis." *Arch Intern Med, 133*, 611–619.
8. Natrajan, K., & Kutlar, A. (2016). Disorders of hemoglobin structure: sickle cell anemia and related abnormalities. In Kaushansky, K., Lichtman, M. A., Prchal, J. T., et al. (Eds.), *Williams Hematology.* (9th ed., pp. 759–788). New York: McGraw-Hill.
9. Serjeant, G. R. (2001). Historical review: the emerging understanding of sickle cell disease. *Br J Haematol, 112*, 3–18.
10. Park, K. W. (2004). Sickle cell disease and other hemoglobinopathies. *Int Anesth Clin, 42*, 77–93.
11. Maron, B. J., Harris, K. M., Thompson, P. D., et al. (2015). Eligibility and disqualification recommendations for competitive athletes with cardiovascular abnormalities: Task Force 14: sickle cell trait. *Circulation, 132*, e343–e345.
12. Rees, D. C., Williams, T. N., & Gladwn, M. T. (2010). Sickle-cell disease. *Lancet, 376*, 2018–2031.
13. Piel, F. B., Patil, A. B., Howes, R. E., et al. (2013). Global epidemiology of sickle haemoglobin in neonates: a contemporary geostatistical model-based map and population estimates. *Lancet, 381*, 142–151.
14. Noronha, S. A., Sadreameli, S. C., & Strouse, J. J. (2016). Management of sickle cell disease in children. *S Med J, 109*(9), 495–502.
15. Shah, A. (2004). Hemoglobinopathies and other congenital hemolytic anemia. *Ind J Med Sci, 58*, 490–493.
16. Wishner, B. C., Ward, K. B., Lattman, E. E., et al. (1975). Crystal structure of sickle-cell deoxyhemoglobin at 5 A resolution. *J Mol Biol, 98*, 179–194.
17. Dykes, G., Crepeau, R. H., & Edelstein, S. J. (1978). Three-dimensional reconstruction of the fibers of sickle cell haemoglobin. *Nature, 272*, 506–510.
18. Dykes, G. W., Crepeau, R. H., & Edelstein, S. J. (1979). Three-dimensional reconstruction of the 14-filament fiber of hemoglobin S. *J Mol Biol, 130*, 451–472.
19. Crepeau, R. H., Edelstein, S. J., Szalay, M., et al. (1981). Sickle cell hemoglobin fiber structure altered by alpha-chain mutation. *Proc Natl Acad Sci U S A, 78*, 1406–1410.
20. Gibbs, N. M., & Larach, D. R. (2013). Anesthetic management during cardiopulmonary bypass. In Hensley, F. A., Gravlee, G. P., & Martin, D. E. (Eds.), *A Practical Approach to Cardiac Anesthesia.* (5th ed., pp. 214–237). Philadelphia: Lippincott, Williams & Wilkins.
21. Kawthalkar, S. M. (2013). Anemias due to excessive red cell destruction. In Kawthalkar, S. M. *Essentials of Hematology.* (2nd ed., pp. 171–184). New Delhi: Jaypee Brothers Medical Publishers.
22. de Jong, K., Larkin, S. K., Styles, L. A., et al. (2001). Characterization of the phosphatidylserine-exposing subpopulation of sickle cells. *Blood, 98*, 860–867.

23. Yasin, Z., Witting, S., & Palascak, M. B. (2003). Phosphatidylserine externalization in sickle red blood cell: associations with cell age, density, and hemoglobin F. *Blood, 102*, 365–370.

24. de Jong, K., Rettig, M. P., Low, P. S., et al. (2002). Protein kinase C activation induces phosphatidylserine exposure on red blood cells. *Biochemistry, 41*, 12562–12567.

25. de Jong, K., & Kuypers, F. A. (2006). Sulfhydral modifications alter scamblase activity in murine sickle cell disease. *Br J Haematol, 133*, 427–432.

26. Manodori, A. B., Barabino, G. A., Lubin, B. H., et al. (2000). Adherence of phosphatidylserine-exposing erythrocytes to endothelial matrix thrombomodulin. *Blood, 95*, 1293–1300.

27. Stuart, M. L., & Setty, B. N. (2001). Hemostatic alterations in sickle cell disease: relationships to disease pathophysiology. *Pediatr Pathol Mol Med, 20*, 27–46.

28. Setty, B. N., Kulkarni, S., & Stuart, M. J. (2002). Role of erythrocyte phosphatidylserine in sickle red cell-endothelial adhesion. *Blood, 99*, 1564–1571.

29. Kuypers, F. A., & Styles, L. A. (2004). The role of secretory phospholipase A2 in acute chest syndrome. *Cell Mol Biol, 50*, 87–94.

30. Neidlinger, N. A., Larkin, S. K., Bhagat, A., et al. (2006). Hydrolysis of phosphatidylserine-exposing red blood cells by secretory phospholipase A2 generates lysophosphatidic acid and results in vascular dysfunction. *J Biol Chem, 281*, 775–781.

31. Hebbel, R. P., & Key, N. S. (2016). Microparticles in sickle cell anaemia: promise and pitfalls. *Br J Haematol, 174*, 16–29.

32. Kato, G. J. (2016). New insights into sickle cell disease: mechanisms and investigational therapies. *Curr Opin Hematol, 23*, 224–232.

33. Benkerrou, M., Alberti, C., Couque, N., et al. (2013). Impact of glucose-6-phosphate dehydrogenase deficiency on sickle cell expression in infancy and early childhood: a prospective study. *Br J Haematol, 163*, 646–654.

34. Noguchi, C. T., Rodgers, G. P., Sergeant, G., et al. (1988). Level of fetal hemoglobin necessary for treatment of sickle cell disease. *N Engl J Med, 318*, 96–99.

35. Diggs, L. W. (1965). Sickle cell crises. *J Clin Pathol, 44*, 1–19.

36. Bartolucci, P., & Galacteros, F. (2012). Clinical management of adult sickle cell disease. *Curr Opin Hematol, 19*, 149–155.

37. Embury, S. H., Hebbel, R. P., Steinberg, M. H., et al. (1994). Pathogenesis of vasoocclusion. In Embury, S. H., Hebbel, R. P., Mohandas, N., et al. (Eds.), *Sickle Cell Disease: Basic Principles and Clinical Practice.* (pp. 311–323). Philadelphia: Lippincott Williams & Wilkins.

38. Jandl, J. H. (1996). *Blood: Textbook of Hematology.* (2nd ed., pp. 531–577). Boston: Little, Brown.

39. Hagar, W., & Vichinsky, E. (2008). Advances in clinical research in sickle cell disease. *Br J Haematol, 141*, 346–356.

40. Styles, L. A., Schalkwijk, C. G., Aarsman, A. J., et al. (1996). Phospholipase A2 levels in acute chest syndrome of sickle cell disease. *Blood, 87*, 2573–2578.

41. Styles, L. A., Aareman, A. J., Vichinski, E. P., et al. (2000). Secretory phospholipase A2 predicts impending acute chest syndrome in sickle cell disease. *Blood, 96*, 3276–3278.

42. Howard, J. (2016). Sickle cell disease: when and how to transfuse. *Hematology Am Soc Hematol Educ Program, 2016*, 625–631.

43. Gangaraju, R., Reddy, V. V. B., & Marquis, M. B. (2016). Fat embolism syndrome secondary to bone marrow necrosis in patients with hemoglobinopathies. *S Med J, 19*(9), 549–553.

44. Morris, C. R., Kuypers, F. A., Larkin, S., et al. (2000). Patterns of arginine and nitrous oxide in patients with sickle cell disease with vaso-occlusive crisis and acute chest syndrome. *J Pediatr Haematol Oncol, 22*, 515–520.

45. Morris, C. R., Kato, G. J., Poljakovic, M., et al. (2005). Dysregulated arginine metabolism, hemolysis-associated pulmonary hypertension, and mortality in sickle cell disease. *JAMA, 294*, 81–90.

46. Hsu, L. L., Champion, H. C., Campbell-Lee, S. C., et al. (2007). Hemolysis in sickle cell mice causes pulmonary hypertension due to global impairment in nitric oxide bioavailability. *Blood, 109*, 3088–3098.

47. Onyekwere, O. C., Campbell, A., Teshome, M., et al. (2008). Pulmonary hypertension in children and adolescence with sickle cell disease. *Pediat Cardiol, 29*(2), 309–312.

48. Wright, J., & Ahmedzai, S. H. (2010). The management of painful crisis in sickle cell disease. *Curr Opin Support Palliat Care, 4*, 97–106.

49. Day, T. G., Drasar, E. R., Fulford, T., et al. (2011). Association between hemolysis and albuminuria in adults with sickle cell anemia. *Haematologica, 97*, 201–205.

50. Kelleher, J. F., Luban, N. L. C., Cohen, B. J., et al. (1984). Human serum parvovirus as a cause of aplastic crisis in sickle cell disease. *Am J Dis Child, 138*, 401–403.

51. Wethers, D. L. (2000). Sickle cell disease in childhood: Part I. laboratory diagnosis, pathophysiology and health maintenance. *Am Fam Physician, 62*, 1013–1020.

52. Agular, C., Vichinsky, E., & Neumayr, L. (2005). Bone and joint disease in sickle cell disease. *Hematol Oncol Clin North Am, 19*, 929–941.

53. Bunn, H. F. (2013). The triumph of good over evil: protection by the sickle gene against malaria. *Blood, 121*, 20–25.

54. Clarke, G. M., & Higgins, T. N. (2000). Laboratory investigation of hemoglobinopathies and thalassemias: review and update. *Clin Chem, 46*, 1284–1290.

55. Bargoma, E. M., Mitsuyashi, J. K., Larkin, S. K., et al. (2005). Serum C-reactive protein parallels secretory phospholipase A2 in sickle cell disease patients with vaso-occlusive crisis or acute chest syndrome. *Blood, 105*, 3384–3385.

56. Célérier, E., González, J. R., Maldonado, R., et al. (2006). Opioid-induced hyperalgesia in a murine model of postoperative pain: role of nitric oxide generated from the inducible nitric oxide synthase. *Anesthesiology, 104*, 546–555.

57. Walters, P. B., Fung, E. B., Killilea, D. W., et al. (2006). Oxidative stress and inflammation in iron-overloaded patients with beta-thalassemia or sickle cell disease. *Br J Haematol, 135*, 254–263.

58. US Department of Health and Human Services, National Institutes of Health, National Heart, Lung, and Blood Institute. (2014). Evidence-based management of sickle cell disease: Expert panel report, 2014. https://www.nhlbi.nih.gov/sites/default/files/media/docs/sickle-cell-disease-report%20020816_0.pdf. Accessed August 3, 2018.

59. Yawn, B. P., Buchanan, G. R., Afenyi-Annan, A. N., et al. (2014). Management of sickle cell disease: summary of the 2014 evidence-based report by expert panel members. *JAMA, 312*, 1033–1048.

60. Chou, S. T. (2013). Transfusion therapy for sickle cell disease: a balancing act. *Hematology Am Soc Hematol Educ Program, 2013*, 439–446.

61. Fung, E. B., Harmatz, P. R., Lee, P. D., et al. (2006). Increased prevalence of iron-overload associated endocrinopathy in thalassemia verses sickle cell disease. *Br J Haematol, 135*, 574–582.

62. Fung, E. B., Harmatz, P. R., Milet, M., et al. (2007). Morbidity and mortality in chronically transfused subjects with thalassemia and sickle cell disease. *Am J Hematol, 82*, 255–265.

63. Marsella, M., & Borgna-Pignatti, C. (2014). Transfusional iron overload and iron chelation therapy in thalassemia major and sickle cell disease. *Hematol Oncol Clin North Am, 28*, 703–727.

64. Arnold, S. D., Bhatia, M., Horan, J., et al. (2016). Haematopoietic stem cell transplantation for sickle cell disease – current practice and new approaches. *Br J Haematol, 174,* 515–525.

65. Cottle, R. N., Lee, C. M., & Bao, G. (2016). Treating hemoglobinopathies using gene-correction approaches: promises and challenges. *Hum Genet, 135,* 993–1010.

66. Bernaudin, F., Socie, G., Kuentz, M., et al. (2007). Long-term results of related, myeloablative stem cell transplantation to cure sickle cell disease. *Blood, 110,* 2749–2756.

67. Panepinto, J. A., Walters, M. C., Carreras, J., et al. (2007). Matched-related donor transplantation for sickle cell disease: report from the Center for International Blood and Transplant Research. *Br J Haematol, 137,* 479–485.

68. Pinto, F. O., & Roberts, I. (2008). Cord blood stem cell transplantation for haemoglobinopathies. *Br J Haematol, 141,* 309–324.

69. Surbek, D., Schoeberlein, A., & Wagner, A. (2008). Perinatal stem cell and gene therapy for hemoglobinopathies. *Semin Fetal Neonatal Med, 13,* 282–290.

70. Paule, I., Sassi, H., Habibi, A., et al. (2011). Population pharmacokinetics and pharmacodynamics of hydroxyurea in sickle cell anemia patients, a basis for optimizing the dosing regimen. *Orphanet J Rare Dis, 6,* 30.

71. Steinberg, M. H., Lu, Z. H., Barton, F. B., et al. (1997). Fetal hemoglobin in sickle cell anemia: determinants of response to hydroxyurea. Multicenter study of hydroxyurea. *Blood, 89,* 1078–1088.

72. Lionnet, F., Arlet, J-B., Bartolucci, P., et al. (2009). Guidelines for management of adult sickle cell disease. *Rev Méd Interne, 30*(Suppl. 3), S162–S223.

73. Nagalla, S., & Ballas S. K. (2012). Drugs for preventing red blood cell dehydration in people with sickle cell disease. *Cochrane Database Syst Rev, 7,* CD003426.

74. Uzun, B., Kekec, Z., & Gurkan, E. (2010). Efficacy of tramadol vs meperidine in vasoocclusive sickle cell crisis. *Am J Emerg Med, 28,* 445–449.

75. Bartolucci, P., El Murr, T., Roudot-Thoraval, F., et al. (2009). A randomized, controlled clinical trial of ketoprofen for sickle-cell disease vaso-occlusive crises in adults. *Blood, 114,* 3742–3747.

76. US Food and Drug Administration. L-glutamine (NCT01179217 - Endari). https://www.fda.gov/Drugs/InformationOnDrugs/ApprovedDrugs/ucm566097.htm. Accessed July 4, 2018.

77. Oder, E., Safo, M., Abdulmalik, O., et al. (2016). New developments in anti-sickling agents: can drugs directly prevent the polymerization of sickle haemoglobin in vivo? *Br J Haematol, 175,* 24–30.

78. Claster, S., & Vichinsky, E. (2003). Managing sickle cell disease. *Br Med J, 327,* 1151–1155.

79. Steinberg, M. H., Ballas, S. K., Brunson, C. Y., et al. (1995). Sickle cell anemia in septuagenarians. *Blood, 86,* 3997–3998.

80. Michlitsch, J., Azimi, M., Hoppe, C., et al. (2009). Newborn screening for hemoglobinopathies in California. *Pediatr Blood Cancer, 52,* 486–490.

81. Hathaway, A. R. (2016). Sickle cell disease in pregnancy. *S Med J, 109*(9), 554–556.

82. Kark, J. A. & Ward, F. T. (1994). Exercise and hemoglobin S. *Semin Hematol, 31*(3), 181–225.

83. Hirsch, R. E., Lin, M. J., Vidugirus, G. J., et al. (1996). Conformational changes in oxyhemoglobin C (Glu beta 8 → Lys) detected by spectroscopic probing. *J Biol Chem, 271,* 372–375.

84. Steinberg, M. H. (2009). Other sickle hemoglobinopathies. In Steinberg, M. H., Forget, B. G., Higgs, D. R., et al. (Eds.), *Disorders of Hemoglobin: Genetics, Pathophysiology and Clinical Management.* (2nd ed., pp. 564–588). Cambridge: Cambridge University Press.

85. Fairbanks, V. F., Gilchrist, G. S., Brimhall, B., et al. (1979). Hemoglobin E trait reexamined: a cause of microcytosis and erythrocytosis. *Blood, 53,* 109–115.

86. Vichinsky, E. (2007). Hemoglobin E syndromes. *Hematology Am Soc Hematol Educ Program, 2007,* 79–83.

87. Randolph, T. R. (2008). Pathophysiology of compound heterozygotes involving hemoglobinopathies and thalassemias. *Clin Lab Sci, 21*(4), 240–248.

88. Lawrence, C., Fabry, M. E., & Nagel, R. L. (1991). The unique red cell heterogeneity of SC disease: crystal formation, dense reticulocytes and unusual morphology. *Blood, 78,* 2104–2112.

89. Platt, O. S., Thorington, B. D., Brambilla, D. J., et al. (1991). Pain in sickle cell disease: rates and risk factors. *N Engl J Med, 325,* 11–16.

90. Steinberg, M. H. (1996). Review: sickle cell disease: present and future treatment. *Am J Med Sci, 312,* 166–174.

91. Monplaisir, N., Merault, G., Poyart, C., et al. (1986). Hemoglobin S Antilles: a variant with lower solubility than hemoglobin S and producing sickle cell disease in heterozygotes. *Proc Natl Acad Sci U S A, 83,* 9363–9367.

92. Nagel, R. L., Daar, S., Romero, J. R., et al. (1998). HbS-Oman heterozygote: a new dominant sickle cell syndrome. *Blood, 92,* 4375–4782.

93. Steinberg, M. (2014). Hemoglobins with altered oxygen affinity, unstable hemoglobins, M-hemoglobins, and dyshemoglobinemias. In Greer, J. P., Arber, D. A., Bertil, G., et al. (Eds.), *Wintrobe's Clinical Hematology.* (Vol. *1,* 13th ed., pp. 1038–1082). Philadelphia: Wolters Kluwer Health/Lippincott Williams & Wilkins.

94. Williamson, D. (1993). The unstable haemoglobins. *Blood Rev, 7,* 146–163.

95. Bunn, H. F. (1986). Hemoglobinopathy due to abnormal oxygen binding. In Bunn, H. F., & Forget, B. G. (Eds.), *Hemoglobin: Molecular, Genetic and Clinical Aspects.* (pp. 595–616). Philadelphia: Saunders.

25

Thalassemias

*Elaine M. Keohane**

OBJECTIVES

After completion of this chapter, the reader will be able to:

1. Describe the hemoglobin defect found in thalassemia.
2. Describe the worldwide geographic distribution of thalassemia and its relationship with the prevalence of malaria.
3. Name the chromosomes that contain the α-globin gene and the β-globin gene clusters and the globin chains produced by each.
4. Describe types of genetic mutations that result in α- and β-thalassemia.
5. Explain the pathophysiologic effects caused by the imbalance of globin chain synthesis in α- and β-thalassemia.
6. Describe four major clinical syndromes of β-thalassemia and the clinical expression of each heterozygous and homozygous form.
7. Recognize the pattern of laboratory findings in heterozygous and homozygous β-thalassemia, including hereditary persistence of fetal hemoglobin (HPFH).
8. Correlate clinical syndromes of α-thalassemia with the number of α genes present.
9. Recognize the laboratory findings associated with various α-thalassemia syndromes.
10. Describe the treatment of transfusion-dependent thalassemia (TDT) and non-transfusion-dependent thalassemia (NTDT), the risks involved, and the reason it is necessary to monitor iron levels.
11. Describe clinical syndromes of thalassemia associated with common structural hemoglobin variants.
12. Discuss the role of the complete blood count, peripheral blood film review, supravital stain, hemoglobin fraction quantification (using hemoglobin electrophoresis, high-performance liquid chromatography, and/or capillary zone electrophoresis), and molecular genetic testing in the diagnosis of thalassemia syndromes.
13. Differentiate β-thalassemia minor from iron deficiency anemia.
14. Given a case history and clinical and laboratory findings, interpret test results to identify the type of thalassemia present.

OUTLINE

*The author extends appreciation to Martha Payne and Rakesh P. Mehta whose work in prior editions provided the foundation for this chapter.

After studying the material in this chapter, the reader should be able to respond to the following case study:

A 24-year-old male medical student in the United States was found to have a hemoglobin level of 10.2 g/dL in a hematology laboratory class. During discussion of the family history with this student, a hematologist at the university discovered that his mother had always been anemic, had periodically been given iron therapy, and had a history of several acute episodes of gallbladder disease (attacks). Both of the student's parents had been born in Sicily. A cousin on his mother's side had two children who died of thalassemia major at the ages of 4 and 5 years and had a third young daughter with thalassemia major who was being treated with regular blood transfusions. The student's laboratory test results were as follows:

	Patient Results	Reference Intervals
RBC ($\times 10^{12}$/L)	5.74	4.60–6.00
HGB (g/dL)	10.2	14.0–18.0
HCT (%)	35	40–54
MCV (fL)	61.0	80–100
MCH (pg)	17.8	26–32
MCHC (g/dL)	29.1	32–36

Peripheral blood RBCs exhibited moderate microcytosis, slight hypochromia, and slight poikilocytosis with occasional target cells, and several RBCs had basophilic stippling. Hb A_2 was 4.9% of total hemoglobin by high-performance liquid chromatography (reference interval, 0% to 3.5%). Serum ferritin level was 320 ng/mL (reference interval, 15 to 400 ng/mL).

1. Why was the family history so important in this case, and what diagnosis did it suggest?
2. What laboratory values helped confirm the diagnosis?
3. From what other disorders should this anemia be differentiated? What laboratory tests would be helpful? Why is differentiation important?
4. If this individual was planning to have children, what genetic counseling should be provided?

DEFINITIONS AND HISTORY

Thalassemias are a diverse group of inherited disorders caused by genetic mutations affecting the globin chain component of the hemoglobin (Hb) tetramer. Thalassemia was first described in 1925 by Cooley and Lee in four children with anemia, splenomegaly, mild hepatomegaly, and mongoloid facies.[1] These characteristics would later become the typical findings in young children with untreated β-thalassemia major, often referred to as *Cooley's anemia*. Seven years later, Whipple and Bradford published a paper outlining detailed autopsy studies of children who died of this disorder.[2] Because of the high incidence of patients of Mediterranean descent with this disorder, Whipple called the disease *Thalassic* (Greek for "great sea") anemia, which was subsequently changed to *thalassemia*.

Thalassemia results from a reduced or absent synthesis of one or more of the globin chains of hemoglobin. A wide variety of mutations in hemoglobin genes lead to clinical outcomes that are wide ranging, with certain mutations causing no anemia and others leading to death in utero, childhood, or early adulthood. Thalassemias are named according to the chain with reduced or absent synthesis. Mutations affecting the α- or β-globin gene are most clinically significant because Hb A ($\alpha_2\beta_2$) is the major adult hemoglobin. The decreased or absent synthesis of one of the chains not only leads to a decreased production of hemoglobin, but also results in an imbalance in the α/β chain ratio.[3] The unaffected gene continues to produce globin chains at normal levels, and the accumulation of the unpaired normal chains damages red blood cells (RBCs) or their precursors, resulting in their premature destruction. This exacerbates the anemia and makes some forms of thalassemia particularly severe.

EPIDEMIOLOGY

The morbidity and mortality due to thalassemia significantly contribute to the global health burden. Across the world, an estimated 56,000 infants are conceived or born with a clinically significant thalassemia each year, with more than half requiring regular transfusions.[4] It is estimated that 5% of the world's population is a carrier of an α-thalassemia mutation and 1.5% is a carrier of a β-thalassemia mutation.[3,5,6] Although thalassemia occurs in all parts of the world, its distribution is concentrated in the "thalassemia belt," which extends from the Mediterranean east through the Middle East and India to Southeast Asia and south to Northern Africa (Figure 24.3).[7] The carrier frequency of β-thalassemia depends on the region, with Sardinia, Cyprus, and Greece having the highest frequency in Europe (6% to 19%) and India, Thailand, and Indonesia having the highest frequency in Asia and Southeast Asia (0.3% to 15%).[7] The carrier frequency of α-thalassemia varies considerably. In Europe, Cyprus has the highest carrier frequency at 14%.[7] The carrier frequency reaches 50% to 60% in Eastern Saudi Arabia and parts of Asia and Africa, and may be as high as 75% to 80% in certain groups in Nepal, India, Thailand, and Papua New Guinea.[7]

The geographic location of the thalassemia belt coincides with areas in which malaria is prevalent (Figure 24.3). This sparked interest in studies to examine the relationship of thalassemia and resistance to malaria. A 2012 meta-analysis of 18 studies on α-thalassemia conducted by Taylor and colleagues showed a decreased risk of severe malaria in α-thalassemia, both in heterozygotes (defined as the - α/αα genotype) and homozygotes (defined as the – α/– α and αα/– – genotypes).[8] Interestingly the protective effect of α-thalassemia was only demonstrated against severe malaria and not against uncomplicated malaria and asymptomatic parasitemia.[8] The researchers were unable to determine the same effect in β-thalassemia due to an insufficient number of published studies.[8] The reasons for the protective effect of thalassemia against malaria are not clear. Some mechanisms under investigation include reduced parasite invasion and growth in thalassemia cells, reduced attachment of infected thalassemia cells to endothelial cells of blood vessels, and greater binding of anti-malarial antibodies to infected cells, thus increasing phagocytosis and immune clearance of parasites.[5]

GENETICS OF GLOBIN SYNTHESIS

The normal hemoglobin molecule is a tetramer of two α-like chains (α or ζ) and two β-like chains (β, γ, δ, or ϵ). Combinations of these chains produce six normal hemoglobins. Three are embryonic hemoglobins: Hb Gower-1 ($\zeta_2\epsilon_2$), Hb Gower-2 ($\alpha_2\epsilon_2$), and Hb Portland ($\zeta_2\gamma_2$). The others are fetal hemoglobin (Hb F [$\alpha_2\gamma_2$]) and two adult hemoglobins: (Hb A [$\alpha_2\beta_2$] and Hb A$_2$ [$\alpha_2\delta_2$]). The α-like globin gene cluster is located on chromosome 16, whereas the β-like globin gene cluster is on chromosome 11. The α-like globin gene cluster contains three functional genes: *HBZ* (ζ-globin), *HBA1* (α_1-globin), and *HBA2* (α_2-globin).[3,9,10] The β-like globin gene cluster contains five functional genes: *HBE* (ϵ-globin), *HBG2* ($^{G}\gamma$-globin), *HBG1* ($^{A}\gamma$-globin), *HBD* (δ-globin), and *HBB* (β-globin).[3,9] These genes are positioned in the order that corresponds to their developmental stage of expression.[9] By 10 weeks' gestation, genes for embryonic ζ and ϵ chains are switched off and silenced, whereas genes for α and γ chains are upregulated (this is called the ζ to α switch on chromosome 16, and the ϵ to γ switch on chromosome 11).[9] The γ chains combine with α chains to form Hb F ($\alpha_2\gamma_2$), the predominant hemoglobin of fetal life. The gene for the β chain is initially activated during the second month of gestation, but β chain production occurs at low levels throughout most of fetal life.[10] Shortly before birth, however, expression of the γ-globin gene is downregulated, whereas expression of the β-globin gene is upregulated (called the γ to β switch).

TABLE 25.1	**Reference Intervals for Normal Hemoglobins in Adults**
Hb A ($\alpha_2\beta_2$)	95%–100%
Hb A$_2$ ($\alpha_2\delta_2$)	0%–3.5%
Hb F ($\alpha_2\gamma_2$)	0%–2%

Therefore by 6 months of age and through adult life, Hb A ($\alpha_2\beta_2$) is the predominant hemoglobin.[3] The gene for the δ chain is activated shortly before birth, but owing to its weak promoter, only produces a relatively small amount of δ chain, resulting in a low level of Hb A$_2$ ($\alpha_2\delta_2$) throughout life (Chapter 7 and Figure 7.6).[3,9] Table 25.1 contains the reference intervals for normal hemoglobins in adults.

γ-globin genes code for two globin chains ($^{G}\gamma$ and $^{A}\gamma$) that differ at position 136 by a single amino acid (glycine and alanine, respectively).[10] Both of these globin chains are found in Hb F, with no functional difference identified between them. Similarly, the α-globin gene loci are duplicated on each chromosome 16 and also code for two globin chains (α_1 and α_2). Either of these genes can contribute to the two α-globin chains in the hemoglobin tetramer, and no functional difference has been identified between the two. Interspersed between the functional genes on these chromosomes are four functionless, gene-like loci, or pseudogenes, that are designated by the prefixed symbol ψ. The purpose of these pseudogenes is unknown.[10] The organization of these genes on chromosomes 16 and 11 is shown in Figure 25.1.

An individual inherits one cluster of the five functional genes on chromosome 11 from each parent. The genotype for normal β chain synthesis is designated β/β. Because two

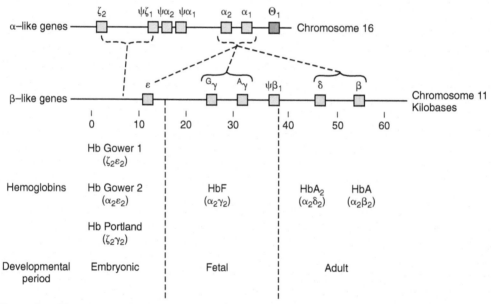

Figure 25.1 Chromosome Organization of Globin Genes and Their Expression During Development. The light blue boxes indicate functional globin genes; the tan boxes indicate pseudogenes. The scale of the depicted chromosomal segments is in kilobases of deoxyribonucleic acid *(DNA)*. The switch from embryonic to fetal hemoglobin *(Hb)* occurs by 10 weeks of gestation, and the switch from fetal to adult hemoglobin begins in the third trimester. (From Sankaran, V. G., Nathan, D. G., Orkin, S. H. [2015]. Thalassemias. In Orkin, S. H., Fisher, D. E., Ginsberg, D., et al. [Eds], *Nathan and Oski's Hematology and Oncology of Infancy and Childhood.* [8th ed., p. 716, Figure 21.2]. Philadelphia: Elsevier/Saunders.)

α-globin genes (α_1 and α_2) are inherited on each chromosome 16, a normal genotype is designated $\alpha\alpha/\alpha\alpha$.

CATEGORIES OF THALASSEMIA

Thalassemias are divided into β-thalassemias, which include all the disorders of reduced globin chain production arising from the β-globin gene cluster on chromosome 11, and α-thalassemias, which involve the genes for the α_1 and α_2 chains on chromosome 16. Various deletional and non-deletional mutations can cause each of these disorders, and individuals with similar clinical manifestations are often heterogeneous at the genetic level.[3,9,10]

β-thalassemias affect mainly β chain production but also may involve δ, $^G\gamma$, $^A\gamma$, and ϵ chains. In β-thalassemias, β^0 is the designation for the various mutations in the β-globin gene in which no β chains are produced. In the homozygous state (β^0/β^0), an individual does not produce Hb A ($\alpha_2\beta_2$). β^+ is the designation for the various mutations in the β-globin gene that result in a partial deficiency of β chains (ranging from 5% to 30% of normal) and a decrease in production of Hb A.[3] Some mutations in the β-globin gene lead to minimal reductions in β chain production and are associated with mild or silent clinical states. The designation β^{silent} for silent carrier has been used for those mutations. The designation $\delta\beta^0$ is used for mutations in the δ- or β-globin genes in which no δ or β chains are produced. In the homozygous state ($\delta\beta^0$/$\delta\beta^0$), no Hb A ($\alpha_2\beta_2$) or Hb A$_2$ ($\alpha_2\delta_2$) is produced. The designation $\delta\beta^{Lepore}$ indicates a fusion of the δ- and β-globin genes that produces Hb Lepore.[3,10]

The most common mutations in α-thalassemia are deletions involving the α_1- and/or α_2-globin genes.[9,11] The designation α^+ is used to indicate a deletion of *either* the α_1- *or* the α_2-globin gene on chromosome 16 (also called the $-\alpha$ *haplotype*). This results in decreased production of α chains from that chromosome. The designation α^0 is used to indicate a deletion of *both* the α_1- and α_2-globin genes on chromosome 16 (also called the $- -$ *haplotype*). This results in no production of α chains from that chromosome.[3,9,10] Non-deletional mutations in the α-globin gene can also result in α-thalassemia, but these are less common.[3,11] The designation α^T is used for these mutations.[10] Major gene designations in thalassemia are summarized in Table 25.2.

GENETIC DEFECTS CAUSING THALASSEMIA

Types of genetic defects that cause a reduced or absent production of a particular globin chain include single nucleotide (or point) mutations, small insertions or deletions, or large deletions.[10,11] The mechanisms by which these mutations interfere with globin chain production include:[3,9,10]

- *Reduced or absent transcription of messenger ribonucleic acid (mRNA)* due to mutations in the promoter region or initiation codon of a globin gene, or to mutations in polyadenylation sites that reduce mRNA stability
- *mRNA processing errors* due to mutations that add or remove splice sites, resulting in no globin chain or altered globin chain production
- *Translation errors* due to mutations that change the codon reading frame (frameshift mutations); substitute an incorrect amino acid codon (missense mutations); add a stop codon, causing premature chain termination (nonsense mutations); or remove a stop codon, resulting in an elongated and unstable mRNA that produces a dysfunctional globin chain

TABLE 25.2 Genetic Designations in Thalassemia

Designation	Definition
Designations for Normal β-Globin and α-Globin Genes	
β	Normal β-globin gene; normal amount of β chain production; one gene located on each chromosome 11
$\alpha\alpha$	Normal α_1- and α_2-globin genes on one chromosome (haplotype $\alpha\alpha$); normal amount of α chain production; two genes located on each chromosome 16
Designations for the Major Thalassemia Genes	
β^0	β-globin gene mutation that results in no β chain production
β^+	β-globin gene mutation that results in decreased β chain production varying from 5% to 30% of normal
β^{silent}	β-globin gene mutation that results in mildly decreased β chain production
$\delta\beta^0$	$\delta\beta$-globin gene deletional or non-deletional mutation that results in no δ or β chain production; accompanied by some increased γ chain production
$\delta\beta^{Lepore}$	$\delta\beta$-globin gene fusion that produces a small amount of fusion product, hemoglobin Lepore, and no normal δ or β chain production; accompanied by some increased γ chain production
HPFH	Hereditary persistence of fetal hemoglobin; $\delta\beta$-globin gene deletional or non-deletional mutation in γ-globin gene promoter that results in no δ or β chain production; accompanied by increased γ chain production
α^0	Deletion of both α-globin genes on one chromosome (haplotype $- -$) that results in no α chain production
α^+	Deletion of one α-globin gene on one chromosome (haplotype $-\alpha$) that results in decreased α chain production
α^T	Non-deletional mutation in one α-globin gene on one chromosome (haplotype $\alpha^T\alpha$) that results in decreased α chain production (*T* denotes thalassemia)

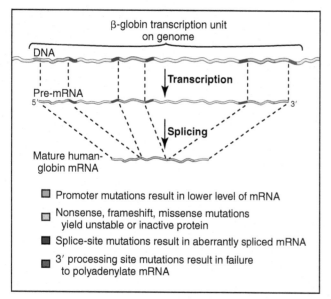

β-globin transcription unit
on genome

DNA

Pre-mRNA
5'   3'

Transcription

Splicing

Mature human-
globin mRNA

■ Promoter mutations result in lower level of mRNA

□ Nonsense, frameshift, missense mutations
    yield unstable or inactive protein

■ Splice-site mutations result in aberrantly spliced mRNA

■ 3' processing site mutations result in failure
    to polyadenylate mRNA

Figure 25.2 The Transcription Unit of the β-Globin Gene. The nucleotide sequence of the deoxyribonucleic acid *(DNA)* template is transcribed into a complementary pre-mRNA (messenger ribonucleic acid). The pre-mRNA is processed by removing introns and splicing together the protein coding exons (orange). The DNA sequences required for expression of a functional β-globin chain are indicated in different colors. Mutations in any of these sequences can lead to decreased or absent β-globin chain production. (From Corden, J. L. [2008]. Gene expression. In Pollard, T. D., & Earnshaw, W. C. [Eds.], *Cell Biology.* [2nd ed., Figure 15.2]. Philadelphia: Elsevier/Saunders.)

- *Deletion of one or more globin genes,* resulting in no production of the corresponding globin chains

All of these heterogeneous genetic mutations cause a reduction or lack of synthesis of one or more globin chains, resulting in the thalassemia syndromes (Figure 25.2).

PATHOPHYSIOLOGY

The clinical manifestations of thalassemia stem from:

1. Reduced or absent production of a particular globin chain, which diminishes hemoglobin synthesis and produces microcytic, hypochromic RBCs; and
2. Unequal production of the α- or β-globin chains, causing an imbalance in the α/β chain ratio; this leads to a markedly decreased survival of RBCs and their precursors.[3,9,10]

The α/β chain imbalance is more significant and determines the clinical severity of the thalassemia.[3,12] The mechanisms and degree of shortened RBC survival are different for β-thalassemia and α-thalassemia.

Mechanisms in β-Thalassemia

In β-thalassemia, unpaired, excess α chains precipitate in developing erythroid precursors forming inclusion bodies; this causes oxidative stress and damage to cellular membranes.[13,14] Apoptosis is triggered, and the damaged and apoptotic erythroid precursors are subsequently phagocytized and destroyed in the bone marrow by activated macrophages.[13] In addition, iron accumulation in the erythroid precursors (discussed below)

and inflammatory cytokines contribute to the apoptosis.[13,14] The premature death of erythroid precursors in the bone marrow is called *ineffective erythropoiesis.*[9,13,14] In this situation, the bone marrow attempts to produce RBCs but is not able to release sufficient viable cells into the circulation. The cells that are released into the periphery are laden with inclusion bodies and are rapidly sequestered and destroyed by macrophages in the spleen (extravascular hemolysis).[9] Therefore in β-thalassemia the anemia is multifactorial and results from ineffective production and increased destruction. Typically, individuals with severe β-thalassemia are asymptomatic during fetal life and through approximately 6 months of age because Hb F ($\alpha_2\gamma_2$) is the predominant hemoglobin. Symptoms usually begin to appear between 6 and 24 months of age, after completion of the γ to β switch.[3,10,15] To compensate for the decreased expression of the β-globin gene, the γ- and/or δ-globin genes are usually upregulated; however, in β-thalassemia major, this increase is insufficient to correct the α/β chain imbalance.[3]

In β-thalassemia major, profound anemia stimulates an increase in erythropoietin (EPO) production by the kidney and results in massive (but ineffective) erythroid hyperplasia mediated through the EPO receptor and JAK2/STAT5 pathway.[3,9,12] In untreated or inadequately treated patients, marked bone changes and deformities occur due to massive bone marrow expansion. Reduction in bone mineral density and thinning of the cortex of bone increases the risk of pathologic fractures.[3,9] In children, radiographs of long bones may exhibit a lacy or lucent appearance.[3] Skull radiographs may demonstrate a typical "hair on end" appearance due to vertical striations of bony trabeculae (Figure 25.3).[3,9,14] A typical facies occurs, with prominence of the forehead (also known as *frontal bossing*), cheekbones, and upper jaw. Extramedullary erythropoiesis causes hepatosplenomegaly, and foci of hematopoietic tissue can appear in other body areas. Sequestration of blood cells in an enlarged spleen can worsen the anemia and can also cause neutropenia and thrombocytopenia.[9] Release of hemoglobin from the excessive destruction of RBCs and their precursors leads to an increase in the level of plasma indirect bilirubin. The bilirubin can diffuse into the tissues, causing jaundice (Chapter 20). Patients also have an increased risk of developing thrombosis.[3,9]

Iron accumulation in various organs is a serious complication in β-thalassemia major and is a significant cause of morbidity and mortality in adults.[3] In children, excess iron causes growth retardation and absence of sexual maturity; in adults, it causes cardiomyopathy, fibrosis and cirrhosis of the liver, and dysfunction of exocrine glands.[3,14,15] The risk of organ damage due to iron accumulation begins to increase after 10 to 11 years of age.[15] On the cellular level, excess iron also promotes more α-globin precipitation and reactive oxygen species (ROS) in erythroid precursors, furthering cellular damage and apoptosis.[12] Iron overload is predominantly due to the regular RBC transfusions required in β-thalassemia major (discussed later). However, the consistently elevated EPO level also promotes the upregulation and secretion of erythroferrone (ERFE) from erythroblasts.[16,17] The ERFE acts on hepatocytes to suppress hepcidin production by a yet unknown mechanism.[3,16,17] The

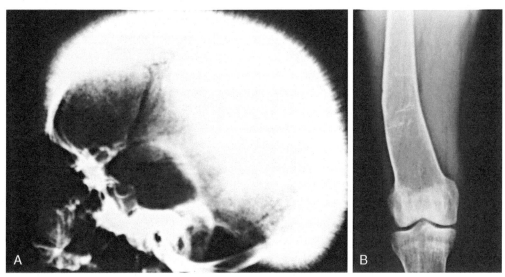

Figure 25.3 Radiologic Abnormalities in a Patient with Homozygous β-Thalassemia Who Receives Blood Transfusions Infrequently (Thalassemia Intermedia). **(A)**, Skull radiograph illustrating the typical "hair on end" appearance. **(B)**, Severe osteoporosis, pseudofractures, thinning of the cortex, and bowing of the femur. (From Sankaran, V. G., Nathan, D. G., Orkin, S. H. [2015]. Thalassemias. In Orkin, S. H., Fisher, D. E., Ginsberg, D., et al. [Eds.], *Nathan and Oski's Hematology and Oncology of Infancy and Childhood.* [8th ed., p. 757, Figure 21.29]. Philadelphia: Elsevier/Saunders.)

low hepicidin level allows more iron absorption by intestinal enterocytes. This mechanism normally serves to provide the additional iron needed to support EPO-stimulated erythropoiesis (Chapter 8).[3,16,17] However, in ineffective erythropoiesis, hyperabsorption of intestinal iron is not needed because iron is continually recycled back into plasma by the massive intramedullary death of erythroid precursors and hemolysis of defective α chain-laden RBCs in circulation. Thus hyperabsorption of iron further adds to the iron overload in β-thalassemia major. In non-transfusion-dependent β-thalassemia, increased ERFE levels may explain the pathologic decrease in hepcidin and the development of iron overload, even when no or very few transfusions are administered.[3,12,16,17] In support of this theory, Ganz and colleagues found increased levels of serum ERFE in patients with transfusion-dependent and non-transfusion-dependent β-thalassemia, with ERFE levels declining after transfusion.[18]

The complex pathophysiology of β-thalassemia major is summarized in Figure 25.4.

Mechanisms in α-Thalassemia

In α-thalassemia, decreased production of α chains can manifest in utero because α chains are a component of both fetal and adult hemoglobins. However, the accumulation of non-α chains has different consequences compared to β-thalassemia. In the fetus and newborn, a decrease in production of α chains results in an excess of γ chains. These γ chains accumulate in proportion to the number of deleted or defective α genes.[9,10] The γ chains are more stable and do not precipitate, but instead form hemoglobin tetramers (γ_4) called *Hb Bart*.[10] After 6 months of age and through adulthood, when the γ to β switch is completed, the decrease in α chain production results in excess β chains. The excess β chains are also relatively stable and form tetramers (β_4), called *Hb H*.[10]

Because Hb H and Hb Bart do not precipitate to any significant degree in developing erythroid precursors in bone marrow, patients with α-thalassemia do not have severe ineffective erythropoiesis.[9] As mature RBCs age in the circulation, however, β_4 tetramers in Hb H eventually precipitate and form inclusion bodies.[9] Macrophages in the spleen recognize and remove these abnormal RBCs from the circulation, and the patient manifests a moderate hemolytic anemia.

In addition to the decreased production and shortened RBC survival mechanisms, a third mechanism is involved in the anemia of α-thalassemia. Hb Bart and Hb H cannot deliver oxygen to tissues due to their very high affinity for oxygen.[10] A fetus cannot survive with only Hb Bart (found with a deletion of all four α-globin genes). The marked tissue hypoxia causes heart failure and massive edema (hydrops fetalis) and hepatomegaly, and the fetus usually dies in utero or shortly after birth.[3] This is discussed in the α-thalassemia section later in the chapter.

β-GLOBIN GENE CLUSTER THALASSEMIA

There is great heterogeneity in the mutations in the β-globin gene cluster that leads to the clinical syndrome of β-thalassemia.[11] More than 280 mutations have been reported in the β-globin gene itself, and more than 300 mutations are known in the entire β-globin cluster, including β-, δ-, and γ-globin genes, individually or in combination.[10,11] A small subset of mutations, however, accounts for the majority of mutant alleles within a single ethnic group or geographic area in which β-thalassemia is found.[3,15] Because multiple mutations are present in each population, most individuals with severe β-thalassemia are compound heterozygotes for two different β-thalassemia mutations.[9] A comprehensive list of hemoglobin

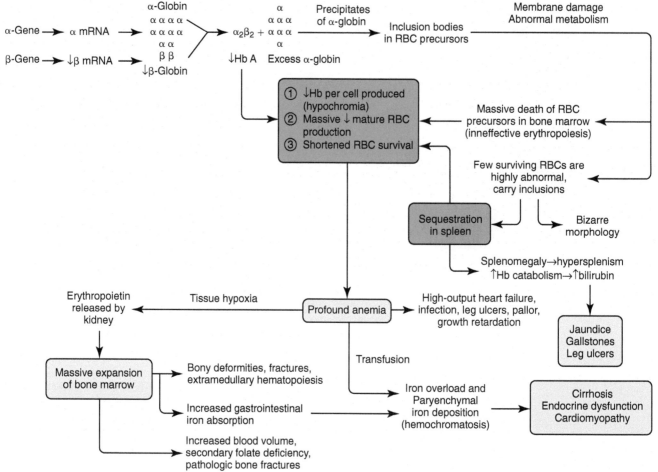

Figure 25.4 **Pathophysiology of Severe Forms of β-Thalassemia.** The diagram outlines the pathogenesis of clinical abnormalities resulting from the primary defect in β-globin chain synthesis. *RBC,* Red blood cell. (From Chapin, J., & Giardina, P. J. [2018]. Thalassemia syndromes. In Hoffman, R., Benz, E. J., Silberstein, L. E., et al. [Eds], *Hematology: Basic Principles and Practice.* [7th ed., p. 550, Figure 40.4]. Philadelphia: Elsevier.)

gene mutations is maintained in the HbVar mutation database, which is available online.[11]

Clinical Syndromes of β-Thalassemia

β-thalassemia is divided into four categories based on clinical manifestations (Table 25.3):[3,10,14]

- β-thalassemia silent carrier (heterozygous state), with *no* hematologic abnormalities or clinical symptoms
- β-thalassemia minor (heterozygous state), with mild hemolytic anemia, microcytic and hypochromic RBCs, and no clinical symptoms
- β-thalassemia major (homozygous or compound heterozygous state), with severe hemolytic anemia, microcytic and hypochromic RBCs, severe clinical symptoms, and transfusion dependence
- β-thalassemia intermedia, with mild to moderate hemolytic anemia, microcytic and hypochromic RBCs, moderate clinical symptoms, and non-transfusion dependence

A simpler clinical classification divides symptomatic thalassemias into two broad groups based on transfusion requirements. *Transfusion-dependent thalassemia (TDT)* includes β-thalassemia major, severe Hb E-β-thalassemia, and α-thalassemia

major (Hb Bart hydrops fetalis). *Non-transfusion-dependent thalassemia (NTDT)* includes β-thalassemia intermedia, mild/moderate Hb E-thalassemia, and α-thalassemia intermedia (Hb H disease).[6,19] In NTDT, occasional transfusions may be required in conditions such as infection, pregnancy, and surgery.[6,14,19] Clinical manifestations of the various mutations depend on whether one or both of the β-globin genes are affected and the extent to which the affected gene or genes are expressed, that is β⁰, β⁺, or β^{silent} (Table 25.2). β-thalassemia is inherited in an autosomal recessive pattern. If both parents are carriers of a β-thalassemia gene mutation, they have a 25% chance of having a child with two mutated β-globin genes (homozygote or compound heterozygote) and clinical manifestations of β-thalassemia major or intermedia.

Silent Carrier State of β-Thalassemia

The designation β^{silent} includes the various heterogeneous β-globin gene mutations that produce only a small decrease in production of the β chains. The silent carrier state (β^{silent}/β) results in nearly normal α/β chain ratios and no hematologic abnormalities.[3,9,10] It is often first recognized inadvertently, when an apparently normal parent with an unknown silent carrier state

TABLE 25.3 Clinical Syndromes of β-Thalassemia with Examples of Genotypes

Genotype	Hb A	Hb A$_2$	Hb F	Hb Lepore
Normal (Normal Hematologic Parameters)				
β/β	N	N	N	0
Silent Carrier State (Asymptomatic; Normal Hematologic Parameters)				
β^{silent}/β	N	N	N	0
Thalassemia Minor (Asymptomatic; Mild Anemia; Microcytic, Hypochromic)				
β$^+$/β	↓	↑	N to Sl ↑	0
β^0/β	↓	↑	N to Sl ↑	0
δβ^0/β	↓	N to ↓	5%–20%	0
δβ^{Lepore}/β	↓	↓	↑	5%–15%
Thalassemia Major (Transfusion-Dependent Thalassemia; Severe Anemia; Microcytic, Hypochromic)				
β$^+$/β$^+$	↓↓	V	↑↑	0
β$^+$/β^0	↓↓↓	V	↑↑	0
β^0/β^0	0	V	↑↑	0
δβ^{Lepore}/δβ^{Lepore}	0	0	80%	20%
Thalassemia Intermedia* (Non–Transfusion-Dependent Thalassemia**; Mild to Moderate Anemia; Microcytic, Hypochromic)				
β^{silent}/β^{silent}	↓	↑	↑	0
β$^+$/β^{silent} or β^0/β^{silent}	↓	↑	↑	0
δβ^0/δβ^0	0	0	100%	0
β^0/δβ^0	0	N	↑↑	0

*Other genotypes are included in this category, such as dominantly inherited β-thalassemia (heterozygous for a very severe β-globin gene mutation) and coinheritance of a triplicated α-globin gene (ααα/αα) with thalassemia minor.

**Patients who are non-transfusion dependent do not require regular transfusions for survival but may need transfusions occasionally, such as during pregnancy, surgery, or infections.

↑, Increased; ↓, decreased; 0, absent; *Hb*, hemoglobin; *N*, normal; *Sl*, slight; *V*, variable.

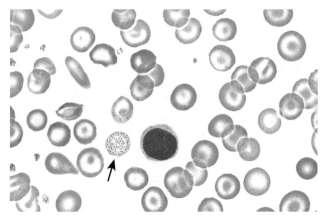

Figure 25.5 Peripheral Blood Film from a Patient with β-thalassemia Minor. Note the microcytic, hypochromic red blood cells, target cells, other poikilocytes, and basophilic stippling (*arrow*). (Wright-Giemsa stain, ×1000.)

(β^{silent}/β) and a parent with β-thalassemia trait (β$^+$/β or β^0/β) have a child with unexpected symptoms of β-thalassemia intermedia due to compound heterozygosity (β$^+$/β^{silent} or β^0/β^{silent}).[10] Some individuals who are homozygous for a silent thalassemia gene mutation (β^{silent}/β^{silent}) have been described.[10,20] They present with a mild β-thalassemia intermedia phenotype with an increased level of Hb F and Hb A$_2$.[10,20]

β-Thalassemia Minor

β-thalassemia minor (also called *β-thalassemia trait*) results when one β-globin gene is affected by a mutation that decreases or abolishes its expression, whereas the other β-globin gene is normal (heterozygous state). It usually presents as a mild, asymptomatic anemia, but the hemoglobin level can range from approximately 11 to 15 g/dL in affected men and 10 to 13 g/dL in affected women.[9,15] The RBC count is within the reference interval or slightly elevated.[3,10] The RBCs are microcytic and hypochromic, with a mean cell volume (MCV) less than 75 fL

and a mean cell hemoglobin (MCH) less than 26 pg.[3] The reticulocyte count is within the reference interval or slightly increased.[3] Some degree of poikilocytosis (including target cells and elliptocytes) and basophilic stippling in the RBCs may be seen on a peripheral blood film (Figure 25.5). The bone marrow shows mild to moderate erythroid hyperplasia, with minimal ineffective erythropoiesis. Hepatomegaly and splenomegaly are seen in a few patients. In the most common β-thalassemia minor syndromes (β^0/β and β$^+$/β), the Hb A level is 92% to 95% and the Hb A$_2$ level is characteristically elevated and can vary from 3.5% to 7.0%.[3,10,15] The Hb F level usually ranges from 1% to 5%.[3,10] Less common types of β-thalassemia minor exist, such as δβ^0/β and δβ^{Lepore}/β. Other rare types have atypical features, such as Dutch β^0-thalassemia minor that shows the expected elevation in Hb A$_2$ level but an Hb F level in the 5% to 20% range,[21] and another mutant found in a Sardinian family in which the Hb A$_2$ level is within the reference interval.[22]

β-Thalassemia Major

β-thalassemia major is characterized by a severe anemia that requires regular transfusion therapy. It is usually diagnosed between 6 months and 2 years of age (after completion of the γ to β switch) when the child's Hb A level does not increase as expected.[3,10]

In untreated β-thalassemia major, the hemoglobin level is below 7 g/dL but can fall as low as 2 to 4 g/dL.[3,10,14] The MCV ranges from 50 to 70 fL, and the MCH from 12 to 20 pg.[9,14,15] The peripheral blood film shows marked microcytosis, hypochromia, anisocytosis, and poikilocytosis, including target cells, teardrop cells, and elliptocytes. Polychromasia and nucleated red blood cells may be observed (Figure 25.6). RBC inclusions are commonly found, including basophilic stippling, Howell-Jolly bodies, and Pappenheimer bodies, the latter as a result of the excess nonheme iron in RBCs. The reticulocyte count is only mildly to moderately elevated and is inappropriately low in relation to the amount of erythroid hyperplasia and hemolysis present.[3] The inappropriate reticulocytosis results from apoptosis of erythroid precursors in the bone marrow (ineffective erythropoiesis).

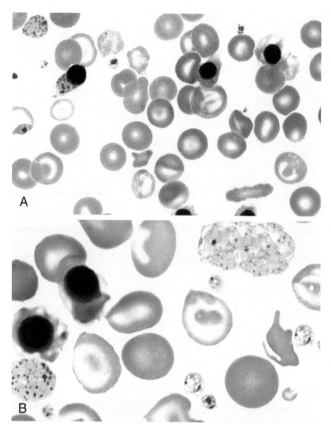

A

B

Figure 25.6 Peripheral Blood Films from a Patient with β-thalassemia Major, (A and B). Note basophilic stippling, microcytosis, hypochromia, target cells, nucleated red blood cells, and red cell fragments. (A, Wright-Giemsa stain, ×500; B, Wright-Giemsa stain, ×1000.) (Adapted from Rodak, B. F., & Carr, J. H. [2017]. *Clinical Hematology Atlas.* [5th ed.]. St. Louis: Elsevier.)

Hb A is absent or decreased, depending on the specific genotype, which determines whether none (β^0/β^0) or a decreased amount (β^+/β^+ or β^0/β^+) of β chains is produced. In β^0/β^0, Hb F is 92% to 95% and Hb A is absent.[14] Hb A is produced only if a β^+ mutation is present and usually ranges from 10% to 30%.[3,14,15] Hb F ranges from 70% to greater than 90%, depending on the genotype and amount of Hb A.[10,14,15] The level of Hb A_2 is variable and can be within or above the reference interval.[3,9,14] Bone marrow shows marked erythroid hyperplasia, with a myeloid-to-erythroid (M:E) ratio of 1:20 (reference interval is 1.5:1 to 3.3:1). As a result of the massive destruction of erythroid cells and release of free hemoglobin, the serum haptoglobin level is reduced or absent, and the serum lactate dehydrogenase activity is markedly elevated (Chapter 20).

Transfusion therapy is the major therapeutic option for patients with thalassemia major and typically is initiated when the hemoglobin drops to less than 7 g/dL and the patient has clinical symptoms.[3,14,23] Typically 10 to 15 mL/kg of leukoreduced RBCs are transfused every 2 to 5 weeks.[3] RBCs that are less than 7 to 10 days old are used for transfusion to allow for maximum donor RBC survival in the patient.[3,14] Extended typing of the patient's RBCs for major blood group antigens (or at least C, c, E, e, and Kell antigens) and transfusion of antigen-matched donor RBCs are recommended to reduce the risk of alloimmunization.[3,9,14,15]

Administration of RBC transfusions at regular intervals began in the mid-1970s. The pretransfusion hemoglobin level is usually maintained between 9 and 10.5 g/dL.[3,14,23] Such transfusion regimens are termed *hypertransfusion* and are used not only to correct the anemia, but also to suppress the marked erythropoiesis. With erythropoiesis suppressed, the marked marrow expansion does not occur; therefore the bone changes do not take place. In addition, the decrease in erythropoiesis reduces the amount of iron absorbed by intestinal enterocytes.[14,17] Children receiving this therapy do not develop hepatosplenomegaly and have much-improved growth and development.[3]

Chronic transfusion regimens, however, lead to iron overload. Because there is no effective physiologic pathway for iron excretion in the body, iron contained in the transfused RBCs accumulates in the body. This iron is stored in organs outside the bone marrow (e.g., liver, heart, pancreas), which results in organ damage. Accumulation of iron in the liver leads to cirrhosis, and the deposition of iron in the heart leads to cardiac dysfunction and arrhythmias. In the past, with transfusion therapy alone, thalassemia patients died in their teens, typically from cardiac failure. Now patients undergo iron chelation therapy with transfusion therapy. Iron-chelating agents bind excess iron so that it can be excreted in urine and stool. Deferoxamine, approved by the US Food and Drug Administration (FDA) in 1982, is usually administered subcutaneously with an infusion pump over 8 to 12 hours.[3,24] However, poor compliance with the regimen is seen in many patients, mainly because of the inconvenience of the infusion pump.[3,9,24] To address this concern, oral chelation agents (deferasirox, taken once daily; and deferiprone, taken 3 times daily) were approved by the FDA in 2005 and 2011, respectively.[24] All three iron-chelating agents have advantages, disadvantages, and side effects and are not effective in all patients; studies comparing the long-term efficacy of these agents are ongoing.[23,24] Combination therapy in which agents are alternated may improve compliance and reduce the side effects.[23,24] Additional oral iron-chelating drugs are in development. Adherence to iron chelation regimens is critical to prevent iron accumulation and subsequent complications of iron overload; its implementation has extended the life expectancy of patients with β-thalassemia major into the fourth and fifth decades and beyond.[3,23]

Hematopoietic stem cell transplantation (HSCT) is the only curative therapy for thalassemia major.[3,25] Young patients (under 14 years of age) who have a human leukocyte antigen (HLA)-identical sibling donor and have not yet developed complications of iron overload have excellent outcomes, with overall survival rates of 90% to 96% and event-free survival rates of 83% to 93%.[25] These rates, however, drop to an overall survival rate of 80% to 82% and event-free survival rate of 74% to 76% in those over 14 years.[25] Because there is only a 25% chance that a sibling will have the identical HLA genotype, this option is not available to all patients. However, HSCT outcomes with well-matched unrelated donors (using high-resolution molecular typing) have been continually improving, thus providing an additional option for those without a matched sibling donor.[23]

Hemoglobin F induction agents, such as hydroxyurea, 5-azacytidine, short chain fatty acids, erythropoietic-stimulating agents, and thalidomide derivatives, have been evaluated for therapy in thalassemia major because of their ability to "switch on" the γ-globin gene to produce more γ chains.[26] The γ chains then combine with the excess α chains to form Hb F, thus partially correcting the α/β chain imbalance. Hydroxyurea therapy has benefited a few β-thalassemia major patients, allowing them to become transfusion independent, but it has not been beneficial in the majority of patients.[3,26] Larger and better-designed studies are needed to determine the efficacy of these agents in reducing the need for transfusions in thalassemia major.[26]

In 2010 a successful ex vivo lentiviral β-globin gene transfer was reported in an adult with severe transfusion-dependent Hb E-β^0-thalassemia.[27] CD34+ hematopoietic stem cells were removed from the patient, transduced with the lentiviral vector encoding β-globin, and reinfused into the patient; as a result, the patient no longer needed transfusions.[27] In 2018 preliminary results were reported for two other clinical trials also using ex vivo lentiviral β-globin gene transfer in 22 patients with severe transfusion-dependent β-thalassemia.[28] Fifteen of these patients (9 with Hb E-β^0-thalassemia, 3 with the β^0/β^0 genotype, and 3 with other non-β^0/β^0 genotypes) no longer needed transfusions, and the other β^0/β^0 patients had a 74% decrease in the number of annual transfusions needed.[28] In the future, gene transfer may become a viable alternative for patients ineligible for HSCT due to the lack of an HLA-identical sibling donor.[14] Other therapies are also being investigated, such as gene editing to correct point mutations in the β-globin gene or to increase expression of the γ-globin gene; JAK2 inhibitors to suppress ineffective erythropoiesis; and mini-hepcidins to prevent iron overload.[3,23]

β-Thalassemia Intermedia

Thalassemia intermedia is a clinical designation for syndromes in which the α/β chain imbalance and symptoms fall between those observed in β-thalassemia minor and β-thalassemia major, but without the need for regular transfusion therapy to maintain the hemoglobin level and quality of life.[3,6,9] Thalassemia intermedia is included in the non-transfusion-dependent thalassemia group.[6,19] Patients with thalassemia intermedia typically maintain a hemoglobin level between 7 and 10 g/dL.[6]

Genotypes of thalassemia intermedia show great heterogeneity. Patients can be homozygous for mutations that cause a mild decrease in β-globin expression. Conversely, they may be compound heterozygous, with one gene causing a mild decrease in β chain production and the other causing a marked reduction in β chain production.[3,9] In rare instances, only one of the β-globin genes carries a mutation, but it is severe enough to cause a significant anemia. These cases are sometimes called *dominantly inherited* β-thalassemia.[10] Some of the thalassemia intermedia phenotypes result from the coinheritance of one or two abnormal β-globin genes with another hemoglobin defect, such as abnormal α-globin genes or unstable hemoglobins.[3,9] The coinheritance of α-thalassemia may permit homozygotes with more severe β-thalassemia mutations to remain transfusion independent because the α/β chain ratio is more balanced

and fewer free α chains are available to precipitate and cause hemolysis.[3] Less severe clinical manifestations also occur when a β-thalassemia mutation is combined with a mutation that increases the expression of the γ-globin gene.[3] The increase in Hb F production ($\alpha_2\gamma_2$) helps to compensate for the reduction in Hb A while helping to correct the α/β balance. Examples of these situations are the deletional forms of $\delta\beta^0$-thalassemia. Individuals homozygous for these mutations, or compound heterozygotes for $\delta\beta^0$-thalassemia and a β-thalassemia mutation, have thalassemia intermedia with increased γ chain and Hb F synthesis.[3,10] Conversely, coinheritance of a triplicated α-globin gene locus ($\alpha\alpha\alpha$) is also a cause of thalassemia intermedia in some individuals heterozygous for β-thalassemia due to the production of more α chains and greater imbalance of the α/β chain ratio.[3,29]

Because of the genetic heterogeneity of β-thalassemia intermedia, the laboratory and clinical features vary. The degree of anemia varies between 7 and 10 g/dL, depending on the extent of the α/β chain imbalance, with an MCV between 50 and 80 fL and an MCH between 16 and 24 pg.[6] Because of the presence of splenomegaly, the platelet and neutrophil counts may be low. The clinical course varies from minimal symptoms (despite moderately severe anemia) to severe exercise intolerance and pathologic fractures.[9]

Patients with thalassemia intermedia also have iron overload, even though they do not receive regular transfusions.[3] As indicated previously, the markedly accelerated ineffective erythropoiesis suppresses hepcidin production by the liver, which results in more iron absorption by intestinal enterocytes.[17] Cardiac, liver, and endocrine complications, however, present 10 to 20 years later in thalassemia intermedia patients than in patients who receive regular transfusions.[3] Regular monitoring for iron overload is recommended after age 10, with periodic chelation therapy to reduce iron levels.[6] Patients also have an increased risk of thrombosis due to the effects of iron overload and α chain precipitation in RBCs, causing platelet and RBC abnormalities and endothelial cell damage.[6,19] This risk is higher after splenectomy.[6,19]

Other Thalassemias Caused by Defects in the β-Globin Gene Cluster

Other thalassemias may be caused by deletion, inactivation, or fusion of a combination of genes of the β-globin gene cluster, such as hereditary persistence of fetal hemoglobin (HPFH), $\delta\beta^0$-thalassemia, and Hb Lepore thalassemia.[3,9,30]

Thalassemias with Increased Levels of Fetal Hemoglobin

HPFH and $\delta\beta^0$-thalassemia are closely related, heterogeneous conditions in which Hb F is expressed at increased levels beyond infancy into adulthood. These conditions have similarities but can be differentiated by the clinical presentation, hemoglobin level, MCV, and amount of Hb F produced.[10]

In HPFH the β-globin gene cluster typically contains a deletion in the $\delta\beta$ region that leads to the increased production of Hb F. However, there are also HPFH conditions that have intact β-globin gene clusters with non-deletional mutations in the promoter region of the γ-globin genes that lead to the increased

Hb F production.[9,10,31] Because individuals with these mutations are characteristically asymptomatic, this condition is of little significance except when it interacts with other forms of thalassemia or structural hemoglobin variants, such as Hb S. The additional γ chains produced are able to replace the missing β chains and help to restore the balance of α and non-α chains (γ or β). Significant variation is seen in heterozygotes for deletional-type HPFH, but these patients typically are asymptomatic, with a normal MCV and Hb F levels of 10% to 35%, depending on the mutation.[3,9] Homozygotes for deletional-type HPFH are also asymptomatic. They have a normal to slightly increased hemoglobin level, 100% Hb F, with slightly hypochromic and microcytic RBCs.[10] The increase in hemoglobin observed in some patients is likely a response to the slight hypoxia induced by the higher oxygen affinity of Hb F compared with Hb A.[3] When assessed using the Kleihauer-Betke acid elution stain (discussed later), the distribution of Hb F in HPFH is usually pancellular (deletional types), but it can be heterocellular (non-deletional types). In contrast, the Hb F distribution in the other β-globin gene cluster thalassemias is always heterocellular.[3,32]

The $\delta\beta^0$-thalassemias are also characterized by deletions in the δ- and β-globin genes and an increase in Hb F in adult life. Non-deletional types have also been described.[9] In this condition, however, the increase in production of the γ chains is not sufficient to completely restore the balance between the α and non-α chains. Heterozygous $\delta\beta^0$-thalassemia individuals ($\delta\beta^0/\beta$) have a decreased level of Hb A, normal or decreased level of Hb A_2, and 5% to 20% Hb F.[9,10] They have a β-thalassemia minor phenotype, with a slight decrease in hemoglobin level and hypochromic, microcytic RBCs. Homozygous $\delta\beta^0$-thalassemia individuals ($\delta\beta^0/\delta\beta^0$) have hypochromic, microcytic RBCs, 100% Hb F, and a β-thalassemia intermedia phenotype (Table 25.3).[9,10]

Hemoglobin Lepore Thalassemia

Hemoglobin Lepore ($\delta\beta^{Lepore}$) is a structural variant and rare type of δβ-thalassemia caused by a fusion of the δβ-globin genes.[11] This mutation occurs during meiosis due to nonhomologous crossover between the δ-globin locus on one chromosome and the β-globin locus on the other chromosome. The Lepore globin chain expressed by the δβ fusion gene contains the first 22 to 87 amino acids of the N-terminus of the δ chain and the last 31 to 97 amino acids of the C-terminus of the β chain, depending on the variant.[11] The δβ fusion gene produces a reduced level of the Lepore globin chain because its transcription is under the control of the δ-globin gene promoter, which is much less active than the β-globin gene promoter.[3] Conversely, in the reciprocal fusion on the other chromosome (called *anti-Lepore*), the β-globin gene locus is intact, so normal production of the β chain occurs.[3,10] In heterozygotes ($\delta\beta^{Lepore}/\beta$), there is a decreased level of Hb A and Hb A_2, an increase in Hb F, and approximately 5% to 15% Hb Lepore.[3,10] The clinical manifestations are similar to those of β-thalassemia minor. In homozygotes ($\delta\beta^{Lepore}/\delta\beta^{Lepore}$), there are no normal δ- or β-globin genes, no production of Hb A and Hb A_2, and approximately 80% Hb F and 20% Hb Lepore.[10] The clinical

manifestations are similar to those of β-thalassemia major[3] (Table 25.3).

Screening for β-Thalassemia Minor

Because of the high carrier frequency of β-thalassemia mutations worldwide, screening has become an important global health issue.[7] Mass screening programs in Italy and Greece combined with prenatal diagnosis have led to a significant reduction in the number of children born with β-thalassemia major.[10] Carrier parents have a 25% risk of having a child with thalassemia major or thalassemia intermedia, depending on the particular β globin gene mutations.[11] Potential β-thalassemia carriers can be initially identified by a mild decrease in hemoglobin concentration and MCV and an increase in Hb A_2, but other causes of microcytic anemias, such as iron deficiency, need to be ruled out.[10] Laboratory diagnosis of thalassemia is covered later in the chapter.

α-THALASSEMIA

In contrast to β-thalassemia, in which point mutations in the β-globin gene cluster are the most common type of mutation, in α-thalassemia large deletions involving the α_1- and/or α_2-globin genes are the predominant genetic defect.[9-11] Non-deletional mutations also occur in α-thalassemia but are uncommon.[10,11] The extent of decreased production of the α chain depends on the specific mutation, the number of α-globin genes affected, and whether the affected α-globin gene is α_2 or α_1.[9] The α_2-globin gene produces approximately 75% of the α chains in normal RBCs, so mutations in the α_2-globin gene generally cause more severe anemia than mutations affecting the α_1-globin gene.[9,10,33] The notation for the normal α-globin gene complex or haplotype is αα, which signifies the two normal genes (α_2 and α_1) on one chromosome 16. A normal genotype is αα/αα.

α-thalassemia is divided into two haplotypes: α^0-thalassemia and α^+-thalassemia. In the α^0-thalassemia haplotype (originally named α-thal-1), a deletion of both α-globin genes on chromosome 16 results in no α chain production from that chromosome. The designation – – is used for the α^0-thalassemia haplotype.[9,10] There are more than 20 known mutations that produce the α^0-thalassemia haplotype and involve deletion of both α-globin genes or the entire α-globin gene cluster (including the ζ-globin gene) on one chromosome.[11,34] The α^0 haplotype (– –) is found in approximately 4% of the population in Southeast Asia, is found less frequently in the Mediterranean region, and occurs infrequently in other parts of the world.[7]

In the α^+-thalassemia haplotype (originally named α-thal-2), a deletional or non-deletional mutation in one of the two α-globin genes on chromosome 16 results in decreased α chain production from that chromosome.[9] The designation – α is used for the deletional mutations, and the designation $\alpha^T\alpha$ is used for the non-deletional mutations. The deletional α^+ haplotype (– α) is by far the most common of the α-thalassemia haplotypes. It is widely distributed throughout the thalassemia belt and central Africa (Figure 24.3), with a carrier frequency reaching 50% to 80% in some regions of Saudi Arabia, India, Southeast Asia, and Africa.[7] The deletional α^+ haplotype $(-\alpha)$ is also found in about 30% of African Americans.[33] The non-deletional α^+ haplotype $(\alpha^T\alpha)$ is relatively uncommon.[10,33] More than 70 different mutations are known, the majority of which are point mutations that affect the predominant α_2 gene.[6,11] The α^T haplotype produces unstable α chains or fewer α chains than the $-\alpha$ haplotype and generally results in a more severe anemia.[10,14,33]

One of the most common non-deletional α-globin gene mutations is Constant Spring $(\alpha_2^{142Stop\rightarrow Gln})$, also called α^{CS} (haplotype $\alpha^{CS}\alpha$).[10,11] It is the result of a point mutation in the α_2-globin gene that changes the stop codon at 142 to a glutamine codon.[10,11,33] As a result, additional bases are added to the end of the mRNA during transcription until the next stop codon is reached. The elongated mRNA is very unstable and produces only a small amount of the α^{CS} chain.[3,34,35] α^{CS} chains (with an additional 31 amino acids added to the C-terminal end) combine with β chains to form Hb Constant Spring, but incorporation of a longer α chain makes the tetramer unstable.[3,35] Because of the instability of both the mRNA and the hemoglobin tetramer, the circulating level of Hb Constant Spring is very low $(<1\%)$.[3,10,35] Consequently, hemoglobin Constant Spring is difficult to detect by alkaline hemoglobin electrophoresis, and when present, is visualized as a faint, slow-moving band near the point of origin.[10]

Clinical Syndromes of α-Thalassemia

α-thalassemia has four clinical syndromes, which are determined by the number of genes affected and the amount of α chains produced (Table 25.4):[3,9,10]
- Silent carrier state
- α-thalassemia minor
- Hb H disease
- Hb Bart hydrops fetalis syndrome

Silent Carrier State

Deletion of one α-globin gene, leaving three functional α-globin genes $(-\alpha/\alpha\alpha)$, is the major cause of the silent carrier state. The α/β chain ratio is nearly normal, and no hematologic abnormalities are present.[9,10] Because one α-globin gene is absent, there is a slight decrease in α chain production. There is a slight excess of γ chains at birth that form tetramers of Hb Bart (γ_4) in the range of 1% to 2%.[9,10] There is no reliable way to diagnose silent carrier state other than genetic analysis. A non-deletional α^+ mutation in one α-globin gene $(\alpha^T\alpha/\alpha\alpha)$ also results in the silent carrier state. In the heterozygous mutation, $\alpha^{CS}\alpha/\alpha\alpha$, Hb Constant Spring is less than 1% of the total hemoglobin.[10]

α-Thalassemia Minor (α-Thalassemia Trait)

Deletion of two α-globin genes is the major cause of α-thalassemia minor. It exists in two forms: homozygous α^+ $(-\alpha/-\alpha)$ or heterozygous α^0 $(--/\alpha\alpha)$.[9,10] This syndrome is asymptomatic and characterized by a mild microcytic anemia with an MCV of less than 80 fL and an MCH of less than 27 pg.[6,14] At birth the proportion of Hb Bart is in the range of

5% to 15%.[10] In adults the production of α and β chains is balanced, so Hb H (β_4) is not usually present. Homozygosity for non-deletional mutations in both α_2-globin genes $(\alpha^T\alpha/\alpha^T\alpha)$ produces a mild to moderate hemolytic anemia, often with jaundice and hepatosplenomegaly.[10,35] In the homozygous mutation, $\alpha^{CS}\alpha/\alpha^{CS}\alpha$, Hb Constant Spring is 5% to 6% of the total hemoglobin and the hemoglobin concentration is 9 to 11 g/dL.[9,10,35]

Hemoglobin H Disease (α-Thalassemia Intermedia)

Deletion of three α-globin genes is the major cause of Hb H disease, in which only one α-globin gene remains to produce α chains $(--/-\alpha)$.[9,10] This genetic abnormality is particularly common in Asians because of the prevalence of the α^0 gene haplotype $(--)$. It is characterized by the accumulation of excess unpaired β chains that form tetramers of Hb H in adults. In the newborn Hb Bart comprises 10% to 40% of the hemoglobin, with the remainder being Hb F and Hb A. After the γ

TABLE 25.4 Clinical Syndromes of α-Thalassemia

Genotype	Hb A	Hb Bart (in Newborn)	Hb H (in Adult)	Hb Constant Spring
Normal (Normal Hematologic Parameters)				
$\alpha\alpha/\alpha\alpha$	N	0	0	0
Silent Carrier State (Asymptomatic; Normal Hematologic Parameters)				
$-\alpha/\alpha\alpha$	N	1%–2%	0	0
$\alpha^{CS}\alpha/\alpha\alpha$	N	1%–3%	0	<1%
α-Thalassemia Minor (Asymptomatic; Mild Anemia; Microcytic, Hypochromic)				
$--/\alpha\alpha$	Sl↓	5%–15%	0	0
$-\alpha/-\alpha$	Sl↓	5%–15%	0	0
$\alpha^{CS}\alpha/\alpha^{CS}\alpha$*	Sl↓	5%–15%	0	<6%
Hb H Disease, α-Thalassemia Intermedia (Non-Transfusion-Dependent Thalassemia, Mild to Moderate Anemia; Microcytic, Hypochromic)**				
$--/-\alpha$	↓	10%–40%	1%–40%	0
$--/\alpha^{CS}\alpha$†	↓	↑↑	↑↑	<1%
Hb Bart Hydrops Fetalis Syndrome, α-Thalassemia Major (Transfusion-Dependent Thalassemia; Severe Anemia; Usually Death in Utero or Shortly after Birth)				
$--/--$	0	80%–90% (remainder Hb Portland)	NA	0

*$\alpha^{CS}\alpha/\alpha^{CS}\alpha$ genotype results in mild to moderate hemolytic anemia with jaundice and hepatosplenomegaly.
**Patients who are non-transfusion dependent do not require regular transfusions for survival but may need transfusions occasionally, such as during pregnancy, surgery, or infections.
†$--/\alpha^{CS}\alpha$ genotype and other non-deletional genotypes $(--/\alpha^T\alpha)$ result in Hb H disease that is moderate to severe and may require more frequent transfusions than the deletional $--/-\alpha$ genotype.
↓, Decreased; ↑↑ increased more than $--/-\alpha$; 0, absent; <, less than; CS, Constant Spring; Hb, hemoglobin; N, normal; NA, not applicable.

to β switch, Hb H replaces most of the Hb Bart, so Hb H is in the range of 1% to 40%, with a reduced amount of Hb A$_2$, traces of Hb Bart, and the remainder Hb A.[9,10,33,34] The non-deletional α$^+$ haplotype, when combined with the α^0 haplotype ($--/\alpha^T\alpha$), generally produces a more severe Hb H disease with a higher level of Hb H than the α^0 interaction with the deletional α$^+$ haplotype ($--/-\alpha$).[10,33,35] Hb H-Hb Constant Spring ($--/\alpha^{CS}\alpha$) is an example.[10,35,36]

Hb H disease is characterized by a mild to moderate, chronic hemolytic anemia with hemoglobin concentrations averaging 7 to 10 g/dL and reticulocyte counts of 3% to 10%, although a wide variability in clinical and laboratory findings exists.[6,9] Patients with deletional Hb H disease generally have higher hemoglobin levels compared to patients with non-deletional types.[6] Bone marrow exhibits erythroid hyperplasia, and the spleen is usually enlarged. Hb H disease is classified as a non-transfusion-dependent thalassemia; that is, patients do not require regular transfusions. However, infection, pregnancy, or exposure to oxidative drugs may cause a hemolytic crisis, requiring transfusions on a temporary basis.[6] Patients may develop iron overload, and the iron status should be monitored starting at age 10 to 15 years.[6]

Hemolytic crises often lead to detection of the disease because individuals with Hb H disease may otherwise be asymptomatic. RBCs are microcytic and hypochromic, with marked poikilocytosis, including target cells and bizarre shapes. Hb H is vulnerable to oxidation and gradually precipitates in the circulating RBCs to form inclusion bodies of denatured hemoglobin.[9] Hb H inclusions alter the shape and viscoelastic properties of the RBCs, contributing to decreased RBC survival. The inclusions are typically removed as the RBC passes through the spleen; however after splenectomy, most RBCs have many inclusions. Hb H inclusions are visualized with supravital staining (discussed in the Laboratory Methods section of this chapter).

Two distinct conditions are associated with Hb H disease and congenital physical and intellectual abnormalities: α-thalassemia retardation-16 (ATR-16) syndrome and α-thalassemia X-linked intellectual disability (ATRX) syndrome. Patients with the ATR-16 syndrome inherit or acquire a large deletion in the short arm of chromosome 16, which removes the ζ- and α-globin genes and all the flanking genes to the terminus of the chromosome.[34] Patients have physical deformities, intellectual disabilities, and Hb H disease.[33,34,36] The ATRX syndrome is due to mutations of the *ATRX* gene located on the X chromosome.[37,38] The ATRX protein is a component of a large complex that regulates expression of various genes, including the α-globin genes.[34,38] The regulation is accomplished by DNA remodeling and/or methylation, thus affecting the transcription, replication, and repair of the target genes.[33,34,38] Therefore when the *ATRX* gene is mutated, patients have decreased α chain production.[33,34,36,38] Affected males with ATRX syndrome have pronounced intellectual disability, physical deformities, developmental delay, and Hb H disease. An acquired Hb H disease with mutations in the *ATRX* gene has been found in myelodysplastic syndrome.[34,38,39]

Hb Bart Hydrops Fetalis Syndrome (α-Thalassemia Major)

Homozygous α^0-thalassemia ($--/--$) results in the absence of all α chain production. It usually results in death in utero or shortly after birth, although a small number survive with aggressive transfusion therapy, including intrauterine transfusions.[3,9,34] It is included in the transfusion-dependent thalassemia category because if the neonate survives, lifelong transfusions are required.[19]

Without intrauterine transfusion, the fetus becomes severely anemic, which leads to cardiac failure and edema in fetal subcutaneous tissues (hydrops fetalis). Hb Bart (γ$_4$) is the predominant hemoglobin, along with a small amount of Hb Portland (ζ$_2$γ$_2$) and traces of Hb H.[3,9] Hb Bart has a very high oxygen affinity; it does not deliver oxygen to the tissues.[9,10,34] The fetus can survive until the third trimester because of Hb Portland, but this hemoglobin cannot support the later stages of fetal growth, and the affected fetus becomes severely anoxic.[3,9] The fetus is delivered prematurely and is usually stillborn or dies shortly after birth. In addition to anemia, edema, and ascites, the fetus has gross hepatosplenomegaly and cardiomegaly.[3,9] At delivery there is a severe microcytic, hypochromic anemia (hemoglobin concentration of 3 to 8 g/dL) with high reticulocyte counts and numerous nucleated RBCs in the peripheral blood.[34] The bone marrow cavity is expanded, and marked erythroid hyperplasia is present, along with foci of extramedullary erythropoiesis.

Hydropic pregnancies are hazardous to the mother, resulting in toxemia and severe postpartum hemorrhage.[9,14,34] Hydropic changes are detected in midgestation by means of ultrasound testing.[40] If both parents carry one α^0-thalassemia haplotype ($--/\alpha\alpha$), prenatal diagnosis of homozygosity can be made by molecular genetic testing of fetal cells from chorionic villus sampling or amniotic fluid.[34] Absence of the α-globin genes establishes the diagnosis. Early termination of the pregnancy prevents the serious maternal complications.[9]

THALASSEMIA ASSOCIATED WITH STRUCTURAL HEMOGLOBIN VARIANTS

Hemoglobin S-Thalassemia

Sickle cell anemia (Hb SS)-α-thalassemia is a genetic abnormality due to the coinheritance of two abnormal β-globin genes for Hb S and an α-thalassemia haplotype. Hb SS-α$^+$-thalassemia is fairly common because the genes for Hb S and the α$^+$-thalassemia haplotype, $-\alpha$, are common in populations of African ancestry. Individuals with Hb SS-α$^+$-thalassemia have a milder anemia with higher hemoglobin levels and lower reticulocyte counts than those with sickle cell anemia alone.[41] In one study Hb SS individuals with the genotypes αα/αα, $-\alpha/\alpha\alpha$, and $-\alpha/-\alpha$ had average hemoglobin concentrations of 8.4, 9.0, and 9.5 g/dL, respectively, and reticulocyte counts of 10.8%, 8.8%, and 6.9%, respectively.[41]

Hb S-β-thalassemia is a compound heterozygous condition that results from the inheritance of a β-thalassemia gene from one parent and an Hb S gene from the other. This syndrome has been reported in the populations of Africa, the Mediterranean area, the Middle East, and India.[10] The clinical expression of Hb S-β-thalassemia depends on the type of β-thalassemia mutation inherited.[9,10] Individuals with Hb S-β$^+$-thalassemia

TABLE 25.5 β-Thalassemia Associated with Structural β-Globin Variants (Compound Heterozygotes)

Genotype	Hb A	Hb A$_2$	Hb F	Other Hb	RBC Morphology	Clinical Manifestations*	Treatment
Hb S-β$^+$-thalassemia	↓↓	↑	N to ↑	Hb S > Hb A	Microcytes, sickle cells, target cells	Ranges from mild to severe anemia with recurrent vasoocclusive crises	Ranges from no treatment to transfusion support and pain control
Hb S-β^0-thalassemia	0	↑	N to ↑	Hb S			
Hb C-β$^+$-thalassemia	↓↓	†	↑	Hb C > Hb A	Microcytes, Hb C crystals, target cells	Ranges from moderate to severe anemia	Usually no treatment needed
Hb C-β^0-thalassemia	0	†	↑	Hb C			
Hb E-β$^+$-thalassemia	↓↓	†	↑↑	Hb E > Hb A	Microcytes, target cells	Ranges from mild to severe anemia with transfusion dependency	Ranges from no treatment to transfusion support
Hb E-β^0-thalassemia	0	†	↑↑	Hb E			

*Clinical manifestations depend on the amount of Hb A produced; compound heterozygotes with the β^0 gene have more severe symptoms.
†Not all methods can quantitate Hb A$_2$ in the presence of the abnormal hemoglobin. High-performance liquid chromatography can separate Hb A$_2$ from Hb C; capillary zone electrophoresis can separate Hb A$_2$ from Hb E.
↑, Increased; ↓, decreased; 0, absent; *Hb,* hemoglobin; *N,* normal; *RBC,* red blood cell.

produce variable amounts of normal β chains. Patients have mostly Hb S with slightly elevated Hb A$_2$ and variable amounts of Hb F and Hb A, depending on the specific abnormal β$^+$ gene inherited. These patients can be distinguished from those with sickle cell anemia by the presence of microcytosis, splenomegaly, an elevated Hb A$_2$ level, and an Hb A level that is less than the Hb S level.

The interaction of β^{silent}-thalassemia (in which β chains are produced at mildly reduced levels) and Hb S results in a condition that may be slightly more severe than sickle cell trait. Typically there is mild hemolytic anemia with splenomegaly. These patients can be distinguished from patients with sickle cell trait by the presence of microcytosis and splenomegaly. Hemoglobin electrophoresis or HPLC confirms this condition when the quantity of Hb S exceeds that of Hb A. In sickle cell trait, Hb A is the predominant hemoglobin.

The combination of β^0-thalassemia and Hb S produces a phenotype similar to sickle cell anemia, with a similar incidence of stroke and a similar life expectancy.[10,42] Both conditions lack Hb A and produce severe painful crises as the predominant symptom. Typically, the microcytosis and elevated Hb A$_2$ level in Hb S-β^0-thalassemia distinguish it from sickle cell anemia.

Hemoglobin C-Thalassemia

Hb C-β-thalassemia produces moderately severe hemolysis, splenomegaly, hypochromia, microcytosis, and numerous target cells. The hemoglobin electrophoresis pattern varies, depending on the type of β-thalassemia gene defect, with higher Hb C concentrations in patients when there is minimal or no β chain production.[10]

Hemoglobin E-Thalassemia

Hb E-β-thalassemia is a significant concern in Southeast Asia and Eastern India, owing to the high prevalence of both genetic mutations.[10] Hb E is due to a point mutation that inserts a splice site in the β-globin gene and results in decreased production of Hb E.[3] In the homozygous state (Hb EE) the clinical symptoms are similar to a mild β-thalassemia (Chapter 24). When the mutations are coinherited in the compound heterozygous

state, there is a marked reduction of β chain production. The clinical symptoms are similar to β-thalassemia intermedia or β-thalassemia major, depending on the particular β-globin gene mutation.[10] Severe Hb E-β-thalassemia manifests a hemoglobin concentration ranging from 4 to 5 g/dL and is classified and managed as a transfusion-dependent thalassemia.[6] Mild and moderate Hb E-β-thalassemias (a hemoglobin concentration of 9 to 12 g/dL and 6 to 7 g/dL, respectively) are classified and managed as non-transfusion-dependent thalassemias.[6]

Table 25.5 summarizes some compound heterozygous states of β-thalassemia combined with a structural β-globin defect.

DIAGNOSIS OF THALASSEMIA

History and Physical Examination

Individual and family histories are paramount in the diagnosis of thalassemia. The ethnic background of the individual should be investigated because of the increased prevalence of specific gene mutations in certain populations. In the clinical examination, findings that suggest thalassemia include pallor (due to the anemia); jaundice (due to the hemolysis); splenomegaly (caused by sequestration of the abnormal RBCs, excessive extravascular hemolysis, and some extramedullary erythropoiesis); and skeletal deformities (due to the massive expansion of the bone marrow cavities). These findings are particularly prominent in untreated or partially treated β-thalassemia major.[10]

Laboratory Methods

Table 25.6 contains a summary of tests for the diagnosis of thalassemia.

Complete Blood Count with Peripheral Blood Film Review

Although most thalassemias result in a microcytic and hypochromic anemia, laboratory results can vary from borderline abnormal to markedly abnormal; this depends on the type and number of globin gene mutations. The hemoglobin and hematocrit are decreased, but the RBC count can be disproportionately high relative to the degree of anemia, which can generate

TABLE 25.6   Laboratory Diagnosis of Thalassemia[3,15,34]

Screening tests	Complete blood count Peripheral blood film review Iron studies (to rule out IDA)	HGB, HCT, MCV, MCH, MCHC: ↓ RETIC: sl to mod ↑ Varying degrees of microcytosis, hypochromia, target cells, anisocytosis, poikilocytosis, RBC inclusions, NRBCs Serum ferritin and serum iron: N to ↑↑
Presumptive diagnosis	Supravital stain Hemoglobin fraction quantification by electrophoresis, HPLC, and/or CZE	α-thal: Hb H inclusions β-thal: Hb A ↓ or 0; Hb A₂ ↑ (carriers); Hb F usually ↑; Hb Lepore and other mutants may be present α-thal: Hb A ↓ or 0 (hydrops fetalis); Hb A₂ ↓; Hb Bart, Hb H, Hb Constant Spring, and other mutants may be present
Definitive diagnosis	Molecular genetic tests* β-thal: >280 mutations** in *HBB* α-thal: >110 mutations** in *HBA1* and/or *HBA2*	β-thal: initial DNA sequence analysis or PCR-based screen for four to six most common mutations if specific ethnic group known; if negative, deletion/duplication analysis, such as MLPA or gene-targeted microarray analysis. α-thal: initial targeted deletional analysis for five most common deletions; if negative, DNA sequence analysis; if negative, deletion/duplication analysis as above.

*Required for prenatal diagnosis, preconception risk assessment/carrier detection in couples, or diagnosis of rare or complex mutations.
**From reference 11 (HbVar database, accessed April 23, 2018).
CZE, Capillary zone electrophoresis; *Hb*, hemoglobin; *HCT*, hematocrit; *HGB*, hemoglobin concentration; *IDA*, iron deficiency anemia; *MCH*, mean cell hemoglobin; *MCHC*, mean cell hemoglobin concentration; *MCV*, mean cell volume; *MLPA*, multiplex ligation-dependent probe amplification; *mod*, moderate; *NRBCs*, nucleated red blood cells; *PCR*, polymerase chain reaction; *RETIC*, reticulocyte count; *RBCs*, red blood cells; *sl*, slight; *thal*, thalassemia; ↓, decreased; ↑, increased; ↑↑, markedly increased.

a very low MCV and MCH. The mean cell hemoglobin concentration (MCHC) is also decreased. The RBC distribution width (RDW) is elevated (reflecting anisocytosis) in untreated β-thalassemia major, but it is often normal in β-thalassemia minor. On a peripheral blood film, the RBCs are typically microcytic and hypochromic, except in silent carrier phenotypes, in which RBCs appear normal. In β-thalassemia minor, α-thalassemia minor, and Hb H disease, the cells are microcytic with target cells and slight to moderate poikilocytosis. In homozygous and compound heterozygous β-thalassemia, extreme poikilocytosis may be present, including target cells and elliptocytes, in addition to polychromasia, basophilic stippling, Howell-Jolly bodies, Pappenheimer bodies, and nucleated RBCs.

Reticulocyte Count

The reticulocyte count is elevated, which indicates that the bone marrow is responding to a hemolytic process. In Hb H disease the typical reticulocyte count is 5% to 10%.[10] In homozygous β-thalassemia it is typically 2% to 8%, disproportionately low relative to the degree of anemia.[3,10] Inadequate reticulocytosis reflects the ineffective erythropoiesis.

Supravital Staining

In Hb H disease, α-thalassemia minor, and silent carrier α-thalassemia, brilliant cresyl blue or new methylene blue stain may be used to induce precipitation of the intrinsically unstable Hb H.[43] Hb H inclusions (denatured β₄ tetramers) typically appear as small, multiple, irregularly shaped greenish-blue bodies that are uniformly distributed throughout the RBC. They produce a pitted pattern on the RBC surface similar to the pattern of a golf ball or raspberry (Figure 25.7). In Hb H disease, almost all RBCs contain Hb H inclusions.[36] In α-thalassemia minor, only a few cells may contain these inclusions, and in silent carrier α-thalassemia, only a rare cell does.

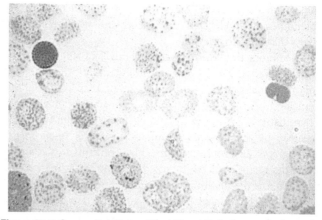

Figure 25.7 Supravital Stain of Red Blood Cells from a Patient with Hemoglobin H Disease. Note the fine, evenly dispersed granular inclusions and the "golf ball" appearance of the cell surface. (Peripheral blood, brilliant cresyl blue stain, ×1000.) (From the American Society for Hematology slide bank.)

These inclusions appear different from Heinz bodies, which are larger and fewer in number and most often appear attached to the inner membrane of the RBC. This test is very sensitive in detecting Hb H in α-thalassemia syndromes.[43]

Assessment of Hemolysis

Because thalassemias have a hemolytic component to their pathophysiology, tests for hemolysis are part of the overall assessment. Typically there is an increase in unconjugated bilirubin and lactate dehydrogenase, and a decrease in haptoglobin (Chapter 20).

Assessment of Normal and Variant Hemoglobins

The major clinical laboratory methods used to identify and quantify normal and variant hemoglobins include hemoglobin electrophoresis, cation-exchange HPLC, and capillary zone electrophoresis (CZE).[44] Each of these methods has advantages and limitations, and no one method is able to identify and quantify all hemoglobin variants. Therefore a combination of at least two of the above methods is used for confirmation of a hemoglobin variant.[45]

Hemoglobin electrophoresis at an alkaline pH has been the traditional tool for thalassemia and hemoglobinopathy diagnosis. In this method the patient's RBC lysate is spotted on a solid support (e.g., agarose) and subjected to an electrical current in an alkaline buffer. Normal and variant hemoglobins will migrate and separate on the support according to their charge. The support is stained, and each hemoglobin band is quantified by scanning densitometry and reported as a percentage of the total hemoglobin.[45] This technique is able to distinguish the common hemoglobins (e.g., Hb A, Hb F, Hb S, and Hb C) and the fast-moving hemoglobins (Hb H and Hb Bart).[44-46] Electrophoresis, however, has several limitations: it is labor intensive, has low resolution, and cannot accurately quantify Hb A_2 and Hb F. In addition, Hb S and Hb C must be confirmed by another method because Hb D and Hb G comigrate with Hb S, and Hb E and Hb O^{Arab} comigrate with Hb C.[45] Methods used for confirmation usually include electrophoresis at an acid pH, HPLC, and CZE, or in the case of Hb S, the hemoglobin solubility test (Figures 24.6 to 24.9). Figure 25.8 shows the relative hemoglobin mobilities in alkaline electrophoresis for various thalassemias and hemoglobinopathies.

In HPLC the patient's RBC lysate in buffer is injected into a cation-exchange column. Both normal and variant hemoglobins will bind to the column. An elution buffer is injected and forms a gradient of varying ionic strength.[45] The various hemoglobin types will be differentially eluted from the column, each having a specific column retention time. As each hemoglobin fraction passes near the end of the column, a detector measures the absorbance of the fraction at 415 nm, which is recorded as a peak on a chromatogram.[45] The area under the peak is used to quantify the hemoglobin fraction, which is reported as a percentage of total hemoglobin. With the availability of fully automated instruments, HPLC has replaced hemoglobin electrophoresis in many laboratories as the routine screening method for analysis of hemoglobins.[44]

The method is ideal for β-thalassemia screening because it can accurately and quickly quantify Hb A, Hb A_2, and Hb F with 100% sensitivity and 90% specificity if no hemoglobin variants are present (Figure 25.9).[46]

The precise and accurate quantification of Hb A_2 is particularly important in screening individuals for β-thalassemia minor (trait). HPLC can also presumptively identify and quantify hemoglobin variants even in low concentration.[44,45] HPLC, however, requires specialized instrumentation and extensive experience and training to accurately interpret the complex chromatograms.[44,45,47] Additional limitations of HPLC include: Hb A_2 and Hb E have the same retention time and therefore cannot be accurately quantified by this method; Hb A_2 can be overestimated in the presence of Hb S due to overlapping peaks and underestimated in the presence of Hb D^{Punjab}; and HPLC is not able to identify all variants.[44-48] A manual microcolumn method is also available for the measurement of Hb A_2.[45]

In CZE the patient's RBC lysate is introduced into a thin silica glass capillary tube in an alkaline buffer. When a current is applied, various hemoglobin fractions migrate to the cathode at different velocities due to electroendosmotic flow.[45] As each hemoglobin fraction passes near the end of the capillary, a detector measures the absorbance of the fraction at 415 nm, which is recorded as a peak on a electrophoretogram. The instrument calculates the percentage of each hemoglobin fraction using an integration of the area under the peak and the migration time.[45] Fully automated systems are available that provide rapid and accurate identification and quantification. The peaks are placed into zones in the electrophoretogram for easier identification, and the method can presumptively identify hemoglobin variants, including those in low concentration (Figure 25.9).[45] An advantage of CZE over HPLC is that it can separate and quantify Hb A_2 in the presence of Hb E.[44,48] However, because there is overlap in the peaks for Hb A_2 and Hb C, it cannot quantify Hb A_2 in the presence of Hb C.[44] As with HPLC, it also cannot detect all variants.[44,45] Complementing electrophoresis, HPLC, and/or CZE results, however, have minimized the limitations of all these methods.[47] Other technologies, such as isoelectric focusing and mass spectrometry, are used in newborn screening programs for detection of common hemoglobin variants.[44,45]

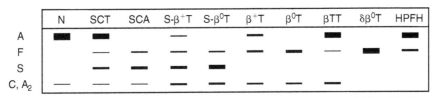

Figure 25.8 Relative Electrophoretic Mobilities at Alkaline pH of Various Hemoglobins *(Hbs)* Important in the Diagnosis of Thalassemia Syndromes and Hemoglobinopathies. *β⁰T*, β⁰-thalassemia major, β⁰/β⁰ (no Hb A, increased Hb F, slight increase in Hb A_2); *β⁺T*, β⁺-thalassemia major, β⁺/β⁺ (decreased Hb A, increased Hb F, slight increase in Hb A_2); *βTT*, β-thalassemia minor (slight decrease in Hb A, increased Hb A_2, some Hb F); *δβ⁰T*, δβ⁰-thalassemia, homozygous, δβ⁰/δβ⁰ (100% Hb F); *HPFH*, hereditary persistence of fetal hemoglobin, heterozygous (mostly Hb A, some Hb F, no Hb A_2); *N*, normal; *SCA*, sickle cell anemia (no Hb A, mostly Hb S, increased Hb F, normal Hb A_2); *SCT*, sickle cell trait (Hb A > Hb S, normal Hb A_2 and Hb F); *S-β⁰T*, sickle cell-β⁰-thalassemia (no Hb A, increased Hb A_2 and F, mostly Hb S); *S-β⁺T*, sickle cell-β⁺-thalassemia (Hb A < Hb S, increased Hb A_2 and Hb F).

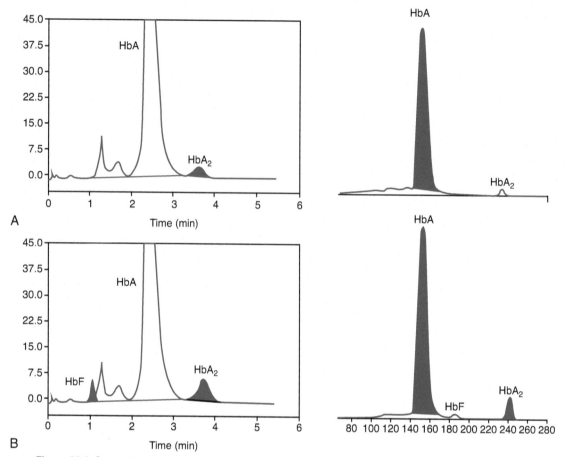

Figure 25.9 Separation and Quantification of Hemoglobin Fractions by High-Performance Liquid Chromatography (Bio-Rad, *left*) and Capillary Electrophoresis (Sebia, *right*). **(A),** Healthy adult with Hb F < 1% and Hb A₂ < 3.5%. **(B),** Adult with β-thalassemia minor with increased Hb F and Hb A₂. (Modified from Giordano, P. C. [2013]. Strategies for basic laboratory diagnostics of the hemoglobinopathies in multiethnic societies: interpretation of results and pitfalls. *Int J Lab Hematol, 35,* p. 472, Figure 3.)

Molecular Genetic Testing

Molecular genetic testing is required to detect specific mutations in globin genes and definitively identify the type of thalassemia. Molecular genetic testing is not usually required in adults with typical findings on the complete blood count (CBC), electrophoresis, and/or HPLC, but it is required for prenatal diagnosis, preconception risk assessment/carrier detection in couples, and diagnosis of rare or complex mutations.[15,34,44,48]

In β-thalassemia, point mutations in the *HBB* gene are the most common abnormality.[11,48] Therefore DNA sequence analysis is a practical initial approach and can identify almost 100% of mutations; however, it is not optimal for detection of deletions.[15,48] Targeted mutation analysis using polymerase chain reaction (PCR)-based methods can also be used for detection and quantification of the four to six most common mutations in genetically homogenous populations if an individual's ethnicity is known.[3,48] If sequencing is not successful, testing can reflex to deletion/duplication analysis, such as multiplex ligation-dependent probe amplification (MLPA) or gene-targeted microarray analysis (Chapter 29).[15,48]

For *HBA1* or *HBA2* mutations in which 95% are deletions, PCR-based targeted mutation analysis, such as GAP-PCR, can be initially performed for the five most common deletional mutations.[34,48] This strategy detects approximately 85% of all deletions.[34] If this analysis is not successful, DNA sequencing of the *HBA1* and *HBA2* genes or deletion/duplication analysis can be performed.[34,48]

When the parents' mutation is known, analysis for the specific mutation in fetal cells can be done on specimens from amniocentesis (at 15 to 18 weeks' gestation), chorionic villus sampling (at 10 to 12 weeks' gestation), or with preimplantation genetic diagnosis using a cell from a 3-day-old embryo after in vitro fertilization.[15,34] Noninvasive methods for detection of the paternal mutation in fetal DNA isolated from maternal circulation are also available.[15,34]

Other Procedures

The classic *alkali denaturation* test is accurate and precise to quantify Hb F in the 0.2% to 50% range.[49] Most human hemoglobins are denatured on exposure to a strong alkali, but Hb F is not. The Hb F can be separated and its concentration compared with that of other hemoglobins. Consistent methodology is required to ensure accurate results.[49] However, automated HPLC is now most often used to quantify Hb F.[45,46]

In the Kleihauer-Betke acid elution slide test, peripheral blood films are ethanol fixed and immersed in a citrate-acid buffer (pH 3.3). Adult hemoglobins are eluted from the RBCs, but Hb F resists acid elution and remains in the cell. When the cells are subsequently stained, RBCs containing Hb F will take up the stain, whereas RBCs containing only adult hemoglobin will appear as "ghosts." This test determines if the Hb F distribution in RBCs is pancellular (found in all RBCs in deletional HPFH cases) or heterocellular (found in some but not all RBCs in β-globin gene cluster thalassemias and non-deletional HPFH cases).[45] The Kleihauer-Betke slide test is also used to estimate the volume of fetal-maternal hemorrhage to determine if an increased dose of Rh immune globulin is needed for an Rh-negative mother who delivers an Rh-positive baby. Because the Kleihauer-Betke slide test is cumbersome to perform and results are difficult to replicate, flow cytometry is becoming the standard test to measure fetal-maternal hemorrhage quickly and accurately.[50]

In underdeveloped countries with limited technology, a single-tube osmotic fragility test has been used to screen populations for thalassemia carriers.[3,9] This is based on the fact that carriers have hypochromic RBCs, resulting in decreased osmotic fragility.[46,51] An aliquot of anticoagulated blood is incubated in 0.375% saline for 5 minutes.[44] Because the solution is hypotonic, normal RBCs will lyse and the solution will clear. However, patients with thalassemia have hypochromic RBCs that will not lyse in 0.375% saline, and the solution will remain turbid. This test is not specific for thalassemia and will be positive for any condition causing hypochromia, including iron deficiency anemia.

Differential Diagnosis of Thalassemia Minor and Iron Deficiency Anemia

RBCs in thalassemia minor are microcytic and hypochromic, and this disease must be differentiated from iron deficiency anemia and other microcytic, hypochromic anemias to avoid unnecessary tests or treatments. An incorrect presumption that a patient has iron deficiency may lead to inappropriate iron therapy or to unnecessary diagnostic procedures, such as colonoscopy, to identify a source of blood loss.

The clinical history is crucial. A family history of thalassemia raises the suspicion for this diagnosis. A history of previously normal hemoglobin levels and RBC indices, significant

bleeding, or pica leads to the diagnosis of iron deficiency (Chapter 17). *Pica* means cravings for nonfood items, such as clay, dirt, or starch. The most common pica symptom in the United States is pagophagia, the craving to chew on ice.

Iron deficiency and β-thalassemia minor are best differentiated using the serum ferritin level, serum iron level, total iron-binding capacity, transferrin saturation, and Hb A₂ level, along with a CBC and examination of a peripheral blood film (Table 17.1).[45,52–54] Additional testing may include soluble transferrin receptor and zinc protoporphyrin levels.

Before the Hb A₂ level is evaluated for β-thalassemia minor, iron deficiency should be ruled out. Low iron levels in patients with β-thalassemia minor reduce the Hb A₂ level, therefore iron stores should be replenished before laboratory analysis for Hb A₂ is undertaken.[45]

A mild erythrocytosis (high RBC count) and marked microcytosis (low MCV) are found more commonly in β-thalassemia minor. In iron deficiency anemia, the RBC count and MCV may be normal or decreased, depending on whether the deficiency is developing or long-standing. The RDW can be normal or increased in both β-thalassemia minor and iron deficiency anemia, with a significant overlap of values; therefore, the RDW alone cannot distinguish these conditions.[52-55] Basophilic stippling can be observed on the peripheral blood film in β-thalassemia minor, which can distinguish it from iron deficiency anemia. Target cells can be found in both conditions, thus their presence does not help discriminate between the two disorders.

More than 40 discrimination indices have been proposed to distinguish β-thalassemia minor from iron deficiency anemia, using an individual parameter or simple calculations based on various parameters, such as the RBC count, hemoglobin concentration, MCV, MCH, RDW, and/or microcytic RBC %/hypochromic RBC % ratio (M/H ratio).[52-55] A 2015 meta-analysis published by Hoffman and colleagues on the 12 most common discrimination indices in the literature found that results were variable among individual studies and populations, and their sensitivity in discriminating β-thalassemia minor and iron deficiency anemia ranged from 62% to 92%.[55] Similar results were found in other studies.[52-54] This leads to a high number of false negative results, thus the use of various discrimination indices in screening for β-thalassemia minor has limited value.[3,9,52-54]

▌ S U M M A R Y

- Thalassemias are a group of heterogeneous disorders in which one or more globin chains are reduced or absent.
- Thalassemias result in a hypochromic, microcytic anemia due to decreased production of hemoglobin. The imbalance of globin chain synthesis causes an excess of the normally produced globin chain that damages the RBCs or their precursors and results in premature hemolysis and ineffective erythropoiesis.
- β-thalassemia is caused by mutations that affect the β-globin gene complex. It is clinically manifested as a silent carrier state, β-thalassemia minor, β-thalassemia intermedia, and β-thalassemia major. Symptomatic thalassemia can also be

classified as transfusion-dependent thalassemia (TDT) or non-transfusion-dependent thalassemia (NTDT), which guides treatment decisions.
- In the silent carrier state (β^silent/β), the blood picture is completely normal. β-thalassemia minor or trait is a heterozygous state with one β-globin gene mutation and a slight reduction in β chain production and Hb A. It results in a mild, asymptomatic, microcytic, hypochromic anemia, usually characterized by an elevated Hb A₂ level, which aids in diagnosis.
- β-thalassemia major is a homozygous or compound heterozygous state with two β-globin gene mutations, resulting in a reduction or absence of β chain production and thus a

reduction in or absence of Hb A. It is a severe anemia characterized by α/β chain imbalance and precipitation of excess α chains in erythroid precursors, causing ineffective erythropoiesis. Patients are transfusion dependent for life. Severe iron overload develops due to repeated transfusions and increased iron absorption by intestinal enterocytes, requiring ongoing iron chelation therapy.

- β-thalassemia intermedia manifests abnormalities with a severity between those of β-thalassemia major and β-thalassemia minor. Patients are non-transfusion dependent but can develop iron overload due to increased iron absorption, requiring periodic iron chelation therapy.
- α-thalassemia is most commonly caused by a deletion of one, two, three, or all four of the α-globin genes, resulting in reduced or absent production of α chains. In the fetus, unpaired γ chains form γ_4 tetramers, called *Hb Bart*. In infancy through adulthood, unpaired β chains form β_4 tetramers, called *Hb H*. Both Hb Bart and Hb H have a high oxygen affinity and are unable to transport oxygen.
- α-thalassemia is divided clinically into a silent carrier state, α-thalassemia minor, Hb H disease, and Hb Bart hydrops fetalis syndrome.
- Silent carrier α-thalassemia is a result of the deletion (or, rarely, a non-deletional mutation) of one of four α-globin genes (–α/αα) or ($\alpha^T\alpha/\alpha\alpha$); it is associated with a normal RBC profile and is asymptomatic. α-thalassemia minor is a result of the deletion of two α-globin genes (–α/–α or – –/αα)

and is clinically similar to β-thalassemia minor except that Hb A_2 is not increased.

- Hb H disease is a result of the deletion of three of the four α-globin genes (– –/– α); Hb H inclusions (β_4 tetramers) precipitate in older circulating RBCs, causing a hemolytic anemia. The RBCs are microcytic and hypochromic, and the disease is clinically similar to β-thalassemia intermedia.
- In Hb Bart hydrops fetalis syndrome, all four of the α-globin genes are deleted (– –/– –). There is severe anemia, and fetal death usually occurs in utero or shortly after birth. The predominant hemoglobin in the fetus is Hb Bart (γ_4).
- The preliminary diagnosis of thalassemia is made from the complete blood count results and RBC morphology, iron studies, supravital staining, and hemoglobin fraction quantification by hemoglobin electrophoresis, high-performance liquid chromatography, and/or capillary zone electrophoresis. Molecular genetic testing is required for definitive diagnosis in prenatal testing, preconception risk assessment/carrier detection in couples, and identification of rare or complex mutations.
- Thalassemia trait must be differentiated from other microcytic, hypochromic anemias, especially iron deficiency anemia. Iron studies are important for this differentiation.

Now that you have completed this chapter, go back and read again the case study at the beginning and respond to the questions presented.

■ REVIEW QUESTIONS

Answers can be found in the Appendix.

1. Thalassemia is caused by:
   a. Structurally abnormal hemoglobins
   b. Absent or reduced synthesis of a polypeptide chain of hemoglobin
   c. Excessive absorption of iron
   d. Reduced or absent protoporphyrin synthesis
2. Thalassemia is more prevalent in individuals from areas along the tropics because it confers:
   a. Resistance to heat in heterozygotes with a thalassemia mutation
   b. Selective advantage against tuberculosis
   c. Resistance to severe malaria in heterozygotes with a thalassemia mutation
   d. Selected advantage against tick-borne illnesses
3. The hemolytic anemia and ineffective erythropoiesis associated with β-thalassemia is due to:
   a. A structurally abnormal hemoglobin
   b. Oxidation of hemoglobin to Heinz bodies
   c. Uncoupling of the RBC membrane from the cytoskeleton
   d. Precipitation of excess α chains in RBCs and their precursors
4. β-thalassemia minor (heterozygous) usually exhibits:
   a. Increased Hb H
   b. 10% to 35% Hb F
   c. No Hb A
   d. Increased Hb A_2

5. RBC morphologic features in β-thalassemia major usually include:
   a. Microcytes, hypochromia, target cells, RBC inclusions, NRBCs
   b. Macrocytes, acanthocytes, target cells, polychromasia, NRBCs
   c. Microcytes, hypochromia, target cells, sickle cells, elliptocytes
   d. Macrocytes, hypochromia, target cells, RBC inclusions, NRBCs
6. β-thalassemia major of the genotype β^0/β^0 can be differentiated from the β^+/β^+ genotype by the amount of:
   a. Hb A
   b. Hb A_2
   c. Hb F
   d. Hb H
7. Homozygotes for deletional-type HPFH are characterized by:
   a. 10% to 35% Hb F with normal RBC morphology
   b. 100% Hb F with slightly hypochromic, microcytic RBCs
   c. 1% Hb F with normal RBC morphology
   d. 5% to 15% Hb F with slightly hypochromic, microcytic RBCs
8. What abnormal hemoglobin is present in adults with α-thalassemia, genotype (– –/α –)?
   a. A_2
   b. F
   c. H
   d. Bart

9. Hb Bart is composed of:
   a. Two α and two β chains
   b. Two ε and two γ chains
   c. Four β chains
   d. Four γ chains

10. When one α gene is deleted (α–/αα), a patient has:
    a. Normal hemoglobin levels
    b. Mild anemia (hemoglobin range 9 to 11 g/dL)
    c. Moderate anemia (hemoglobin range 7 to 9 g/dL)
    d. Marked anemia requiring regular transfusions

11. In which part of the world is the α gene mutation causing Hb Bart hydrops fetalis (– –/– –) most common?
    a. Northern Africa
    b. Mediterranean
    c. Middle East
    d. Southeast Asia

12. A patient with a hemoglobin concentration of 8.0 g/dL and an MCV of 62 fL had microcytes, target cells, and a few sickle cells on his peripheral blood film. High-performance liquid chromatography showed 25% Hb A, 65% Hb S, 6% Hb A_2, and 4% Hb F. These results are most compatible with:
    a. Sickle cell trait
    b. Sickle cell anemia
    c. Hb S-β^0-thalassemia
    d. Hb S-β^+-thalassemia

13. Hb H inclusions in a supravital stain preparation appear as:
    a. A few large, blue, round bodies in the RBCs with aggregated reticulum
    b. Uniformly stained blue cytoplasm in the RBC
    c. Small, evenly distributed, greenish-blue granules that pit the surface of RBCs
    d. Uniform round bodies that adhere to the inner RBC membrane

14. Which of the following laboratory findings is *inconsistent* with β-thalassemia minor?
    a. A slightly elevated RBC count and marked microcytosis
    b. Target cells and basophilic stippling on the peripheral blood film
    c. Hemoglobin level of 10 to 13 g/dL
    d. Elevated MCHC and spherocytic RBCs

15. A 9-month-old infant of Asian heritage is seen for severe fatigue and pallor. Her hemoglobin concentration is 6.5 g/dL with an MCV of 59 fL; microcytosis, hypochromia, poikilocytosis, basophilic stippling, Howell Jolly bodies, Pappenheimer bodies, and nucleated RBCs are noted on the peripheral blood film. High-performance liquid chromatography showed 0% Hb A, 96% Hb F, and 4% Hb A_2. These findings should lead the physician to suspect:
    a. β-thalassemia major, β^0/β^0
    b. β-thalassemia major, β^+/β^+
    c. Severe iron deficiency anemia
    d. Homozygous α-thalassemia (– –/– –)

REFERENCES

1. Cooley, T. B., & Lee, P. (1925). A series of cases of splenomegaly in children with anemia and peculiar bone changes. *Trans Am Pediatr Soc, 37*, 29–33.
2. Whipple, G. H., & Bradford, W. L. (1932). Racial or familial anemia of children associated with fundamental disturbances of bone and pigment metabolism (Cooley-von Jaksch). *Am J Dis Child, 44*, 336–365.
3. Chapin, J., & Giardina, P. J. (2018). Thalassemia syndromes. In Hoffman, R., Benz, E. J., Silberstein, L. E., et al. (Eds.), *Hematology: Basic Principles and Practice*. (7th ed., pp. 546–570). Philadelphia: Elsevier.
4. Modell, B., & Darlison, M. (2008). Global epidemiology of haemoglobin disorders and derived service indicators. *Bull World Health Org, 86*, 480–487.
5. Goheen, M. M., Campino, S., & Cerami, C. (2017). The role of the red blood cell in host defense against falciparum malaria: an expanding repertoire of evolutionary alterations. *Br J Haematol, 179*, 543–556.
6. Taher, A., Vichinsky, E., Musallam, K., et al. (2013). *Guidelines for the Management of Non-Transfusion-Dependent Thalassaemia (NTDT)*. Nicosia, Cyprus: Thalassaemia International Federation.
7. Weatherall, D. J., & Clegg, J. B. (2001). Inherited haemoglobin disorders: an increasing global health problem. *Bull World Health Organ, 79*, 704–712.
8. Taylor, S. M., Parobek, C. M., & Fairhurst, R. M. (2012). Impact of haemoglobinopathies on the clinical epidemiology of malaria: a systematic review and meta-analysis. *Lancet Infect Dis, 12*, 457–468.
9. Borgna-Pignatti, C., & Galanello, R. (2014). Thalassemias and related disorders: quantitative disorders of hemoglobin synthesis. In Greer, J. P., Arber, D. A., Glader, B., et al. (Eds.), *Wintrobe's Clinical Hematology*. (13th ed., pp. 862–913). Philadelphia: Lippincott Williams & Wilkins.
10. Weatherall, D. J. (2016). The thalassemias: disorders of globin synthesis. In Kaushansky, K., Lichtman, M. A., Prchal, J. T., et al. (Eds.), *Williams Hematology*. (9th ed., pp. 725–758). New York: McGraw-Hill.
11. Patrinos, G. P., Giardine, B., Riemer, C., et al. (2004). Improvements in the HbVar database of human hemoglobin variants and thalassemia mutations for population and sequence variation studies. *Nucl Acids Res, 32*(Database issue), D537–541. http://globin.cse.psu.edu/hbvar/menu.html. Accessed April 18, 2018.
12. Camaschella, C., & Nai, A. (2016). Ineffective erythropoiesis and regulation of iron status in iron loading anaemias. *Br J Haematol, 172*, 512–523.
13. Ribeil, J.-A., Arlet, J.-B., Dussiot, M., et al. (2013). Ineffective erythropoiesis in β-thalassemia. *Sci World J, 394295*. doi:10.1155/2013/394295.
14. Cappellini, M. D., Cohen, A., Porter, J., et al. (2014). *Guidelines for the Management of Transfusion Dependent Thalassemia (TDT)*. 3rd ed. Nicosia, Cyprus: Thalassaemia International Federation.
15. Origa, R. Beta-thalassemia. 2000 Sep 28 [Updated 2018 Jan 25]. In: Adam, M. P., Ardinger, H. H., Pagon, R. A., et al., editors. *GeneReviews®* [Internet]. Seattle (WA): University of Washington, Seattle; 1993-2018. https://www.ncbi.nlm.nih.gov/books/NBK1426/. Accessed April 23, 2018.
16. Kautz, L., Jung, G., Du, X., et al. (2015). Erythroferrone contributes to hepcidin suppression and iron overload in a mouse model of β-thalassemia. *Blood, 126*, 2031–2037.
17. Kim, A., & Nemeth, E. (2015). New insights into iron regulation and erythropoiesis. *Curr Opin Hematol, 22*, 199–205.
18. Ganz, T., Jung, G., Naeim, A., et al. (2017). Immunoassay for human serum erythroferrone. *Blood, 130*, 1243–1246.

19. Musallam, K. M., Rivella, S., Vichinsky, E., et al. (2013). Non-transfusion-dependent thalassemias. *Haematologica, 98,* 833–844.

20. Basran, R. K., Reiss, U. M., Luo, H-Y., et al. (2008). β-Thalassemia intermedia due to compound heterozygosity for two β-globin gene promoter mutations, including a novel TATA box deletion. *Pediatr Blood Cancer, 50,* 363–366.

21. Gilman, J. G., Huisman, T. H., & Abels, J. (1984). Dutch beta 0-thalassaemia: a 10 kilobase DNA deletion associated with significant gamma-chain production. *Br J Haematol, 56,* 339–348.

22. Oggiano, L., Pirastu, M., Moi, P., et al. (1987). Molecular characterization of a normal Hb A$_2$ beta-thalassaemia determinant in a Sardinian family. *Br J Haematol, 67,* 225–229.

23. Cappellini, M. D., Porter, J. B., Viprakasit, V., et al. (2018). A paradigm shift on beta-thalassaemia treatment: how will we manage this old disease with new therapies? *Blood Rev, 32*(4), 300–311.

24. Marsella, M., & Borgna-Pignatti, C. (2014). Transfusional iron overload and iron chelation therapy in thalassemia major and sickle cell disease. *Hematol Oncol Clin North Am, 28,* 703–727.

25. Baronciani, D., Angelucci, E., Potschger, U., et al. (2016). Hemopoietic stem cell transplantation in thalassemia: a report from the European Society for Blood and Bone Marrow Transplantation Hemoglobinopathy Registry, 2000–2010. *Bone Marrow Transplant, 51,* 536–541.

26. Musallam, K. M., Taher, A. T., Cappellini, M. D., et al. (2013). Clinical experience with fetal hemoglobin induction therapy in patients with β-thalassemia. *Blood, 121,* 2199–2212.

27. Cavazzana-Calvo, M., Payen, E., Negre, O., et al. (2010). Transfusion independence and *HMGA2* activation after gene therapy of human β-thalassaemia. *Nature, 467,* 318–322.

28. Thompson, A. A., Walters, M. C., Kwiatkowski, J., et al. (2018). Gene therapy in patients with transfusion-dependent β-thalassemia. *N Engl J Med, 378,* 1479–1493.

29. Oron, V., Filon, D., Oppenheim, A., et al. (1994). Severe thalassaemia intermedia caused by interaction of homozygosity for alpha-globin gene triplication with heterozygosity for beta zero-thalassaemia. *Br J Haematol, 86,* 377–379.

30. Bollekens, J. A., & Forget, B. G. (1991). Delta beta thalassemia and hereditary persistence of fetal hemoglobin. *Hematol Oncol Clin North Am, 5,* 399–422.

31. Tuan, D., Feingold, E., Newman, M., et al. (1983). Different 3' end points of deletions causing delta beta-thalassemia and hereditary persistence of fetal hemoglobin: implications for the control of gamma-globin gene expression in man. *Proc Natl Acad Sci U S A, 80,* 6937–6941.

32. Stephens, A. D., Angastiniotis, M., Baysal, E., et al. (2012). ICSH recommendations for measurement of haemaglobin F. *Int J Lab Hematol, 34,* 14–20.

33. Chui, D. H. K., Fucharoen, S., Chan, V. (2003). Hemoglobin H disease: not necessarily a benign disorder. *Blood, 101,* 791–800.

34. Origa, R., & Moi, P. Alpha-Thalassemia. 2005 Nov 1 [Updated 2016 Dec 29]. In: Adam, M. P., Ardinger, H. H., Pagon, R. A., et al. (Eds.), *GeneReviews®* [Internet]. Seattle (WA): University of Washington, Seattle; 1993-2018. https://www.ncbi.nlm.nih.gov/books/NBK1435/. Accessed April 23, 2018.

35. Singsanan, S., Fucharoen, G., Savongsy, O., et al. (2007). Molecular characterization and origins of Hb Constant Spring and Hb Pakse in Southeast Asian populations. *Ann Hematol, 86,* 665–669.

36. Fucharoen, S., & Viprakasit, V. (2009). Hb H disease: clinical course and disease modifiers. *Am Soc Hematol Educ Program,* 26–34.

37. Wilkie, A. O., Zeitlin, H. C., Lindenbaum, R. H., et al. (1990). Clinical features and molecular analysis of the alpha thalassemia/mental retardation syndromes. II. Cases without detectable abnormality of the alpha globin complex. *Am J Hum Genet, 46,* 1127–1140.

38. Higgs, D. R. (2004). Gene regulation in hematopoiesis: new lessons from thalassemia. *Hematology Am Soc Hematol Educ Program,* 1–13.

39. Nelson, M. E., Thurmes, P. J., Hoyer, J. D., et al. (2005). A novel 5' ATRX mutation with splicing consequences in acquired α thalassemia-myelodysplastic syndrome. *Haematologica, 90,* 1463–1470.

40. Ko, T. M., Tseng, L. H., Hsu, P. M., et al. (1995). Ultrasonographic scanning of placental thickness and the prenatal diagnosis of homozygous alpha-thalassaemia 1 in the second trimester. *Prenat Diagn, 15,* 7–10.

41. Steinberg, M. H., Rosenstock, W., Coleman, M. B., et al. (1984). Effects of thalassemia and microcytosis on the hematologic and vasoocclusive severity of sickle cell anemia. *Blood, 63,* 1353–1360.

42. Quinn, C. T., Rogers, Z. R., & Buchanan, G. R. (2004). Survival of children with sickle cell disease. *Blood, 103,* 4023–4027.

43. Pan, L. L., Eng, H. L., Kuo, C. Y., et al. (2005). Usefulness of brilliant cresyl blue staining as an auxiliary method of screening for alpha-thalassemia. *J Lab Clin Med, 145,* 94–97.

44. Gallivan, M. V. E., & Giordano, P. C. (2012). Analysis of hemoglobinopathies, hemoglobin variants and thalassemias. In Kottke-Marchant, K., & Davis, B. H. (Eds.), *Laboratory Hematology Practice.* West Sussex, UK: Wiley-Blackwell.

45. Stephens, A. D., Angastiniotis, M., Baysal, E., et al. (2012). ICSH recommendations for the measurement of haemoglobin A$_2$. *Int J Lab Hematol, 34,* 1–13.

46. Giordano, P. C. (2013). Strategies for basic laboratory diagnostics of the hemoglobinopathies in multi-ethnic societies: interpretation of results and pitfalls. *Int J Lab Hematol, 35,* 465–479.

47. Keren, D. F., Hedstrom, D., Gulbranson, R., et al. (2008). Comparison of Sebia Capillarys capillary electrophoresis with the Primus high-pressure liquid chromatography in the evaluation of hemoglobinopathies. *Am J Clin Pathol, 130,* 824–831.

48. Sabath, D. E. (2017). Molecular diagnosis of thalassemias and hemogloniopathies. *Am J Clin Pathol, 148,* 6–15.

49. Wild, B. J., & Bain, B. J. (2004). Detection and quantitation of normal and variant haemoglobins: an analytic review. *Ann Clin Biochem, 41,* 355–369.

50. Mundee, Y., Bigelow, N. C., Davis, B. H., et al. (2000). Simplified flow cytometric method for fetal hemoglobin containing red blood cells. *Cytometry, 42,* 389–393.

51. Singh, S. P., & Gupta, S. C. (2008). Effectiveness of red cell osmotic fragility test with varying degrees of saline content in detection of beta-thalassemia trait. *Singapore Med J, 49,* 823–826.

52. Beyan, C., Kaptan, K., & Ifran, A. (2007). Predictive value of discrimination indices in differential diagnosis of iron deficiency anemia and beta-thalassemia trait. *Eur J Haematol, 78,* 524–526.

53. Ntaois, G., Chatzinikolaou, A., Saouli, Z., et al. (2007). Discrimination indices as screening tests for β-thalassemia trait. *Ann Hematol, 86,* 487–491.

54. Nalbantoglu, B., Guzel, S., Buyukyalcin, V., et al. (2012). Indices used in differentiation of thalassemia trait from iron deficiency anemia in pediatric population. Are they reliable? *Pediatr Hematol Oncol, 29,* 472–478.

55. Hoffmann, J. J. M. L., Urrechaga, E., & Aguirre, U. (2015). Discriminant indices for distinguishing thalassemia and iron deficiency in patients with microcytic anemia: a meta-analysis. *Clin Chem Lab Med, 53,* 1883–1894.

26

Nonmalignant Leukocyte Disorders

Steven Marionneaux*

OBJECTIVES

After the completion of this chapter, the reader will be able to:

1. Compare the genetic defects, pathologic mechanisms, and clinical and hematologic findings in primary immunodeficiency disorders.
2. Explain how Pelger-Huët cells might be confused with the presence of a neutrophilic left shift.
3. Discuss the peripheral blood film findings in Alder-Reilly anomaly and May-Hegglin anomaly and how these might be confused with morphologically similar conditions.
4. Describe the inherited enzyme deficiencies in the lysosomal storage diseases and associated clinical and laboratory findings.

5. Define *neutrophilia, neutropenia, lymphocytosis, lymphocytopenia, monocytosis, monocytopenia, eosinophilia, eosinopenia,* and *basophilia.*
6. List acquired conditions associated with changes in the number of circulating leukocyte subpopulations.
7. Compare in vivo and in vitro changes in leukocyte morphology with normal cells.
8. Outline the pathogenesis and clinical and laboratory features of infectious mononucleosis.

OUTLINE

Congenital Defects of Leukocyte Number and Function
  Severe Combined Immune Deficiency
  Wiskott-Aldrich Syndrome
  22q11 Syndromes
  Bruton Tyrosine Kinase Deficiency
  Chédiak-Higashi Syndrome
  Congenital Defects of Phagocytes
  Leukocyte Adhesion Disorders
  Defects of Respiratory Burst
  WHIM Syndrome
Morphologic Abnormalities of Leukocytes
  Pelger-Huët Anomaly
  Pseudo- or Acquired Pelger-Huët Anomaly
  Neutrophil Hypersegmentation
  Alder-Reilly Anomaly

  May-Hegglin Anomaly
  Lysosomal Storage Diseases
Quantitative Abnormalities of Leukocytes
  Neutrophils
  Eosinophils
  Basophils
  Monocytes
  Lymphocytes
Secondary Morphological Changes
  Neutrophils
  Eosinophils and Basophils
  Monocytes
  Lymphocytes
Infectious Mononucleosis

*The author extends appreciation to Anne Steine-Martin, whose work in prior editions provided the foundation for this chapter.

CASE STUDY

After studying the material in this chapter, the reader should be able to respond to the following case study:

A 25-year-old female was seen by her primary care physician complaining of fatigue. Physical exam revealed pale conjunctiva. The remainder of the exam was unremarkable. The patient admitted to experiencing heavier than normal bleeding during menses. CBC results:

WBC	8.1×10^9/L
Hemoglobin	8.6 g/dL
MCV	65 fL
MCHC	29 %
Platelets	172×10^9/L

Because of the low MCV, a blood film review was performed. There appeared to be immature granulocytes present, (eosinophils and basophils were normal) which required performing a manual differential:

Cell	%
Segmented neutrophils	9
Band neutrophils	21
Metamyelocytes	16
Myelocytes	14
Lymphocytes	30
Monocytes	7
Eosinophils	2
Basophils	1

1. Do you agree with the cell on top being classified as a myelocyte? If not, provide an explanation in morphologic terms.
2. The patient was subsequently diagnosed with iron deficiency anemia. If cells identified as band neutrophils and metamyelocytes appeared very much like

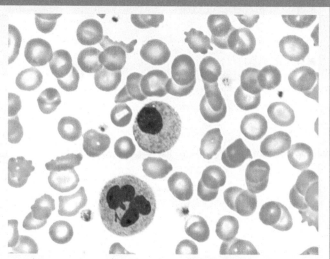

Figure 26.1 Peripheral Blood Film for the Patient in the Case Study. The cell on the top was classified as a myelocyte. The other immature neutrophils reported in the differential (not shown) appeared similar in morphology. The cell on the bottom was classified as a neutrophil. (Wright-Giemsa stain, X1000.) (Courtesy Nicholas Brehl, Indiana University, Indianapolis, IN.)

the cell depicted, except for some nuclear indentations, what other hematologic diagnosis is suspected?
3. Provide an approach to correcting the results of the WBC differential that does not require repeating the test.
4. What are clinical implications of reporting the manual differential results above if a left shift does not actually exist?

This chapter concentrates on leukocyte disorders that are not caused by clonal or neoplastic changes in hematopoietic precursor cells. The causes can be genetic or acquired and involve one or more lineages: neutrophil, lymphocyte, monocyte, eosinophil, and basophil, affecting the number of circulating cells, morphology, or both. Many of these disorders are associated with significant clinical manifestations, although some are benign in nature.

CONGENITAL DEFECTS OF LEUKOCYTE NUMBER AND FUNCTION

There are more than 350 primary immunodeficiency disorders, each caused by genetic abnormalities that disrupt normal function of innate or adaptive immune systems.[1] Cellular functions, number of cells or both are affected, and the resulting clinical manifestations are often severe and widespread. This chapter highlights some of the more common and well-known diseases with significant peripheral blood film abnormalities.

Severe combined immune deficiency (SCID) is a group of genetic immunodeficiencies affecting both cellular and humoral immunity. Almost all patients with SCID have a marked decrease in circulating T cells, poorly functioning B cells, hypogammaglobulinemia, and profound clinical manifestations. Left untreated, most patients die within the first two years of life. Two examples of SCID are γc deficiency and adenosine deaminase (ADA) deficiency.

Severe Combined Immune Deficiency

Gamma chain deficiency, or X-linked SCID, is the most common form of SCID and is caused by mutations in the *IL2RG* gene located at Xq13.1.[2] *IL2RG* normally codes for the common γ chain in leukocyte receptors that bind with interleukins 2, 4, 7, 9, 15 and 21. These interleukins normally provide growth, differentiation and survival signals for B, T and NK cells. These signals are disrupted becasue of altered leukocyte receptors in γc deficiency. Patients become symptomatic between 3 to 6 months of age as protective maternal immunoglobulins are depleted, presenting without tonsils or lymph nodes along with severe life-threatening recurring infections. Circulating T and natural killer (NK) lymphocytes are nearly absent. B cells are adequate in number but are dysfunctional. Children with γc deficiency fail to thrive and death usually occurs before age 2 unless treatment with hematopoietic stem cell transplant is successful.[3] Gene therapy has been effective in clinical trials; however, there is a significant risk of leukemic transformation.

Autosomal recessive adenosine deaminase ADA deficiency represents 10% to 20% of SCID cases and is caused by one of many mutations in the *ADA* gene located at chromosome 20q13.12.[4] Adenosine deaminase is a key component of the metabolic breakdown of adenosine triphosphate (ATP) and

RNA. ADA deficiency results in an intra- and extracellular accumulation of adenosine, which is lymphotoxic, leading to profound decreases in T, B, and NK cells. Patients experience a range of recurring, life-threatening bacterial, viral, and fungal infections beginning early in life. In addition, there are skeletal abnormalities, neurologic deficits, and skin rashes. As with X-linked SCID, stem cell transplant and gene therapy (experimental) are used to reconstitute the failed immune system.

Wiskott-Aldrich Syndrome

Wiskott-Aldrich syndrome (WAS), is classified as a combined immunodeficiency.[1] It is a rare X-linked disease caused by one of more than 400 mutations in the *WAS* gene, which results in decreased levels of WASp protein.[5] WASp is important in cytoskeletal remodeling and nuclear transcription in hematopoietic cells. T cells are decreased; B cells, T cells and NK cells, neutrophils and monocytes are dysfunctional which leads to bacterial, viral and fungal infections. There is a risk of bleeding due to thrombocytopenia and small abnormal platelets. Therapies using eltrombopag and romiplostim have been somewhat successful in increasing the platelet count in WAS hematopoietic stem cell transplant is potentially curative; however, up to 55% of transplanted patients develop significant autoimmune cytopenias.[5] Gene therapy has been successful in clinical trials, although there is a substantial risk for the development of acute leukemia.[6]

22q11 Syndromes

22q11 deletion syndromes, also classified as combined immunodeficiency, include DiGeorge syndrome, autosomal dominant Opitz GBBB, Sedlackova syndrome, Caylor cardiofacial syndrome, Shprintzen syndrome, and conotruncal anomaly face syndrome.[1,7] All the disorders within the 22q11 deletion syndrome have variable degrees of immunodeficiency because of the absence or decreased size of the thymus and low numbers of T lymphocytes. The underlying genetic abnormality is a microdeletion in chromosome band 22q11.2, most likely involving *TBX1* and occurs in approximately 1 in 3000 to 6000 births.[8] The 22q11 deletion is associated with a broad range of problems such as cardiac defects, palatal abnormalities, distinctive facial features, developmental delays, psychiatric disorders, short stature, kidney disease, and hypocalcemia. Hematologic issues include thrombocytopenia and large platelets, autoimmune cytopenias, and increased risk of malignancy. Patients are often treated with thymic tissue transplantation or fully matched peripheral blood T cell transplantation, however, the death rate is high and many succumb to the disease before 1 year of age.

Bruton Tyrosine Kinase Deficiency

Classified as an antibody deficiency, Bruton tyrosine kinase (BTK) deficiency (X-linked agammaglobulinemia) is a primary immunodeficiency disease characterized by reductions in all serum immunoglobulin isotypes and profoundly decreased or absent B cells.[1] BTK deficiency is caused by a mutation in the gene encoding Bruton tyrosine kinase, resulting in decreased production of BTK, which is important for B cell development,

differentiation, and signaling.[1,9] Without BTK, lymphocytes fail to fully mature, leading to severe hypogammaglobulinemia and an inability to produce specific antibodies. Infants with BTK deficiency display symptoms between 4 and 6 months, once maternal antibodies have cleared. Recurring life-threatening bacterial infections ensue. Risk of fungal and viral (except enterovirus) infection is low because of normal T cell function. Treatment consists of immunoglobulin replacement therapy.

Chédiak-Higashi Syndrome

Chédiak-Higashi syndrome is a rare autosomal recessive disease of immune dysregulation. Only 500 cases had been reported worldwide as of 2008.[10] Chédiak-Higashi syndrome is associated with a mutation in the *CHS1 LYST* gene on chromosome 1q42.1-2 that encodes for a protein that regulates the morphology and function of lysosome-related organelles.[10,11] Many types of cells in the body are affected and exhibit abnormally large lysosomes, which contain fused dysfunctional granules. Clinical manifestations begin in infancy with partial albinism and severe recurrent life-threatening bacterial infections. Hematologic findings in Chédiak-Higashi syndrome include giant lysosomal granules in granulocytes, monocytes, and lymphocytes (Figure 26.2). These fused granules result in leukocyte dysfunction. Patients often have bleeding issues as a result of abnormal dense granules in platelets. Death occurs before the age of 10 years.

Pseudo-Chédiak-Higashi granules are cytoplasmic inclusions that resemble the fused lysosomal granules in Chédiak-Higashi syndrome. Pseudo-Chédiak-Higashi granules have been reported in patients with acute myeloid leukemia, chronic myeloid leukemia, and myelodysplastic syndrome (MDS).[12-14]

Congenital Defects of Phagocytes

The congenital neutropenias (CNs) are a rare group of genetic diseases characterized by low neutrophil count, increased risk of infection, organ dysfunction, and a high rate of leukemic transformation.[15,16] CNs usually present in the first year of life as recurrent fevers caused by bacterial and fungal infections, which are often life threatening. Improvements in treatment, including antibiotic prophylaxis and use of granulocyte colony-stimulating factor (G-CSF), have decreased morbidity and mortality rates; however, higher doses of G-CSF have been associated with increased risk of malignant transformation.[17] Twenty-four genes have been identified as causing CN.[15] Some more common and better known CNs are described in Table 26.1

Leukocyte Adhesion Disorders (Defects of Motility)

As leukocytes leave circulation to move to a site of infection, they adhere to endothelial cells and the tissue matrix and roll along vessel walls. Selectins and other adhesion molecules expressed on endothelial cells and leukocytes mediate this process, interacting with ligands on the surface of leukocytes to slow the speed of the leukocytes in circulation.[18] Ligand binding induces high-affinity attachment of integrins with endothelial cell receptors. Leukocyte adhesion disorders (LADs) are rare autosomal recessive inherited conditions resulting in the inability of neutrophils and monocytes to move from circulation to

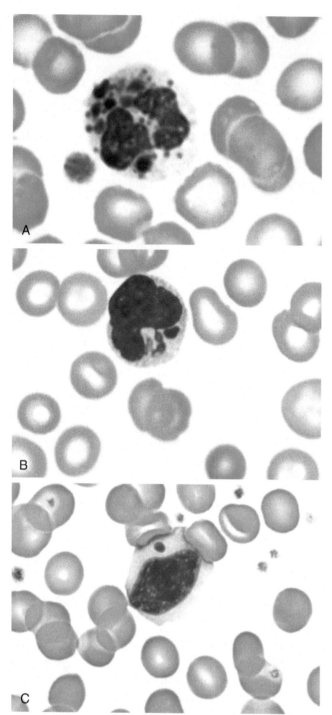

Figure 26.2 Cells from a Patient with Chédiak-Higashi Syndrome. (A), Neutrophil with large dark lysosomal granules. **(B),** Monocyte with large azure granules. **(C),** Lymphocyte with one large azure granule. (Peripheral blood, Wright-Giemsa stain, ×1000.)

the site of inflammation (called extravasation).Consequences of these disorders are recurrent severe bacterial and fungal infections. Hematopoietic stem cell transplant is the only curative treatment.

LAD I is caused by a mutation in *ITGB2,* the gene encoding the CD18 subunit of β_2 integrins, resulting in either a decreased or truncated form of the β_2 integrin, which is necessary for adhesion to endothelial cells, recognition of bacteria, and

outside-in signaling.[19,20] These activities are compromised in individuals with LAD 1. Shortly after birth, patients suffer from recurrent infections, often affecting skin and mucosal infections. Lymphadenopathy, splenomegaly, and neutrophilia are common findings. The clinical severity, including number of infections and survival, depends on the amount of β_2 integrins produced.[20] Infant mortality rate is high in LAD I.

LAD II presents in a similar manner as LAD 1, however leukocytes have normal β_2 integrins. There are molecular defects in *SLC35C1,* which codes for a fucose transporter that moves fucose from the endoplasmic reticulum to the Golgi region. Fucose is needed for posttranslational fucosylation of glycoconjugates, which are required for synthesis of selectin ligands.[21] In LAD II, selectin synthesis is compromised. Clinically, LAD II patients have recurring infections, neutrophilia, growth retardation, a coarse face, and other physical deformities. In LAD II the defective fucose transporter leads to an inability to produce functional selectins and defective leukocyte recruitment, which leads to recurring infections. Other clinical findings related to defective fucose transport are absence of blood group H antigen, growth retardation, and neurologic defects.[22]

LAD III is caused by mutations in *Kindlin-3.*[23] Kindlin-3 protein along with talin are required for activation of β integrin and leukocyte rolling. In LAD III, leukocytes and platelets have normal expression of integrins; however, there is failure in response to external signals that normally results in leukocyte activation. Clinically, LAD III patients experience a mild LAD I-like immunodeficiency with recurrent infections. Additionally, there is decreased platelet integrin GPIIbβ3 (glycoprotein IIb/IIIa), resulting in bleeding similar to that seen in Glanzmann thrombasthenia.

Like LAD, Shwachman-Diamond syndrome (SDS) is a defect in leukocyte motility. SDS is a rare autosomal recessive disease caused by mutations in the *SBDS* gene located at 7q11.22.[24] This affects the SBDS protein product which has an important role in ribosomal maturation, cell proliferation and bone marrow microenvironment.[25] Patients are usually diagnosed in infancy with exocrine pancreatic insufficiency associated malabsorption, malnutrition, chronic steatorrhea, and failure to thrive. There is bone marrow failure, including cytopenias, myelodysplasia, and an increased risk of acute leukemia. Patients also suffer from recurring infections, skeletal abnormalities, skin and dental problems, and cognitive issues. Hematopoietic stem cell transplant is an option for patients with bone marrow failure, myelodysplastic syndrome (MDS), and acute leukemia.

Defects of Respiratory Burst

Chronic granulomatous disease (CGD) is a rare condition caused by the decreased ability of neutrophils to undergo a respiratory burst after phagocytosis of foreign organisms. Approximately 60% of cases are X-linked recessive and 40% are autosomal recessive.[26] X-linked recessive patients experience a more severe disease course and have shorter lifespans than autosomal recessive patients. CGD is caused by mutations in genes responsible for proteins that make up the reduced form of nicotinamide adenine dinucleotide phosphate (NADPH)

TABLE 26.1 Congenital Neutropenias

Name	Gene	Gene Location	Inheritance	Hematologic/Clinical Features
Elastase deficiency	ELANE	19p13.3	Dominant	Severe/permanent neutropenia, bone marrow maturation arrest. Recurring infections. Risk for MDS/leukemia
Cyclic neutropenia (SCN1)	ELANE	19p13.3	Dominant	Neutropenia cycles every 21 days along with mouth ulcers, fevers, and bacterial infections
Kostmann disease (SCN3)	HAX1	1q21.3	Recessive	Cognitive and neurologic defects, recurring infections, seizures, risk for MDS/leukemia
X-linked neutropenia	WAS	Xp11.4-p11.21	X-linked	Severe/permanent neutropenia, maturation arrest, recurring infections, monocytopenia
Glycogen storage type Ib	SLC37A4	11q23.3	Recessive	Hypoglycemia, lactic acidosis, hyperlipidemia, hepatomegaly, increased risk of infection

MDS, Myelodysplastic syndrome.

oxidase. Under normal conditions, phagocytosis of foreign organism leads to phosphorylation and binding of cytosolic $p47_{phos}$ and $p67_{phos}$.[17] Primary granules containing antibacterial neutrophil elastase and cathepsin G and secondary granules containing the cytochrome complex $gp91_{phox}$ and $gp22_{phox}$ migrate to the phagolysosome. NADPH oxidase forms when $p47_{phos}$ and $p67_{phos}$ along with $p40_{phox}$ and RAC2 combine with the cytochrome complex. Superoxide is generated in the phagolysosome when an electron from NADPH is added to oxygen. NADPH has additional regulatory functions in the generation of other antimicrobial agents. Most cases of CGD are due to mutations in gp91phox or p47. The genes implicated in CGD and protein products are listed in Table 26.2.

CGD patients experience life-threatening catalase-positive bacterial and fungal infections. Advancements in care, including the routine use of prophylactic antibiotics and azole antifungals, have improved the clinical course of the disease and increased survival rates.[27,28] CGD is diagnosed through a test that uses a fluorescent probe dihydrorhodamine to measure intracellular production of reactive oxygen species.[26]

WHIM Syndrome

WHIM (warts, hypogammaglobulinemia, infections, and myelokathexis syndrome) is classified as a defect in intrinsic and innate immunity. WHIM results from mutations in the *CXCR4* gene located at 2q22.[29] Normal CXCR4 protein regulates movement of white blood cells between the bone marrow and peripheral blood. Neutrophils accumulate in the bone marrow (myelokathexis),

TABLE 26.2 Genes Involved in Chronic Granulomatous Disease

Inheritance	Gene	Location	Protein Product
XLR	CYBB	Xp21.1	$gp91^{phox}$
AR	CYBA	16q24	$p22^{phox}$
AR	NCF1	7q11.23	$P47^{phox}$
AR	NCF2	1q25	$p67^{phox}$
AR	NCF4	22q13.1	$P40^{phox}$

AR, Autosomal recessive; *XLR,* sex-linked recessive.

which results in low numbers of circulating neutrophils. The retained neutrophils in the marrow exhibit degenerative, pyknotic, morphologic changes. In addition to neutropenia, lymphopenia, monocytopenia, and hypogammaglobulinemia are present. As a result, patients experience recurrent bacterial infections and are highly susceptible to human papillomavirus (HPV) infection, which leads to warts, which can be widespread and resistant to treatment. Treatment consists of antibiotic prophylaxis, immunoglobulin replacement therapy, and G-CSF.[30] CXCR4 receptor antagonist is a targeted treatment proving to be effective at increasing neutrophil and lymphocyte counts.

MORPHOLOGIC ABNORMALITIES OF LEUKOCYTES WITHOUT ASSOCIATED IMMUNODEFICIENCY

Pelger-Huët Anomaly

Pelger-Huët anomaly (PHA), also known as true or congenital PHA, is an autosomal dominant disorder characterized by decreased nuclear segmentation and distinctive coarse chromatin clumping pattern. PHA potentially affects all leukocytes, although morphologic changes are most obvious in mature neutrophils.[31] The prevalence of PHA is approximately 1 in 4785 in the United States.[31] The disorder is a result of a mutation in the *lamin* β*-receptor* gene.[2] The lamin β receptor is an inner nuclear membrane protein that combines β-type lamins and heterochromatin and plays a major role in leukocyte nuclear shape changes that occur during normal maturation. Mutations in the *lamin* β*-receptor* gene result in the morphologic changes characteristic of PHA. Pelger-Huët (PH) nuclei may appear round, ovoid, or peanut shaped. Bilobed forms—the characteristic spectacle-like ("pince-nez") morphology with the nuclei attached by a thin filament can also be seen (Figure 26.3). Reports of patients with homozygous PHA are rare. Virtually all identified cases are heterozygotes, in which greater than 68% of neutrophils exhibit PH morphology.[32] Neutrophils in PHA appear to function normally.[33] In heterozygous PHS, individuals are clinically normal, while in homozygous PHS, cognitive impairment, heart defects, and skeletal abnormalities may occur.[31,24]

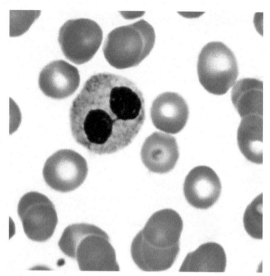

Figure 26.3 Pelger-Huët Cell. Pince-nez form with two rounded segments connected by a filament. Notice the dense chromatin pattern. (Peripheral blood, Wright-Giemsa stain, ×1000.)

Pseudo- or Acquired Pelger-Huët Anomaly

Neutrophils with similar morphology to PHA can be seen in patients with MDS, acute myeloid leukemia, and myeloproliferative neoplasm. Acquired or pseudo-PHA neutrophils are also associated with severe bacterial infections, HIV, tuberculosis, and mycoplasma pneumonia.[33] Drugs known to induce PHA morphology include immunosuppressants, chemotherapies, valproate, sulfisoxazole, fluconazole, ganciclovir, hematopoietic growth factors, and ibuprofen.[3,35]

Because nuclei of PHA neutrophils are round, oval, or peanut shaped, cells may be misclassified as myelocytes, metamyelocytes, or band neutrophils in the white blood cell (WBC) differential. This can lead to unnecessary tests, misdiagnosis, and inappropriate treatment. Because PHA neutrophils maintain normal function and their presence is not associated with inflammation, infection, or other causes of a neutrophilic left shift, it is recommended that PHA neutrophils be classified as segmented neutrophils with an appropriate interpretive comment.[36] There are morphologic differences between PHA neutrophils and normal neutrophils that can aid in differentiating between the two. Cell size is smaller, the nucleus/cytoplasm (N/C) ratio of PHA neutrophils is lower, and chromatin is darker, more coarse, and more densely clumped than band neutrophils, metamyelocytes, and myelocytes. Metamyelocytes and myelocytes generally show some degree of cytoplasmic basophilia, whereas PHA neutrophils exhibit nearly colorless cytoplasm except for that imparted by normal cytoplasmic granulation. Pseudo-PHA cells can exhibit hypogranularity in MDS.

Differentiating between true and pseudo-PHA can be challenging. It is important to consider the number of cells exhibiting characteristic morphology. In true PHA the number of affected cells is higher than in pseudo-PHA (>68% vs. <35%, respectively).[32,37] In true PHA, all WBC lineages can be affected in terms of nuclear shape and chromatin structure. In pseudo-PHA the phenomenon is restricted to neutrophils, except in MDS where monocytes, eosinophils, and basophils may be

affected. Furthermore, if true PHA is suspected, careful examination of peripheral blood films of family members may reveal characteristic morphology. Clinical correlation can also help to differentiate true and pseudo-PHA.

Neutrophil Hypersegmentation

Normal neutrophils contain three to five lobes that are separated by filaments. Hypersegmented neutrophils have more than five lobes and are most often associated with megaloblastic anemia, in which hypersegmented neutrophils are usually larger than normal (Figure 26.4). Hypersegmented neutrophils can also be seen in MDS where they represent a form of dysplasia. Less often hypersegmented neutrophils can be found in hereditary neutrophil hypersegmentation. In this disorder individuals are asymptomatic and have no signs of megaloblastic anemia.

Alder-Reilly Anomaly

Alder-Reilly anomaly (AR) is a rare inherited disorder characterized by granulocytes (monocytes and lymphocytes less often) with large, darkly staining metachromatic cytoplasmic granules (Figure 26.5). AR anomaly was initially reported in patients with gargoylism; however, it can be seen in otherwise healthy individuals.[38] The characteristic granulation, called Reilly bodies, is also found in the mucopolysaccharidoses (MPSs). The cytoplasmic granules contain partially digested mucopolysaccharides. Leukocyte function is not affected in AR. AR bodies in neutrophils may resemble heavy toxic granulation, however, Reilly bodies can also be present in monocytes and lymphocytes, whereas toxic granulation occurs only in neutrophils. Also, neutrophilia with left shift, Döhle bodies, or both often accompany toxic granulation. These are not associated with AR.

May-Hegglin Anomaly

May-Hegglin anomaly is a rare, autosomal dominant disorder characterized by variable thrombocytopenia, giant platelets, and

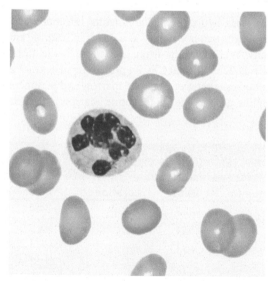

Figure 26.4 Hypersegmented Neutrophil. (Peripheral blood, Wright-Giemsa stain, ×1000.) (From Rodak, B. F., & Carr, J. H. [2017]. *Clinical Hematology Atlas.* [5th ed.]. St. Louis: Saunders.)

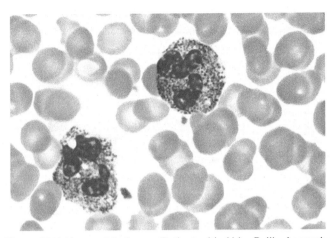

Figure 26.5 Neutrophils from a Patient with Alder-Reilly Anomaly. Note the dark granules present in both cells. Such granules may also be seen in eosinophils and basophils. (Peripheral blood, Wright-Giemsa stain, ×1000.) (Courtesy Dennis R. O'Malley, US Labs, Irvine, CA.)

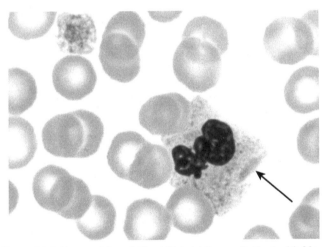

Figure 26.6 Neutrophil and Giant Platelet from a Patient with May-Hegglin Anomaly. Note the large, elongated, bluish inclusion in the neutrophil cytoplasm. (Peripheral blood, Wright-Giemsa stain, ×1000.)

large Döhle body-like inclusions in neutrophils, eosinophils, basophils, and monocytes (Figure 26.6). May-Hegglin anomaly is caused by a mutation in the *MYH9* gene on chromosome 22q12-13.[39] There is disordered production of myosin heavy chain type IIA, which affects megakaryocyte maturation and platelet fragmentation when shedding from megakaryoytes

The basophilic Döhle body-like leukocyte inclusions in May-Hegglin anomaly are composed of precipitated myosin heavy chains. True Döhle bodies consist of lamellar rows of rough endoplasmic reticulum. Most individuals with May-Hegglin anomaly are asymptomatic, but a few have mild bleeding tendencies related to the degree of thrombocytopenia.

Lysosomal Storage Diseases

Lysosomal storage disorders (LSDs) are a group of more than 50 inherited enzyme deficiencies resulting from mutations in genes that code for the production of lysosomal enzymes.[40] The result is flawed degradation of phagocytized material and buildup of undigested substrates within lysosomes. This causes cell dysfunction, cell death, and a range of clinical symptoms. All cells containing lysosomes can be affected. LSDs are classified according to the underdegraded macromolecule that accumulates in the cell. The categories include sphingolipidoses, oligosaccharidoses, mucolipidoses, mucopolysaccharidoses (MPS), lipoprotein storage disorders, and lysosomal transport defects. More common LSDs are presented.

Mucopolysaccharidoses

The MPS are a family of inherited disorders of mucopolysaccharide or glycoaminoglycan (GAG) degradation. Each MPS is caused by deficient activity of an enzyme necessary for the degradation of dermatan sulfate, heparan sulfate, keratan sulfate, and/or chondroitin sulfate. The partially degraded material builds up in lysosomes and results in serious physical and cognitive problems and shortened survival. Table 26.3 provides genetic and clinical information about MPS subtypes along with the deficient enzymes and accumulated substrates.

The peripheral blood of a patient with MPS may show metachromatic Reilly bodies in neutrophils, monocytes, and lymphocytes. Macrophages in the bone marrow can also demonstrate cytoplasmic metachromatic material. Diagnosis relies on assays that measure the specific enzymes involved. MPS treatment consists of enzyme replacement therapy or hematopoietic stem cell transplantation (Hurler patients only). Emerging therapies include additional enzyme replacement therapies, improved antiinflammatories, gene therapy, nanoparticles, and substrate reduction therapy.[41]

The sphingolipidoses are inherited disorders in which lipid catabolism is defective (Figure 26.7). Two of these disorders, Gaucher and Neimann-Pick diseases are characterized by macrophages with distinctive morphology.

Gaucher Disease

Gaucher disease is the most common of the lysosomal lipid storage diseases. It is an autosomal recessive disorder caused by a defect or deficiency in the catabolic enzyme β-glucocerebrosidase (gene located at *1q21-q22*), which is necessary for glycolipid metabolism. As a result, there is an accumulation of unmetabolized substrate sphingolipid glucocerebroside in macrophages throughout the body, including osteoclasts in bone and microglia in the brain. At least 1 in 17 Ashkenazi Jews are carriers.[42] More than 400 genetic mutations have been reported, and although some correlations have been found with specific mutations and disease severity and course, most cases (phenotypes) cannot be predicted by genotype.[43]

There are three types of Gaucher disease and type I is by far the most common. Neurologic symptoms are key factors to differentiate the subtypes. The phenotype is quite heterogeneous, with some patients being asymptomatic, whereas others experience a multitude of clinical problems. Demographic and clinical information associated with the three types of Gaucher disease are provided in Table 26.4.

Bone marrow replacement by Gaucher cells contribute to anemia and thrombocytopenia, which are common findings in these patients. Gaucher cells are distinctive macrophages, single

TABLE 26.3   Mucopolysaccharidoses Disorders

Name	Subtype	Enzyme Deficiency	AS	Genetics	Clinical Features
MPS I	Hurler syndrome	α-l-iduronidase	DS + HS	*IDUA* 4p16.3	Coarse facies, short stature, corneal clouding, joint stiffening, umbilical hernia, dysostosis multiplex, hepatosplenomegaly, frequent upper respiratory infections, cognitive impairment; death before 10 y
MPS I	Scheie syndrome	α-l-iduronidase	DS + HS	*IDUA* 4p16.3	Hepatomegaly, joint contractures, cardiac valve abnormalities, corneal clouding; prolonged survival but with disability
MPS II	Hunter syndrome	Iduronate sulfatase	DS + HS	*IDS* Xq28	Coarse facial features, short stature, skeletal deformities, joint stiffness, mental retardation
MPS III A	Sanfilippo syndrome	Heparan *N*-sulfatase	HS	*SGSH* 17q25.3	Hirsutism, coarse facial features, behavioral problems, aggressive behavior, speech delay, hepatomegaly; most die before 20 y
MPS III B	Sanfilippo syndrome	α-*N*-acetylglucosaminidase	HS	*NAGLU* 17q21.2	Cardiomegaly, coarse facial features, progressive dementia, convulsions, survive into 20s, 30s
MPS III C	Sanfilippo syndrome	Heparan acetyl-CoA: α-glucosaminidase *N*-acetyltransferase	HS	*HGSNAT* 8p11.21	Delayed psychomotor development, behavioral problems, sleeping/hearing problems, coarse facial features, recurrent infection, diarrhea, epilepsy, and retinitis pigmentosa
MPS IV A	Morquio syndrome	Galactose-6-sulfatase	KS + CS	*GALNS* 16q24.3	Musculoskeletal abnormalities, short stature, pulmonary and cardiac dysfunction, hearing loss corneal clouding; most die before 30 y
MPS IV B	Morquio syndrome	β-Galactosidase	KS	*GLB1* 3p22.3	Musculoskeletal abnormalities, short stature, pulmonary and cardiac dysfunction, hearing loss corneal clouding; most die before 30 y

AS, accumulated substrate; *CS*, Chondroitin-6-sulfate; *DS*, dermatan sulfate; *HS*, heparin sulfate; *KS*, keratan sulfate.
Adapted from Wraith, J. E., & Jones, S. (2014). Mucopolysaccharidosis type I. *Pediatr Endocrinol Rev, 12*(1), 102–106; Francisca, M., Coutinho, L., & Alves, S. (2015). From bedside to cell biology: A century of history on lysosomal dysfunction. *Gene, 555*(1), 50–58; Meyer, A., Kossow, K., Gal, A., et al. (2007). Scoring evaluation of the natural course of mucopolysaccharidosis type IIIA (Sanfilippo syndrome type A). *Pediatrics, 120*(5), 1255–1261; and Morrone, A., Caciotti, A., Atwood, R., et al. (2014). Morquio A syndrome-associated mutations: A review of alterations in the GALNS gene and a new locus-specific database. *Human Mutation, 35*(11), 1271–1279.

or in clusters, exhibiting abundant fibrillar blue-gray cytoplasm with a striated or wrinkled appearance (sometimes described as onion skin-like) (Figure 26.8). Gaucher cells stain positive with trichrome, aldehyde fuchsin, periodic acid-Schiff (PAS) and acid phosphatase.[40] A commercially available test for β-glucosidase (glucocerebrosidase) is available to confirm diagnosis. Genetic testing is sometimes used in Ashkenazi Jews to screen for the most common mutations, including N370S, 84GG, IVS2 + 1G> A, and L444P.[40] In all three forms of Gaucher disease, there is a fifteenfold increase for developing hematologic malignancies such as plasma cell neoplasm, chronic lymphocytic leukemia, non-Hodgkin lymphoma, and acute leukemia.[44]

Treatment of Gaucher disease includes enzyme replacement therapy with recombinant glucocerebrosidase. Agents are also available to reduce glucocerebroside. Allogeneic stem cell transplantation offers the potential for cure; however, treatment-related mortality rate is high and no studies have determined the safety or efficacy of transplant compared with standard of care therapies.[45] Pseudo-Gaucher cells can be found in bone marrow of some patients with thalassemia,[46] chronic myeloid leukemia,[47] acute lymphoblastic leukemia,[48] non-Hodgkin lymphoma,[49] and plasma cell neoplasms.[50,51] In these diseases, pseudo-Gaucher cells most likely form as a result of excessive cell turnover, which overwhelms the glucocerebrosidase enzyme, rather than a true decrease in the enzyme. Electron microscopy shows that pseudo-Gaucher cells do not contain the tubular inclusions described in Gaucher cells.

Niemann-Pick Disease

Niemann-Pick disease (NP) is characterized by an accumulation of fat in cellular lysosomes of vital organs, which impairs their function, leading to a range of clinical findings. NP has three subtypes. Types A and B are caused by recessive mutations in the *SMPD1* gene located within the chromosomal region 11p15.4. This results in a deficiency of lysosomal hydrolase enzyme acid sphingomyelinase (ASM) and a subsequent buildup of the substrate sphingomyelin in the liver, spleen, and lungs.[40] More than 180 mutations in *SMPD1* have been reported.[40] Foam cells and sea-blue histiocytes can be seen in the bone marrow. Foam cells are macrophages with cytoplasm packed with lipid-filled lysosomes that appear as small vacuoles (foam) after staining (Figure 26.9). Sea blue histiocytes are macrophages with lipofuscin-, glycophospholipid-, and sphingomyelin contained in -cytoplasmic granules, 1 to 3 μ in diameter, that appear blue with Wright stain. Type A (acute neuronopathic form) NP mostly affects Eastern European Jews. Type A presents in infancy and is associated with failure to thrive, lymphadenopathy, hepatosplenomegaly, vision problems, and rapid neurodegenerative decline that results in death, usually by 4 years of age. In type A, there is less than 5% of normal sphingomyelinase activity. In type B (the non-neuronopathic form) there is approximately 10%

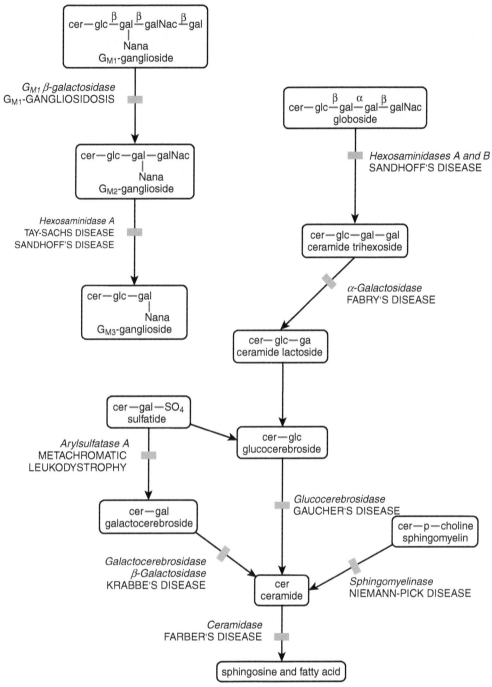

Figure 26.7 Pathways and Diseases of Sphingolipid Metabolism. (From Orkin, S. H., Fisher, D. E., & Look, A. T., et al. [2009]. *Nathan and Oski's hematology of infancy and childhood.* [7th ed.]. Philadelphia: Saunders.)

TABLE 26.4	Clinical Subtypes of Gaucher Disease		
	Type I: Non-Neuronopathic	**Type II: Acute Neuronopathic**	**Type III: Subacute Neuronopathic**
Age at presentation	Childhood/adulthood	Infancy	Childhood/adulthood
Hepatosplenomegaly	$+ \rightarrow +++$	$+$	$+ \rightarrow +++$
Skeletal abnormality	$- \rightarrow +++$	$-$	$++ \rightarrow +++$
CNS disease	$-$	$+++$	$+ \rightarrow +++$
Life span	6–80 + years	<2 years	2–60 years
Ethnicity	Ashkenazi Jews	Panethnic	Panethnic, Swedes

CNS, Central nervous system.
Note: Absence and severity of features are indicated by − to +++.

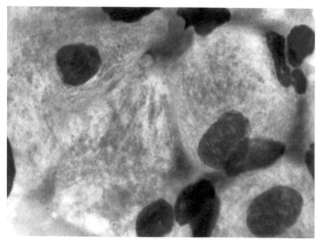

Figure 26.8 Characteristic Macrophages in Patient with Gaucher Disease. Note cytoplasmic striations in the cytoplasm. (Bone marrow, hematoxylin and eosin stain, ×1000.) (From Rodak, B. F., & Carr, J. H. [2013]. *Clinical Hematology Atlas.* [4th ed.]. St. Louis: Saunders.)

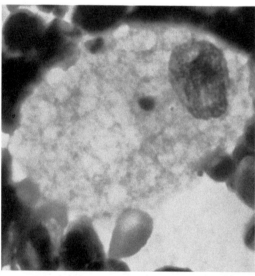

Figure 26.9 Niemann-Pick Cell. Note eccentric nucleus and bubble-like pattern of storage deposit in the cytoplasm. (Bone marrow, hematoxylin and eosin stain, ×1000.) (From Rodak, B. F., & Carr, J. H. [2017]. *Clinical Hematology Atlas.* [5th ed.]. St. Louis: Saunders.)

to 20% normal enzyme activity.[52] Type B NP is more common in individuals of Northern African descent and presents in the first decade to adulthood with a variable clinical course. Although there is no neurocognitive impairment, patients experience massive hepatosplenomegaly, heart disease, and pulmonary insufficiency.[53] Diagnosis of types A and B NP is based on enzymatic quantitation of sphingomyelinase activity in cell or tissue extracts. Genetic testing screens for three genes responsible for more than 90% of cases in the Ashkenazi Jewish population and one gene in approximately 90% of type B patients from North Africa.[40,53] Treatment primarily consists of enzyme replacement therapy, although it is ineffective at slowing the progression of neurologic disease in type A patients.

Type C NP is an autosomal recessive lipidosis in which mutations in *NPC1* or *NP2* gene (95% and 5% of cases, respectively) causes impaired cellular trafficking and homeostasis of cholesterol.[54] The result is buildup of unesterified cholesterol in lysosomes. The clinical presentation in type C NP is heterogeneous

with regard to age of onset and type and severity of neurologic and psychiatric symptoms, as well as visceral involvement.[40,54] Early diagnosis is important because substrate reduction therapy can slow the progression of neurologic damage[55]; however, because of its heterogeneous presentation, diagnosis is often challenging. A suspicion index tool for type C disease has been found to be highly sensitive and specific for arriving at a presumptive diagnosis.[56] Confirmation is obtained through genetic testing or biochemical staining of cultured fibroblasts with filipin to demonstrate unesterified cholesterol in cellular vesicles. Therapy focuses on symptom relief. The prognosis in type C NP is poor, with most patients dying before the age of 25 years.[57]

QUANTITATIVE ABNORMALITIES OF LEUKOCYTES

Neutrophils

Normal relative neutrophil count in adults, bands plus segmented forms, is approximately 50% to 70%. Normal absolute neutrophil count (ANC) is approximately 2 to 7.7×10^9/L. In patients with a neutrophilic left shift (presence of immature cells in the myelocytic cell line), some clinicians prefer to include metamyelocytes and myelocytes in addition to band and segmented forms when calculating the ANC.

Neutrophilia

An absolute increase in neutrophils greater than 7.0×10^9/L in adults or 8.5×10^9/L in children is called neutrophilia. Neutrophilia can occur as a result of catecholamine-induced shift in neutrophils from the marginal pool (cells normally adhering to vessel walls) to the circulating pool. More often, neutrophilia occurs when there is an increase in bone marrow production of the neutrophil series or there is a transfer of neutrophils from the bone marrow storage pool to the circulating pool. Neutrophilia is often accompanied by a left shift. Box 26.1 lists conditions and drugs associated with neutrophilia.

The term *leukemoid reaction* refers to a reactive neutrophilic leukocytosis greater than 50×10^9/L with a shift to the left. Leukemoid reactions are usually caused by acute and chronic infections, metabolic disease, or inflammation or occur as part of an inflammatory response to malignancy. When there is a suspected leukemoid reaction, chronic myelogenous (myeloid) leukemia should be ruled out. Distinguishing features between the two are listed in Table 26.5.

The term *leukoerythroblastic reaction* refers to the simultaneous presence of immature neutrophils, nucleated red blood cells, and teardrop red blood cells (RBCs). A leukoerythroblastic reaction is sometimes accompanied by neutrophilia. A leukoerythroblastic reaction suggests either (1) a space-occupying lesion in the bone marrow such as metastatic tumor, fibrosis, lymphoma, or leukemia, or a marked increase in one of the normal marrow cells (e.g., erythroid hyperplasia seen in hemolytic anemia); or (2) primary myelofibrosis.

Neutropenia

Neutropenia is defined as a decrease in the ANC to less than 2.0×10^9/L in white adults or 1.3×10^9/L in black adults. The risk of infection increases as the ANC falls to less than 1.0×10^9/L. Severe

BOX 26.1 Causes of Neutrophilia

- Emotional stress
- Strenuous exercise
- Trauma/injury
- Pregnancy: labor and delivery
- Eclampsia
- Surgery
- Infections: bacterial, some viral
- Burns
- Myocardial infarction
- Pancreatitis
- Vasculitis
- Colitis
- Autoimmune disease
- Acute hemorrhage
- Chronic blood loss
- Hemolysis
- Smoking
- Chronic blood loss
- Metabolic ketoacidosis
- Uremia
- Leukocyte adhesion deficiency
- Familial cold urticaria
- Hereditary neutrophilia
- Leukemia
- Chronic myeloproliferative neoplasm
- Steroids
- Lithium
- Colony-stimulating factors (granulocyte CSF)
- Cortisol
- Epinephrine

Adapted from Dale, D. C., & Welte, K. (2016). Neutropenia and neutrophilia. In: Kaushansky, K., Lichtman, M. A., Prchal, J. T., et al. (Eds.), *Williams Hematology.* (9th ed., pp. 991–1004). New York: McGraw-Hill; and Reichard, K. (2010). Non-neoplastic granulocytic and monocytic disorders, excluding neutropenia. In Foucar, K., Reichard, K., & Czuchlewski, D. (Eds.), *Bone Marrow Pathology.* (3rd ed., Vol 1, pp. 180–205). Chicago: American Society for Clinical Pathology Press.

TABLE 26.5 Distinguishing Features between Leukemoid Reaction and Chronic Myeloid Leukemia

	Leukemoid Reaction	Chronic Myeloid Leukemia
Eosinophils & basophils	Normal count and morphology	Often elevated; may show mixed granulation
Neutrophil morphology	Toxic granulation and Döhle bodies often	May see pseudo-Pelger-Huët forms
Platelet count	Normal	Elevated early; decreased late
Platelet morphology	Normal	Possible giant, hypogranular, and/or bizarre forms
Hemoglobin	Normal	Often anemic
LAP score	Elevated	Decreased
Genetics	Normal	Positive for t(9;22); *BCR-ABL*

LAP, Leukocyte alkaline phosphatase.

neutropenia ($<0.5 \times 10^9$/L) further increases the risk. *Agranulocytosis* refers to a neutrophil count of less than 0.1×10^9/L. Some causes of neutropenia are (1) increased rate of removal or destruction of peripheral blood neutrophils ; (2) fewer neutrophils released from the bone marrow to the blood because of decreased production or ineffective hematopoiesis, where neutrophils are present in the bone marrow but not released into circulation because they are defective; (3) decreased ratio of circulating versus marginal pool of neutrophils; or (4) a combination of these.

Acquired Neutropenia

Acquired forms of neutropenia include are much more common than congenital syndromes. Box 26.2 provides a list of acquired causes of neutropenia.

BOX 26.2 Causes of Acquired Neutropenia

Drugs
- Anticancer
- Analgesics/antiinflammatories: acetaminophen, aspirin, diclofenac, ibuprofen, indomethacin, linezolid, naproxen, sulfasalazine
- Antibiotics: β-lactams, cephalosporins, chloramphenicol, clindamycin, gentamicin, penicillin, sulfonamides, trimethoprim-sulfamethoxazole, tetracycline, vancomycin
- Antivirals: acyclovir, ganciclovir, abacavir, zidovudine
- Antifungals: terbinafine, Amphotericin B
- Anticonvulsants: carbamazepine, phenytoin, valproate
- Antihistamines: brompheniramine, chlorphenamine, cimetidine, famotidine, ranitidine
- Antimalarials: chloroquine, dapsone, quinine
- Antithyroids: propylthiouracil, methimazole, carbimazole
- Cardiovascular: amiodarone, captopril, clopidogrel, flecainide, furosemide, methyldopa, procainamide, propranolol, quinidine, spironolactone, thiazide diuretics, ticlopidine
- Antianxiety/hypnotics: benzodiazepines, meprobamate
- Psychotropics: amitriptyline, amoxapine, clozapine, doxepin, olanzapine, phenothiazines, risperidone
- Hypoglycemics: chlorpropamide, tolbutamide
- Phenothiazines: chlorpromazine, phenothiazines

Other
- Levamisole (adulterated cocaine)
- Immunologic
- Radiation
- Toxins
- Overwhelming infections
- Splenomegaly
- Hemodialysis
- Aplastic anemia
- Copper deficiency
- Alcoholism
- Tumor metastasis to bone marrow/space-occupying lesion
- Hematologic malignancy
  - Myelodysplastic syndrome
  - Large granular lymphocyte syndrome
  - Leukemia
  - Plasma cell neoplasm

Adapted from Andres, E., & Maloisel, F. (2008). Idiosyncratic drug-induced agranulocytosis or acute neutropenia. *Curr Opin Hematol, 15*(1), 15–21; Andrès, E., & Mourot-Cottet, R. (2017). Non-chemotherapy drug-induced neutropenia—an update. *Exp Opin Drug Saf, 16*(11), 1235–1242; Gibson, C., & Berliner, N. (2014). How we evaluate and treat neutropenia in adults. *Blood, 124*(8), 1251–1258; and Pick, A. M., & Nystrom, K. K. (2014). Nonchemotherapy drug-induced neutropenia and agranulocytosis: could medications be the culprit? *J Pharm Pract, 27*(5), 447–452.

Drug-induced neutropenia. Medications are the most common causes of acquired neutropenia. Neutropenia has been associated with almost all classes of drugs and is a result of myeloid suppression or immunologic response. Many agents used to treat cancer are known to induce neutropenia, including traditional myelosuppressive chemotherapeutics, targeted therapies, and immunotherapies. Nonchemotherapy drug-induced neutropenia and agranulocytosis most often present as idiosyncratic reactions. The annual rate of occurrence of drug-induced agranulocytosis is 2.3 to 15.4 cases per million in the United States.[58] The mortality rate is 10% to 16%.[58]

Immune neutropenia. In neonatal alloimmune neutropenia (NAN), maternal immunoglobulin G (IgG) crosses the placenta and binds to paternal human neutrophil antigens (HNA) found on fetal leukocytes. Antibody-coated neutrophils are removed from circulation by the reticuloendothelial system, resulting in an ANC of less than 0.5×10^9/L. Of the nine HNA located on Fcγ-receptor IIIb (FcγRIIIb), HNA-1a, -1b, -1c, -1d, and -2 are most often implicated in NAN.[59,60] The incidence of NAN is not well defined; it varies from .02% to 0.8% of live births.[61-63] Resulting infections are most often not life threatening, and neutropenia resolves within 6 months after clearance of material IgG.

Autoimmune neutropenia (AIN) is associated with IgG autoantibodies against one or more HNA. Primary AIN usually presents around 7 to 9 months of age.[64] The disease tends to be self-limiting, and 90% of patients spontaneously recover by 2 years of age.[64,65] Secondary AIN is more common in adults and is associated with connective tissue disorders, Felty syndrome, hematologic neoplasms, solid tumors, primary immunodeficiencies, bacterial and viral infections, and posttransplantation complications and as idiosyncratic reactions to a number of medications.[64,66] Immunologic mechanisms involved in drug-induced neutropenia include formation of immune complexes, haptens, drug-induced formation of neutrophil autoantibodies, and T-lymphocyte toxicity.[66]

Eosinophils

Several factors influence the number of eosinophils in circulation: bone marrow proliferation rate and release into the bloodstream, movement from the blood into extravascular tissues, and cell survival and destruction after eosinophils have moved into the tissues.

Eosinophilia

Eosinophilia is defined as an absolute eosinophil count greater than 0.4×10^9/L. A major function of eosinophils is degranulation, where substances are released that damage an offending organism (i.e., parasites) or target cell. Nonmalignant causes of eosinophilia are generally a result of cytokine stimulation, especially from interleukin-3 and interleukin-5 (IL-3 and IL-5).[67,68] Eosinophilia is associated with parasitic infections, especially helminths. It is also associated with allergic reactions, including asthma, rhinitis, urticaria, and atopic dermatitis; scabies infestation, scarlet fever, HIV, primary biliary cirrhosis, hepatitis, autoimmune disorders, drug reactions, and some hematologic neoplasms.[68-70]

Eosinopenia is defined as an absolute eosinophil count of less than 0.09×10^9/L and can be difficult to detect because the reference interval is low. Eosinopenia often accompanies other cytopenias in conditions that result in marrow hypoplasia, specifically involving leukocytes. Eosinopenia has been reported in autoimmune disorders, steroid therapy, stress, sepsis, and acute inflammatory states.[71,72]

Basophils

Basophilia is defined as an absolute basophil count greater than 0.15×10^9/L and is associated with chronic myeloid leukemia, allergic rhinitis, hypersensitivity to drugs or food, chronic infections, hypothyroidism, chronic inflammatory conditions, radiation therapy, and bee stings.[73,74]

Monocytes

Monocytosis is defined as an absolute monocyte count greater than 1.0×10^9/L in adults and greater than 3.5×10^9/L in neonates. Monocytosis is associated with numerous conditions because of their role in acute and chronic inflammation and infections, immunologic conditions, hypersensitivity reactions, and tissue repair. Monocytosis is often the first sign of recovery after myelosuppression. It is also seen in congenital cyclic neutropenia, where monocytosis occurs during periods of neutropenia in the 21-day cycle. A list of conditions associated with monocytosis is provided in Box 26.3.

Monocytopenia, defined as an absolute monocyte count of less than 0.2×10^9/L, is very rare in conditions that do not

---

BOX 26.3 Conditions Associated With Monocytosis

- Infection
  - Tuberculosis
  - Brucellosis
  - Leishmaniasis
  - Fungal
  - Subacute bacterial endocarditis
  - Malaria
- Recovery from acute infection
- Recovery from myelosuppression
- Immunologic/autoimmune
  - Systemic lupus erythematosus
  - Rheumatoid arthritis
  - Autoimmune neutropenia
  - Inflammatory bowel disease
  - Myositis
  - Sarcoidosis
- Cyclic neutropenia
- Postsplenectomy
- Drugs
  - Colony-stimulating factors
  - Olanzapine
- Malignancy
  - Hodgkin disease
  - Myelodysplastic/myeloproliferative neoplasms
  - Myelodysplastic syndromes
  - Acute myeloid leukemia involving the monocyte lineage

Adapted from Lynch, D. T., & Foucar, K. F. (2016). Ask the hematopathologists: diagnostic approach to monocytosis. *Hematologist*, *13*(4), 4; Robinson, R. L., Burk, M. S., & Raman, S. (2003). Fever, delirium, autonomic instability, and monocytosis associated with olanzapine. *J Postgrad Med*, *49*(1), 96; and Tsolia, M., Drakonaki, S., Messaritaki, A., et al. (2002). Clinical features, complications and treatment outcome of childhood brucellosis in central Greece. *J Infect*, *44*(4), 257–262.

also involve cytopenias of other lineages, such as aplastic anemia or chemotherapy-induced cytopenias. Monocytopenia has been found in patients receiving steroid therapy[75] or hemodialysis and in sepsis.[76] Viral infections, especially those caused by the Epstein-Barr virus (EBV), can also cause monocytopenia.[77] Profound monocytopenia is associated with hairy cell leukemia.[78]

Lymphocytes

Identification of lymphocytosis varies with the age of the individual. Children between 2 weeks and 8 to 10 years of age have higher absolute lymphocyte counts than adults. In adults, lymphocytes represent 20% to 40% of circulating leukocytes. Lymphocytosis in children is defined as an absolute lymphocyte count greater than 10.0×10^9/L, whereas in adults it is defined as a count greater than 5.0×10^9/L. Newborns have lymphocyte counts similar to those of adults.

Lymphocytosis is usually accompanied by changes in lymphocyte morphology. See Table 26.6 for a list of disorders associated with reactive lymphocytosis.

Lymphocytopenia in children is defined as an absolute lymphocyte count less than 2.0×10^9/L, whereas in adults it is defined as a count less than 1.0×10^9/L. Nonmalignant causes of lymphocytopenia can be subdivided into inherited and acquired and are listed in Table 26.6.

SECONDARY MORPHOLOGICAL CHANGES

Neutrophils

Physiologic response to infection, inflammation, stress, or administration of recombinant colony-stimulating factor (CSF) results in neutrophilia, often with a shift to the left and occasionally with the presence of blasts. The severity of infection, inflammation, or dose of CSF influences ANC and level of immaturity of neutrophils released into circulation. Additionally, neutrophils may exhibit changes in morphology such as toxic granulation, Döhle bodies, and cytoplasmic vacuoles. Toxic granulation appears as dark, blue-black granules in the cytoplasm of neutrophils, usually in segmented and band forms. Toxic granules are peroxidase positive and reflect an increase in acid mucosubstance within primary, azurophilic granules that may enhance bactericidal activity.[79] There is a positive correlation between level of C-reactive protein (an acute phase protein) and the number of neutrophils with toxic granulation; therefore toxic granulation is suggestive of inflammation.[7,80] In addition, toxic granulation can be seen in various infections as well as in patients who have received G-CSF.[81] Toxic granulation can mimic granulation found in Alder-Reilly anomaly. One helpful defining characteristic of toxic granulation is that in most cases, not all neutrophils are equally affected (Figure 26.10). Table 26.7 highlights reactive neutrophil morphologic changes and associated conditions.

Döhle bodies are cytoplasmic inclusions consisting of remnants of ribosomal ribonucleic acid (RNA) arranged in parallel rows.[82] Döhle bodies are typically found in band and segmented neutrophils (Figure 26.11) and can appear together

TABLE 26.6 Causes of Nonmalignant Lymphocytosis and Lymphocytopenia	
Lymphocytosis	**Lymphocytopenia**
Reactive Morphology	Congenital Immunodeficiencies
Infections	• Severe combined immunodeficiency disease
• Infectious mononucleosis	• Common variable immune deficiency
• Cytomegalovirus infection	• Ataxia-telangiectasia
• Hepatitis	• Wiskott-Aldrich syndrome
• Acute HIV infection	• Others
• Adenovirus	Infections
• Chickenpox	• Acquired immunodeficiency syndrome
• Herpes	• Severe acute respiratory syndrome
• Influenza	• West Nile
• Paramyxovirus (mumps)	• Hepatitis
• Rubella (measles)	• Influenza
• Roseola	• Herpes
• β-Hemolytic streptococci	• Measles
• Brucellosis	• Tuberculosis
• Paratyphoid fever	• Typhoid fever
• Toxoplasmosis	• Pneumonia
• Typhoid fever	• Rickettsiosis
• Listeria	• Ehrlichiosis
• Mycoplasma	• Sepsis
• Syphilis	• Malaria
Other	Other
• Idiosyncratic drug reactions	• Immunosuppressive agents
• Postvaccination	• Stevens-Johnson syndrome
• Sudden onset of stress from myocardial infarction	• Chemotherapy
• Allergic reaction	• Radiation
• Hyperthyroidism	• Aplastic anemia
• Malnutrition	• Platelet or stem cell apheresis
	• Major surgery
Nonreactive Morphology	• Autoimmune disease
• Bordetella pertussis (whooping cough)	• Hodgkin lymphoma
• Polyclonal B-lymphocytosis	• Advanced cancers
	• Primary myelofibrosis
	• Protein-losing enteropathy
	• Renal failure
	• Ethanol abuse
	• Zinc deficiency

Adapted from Vasu, S., & Caligiuri, M. A. (2016). Lymphocytosis and lymphocytopenia. In: Kaushansky, K., Lichtman, M. A., Prchal, J. T., et al. (Eds.), *Williams Hematology*. (9th ed., pp. 1199–1210). New York: McGraw-Hill; and Foucar, K. (2010). Non-neoplastic disorders of lymphoid cells. In Foucar, K., Reichard, K., & Czuchlewski, D. (Eds.), *Bone Marrow Pathology*. (3rd ed., Vol 2, pp. 448–473). Chicago: American Society for Clinical Pathology Press.

with toxic granulation. They are intracytoplasmic, pale blue round or elongated inclusions between 1 and 5 μm in diameter. Döhle bodies are usually located close to cellular membranes. A delay in preparing the blood film after collection may affect Döhle body appearance in that they are more grey than blue or in some cases may not be visible. Döhle bodies are relatively

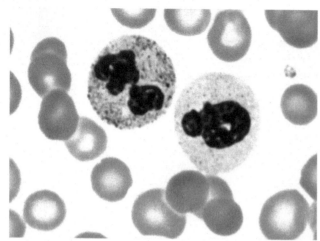

Figure 26.10 Toxic Granulation. Note that one neutrophil contains toxic granulation and the other does not. Also note that the toxic granules are clustered in some areas of the cytoplasm. Both of these findings help in distinguishing toxic granulation from poor staining or from the dark granules seen in Alder-Reilly anomaly. (Peripheral blood, Wright-Giemsa stain, ×1000.)

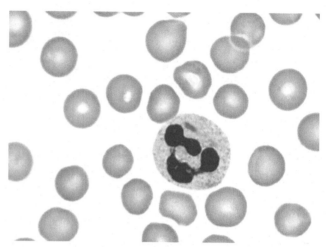

Figure 26.11 Neutrophil Containing a Döhle Body. (Peripheral blood, Wright-Giemsa stain, ×1000.)

TABLE 26.7   Reactive Morphologic Changes in Neutrophils

Reactive Change	Appearance	Associated with
Toxic granulation	Dark, blue-black cytoplasmic granules	Inflammation, infection, G-CSF
Döhle bodies	Intracytoplasmic pale blue round or elongated bodies between 1 and 5 μm in diameter, usually adjacent to cellular membranes.	Infection, G-CSF, pregnancy, burns
Cytoplasmic vacuoles	Small to large circular clear areas in cytoplasm, rarely may contain organism	Bacterial infection, autophagocytosis secondary to drug ingestion, acute alcoholism, or excess storage of sample before making blood film

G-CSF, Granulocyte colony-stimulating factor.

nonspecific. Their presence has been associated with a wide range of conditions, including bacterial infections, sepsis, and pregnancy.[82,83] Döhle bodies are similar in appearance to the inclusions found in May-Hegglin anomaly. However, in May-Hegglin anomaly, Döhle body-like inclusions can also be seen in eosinophils, basophils, and monocytes.

Cytoplasmic vacuolation of neutrophils is encountered less often than toxic granules and Döhle bodies. Vacuoles generally reflect phagocytosis, either of self (autophagocytosis) or of extracellular material (Figure 26.12). Autophagocytic vacuoles tend to be small (approximately 2 μm) and distributed throughout the cytoplasm. Autophagocytosis can be induced by specimen storage in ethylene diamintetraacetic (EDTA) for more than 2 hours,

autoantibodies, acute alcoholism, and exposure to high doses of radiation.[84-86] Phagocytic vacuoles induced by either bacteria or fungi are suggestive of sepsis. When phagocytic vacuoles are seen, a careful examination sometimes reveals organisms within the vacuoles. Phagocytic vacuoles tend to be large (up to 6 μm) and often accompanied by toxic granulation.

Cases of ehrlichiosis and anaplasmosis have been increasing in the United States over the past decade.[85] *Ehrlichia* and *Anaplasma* are small, obligate, intracellular bacteria transmitted by ticks to humans and other vertebrate hosts. These organisms grow as a cluster (morulae) in neutrophils (*Anaplasma phagocytophilum* and rarely in *Ehrlichia ewingii*) (Figure 26.13A) and in monocytes (*Ehrlichia chaffeensis*) (Figure 26.13B). Leukopenia, thrombocytopenia, and elevated liver enzymes are common laboratory findings, and anemia occurs in about half the cases ofehrlichiosis.[88] Intracellular aggregates of purple colored particles (morulae) in neutrophils or monocytes may occasionally be detected in the first week of infection on a Wright-Giemsa stained peripheral blood film or a buffy coat preparation. Morulae can be mistaken for Döhle bodies in neutrophils. Polymerase chain reaction testing is often required to confirm diagnosis.[87] Early detection is essential because antibiotic treatment with doxycycline is effective and can prevent serious complications.

Pyknotic nuclei in neutrophils generally indicate imminent cell death. In a pyknotic nucleus, water has been lost and the chromatin becomes dense and dark; however, chromatin or filaments can still be seen between nuclear lobes (depending on whether the cell is a band or segmented form).[89,90]

Necrotic nuclei are found in dead neutrophils. They are rounded nuclear fragments with no filaments and no chromatin pattern (Figure 26.14). Increased numbers of pyknotic or necrotic cells suggest that an extended amount of time has elapsed between blood collection and blood film preparation.

Cytoplasmic swelling of neutrophils is a result of osmotic swelling of the cytoplasm or by increased adhesion to the glass slide in stimulated neutrophils. Regardless of the cause, the result is a variation in neutrophil size or neutrophil anisocytosis (Figure 26.15).

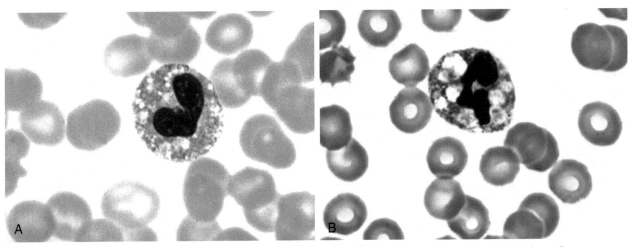

Figure 26.12 Cytoplasmic vacuoles. (A), Band neutrophil with autophagocytic vacuoles. Note their small size. **(B),** Neutrophil with phagocytic vacuoles. Note their larger size. Other evidence of toxicity in this cell is the pyknotic nucleus. (Peripheral blood, Wright-Giemsa stain, ×1000.)

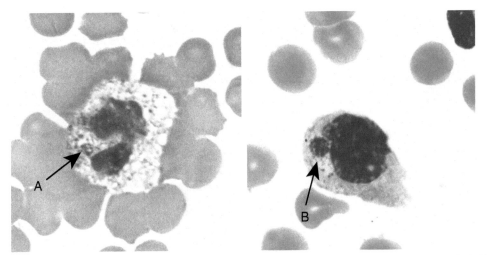

Figure 26.13 Intracellular Organisms. (A), *Anaplasma phagocytophilum* in a neutrophil. **(B),** *Ehrlichia chaffeensis* in a monocytic cell. (Peripheral blood, Wright-Giemsa stain, ×1000.) (Courtesy J. Stephen Dumler, The Johns Hopkins Medical Institution, Baltimore, MD.)

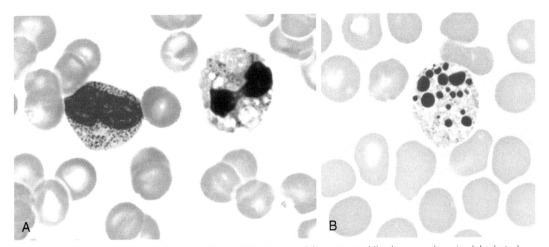

Figure 26.14 Pyknotic and Necrotic Cells. (A), Upper cell is a neutrophil whose nucleus is dehydrated, which makes it very dark and dense. Note that there is still a filament between the segments. This is referred to as a pyknotic cell. The cell is also vacuolated. **(B),** Neutrophil that has died. Note that the nucleus has disintegrated into numerous rounded spheres of DNA with no filaments. This is referred to as a necrotic or necrobiotic cell. (Peripheral blood, Wright-Giemsa stain, ×1000.) (B from Carr, J. H., & Rodak, B. F. [2009]. *Clinical Hematology Atlas.* [3rd ed.]. St. Louis: Saunders.)

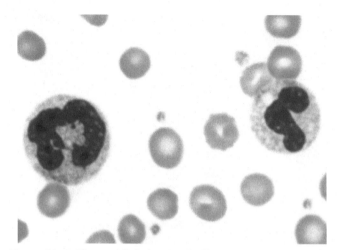

Figure 26.15 Neutrophil Anisocytosis. The neutrophil to the left is larger than the other neutrophil. This is often caused by cytoplasmic swelling. (Peripheral blood, Wright-Giemsa stain, ×1000.)

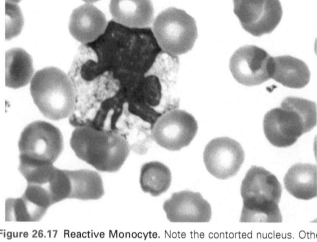

Figure 26.17 Reactive Monocyte. Note the contorted nucleus. Other evidence of toxicity is the several vacuoles in the cytoplasm. (Peripheral blood, Wright-Giemsa stain, ×1000.)

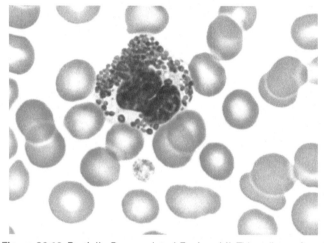

Figure 26.16 Partially Degranulated Eosinophil. This cell was found on the blood film for a patient with trichinosis. (Peripheral blood, Wright-Giemsa stain, ×1000.)

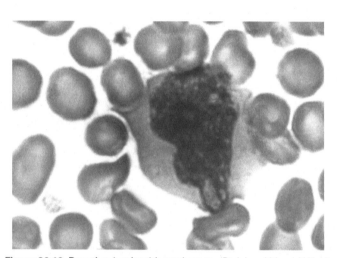

Figure 26.18 Reactive (variant) Lymphocyte. (Peripheral blood, Wright-Giemsa stain, ×1000.)

Eosinophils and Basophils

Eosinophils can sometimes appear hypogranular (Figure 26.16). Hypogranular eosinophils have been associated with acute lymphoblastic leukemia and hypereosinophilic syndrome.[91,92] In vitro disruption of the cellular membrane may occur during the process of making the blood film as eosinophils are fragile. To promote accuracy, it is recommended that fractured eosinophils be counted as eosinophils in the manual WBC differential.[35]

Basophil granules are water soluble, and it is not uncommon for them to be partially or completely washed away during staining.[93] Sometimes few or no granules remain; only a pinkish tinge in or around the cell is seen. This can hamper proper identification of basophils when performing manual WBC differentials.

Monocytes

Reactive changes in monocytes are an uncommon finding. Reactive monocytes exhibit thin, band-like, or segmenting nuclei (Figure 26.17). Reactive changes also include increased cytoplasmic volume, irregular cytoplasmic borders, and changes in granule size and coloration. Reactive monocytes have been associated with infection, recovery from myelosuppression, and administration of granulocyte-macrophage CSF.

Lymphocytes

Lymphocytes that exhibit reactive morphology have been classified using various terms, including *reactive, variant, atypical, transformed, effector, plasmacytoid, Turk cells, Downey,* and *immunoblasts.* The International Council for Standardization in Hematology (ICSH) recommends using *reactive* when the lymphocyte exhibits morphology consistent with a benign etiology and *abnormal* when lymphocyte morphology suggests a malignant or clonal etiology.[36]

Reactive changes in lymphocyte morphology occur as lymphocytes are stimulated when interacting with antigens in peripheral lymphoid organs (Figures. 26.18 and 26.19). B and T lymphocyte activation results in the transformation of small, resting lymphocytes into proliferating larger cells. These reactive lymphocytes spill into peripheral circulation. Reactive lymphocytes often present as a heterogeneous population of various

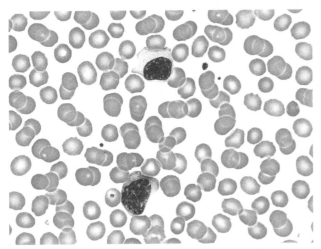

Figure 26.19 Reactive (Variant) Lymphocytes. Cells from a patient with infectious mononucleosis. (Peripheral blood, Wright-Giemsa stain, ×1000.)

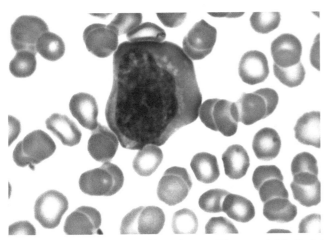

Figure 26.20 Reactive (Variant) lymphocyte (Plasmacytoid). (Peripheral blood, Wright-Giemsa stain, ×1000.)

shapes and sizes. There is variation in the nuclear to cytoplasmic ratio, nuclear shape, and chromatin pattern, which is clumped, but some cells may contain less condensed chromatin. Nucleoli may be visible. An increase in basophilic cytoplasm that varies in intensity within and between cells is a common finding. The cytoplasm may be indented by surrounding RBCs; however, other cells, including blasts, may also show similar indentation. A *plasmacytoid lymphocyte* is a type of reactive lymphocyte that has some morphologic features of plasma cells (Figure 26.20). If such cells are numerous, lymphoma or Waldenstrom's macroglobulinemia may be suspected. True plasma cells are not commonly encountered on blood film review.

INFECTIOUS MONONUCLEOSIS

Most humans are subclinically infected with Epstein-Barr virus. EBV has been associated with several benign and malignant diseases but has been proven to be the causative agent in only a few, including infectious mononucleosis (IM). When primary infection with EBV occurs in childhood, it often goes unnoticed.

Early childhood infection with EBV is not usually identified as the symptoms are generally mild and overlap with other viral syndromes. The incubation period of IM is approximately 3 to 7 weeks, and during this time EBV preferentially infects B lymphocytes through attachment of viral envelope glycoprotein 350/220 to CD21 (C3d complement receptors).[94] The oropharynx epithelial cells are also infected, but the mechanism is unclear because these cells do not express CD21. The cellular response in IM is important in the control of the infection and is characterized by proliferation and activation of NK lymphocytes, CD4+ T cells, and CD8+ memory cytotoxic T cells (EBV-CTLs) in response to B cell infection. Most of the circulating reactive lymphocytes represent activated T cells.

Common clinical manifestations of IM include sore throat, dysphagia, fever, chills, cervical lymphadenopathy, fatigue, and headache. An absolute lymphocytosis is present with up to 50% or more reactive forms. Complications are generally mild and include hepatosplenomegaly (and elevated transaminases), hemolytic anemia, and moderate thrombocytopenia. In rare cases patients develop aplastic anemia, disseminated intravascular coagulation, thrombotic thrombocytopenic purpura, hemolytic uremic syndrome, Guillain-Barré syndrome, or other neurologic complication.[95] The incidence of clinically apparent IM in the United States is 500 cases per 100,000 annually. The highest frequency of clinically overt IM is in young adults aged 15 to 24 years, although IM has been reported in patients 3 months to 70 years of age.[96]

Heterophile antibodies stimulated by EBV that cross-react with antigens found on sheep and horse RBCs. Rapid screening procedures detect heterophile antibodies. However, not everyone with IM will produce heterophile antibodies, especially children. Definitive testing (if needed) for EBV infection includes a panel of antigen and antibody tests for viral capsid antigen (VCA), Epstein-Barr nuclear antigen (EBNA), and IgG/IgM antibodies against VCA and EBNA. Cytomegalovirus can cause a mononucleosis syndrome with similar clinical features. Clinical and laboratory findings associated with IM are summarized in Box 26.4.

BOX 26.4 **Infectious Mononucleosis: Clinical and Laboratory Findings**	
Clinical Manifestations	**Laboratory Test Results**
Common	• WBC count: 10–30 × 10⁹/L (or higher)
• Sore throat	because of an absolute lymphocytosis
• Dysphagia	• Reactive lymphocyte morphology
• Fever	• Positive heterophile antibody test
• Chills	• Positive EBV-specific antigen & anti-
• Cervical lymphadenopathy	body tests
• Fatigue	
• Headache	
Less Common	
• Hepatomegaly	
• Elevated transaminases	
• Splenomegaly	
• Hemolytic anemia	
• Thrombocytopenia	

EBV, Epstein-Barr virus; *WBC,* white blood cell

SUMMARY

- The primary immunodeficiency disorders are a group of inherited diseases of the innate or adaptive immune system that often result in severe clinical manifestations.
- Both γc deficiency and adenosine deaminase (ADA) deficiency are examples of severe combined immune deficiency (SCID), characterized by defects in cellular and humoral immunity, with a wide range of severe clinical symptoms and death within the first few years of life.
- Wiskott-Aldrich syndrome is a combined immunodeficiency disease with numerous hematologic and clinical findings and increased risk for leukemic transformation.
- DiGeorge syndrome is a disease characterized by a severe decrease in T cells, physical abnormalities, neurologic/psychiatric issues, and hematologic manifestations.
- Bruton tyrosine kinase (BTK) deficiency (X-linked agammaglobulinemia) results in a profound decrease in B cells, hypogammaglobulinemia, and severe, life-threatening infections.
- Chédiak-Higashi syndrome is an extremely rare condition affecting various cells in the body where granules fuse within lysosomes, disrupting normal function, leading to a wide range of serious clinical symptoms and early death.
- The congenital neutropenias manifest early in life as recurrent life-threatening bacterial and fungal infections with increased risk for leukemic transformation.
- Leukocyte adhesion disorders arise as a result of impaired ability of neutrophils and monocytes to move to sites of infection. Clinical findings include recurring severe infections, organomegaly, and neurologic defects.
- Shwachman-Diamond syndrome is characterized by exocrine pancreatic insufficiency, digestive issues, infections, physical anomalies, neurologic defects, bone marrow failure, and increased risk of leukemia.
- Chronic granulomatous disease results from a failure in the neutrophil respiratory burst after ingestion of organisms. Patients suffer from severe recurrent infections; however, advances in the use of antimicrobial agents have been effective at improving the clinical condition.
- WHIM (warts, hypogammaglobulinemia, infections, and myelokathexis syndrome) is a disorder of white blood cell (WBC) movement from the bone marrow to blood resulting in leukopenia, hypogammaglobulinemia, bacterial infections, human papillomavirus infection, and warts.
- Pelger-Huët anomaly is a genetic disorder resulting in hypolobulated mature leukocytes. These cells can be confused with immature neutrophils. An acquired form of hyposegmentation called pseudo-Pelger-Huët is associated with hematologic neoplasms and other disorders.
- Alder-Reilly anomaly is a manifestation of mucopolysaccharidosis characterized by metachromatic granules in leukocytes, which can be confused with toxic granulation.
- May-Hegglin anomaly is characterized by thrombocytopenia, giant platelets, and Döhle body-like inclusions in leukocytes. Most cases are asymptomatic.
- Lysosomal storage disorders are congenital deficiencies of lysosomal enzymes and impaired digestion of macromolecules, which accumulate and impair cellular functions.
- The mucopolysaccharidoses are associated with a specific defect in an enzyme necessary for the degradation of glycoaminoglycan (GAG). Partially digested GAGs build up and disrupt cellular functions leading to serious physical and neurologic problems.
- Gaucher disease is characterized by a deficiency in β-glucocerebrosidase and accumulation of cell sphingolipids leading to a range of clinical manifestations and increased risk for malignant transformation
- Niemann-Pick disease is caused by a deficiency in sphingomyelinase and buildup of fats in various organs in the body, resulting in neurologic defects, organomegaly, failure to thrive, and early death.
- Reactive changes in neutrophils include a left shift, Döhle bodies, toxic granulation, and vacuoles.
- Reactive morphology in monocytes includes segmenting nuclei, changes in granule color and size, and irregular cytoplasmic borders.
- Reactive changes in lymphocytes include increased size, increased basophilic cytoplasm, and morphologic heterogeneity.

Now that you have completed this chapter, go back and read again the case study at the beginning and respond to the questions presented.

REVIEW QUESTIONS

Answers can be found in the Appendix.

1. Which of the following inherited leukocyte disorders is caused by a mutation in the lamin B receptor?
   a. Pelger-Huët anomaly
   b. Chédiak-Higashi disease
   c. Alder-Reilly anomaly
   d. May-Hegglin anomaly

2. Which of the following inherited leukocyte disorders involves mutations in nonmuscle myosin heavy-chain IIA?
   a. Pelger-Huët anomaly
   b. Chédiak-Higashi disease
   c. Alder-Reilly anomaly
   d. May-Hegglin anomaly

3. Which of the following inherited leukocyte disorders might be seen in Hurler syndrome?
   a. Pelger-Huët anomaly
   b. Chédiak-Higashi disease
   c. Alder-Reilly anomaly
   d. May-Hegglin anomaly

4. Which of the following lysosomal storage diseases is characterized by macrophages with striated cytoplasm and storage of glucocerebroside?
   a. Sanfilippo syndrome
   b. Gaucher disease
   c. Fabry disease
   d. Niemann-Pick disease

5. The neutrophils in chronic granulomatous disease are incapable of producing:
   a. Hydrogen peroxide
   b. Hypochlorite
   c. Superoxide
   d. All of the above

6. Individuals with X-linked SCID have a mutation that affects their ability to synthesize:
   a. Deaminase
   b. Oxidase
   c. IL-2 receptor
   d. IL-8 receptor

7. An absolute lymphocytosis with reactive lymphocytes suggests which of the following conditions?
   a. DiGeorge syndrome
   b. Bacterial infection
   c. Parasitic infection
   d. Viral infection

8. What leukocyte cytoplasmic inclusion is composed of ribosomal RNA?
   a. Primary granules
   b. Toxic granules
   c. Döhle bodies
   d. Howell-Jolly bodies

9. The expected complete blood cell count (CBC) results for women in active labor would include:
   a. High total white blood cell (WBC) count with increased lymphocytes
   b. High total WBC count with a slight shift to the left in neutrophils
   c. Normal WBC count with increased eosinophils
   d. Low WBC count with increased monocytes

10. Which of the following is true of an absolute increase in lymphocytes with reactive morphology?
   a. The population of lymphocytes appears morphologically homogeneous.
   b. They are usually effector B cells.
   c. The reactive lymphocytes have increased cytoplasm with variable basophilia.
   d. They are most commonly seen in bacterial infections.

REFERENCES

1. Picard, C., Bobby Gaspar, H., Al-Herz, W. et al. (2018). International Union of Immunological Societies: 2017 primary immunodeficiency diseases committee report on inborn errors of immunity. *J Clin Immunol, 38,* 96–128.

2. Puck, J. M., Deschenes, S. M., Porter, J. C., et al. (1993). The interleukin-2 receptor γ chain maps to Xq13.1 and is mutated in X-linked severe combined immunodeficiency, SCIDX1. *Hum Mol Genet, 2*(8), 1099–1104.

3. Allenspach, E., Rawlings, D. J., & Scharenberg, A. M. (2016) X-linked severe combined immunodeficiency. In Adam, M. P., Ardinger, H. H., Pagon, R. A., et al. (Eds.), *GeneReviews®* [Internet]. Seattle (WA): University of Washington, Seattle; 1993R–2016. https://www.ncbi.nlm.nih.gov/books/NBK1410/. Accessed July 17, 2018.

4. Bradford, K. L., Moretti, F. A., Carbonaro-Sarracino, D. A., et al. (2017). Adenosine deaminase (ADA)-deficient severe combined immune deficiency (SCID): molecular pathogenesis and clinical manifestations. *J Clin Immunol, 37,* 626–637.

5. Candotti, F. J. (2018). Clinical manifestations and pathophysiological mechanisms of the Wiskott-Aldrich syndrome. *Clin Immunol, 38,* 13–27.

6. Braun, C. J., Witzel, M., Paruzynski, A., et al. (2014). Gene therapy for Wiskott-Aldrich syndrome—long-term reconstitution and clinical benefits, but increased risk for leukemogenesis. *Rare Diseases, 2*(1), e947749.

7. Morsheimer, M., Brown Whitehorn, T. F., Heimall, J., et al. (2017). The immune deficiency of chromosome 22q11.2 deletion syndrome. *Am J Med Genet Part A, 173,* 2366–2372.

8. Lambert, M. P., Arulselvan, A., Schott, A., et al. (2017). The 22q11.2 deletion syndrome: cancer predisposition, platelet abnormalities and cytopenias. *Am J Med Genet,* 1–7.

9. Shillitoe, B., & Gennery, A. (2017). X-linked agammaglobulinemia: outcomes in the modern era. *Clin Immunol, 183,* 54–62.

10. Kaplan, J., De Domenico, I., & Ward, D. M. (2008). Chediak-Higashi syndrome. *Curr Opin Hematol, 15*(1), 22–29.

11. Introne, W., Boissy, R. E., & Gahl, W. A. (1999). Clinical, molecular, and cell biological aspects of Chediak-Higashi syndrome. *Mol Genet Metab, 68*(2), 283–303.

12. Daneshbod, Y., & Medeiros, L. J. (2016). Pseudo Chediak-Higashi anomaly in acute monoblastic leukemia. *Blood, 128*(21), 2583.

13. La Gioia, A., Bombara, M., Fiorini, F., et al. (2017). Pseudo-Chédiak-Higashi granules and other unusual cytoplasmic inclusions in refractory anaemia with excess blasts-2. *Br J Haematol, 176,* 156.

14. Tsai, I. M., Tsai, C. C., & Ladd, D. J. (1977). Pseudo-Chediak-higashi anomaly in chronic myelogenous leukemia with myelofibrosis. *Am J Clin Pathol, 67*(6), 608–609.

15. Donadieu, J., Beaupain, B., Fenneteau, O., et al. (2017). Congenital neutropenia in the era of genomics: classification, diagnosis, and natural history. *Br J Haematol, 179,* 557–574.

16. Hauck, F, & Klein, C. (2013). Pathogenic mechanisms and clinical implications of congenital neutropenia syndromes. *Curr Opin Allergy Clin Immunol, 13*(6), 596–606.

17. Rosenberg, P. S., Alter, B. P., Bolyard, A. A., et al. (2006). The incidence of leukemia and mortality from sepsis in patients with severe congenital neutropenia receiving long-term G-CSF therapy. *Blood, 107*(12), 4628–4635.

18. Lawrence, M. B., Kansas, G. S., Kunkel, E. J., et al. (1997). Threshold levels of fluid shear promote leukocyte adhesion through selectins (CD62L,P,E). *J Cell Biol, 136*(3), 717–727.

19. Harris, E. S., McIntyre, T. M., Prescott, S. M. et al.. (2000). The leukocyte integrins. *J Biol Chem, 275*(31), 23409–23412.

20. Schmidt, S., Moser, M., & Sperandio, M. (2013). The molecular basis of leukocyte recruitment and its deficiencies. *Mol Immunol, 55*(1), 49–58.

21. Sperandio, M., Gleissner, C. A., & Ley, K. (2009). Glycosylation in immune cell trafficking. *Immunol Rev, 230*(1), 97–113.

22. Gazit, Y., Mory, A., Etzioni, A., et al. (2010). Leukocyte adhesion deficiency type II: long-term follow-up and review of the literature. *J Clin Immunol, 30*(2), 308–313.

23. Moser, M., Nieswandt, B., Ussar, S., et al. (2008). Kindlin-3 is essential for integrin activation and platelet aggregation. *Nat Med, 14*(3), 325–330.

24. Myers, K. (2014). Shwachman-Diamond syndrome. In Adam, M. P., Ardinger, H. H., Pagon, R. A., et al. (Eds.), *GeneReviews®* [Internet]. Seattle (WA): University of Washington, Seattle; 1993–2017. https://www.ncbi.nlm.nih.gov/books/NBK1756/. Accessed July 17, 2018.

25. Nelson, A. & Myers, K. (2018) Diagnosis, treatment and molecular pathology of Shwachman-Diamond syndrome. *Hematol Oncol Clin North Am, 32*(4), 687–700.

26. Chiriaco, M., Salfa, I., Di Matteo, G., et al. (2016). Chronic granulomatous disease: clinical, molecular, and therapeutic aspects. *Pediatr Allergy Immunol, 27*(3), 242–253.

27. Arnold, D. E., & Heimall, J. R. (2017). A review of chronic granulomatous disease. *Adv Ther, 34*(12), 2543–2557.

28. Dinauer, M. C. (2016). Primary immune deficiencies with defects in neutrophil function. *Hematology Am Soc Hematol Educ Program, 2016*(1), 43–50.

29. Dotta, L., Tassone, L., & Badolato, R. (2011). Clinical and genetic features of warts, hypogammaglobulinemia, infections and myelokathexis (WHIM) syndrome. *Curr Mol Med, 11*(4), 317–325.

30. Badolato, R., Donadieu, J., & the WHIM Research Group. (2017). How I treat warts, hypogammaglobulinemia, infections, and myelokathexis syndrome. *Blood, 130*(23), 2491–2498.

31. Colella, R., & Hollensead, S. C. (2012). Understanding and recognizing the Pelger-Huët anomaly. *Am J Clin Pathol, 137*(3), 358–366.

32. Skendzel, L. P., & Hoffman, G. C. (1962). The Pelger anomaly of leukocytes: forty-one cases in seven families. *Am J Clin Pathol, 37*, 294–301.

33. Johnson, C. A., Bass, D. A., Trillo, A. A., et al. (1980). Functional and metabolic studies of polymorphonuclear leukocytes in the congenital Pelger-Huët anomaly. *Blood, 55*(3), 466–469.

34. Cunningham, J. M., Patnaik, M. M., Hammerschmidt, D. E., et al. (2009). Historical perspective and clinical implications of the Pelger-Huët cell. *Am J Hematol, 84*(2), 116–119.

35. Wang, E. (2011). Pseudo-Pelger Huet anomoly induced by medications. *Am J Clin Pathol, 135*, 291–303.

36. Palmer, L., Briggs, C., McFadden, S., et al. (2015), ICSH recommendations for the standardization of nomenclature and grading of peripheral blood cell morphological features. *Int J Lab Hematol, 37*, 287–303.

37. Shetty, V. T., Mundle, S. D., & Raza, A. (2001). Pseudo Pelger-Huët anomaly in myelodysplastic syndrome: hyposegmented or apoptotic neutrophil? *Blood, 98*(4), 1273–1275.

38. Brunning, R. D. (1970). Morphologic alterations in nucleated blood and marrow cells in genetic disorders. *Hum Pathol, 1*, 99–124.

39. Kunishima, S., Kojima, T., Tanaka, T., et al. (1999). Mapping of a gene for May-Hegglin anomaly to chromosome 22q. *Hum Genet, 105*(5), 379–383.

40. Ferreira, C. R., & Gahl, W. A. (2017). Lysosomal storage diseases. *Transl Sci Rare Dis, 2*, 1–71.

41. Giugliani, R., Federhen, A., Vairo, F., et al. (2016). Emerging drugs for the treatment lef of mucopolysaccharidoses. *Expert Opin Emerg Drugs, 21*(1), 9–26.

42. Beutler, E., Nguyen, N. J., Henneberger, M. W., et al. (1993). Gaucher disease: gene frequencies in the Ashkenazi Jewish population. *Am J Hum Genet, 52*(1), 85–88.

43. Stenson, P. D., Mort, M., Ball, E. V., et al. (2014). The human gene mutation database: building a comprehensive mutation repository for clinical and molecular genetics, diagnostic testing and personalized genomic medicine. *Hum Genet, 133*(1), 1–9.

44. Rosenbloom, B. E., Weinreb, N. J., Zimran, A., et al. (2005). Gaucher disease and cancer incidence: a study from the Gaucher Registry. *Blood, 105*(12), 4569–4572.

45. Somaraju, U. R., & Tadepalli, K. (2017). Hematopoietic stem cell transplantation for Gaucher disease. *Cochrane Database Syst Rev, 10*: CD006974.

46. Sharma, P., Khurana, N., & Singh, T. (2007). Pseudo-Gaucher cells in Hb E disease and thalassemia intermedia. *Hematology, 12*(5), 457–459.

47. Helbig, G., Janikowska, A., & Kyrcz-Krzemien, S. (2015). Aggregates of pseudo-Gaucher cells after treatment of chronic myeloid leukemia in blastic phase. *Int J Hematol, 101*(1), 3–4.

48. Carrington, P. A., Stevens, R. F., & Lendon, M. (1992). Pseudo-Gaucher cells. *J Clin Pathol, 45*(4), 360.

49. Cozzolino, L., Picardi, M., Pagliuca, S., et al. (2016). B-cell non-Hodgkin lymphoma and pseudo-Gaucher cells in a lymph node fine needle aspiration. *Cytopathology, 27*(2), 134–136.

50. Shenjere, P., B., & Banerjee, S. B. (2008). Pseudo-Gaucher cells in multiple myeloma. *Int J Surg Pathol, 16*(2), 176–179.

51. Dubois-Galopin, F., & Berger, M. G. (2010). Waldenström macroglobulinemia with pseudo-Gaucher cells. *Blood, 116*(18), 3388.

52. Schuchman, E. H. (2009). The pathogenesis and treatment of acid sphingomyelinase-deficient Niemann-Pick disease. *Int J Clin Pharmacol Ther, 47*(Suppl. 1), S48–S57.

53. Schuchman, E. H., & Desnick, R. J. (2017). Types A and B Niemann-Pick disease. *Mol Genet Metab, 120*, 27–33.

54. McKay Bounford, K., & Gissen, P. (2014). Genetic and laboratory diagnostic approach in Niemann Pick disease type C. *J Neurol, 261*(Suppl. 2), 569–575.

55. Mengel, E., Klünemann, H. H., Lourenço, C. M., et al. (2013). Niemann-Pick disease type C symptomatology: an expert-based clinical description. *Orphanet J Rare Dis, 8*, 166.

56. Wijburg, F.A., Sedel, F., Pineda, M., et al. (2012). Development of a suspicion index to aid diagnosis of Niemann-Pick disease type C. *Neurology. 78*(20), 1560–1567.

57. Evans, W. R. H., & Hendriksz, C. J. (2017). Niemann-Pick type C disease – the tip of the iceberg? A review of neuropsychiatric presentation, diagnosis and treatment. *BJPsych Bull, 41*(2), 109–114.

58. Andrès, E., & Mourot-Cottet, R. (2017). Non-chemotherapy drug-induced neutropenia - an update. *Expert Opin Drug Saf, 16*(11), 1235–1242

59. Reil, A., Sachs, U. J., Siahanidou, T., et al. (2013). HNA-1d: a new human neutrophil antigen located on Fcγ receptor IIIb associated with neonatal immune neutropenia. *Transfusion, 53*, 2145–2151

60. van den Tooren-de Groot, R., Ottink, M., Huiskes, E., et al. (2014). Management and outcome of 35 cases with foetal/neonatal alloimmune neutropenia. *Acta Paediatr, 103*, e467–e474.

61. BUX, J., Jung, K. D., Kauth, T., et al. (1992). Serological and clinical aspects of granulocyte antibodies leading to alloimmune neonatal neutropenia. *Transfus Med, 2*, 143–149.

62. Żupańska, B., Uhrynowska, M., Guz, K., et al. (2001). The risk of antibody formation against HNA1a and HNA1b granulocyte antigens during pregnancy and its relation to neonatal neutropenia. *Transfus Med, 11*, 377–382.

63. Williams, B. A., & Fung, Y. (2006). Alloimmune neonatal neutropenia: can we afford the consequences of a missed diagnosis? *J Paediatr Child Health, 42,* 59–61.

64. Afzal, W., Owlia, M. B., Hasni., et al. (2017). Autoimmune neutropenia updates: etiology, pathology, and treatment. *South Med J, 110*(4), 300–307.

65. Dale, D. C. (2017). How I manage children with neutropenia. *Br J Haematol, 178,* 351–363.

66. Autrel-Moignet, A., & Lamy, T. (2014). Autoimmune neutropenia. *Presse Med, 43*(4), e105–e118.

67. Korenaga, M., Hitoshi, Y., Yamaguchi, N., et al. (1991). The role of interleukin-5 in protective immunity to *Strongyloides venezuelensis* infection in mice. *Immunology, 72*(4), 502–507.

68. Simon, D., & Simon, H. U. (2007). Eosinophilic disorders. *J Allergy Clin Immunol, 119*(6), 1291–1300.

69. Simon, D., Braathen, L. R., & Simon, H. U. (2004). Eosinophils and atopic dermatitis. *Allergy, 59*(6), 561–570.

70. Filley, W. V., Holley, K. E., Kephart, G. M., et al. (1982). Identification by immunofluorescence of eosinophil granule major basic protein in lung tissues of patients with bronchial asthma. *Lancet, 2*(8288), 11–16.

71. Abidi, K., Khoudri, I., Belayachi, J., et al. (2008). Eosinopenia is a reliable marker of sepsis on admission to medical intensive care units. *Crit Care, 12*(2), R59.

72. Abidi, K., Belayachi, J., Derras, Y., et al. (2011). Eosinopenia, an early marker of increased mortality in critically ill medical patients. *Intensive Care Med, 37*(7), 1136–1142.

73. Jimenez, C., Gasalla, R., et al. (1987). Incidence and clinical significance of peripheral and bone marrow basophilia. *J Med, 18*(5–6), 293–303.

74. May, M. E., & Waddell, C. C. (1984). Basophils in peripheral blood and bone marrow. A retrospective review. *Am J Med, 76*(3), 509–511.

75. Chakraborty, A., Blum, R. A., Cutler, D. L., et al. (1999). Pharmacoimmunodynamic interactions of interleukin-10 and prednisone in healthy volunteers. *Clin Pharmacol Ther, 65*(3), 304–318.

76. Nockher, W. A., Wiemer, J., & Scherberich, J. E. (2001). Haemodialysis monocytopenia: differential sequestration kinetics of CD14+CD16+ and CD14++ blood monocyte subsets. *Clin Exp Immunol, 123*(1), 49–55.

77. Savard, M., & Gosselin, J. (2006). Epstein-Barr virus immunosuppression of innate immunity mediated by phagocytes. *Virus Res, 119*(2), 134–145.

78. Bethel, K. (2003). Pathology of hairy-cell leukaemia. *Best Pract Res Clin Haematol, 16*(1), 15–31.

79. van de Vyver, A., Delport, E. F., Esterhuizen, M., et al. (2010). The correlation between C-reactive protein and toxic granulation of neutrophils in the peripheral blood. *S Afr Med J, 100*(7), 442–444.

80. Kabutomori, O., Iwatani, Y., & Kanakura, Y. (2000). Toxic granulation neutrophils and C-reactive protein. *Arch Intern Med, 160*(21), 3326–3327.

81. Kabutomori, O., Kanakura, Y., & Watani, Y. (2002). Induction of toxic granulation in neutrophils by granulocyte colony-stimulating factor. *Eur J Haematol, 69*(3), 187–188.

82. Prokocimer, M., & Potasman, I. (2008). The added value of peripheral blood cell morphology in the diagnosis and management of infectious diseases—part 1: basic concepts. *Postgrad Med J, 84,* 579–585.

83. Abernathy, M. R. (1966). Döhle bodies associated with uncomplicated pregnancy. *Blood, 27*(3), 380–385.

84. Boxer, L. A., & Stossel, T. P. (1974). Effects of anti-human neutrophil antibodies in vitro. quantitative studies. *J Clin Invest, 53*(6), 1534–1545.

85. Davidson, R. J., & McPhie, J. L. (1980). Cytoplasmic vacuolation of peripheral blood cells in acute alcoholism. *J Clin Pathol, 33*(12), 1193–1196.

86. Holley, T. R., Van Epps, D. E., Harvey, R. L., et al. (1974). Effect of high doses of radiation on human neutrophil chemotaxis, phagocytosis and morphology. *Am J Pathol, 75*(1), 61–72.

87. Dahlgren, F. S., Mandel, E. J., Krebs, J. W., et al. (2011). Increasing incidence of *Ehrlichia chaffeensis* and *Anaplasma phagocytophilum* in the United States, 2000-2007. *Am J Trop Med Hyg, 85*(1), 124–131.

88. Ismail, N., Bloch, K. C., & McBride, J. W. (2010). Human ehrlichiosis and anaplasmosis. *Clin Lab Med, 30*(1), 261–292.

89. Taneja, R., Parodo, J., Jia, S. H., et al. (2004). Delayed neutrophil apoptosis in sepsis is associated with maintenance of mitochondrial transmembrane potential and reduced caspase-9 activity. *Crit Care Med, 32*(7), 1460–1469.

90. Son, Y. O., Jang, Y. S., Heo, J. S., et al. (2009). Apoptosis-inducing factor plays a critical role in caspase-independent, pyknotic cell death in hydrogen peroxide-exposed cells. *Apoptosis, 14*(6), 796–808.

91. Catovsky, D., Bernasconi, C., Verdonck, P. J., et al. (1980). The association of eosinophilia with lymphoblastic leukaemia or lymphoma: a study of seven patients. *Br J Haematol, 45*(4), 1365–2141.

92. Kim, H., Lee, Y., Lee, D., et al. (1999). A case of idiopathic hypereosinophilic syndrome with hypersegmented and hypogranular eosinophils. *Clin Lab Haematol, 21*(6), 427–430.

93. Scordino, T. (2016). Basophil with washed out granules. ASH Image Bank. https://imagebank.hematology.org/image/60505/basophil-with-washed-out-granules?type = atlas. Accessed January 23, 2019.

94. Fingeroth, J. D., Weis, J. J., Tedder, T. F., et al. (1984). Epstein-Barr virus receptor of human B lymphocytes is the C3d receptor CR2. *Proc Natl Acad Sci U S A, 81*(14), 4510–4514.

95. Luzuriaga, K., & Sullivan, J. L. (2010). Infectious mononucleosis. *N Engl J Med, 362*(21), 1993–2000.

96. Crawford, D. H., Macsween, K. F., Higgins, C. D., et al. (2006). A cohort study among university students: identification of risk factors for Epstein-Barr virus seroconversion and infectious mononucleosis. *Clin Infect Dis, 43*(3), 276–282.

Introduction to Hematologic Neoplasms

Elaine M. Keohane*

OBJECTIVES

After completion of this chapter, the reader will be able to:

1. Describe the difference between a leukemia and lymphoma.
2. Compare and contrast acute versus chronic leukemias.
3. Describe etiologic factors associated with hematologic neoplasms to include environmental exposures, viruses, and hereditary cancer predisposition syndromes.
4. Describe the difference between the French-American-British (FAB) and World Health Organization (WHO) systems of classification of hematologic neoplasms.
5. Describe how mutations in genes for key hematopoietic cell proteins and processes can lead to malignant transformation.
6. Compare and contrast oncogenes and tumor suppressor genes in terms of their normal functions, mechanisms by which each produces malignant transformation, effect of mutations on cells, and whether they act in a dominant or recessive manner, and provide an example of each.
7. Explain how mutation or loss of DNA repair genes can result in malignant transformation.
8. Explain why localized treatments are rarely used for hematologic neoplasms.
9. Briefly describe various types of therapies used for hematologic neoplasms.

OUTLINE

General Characteristics of Hematologic Neoplasms
Incidence, Prevalence, and Etiology
Classification Schemes
Molecular Pathogenesis
    Cellular Processes Perturbed in Hematologic Neoplasms
    Epigenetic Mechanisms
    Oncogenes

    Tumor Suppressor Genes
    DNA Repair Genes
Therapy
    Chemotherapy
    Radiation Therapy
    Supportive Therapy
    Targeted Therapy
    Hematopoietic Stem Cell Transplantation

CASE STUDY

After studying the material in this chapter, the reader should be able to respond to the following case study:

A 66-year-old previously healthy man presented to his primary care physician with a 5-day history of progressive weakness, fever, and bruising. Physical examination was unremarkable except for generalized ecchymoses. A complete blood count (CBC) was ordered and the WBC count was 3.2×10^9/L, the absolute neutrophil count (ANC) was 0.5×10^9/L, hemoglobin concentration was 8.9 g/dL, and the platelet count was 12×10^9/L. In the differential count, 44% of the white blood cells were similar to those in Figure 27.1, and a markedly decreased number of platelets and neutrophils were observed on his peripheral blood film.

1. Describe the nucleated cells in the figure, indicate how you would report them in the differential count, and identify the inclusions at the arrows and their significance.

2. What is the most likely diagnosis?
3. What additional laboratory testing should be performed to confirm the identity of the cells and the diagnosis?
4. Correlate the findings of weakness, fever, and ecchymoses with the applicable CBC results.
5. Discuss molecular mechanisms that can cause maturation arrest in acute leukemia.

Continued

The author extends appreciation to Peter D. Emanuel whose work in prior editions provided the foundation for this chapter.

CASE STUDY—cont'd

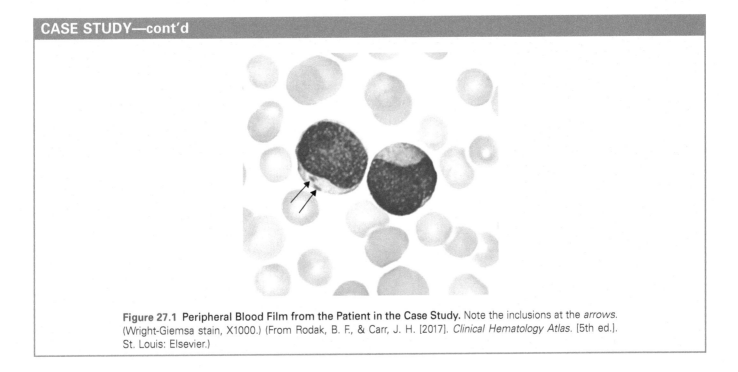

Figure 27.1 Peripheral Blood Film from the Patient in the Case Study. Note the inclusions at the *arrows.* (Wright-Giemsa stain, X1000.) (From Rodak, B. F., & Carr, J. H. [2017]. *Clinical Hematology Atlas.* [5th ed.]. St. Louis: Elsevier.)

GENERAL CHARACTERISTICS OF HEMATOLOGIC NEOPLASMS

Hematologic neoplasms result from abnormal growth of cells of the hematopoietic system. In the context of this and the chapters that follow, discussion focuses on malignant neoplasms or hematologic malignancies. They are acquired genetic diseases; that is, most patients are not born with the condition but acquire it sometime later.

Hematologic neoplasms were the first human cancers in which a consistent genetic defect was identified. In 1960 Nowell and Hungerford published an abstract that described a consistent shortened chromosome in seven patients with chronic myeloid (myelogenous) leukemia (CML).[1] This shortened chromosome was later named the Philadelphia chromosome for the city in which it was discovered. In 1973 Rowley reported the t(9;22) translocation in CML[2] and in 1982 Taub and colleagues reported the t(8;14) translocation in Burkitt lymphoma.[3] Since then, with development of increasingly sensitive methods, a multitude of other mutations have been and continue to be identified in hematologic neoplasms.

Hematologic neoplasms include *leukemias, lymphomas,* and *myelodysplastic syndromes* (previously called preleukemias), which are broad terms that refer to large heterogeneous groups of disorders. They initiate in a hematopoietic cell as a result of acquisition of one or more mutations in key genes that regulate cell growth (proliferation), survival, differentiation, or maturation. They occur in hematopoietic cells of all lineages and at various stages of their development.

Most hematologic neoplasms are not localized but rather are systemic at initiation of the malignant process. Leukemias originate in bone marrow, and leukemia cells readily pass into peripheral blood, but they can also infiltrate lymphoid tissues (spleen, liver, lymph nodes) as well as other organs and tissues of the body. Lymphomas are solid tumors of lymphoid cells that usually originate in the lymphatic system and proliferate in lymph nodes and other lymphoid organs and tissues. Lymphoma cells also can circulate in peripheral blood. With rare exceptions, most treatments for hematologic neoplasms given with curative intent are not localized, such as radiation or surgery, but must by nature be systemic-type treatments.

Leukemias are divided into lymphoid and myeloid lineages, and further into acute (precursor cell) and chronic (mature cell) categories. In acute leukemias, onset is sudden, progression is rapid, and the outcome is fatal in weeks or months if left untreated. The white blood cell (WBC) count is variable, and there is an excess accumulation of precursor hematopoietic cells or blasts of a specific lineage in bone marrow and peripheral blood because of a block in differentiation (maturation arrest). In chronic leukemias, onset is insidious and progression is slower, with a longer survival compared with acute leukemia. The WBC count is usually elevated, and there is a proliferation and accumulation of mature and maturing cells of a specific lineage. In all untreated leukemias, most normal hematopoietic cells in bone marrow are eventually replaced by leukemia cells, thus affecting normal bone marrow function. Because of the rapid expansion of blasts in bone marrow in acute leukemia, bleeding as a result of thrombocytopenia, fever caused by neutropenia-induced infection, and fatigue as a result of decreased hemoglobin concentration are often found at presentation. Symptoms of chronic leukemias at presentation are generally nonspecific and variable; some patients may be asymptomatic and diagnosed after an incidental finding of an elevated WBC count or abnormal peripheral blood film. Table 27.1 compares acute and chronic leukemias.

This chapter presents an overview of hematologic neoplasms as an introduction to the chapters that follow. In addition to the complete blood cell count, peripheral blood film examination (Chapter 13), and bone marrow examination by aspiration and

TABLE 27.1　General Characteristics of Acute and Chronic Leukemia

	Acute Leukemia	Chronic Leukemia
Predominant cell type	Precursor cell or blast	Mature
Onset	Sudden	Insidious
Symptoms at presentation	Fever (as a result of neutropenia-induced infection) Mucocutaneous bleeding (as a result of thrombocytopenia) Fatigue (as a result of anemia)	Variable, nonspecific; some asymptomatic
White blood cell count	Variable	Increased
Progression without treatment	Rapid; weeks to months	Slower; months to years

biopsy (Chapter 14), laboratory methods used to diagnose and monitor hematologic neoplasms include immunophenotyping by flow cytometric analysis (Chapter 28), molecular diagnostics (Chapter 29), and cytogenetics (Chapter 30). Specific hematologic neoplasms that are covered include acute lymphoblastic and myeloid leukemias (Chapter 31), myeloproliferative neoplasms (Chapter 32), myelodysplastic syndromes (Chapter 33), and mature lymphoid neoplasms (Chapter 34).

INCIDENCE, PREVALENCE, AND ETIOLOGY

The National Cancer Institute Surveillance, Epidemiology, and End Results Program (SEER) projected an estimated 60,300 new cases of leukemia, 74,680 cases of non-Hodgkin lymphoma, and 8500 cases of Hodgkin lymphoma for 2018 in the United States, representing 3.5%, 4.3%, and 0.5% of all cancers, respectively.[4-6] SEER estimated the prevalence of leukemia and lymphoma in the United States to be 1.3 million people in 2015.[4-6] Certain types of leukemia are more prevalent in a particular age group; for example, acute lymphoblastic leukemia is more common in young children, whereas chronic lymphocytic leukemia and myelodysplastic syndrome are more common in older adults.

For most hematologic neoplasms, causes directly related to development of the malignancy are unknown. There are, however, a few exceptions. Environmental toxins can induce genetic changes, leading to a malignant phenotype. Environmental exposures known to lead to hematologic neoplasms include radiation exposure, as experienced by survivors of atomic explosions, and exposure to organic solvents, such as benzene. In addition, as more cancer survivors live longer, it is clear that some alkylating agents and other types of chemotherapy used to treat various cancers can induce deoxyribonucleic acid (DNA) damage in hematopoietic cells, leading to hematologic neoplasms.

Some viruses have been implicated in hematologic neoplasms as a result of their ability to insert into host cell genomes, cause genetic and epigenetic changes, and/or produce oncoproteins that interfere with normal cell processes that protect cells from malignant transformation.[7] Examples include human T cell lymphotropic virus type 1 (HTLV-1), a retrovirus that invades CD4$^+$ lymphocytes and can cause adult T cell leukemia/lymphoma,[8] and Epstein-Barr virus, a DNA virus that invades mainly B lymphocytes and has been implicated as a contributing causal factor in Burkitt and other non-Hodgkin lymphomas and in a subset of classic Hodgkin lymphoma.[9] In addition, immunosuppression resulting from HIV-1 infection also causes an increased risk of non-Hodgkin lymphoma.[10]

In hereditary cancer predisposition syndromes, germline mutations in more than 60 different genes impart an increased risk of developing a hematologic neoplasm to varying degrees.[11] Some examples include congenital bone marrow failure syndromes (Chapter 19), such as Fanconi anemia (caused by mutation in one of the *FA* genes needed for DNA repair) and dyskeratosis congenita (caused by mutation in genes for telomere maintenance).[11] Other examples include Li-Fraumeni syndrome (caused by mutations in *TP53*) and ataxia telangiectasia (caused by mutations in *ATM*).[11] TP53 (also called the *molecular policeman*) is a nuclear transcription factor that promotes cell cycle arrest and apoptosis or programmed cell death (Chapter 3) when damaged cellular DNA cannot be repaired; ATM kinase is a component of the DNA damage response signaling pathway.[12,13] These proteins are part of a highly complex system to prevent cells with damaged DNA from progressing through the cell cycle (Chapter 3). When mutated or deleted, they help sustain malignant cell phenotypes. Down syndrome (trisomy 21) is another condition that increases the risk of leukemia, but the genetic mechanisms involved are not fully understood.[14]

CLASSIFICATION SCHEMES

The French-American-British (FAB) classification of acute leukemias was devised in the 1970s and 1980s. FAB schemas were based largely on morphologic characteristics and relied heavily on examination of routine histologic stain preparations to distinguish lymphoid neoplasms from myeloid neoplasms (Figure 31.2). Although these types of diagnostic criteria have not been abandoned, a more precise World Health Organization (WHO) classification of hematologic neoplasms is now being used.[15,16] WHO periodically convenes an expert panel of hematopathologists, geneticists, and clinicians to determine consensus opinion on the classification scheme for hematologic neoplasms. Published in 2001 and updated in 2008 and 2016, in collaboration with the Society for Hematopathology and the European Association for Haematopathology, the classification considers clinical features, morphology, immunophenotyping, cytogenetics, and molecular genetics. The classification uses broad categories of mature lymphoid neoplasms, myeloid neoplasms, and acute leukemia that will be discussed in detail in the chapters that follow.[15,16]

MOLECULAR PATHOGENESIS

Cellular Processes Perturbed in Hematologic Neoplasms

Cellular processes involved in hematopoiesis and its regulation are highly complex (Chapter 4), and mutations can cause dysregulation in stimulatory as well as inhibitory pathways. The types of mutations found in hematologic neoplasms include chromosomal rearrangement (such as translocation or inversion), gain or loss of chromosomes (aneuploidy), total or partial gene deletion, point mutation, insertion, or gene duplication/amplification (Chapters 29 and 30). Mutations may change or delete the DNA code of essential genes for hematopoiesis or may disrupt regulatory mechanisms involved in their expression. The latter are called *epigenetic* mechanisms because the DNA sequence of the gene itself is not altered, but there is a heritable abnormality in how that gene is expressed (discussed later).

Leukemogenesis (initiation and maintenance of leukemia) is a stepwise process in which a hematopoietic cell accumulates multiple, independent mutations or "multihits" that affect various cellular pathways, which eventually transforms it into a malignant clone. There are exceptions, however, such as in CML in which apparently only one genetic mutation, the t(9;22) translocation with fusion of the *BCR-ABL1* genes, is required for initiation of the leukemia (Chapter 32).[17,18] However, this initiating mutation in CML causes genetic instability in the cell and as the malignant clone rapidly proliferates, additional mutations accumulate causing more genetic defects, including a block in differentiation, which leads to the terminal blast transformation stage.[19]

In hematologic neoplasms, mutations or deletions disrupt key genes coding for various cellular proteins (Box 27.1) and processes and may result in one or more of the following:[20]

- Uncontrolled proliferation caused by mutation in genes coding for *signal transduction proteins* or *growth factor receptors*; this leads to activation without stimulus and without ability to suppress the response.
- Loss of DNA repair capability and cell cycle control as a result of inactivating mutation or deletion of genes coding for *DNA repair* proteins, *cell cycle proteins* that regulate the cell cycle, or *checkpoint control proteins* that arrest the cell cycle when DNA is damaged; inactivation or loss of one or more of these proteins allows cells with damaged DNA to progress through the cell cycle and proliferate.
- Block in differentiation due to mutation in genes coding for *nuclear transcription factors* or aberrant changes in their *epigenetic regulation*; this leads to maturation arrest or dysplastic changes.
- Continued cell survival and inhibition of apoptosis as a result of mutation or deletion of genes coding for *proapoptotic* and other related proteins; this leads to persistence of *leukemic stem cells* that retain self-renewal properties. In the hematopoietic environment, apoptosis is essential to contain and control the massive cell expansion that occurs in the hematopoietic system during times of stress, infection, hemolysis, or hemorrhage.

Epigenetic Mechanisms

Epigenetic mechanisms control how genes are expressed and silenced (Table 27.2). They are important for normal gene expression in all types of cells and are critical for complex processes such as embryogenesis and cell differentiation. Heritable aberrant epigenetic changes can occur in hematopoietic cells and those changes are retained in their progeny. Aberrant epigenetic mechanisms can initiate and maintain many hematologic neoplasms. Examples include (1) hyper- and hypomethylation of CpG islands in gene promoters and other noncoding DNA regions by DNA methyltransferases (DNMTs) that inhibit gene transcription or cause inappropriate gene expression; (2) mutations in histone acetyltransferases or excessive recruitment of histone deacetylases to transcription sites that keep DNA chromatin in a closed inactive state so genes are unavailable for transcription, replication, and repair; and (3) microRNAs (miRNAs, small 22-nucleotide RNA segments) that inhibit gene expression by specifically binding to targeted messenger RNA (mRNA) transcripts, blocking their translation to protein, and causing their destabilization and degradation.[21,22] Examples of transcriptional epigenetic repression of hematopoietic genes causing a block in differentiation are the t(8;21) translocation and fusion of the core-binding transcription factor gene, *RUNX1*, with the *RUNX1T1* gene in acute myeloid leukemia, and the t(15;17) translocation and fusion of the retinoic acid receptor gene, *RARA*, with the *PML* gene in acute promyelocytic leukemia (Chapter 31). Hypermethylation is also a common method of silencing tumor suppressor genes (discussed later).

Oncogenes

Oncogenes originally were identified in tumor-forming retroviruses but are derived from normal human cellular homologues called protooncogenes. The DNA sequence of protooncogenes is highly conserved and the protein products they encode are essential for normal cellular function. They are important in signaling pathways, cell proliferation, cell differentiation, and apoptosis. Mutation of a protooncogene can convert it to an oncogene with leukemogenic potential. These are considered

---

BOX 27.1   Examples of Cell Proteins Altered in Hematologic Neoplasms

Cell cycle regulatory proteins	Nuclear transcription factors
Checkpoint control proteins	Pro- and anti-apoptotic proteins
DNA repair proteins	Signal transduction proteins
Growth factor receptors	

TABLE 27.2   Examples of Epigenetic Mechanisms That Control Gene Expression

DNA methylation	Hypermethylation of CpG islands in gene promoters and other noncoding DNA regions by DNA methyltransferases prevents gene transcription and expression.
Histone acetylation	Histone acetyltransferases keep DNA chromatin in an open configuration so transcription can occur. Histone deacetylases (HDACs) keep DNA chromatin in a closed configuration so genes are unavailable for transcription, replication, and repair.
microRNAs (miRNAs)	miRNAs (small 22 nucleotide RNA segments) inhibit gene expression by specifically binding to targeted mRNA transcripts, blocking their translation to protein, and causing their destabilization and degradation.

dominant disorders because only one mutated copy of the oncogene is required to contribute to leukemogenesis. Activation of the dominant oncogene alters the gene product or its expression and transforms the cell into a malignant phenotype, even in the presence of a residual normal allele. Most chromosome translocations in leukemias involve oncogenes. Mutations cause constitutive (continuous) and unregulated activation of the oncogene and therefore are called *gain-of-function* mutations. In hematologic neoplasms the type of protooncogenes usually involved are signal transducers (such as tyrosine kinases), growth factor receptors, or transcription factors.

Mutations that activate protooncogenes can be qualitative or quantitative. Qualitative alterations involve a structural change to the protooncogene and production of an *abnormal protein product*. The structural change results in dysregulation and constitutive activation of the abnormal oncogene product. A common qualitative mutation is a *translocation* that results in a chimeric fusion gene, such as the t(9;22) translocation forming the *BCR-ABL1* fusion gene in CML and in some cases of acute lymphoblastic leukemia. The abnormal fusion gene is transcribed and translated to the BCR-ABL1 fusion protein with dysregulated tyrosine kinase activity that is inappropriately expressed (Chapter 32). Other genetic mechanisms that cause dysregulation of a tyrosine kinase include *point mutations,* such as the *JAK2* p.Val617Phe (c.1849G>T) mutation in polycythemia vera (Chapter 32), or an *internal tandem* duplication such as the *FLT3*-ITD mutation in acute myeloid leukemia (Chapter 31). *JAK2* encodes a nonreceptor tyrosine kinase associated with the intracellular domain of growth factor receptors, such as the erythropoietin receptor, and normally transmits an intracellular signal for proliferation when the appropriate growth factor ligand binds to the extracellular domain of the receptor. *FLT3* codes for a receptor tyrosine kinase preferentially expressed on the membrane of hematopoietic stem and progenitor cells that promotes hematopoietic cell proliferation and differentiation when bound with its ligand. The common feature of these examples is constitutive activation of the mutated kinase and its intracellular signaling for proliferation in the absence of ligand binding, with an inability to suppress or turn off the signal.

In quantitative mutations, there is an *overexpression of a normal protooncogene* in a hematopoietic cell. An example of this type of mechanism is found in B-lymphoid neoplasms in which a protooncogene becomes oncogenic by translocation next to the promoter of the immunoglobulin heavy chain (IGH) locus on chromosome 14. The IGH gene is normally actively transcribed in B-lymphoid cells, so when a normal protooncogene comes under the control of the IGH promoter, there is an *overexpression* of its normal protooncogene product. Examples include the t(14;18) translocation in follicular lymphoma with overexpression of the *BCL2* gene, normally located on chromosome 18, or t(11;14) translocation in mantle cell lymphoma with overexpression of the *CCND1* gene, normally located on chromosome 11, that codes for cyclin D1. BCL2 protein inhibits apoptosis and cyclin D1 regulates the cell cycle (Chapter 3). Excess production of either of these proteins causes dysregulation in apoptosis or the cell cycle contributing to malignant transformation.

Another mechanism that result in overexpression of a normal protooncogene product is *gene amplification*. By increasing the gene copy number in each cell, there is an increased production of the protein product and oncogenic potential. This mechanism, however, is uncommon in hematologic neoplasms. Gene expression can also be increased by aberrant epigenetic mechanisms and by an increase in the number of chromosomes, such as in trisomy (presence of three copies of a chromosome and three copies of its coded genes, instead of the normal two copies).

Tumor Suppressor Genes

Tumor suppressor genes are so named because they code for proteins that protect cells from malignant transformation. These gene products differ from oncogenes in that they normally slow down cell division or promote apoptosis. Whereas protooncogenes become oncogenic when activated, tumor suppressor genes promote malignant transformation when they are inactivated or deleted. They do not act in a dominant fashion as in oncogenes; rather, cells are transformed into a malignant phenotype only after both alleles are deleted or inactivated (*loss-of-function* mutations), the so-called two-hit mechanism proposed by Knudson.[23] Mechanisms for loss of function of tumor suppressor genes include gene deletion, inactivating mutation, or epigenetic silencing.

Numerous tumor suppressor genes have now been identified, and many have been found to be associated with autosomal dominant familial cancer predisposition syndromes. Some well-known examples of loss or inactivation of tumor suppressor genes include *TP53* in Li-Fraumeni syndrome (discussed previously), *RB1* involved in familial retinoblastoma, and *WT1* in Wilms tumor. More importantly, these tumor suppressor genes are deleted or inactivated in many sporadic (non-familial) cancers, including hematologic neoplasms, which leads to accumulation of additional mutations, and a more clinically aggressive state. An example is chronic lymphocytic leukemia, which has a more aggressive course when the *TP53* gene is deleted or mutated, warranting a different approach to therapy (Chapter 34).[24]

Table 27.3 compares characteristics of oncogenes and tumor suppressor genes.

DNA Repair Genes

Mutations in *DNA repair genes* are also involved in hematologic neoplasms. Mutations in these genes cause genetic instability and increased mutation rates, leading to an increased risk of malignant transformation. An example is the Fanconi anemia gene, *FA,* which is important for maintaining genomic stability in hematopoietic tissues (discussed previously).

Regardless of the type of chromosome or genetic abnormality, oncogene activation or the loss of tumor suppressor or DNA repair genes have adverse molecular effects on proliferation, differentiation, maturation, survival, apoptosis, cell cycle control, and/or DNA repair mechanisms in hematopoietic cells, and an increased risk of malignant transformation. The list of chromosomal and molecular aberrations known to occur in various

TABLE 27.3 Comparison of Oncogenes and Tumor Suppressor Genes

	Oncogenes	Tumor Suppressor Genes
Normal functions	Promote cell proliferation and differentiation, signal transduction, apoptosis	Detect damaged DNA and delay cell cycle to allow for DNA repair or apoptosis
Effect of mutations	Leukemogenic when inappropriately activated (gain-of-function mutation); causes constitutive (continuous), dysregulated, and/or overexpression of oncogene product	Leukemogenic when inactivated or deleted (loss-of-function mutation); causes inability to prevent cells with damaged DNA from progressing through the cell cycle; helps sustain malignant phenotypes
Genetics	Dominant; only one mutant allele needed for leukemogenesis	Recessive; deletion or inactivation of both alleles needed for leukemogenesis
Examples of mutations	Chromosomal rearrangement (translocation, inversion), point mutation, internal tandem duplication, gene amplification	Deletion, inactivating mutation, epigenetic silencing
Examples relevant to hematologic neoplasms	ABL1 JAK2 BCL2	TP53 RB1 WT1

BOX 27.2 General Categories of Therapy for Hematologic Neoplasms

Chemotherapy
  Cell cycle effects: phase specific or phase nonspecific agents
  Biochemical mode of action: alkylating agents, plant alkaloids, antimetabolites, antitumor antibiotics, glucocorticoids
Radiation therapy
Supportive therapy
  Growth factors and cytokines
Targeted therapy
  Targeted molecular therapy
  Immunotherapy
  Cellular therapy
Hematopoietic stem cell transplantation
  Syngeneic
  Allogeneic
  Autologous

hematologic neoplasms continues to grow on an almost daily basis. Indexing this list is far beyond the scope of this chapter, but specific examples will be discussed in the chapters that follow.

THERAPY

Treatment for leukemia and lymphoma may involve chemotherapy, radiation, supportive therapy, targeted therapies, and hematopoietic stem cell transplant (Box 27.2). Research in leukemia-specific therapy using molecular targets and immuno- and cellular therapy is ongoing and rapidly advancing. New schemes for risk stratification and treatment modalities have resulted in prolonged survival and cures for conditions that were uniformly fatal with conventional treatment. In contrast to many solid tumors, numerous hematologic neoplasms now have cure rates that are substantially higher than they were two or three decades ago. Many new and exciting therapies that are less toxic are now under development or are already employed in patient settings. These therapies are bringing more optimism to the care of patients with hematologic neoplasms. Selection of the best therapy must start, however, with an accurate diagnosis. Even the most effective therapies do not work if they are applied in the wrong circumstances.

Curative treatment strategies are now a realistic goal for patients with Hodgkin lymphoma, chronic myeloid leukemia, hairy cell leukemia, and some forms of non-Hodgkin lymphoma and for children with acute lymphoblastic leukemia. Cure may be attainable in other patients with acute lymphoblastic or myeloid leukemia, and long-term remissions may be achievable in adults with multiple myeloma. For patients with other hematologic neoplasms such as mantle cell lymphoma, chronic lymphocytic leukemia, or a therapy-related leukemia, cure remains elusive, and therapy must be directed more toward attaining remissions or providing supportive care.

Chemotherapy

Chemotherapy is oral or parenteral cancer treatment with compounds that possess antitumor properties. Methods of action of chemotherapy drugs vary considerably. Chemotherapy agents can be classified in two ways: by their effects on the cell cycle and by their biochemical mechanism of action. Some chemotherapy drugs can affect cells only in specific phases of the cell cycle (phase specific), whereas other drugs act during any phase of the cell cycle (phase nonspecific). A general biochemical classification of chemotherapy agents includes alkylating agents, plant alkaloids, antimetabolites, antitumor antibiotics, and glucocorticoids. Chemotherapy drugs are usually given in combination according to various published protocols or in the context of a clinical trial.

Chemotherapy is usually administered in three phases: induction, consolidation, and maintenance. The goal of induction is to rapidly decrease the tumor burden and achieve remission. There are different types of remission depending on the leukemia and the sensitivity of methods used for detection of malignant cells. For example, a *hematologic* remission in acute leukemia may include a normocellular bone marrow, recovery of peripheral blood cell counts, and no microscopic evidence of leukemia cells, whereas a *cytogenetic* remission is the absence of the cytogenetic defect determined by karyotyping methods (Chapter 30). A *molecular* remission is the absence of leukemia cell nucleic acid sequences using highly sensitive molecular methods capable of detecting one leukemia cell among 10^5 or 10^6 normal cells (Chapter 29). After hematologic remission is achieved, millions of leukemia cells may still be undetected in the body (called *minimal residual disease*), so a consolidation phase is done with different chemotherapy agents to further reduce the number of leukemia cells. A maintenance phase may be incorporated in the treatment plan, which is continued for a longer period with less intensive agents to eradicate any remaining leukemia cells to prevent a relapse.

Chemotherapy agents affect both malignant and normal cells. Their effects are most pronounced on rapidly dividing cells, such as those in gastrointestinal mucosa and bone marrow. This limits dosage and usually determines the maximum tolerated dose for a patient. Neutrophil and platelet counts are routinely monitored because they are the first cells to decrease after chemotherapy because of their shorter life spans.

Radiation Therapy

Radiation kills cells by producing unstable ions that damage DNA and may cause instant or delayed death of cells. Toxic effects of radiotherapy can occur during therapy or much later. Complications can be reduced through use of combined anterior and posterior treatment ports and application of maximal shielding techniques to prevent damage to normal tissues. The hematopoietic system, gastrointestinal tract, and skin are most often affected during radiotherapy. Spinal and pelvic irradiation can cause marrow suppression, sometimes lowering blood counts to life-threatening levels. Toxic effects are usually reversible when radiation is stopped.

Supportive Therapy

Numerous substances that are naturally produced in the human body have now been developed using recombinant technologies. Some are commercially produced and cleared by the US Food and Drug Administration (FDA) for supportive care of cancer patients, including those with hematologic neoplasms. Growth factors and colony-stimulating factors (CSFs), a class of cytokines, normally act in the bone marrow microenvironment to stimulate blood cell formation (Chapter 4). Erythropoietin promotes red blood cell formation and recombinant forms are administered to cancer patients with anemia induced by chemotherapy. Similarly, granulocyte colony-stimulating factor (G-CSF) and granulocyte-macrophage colony-stimulating factor (GM-CSF) are used to rapidly expand the number of mature neutrophils to fight or prevent infection. Recombinant forms of G-CSF and GM-CSF are administered to cancer patients with chemotherapy-induced neutropenia. These agents not only have improved patients' quality of life but also have allowed more efficient and effective delivery of chemotherapy regimens by preventing delays of or dosage reductions in chemotherapy courses as a result of low blood cell counts.

Targeted Therapy

As more has been learned about specific genetic lesions that cause hematologic neoplasms, researchers have worked to develop targeted therapies that act specifically on malignant cells and leave normal cells untouched. As a result of these advances, cancer therapy is realizing the dream of targeted therapeutics and is moving away from nonspecific therapies such as chemotherapy and radiation. In 2001 the FDA cleared imatinib mesylate for treatment of chronic-phase CML as the first rationally designed molecular targeted therapy for a cancer.[25] The t(9;22) translocation in CML results in production of the BCR-ABL1 fusion protein with constitutive and unregulated tyrosine kinase activity. Imatinib is an orally administered, small, tyrosine kinase inhibitor (TKI) molecule that binds to the ABL1 domain of the BCR-ABL1 fusion protein and selectively blocks its tyrosine kinase activity.[25,26] It reduces the massive cell proliferation and induces apoptosis of CML cells and remission with very few side effects.[26] Imatinib is now the first-line treatment for chronic-phase CML and has resulted in long-term remissions of 10 years and longer (Chapter 32).[25,26] Newer and more potent TKIs have also been developed (such as dasatinib and nilotinib) to treat imatinib resistance that develops in some CML patients; these second generation drugs have also been FDA cleared for first-line treatment in CML.[25,26] Imatinib is also used in combination with chemotherapeutic agents to treat *BCR-ABL1* positive acute lymphoblastic leukemia.[27] Other TKIs are in development and their effectiveness and safety are being evaluated in other hematologic neoplasms with dysregulated kinases, such as JAK2 inhibitors in polycythemia vera and FLT3 inhibitors in acute myeloid leukemia.[28,29]

In acute promyelocytic leukemia (APL), the t(15;17) translocation results in fusion of the retinoic acid receptor gene, *RARA*, with the *PML* gene. RARA protein is a ligand-dependent transcription factor that, when bound to retinoic acid, upregulates expression of target genes required for myeloid differentiation.[30] However, RARA in the PML-RARA fusion protein does not respond to retinoic acid, resulting in silencing of transcription of genes needed for differentiation, and a block in maturation beyond the promyelocytic stage.[30] Now the prognosis of patients with APL is dramatically improved with the availability of differentiation therapy using all-trans retinoic acid (ATRA) as first-line treatment along with chemotherapeutic agents (Chapter 31). ATRA binds to RARA in the fusion protein and overcomes the block, allowing transcription and expression of genes needed for myeloid differentiation and maturation.[30]

In lymphoid neoplasms, treatment includes immunotherapy using monoclonal antibodies for targeted therapeutic strategies. Monoclonal antibodies generally must be delivered intravenously or subcutaneously. An example is rituximab (anti-CD20), which binds to the CD20 antigen present on malignant cells in many B-lymphoid neoplasms and has shown efficacy in non-Hodgkin lymphoma and chronic lymphocytic leukemia.[31] The antibody targets CD20$^+$ lymphocytes for destruction by antibody-mediated and complement-mediated cytotoxicity.[31] Additional modifications of immunotherapy are now being developed, such as the bispecific T cell engager (BiTE) monoclonal antibody, blinatumomab.[32] It can bind both CD19 and CD3, bringing CD3$^+$ T-lymphoid cells closer to CD19$^+$ B-lymphoid cells to promote their destruction by cytokines.[32] It has shown efficacy in relapsed or refractory non-Hodgkin lymphoma and precursor acute lymphoblastic leukemia.[32] Monoclonal antibodies can also be conjugated with toxins (called *immunoconjugates*) to kill target cells. An example is inotuzumab ozogamicin, an anti-CD22 monoclonal antibody conjugated with calicheamicin, an antibiotic with cytotoxic activity.[33] The conjugated antibody binds to CD22$^+$ B-lymphoid cells bringing the toxin close to the cell where it rapidly enters, binds to and damages DNA, and induces apoptosis.[33] It has been used with encouraging results in relapsed or refractory acute lymphoblastic leukemia.[33]

Cellular therapy is also being implemented with high efficacy in patients with high-risk hematologic neoplasms. One such therapy uses CD19-specific chimeric antigen receptor T (CAR-T) cells in which patient T cells are collected by pheresis and are genetically engineered ex vivo using lentiviral or retroviral vectors to express protein complexes that recognize only the patient's leukemia cells.[34] Engineered CAR-T cells then specifically bind to patient's leukemia cells and target them for destruction.[34] CAR-T cells have been successful in achieving remission in high-risk, refractory or relapsed acute lymphoblastic leukemia and non-Hodgkin lymphoma.[34] Gene editing technologies, such as CRISPR/Cas9 targeted nuclease, are also being used to improve the potency and safety of CAR-T cells.[34]

Epigenetic therapies are also used in hematologic neoplasms to reverse epigenetic silencing of gene transcription. For example, histone deacetylase inhibitors (HDACi) are being used in cutaneous T cell lymphoma to prevent deacetylation allowing chromatin to open so repressed genes can be transcribed and expressed.[21,35] Likewise, hypomethylating treatment (HMT), using drugs that remove methyl groups from gene promoters allowing expression of genes, is used in high-risk myelodysplastic syndromes.[21,36]

These and other targeted therapies will be discussed in more detail in chapters covering specific hematologic neoplasms. Development and optimization of targeted therapies is an area of intense research and their use will continue to improve patient outcomes and survival as they more specifically target malignant cells and not patient's normal cells.

Hematopoietic Stem Cell Transplantation

As more has been learned about hematopoietic stem cells, the therapeutic method of *bone marrow transplantation* has evolved to be more aptly termed *hematopoietic stem cell transplantation* (HSCT), because different sources in addition to bone marrow can be used to obtain hematopoietic stem cells. Along with bone marrow, peripheral blood and umbilical cord blood (UCB) are rich sources. Bone marrow is harvested through multiple needle aspirations typically from the posterior iliac crests, and it is done

in a sterile surgical environment usually under general or regional anesthesia.[37] Collection of peripheral blood stem cells (PBSCs) is less invasive in that they are harvested by pheresis after mobilization out of bone marrow by cytokines and chemokines such as G-CSF and plerixafor.[37] UCB is collected by inserting a sterile needle into the umbilical vein after the infant is delivered and the cord is clamped and cut, either before or after delivery of the placenta.[37] Regardless of the source, hematopoietic stem cells are considered *adult stem cells,* even when they come from umbilical cord blood, as opposed to *embryonic stem cells,* which are the subject of considerable ethical debate. Stem cell transplantation still remains an expensive and difficult treatment alternative.

When the decision to transplant has been made and a donor has been found, an extensive hospital stay is usually required. Pretransplantation conditioning regimens use high-dose therapy to kill patient's malignant cells and normal bone marrow cells. This regimen reduces the body's immunity to dangerously low levels and necessitates special protective isolation. Granulocyte counts approaching zero are commonly seen immediately before and after transplantation. After infusion of donor hematopoietic stem cells, the recipient remains in a severely immunosuppressed condition for 2 weeks or longer. Strict isolation at this point is crucial. Prophylactic antibiotics and intravenous nutrition are also essential to keep the patient alive until marrow engraftment. Recovery of granulocytes, reticulocytes, and platelets to normal levels is monitored closely in peripheral blood. Evaluation and management of red blood cell and platelet transfusions are crucial components of stem cell transplantation. After discharge, peripheral blood cell counts and bone marrow continue to be monitored to measure the progress of engraftment of donor stem cells.

Hematopoietic stem cell transplants for treatment of malignant disease have come from donors of three general types: (1) *syngeneic* or from an identical twin; (2) *allogeneic,* usually from an HLA-identical sibling or HLA-matched unrelated donor; or (3) *autologous,* in which the patient's own marrow or peripheral blood stem cells are used (Figure 27.2). Most stem cell donors are allogeneic, but for optimal outcomes, it is important to match as many HLA antigens as possible. Within any given family, there can be only four HLA haplotypes (two maternal and two paternal), and there is one chance in four that a sibling will be HLA identical. If an HLA-identical sibling or fully HLA-matched unrelated donor is not available, HLA-partially matched, related or unrelated donors have been used.

Even with continued improvement in technique and supportive care, hematopoietic stem cell transplantation carries many risks. Death after transplantation is caused by complications of the conditioning regimens, such as infections or bleeding from bone marrow suppression; graft-versus-host disease; regrowth of malignant cells; and/or failure of donor stem cells to engraft.

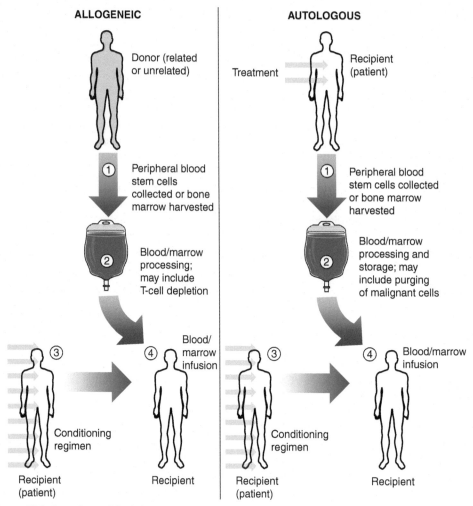

Figure 27.2 Overview of Peripheral Blood Stem Cell or Bone Marrow Transplantation Protocols in Allogeneic and Autologous Donors.

SUMMARY

- Most neoplasms of the hematopoietic system are acquired genetic diseases. They include leukemias, lymphomas, and myelodysplastic syndromes.
- Leukemias originate in bone marrow and leukemia cells readily pass into peripheral blood, but they can also infiltrate lymphoid tissues (spleen, liver, lymph nodes) as well as other organs and tissues of the body. Lymphomas are solid tumors of lymphoid cells that usually originate in the lymphatic system and proliferate in lymph nodes and other lymphoid organs and tissues.
- Leukemias are divided into lymphoid and myeloid lineages, and further into acute (precursor cell) and chronic (mature cell) categories. In acute leukemias, onset is sudden, progression is rapid, and the outcome is fatal in weeks or months if left untreated. In chronic leukemias, onset is insidious and progression is slower with a longer survival compared with acute leukemia.
- For most hematologic neoplasms, causes directly related to development of the malignancy are unknown, but a few exceptions exist. Some known causes include environmental

toxins, certain viruses, previous chemotherapy, and familial predisposition.
- Classification schemes for hematologic neoplasms include the older French-American-British (FAB) system, based primarily on morphology and cytochemical staining, and the World Health Organization (WHO) system, which retains some elements of the FAB scheme but emphasizes molecular and cytogenetic abnormalities.
- Types of mutations found in hematologic neoplasms include chromosomal rearrangement (such as translocation or inversion), gain or loss of chromosomes (aneuploidy), total or partial gene deletion, point mutation, insertion, or gene duplication/amplification.
- Hematologic neoplasms illustrate that a single mutation, or more commonly a series of mutations, can lead to malignant transformation by disrupting the molecular machinery of hematopoietic cells.
- Most chromosomal translocations in leukemias involve oncogenes. Activation of the dominant transforming oncogene alters its gene product or its expression and transforms the

cell into a malignant phenotype, even in the presence of a residual normal allele.

- In contrast to oncogenes, tumor suppressor genes contribute to the malignant process only if both alleles have been lost or otherwise inactivated.
- Activation of oncogenes or the loss of tumor suppressor or DNA repair genes have adverse molecular effects on proliferation, survival, differentiation, and/or maturation of hematopoietic cells.
- Most hematologic neoplasms are not localized, but rather are systemic at initiation of the malignant process. Therefore with rare exceptions, most treatments for hematologic neoplasms given with curative intent are not localized, such as radiation or surgery, but must by nature be systemic treatments.
- Current treatments for hematologic neoplasms can be generally divided into the following categories: chemotherapy, radiation therapy, supportive therapy, targeted therapy, and hematopoietic stem cell transplantation.

Now that you have completed this chapter, go back and read again the case study at the beginning and respond to the questions presented.

REVIEW QUESTIONS

Answers can be found in the Appendix.

1. Lymphomas differ from leukemias in that they are:
   a. Solid tumors
   b. Not considered systemic diseases
   c. Never found in peripheral blood
   d. Do not originate from hematopoietic cells
2. Which one of the following viruses is known to *cause* lymphoid neoplasms in humans?
   a. HIV-1
   b. HTLV-1
   c. Hepatitis B
   d. Parvovirus B
3. Loss-of-function of tumor suppressor genes increase the risk of hematologic neoplasms by:
   a. Suppressing cell division
   b. Activating tyrosine kinases which promote proliferation
   c. Promoting excessive apoptosis of hematopoietic cells
   d. Allowing cells with damaged DNA to progress through the cell cycle
4. Oncogenes are said to act in a dominant fashion because:
   a. Leukemia is a dominating disease that is systemic
   b. The oncogene product is a gain-of-function mutation
   c. A mutation in only one allele is sufficient to promote a malignant phenotype
   d. They are inherited by autosomal dominant transmission
5. Which one of the following is NOT one of the cellular abnormalities produced by oncogenes:
   a. Constitutive activation of a growth factor receptor
   b. Constitutive activation of a signaling protein
   c. Acceleration of DNA catabolism
   d. Dysregulation of apoptosis
6. Which one of the following is an example of a tumor suppressor gene?
   a. *ABL1*
   b. *RARA*
   c. *TP53*
   d. *JAK2*
7. G-CSF is provided as supportive treatment during leukemia treatment regimens to:
   a. Suppress GVHD
   b. Overcome anorexia
   c. Prevent anemia
   d. Reduce the risk of infection
8. Imatinib is an example of what type of leukemia treatment?
   a. Supportive care
   b. Chemotherapy
   c. Bone marrow conditioning agent
   d. Targeted therapy
9. Which one of the following is FALSE about epigenetic mechanisms?
   a. Epigenetic mechanisms control how genes are expressed and silenced.
   b. Micro RNAs can bind to specific mRNAs and block their translation.
   c. Hypermethylation of CpG islands in gene promoters result in their overactivation.
   d. Histone deacetylases keep chromatin of target genes in a closed inactive state.
10. Which one of the following is NOT a source of hematopoietic stem cells for transplantation:
    a. Spleen
    b. Bone marrow
    c. Peripheral blood
    d. Umbilical cord blood

REFERENCES

1. Nowell, P. C., & Hungerford, D. A. (1960). A minute chromosome in human granulocytic leukemia (Abstract). *Science, 132,* 1497.
2. Rowley, J. D. (1973). A new consistent chromosomal abnormality in chronic myelogenous leukemia identified by quinacrine fluorescence and Giemsa staining. *Nature, 243,* 290–293.
3. Taub, R., Kirsch, I., Morton, C., et al. (1982). Translocation of the c-myc gene into the immunoglobulin heavy chain locus in human Burkitt lymphoma and murine plasmacytoma cells. *Proc Natl Acad Sci USA, 79,* 7837–7841.
4. National Cancer Institute, Surveillance, Epidemiology, and End Results Program (SEER). Cancer Stat Facts: Leukemia. https://seer.cancer.gov/statfacts/html/leuks.html. Accessed May 15, 2018.

5. National Cancer Institute, Surveillance, Epidemiology, and End Results Program (SEER). Cancer Stat Facts: Non-Hodgkin Lymphoma. https://seer.cancer.gov/statfacts/html/nhl.html. Accessed May 15, 2018.

6. National Cancer Institute, Surveillance, Epidemiology, and End Results Program (SEER). Cancer Stat Facts: Hodgkin Lymphoma. https://seer.cancer.gov/statfacts/html/hodg.html. Accessed May 15, 2018..

7. Luo, G. G., & Ou, J.-H. J. (2015). Oncogenic viruses and cancer. *Virol Sin, 30*(2), 83–84.

8. Qayyum, S., & Choi, J. K. (2014). Adult T-cell leukemia/lymphoma. *Arch Pathol Lab Med, 138*(2), 282–286.

9. Vockerodt, M., Yap, L-F., Shannon-Lowe, C., et al. (2015). The Epstein–Barr virus and the pathogenesis of lymphoma. *J Pathol, 235,* 312–322.

10. Krishnan, A., & Zaia, J. A. (2014). HIV-associated non-Hodgkin lymphoma: viral origins and therapeutic options. *Hematology Am Soc Hematol Educ Program, 2014,* 584–589.

11. Malkin, D., Nichols, K. E., Zelley, K., et al. (2014). Predisposition to pediatric and hematologic cancers: a moving target. *Am Soc Clin Oncol Educ Book, 2014,* e44–55.

12. Ozaki, T., & Nakagawara, A. (2011). Role of p53 in cell death and human cancers. *Cancers, 3,* 994–1013.

13. Marechal, A., & Zou, L. (2013). DNA damage sensing by the ATM and ATR kinases. *Cold Spring Harb Perspect Biol, 5,* a012716.

14. Hasle, H., Clemmensen, I. H., & Mikkelsen, M. (2000). Risks of leukaemia and solid tumours in individuals with Down's syndrome. *Lancet, 355,* 165–169.

15. Swerdlow, S. H., Campo, E., Pileri, S. A., et al. (2016). The 2016 revision of the World Health Organization classification of lymphoid neoplasms. *Blood, 127,* 2375–2390.

16. Arber, D. A., Orazi, A., Hasserjian, R., et al. (2016). The 2016 revision to the World Health Organization classification of myeloid neoplasms and acute leukemia. *Blood, 127,* 2391–2405.

17. Stam, K., Heisterkamp, N., & Grosveld, G. (1985). Evidence of a new chimeric bcr/c-abl mRNA in patients with chronic myelocytic leukemia and the Philadelphia chromosome. *N Engl J Med, 313*(23), 1429–1433.

18. Daley, G. Q., Van Etten, R. A., & Baltimore, D. (1990). Induction of chronic myelogenous leukemia in mice by the P210bcr/abl gene of the Philadelphia chromosome. *Science, 247,* 824–830.

19. Calabretta, B., & Perrotti, D. (2004). The biology of CML blast crisis. *Blood, 103,* 4010–4022.

20. Lodish, H., Birk, A., Kaiser, C. A., et al. (2016). Cancer. In *Molecular Cell Biology.* (8th ed., pp. 1135–1166). New York: W.H. Freeman MacMillan.

21. Fong, C. Y., Morison, J., & Dawson, M. A. (2014). Epigenetics in the hematologic malignancies. *Haematologica, 99*(12), 1772–1783.

22. Weiss, C. N., & Ito, K. (2017). A macro view of microRNAs: the discovery of microRNAs and their role in hematopoiesis and hematologic disease. *Int Rev Cell Mol Biol, 334,* 99–175.

23. Knudson, A. G. (1985). Hereditary cancer, oncogenes, and antioncogenes. *Cancer Res, 45,* 1437–1443.

24. Zenz, T., Eichhorst, B., Busch, R., et al. (2010). TP53 mutation and survival in chronic lymphocytic leukemia. *J Clin Oncol, 28*(29), 4473–4479.

25. Druker, B. J. (2008). Translation of the Philadelphia chromosome into therapy for CML. *Blood, 112,* 4808–4817.

26. Hochhaus, A., Larson, R. A., Guilhot, F., et al. (2017). Long-term outcomes of imatinib treatment for chronic myeloid leukemia. *N Eng J Med, 376,* 917–927.

27. Schultz, K. R., Bowman, W. P., Aledo, A., et al. (2009). Improved early event-free survival with imatinib in Philadelphia chromosome-positive acute lymphoblastic leukemia: a children's oncology group study. *J Clin Oncol, 27,* 5175–5181.

28. Springuel, L., Renauld, J. C., & Knoops, L. (2015). JAK kinase targeting in hematologic malignancies: a sinuous pathway from identification of genetic alterations towards clinical indications. *Hematologica, 100,* 1240–1253.

29. Grunwald, M. R., & Levis, M. J. (2013). FLT3 inhibitors for acute myeloid leukemia: a review of their efficacy and mechanisms of resistance. *Int J Hematol, 97,* 683–694.

30. Downing, J. R. (2008). Targeted therapy in leukemia. *Mod Pathol, 21,* S2–S7.

31. Feugier, P. (2015). A review of rituximab, the first anti-CD20 monoclonal antibody used in the treatment of B non-Hodgkin's lymphomas. *Future Oncol, 11*(9), 1327–1342.

32. Goebeler, M. E., & Bargou, R. (2016). Blinatumomab: a CD19/CD3 bispecific T cell engager (BiTE) with unique anti-tumor efficacy. *Leuk Lymphoma, 57,* 1021–1032.

33. Kantarjian, H. M., DeAngelo, D. J., Stelljes, M., et al. (2016). Inotuzumab ozogamicin versus standard care for acute lymphoblastic leukemia. *N Engl J Med, 375*(8), 740–753.

34. Perales, M. A., Kebriaei, P., Kean, L. S., et al. (2018). Building a safer and faster CAR: seatbelts, airbags, and CRISPR. *Biol Blood Marrow Transplant, 24*(1), 27–31.

35. Duvic, M. (2015). Histone deacetylase inhibitors for cutaneous T-cell lymphoma. *Dermatol Clin, 33,* 757–764.

36. Voso, M. T., Lo-Coco, F., & Fianchi, L. (2015). Epigenetic therapy of myelodysplastic syndromes and acute myeloid leukemia. *Curr Opin Oncol, 27,* 532–539.

37. Rowley, S. D., & Donato, M. L. (2018). Practical aspects of hematologic stem cell harvesting and mobilization. In Hoffman, R., Benz, E. J., Silberstein, L. E., et al. (Eds.), *Hematology: Basic Principles and Practice.* (7th ed., pp. 1517–1530). Philadelphia: Elsevier.

Flow Cytometric Analysis in Hematologic Disorders

Magdalena Czader

OBJECTIVES

After completion of this chapter, the reader will be able to:

1. Describe the technique of flow cytometry, including specimen selection and preparation, instrumentation, data collection, and a design of an antibody panel.
2. Discuss the pattern recognition approach to analysis of flow cytometric data for diagnosis and follow-up of hematologic malignancies.
3. Identify basic cell populations defined by flow cytometric parameters.
4. Recognize key immunophenotypic features of normal bone marrow, peripheral blood, and lymph node tissue, and specimens from patients with acute leukemia or lymphoma.
5. Discuss applications of flow cytometry beyond the immunophenotyping of hematologic malignancies.

OUTLINE

CASE STUDIES

After studying the material in this chapter, the reader should be able to respond to the following case studies:

Case 1

A 58-year-old man had a 5-month history of extensive right cervical lymphadenopathy and night sweats. His complete blood count (CBC) results were within normal limits. Physical examination showed additional bilateral axillary lymphadenopathy. The cervical lymph node was excised. Histologic examination revealed nodular architecture with predominantly medium-sized lymphoid cells with irregular nuclear outlines. Flow cytometric data are presented in Figure 28.1.

1. What cell population predominates on the forward scatter (FS)/side scatter (SS) scattergram?
2. List antigens positive in this population.
3. Does the pattern of light chain expression support the diagnosis of lymphoma?

Case 2

A 3-year-old girl was brought to the physician because of fatigue and fevers. The CBC revealed a WBC count of 3×10^9/L, HGB level of 8.3 g/dL, and platelet count of 32×10^9/L. Review of the peripheral blood film showed rare undifferentiated blasts with occasional cytoplasmic blebs. No granules

Continued

CASE STUDIES—cont'd

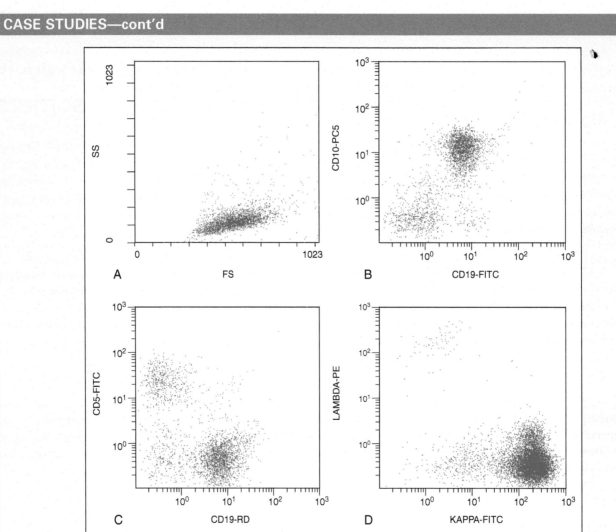

Figure 28.1 Scattergrams Showing Immunophenotypic Features of Lymphoid Cells from the Patient in Case 1. *FITC*, Fluorescein isothiocyanate; *FS*, forward scatter; *RD*, rhodamine; *SS*, side scatter.

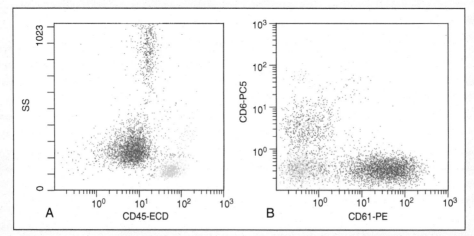

Figure 28.2 Predominant Bone Marrow Population for the Patient in Case 2. *ECD*, Phycoerythrin–Texas red; *PE*, phycoerythrin; *SS*, Side scatter.

or Auer rods were identified. Bone marrow examination showed a marked increase in blasts (79%) and decreased trilineage hematopoiesis. Flow cytometric analysis was performed. In addition to the markers shown in Figure 28.2, the population of interest was positive for CD34, CD33, CD41, and HLA-DR.

1. What abnormal features are observed on the CD45/SS scattergram?
2. What is the most likely diagnosis considering the constellation of markers expressed by the predominant population?

Flow cytometry was originally designed to measure physical properties of cells based on their ability to deflect light. Over the years it has evolved to include detection of fluorescent signals emitted by dyes bound directly to specific molecules or attached to proteins through monoclonal antibodies. The development of monoclonal antibodies is the most significant factor contributing to today's broad application of flow cytometry. Although the term *flow cytometry* implies the measurement of a cell, this technique is also applied to study other particles, including chromosomes, microorganisms, and proteins. The main advantage of flow cytometry over other techniques of cell analysis is its ability to rapidly and simultaneously analyze multiple parameters in a large number of cells. When one adds the capability of identifying and quantifying rare-event cells in a heterogeneous cell population, the value of flow cytometry to clinical hematology becomes obvious. This technique not only is applied to analysis of cell lineage in acute leukemia or a detection of clonality in lymphoid populations but also makes it possible to discern abnormal populations in chronic myeloid neoplasms, quantitate minimal residual disease, and monitor immunodeficiency states. Immunophenotypes that originally were used to supplement morphologic classification frequently correlate with specific cytogenetic or molecular abnormalities. As recommended by the World Health Organization classification of hematopoietic neoplasms,[1] current diagnostic algorithms integrate morphologic, immunophenotypic, and genotypic information. This approach emphasizes the central role that flow cytometry plays in a hematopathology laboratory.

This chapter is focused on the use of flow cytometry in a routine hematopathology laboratory. The chapter follows a "life" of a flow cytometric specimen that begins with specimen processing and ends with a final diagnosis. The discussion is divided into preanalytical (specimen processing), analytical (flow cytometric instrumentation and analysis), and postanalytical (immunophenotypic features of hematopoietic disorders) sections.

SPECIMEN PROCESSING

Flow cytometric analysis is particularly useful in diagnosing hematologic disorders. The specimens most commonly analyzed are bone marrow, peripheral blood, and lymphoid tissues. In addition, immunophenotyping is often performed on body cavity fluids and solid tissues when they are suspected to harbor a hematologic malignancy.[2]

Prolonged transport or transport under inappropriate conditions may render a specimen unsuitable for analysis. Peripheral blood and bone marrow specimens should be processed within 24 to 48 hours from the time of collection, dependent on the anticoagulant. Certain specimens, such as body cavity fluids or samples from neoplasms with a high proliferative activity, may require even more rapid processing.

When cells are suspended in a fluid, as in peripheral blood and bone marrow, minimal sample preparation is required. These specimens are collected into a tube or container with an anticoagulant, most commonly heparin or EDTA, and are transported to a flow cytometry laboratory at room temperature. Bone marrow biopsy specimens and solid tissue specimens, including core biopsy specimens, are submitted in culture media to maintain viability or on saline-moistened gauze. Tissue fragments are mechanically dissociated to yield a cell suspension, usually by mincing with a scalpel. Cellularity of a flow cytometry sample obtained from small biopsy specimens can be variable. Therefore when only a small biopsy specimen such as from a core needle biopsy can be obtained, a concurrent fine needle aspiration biopsy specimen is the preferred material for flow cytometry.[3]

To obtain a pure population of nucleated cells, red blood cells (RBCs) are lysed. Cellularity and viability of a specimen are routinely assessed before a sample is stained. Cell count can be obtained using automated cell counters or flow cytometry. A specimen is stained with propidium iodide or 7-amino actinomycin to test viability. A cytocentrifuge slide (Chapter 15) can be prepared for a morphologic inspection of a cell suspension.

As soon as these steps are completed, a sample is stained with a cocktail of fluorochrome-conjugated monoclonal antibodies. The analysis of intracytoplasmic markers requires an additional fixation and permeabilization step to allow antibodies to pass through a cell membrane. Typically a predetermined panel of antibodies may be used to detect membrane-bound and intracellular markers. In individual cases, particularly in patients with prior diagnoses and low cellularity samples, customized antibody panels may be used. Simultaneous analysis of multiple markers, known as *multicolor* or *multiparameter flow cytometry*, has numerous advantages. It facilitates visualization of antigen expression and maturation patterns, which are often disturbed in hematopoietic malignancies. In addition, regardless of a complexity of a specimen, analysis can be accomplished using few tubes and with a lower total number of cells, which saves reagents, time, and data storage. There is no consensus on the standardized panel of antibodies to be used in routine flow cytometric evaluation. The US-Canadian Consensus Project in Leukemia/Lymphoma Immunophenotyping recommends the comprehensive approach with multiple markers for myeloid and lymphoid lineage.[4] Selected markers commonly analyzed by flow cytometry are presented in Table 28.1.

FLOW CYTOMETRY: PRINCIPLE AND INSTRUMENTATION

The most significant discovery that led to the advancement of flow cytometry and its subsequent widespread application in clinical practice was the development of monoclonal antibodies.[5] In the original *hybridoma* experiments, lymphocytes with predetermined antibody specificity were cocultured with a myeloma cell line to form immortalized hybrid cells producing specific monoclonal antibodies. For this discovery, which not only fueled the development of flow cytometry but also had innumerable research and, more recently, clinical applications, Köhler and Milstein received a Nobel Prize in 1984. Over the years, numerous antibodies were produced and tested for their lineage specificity. Categorization of these antibodies and associated antigens is accomplished through workshops on human leukocyte differentiation antigens that have been held regularly since 1982. These workshops provide a forum for reporting new antigens and antibodies and define a cluster of antibodies recognizing the same antigen, called *cluster of differentiation* (CD) (Table 28.2; Table 28.1). Consecutive numbers are assigned

TABLE 28.1 Lineage-Associated Markers Commonly Analyzed in Routine Flow Cytometry

Lineage	Markers	Lineage	Markers
Immature	CD34	B lymphocytes	CD19
	CD117		CD20
	Terminal deoxynucleotidyl transferase		CD22
			κ Light chain
Granulocytic/monocytic	CD33		λ Light chain
	CD13	T lymphocytes	CD2
	CD15		CD3
	CD14		CD4
Erythroid	CD71		CD5
	Glycophorin A		CD7
			CD8
Megakaryocytic	CD41		
	CD42		
	CD61		

TABLE 28.2 Hematolymphoid Antigens Commonly Used in Clinical Flow Cytometry

Cluster of Differentiation	Function	Cellular Expression
CD1a	T cell development	Precursor T cells
CD2	T cell activation	Precursor and mature T cells, NK cells
CD3	Antigen recognition	Precursor and mature T cells
CD4	Coreceptor for HLA class II	Precursor T cells, helper T cells, monocytes
CD5	T cell signaling	Precursor and mature T cells, subset of B cells
CD7	T cell activation	Precursor and mature T cells, NK cells
CD8	Coreceptor for HLA class I	Precursor T cells, suppressor/cytotoxic T cells, subset of NK cells
CD10	B cell regulation	Precursor B cells, germinal center B cells, granulocytes
CD11b	Cell adhesion	Granulocytic and monocytic lineage, NK cells
CD13	Monocyte adhesion to endothelial cells	Granulocytic and monocytic lineage
CD14	Monocyte activation	Mature monocytes
CD15	Ligand for selectins	Granulocytic and monocytic lineage
CD16	Low-affinity IgG Fc receptor	Granulocytic and monocytic lineage, NK cells
CD18	Cell adhesion and signaling	Granulocytic and monocytic lineage
CD19	B cell activation	Precursor and mature B cells
CD20	B cell activation	Precursor and mature B cells
CD22	B cell activation and adhesion	Precursor and mature B cells
CD31	Cell adhesion	Megakaryocytes, platelets, leukocytes
CD33	Cell proliferation and survival	Granulocytic and monocytic lineage
CD34	Cell adhesion	Hematopoietic stem cells
CD36	Cell adhesion	Megakaryocytes, platelets, erythroid precursors, monocytes
CD38	Cell activation and proliferation	Hematopoietic cells, including activated lymphocytes and plasma cells
CD41	Cell adhesion	Megakaryocytes, platelets
CD42b	Receptor for von Willebrand factor	Megakaryocytes, platelets
CD45	T and B cell receptor activation	Hematopoietic cells
CD56	Cell adhesion	NK cells, subset of T cells
CD61	Cell adhesion	Megakaryocytes, platelets
CD62P	Homing	Platelets
CD63	Cell development, activation, growth, and motility	Platelets
CD64	High-affinity IgG Fc receptor	Granulocytic and monocytic lineage
CD71	Iron uptake	High density on erythroid precursors, low to intermediate density on other proliferating cells
CD79a	B cell receptor signal transduction	Precursor and mature B cells
CD117	Stem cell factor receptor	Hematopoietic stem cells, mast cells

Ig, Immunoglobulin; *NK,* natural killer.

to each new reported antigen. The Tenth International Conference on Human Leukocyte Differentiation Antigens listed over 370 clusters of differentiation.[6]

Monoclonal antibodies have numerous diagnostic applications and are increasingly used in immunotherapy. Common routine diagnostic methods using monoclonal antibodies are immunohistochemistry, immunofluorescence, and Western blot. These methods study cellular proteins in fixed tissues, or in cellular extracts; however, they do not examine antigens in their native state and cannot decipher composite cell populations with a complex antigen makeup. In contrast, flow cytometry can define antigen expression on numerous viable cells. Multiple antigens can be detected simultaneously on an individual cell.[7] This is accomplished by the conjugation of monoclonal antibodies to a variety of fluorochromes that can be detected directly by a flow cytometer. In a flow cytometer, particles stained with such monoclonal antibodies are suspended in fluid and pass one by one in front of a light source. As antibodies with fluorochromes are illuminated, they emit fluorescent signals registered by detectors. These results are later converted to digital output and analyzed using flow cytometry software.

The flow cytometer consists of fluidics, a light source (laser), a detection system, and a computer. A brief discussion of these basic components is presented in the following paragraph. To be analyzed individually, cells must pass separately, one by one, through the illumination and detection system of a flow cytometer. This is accomplished by injecting a cell suspension into a stream of sheath fluid. This technique, called *hydrodynamic focusing*, creates a central core of individually aligned cells surrounded by a sheath fluid (Figure 28.3). The central alignment is essential for consistent illumination of cells as they pass before a laser light source.

A laser is composed of a tube filled with gas, most commonly argon or helium-neon, and a power supply. Current is applied to the gas to raise electrons of a gas to an excited state. When electrons return to a ground state, they emit photons of light. Through an amplification system, a strong beam of light with light waves of identical direction, polarization plane, and wavelength is produced. This narrow coherent beam of light is used to illuminate individual cells, each stained with antibodies conjugated to specific fluorochromes.

After absorption of laser light, the electrons of fluorochromes are raised from a ground state to a higher energy state (Figure 28.4). The return to the original ground level is accompanied by a loss of energy, emitted as light of a specific wavelength. Flow cytometers are equipped with several photodetectors, each specific for light of a unique color (wavelength). The fluorescence from an individual cell is partitioned into different wavelengths through a series of filters (dichroic mirrors) and directed to the corresponding photodetector. Thus fluorescent signals derived from different fluorochromes attached to particular antibodies are registered separately.

In addition to fluorescence, scatter signals are recorded. The detector situated directly in line with the illuminating laser beam measures forward scatter (FS or FSC), which is proportional to particle volume or size. A photodetector located to the side measures side scatter (SS or SSC), which reflects surface complexity and internal structures such as granules and vacuoles. FS, SS, and fluorescence are displayed simultaneously on the instrument screen and registered by the computer.

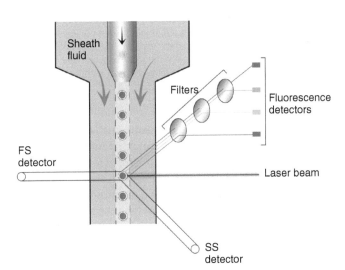

Figure 28.3 Diagram of a Flow Cytometer. As cells are injected into pressurized sheath fluid, they are positioned in the center of the stream and one by one exposed to the laser light. Forward scatter *(FS)* and side scatter *(SS)* are collected by separate detectors.

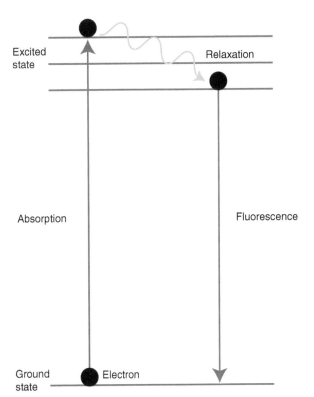

Figure 28.4 Jablonski Diagram Showing a Principle of Fluorescence. When electrons absorb energy, they are raised to the excited state. Subsequently, on their return to ground state, the absorbed energy is emitted in a form of fluorescence.

ANALYSIS OF FLOW CYTOMETRIC DATA

Concept of Gating

Cell populations with similar physical properties such as size, cytoplasmic complexity, and expression of a specific antigen form *clusters* on data displays generated by flow cytometers. A *gate* is an electronic boundary used by an operator to delineate cell clusters. Thus gating is a process of selecting a population of interest as defined by one or more flow cytometric parameters.

Gating can be applied at the time of data acquisition (live gate) or at the time of analysis. For diagnostic purposes, data are collected ungated; that is, all events detected by the flow cytometer are recorded. This allows comprehensive testing and retention of positive and negative internal controls. In addition, unexpected abnormal populations can be detected. Gating is most commonly applied after a specimen is run through a flow cytometer, when a target population is already known. In contrast, live gating focuses on the acquisition of data for a specific cell population as defined by flow cytometric parameters. For example, one can collect data only on CD19$^+$ B cells to facilitate detection of a small population of monoclonal B cells.

Analysis of Flow Cytometric Data

As with microscopic examination, an evaluation of flow cytometric data is based on an inspection of visual patterns. First, data are scanned to detect abnormal populations. Subsequent analysis focuses on antigenic properties of abnormal cells.

Analysis begins with inspection of dot plots presenting cell size, cytoplasmic complexity, and expression of panhematopoietic antigen CD45. As in microscopic examination at low magnification, an operator detects specific cell populations based on their physical properties (Figure 28.5). The identification of particular populations can be confirmed and further resolved on the scattergram of CD45 antigen and SS (Figure 28.6). This display also provides information on a relative proportion of specific cell populations in a flow cytometric sample. Lymphocytes show the highest density of CD45, with approximately 10% of the cell membrane occupied by this antigen. Granulocytic series show intermediate CD45 density; late erythroid precursors and megakaryocytes are negative for CD45. The CD45/SS display is particularly useful for detection of blasts, which overlap with lymphocytes, monocytes, or both on the FS/SS display.[8]

The FS/SS and CD45/SS displays allow the initial identification of the target population. Further analysis focuses on patterns of antigen expression, including qualitative data (antigen presence or absence) and fluorescence intensity as a relative measure of an antigen density.

CELL POPULATIONS IDENTIFIED BY FLOW CYTOMETRY

Surface and cytoplasmic markers expressed in hematologic malignancies resemble those of normal hematopoietic cell differentiation. Often, neoplastic cells are arrested at a particular stage of development and show aberrant antigen expression. Diagnosis

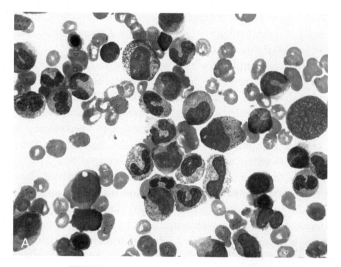

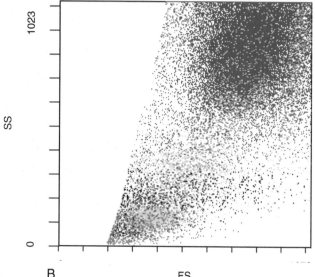

Figure 28.5 Main Cell Subpopulations of Normal Bone Marrow. (A), Bone marrow is composed of a heterogeneous population of cells of different sizes and variable complexity of cytoplasm (Wright-Giemsa stain, ×1000). **(B),** Dot plot of forward scatter (*FS*, cell size) versus side scatter (*SS*, internal complexity) reflects the heterogeneity of bone marrow subpopulations. Lymphocytes are smallest with negligible amount of agranular cytoplasm and are located closest to the origins of the axes *(aqua)*. Monocytes are slightly larger with occasional granules and vacuoles *(green)*. Granulocytic series shows prominent granularity *(navy)*.

and classification of hematologic neoplasms is based on the knowledge of normal hematopoietic maturation pathways.

In the past, differentiation of hematopoietic cells was defined by morphologic criteria. Over time it became clear that specific morphologic stages of development are accompanied by distinct changes in immunophenotype. Approximate morphologic-immunophenotypic correlates exist; however, because hematopoiesis is a continuous process, transitions between various developmental phases are not discrete.

All hematopoietic progeny are derived from pluripotent stem cells. These cells are morphologically unrecognizable and are defined by their functional and antigenic characteristics. They usually express a combination of CD34, CD117 *(c-kit)*, CD38,

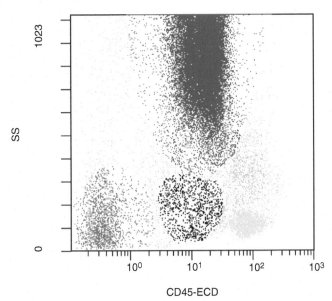

Figure 28.6 Scattergram Showing Differential Densities of Pan-Hematopoietic Marker CD45 on Bone Marrow Leukocytes. Lymphocytes *(aqua)* and monocytes *(green)* show highest density of CD45 antigen. Intermediate expression of CD45 is seen in the granulocytic population *(navy)* and blasts *(black)*. Erythroid precursors *(red)* are CD45−. *ECD,* Phycoerythrin–Texas red; *SS,* side scatter.

and HLA-DR antigens.[9] As hematopoietic cells mature, they lose stem cell markers and acquire lineage-specific antigens. A brief discussion of the maturation sequence of major hematopoietic cell lineages is presented in the following sections.

Granulocytic Lineage

The developmental stages of granulocytic lineage defined by the expression of specific antigens, correspond closely to the morphologic sequence.[10] The first morphologically recognizable cell committed to the granulocytic lineage is a myeloblast (Chapter 9). A myeloblast is characterized by an expression of immature cell markers CD34, CD38, HLA-DR, and stem cell factor receptor CD117. Pan-myeloid markers CD13 and CD33, present on all myeloid progeny, are first expressed at this stage. As a myeloblast matures to a promyelocyte, it loses CD34 and HLA-DR and acquires CD15 antigen. Further maturation to a myelocyte stage leads to an expression of CD11b, a temporary loss of CD13, and a gradual decrease in the density of CD33. Finally, as granulocytic cells near a band stage, CD16 is acquired, and the density of CD13 increases.

Monocytic Lineage

The earliest immunophenotype stage of monocytic development is defined by a gradual increase in the density of CD13, CD33, and CD11b antigens. Subsequent acquisition of CD15 and CD14 marks the transition to a promonocyte and mature monocyte. In contrast to the granulocytic series, strong expression of CD64 and HLA-DR antigens persists throughout monocytic maturation.

Erythroid Lineage

The majority of erythroid precursors do not express pan-hematopoietic marker CD45. The earliest marker of erythroid

differentiation is the transferrin receptor, CD71. The density of this antigen increases starting in the pronormoblast stage and is rapidly downregulated in reticulocytes.[11] In contrast, glycophorin A (CD235a), although present on reticulocytes and erythrocytes, first appears at the basophilic normoblast stage.

Megakaryocytic Lineage

The maturation sequence of megakaryocytes is less well defined. CD41 and CD61, referred to as glycoprotein IIb/IIIa complex, appear as the first markers of megakaryocytic differentiation. These antigens are present on a small subset of CD34+ cells believed to represent early megakaryoblasts.[9] CD31 and CD36, although not entirely specific for megakaryocytic lineage, also are present on megakaryoblasts. Subsequent maturation to megakaryocytes and platelets is characterized by the appearance of additional glycoproteins, CD42, CD62P, and CD63.

Lymphoid Lineage

The B and T lymphocytes are derived from lymphoid progenitors that express CD34, terminal deoxynucleotidyl transferase (TdT), and HLA-DR. Lymphoid differentiation is characterized by a continuum of changes in the expression of surface and intracellular antigens. The earliest B cell markers include CD19, cytoplasmic CD22, and cytoplasmic CD79.[12] As B cell precursors mature, they acquire the CD10 antigen. The appearance of the mature B cell marker CD20 coincides with the decrease in the expression of CD10. Another specific immature B cell marker is the cytoplasmic μ chain that eventually is transported to the surface and forms the B cell receptor. At this stage, the immunoglobulin chains in so-called naive B cells have become rearranged. The normal mature B cell population shows a mix of κ and λ light chain–expressing cells. The exclusive expression of only κ or λ molecules is a marker of clonality, seen often in mature B cell neoplasms. The differentiation of mature naive B cells, often recapitulated by B cell malignancies, is discussed in detail in Chapter 34.

Similar to B cell precursors, immature T cells express CD34 and TdT.[13] The first markers associated with T cell lineage are CD2, CD7, and cytoplasmic CD3. CD2 and CD7 are also present in natural killer (NK) cells and, along with the CD56 molecule, are used to detect NK cell–derived neoplasms. In T cells the expression of CD2, CD7, and cytoplasmic CD3 is followed by the appearance of CD1a and CD5 and coexpression of CD4 and CD8 antigens. Finally, the CD3 antigen appears on a cell surface, and CD4 or CD8 is lost. The sequential transition from double-negative (CD4−CD8−) through double-positive (CD4+CD8+) stages generates a population of mature helper (CD4+) and suppressor (CD8+) T cells. T cell differentiation occurs in a thymus.

FLOW CYTOMETRIC ANALYSIS OF MYELOID NEOPLASMS (ACUTE MYELOID LEUKEMIAS AND CHRONIC MYELOID NEOPLASMS)

In myeloid malignancies, flow cytometry is used for initial diagnosis, follow-up, and prognostication. Specific immunophenotypes are associated with select cytogenetic abnormalities. Because most myeloid malignancies are stem cell disorders, evaluation of blast population and maturing myeloid component is considered mandatory. Almost invariably, blasts are characterized by a low-density expression of CD45 antigen. In normal bone marrow a blast gate includes a relatively low number of cells showing the immature myeloid immunophenotype (Figure 28.6). In acute myeloid and lymphoblastic leukemias, this region becomes densely populated by immature cells, which reflects the increased number of blasts seen in a bone marrow (Figure 28.7). The location of the immature population on the CD45/SS displays depends on the subtype of acute myeloid leukemia (AML). In this chapter the immunophenotypic features of AML and chronic

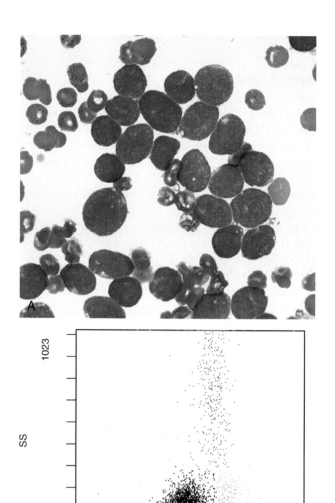

Figure 28.7 Bone Marrow Specimen Showing Acute Leukemia. Note uniform cytologic and flow cytometric characteristics. **(A),** Bone marrow aspirate from a patient with acute lymphoblastic anemia (Wright-Giemsa stain, ×500). **(B),** CD45 versus side scatter (SS) plot shows a homogeneous population of blasts with a marked decrease in normal hematopoietic elements. Compare with the heterogeneous pattern of normal bone marrow in Figure 28.5. *ECD,* Phycoerythrin–Texas red.

myeloid neoplasms are discussed in the context of the World Health Organization classification, which introduced categories defined by recurrent cytogenetic abnormalities.[1] These leukemias often show specific immunophenotypes and are discussed separately in the following sections.

Acute Myeloid Leukemias With Recurrent Cytogenetic Abnormalities

In most cases, AML with t(8;21)(q22;q22.1); *RUNX1/RUNX1T1* shows an immature myeloid immunophenotype with high-density CD34 and coexpression of CD19 and other B cell markers (Figure 28.8).[14] In addition, numerous myeloid antigens, including CD13, myeloperoxidase and often weak CD33, are expressed. Often there is asynchronous coexpression of CD34 and CD15. TdT is commonly present.

AML with inv (16)(p13.1q22) or t(16;16)(p13.1;q22);*CBFB/MYH11* is characterized by the presence of immature cells with expression of CD34, CD117, and TdT, and subpopulations of maturing cells showing monocytic (CD14, CD11b, CD4) and granulocytic (CD15) markers.[15] The aberrant coexpression of CD2 on the monocytic population is common.

Acute promyelocytic leukemia with *PML/RARA* shows a specific immunophenotype. In contrast to most less-differentiated acute myeloid leukemias, the majority of cases of acute promyelocytic leukemia manifest with high SS, which reflects the granular cytoplasm of leukemic cells (Figure 28.9). The constellation of immunophenotypic features used to diagnose acute promyelocytic leukemia includes lack of CD34, HLA-DR and leukocyte integrin antigens (CD11a, CD11b, CD18), presence of homogeneous strong CD33 along with myeloperoxidase and CD117, and variable CD13 and CD15.[16]

AMLs with t(9;11)(p21.3;q23.3); *KMT2A/MLLT3* in adults most commonly present with monocytic differentiation. The immunophenotypic features are nonspecific and can be seen in any acute myelomonocytic or monocytic leukemia (negative for CD34 and positive for CD33, CD13, CD14, CD4, CD11b, and CD64).

Acute Myeloid Leukemias, Not Otherwise Specified

In the least-differentiated AMLs—AML with minimal differentiation and AML without maturation—blasts are present in the region of low-density CD45 antigen and display low SS reflecting their relatively agranular cytoplasm. Even the least differentiated AML with minimal differentiation is usually positive for myeloid markers. The expression of CD13, CD33, and CD117 is common. Primitive hematopoietic antigens such as CD34, HLA-DR, and even TdT are often seen. Myeloperoxidase is absent or is expressed in only a few cells. The immunophenotypic profile of AML with maturation is similar, but more mature myeloid markers such as CD15 and myeloperoxidase are often expressed.

Occasionally, aberrant coexpression of antigens is seen. Simultaneous expression of early and late markers of myeloid differentiation on the leukemic blasts is not uncommon (asynchronous antigen expression). Similarly, markers specific for other lineages, such as lymphoid lineage, may be seen on

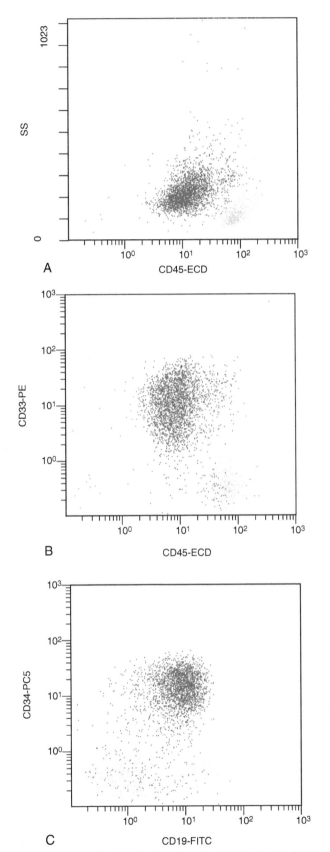

Figure 28.8 Acute Myeloid Leukemia with t(8;21)(q22;q22);*RUNX1-RUNX1T1.* **(A),** CD45 versus side scatter *(SS)* showing increase in blasts *(red)* with residual lymphocytes *(aqua).* **(B** and **C),** Blasts are positive for CD33 and CD34 with characteristic coexpression of CD19 antigen. *ECD,* Phycoerythrin–Texas red; *FITC,* fluorescein isothiocyanate.

myeloid blasts. The most common example is CD7 antigen, which is typically considered a T/NK cell–associated marker (Figure 28.10).

Acute myelomonocytic leukemia and acute monoblastic leukemia usually show higher expression of CD45, similar to normal monocytic precursors. In addition, in acute myelomonocytic leukemia, a population of primitive myeloid blasts is often seen (Figure 28.11). Acute monoblastic and monocytic leukemias express myeloid markers and antigens associated with monocytic lineage, such as CD14, CD4, CD11b, and CD64. Although CD14 is present on all mature monocytes, it may be absent in monocytic leukemias.[17] More immature monocytic markers, such as CD64, are more consistently expressed.

In pure erythroid leukemia leukemic cells are positive for erythroid markers such as CD71, glycophorin A, and hemoglobin. However, in more immature erythroid leukemias, glycophorin A and hemoglobin may be absent. In these cases, the diagnosis is based on the absence of myeloid markers, high expression of CD71, and scatter characteristics.

Acute megakaryoblastic leukemia usually shows low SS and low to absent CD45. Early megakaryocytic markers, CD41 and CD61, are often expressed (Figure 28.2).[18] Occasionally, the late megakaryocytic marker CD42b is present. The expression of stem cell markers CD34 and HLA-DR on the population of leukemic megakaryoblasts varies. Myeloid markers may be positive.

Myeloproliferative Neoplasms and Myelodysplastic Syndromes

The knowledge of antigen expression in the normal differentiation of myeloid lineages allows us to define the aberrant expression patterns commonly seen in chronic myeloid neoplasms. The abnormalities detected by flow cytometry reflect morphologic features (e.g., hypogranulation of neutrophils in myelodysplastic syndrome detected by low SS) and show changes in antigen expression. Qualitative (presence or absence of a particular antigen) and quantitative abnormalities (differences in the number of antigen molecules) can be used for diagnostic purposes. The interested reader is referred to review articles discussing the details of immunophenotyping in myelodysplastic syndromes and myeloproliferative neoplasms.[19-23] A few examples are highlighted to illustrate the role of flow cytometry in diagnosing these diseases.

SS abnormalities related to hypogranular neutrophils are seen in approximately 70% of myelodysplastic syndromes (Figure 28.12). In high-grade myelodysplastic syndrome and myeloproliferative neoplasms undergoing transformation, the increase in immature cells is seen. Blasts have a variety of aberrant immunophenotypic features, most commonly coexpression of CD7 and CD56 antigens. Blasts and maturing granulocytic precursors may show asynchronous expression of myeloid markers, including retention of CD34 and HLA-DR in late stages of maturation or late myeloid markers presenting early in differentiation, such as CD15 on myeloblasts. Asynchronous coexpression of markers can also be seen in monocytic and erythroid lineages. Aberrant immunophenotypes are seen in 98% of cases of myelodysplastic syndrome. More importantly,

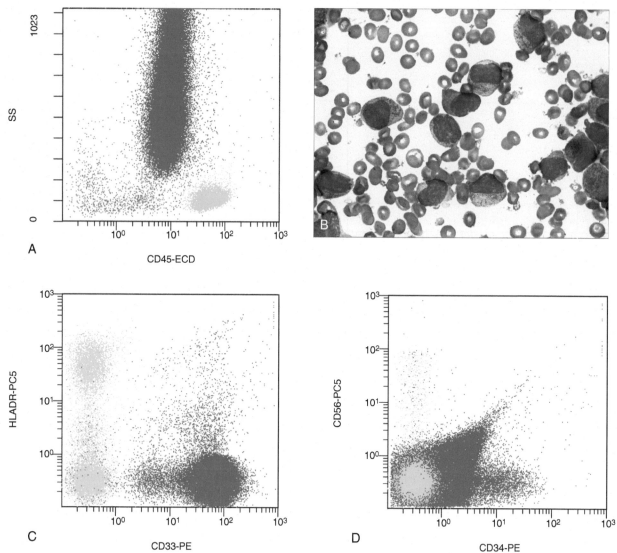

Figure 28.9 Acute Promyelocytic Leukemia with *PML-RARA.* **(A),** Typical side scatter *(SS)* pattern in acute promyelocytic leukemia corresponding to prominent granularity of leukemic cells *(red).* Residual lymphocytes are shown in aqua. **(B),** Numerous leukemic promyelocytes with distinct granules and occasional Auer rods (Wright-Giemsa stain, ×1000). **(C),** Leukemic cells show high-density expression of CD33 antigen and lack HLA-DR. **(D),** Similarly, CD34 antigen is absent or present in only a few leukemic cells. *ECD,* Phycoerythrin–Texas red; *PC5,* phycoerythrin-cyanine 5; *PE,* phycoerythrin; *SS,* side scatter.

immunophenotypic abnormalities can be seen in cases with minimal or no morphologic dysplasia.[19] Other studies underscore the significance of immunophenotypic abnormalities in predicting the outcome after stem cell transplantation.[23]

The utility of flow cytometry in myeloproliferative neoplasms is less well established. Specifically, the application of flow cytometry as a diagnostic tool in chronic myeloid leukemia is limited to an accelerated or blast phase, in which a lineage of a blast population needs to be determined. In a chronic phase the presence of *BCR-ABL1* rearrangement (Philadelphia chromosome) demonstrated by conventional karyotyping or molecular studies remains the defining feature of this disease. Other myeloproliferative neoplasms are not well studied. In general, flow cytometric abnormalities are seen in most cases with abnormal karyotype.[21] No consistent set of

immunophenotypic features that can be routinely used in the workup of myeloproliferative states has been described.

FLOW CYTOMETRIC ANALYSIS OF LYMPHOID NEOPLASMS (LYMPHOBLASTIC LEUKEMIA/LYMPHOMA AND MATURE LYMPHOID NEOPLASMS)

Similar to myeloid neoplasms, a diagnosis of lymphoid malignancies relies on the expression of lineage-associated markers corresponding to specific stages of lymphoid development. No single marker can be used for lineage assignment, and a diagnosis is typically based on the presence of several B cell or T cell antigens. The sentinel feature of mature B and T cells is the

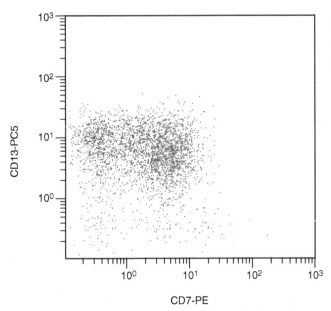

Figure 28.10 Myeloblasts of Acute Myeloid Leukemia Show Aberrant Coexpression of CD7 Antigen. *PE,* Phycoerythrin; *PC5,* phycoerythrin-cyanine 5.

presence of surface receptor complexes. The immune system responds to a wide array of antigens; in healthy individuals, B and T cells express a great diversity of surface immunoglobulin and T cell receptor complexes (polyclonal populations). A neoplastic lymphoid population is characterized by an expression of a monoclonal B or T cell receptor. In most cases a clonality confirms the malignant nature of lymphoid proliferation. In contrast, lymphoid precursors are generally negative for surface immunoglobulin and T cell receptors and instead carry immature markers. In lymphoblastic (precursor-derived) neoplasms, an expansion of a population with homogeneous marker expression, rather than clonality, is diagnostic of malignancy. The following section presents the key immunophenotypic features of lymphoblastic leukemias and lymphomas. Selected examples of associations between the immunophenotype and the genotype are discussed.

B Lymphoblastic Leukemia/Lymphoma

B lymphoblastic leukemia/lymphoma (B-LL) is derived from lymphoblasts and is positive for CD19, CD22, CD79a, HLA-DR,

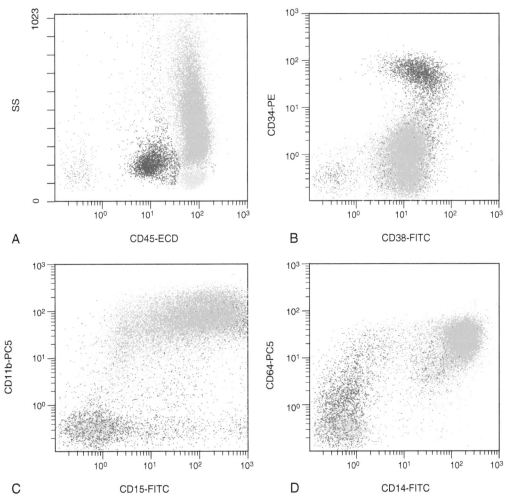

Figure 28.11 Peripheral Blood Immunophenotyping in Acute Myelomonocytic Leukemia. (A), CD45 versus side scatter *(SS)* display shows myeloid blasts *(red)* and a monocytic population *(green).* **(B–D),** Primitive leukemic blasts are positive for CD34 and negative for CD14. In contrast, monocytic population does not express CD34 and shows positivity for mature monocyte marker CD14 and characteristic monocytic pattern of CD11b and CD15 expression. *ECD,* Phycoerythrin–Texas red; *FITC,* fluorescein isothiocyanate; *PC5,* phycoerythrin-cyanine 5.

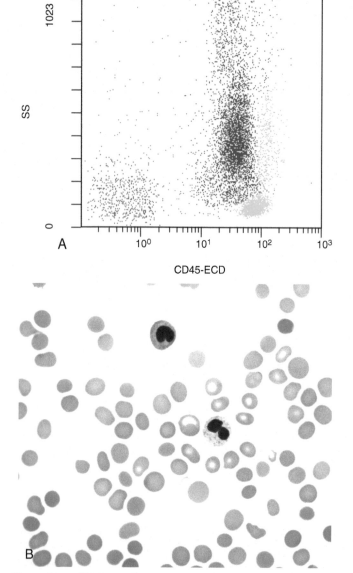

Figure 28.12 Myelodysplastic Syndrome. (A), Low side scatter *(SS)* of hypogranular neutrophils seen in most cases of myelodysplastic syndrome *(navy)*. **(B),** Corresponding photomicrograph of markedly dysplastic, hypogranular neutrophils in myelodysplastic syndrome (Wright-Giemsa stain, ×1000). *ECD,* Phycoerythrin–Texas red.

and TdT (Figure 28.13). The expression of CD34 and CD10 is often seen. Surface immunoglobulin light chains are not present. Cytoplasmic μ chain or surface immunoglobulin M (IgM) may be detected, however. Because B-LL can arise at any stage of B cell differentiation, the presence of several specific markers usually defines early precursor, intermediate, and pre-B stages. Often, immunophenotypes correlate with the cytogenetic and clinical features. In routine practice, confirmation of cytogenetic abnormality using conventional karyotyping or molecular techniques is necessary.

B Lymphoblastic Leukemia/Lymphoma with t(v;11q23);*KMT2A*–Rearranged

KMT2A gene rearrangements occur most often in infant B-LL. In contrast to other B-LLs, blasts in this leukemia are negative for CD10 antigen.[24] CD19, CD34, TdT, and occasionally myeloid markers are present. The more mature B cell marker CD20 is absent.

B Lymphoblastic Leukemia/Lymphoma with t(9;22)(q34;q11.2);*BCR-ABL1*

Philadelphia chromosome, t(9;22);*BCR-ABL1*, is a hallmark of chronic myeloid leukemia but also can occur in de novo pediatric and adult B-LL. These cases benefit from an addition of tyrosine kinase inhibitor to the chemotherapy regimen, and it is important to identify them promptly. Most *BCR-ABL1*–positive cases have a classic intermediate or common B-LL immunophenotype with the expression of CD19, CD10, CD34, and TdT. The presence of myeloid markers CD13 and CD33 and the lack or decreased expression of CD38 antigen on leukemic blasts are common. The density of antigens and their homogeneous or heterogeneous expression within leukemic populations correlates closely with the presence of *BCR-ABL1*.[25]

B Lymphoblastic Leukemia/Lymphoma, *BCR-ABL1*-like

BCR-ABL1-like B-LL does not have *BCR-ABL1* rearrangement; however, it shows a gene expression pattern similar to *BCR-ABL1*–positive cases[1] and often has rearrangements of other tyrosine kinases. It occurs in 10% to 25% of patients diagnosed with B-LL. Diagnosis can be challenging without gene expression profiling. Flow cytometry can be used as a screening tool to identify overexpression of CRLF2 protein (Figure 28.13D), which is seen in approximately 40% to 50% of *BCR-ABL*-like B-LL cases. Patients with this leukemia are treated using regimens including tyrosine kinase inhibitors.

T Lymphoblastic Leukemia/Lymphoma

T lymphoblastic leukemia/lymphoma (T-LL) is derived from immature cells committed to T cell lineage. T-LL expresses a combination of markers reflecting the stage of T cell differentiation. CD3 is the most specific T cell marker. As with normal T cells, this antigen is seen initially in the cytoplasm before appearing on the cell surface. Other T cell antigens include CD2, CD7, CD5, CD1a, CD4, and CD8. Usually a series of these antigens is detected, recapitulating the T cell differentiation (Figure 28.14). CD34 and CD10 may be present. As in other lymphoid neoplasms, the panel of markers determines the lineage.

Mature Lymphoid Neoplasms

B and T cell lymphomas display immunophenotypes resembling their normal counterparts. The immunophenotypic features of lymphomas are discussed in detail in Chapter 34 and are summarized in Table 34.6. The flow cytometric workup of lymphomas is facilitated by the *clonal* origin of mature lymphoid neoplasms, which implies that the malignant population is derived from a single cell. Therefore all neoplastic cells typically show similar genetic and immunophenotypic features. This stands in strong contrast to variable immunophenotypes of normal lymphoid populations, reflecting a process of antigen-driven selection.

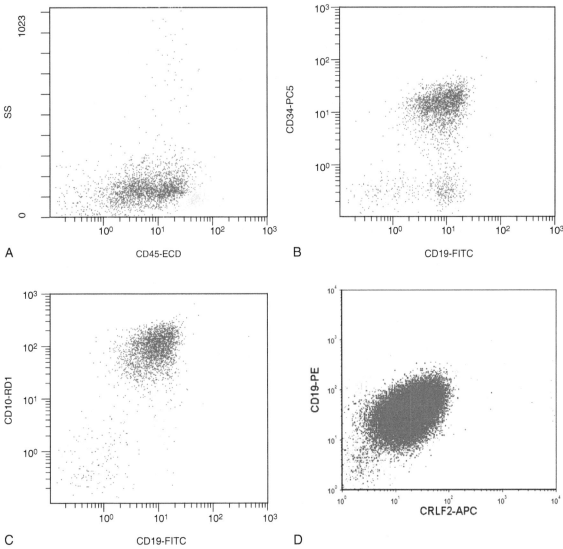

Figure 28.13 B Lymphoblastic Leukemia/Lymphoma. **(A),** Low-density CD45 antigen characteristic of the blast population. **(B),** Uniform expression of CD34 and CD19 on leukemic blasts. **(C),** High-density CD10 on CD19+ blasts. **(D),** Leukemic blasts positive for CRLF2 antigen are seen in a proportion of cases of B lymphoblastic leukemia/lymphoma, *BCR-ABL1*-like. *APC,* Allophycocyanin; *ECD,* phycoerythrin–Texas red; *FITC,* fluorescein isothiocyanate; *PC5,* phycoerythrin-cyanine 5; *PE,* phycoerythrin; *SS,* Side scatter.

Mature B Cell Neoplasms

Normal precursor B cells randomly rearrange immunoglobulin heavy and light chain genes. As a result, a mature B cell population expresses a mix of heavy and light chains (Figure 28.15A). In contrast, a monoclonal (monotypic) surface light chain expression, exclusively κ or λ, is seen in most B cell lymphomas (Figure 28.15B). Light chain monoclonality along with the expression of pan–B cell markers is diagnostic of B cell lymphoma. Rarely, lymphomas may lose the expression of surface light chains, a feature not seen in normal mature B cells.[26] In most cases of plasma cell myeloma, neoplastic plasma cells lack surface immunoglobulin light chains and express only cytoplasmic κ or λ.

Mature T Cell Neoplasms

In T cells, similar to B cells, clonality in most cases indicates malignancy. In the majority of laboratories the clonality of

T cells is confirmed by using a molecular analysis of T cell receptor genes. However, flow cytometry can also be used to detect clonality in most cases of T cell lymphoma.[27] This technique uses a broad array of antibodies against variable regions of T cell receptors. Because this methodology is not widely available, often a diagnosis of T cell lymphoma is based on an aberrant T cell immunophenotype. In most cases a loss or atypical expression of a lymphoid marker can be shown using flow cytometry. For example, mycosis fungoides/Sézary syndrome is characterized by a mature T cell immunophenotype with expression of CD2, surface CD3, CD5, and CD4 and with a loss of the CD7 antigen (Figure 28.16). Over the years it has been shown that the aberrant immunophenotype is a reliable diagnostic feature when the neoplastic population is sizeable. However, small numbers of T cells with unusual antigen makeup can appear in inflammatory conditions[28]; thus the

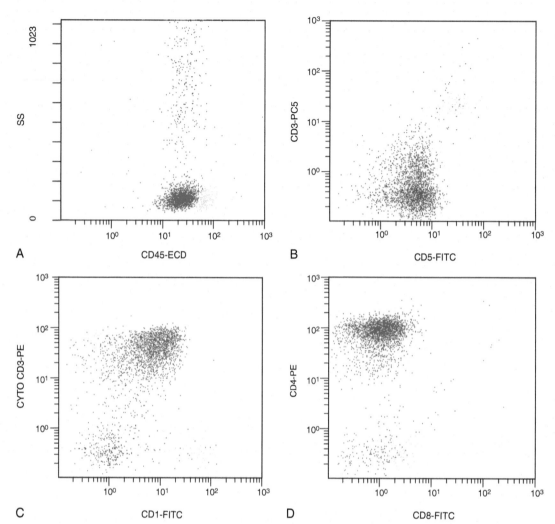

Figure 28.14 T Lymphoblastic Leukemia/Lymphoma. (A), Predominant population in the blast gate. (**B** and **C**), Although CD3 antigen is absent from the surface of leukemic cells, it is present in blast cytoplasm, confirming the precursor T cell origin of the leukemia. (**C**), Note residual normal T cells *(aqua)* positive for surface CD3 and CD5 antigens. (**D**), Simultaneous expression of CD4 and CD8 antigens. *ECD,* Phycoerythrin–Texas red; *FITC,* fluorescein isothiocyanate; *PC5,* phycoerythrin-cyanine 5; *PE,* phycoerythrin; *SS,* side scatter.

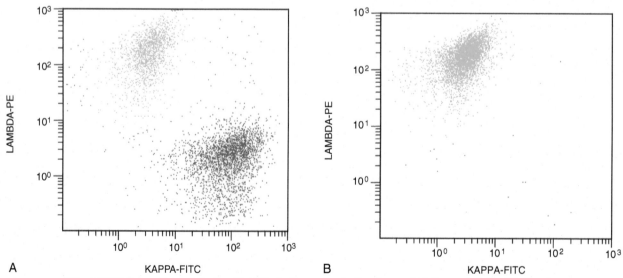

Figure 28.15 Comparison of Surface Light Chain Expression in Reactive and Malignant B Cells. (A), Reactive B cells show heterogeneous expression of κ and λ. **(B),** B cell lymphomas are monoclonal (monotypic), with the entire lymphoma population expressing only one type of light chain. *FITC,* Fluorescein isothiocyanate; *PE,* phycoerythrin.

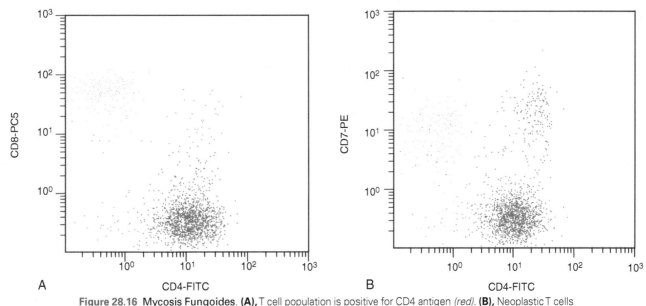

Figure 28.16 Mycosis Fungoides. **(A),** T cell population is positive for CD4 antigen *(red).* **(B),** Neoplastic T cells show loss of CD7 *(green). FITC,* Fluorescein isothiocyanate; *PC5,* phycoerythrin-cyanine 5; *PE,* phycoerythrin.

aberrant immunophenotype alone cannot be considered pathognomonic of T cell malignancy.

OTHER APPLICATIONS OF FLOW CYTOMETRY BEYOND IMMUNOPHENOTYPING OF HEMATOLOGIC MALIGNANCIES

The immunophenotyping of hematolymphoid neoplasms is one of many applications of flow cytometry. Other common applications include a diagnosis and monitoring of immunodeficiency states, diagnosis of paroxysmal nocturnal hemoglobinuria (PNH), stem cell enumeration, cell cycle analysis, detection of fetal hemoglobin, and monitoring of sepsis.

Select primary (inherited) and secondary (acquired) immunodeficiencies can be diagnosed using flow cytometry. Both a loss of specific antigens (e.g., CD11/CD18 in leukocyte adhesion deficiency) and functional defects (e.g., oxidative burst evaluation in chronic granulomatous disease) can be assayed by flow cytometry.

Human immunodeficiency virus (HIV) infection causes a progressive decrease in the number of CD4$^+$ helper T cells. The absolute number of helper T cells in peripheral blood correlates with the stage of the disease and with patient prognosis. The enumeration of T cells and their subsets is easily accomplished by flow cytometry using antibodies against CD4 and CD8 antigens. The absolute numbers are derived by performing a routine white blood cell (WBC) count on the concurrent peripheral blood specimen or by running calibrating beads simultaneously with the patient specimen. The CD4:CD8 ratio in healthy individuals is typically greater than 1. There is a significant decrease in numbers of CD4-positive T cells in HIV-positive patients, resulting in a reversed CD4:CD8 ratio. Because the CD4 lymphocyte depletion is associated with various infections, the absolute number of CD4 positive lymphocytes serves also as a guide for antibiotic prophylaxis in HIV-positive patients.

The diagnostic approach to PNH is a prime example of how an application of flow cytometry increases understanding of hematologic disorders and directly contributes to clinical decision making (Chapter 21).[29] Before the development of the flow cytometric assays, PNH diagnosis was based on detection of increased susceptibility of RBCs to lysis by the Ham or sucrose hemolysis tests, both of which showed inconsistent sensitivity. Flow cytometry significantly improved the sensitivity and specificity of PNH testing. The decreased expression of glycosylphosphatidylinositol-anchored proteins on RBCs, granulocytes, and monocytes of PNH patients can be measured by flow cytometry. The loss of these proteins is diagnostic of PNH and correlates with clinical symptoms. Typically, several markers are investigated simultaneously including CD59, CD24, CD14 and aerolysin. The latter is not present on human cells in vivo; however, it binds to glycosylphosphatidylinositol anchors in an in vitro assay (Figure 28.17).

Another important application of flow cytometry is cell sorting. During sorting, a heterogeneous cell population is physically divided into subsets according to their physical or immunophenotypic properties. High-speed sorting is achieved by charging droplets containing individual cells of interest. As the charged droplet passes through the electrostatic field, it is isolated from the remainder of the sample and collected into a separate container. The primary clinical application of cell sorting is in stem cell transplantation. More recently cell sorting has been used to isolate rare cells for genetic analysis.

Initially, flow cytometry was primarily confined to the hematopathology and research laboratories. Over the years, its use expanded to bone marrow transplantation, transfusion medicine, coagulation, microbiology, molecular pathology, and drug development. Examples of these applications include tissue typing, molecular testing for neoplasia-associated

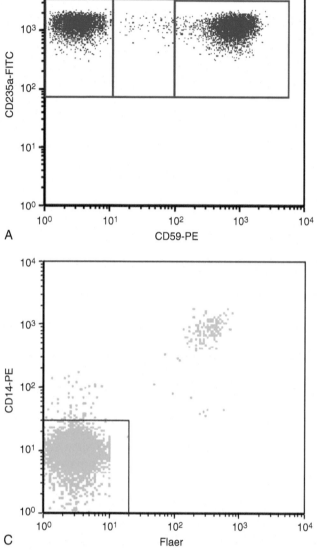

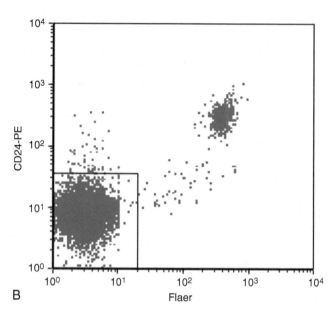

Figure 28.17 Diagnosis of Paroxysmal Nocturnal Hemoglobinuria (PNH) is Based on the Decreased Expression of Glycosylphosphatidylinositol (GPI)–Linked Molecules. Different levels of GPI-anchored proteins are best visualized in red blood cells (RBCs) using an antibody against CD59 antigen. **(A),** RBCs from a patient diagnosed with PNH. Three populations of RBCs are seen with variable expression of CD59 molecule. Type I cells show normal level of CD59 expression *(rightmost box)*. A few cells show a slight decrease in CD59 level (type II cells). A prominent population of RBCs negative for CD59 antigen is also seen (type III cells, *leftmost box*). **(B),** Granulocytes in PNH show a complete loss of CD24 and FLAER (in *black box*). A small population of normal granulocytes positive for CD24 and FLAER is also seen. **(C),** PNH monocytes negative for CD14 and FLAER, and a few normal monocytes positive for both antigens are seen. *FITC,* Fluorescein isothiocyanate; *FLAER,* fluorescent aerolysin; *PE,* phycoerythrin.

translocations, evaluation of drug response, such as monitoring platelet activation after antiplatelet therapy or after cellular therapies such as chimeric antigen receptor (CAR) T cells after infusion.

Flow cytometry is a mature field that in recent years experienced a revival with a focus on high-throughput testing for simultaneous analysis of multiple biologic constituents. New approaches to a single cell analysis such as spectral flow cytometry and an integration of mass spectrometry with single cell fluidics provide a superior resolution and expand the number of parameters that can be measured in any given cell. These methodologies are still predominantly research tools; however, they have opened new avenues to diagnostic immunophenotyping in hematopathology.[30,31]

■ SUMMARY

- Flow cytometry measures physical, antigenic, and functional properties of particles suspended in a fluid.
- Multiparameter flow cytometry is a technique routinely used for a diagnosis and follow-up of hematologic disorders.
- The characterization of complex specimens is achieved through analysis of multiple parameters in individual cells and the simultaneous display of data for thousands of cells. The cell size, cytoplasmic complexity, and immunophenotypic features

detected by monoclonal antibodies conjugated to various fluorochromes are analyzed in clinical specimens.
- A key starting point in flow cytometric analysis is a fresh high-quality specimen.
- A flow cytometer consists of fluidics, a light source (laser), multiple detectors, and a computer.
- As with microscopic examination, an evaluation of flow cytometric data is based on the inspection of visual patterns.

Initially the entire sample is scanned for the presence of abnormal populations. Subsequently, detailed immunophenotypic features of cell subsets are studied.

- The immunophenotyping of hematologic specimens is based on knowledge of the maturation patterns of hematopoietic cells. In comparison to normal cells, malignant myeloid and lymphoid cells and cell populations in nonneoplastic hematologic disorders show significant qualitative and quantitative differences in antigen expression.
- Flow cytometric analysis of acute leukemia determines a lineage of leukemic cells. In select entities, immunophenotype corresponds to the underlying genetic lesion.

- Immunophenotyping of myelodysplastic syndromes and chronic myeloproliferative neoplasms is an advanced application of clinical flow cytometry.
- The clonality of mature B cell and T cell neoplasms can be detected by flow cytometry.
- Flow cytometric analysis is used for diagnosis and monitoring of immunodeficiencies, stem cell enumeration, detection of fetal hemoglobin, tissue typing, molecular analysis, and drug testing.

Now that you have completed this chapter, go back and read again the case studies at the beginning and respond to the questions presented.

REVIEW QUESTIONS

Answers can be found in the Appendix.

1. What is the most common clinical application of flow cytometry?
   a. Diagnosis of platelet disorders
   b. Detection of fetomaternal hemorrhage
   c. Diagnosis of leukemias and lymphomas
   d. Differentiation of anemias

2. Which of the following is true of CD45 antigen?
   a. It is present on every cell subpopulation in the bone marrow.
   b. It is expressed on all hematopoietic cells, with the exception of megakaryocytes and late erythroid precursors.
   c. It is not measured routinely in flow cytometry.
   d. It may be present on nonhematopoietic cells.

3. Erythroid precursors are characterized by the expression of:
   a. CD71
   b. CD20
   c. CD61
   d. CD3

4. In Figure 28.2A, the cell population colored in aqua represents:
   a. Monocytes
   b. Nonhematopoietic cells
   c. Granulocytes
   d. Lymphocytes

5. Antigens expressed by B-LL include:
   a. CD3, CD4, and CD8
   b. CD19, CD34, and CD10
   c. There are no antigens specific for B-LL.
   d. Myeloperoxidase

6. Which of the following is true of flow cytometric gating?
   a. It is best defined as selection of a target population for flow cytometric analysis.
   b. It can be done only at the time of data acquisition.
   c. It can be done only at the time of final analysis and interpretation of flow cytometric data.
   d. It is accomplished by adjusting flow rate.

7. Collection of ungated events:
   a. Facilitates comprehensive analysis of all cells
   b. Does not help in detection of unexpected abnormal populations
   c. Allows the collection of data on a large number of rare cells
   d. Is used for leukemia diagnosis only

8. Mycosis fungoides is characterized by:
   a. Loss of certain antigens compared with the normal T cell population
   b. Polyclonal T cell receptor
   c. Immunophenotype indistinguishable from that of normal T cells
   d. Expression of CD3 and CD8 antigens

9. Mature granulocytes show the expression of:
   a. CD15, CD33, and CD34
   b. CD15, CD33, and CD41
   c. CD15, CD33, and CD13
   d. CD15, CD33, and CD7

10. During the initial evaluation of flow cytometric data, cell size, cytoplasmic complexity, and expression of CD45 antigen are used to define cell subpopulations. Which of the following parameters defines cytoplasmic complexity/granularity?
    a. SS
    b. FS
    c. CD45
    d. HLA-DR

11. The most important feature of the mature neoplastic B cell population is:
    a. The presence of a specific immunophenotype with expression of CD19 antigen
    b. A clonal light chain expression (i.e., exclusively κ- or λ-positive population)
    c. A clonal T cell receptor expression
    d. Aberrant expression of CD5 antigen on CD19$^+$ cells

REFERENCES

1. Swerdlow, S. H., Campo, E., Harris, N. L., et al. (Eds.). (2016). *WHO Classification of Tumours of Haematopoietic and Lymphoid Tissues.* (Revised 4th ed.). Lyon, France: IARC Press.

2. Czader, M., & Ali, S. Z. (2003). Flow cytometry as an adjunct to cytomorphologic analysis of serous effusions. *Diagn Cytopathol, 29,* 74–78.

3. Czader, M., Chiu, A., Perkins, S., et al. (2014). Core Needle Biopsy in Lymphoma Diagnosis: A Multi-Institutional Study. *Mod Pathol, 27*(Suppl. 2), 344A.

4. Wood, B. L., Arroz, M., Barnett, D., et al. (2007). 2006 Bethesda International Consensus recommendations on the immunophenotypic analysis of hematolymphoid neoplasia by flow cytometry: optimal reagents and reporting for the flow cytometric diagnosis of hematopoietic neoplasia. *Cytometry B Clin Cytom, 72,* S14–S22.

5. Köhler, G., & Milstein, C. (1975). Continuous cultures of fused cells secreting antibody of predefined specificity. *Nature, 256,* 495–497.

6. Human Cell Differentiation Molecules. http://hcdm.org. Accessed February 19, 2018.

7. Rajab, A., Axler, O., Leung, J., et al. (2017). Ten-color 15-antibody flow cytometry panel for immunophenotyping of lymphocyte population. *Int J Lab Hematol, 39*(Suppl. 1), 76–85.

8. Borowitz, M. J., Guenther, K. L., Shults, K. E., et al. (1993). Immunophenotyping of acute leukemia by flow cytometric analysis: use of CD45 and right-angle light scattered to gate on leukemic blasts in three-color analysis. *Am J Clin Pathol, 100,* 534–540.

9. Macedo, A., Orfao, A., Ciudad, J., et al. (1995). Phenotypic analysis of CD34 subpopulations in normal human bone marrow and its application for the detection of minimal residual disease. *Leukemia, 9,* 1896–1901.

10. Terstappen, L. W., Safford, M., & Loken, M. R. (1990). Flow cytometric analysis of human bone marrow: III. Neutrophil maturation. *Leukemia, 4,* 657–663.

11. Loken, M. R., Shah, V. O., Dattilio, K. L., et al. (1987). Flow cytometric analysis of human bone marrow: I. Normal erythroid development. *Blood, 69,* 255–263.

12. Ciudad, J., Orfao, A., Vidriales, B., et al. (1998). Immunophenotypic analysis of CD19+ precursors in normal human adult bone marrow: implications for minimal residual disease detection. *Haematologica, 83,* 1069–1075.

13. Terstappen, L. W., Huang, S., & Picker, L. J. (1992). Flow cytometric assessment of human T cell differentiation in thymus and bone marrow. *Blood, 79,* 666–677.

14. Andrieu, V., Radford-Weiss, I., Troussard, X., et al. (1996). Molecular detection of t(8;21)/AML1-ETO in AML M1/M2: correlation with cytogenetics, morphology and immunophenotype. *Br J Haematol, 92,* 855–865.

15. Adriaansen, H., Boekhorst, P. A. W., Hagemeijer, A. M., et al. (1993). Acute myeloid leukemia M4 with bone marrow eosinophilia (M4Eo) and inv(16)(p13q22) exhibits a specific immunophenotype with CD2 expression. *Blood, 81,* 3043–3051.

16. Lo Coco, F., Avvisati, G., Diverio, D., et al. (1991). Rearrangements of the RAR-alpha gene in acute promyelocytic leukaemia: correlations with morphology and immunophenotype. *Br J Haematol, 78,* 494–499.

17. Krasinskas, A. M., Wasik, M. A., Kamoun, M., et al. (1998). The usefulness of CD64, other monocyte-associated antigens, and CD45 gating in the subclassification of acute myeloid leukemias with monocytic differentiation. *Am J Clin Pathol, 110,* 797–805.

18. Helleberg, C., Knudsen, H., Hansen, P. B., et al. (1994). CD34+ megakaryoblastic leukaemic cells are CD38−, but CD61+ and glycophorin A+: improved criteria for diagnosis of AML-M7? *Leukemia, 11,* 830–834.

19. Stetler-Stevenson, M., Arthur, D. C., Jabbour, N., et al. (2001). Diagnostic utility of flow cytometric immunophenotyping in myelodysplastic syndrome. *Blood, 98,* 979–987.

20. Porwit, A., van de Loosdrecht, A.A., Bettelheim, P., et al. (2014). Revisiting guidelines for integration of flow cytometry results in the WHO classification of myelodysplastic syndromes-proposal from the International/European LeukemiaNet Working Group for Flow Cytometry in MDS. *Leukemia, 28,* 1793–1798.

21. Kussick, S. J., & Wood, B. L. (2003). Four-color flow cytometry identifies virtually all cytogenetically abnormal bone marrow samples in the workup of non-CML myeloproliferative disorders. *Am J Clin Pathol, 120,* 854–865.

22. Zhang, S., Zhou, J., Nassiri, M., et al. (2013). Diagnostic approach to myelodysplastic syndrome. In Sayar, H., (Ed.), *Myelodysplastic Syndrome* (pp. 25–60). Hauppauge, NY: Nova Science Publishers.

23. Wells, D. A., Benesch, M., Loken, M. R., et al. Myeloid and monocytic dyspoiesis as determined by flow cytometric scoring in myelodysplastic syndrome correlates with the IPSS and with outcome after hematopoietic stem cell transplantation. *Blood, 102,* 394–403.

24. Harbott, J., Mancini, M., Verellen-Dumoulin, C., et al. (1998). Hematological malignancies with a deletion of 11q23: cytogenetic and clinical aspects. *Leukemia, 12,* 823–827.

25. Tabernero, M. D., Bortoluci, A. M., Alaejos, I., et al. (2001). Adult precursor B-ALL with *BCR/ABL* gene rearrangements displays a unique immunophenotype based on the pattern of CD10, CD34, CD13 and CD38 expression. *Leukemia, 15,* 406–414.

26. Li, S., Eshleman, J. R., & Borowitz, M. J. (2002). Lack of surface immunoglobulin light chain expression by flow cytometric immunophenotyping can help diagnose peripheral B cell lymphoma. *Am J Clin Pathol, 118,* 229–234.

27. Beck, R. C., Stahl, S., O'Keefe, C. L., et al. (2003). Detection of mature T cell leukemias by flow cytometry using anti T cell receptor V beta antibodies. *Am J Clin Pathol, 120,* 785–794.

28. Alaibac, M., Pigozzi, B., Belloni-Fortina, A., et al. (2003). CD7 expression in reactive and malignant human skin T-lymphocytes. *Anticancer Res, 23,* 2707–2710.

29. Dezern A. E., & Borowitz, M. J. (2018). ICCS/ESCCA consensus guidelines to detect GPI-deficient cells in paroxysmal nocturnal hemoglobinuria (PNH) and related disorders part 1 - clinical utility. *Cytometry B Clin Cytom, 94,* 16–22.

30. Sander, C. K., & Mourant, J. R. (2013). Advantages of full spectrum flow cytometry. *J Biomed Opt, 18,* 037004.

31. Behbehani, G. K. (2017). Applications of Mass Cytometry in Clinical Medicine: The Promise and Perils of Clinical CyTOF. *Clin Lab Med, 37,* 945–964.

Molecular Diagnostics in Hematopathology

*Cynthia L. Jackson, Shashi Mehta**

OBJECTIVES

After completion of this chapter, the reader will be able to:

1. Describe the structure of DNA, including the composition of a nucleotide, the double helix, and the antiparallel complementary strand orientation.
2. Predict the nucleotide sequence of a complementary strand of DNA or RNA given the nucleotide sequence of a DNA template.
3. Explain the relationship between DNA structure and protein structure.
4. Discuss the process of DNA replication, including replication origin, replication fork, primer, DNA polymerase, Okazaki fragments, and leading and lagging strands.
5. Determine the appropriate patient specimen required for DNA isolation to identify an inherited or somatic mutation.
6. Discuss common methods of DNA and RNA isolation.
7. Explain the principle of the polymerase chain reaction (PCR), reverse transcriptase PCR, nucleic acid hybridization and Southern blotting, and cleavage-based signal amplification methods.

8. Compare and contrast the methods for detecting amplified target DNA, including gel electrophoresis using intercalating dyes, capillary gel electrophoresis, and restriction fragment length polymorphism methods.
9. Compare and contrast qualitative real-time PCR and end-point PCR.
10. Discuss the principle and use of quantitative real-time PCR for monitoring minimal residual disease.
11. Explain the principle and clinical applications of traditional Sanger DNA sequencing, and contrast this method with pyrosequencing and next-generation sequencing (massively parallel sequencing).
12. Describe the use of microarray-based comparative genomic hybridization (aCGH) and single nucleotide polymorphism array (SNP-A) karyotyping for the detection of chromosome copy number alterations.

OUTLINE

*The authors extend appreciation to Mark E. Lasbury whose work in prior editions provided the foundation for this chapter.

CASE STUDY

After studying the material in this chapter, the reader should be able to respond to the following case study:

A 55-year-old man presented to his hematologist for a follow-up visit for a 3-year history of thrombocytosis thought to be reactive in the setting of chronic retained kidney stones. He had a basal cell carcinoma removed a year ago, and he states that his dermatologist was satisfied with the removal. He also has a history of chronic back pain from a herniated disk, which he elected to treat conservatively. He reports overall good quality of life with the exception of occasional right toe numbness. In the current visit his spleen is slightly palpable. The following are the results of his complete blood count (CBC):

	Patient Results	Reference Intervals
WBC ($\times 10^9$/L)	13.6	3.6–10.6
RBC ($\times 10^{12}$/L)	5.70	4.60–6.00
HGB (g/dL)	17.2	14.0–18.0
HCT (%)	51.4	40–54
PLT ($\times 10^9$/L)	605	150–450

Based on the CBC results a bone marrow biopsy was done, which showed a hypercellular marrow with trilineage hematopoiesis and hyperplasia of granulocytes. A reticulin stain of the bone marrow showed a grade 2/3 fibrosis. Given the clinical history and laboratory results a myeloproliferative neoplasm, such as polycythemia vera, was considered. The hematologist ordered an erythropoietin level, which was 3.0 mU/mL (reference interval 4.0 to 19.5 mU/mL), and a real-time PCR Taqman probe assay for the *JAK2* p.Val617Phe (c.1849G>T) mutation. Figure 29.1 illustrates the assay results.

1. What type of specimen is appropriate for *JAK2* mutation testing?
2. Based on the real-time PCR curves with wild-type and mutant probes, in which reaction does the patient specimen amplify?
3. Does the patient have a *JAK2* p.Val617Phe mutation; if so, is it heterozygous or homozygous?
4. Based on the test results, what is the probable diagnosis?

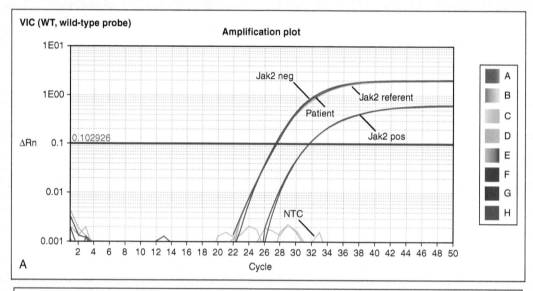

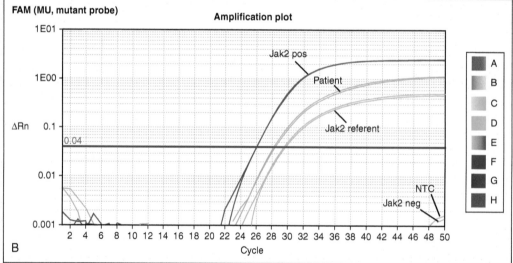

Figure 29.1 Results of the Real-Time PCR Taqman Hydrolysis Probe Assay for the *JAK2* p.Val617Phe (c.1849G>T) Mutation for the Patient in the Case Study. (A), Real-time amplification curves with a probe complementary to the wild-type allele (labeled VIC). Curves are shown for the positive control (Jak2 Pos), negative control (Jak2 Neg, wild-type), no-template control (NTC), referent (sensitivity) control, and the patient. **(B),** Real-time amplification curves with a probe complementary to the mutant allele (labeled FAM). Curves are shown for the positive control (Jak2 Pos), negative control (Jak2 Neg, wild-type), no-template control (NTC), referent (sensitivity) control, and the patient.

Continued

Specimen	Vic (WT)	Fam (MU)	Ratio (MU/WT)	Average
Negative control	2.973	0.804	0.270	
Negative control	2.986	0.756	0.253	0.262
Positive control	1.073	3.395	3.130	
Positive control	1.109	3.359	3.061	3.096
No template control	0.066	0.026	0.394	
No template control	0.069	0.027	0.391	
Sensitivity control	2.999	1.074	0.358	
Sensitivity control	2.989	1.077	0.359	0.359
Patient	3.06	2.695	0.881	0.898
Patient	3.008	2.75	0.914	

C

Figure 29.1, cont'd (C), Table of the fluorescent values after 35 cycles of PCR showing the relative ratio of FAM/VIC fluorescence for each of the specimens. Specimens with a FAM/VIC ratio greater than the sensitivity or referent control are considered mutant.

Molecular biology techniques enhance the diagnostic team's ability to predict or identify an increasing number of diseases in the clinical laboratory. Molecular techniques also enable clinicians to monitor disease progression during treatment, make accurate prognoses, and predict the response to therapeutics. The short interval required to perform molecular diagnostic tests and analyze their results is an additional positive aspect of this type of testing, resulting in more efficient patient management, especially in cases of infection.

Five main areas of hematopathologic molecular testing include detection of mutations, gene rearrangements, and chromosomal abnormalities for diagnosis and prognosis of hematologic malignancies (Box 29.1); detection and quantification of minimal residual disease to monitor treatment of hematologic malignancies; detection of mutations in inherited hematologic disorders (Box 29.2); pharmacogenetic testing to detect genetic variation affecting certain drug therapies (Box 29.3); and identification of hematologically important infectious diseases (Box 29.4).

STRUCTURE AND FUNCTION OF DNA

The Central Dogma: DNA to RNA to Protein

Most of the stored information needed to carry out cell processes resides in deoxyribonucleic acid (DNA); therefore proper cellular storage, maintenance, and replication of DNA are necessary to ensure homeostasis. Because molecular testing takes advantage of DNA structure and replication, a review of molecular biology is helpful.

The central dogma in genetics is that information stored in DNA is *replicated* to daughter DNA, *transcribed* to messenger

BOX 29.1 Major Hematologic Malignancies in Which Molecular Methods Are Performed for Diagnosis and Monitoring Minimal Residual Disease

For Diagnosis:
Acute leukemias
  Myeloid
  Lymphoblastic
Myeloproliferative neoplasms
  Chronic myeloid (myelogenous) leukemia
  Polycythemia vera
  Essential thrombocythemia
  Primary myelofibrosis
Myelodysplastic syndromes
Mature lymphoid neoplasms
  Chronic lymphocytic leukemia
  Lymphomas

For Monitoring Minimal Residual Disease:
Acute leukemias
  Quantification of fusion mRNA transcripts due to translocations
  Quantification of specific B and T cell receptor rearrangements
Chronic myeloid leukemia
  Quantification of fusion messenger ribonucleic acid (mRNA) transcripts due to translocation

ribonucleic acid (mRNA), and *translated* into a functional protein (Figure 29.2). This process is essential to carry out cellular functions while preserving a record of the stored DNA information. In eukaryotes the initial DNA sequence is composed of *translated* exons separated by *untranslated* introns. The introns

Erythrocyte disorders
   Hemoglobinopathies/thalassemias
   Membrane abnormalities
   Enzyme deficiencies
   Erythropoietic porphyrias
Leukocyte disorders
   Quantitative disorders
   Functional disorders
   Storage disorders
Platelet disorders
   Quantitative disorders
   Functional disorders
Bone marrow failure syndromes
   Coagulopathies
   Thrombophilia

Warfarin sensitivity
   Cytochrome P450 2C9 variants, CYP2C9*2, CYP2C9*3
   VKORC1 variants
Clopidogrel sensitivity
   Cytochrome P450 2C19 variants, CYP2C19*17, others
Thiopurine sensitivity
   Thiopurine S-methyltransferase, TPMT*2, TPMT*3C, TPMT*3A
Imatinib resistance
   ABL1 mutation analysis

Parasitic pathogens
   Plasmodium
   Filaria
   Babesia
   Leishmania
   Trypanosoma
Fungal pathogens
Bacterial pathogens
Viral pathogens
   Parvovirus B19
   Cytomegalovirus
   Epstein-Barr virus
   Human immunodeficiency virus types 1 and 2
   Human T-cell lymphotropic virus type 1

Modified from Paessler, M., & Bagg, A. (2005). Use of molecular techniques in the analysis of hematologic diseases. In Hoffman, R., Benz, E. J. Jr, Shattil, S. J., et al (Eds.), *Hematology: Basic Principles and Practice.* (4th ed., pp. 2713–2726). Philadelphia: Churchill Livingstone.

are enzymatically excised following transcription from DNA to RNA, and the mature mRNA sequence is then translated. Translation is an enzymatic process wherein mRNA three-nucleotide base sequences, called *codons,* drive the addition of encoded amino acids to the growing peptide. The mature

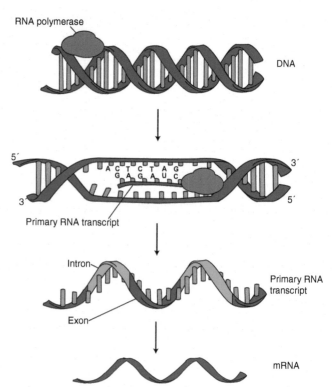

Figure 29.2 Transcription of DNA to Messenger RNA. RNA polymerase binds to a sequence of DNA called the *promoter region,* which causes the DNA strands to separate. Using one of the DNA strands as a template, RNA polymerase moves along and simultaneously reads (transcribes) the DNA strand, forming the primary messenger RNA (mRNA) transcript by joining the complementary ribonucleotides. The primary mRNA transcript consists of sequences called *exons,* which provide coding information, and *introns,* which are excised from the mature mRNA. The spliced mRNA then leaves the nucleus and enters the cytoplasm, where ribosomes translate the mRNA into protein.

protein then carries out its cellular function, which may be structural or may involve recognition, regulation, or enzymatic activity.

The structural units that carry DNA's message are called *genes.* The human β-globin gene (*SBB*), part of the hemoglobin molecule, provides a good example of replication and transcription, because it was one of the first sequenced and demonstrates the result of aberrant sequence maintenance. A normal (or wild-type) β-globin gene contains a sequence of bases that code for a β-globin peptide of 146 amino acids (Chapter 7). In hemoglobin S (Hb S) one inherited mutation changes a single DNA base. This is called a *point mutation.* The mutation occurs in the sequence that codes for the sixth amino acid of β-globin, and it substitutes the amino acid valine for glutamic acid in the growing peptide. Valine modifies the overall charge, producing a protein that polymerizes in a low-oxygen environment. This leads to sickled erythrocytes, circulatory ischemia and its sequelae, and chronic hemolytic anemia (Chapter 24).[1] Mutation in one of the two copies (*alleles*) of this gene inherited from the parents results in a *heterozygous* condition, or sickle cell trait. Heterozygotes are asymptomatic, with rare exceptions (i.e., during times of extreme physical stress or low-oxygen conditions). If both alleles are mutated, there is overt *homozygous* sickle cell disease, and the symptoms are usually severe.

Every active gene is translated. Human somatic (nongamete) cells contain 20,000 to 25,000 genes in 2 meters of DNA, with approximately 3 billion DNA base pairs.[2] Significant packing takes place to reduce the volume of the nucleic acid to the size of chromosomes (Figure 30.3).

DNA at the Molecular Level

DNA is a duplex molecule composed of two complementary, hydrogen-bonded *nucleotide* strands (Figure 29.3). Deoxyribonucleotides and ribonucleotides are the building blocks of DNA and RNA, respectively. Each nucleotide is composed of a 5-carbon sugar (pentose), a nitrogenous base, and a phosphate group. The numbers one prime (1′) to five prime (5′) designate the pentose's carbons. In DNA the pentose is a ribose in which the hydroxyl group on the 2′ carbon is replaced by a hydrogen molecule, hence 2′-deoxyribose (Figure 29.4A). In RNA the 2′ ribose retains the 2′ hydroxyl group. The hydroxyl group present on the 3′ carbon of the sugar is crucial for polymerization of the nucleotide monomers to form the nucleic acid strand.

The nitrogenous base is linked to the sugar by a glycosidic bond at the 1′ carbon. Four different bases form DNA, but the linkage to the sugar is the same for each. The phosphate group is linked to the sugar at the 5′ carbon by a phosphodiester bond (Figure 29.4B–C). The phosphate group is also crucial for addition of nucleotides to the growing polymer. A sugar, whether ribose or deoxyribose, linked to a nitrogenous base but without a phosphate group, is called a *nucleoside*. A nucleoside cannot be incorporated into DNA, and neither can a nucleotide consisting of only one phosphate group (deoxynucleotide monophosphate, or dNMP). To be incorporated into a growing strand of DNA, the nucleotide must have three phosphate groups linked to one another, referred to as α-, β-, and γ-phosphates, with the α-phosphate linked to the sugar (Figure 29.5).

Synthesis of a DNA strand requires the enzyme DNA polymerase. This enzyme recognizes the hydroxyl group on the 3′ carbon of the deoxyribose. It then forms a phosphodiester bond between the 3′ hydroxyl group of the last nucleotide and the 5′ α-phosphate group of the next nucleotide to be added

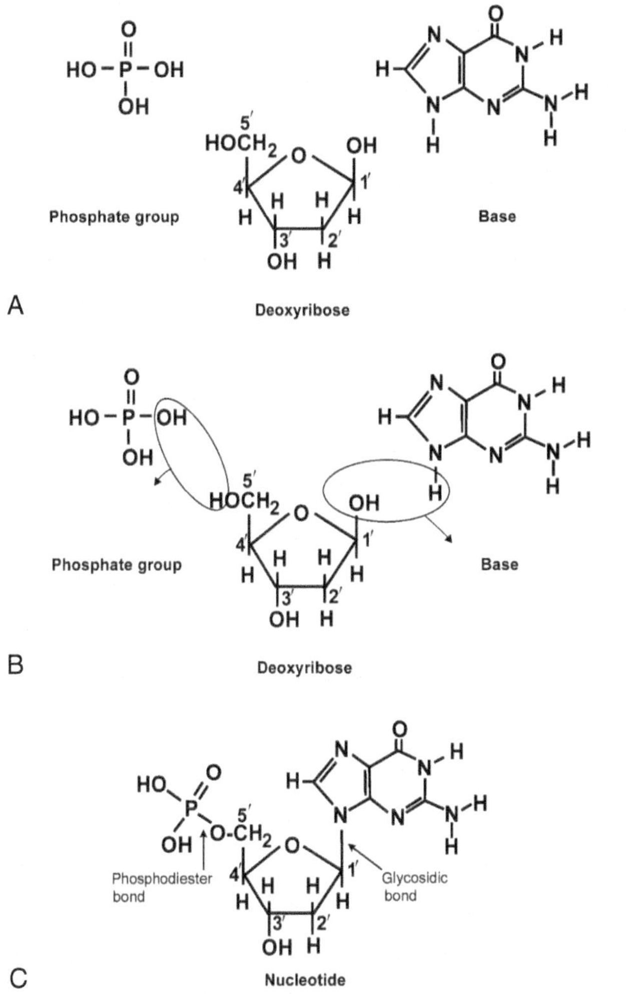

Figure 29.4 DNA Nucleotide Structure. **(A),** The pentose sugar, deoxyribose, a phosphate group, and a nitrogenous base compose a DNA nucleotide. The carbons of the deoxyribose molecule are numbered 1′ through 5′. The hydroxyl group on the 2′ carbon of ribose is replaced by a hydrogen molecule, making the structure a deoxyribose. **(B),** A nucleotide results from the formation of a glycosidic bond between the nitrogenous base and the hydroxyl group on the 1′ carbon of deoxyribose and a phosphodiester bond between the phosphate group and the hydroxyl group on the 5′ carbon of deoxyribose. **(C),** A nucleotide illustrating the glycosidic and phosphodiester bonds.

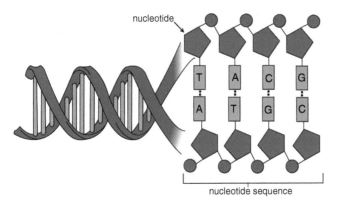

Figure 29.3 DNA Structure. DNA is a double-stranded helical macromolecule consisting of nucleotide subunits joined in sequence by deoxyribose molecules (pentagons) and phosphate radicals (circles). The bases thymine (T), adenine (A), cytosine (C), and guanine (G) are illustrated in their standard pairs: thymine to adenine, cytosine to guanine.

(Figure 29.5). Polymerization of subsequent nucleotides forms a DNA strand.

DNA consists of two strands that are antiparallel and complementary (Figure 29.6). One strand begins with a phosphate group attached to the 5′ carbon of the first nucleotide and ends with the hydroxyl group on the 3′ carbon of the last nucleotide. This strand is in the 5′ to 3′ direction. The other strand runs in the 3′ to 5′ direction, or antiparallel. Nucleotide sequences composing these strands provide the encoded messages of the genes. Therefore addition of nucleotides to a DNA strand is highly regulated.

One regulation mechanism arises from the complementary characteristic of the nucleotides. A nucleotide's identity depends on the type of its nitrogenous base. There are two categories of nitrogenous bases in nucleic acids: purines and

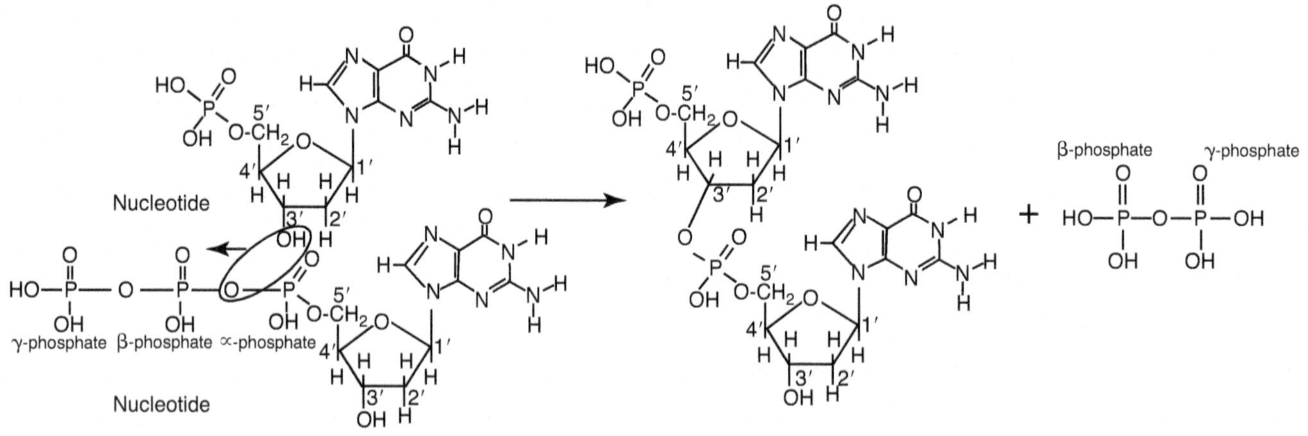

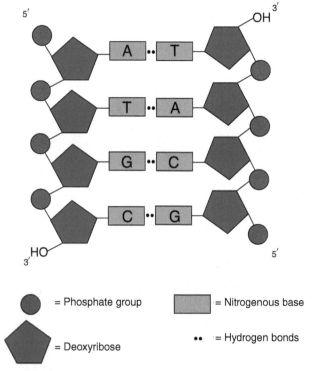

Figure 29.5 **Action of DNA Polymerase.** The enzyme DNA polymerase catalyzes the formation of a phosphodiester bond between the hydroxyl group on the 3′ carbon of one nucleotide with the phosphate group on the 5′ carbon of the downstream nucleotide (*circled area on left*). The α-phosphate group is split with release of the β- and γ-phosphates.

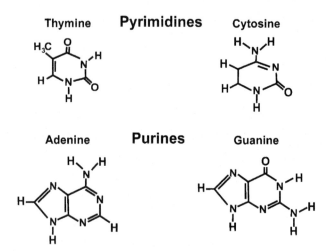

● = Phosphate group   ▭ = Nitrogenous base

⬠ = Deoxyribose   •• = Hydrogen bonds

Figure 29.6 **DNA Structure Showing Two Antiparallel and Complementary Strands.** One strand begins with a 5′ phosphate group and ends with a 3′ hydroxyl group. This strand is read in the 5′ to 3′ direction. The other strand begins with a 3′ hydroxyl group and ends with a 5′ phosphate group. This strand is shown in the 3′ to 5′ orientation.

Figure 29.7 **Structure of Pyrimidines and Purines.** The single-ringed pyrimidines (thymine and cytosine) and the double-ringed purines (adenine and guanine) are the code-carrying nitrogenous bases of DNA.

pyrimidines (Figure 29.7). Adenine (A) and guanine (G) are double-ringed purines, whereas thymine (T) and cytosine(C) are single-ringed pyrimidines. Adenine forms hydrogen bonds at two points with thymine (A:T), whereas guanine forms hydrogen bonds at three points with cytosine (G:C). If a strand has a 5′-CTAG-3′ sequence, the complementary nucleotides on the 3′ to 5′ strand are 3′-GATC-5′. Hydrogen bonds between A:T and G:C hold the strands together (Figure 29.8). In RNA the pyrimidine uracil (U) takes the place of thymine and can form hydrogen bonds with adenine. RNA is most often single stranded but can have significant secondary structure.

DNA resembles a ladder, with the repeating sugar and phosphate groups forming the sides of the ladder and the bases forming the rungs. The pairing of a double-ringed purine on one strand with a single-ringed pyrimidine on the other maintains a consistent distance between the DNA strands. This makes DNA flexible, which allows the molecule to twist into a helix. Twisting stabilizes the molecule and protects the bases from their environment.

Transcription and Translation

Transcription is the process of conversion of the DNA nucleotide code to mRNA by the enzyme RNA polymerase, which recognizes initiation sequences called *promoters*. Promoters lie upstream of coding sequences and bind RNA polymerase, which separates the DNA strands. The enzyme then slides along the 3′ to 5′ template DNA strand, "reading" the code and polymerizing (assembling) the complementary ribonucleotides in

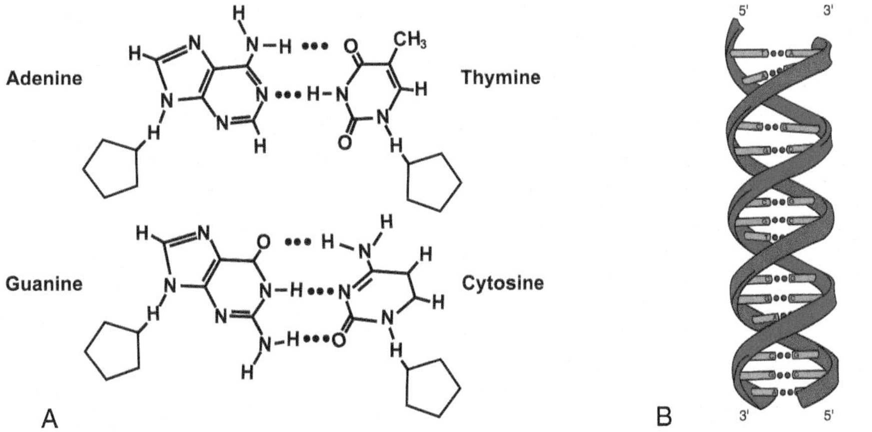

Figure 29.8 Hydrogen Bonding of Complementary DNA Strands. (A), The purine adenine forms two hydrogen bonds with the pyrimidine thymine. The purine guanine forms three hydrogen bonds with the pyrimidine cytosine. **(B),** The two strands maintain a consistent distance from each other, which allows DNA to twist into a helix.

the 5' to 3' direction. As the complementary ribonucleotides form hydrogen bonds with the bases of the exposed DNA strand, the RNA polymerase creates phosphodiester bonds to extend the single-stranded primary RNA transcript (Figure 29.2). If the nucleotide sequence of the template DNA strand is 3'-CTAG-5', the primary RNA transcript is 5'-GAUC-3', in which uracil is substituted for thymine.

Primary mRNA transcripts are composed of introns and exons. Introns are untranslated intervening sequences located between the coding portions of genes. Their many functions are being actively investigated, particularly their role in regulation of gene expression and alternative splicing.[3] Exons are sequences that encode the gene product. Before mRNA can serve as a translation template, introns must be excised from the primary transcript and the exons adjoined. The mature mRNA is completed by the addition of a 5' cap and a tail of many repeated adenine nucleotides (polyA tail).[4] The mature mRNA leaves the nucleus and enters the cytoplasm to be translated by ribosomes.

Ribosomes translate the mRNA code into a peptide sequence. Complexes of proteins and structural ribosomal RNAs (rRNAs) form both large and small ribosome subunits. Mature cytoplasmic mRNA is bound by the small ribosomal subunit at the translation initiation site. At this point another series of elements is introduced, transfer RNAs (tRNAs), each bound to its specific amino acid. Because there are 20 natural amino acids, there are 20 tRNAs. Each tRNA has a specific nucleic acid sequence located at the point of interaction with the mRNA, complementary to the nucleotide sequence of the mRNA. Each tRNA interacting sequence (anticodon) complements a specific three-nucleotide sequence (codon) of the mRNA.

The mRNA codon AUG is the most common translation initiation site and codes for the amino acid methionine. The first step in translation is hydrogen bonding of the tRNA (with a bound methionine) to the initiation codon of the mRNA. The appropriate tRNA is then bonded to the adjacent codon, and a peptide bond is catalyzed between the two amino acids. The peptide bond forms between the carboxyl terminus of the methionine in the existing peptide chain and the amino terminus

of the amino acid to be added. Hydrogen bonding of tRNAs to the codons and the formation of the peptide bonds are mediated by the ribosome. With the addition of more amino acids, translation proceeds until a termination codon is reached. Three termination codons exist that do not code for any amino acid and terminate translation: UAA, UAG, and UGA. The ribosome then dissociates, and the peptide folds into its functional shape.

DNA Replication and the Cell Cycle

After cells carry out their functions, they either divide by mitosis or die by apoptosis, also called programmed cell death. The cell cycle progresses through a defined sequence of G1 (gap 1), S (DNA synthesis), G2 (gap 2), and M (mitosis) phases with various checkpoints along the cycle (Chapter 3 and Figure 3.5). The checkpoints have complex mechanisms to stop the progression of the cell cycle if a problem is detected, at which point the cell will undergo apoptosis. Some cells exit the cell cycle during the G_1 phase and enter a phase called G_0 (quiescence). Cells in G_0 normally do not reenter the cell cycle and remain alive, performing their function until apoptosis occurs.

DNA replication during the S phase requires a complex orchestration of events; this discussion focuses on those events that are exploited for molecular diagnostic testing. Contained within the double-stranded DNA helix are multiple origins of replication. At each origin the enzyme helicase disrupts the hydrogen bonds, untwisting and separating the DNA strands, producing two replication forks. Here a deoxyribonucleotide (deoxynucleotide triphosphate, or dNTP) polymerizes to form new complementary strands (Figure 29.9). DNA replication occurs bidirectionally from the two replication origin sites. Each DNA strand in the replication fork serves as a template for the formation of a daughter or complementary strand through the activity of DNA polymerase.[5] The DNA polymerase substrate is the free hydroxyl group located on the 3' carbon of a deoxyribonucleotide. DNA polymerase recognizes this group and catalyzes the joining of the complementary deoxyribonucleotide. DNA polymerase reads the DNA template in the 3' to 5'

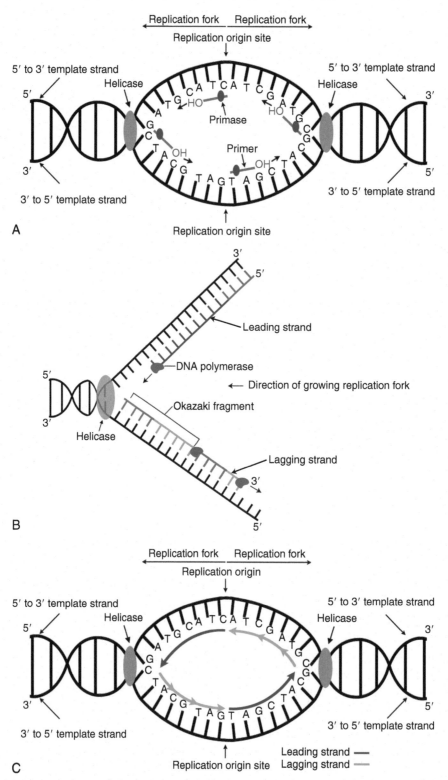

Figure 29.9 DNA Replication. (A), Primases synthesize RNA primers that anneal to the single-stranded template strands. The primers must be oriented in such a way that the hydroxyl group on the 3' end of the primers is available for deoxyribonucleotide addition by DNA polymerase. **(B),** DNA polymerase extends the primer located on the 5' to 3' coding strand, producing the complementary leading strand (blue). On the 3' to 5' template strand, DNA polymerase extends the primers, producing Okazaki fragments. The primer ribonucleotides (red) are replaced with deoxynucleotides by DNA polymerase to produce the complementary lagging strand (green). **(C),** Bidirectional DNA replication, in which the 5' to 3' parent strand serves as the template for producing the continuous leading strands on a replication fork to the left of an origin. The 3' to 5' parent lestrand is the template for the lagging strands, which are produced in a discontinuous manner. The continuous and discontinuous strands are reversed on the replication fork to the right.

direction, and the complementary strand is synthesized in the 5′ to 3′ direction.

A primer is required to provide the free 3′ hydroxyl group that is necessary for DNA polymerase activity. The enzyme primase synthesizes short RNA polymers complementary to the template that serve as primers to initiate DNA synthesis. At the replication origin the primer hybridizes to the 3′ end of the 5′ to 3′ (top) template strand (Figure 29.9). Then DNA polymerase recognizes the free hydroxyl group on the 3′ carbon of the last nucleotide in the primer and catalyzes the formation of phosphodiester bonds between the correct complementary nucleotide triphosphate and the primer, releasing the β- and γ-phosphate groups. DNA polymerase continues adding deoxyribonucleotides along the replication fork, going to the left of the replication origin, producing the complementary strand called the *leading strand.*

The second template strand, called the *lagging strand,* is also read in the 3′ to 5′ direction. To form a complementary strand, a primer hybridizes to the exposed 3′ end of the replication fork. To proceed in the 5′ to 3′ direction, nucleotides are added in fragments toward the origin of replication. As the left replication fork extends to open more of the template strands for replication, additional primers are hybridized, and DNA polymerase uses the primers to initiate the formation of the complementary strand, continuing until it meets a previously hybridized primer.

DNA polymerase not only joins nucleotides, but also degrades the RNA primers and fills in the correct complementary deoxyribonucleotides. Because the replication of the lagging strand produces many small fragments, it is called *discontinuous replication*, and the fragments are called *Okazaki fragments.* Finally, the enzyme ligase joins the discontinuous fragments. The replication fork to the right (downstream) is replicated in the same fashion, although the lagging strand is now formed complementary to the top (5′ to 3′) strand, and the leading strand is formed from the 3′ to 5′ strand; the opposite of the situation described occurs for the left replication fork (Figure 29.9).

The cell cycle is highly regulated. At certain critical points within the cycle, decisions are made to continue or begin cell death via apoptosis. This decision may depend on the state of the DNA replicated. Normally the cell detects errors made during replication and either corrects them or begins apoptosis. This prevents the persistence of daughter cells with genetic errors. If the sensing molecules fail, cell division may continue. Debilitating mutations that mediate cell cycle control may result in tumor formation. In summary, DNA synthesis and accurate cell cycle control demand that the integrity of the nucleotide sequence be maintained during DNA replication.

MOLECULAR DIAGNOSTIC TESTING OVERVIEW

DNA or RNA sequences are used to diagnose and monitor solid tumors, acute leukemia, myeloproliferative neoplasms, myelodysplastic syndromes, inherited hematologic disorders, and viral, parasitic, and bacterial infections. Molecular diagnostic testing exploits the enzymes and processes of DNA replication.

Most molecular testing methods use replication – for example, polymerase chain reaction (PCR) – to make millions of *amplicons* (copies) of a DNA sequence of interest. Further, creation of synthetic DNA requires the use of short sequences used as either primers or probes to locate specific DNA or RNA sequences within vast populations of nucleic acids.

Specific mutations are associated with hematologic disease. These are detected primarily by allele-specific amplification methods, Sanger sequencing, next-generation sequencing, and occasionally by restriction fragment length polymorphism analysis of amplified DNA. Messenger and ribosomal RNA also may be amplified through a process called *reverse transcriptase PCR* (RT-PCR). Using mRNA as the target, the existence of mutations that are being actively translated can be detected. Assessment of mRNA shows whether a mutation is expressed in a certain cell type or tissue and can be used to quantitatively determine the level of transcription of a gene. It can also be used to detect and monitor chromosome translocations that produce novel chimeric mRNA transcripts in conditions in which the breakpoints are too widely separated to be detected by PCR amplification of DNA.

Most molecular tests use DNA amplification (e.g., PCR), generating multiple amplicons of the target sequence. Amplification is meant to be specific to the sequence of interest in the specimen being tested; however, it will amplify any DNA that is present in the reaction. Consequently it is critical to eliminate contamination of newly isolated target DNA with amplicons from previously amplified specimens. Contamination can be avoided by designating separate laboratory locations for each step, having a unidirectional work flow, and employing appropriate controls. Operators routinely use ultraviolet (UV) light and bleach to induce strand breaks in contaminating DNA on work surfaces, and a uracil-N-glycosylase system that destroys previously amplified DNA can also be incorporated into the PCR reactions.

In genetically based hematologic disease, sequence variants can occur that do not affect function. Individuals vary in genetic sequences coding for identical proteins. Such single nucleotide polymorphisms (SNPs) are commonly detected but might not be associated with disease. With these caveats in mind, several techniques are presented, and an example from hematopathology is given for each. Box 29.5 is a summary of molecular methods with hematopathology applications.

NUCLEIC ACID ISOLATION

Isolating DNA from Clinical Specimens

Most molecular diagnostic tests begin with isolation of DNA or RNA from a patient specimen. To test for a mutation in patient DNA, the patient's DNA is isolated. To test for microorganism DNA, as in an infection, DNA is also isolated from the patient specimen because it will include the organism DNA. The preferred nucleic acid for clinical diagnosis is DNA because it is inherently more stable than RNA and is less labor intensive to isolate.

The molecular laboratory isolates nucleic acid from a wide variety of clinical specimen types. Patient specimens for human

BOX 29.5 Molecular Methods with Hematopathology Applications

Nucleic acid isolation
    DNA
    RNA
Nucleic acid hybridization and Southern blotting
Amplification of nucleic acid
    Polymerase chain reaction (PCR)
    Reverse transcriptase PCR
Detection of amplified DNA
    Gel electrophoresis
    Restriction endonuclease methods
Cleavage-based signal amplification
Real-time PCR
    Qualitative
    Quantitative
    Minimal residual disease in leukemia
    Mutation enrichment strategies
Nucleic acid sequencing
    DNA sequencing by capillary electrophoresis
    Next-generation sequencing
Chromosomal microarrays
Pathogen detection and infectious disease load
Current developments
    Mass spectrometry
    Digital PCR
    Detection of circulating tumor DNA (liquid biopsy)
    miRNAs

DNA isolation may include peripheral blood, bone marrow, tissue biopsy specimens (both fresh and formalin fixed, paraffin embedded), needle aspirates, body fluids, saliva, and cheek swabs. Blood, saliva, or cheek swab specimens are all appropriate for identifying an inherited defect, although blood is the most common specimen type. Every nucleated cell contains a full complement of DNA. If individuals inherit a mutation, it is present in the DNA of all their nucleated cells, both gamete and nongamete (somatic) cells. Thus the DNA in the nucleus of white blood cells (WBCs) can reveal inherited mutations. In solid tumors somatic (acquired) mutations are detected by analyzing DNA from the suspect tissue. For identification of infectious disease organisms by molecular techniques, DNA must also be isolated from the affected tissues. Peripheral blood is adequate for infections with viruses (e.g., the human immunodeficiency virus [HIV] and cytomegalovirus [CMV]) that infect blood cells, whereas cerebrospinal fluid is required for meningeal infections.

Whole blood is preferentially collected in an ethylenediaminetetraacetic acid (EDTA) tube to prevent clotting and to inhibit enzymes that may digest DNA, although other tubes may also be acceptable. The red blood cells (RBCs) are removed by taking advantage of the differential lysis in a hypotonic buffer due to differing osmotic fragility between white and red blood cells. Incubation in hypotonic buffer will result in the RBCs lysing before the WBCs, thus allowing the WBCs to be removed from the hemoglobin and lysed RBCs by centrifugation. Hemoglobin is a potent inhibitor of PCR and other downstream procedures.[6]

DNA from tissue suspected of being malignant can be isolated from formalin-fixed, paraffin-embedded tissue sections mounted on glass microscope slides or whole sections cut directly into a microfuge tube. Tissue is obtained from the entire section or from a portion of the section by microdissection, either by scraping or by laser. The tissue is degraded by an enzyme called *proteinase K* to break open the cells and release the DNA. The specimen is then purified using an automated or manual extraction kit as described below.[7] In addition to paraffin-embedded specimens, fresh or frozen tissue specimens are appropriate for DNA isolation. Quickly thawing and mincing the frozen tissue prepares the specimen for DNA isolation. The minced tissue is mixed with an extraction buffer to release the DNA from the cells, and it is then purified.

There are a number of automated extraction systems, in addition to manual extraction kits, available for DNA extraction. Most of these systems use a solid phase extraction system that takes advantage of the binding of DNA to silica under high-salt conditions. Manual kits use columns that can be spun in a microcentrifuge, with the eluent collected in microfuge tubes. Cells that have been lysed and protease treated are applied to a column in a high-salt buffer. The column is washed to remove impurities, and the DNA is eluted in a low-ionic-strength buffer and collected in a microfuge tube.[8] Automated extractors have reagents packaged in sets and can be programmed to extract and purify the DNA automatically. There are a variety of models to choose from, depending on the number and type of specimens. Isolated DNA can be stored at $-20°$ C. If a delay in the molecular testing is necessary, the isolated DNA specimen can be stored at $-80°$ C indefinitely.

Isolating RNA from Clinical Specimens

RNA isolation poses greater technical challenges than DNA isolation. Ubiquitous ribonucleases (RNases) degrade RNA. These enzymes are the body's primary defense against pathogens and are found on mammalian epidermal surfaces; therefore they contaminate all laboratory surfaces.[9] Clinical laboratories that isolate RNA must be RNase free, which necessitates additional precautions and decontamination steps.[10]

Isolated total RNA includes mRNA, rRNA, and tRNA, all of which participate in protein synthesis. Depending on cell type, mRNA may comprise only 3% to 5% of the total cellular RNA; therefore a large-volume specimen may be needed to obtain adequate mRNA. The mRNA does not represent all the information stored in the DNA, only those genes being expressed. Consequently mRNA provides quantitative information on the genes being expressed in a cell at the time the specimen was collected.

RNA may be purified using either liquid or solid phase procedures. The steps of RNA isolation using a liquid phase method are (1) RNA release by cell lysis combined with RNase inhibition by homogenization or incubation in a strongly denaturing solution containing chemical agents such as urea or guanidine isothiocyanate; (2) protein and DNA removal; and (3) RNA precipitation using alcohols. In step 2, extraction is performed using acidic phenol chloroform and guanidine isothiocyanate.

These steps separate the DNA and protein into the organic phase, while the RNA remains in the aqueous phase. RNA resists an acidic pH, whereas DNA is readily depurinated because acid cleaves the bond between the purine base and the deoxyribose sugar. Therefore acidic phenol preferentially isolates and preserves RNA, whereas the genomic DNA (all the DNA) is partitioned along with contaminating proteins, lipids, and carbohydrates. Precipitating the RNA from the aqueous phase requires the addition of salt to neutralize the charge of the phosphodiester backbone and ethanol to make the nucleic acid insoluble.[11] Purification of RNA using column-based methods is similar to DNA except that the RNA is suspended in a high-salt buffer that preferentially binds RNA greater than 200 nucleotides to the column to remove smaller RNAs, such as tRNA and 5S RNA.

NUCLEIC ACID HYBRIDIZATION AND SOUTHERN BLOTTING

Once used in a number of molecular tests, including B and T cell clonality assays and the detection of chromosome translocations, Southern blots are now largely used for specimens that do not provide a result using standard PCR methods or for research applications. Southern blots can only be performed on high-quality genomic DNA or PCR amplicons. Briefly, DNA is digested with a restriction enzyme, size fractionated using agarose gel electrophoresis, denatured to become single stranded, and then finally transferred to a solid support, typically a nylon or nitrocellulose membrane. DNA fragments of interest are then detected with a labeled complementary probe (Figure 29.10).[12,13]

AMPLIFICATION OF NUCLEIC ACIDS BY POLYMERASE CHAIN REACTION

Polymerase Chain Reaction for Amplifying DNA

PCR is the principal technique in the clinical molecular laboratory. PCR is an enzyme-based method for amplifying a specific target sequence to allow its detection from a small amount of highly complex material.[14] As an example, sickle cell anemia results from a single β-globin gene nucleotide substitution (point mutation) in which adenine is replaced by thymine (*HBB* c.20A>T). Detecting this mutation from among 3 billion base pairs in the human genome would be like finding a needle in a haystack if only a few cells were assessed. When millions of β-globin copies are produced in PCR, however, the mutation is easily detected.[15] There are two categories of PCR reactions: end-point PCR and real-time PCR. Amplification for both categories is basically the same. The major difference is in the method of detection of the PCR product. With end-point PCR, the amplification products must be detected at the end of the amplification phase (when all the amplification cycles are completed) using another technique, such as gel electrophoresis. In real-time PCR, the amplicons are detected during each PCR cycle using fluorescence detection. Detection methods are described later in the chapter.

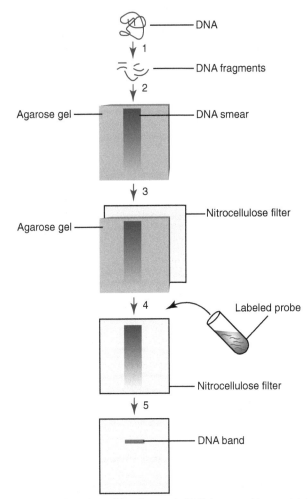

Figure 29.10 Southern Blot Steps. *1,* DNA is cut with a restriction endonuclease which produces many restriction fragments. *2,* DNA fragments are separated on an agarose gel. *3,* DNA fragments are transferred to a nitrocellulose filter. *4,* A labeled probe is hybridized to the DNA fragments on the filter. *5,* Autoradiography is used to visualize the hybridized DNA probe, the detection of which indicates the presence of the given DNA sequence in the specimen.

As with natural DNA replication, PCR amplification requires primers that anneal (bind) to complementary nucleotide sequences on either side of the target region. In testing for the sickle cell mutation, for example, selected primers flank (i.e., bind on either side of) the β-globin gene sequence containing the mutation. The total base pair (bp) length of the primer sequences plus the target sequence can vary, but in this example, it is 110 bp for the β-globin gene, a typical sequence length for many PCR assays (Figure 29.11).[15] Besides primers the PCR master mix reagents include a heat-insensitive DNA polymerase (e.g., Taq polymerase) isolated from the thermophilic bacterium *Thermus aquaticus* and a mixture of the four deoxyribonucleotides – deoxyadenosine triphosphate (dATP), deoxythymidine triphosphate (dTTP), deoxyguanosine triphosphate (dGTP), and deoxycytidine triphosphate (dCTP) – in a magnesium-containing buffer.

The DNA is first denatured at 95° C, which separates the strands; then cooled to the primer annealing (binding) temperature

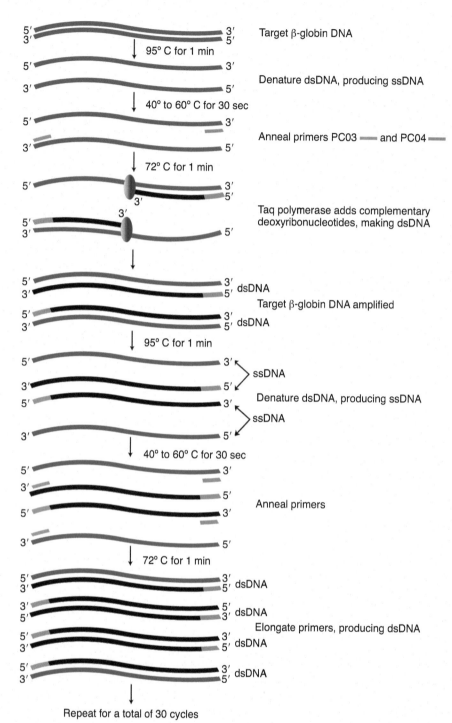

Figure 29.11 Application of PCR to Target β-Globin DNA Amplification. PCR amplifies the target DNA, making millions of copies of the target DNA after 30 cycles. Flanking forward and reverse primers (PCO3 and PCO4) are used to amplify the target β-globin DNA segment. One primer (PCO3, orange) anneals to the 3′ end of the 3′ to 5′ DNA strand. The other primer (PCO4, green) anneals to the 3′ end of the 5′ to 3′ DNA strand. These primers provide the 3′-OH end for extension in the 5′ to 3′ direction during the PCR reaction and set the boundaries for the size of the amplicon. *dsDNA,* double-stranded DNA; *ssDNA,* single-stranded DNA.

of 40° C to 60° C; and then warmed to 72° C to promote specific chain extension, in which nucleotides are added to the primers by DNA polymerase. The annealing temperature is optimized for each set of primers. A thermocycler is used to accurately produce and monitor the rapid temperature changes.

Once double-stranded DNA is denatured, one primer anneals to the 3′ end of the 5′ to 3′ strand and the other primer to the 3′ end of the complementary 3′ to 5′ strand. Both primers possess a free 3′ hydroxyl group. The DNA polymerase recognizes this hydroxyl group, reads the template, and catalyzes formation of the phosphodiester bond joining the first complementary deoxyribonucleotide to the primer. The polymerase rapidly continues down the template strands at 1000 nucleotides per second, extending the complementary strand in the 5′ to 3′ direction to eventually produce complete daughter strands that continue to the 5′ end of the template.[16] This completes one PCR cycle. In the second cycle the temperature changes are repeated, and the first-cycle products become the template for additional daughter strands. After the second cycle, daughter strands are produced that are bounded by the primer sequences at the 5′ and 3′ ends, resulting in a fragment of DNA of the desired length. After 25 to 40 subsequent cycles, double-stranded DNA of specific length and sequence, called an *amplicon,* is reproduced millions of times.[17,18]

Primer annealing accounts for PCR specificity, and primer design is crucial for achieving confidence in the test results regardless of the application. Wherever primers anneal, specifically or nonspecifically, they become starting points for extension by DNA polymerase.

Commercial kits contain primer sets that have been tested for annealing specificity, but care must be taken to use the optimal annealing temperature. Even if the primer is properly designed, it can anneal to noncomplementary regions if the annealing temperature is too low. Several online primer design programs are available from genome centers and company websites. One such program that can help determine the uniqueness, and therefore specificity, of the primers is the Basic Local Alignment Sequence Tool (BLAST).[19] These programs will also analyze pairs of primers to avoid complementarity between the primers themselves; this prevents primer hybridization to each other, which forms undesirable primer dimers.

Controls are essential for the accurate interpretation of a PCR result. The three controls required for PCR are the negative, positive, and no-DNA or no-template (NTC) controls. All three are included in each run. In addition, in most applications, a sensitivity control will be included that consists of a low positive specimen at the lowest concentration detected (LOD). The negative control consists of DNA known to lack the sequence of interest; the positive control contains the target sequence. Comparison of the amplification in the patient specimen to results in the negative and positive controls determines whether the target DNA sequence is present in the patient's DNA. The no-template control detects master mix contamination. Amplification in the no-template control indicates DNA contamination, which renders the entire test result unreliable.[20]

Reverse Transcription Polymerase Chain Reaction for Amplifying RNA

Some hematology molecular tests, such as those for translocations, require mRNA as the starting material. Genetically altered mRNA sequences often translate to an altered protein. The classic example is the Philadelphia chromosome (Ph′), carrying the chromosome translocation t(9;22)(q34;q11.2) (Chapter 32). This translocation is present in 95% of chronic myeloid (myelogenous) leukemia (CML) cases; in 20% of adult acute lymphoblastic leukemia (ALL) cases; in 5% of pediatric ALL cases; and in rare instances in acute myeloid leukemia.[21,22] Ph′ results from a reciprocal translocation of the *ABL1* gene on

chromosome 9 to the breakpoint cluster region *(BCR)* of chromosome 22, producing a *BCR-ABL1* hybrid or chimeric gene (Figure 29.12A).[23,24] Transcription of *BCR-ABL1* produces a chimeric mRNA made up of exons from both the *BCR* and *ABL1* genes. Translation generates a fusion protein with tyrosine kinase activity that alters normal cell cycle control, resulting in unrestrained cell proliferation.[25] RT-PCR of the chimeric mRNA is the standard method to detect this mutation (Figure 29.12B). Although the mutation is present at the DNA level, the nucleotide position at which the two chromosome sections join is variable. The DNA also includes untranslated introns, which make the chimera too long to replicate. The physiologic excision and splicing of mRNA yields a much shorter target that is more easily amplified.

In RT-PCR, the *reverse* transcriptase enzyme produces complementary DNA (cDNA) from mRNA present in a total RNA specimen extracted from patient specimens such as blood or bone marrow (Figure 29.12B). PCR subsequently amplifies the cDNA.

The first step is to transcribe the RNA into DNA using reverse transcriptase and a primer to produce an RNA-cDNA hybrid. The primer can be oligo(dT), a series of thymine nucleotides complementary to the string of adenine nucleotides on the 3′ end of most mRNAs, called the *polyA tail;* a set of short random primers that prime the cDNA synthesis more evenly; or a specific primer for the gene of interest. The primer anneals to the complementary sequence of the mRNA. Reverse transcriptase recognizes the 3' hydroxyl group on the last nucleotide of the primer and reads the mRNA template strand, then adds the correct complementary deoxyribonucleotide. Reverse transcriptase continues along the mRNA template strand, joining the complementary deoxyribonucleotides to the growing cDNA strand to form the mRNA-cDNA hybrid. Subsequently heat denaturation breaks the hydrogen bonds between the mRNA-cDNA hybrid, separating the two strands. The cDNA strand then acts as a template for replication by DNA polymerase. The cDNA synthesis can be done separately from the PCR amplification step in a two-step procedure or combined with the PCR in a single reaction. For example, with the *BCR-ABL1* translocation, the single-stranded cDNA is amplified as in DNA-based PCR using one primer specific for a target sequence in the *BCR* gene and a second primer specific for the *ABL1* gene. DNA polymerase extends the primers, forming a double-stranded cDNA of a specific region of the target chimeric gene. Only the cDNA containing the translocation, and therefore both primer binding sites, will be amplified, resulting in millions of copies of the *BCR-ABL1* sequence.[26,27]

DETECTION OF AMPLIFIED DNA

Although many molecular tests are now performed using real-time PCR, there are still circumstances in which amplicons are produced using end-point PCR and the product must be detected using downstream techniques. PCR-amplified target DNA may be detected by gel electrophoresis using fluorescent dyes; can be combined with restriction enzyme digestion of the amplicons followed by gel electrophoresis; or by DNA sequencing by capillary electrophoresis (discussed later in the chapter).

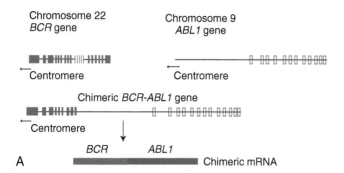

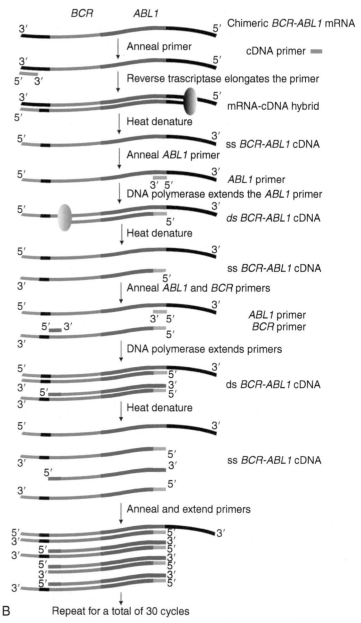

Figure 29.12 Formation and Detection of *BCR-ABL1* mRNA. (A), The *BCR* gene is present on chromosome 22, and the *ABL1* gene is located on chromosome 9. The Ph' chromosome results from the translocation of the *ABL1* gene to chromosome 22, which places the *ABL1* gene next to the *BCR* gene and produces a chimeric *BCR-ABL1* gene. The transcription of the *BCR-ABL1* gene produces a chimeric messenger RNA (mRNA) consisting of a portion of the *BCR* gene and a portion of the *ABL1* gene. **(B),** Reverse transcriptase polymerase chain reaction (RT-PCR) produces complementary DNA (cDNA) from messenger RNA (mRNA). This diagram shows the RT-PCR steps used to produce amplified *BCR-ABL1* cDNA. Initially a gene-specific primer or short random primers anneal to the chimeric *BCR-ABL1* mRNA. Reverse transcriptase elongates the primer, producing an mRNA-cDNA hybrid. Heat denaturation breaks the hydrogen bonds, holding the hybrid molecule together, releasing the single-stranded (ss) *BCR-ABL1* cDNA. Next, a primer specific for the *ABL1* gene is annealed to the cDNA. DNA polymerase elongates the primer, producing the double-stranded (ds) *BCR-ABL1* cDNA. The cDNA becomes single stranded by heat denaturation. Then the *ABL1* primer, in addition to a primer specific for the *BCR* gene, anneal to the ss cDNA. DNA polymerase elongates the primers, producing ds *BCR-ABL1* cDNA. The cycle is repeated 20 to 40 times, producing millions of copies of the ds *BCR-ABL1* cDNA.

Gel Electrophoresis

Nucleic acid phosphate groups confer a net negative charge to DNA fragments. Consequently, in electrophoresis, the rate at which DNA fragments (amplicons) migrate through gels is proportional to their mass only and, unlike proteins, not their relative charge. DNA fragment mass is a function of the length in base pairs (bp) or kilobase pairs (kb, $1000\times$ bp). Fragments are sieved through an agarose or a polyacrylamide gel matrix by passing a current through the gel as it is bathed in a buffered conducting salt solution. Electrophoresis gel pore diameter is a function of gel concentration. The pores of an agarose gel are larger than the pores of a polyacrylamide gel. When larger fragments (500 bp to 50 kb) are to be separated, an agarose gel is most effective. For smaller DNA fragments (5 to 1000 bp), a polyacrylamide gel is used.[28]

An electrical current moves the negatively charged fragments toward the positive electrode (anode). Smaller fragments move faster and migrate farther than larger fragments. A size marker, composed of fragments of known masses (sizes), measured in base pairs or kilobase pairs, runs alongside the patient and control lanes and is used to determine the mass (size) of any DNA fragments in the patient and control specimens (Figure 29.13). Fluorescent dyes such as Gel Red (which intercalate between the base pairs of the DNA helix) or SYBR green (which binds to the minor groove of the DNA helix) are used to visualize the DNA fragments of the patient, controls, and size markers in the gel after exposure to UV light. The size of the bands in the patient and control lanes is determined by comparing the distance migrated in the gel with the distance migrated by the bands of the size markers. Gel electrophoresis

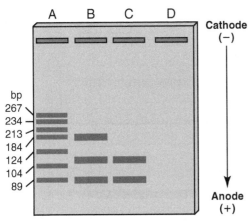

Figure 29.13 DNA Electrophoresis on a Slab Gel. (A), Molecular size marker (ladder); **(B),** positive control; **(C),** negative control; **(D),** no-DNA control. DNA specimens are placed in wells at the cathode (negative pole) and migrate to the anode (positive pole) due to the negative charge of the DNA molecules. By comparing the bands present in the gel with the molecular size markers, the mass of each band, measured in base pairs, is determined. For example, in the positive control specimen, the three bands are 184, 110, and 89 bp. Positive, negative, and no-DNA controls must be used when performing gel electrophoresis. The positive control contains the target DNA sequence, and the negative control lacks this sequence. The no-DNA control specimen lacks DNA. No banding should be present in the no-DNA control. If bands are present, contamination of specimens occurred during the testing process.

is appropriate when the goal is qualitative; that is, to determine the presence or absence of the target DNA.

Another method of fractionating DNA fragments by mass (size) is capillary gel electrophoresis. In this type of electrophoresis, long fused silica capillaries filled with derivatized acrylamide polymer are used for separation of single-stranded, negatively charged DNA fragments on the basis of size or number of base pairs. Specimen is applied to the capillary using electrokinetic injection, and the DNA fragments are separated using a high voltage as they migrate through the capillary from the negative electrode to the positive electrode. Smaller DNA fragments move faster through the polymer in the capillary compared to larger fragments. Detection of the separated fragments occurs by incorporating a fluorescent label into the PCR-amplified DNA. Before reaching the positive electrode the fluorescently labeled DNA fragments cross the path of a laser beam and detector. When the laser beam hits a fluorescent DNA fragment, light is emitted at a specific wavelength. The light emission is read by the detector, and the signal produces a peak on an electropherogram (Figure 29.14).

Capillary electrophoresis offers a number of advantages over traditional gel electrophoresis. Injection, separation, and detection of the fragments are automated. Separation can be quite rapid with excellent resolution. Time of fragment elution and peak height information are stored for easy retrieval. Size ladders can be labeled with different fluorescent dyes and run in the same capillary as the specimen providing more accurate sizing.[29] This method of separation is used in a number of applications, including B and T cell clonality testing, bone marrow engraftment analysis, and screening for the internal tandem duplication mutation in the *FLT3* gene in acute myeloid leukemia (Chapter 31).[30]

Restriction Endonuclease Methods

One method to determine whether an amplified target DNA fragment contains a mutation of interest uses enzymes derived from bacteria called *restriction endonucleases* (also known as restriction enzymes). Each restriction enzyme recognizes a specific nucleotide sequence and cuts both strands of the target DNA at the sequence, producing restriction fragments. The number of restriction fragments produced depends on the number of restriction sites present in the amplified target.[31,32] Enzyme action at one restriction site produces two restriction fragments, action at two restriction sites produces three restriction fragments, and so on.

A restriction enzyme detects even a single base substitution if the mutation alters the recognition sequence and prevents digestion at the site or creates a new site resulting in an additional fragment. A restriction fragment length polymorphism (RFLP) is a mutation or polymorphism-induced change in the

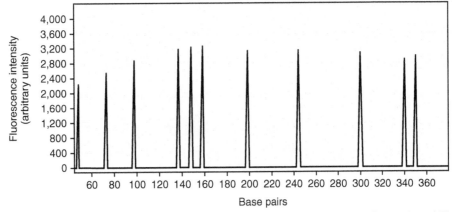

Figure 29.14 An Electropherogram of Capillary Gel Electrophoresis Showing the Separation of Fluorescently Labeled DNA Fragments by Size (Number of Base Pairs). Fragments migrate through the matrix in the capillary from the negative to the positive pole and emerge from the capillary in size order (smaller fragments first). Before reaching the positive electrode, the fluorescently labeled DNA fragments are detected by passing one at a time between a laser beam and the detector. Each fragment is represented by a peak on the electropherogram.

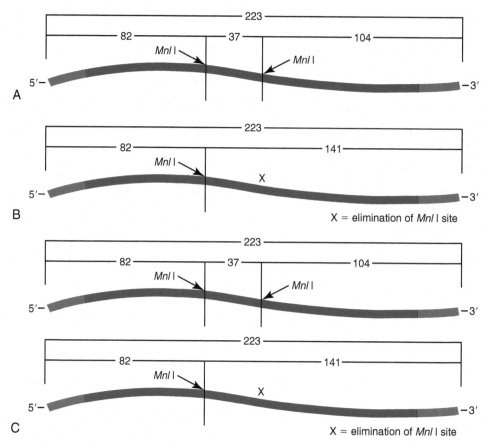

Figure 29.15 Diagram of the Amplified Target Sequence of the Coagulation Factor V (*F5*) Gene (223 bp) in a PCR-Restriction Fragment Length Polymorphism (RFLP) Method to Detect the *F5* Leiden Mutation (c.1691G>A, also called c.1601G>A [p.Arg534Gln]). After digestion of the 223 bp PCR product with the restriction enzyme, *Mnl* I, the size (mass) of the fragments are detected by capillary or gel electrophoresis. Red areas on the fragments represent primer binding sites. **(A),** The amplified target sequence for the normal (wild-type) *F5* gene contains two restriction sites for *Mnl* I, so three restriction fragments of 37, 82, and 104 bp are produced. **(B),** In the *F5* Leiden mutation, the substitution of an A for a G in position 1691 of the *F5* gene eliminates one of the restriction sites for *Mnl* I. Thus the mutated *F5* Leiden gene possesses only one restriction site for *Mnl* I. In individuals homozygous for the mutation, only two restriction fragments of 82 and 141 bp are produced. **(C),** An individual who is heterozygous for the *F5* Leiden mutation has a normal and a mutated *F5* gene. *Mnl* I produces four restriction fragments of 37, 82, 104, and 141 bp.

restriction enzyme recognition site of the target DNA template that alters the length (number of base pairs) of the restriction fragments. A mutation in the coagulation factor V gene (*F5* Leiden mutation, c.1619G>A, also called c.1601G>A [p.Arg534Gln]) is an example of an RFLP used in a PCR-based mutation detection assay (Figure 29.15).[33,34]

CLEAVAGE-BASED SIGNAL AMPLIFICATION

Cleavage-based amplification is an isothermal signal amplification method marketed as the Invader assay (Hologic). In the primary reaction the 3′ end of a test probe and an Invader oligo probe anneal to complementary sequences on the target DNA template, forming a specific substrate site recognized by a cleavase enzyme (Figure 29.16). The 5′ end of the test probe (5′ flap) does not anneal to the target. The cleavase enzyme cuts and releases the 5′ flap of the test probe. In a coupled secondary reaction the 5′ flap of the test probe anneals to a complementary signal probe that has a fluorescence resonance energy transfer

(FRET) reporter. The signal probe and reporter (called a *FRET cassette*) are specific for the 5′ flap of the test probe. The FRET reporter is a fluorescent dye bound to the signal probe in close proximity to a quencher; the quencher prevents the reporter dye from emitting a fluorescent signal. The combination of the 5′ flap of the test probe and the FRET cassette forms another specific substrate site for the cleavage enzyme. Cleavage of the 5′ end of the FRET cassette results in separation of the fluorescent reporter from the quencher and production of a fluorescent signal. Repeated binding and cleavage result in signal amplification. Two reactions are done simultaneously using different fluorescent molecules for detection of either the wild-type or mutant sequence. Because the mutant sequence is different from the wild-type sequence, the wild-type test probe will not anneal to the mutant target, and no fluorescent signal will occur. This technique can be used to detect single base pair changes, small insertions, and deletions. It also has been approved by the US Food and Drug Administration (FDA) for the detection of pathogenic variants associated with thrombophilia, including

Mutant target DNA plus mutant (MUT) test probe

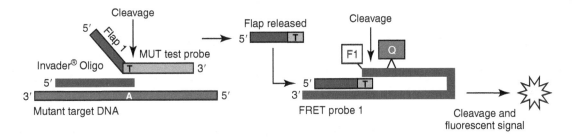

Mutant target DNA plus wild-type (WT) test probe

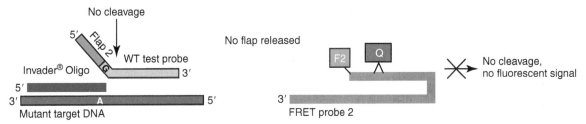

Figure 29.16 Cleavage-Based Signal Amplification. Cleavage-based DNA signal amplification assays use a cleavase enzyme to recognize and cleave specific structures formed by the addition of two oligonucleotide probes to a nucleic acid target. Two oligonucleotide probes (a test probe and an Invader oligo probe) hybridize in tandem to the target DNA to form an overlapping structure. The 5′ end of the test probe includes a 5′ flap that does not hybridize to the target DNA. The 3′ nucleotide of the bound Invader oligo overlaps the test probe. The cleavase enzyme recognizes this overlapping structure and cleaves off the unpaired 5′ flap of the test probe, releasing it as a target-specific product. In the secondary reaction, each released 5′ flap anneals to a fluorescence resonance energy transfer (FRET) probe to create another overlapping structure that is recognized and cleaved by the cleavase enzyme. When the FRET probe is cleaved, the fluorophore (F) and quencher (Q) on the FRET probe are separated, generating a detectable fluorescence signal. The initial and secondary reactions run concurrently in the same well. Two different fluorescent labels are used, one to identify the presence of the wild-type allele and one to identify the presence of the mutant allele.

the factor V (*F5*) Leiden mutation (c.1619G>A, also called c.1601G>A [p.Arg534Gln]) and the prothrombin (*F2*) G20210A (c.*97G>A) mutation.[35]

REAL-TIME POLYMERASE CHAIN REACTION

In contrast to end-point PCR, real-time PCR measures the change in nucleic acid amplification as replication progresses using fluorescent marker dyes. There are several commercially available instruments that vary in their capacity, specimen volume, and optics.[36] There is a variety of choices in the optics for fluorescent detection. A tungsten lamp is commonly used for excitation, and different filters are used to select the excitation and emission wavelength. Light-emitting diodes (LEDs) or lasers for excitation can also be coupled with emission detection, depending on the instrument. Real-time PCR can be used in quantitative or qualitative assays. The time interval (expressed as the number of replication cycles) required to reach a selected fluorescence threshold is proportional to the copy number of target molecules in the original specimen.[37] The PCR cycle at which amplification crosses the threshold is denoted as the *Ct*

for threshold value or the *Cp* for crossing point value. Importantly these values are calculated from the exponential portion of the amplification curve. The Ct value is inversely related to the amount of target, so that the more starting DNA or cDNA present in the reaction, the lower the number of PCR cycles required to reach the threshold and exponential phase of the reaction (Figure 29.17).

Real-time PCR requires the use of fluorescent detection, and there are several different options available. The simplest and the most straightforward option is to add a fluorescent dye, such as SYBR green, to the PCR reaction. These dyes bind to double-stranded DNA so that the fluorescence increases in proportion to the number of copies of the PCR product. The disadvantage of this approach is that these dyes do not differentiate between specific and nonspecific PCR amplicons, so the PCR reaction must be free of mispriming and primer dimers (primers that partially anneal to one another and are extended by the polymerase, forming very short amplicons). A more specific method of detection adds a probe in addition to the forward and reverse PCR primers, which also binds to the amplicon, providing additional specificity.

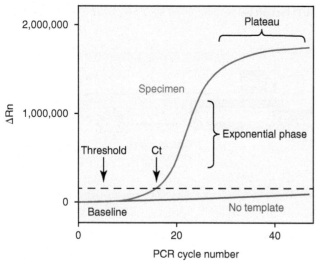

Figure 29.17 Real-Time PCR Amplification Curve. Note the important features of the curve, including the threshold Ct value and the exponential phase of the curve.

There are several methods commonly used, including hybridization probes, Taqman probes, and molecular beacon and Scorpion probes. Hybridization probes use two oligonucleotide probes that bind to the amplicon adjacent (within one to five bases) to one another. One of the oligos has a 3′ donor fluorophore and the other a 5′ acceptor. The 3′ fluorophore is excited, and the energy is transferred to the acceptor, which then fluoresces at a detectable wavelength. This is called fluorescence resonance energy transfer.[38] Hybridization probe technology in combination with melting curve analysis is used in some commercial thrombophilia assays.

Taqman probes consist of a single oligonucleotide that anneals between the forward and reverse primers. This probe contains a fluorophore on the 5′ end and a quencher on the 3′ end. This method takes advantage of the 5′ to 3′ exonuclease activity of DNA polymerase. As the amplicon is synthesized by DNA polymerase, the probe is degraded. This separates the fluorophore from the quencher and results in fluorescence. As the number of amplicons increases, there is more target to anneal to the probe and greater fluorescence as the probes are degraded.[39] Molecular beacons and Scorpion probes use a hairpin structure to juxtapose the reporter and quencher. When the probe binds to the target, the hairpin unfolds and separates the fluorophore from the quencher, and fluorescence is detected.[40]

Qualitative Real-Time Polymerase Chain Reaction

Taqman assays are used to detect point mutations, such as a common point mutation in hereditary hemochromatosis, *HFE* C282Y (c.845G>A [p.Cys282Tyr]) (Chapter 17). Two Taqman probes are synthesized with a different fluorescent label, complementary to either the wild-type or mutant sequence. If the sequence is complementary to the target, the probe will be degraded as described above, and fluorescence will be produced. If the sequence contains a mismatch, the probe will be displaced and the fluorescence will remain quenched (Figure 29.18). Real-time PCR can also be combined with sequence-specific primer PCR (SSP-PCR) to detect point mutations or SNPs.

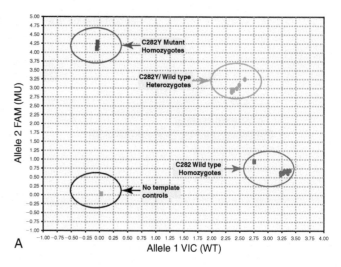

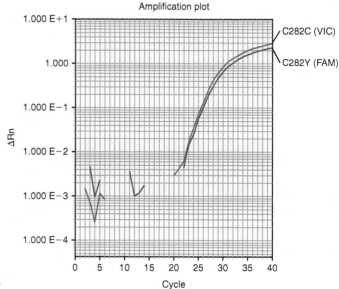

Figure 29.18 Qualitative Real-Time PCR for Hereditary Hemochromatosis, *HFE* **C282Y Gene Mutation Detection (c.845G>A [p.Cys282Tyr]).** The mutation replaces the amino acid cysteine (C) with tyrosine (Y) in position 282 of the HFE protein. The method uses two Taqman amplification probes, one for the wild type (normal) and one for the mutant allele, each labeled with a different fluorescent reporter. **(A),** Taqman allelic discrimination plot demonstrating the three genotypic populations for the *HFE* gene and no template controls. The scatter plots are derived from the total fluorescence of the amplification curve for both fluorescent probes. The genotype can be determined from the position on the scatter plot. **(B),** Real-time PCR amplification curves of a heterozygous C282C/Y mutant patient showing fluorescence with the two Taqman probes: VIC for the wild type and FAM for the mutant allele.

This method takes advantage of the fact that the 3′ end of a primer in PCR must match the template sequence exactly to be extended by the polymerase. This is in contrast to the 5′ end of the primer, which can have additional nucleotides added. By using primers complementary to either the wild-type or mutant nucleotide, the presence or absence of a mutation can be determined by the reaction that produces the PCR product.[41] There are several modifications of this technique. One widely used technique, called SnaPshot, uses dideoxynucleotides, each labeled with a different fluorophore and primers of different size in a multiplex reaction to detect several different nucleotide changes simultaneously. The different-sized PCR products are then identified by size fractionation using capillary gel electrophoresis.[42,43] There are other variations on this technique that are not discussed here. It is clear, however, that there are an increasing number of applications of real-time PCR in hematology, and multiple different techniques can be used to detect the same mutation. Applications of these techniques include the detection of resistance mutations in viruses or bacteria, in addition to somatic mutations in cancer cells and germline mutations in genetic diseases.

Quantitative Real-Time Polymerase Chain Reaction

Real-time quantitative PCR can be done in two ways: relative quantitation, which normalizes to a reference gene used when measuring gene expression, or absolute quantitation, in which a standard curve of a known copy number of diluted standards is run along with the patient specimens. Once the relationship between the copy number of the standards and the Ct value is determined using the standard curve, the copy number of

the patient specimen can be determined from the crossing point value. This assay is used to monitor residual disease in chronic myeloid leukemia by quantifying the amount of the *BCR-ABL1* transcript (Figure 29.19) (Chapter 32), and also viral loads in infectious disease.[44,45] For *BCR-ABL1* quantification a normalized copy number (NCN) is generated by dividing the *BCR-ABL1* copies by the control gene copy number. If an international standard is included in the assay, the NCN value can be converted to an International Standard NCN (ISNCN). This value should be reproducible across different laboratories and is the preferred value to be used to follow patients being treated with tyrosine kinase inhibitors.[46,47]

High-resolution melting curve (HRM) analysis is a real-time PCR method that uses the quantitative analysis of the melting curve to detect sequence differences in PCR amplicons. Melting curves are often run in conjunction with real-time PCRs to confirm specificity of the product by heating the amplicon in increasing intervals from 65° C to 95° C and measuring the fluorescence. When the double-stranded DNA melts, the fluorescence will sharply decrease. High-resolution melt curves use

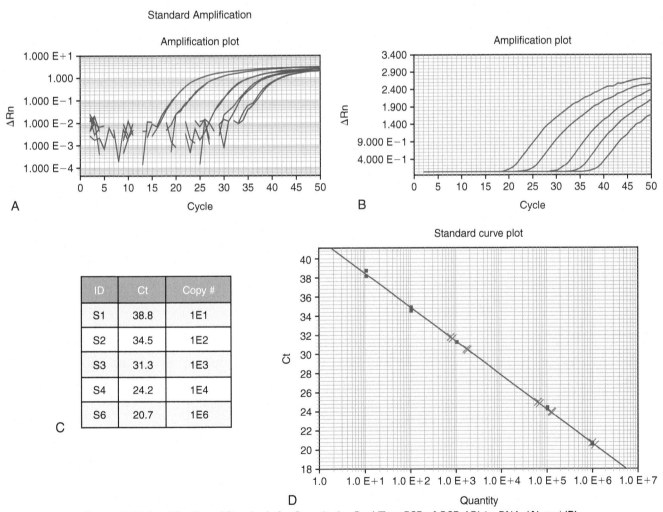

Figure 29.19 Amplification of Standards for Quantitative Real-Time PCR of *BCR-ABL1* mRNA. (A), and **(B),** Amplification curves for a series of standards of known copy number. **(C),** Table listing the Ct value and copy number of the standards containing known copy numbers of *BCR-ABL1* transcripts. **(D),** Graph of the Ct value versus the log of the copy number of the standards to generate a standard curve.

narrower temperature increments and a saturating fluorescent dye to determine the melting curve. This allows the determination of sequence differences in PCR amplicons. This method requires a thermocycler with good temperature stability and a software package for HRM analysis. The advantage of HRM is that it will detect any sequence difference in an amplicon, and the exact mutation does not have to be known in advance.[48]

Minimal Residual Disease in Leukemia

Various therapies reduce leukemia cells to undetectable levels when assessed by visual examination of a peripheral blood film or bone marrow smear. However, residual leukemia cells may still be present in the patient after treatment that are not detected by conventional morphology assessment; this is called *minimal residual disease* (MRD).[49] More sensitive methods are required to detect MRD. Real-time quantitative PCR provides the opportunity to follow disease burden and to measure MRD in leukemia, a key indicator of treatment efficacy, clinical remission, and prognosis.[47]

Real-time quantitative PCR identifies the specific nucleic acid sequence in residual leukemia cells and helps guide the types and intensity of therapy, with the goal of *molecular remission*. Real-time reverse transcriptase quantitative PCR to assess the fusion transcript levels in CML is regarded as the gold standard for the detection and quantification of MRD. Subsequent to remission, periodic real-time quantitative PCR assays are used to detect early relapse and drug resistance, enabling the hematologist to initiate appropriate follow-up therapy.[50]

Real-time quantitative PCR is able to detect a few malignant cells within a population of a million cells, providing unparalleled sensitivity. Current assays to assess MRD can detect one leukemia cell among 10^5 to 10^6 normal cells. Current applications include detection of *BCR-ABL1* transcripts in CML and some acute leukemias (Figure 29.20); *JAK2* mutations in the myeloproliferative neoplasms, such as polycythemia vera, essential thrombocythemia, and primary myelofibrosis (Chapter 32); the t(15;17) or *PML-RARA* fusion transcript in acute promyelocytic leukemia (Chapter 31); and gene rearrangements in mature lymphoid neoplasms (Chapter 34).[51]

A major issue with quantitative assays has been the lack of reproducibility between different laboratories due to the specimen type and quality, the choice of housekeeping gene for normalization, and the specific assay used. An international standard for *BCR-ABL1* quantification has been developed and made available by the World Health Organization (WHO). This standard serves as a universal standard and allows for interlaboratory comparison.[52]

Mutation Enrichment Strategies

In order to detect low levels of disease or emerging resistance, it is helpful to be able to enrich for the presence of the mutation. There are currently several methods to accomplish this, all of which seek to selectively amplify the mutant sequence in the presence of an excess of wild-type sequence. Peptide-nucleic acid (PNA) and locked nucleic acid (LNA) both contain normal nucleotide bases for hybridization but different backbones from

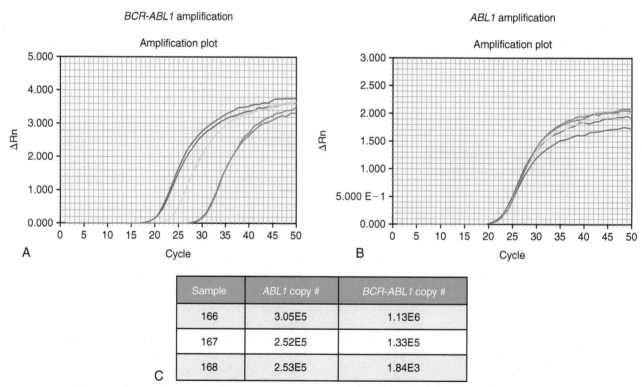

Sample	ABL1 copy #	BCR-ABL1 copy #
166	3.05E5	1.13E6
167	2.52E5	1.33E5
168	2.53E5	1.84E3

Figure 29.20 Quantitative Real-Time PCR for the *BCR-ABL1* mRNA. (A), Real-time PCR amplification for *BCR-ABL1* transcripts. **(B),** Real-time PCR amplification for the control gene, *ABL1*, as a measure of specimen quality. **(C),** Table listing the copy numbers for *ABL1* and *BCR-ABL1* for three specimens derived from standard curves, such as the one illustrated in Figure 29.19.

the phosphodiester backbone of DNA and RNA.[53] This gives these probes the ability to hybridize more tightly when used as probes in PCR reactions. When the probes span and match the wild-type sequence, they can inhibit the amplification of the wild-type allele, thus enriching for the mutant allele.[54]

COLD-PCR (**co**amplification at **l**ower **d**enaturation temperature–**PCR**) is another mutation enrichment technique based on PCR amplification. COLD-PCR is based on the principle that DNA containing a mismatch will melt at a slightly lower temperature than completely matched sequences. Designing the PCR cycle temperatures to maximize that difference results in a preferential amplification of the mutant sequence in a mixed specimen of mutant and wild-type DNA, even when the mutant is in very low concentration. This is accomplished by carrying out the denaturation step at the temperature that will have mutant-wild-type heteroduplexes in a single-stranded state, whereas wild-type homoduplexes will not yet have denatured.[55] All of these methods, although useful to enrich for mutant alleles, are technically demanding and therefore are not yet in widespread use in molecular laboratories.

NUCLEIC ACID SEQUENCING

DNA Sequencing by Capillary Electrophoresis

The ability to read the sequence of the nucleic acid has been just as important as PCR in the development of molecular biology. A combination of these two important techniques (cycle sequencing) has made DNA sequencing an integral part of molecular diagnostics. In cycle sequencing the order of the nucleotide bases is determined after amplification.[56] Cycle sequencing is applied in molecular testing to assess amplified sequences for insertions, deletions, or point mutations, such as *CEBPA* mutations that occur in some cases of AML (Chapter 31) or *JAK2* exons 12-15 mutations that occur in some cases of *BCR-ABL1*-negative myeloproliferative neoplasms (Chapter 32).[57,58]

Cycle sequencing is based on dideoxynucleotide terminator sequencing.[59] Addition of nucleotides to a growing DNA polymer requires a 3′ hydroxyl group on the last added nucleotide and a triphosphate group on the 5′ end of the next nucleotide to be added (Figure 29.5). If a nucleotide lacks the 3′ hydroxyl group, it can be incorporated into the newly synthesized strand of the DNA but cannot be extended, so the fragment terminates at the "defective" base. If low concentrations of the terminators – dideoxyadenosine triphosphate, dideoxycytosine triphosphate, dideoxyguanine triphosphate, and dideoxythymine triphosphate – are included in the single primer PCR master mix used for sequencing, over a number of cycles a series of DNA fragments is produced that terminate at each successive base with each fragment differing in length by one nucleotide. This is called a *ladder* or *nested series* of fragments.

In the dye terminator method each of the four dideoxynucleotides in the PCR reaction is labeled with a different fluorescent dye so that each DNA fragment terminates in a labeled dideoxynucleotide corresponding to the sequence of the target DNA (Figure 29.21A). The specific fluorescent color of the DNA fragment identifies the terminal nucleotide. Alternatively, in the dye primer method, the primers are labeled with four

different fluorescent dyes (corresponding to each nucleotide), and in separate tubes each labeled primer is subjected to PCR with unlabeled dideoxynucleotides (Figure 29.21B). As in the dye terminator method, the specific fluorescent color of the DNA fragments corresponds to the terminal nucleotide.

Fluorescently labeled fragments are subjected to capillary electrophoresis (described earlier in the chapter). DNA fragments migrate through the capillary and separate based on their size. Near the end of the capillary, fragments pass one by one through the beam of a laser in an order based on their length (with the shortest fragments emerging first). A detector reads the specific fluorescent color of each fragment and displays the signal as a peak on an electropherogram; this allows the sequence to be read (Figure 29.21C).

In order to unambiguously read the nucleotide at each position, the PCR reaction for cycle sequencing contains only a single primer that produces single-sided PCR. Two separate reactions are typically carried out, one using the forward primer and a second using the reverse primer. This produces complementary sequences from both strands. After the cycle sequencing reactions, the nested products are purified and denatured before loading on the capillary sequencer. Injection, separation, and detection are automated, but the operator can set the parameters, such as amount of specimen injected, length of capillaries, and type of polymer. Capillary DNA sequencing instruments are equipped with base calling software that will read the base sequence of the DNA fragment sequenced. Software packages will also identify alterations in the sequence, such as SNPs, point mutations, and insertions or deletions based on comparison to a specific reference sequence.

Pyrosequencing is another sequencing method that is useful for the determination of point mutations and short sequence analysis. This method uses a "sequencing by synthesis" principle and the detection of pyrophosphate release upon nucleotide incorporation. Nucleotides are added sequentially to a single-stranded template, and when the complementary base is added, it is incorporated, resulting in pyrophosphate release. The pyrophosphate released is then converted to adenosine triphosphate (ATP) by sulfurylase in the presence of adenosine 5′ phosphosulfate. This reaction is coupled to the luminescent conversion of luciferin to oxyluciferin by the enzyme luciferase, resulting in the release of light. Luminescent reactions resulting from the incorporation of nucleotides are represented as peaks on a pyrogram. The intensity of the light determines if there are multiple nucleotides that are identical because the peak height in the pyrogram will be proportional to the number of nucleotides.[60]

Sanger DNA sequencing has been considered the gold standard for the detection of germline point mutations and single nucleotide polymorphisms. With a point mutation, for example, sequencing of either strand will show whether the mutation (e.g., adenine to thymine) is present by comparison of the sequence to the reference sequence. Each cell has two copies (alleles) of somatic genes; therefore sequencing will produce a nested series of fragments from each allele. If the patient is a homozygote, the two nested series of fragments will be

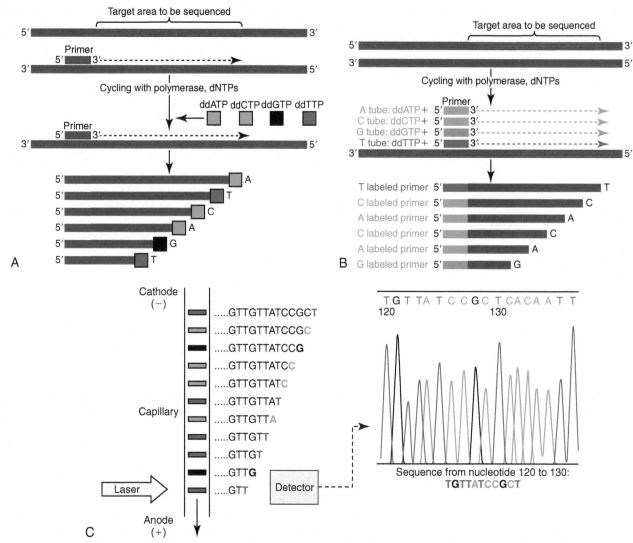

Figure 29.21 Dideoxy Chain Termination (Sanger) DNA Sequencing. Cycle sequencing of a DNA template produces a nested series of fragments that differ by one nucleotide each. The template is amplified by polymerase chain reaction (PCR) using a single primer sequence (single-sided PCR). The PCR master mix includes small amounts of dideoxynucleotides. When a dideoxynucleotide is incorporated into the growing DNA polymer, chain extension terminates. **(A),** Dye terminator method, in which each of the four dideoxynucleotides are labeled with a different fluorescent dye. The identity of the terminal nucleotide corresponds to its specific fluorescent color. **(B),** Dye primer method, in which the primer is labeled with four different fluorescent dyes, corresponding to each nucleotide. Again, the identity of the terminal nucleotide corresponds to the specific color of the primer. **(C),** Capillary gel electrophoresis, in which fluorescently labeled fragments pass between a laser and detector in size order (smallest fragments first). The fluorescent color of the fragment identifies the terminal nucleotide. The signals appear as peaks on an electropherogram, with each peak representing a specific terminal nucleotide in sequence order.

identical, whether wild type or mutant. If the patient is a heterozygote, both wild-type and mutant fragments will be produced in the single-sided PCR, generating two nested series of fragments. In analysis of this sequence, both signals will be present at the position of the mutation, but half the templates will contain each sequence.

Next-Generation Sequencing

Next-generation sequencing (NGS), also known as massively parallel sequencing (MPS), is a technique that is being increasingly applied in all areas of molecular diagnostics, including

hematology.[61,62] Large-scale sequencing efforts, such as The Cancer Genome Atlas (TCGA) and The 1000 Genomes Project, have greatly expanded the number of clinically relevant genes and gene variants.[63,64] Important variants have been identified in oncogenes, tumor suppressors, receptors and other signaling molecules, and in metabolic enzymes. Many of these genes have diagnostic, prognostic, or therapeutic implications in hematologic malignancies.[65] As the number of clinically significant variants has increased, so has the need for a unified platform for testing. Therefore NGS is playing an increasingly important role in clinical practice. The technology is still evolving, but the most commonly used and currently available methods sequence short fragments multiple times and use bioinformatics to reassemble the sequence and detect sequence variants. Most clinical NGS tests for hematologic malignancies and genetic diseases involve the selection of a panel of clinically relevant genes for testing.[66,67] These panels can detect single nucleotide variants, small insertions and deletions (indels), and in some cases, copy number variants. There are also RNA-based panels for the detection of fusion genes resulting from translocations.

The process of NGS can be divided into several steps, including template and library preparation, sequencing and detection, and finally, data analysis and assembly (Figure 29.22). Currently available commercial systems use a variety of methods. There are two common methods of template selection: amplicon based or capture based.[61,62] Amplicon-based target selection uses multiplex PCR reactions to amplify the sequences of interest, whereas capture-based target selection first uses baits to hybridize and capture the targets of interest, followed by PCR amplification. The libraries are prepared by the addition of indexing primers to identify each specimen. One commonly used method for sequencing involves immobilization of molecules on a solid phase followed by amplification to produce clonally amplified clusters. Sequencing by synthesis reactions is carried out using cyclic reversible terminators in four colors and fluorescent detection by lasers after each base addition. A second commonly used method also amplifies the sequencing template, but uses emulsion PCR to accomplish it. The sequencing technology takes advantage of the hydrogen ion released when a base is added and uses semiconductor technology to translate the release of a hydrogen ion into a nucleotide sequence by the sequential addition of bases and the measurement of the voltage produced when the correct nucleotide base is added. Both methods use proprietary software and alignment to a reference sequence to produce the final template sequence. There are also numerous programs available as open source or from commercial vendors for analysis.

As with any assay there are quality measures that are evaluated. All NGS sequencing reactions are given a quality score (Q score) and the number of reads (the number of times a target is sequenced) is evaluated. The variant allele fraction (VAF) is also evaluated to confirm it is above the limit of detection. Several consensus documents have been issued with respect to NGS including laboratory standards by the College of American Pathologists (CAP)[68], joint standards and guidelines on validating oncology panels and bioinformatics pipelines by CAP and the Association for Molecular Pathology (AMP),[69,70] as well as joint standards and guidelines for interpreting and reporting sequence variants in cancer by CAP, AMP, and the American Society of Clinical Oncology.[71] Current clinical applications for NGS have been mainly limited to the sequencing of panels of genes associated with a particular disease. This makes the bioinformatics analyses more manageable and limits the number of variants of unknown significance (VUS) that are identified. NGS clinical assays have been developed for many different hematologic diseases including myeloid, lymphoid, and erythroid malignancies.[72–75] In addition to sequencing panels of genes, this technology has been used to sequence whole genomes, exomes (the coding exons), as well as RNA sequencing (RNAseq).[76–78] This technology is also being applied to the determination of epigenome modifications such as methylation that affects gene regulation and expression.[79] NGS will continue to play an increasingly important role in molecular diagnostics.

CHROMOSOMAL MICROARRAYS

Chromosomal microarray analysis is a methodology used to measure gains and losses of genomic DNA. The advantage of a microarray, compared to conventional karyotyping, is that it is a higher-resolution method and will detect genetic changes that cannot be observed by karyotyping (Chapter 30). In addition, chromosomal microarrays have the advantage of also detecting aneuploidy and large chromosomal duplications and insertions.

There are two different types of chromosomal microarrays: comparative genomic hybridization (aCGH) and single nucleotide polymorphism array (SNP-A) karyotyping. Both types of arrays can identify variation in copy number. Due to differences in methodology, however, they detect different types of variants (Figures 29.23, 30.26, and 30.27).

In array-based assays, the specimen DNA is isolated, denatured, and hybridized to a chip or an array containing thousands of probes with known sequences. For comparative genome hybridization the patient DNA and a control DNA are labeled with different fluorescent dyes, and after hybridization the relative intensity of the two fluorescent signals is used to determine if there are any genomic gains or losses. Duplications result in a higher-intensity fluorescence relative to control, and deletions result in a lower-intensity fluorescence. CGH is most useful in the detection of relatively large duplications or deletions.[80]

In SNP arrays only the patient DNA is labeled, denatured, and hybridized to an array containing probes with known SNPs. Again, the signal intensity is used to determine the copy number. SNP arrays are able to detect runs of homozygosity that can indicate uniparental disomy or consanguinity.[81] Because each of these methods has both advantages and disadvantages, array platforms have been developed that contain both types of sequences: SNPs and larger clones used in CGH. This provides a more uniform coverage over the entire genome. Array procedures have improved such that in addition to DNA isolated from peripheral blood, DNA isolated from formalin-fixed paraffin-embedded specimens can also be used. In certain situations arrays are replacing. or are used as an adjunct to, conventional karyotyping and fluorescence in situ hybridization (FISH) (Chapter 30). Arrays are useful to detect copy number variants but do not detect balanced translocations.[81]

PATHOGEN DETECTION AND INFECTIOUS DISEASE LOAD

Box 29.4 contains a list of hematologically important pathogens detected by molecular methods. Real-time quantitative PCR can detect and quantify a number of blood-borne viruses: hepatitis B and C viruses, human papillomavirus, CMV,

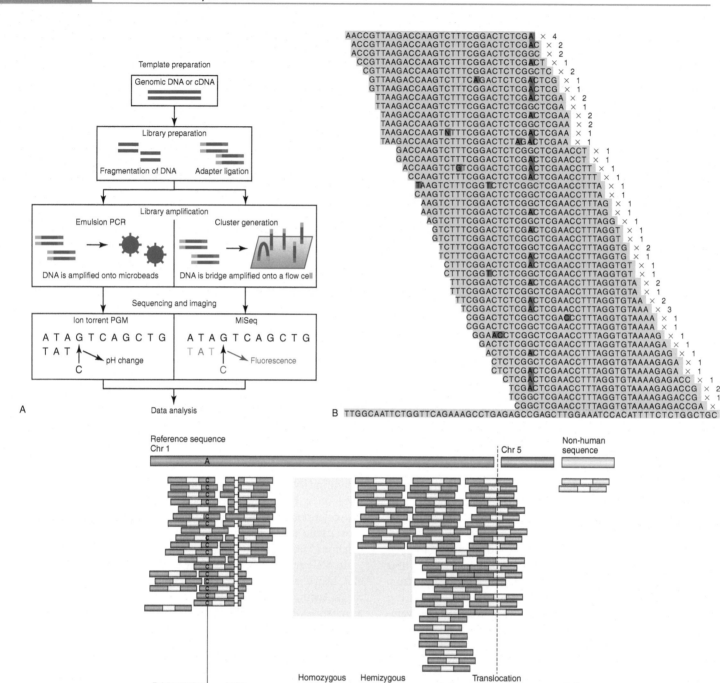

Figure 29.22 Next-Generation Sequencing. (A), Diagram of the procedure for next-generation sequencing (NGS) using the two most common technologies. **(B),** An illustration of a number of NGS reads for a 32-nucleotide sequence aligned with the genomic reference sequence in blue on the bottom (sequence mismatches are in red). The center of the alignment shows a variant present in the heterozygous state. **(C),** Sequenced fragments are depicted as bars with colored tips representing the sequenced ends and the unsequenced portion of the fragment in gray. Reads are aligned to the reference genome (e.g., mostly chromosome 1 in this example). The colors of the sequenced ends show where they align. Different types of genomic alterations can be detected. *Left to right,* Point mutations (in this example, A to C) and small insertions and deletions (indels) (in this example, a deletion shown by a dashed line) are detected by identifying multiple reads that show nonreference sequence; changes in sequencing depth (relative to a normal control) are used to identify copy number changes (shaded boxes represent absent or decreased reads in a tumor specimen); paired-ends that map to different genomic loci (in this case, chromosome 5) are evidence of rearrangements; and sequences that map to nonhuman sequences are evidence for the potential presence of genomic material from pathogens. (**A** from Grada, A. & Weinbrecht, K. [2013]. Next-generation sequencing: methodology and application. *J Invest Dermatol, 133,* 248–251; **B** from Almomani, R., van der Heijden, J., Ariyurek, Y., et al. [2011]. Experiences with array-based sequence capture; toward clinical applications. *Eur J Hum Genet, 19,* 50–55; **C** from Meyerson, M., Gabriel, S., & Getz, G. [2010]. Advances in understanding cancer genomes through second generation sequencing. *Nat Rev Genet, 11,* 685–696.)

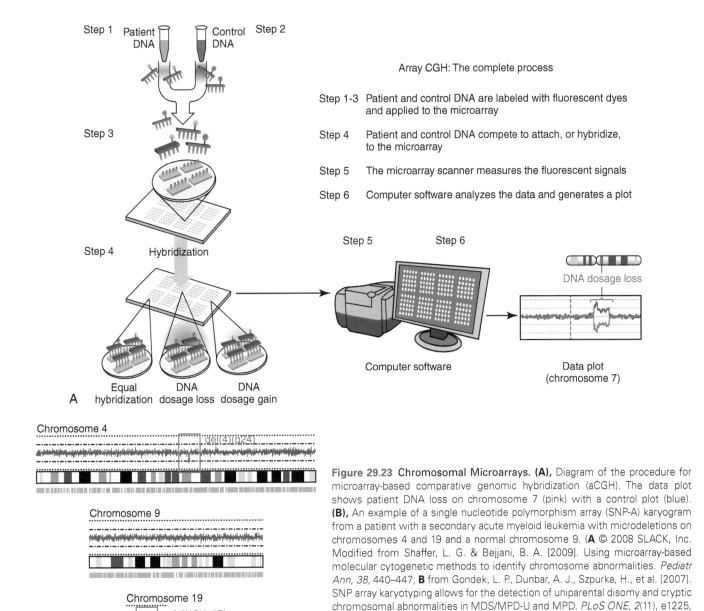

Figure 29.23 Chromosomal Microarrays. (A), Diagram of the procedure for microarray-based comparative genomic hybridization (aCGH). The data plot shows patient DNA loss on chromosome 7 (pink) with a control plot (blue). **(B),** An example of a single nucleotide polymorphism array (SNP-A) karyogram from a patient with a secondary acute myeloid leukemia with microdeletions on chromosomes 4 and 19 and a normal chromosome 9. (**A** © 2008 SLACK, Inc. Modified from Shaffer, L. G. & Bejjani, B. A. [2009]. Using microarray-based molecular cytogenetic methods to identify chromosome abnormalities. *Pediatr Ann, 38,* 440–447; **B** from Gondek, L. P., Dunbar, A. J., Szpurka, H., et al. [2007]. SNP array karyotyping allows for the detection of uniparental disomy and cryptic chromosomal abnormalities in MDS/MPD-U and MPD. *PLoS ONE, 2*(11), e1225, doi:10.1371/journal.pone.0001225.)

Epstein-Barr virus, and HIV.[82,83] Human bacterial pathogens, such as β-hemolytic *Streptococcus* from throat swabs, anaerobes from wound swabs, and bacteria from urine or other body fluids, can be detected within hours of collection. Antibacterial therapy can be initiated based upon the rapid results of molecular susceptibility testing. Real-time quantitative PCR is the reference method for detection and quantification of methicillin-resistant *Staphylococcus aureus* (MRSA), vancomycin-resistant *Enterococcus*, and opportunistic *Clostridium difficile*. Molecular diagnostic techniques are effective in identifying and monitoring malarial and other blood-borne parasites. The challenge to primer and probe developers is to select sequences that are specific enough to avoid false positives caused by nonpathogenic strains, sensitive enough to positively identify

infectious strains, and flexible enough to remain effective as pathogenic microorganisms mutate and evolve. There are currently multiple FDA-approved assays for the detection of viral, bacterial, and parasitic pathogens. A current listing of these tests can be found in the test directory on the Association for Molecular Pathology website (https://www.amp.org).

Clinical relevance is important when assessing infectious disease using molecular techniques. These methods allow millions of copies to be generated from a single DNA or RNA sequence from a microorganism or virus. Theoretically, the presence of a single organism can lead to a positive test result, but a single organism may not be clinically relevant. Standard curves of template number are crucial to data interpretation. Also, because DNA survives the organism, a positive result on a test for a given sequence does not guarantee that the organism was viable at the time of sampling.

CURRENT DEVELOPMENTS

Molecular diagnostics is a rapidly growing area of the clinical laboratory, and the technology continues to develop. It promises to revolutionize laboratory techniques in all disciplines, and the technologies of genomics are being extended to proteomics (the molecular analysis of proteins) and metabolomics (the molecular analysis of metabolism). Methods continue to be automated and miniaturized, providing ever greater sensitivity and reliability coupled with short turnaround time and technical simplification. In many situations assays are moving from single analyte assays to multiplex assays detecting panels of analytes. In the case of leukemias such as AML, mutations in multiple genes are incorporated into the WHO guidelines.[65] Methods such as NGS, described previously, are being applied to detect multiple mutations simultaneously.

Another technique being applied to the detection of mutation panels is matrix-assisted laser desorption/ionization-time of flight (MALDI-TOF) mass spectrometry. This methodology uses PCR coupled to a single-base extension reaction that adds labeled nucleotides so that the extension products containing different mutations have different masses. These reactions are also multiplexed to increase throughput, detecting hundreds of mutations in a single panel assay.[84]

Digital PCR (ddPCR) is a technique with very high sensitivity that can be used to detect resistance mutations to tyrosine kinase inhibitors used to treat CML (e.g., the T315I resistance mutation in the *BCR-ABL1* gene)[85] (Chapter 32) or to quantify virus copy number.[86] This technique uses various methods, for example, a droplet generator to create nanoliter droplets that partition template molecules, which are then amplified by PCR. The amplicons are detected by fluorescence and either read by a droplet reader or by some other detection mechanism. For translocation detection, wells containing an amplified housekeeping gene, translocation product, or both are then quantified. This method is extremely sensitive, detecting a few molecules per specimen, and can be applied to both DNA and RNA applications.[87]

Circulating tumor DNA is a promising technique using a minimally invasive specimen type for the monitoring of genetic alterations in solid tumors (e.g., lymphomas), which may shed DNA into the blood stream. This technique, known as "liquid biopsy," can potentially be used instead of a tissue biopsy to monitor for residual disease or the development of resistance to targeted drug therapy. The circulating tumor DNA can be tested using a variety of downstream techniques, including real-time PCR, digital PCR, or next-generation sequencing.[88]

Small microRNAs (miR, ~290 nucleotides long) that were once thought to be insignificant are evolving as biomarkers for the progression of hematologic malignancies. The dysregulation of miRs affects normal hematopoiesis, and their atypical expression is beginning to be established in T and B cell leukemias and lymphomas.[89] These miRs target genes in the 3′ UTR (3′ untranslated region) and are hypothesized to inhibit the translation of mRNAs to proteins.[90] These miRs can be detected by many molecular-based techniques, such as PCR, NGS, and microarray technology. Their clinical role in hematologic cancer therapy as a prognostic marker is now starting to be recognized. An overexpression of miR-21 has been demonstrated in CLL patients who are fludarabine nonresponders and in drug resistance in patients with plasma cell myeloma.[91,92] The overexpression of plasma miR-155 is also correlated to the identification of B-CLL in patients.[93] The listed studies demonstrate that the ability to measure the expression of miR has expanded the repertoire of diagnostic, prognostic, and therapeutic efficacy markers in hematologic malignancies.

In the future, molecular technologies will increase the efficiency and sensitivity for detection of all types of genome alterations, including point mutations, insertion and deletion mutations, copy number variants, and chromosome rearrangements. These new or improved techniques will facilitate the discovery of new chromosome rearrangements, in addition to the diagnosis of microbial infections. This will result in refined classification and improved treatment of hematologic diseases.

SUMMARY

- DNA directs cell function, as described by the central dogma. DNA retains the genetic code and reproduces itself through replication.
- The genetic code is transcribed from DNA to mRNA. The mRNA consists of coding exons and noncoding introns that are excised after transcription. The processed mRNA then transports the code from the nucleus to the cytoplasm, where it is translated to a peptide by the cytoplasmic ribosomes.
- DNA consists of a five-carbon sugar (deoxyribose), a phosphate group, and a nitrogenous base. Bases are either purines or pyrimidines. The purines are adenine (A) and guanine (G); the pyrimidines are thymine (T) and cytosine (C).
- DNA is a double-stranded molecule held together by hydrogen bonding between the bases, A to T and G to C. Heat denatures double-stranded DNA by breaking the hydrogen bonds,

producing single-stranded DNA. DNA strands are antiparallel; that is, 5′ to 3′ strands anneal to 3′ to 5′ complementary strands.
- DNA replication occurs in the 5′ to 3′ direction and requires a template, primer, 4 nucleotides (A, C, G, T), and DNA polymerase to add nucleotides which are complementary to the template.
- RNA is a single-stranded molecule that contains the sugar ribose instead of deoxyribose and the pyrimidine uracil in place of thymine.
- During transcription RNA polymerase recognizes a sequence of deoxyribonucleotides, called the *promoter*, within DNA. RNA polymerase binds to the promoter, separates the DNA strands, and begins adding ribonucleotides which are complementary to the DNA template, forming a primary RNA transcript consisting of introns and exons. The exons provide

the coding information. The introns are excised and the exons are spliced together forming a mature mRNA which enters the cytoplasm and is translated to protein by ribosomes.

- Translation depends on tRNA, small RNA molecules designed to transport and add amino acids to growing peptide chains in cytoplasmic ribosomes.

- Five areas of hematopathologic molecular testing include detection of mutations, gene rearrangements, and chromosomal abnormalities for diagnosis and prognosis of hematologic malignancies; detection and quantification of minimal residual disease to monitor treatment of hematologic malignancies; detection of mutations in inherited hematologic disorders; pharmacogenetic testing to detect genetic variation affecting certain drug therapies; and identification of hematologically important infectious diseases.

- Peripheral blood, bone marrow, tissue biopsy specimens (both fresh and formalin fixed paraffin embedded), fine-needle aspirates, body fluids, saliva, and cheek swabs are specimens used for DNA and RNA isolation.

- Specific DNA sequences are amplified by end-point polymerase chain reaction (PCR) and real-time PCR. RNA targets can be amplified by PCR by first converting the RNA target to complementary DNA, or cDNA.

- In end-point PCR, amplified DNA is detected by gel electrophoresis (slab gel or automated capillary gel electrophoresis) or DNA sequencing. End-point PCR can also be combined with restriction enzyme digestion of amplicons, followed by detection of the restriction fragments by one of the methods mentioned above. In real-time PCR, the amplicons are detected during the PCR cycles by fluorescence detection. Cleavage-based signal amplification is a non-PCR technology that identifies a DNA target by amplifying a signal from that target.

- Real-time PCR can be used qualitatively to determine the presence or absence of a target or can quantify the copy number of a target DNA or RNA. PCR can be used to amplify RNA targets by first converting them to cDNA with reverse transcriptase.

- The dideoxy chain termination (Sanger) method for DNA sequencing is based on the principle that synthesis of a DNA polymer is terminated upon incorporation of a dideoxynucleotide. The target DNA template is amplified over a number of cycles, which produces a series of DNA fragments that terminate at each successive base, with each fragment differing in length by one nucleotide. DNA fragments are detected by labeling either the dideoxynucleotide or the primer with a fluorescent dye. Other methods for DNA sequencing include pyrosequencing and next-generation sequencing (NGS).

- NGS is a parallel sequencing technique in which multiple molecules are sequenced simultaneously. This technique can be used to sequence panels of genes to identify mutations and small insertions and deletions (indels).

- Chromosomal microarrays measure gains and losses of genomic DNA. They provide much greater sensitivity in detecting small genomic changes compared to conventional karyotyping. There are two types: microarray-based comparative genomic hybridization (aCGH) and single nucleotide polymorphism array (SNP-A) karyotyping. CGH requires the use of a control DNA.

- Molecular testing permits clinicians to make more accurate diagnostic, therapeutic, and prognostic decisions. It also allows a more sensitive assessment of minimal residual disease and therapeutic efficacy, resulting in better patient management.

Now that you have completed this chapter, go back and read again the case study at the beginning and respond to the questions presented.

REVIEW QUESTIONS

Answers can be found in the Appendix.

1. If the DNA nucleotide sequence is 5′-ATTAGC-3′, then the mRNA sequence transcribed from this template is:
   a. 5′-GCUAAU-3′
   b. 5′-AUUAGC-3′
   c. 5′-TAATCG-3′
   d. 5′-UAAUCG-3′

2. Cells with damaged DNA and mutated or nonfunctioning cell cycle regulatory proteins:
   a. Are arrested in G1 and the DNA is repaired
   b. Continue to divide, which leads to tumor progression
   c. Divide normally, producing identical daughter cells
   d. Go through apoptosis

3. To start DNA replication, DNA polymerase requires an available 3′ hydroxyl group found on the:
   a. Leading strand
   b. mRNA
   c. Parent strand
   d. Primer

4. Ligase joins Okazaki fragments of the:
   a. 5′ to 3′ template strand
   b. Lagging strand
   c. Leading strand
   d. Primer fragments

5. A 40-year-old patient enters the hospital with a rare form of cancer caused by faulty cell division regulation. This cancer localized in the patient's spleen. An ambitious laboratory developed a molecular test to verify the type of cancer present. This molecular test would require patient specimens taken from which two tissues?
   a. Abnormal growths found on the skin and in the bone marrow
   b. Normal splenic tissue and cancerous tissue
   c. Cancerous tissue in spleen and bone marrow
   d. Peripheral blood and cancerous tissue in the spleen

6. One main difference between PCR and reverse transcriptase PCR is that:
   a. PCR requires primers
   b. PCR uses reverse transcriptase to elongate the primers
   c. Reverse transcriptase PCR uses cDNA as a template
   d. Reverse transcriptase PCR requires ligase to amplify the target DNA

7. Which one of the following statements about gel electrophoresis is FALSE?
   a. The gel is oriented in the chamber with the wells at the positive terminal.
   b. A buffer solution is required to maintain the electrical current.
   c. The matrix of a polyacrylamide gel is tighter than that of an agarose gel.
   d. The larger DNA fragments will be closest to the wells of the gel.

8. In which of the following applications would it be most appropriate to use NGS technology?
   a. Testing for a point mutation in the *FV* gene
   b. Testing for the *BCR-ABL1* translocation in CML
   c. Sequencing a B cell lymphoma genome
   d. Determining the karyotype in AML

9. One major difference between endpoint PCR and real-time PCR is that:
   a. End-point PCR requires thermostable DNA polymerase, deoxynucleotides, and primers
   b. End-point PCR requires a separate step to detect the amplicons formed in the reaction
   c. Real-time PCR uses capillary gel electrophoresis to detect amplicons during PCR cycling
   d. Real-time PCR detects and quantifies amplicons using cleavage-based signal amplification

10. Which of the following statements about minimal residual disease is TRUE?
    a. Clinical remission of hematologic cancers is determined by molecular techniques such as PCR and flow cytometry.
    b. Real-time quantitative PCR-determined copy number of *BCR-ABL1* transcripts will always be lower in molecular remission than in clinical remission.
    c. Qualitative PCR that uses a known copy number of a target sequence is of use in determining minimal residual disease levels.
    d. Minimal residual disease assessment can aid physicians in making treatment decisions but does not yet offer insights into prognosis.

REFERENCES

1. Rees, D. C., Williams, T. N., & Gladwin, M. T. (2010). Sickle-cell disease. *Lancet*, *376*(9757), 2018–2031.
2. National Human Genome Research Institute. *A Brief Guide to Genomics*. https://www.genome.gov/18016863/a-brief-guide-to-genomics/. Accessed May 10, 2018.
3. Hubé, F., & Francastel, C. (2015). Mammalian introns: when the junk generates molecular diversity. *Int J Mol Sci*, *16*(3), 4429–4452.
4. Lewin, B. (2008). Messenger RNA. In *Genes IX*. (3rd ed., pp. 127–150). Sudbury, Mass: Jones & Bartlett.
5. Lodish, H., Berk, A., Kaiser, C. A., et al. (2016). Fundamental molecular genetic mechanisms. In *Molecular Cell Biology* (8th ed., pp. 167–222). New York, NY: WH Freeman.
6. Bartlett, J. M. S., & White, A. (2003). Extraction of DNA from whole blood. In Bartlett, J. M. S., & Stirling, D. (Eds.), *PCR Protocols*. (2nd ed., pp. 29–31). Totowa, NJ: Humana Press.
7. Shimizu, H., & Burns, J. C. (1995). Extraction nucleic acids: sample preparation from paraffin-embedded tissues. In Innis, M. A., Gelfand, D. H., & Sninsky, J. J. (Eds.), *PCR Strategies* (pp. 32–38). San Diego: Academic Press.
8. Cao, W., Hashibe, M., Rao, J. Y., et al. (2003). Comparison of methods for DNA extraction from paraffin-embedded tissues and buccal cells. *Cancer Detect Prevent*, *27*, 397–404.
9. Harder, J., & Schroder, J. M. (2002). RNase 7, a novel innate immune defense antimicrobial protein of healthy human skin. *J Biol Chem*, *277*, 46779–46784.
10. Bogner, P. N., & Killeen, A. A. (2006). Extraction of nucleic acids. In Coleman, W. B., & Tsongalis, G. J. (Eds.), *Molecular Diagnostics for the Clinical Laboratorian*. (pp. 25–30). Totowa, NJ: Humana Press.
11. Killeen, A. A. (2004). Methods in molecular pathology. In *Principles of Molecular Pathology* (pp. 89–139). Totowa, NJ: Humana Press.
12. Southern, E. M. (1975). Detection of specific sequences among DNA fragments separated by gel electrophoresis. *J Mol Biol*, *98*, 503–517.
13. Yuen, E., & Brown, R. D. (2005). Southern blotting of IgH rearrangements in B-cell disorders. In Brown, R. D., & Ho, P. (Eds.), *Multiple Myeloma*. (pp. 85–103). Totowa, NJ: Humana Press.
14. Mullis, K. B., & Faloona, F. A. (1987). Specific synthesis of DNA in vitro via a polymerase-catalyzed chain reaction. *Methods Enzymol*, *155*, 335–350.
15. Saiki, R. K., Scharf, S., Faloona, F., et al. (1985). Enzymatic amplification of β-globin genomic sequences and restriction site analysis for diagnosis of sickle cell anemia. *Science*, *230*, 1350–1354.
16. Studwell, P. S., & O'Donnell, M. (1990). Processive replication is contingent on the exonuclease subunit of DNA polymerase III holoenzyme. *J Biol Chem*, *265*, 1171–1178.
17. Saiki, R. K., Gelfand, D. H., Stoffel, S., et al. (1988). Primer-directed enzymatic amplification of DNA with a thermostable DNA polymerase. *Science*, *239*, 487–491.
18. Cha, R. S., & Thilly, W. G. (1995). Specificity, fidelity and efficiency of PCR. In Dieffenbach, C. W., & Dveksler, G. S. (Eds.), *PCR Primer: A Laboratory Manual*. (pp. 37–52). Cold Spring Harbor, NY: Cold Spring Harbor Press.
19. Altschul, S. F., Gish, W., Miller, W., et al. (1990). Basic local alignment search tool. *J Mol Biol*, *215*, 403–410.
20. Mifflin, T. E. (2003). Setting up a PCR laboratory. In Dieffenbach, C. W., & Dveksler, G. S. (Eds.), *PCR Primer: A Laboratory Manual*. (2nd ed., pp. 5–14). Cold Spring Harbor, NY: Cold Spring Harbor Laboratory Press.
21. Najfeld, V. (2018). Conventional and molecular cytogenomic basis of hematologic malignancies. In Hoffman, R., Benz, E. J., Silberstein, L. E., et al. (Eds.), *Hematology: Basic Principles and Practice*. (7th ed., pp. 774–848). Philadelphia, PA: Elsevier.
22. Bhatt, V. R., Akhtari, M., Bociek, R, G., et al. (2014). Allogeneic stem cell transplantation for Philadelphia chromosome-positive acute myeloid leukemia. *J Natl Compr Canc Netw*, *12*, 963–968.

23. Bartram, C. R., de Klein, A., Hagemeijer, A., et al. (1983). Translocation of the *c-abl* oncogene correlates with the presence of a Philadelphia chromosome in chronic myelocytic leukemia. *Nature, 306,* 277–280.

24. Heisterkamp, N., Stephenson, J. R., Groffen, J., et al. (1983). Localization of the *c-abl* oncogene adjacent to a translocation break point in chronic myelocytic leukemia. *Nature, 306,* 239–242.

25. Clark, S. S., McLaughlin, J., Crist, W. M., et al. (1987). Unique forms of the abl tyrosine kinase distinguish Ph1-positive CML from Ph1-positive ALL. *Science, 235,* 85–88.

26. Preudhomme, C., Revillion, F., Merlat, A., et al. (1999). Detection of BCR-ABL transcripts in chronic myeloid leukemia (CML) using a "real-time" quantitative RT-PCR assay. *Leukemia, 13,* 957–964.

27. Luu, M. H., & Press, R. D. (2013). BCR-ABL PCR testing in chronic myelogenous leukemia: molecular diagnosis for targeted cancer therapy and monitoring. *Expert Rev Mol Diagn, 13,* 749–762.

28. Sambrook, J., & Russell, D. W. (2001). Gel electrophoresis of DNA and pulsed-field agarose gel electrophoresis. In Sambrook, J., & Russell, D. W. (Eds.), *Molecular Cloning: A Laboratory Manual.* (3rd ed., pp. 5.4–5.86). Cold Spring Harbor, NY: Cold Spring Harbor Laboratory Press.

29. Dubrow, R. S. (1992). Capillary gel electrophoresis. In Grossman, P. D., & Colburn, J. C. (Eds.), *Capillary Gel Electrophoresis Theory and Practice.* (pp. 146–154). San Diego: Academic Press.

30. Van Dongen, J., Langerak, A. W., Bruggemann, M., et al. (2003). Design and standardization of PCR primers and protocols for the detection of immunoglobulin and T cell receptor gene rearrangements in suspect lymphoproliferations. Report of the BIOMED-2 Concerted Action BMH4-CT98-3936. *Leukemia, 12,* 2257–2317.

31. Nathans, D., & Smith, H. O. (1975). Restriction endonucleases in the analysis and restructuring of DNA molecules. *Annu Rev Biochem, 44,* 273–293.

32. Ross, D. W. (1990). Restriction enzymes. *Arch Pathol Lab Med, 114,* 906.

33. De Stefano, V., Finazzi, G., & Mannucci, P. M. (1996). Inherited thrombophilia: pathogenesis, clinical syndromes, and management. *Blood, 87,* 3531–3544.

34. Liu, X. Y., Nelson, D., Grant, C., et al. (1995). Molecular detection of a common mutation in coagulation F5 causing thrombosis via hereditary resistance to activated protein C. *Diagn Mol Pathol, 4,* 191–197.

35. Kwiatkowski, R. W., Lyamichev, V., de Arruda, M., et al. (1999). Clinical, genetic and pharmacogenetic applications of the Invader assay. *Mol Diagn, 4,* 353–364.

36. Templeton, K. E., & Claas, E. C. J. (2003). Comparison of four real-time PCR detection systems. In Dieffenbach, C. W., & Dveksler, G. S. (Eds.), *PCR Primer: A Laboratory Manual.* (2nd ed., pp. 187–198). Cold Spring Harbor, NY: Cold Spring Harbor Laboratory Press.

37. van der Velden, V. H. J., Hochhaus, A., Cazzaniga, G., et al. (2003). Detection of minimal residual disease in hematologic malignancies by real-time quantitative PCR: principles, approaches, and laboratory aspects. *Leukemia, 17,* 1013–1034.

38. Ahmad, A. I., & Ghasemi, J. B. (2007). New FRET primers for quantitative real-time PCR. *Anal Bioanal Chem, 387,* 2737–2743.

39. Luthra, R., & Medeiros, L. J. (2006). TaqMan reverse transcriptase-polymerase chain reaction coupled with capillary electrophoresis for quantification and identification of bcr-abl transcript type. *Methods Mol Biol, 335,* 135–145.

40. Tan, W., Wang, K., & Drake, T. J. (2004). Molecular beacons. *Curr Opin Chem Biol, 8,* 547–553.

41. Rudert, W. A., Braun, E. R., & Faas, S. J. (1997). Double labeled fluorescent probes for 5′ nuclease assays: purification and performance evaluation. *BioTechniques, 22,* 1140–1145.

42. Fanis, P., Kousiappa, I., Phylactides, M., et al. (2014). Genotyping of BCL11A and HBSIL-MYB SNPs associated with fetal haemoglobin levels: a SNaPshot minisequencing approach. *BMC Genomics, 15,* 108. doi:10.1186/1471-2164-15-108.

43. Latini, F. R., Gazito, D., Amoni, C. P., et al. (2014). A new strategy to identify rare blood donors: single polymerase chain reaction multiplex SNaPshot reaction for detection of 16 blood group alleles. *Blood Transfus, 12*(Suppl. 1), s256–s263.

44. Jennings, L. J., Smith, F. A., Halling, K. C., et al. (2012). Design and analytic validation of BCR-ABL1 quantitative reverse transcription polymerase chain reaction assay for monitoring minimal residual disease. *Arch Pathol Lab Med, 136,* 33–40.

45. Wittek, M., Stürmer, M., Doerr, H. W., et al. (2007). Molecular assays for monitoring HIV infection and antiretroviral therapy. *Expert Rev Mol Diagn, 7,* 237–746.

46. Gabert, J., Beillard, E., van der Velden, V. H., et al. (2003). Standardization and quality control of "real-time" quantitative reverse transcriptase polymerase chain reaction of fusion transcripts for residual disease detection in leukemia: a Europe Against Cancer program. *Leukemia, 17,* 2318–2357.

47. Press, R. D., Kamel-Reid, S., & Ang, D. (2013). BCR-ABL1 RT-qPCR for monitoring the molecular response to tyrosine kinase inhibitors in chronic myeloid leukemia. *J Mol Diagn, 15,* 565–576.

48. Wittwer, C., Gudrun, H. R., Gundry, C. N., et al. (2003). High-resolution genotyping by amplicon melting analysis using LC Green. *Clin Chem, 49,* 853–860.

49. Kantarjian, H., Schiffer, C., Jones, D., et al. (2008). Monitoring the response and course of chronic myeloid leukemia in the modern era of BCR-ABL tyrosine kinase inhibitors: practical advice on the use and interpretation of monitoring methods. *Blood, 111,* 1774–1780.

50. Parker, W. T., Lawrence, R. M., Ho, M., et al. (2011). Sensitive detection of BCR-ABL1 mutations with chronic myeloid leukemia after imatinib resistance is predictive of outcome during subsequent therapy. *J Clin Oncol, 29,* 4250–4259.

51. Lobetti-Bodoni, C., Mantoan, B., Monitillo, L., et al. (2013). Clinical implications and prognostic role of minimal residual disease detection in follicular lymphoma. *Ther Adv Hematol, 4,* 189–198.

52. White, H. E., Matejtschuk, P., Rigsby, P., et al. (2010). Establishment of the first World Health Organization International Genetic Reference Panel for quantitation of BCR-ABL mRNA. *Blood, 116,* e111–e117.

53. Porcheddu, A., & Giacomelli, G. (2005). Peptide nucleic acids (PNAs), a chemical overview. *Curr Med Chem, 12,* 2561–2599.

54. Oh, J. E., Lim, H. S., An, C. H., et al. (2010). Detection of low-level KRAS mutations using PNA-mediated asymmetric PCR clamping and melting curve analysis with unlabeled probes. *J Mol Diagn, 12,* 418–424.

55. Milbury, C. A., Li, J., Liu, P., et al. (2011). COLD-PCR: improving the sensitivity of molecular diagnostics assays. *Expert Rev Mol Diagn, 11,* 159–169.

56. Buckingham, L. (2012). DNA sequencing. In Buckingham, L. (Ed.), *Molecular Diagnostics: Fundamentals, Methods, and Clinical Applications.* (2nd ed., pp. 222–240). Philadelphia, PA: FA Davis.

57. Behdad, A., Weigelin, H. C., Elenitoba-Johnson, K. S., et al. (2015). A clinical grade sequencing-based assay for *CEBPA* mutation testing: report of a large series of myeloid neoplasms. *J Mol Diagn, 17*(1), 76–84.

58. Alghasham, N., Alnouri, Y., Abalkhail, H., et al. (2016). Detection of mutations in *JAK2* exons 12-15 by Sanger sequencing. *Int J Lab Hematol, 38*(1), 34–41.

59. Sanger, F., Nicklen, S., & Coulson, A. R. (1977). DNA sequencing with chain-terminating inhibitors. *Proc Natl Acad Sci U S A, 74,* 5463–5467.

60. Fakhrai-Rad, H., Pourmand, N., & Ronaghi, M. (2002). Pyrosequencing: an accurate detection platform for single nucleotide polymorphisms. *Hum Mutat, 19,* 479–485.

61. Goodwin, S., McPherson, J. D., & McCombie, W. R. (2016). Coming of age: ten years of next-generation sequencing technologies. *Nat Rev Genet, 17,* 333–351.

62. Levy, S. E., & Myers, R. M. (2016). Advancements in next-generation sequencing. *Annu Rev Genomics Hum Genet, 17,* 95–115.

63. The Cancer Genome Atlas. National Cancer Institute, National Human Genome Research Institute. https://cancergenome.nih.gov. Accessed April 22, 2018.

64. The 1000 Genomes Consortium. (2015). A global reference for human genetic variation. *Nature, 526,* 68–74.

65. Swerdlow, S. H., Campo, E., Harris, N. L., et al. (2017). *WHO Classification of Tumours of Haematopoietic and Lymphod Tissues* (Revised 4th ed.). Lyon: IARC.

66. He, J., Abdel-Wahab, O., Nahas, M. K., et al. (2016). Integrated genomic DNA/RNA profiling of hematologic malignancies in the clinical setting. *Blood, 127*(24), 3004–3014.

67. Kluk, M. J., Lindsley, R. C., Aster, J. C., et al. (2016). Validation and implementation of a custom next-generation sequencing clinical assay for hematologic malignancies. *J Mol Diagn, 18*(4), 507–515.

68. Aziz, N., Zhao, Q., Bry, L., et al. (2015). College of American Pathologists' laboratory standards for next-generation sequencing clinical tests. *Arch Pathol Lab Med, 139,* 481–493.

69. Jennings, L. J., Arcila, M. E., Corless, C., et al. (2017). Guidelines for the validation of next-generation sequencing based oncology panels: a joint consensus recommendation of the Association for Molecular Pathology and College of American Pathologists. *J Mol Diagn, 19*(3), 341–365.

70. Roy, S., Coldren, C., Karunamurthy, A., et al. (2018). Standards and guidelines for validating next-generation sequencing bioinformatics pipelines: a joint recommendation of the Association for Molecular Pathology and the College of American Pathologists. *J Mol Diagn, 20*(1), 4–27.

71. Li, M. M., Datto, M., Duncavage, E. J., et al. (2017). Standards and guidelines for the interpretation and reporting of sequence variants in cancer. A joint consensus recommendation of the Association for Molecular Pathology, American Society of Clinical Oncology, and College of American Pathologists. *J Mol Diagn, 19*(1), 4–23.

72. Stamatopoulos, B., Timbs, A., & Bruce, D. (2017). Targeted deep sequencing reveals clinically relevant subclonal *IGHV* rearrangements in chronic lymphocytic leukemia. *Leukemia, 31,* 837–845.

73. Patnaik, M. M., Lasho, T. L., Finke, C. M., et al. (2016). Predictors of survival in refractory anemia with ring sideroblasts and thrombocytosis (RARS-T) and the role of next generation sequencing. *Am J Hematol, 91,* 492–498.

74. Mata, E., Diaz-Lopez, A., Martin-Moreno, A. M., et al. (2017). Analysis of the mutational landscape of classic Hodgkin lymphoma identifies disease heterogeneity and potential therapeutic targets. *Oncotarget, 8*(67), 111386–111395.

75. Bartels, S., Schipper, E., Hasemeier, B., et al. (2016). Routine clinical mutation profiling using next generation sequencing and a customized gene panel improves diagnostic precision in myeloid neoplasms. *Oncotarget, 7*(21), 30084–30093.

76. Oberg, J. A., Glade Bender, J. L., Sulis, M. L., et al. (2016). Implementation of next generation sequencing into pediatric hematology-oncology practice: moving beyond actionable alterations. *Genome Med, 8,* 133–151.

77. Ferreira, P. G., Jares, P., Rico, D., et al. (2014). Transcriptome characterization by RNA sequencing identifies a major molecular and clinical subdivision in chronic lymphocytic leukemia. *Genome Res, 24,* 212–226.

78. Koboldt, D. C., Steinberg, K. M., Larson, D. E., et al. (2013). The next-generation sequencing revolution and its impact on genomics. *Cell, 155,* 27–38.

79. Rivera, C. M., & Ren, B. (2013). Mapping human epigenomes. *Cell, 155,* 39–55.

80. Shao, L., Kang, S-H., Li, J., et al. (2010). Array comparative genomic hybridization detects chromosomal abnormalities in hematological cancers that are not detected by conventional cytogenetics. *J Mol Diagn, 12,* 670–679.

81. Hagenkord, J., & Chang, C. C. (2009). The reward and challenges of array-based karyotyping for clinical oncology applications. *Leukemia, 23,* 829–833.

82. Kwong, Y. L., Pang, A. W., Leung, A. Y., et al. (2014). Quantification of circulating Epstein-Barr virus DNA in NK/T-cell lymphoma treated with the SMILE protocol: diagnostic and prognostic significance. *Leukemia, 28,* 865–870.

83. Chevaliez, S., Bouvier-Alias, M., Rodriguez, C., et al. (2013). The COBAS Ampliprep/COBAS TaqMan HCV test v2.0, real-time PCR assay accurately quantifies hepatitis C virus genotype 4 RNA. *J Clin Microbiol, 51,* 1078–1082.

84. Dunlap, J., Beadling, C., Warrick, A., et al. (2012). Multiplex high-throughput gene mutation analysis in acute myeloid leukemia. *Hum Pathol, 43,* 2167–2176.

85. Jennings, L. J., George, D., Czech, J., et al. (2014). Detection and quantification of BCR-ABL1 fusion transcripts by droplet digital PCR. *J Mol Diagn, 16,* 174–179.

86. Hall Sedlak, R., & Jerome, K. R. (2014). The potential advantages of digital PCR for clinical virology diagnostics. *Expert Rev Mol Diagn, 14,* 501–507.

87. Huggett, J. F., Cowen, S., & Foy, C. A. (2015). Considerations for digital PCR as an accurate molecular diagnostic tool. *Clin Chem, 61*(1), 79–88.

88. Wood-Bouwens, C., Lau, B. T., Hande, C. M., et al. (2017). Single-color digital PCR provides high-performance detection of cancer mutations from circulating DNA. *J Mol Diagn, 19*(5), 697–710.

89. Zhao, H., Wang, D., Du, W., et al. (2010). MicroRNA and leukemia: tiny molecule, great function. *Crit Rev Oncol Hematol, 74,* 149–155.

90. Undi, R. B., Kandi, R., & Gutti, R. K. (2013). MicroRNA as haematopoiesis regulators. *Adv Hematol, 2013,* 1–20.

91. Ferracin, M., Zagatti, B., Rizzotto, L., et al. (2010). MicroRNAs involvement in fludarabine refractory chronic lymphocytic leukemia. *Mol Cancer, 9,* 123.

92. Ma, J., Liu, S., & Wang, Y. (2014). MicroRNA-21 and multiple myeloma: small molecule and big function. *Med Oncol, 31,* 94.

93. Ferraioli, A., Shanafelt, T. D., Shimizu, M., et al. (2013). Prognostic value of miR-155 in individuals with monoclonal B-cell lymphocytosis and patients with B chronic lymphocytic leukemia. *Blood, 122,* 1891–1899.

Cytogenetics/Cytogenomics

Gail H. Vance

OBJECTIVES

After completion of this chapter, the reader will be able to:

1. Describe chromosome structure and the methods used in G-banded chromosome identification.
2. Explain the basic laboratory techniques for preparing chromosomes for analysis.
3. Differentiate between numeric and structural chromosome abnormalities.
4. Discuss the importance of karyotype in the diagnosis of hematologic cancer.
5. Explain the basic technique of fluorescence *in situ* hybridization (FISH).
6. Discuss the advantage of using FISH analysis in conjunction with G-banded analysis of cells.
7. Describe the types of chromosomal abnormalities that are detectable with cytogenetic methods.
8. Given a diagram of a G-banded chromosome and be able to name the chromosome structures identifiable by light microscopy.
9. Given the designation of a chromosome mutation, be able to determine whether the abnormality is numeric or structural, which chromosomes are affected, what type of abnormality it is, and what portion of the chromosome is affected.
10. Define chromosomal microarray analysis and understand the genomic nature of this test.

OUTLINE

CASE STUDY

After studying the material in this chapter, the reader should be able to respond to the questions from the following case study:

A 54-year-old man came to his physician with a history of fatigue, weight loss, and increased bruising over a 6-month period. His WBC count was elevated at 200×10^9/L. A bone marrow aspirate was sent for cytogenetic analysis. G-banded chromosome analysis of 20 cells from bone marrow cultures showed all cells to be positive for the Philadelphia chromosome, t(9;22)(q34;q11.2), as seen in chronic myeloid leukemia (Figure 30.1). FISH studies using the *BCR* and *ABL1* gene probes (Abbott Molecular, Des Plaines, IL) produced dual fusion signals, one located on the derivative chromosome 9 and one on the derivative chromosome 22, characteristic of the translocation between chromosomes 9 and 22 leading to the rearrangement of *BCR* and *ABL1* oncogenes (Figure 30.2). The patient was treated with imatinib mesylate for the next 2 months. Another cytogenetic study was performed on a second bone marrow aspirate. This analysis showed that 12 of 20 cells analyzed were normal, 46,XY[12]; however,

Continued

CASE STUDY—cont'd

there were still 8 cells positive for the Philadelphia chromosome, 46,XY,t(9;22)(q34; q11.2)[8].

1. What is G-banded chromosome analysis?
2. Is the described mutation an example of a numeric or a structural abnormality? What type? Which chromosomes are involved? Explain.
3. What is FISH, and how does it complement standard chromosome analysis?

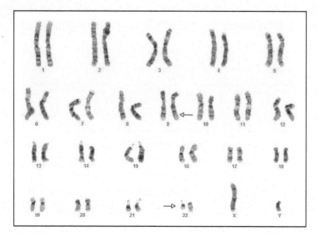

Figure 30.1 Karyogram for the Patient in the Case Study. Shows a translocation between chromosomes 9 and 22, which is characteristic of chronic myelogenous leukemia. (Courtesy the Cytogenetics Laboratory, Indiana University School of Medicine, Indianapolis, IN.)

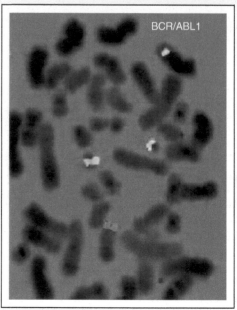

Figure 30.2 Bone Marrow Metaphase Cell from the Patient in the Case Study. Cell is hybridized with probes for BCR (green) and ABL1 (red) (Abbott Molecular, Des Plaines, IL). The fusion signals (yellow) represent the translocated chromosomes 9 and 22 (der(9) and der(22)). (Courtesy the Cytogenetics Laboratory, Indiana University School of Medicine, Indianapolis, IN.)

Human cytogenetics is the study of chromosomes, their structure, and their inheritance. There are approximately 23,000 genes in the human genome, most of which reside on the 46 chromosomes normally found in each somatic cell.[1]

Chromosome disorders are classified as structural or numeric and involve the loss, gain, or rearrangement of either a piece of a chromosome or the entire chromosome. Because each chromosome contains thousands of genes, a chromosomal abnormality that is observable by light microscopy involves, on average, 3 to 5 megabases (Mb) of DNA and represents the disruption or loss of hundreds of genes. Such disruptions often have a profound clinical effect.

Chromosomal abnormalities are observed in approximately 0.65% of all live births.[2] The gain or loss of an entire chromosome, other than a sex chromosome, is usually incompatible with life and accounts for approximately 50% of first-trimester spontaneous abortions.[3] In leukemia, cytogenetic abnormalities are observed in more than 50% of bone marrow specimens.[4] These recurring abnormalities often define the leukemia and frequently indicate clinical prognosis.

REASONS FOR CHROMOSOME ANALYSIS

Chromosome analysis is an important diagnostic procedure in clinical medicine. Not only are chromosomal anomalies major causes of reproductive loss and birth defects, but also nonrandom chromosome abnormalities are recognized in many forms of cancer.

Physicians who care for patients of all ages may order chromosome analysis or karyotyping for patients with intellectual disability, infertility, ambiguous genitalia, short stature, fetal loss,

risk of genetic or chromosomal disease, and cancer (Table 30.1). In the following discussion basic cytogenetic concepts are presented. Supplementation of this chapter with the material in Chapter 29 is recommended.

CHROMOSOME STRUCTURE

Cell Cycle

The cell cycle is divided into four stages: G_1, the growth period before synthesis of deoxyribonucleic acid (DNA); S phase, the period during which DNA synthesis takes place; G_2, the period after DNA synthesis; and M, the period of mitosis, or cell division, the shortest phase of the cell cycle (Figure 3.5). During mitosis, chromosomes are maximally condensed. While in mitosis, cells can be chemically treated to arrest cell progression through the cycle so that the chromosomes may be isolated and analyzed.

Chromosome Architecture

A chromosome is formed from a double-stranded DNA molecule that contains a series of genes. The complementary double-helix structure of DNA was established in 1953 by Watson and Crick.[5] The backbone is a sugar-phosphate-sugar polymer. The sugar is deoxyribose. Attached to the backbone and filling the center of the helix are four nitrogen-containing bases. Two of these, adenine (A) and guanine (G), are purines; the other two, cytosine (C) and thymine (T), are pyrimidines (Figure 29.6).

The chromosomal DNA of the cell resides in the cell's nucleus. This DNA and its associated proteins are referred to as

TABLE 30.1 Common Translocations in Hematopoietic and Lymphoid Neoplasia and Sarcoma[a]

Tumor Type	Karyotype	Genes
Myeloid Leukemias		
CML (and pre-B-ALL) (Box 31.1)	t(9;22)(q34;q11.2)	BCR/ABL1
B Cell Leukemias/Lymphomas		
B lymphoblastic leukemia	t(12;21)(p13;q22)	ETV6/RUNX1
	t(1;19)(q23.3;p13.3)	PBX1/TCF3
	t(4;11)(q21;q23)	AFF1/KMT2A
Burkitt lymphoma	t(8;14)(q24;q32.3)	MYC/IGH
	t(2;8)(p12;q24)	IGK/MYC
	t(8;22)(q24;q11.2)	MYC/IGL
Mantle cell lymphoma	t(11;14)(q13;q32.3)	CCND1/IGH
Follicular lymphoma	t(14;18)(q32.3;q21.3)	IGH/BCL2
Diffuse large B cell lymphoma	t(3;14)(q27;q32.3)	BCL6/IGH
Lymphoplasmacytic lymphoma	t(9;14)(p13.2;q32.3)	PAX5/IGH
MALT lymphoma	t(14;18)(q32.3;q21)	IGH/MALT1
	t(11;18)(q22;q21)	BIRC3/MALT1
	t(1;14)(p22;q32.3)	BCL10/IGH
T Cell Leukemias/Lymphomas		
T lymphoblastic leukemia	del(1)(p32p32)	STIL/TAL1
	t(7;11)(q34;p13)	TRB/LMO2
ALCL	t(2;5)(p23;q35.1)	ALK/NPM1
Sarcomas and Tumors of Bone and Soft Tissue		
Alveolar rhabdomyosarcoma	t(2;13)(q36.1;q14.1)	PAX3/FOXO1A
	t(1;13)(p36.13;q14.1)	PAX7/FOXO1A
Ewing sarcoma/PNET	t(11;22)(q24;q12.2)	FLI1/EWSR1
	t(21;22)(q22.3;q12.2)	ERG/EWSR1
	t(7;22)(p22;q12.2)	ETV1/EWSR1
Clear cell sarcoma	t(12;22)(q13;q12.2)	ATF1/EWSR1
Myxoid liposarcoma	t(12;16)(q13;p11.2)	DDIT3/FUS
	t(12;22)(q13;q12.2)	DDIT3/EWSR1
Synovial sarcoma	t(X;18)(p11.2;q11.2)	SSX1 or SSX2/SS18
Alveolar soft part sarcoma	t(X;17)(p11.2;q25)	TFE3/ASPSCR1

[a]Modified per the Hugo Nomenclature Database, January, 2018.
ALCL, Anaplastic large cell leukemia; *ALL,* acute lymphoblastic leukemia; *AML,* acute myeloid leukemia; *CML,* chronic myeloid leukemia; *CMML,* chronic myelomonocytic leukemia; *MALT,* mucosa-associated lymphoid tissue; *PNET,* primitive neuroectodermal tumor.

chromatin. During the cell cycle, at mitosis, the nuclear chromatin condenses approximately 10,000-fold to form chromosomes.[6] Each chromosome results from progressive folding, compression, and compaction of the entire nuclear chromatin. This condensation is achieved through multiple levels of helical coiling and supercoiling (Figure 30.3).

Metaphase Chromosomes

Metaphase is the stage of mitosis in which the chromosomes align on the equatorial plate. Electron micrographs of metaphase

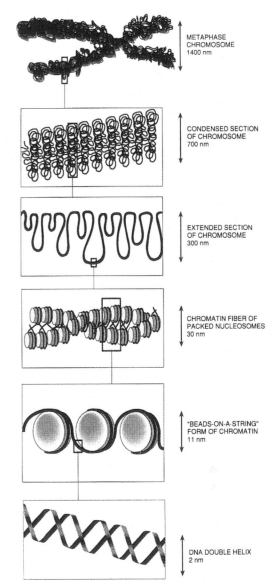

Figure 30.3 Chromosome Structure. The folding and twisting of the DNA double helix. (From Gelehrter, T. D., Collins, F.S., Ginsberg, D. [1998]. *Principles of Medical Genetics,* 2nd ed, Philadelphia: Lippincott Williams & Wilkins.)

chromosomes have provided models of chromosome structure. In the "beads-on-a-string" model of chromatin folding, the DNA helix is looped around a core of histone proteins.[7] This packaging unit is known as a *nucleosome* and measures approximately 11 nm in diameter.[8] Nucleosomes are coiled into twisted forms to create an approximately 30-nm chromatin fiber. This fiber, called a *solenoid,* is condensed further and bent into a loop configuration. These loops extend at an angle from the main chromosome axis.[9]

CHROMOSOME IDENTIFICATION

Chromosome Number

In 1956 Tijo and Levan[10] identified the correct number of human chromosomes as 46. This is the *diploid* chromosome number and is determined by counting the chromosomes in dividing somatic cells. The designation for the diploid number

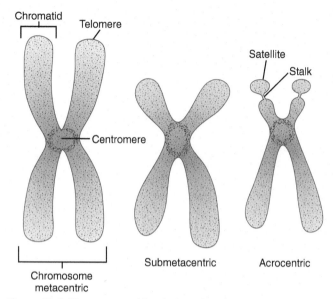

Figure 30.4 Chromosome Morphology. The three shapes of chromosomes are metacentric, submetacentric, and acrocentric. This figure also shows the position of the centromere and telomere, in addition to the two sister chromatids that comprise a metaphase chromosome.

is *2n.* Gametes (ova and sperm) have half the diploid number (23). This is called the *haploid* number of chromosomes and is designated as *n.* Different species have different numbers of chromosomes. The reindeer has a relatively high chromosome number for a mammal (2n = 76), whereas the Indian muntjac, or barking deer, has a very low chromosome number (2n = 7 in the male and 2n = 6 in the female).[11]

Chromosome Size and Type

In the 1960s, before the discovery of banding, chromosomes were categorized by overall size and the location of the centromere (primary constriction) and were assigned to one of seven groups: A through G. Group A includes chromosome pairs 1, 2, and 3. These are the largest chromosomes, and their centromeres are located in the middle of the chromosome; that is, they are metacentric. Group B chromosomes, pairs 4 and 5, are the next largest chromosomes; their centromeres are off center, or submetacentric. Group G consists of the smallest chromosomes, pairs 21 and 22, whose centromeres are located at one end of the chromosomes and are designated as acrocentric (Figure 30.4).

TECHNIQUES FOR CHROMOSOME PREPARATION AND ANALYSIS

Chromosome Preparation

Tissues used for chromosome analysis contain cells with an inherently high mitotic rate (bone marrow cells) or cells that can be stimulated to divide in culture (peripheral blood lymphocytes). Special harvesting procedures are established for each tissue type. Mitogens such as phytohemagglutinin or pokeweed mitogen are added to peripheral blood cultures. Phytohemagglutinin primarily stimulates T cells to divide,[12] whereas pokeweed preferentially stimulates B lymphocytes.[13]

Chromosomes may be obtained from replicating cells by arresting the cell in metaphase. Cells from the peripheral blood or bone marrow are cultured in media for 24 to 72 hours. In standard peripheral blood cultures, because the cells are terminally differentiated, a mitogen is added to stimulate cellular division. Neoplastic cells are spontaneously dividing and generally do not require stimulation with a mitogen. After the cell cultures have grown for the appropriate period, Colcemid, an analogue of colchicine, is added to disrupt the mitotic spindle fiber attachment to the chromosome. Following culture and treatment with Colcemid, cells are exposed to a hypotonic (potassium chloride) solution that lyses red cells and causes the chromosomes to spread apart from one another. A fixative of 3:1 methanol and acetic acid is added that "hardens" cells and removes proteinaceous material. Cells are dropped onto cold, wet glass slides to achieve optimal dispersal of the chromosomes. The slides are then aged, typically by exposure to heat, before banding.

Chromosome Banding

Analysis of each chromosome is made possible by staining with a dye. The name chromosome is derived from the Greek words *chroma,* meaning "color," and *soma,* meaning "body." Hence *chromosome* means "colored body." In 1969 Caspersson and colleagues[14] were the first investigators to stain chromosomes successfully with a fluorochrome dye. Using quinacrine mustard, which binds to adenine-thymine-rich areas of the chromosome, they were able to distinguish a banding pattern unique to each chromosome. This banding pattern, called *Q-banding,* differentiates the chromosome into bands of differing widths and relative brightnesses (Figure 30.5). The most brightly fluorescent bands of the 46 human chromosomes include the distal end of the Y chromosome, the centromeric regions of chromosomes 3 and 4, and the short arms of the acrocentric chromosomes (13, 14, 15, 21, and 22).

Other stains are used to identify chromosomes, but in contrast to Q-banding, these methods normally necessitate some pretreatment of the slide to be analyzed. Giemsa (G) bands are obtained by pretreating the chromosomes with the proteolytic enzyme trypsin. *GTG banding* means "G banding by Giemsa with the use of trypsin." Giemsa, like quinacrine mustard, stains AT-rich areas of the chromosome. The dark bands are called *G-positive*(+) bands. Guanine-cytosine-rich areas of the chromosome have little affinity for the dye and are referred to as *G-negative*(−) bands. G+ bands correspond with the brightly fluorescing bands of Q-banding (Figures 30.6 and 30.7). G-banding is the most common method used for staining chromosomes.

C-banding stains the centromere (primary constriction) of the chromosome and the surrounding condensed heterochromatin. Constitutive heterochromatin is a special type of late-replicating repetitive DNA that is located primarily at the centromere of the chromosome. In C-banding the chromosomes are treated first with an acid and then with an alkali (barium hydroxide) before Giemsa staining. C-banding is most intense in human chromosomes 1, 9, and 16 and the Y chromosome. Polymorphisms from different individuals are also observed in the C-bands. These polymorphisms have no clinical significance (Figure 30.8).

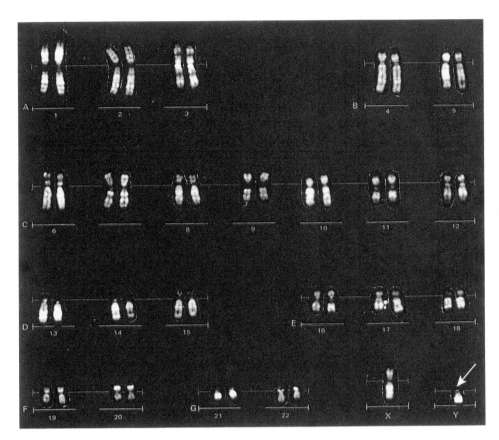

Figure 30.5 Q-Banded Preparation. Note the intense brilliance of Yq. (Courtesy Cytogenetics Laboratory, Indiana University School of Medicine, Indianapolis, IN.)

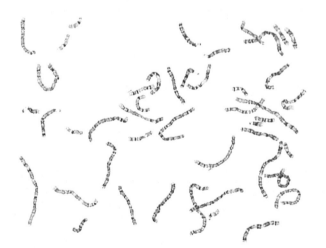

Figure 30.6 Normal Male Metaphase Chromosomes.

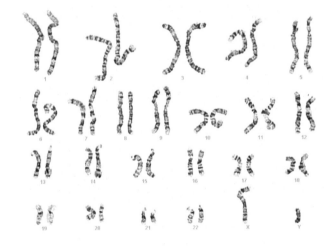

Figure 30.7 Normal Male Karyogram, GTG-Banded Preparations. (Courtesy Cytogenetics Laboratory, Indiana University School of Medicine, Indianapolis, IN.)

Specific chromosomal regions that are associated with the nucleoli in interphase cells are called *nucleolar organizer regions* (NORs). NORs contain tandemly repeated ribosomal nucleic acid (RNA) genes. NORs can be differentially stained in chromosomes by a silver stain in a method called *AG-NOR-banding*.

Chromosome banding is visible after chromosome condensation, which occurs during mitosis. The banding pattern observed depends on the degree of condensation. By examination of human chromosomes early in mitosis, it has been possible to estimate a total haploid genome (23 chromosomes) with approximately 2000 AT-rich (G+) bands.[15] The later the stage of mitosis, the more condensed the chromosome and the fewer total G+ bands observed.

Metaphase Analysis

After banding, prepared slides with dividing cells are scanned under a light microscope with a low-power objective lens (10×). When a metaphase cell has been selected for analysis, a 63× or 100× oil immersion objective lens is used. Each metaphase cell is analyzed first for a chromosome number. Then each chromosome pair is analyzed for its banding pattern. A normal somatic cell

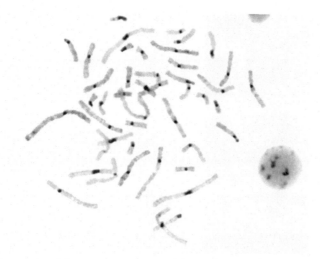

Figure 30.8 C-Banded Male Metaphase Chromosomes. Note the stain at the centromere and heterochromatic regions of the chromosomes. (Courtesy Cytogenetics Laboratory, Indiana University School of Medicine, Indianapolis, IN.)

contains 46 chromosomes, which includes two sex chromosomes and 22 pairs of autosomes (chromosomes 1 through 22). The laboratory scientist records his or her summary of the analysis using chromosome nomenclature. This summary is called a *karyotype.* Any variation in number and banding pattern is recorded by the laboratory scientist. At least 20 metaphase cells are analyzed from leukocyte cultures. If abnormalities are noted, the laboratory scientist may need to analyze additional cells. Computer imaging or photography is used to confirm and record the microscopic analysis. A picture of all the chromosomes aligned from 1 to 22 including the sex chromosomes is called a *karyogram.*

Fluorescence *in situ* Hybridization

The use of molecular methods coupled with standard karyotype analysis has improved chromosomal mutation detection

beyond that of the light microscope. DNA or RNA probes labeled with either fluorescent or enzymatic detection systems are hybridized directly to metaphase or interphase cells on a glass microscope slide. These probes usually belong to one of three classes: probes for repetitive DNA sequences, primarily generated from centromeric DNA; whole-chromosome probes that include segments of an entire chromosome; and specific loci or single-copy probes.

Fluorescence *in situ* hybridization (FISH) is a molecular technique commonly used in cytogenetic laboratories. FISH studies are a valuable adjunct to the diagnostic workup. In FISH, the DNA or RNA probe is labeled with a fluorophore. Target DNA is treated with heat and formamide to denature the double-stranded DNA, which renders it single stranded. The target DNA anneals to a similarly denatured, single-stranded, fluorescently labeled DNA or RNA probe with a complementary sequence. After hybridization the unbound probe is removed through a series of stringent washes, and the cells are counterstained for visualization (Figure 30.9).

In situ hybridization with centromere or whole-chromosome painting probes can be used to identify individual chromosomes (Figure 30.10). Marker chromosomes represent chromatin material that has been structurally altered and cannot be identified by a G-band pattern. FISH using a centromere or paint probe, or both, is often helpful in identifying the chromosome of origin (Figure 30.11).[16] Specific loci probes can be used to detect both structural and numeric abnormalities but are especially helpful in identifying chromosomal translocations or inversions.

The FISH procedure has many advantages and has advanced the detection of chromosomal abnormalities beyond that of G-banded analysis. Both dividing (metaphase) and nondividing (interphase) cells can be analyzed with FISH. Performance of FISH on uncultured cells, such as bone marrow smears, provides a quick test result that can be reported within 24 hours. Also, in cultured bone marrow samples submitted for G-band

General FISH Protocol

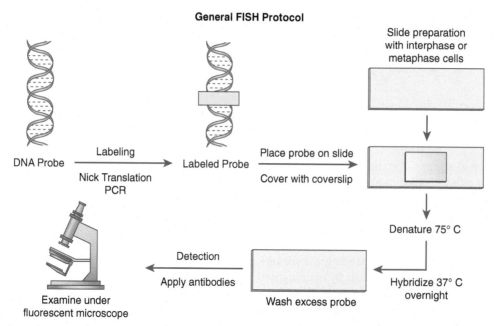

Figure 30.9 General Protocol for Fluorescence *in Situ* Hybridization *(FISH).* *PCR,* Polymerase chain reaction.

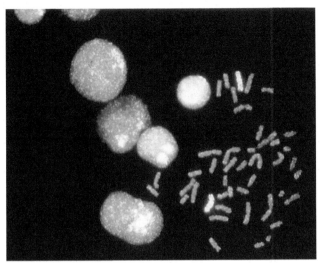

Figure 30.10 Metaphase Preparation is "Painted" with Multiple Probes for Chromosome 7, Producing a Fluorescent Signal. (Courtesy Cytogenetics Laboratory, Indiana University School of Medicine, Indianapolis, IN.)

Locus-specific probes
Chromosome paint probes
Centromere probes

Detection of numerical chromosome abnormalities	Detection of structural chromosome abnormalities
Trisomy Monosomy Polyploidy	Deletions Duplications Inversions Translocations Ring chromosomes Marker chromosomes Dicentric chromosomes

Figure 30.11 Fluorescence *in Situ* Hybridization in the Clinical Laboratory.

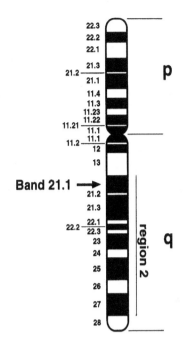

Figure 30.12 Banding Pattern of the Human X Chromosome at the 550 Average Band Level. Arrow indicates the location of Xq21.1.

CYTOGENETIC NOMENCLATURE

Banding techniques enabled scientists to identify each chromosome pair by a characteristic banding pattern. In 1971 a Paris conference for nomenclature of human chromosomes was convened to designate a system to describe the regions and specific bands of the chromosomes. The chromosome arms were designated *p* (petite) for the short arm and *q* for the long arm. The regions in each arm and the bands contained within each region were numbered consecutively, from the centromere outward to the telomere or end of the chromosome. To designate a specific region of the chromosome, the chromosome number is written first, followed by the designation of either the short or long arm, then the region of the arm, and finally the specific

analysis, the number of dividing cells may be insufficient for cytogenetic diagnosis. In such cases FISH performed on interphase (nondividing) cells with probes for a specific translocation or structural abnormality may provide the diagnosis. FISH also may be performed on paraffin-embedded tissue sections, specimens obtained by fine needle aspiration, and touch preparations from lymph nodes or solid tumors.

band. *Xq21* designates the long arm of the X chromosome, region 2, band 1. To designate a sub-band, a decimal point is placed after the band designation, followed by the number assigned to the sub-band, as in Xq21.1 (Figure 30.12).

Cytogenetic (and FISH) nomenclature represents a uniform code used by cytogeneticists around the world to communicate chromosome abnormalities. In this nomenclature each string begins with the modal number of chromosomes, followed by the sex chromosome designation. A normal male karyotype is designated 46,XY, and a normal female karyotype is designated 46,XX. If abnormalities are observed in the cell, the designation is written to include abnormalities of modal chromosome number, sex chromosomes, and then the autosomes. A cell from a bone marrow specimen with trisomy of chromosome 8 (three copies of chromosome 8) in a male is written as 47,XY,+8 (no intervening spaces). The number of cells with this abnormality is indicated in brackets. If 20 cells were examined, trisomy 8 was found in 10 cells, and the remainder were normal, the findings would be written as 47,XY,+8[10]/46,XY[10].

Translocations (exchange of material between two chromosomes) are designated *t*, with the lowest chromosome number listed first. Thus a translocation between the short arm of chromosome 12 at band p13 and the long arm of chromosome 21 at band q22 is written as t(12;21)(p13;q22). A semicolon is used to separate the chromosomes and the band designations. A translocated chromosome is called a *derivative chromosome*. Using the previous example, chromosomes 12 and 21 are referred to as der(12) and der(21). Deletions are written with the abbreviation *del* preceding the chromosome. A deletion of the long arm of chromosome 5 at band 31 is written as del(5)(q31). No spaces are entered in these designations except between abbreviations.[17]

CHROMOSOME ABNORMALITIES

There are many types of chromosome abnormalities, such as deletions, inversions, ring formations, trisomies, and polyploidy. All these defects can be grouped into two major categories: defects involving an abnormality in the *number* of chromosomes and defects involving *structural* changes in one or more chromosomes.

Numeric Abnormalities

Numeric abnormalities often are subclassified as aneuploidy or polyploidy. *Aneuploidy* refers to any abnormal number of chromosomes that is not a multiple of the haploid number (23 chromosomes). The common forms of aneuploidy in humans are trisomy (the presence of an extra chromosome) and monosomy (the absence of a single chromosome). Aneuploidy is the result of nondisjunction, the failure of chromosomes to separate normally during cell division. Nondisjunction can occur during either of the two types of cell division: mitosis or meiosis. During normal mitosis a cell divides once to produce two cells that are identical to the parent cell. In mitosis each daughter cell contains 46 chromosomes. Meiosis is a special type of cell division that generates male and female gametes (sperm and ova). In contrast to mitosis, meiosis entails two cell divisions: meiosis I and meiosis II. The end result is a cell with 23 chromosomes, which is the haploid number (n).

In polyploidy the chromosome number is higher than 46 but is always an exact multiple of the haploid chromosome number of 23. A karyotype with 69 chromosomes is called *triploidy (3n)* (Figure 30.13). A karyotype with 92 chromosomes is called *tetraploidy (4n).*

In cancer numeric abnormalities in the karyotype may be classified further based on the modal number of chromosomes in a neoplastic clone. *Hypodiploid* refers to a cell with fewer than 45 chromosomes; *near-haploid* cells have from 23 up to approximately 34 chromosomes (Figure 30.14); *hyperdiploid* cells have more than 46 chromosomes. *High hyperdiploidy* refers to a chromosome number of more than 50.[18] Finally, the term *pseudodiploid* is used to describe a cell with 46 chromosomes and structural abnormalities.[17]

Structural Abnormalities

Structural rearrangements result from breakage of a chromosome region, with loss or subsequent rejoining in an abnormal

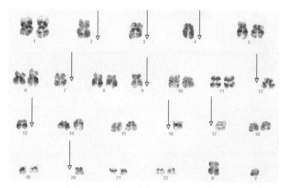

Figure 30.14 Hypodiploid karyotype with 36 Chromosomes. Arrows indicate missing chromosomes.). (Courtesy the Cytogenetics Laboratory, Indiana University School of Medicine, Indianapolis, IN.)

combination. Structural rearrangements are defined as *balanced* (no loss or gain of genetic chromatin) or *unbalanced* (gain or loss of genetic material). Structural rearrangements of single chromosomes include inversions, deletions, isochromosomes, ring formations, insertions, translocations, and duplications. Inversions (inv) involve one or two breaks in a single chromosome, followed by a 180-degree rotation of the segment between the breaks with no loss or gain of material. If the chromosomal material involves the centromere, the inversion is called *pericentric.* If the material that is inverted does not include the centromere, the inversion is called *paracentric* (Figure 30.15).

Interstitial *deletions* arise after two breaks in the same chromosome arm and loss of the segment between the breaks. Terminal deletions (loss of chromosomal material from the end of a chromosome) and interstitial deletions involve the loss of genetic material. The clinical consequence to the individual with a deletion depends on the extent and location of the deleted chromosomal material (Figure 30.16).

Isochromosomes arise from either abnormal division of the centromeres, in which division is perpendicular to the long axis of the chromosome rather than parallel to it, or from breakage and reunion in chromatin adjacent to the centromere. Each resulting daughter cell has a chromosome in which the short arm or the long arm is duplicated.

Ring chromosomes can result from breakage and reunion of a single chromosome, with loss of chromosomal material outside

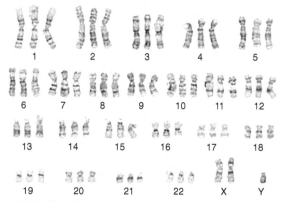

Figure 30.13 Triploid Karyotype, 69,XXY. (Courtesy Cytogenetics Laboratory, Indiana University School of Medicine, Indianapolis, IN.)

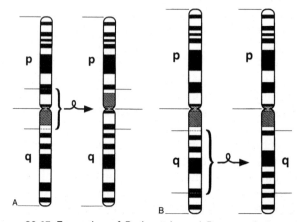

Figure 30.15 Examples of Pericentric and Paracentric Inversion. (A), Pericentric inversion involves the centromere. **(B),** Paracentric inversion occurs in either the short or long arm of the chromosome.

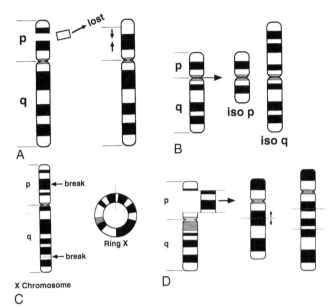

Figure 30.16 Structural Abnormalities of Chromosomes. (A), Interstitial deletion. (B), Isochromosome. (C), Ring chromosome. (D), Insertion.

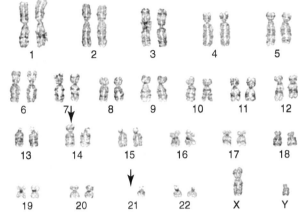

Figure 30.17 Balanced Robertsonian Translocation Between Chromosomes 14 and 21. The nomenclature for this karyogram is written 45,XY,der(14;21)(q10;q10). (Courtesy Cytogenetics Laboratory, Indiana University School of Medicine, Indianapolis, IN.)

the break points. Alternatively one or both telomeres (chromosome ends) may join to form a ring chromosome without significant loss of chromosomal material.

Insertions involve movement of a segment of a chromosome from one location of the chromosome to another location of the same chromosome or to another chromosome. The segment is released as a result of two breaks, and the insertion occurs at the site of another break.

Duplication means partial trisomy for part of a chromosome. This can result from an unbalanced insertion or unequal crossing over in meiosis or mitosis.

Translocations occur when there is breakage in two chromosomes and each of the broken pieces reunites with another chromosome. If chromatin is neither lost nor gained, the exchange is called a *balanced reciprocal translocation*. A reciprocal translocation is balanced if all chromatin material is present. The loss or gain of chromatin material results in partial monosomy or trisomy for a segment of the chromosome, which is designated an *unbalanced rearrangement*.

Another type of translocation involving breakage and reunion near the centromeric regions of two acrocentric chromosomes is known as a *robertsonian translocation*. Effectively this is a fusion between two whole chromosomes rather than an exchange of material, as in a reciprocal translocation. These translocations are among the most common balanced structural rearrangements seen in the general population, with a frequency of 0.09% to 0.1%.[19] All five human acrocentric autosomes (13, 14, 15, 21, and 22) are capable of forming a robertsonian translocation. In this case the resulting balanced karyotype has only 45 chromosomes, which includes the translocated chromosomes (Figure 30.17).

CANCER CYTOGENETICS

Cancer cytogenetics is a field that has been built upon discovery of nonrandom chromosome abnormalities in many types of cancer.

In hematologic neoplasias specific structural rearrangements are associated with distinct subtypes of leukemia that have characteristic morphologic and clinical features. Cytogenetic analysis of malignant cells can help determine the diagnosis and often the prognosis of a hematologic malignancy, assist the oncologist in the selection of appropriate therapy, and aid in monitoring the effects of therapy. Bone marrow is the tissue most frequently used to study the cytogenetics of a hematologic malignancy. Unstimulated peripheral blood and bone marrow trephine biopsy samples also may be analyzed. Cytogenetic analysis of cancers involving other organ systems may be performed using solid tissue obtained during surgery or by needle biopsy. Chromosomal defects in cancer include a wide range of numeric abnormalities and structural rearrangements, as discussed earlier (Table 30.1).

Cancer results from multiple and sequential genetic mutations occurring in a somatic cell. At some juncture a critical mutation occurs, and the cell becomes self-perpetuating or clonal. A *clone* is a cell population derived from a single progenitor.[17] A cytogenetic clone exists if two or more cells contain the same structural abnormality or supernumerary marker chromosome, or if three or more cells are missing the same chromosome. The primary aberration, or stemline, of a clone is a cytogenetic abnormality that is frequently observed as the sole abnormality associated with the cancer. The secondary aberration, or sideline, includes abnormalities additional to the primary aberration.[17] In chronic myeloid leukemia the primary aberration is the Philadelphia chromosome resulting from a translocation between the long arms of chromosomes 9 and 22, t(9;22)(q34;q11.2). A sideline of this clone would include secondary abnormalities, such as trisomy for chromosome 8, written as +8,t(9;22)(q34;q11.2).

Leukemia

Leukemias are clonal proliferations of malignant leukocytes that arise initially in the bone marrow before disseminating to the peripheral blood, lymph nodes, and other organs. They are broadly classified by the type of blood cell giving rise to the clonal proliferation (lymphoid or myeloid) and by the clinical course of the disease (acute or chronic). The four main leukemia categories are acute lymphoblastic leukemia (ALL), acute myeloid leukemia

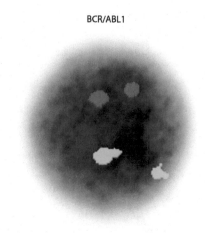

Figure 30.18 Normal Bone Marrow Interphase Cell Hybridized with the *BCR* (green) and *ABL1* (red) Genes (Abbott Molecular, Des Plaines, IL). The two red and two green signals represent the genes on the normal chromosomes 9 and 22. (Courtesy Cytogenetics Laboratory, Indiana University School of Medicine, Indianapolis, IN.)

BOX 30.1   Acute Myeloid Leukemia (AML) with Recurrent Genetic Abnormalities[a]

AML with t(8;21)(q22;q22); *RUNX1T1/RUNX1*
AML with inv(16)(p13.1q22) or t(16;16)(p13.1;q22); *MYH11/CBFB*
APL with t(15;17)(q24.1;q21.1); *PML/RARA*
AML with t(9;11)(p22;q23); *MLLT3/ KMT2A (MLL)*
AML with t(6;9)(p23;q34); *DEK/NUP214*
AML with inv(3)(q21q26.2) or t(3;3)(q21.3;q26.2); *RPN1/MECOM*
AML (megakaryoblastic) with t(1;22)(p13.3;q13.2); *RBM15/MKL1*
AML with *BCR/ABL1*
AML with mutated *NPM1* (5q35.1)
AML with biallelic mutations of *CEBPA* (19q13.1)
AML with mutated *RUNX1* (21q22.1)

Modified from Arber D.A., Orazi A., Hasserjian R., et al. (2016) The 2016 revision to the World Health Organization classification of myeloid neoplasms and acute leukemia. *Blood, 127,* 2391–2405.
[a]Updated per Hugo Nomenclature Database, January, 2018.

(AML), chronic lymphocytic leukemia (CLL), and chronic myeloid leukemia (CML). The World Health Organization (WHO) classification for myeloid malignancies has categorized AML into eight subtypes: AML with recurrent genetic abnormalities; AML with myelodysplasia-related changes; therapy-related myeloid neoplasms; AML not otherwise specified; myeloid sarcoma; myeloid proliferations related to Down syndrome; blastic plasmacytoid dendritic cell neoplasm and acute leukemias of ambiguous lineage. (Chapter 31).[20] "AML with recurrent genetic abnormalities" is a classification based on the cytogenetic and molecular mutations observed (Box 30.1). Some of the divisions of the French-American-British (FAB) classification[21] are included in the "not otherwise classified" category.

Chronic Myeloid Leukemia

The first malignancy to be associated with a specific chromosome defect was CML, in which approximately 95% of patients were found to have the Philadelphia chromosome translocation, t(9;22)(q34;q11.2) by G-banded analysis.[22,23] The Philadelphia chromosome (derivative chromosome 22) is characterized by a balanced translocation between the long arms of chromosomes 9 and 22. At the molecular level, the gene for *ABL1*, an oncogene on chromosome 9, joins a gene on chromosome 22 named *BCR*. The result of the fusion of these two genes is a new fusion protein of about 210 kD with growth-promoting capabilities that override normal cell regulatory mechanisms (Figures 30.18 and 30.19) (Chapter 32).[24] The fusion protein activates tyrosine kinase signaling to drive proliferation of the cell. This signaling can be blocked by imatinib mesylate or another tyrosine kinase inhibitor.[25] The patient's response to imatinib is monitored by cytogenetic analysis and FISH.

At diagnosis the characteristic karyotype is the presence of the Philadelphia chromosome in all cells analyzed. After treatment with imatinib for several months, the karyotype typically has a mixture of abnormal and normal cells indicating the patient's response to therapy. A complete cytogenetic response is defined as a bone marrow karyotype with only normal cells. The therapeutic response is often monitored using peripheral blood instead of a bone marrow aspirate. In contrast to the bone marrow,

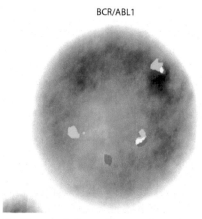

Figure 30.19 Abnormal Bone Marrow Interphase Cell with One *BCR* (green) and One *ABL1* (red) Signal (Abbott Molecular, Des Plaines, IL) representing the normal chromosomes and two fusion signals from the derivative chromosomes 9 and 22. (Courtesy Cytogenetics Laboratory, Indiana University School of Medicine, Indianapolis, IN.)

the peripheral blood does not contain spontaneously dividing cells. As a result chromosomal analysis of a specimen of unstimulated peripheral blood may be unsuccessful because of the absence of dividing cells. In these cases FISH with probes for the specific abnormality is performed on 200 or more interphase (nondividing) cells of the peripheral blood specimen to search for chromosomally abnormal cells. The detection of cytogenetic abnormalities in interphase (nondividing) cells is an important advantage of FISH technology.

Acute Leukemia

The Philadelphia chromosome is also observed in acute leukemia. It is seen in about 25% of adults with ALL, 2% to 5% of children with ALL, and 1% of patients with AML.[26–28] In childhood ALL the chromosome number is critical for predicting the severity of the leukemia. Children whose leukemic cells contain more than 50 chromosomes (high hyperdiploid karyotype) have the best prognosis for complete recovery with therapy. Recurring translocations observed in ALL include t(4;11)(q21;q23), t(12;21)(p13;q22), and t(1;19)(q23;p13.3). Each translocation is associated with a prognostic outcome, which assists oncologists in determining the patient's therapy. The t(4;11) translocation is the one most commonly found in infants with acute lymphoblastic leukemia. Rearrangements of the *AFF1* gene on chromosome 4 and the *KMT2A* (formerly *MLL*) gene on chromosome 11 occur in this translocation.[29,30] Disruption of the *KMT2A* gene is seen in both ALL and AML (Figures 30.20 and 30.21).

The AMLs are subdivided into several morphologic classifications, ranging from M0 to M7 according to the FAB classification (Chapter 31).[31,32] Characteristic chromosome translocations are associated with some subgroups and were incorporated into the WHO classification. Among them is a translocation between the long arms of chromosomes 8 and 21, t(8;21)(q22;q22), which is representative of AML with maturation. Acute promyelocytic leukemia is associated with a translocation between the long arms of chromosomes 15 and 17, t(15;17)(q24;q21) (Figure 30.22). A pericentric inversion of chromosome 16, inv(16)(p13.1q22), is

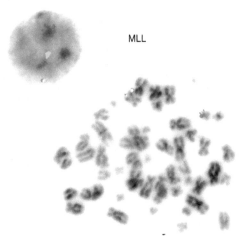

Figure 30.20 Bone Marrow Metaphase Cell with Fusion *KMT2A (MLL)* Signal on the Normal Chromosome 11 and Split Red and Green Signals on the Translocated Chromosomes, Representing a Disruption of the *KMT2A (MLL)* Gene. (Courtesy Cytogenetics Laboratory, Indiana University School of Medicine, Indianapolis, IN.)

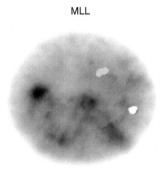

Figure 30.21 Bone Marrow Interphase Cell with a Fusion Signal (Normal Chromosome 11) and Split Red and Green Signals from the *KMT2A (MLL)* Gene Representing a Rearrangement. (Courtesy Cytogenetics Laboratory, Indiana University School of Medicine, Indianapolis, IN.)

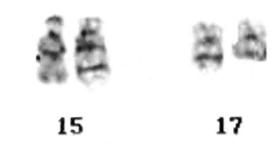

Figure 30.22 Bone Marrow Metaphase Chromosomes 15 and 17 Homologues Showing a Translocation between the Long Arms of Chromosomes 15 and 17, t(15;17)(q24.1;q21.1), Diagnostic of Acute Promyelocytic Leukemia. The abnormal chromosomes are on the right. (Courtesy Cytogenetics Laboratory, Indiana University School of Medicine, Indianapolis, IN.)

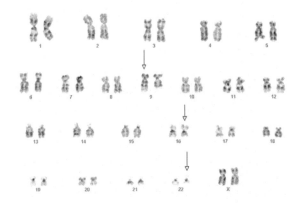

Figure 30.23 Bone Marrow Karyogram for a Patient with Acute Myeloid Leukemia (AML) Showing a Translocation, t(9;22)(q34;q11.2), and an Inverted Chromosome 16, inv(16)(p13.1q22). (Courtesy Cytogenetics Laboratory, Indiana University School of Medicine, Indianapolis, IN.)

seen in AML with increased eosinophils. The inversion juxtaposes the core the binding factor beta (*CBFB*) gene on 16q with the myosin heavy chain gene (*MYH11*) on 16p to form a new fusion protein (Figure 30.23).[33] These recurring translocations have enabled researchers to localize genes important for cell growth and regulation. As with acute lymphoblastic leukemia, the specific translocation in AML often predicts the patient's prognosis and response to therapy. Understanding the molecular consequences of the cytogenetic mutations, such as the *BCR/ABL1* translocation, provides the fundamental information for the development of targeted therapies.

Solid Tumors

Just as recurring structural and numeric chromosome defects have been observed in the hematologic malignancies, a wide range of nonrandom abnormalities have also been found in solid tumors. Most of these abnormalities confer a proliferative advantage on the malignant cell and serve as useful prognostic indicators. Amplification (increased copy number) of the gene *HER2* (also called *ERBB2*) on chromosome 17, a transmembrane growth factor receptor, is associated with an aggressive form of invasive breast cancer.[34,35] FISH with probes for the *HER2* gene and an internal control (17 centromere) can determine if there is gene amplification in the tumor (Figure 30.24).[36] If FISH testing shows amplification to be present, the patient is eligible for

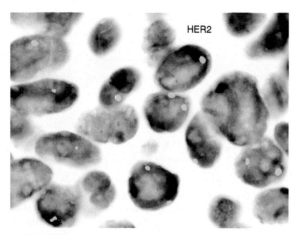

Figure 30.24 Normal Interphase Nuclei from a Paraffin-Embedded Tissue Section Hybridized with Probes for *HER2* (red) and the Chromosome 17 Centromere (green) (Abbott Molecular, Des Plaines, IL). Two green and two red signals are seen per cell.

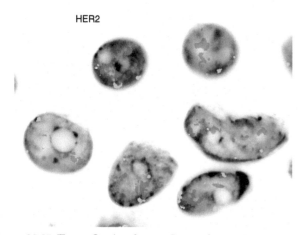

Figure 30.25 Tissue Section from a Breast Cancer Demonstrating Amplification of HER2. The tissue was hybridized with fluorescence *in situ* hybridization probes for *HER2* (red) and the chromosome 17 centromere probe (green) (Abbott Molecular, Des Plaines, IL). The number of *HER2* signals exceeds the number of centromere signals, which indicates selective amplification of *HER2*.

targeted therapy with a monoclonal antibody, trastuzumab (Figure 30.25).[37] FISH for *HER2* typically is performed on tissue sections from the paraffin-embedded tumor block.

CHROMOSOMAL MICROARRAY ANALYSIS

Chromosomal microarray (CMA) is a fluorescence-based molecular technique for submicroscopic analysis of genomic DNA. CMA testing increases the detection of clinically significant imbalances over a karyotype.[38] CMA is performed using a glass slide or chip platform. Chromosomal microarrays, like standard cytogenetic analysis, look at the entire genome but with higher levels of resolution (base pair or kilobase level) determined by the number and composition of targets on the array. Using a single nucleotide polymorphism (SNP)-based array, the patient's DNA is hybridized to a chip composed of greater than 2 million markers that detect copy number variation (gains and losses) and single nucleotide polymorphisms. SNP probes detect

position-specific markers that have different forms (polymorphic). Analysis of the SNP data from a specimen allows for detection of copy neutral loss of heterozygosity or uniparental disomy, in addition to gains and losses of genomic DNA. Regions of imbalance (copy gain or copy loss) in the patient's specimen are assessed relative to a reference control. The yield of detection of abnormalities is increased from an average of 3% to 11% due to the high resolution of the array (Figures 30.26 and 30.27).[38–40] This technique is presently used primarily for diagnosis of constitutional (inherited) disorders, but applications for cancer have recently been instituted in some laboratories.[41]

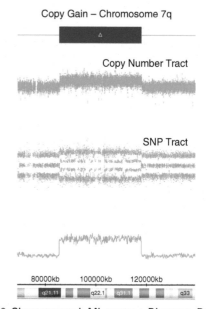

Figure 30.26 Chromosomal Microarray Diagram Demonstrating Approximately a 32.4 Mb Gain of Genetic Material between Bands 7q21 and 7q31. (Courtesy Cytogenetics Laboratory, Indiana University School of Medicine, Indianapolis, IN.)

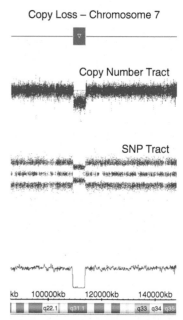

Figure 30.27 Chromosomal Microarray Diagram Demonstrating Approximately a 4.6 Mb Loss at Band 7q31.1. (Courtesy Cytogenetics Laboratory, Indiana University School of Medicine, Indianapolis, IN.)

SUMMARY

- Cytogenetics is the study of chromosome structure and inheritance.
- Chromosome disorders are secondary to structural or numeric chromosomal abnormalities involving the rearrangement or the loss or gain of a piece of a chromosome or the entire chromosome.
- Nonrandom chromosome abnormalities are observed in constitutional genetic syndromes as well as cancer.
- A chromosome is composed of a double helix strand of DNA. Attached to the backbone of deoxyribose are adenine (A), guanine (G), cytosine (C), and thymine (T).
- During mitosis, cells can be chemically treated to arrest cell progression in metaphase so that chromosomes can be analyzed.
- Q-banding differentiates chromosomes into bands of different widths and relative brightness, revealing a banding pattern unique to each individual chromosome.
- Other stains used to identify chromosomes may require pretreatment of the slide for analysis. These include G-banding, C-banding, and AG-NOR-banding.
- FISH, a molecular cytogenetic technique, uses DNA or RNA probes and fluorescence microscopy to identify individual chromosomes and targeted chromosomal loci. Metaphase and interphase cells may be analyzed by FISH.

- Tissues used for chromosome analysis typically include bone marrow cells and peripheral blood lymphocytes, amniotic fluid, non-neoplastic tissue, and tumors.
- A normal cell contains 46 chromosomes, which include 2 sex chromosomes (XX or XY).
- Defects in chromosomes can be categorized as numeric or structural. Numeric abnormalities can be subclassified as aneuploidy and polyploidy.
- Structural rearrangements include inversions, deletions, isochromosomes, ring formations, insertions, translocations, and duplications.
- Specific structural rearrangements are associated with distinct subtypes of leukemias and may assist in diagnosis, prognosis, and monitoring of therapy. Solid tumors also may be analyzed using cytogenetic analysis.
- Chromosomal microarray testing uses a microarray platform to detect abnormalities at a submicroscopic level of resolution. The higher resolution increases the detection of chromosomal abnormalities.

Now that you have completed this chapter, go back and read again the case study at the beginning and respond to the questions presented.

REVIEW QUESTIONS

Answers can be found in the Appendix.

1. *G-banding* refers to the technique of staining chromosomes:
   a. To isolate those in the G group (i.e., chromosomes 21 and 22)
   b. In the G0 or resting stage
   c. Using Giemsa stain
   d. To emphasize areas high in guanine residues
2. Which of the following compounds is used to halt mitosis in metaphase for chromosome analyses?
   a. Imatinib
   b. Fluorescein
   c. Trypsin
   d. Colchicine
3. One arm of a chromosome has 30 bands. Which band would be nearest the centromere?
   a. Band 1
   b. Band 15
   c. Band 30
4. Which of the following is *not* an advantage of the use of FISH?
   a. It can be used on nondividing cells.
   b. It can be used on paraffin-embedded tissue.
   c. It can detect mutations that do not result in abnormal banding patterns.
   d. It must be performed on dividing cells.

5. Which of the following types of mutations would likely *not* be detectable with cytogenetic banding techniques?
   a. Point mutation resulting in a single amino acid substitution
   b. Transfer of genetic material from one chromosome to another
   c. Loss of genetic material from a chromosome that does not appear on any other chromosome
   d. Duplication of a chromosome resulting in 3n of that genetic material
6. Which of the following describes a chromosomal deletion?
   a. Point mutation resulting in a single amino acid substitution
   b. Transfer of genetic material from one chromosome to another
   c. Loss of genetic material from a chromosome that does not appear on any other chromosome
   d. Duplication of a chromosome resulting in 3n of that genetic material

   The chromosome analysis performed on a patient's leukemic cells is reported as 47, XY,+4,del(5)(q31)[20]. Answer questions 7 to 9 based on this description.
7. This patient's cells have which of the following mutations?
   a. Loss of the entire number 31 chromosome
   b. Loss of the entire number 5 chromosome
   c. Loss of a portion of the short arm of chromosome 4
   d. Loss of a portion of the long arm of chromosome 5

8. What other mutation is present in this patient's cells?
   a. Polyploidy
   b. Tetraploidy
   c. An extra chromosome 4
   d. Four copies of chromosome 5
9. This patient's leukemic cells demonstrate:
   a. Structural chromosomal defects only
   b. Numeric chromosomal defects only
   c. Both structural and numeric chromosomal defects

10. *Aneuploidy* describes the total chromosome number:
    a. That is a multiple of the haploid number
    b. That reflects a loss or gain of a single chromosome
    c. That is diploid but has a balanced deletion and duplication of whole chromosomes
    d. In gametes; *diploid* is the number in somatic cells

REFERENCES

1. International Human Genome Sequencing Consortium. (2004). Finishing the euchromatic sequence of the human genome. *Nature, 431,* 931–945.
2. Benn, P. (2010). Prenatal diagnosis of chromosomal abnormalities through amniocentesis. In Milunsky, A., & Milunsky, J. M. (Eds.), *Genetic disorders and the fetus* (6th ed., pp. 194–195). Baltimore: Wiley-Blackwell.
3. Boué, J., Boué, A., & Lazar, P. (1975). Retrospective and prospective epidemiological studies of 1500 karyotyped spontaneous human abortions. *Teratology, 12,* 11–26.
4. Rowley, J. D. (2008). Chromosomal translocations: revisited yet again. *Blood, 112,* 2183–2189.
5. Watson, J. D., & Crick, F. H. C. (1983). Molecular structure of nucleic acids: a structure for deoxyribose nucleic acid. *Nature, 171,* 737–738.
6. Earnshaw, W. C. (1988). Mitotic chromosome structure. *Bioessays, 9,* 147–150.
7. Olins, A. L., & Olins, D. E. (1974). Spheroid chromatin units. *Science, 183,* 330–332.
8. Oudet, P., Gross-Bellard, M., & Chambon, P. (1975). Electron microscopic and biochemical evidence that chromatin structure is a repeating unit. *Cell, 4,* 281–300.
9. Rattner, J. B. (1988). Chromatin hierarchies and metaphase chromatin structure. In Adolph, K. W., (Ed.), *Chromosomes and chromatin* (Vol. 3, p. 30). Boca Raton, Fl: CRC Press.
10. Tijo, J. H., & Levan, A. (1956). The chromosome number of man. *Hereditas, 42,* 1–6.
11. Hsu, T. C. (1979). *Human and mammalian cytogenetics* (pp. 6–7). New York, NY: Springer-Verlag.
12. Nowell, P. C. (1960). Phytohemagglutinin: an initiator of mitosis in culture of normal human leukocytes. *Cancer Res, 20,* 462–466.
13. Farnes, P., Barker, B. E., Brownhill, L. E., et al. (1964). Mitogenic activity of *Phytolacca americana* (pokeweed). *Lancet, 2,* 1100–1101.
14. Caspersson, T., Zech, L., Modest, E. J., et al. (1969). Chemical differentiation with fluorescent alkylating agents in *Vicia faba* metaphase chromosomes. *Exp Cell Res, 58,* 128–140.
15. Yunis, J. J. (1979). Cytogenetics. In Henry, J. B., (Ed.). *Clinical diagnosis and management by laboratory methods* (16th ed., p. 825). Philadelphia, PA: Saunders.
16. Plattner, R., Heerema, N. A., Yurov, Y. B., et al. (1993). Efficient identification of marker chromosomes in 27 patients by stepwise hybridization with alpha satellite DNA probes. *Hum Genet, 91,* 131–140.
17. McGowan-Jordan, J, Simons, A., Schmid, M., (Eds.). (2016). ISCN 2016. *An international system for human cytogenetic nomenclature.* Basel, Switzerland: S. Karger.
18. Moorman, A. V., Richards, S. M., Martineau, M., et al. (2003). Outcome heterogeneity in childhood high-hyperdiploid acute lymphoblastic leukemia. *Blood, 102,* 2756–2762.
19. Turleau, C., Chavin-Colin, F., & de Grouchy, J. (1979). Cytogenetic investigation in 413 couples with spontaneous abortions. *Eur J Obstet Gynecol Reprod Biol, 9,* 65–74.
20. Arber, D. A., Orazi, A., Hasserjian, R., et al. (2016). The 2016 revision to the World Health Organization classification of myeloid neoplasms and acute leukemia. *Blood, 127,* 2391–2405.
21. Bennett, J. M., Catovsky, D., Daniel, M. T., et al. (1976). Proposals for classification of the acute leukaemias. French-American-British (FAB) Co-operative Group. *Br J Haematol, 33,* 451–458.
22. Nowell, P. C., & Hungerford, D. A. (1960). A minute chromosome in human chronic granulocytic leukemia. *Science, 132,* 1497 (abstract).
23. Rowley, J. D. (1973). A new consistent chromosomal abnormality in chronic myelogenous leukemia identified by quinacrine fluorescence and Giemsa staining. *Nature, 243,* 290–293.
24. Ben-Neriah, Y., Daley, G. Q., Mes-Masson, A., et al. (1986). The chronic myelogenous leukemia–specific P210 protein is the product of the *BCR/ABL* hybrid gene. *Science, 233,* 212–214.
25. Druker, B. J., Tamura, S., Buchdunger, E., et al. (1996). Effects of a selective inhibitor of the Abl tyrosine kinase on the growth of BCR-ABL positive cells. *Nat Med, 2,* 561–566.
26. Moorman, A. V., Harrison, C. J., Buck, G. A. N., et al. (2007). Karyotype is an independent prognostic factor in adult acute lymphoblastic leukemia (ALL): analysis of cytogenetic data from patients treated on the Medical Research Council (MRC) UKALLXII/Eastern Cooperative Oncology Group (ECOG) 2993 trial. *Blood, 109,* 3189–3197.
27. Hunger, S. P., Mulligan, C. G. (2015). Acute lymphoblastic leukemia in children. *N Engl J Med, 373,* 1541–1552.
28. Crist, W., Carroll, A., Shuster, J., et al. (1990). Philadelphia chromosome positive acute lymphoblastic leukemia: clinical and cytogenetic characteristics and treatment outcome. A Pediatric Oncology Group study. *Blood, 76,* 489–494.
29. Morrissey, J., Tkachuk, D. C., Milatovich, A., et al. (1993). A serine/proline-rich protein is fused to HRX in t(4;11) acute leukemias. *Blood, 81,* 1124–1131.
30. Hayne, C. C., Winer, E., Williams, T., et al. (2006). Acute lymphoblastic leukemia with a 4;11 translocation analyzed by multimodal strategy of conventional cytogenetics, FISH, morphology, flow cytometry, molecular genetics and review of the literature. *Exp Mol Pathol, 81,* 62–71.
31. Bennett, J. M., Catovsky, D., Daniel, M. T., et al. Proposed revised criteria for the classification of acute myeloid leukemia: a report of the French-American-British Cooperative Group. *Ann Intern Med, 103,* 620–625.
32. Bennett, J. M., Catovsky, D., Daniel, M. T., et al. (1985). Criteria for the diagnosis of acute leukemia of megakaryocytic lineage (M7): a report of the French-American-British Cooperative Group. *Ann Intern Med, 103,* 460–462.

33. Claxton, D. F., Liu, P., Hsu, H. B., et al. (1994). Detection of fusion transcripts generated by the inversion 16 chromosome in acute myelogenous leukemia. *Blood, 83,* 1750–1756.

34. Slamon, D. J., Godolphin, W., Jones, L. A., et al. (1989). Studies of the HER-2 proto-oncogene in human breast and ovarian cancer. *Science, 244,* 707–712.

35. Perez, E. A., Roche, P. C., Jenkins, R. B., et al. (2002). HER2 testing in patients with breast cancer: poor correlation between weak positivity by immunohistochemistry and gene amplification by fluorescence in situ hybridization. *Mayo Clin Proc, 77,* 148–154.

36. Wolff, A. C., Hammond, M. E. H., Hicks, D. G., et al. (2013). Recommendations for Human Epidermal Growth Factor Receptor 2 Testing in Breast Cancer: American Society of Clinical Oncology/College of American Pathologists clinical practice guideline update. *J Clin Oncol, 31*(31), 3997–4015.

37. Slamon, D. J., Leyland-Jones, B., Shak, S., et al. (2001). Use of chemotherapy plus a monoclonal antibody against HER2 for metastatic breast cancer that overexpresses HER2. *N Engl J Med, 344,* 783–792.

38. Miller, D. T., Adam, M. P., Aradhya, S., et al. (2010). Consensus statement: chromosomal microarray is the first-tier clinical diagnostic test for individuals with developmental disabilities or congenital anomalies. *Am J Hum Genet, 86,* 749–764.

39. Kearney, H. M., Thorland, E. C., Brown, K. K., et al. (2011). American College of Medical Genetics standards and guidelines for interpretation and reporting of postnatal constitutional copy number variants. *Genet Med, 13,* 680–685.

40. Kearney, H. M., South, S. T., Wolff, D. J., et al. (2011). American College of Medical Genetics recommendations for the design and performance expectations for clinical genomic copy number microarrays intended for use in the postnatal setting for detection of constitutional abnormalities. *Genet Med, 13,* 676–679.

41. Cooley, L. D., Lebo, M., Li, M. M., et al. (2013). American College of Medical Genetics and Genomics technical standards and guidelines: microarray analysis for chromosome abnormalities in neoplastic disorders. *Genet Med, 15,* 484–494.

Acute Leukemias

*Reeba A. Omman, Ameet R. Kini**

CASE STUDY

After studying the material in this chapter, the reader should be able to respond to the following case study:

A 5-year-old child was seen by her family physician because of weakness and headaches. She had been in good health except for the usual communicable diseases of childhood. Physical examination revealed a pale, listless child with multiple bruises. The WBC count was 15×10^9/L, the hemoglobin was 8 g/dL, and the platelet count was 90×10^9/L. She had "abnormal cells" in her peripheral blood (Figure 31.1). Cytogenetic studies revealed hyperdiploidy.

1. What is the most likely diagnosis?
2. What characteristics of this disease indicate a positive prognosis?
3. What prognosis is associated with the hyperdiploidy?

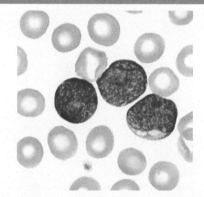

Figure 31.1 Peripheral Blood Film for the Patient in the Case Study. (Wright-Giemsa stain, ×1000.) (From Rodak, B. F., & Carr, J. H. [2017]. *Clinical Hematology Atlas.* [5th ed.]. St. Louis: Elsevier.)

*The authors extend appreciation to Bernadette F. Rodak, Woodlyne Roquiz, and Pranav Gandhi, whose work in prior editions provided the foundation for this chapter.

INTRODUCTION

The broad term *leukemia* is derived from the ancient Greek words *leukos* (λευκός), meaning "white," and *haima* (αἷμα), meaning "blood."[1] As defined today, acute leukemia refers to the rapid, clonal proliferation in the bone marrow of lymphoid or myeloid progenitor cells known as *lymphoblasts* and *myeloblasts,* respectively. When proliferation of blasts overwhelms the bone marrow, blasts are seen in the peripheral blood and the patient's symptoms reflect suppression of normal hematopoiesis.

For most cases of acute leukemia, the causes directly related to the development of the malignancy are unknown. The exceptions that exist are certain toxins that can induce genetic changes leading to a malignant phenotype. Environmental exposures known to lead to hematopoietic malignancies include radiation and exposure to organic solvents, such as benzene. Rarely, leukemias can be seen in patients with known familial cancer predisposition syndromes. Alkylating agents and other forms of chemotherapy used to treat various forms of cancer can induce deoxyribonucleic acid (DNA) damage in hematopoietic cells, leading to therapy-related leukemias.

Regardless of the mechanism of initial genetic damage, the development of leukemia is currently believed to be a stepwise progression of mutations or "multiple hits" involving mutations in genes that give cells a proliferative advantage, in addition to mutations that hinder differentiation.[2,3] These mutations result in transformation of normal hematopoietic stem cells or precursors into leukemic stem cells (LSCs). The LSCs then initiate, proliferate, and sustain the leukemia.[4]

CLASSIFICATION SCHEMES FOR ACUTE LEUKEMIAS

The French-American-British (FAB) classification of the acute leukemias was devised in the 1970s and was based on morphologic examination along with cytochemical stains to distinguish lymphoblasts from myeloblasts (Figure 31.2). The use of cytochemical stains continues to be a useful adjunct for differentiation of hematopoietic diseases, especially acute leukemias. The details of the cytochemical stains are addressed at the end of this chapter. In addition to morphologic and cytochemical stains, techniques commonly used to diagnose hematopoietic malignancies include flow cytometry and genetic/molecular studies. Findings of these techniques are discussed throughout the chapter in relation to specific leukemias.

Hematologists and pathologists are now moving toward more precise classification of many of the leukocyte neoplasms based on recurring chromosomal and genetic lesions found in many patients. These lesions are related to disruptions of oncogenes, tumor suppressor genes, and other regulatory elements that control proliferation, maturation, apoptosis, and other vital cell functions. In 2001 the World Health Organization (WHO) published new classification schemes for nearly all of the tumors of hematopoietic and lymphoid tissues,[5] and in some cases WHO melded the older morphologic schemes with the newer schemes. For instance, in the WHO classification scheme for acute myeloid leukemias (AMLs), there are some remnants of the old FAB classification, but new classifications were introduced for leukemias associated with consistently recurring chromosomal translocations. According to the WHO classification, a finding of at least 20% blasts in the bone marrow is required for diagnosis of the majority of acute leukemias, and testing must be performed to detect the presence or absence of genetic anomalies. The most recent (2017) WHO classification was released due to further insights into the molecular biology of the entities, with updates reflected in some of the classifications.[6] In-depth discussion of each of the subclassifications is beyond the scope of this book; only the most common subtypes of acute lymphoblastic leukemia and acute myeloid leukemia are described.

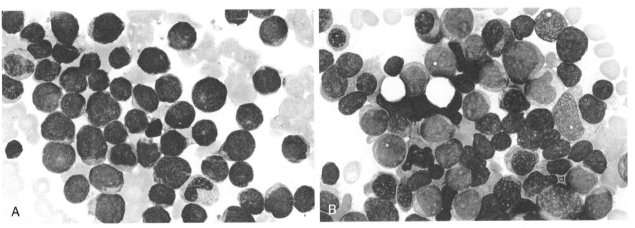

Figure 31.2 Lymphoblasts and Myeloblasts. (A), Lymphoblasts have a diameter two to three times the normal lymphocyte diameter, scant blue cytoplasm, coarse chromatin, deeper staining than myeloblasts, and inconspicuous nucleoli. **(B),** Myeloblasts have a diameter three to five times the lymphocyte diameter, moderate gray cytoplasm, uniform fine chromatin, two or more prominent nucleoli, and possibly Auer rods. (A and B, Bone marrow, Wright-Giemsa stain, ×500.)

ACUTE LYMPHOBLASTIC LEUKEMIA

Acute lymphoblastic leukemia (ALL) is primarily a disease of childhood and adolescence, accounting for 25% of childhood cancers and up to 75% of childhood leukemia.[7] The peak incidence of ALL in children is between 2 and 5 years of age.[8] Although ALL is rare in adults, risk increases with age; most adult patients are older than 50 years of age. The subtype of ALL is an important prognostic indicator for survival.[6] Adults have a poorer outlook: 80% to 90% experience complete remission, but the cure rate is less than 40%.[9,10]

Patients with B cell ALL typically present with fatigue (caused by anemia), fever (caused by neutropenia and infection), and mucocutaneous bleeding (caused by thrombocytopenia). Lymphadenopathy, including enlargement, is often a symptom.[11] Enlargement of the spleen (splenomegaly) and of the liver (hepatomegaly) may be seen. Bone pain often results from intramedullary growth of leukemic cells.[11] Eventual infiltration of malignant cells into the meninges, testes, or ovaries occurs frequently, and lymphoblasts can be found in the cerebrospinal fluid.[12]

In T cell ALL, there may be a large mass in the mediastinum leading to compromise of regional anatomic structures. Similar to B-ALL, T-ALL may present with anemia, thrombocytopenia, organomegaly, and bone pain, although the degree of leukopenia is often less severe.[13]

World Health Organization Classification

B-lymphoblastic leukemia/lymphoma (B-ALL) is subdivided into nine subtypes that are associated with recurrent cytogenetic abnormalities.[6] These entities are linked with unique clinical, phenotypic, or prognostic features (Box 31.1). Cases of B cell ALL that do not exhibit the specific genetic abnormalities are classified as B-lymphoblastic leukemia/lymphoma, not otherwise specified. Although 50% to 70% of patients with T-lymphoblastic leukemia/lymphoma have abnormal gene rearrangements, none of the abnormalities is clearly associated with specific biologic features. The 2017 WHO classification also subcategorizes T-ALL into early T-cell precursor lymphoblastic leukemia, which has limited early T cell differentiation.[6]

Morphology

Lymphoblasts vary in size but fall into two morphologic types. The most common type seen is a small lymphoblast (1.0 to 2.5 times the size of a normal lymphocyte) with scant blue cytoplasm and indistinct nucleoli (Figure 31.2); the second type of lymphoblast is larger (two to three times the size of a lymphocyte) with prominent nucleoli and nuclear membrane irregularities (Figure 31.3).[13] These cells may be confused with the blasts of AML.

Prognosis

Prognosis in ALL has improved dramatically over the past decades as a result of improvement in algorithms for treatment.[13] The prognosis for ALL depends on age at the time of diagnosis, lymphoblast load (tumor burden), immunophenotype, and genetic abnormalities. Children rather than infants or teens do the best. Chromosomal translocations are the strongest predictor of adverse treatment outcomes for children and adults. Peripheral blood lymphoblast counts greater than 20 to 30 $\times$ 10^9/L, hepatosplenomegaly, and lymphadenopathy all are associated with a worse outcome. The effects of other variables previously associated with a poorer prognosis, such as sex and ethnic group, have been eliminated when patients have been given equal access to treatment in trials carried out at a single institution.[14]

Immunophenotyping

Although morphology is the first tool used to distinguish ALL from AML, immunophenotyping and genetic analysis are the most reliable indicators of a cell's origin. Because both B and T cells are derived from lymphoid progenitors, both usually express CD34, terminal deoxynucleotidyl transferase (TdT), and human leukocyte antigen, DR subregion (HLA-DR). Four

---

BOX 31.1   2017 WHO Classification of B-Lymphoblastic Leukemia/Lymphoma with Recurrent Genetic Abnormalities[6]

B-lymphoblastic leukemia/lymphoma with t(9;22)(q34.1;q11.2); *BCR-ABL1*

B-lymphoblastic leukemia/lymphoma with t(v;11q23.3); *KMT2A (MLL)* rearranged

B-lymphoblastic leukemia/lymphoma with t(12;21)(p13.2;q22.1); *TEL-AML1 (ETV6-RUNX1)*

B-lymphoblastic leukemia/lymphoma with hyperdiploidy

B-lymphoblastic leukemia/lymphoma with hypodiploidy

B-lymphoblastic leukemia/lymphoma with t(5;14)(q31.1;q32.1); *IGH/IL3*

B-lymphoblastic leukemia/lymphoma with t(1;19)(q23;p13.3); *TCF3-PBX1 (E2A-PBX1)*

B-lymphoblastic leukemia/lymphoma, *BCR-ABL1*-like

B-lymphoblastic leukemia/lymphoma with iAMP21

WHO, World Health Organization

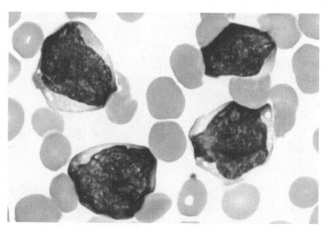

Figure 31.3 Peripheral Blood Film from a Patient with Acute Lymphoblastic Leukemia. Note large lymphoblasts with prominent nucleoli and membrane irregularities. (Wright-Giemsa stain, ×1000.) (From Rodak, B. F., & Carr, J. H. [2017]. *Clinical Hematology Atlas.* [5th ed.]. St. Louis: Elsevier.)

TABLE 31.1   Immunophenotypic Characteristics of Acute Lymphoblastic Leukemia (ALL)

ALL Subtype	Immunophenotype
Early (pro/pre-pre) B-ALL	CD34, CD19, cytoplasmic CD22, TdT
Intermediate (common) B-ALL	CD34, CD19, CD10, cytoplasmic CD22, TdT
Pre-B-ALL	CD34, CD19, cytoplasmic CD22, cytoplasmic μ, TdT (variable)
T-ALL	CD2, CD3, CD4, CD5, CD7, CD8, TdT

types of ALL have been identified by immunologic methods: early B-ALL (pro-B, or pre-pre-B), intermediate (common) B-ALL, pre-B-ALL, and T-ALL (Table 31.1). B-ALL is characterized by specific B cell antigens that are expressed at different stages of B cell development. In general, B cells express CD19, CD20, CD22, CD24, C79a, CD10, cytoplasmic μ, and PAX-5 (B cell specific activator protein). The degree of differentiation of B-lineage lymphoblasts often correlates with genetics and plays an important role in treatment decisions.[6,13,15] In the earliest stage of differentiation (pre-pre-B or pro-B), blasts express CD34, CD19, cytoplasmic CD22, and TdT. The incidence of pro-B-ALL is about 5% in children and 11% in adults. In intermediate, or *common*, B-ALL, CD10 is expressed. The most mature B-ALL is called *pre-B-ALL,* in which CD34 is typically negative, but there is characteristic expression of cytoplasmic μ heavy chain. Pre-B-ALL accounts for 15% of childhood cases and 10% of adult B-ALL.[16]

T-ALL is seen most often in teenaged males with a mediastinal mass, elevated peripheral blast counts, meningeal involvement, and infiltration of extra marrow sites.[17,18] The common T cell markers CD2, CD3, CD4, CD5, CD7, and CD8 are usually present. Most cases express TdT. A distinct subtype of T-ALL, ETP-ALL (early T cell precursor ALL) often shows expression of myeloid makers and is thought to be derived from T cell precursor cells that have the capacity for myeloid differentiation.[6] Early studies showed poor response to therapy in ETP-ALL; however, more recent studies have suggested that the prognosis is the same as with other T-ALL with optimal therapy.[6]

Genetic and Molecular Findings

Cytogenetic abnormalities are seen in the majority of B and T cell ALL, which produce changes that affect normal B and T cell development and underlie the pathogenesis of these neoplasms. A majority of T-ALL have been shown to have gain-of-function mutations involving the *NOTCH1* gene, which alters the Notch receptor signaling pathway responsible for normal T cell development.[19]

In T-ALL, however, the cytogenetic alterations show less specificity and less correlation with the prognosis and treatment outcome than in B-ALL. B-lymphoblastic leukemia/lymphoma with the t(9;22)(q34;q11.2);*BCR-ABL1* mutation (Philadelphia chromosome–positive ALL) has the worst prognosis among ALLs. It is more common in adults than in children. Imatinib, which has shown success in treating chronic myeloid leukemia, has improved survival (Chapter 32).

B-lymphoblastic leukemia/lymphoma with t(v;11q23); *KMT2A(MLL)*-rearranged is more common in very young infants, and the translocation may even occur in utero.[20] This leukemia has a very poor prognosis. About 25% of childhood ALL cases show a t(12;21)(p13.2;q22.1);*ETV6-RUNX1* translocation and appear to derive from a B cell progenitor rather than the hematopoietic stem cell.[21] This translocation is rare in adults. In children it carries an excellent prognosis, with a cure rate of over 90%. Hyperdiploidy in B-lymphoblastic leukemia/lymphoma is common in childhood B-ALL, accounting for 25% of cases, but it is much less common in adults. This genotype is associated with a very favorable prognosis in children. Conversely, hypodiploidy (less than 46 chromosomes) conveys a poor prognosis in both children and adults.

ACUTE MYELOID LEUKEMIA

AML is the most common type of leukemia in adults, and the incidence increases with age. AML is less common in children. The FAB classification of AML was based on morphology and cytochemistry; the WHO classification relies heavily on molecular characterization and cytogenetics (Chapters 29 and 30).[6]

Clinical Presentation

The clinical presentation of AML is nonspecific but reflects decreased production of normal bone marrow elements. Most patients with AML have a total white blood cell (WBC) count between 5 and 30×10^9/L, although the WBC count may range from 1 to 200×10^9/L. Myeloblasts are present in the peripheral blood in 90% of patients. Anemia, thrombocytopenia, and neutropenia give rise to the clinical findings of pallor, fatigue, fever, bruising, and bleeding. In addition, disseminated intravascular coagulation and other bleeding abnormalities can be significant.[22] Infiltration of malignant cells into the gums and other mucosal sites and skin also can be seen.

Splenomegaly is seen in half of AML patients, but lymph node enlargement is rare. Cerebrospinal fluid involvement in AML is rare and does not seem to be as ominous a sign as in ALL. Patients with AML tend to have few symptoms related to the central nervous system, even when it is infiltrated by blasts.

Common abnormalities in laboratory test results include hyperuricemia (caused by increased cellular turnover), hyperphosphatemia (due to cell lysis), and hypocalcemia (the latter two are also involved in progressive bone destruction). Hypokalemia is also common at presentation. During induction chemotherapy, especially when the WBC count is quite elevated, tumor lysis syndrome may occur. Tumor lysis syndrome is a group of metabolic complications that can occur in patients with malignancy, most notably lymphomas and leukemias, with and without treatment of the malignancy. These complications are caused by the breakdown products of dying cancer cells, which in turn cause acute uric acid nephropathy and renal failure. Tumor lysis syndrome is characterized by hyperkalemia, hyperphosphatemia, hyperuricemia and hyperuricosuria, and hypocalcemia.[23] The hyperkalemia alone can be life-threatening. Aggressive prophylactic measures to prevent or reduce the clinical manifestations of tumor lysis syndrome are critical.[24]

Subtypes of Acute Myeloid Leukemia and Related Precursor Neoplasms

Laboratory diagnosis of AML begins with a complete blood count, peripheral blood film examination, and bone marrow aspirate and biopsy specimen examination. The total WBC count may be normal, increased, or decreased; anemia is usually present, along with significant thrombocytopenia. The bone marrow is usually hypercellular, and greater than 20% of cells typically are marrow blasts, although if certain genetic abnormalities are present, the 20% blast threshold is not necessary for the diagnosis of AML.[6] Each category is discussed, and a summary of the classification is presented in Box 31.2.

The 2017 WHO classification for myeloid malignancies has categorized AMLs with recurrent cytogenetic abnormalities into subgroups based on the primary cytogenetic aberrations along with a few new entities (Box 31.3).[6]

AML with Recurrent Genetic Abnormalities

Acute myeloid leukemia with t(8;21)(q22;q22.1);RUNX1/RUNX1T1 The t(8;21)(q22;q22.1); *RUNX1/RUNX1T1* mutation is found in about 5% of AML cases. Seen predominantly in children and young adults, AML with this translocation has

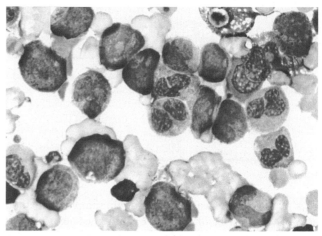

Figure 31.4 Bone Marrow Aspirate from a Patient with Acute Myeloid Leukemia with t(8;21). Note myeloblasts with granular cytoplasm and some maturation. (Wright-Giemsa stain, ×500.) (From Rodak, B. F., & Carr, J. H. [2017]. *Clinical Hematology Atlas.* [5th ed.]. St. Louis: Elsevier.)

myeloblasts with dysplastic granular cytoplasm, Auer rods, and some maturation (Figure 31.4), similar to the FAB M2 classification (discussed later in the chapter). Various anomalies, such as pseudo–Pelger-Huët cells and hypogranulation, can be seen. Eosinophilia is possible. Prognosis is generally favorable but may be negatively affected if unfavorable additional abnormalities, such as monosomy 7, occur.[25] The diagnosis of this subtype is based on the genetic abnormality, regardless of blast count.[6]

Acute myeloid leukemia with inv(16)(p13.1q22) or t(16;16)(p13.1;q22);CBFB-MYH11. Accounting for approximately 5% to 8% of all AML cases, core-binding factor (CBF) AML occurs at all ages, but it is found predominantly in younger patients.[6] The genetic aberration is sufficient for diagnosis regardless of blast count.[6,26] Myeloblasts, monoblasts, and promyelocytes are seen in the peripheral blood and bone marrow. In the bone marrow there may be eosinophilia with dysplastic changes (Figure 31.5). The incidence of extramedullary disease is higher than in most types of AML, and the central nervous system is a common site for relapse.[6,26] The remission rate is good, but only one half of patients are cured.[26]

Acute promyelocytic leukemia with PML-RARA. Acute promyelocytic leukemia comprises 5% to 10% of AML cases. It occurs in all age groups but is seen most commonly in young adults. This disorder is characterized by a differentiation block at the promyelocytic stage. The abnormal promyelocytes are considered to be comparable to blasts for the purpose of diagnosis. Detection of the 15;17 translocation is sufficient for diagnosis regardless of blast count.[6,25] Characteristic of this presentation are the abnormal hypergranular promyelocytes, some with Auer rods (Figure 31.6). When promyelocytes release primary granule contents, their procoagulant activity initiates disseminated intravascular coagulation; however, thromboembolic events may occur at presentation and during treatment.[27] In one variant of APL, the granules are so small that because of the limits of light microscopy, the cells give the appearance of

---

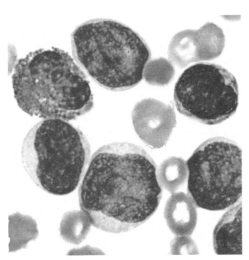

Figure 31.5 Peripheral Blood Film from a Patient with Acute Myeloid Leukemia with inv(16). There is an increase in myeloid and monocytic lines. Eosinophilia may also be present. (Wright-Giemsa stain, ×1000.) (From Rodak, B. F., & Carr, J. H. [2017]. *Clinical Hematology Atlas.* [5th ed.]. St. Louis: Elsevier.)

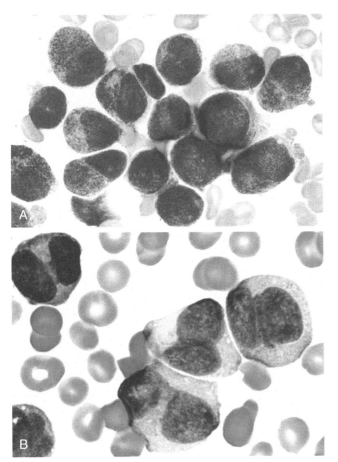

Figure 31.6 Peripheral Blood Films from a Patient with Acute Myeloid Leukemia with t(15;17) or Promyelocytic Leukemia. **(A),** Low-power view of the more common hypergranular variant. (Wright-Giemsa stain, ×500.) **(B),** Oil immersion view of the microgranular variant showing bilobed nuclear features. (Wright-Giemsa stain, ×1000.) (B from Rodak, B. F., & Carr, J. H. [2017]. *Clinical Hematology Atlas.* [5th ed.]. St. Louis: Elsevier.)

having no granules. This microgranular variant, accounting for 30% to 40% of APL cases, may be confused with other presentations of AML, but the presence of occasional Auer rods, the "butterfly" or "coin-on-coin" nucleus, and the clinical presentation are clues. The treatment of APL is significantly different from all other types of acute myeloid leukemia, and it is therefore important to arrive at an accurate diagnosis. Treatment includes all-*trans*-retinoic acid (ATRA) and arsenic trioxide.[28] ATRA is a vitamin A analogue and induces differentiation of the malignant promyelocytes. In adults who achieve a complete remission, the prognosis is better than for any other type of AML.[25] There are a few variant *RARA* translocations that confer a less favorable prognosis because the cells do not respond to ATRA therapy.[6]

Acute myeloid leukemia with t(9;11)(p22;q23);KMT2A (MLL)-MLLT3. AML with t(9;11)(p22;q23);*KMT2A (MLL)-MLLT3* represents a specific subgroup of the previous classification of AML with 11q23 abnormalities, and AMLs with other *KMT2A (MLL)* abnormalities should not be placed in this group.[29] AML with t(9;11) is a rare leukemia (6% of AML cases) that presents with an increase in monoblasts and immature monocytes (Figure 31.7). The blasts are large with abundant cytoplasm and fine nuclear chromatin. The cells may have motility, with pseudopodia seen frequently. Granules and vacuoles can be observed in the blasts. Typically this disease occurs in children and may be associated with gingival and skin involvement and/or disseminated intravascular coagulation.

Acute myeloid leukemia with t(6;9)(p23;q34);DEK-NUP214, acute myeloid leukemia with inv(3)(q21.3q26.2) or t(3;3)(q21.3; q26.2);GATA2, MECOM (RPN1-EVI1), acute myeloid leukemia (megakaryoblastic) with t(1;22)(p13.3;q13.1);RBM15-MKL1 and acute myeloid leukemia with BCR-ABL1. These are rare leukemias included in the 2017 WHO classification.[6] Detailed description of these entities is beyond the scope of this chapter.

Acute myeloid leukemia with mutated NPM1, acute myeloid leukemia with biallelic mutations of CEBPA, and acute myeloid leukemia with mutated RUNX1. These three additional entities with gene mutations were added in the 2017 WHO classification.[6]

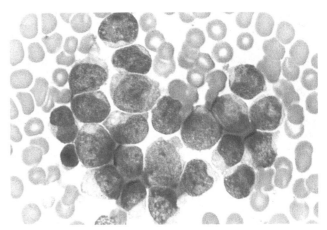

Figure 31.7 Bone Marrow Aspirate of a Patient with Acute Myeloid Leukemia with t(9;11) Abnormalities. Both monoblasts and immature monocytes are increased. (Wright-Giemsa stain, ×500.)

Acute myeloid leukemia with mutated *NPM1* (often leukemia with monocytic features) and AML with biallelic mutations of *CEBPA* are associated with a better prognosis.[6,30] *RUNX1* mutations are associated with worse overall survival.[31–34]

Acute Myeloid Leukemia with Myelodysplasia-Related Changes

AML with myelodysplasia affects primarily older adults and has a poor prognosis. This subcategory of AML with myelodysplasia-related changes incorporates leukemias with at least 20% blasts, multilineage dysplasia, a history of myelodysplastic syndrome (MDS) or MDS/myeloproliferative neoplasm (MPN), or a specific MDS-associated cytogenetic abnormality except del(9q). There must also be absence of AML with recurrent genetic abnormalities, *NPM1* and biallelic mutation of *CEBPA*. There must be morphologic criteria for multilineage dysplasia, defined as greater than 50% dysplasia in at least two cell lineages.[6] Significant dysplastic morphology includes pancytopenia with neutrophil hypogranulation or hypergranulation, pseudo–Pelger-Huët cells, and unusually segmented nuclei. Erythrocyte precursors have vacuoles, karyorrhexis, megaloblastoid features, and ring sideroblasts. There may be dysplastic micromegakaryocytes and dysplastic megakaryocytes. Genetic findings are similar to those found in MDS, with complex karyotypes and −7/del(7q) and −5/del(5q) being the most common.[6,35]

Therapy-Related Myeloid Neoplasms (t-MNs)

t-MNs are further classified into therapy-related MDS (t-MDS), AML (t-AML) and myelodysplastic/myeloproliferative neoplasms (t-MDS/MPN).[6] Treatment with alkylating agents, radiation, or topoisomerase II inhibitors has been associated with the development of a secondary AML, MDS, or MDS/MPN.[6,25,36,37] These therapy-related neoplasms account for 10% to 20% of AMLs, MDSs, and MDSs/MPNs. Generally these disorders occur following treatment for a prior malignancy, but they have also been associated with intensive treatment of patients with nonmalignant disorders requiring cytotoxic therapy.[6,36,38] Therapy-related myeloid neoplasms are similar in morphology to AML with myelodysplasia, monocytic/monoblastic leukemia, or AML with maturation, and the prognosis is generally poor, although therapy-related neoplasms with the t(15;17) and inv(16) mutations behave more like the de novo counterparts.[6,25]

Acute Myeloid Leukemia, Not Otherwise Specified

Because the leukemias in the "not otherwise specified" category do not fit easily into the WHO subtypes described earlier, they are grouped according to morphology, flow cytometric phenotyping (Chapter 28), and limited cytochemical reactions, as in the FAB classification. The FAB classification was based on the cell of origin, degree of maturity, cytochemical reactions, and limited cytogenetic features (Table 31.2).[39,40] A blast percentage of at least 20% in the peripheral blood or bone marrow is required for diagnosis. This category accounts for about 25% of all AML, but as more genetic subgroups are recognized, the number in this group will diminish.[29]

Acute myeloid leukemia with minimal differentiation. The blasts in AML with minimal differentiation are CD13[+], CD33[+],

TABLE 31.2 French-American-British (FAB) Classification of the Acute Myeloid Leukemias[39,40]

Subtype	Description
M0	Acute myeloid leukemia, minimally differentiated
M1	Acute myeloid leukemia without maturation
M2	Acute myeloid leukemia with maturation
M3	Acute promyelocytic leukemia
M4	Acute myelomonocytic leukemia
M4eo	Acute myelomonocytic leukemia with eosinophilia
M5a	Acute monocytic leukemia, poorly differentiated
M5b	Acute monocytic leukemia, well differentiated
M6	Acute erythroleukemia
M7	Acute megakaryocytic leukemia

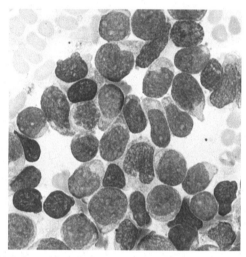

Figure 31.8 Bone Marrow Aspirate of a Patient with Acute Myeloid Leukemia, Minimally Differentiated (French-American-British Classification M0). Blasts lack myeloid morphologic features and yield negative results with myeloperoxidase and Sudan black B staining. Auer rods are not seen. CD34 is frequently present. (Wright-Giemsa stain, ×500.) (From Carr, J. H., & Rodak, B. F. [2013]. *Clinical Hematology Atlas.* [4th ed.]. St. Louis: Elsevier.)

CD34[+], and CD117[+] (Figure 31.8).[6,41] Auer rods typically are absent, and there is no clear evidence of cellular maturation. The cells yield negative results with the cytochemical stains myeloperoxidase and Sudan black B. These cases account for less than 5% of AML, and patients are generally either infants or older adults.

Acute myeloid leukemia without maturation. Closely aligned with the blasts in minimally differentiated AML, the blasts in AML without maturation are also CD13[+], CD33[+], with CD117 and CD34 being positive in the majority of cases (Figure 31.9).[6] Blasts may comprise 90% of nonerythroid cells in the bone marrow, and fewer than 10% of the leukocytes show maturation to the promyelocyte stage or beyond. At least 3% of blasts give positive results with myeloperoxidase or Sudan black B stains.[6,25]

Acute myeloid leukemia with maturation. AML with maturation is a common variant that presents with greater than 20% blasts, at least 10% maturing cells of neutrophil lineage (Figure 31.10), and fewer than 20% precursors with monocytic lineage. Auer rods are often present.[6]

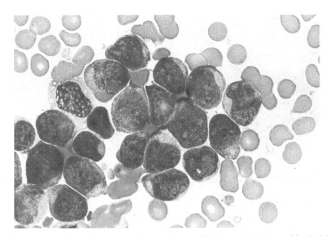

Figure 31.9 Bone Marrow Aspirate from a Patient with Acute Myeloid Leukemia without Maturation (French-American-British Classification M1). Blasts constitute 90% of the nonerythroid cells; there is less than 10% maturation of the granulocytic series beyond the promyelocyte stage. (Wright-Giemsa stain, ×500.)

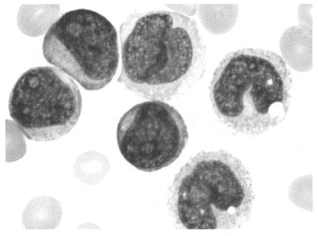

Figure 31.11 Peripheral Blood Film from a Patient with Acute Myelomonocytic Leukemia. Both myeloid and monocytic cells are present. Monocytic cells comprise at least 20% of all marrow cells, with monoblasts and promonocytes present. (Wright-Giemsa stain, ×1000.) (From Rodak, B. F., & Carr, J. H. [2017]. *Clinical Hematology Atlas.* [5th ed.]. St. Louis: Elsevier.)

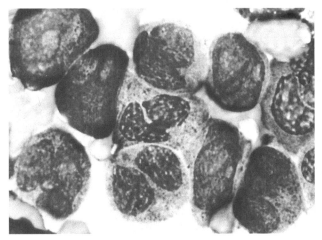

Figure 31.10 Bone Marrow Aspirate from a Patient with Acute Myeloid Leukemia with Maturation. Blasts constitute 20% or more of the nucleated cells of the bone marrow, and there is maturation beyond the promyelocyte stage in more than 10% of the nonerythroid cells. (Wright-Giemsa stain, ×1000.)

Acute myelomonocytic leukemia. Acute myelomonocytic leukemia is characterized by a significantly elevated WBC count and the presence of myeloid and monocytoid cells in the peripheral blood and bone marrow (Figure 31.11). Monocytic cells (monoblasts and promonocytes) constitute at least 20% of all marrow cells, as do neutrophils and their precursors. The monoblasts are large with abundant cytoplasm containing small granules and pseudopodia. The nucleus is large and immature and may contain multiple nucleoli. Promonocytes also are present and may have contorted nuclei. The cells are positive for the myeloid antigens CD13 and CD33 and the monocytic antigens CD14, CD4, CD11b, CD11c, and CD64. Nonspecific cytogenetic changes are found in most cases.[6]

Acute monoblastic and monocytic leukemias. In these leukemias, which are divided into monoblastic and monocytic based on the degree of maturity of the monocytic cells present

in the marrow and peripheral blood, more than 80% of the marrow cells are of monocytic origin. These cells are CD14[+], CD4[+], CD11b[+], CD11c[+], [+]and CD64. Blasts are large with abundant, often agranular cytoplasm and large prominent nucleoli (Figure 31.12A). When some evidence of maturation is present, the cells are called *promonocytes.* Promonocytes in monocytic leukemias with differentiation are considered to be blast equivalents (Figure 31.12B). Nonspecific esterase testing usually yields positive results. Acute monoblastic/monocytic leukemia comprises fewer than 5% of cases of AML and is most common in younger individuals. Extramedullary involvement, including cutaneous and gingival infiltration, and bleeding disorders are common. Nonspecific cytogenetic abnormalities are seen in most cases.[6,42]

Pure erythroid leukemia. One of the major changes in the 2017 WHO classification is the removal of acute erythroleukemia (erythroid/myeloid type) – most of these cases will now be classified as MDS with excess blasts.[6]

Pure erythroid leukemia remains as M6, the only acute erythroid leukemia.[6] In this leukemia 80% or more of the bone marrow cells are erythroid, and greater than 30% are proerythroblasts.[43–45] The myeloblast component is not significant. Complex rearrangements and hypodiploid chromosome number are common. Chromosomes 5 and 7 are frequently affected.[6]

The red blood cell (RBC) precursors have significant dysplastic features, such as multinucleation, megaloblastoid asynchrony, and vacuolization. The nucleated RBCs in the peripheral blood may account for more than 50% of the total number of nucleated cells. Ring sideroblasts, Howell-Jolly bodies, and other inclusions may be present (Figure 31.13). Abnormal megakaryocytes may be seen. Pure erythroid leukemia has an aggressive and rapid clinical course.[6]

Acute megakaryoblastic leukemia. Patients with acute megakaryoblastic leukemia usually have cytopenias, although

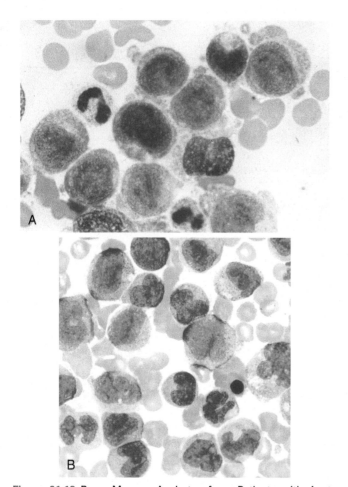

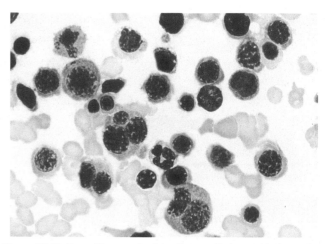

Figure 31.13 Bone Marrow Aspirate from a Patient with Acute Erythroid Leukemia. Erythroid precursors showing dysplastic features, including multinucleation and megaloblastic asynchrony. (Wright-Giemsa stain, ×500.) (From Rodak, B. F., & Carr, J. H. [2017]. *Clinical Hematology Atlas.* [5th ed.]. St. Louis: Elsevier.)

Figure 31.12 Bone Marrow Aspirates from Patients with Acute Monoblastic Leukemia and Acute Monocytic Leukemia. (A), Acute monoblastic leukemia with more than 80% of the bone marrow cells of monocytic origin. (Wright-Giemsa stain, ×500.) **(B),** Acute monocytic leukemia with promonocytes. Promonocytes are considered blast equivalents. (Wright Giemsa stain, ×500.) (B from Carr, J. H., & Rodak, B. F. [2013]. *Clinical Hematology Atlas.* [4th ed.]. St. Louis: Elsevier.)

some may have thrombocytosis. Dysplastic features are often present in all cell lines. Diagnosis requires the presence of at least 20% blasts, of which at least 50% must be of megakaryocyte origin. This category excludes AML with MDS-related changes and Down syndrome–related cases, in addition to those with recurrent genetic abnormalities, as discussed previously.

Megakaryoblast diameters vary from that of a small lymphocyte to three times their size. Chromatin is delicate with prominent nucleoli. Immature megakaryocytes may have light blue cytoplasmic blebs (Figure 31.14A). Megakaryoblasts are identified by immunostaining, using antibodies specific for cytoplasmic von Willebrand factor or platelet membrane antigens CD41

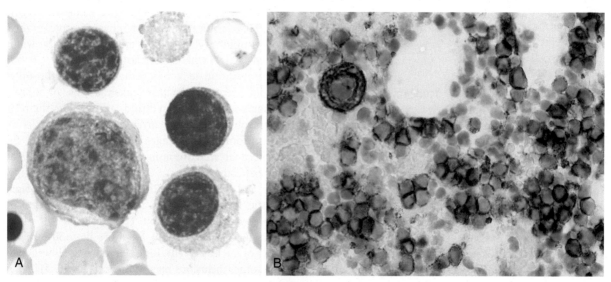

Figure 31.14 Peripheral Blood Film (A) and Bone Marrow Aspirate (B) from a Patient with Acute Megakaryocytic Leukemia. (A), Note the heterogeneity of blasts, one small with scant cytoplasm, two with cytoplasmic blebbing, and one quite large. (Wright-Giemsa stain, ×1000.) **(B),** Positive reaction for CD42b. (Immunostain, ×1000.) (B from Carr, J. H., & Rodak, B. F. [2013]. *Clinical Hematology Atlas.* [4th ed.]. St. Louis: Elsevier.)

(glycoprotein IIb), CD42b (glycoprotein Ib) (Figure 31.14B), or CD61 (glycoprotein IIIa).[6]

Myeloid Sarcoma

Myeloid sarcoma refers to extramedullary proliferation of blasts of one or more myeloid lineages that disrupts tissue architecture. Tissue architecture must be effaced for the neoplasm to qualify for this diagnosis. Tissues commonly affected include skin, gastrointestinal tract and lymph nodes.[6,25]

Myeloid Proliferations Related to Down Syndrome

Unique patterns of malignancy occur in persons with trisomy 21 resulting in Down syndrome. Approximately 10% of newborns with Down syndrome present with transient abnormal myelopoiesis, which is morphologically indistinguishable from AML. Both conditions are associated with *GATA1* mutations.[46–48] Spontaneous remission generally occurs within a few months. Among individuals with Down syndrome, there is a fiftyfold increased incidence of AML during the first 5 years of life compared with individuals without Down syndrome. The leukemia is of megakaryocytic lineage, and young children respond well to chemotherapy, although older children do not fare as well.[6,49]

Blastic Plasmacytoid Dendritic Cell Neoplasm

Blastic plasmacytoid cell neoplasm is a rare clinically aggressive tumor derived from precursors of plasmacytoid dendritic cells. It presents with skin lesions and may ultimately progress to involve peripheral blood and bone marrow.[6,29]

ACUTE LEUKEMIAS OF AMBIGUOUS LINEAGE

Acute leukemias of ambiguous lineage (ALALs) include leukemia in which there is no clear evidence of differentiation along a single cell line; leukemias of this type are commonly referred to as *acute undifferentiated leukemias* (AULs). Other cases of ALAL that demonstrate a multiplicity of antigens in which it is not possible to determine a specific lineage are called *mixed phenotype acute leukemias* (MPALs). The 2008 WHO classification significantly revised the criteria for this designation. This revision was maintained in the 2017 WHO classification and is shown in Box 31.4.[6,50]

BOX 31.4 WHO Classification of Acute Leukemia of Ambiguous Lineage (ALAL).[6]

Acute undifferentiated leukemia (AUL) – synonyms: ALAL without differentiation, primitive acute leukemia, stem cell leukemia

Mixed phenotype acute leukemia (MPAL) – synonyms: biphenotypic acute leukemia, bilineal leukemia, mixed lineage acute leukemia, dual lineage acute leukemia, hybrid acute leukemia:
  MPAL with t(9;22)(q34.1;q11.2);*BCR-ABL1*
  MPAL with t(v;11q23);*KMT2A (MLL)*-rearranged
  MPAL B/myeloid, not otherwise specified
  MPAL T/myeloid, not otherwise specified
  MPAL, not otherwise specified, rare types
Acute leukemias of ambiguous lineage, not otherwise specified

---

CYTOCHEMICAL STAINS AND INTERPRETATIONS

Techniques such as flow cytometry, cytogenetic analysis, and molecular testing are now commonly used in the diagnosis of acute leukemias. However, older techniques, such as cytochemical stains, still retain their importance. An advantage of cytochemical stains is that they are relatively inexpensive and can be performed by laboratories throughout the world, including in areas where resources and access to advanced techniques are limited. The cytochemical stains are summarized in Table 31.3.

Myeloperoxidase

Myeloperoxidase (MPO) (Figures 31.15 and 31.16) is an enzyme found in the primary granules of granulocytic cells (neutrophils, eosinophils, and, to a certain extent, monocytes). Lymphocytes do not exhibit MPO activity. This stain is useful for differentiating the blasts of AML from those of ALL.

TABLE 31.3 Acute Leukemia Cytochemical Reaction Chart

Condition	MPO	SBB	NASDA	ANBE	ANAE
ALL	–	–	–	–/+ (focal)	–/+ (focal)
AML	+	+	+	–	–
AMML	+	+	+	+ (diffuse)	+ (diffuse)
AMoL	–	–/+	–	+ (diffuse)	+ (diffuse)
Megakaryocytic leukemia	–	–	–	–	+ (localized)

+, Positive reaction; –, negative reaction; –/+, negative or positive reaction; *ALL*, acute lymphoblastic leukemia; *AML*, acute myeloid leukemia; *AMML*, acute myelomonocytic leukemia; *AMoL*, acute monocytic leukemia; *ANAE*, α-naphthyl acetate esterase; *ANBE*, α-naphthyl butyrate esterase; *MPO*, myeloperoxidase; *NASDA*, naphthol AS-D chloroacetate esterase; *SBB*, Sudan black B.

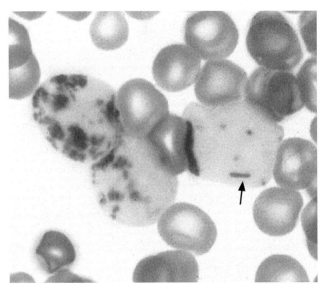

Figure 31.15 Positive Reaction to Myeloperoxidase Stain in Early Myeloid Cells. Note Auer rod at *arrow.* (Bone marrow, myeloperoxidase stain, ×1000.)

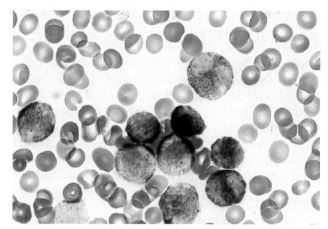

Figure 31.16 Strong Positive Reaction to Myeloperoxidase Stain in Leukemic Promyelocytes. From a patient with acute promyelocytic leukemia. (Bone marrow, myeloperoxidase stain, ×1000.)

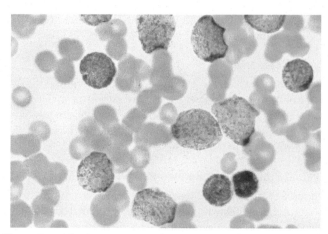

Figure 31.17 Sudan Black B Reaction. Positivity increases with the maturity of the granulocytic cell. (Bone marrow, Sudan black B stain, ×1000.)

Interpretation

MPO is present in the primary granules of most granulocytic cells, beginning at the promyelocyte stage and continuing throughout maturation. Leukemic myeloblasts are usually positive for MPO. In many cases of the AMLs (without maturation, with maturation, and promyelocytic leukemia), it has been found that more than 80% of the blasts show MPO activity. Auer rods found in leukemic blasts and promyelocytes test strongly MPO positive.

In contrast, lymphoblasts in ALL and lymphoid cells are MPO negative. It is important that the reaction only in the blast cells be used as the determining factor for the differentiation of acute leukemias. This is true for MPO and for other cytochemical stains used in determining cell lineage described in this chapter: maturing granulocytes are MPO positive; this is a normal finding and has little or no diagnostic significance.

Sudan Black B

Sudan black B (SBB) staining (Figure 31.17) is another useful technique for the differentiation of AML from ALL. SBB stains cellular lipids. The staining pattern is quite similar to that of MPO; SBB staining is possibly a little more sensitive for the early myeloid cells.

Interpretation

Granulocytes (neutrophils) show a positive reaction to SBB from the myeloblast through the maturation series. The staining becomes more intense as the cell matures as a result of the increase in the numbers of primary and secondary granules. Monocytic cells can demonstrate negative to weakly positive staining due to various changes that occur during differentiation. Lymphoid cells generally do not stain.

Esterases

Esterase reactions are used to differentiate myeloblasts and neutrophilic granulocytes from cells of monocytic origin. Nine

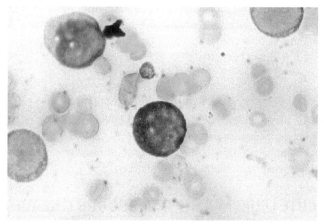

Figure 31.18 Positive Reaction to AS-D Chloroacetate Esterase Stain. Two granulocytic cells with positive reaction. (Bone marrow, AS-C chloroacetate esterase stain, ×1000.)

isoenzymes of esterases are present in leukocytes. Two substrate esters commonly used are α-naphthyl acetate and α-naphthyl butyrate (both nonspecific). Naphthol AS-D chloroacetate (specific) also may be used. "Specific" refers to the fact that only granulocytic cells show staining, whereas nonspecific stains also may produce positive results in other cells.

Interpretation

Esterase stains can be used to distinguish acute leukemias that are granulocytic from leukemias that are primarily of monocytic origin. When naphthol AS-D chloroacetate is used as a substrate, the reaction is positive in the granulocytic cells and negative to weak in the monocytic cells (Figure 31.18). Chloroacetate esterase is present in the primary granules of neutrophils. Leukemic myeloblasts generally show a positive reaction. Auer rods also show positivity.

α-Naphthyl acetate, in contrast to naphthol AS-D chloroacetate, reveals strong esterase activity in monocytes that can be inhibited with the addition of sodium fluoride.[51,52] Granulocytes and lymphoid cells generally show a negative result on nonspecific esterase staining (Figure 31.19).

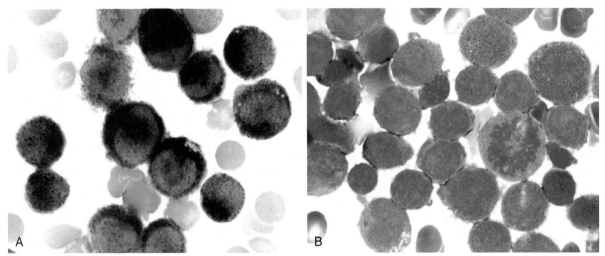

Figure 31.19 α-Naphthyl Acetate Esterase Positivity in Cells of Monocytic Origin (A) and Inhibition of Reaction with Sodium Fluoride (B). (A), Positive reaction with α-naphthyl acetate esterase stain in immature monocytic cells. (Bone marrow, α-naphthyl acetate esterase stain, ×1000.) **(B),** Same specimen with addition of sodium fluoride to the stain. The esterase reaction in the immature monocytic cells is inhibited. (Bone marrow, α-naphthyl acetate esterase stain and sodium fluoride, ×1000.)

A diffuse positive α-naphthyl butyrate esterase reaction is seen in monocytes. α-Naphthyl butyrate is less sensitive than α-naphthyl acetate, but it is more specific. Granulocytes and lymphoid cells generally show a negative reaction (Figure 31.20), although a small positive dot may be seen in lymphocytes. In myelomonocytic leukemia, positive AS-D chloroacetate activity and positive α-naphthyl butyrate or α-naphthyl acetate activity should be seen because myeloid and monocytic cells are present. In myelomonocytic leukemia, at least 20% of the cells must show monocytic differentiation that is nonspecific esterase positive and is inhibited by sodium fluoride. In the pure monocytic leukemias, 80% or more of the blasts are nonspecific esterase positive and specific esterase negative.

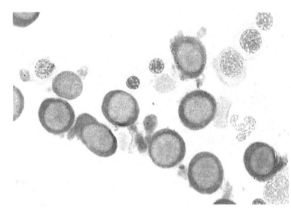

Figure 31.20 α-Naphthyl Butyrate Esterase Positivity in Cells of Monocytic Origin. From a patient with acute monoblastic/monocytic leukemia. Note the negative reaction of myeloid and erythroid precursors. (Bone marrow, α-Naphthyl butyrate esterase stain, ×1000.)

SUMMARY

- The development of leukemia is currently believed to be a stepwise progression of mutations, or "multiple hits," involving mutations that give leukemic stem cells a proliferative advantage and also hinder differentiation.
- For most acute leukemias, causes directly related to the development of the malignancy are unknown, but a few exceptions exist. Some known causes include environmental toxins, certain viruses, previous chemotherapy, and familial predisposition.
- There are several classification schemes for leukocyte neoplasia, including the FAB system, based primarily on morphology and cytochemical staining, and the WHO system, which retains some elements of the FAB scheme but emphasizes molecular and cytogenetic changes.
- Only half of patients with ALL have leukocytosis, and many do not have circulating lymphoblasts, but neutropenia, thrombocytopenia, and anemia are usually present.

- In children ALL is a disease in which the "good prognosis" subtypes are associated with a 95% rate of complete remission, but adults with ALL have a poorer outlook.
- Infiltration of malignant cells into the meninges can occur, with lymphoblasts found in the cerebrospinal fluid, testes, and ovaries.
- Prognosis in ALL depends primarily on age at the time of diagnosis, lymphoblast load (tumor burden), and immunophenotype. Chromosomal translocations seem to be the strongest predictor of adverse treatment outcomes for children and adults.
- The t(12;21) marker is found in a significant number of patients with childhood ALL.
- There are two main subtypes of ALL according to the WHO classification system: B-lymphoblastic leukemia/lymphoma and T-lymphoblastic leukemia/lymphoma.
- Tumor lysis syndrome is an increasingly common complication of treatment, especially in patients with a high tumor burden.

- Although morphology is the first tool in distinguishing ALL from AML, immunophenotyping is often the only reliable indicator of a cell's origin.
- The incidence of AML in adults increases with age.
- The clinical presentation of a patient with AML is nonspecific and reflects the decreased production of normal bone marrow elements, an elevated WBC count, and the presence of myeloblasts. Anemia, thrombocytopenia, and neutropenia give rise to the clinical findings of pallor, fatigue, bruising and bleeding, and fever with infections.
- The classification of AML is complicated by the presence or absence of multiple cell lines defined as "myeloid" in origin, specific cells within these cell lines, and specific karyotype abnormalities.
- Leukemias with ambiguous lineage include leukemias in which there is no clear evidence of differentiation along a single cell line.
- Cytochemical techniques are often used in conjunction with morphologic analysis, immunohistochemical methods, flow cytometry, cytogenetic analysis, and molecular biologic techniques in establishing a diagnosis.
- Cytochemical reactions may be enzymatic or nonenzymatic. Fresh smears must be used to detect enzymatic activity, whereas nonenzymatic procedures may be performed on specimens that have been stored at room temperature.
- MPO stains primary granules and is useful in differentiating granulocytic from lymphoid cells.
- SBB stains lipids and results parallel those with the MPO stain.
- Esterases help differentiate granulocytes and their precursors from cells of monocytic origin. Butyrate esterase testing gives positive results in monocytes but not in granulocyte precursors, whereas naphthol AS-D chloroacetate esterase stains granulocyte precursors.

Now that you have completed this chapter, go back and read again the case study at the beginning and respond to the questions presented.

REVIEW QUESTIONS

Answers can be found in the Appendix.

1. According to the WHO classification, except in leukemias with specific genetic anomalies, the minimal percentage of blasts necessary for a diagnosis of acute leukemia is:
   a. 10%
   b. 20%
   c. 30%
   d. 50%

2. A 20-year-old patient has an elevated WBC count with 70% blasts, 4% neutrophils, 5% lymphocytes, and 21% monocytes in the peripheral blood. Eosinophils with dysplastic changes are seen in the bone marrow. AML with which of the following karyotypes would be most likely to be seen?
   a. AML with t(8;21)(q22;q22)
   b. AML with t(16;16)(p13;q22)
   c. APL with *PML-RARA*
   d. AML with t(9;11)(p22;q23)

3. Which of the following would be considered a sign of potentially favorable prognosis in children with ALL?
   a. Hyperdiploidy
   b. Presence of CD19 and CD20
   c. Absence of trisomy 8
   d. Presence of *BCR/ABL* gene

4. Signs and symptoms of cerebral infiltration with blasts are more commonly seen in:
   a. AML with recurrent cytogenetic abnormalities
   b. Therapy-related myeloid neoplasms
   c. AML with myelodysplasia-related changes
   d. ALL

5. An oncology patient exhibiting signs of renal failure with seizures after initial chemotherapy may potentially develop:
   a. Hyperleukocytosis
   b. Tumor lysis syndrome
   c. Acute leukemia secondary to chemotherapy
   d. Myelodysplasia

6. Disseminated intravascular coagulation is more often seen in association with leukemia characterized by which of the following mutations?
   a. t(12;21)(p13;q22)
   b. t(9;22)(q34;q11.2)
   c. inv(16)(p13;q22)
   d. t(15;17)(q22;q12)

7. Which of the following leukemias affects primarily children, is characterized by an increase in monoblasts and monocytes, and often is associated with gingival and skin involvement?
   a. Pre-B-lymphoblastic leukemia
   b. Pure erythroid leukemia
   c. AML with t(9;11)(p22;q23)
   d. APL with *PML-RARA*

8. A 20-year-old patient presents with fatigue, pallor, easy bruising, and swollen gums. Bone marrow examination reveals 82% cells with delicate chromatin and prominent nucleoli that are CD14$^+$, CD4$^+$, CD11b$^+$, and CD36$^+$. Which of the following acute leukemias is likely?
   a. Minimally differentiated leukemia
   b. Leukemia of ambiguous lineage
   c. Acute monoblastic/monocytic leukemia
   d. Acute megakaryoblastic leukemia

9. Pure erythroid leukemia is a disorder involving:
   a. Pronormoblasts only
   b. Pronormoblasts and basophilic normoblasts
   c. All forms of developing RBC precursors
   d. Equal numbers of pronormoblasts and myeloblasts

10. A patient with normal chromosomes has a WBC count of $3.0 \times 10^9/L$ and dysplasia in all cell lines. There are 60% blasts of varying sizes. The blasts stain positive for CD61. The most likely type of leukemia is:
    a. Acute lymphoblastic
    b. Acute megakaryoblastic
    c. Acute monoblastic
    d. APL with *PML-RARA*

11. SBB stains which of the following component of cells?
    a. Glycogen
    b. Lipids
    c. Structural proteins
    d. Enzymes

12. The cytochemical stain α-naphthyl butyrate is a nonspecific esterase stain that shows diffuse positivity in cells of which lineage?
    a. Erythroid
    b. Monocytic
    c. Granulocytic
    d. Lymphoid

REFERENCES

1. Anderson, D. M., Novak, P. D., Elliot, M. A., et al. (1994). Leukemia. *Mosby's Medical, Nursing & Allied Health Dictionary.* (4th ed.). Mosby-Yearbook: St. Louis.

2. Bachas, C., Schuurhuis, G. J., Hollink, I. H., et al. (2010). High-frequency type I/II mutational shifts between diagnosis and relapse are associated with outcome in pediatric AML: implications for personalized medicine. *Blood, 116*(15), 2752–2758.

3. Reilly, J. T. (2005). Pathogenesis of acute myeloid leukaemia and inv(16)(p13;q22): a paradigm for understanding leukaemogenesis? *Br J Haematol, 128*(1), 18–34.

4. Lane, S. W., & Gilliland, D. G. (2010). Leukemia stem cells. *Semin Cancer Biol, 20*(2), 71–76.

5. International Agency for Research on Cancer. (2001). *World Health Organization Classification of Tumours: Pathology and Genetics of Tumours of Haematopoietic and Hymphoid Tissues.* Lyon, France: IARC Press.

6. Swerdlow, S. H., Campo, E., Harris, N. L., et al. (Eds). (2017). *WHO Classification of Tumours of Haematopoietic and Lymphoid Tissues Revised* (4th ed.). *Volume 2.* Lyon: IARC.

7. Stanulla, M., & Schrauder, A. (2009). Bridging the gap between the north and south of the world: the case of treatment response in childhood acute lymphoblastic leukemia. *Haematologica, 94*(6), 748–752.

8. Inaba, H., Greaves, M., & Mullighan, C. G. (2013). Acute lymphoblastic leukaemia. *Lancet. 9881,* 1943–1955.

9. Pui, C. H., & Evans, W. E. (2006). Treatment of acute lymphoblastic leukemia. *N Engl J Med, 354*(2), 166–178.

10. Advani, A., Jin, T., Bolwell, B., et al. (2009). A prognostic scoring system for adult patients less than 60 years of age with acute lymphoblastic leukemia in first relapse. *Leuk Lymphoma, 50*(7), 1126–1131.

11. Redaelli, A., Laskin, B. L., Stephens, J. M., et al. (2005). A systematic literature review of the clinical and epidemiological burden of acute lymphoblastic leukaemia (ALL). *Eur J Cancer Care (Engl), 14*(1), 53–62.

12. Hutter, J. J. (2010). Childhood leukemia. *Pediatr Rev, 31*(6), 234–241.

13. Onciu, M. (2009). Acute lymphoblastic leukemia. *Hematol Oncol Clin North Am, 23*(4), 655–674.

14. Pilozzi, E., Pulford, K., Jones, M., et al. (1998). Co-expression of CD79a (JCB117) and CD3 by lymphoblastic lymphoma. *J Pathol, 186*(2), 140–143.

15. Thomas, D. A., O'Brien, S., & Kantarjian, H. M. (2009). Monoclonal antibody therapy with rituximab for acute lymphoblastic leukemia. *Hematol Oncol Clin North Am, 23*(5), 949–971.

16. Dinner, S., Burbaxani, S., Jain, N., et al. (2018). Acute lymphoblastic leukemia in adults. In Hoffman, R., Benz, E. J. Jr., Silberstein, L.E., et al. (Eds.), *Hematology: Basic Principles and Practice.* (7th ed., pp. 1029–1054). Philadelphia: Elsevier.

17. Attarbaschi, A., Mann, G., Dworzak, M., et al. (2002). Mediastinal mass in childhood T-cell acute lymphoblastic leukemia: significance and therapy response. *Med Pediatr Oncol, 39*(6), 558–565.

18. Goldberg, J. M., Silverman, L. B., Levy, D. E., et al. (2003). Childhood T-cell acute lymphoblastic leukemia: the Dana-Farber Cancer Institute acute lymphoblastic leukemia consortium experience. *J Clin Oncol, 21*(19), 3616–3622.

19. Van Vlierberghe, P., & Ferrando, A. (2012). The molecular basis of T cell acute lymphoblastic leukemia. *J Clin Invest, 122*(10), 3398–3406.

20. Gale, K. B., Ford, A. M., Repp, R., et al. (1997). Backtracking leukemia to birth: identification of clonotypic gene fusion sequences in neonatal blood spots. *Proc Natl Acad Sci U S A, 94*(25), 13950–13954.

21. Castor, A., Nilsson, L., Astrand-Grundstrom, I., et al. (2005). Distinct patterns of hematopoietic stem cell involvement in acute lymphoblastic leukemia. *Nat Med, 11*(6), 630–637.

22. Uchiumi, H., Matsushima, T., Yamane, A., et al. (2007). Prevalence and clinical characteristics of acute myeloid leukemia associated with disseminated intravascular coagulation. *Int J Hematol, 86*(2), 137–142.

23. Montesinos, P., Lorenzo, I., Martin, G., et al. (2008). Tumor lysis syndrome in patients with acute myeloid leukemia: identification of risk factors and development of a predictive model. *Haematologica, 93*(1), 67–74.

24. Cairo, M. S., & Bishop, M. (2004). Tumour lysis syndrome: new therapeutic strategies and classification. *Br J Haematol, 127*(1), 3–11.

25. Heerema-McKenney, A., & Arber, D. A. (2009). Acute myeloid leukemia. *Hematol Oncol Clin North Am, 23*(4), 633–654.

26. Mrozek, K., Marcucci, G., Paschka, P., et al. (2008). Advances in molecular genetics and treatment of core-binding factor acute myeloid leukemia. *Curr Opin Oncol, 20*(6), 711–718.

27. Stein, E., McMahon, B., Kwaan, H., et al. (2009). The coagulopathy of acute promyelocytic leukaemia revisited. *Best Pract Res Clin Haematol, 22*(1), 153–163.

28. Nasr, R., Lallemand-Breitenbach, V., Zhu, J., et al. (2009). Therapy-induced PML/RARA proteolysis and acute promyelocytic leukemia cure. *Clin Cancer Res, 15*(20), 6321–6326.

29. Vardiman, J. W., Thiele, J., Arber, D. A., et al. (2009). The 2008 revision of the World Health Organization (WHO) classification of myeloid neoplasms and acute leukemia: rationale and important changes. *Blood, 114*(5), 937–951.

30. Falini, B., Mecucci, C., Tiacci, E., et al. (2005). Cytoplasmic nucleophosmin in acute myelogenous leukemia with a normal karyotype. *N Engl J Med, 352*(3), 254–266.

31. Tang, J. L., Hou, H. A., Chen, C. Y., et al. (2009). AML1/RUNX1 mutations in 470 adult patients with de novo acute myeloid leukemia: prognostic implication and interaction with other gene alterations. *Blood, 114*(26), 5352–5361.

32. Gaidzik, V. I., Bullinger, L., Schlenk, R. F., et al. (2011). RUNX1 mutations in acute myeloid leukemia: results from a comprehensive genetic and clinical analysis from the AML study group. *J Clin Oncol, 29*(10), 1364–1372.

33. Schnittger, S., Dicker, F., Kern, W., et al. (2011). RUNX1 mutations are frequent in de novo AML with noncomplex karyotype and confer an unfavorable prognosis. *Blood, 117*(8), 2348–2357.

34. Mendler, J. H., Maharry, K., Radmacher, M. D., et al. (2012). RUNX1 mutations are associated with poor outcome in younger and older patients with cytogenetically normal acute myeloid leukemia and with distinct gene and MicroRNA expression signatures. *J Clin Oncol, 30*(25), 3109–3118.

35. Ngo, N., Lampert, I. A., & Naresh, K. N. (2008). Bone marrow trephine findings in acute myeloid leukaemia with multilineage dysplasia. *Br J Haematol, 140*(3), 279–286.

36. Czader, M., & Orazi, A. (2009). Therapy-related myeloid neoplasms. *Am J Clin Pathol, 132*(3), 410–425.

37. Vardiman, J. W. (2010). The World Health Organization (WHO) classification of tumors of the hematopoietic and lymphoid tissues: an overview with emphasis on the myeloid neoplasms. *Chem Biol Interact, 184*(1-2), 16-20.

38. Anderson, L. A., Pfeiffer, R. M., Landgren, O., et al. (2009). Risks of myeloid malignancies in patients with autoimmune conditions. *Br J Cancer, 100*(5), 822–828.

39. Bennett, J. M., Catovsky, D., Daniel, M. T., et al. (1976). Proposals for the classification of the acute leukaemias. French-American-British (FAB) co-operative group. *Br J Haematol, 33*(4), 451–458.

40. Bennett, J. M., Catovsky, D., Daniel, M. T., et al. (1985). Proposed revised criteria for the classification of acute myeloid leukemia. A report of the French-American-British Cooperative Group. *Ann Intern Med, 103*(4), 620–625.

41. Kaleem, Z., Crawford, E., Pathan, M. H., et al. (2003). Flow cytometric analysis of acute leukemias. Diagnostic utility and critical analysis of data. *Arch Pathol Lab Med, 127*(1), 42–48.

42. Villeneuve, P., Kim, D. T., Xu, W., et al. (2008). The morphological subcategories of acute monocytic leukemia (M5a and M5b) share similar immunophenotypic and cytogenetic features and clinical outcomes. *Leuk Res, 32*(2), 269–273.

43. Kowal-Vern, A., Cotelingam, J., & Schumacher, H. R. (1992). The prognostic significance of proerythroblasts in acute erythroleukemia. *Am J Clin Pathol, 98*(1), 34–40.

44. Lessard, M., Struski, S., Leymarie, V., et al. (2005). Cytogenetic study of 75 erythroleukemias. *Cancer Genet Cytogenet, 163*(2), 113–122.

45. Liu, W., Hasserjian, R. P., Hu, Y., et al. (2011). Pure erythroid leukemia: a reassessment of the entity using the 2008 World Health Organization classification. *Mod Pathol, 24*(3), 375–383.

46. Greene, M. E., Mundschau, G., Wechsler, J., et al. (2003, Nov-Dec). Mutations in GATA1 in both transient myeloproliferative disorder and acute megakaryoblastic leukemia of Down syndrome. *Blood Cells Mol Dis, 31*(3), 351–356.

47. Hitzler, J. K., Cheung, J., Li, Y., et al. (2003). GATA1 mutations in transient leukemia and acute megakaryoblastic leukemia of Down syndrome. *Blood, 101*(11), 4301–4304.

48. Magalhaes, I. Q., Splendore, A., Emerenciano, M., et al. (2006). GATA1 mutations in acute leukemia in children with Down syndrome. *Cancer Genet Cytogenet, 166*(2), 112–116.

49. Xavier, A. C., Ge, Y., & Taub, J. W. (2009). Down syndrome and malignancies: a unique clinical relationship: a paper from the 2008 william beaumont hospital symposium on molecular pathology. *J Mol Diagn, 11*(5), 371–380.

50. Swerdlow, S. H., Campo, E., Harris, N. L., et al. (2008). *WHO Classification of Tumours of Haematopoietic and Lymphoid Tissues.* (4th ed.). Lyon, France: IARC Press.

51. Scott, C. S., Den Ottolander, G. J., Swirsky, D., et al. (1993). Recommended procedures for the classification of acute leukaemias. International Council for Standardization in Haematology (ICSH). *Leuk Lymphoma, 11*(1-2), 37–50.

52. Head, D. R. (1996). Revised classification of acute myeloid leukemia. *Leukemia, 10*(11), 1826–1831.

Myeloproliferative Neoplasms

Tim R. Randolph

OBJECTIVES

After completion of this chapter, the reader will be able to:

1. Define myeloproliferative neoplasms (MPNs), list the most common diseases included in the World Health Organization (WHO) classification of MPNs, and recognize their abbreviations.
2. Define chronic myeloid leukemia (CML) and describe the cell lines involved, the clinical phases, and the expected clinical manifestations, key peripheral blood and bone marrow findings, and diagnostic criteria applicable to each stage.
3. Discuss the cytogenetics, molecular genetics, and molecular pathophysiology of CML and relate it to treatment approaches, monitoring minimal residual disease, and mechanisms of drug resistance.
4. Define polycythemia vera (PV) and describe the cell lines involved, clinical manifestations, key peripheral blood and bone marrow findings, and the diagnostic criteria.
5. Discuss the *JAK2* mutation and the proposed pathogenic mechanism in PV.
6. Discuss the progression of PV and treatment modalities to include JAK inhibitors.
7. Define essential thrombocythemia (ET) and describe the cell lines involved, clinical manifestations, key

peripheral blood and bone marrow findings, and diagnostic criteria.
8. Discuss common mutations, pathophysiology, and two complications that may occur in patients with ET.
9. Define primary myelofibrosis (PMF) and describe the cell lines involved; clinical manifestations; key pathologic features in peripheral blood, bone marrow, and tissues; and diagnostic criteria.
10. Describe the mutations that occur in PMF and relate them to disease progression and current therapy.
11. Briefly discuss the potential interrelationships between the mutations and hypotheses for disease development and progression among between ET, PV, and PMF.
12. Briefly describe the other myeloproliferative disorders outlined in this chapter.
13. Given complete blood count and cytogenetic, molecular, and other laboratory results, recognize the findings consistent with each major MPN.
14. Recommend follow-up testing for suspected MPN and interpret the results of testing.

OUTLINE

Chronic Myeloid Leukemia
  Incidence
  Cytogenetics of the Philadelphia Chromosome
  Molecular Genetics
  Pathogenetic Mechanism
  Peripheral Blood and Bone Marrow
  Other Laboratory Findings
  Progression
  Related Diseases
  Treatment
Polycythemia Vera
  Incidence
  Pathogenic Mechanism
  Diagnosis
  Peripheral Blood and Bone Marrow
  Clinical Presentation
  Treatment and Prognosis

Essential Thrombocythemia
  Incidence
  Pathogenic Mechanism
  Clinical Presentation
  Diagnosis
  Peripheral Blood and Bone Marrow
  Treatment and Prognosis
Primary Myelofibrosis
  Myelofibrosis
  Hematopoiesis and Extramedullary Hematopoiesis
  Pathogenic Mechanism
  Incidence and Clinical Presentation
  Peripheral Blood and Bone Marrow
  Immune Response
  Treatment and Prognosis
Summary of Current Therapy of Non-*BCR-ABL1*, Primary MPNs

Interconnection among Essential Thrombocythemia, Polycythemia Vera, and Primary Myelofibrosis
Other Myeloproliferative Neoplasms
  Chronic Neutrophilic Leukemia
  Chronic Eosinophilic Leukemia, Not Otherwise Specified

Myeloid/Lymphoid Neoplasms with Eosinophilia and
  Rearrangement of *PDGFRA*, *PDGFRB*, or *FGFR1*
  or with *PCM1-JAK2*
Mastocytosis
Myeloproliferative Neoplasm, Unclassifiable

CASE STUDY

After studying the material in this chapter, the reader should be able to respond to the following case study:

A 34-year-old woman came to the physician with a 2-month history of increasing weakness, persistent nonproductive cough, fever and chills accompanied by night sweats, and a 13-pound weight loss over a 6-month period. Results of chest radiographs and purified protein derivative test (for tuberculosis) were negative. The patient was treated with ciprofloxacin and her cough improved, but she continued to grow weaker and was able to consume only small quantities of food. The patient appeared pale and cachectic. Tenderness and fullness were present in the left upper quadrant, and the spleen was palpable below the umbilicus. No hepatomegaly or peripheral adenopathy was noted. Her laboratory results were as follows:

White blood cells (WBCs)	248×10^9/L
Hemoglobin (HGB)	9.5 g/dL
Hematocrit (HCT)	26.3%
Platelets	449×10^9/L
Segmented neutrophils	44%
Band neutrophils	4%
Lymphocytes	10%
Eosinophils	3%

Basophils	7%
Myelocytes	30%
Promyelocytes	1%
Myeloblasts	1%
Nucleated red blood cells	2 per 100 WBCs
Reticulocytes	3%
Leukocyte alkaline phosphatase (LAP) score	20 (reference interval, 40–130)
Lactate dehydrogenase	692 IU (reference interval, 140–280 IU)
Uric acid	8.1 mg/dL (reference interval, 4–6 mg/dL)

1. What is the significance of the elevated WBC count and abnormal WBC differential?
2. How does the LAP score aid in the diagnosis?
3. Justify the use of cytogenetic studies in a patient with test results similar to those in this case study.
4. Predict the results of the cytogenetic studies.
5. Describe the molecular mutation resulting from the cytogenetic abnormality.
6. What is the usual treatment for this disorder?
7. Briefly discuss mechanisms of drug resistance.

The myeloproliferative neoplasms (MPNs) are clonal hematopoietic disorders caused by genetic mutations in the hematopoietic stem cells (HSCs) that result in expansion, excessive production, and accumulation of mature erythrocytes, granulocytes, and platelets. Each MPN is characterized by the clonal expansion of one or more myeloid cell lines, but one cell line dominates. The MPNs have the propensity to transform into other MPNs or progress into acute leukemias (ALs). Myeloproliferation largely is due to hypersensitivity or independence of normal cytokine regulation resulting from genetic mutations that reduces cytokine levels through negative feedback systems normally induced by mature cells.[1,2] Further evidence suggests that the fate of HSCs and hematopoietic progenitor cells (HPCs) in the MPNs is partially controlled by their interaction with the bone marrow (BM) stroma and the BM microenvironment, including adhesion molecules, chemokines, chemokine receptors, and both soluble and membrane-bound factor receptors.[3] In addition, evidence suggests that the three *BCR-ABL1* negative primary MPNs may be preceded by or coexist with chronic inflammation, which may predispose to the development of other cancers.[4,5]

Cellular expansion occurs in varying combinations in the bone marrow, peripheral blood, and tissues. MPNs are predominantly chronic with accelerated, subacute, or acute phases. In certain patients it is difficult to make a clear delineation between subacute and chronic phases using clinical and morphologic findings. As originally described by Damasek in 1951, the MPNs have pathogenetic similarities, as well as common clinical and laboratory features resulting in the classification of MPNs.[6]

The World Health Organization (WHO) has classified the MPNs into four predominant disorders: chronic myeloid leukemia (CML); polycythemia vera (PV), also known as *polycythemia rubra vera*; essential (primary) thrombocythemia (ET); and primary myelofibrosis (PMF), formerly known as *agnogenic myelofibrosis with myeloid metaplasia* and *chronic idiopathic myelofibrosis*. Several other less common MPN conditions have been described and are classified as chronic neutrophilic leukemia (CNL); chronic eosinophilic leukemia, not otherwise specified (CEL-NOS); and MPN, unclassified (MPN-U). PMF is further subdivided into PMF, prefibrotic/early stage and PMF, overt fibrotic stage.[7] ET, PV, and PMF are genetically related based on the presence of the Janus kinase 2 (*JAK2*) mutation in most cases and the absence of the Philadelphia chromosome (Ph) or *BCR-ABL1* fusion gene in all cases. Each of these three MPNs present with proliferation of one primary myeloid element: thrombocytosis in ET; erythrocytosis in PV; and neutrophilia, a left shift, and eventual fibrosis in PMF. ET and PV are very closely related because they share several driver mutations. PMF is a combination of overproduction of hematopoietic cells and stimulation of fibroblast production leading to ineffective hematopoiesis with resultant peripheral blood cytopenias. CML is characterized by neutrophilia, a significant left shift to include all stages of myeloid development, and the presence of the Ph translocation and/or the *BCR-ABL1* fusion gene. The critical changes from the original French-American-British (FAB) classification to the WHO classification system for the MPNs include the following: (1) Ph and/or the *BCR-ABL1* fusion gene is required for a diagnosis of CML; (2) minimum BM blast count threshold to differentiate MPNs from ALs is reduced from 30% to 20%; and (3) eosinophil disorders have been reclassified. Ph- and *BCR-ABL1*-negative cases with myelodysplastic and myeloproliferative features are included in the WHO myelodysplastic syndrome (MDS)/MPN group and called *atypical CML (aCML)*. In the category of MPNs, few changes were made from the 2008 to the 2016 classification system. The major changes include integration of new mutations to distinguish subtypes, some distinct morphologic features, and the elimination of mastocytosis as a MPN subgroup.[7]

MPNs present as stable chronic disorders that may transform first to a subacute and then to an aggressive cellular growth phase, such as acute myeloid leukemia (AML) or acute lymphoblastic leukemia (ALL). They may manifest a depleted cellular phase, such as BM hypoplasia, or exhibit clinical symptoms and morphologic patterns characteristic of subacute disease followed by a more aggressive cellular expression. Familial MPNs have been described in families in which two or more members are affected.[8]

CHRONIC MYELOID LEUKEMIA

CML is an MPN arising from a single genetic translocation in a pluripotential HSC producing a clonal overproduction of the myeloid cell line, resulting in a preponderance of immature cells in the neutrophilic line. CML begins with a chronic clinical phase and, if untreated, progresses to an accelerated phase in 3 to 4 years and often terminates as an AL (blast crisis phase). Progression to AL can be of the myeloid type (AML) or the lymphoid type (ALL). The clinical features are frequent infection, anemia, bleeding, and splenomegaly, all secondary to massive pathologic accumulation of myeloid progenitor cells in bone marrow, peripheral blood, and extramedullary tissues. Neutrophilia with all maturational stages present, basophilia, eosinophilia, and often thrombocytosis are noted in peripheral blood. The clonal origin of hematopoietic cells in CML has been verified in studies of females heterozygous for glucose-6-phosphate dehydrogenase. Only one isoenzyme is active in affected cells, whereas two isoenzymes are active in nonaffected cells.[9]

Incidence

CML occurs at all ages but is seen predominantly in those aged 46 to 53 years. It represents about 20% of all cases of leukemia, is slightly more common in men than in women, and carried a mortality rate of 1.5 per 100,000 per year in the era before the development of imatinib mesylate. Imatinib is a tyrosine kinase inhibitor that has changed the prognosis and treatment for CML and is described in detail later.

Symptoms associated with clinical onset are usually of minimal intensity and include fatigue, decreased tolerance of exertion, anorexia, abdominal discomfort, weight loss, and symptomatic effects from splenic enlargement.

Cytogenetics of the Philadelphia Chromosome

A unique chromosome, the Philadelphia chromosome, is present in proliferating HSCs and their progeny in CML and must be identified to confirm the diagnosis. Although the cause of Ph formation is unknown, it appears more often in populations exposed to ionizing radiation.[10,11] In most patients a cause cannot be identified. Appearance of Ph in donor cells after allogeneic BM transplantation indicates the possibility of a transmissible agent.[12] Ph was first identified as a short chromosome 22 in 1960 by Nowell and Hungerford in Philadelphia.[13] In 1973 Rowley, of the University of Illinois at Chicago, discovered that Ph is a reciprocal translocation between the long arms of chromosomes 9 and 22 (Chapter 30).[14] This acquired somatic mutation specifically reflects the translocation of an *ABL1* proto-oncogene from band q34 of chromosome 9 to the breakpoint cluster region (BCR) of band q11 of chromosome 22, resulting in a unique chimeric gene, *BCR-ABL1*.[15] This new gene produces a 210-kD BCR-ABL1 fusion protein (p210BCR-ABL1) that expresses enhanced tyrosine kinase activity from the ABL1 moiety compared with its natural enzymatic counterpart.

Molecular Genetics

The t(9;22) translocation that produces the *BCR-ABL1* chimeric gene has been identified in four primary molecular forms that produce three versions of the BCR-ABL1 chimeric protein: p190, p210, and p230 (Figure 32.1). The four genetic variations are based on the area of the *BCR* gene that houses the breakpoint on chromosome 22, because the breakpoint on chromosome 9 occurs in the same location. The wild-type (normal) *ABL1* gene on chromosome 9 is a relatively large gene of approximately 230 kilobases (kb) containing 11 exons. The breakpoint consistently occurs 5′ of the second exon such that exons 2 to 11 are contributed to the *BCR-ABL1* fusion gene.[15]

There are four *BCR* genes in the human genome: *BCR1*, *BCR2*, *BCR3*, and *BCR4*. It is the *BCR1* gene that is involved in the Philadelphia translocation. The wild-type (normal) *BCR1* gene is approximately 100 kb with 20 exons. In 1984 Groffen and colleagues identified the BCR on chromosome 22 as a 5-exon region involving exons 12 to 16 that was the area of breakage in the traditional t(9;22) translocation.[16] This area was later termed the *major BCR*. Two other areas of breakage were identified on chromosome 22, one near the 5′ (head) of the *BCR1* gene, called the *minor BCR*, and one in the 3′ end (tail) of the *BCR1* gene, termed the *micro BCR*. Therefore two areas of breakage in the major BCR, one breakpoint area in the minor BCR, and one breakpoint region in the micro BCR produce four versions of the *BCR* gene that combine with exons 2 to 11 of the *ABL1* gene to form four versions of the *BCR-ABL1* chimeric gene.

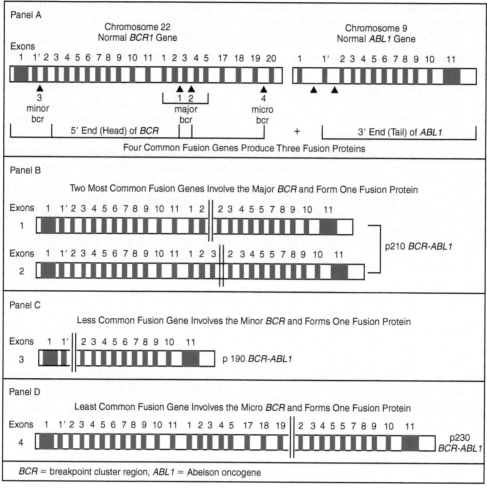

Figure 32.1 Molecular Biology of the *BCR-ABL1* Fusion Gene. **(A),** Normal *BCR1* gene on chromosome 22 and *ABL1* gene on chromosome 9. **(B),** Two *BCR* fusion gene products from the major *BCR*. **(C),** Fusion gene product from the minor *BCR*. **(D),** Fusion gene product from the micro *BCR*.

Within the major BCR, two specific breakpoints account for the t(9;22) translocation involved in the development of CML. Breakage in the *BCR1* gene in the major BCR contributes exons 1 to 13 or 1 to 14, whereas the *ABL1* gene contributes exons 2 to 11. Because the two breakpoints in the major BCR differ by only one exon, the chimeric protein product is essentially the same size and is designated as the p210 protein. Breakage in the minor BCR contributes only exon one from *BCR1*, which joins with the same exons 2 to 11 of *ABL1* to produce a p190 protein. The micro BCR breakpoint contributes exons 2 to 19 from *BCR1*, which fuse with *ABL1* exons 2 to 11, producing the p230 protein. Therefore the four possible *BCR1* breakpoints produce four different chimeric genes, resulting in a total of three different protein products.[17]

Pathogenetic Mechanism

To understand the aberrant function of the *BCR-ABL1* fusion protein, it is first helpful to understand both the normal BCR and ABL1 proteins. The wild-type ABL1 protein, when in its usual location on chromosome 9, codes for p125, which exhibits normal tyrosine kinase activity. The *BCR1* gene produces p160, expresses serine and threonine kinase activity, and is thought to function in the regulation of cell growth. Protein kinases are enzymes that catalyze the transfer of phosphate groups from adenosine triphosphate (ATP), guanosine triphosphate (GTP), and other phosphate donors to receiver proteins. A tyrosine kinase transfers the phosphate group to a tyrosine amino acid on the receiver protein. For the kinase activity of the ABL1 protein to occur, the ABL1 protein must first be phosphorylated. This is often accomplished through autophosphorylation. The ABL1 protein has three primary domains called *SH1, SH2,* and *SH3* that together express and regulate the kinase activity. SH1 is the binding site for ATP; SH2 is the docking point for phosphate receiver proteins; and SH3 is the domain that controls the phosphorylation activity. When ATP binds to the ATP binding site, the phosphate is transferred to the SH2 region of the ABL protein, which initiates a conformational change that alters the tertiary structure of the protein and exposes the active site of the kinase enzyme. When a second ATP binds the ATP binding site and a receiver protein docks in the SH2 domain, the phosphate group is transferred to the receiver protein. In most

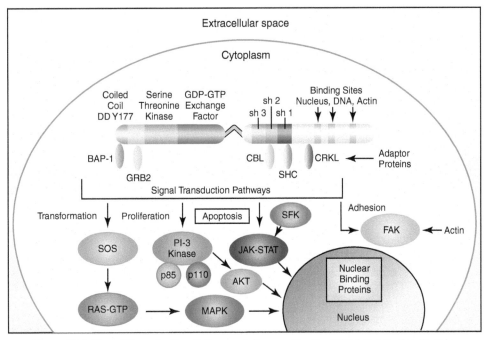

Figure 32.2 Signal Transduction Pathways Influenced by the BCR-ABL1 Fusion Protein.

physiologically normal intracellular pathways, protein phosphorylation activates the receiver proteins (Figure 32.2). This phosphorylation initiates a cascade of phosphorylation events, each activating the next protein until a transcription factor becomes activated. These activation cascades, called *signal transduction pathways*, are designed to activate genes necessary to control cell proliferation, differentiation, and natural cell death, called *apoptosis*. There are several signal transduction pathways activated by the ABL1 tyrosine kinase that function in concert to activate these genes in a precise order and at the required level of activation to control these cellular events.[17,18]

In the case of CML, the *BCR-ABL1* translocation occurs next to the SH3 domain of the *ABL1* moiety, which is designed to control the rate and timing of phosphorylation. Therefore the BCR-ABL1 tyrosine kinase loses the ability to shut off kinase activity and is said to have constitutive tyrosine kinase activity. The BCR-ABL1 enzyme continuously adds phosphate groups to tyrosine residues on cytoplasmic proteins, activating several signal transduction pathways. These pathways stimulate gene expression, keeping the myeloid cells proliferating, reducing differentiation, reducing adhesion of cells to BM stroma, and virtually eliminating apoptosis. The result is increased clonal proliferation of myeloid cells secondary to a reduction in or loss of sensitivity to protein regulators.[19] There is an increase in growth factor–independent cellular proliferation from activation of the *RAS* gene and a decrease in or resistance to apoptosis. New clones of stem cells vulnerable to additional genetic changes lead to the accelerated and blast phases of CML. In addition, the BCR-ABL1 protein localizes in the cytoplasm rather than in the nucleus, as does the normal ABL1 protein. The mutation affects maturation and differentiation of

hematopoietic and lymphopoietic cells, whose progeny eventually dominates in the affected individual. Progeny cells that exhibit this chromosome include neutrophils, eosinophils, basophils, monocytes, nucleated erythrocytes, megakaryocytes, and B lymphocytes.[18-20]

In addition, the loss of genetic segments in the 5′ end of the *ABL1* gene results in an altered protein-binding affinity for F-actin, which leads to a reduction in contact binding of hematopoietic CML cells to stromal cells, causing premature release of cells into the circulation.[21] Abnormal adhesion between stem cells and stroma may dysregulate hematopoiesis. One action of interferon-α therapy is to reverse the loss of adhesion of CML progenitor cells, which reduces the premature release of these cells into the circulation.[20]

Apoptotic functions are lost because the BCR-ABL1 fusion protein has a propensity to be sequestered in the cytoplasm, which has antiapoptotic functions. The p210 is necessary for CML transformation of the HSC.

The *BCR-ABL1* fusion gene is also identified with Philadelphia chromosome-positive ALL. The chromosome appears in 20% of adults and 2% to 5% of children with this disease. The minor chimeric *BCR-ABL1* gene that transcribes and translates to a p185/p190 protein is present in 50% of Philadelphia chromosome-positive ALL cases in adults and 75% of Philadelphia chromosome-positive ALL cases in children. The micro *BCR*, when fused with the *ABL1* gene, produces a large p230 protein that is associated with CNL and is the least common version found.

Peripheral Blood and Bone Marrow

There are dramatic morphologic changes in the peripheral blood and BM that reflect the expansion of the granulocyte

TABLE 32.1   Common Morphologic Changes in Chronic Myeloid Leukemia

Peripheral Blood

Erythrocytes	Normal or decreased
Reticulocytes	Normal
Nucleated red blood cells	Present
Total white blood cells	Increased
Lymphocytes	Normal or increased
Neutrophils	Increased
Basophils	Increased
Eosinophils	Increased
Myelocytes	Increased
Leukocyte alkaline phosphatase	Decreased
Platelets	Normal or increased

Bone Marrow

Cellularity	Increased
Granulopoiesis	Increased
Erythropoiesis	Decreased
Megakaryopoiesis	Increased or normal
Reticulin	Increased

Macrophages

Gaucher-like	Sea blue
Green-gray crystals	Increased

Megakaryocytes

Small	Increased

Extramedullary Tissue

Splenomegaly	Present
Sinusoidal	Present
Medullary	Present
Hepatomegaly	Present
Sinusoidal	Present
Portal tract	Present
Local infiltrates	Present

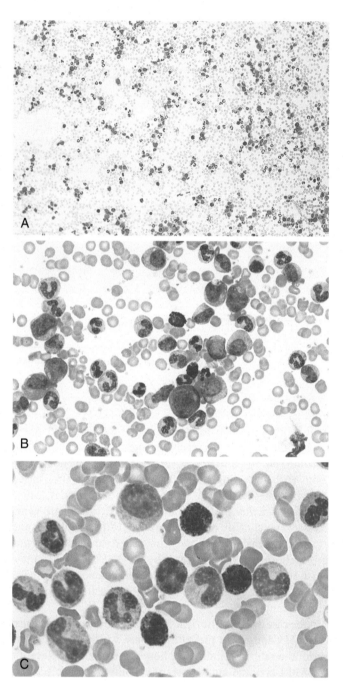

Figure 32.3 Peripheral Blood Films from a Patient in the Chronic Phase Chronic Myeloid Leukemia. (A), Leukocytosis is evident at scanning power (Wright-Giemsa stain, ×100.) **(B),** Bimodal population of segmented neutrophils and myelocytes (Wright-Giemsa stain, ×500.) **(C),** Increased basophils and immature neutrophils (Wright-Giemsa stain, ×1000.)

pool, particularly in the later maturational stages. Table 32.1 lists the qualitative changes in the peripheral blood, bone marrow, and extramedullary tissues that are commonly observed at the time of diagnosis. A dramatic left shift is noted that extends down to the promyelocyte stage and occasionally even produces a few blasts in the peripheral blood. The platelet count is often elevated, reflecting the myeloproliferative nature of the disease. Extramedullary granulopoiesis may involve sinusoids and medullary cords in the spleen and sinusoids, portal tract zones, and solid areas of the liver.

Figure 32.3 illustrates a common pattern in the peripheral blood film of chronic phase CML at the time of diagnosis. Leukocytosis is readily apparent at scanning microscopic powers. Segmented neutrophils, bands, metamyelocytes, and myelocytes predominate, and immature and mature eosinophils and basophils are increased. Myeloblasts and promyelocytes are present at a rate of approximately 1% and 5%, respectively. Lymphocytes and monocytes are present and often show an absolute increase in number but a relative decrease in percentage.

Nucleated red blood cells (NRBCs) are rare. Platelets are normal or increased, and some may exhibit abnormal morphology.

BM changes are illustrated in Figure 32.4. An intense hypercellularity is present as a result of granulopoiesis, marked by broad zones of immature granulocytes, usually perivascular or periosteal, differentiating into more centrally placed mature granulocytes. Normoblasts appear reduced in number. Megakaryocytes are normal or increased in number and, when increased, may appear in clusters and exhibit dyspoietic cytologic

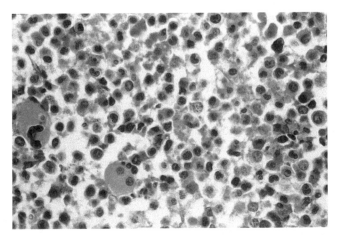

Figure 32.4 Bone Marrow Biopsy Specimen from a Patient in the Chronic Phase of Chronic Myeloid Leukemia. Note the hypercellularity with increased granulocytes and megakaryocytes. (Hematoxylin and eosin stain, ×400.)

changes. They often appear small with reduced nuclear size (by approximately 20%) and reduced nuclear lobulations. Reticulin fibers are increased in approximately 20% of patients. Increased megakaryocyte density is associated with an increase in myelofibrosis.[22] The presence of pseudo-Gaucher cells (Chapter 26) usually occurs.

Other Laboratory Findings

Hyperuricemia and uricosuria from increased cell turnover may be associated with secondary gout, urinary uric acid stones, and uric acid nephropathy. Approximately 15% of patients exhibit total white blood cell (WBC) counts greater than 300×10^9/L.[23] Symptoms in these patients are secondary to vascular stasis and possible intravascular consumption of oxygen by the leukocytes. Symptoms are reversible with the lowering of the total WBC count.[24]

In patients with typical peripheral blood findings discussed earlier, diagnosis of CML is confirmed by demonstrating the presence of the t(9;22) translocation by cytogenetic analysis (Figure 30.1), detection of the *BCR-ABL1* fusion gene using fluorescence in situ hybridization (Figures 30.2 and 30.21), and/or detecting the BCR-ABL1 fusion transcript by qualitative reverse transcriptase polymerase chain reaction (Figure 29.12).

Although molecular techniques are more commonly used to diagnose CML, initial testing of the cells for leukocyte alkaline phosphatase (LAP) enzyme activity may be useful in some setting for preliminary differentiation of CML from a leukemoid reaction caused by severe infection (Chapter 26).

LAP is an enzyme found in the membranes of secondary granules of neutrophils. To perform the LAP a blood film is incubated with a naphthol-phosphate substrate and diazo dye at an alkaline pH. The LAP enzyme hydrolyzes the substrate, and the liberated naphthol reacts with the dye, producing a colored precipitate on the granules. The slide is examined microscopically and 100 segmented neutrophils and bands are counted and rated from 0 to 4+ based on the intensity of the

staining. The LAP score is calculated by multiplying each score by the number of cells, and adding the products. For example, 5 cells with 4+ staining, 5 cells with 3+, 25 cells with 2+, 45 cells with 1+, and 20 cells with 0 staining calculates to a LAP score of 130. Because scoring is subjective, the mean score of two examiners is reported, and they should agree within 10%.

A sample reference interval for the LAP score is 15 to 170, but every laboratory establishes its own. The LAP score is decreased in untreated CML, and normal or increased in leukemoid reactions. Individuals with PV or those in the third trimester of pregnancy can also have higher LAP scores.

Progression

In the preimatinib era, most cases of this disease would eventually transform into AL.[25] Before blastic transformation, some patients proceed through an intermediate *metamorphosis* or *accelerated* phase. Disease progression is accompanied by an increase in the frequency and number of clinical symptoms, adverse changes in laboratory values, and poorer response to therapy than in the chronic phase. Additional chromosome abnormalities reflect evolution of the malignant clone and may appear associated with enhanced dyshematopoietic cell maturation patterns and increases in morphologic and functional abnormalities in blood cells. There is often an increasing degree of anemia and, in the peripheral blood, fewer mature leukocytes, more basophils, and fewer platelets, with a greater proportion of abnormal platelets, micromegakaryocytes, and megakaryocytic fragments. The circulating blast count increases to 10% to 19%. This total blast percentage, or a combination of 20% blasts and promyelocytes, has been proposed as a diagnostic criterion for the accelerated phase.[26]

Blast crisis involves the peripheral blood, bone marrow, and extramedullary tissues. Based on AL definitions, blasts constitute more than 20% of total BM cellularity, and the peripheral blood exhibits increased blasts. Blast crisis leukemia usually is AML or ALL, but origins from other hematopoietic clonal cells are possible. Extramedullary growth may occur as lymphocytic or myeloid cell proliferations; the latter are often referred to as *granulocytic sarcoma*. Extramedullary sarcoma is observed at many sites or locations in the body and may precede a marrow blast crisis. The clinical symptoms of blast crisis mimic those of AL, including severe anemia, leukopenia of all WBCs except blasts, and thrombocytopenia. Chromosome abnormalities such as additional Philadelphia chromosomes, isochromosome 17, trisomy 8, loss of Y chromosome, and trisomy 19 accumulate with disease progression.[27,28] These generally occurred in approximately 75% of patients in the preimatinib era.

Related Diseases

Several diseases exist that are clinically similar to CML but do not exhibit the Philadelphia chromosome and express only a few pseudo-Gaucher cells. CNL is another MPN that manifests with peripheral blood, bone marrow, and extramedullary infiltrative patterns similar to those of CML, except that only neutrophilic granulocytes are present and fewer than 10% of peripheral blood neutrophils are immature.[29] Similarly, chronic monocytic leukemia involves a comparable expansion of monocytes, including functional monocytes.[30]

Juvenile myelomonocytic leukemia and adult chronic myelomonocytic leukemia are classified by the WHO as myelodysplastic/myeloproliferative diseases because of the overlap in clinical, laboratory, or morphologic findings. Juvenile myelomonocytic leukemia occurs in children younger than 4 years of age and is accompanied by an expansion in the number of monocytes and granulocytes, including immature granulocytes, and manifestations of dyserythropoiesis.[31]

Ph is sometimes found in patients with AML and ALL. It is understood that some of these cases likely represent undiagnosed CML that rapidly progressed to an AL before diagnosis. However, because rapidly dividing malignant cells are more prone to genetic mutation, the presence of Ph in ALs may reflect a late-stage mutation that contributed little to AL leukemogenesis.

Treatment

Early treatment approaches for CML were unable to produce remission, so the goal of therapy became the reduction of tumor burden. The first forms of therapy for CML included alkylating agents such as nitrogen mustard,[32] introduced in the late 1940s, and busulfan,[33] which came into use in the early 1950s. Later, busulfan in combination with 6-thioguanine was used to achieve the goal of tumor burden reduction. Other drugs like hydroxyurea and 6-mercaptopurine were introduced later and found to improve patient survival. The discovery of interferon-α in 1983 dramatically improved outcomes of patients with CML by inducing the suppression of the Philadelphia chromosome, reducing the rate of cellular progression to blast cells, and increasing the frequency of long-term patient survival especially when combined with cytarabine.[34,35] Using former cytoreductive treatment approaches, most patients would experience disease progression and eventually succumb to their disease.

BM and stem cell transplantation with either autologous or allogeneic HSCs have been reported as curative, especially in patients younger than age 55. Relapses occur, but long-term, disease-free survival is possible. Optimal survival occurs when the patient is treated during the chronic phase within 1 year of diagnosis and is younger than age 50. Treatment requires ablative chemotherapy followed by transplantation of mobilized normal progenitor cells that exhibit CD34+ surface markers. Allogeneic BM transplants are more successful in patients up to age 55 when donors are matched for HLA antigens A, B, and DR. Donor-matched lymphocyte infusions after allogeneic transplantation of marrow from a sibling donor may assist in producing complete remissions.[36]

Current therapies involve the use of synthetic proteins that bind the abnormal BCR-ABL1 protein, blocking the constitutive tyrosine kinase activity and reducing signal transduction activation. Imatinib mesylate was the first synthetic tyrosine kinase inhibitor designed to selectively bind the ATP binding site and thus inhibit the tyrosine kinase activity of the BCR-ABL1 fusion protein. When imatinib binds the ATP binding site, ATP is unable to bind to provide the phosphate group necessary for kinase activity. Imatinib binds the BCR-ABL1 protein in the inactive conformation, which precedes the autophosphorylation necessary to generate the kinase active site (Figure 32.5).[37] Imatinib has also been shown to bind the ATP binding site of other tyrosine kinases, including TEL/ABL1, stem cell factor receptor (a-KIT, b-KIT, c-KIT), and platelet-derived growth factor receptor (PDGFR), lymphocyte-specific kinase (Lck), vascular endothelial growth factor receptor-1 (VEGFR-1), VEGFR-2, VEGFR-3, colony-stimulating factor receptor-1 (CSFR-1), nicotinamide adenine dinucleotide phosphate (NAD[P]H) dehydrogenase, quinone 2 (NQ02), and c-Raf in most tissues. Therefore imatinib may be a useful treatment option in other conditions but it raises questions about clinical efficacy and toxicity.[38]

Goals of therapy include complete hematologic, cytogenetic, and molecular remission as indicated by a normalized complete blood count (CBC) and differential, absence of Ph by karyotype analysis, and absence of measurable BCR-ABL1 transcripts, respectively. Complete remission from imatinib therapy is induced in part by the reactivation of apoptotic pathways.[39] The effectiveness of imatinib therapy and stem cell transplantation is best monitored by measuring BCR-ABL1 transcripts using quantitative real-time reverse transcriptase polymerase chain reaction (RT-PCR). These monitoring tools are used to determine the extent of molecular remission. The most sensitive measure of the effectiveness of imatinib therapy is the number of log reductions of BCR-ABL1 transcripts using real-time RT-PCR.[40] Remission milestones indicating effective imatinib therapy are complete hematologic remission in 3 to 6 months, complete cytogenetic response in 6 months to 1 year, and a 2- to 3-log reduction in BCR-ABL1 transcripts. When real-time RT-PCR is used, the greatest log reduction possible is a more than 4 log reduction, which represents the maximum sensitivity of the assay. However, discontinuation of imatinib therapy in patients who achieve a more than 4-log reduction usually results in relapse.

Although imatinib has proven to be a successful form of therapy, a major limitation is the development of imatinib resistance resulting in relapse. Approximately 25% to 30% of patients with newly diagnosed CML will discontinue imatinib therapy within 5 years because of lack of remission, resistance, or toxicity.[41] The two major categories of imatinib resistance are primary and secondary. Primary resistance is defined as the inability to reach the remission milestones. This form of resistance accounts for most treatment failures and probably results from the presence of mutations other than the BCR-ABL1 mutation at the time of diagnosis. Secondary resistance involves the loss of a previous response and occurs at a rate of 16% at 42 months. The majority of cases of imatinib resistance result from two primary causes: acquisition of additional BCR-ABL1 mutations and expression of point mutations in the ATP binding site. Additional BCR-ABL1 mutations can occur through the usual translocation of the remaining unaffected chromosomes 9 and 22, which converts the HSC from heterozygous to homozygous for the BCR-ABL1 mutation. A double

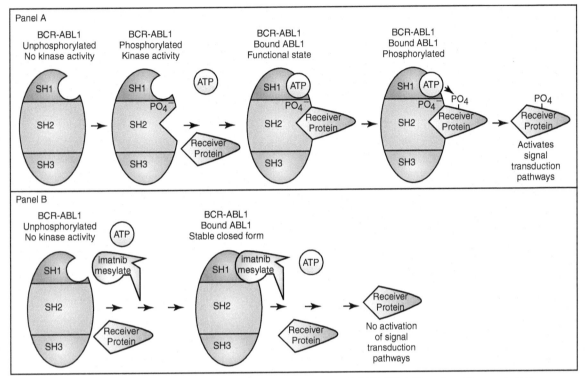

Figure 32.5 Mechanism of Imatinib Mesylate Inhibition of BCR-ABL1 Tyrosine Kinase Activity. **(A),** Mechanism of tyrosine kinase activity of the BCR-ABL1 fusion protein. **(B),** Mechanism of tyrosine kinase inhibition by imatinib mesylate. *ATP,* Adenosine triphosphate.

dose of *BCR-ABL1* can also be acquired from gene duplication during mitosis and accounts for 10% of secondary mutations. An additional *BCR-ABL1* mutation will double the tyrosine kinase activity, making the imatinib dosage inadequate. In these cases higher doses of imatinib will restore remission in most patients (Figure 32.6). The majority of patients who do not respond to higher doses of imatinib express point mutations in the ATP binding site. More than 60 mutations have been identified in the ATP binding site, and these account for the remaining 50% to 90% of secondary mutations. Mutations in the ATP binding site reduce the binding affinity of imatinib, producing some level of resistance (Figure 32.7). Three second-generation tyrosine kinase inhibitors—dasatinib, nilotinib and bosutinib—overcome the ATP binding site mutations because they have a much higher binding affinity than imatinib.[41-43]

Dasatinib binds the ABL1 portion of the BCR-ABL1 protein with an affinity of imatinib and it binds both the active and inactive conformations. Dasatinib also inhibits SRC family kinases (SFK), c-kit, PDGFR, and epherin A receptor kinase.[38] It is effective against all imatinib resistant mutants currently identified except the T315I mutation. Dasatinib can be used as first-line therapy and to rescue patients resistant to imatinib therapy unless the T315I mutation has been identified.

Nilotinib binds to the ATP binding site of the ABL1 protein in the inactive conformation with 30 times greater potency than imatinib. Structurally, nilotinib is a derivative of imatinib and binds more specifically than imatinib to ABL1, stabilizing the

ABL1 protein. Nilotinib also binds PDGFR and kit family kinases.[38] Like dasatinib, nilotinib can be used as first-line therapy and to rescue patients with imatinib resistance against all mutants currently identified except the T315I mutation.

Bosutinib binds both the active and inactive conformations of ABL1 and is 10 times more potent than imatinib. It inhibits ABL1 and SRC kinases, fibroblast growth factor receptor (FGFR), and mitogen-activated protein kinase (MAPK) but does not significantly inhibit PDGFR or c-kit. Like dasatinib and nilotinib it is effective against most imatinib-resistant mutants except the T315I mutation, showing a complete hematologic response in 83% and a complete cytogenetic response in 23% of imatinib- and dasatinib-resistant patients. Because the T315I mutation is not treatable by any of the first- and second-generation tyrosine kinase inhibitors (TKIs), other non-TKI therapies have also been developed. Preliminary results suggest that second-generation TKIs may prove to be a superior first-line therapy for new CML patients than inatinib.[38]

All three second-generation TKIs are approved by the US Food and Drug Administration for first-line therapy and are effective at rescuing patients resistant to imatinib, except patients (about 15%) who have developed the T315I mutation. The T315I mutation places a large, bulky isoleucine residue in the center of the ATP binding site, and all four FDA-approved tyrosine kinase inhibitors are resistant to this mutation. However, a third-generation tyrosine kinase inhibitor, ponatinib, inhibits the T315I mutation.[41-43]

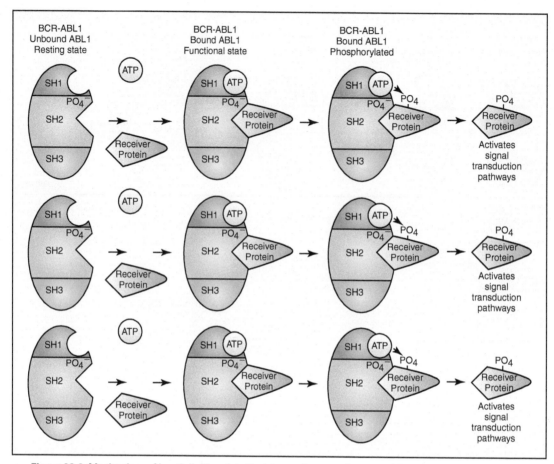

Figure 32.6 Mechanism of Imatinib Mesylate Resistance due to an Increased Copy Number of *BCR-ABL1* Genes. The increased copies produce more BCR-ABL1 fusion proteins, which results in an increased tyrosine kinase activity requiring a higher dosage of imatinib to restore remission. *ATP,* Adenosine triphosphate.

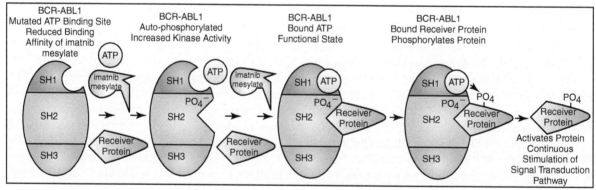

Figure 32.7 Mechanism of Imatinib Mesylate Resistance as a Result of Point Mutations in the Adenosine Triphosphate *(ATP)* Binding Site. The mutations reduce the binding affinity of imatinib, allowing ATP to bind; this restores the increased tyrosine kinase activity that drives the phenotype and pathogenesis of the disease.

Ponatinib was FDA approved in 2012 as a rescue therapy for patients resistant to imatinib, dasatinib, and nilotinib when administered as a 45-mg tablet taken once a day. In addition to inhibiting the T315I mutation, it can also inhibit a wide range of tyrosine kinases, including PDGFR, c-kit, SFK, FGFR, VEGFR-1, VEGFR-2, VEGFR-3, Flt-3, RET, and ARG.[38,44] The newest third-generation TKI in clinical trials is bafetinib.

Because all the first- and second-generation TKIs are ineffective against the T315I mutation, other non-TKI therapies have also been developed, some of which bind the A loop (receiver protein binding site), that will also inhibit tyrosine kinase activity and overcome the T315I mutation.[41-43]

Homoharringtonine was originally discovered and used for CML therapy before the development of TKIs. It was reintroduced as a supplemental therapy to TKIs to rescue patients who developed TKI resistance. Homoharringtonine is a plant alkaloid that induces apoptosis, inhibits protein synthesis and upregulates B cell chronic lymphocytic leukemia/lymphoma (BCL-2)-associated X protein (BAX) and caspase-mediated cleavage of poly (ADP) ribose polymerase (PARP).[38]

Omacetaxine is a semisynthetic derivative of homoharringtonine and was FDA approved as rescue therapy in 2012. It was designed for more efficient manufacturing compared with homoharringtonine. Omacetaxine is administered as 1.25 mg/m^2 subcutaneous injection twice daily for 14 days of a 28-day cycle for the induction phase and 1.25 mg/m^2 subcutaneous injection twice daily for 7 days of a 28-day cycle for maintenance. Omacetaxine has been shown to induce apoptosis but by downregulating myeloid cell leukemia sequence-1 (Mcl-1), which is *BAX* independent.[38]

The development of a care plan for treating patients with newly diagnosed CML is an ongoing commitment requiring not only the formulation of alternative approaches to achieve and maintain complete cellular remission but also the establishment of laboratory monitoring parameters to follow that confirm long-term success of therapy. Historically, chemotherapy has provided cellular remission but usually has not prevented clinical progression to accelerated or blast phases. BM transplantation is the preferred approach for curative treatment available for patients who qualify. However, the long-term success (cure) rate remains at 50% to 70%, and most patients will not qualify. For a patient to qualify for transplantation, the patient must be younger than 50 years of age, in the first year of the disease, have CML that is still in the chronic phase, and have an available histocompatible donor. For nearly 20 years, imatinib has been considered first-line therapy for all patients with newly diagnosed CML. For the small subset of patients who qualify for HSC transplantation, imatinib is used to induce hematologic remission before transplantation. For all other CML patients, imatinib has been used as first-line therapy unless remission is not achieved (primary resistance) or until relapse occurs after remission (secondary resistance). Once the cause of relapse has been determined by cytogenetic and molecular testing, either a higher dosage of imatinib can be given (for an additional *BCR-ABL1* mutation) or a second- or third-generation tyrosine kinase inhibitor (dasatinib, nilotinib, bosutinib) can be prescribed, unless the mutation is the T315I mutation in the ATP binding site. If the T315I mutation is detected, the patient can be given ponatinib or an A-loop inhibitor (ONO12380) or other drugs like omacetaxine, MK 0457, or BIRB-796 that inhibit the T315I mutation.[43] Physicians are beginning to prescribe dasatinib, nilotinib, and bosutinib as first-line therapy to replace imatinib in hopes that tyrosine kinase inhibitors with higher binding affinities will extend remissions by reducing the rate of mutation-induced relapses. Among the second-generation TKIs, bosutinib shows the most promise because it demonstrates high potency, has the ability to overcome most P-loop mutations (except T315I), and shows fewer side effects like neutropenia, thrombocytopenia, cardiotoxicity, and pancreatitis compared with nilotinib and dasatinib. Ponatinib and A-loop inhibitors can be used to rescue patients treated with second-generation tyrosine kinase inhibitors, particularly those who develop the T315I mutation.[41]

POLYCYTHEMIA VERA

PV is a neoplastic clonal MPN that commonly manifests with panmyelosis in the BM and increases in erythrocytes, granulocytes, and platelets in the peripheral blood.[2] Splenomegaly is common. The disease arises in a HSC and is clonal in nature.[45]

Incidence

The annual incidence of PV varies by country, with Japan reporting 2 cases per million, Australia and Europe 13 cases per million, and the United States averaging 8 to 10 cases per million. PV rarely occurs in children and occurs most often between the ages of 40 and 60 years, with a peak incidence after the age of 60 years. It occurs more often in men than women and more often in whites than blacks and is more common in people of Jewish descent.[46] A familial predisposition for PV may exist because it has been reported in several members of the same family.

Pathogenic Mechanism

In PV, neoplastic clonal stem cells are hypersensitive to, or function independently of, erythropoietin for cell growth. Trace levels of erythropoietin in serum stimulate the growth of erythroid progenitor cells in in vitro colony-forming growth systems. There is preservation of hypersensitive and normosensitive erythroid colony-forming units, however, which indicates some level of normal hematopoiesis.[47] Adverse clinical progression seems to correlate with the propagation of the erythropoietin-sensitive colony-forming units.[48]

Understanding of the pathologic mechanism explaining this phenomenon in PV was significantly advanced in 2005 with the discovery of a consistent mutation in the *JAK2* gene. The normal JAK2 protein is a tyrosine kinase enzyme much like the ABL1 moiety of the *BCR-ABL1* fusion gene found in CML. Normally the JAK2 protein is closely associated with cytokine receptors and functions near the cell membrane. When a cytokine receptor binds its ligand, the JAK2 protein becomes activated through transphosphorylation when bound to the cytoplasmic region of the receptor. Once activated, the kinase activity of JAK2 phosphorylates **s**ignal **t**ransducers and **a**ctivators of **t**ranscription (STAT) proteins, eventually generating transcription proteins that bind promotor regions and signal gene expression. The JAK-receptor complex also activates other signaling pathways.[49]

The normal JAK2 protein controls transphosphorylation through conformational inhibition. JAK2 has seven domains (JH1-JH7), but two domains (JH1 and JH2) control the kinase activity. JH1 has kinase activity and JH2 (pseudokinase) does not. Normally, JH2 folds and interacts with the JH1 domain to inhibit kinase activity and to modulate or regulate receptor signaling.[49] Mutations in the JH2 domain removes this inhibitory function.

The specific *JAK2* mutation, *JAK2* V617F, is detected in more than 95% of patients with PV and is found on chromosome band 9p24. Shortly after the *JAK2* V617F mutation was reported, several groups corroborated the finding using other approaches and reported that the mutation is acquired, clonal, present in the HSC, constitutively active, and capable of activating the erythropoietic signal transduction pathway in the absence of erythropoietin.[50,51] The point mutation replaces guanine with thymine at exon 14 of the gene, which changes the amino acid at position 617 from valine to phenylalanine in the pseudokinase domain. This one amino acid change prevents the inhibition conformation of the tyrosine kinase, causing it to remain in the active conformation. More specifically, the phenylalanine mutation in the kinase domain is unable to bind the corresponding amino acid in the pseudokinase domain, as can the valine in the wild-type counterpart, which prevents the protein from folding into the inactive conformation (Figure 32.8).[52,53]

Normally, erythropoietin is released from the kidney into the blood in response to hypoxia and binds to erythropoietin receptors on the surface of erythroid precursor cells. The resulting conformational change in the erythropoietin receptor causes two erythropoietin receptors to dimerize. This produces a docking point for the head of the inactive JAK2 protein at a domain on JAK2 known as FERM (Band-4.1, ezrin, radixin, and moesin). Docking of JAK2 stimulates a phosphorylation event, causing a conformational change, and the valine releases from the pseudokinase domain, converting it to an active tyrosine kinase. JAK2 can also bind to several other receptors, including myeloproliferative leukemia (MPL, also known as thrombopoietin receptor [TPO-R]), granulocyte colony-stimulating factor receptor (GCSF-R), prolactin receptor, growth hormone receptor, granulocyte-macrophage colony-stimulating factor receptor (GM-CSF-R), interleukin-3 receptor (IL-3-R), IL-5-R, and interferon-γ2 receptor (INF-γ2-R).[3] The diversity in ligand receptor binding of *JAK2* explains the range of myeloid proliferation observed in the MPNs in which the *JAK2* mutation is found: PV (erythroid), ET (thrombopoietic), and neutrophilic (PMF). Once activated, JAK2 phosphorylates several cytoplasmic proteins, but the

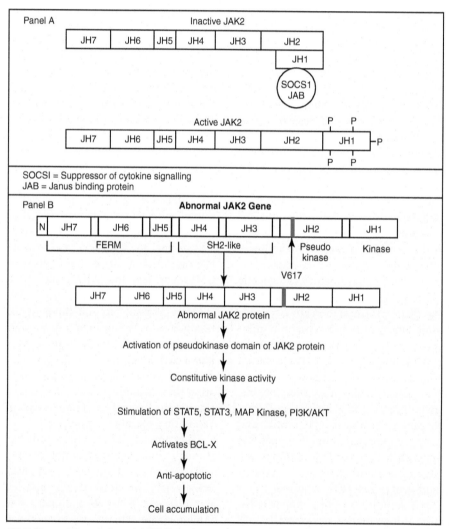

Figure 32.8 Normal Regulation of JAK2 Function and Loss of Regulation from the *JAK2* V617F Mutation. **(A),** Normal function of the JAK2 protein and regulation of phosphorylation by *JAK2* intrachain folding and the binding of JAK2 inhibitors SOCS1 and JAB proteins. **(B),** The *JAK2* V617F mutation and the loss of normal JAK2 folding and inhibitor binding resulting in phosphorylation, activation, and the stimulation of STAT, MAP kinase, and PI3K/AKT signal transduction pathways.

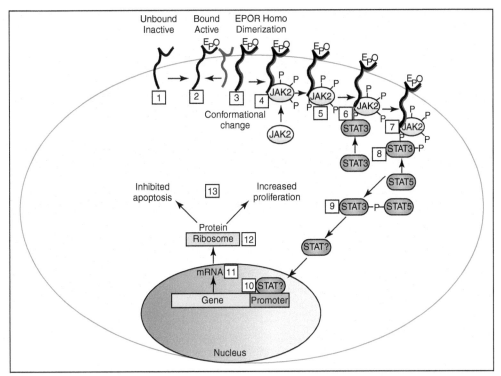

Figure 32.9 Normal Erythropoiesis Involving Erythropoietin Binding to Erythropoietin Receptors and Stimulation of the JAK-STAT Pathway via the Normal JAK2 Protein. The numbers in the figure represent the sequence of events in the signal transduction pathway.

STAT proteins are the main targets. A cascade of phosphorylation reactions through the STAT proteins produce activated transcription factors that activate a host of genes designed to drive and control cell proliferation and differentiation while also initiating apoptosis (Figure 32.9). Constitutive tyrosine kinase activity of the mutated JAK2 protein causes continuous activation of several signal transduction pathways that are normally activated after erythropoietin stimulation via the erythropoietic receptor. Mutated JAK2 is active and will phosphorylate STAT proteins in the absence of erythropoietin or will overphosphorylate in its presence (Figure 32.10). HSCs that bear the *JAK2* mutation are resistant to erythropoietin-deprivation apoptosis by upregulation of BCL-X, an antiapoptotic protein. PV progenitor cells do not divide more rapidly but accumulate because they do not die normally.[54-56] In addition to the role of mutated JAK2 in the abrogation of STAT signaling, it has also been shown to influence chromatin structure[57,58] and to decrease methyltransferase activity.[59] Lastly, it is unclear how the *JAK2* (V617F) mutation can result in three different conditions when it is found in nearly all patients with PV and in about half of patients with ET and PMF. Because most patients with ET are heterozygous for *JAK2*, whereas PV patients tend to be homozygous, it is possible that dosage effect of the *JAK2* mutation may play an important role in determining disease phenotype.[53] In addition, the suspicion of a pre-*JAK2* mutation in the MPNs negative for *JAK2* and the discovery of the mutated *MPL* suggest the following mutational sequence.[60]

- A pre-*JAK2* mutation produces a hyperproliferative clone with increased susceptibility to additional mutations. Either the *MPL* or *JAK2* mutation occurs, triggering the ET phenotype.

The *JAK2* mutation may produce preferential triggering of the MPL receptor over the ETO receptor because MPL receptors have a higher density on the HSC surface.

- When a second *JAK2* mutation occurs, sufficient JAK2 proteins exist to trigger the erythropoietin receptors (EPO-R), converting the disease phenotype to PV.
- Additional mutations evolve the phenotype to that of PMF, but thrombocytosis remains because of chemokines released in response to the fibrosis.

Because approximately 5% of PV patients do not possess the *JAK2* V617F mutation and because PV has a familial predisposition, it is thought that other mutations must be involved in the pathogenesis of PV and some must precede and possibly predispose the *JAK2* V617F mutation. Since the original discovery of a mutation in the thrombopoietic receptor gene *MPL* in 2006,[61] several gain-of-function mutations have been identified. Most *MPL* mutations occur in exon 10 where tryptophan 515 is substituted for a leucine, lysine, asparagine, or alanine.[61-64] Tryptophan 515 is located on the cytosolic side of the membrane and is key in transducing the signal that thrombopoietin (TPO) has bound to the receptor. These mutations cause the MPL receptor to be hypersensitive to TPO and in some cases to assume the active conformation in the absence of TPO. A similar mutation, *MPL* S505N, was initially described in familial PV but has since been found in sporadic MPN.[61,64] These types of *MPL* mutations have since been identified in up to 15% of *JAK2* V617F–negative ET and PMF patients.[65]

In 2007 a second type of *JAK2* mutation was identified in exon 12, usually between amino acid residues 536 and 547, also resulting in a gain of function similar to the *JAK2* V617F.[66]

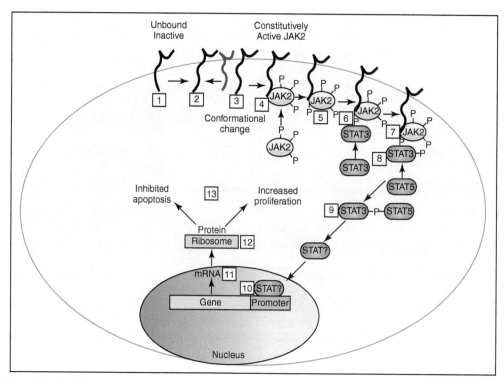

Figure 32.10 Stimulation of Erythropoiesis in the Absence of Erythropoietin that is Driven by a Constitutively Phosphorylated and Activated JAK2 Protein Resulting from the *JAK2* V617F Mutation. The numbers in the figure represent the sequence of events in the signal transduction pathway.

Exon 12 is not located in the pseudokinase domain, but it is hypothesized that the mutation can modify the structure of the JH2 domain, rendering the protein incapable of forming the inactive conformation.[53] *JAK2* exon 12 mutations have been found in 3% of patients with PV and are not associated with ET or PMF but can be found in patients who progress to secondary myelofibrosis.[66,67]

Experts hypothesize that mutations in signaling molecules alone are insufficient to initiate MPNs, suggesting that other mutations are necessary before *JAK2* V617F to induce disease and later to drive progression. Four lines of evidence support this hypothesis: (1) Familial MPN expresses a classic PV or ET phenotype in the absence of *JAK2* V617F or *MPL* W515L mutations and transmits in an autosomal dominant fashion; (2) in some ET and PV clones that were erythropoietin independent, *JAK2* V617F was identified in a minority of cells, indicating that a pre–*JAK2* mutation drove the disease; (3) approximately 50% of patients who developed AL from a *JAK2* V617F form of MPN expressed wild-type *JAK2*, suggesting a line of clonal evolution independent of *JAK2*; and (4) in patients with PV and ET at diagnosis, the *JAK2* V617F allele burden in HSCs was low compared with the allele burden in later stages of hematopoiesis, suggesting that *JAK2* V617F confers a weak proliferative advantage to HSCs.[53]

Three reports in 2010 identified a germline haplotype block that predisposes patients to *JAK2* mutations.[68-70] This haplotype block was identified as a single nucleotide polymorphism (rs10974944) located in intron 12 of the *JAK2* gene, increasing the development of MPN by three- to fourfold.[52]

Also in 2010, mutations were discovered in the adapter protein LNK (also known as Src homology 2 B3–SH2B3), which downregulates JAK-STAT signaling pathways by regulating JAK2 activation. Approximately 3% to 6% of patients with MPN bear an *LNK* mutation,[71,72] with approximately 13% of mutations appearing in the blast phase versus the chronic phase of the disease.[73] After the binding of the corresponding ligand to its receptor, LNK binds to EPO-R, thrombopoietin receptor (MPL), and JAK2 to downregulate the JAK-STAT pathway as a negative modulator. Mutations in *LNK* produce a loss of function that removes a level of inhibitory control, increasing the proliferation of erythrocytes and thrombocytes. This loss of function mutation is accentuated in the presence of *JAK2* V617F and *MPL* W515L mutations, resulting in the PV and ET phenotypes, respectively.[52] More recently, somatic mutations have been identified in genes that control DNA methylation in patients with PV and other MPNs. The most notable are *TET2* (ten eleven translocation 2), *IDH1* (isocitrate dehydrogenase 1), and *IDH2*. *TET2* is one of three members of the *TET* family of genes (*TET1* and *TET3*) and the only one identified with sequence alterations. *TET2* appears to be highly mutagenic for three reasons: (1) Mutations have been identified in all types of myeloid disorders, including MPNs, MDSs, and AMLs; (2) mutations have been found in all coding regions of the gene; and (3) mutations are often biallelic (homozygous).[74] *TET2* catalyzes the reaction that oxidizes the 5-methyl group of cytosine (5-mC) to 5-hydroxymethycytosine (5-hmC).[75] It is hypothesized that 5-hmC serves as an intermediate base in the demethylation of DNA. Methylation of histones serves to silence genes.

Therefore *TET2* mutations produce a loss-of-function effect, resulting in hypermethylation and a loss of gene activation (inactivation of tumor suppressor genes).[52] In addition, it appears that *TET2* mutations precede *JAK2* mutations based on three observations: (1) *TET2* mutations are expressed in CD34[+] HSCs; (2) *TET2* mutations have been identified in all forms of myeloid disorders; and (3) all patients with both *TET2* and *JAK2* mutations produced clones with both mutations and clones that were *TET2* positive and *JAK2* negative but none that were *JAK2* positive and *TET2* negative. Therefore *TET2* mutations may create abnormal clones that predispose to *JAK2* mutations.[74] *TET2* mutations have been identified in 9.8% to 16% of PV, 4.4% to 5% of ET, and 7.7% to 17% of PMF patients.[52]

Mutations in the genes that code for the citric acid cycle enzymes isocitrate dehydrogenase 1 (IDH1) and isocitrate dehydrogenase 2 (IDH2) have been associated with hypermethylation of DNA in patients with MPN and AML.[76] Normally these enzymes function to convert isocitrate to α-ketoglutarate, requiring the reduction of NAD(P)[+] to NADPH as the energy source. In patients with MPNs, mutations in *IDH1/2* occur most often at the *IDH2* R140 residue, the *IDH1* R132 residue, and the *IDA2* R172 residue.[77] These mutations are thought to alter enzyme function, causing the conversion of α-ketoglutarate to 2-hydroxyglutarate (2-HG).[78] It is hypothesized that because *TET2* is dependent on α-ketoglutarate, the *IDH1/2* mutations would result in less α-ketoglutarate, thus impairing the function of *TET2* and exacerbating the hypermethylation function of mutated *TET2* protein products.[76] *IDH1/2* mutations occur most often (21.6% of patients) in late-stage PV and ET patients during blast transformation, compared with an incidence of 1% to 5% in patients with early PV (1.9%), ET (0.8%), and PMF (4.2%).[61] As expected, *IDH1/2* mutations are associated with adverse overall survival, raising the potential of using *IDH1/2* mutational analysis or 2-HG detection as indicators of poor prognosis.

Mutations in two additional genes involved in epigenetic modification, *EZH2* and *ASXL1*, have been implicated in MPN, MDS, and MDS/MPN and, along with *TET2*, may precede *JAK2* V617F mutations. *EZH2* and *EZH1* function as two of several proteins that form the polychrome repressive complex 2 (PRC2) that regulates chromatin structure. More specifically, *EZH1* and *EZH2* provide the functional domain for the PRC2 complex to methylate histone H3 at lysine 27.[79] The array of mutations noted in *EZH2* to date function to either eliminate protein production or abrogate methyltransferase activity. Mutations in *EZH2* have been identified in 3% of PV patients, 13% of PMF patients, 12.3% of MDS/MPN patients, and 5.8% to 23% of MDS patients.[80,81] *ASXL1* (additional sex combs–like 1) mutations have been identified in most myeloid malignancies and at a frequency similar to *TET2*.[53] *ASXL1* normally functions in conjunction with *ASXL2* and *ASXL3* to deubiquinate histone H2 to balance the activity of PRC1 to monoubiquinate target genes to modify chromatin structure.[82,83] Ubiquination tags proteins for natural removal, thus regulating their function. The function of *ASXL1* in hematopoiesis is poorly understood, but the loss of function mutations have been identified in less than 7% of PV and ET and from 19% to 40% in PMF.[84,85]

Disease progression to blast crisis occurs in less than 10% of PV and ET patients, but several genetic mutation are implicated in this transformation.[86-88] In addition to those that modulate epigenetic changes previously discussed (*IDH1/2* and *TET2*), mutations in *TP53* and *RUNX1* are involved in blast transformation. *TP53* produces the P53 protein that is known to be a tumor suppressor gene. P53 controls cell cycle checkpoints and apoptosis, and loss-of-function mutations are implicated in a host of cancers, including disease progression in the classic MPNs. *TP53* mutations have not been identified in MPNs in the chronic phase but have been found in 20% of patients with MPNs who have progressed to AML.[89-91] The protein product of the *RUNX1/AML1* gene is a transcription factor that is important in hematopoiesis. *RUNX1* mutations were identified in 30% of post-MPN-AML patients, making it a candidate for the most common mutation involved in MPN transformation to AML.[53]

Diagnosis

Based on WHO standards, the diagnosis of PV requires that three major criteria and one minor criterion be met or that the patient meet the previous higher hemoglobin (HB) level of 18.5g/dL in men but not the BM criteria. The three major criteria are (1) an elevated HGB, hematocrit (HCT), or red cell mass (RCM) level (HGB > 16.5 g/dL in men and HGB > 16.5 g/dL in women *or* HCT > 49% in men and HCT > 48% in women *or* RCM > 25% of the mean normal); (2) BM showing hypercellularity for age with trilineage growth (panmyelosis) including prominent erythroid, granulocytic proliferation with pleomorphic, mature megakaryocytes; and (3) the identification of the *JAK2* V617F mutation or the *JAK2* exon 12 mutation. The one minor criteria is low serum erythropoietin levels.[7] Additional diagnostic features of PV include an arterial oxygen saturation of 92% (normal) or greater and splenomegaly. Other features of PV are thrombocytosis of greater than 400×10^9 platelets/L; leukocytosis of greater than 12×10^9 cells/L without fever or infection; and increases in LAP, serum vitamin B_{12}, or unbound vitamin B_{12} binding capacity.[92,93] WHO criteria for the diagnosis of PV are summarized in Box 32.1.

It is not always easy to assign an early diagnosis of PV. Erythrocytosis secondary to hypoxia or erythropoietin-producing neoplasms are the most difficult to diagnose correctly. In individuals with these conditions, the BM exhibits erythroid hyperplasia without granulocytic or megakaryocytic hyperplasia. Patients with stress or spurious erythrocytosis exhibit increased HB and HCT without increased erythrocyte mass or splenomegaly.

Peripheral Blood and Bone Marrow

Common peripheral blood, bone marrow, and tissue findings in the early or proliferative phase of PV are listed in Table 32.2. Figures 32.11 and 32.12 show common morphologic patterns in peripheral blood and BM morphologic and cellular changes. Not only are quantitative changes seen, but BM normoblasts may collect in large clusters, megakaryocytes are enlarged and exhibit lobulated nuclei, and BM sinuses are enlarged without fibrosis. Pseudo-Gaucher cells are rare. Approximately 80% of

---

BOX 32.1 WHO Diagnostic Criteria[7]

Polycythemia Vera

Major Criteria

1. Hemoglobin >16.5 g/dL in men and >16.0 g/dL in women OR
   Hematocrit >49% in men and >48% in women OR
   Increased red blood cell (RBC) mass mean normal
2. Bone marrow showing hypercellularity for age with trilineage growth (panmyelosis) including prominent erythroid, granulocytic, and megakaryocytic proliferation with pleomorphic, mature megakaryocytes (difference is size)
3. Presence of *JAK2V617F* or *JAK2* exon 12 mutation

Minor Criterion

1. Subnormal serum erythropoietin level

Pre-Primary Myelofibrosis

Major Criteria

1. Megakaryocytic proliferation and atypia, without reticulin fibrosis >grade 1, accompanied by increased age-adjusted BM cellularity, granulocytic proliferation, and often decreased erythropoiesis.
2. Not meeting the WHO criteria for *BCR-ABL1* + CML, PV, ET, MDS, or other myeloid neoplasms
3. Presence of *JAK2, CALR, or MPL* mutation or in the absence of these mutations, presence of another clonal marker, or absence of minor reactive BM reticulin fibrosis

Minor Criteria

1. Presence of at least one of the following, confirmed in two consecutive determinations
   a. Anemia not attributed to a comorbid condition
   b. Leukocytosis >11 × 10^9/L
   c. Palpable splenomegaly
   d. LDH increased to above upper limit of institutions reference range
   Diagnosis of pre-PMF requires meeting all three major criteria, and at least one minor criteria.

Primary Myelofibrosis (Overt)

Major Criteria

1. Megakaryocytic proliferation and atypia, accompanied by either reticulin and/or collagen fibrosis grades 2 or 3

2. Not meeting the WHO criteria for *BCR-ABL1* + CML, PV, ET, MDS, or other myeloid neoplasms
3. Presence of *JAK2, CALR, or MPL* mutation or in the absence of these mutations, presence of another clonal marker, or absence of minor reactive BM myelofibrosis

Minor Criteria

1. Presence of at least one of the following, confirmed in two consecutive determinations
   a. Anemia not attributed to a comorbid condition
   b. Leukocytosis >11 × 10^9/L
   c. Palpable splenomegaly
   d. LDH increased to above upper limit of institutions reference range
   e. Leukoerythroblastosis
   Diagnosis of pre-PMF requires meeting all three major criteria, and at least one minor criteria.

Chronic Neutrophilic Leukemia

1. Peripheral blood leukocytosis
   Bands and segmented neutrophils white blood cells (WBC)
   Immature granulocytes (promyelocytes, myelocytes, metamyelocytes) of WBC
   Myeloblasts rarely observed
   Monocyte count <1 × 10^9/L
   No dysgranulopoiesis
2. Hypercellular BM
   Neutrophilic granulocytes increased in percentage and number
   Myeloblasts of nucleated cells
   Neutrophil maturation appears normal
3. Not meeting WHO criteria for *BCR-ABL1* + CML, PV, ET, or PMF
4. No rearrangement of *PDGFRA, PDGFRB, FGFR1,* or *PCM1-JAK2*
5. Presence of *CSF3R T618I* or other activating *CSF3R* mutation
6. If *CSF3R T618I* is absent, persistent neutrophilia for at least 3 months, splenomegaly, no identifiable cause of reactive neutrophilia including the absence of a plasma cell neoplasm OR demonstration of clonality of myeloid cells by cytogenetic or molecular studies.

BM, Bone marrow; *CML,* chronic myeloid leukemia; *ET,* essential thrombocytopenia; *LDH,* lactate dehydrogenase; *MDS,* myelodysplastic syndrome; *PMF,* primary myelofibrosis; *PV,* polycythemia vera; *WHO,* World Health Organization.

---

patients manifest BM panmyelosis, and 100% of BM volume may exhibit hematopoietic cellularity. Although the BM pattern may mimic that of other MPNs, the peripheral blood cells appear normal, with normocytic, normochromic erythrocytes; mature granulocytes; and normal-sized, granulated platelets. The other 20% of patients exhibit lesser degrees of cellularity in the BM and peripheral blood. Splenomegaly, hepatomegaly, generalized vascular engorgement, and circulatory disturbances increase the risk of hemorrhage, tissue infarction, and thrombosis.

Clinical Presentation

PV often presents with a history of mild symptoms occurring for several years, although some patients are diagnosed serendipitously from laboratory values of asymptomatic patients. PV

initially manifests in a proliferative phase independent of normal regulatory mechanisms that is associated with increased red blood cell (RBC) mass. The increased RCM produces blood hyperviscosity, often resulting in cardiovascular disease. In the early stages of the disease, before treatment, extended periods of high HCT (>60%) and hyperviscosity produce hypertension in about 50% of patients with PV. Presenting symptoms are associated with hyperviscosity and hyperproliferation and include headache, weakness, pruritis, weight loss, and fatigue. Pruritis has been associated with elevated blood histamine and is often not associated with a visible rash.

About half of PV patients have thrombocytosis and one-third experience thrombotic or hemorrhagic episodes. PV patients older than 60 years of age or those associated with a history of thrombosis are considered high risk for thrombotic

TABLE 32.2 Common Morphologic Changes in Polycythemia Vera

Peripheral Blood

Hemoglobin	Increased
Hematocrit	Increased
Red blood cell volume	Increased
Erythrocyte morphology	Normocytic/normochromic
Total white blood cells	Increased
Granulocytes	Increased
Platelets	Increased
Leukocyte alkaline phosphatase	Normal or increased

Bone Marrow

Normoblasts	Increased
Granulocytes	Increased
Megakaryocytes	Increased
Reticulin	Increased

Extramedullary Tissue

Splenomegaly	Present
Sinusoidal	Present
Medullary	Present
Hepatomegaly	Present
Sinusoidal	Present

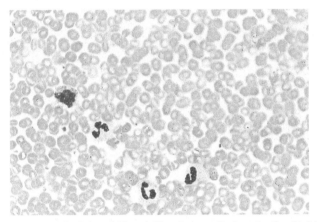

Figure 32.11 Peripheral Blood Film from a Patient in the Stable Phase of Polycythemia Vera. Note the essentially normocytic, normochromic erythrocytes. (Wright-Giemsa stain, ×500.)

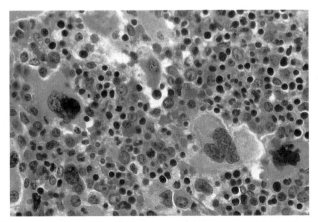

Figure 32.12 Bone Marrow Biopsy Specimen from a Patient in the Stable Phase of Polycythemia Vera. Note the panmyelosis. (Hematoxylin and eosin stain, ×400.)

or hemorrhagic events. Similarly, PV patients have an intermediate risk if concomitant risk factors exist, including uncontrolled hypertension, diabetes, smoking, obesity, or hypercholesterolemia. Thrombotic risk is reduced if the calreticulin (*CALR*) mutation is identified, especially in ET patients.[94] Other thrombosis-related events like myocardial infarctions, retinal vein thrombosis, thrombophlebitis, and cerebral ischemia can occur at any stage of the disease and occasionally are the first indication of the disease.

The stable phase of PV can progress to a spent phase in a few patients, usually within 10 years from diagnosis. In the spent phase, patients experience progressive splenomegaly (palpable spleen) or hypersplenism (large spleen with BM hyperplasia and peripheral blood cytopenias) and pancytopenia. They may also exhibit the triad of BM fibrosis, splenomegaly, and anemia with teardrop-shaped poikilocytes. The latter pattern is called *postpolycythemic myeloid metaplasia* and develops in about 30% of PV patients within 20 years. This phase of PV is morphologically similar to PMF and must be carefully differentiated. Peripheral WBC and RBC counts vary, and nucleated erythrocytes, immature granulocytes, and large platelets are present. Usually, splenomegaly is secondary to extramedullary hematopoiesis.[95] Myelofibrosis occurs within the BM and may come to occupy a significant proportion of BM volume, with subsequent ineffective hematopoiesis.[96]

Treatment and Prognosis

Treatment options for PV can be placed into three groups: therapeutic phlebotomy, myelosuppressive therapy, and targeted molecular therapy. The treatment of choice for PV in the early stages of the disease is therapeutic phlebotomy at a frequency necessary to maintain the HCT at less than 45% for men and 42% for women. Therapeutic phlebotomy decreases erythrocyte counts to reduce blood viscosity, thus restoring normal blood flow and ameliorating the associated symptoms of headache, weakness, fatigue, and pruritus. Blood removal also reduces available iron, which inhibits erythropoiesis delaying the return of erythrocytosis. Low-dose aspirin has been found to be efficacious to minimize thrombosis in all risk categories.[97]

The alkylating agent hydroxyurea is recommended in high-risk patients with PV and can be substituted with INF-γ in younger patients[98,99] and busulfan in older patients who develop intolerance or resistance to hydroxyuria.[100] The risk of thrombosis and bleeding is increased in patients treated with phlebotomy alone, so the use of alkylating myelosuppressive agents may be required to control these complications. Patients with both early and advanced PV may show clinical, peripheral blood, bone marrow, and extramedullary features that mimic those of other MPNs. Some patients may manifest a temporary disease pattern similar to myelodysplasia, whereas others may exhibit cell morphology suggesting transformation to AL, making the disease difficult to classify.

Treatment with modern JAK inhibitors like ruxolitinib has provided important benefits to patients with PV. Ruxolitinib binds with high affinity to the ATP-binding site of the active form of JAK1, JAK2, JAK3, and wild-type JAK proteins as well as the *JAK2* V617F mutation. In addition, ruxolitinib was tested against 26 other tyrosine kinases and found to have a low binding affinity for all 26 proteins.[38] A total of 34 patients intolerant or refractory to hydroxyurea were enrolled in the phase II study and treated with ruxolitinib at a dose of 10 mg twice a day. Of the 34 patients, 15 (45%) had a complete remission.[101] In addition, 32 patients (97%) achieved phlebotomy independence, and 27 patients (80%) achieved a 50% decrease in spleen size, as well as a reduction in pruritus, bone pain, and night sweats.[102]

Lestaurtinib is a tyrosine kinase inhibitor that binds FLT3, JAK2, and TRKA, TRKB and TRKC. Lestaurtinib was studied on 27 PV and 12 ET patients refractory or intolerant to hydroxyurea, and the outcomes were less promising. In 15 of the 39 patients who completed 18 weeks of treatment, 83% (15/18) achieved some degree of spleen size reduction, 60% (3/5) had a reduction in phlebotomy requirements, 20% (3/15) had a 15% decrease in *JAK2* allele burden, and 15% developed thrombosis; gastrointestinal events were common.[103,104]

About half of PV patients will survival 15 months without treatment, and survival is extended to 14 years with phlebotomy as the only treatment. PV in the spent phase transitions into AL in 5% to 10% of patients. Age, abnormal karyotype, leukocytosis, and a history of thrombosis are factors that adversely affect survival. The median survival for PV patients stratified by risk into high-, medium-, and low-risk groups using criteria of age, WBC count and thrombosis is 10.9, 18.9, and 27.8 years, respectively.[94] Overall median survival exceeds 10 to 20 years.[105] However, the disease progresses to AL in 15% of patients. The use of myelosuppressive therapy increases the risk, whereas only 1% to 2% of patients treated with phlebotomy alone experience leukemic transformation.

ESSENTIAL THROMBOCYTHEMIA

Essential thrombocythemia is a clonal MPN with increased megakaryopoiesis and thrombocytosis, usually with a count greater than 600×10^9/L and sometimes with a count greater than 1000×10^9/L.[106] However, WHO criteria require a sustained thrombocytosis with a platelet count of 400×10^9/L or greater. Over the years, ET has been known as *primary thrombocytosis, idiopathic thrombocytosis,* and *hemorrhagic thrombocythaemia.*[107]

Incidence

In the absence of a well-defined diagnostic algorithm, determining the true incidence of ET has been difficult. When the diagnostic system developed by the Polycythemia Vera Study Group (PVSG) is applied, however, the incidence is estimated to be between 0.6 and 2.5 cases per 100,000 persons per year. Prevalence rates have been reported of 38 to 57 out of 100,000 people, with women affected more often than men.[94] The majority of cases occur in individuals between the ages of 50 and 60 years, but a second peak occurs primarily in women in the childbearing years, approximately 30 years of age.[107]

Pathogenic Mechanism

Most of the mutations described in PV also occur in ET. Three mutations in particular, *JAK2, MPL,* and *CALR,* are considered driver mutations for ET and occur at a rate of 64.1% *(JAK2),* 4.3% *(MPL),* and 15.5% *(CALR).* Some ET patients are negative for both *JAK2* and *MPL,* but 10% to 15% of these cases are positive for the *CALR* mutation. The remaining ET patients, about 16%, are negative for all three driver mutations and are referred to as triple negative. Most triple negative patients have been found to express new somatic mutations in *JAK2* and *MPL* or an uncommon hereditary version.[108] Mutations in the EPO and G-CSF cytokine receptors may activate *JAK2* in *JAK2* (V617F)–negative patients.

In ET one *JAK2* V617F mutation is more common, but in PV two *JAK2* V617F mutations are more common. Therefore *JAK2* V617F burden is thought to be critical in the transformation of ET to PV and in disease progression in PV.

As previously discussed, two *MPL* mutations (MPLW515L and MPLW515K) occur in approximately 4% of patients with *JAK2* (V617F)–negative ET and 10% with PMF. This mutation results in cytokine-independent growth and constitutive downstream signaling pathways and favors the ET phenotype.[49]

CALR, like *JAK2* and *MPL,* modulates the JAK-STAT pathway. Two type 1 and two type 2 mutations have been described in *CALR.* ET patients with a *CALR* mutation show 45% type 1 mutations and 39% type 2 mutations. These mutations occurred in the last exon that codes for the C-terminal amino acids. CALR proteins normally locate to the endoplasmic reticulum, but these mutations alter the subcellular localization. The *CALR* mutation was associated with a higher platelet count, but patients experience thrombosis rates half those of ET patients with a *JAK2* mutation. ET patients with the *CALR* mutation have lower WBC and HB levels compared with ET patients with a *JAK2* mutation, and most do not progress to PV.[108]

Several other mutations previously discussed with PV also occur in ET, including *TET2* (4.4% to 5%), *ASXL1* (5.6%), *LNK* (3% to 6%), and *IDH1/2* (0.8%).[52] The manner in which these mutations alter normal cellular functions is similar to PV, as previously described.

Clinical Presentation

In more than half of patients diagnosed with ET, the disorder is discovered in the laboratory by virtue of an unexpectedly elevated platelet count on a routine complete blood count; the remaining patients see a physician because of vascular occlusion or hemorrhage. Vascular occlusions are often the result of microvascular thromboses in the digits or thromboses in major arteries and veins that occur in a variety of organ systems, including splenic or hepatic veins, as in Budd-Chiari syndrome. Repeated splenic infarcts can result in splenic atrophy. Thrombosis can result in pulmonary emboli and neurologic complications like headache, paresthesis of the extremities, visual impairments, and tinnitus. Arterial thrombi can cause myocardial infarction, transient ischemic attack, and cerebral vascular accident.[94] Bleeding occurs most often from mucous membranes in the gastrointestinal, skin, urinary, and upper respiratory tracts.

A minimally palpable spleen is seen in about half of ET patients that can result in abdominal fullness. Fatigue, weight loss, and night sweats can also occur along with Raynaud syndrome and gout.[94]

Diagnosis

ET must be differentiated from secondary or reactive thrombocytoses and from other MPNs. Thrombocytosis may be secondary to chronic active blood loss, hemolytic anemia, chronic inflammation or infection, or nonhematogenous neoplasia. The identification of the *JAK2* V617F and *MPL* W515K/L mutations exclude cases of reactive thrombocytosis.

The newest WHO group requires four major and one minor diagnostic criteria for the diagnosis of ET. WHO major diagnostic criteria include the following: (1) megakaryocyte proliferation with large and mature morphology, little to no granulocyte or erythroid proliferation; (2) rarely, minor (grade 1) increase in reticulin fibers; (3) must not meet any criteria for *BCR-ABL1*-positive CML, PV, PMF, MDS or other myeloid neoplasms; and (4) must demonstrate *JAK2* V617F, *CALR,* or *MPL* mutations. Minor criteria include presence of a clonal marker or absence of evidence of reactive thrombocytosis. Based on WHO standards, a diagnosis of ET requires meeting all four major criteria or the first three major criteria and one minor criteria.[7]

Careful analysis of the BM biopsy specimen is useful in distinguishing ET from MDSs associated with the del(5q) mutation, refractory anemia with ringed sideroblasts with thrombocytosis, and the prefibrotic phase of PMF.

Peripheral Blood and Bone Marrow

The most consistent finding in the peripheral blood is thrombocytosis that must exceed 400×10^9/L to meet WHO criteria but often ranges from 1000 to 5000×10^9/L. Platelets often appear normal, but giant bizarre platelets, platelet aggregates, micromegakaryocytes, and megakaryocyte fragments can also be observed. Figure 32.13 shows a peripheral blood film that exhibits early-phase thrombocytosis with variation in platelet diameter and shape, including giantism, agranularity, and pseudopods. Commonly, platelets are present in clusters and tend to accumulate near the thin edge of the blood film. Abnormal platelet function testing can occur.

In the early stages of the disease most patients are not anemic unless bleeding induces anemia. Erythrocytes are normocytic and normochromic, unless iron deficiency is present secondary to excessive bleeding. Significant bleeding can also stimulate reticulocytosis, producing polychromasia on the peripheral blood smear. Splenic infarction can result in Howell-Jolly bodies, nucleated erythrocytes, and poikilocytosis. About one-third of patients will present with a mild erythrocytosis, which must be distinguished from PV.

Leukocytosis is usually present and ranges from 22 to 40×10^9/L. Segmented neutrophils may be increased, and occasionally metamyelocytes and myelocytes are seen. Basophils and eosinophils are usually normal but can be mildly elevated.

Early-phase BM has marked megakaryocytic hypercellularity, clustering of megakaryocytes, and increased megakaryocyte diameter with nuclear hyperlobulation and density (Figure 32.14). Special studies reveal increased numbers of smaller and less mature megakaryocytes.[109] Increased granulopoiesis and erythropoiesis may contribute to BM hypercellularity, and, in about 25% of patients, reticulin fibers may be increased. However, significant fibrosis is usually not seen.[49] The major peripheral blood, bone marrow, and extramedullary findings are listed in Table 32.3.

A diagnosis of ET is questionable in patients with a platelet count of more than 400×10^9/L if certain features are observed on the BM biopsy specimen. For example, increased erythropoiesis or granulopoiesis in the BM is a questionable finding for ET and suggests an alternative diagnosis of PV or PMF, respectively, especially if bizarre or significantly atypical megakaryocytes are also identified. Dyserythropoiesis or dysgranulopoiesis suggests a myelodysplastic disorder and should prompt an investigation for (del)5q, (inv)3, or t(3;3).[107]

Treatment and Prognosis

Patients with thrombocytosis without a history of thrombosis or cardiovascular risk factors may not require treatment,

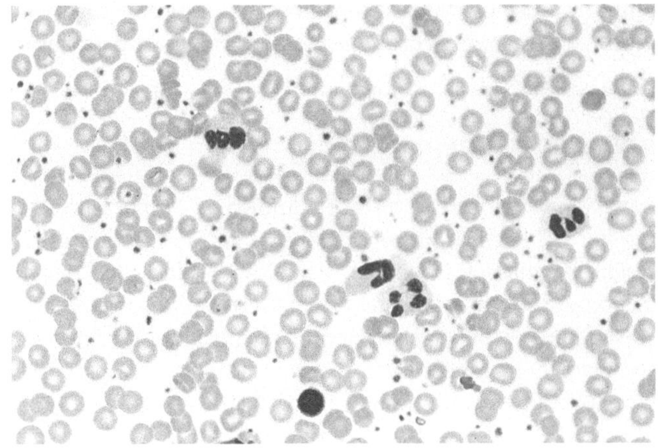

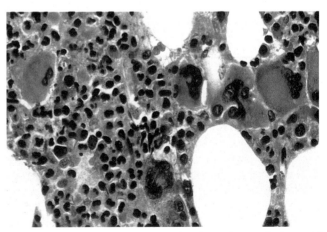

Figure 32.13 Peripheral Blood Film from a Patient in the Stable Phase of Essential Thrombocythemia. Note the increased numbers of platelets and mature neutrophils. (Wright-Giemsa stain, ×500.)

Figure 32.14 Bone Marrow Biopsy Specimen from a Patient with Essential Thrombocythemia. Note the marked number of megakaryocytes. (Hematoxylin and eosin stain, ×400.)

TABLE 32.3   Common Morphologic Changes in Essential Thrombocythemia

Peripheral Blood	
Hemoglobin	Slightly decreased
Hematocrit	Slightly decreased
Red blood cell volume	Normal
Total white blood cells	Normal or slightly increased
Neutrophils	Normal or slightly increased
Platelets	Increased
Platelet function	Decreased
Bone Marrow	
Normoblasts	Normal or increased
Granulocytes	Normal or slightly increased
Megakaryocytes	
Clusters	Present
Large	Present
Hyperlobulated	Present
Dense nuclei	Present
Variability in size	Increased
Reticulin	Normal or slightly increased
Extramedullary Tissue	
Splenomegaly	Present
Sinusoidal	Present
Medullary	Present
Megakaryocytic proliferation	Present

otherwise treatment is initiated to reduce the platelet count and control thrombosis. Treatment involves prevention or early alleviation of hemorrhagic or vasoocclusive complications that occur as the platelet count increases. Plateletpheresis can be used to quickly reduce the platelet count, but cytoreductive therapy is needed for ongoing control. The production of platelets must be reduced by suppressing marrow megakaryocyte production with an alkylating agent like hydroxyurea or anagrelide. Hydroxyurea is preferred in ET patients with concomitant thrombocytosis and leukocytosis because it targets both cell lines, whereas anagrelide is preferred if only the platelet count is elevated because of fewer side effects compared with hydroxyurea.[49] Clinical trials are underway to evaluate two long-acting formulations of anagrelide.[94] As observed in PV, ET patients treated with hydroxyurea may incur an increased risk for disease transformation to AL or myelofibrosis. However, malignant transformation occurs at a frequency of less than 5%.[105] Hydroxyurea therapy may achieve a desired reduction of peripheral platelets without the risk of complications experienced with myelosuppressive agents. This may relate to the youth of ET patients, in whom the risk of leukemic transformation seems relatively low. For patients who develop intolerance or resistance to hydroxyurea, cytoreduction can be achieved with interferon-α in younger patients[98] and busulfan in older patients.[110] Low-dose aspirin is also recommended to prevent thrombosis and is particularly recommended for intermediate- and high-risk patients or those with the *JAK2* V617F mutation.[94,105]

JAK2 inhibitors are being investigated in ET patients who are refractory or intolerant to hydroxyurea or are otherwise

high risk. Ruxolitinib was studied in 39 patients with ET at a dose of 25 mg twice daily. In all 39 patients, the median platelet count reduced from 884 to 558 × 10^9/L, and the 11 patients who had leukocytosis achieved a normal WBC count after 6 months of treatment. Four patients who demonstrated splenomegaly had spleen size reduction; 40% to 75% of patients had a 50% or greater improvement in one or more of the following: pruritus, bone pain, night sweats, and peripheral tingling/numbness. Only 13% (5 patients), achieved complete remission. However, a follow-up report at 10.4 months of treatment indicated that 92% were still participating in the study, no grade 3 or 4 hematologic complications were noted, and although cytopenias were identified in 10% to 20%, they were grade 2 (mild).[102]

Lestaurtinib was studied in 27 patients with PV and 12 patients with ET who were refractory or intolerant to hydroxyurea. In 15 of the 39 patients who completed 18 weeks of treatment, 83% (15/18) achieved some degree of spleen size reduction, 20% (3/15) had a 15% decrease in *JAK2* allele burden, and 15% developed thrombosis and had frequent gastrointestinal events.[103,104]

Patients with ET experience relatively long survival provided they remain free of serious thromboembolic or hemorrhagic complications. Clinical symptoms associated with thromboembolic vasoocclusive events include the syndrome of erythromelalgia (throbbing and burning pain in the hands and feet, accompanied by mottled redness of areas), transient ischemic attacks, seizures, and cerebral or myocardial infarction. Other symptoms include headache, dizziness, visual disturbances, and dysesthesias (decreased sensations). Hemorrhagic complications include bleeding from oral and nasal mucous membranes or gastrointestinal mucosa and the appearance of cutaneous ecchymoses (Chapter 38).

The median survival for patients with ET is 20 years, including cases in which the process arises in younger patients.[107,111] Risk stratification placed low-risk patients with a long-term survival that did not reach median, intermediate-risk patients had a median survival of 24.5 years and high-risk patients' survival was 13.8 years. ET patients progressed to PMF at a rate of 10% and AL at a rate of 5%. The *JAK2* mutation increased the risk of transformation into polycythemia vera.[93] The most common cause of death is thrombosis and bleeding. Patients whose cells manifest chromosome abnormalities may have a poorer prognosis.

PRIMARY MYELOFIBROSIS

Primary myelofibrosis, previously known as *chronic idiopathic myelofibrosis, agnogenic myelofibrosis,* and *myelofibrosis with myeloid metaplasia,* is a clonal HSC MPN[112] in which there is splenomegaly and ineffective hematopoiesis associated with areas of marrow hypercellularity (leukoerythroblastosis), extramedullary hematopoiesis, fibrosis, and increased megakaryocytes. It is the least common but most aggressive form of MPN. PMF can form de novo or as an evolutionary consequence of PV or ET. Megakaryocytes are enlarged with pleomorphic nuclei, coarse segmentation, and areas of hypochromia. The peripheral blood film exhibits immature granulocytes and normoblasts, dacryocytes (teardrop-shaped RBCs), and other bizarre RBC shapes.

PMF clonality was manifest in studies in which cytogenetic abnormalities were detected in normoblasts, neutrophils, macrophages, basophils, and megakaryocytes. Female patients heterozygous for glucose-6-phosphate dehydrogenase isoenzymes have PMF cells of a single enzyme isotype, whereas tissue cells, including marrow fibroblasts, contain both enzyme isotypes.[112]

Myelofibrosis

Fibroblasts are normally found in the BM and produce collagen to provide structural support for HSCs. In PMF a reactive process causes overproduction of collagen that eventually disrupts the normal architecture of the BM and replaces hematopoietic tissue resulting in pancytopenia. The myelofibrosis in this disease consists of three of the five types of collagen: I, III, and IV. Increases in type III collagen are detected by silver impregnation techniques, increases in type I by staining with trichrome, and increases in type IV by the presence of osteosclerosis, which may be diagnosed from increased radiographic bone density.[113] In approximately 30% of patients, biopsy specimens show no fibrosis. Increases in these collagens are not a part of the clonal proliferative process but are considered secondary to an increased release of fibroblastic growth factors, such as platelet-derived growth factor (PDGF), transforming growth factor-α and -β (TGF-α/-β), tumor necrosis factor-α (TNF-α), IL-1α, and IL-1β. Vascular endothelial growth factor (VEGF), PDGF, fibroblast growth factor (FGF), epidermal growth factor (EGF), hepatocyte growth factor (HGF), and insulin-like growth factor (IGF) are contained in the α-granules of megakaryocytes and platelets, and collectively stimulate the growth and proliferation of endothelial cells, blood vessels, and fibroblasts. The abnormal release or leakage of PDGF from the platelet results in reduced platelet concentrations of PDGF and increased levels of serum PDGF that are characteristic of PMF. PDGF does not stimulate synthesis of collagen, laminin, or fibronectin, but TGF-β stimulates increased expression of genes for fibronectin and collagen, whereas it decreases synthesis of collagenase-like enzymes. Thus the net effect is the accumulation of BM stromal elements.[114] Marrow fibrosis causes expansion of marrow sinuses and vascular volume, with an increased rate of blood flow. BM fibrosis is not the sole criterion for the diagnosis of PMF because increases in marrow fibrosis may reflect a reparative response to injury from benzene or ionizing radiation, may be a consequence of immunologically mediated injury, or may represent a reactive response to other hematologic conditions.

Type IV collagen and laminin normally are discontinuous in sinusoidal membranes but appear as stromal sheets in association with neovascularization and endothelial cell proliferation in regions of fibrosis. In addition, deposition of type VII collagen is observed, and this may form a linkage between type I fibers, type III fibers, and type I plus type III fibers.[115]

Hematopoiesis and Extramedullary Hematopoiesis

Extramedullary hematopoiesis, clinically recognized as hepatomegaly or splenomegaly, seems to originate from release of clonal stem cells into the circulation.[116] The cells accumulate in the spleen, liver, or other organs, including adrenals, kidneys, lymph nodes, bowel, breasts, lungs, mediastinum, mesentery, skin, synovium, thymus, and lower urinary tract. The cause of extramedullary hematopoiesis is unknown. In experimental animal models, chemicals, hormones, viruses, radiation, and immunologic factors have been implicated. The disease is associated with an increase in circulating hematopoietic cells, but fibroblasts are a secondary abnormality and not clonal.[112] B and T cells may be involved.[117] There is an increase in circulating unilineage and multilineage HPCs,[118] and the number of CD34$^+$ cells may be 300 times normal.[119] The increase in circulating CD34$^+$ cells separates PMF from other MPNs and predicts the degree of splenic involvement and risk of conversion to AL.

Body cavity effusions containing hematopoietic cells may arise from extramedullary hematopoiesis in the cranium, the intraspinal epidural space, or the serosal surfaces of pleura, pericardium, and peritoneum. Portal hypertension, with its attendant consequences of ascites, esophageal and gastric varices, gastrointestinal hemorrhage, and hepatic encephalopathy, arises from the combination of a massive increase in splenoportal blood flow and a decrease in hepatic vascular compliance secondary to fibrosis around the sinusoids and hematopoietic cells within the sinusoids.[120]

Pathogenetic Mechanism

As with ET and PV, most patients with PMF have a somatic mutation in one of three driver genes; *JAK2* (V617F), *CALR*, or *MPL*, that affect the JAK-STAT pathway. About 60% of PMF patients bear the *JAK2* (V617F) mutation; 30% have a mutation in *CALR*; and 5% have an *MPL* mutation.[52,121] A small number of PMF patients are negative for all three driver mutations (termed triple negative) and have a worse prognosis. Mutations in genes that regulate epigenetic modification rather than the JAK-STAT pathway have also been identified in PMF, including *TET2* (7.7% to 17%), *ASXL1* (13% to 23%), DNA methyltransferase 3A (*DNMT3A*), and enhancer of Zeste homolog 2 (*EZH2*).[52,121] In addition, 6% of patients with PML expressed a *CBL* mutation that is more typically found in juvenile myelomonocytic leukemia (JMML) or chronic myelomonocytic leukemia (CMML).[122] Lastly, other mutations previously discussed (*LNK* [3% to 6%], *EZH2* [13%], and *IDH1/2* [4.2%]) have also been identified in PML.[52]

Incidence and Clinical Presentation

PMF occurs in patients older than age 60 and equally in both genders. The disease may be asymptomatic and usually progresses as a slow, chronic condition. On occasion it can follow as a rapid, acute course marked by rapid fibrosis formation and the associated pancytopenia. Symptoms result from anemia, myeloproliferation, or splenomegaly and include fatigue, weakness, shortness of breath, palpitations, loss of appetite, weight loss, night sweats, pruritis, pain in the extremities and bones, bleeding, and discomfort or pain in the left upper quadrant associated with splenomegaly. Major hemolytic episodes occur in 15% of PMF patients during the course of their disease and

10% of patients demonstrate hemosiderinuria and decreased blood haptoglobin levels suggesting intravascular hemolysis. Some patients develop bleeding diathesis resulting from a combination of thrombocytopenia, abnormal platelet function, and hemostatic abnormalities suggestive of chronic disseminated intravascular coagulation (DIC).[123]

Peripheral Blood and Bone Marrow

PMF presents with a broad range of changes in laboratory test values and peripheral blood film results that reflect both quantitative and qualitative abnormalities. In the early stages, anemia, leukocytosis with a left shift, and thrombocytosis are identified that are consistent with a MPN. However, as the fibrosis develops in the bone marrow, blood cell counts fall and pancytopenia eventually develops, along with leukoerythroblastosis, anisocytosis, and poikilocytosis. Examination of the BM biopsy specimen provides most of the information for diagnosis. Changes commonly observed in peripheral blood and BM examinations are summarized in Table 32.4.

Abnormalities in erythrocytes noted on peripheral blood films include the presence of dacryocytes, other bizarre shapes, nucleated RBCs, and polychromatophilia in the context of a normocytic and normochromic anemia. Between 35% to 54% of PMF patients have a HB of less than 10 g/dL.[124] Reticulocytosis is common ranging from 2% to 15%.

Granulocytes can be increased, normal, or decreased in number at presentation but fall as the disease progresses. The differential will indicate immature granulocytes producing a left shift, blasts (<5%), and cells with nuclear or cytoplasmic anomalies. Eosinophilia, basophilia, and pseudo-Pelger-Huët anomaly can also be identified. LAP is variable but often elevated or normal.

Platelets may be normal, increased, or decreased in number, with a mixture of normal and abnormal morphologic features (Figure 32.15). Thrombocytosis is more common early in the disease and thrombocytopenia in the later stages. Micromegakaryocytes may be observed (Figure 32.16) with naked micromegakaryocytic nuclei, megakaryocyte fragments, and cytoplasmic blebbing.

BM biopsy specimens are difficult to obtain and often yield a dry tap. If an aspirate is obtained, the sample will often appear

TABLE 32.4 Common Morphologic Changes in Primary Myelofibrosis	
Peripheral Blood	
Hemoglobin	Normal or decreased
Anisocytosis	Present
Poikilocytosis	Present
Teardrop-shaped erythrocytes	Present
Nucleated red blood cells	Present
Polychromasia	Normal or increased
Total white blood cells	Normal, decreased, or increased
Immature granulocytes	Increased
Blasts	Present
Basophils	Present
Leukocyte anomaly	Present
Leukocyte alkaline phosphatase	Increased, normal, or decreased
Platelets	Increased, normal, or decreased
Abnormal platelets	Present
Megakaryocytes	Present
Bone Marrow	
Cellularity	Increased
Granulopoiesis	Increased
Megakaryocytes	Increased
Erythropoiesis	Normal or increased
Myelofibrosis	Increased
Sinuses	Increased
Dysmegakaryopoiesis	Present
Dysgranulopoiesis	Present
Extramedullary Tissue	
Splenomegaly	Present
Sinusoidal	Present
Medullary	Present
Hepatomegaly	Present
Sinusoidal	Present
Portal tract	Present
Local infiltrates	Present
Other tissues	Present

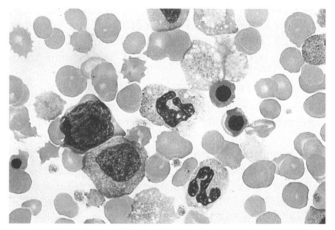

Figure 32.15 Peripheral Blood Film from a Patient with Primary Myelofibrosis. Note the nucleated red blood cells, giant platelets, and immature myeloid cells. (Wright-Giemsa stain, ×1000.)

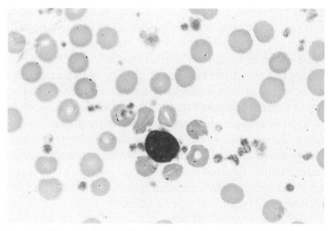

Figure 32.16 Peripheral Blood Film from a Patient with Primary Myelofibrosis. Note the increased platelets and a micromegakaryocyte. (Wright-Giemsa stain, ×1000.)

normal, making a biopsy critical to assess fibrosis. The BM biopsy specimen exhibits intense fibrosis, granulocytic and megakaryocytic hypercellularity, dysmegakaryopoiesis, dysgranulopoiesis, and numerous dilated sinuses containing luminal hematopoiesis.

Immune Response

Humoral immune responses are altered in approximately 50% of patients and include the appearance of autoantibodies to erythrocyte antigens, nuclear proteins, gamma globulins, phospholipids, and organ-specific antigens.[125] Circulating immune complexes, increased proportions of marrow-reactive lymphocytes, and the development of amyloidosis are evidence for active immune processes. Collagen disorders coexist with PMF, which suggests that immunologic processes may stimulate marrow fibroblast activity.

Treatment and Prognosis

A diverse spectrum of therapies has been implemented to alleviate symptoms or modify clinical problems in patients with PMF. None has been disease modifying, so treatment approaches have historically been palliative. Treatment has been targeted at the amelioration of anemia, hepatosplenomegaly, and constitutional symptoms. Between 34% and 54% of PMF patients present with a HGB of less than 10 g/dL.[124,126] Severe anemia has been treated with androgen therapy, prednisone, danazol,[127] thalidomide,[128,129] or lenalidomide,[130] and hemolytic anemia with glucocorticosteroids. Approximately 20% of patients respond with an average duration of 1 to 2 years. Thalidomide and lenalidomide must be used with caution because of the occurrence of neuropathies and myelosuppression, particularly if the patient has been identified with del(5q31).[131] Pomalidomide has been found to produce anemia and symptom relief without neuropathy and myelosuppression.[132]

Splenomegaly is present in 90% of patients with PMF, and 50% have hepatomegaly.[124,126] The most common first-line therapy for splenomegaly is hydroxyurea, but caution must be exercised so as not to exacerbate preexisting cytopenias.[133,134] Splenectomy and local radiation to the spleen and liver have been used in patients refractory to hydroxyurea, but patients must be carefully monitored for postoperative thrombosis, bleeding, infections, and cytopenias.[135]

The most common constitutional symptoms encountered by patients with PMF include fatigue (84%), bone pain (47%), night sweats (56%), pruritus (50%), and fever (18%).[136,137] However, treatments to alleviate these symptoms are minimally effective.

The development and testing of JAK inhibitors were directed at PMF because the symptoms and outcomes are worse compared with those of PV and ET. Among the JAK2 inhibitors tested, the four that showed the most promise were two JAK1/2 inhibitors, ruxolitinib and momelotinib; one JAK2 inhibitor, fedratinib; and one non-JAK inhibitor, lestaurtinib.

Ruxolitinib, when administered to patients with advanced PMF at maximum tolerated doses daily, resulted in clinical improvement for some patients.[138] Partial or complete molecular response to the JAK2 clone was achieved in nearly 10% of PMF patients treated with ruxolitinib. Ruxolitinib decreased spleen size, producing clinically significant symptom relief but did not affect JAK2 V617F allele burden. However, ruxolitinib produced anemia (23%) and thrombocytopenia (20%) along with a lowering of elevated WBC counts.[38,138,139]

Momelotinib is also a JAK1/2 inhibitor that has been found to have limited inhibitory effect against JAK3. All patients reported some degree of splenic reduction and most reported symptom relief. The most common symptom improvements included lessening of fatigue, pruritis, night sweats, cough, and bone pain and fewer bouts of fever. Momelotinib produced few hematologic toxicities, but some elevations in pancreatic and liver enzymes were reported.[103,140]

Fedratinib is a tyrosine kinase inhibitor that has been found to inhibit JAK2, FLT3, and RET (rearranged during transfection) and to a lesser extent, JAK3. When administered at the maximum tolerated dose, fedratinib produced clinical improvement in 66% of PMF patients. The majority of patients with leukocytosis and/or thrombocytosis experienced normalization of counts and a 50% reduction in JAK2 allele burden.[141]

Lestaurtinib is a JAK2/FLT3 selective inhibitor that has been the most disappointing in clinical trials. Patients did not report clinical improvement, nor was a significant reduction in JAK2 allele burden or reductions in proinflammatory cytokines noted.[103,140]

Pacritinib is also a JAK2/FLT3 inhibitor, but it does not produce inhibition to JAK1. In clinical trials pacritinib did induce reduction in spleen size and symptom relief, but diarrhea was a common yet manageable complaint. Nonetheless, pacritinib is a potential treatment option for myelofibrosis patients with preexisting anemia and thrombocytopenia.[142]

Reduction of myelofibrosis and of marrow and tissue hypercellularity has been accomplished with busulfan hydroxyurea and, in a few patients, interferon-α and interferon-γ. Radiotherapy is considered for patients with severe splenic pain, patients with massive splenomegaly who are not clinical candidates for splenectomy, patients with ascites secondary to serosal implants (metastatic nodules), and patients with localized bone pain and localized extramedullary fibrohematopoietic masses in other areas, especially in the epidural space. Splenectomy is performed to end severe pain, excessive transfusion requirements, or severe thrombocytopenia and to correct severe portal hypertension.

Chemotherapy is partially successful in reducing the number of CD34+ cells and immature hematopoietic cells, marrow fibrosis, and splenomegaly.[143] Single-agent chemotherapy is most helpful in the early clinical phases of the disease, and agents such as busulfan, 6-thioguanine, and chlorambucil, alone or in combination with other chemotherapy, are useful. Other therapies include interferon-α, hydroxyurea, and combinations of the previously mentioned drugs.[144] The most successful treatment to date for patients younger than age 60 is allogeneic stem cell transplantation. Five-year survival approaches 50% in patients undergoing transplantation, but 1-year mortality is 27%, and graft-versus-host disease occurs in 33%.[145]

Average survival from the time of diagnosis is about 5 years, but patients have lived as long as 15 years. During this time, increasing numbers and pleomorphy of megakaryocytes lead to progressive marrow failure. Marrow blasts may increase. Adverse prognostic indicators include more severe anemia and thrombocytopenia, greater hepatomegaly, unexplained fever, and hemolysis. Mortality is associated with infection, hemorrhage, postsplenectomy complications, cardiac failure, and transformation to AL.[123]

SUMMARY OF CURRENT THERAPY OF NON-*BCR-ABL1*, PRIMARY MPNS

JAK2 inhibitors are most effective in patients with PMF in part because of the more severe symptoms in PMF compared with PV and ET. Ruxolitnib, fedratinib, and momelotinib appear to have a significant effect on decreasing splenomegaly—one of the more serious symptoms in PMF patients—within the first cycle of therapy, which peaks in 3 months. Splenic responses are dose dependent, durable through 12 treatment cycles, and limited by concomitant myelosuppression. Splenomegaly quickly returns with cessation of *JAK2* inhibitors either within days for ruxolitnib or within weeks for fedratinib, largely because of their respective half-lives and possibly mode of action. The same three *JAK2* inhibitors improve constitutional symptoms and appear to be durable. Treatment-related anemia is associated more with some JAK1/2 inhibitors (ruxolitnib) than others (momelotinib) and is also associated with some *JAK2* inhibitors (fedratinib).[105]

In contrast, adverse events are dissimilar across the JAK inhibitors. For example, gastrointestinal events occur more often with the *JAK2* inhibitor (fedratinib) and with the non–*JAK2* inhibitor (lestaurtinib), which might be due to the off-target *FLT3* inhibition. Acute relapse of symptoms with drug discontinuation is seen in only one particular JAK1/2 inhibitor (ruxolitnib), which may be due to a "cytokine flare." Lastly, only one of the JAK1/2 inhibitors (momelotinib) produces first-dose symptoms of transient hypotension, flushing, and light-headedness. Future JAK inhibitor treatment may start with an induction dose to maximize response, followed by a maintenance dose with the addition and removal of other therapies tailored to the unique symptoms of each patient. For example, treatment-related myelosuppression could be ameliorated with pomalidomide, androgens, erythropoietin, and transfusions, and constitutional symptoms can also be managed through a host of traditional therapies. Outcomes in PV and ET are not as impressive, and the need to modulate symptoms is not as critical. Nonetheless, the *JAK2* inhibitor fedratinib is most useful because of its ability to normalize leukocytosis and thrombocytosis.[105,146]

INTERCONNECTION AMONG ESSENTIAL THROMBOCYTHEMIA, POLYCYTHEMIA VERA, AND PRIMARY MYELOFIBROSIS

The discovery of the *JAK2* V617F mutation has advanced our understanding of the MPNs but has also raised questions about the interconnection of three of the primary myeloproliferative conditions: ET, PV, and PMF. Why is the *JAK2* mutation found in more than 90% to 95% of patients with PV but in only 50% to 60% of patients with ET and PMF, and how can the same mutation produce three distinct phenotypes?

Currently four hypotheses exist to account for this apparent discordance. One prevailing thought suggests that the resulting phenotype is dependent on the stage of differentiation of the HSC. For example, if the HSC has developed a predilection toward platelet development at the time of the *JAK2* mutation, ET will develop. Reports have described differences in differentiation programs[147,148] and in *JAK2* mutations among ET, PV, and PMF.[149] A second hypothesis proposes that the genetic background of the patient predisposes the patient to a particular phenotype. Mutations in the erythropoietin receptor, thrombopoietin receptor (MPL), and granulocyte colony-stimulating factor receptor have all been implicated.[150] The third hypothesis suggests that the phenotype depends on the level of *JAK2* tyrosine kinase activity, called the *dosage effect*. Patients diagnosed with PV had greater tyrosine kinase activity than patients presenting with an ET phenotype. Experiments in which erythroid progenitors were collected from these patients and tested in colony-forming assays indicated that nearly all the cell cultures developing a PV phenotype were homozygous for the *JAK2* mutation, whereas the ET phenotype was identified in the vast majority of cell cultures expressing a heterozygous genotype.[60,151] This phenomenon was corroborated in experiments with transgenic mice.[152,153] The last hypothesis proposes that a pre-*JAK2* mutation produces a premalignant clone,[154-156] predisposing the HSC to a particular phenotype, and that the *JAK2* mutation drives the malignant transformation. Groups have reported mutations coexisting with the *JAK2* V617F mutation, like *BCR-ABL1*[157,158] *MPL* mutations,[159] and another version of the *JAK2* mutation.[160,161] Familial MPN provides the strongest support for a pre-*JAK2* mutation.[162,163]

The most appealing model includes all the hypotheses previously presented and suggests that ET, PV, and PMF may represent a continuum of diseases. It seems reasonable to assume that a pre-*JAK2* mutation occurs in the HSC most if not all of the time to create a hyperproliferative clone that predisposes to additional mutations like the *JAK2* mutation. The pre-*JAK2* mutation can be familial, congenital, or somatic. Because MPL is expressed in high levels on megakaryocyte precursors, one *JAK2* V617F mutation (heterozygous) is sufficient to induce MPL signaling and thus stimulate megakaryocyte production. This could lead to the ET phenotype. In contrast, the erythropoietin receptor is expressed in low density on the surface of erythroid precursors, which requires the higher amount of *JAK2* V617F tyrosine kinase that is produced by two *JAK2* mutations (homozygous). This could lead to the PV phenotype. Because MPL stimulation begins with the first *JAK2* mutation and continues with the second *JAK2* mutation, the MPL receptor undergoes continuous stimulation. It has been found that excessive thrombopoietin stimulation leads to myelofibrosis, which may result in a progression to PMF.[164] The identification of additional mutations in the *BCR-ABL1*-negative MPNs, including negative regulators of signaling pathways (*LNK*, *c-CBL*,

SOCs), tumor suppressor genes (IZF1, TP53), and epigenetic regulators (TET2, IDH1/2, ASXL1, EZH2) combines to set the disease on a particular course. JAK2 and MPL mutations serve as drivers for the disease, but mutations in the negative regulators of signaling pathways may synergize with the driver mutations. Mutations in the epigenetic regulator genes may be early events that precede JAK2 but can also appear late to promote progression. Tumor suppressor gene mutations tend to occur during phases of disease progression.[53] More than likely, most, if not all, of the hypotheses previously described function together to drive the BCR-ABL1-negative MPNs down a particular phenotype and through the phases of clonal expansion and disease progression.

OTHER MYELOPROLIFERATIVE NEOPLASMS

Chronic Neutrophilic Leukemia

CNL is a clonal disorder in which a hyperproliferation of neutrophilic cells in the BM produces sustained neutrophilia in the peripheral blood and hepatosplenomegaly. CNL must be differentiated from CML, myelodysplasia, a reactive neutrophilic process, and other MPNs.[165] A monocyte count of 1×10^9/L or less and 10% WBCs or less on the differential distinguishes CNL from myelodysplasia and the absence of basophilia and Ph distinguishes CNL from CML. Absence of MPN driver mutations (JAK2, MPL, or CALR) and meeting WHO diagnostic criteria differentiates CNL from other MPNs. The presence of CSF3R T618I or other activating CSF3R mutation and the remaining WHO diagnostic criteria distinguish CNL from reactive neutrophilia. The BM is hypercellular because of increased neutrophilic granulocyte proliferation but dysplasia is absent.[2]

Incidence

The incidence of CNL is not known, but it is a rare disorder of which about 150 cases have been reported. However, if the WHO criteria had been applied in these cases, many might have been reclassified as reactive rather than neoplastic conditions.[165] The median age at diagnosis is 67 years and men and women are equally affected.

Clinical Presentation

At the time of diagnosis most patients are asymptomatic, but fatigue, weight loss, easy bruising, bone pain, and night sweats can occur. Hepatosplenomegaly is the most common finding, but 25% to 30% of patients report bleeding from mucocutaneous sites like the gastrointestinal tract. Other symptoms include gout from WBC turnover and pruritus that may be associated with neutrophil infiltration of tissues and organs.[165]

Peripheral Blood and Bone Marrow

Patients have a WBC count of more than 25×10^9/L (WHO criteria) with a slight left shift. Neutrophils dominate (>80%, WHO criteria), but the increase in bands, metamyelocytes, myelocytes, and promyelocytes in combination usually comprise fewer than 5% of WBCs but can be as many as 10%. Neutrophils do not appear dysplastic, but they often contain toxic granules. RBC count and platelet morphology are normal in the peripheral blood. Thrombocytopenia can develop as the disease progresses largely because of splenomegaly.[165]

The BM reflects the peripheral blood in that it is hypercellular with predominantly a proliferation of neutrophils, including myelocytes, metamyelocytes, bands, and segmented neutrophils. The myeloid-to-erythroid ratio is at least 20:1. RBCs and platelets are normal in number, and no cell line exhibits significant dysplastic morphology.[165]

Diagnosis

WHO criteria requires that the WBC count must be greater than 25×10^9/L, with greater than 90% mature neutrophils (bands and segmented neutrophils), fewer than 10% immature neutrophilic cells, and rare blasts in the peripheral blood. The monocyte count must be less than 1×10^9/L, with no dysgranulopoiesis observed. The BM is hypercellular with an increase in normal-appearing neutrophilic cells with fewer than 5% myeloblasts (WHO criteria). Megakaryocytes are normal or slightly left shifted. Splenomegaly must be present and is often accompanied by hepatomegaly. Reactive neutrophilia must be excluded by eliminating infection, inflammation, and tumors as a cause of the neutrophilia. A diagnosis of CNL can still be made in the presence of a reactive process if clonality of the myeloid line can be documented by karyotyping or molecular analysis. There must be no evidence of the Philadelphia chromosome, BCR-ABL1 mutation, or rearrangements of the PDGFRA, PDGFRB, FGRF1, or PCM1-JAK2 genes. The CSF3R T618I or other activating CSF3R mutation must be present. In the rare instance where the CSF3R T618I is absent, the following must be present: persistent neutrophilia for 3 months; splenomegaly; and no identifiable cause of reactive neutrophilia, including the presence of a plasma cell neoplasm or demonstration of clonality of myeloid cells by cytogenetic or molecular studies.[7] Lastly, there can be no evidence of PV, PMF, ET, MDS, or MDS/MPN disorders.[165]

Genetics

Approximately 90% of CNL patients have a normal karyotype, but chromosomal abnormalities are identified, particularly as the disease progresses, including +8, +9, +21, del(20q), del(11q), and del(12p). The Philadelphia chromosome or a BCR-ABL1 mutation cannot be expressed in CNL; otherwise, a diagnosis of CML is required. JAK2 mutations have been identified, but rarely.[165] As stated earlier, there must be no rearrangements of the PDGFRA, PDGFRB, FGRF1, or PCM1-JAK2 genes, and the CSF3R T618I mutation or other activating CSF3R mutation should be present.

Therapy

First-line therapy for CNL is hydroxyurea followed by α-interferon for treatment failures. Therapeutic responses generally last about 12 months. The only curative treatment is allogeneic stem cell transplant for those who qualify.

Prognosis

CNL is a slow, smoldering condition, and patient survival ranges from as short as 6 months to longer than 20 years.

Median survival is 2 years. CNL progresses to an accelerated phase that exhibits progressive neutrophilia, anemia, thrombocytopenia, and splenomegaly that are unresponsive to treatment.[166] Blasts and other immature cells can be present in the peripheral blood, and some patients develop myelodysplasia that can transform into AML.[165]

Chronic Eosinophilic Leukemia, Not Otherwise Specified

Chronic eosinophilic leukemia (CEL) is a clonal proliferation of eosinophils from eosinophil precursors that dominate in the BM and peripheral blood. Eosinophils are found in other peripheral tissues, including heart, lungs, central nervous system, gastrointestinal tract, and skin. Hepatosplenomegaly occurs in approximately 30% to 50% of patients. Infiltrating eosinophils degranulate to release cytokines, enzymes, and other granular proteins that damage the surrounding tissue, which results in organ dysfunction.[167]

Clinical Presentation

Although some patients may be asymptomatic when found to have eosinophilia, most have signs and symptoms of fever, fatigue, cough, angioedema, muscle pain, and pruritus. A more severe sequela of CEL involves the heart. Fibrosis can form in the heart (endomyocardial fibrosis), which can evolve into cardiomegaly. Within the heart, scar tissue may form in the mitral and tricuspid valves, affecting valve function and predisposing to thrombi formation. Other serious complications include peripheral neuropathy, central nervous system dysfunction, pulmonary symptoms from eosinophilic infiltrates, and rheumatologic problems.[167]

Peripheral Blood and Bone Marrow

Peripheral eosinophilia must be observed, with the majority of eosinophils appearing normal. Some evidence of eosinophil abnormality is found, however, and includes the presence of eosinophilic myelocytes and metamyelocytes, hypogranulation, and vacuolization. Neutrophilia is a common finding; other features such as mild monocytosis, basophilia, and the presence of blasts are less common. The BM is hypercellular because of eosinophilic proliferation and can demonstrate Charcot-Leyden crystals. Myeloblast numbers are elevated but less than the 20% threshold necessary to classify the disorder as an AL. Erythrocytes and megakaryocytes are normal in number but sometimes demonstrate dysplastic morphologic features. BM fibrosis occurs as a result of the release of eosinophilic basic protein and eosinophilic cationic proteins from the eosinophil granules. BM fibrosis contributes to the premature release of eosinophils into the circulation, and they deposit in a variety of tissues.[167]

Diagnosis

The diagnosis of CEL-NOS requires eosinophilia with a count of more than 1.5×10^9 cells/L and the presence of malignant features and the elimination of reactive eosinophilia and other malignancies that have concomitant eosinophilia. Reactive conditions like parasitic infections, allergies, Loeffler syndrome (pulmonary disease), cyclical eosinophilia, angiolymphoid hyperplasia of the skin, collagen vascular disorders, and Kimura disease must be excluded in the differential diagnosis. Likewise, other malignancies that can produce a concomitant eosinophilia include T cell lymphoma, Hodgkin lymphoma, systemic mastocytosis, chronic myelomonocytic leukemia, atypical CML, and ALL. These disorders lead to the release of a variety of interleukins that can drive a secondary eosinophil reaction. No single genetic abnormality is specific for CEL-NOS, but the diagnosis requires myeloblasts in the blood (1% to 2%) or an increase in myeloblasts the BM (>5%) and/or nonspecific cytogenetic abnormalities such as trisomy 8, isochromosome 17[i(17q)], or rearrangements of *JAK2*, *ABL1*, and *FLT3*. This criteria excludes *PCM1-JAK2* that is observed in the group of disorders called myeloid/lymphoid neoplasms with eosinophilia and rearrangement of *PDGFRA*, *PDGFRB*, or *FGFR1* or with *PCM1-JAK2*, which will be discussed next.[168]

Treatment

No standard of care has been established for patients with CEL-NOS. Hydroxyurea can be used to control leukocytosis, eosinophilia, and splenomegaly and α-interferon has been used for refractory patients producing hematologic and cytogenetic remissions in some patients. Allogeneic HSC transplantation has produced long-term remission in a few patients.

Prognosis

Survival is variable, but the prognosis is considered poor. In a small case series of 10 participants with CEL-NOS, the median survival was 22 months, with 50% transforming to AML.[168] Features of dysplasia, an increase in karyotype abnormalities, or an increase in blasts indicates an unfavorable prognosis.[167]

Myeloid/Lymphoid Neoplasms with Eosinophilia and Rearrangement of PDGFRA, PDGFRB, or FGFR1 or with PCM1-JAK2

Myeloid/lymphoid neoplasms with eosinophilia and rearrangement of *PDGFRA*, *PDGFRB*, or *FGFR1* or with *PCM1-JAK2* were segregated into their own category for three primary reasons: (1) Each disorder has as underlying neoplasm of either the myeloid or lymphoid type; (2) these conditions usually have an associated eosinophilia; (3) the mutations listed result in a constitutive activation of a tyrosine kinase and respond to tyrosine kinase inhibitors like imatinib and ponatinib.[168]

The most common mutation involving *PDGFRA* is a fusion gene involving *FIP1L1-PDGFRA*, which occurs more often in men. This fusion gene and most of the other *PDGFRA* rearrangements respond well to imatinib. Most patients achieve complete hematologic remission and complete molecular remission on imatinib therapy. Imatinib resistance is rare, but when it does occur it is usually attributed to a specific mutation (T674I) that occurs in the ATP binding site of *PDGFRA* similar to the T315I mutation in the *BCR-ABL1* fusion gene. Discontinuation of imatinib therapy has been investigated with some patients relapsing and others maintaining a durable remission.[168]

Although more than 30 distinct fusion genes have been identified with *PDGFRB*, the most common rearrangement is *ETV6-PDGFRB*. Like the fusion genes associated with *PDGFRA*, those involving *PDGFRB* are also sensitive to imatinib and consistently produce complete hematologic remission. Eosinophilia is common but not required and many patients express features that resemble CMML, atypical CML, juvenile CML or, rarely, AML. Long-term remissions are common and loss of complete hematologic or molecular remission has yet to occur.[168]

Fourteen different fusion genes have been associated with *FGFR1*, with t(8;13), t(8;9), and t(6;8) being the most common. Patients present with a myeloproliferative syndrome with variable eosinophilia or with a leukemia/lymphoma picture. The t(8;13) fusion gene is associated with a high incidence of T-lymphoblastic lymphoma transformation. The t(8;9) and t(6;8) fusion genes are often associated with features of CMML, whereas other times the t(6;8) mutation resembles a PV phenotype without eosinophilia. The clinical course is more aggressive and not responsive to imatinib, nilotinib, or dasatinib with minimal response to ponatinib. Chemotherapy did not produce sustained complete remission, leaving allogeneic HSC transplant as the only treatment with the potential for long-term remission or cure.[168]

In 2016 the WHO group proposed to add the *PCM1-JAK2* fusion gene, t(8;9), to this category of disease. Two other less common rearrangements have been described involving *ETV6-JAK2*, t(9;12), and *BCR-JAK2*, t(9;9). Patients present with features of a chronic myeloid neoplasm with either eosinophilia or BM fibrosis 50% to 70% of the time. The clinical course is aggressive, with rapid transformation to AML or occasionally ALL. Treatment with ruxolitinib has produced complete hematologic remission, but it is usually short lived, with relapse occurring after 18 to 24 months. Like the *FGFR1* rearrangements, allogeneic stem cell transplantation offers the best hope of long-term survival and potential for cure in patients with the *PCM1-JAK2* fusion gene.[168]

Idiopathic hypereosinophilic syndrome is a diagnosis reserved for patients with eosinophilia who do not meet the diagnostic criteria for a reactive process; myeloid or lymphoid neoplasms with eosinophilia (*PDGFRA, PDGFRB, FGFR1,* or *PCM1-JAK2* negative); CML (*BCR-ABL1* negative); chronic mastocytosis (*KIT* D816V negative), AML (blasts >20% and inv[16], t(16;16), *CBFB-MYH11* negative); chronic eosinophilic leukemia, not otherwise specified (see previous criteria); or lymphocyte-variant hypereosinophilia (abnormal cytokine-producing T cells).[168]

Mastocytosis

Mastocytosis is no longer considered a subgroup of the MPNs but will still be discussed in this chapter. Mastocytosis is a heterogeneous group of disorders caused by a clonal neoplastic proliferation of mast cells (MCs), which accumulate in one or more organ systems, but it can present differently and manifest in a range of severities. The WHO group has classified mastocytosis into three subcategories: cutaneous mastocytosis (CM), systemic mastocytosis (SM), and localized MC tumors.[169]

Incidence

Mastocytosis can occur at any age, with CM seen most often in children. Babies can be born with cutaneous mastocytosis, and half of affected children develop the disease before 6 months of age. In contrast, SM generally occurs after the second decade of life. Approximately 80% of patients with mastocytosis have skin involvement regardless of the type of mastocytosis diagnosed. CM occurs in the skin; SM usually involves the BM and other organ systems like the spleen, lymph nodes, liver, and gastrointestinal tract; and MC leukemia is characterized by MCs in the peripheral blood.[170]

Clinical Presentation

Patients present with urticarial lesions (wheel and flare) that may become activated when stroked on physical examination. Skin lesions also tend to have melanin pigmentation. Four categories of symptom severity have been described in mastocytosis: constitutional systems like fatigue and weight loss; skin manifestations; mediator-related systemic events such as abdominal pain, gastrointestinal distress, headache, and respiratory symptoms; and musculoskeletal complaints like bone pain, arthralgias, and myalgias. Hematologic findings include anemia, leukocytosis, eosinophilia, neutropenia, and thrombocytopenia. In patients with SM with associated clonal hematologic non–mast-cell-lineage disease, the most common associated hematologic finding is chronic myelomonocytic leukemia, but any myeloid or lymphoid malignancy can occur, although myeloid versions predominate.[170]

Diagnosis

The typical skin lesion is the first diagnostic clue to mastocytosis. CM occurs in three forms: macropapular CM (also known as urticaria pigmentosa), diffuse cutaneous mastocytosis, and localized mastocytosis of the skin, all of which occur predominantly in children. In macropapular CM (urticaria pigmentosa), MCs are confined to the skin and form aggregates in the dermis, whereas in diffuse cutaneous mastocytosis, MCs are found in more than one cutaneous location. CM is usually found in children and has a good prognosis often resulting in natural lesion disappearance during puberty. In contrast, SM often develops in adults and MCs are identified in various internal organs and in the bone marrow. To establish a diagnosis of SM either one major and one minor criterion are met or three minor criteria are fulfilled. Major criteria involves multifocal dense infiltrates of MCs (≥15 MCs in aggregates) in BM biopsy specimens and/or in sections of other extracutaneous organs. Minor criteria include the following: (1) More than 25% of MCs are atypical cells (type I or type II) on BM smears or are spindle-shaped in MC infiltrates detected on sections of visceral organs; (2) MCs must express a *KIT* mutation at codon 816 in the BM or other extracutaneous organ; (3) MCs in BM, blood, or extracutaneous organs must express CD2 and/or CD25; and (4) total serum tryptase must be greater than 20 ng/mL. Key diagnostic features distinguish the five types of systemic mastocytosis: indolent systemic mastocytosis (ISM); smoldering systemic mastocytosis (SSM); systemic mastocytosis with an associated hematologic (non-MC lineage) neoplasm

(SM-AHN), aggressive systemic mastocytosis (ASM); and mast cell leukemia (MCL). ISM is characterized by a low MC burden. SSM is new to the 2016 WHO classification and exhibits a prognosis that is less favorable than ISM but more favorable than ASM or MCL.[169] SM-AHM presents with myelodysplastic syndrome, MPN, AML, lymphoma, or another hematopoietic neoplasm. ASM usually does not manifest with skin lesions or MCs in circulation but does have MCs in bone marrow, dysplastic hematopoietic changes, and/or hepatosplenomegaly. ASM has been subdivided into two variants: untransformed variant and variant in transformation (ASM-t) in which BM MCs are between 5% to 20%. MCL is characterized by more than 20% atypical MCs in the bone marrow. MCL is subdivided into two types: classical MCL, where more than 10% MCs are found in the peripheral blood; and aleukemic MCL, in which less than 10% MCs are found in the peripheral blood. Recently it has been proposed to further subdivide MCL leukemia into acute MCL (with organ damage) and chronic MCL (without organ damage).[169] MC sarcoma presents as a single unifocal MC tumor with high-grade pathologic characteristics. Extracutaneous mastocytoma also exhibits a unifocal MC tumor, but it is pathologically low grade.[170] A provisional subentity of SM termed bone marrow mastocytosis is being discussed and presents with no skin lesions, a low MC burden, and a good prognosis. Concurrently, extracutaneous mastocytoma was removed from the classification system because of its rarity.[169]

Genetics

The most common genetic mutation in patients with mastocytosis involves codon 816 in the *KIT* gene and occurs in about 95% of adults and 33% of children with systemic mastocytosis. This mutation replaces aspartic acid with valine, which alters the tyrosine kinase receptor activity so as to cause constitutive kinase activity in the absence of ligand. Usually the mutation is somatic, but a few cases of familial *KIT* mutations have been reported. Additional mutations can push proliferation of hematopoietic clones, causing SM with associated clonal hematologic non–mast-cell-lineage disease. These include mutations of *RUNX1/RUNX1T* in AML, *JAK1* in MPN, and *FIP1L1/PDGFRA* in myeloid neoplasms with eosinophilia.[170]

Prognosis

CM in children has a favorable prognosis and may regress spontaneously around puberty. Milder versions like CM and indolent CM follow a benign course and are associated with a normal life span. Hematologic involvement usually evolves into the corresponding hematologic disease. Patients with aggressive systemic mastocytosis, mast cell leukemia, and mast cell sarcoma are often treated with cytoreductive chemotherapy but may survive only a few months after diagnosis. Signs and symptoms that predict a poorer prognosis include elevated lactate dehydrogenase and alkaline phosphatase, anemia, thrombocythemia, abnormal peripheral blood morphology, BM hypercellularity, and hepatosplenomegaly.[170]

Myeloproliferative Neoplasm, Unclassifiable

The category *myeloproliferative neoplasm, unclassifiable* is designed to capture disorders that clearly express myeloproliferative features but either fail to meet the criteria of a specific condition or have features that overlap two or more specific conditions. Most patients with MPN-U fall into one of three groups: patients with an early stage of PV, ET, or PMF in which the criteria that define the disorders are not yet fully developed; patients presenting with features indicative of advanced disease resulting from clonal evolution that masks the potential underlying condition; and patients who have clear evidence of an MPN but who have a concomitant condition like a second neoplasm or an inflammatory condition that alters the MPN features. MPN-U may account for as many as 10% to 15% of MPN disorders, but caution should be exercised so that morphologic changes caused by the patient's cytotoxic drug therapy or growth factor therapy or poor collection of samples are not confused with the features of MPN-U. In patients with MPN-U in the early stages of development or with a concomitant disorder like inflammation, the MPN-U may be reclassified to a specific category of MPN once the disease begins to express typical features or the secondary condition subsides. Likewise, in patients with an advanced MPN, the disorder may be reclassified as an AL once the blast criterion of more than 20% blasts in the BM is met.[171]

SUMMARY

- Myeloproliferative neoplasms (MPNs) are clonal hematopoietic stem cell disorders that result in excessive production and overaccumulation of erythrocytes, granulocytes, and platelets in some combination in bone marrow, peripheral blood, and body tissues.
- Within the classification of MPN, the four major conditions are chronic myeloid leukemia (CML), polycythemia vera (PV), essential thrombocytopenia (ET), and primary myelofibrosis (PMF).
- In CML there are large numbers of myeloid precursors in the bone marrow, peripheral blood, and extramedullary tissues.

- The peripheral blood exhibits leukocytosis with increased myeloid series, particularly the later maturation stages, often with increases in eosinophils and basophils.
- The leukocyte alkaline phosphatase (LAP) score is dramatically decreased in CML.
- The Philadelphia chromosome, t(9;22), either at the chromosomal or molecular level *BCR-ABL1*, must be present in all cases of CML.
- In CML the bone marrow (BM) exhibits intense hypercellularity with a predominance of myeloid precursors. Megakaryocyte numbers are normal to increased.

- Patients with CML can progress from a chronic stable phase through an accelerated phase into transformation to acute leukemia.
- BM transplantation has been successful in CML, and imatinib mesylate, a tyrosine kinase inhibitor, produces remission in most cases.
- Approximately 4% of CML patients given imatinib as first-line therapy develop imatinib resistance.
- Dosage escalation or administration of second- or third-generation tyrosine kinase inhibitors restores remission in most patients with imatinib resistance, except those with the T315I mutation.
- PV manifests with panmyelosis in the BM with increases in erythrocytes, granulocytes, and platelets.
- Based on the World Health Organization (WHO) standards, the diagnosis of PV requires that three major criteria and one minor criterion be met or that the patient meet the previous higher hemoglobin level of 18.5 g/dL in men but not the BM criteria. The clinical diagnosis of PV requires a hemoglobin of greater than 16.5 g/dL in men and women (or elevated hematocrit or elevated red cell mass—major criteria 1); BM hypercellularity and panmyelosis (major criteria 2); and the presence of *JAK2* V617F or another mutation in the *JAK2* gene. The one minor criteria is low serum erythropoietin levels.
- The *JAK2* V617F mutation is found in 95% of PV patients and contributes to the pathogenesis of the disease.
- PV is currently treated with phlebotomy, hydroxyurea, and low-dose aspirin; and in the future *JAK2* inhibitors will be a treatment alternative.
- ET involves an increase in megakaryocytes with a sustained platelet count greater than 400×10^9/L.
- Other diagnostic criteria include normal red blood cell (RBC) mass, stainable iron in the bone marrow, absence of the Philadelphia chromosome, lack of marrow collagen fibrosis, absence of splenomegaly or leukoerythroblastic reaction, and absence of any known cause of reactive thrombocytosis.

- In the early phases of ET, peripheral blood shows increased numbers of platelets with abnormalities in size and shape. BM megakaryocytes are increased in number and in size.
- Complications of ET include thromboembolism and hemorrhage.
- The *JAK2* V617F mutation is observed in 50% to 60% of patients with ET and PMF and contributes to the pathogenesis of the disorders.
- PMF manifests with ineffective hematopoiesis, sparse areas of marrow hypercellularity (especially with increased megakaryocytes), BM fibrosis, splenomegaly, and hepatomegaly.
- The peripheral blood in PMF exhibits immature granulocytes and nucleated RBCs; teardrop-shaped cells are a common finding.
- Platelets may be normal, increased, or decreased in number with abnormal morphology. Micromegakaryocytes may be present.
- Immune responses are altered in about 50% of patients.
- Treatment of PMF includes a variety of approaches, including transfusions, hydroxyurea, interferon-γ, busulfan, androgens, erythropoietin, and others.
- JAK inhibitors improve splenomegaly and constitutional symptoms in patients with PMF to a greater degree than in ET or PV.
- Other MPNs include chronic neutrophilic leukemia (CNL); chronic eosinophilic leukemia, not otherwise specified (CEL-NOS); myeloid/lymphoid neoplasms with eosinophilia and rearrangement of *PDGFRA*, *PDGFRB*, or *FGFR1* or with *PCM1-JAK2*; and unclassifiable MPN.
- Mastocytosis is no longer considered an MPN and is divided into three subcategories: cutaneous mastocytosis (CM), systemic mastocytosis (SM), and localized mast cell tumors.

Now that you have completed this chapter, go back and read again the case study at the beginning and respond to the questions presented.

REVIEW QUESTIONS

Answers can be found in the Appendix.

1. A peripheral blood film that shows increased neutrophils, basophils, eosinophils, and platelets is highly suggestive of:
   a. AML
   b. CML
   c. MDS
   d. Multiple myeloma

2. Which of the following chromosome abnormalities is associated with CML?
   a. t(15;17)
   b. t(8;14)
   c. t(9;22)
   d. Monosomy 7

3. A patient has a WBC count of 30×10^9/L and the following WBC differential:
   Segmented neutrophils—38%
   Bands—17%
   Metamyelocytes—7%
   Myelocytes—20%
   Promyelocytes—10%
   Eosinophils—3%
   Basophils—5%
   Which of the following test results would be helpful in determining whether the patient has CML?
   a. Nitroblue tetrazolium reduction product increased
   b. Myeloperoxidase increased
   c. Periodic acid–Schiff staining decreased
   d. FISH positive for *BCR-ABL1* fusion

4. A patient in whom CML has previously been diagnosed has circulating blasts and promyelocytes that total 30% of leukocytes. The disease is considered to be in what phase?
   a. Chronic stable phase
   b. Accelerated phase
   c. Transformation to acute leukemia
   d. Temporary remission

5. The most common mutation found in patients with primary PV is:
   a. *BCR-ABL1*
   b. Philadelphia chromosome
   c. *JAK2* V617F
   d. t(15;17)

6. The peripheral blood in PV typically manifests:
   a. Erythrocytosis only
   b. Erythrocytosis and thrombocytopenia
   c. Erythrocytosis, thrombocytosis, and granulocytosis
   d. Anemia and thrombocytopenia

7. A patient has a platelet count of 700×10^9 /L with abnormalities in the size, shape, and granularity of platelets; a WBC count of 12×10^9 /L; and hemoglobin of 11 g/dL. The Philadelphia chromosome is not present. The most likely diagnosis is:
   a. PV
   b. ET
   c. CML
   d. Leukemoid reaction

8. Complications of ET include all of the following *except*:
   a. Thrombosis
   b. Hemorrhage
   c. Seizures
   d. Infections

9. Which of the following patterns is characteristic of the peripheral blood in patients with PMF?
   a. Teardrop-shaped erythrocytes, nucleated RBCs, immature granulocytes
   b. Abnormal platelets only
   c. Hypochromic erythrocytes, immature granulocytes, and normal platelets
   d. Spherocytes, immature granulocytes, and increased numbers of platelets

10. The myelofibrosis associated with PMF is a result of:
    a. Apoptosis resistance in the fibroblasts of the bone marrow
    b. Impaired production of normal collagenase by the mutated cells
    c. Enhanced activity of fibroblasts as a result of increased stimulatory cytokines
    d. Increased numbers of fibroblasts as a result of cytokine stimulation of the pluripotential stem cells

REFERENCES

1. Delhommeau, F., Pisani, D. F., James, C., et al. (2006). Oncogenic mechanisms in myeloproliferative disorders. *Cell Mol Life Sci, 63*(24), 2939–2953.
2. Campbell, P. J., & Green, A. R. (2006). The myeloproliferative disorders. *N Engl J Med, 355*(23), 2452–2466.
3. Schmitt-Graeff, A. H., Nitschke, R., & Zeiser, R. (2015). The hematopoietic niche in myeloproliferative neoplasms. *Mediators Inflamm*, http://dx.doi.org/10.1155/2015/347270. Accessed January 23, 2019.
4. Hasselbalch, H. C., & Bjorn, M. E. (2015). MPNs as inflammatory diseases: the evidence, consequences, and perspectives. *Mediators Inflamm*, http://dx.doi.org/10.1155/2015/102476. Accessed January 23, 2019.
5. Hermouet, S., Bigot-Corbel, E., & Gardie, B. (2015). Pathogenesis of myeloproliferative neoplasms: role and mechanisms of chronic inflammation. *Mediators Inflamm*, http://dx.doi.org/10.1155/2015/145293.Accessed January 23, 2019.
6. Dameshek, W. (1951). Some speculations on the myeloproliferative syndromes. *Blood, 6*, 372.
7. Arber, D., Orazi, A., Hasserjian, R., et al. (2016). The 2016 revision to the World Health Organization classification of myeloid neoplasms and acute leukemia. *Blood. 127*, 2391–2405.
8. Gilbert, H. S. (1998). Familial myeloproliferative disease. *Ballieres Clin Haematol, 11*, 849–858.
9. Barr, R. D., & Fialkow, P. J. (1973). Clonal origin of chronic myelocytic leukemia. *N Engl J Med, 289*, 307–309.
10. Bizzozzero, O. J., Johnson, K. G., & Ciocco, A. (1966). Radiation-related leukemia in Hiroshima and Nagasaki, 1946-1964: I. Distribution, incidence, and appearance time. *N Engl J Med, 274*, 1095–1101.
11. Brown, W. M., & Doll, R. (1965). Mortality from cancer and other causes after radiotherapy for ankylosing spondylitis. *BMJ, 5474*, 1327–1332.
12. Marmont, A., Frassoni, F., Bacigalupo, A., et al. (1984). Recurrence of Ph¹-positive leukemia in donor cells after marrow transplantation for chronic granulocytic leukemia. *N Engl J Med, 310*, 903–906.
13. Nowell, P., & Hungerford, D. A. (1960). A minute chromosome in human granulocytic leukemia. *Science, 132*, 1497–1499.
14. Rowley, J. D. (1973). A new consistent chromosome abnormality in chronic myelogenous leukemia identified by quinacrine fluorescence and Giemsa banding. *Nature, 243*, 290–293.
15. Stam, K., Heisterkamp, N., Grosveld, G., et al. (1985). Evidence of a new chimeric bcr/c-abl mRNA in patients with chronic myelocytic leukemia and the Philadelphia chromosome. *N Engl J Med, 313*, 1429–1433.
16. Groffen, J., Stephenson, J. R., Heisterkamp, N., et al. (1984). Philadelphia chromosomal breakpoints are clustered within a limited region, bcr, on chromosome 22. *Cell, 36*(1), 93–99.
17. Randolph, T. R. (2005). Chronic myelocytic leukemia part I: history, clinical presentation, and molecular biology. *Clin Lab Sci, 18*(1), 38–48.
18. Faderl, S., Talpaz, M., Estrov, Z., et al. (1999). Mechanisms of disease: the biology of chronic myeloid leukemia. *N Engl J Med, 341*(3), 164–172.
19. Epner, D. E., & Koeffler, H. P. (1990). Molecular genetic advances in chronic myelogenous leukemia. *Ann Intern Med, 113*, 3–6.
20. Douer, D., Levine, A. M., Sparkes, R. S., et al. (1981). Chronic myelocytic leukemia: a pluripotent haemopoietic cell is involved in the malignant clone. *Br J Haematol, 49*, 615–619.

21. Bhatia, R., & Verfaillie, C. M. (1998). The effects of interferon-alpha on beta-1 integrin mediated adhesion and growth regulation in chronic myelogenous leukemia. *Leuk Lymphoma, 28,* 241–254.

22. Georgii, A., Buesche, G., & Krept, A. (1998). The histopathology of chronic myeloproliferative disorders: review. *Ballieres Clin Haematol, 11,* 721–749.

23. Lichtman, M. A., & Rowe, J. M. (1982). Hyperleukocytic leukemias: rheological, clinical and therapeutic considerations. *Blood, 60,* 279–283.

24. Lichtman, M. A., Heal, J., & Rowe, J. M. (1987). Hyperleukocytic leukemia. *Ballieres Clin Haematol, 1,* 725–746.

25. Muehleck, S. D., McKenna, R. D., Arthur, D. C., et al. (1984). Transformation of chronic myelogenous leukemia: clinical, morphologic and cytogenetic features. *Am J Clin Pathol, 82,* 1–14.

26. Vardiman, J. W., Melo, J. V., Baccarani, M., et al. (2008). Chronic myelogenous leukemia. BCR-ABL1 positive. In Swerdlow, S. H., Campo, E., Harris, N. L., et al. (Eds.), *WHO Classification of Tumours of Haematopoietic and Lymphoid Tissues.* (4th ed., pp. 32–37). Lyon, France: IARC Press.

27. Bernstein, R. (1988). Cytogenetics of chronic myelogenous leukemia. *Semin Hematol, 25,* 20–34.

28. Sandberg, A. A. (1978). Chromosomes in the chronic phase of CML. *Virchows Arch B Cell Pathol, 29,* 51–55.

29. Bareford, D., & Jacobs, P. (1980). Chronic neutrophilic leukemia. *Am J Clin Pathol, 73,* 837.

30. Bearman, R. M., Kjeldsburg, C. R., Pangalis, G. A., et al. (1981). Chronic monocytic leukemia in adults. *Cancer, 48,* 2239–2255.

31. Thomas, W. J., North, R. B., Poplack, D. G., et al. (1981). Chronic myelomonocytic leukemia in childhood. *Am J Hematol, 10,* 181–194.

32. Wintrobe, M. M., Huguley, C. M., McLennan, M. T., et al. (1947). Nitrogen mustard as a therapeutic agent for Hodgkin's disease, lymphosarcoma and leukemia. *Ann Intern Med, 27,* 529–539.

33. Galton, D. A. (1953). The use of myleran in chronic myeloid leukemia: results of treatment. *Lancet, 264,* 208–213.

34. Lion, T., Gaiger, A., Henn, T., et al. (1995). Use of quantitative polymerase chain reaction to monitor residual disease in chronic myelogenous leukemia during treatment with interferon. *Leukemia, 9,* 1353–1360.

35. Guilhot, F., Chastang, C., Michallet, M., et al. (1997). Interferon alpha 2b combined with cytarabine versus interferon alone in chronic myelogenous leukemia. *N Engl J Med, 337,* 223–229.

36. O'Brien, S. G. (1997). Autografting for chronic myeloid leukemia. *Baillieres Clin Haematol, 10,* 369–388.

37. Atwell, S., Adams, J. M., Badger, J., et al. (2004). A novel mode of Gleevec binding is revealed by the structure of spleen tyrosine kinase. *J Biol Chem, 279*(53), 55827–55832.

38. Green, M. R., Newton, M. D., & Fancher, K. M. (2016). Off-target effects of BCR-ABL and JAK2 inhibitors. *Am J Clin Oncol, 39,* 76–84.

39. Druker, B. J., Talpaz, M., Resta, D. J., et al. (2001). Efficacy and safety of a specific inhibitor of the BCR-ABL tyrosine kinase in chronic myeloid leukemia. *N Engl J Med, 344,* 1031–1037.

40. Lin, F., Drummond, M., O'Brien, S., et al. (2003). Molecular monitoring in chronic myeloid leukemia patients who achieve complete remission on imatinib. *Blood, 102,* 1143.

41. Bhamidipati, P. K., Kantarjian, H., Cortex, J., et al. (2013). Management of imatinib-resistant patients with chronic myeloid leukemia. *Ther Adv Hem, 4*(2), 103–117.

42. Nardi, A., Azam, M., & Daley, G. O. (2004). Mechanisms and implications of imatinib resistance mutations in BCR-ABL. *Curr Opin Hematol, 11,* 35–43.

43. Kantarjian, H. M., Talpaz, M., Giles, F., et al. (2006). New insights into the pathophysiology of chronic myeloid leukemia and imatinib resistance. *Ann Intern Med, 145,* 913–923.

44. Narayanan, V., Pollyea, D. A., Gutman, J. A., et al. (2013). Ponatinib for the treatment of chronic myeloid leukemia and Philadelphia chromosome-positive acute lymphoblastic leukemia. *Drugs Today, 49*(4), 261–269.

45. Gilliland, D. G., Blanchard, K. L., Levy, J., et al. (1991). Clonality in myeloproliferative disorders: analysis by means of the po-lymerase chain reaction. *Proc Natl Acad Sci U S A, 88,* 6848–6852.

46. Tefferi, A., & Barbui, T. (2017). Polycythemia vera and essential thrombocythemia: 2017 update on diagnosis, risk-stratification, and management. *Am J Hematol, 92*(1), 95–108.

47. Prchal, J. F., Adamson, J. W., Murphy, S., et al. (1978). Polycythemia vera: the in vitro response of normal and abnormal stem cell lines to erythropoietin. *J Clin Invest, 61,* 1044–1047.

48. Adamson, J. W., Singer, J. W., Catalano, P., et al. (1980). Polycythemia vera: further in vitro studies of hematopoietic regulation. *J Clin Invest, 66,* 1363–1368.

49. Beer, P. A., & Green, A. R. (2016). Essential thrombocythemia. In Kaushansky, K., Lichtman, M. A., Prchal, J. T., et al. (Eds.), *Williams Hematology.* (9th ed., pp. 1307–1318). New York: McGraw-Hill.

50. Tefferi, A., Thiele, J., & Vardiman, J. W. (2009). The World Health Organization classification system for myeloproliferative neoplasms: order out of chaos. *Cancer, 115*(17), 3842–3847.

51. Kralovicics, R., Guan, Y., & Prchal, J. T. (2002). Acquired uniparental disomy of chromosome 9p is a frequent stem cell defect in polycythemia vera. *Exp Hematol, 30*(3), 229–236.

52. Wahab-Abdel, O. (2011). Genetics of the myeloproliferative neoplasms. *Curr Opin Hematol, 18,* 117–123.

53. Vainchenker, W., Delhommeau, F., Constantinescu, S. N., et al. (2011). New mutations and pathogenesis of myeloproliferative neoplasms. *Blood, 118*(7), 1723–1735.

54. James, C., Ugo, V., Le Couedic, J. P., et al. (2005). A unique clonal JAK2 mutation leading to constitutive signalling causes polycythemia vera. *Nature, 434,* 1144–1148.

55. Baxter, E. J., Scott, L. M., Campbell, P. J., et al. (2005). Acquired mutation of the tyrosine kinase JAK2 in human myeloproliferative disorders. *Lancet, 365,* 1054–1061.

56. Levine, R. L., Wadleigh, M., Cools, J., et al. (2005). Activating mutation in the tyrosine kinase JAK2 in polycythemia vera, essential thrombocythemia, and myeloid metaplasia with myelofibrosis. *Cancer Cell, 7,* 387–397.

57. Shi, S., Calhgoun, H. C., Xai, F., et al. (2006). JAK signaling globally counteracts heterochromatic gene silencing. *Nat Genet, 38*(9), 1071–1076.

58. Shi, S., Larson, K., Guo, D., et al. (2008). Drosophila STAT is required for directly maintaining HP1localization and heterochromatin stability. *Nat Cell Biol, 10*(4), 489–496.

59. Liu, F., Zhao, X., Pema, F., et al. (2011). JAK2V617F-mediated phosphorylation of PRMT5 downregulates its methyltransferase activity and promotes myeloproliferation. *Cancer Cell, 19*(2), 283–294.

60. Dupont, S., Masse, A., & James, C., et al. (2007). The JAK2 617 V>F mutation triggers erythrocyte hypersensitivity and terminal erythroid amplification in primary erythroid cells from patients with polycythemia vera. *Blood, 110,* 1013–1021.

61. Pikman, Y., Lee, B. H., Mercher, T., et al. (2006). MPLW515L is a novel somatic activating mutation in myelofibrosis with myeloid metaplasia. *PLoS Med, 3,* e270.

62. Beer, P. A., Campbell, P. J., Scott, L. M., et al. (2008). MPL mutations in myeloproliferative disorders; analysis of the PT-1 cohort. *Blood, 112*(1), 141–149.

63. Boyd, E. M., Bench, A. J., Goday-Fernandez, A., et al. (2010). Clinical utility of routing MPL exon 10 analysis in the diagnosis of essential thrombocythaemia and primary myelofibrosis. *Br J Haematol, 149*(2), 250–257.

64. Chaligne, R., Tonetti, C., Besancenot, R., et al. (2008). New mutations in MPL in primitive myelofibrosis: only the MPL W515L mutations promote a G1/S-phase transition. *Leukemia, 22*(8), 1557–1566.

65. Pietra, D., Brisci, A., Rumi, E., et al. (2011). Deep sequencing reveals double mutations in cis of MPL exon 10 in myeloproliferative neoplasms. *Haematologica, 96*(4), 607–611.

66. Scott, L. M., Tong, W., Levine, R. L., et al. (2007). JAK2 exon 12 mutations in polycythemia vera and idiopathic erythrocytosis. *N Engl J Med, 356*, 459–468.

67. Passamonti, F., Elena, C., Schnittger, S., et al. (2011). Molecular and clinical features of the myeloproliferative neoplasm associated with JAK2 exon 12 mutations. *Blood. 117*, 2813–2816.

68. Jones, A. V., Chase, A., Silver, R. T., et al. (2009). JAK2 haplotype is a major risk factor for the development of myeloproliferative neoplasms. *Nat Genet, 41*, 446–449.

69. Kilpivaara, O., Mukherjee, S., Schram, A. M., et al. (2009). A germline JAK2 SNP is associated predisposition to the development of JAK2(V617F)-positive myeloproliferative neoplasms. *Nat Genet, 41*, 455–459.

70. Olcaydu, D., Harutyunyan, A., Jager, R., et al. (2009). A common JAK2 haplotype confers susceptibility to myeloproliferative neoplasms. *Nat Genet, 41*, 450–454.

71. Lasho, T. L., Pardanani, A., & Tefferi, A. (2010). LNK mutations in JAK2 mutation-negative erythropoiesis. *N Engl J Med, 363*, 1189–1190.

72. Oh, S. T., Simonds, E. F., Jones, C., et al. (2010). Novel mutations in the inhibitory adaptor protein LNK drive JAK-STAT signaling in patients with myeloproliferative neoplasms. *Blood, 116*, 988–992.

73. Pardanani, A., Lasho, T., Finke, C., et al. (2010). LNK mutation studies in blast-phase myeloproliferative neoplasms, and in chronic-phase disease with TET2, IDH, JAK2 or MPL mutations. *Leukemia, 24*(10), 1713–1718.

74. Delhommeau, F., Dupont, S., Della Valle, V., et al. (2009). Mutations in TET2 in myeloid cancers. *N Engl J Med, 360*, 2289–2301.

75. Tahiliani, M., Koh, K. P., Shen, Y., et al. (2009). Conversion of 5-methylcytosine to 5-hydroxymethylcytosine in mammalian DNA by MLL partner TET1. *Science, 324*, 930–935.

76. Figueroa, M., Abdel-Wahab, O., Lu, C., et al. (2010). Leukemic IDH1 and IDH2 mutations result in a hypermethylation phenotype, disrupt TET2 function, and impair hematopoietic differentiation. *Cancer Cell, 18*, 553–567.

77. Tefferi, A., Lasho, T. L., Abdel-Wahab, O., et al. (2010). IDH1 and IDH2 mutation studies in 1473 patients with chronic-, fibrotic-, or blast-phase essential thrombocythemia, polycythemia vera or myelofibrosis. *Leukemia, 24*, 1302–1309.

78. Dang, L., White, D. W., Gross, S., et al. (2009). Cancer-associated IDH1 mutations produce 2-hydroxyglutarate. *Nature, 462*, 739–744.

79. Cao, R. & Zhang, Y. (2004). The functions of E(Z)/EZH2- mediated methylation of lysine 27 in histone H3. *Curr Opin Genet Dev, 14*(2), 155–164.

80. Ernest, T., Chase, A. J., Score, J., et al. (2010). Inactivating mutations of the histone methyltransferase gene EZH2 in myeloid disorders. *Nat Genet, 42*, 722–776.

81. Nikoloski, G., Langemeijer, S. M., Kuiper, R. P., et al. (2010). Somatic mutations of the histone methyltransferase gene EZH2 in myelodysplastic syndromes. *Nat Genet, 42*, 665–667.

82. Sauvageau, M., & Sauvaheau, G. (2010). Polycomb group proteins: multi-faceted regulators of somatic stem cells and cancer. *Cell Stem Cell, 7*(3), 299–313.

83. Scheuermann, J. C., de Ayala Alonso, A. G., Oktaba, K., et al. (2010). Histone H2A deubiquitinas activity of the Polycomb repressor complex PR-DUB. *Nature, 465*(7295), 243–247.

84. Carbuccia, N., Murati, A., Trouplin, A., et al. (2009). Mutations of ASXL1 gene in myeloproliferative neoplasms. *Leukemia, 23*(11), 2183–2186.

85. Tefferi, A. (2010). Novel mutations and their functional clinical relevance in myeloproliferative neoplasms: JAK2, MPL, TET2, ASXL1, CBL, IDH and IKZF1. *Leukemia, 24*(6), 1128–1138.

86. Najean, Y., & Rain, J. D. (1997). The very long-term evolution of polycythemia vera: an analysis of 318 patients initially treated by phlebotomy or 32P between 1969 and 1981. *Semin Hematol, 34*(1), 6–16.

87. Campbell, P. J., Baxter, E. J., Beer, P. A., et al. (2006). Mutation of JAK2 in the myeloproliferative disorders: timing, clonality studies, cytogenetic associations, and role in leukemic transformation. *Blood, 108*(10), 3548–3555.

88. Mesa, R. A., Li, C. Y., Ketterling, R. P., et al. (2005). Leukemic transformation in myelofibrosis with myeloid metaplasia: a single-institution experience with 91 cases. *Blood, 105*(3), 973–977.

89. Beer, P. A., Delhommeau, F., LeCouedic, J. P., et al. (2010). Two routes to leukemic transformation after a JAK2 mutation-positive myeloproliferative neoplasm. *Blood, 115*(14), 2891–2900.

90. Harutyunyan, A., Klampfl, T., Cazzola, M., et al. (2011). p53 lesions in leukemic transformation. *N Engl J Med, 364*(5), 488–490.

91. Beer, P. A., Ortmann, C. A., Campbell, P. J., et al. (2010). Independently acquired biallelic JAK2 mutations are present in a minority of patients with essential thrombocythemia. *Blood, 116*(6), 1013–1014.

92. Berlin, N. (1975). Diagnosis and classification of the polycythemias. *Semin Hematol, 12*, 339–351.

93. Berk, P. D., Goldberg, J. N., Donovan, P. B., et al. (1986). Therapeutic recommendations in polycythemia vera based on Polycythemia Vera Study Group protocols. *Semin Hematol, 23*, 132–143.

94. Aruch, D., & Mascarenhas J. (2016). Contemporary approach to essential thrombocythemia and polycythemia vera. *Curr Opin Hematol, 23*, 150–160.

95. Wolf, B. C., Bank, P. M., Mann, R. B., et al. (1988). Splenic hematopoiesis in polycythemia vera: a morphologic and immunohistologic study. *Am J Clin Pathol, 89*, 69–75.

96. Ellis, J. T., Peterson, P., Geller, S. A., et al. (1986). Studies of the bone marrow in polycythemia vera and the evolution of myelofibrosis and second hematologic malignancies. *Semin Hematol, 23*, 144–155.

97. Landolfi, R., Marchioli, R., Kutti, J., et al. (2004). Efficacy and safety of low-dose aspirin in polycythemia vera. *N Engl J Med, 350*, 114–124.

98. Quintas-Cardama, A., Kantarjian, H., Manshouri, T., et al. (2009). Pegylated interferon alfa-2a yields high rates of hematologic and molecular response in patients with advanced essential thrombocythemia and polycythemia vera. *J Clin Oncol, 27*, 5418–5424.

99. Kiladjian, J. J., Cassinat, B., Chevret, S., et al. (2008). Pegylated interferon-alfa-2a induces complete hematologic and molecular responses with low toxicity in polycythemia vera. *Blood, 112*, 3065–3072.

100. "Leukemia and Hematosarcoma" Cooperative Group, European Organization for research on Treatment of Cancer (E.O.R.T.C.). (1981). Treatment of polycythaemia vera by radiophosphorus or busulphan: a randomized trial. *Br J Cancer, 44*, 75–80.

101. Barosi, G., Birgegard, G., Finazzi, G., et al. (2009). Response criteria for essential thrombocythemia and polycythemia vera: results of a European LeukemiaNet consensus conference. *Blood, 113*, 4829–4833.

102. Verstovsek, S., Passamonti, F., Rambaldi, A., et al. (2009). A phase 2 study of INCB018424, an oral, selective JAK1/JAK2 inhibitor, in patients with advanced polycythemia vera (PV) and essential thrombocythemia (ET) refractory to hydroxyurea. *Blood, 113*, 4829–4833.

103. Scherber, R., & Mesa, R. A. (2011). Future Therapies for the Myeloproliferative Neoplasms. *Curr Hematol Malig Rep, 6*, 2–27.

104. Moliterno, A. R., Hexner, E., Roboz, G. J., et al. (2009). An open-label study of CEP-701 in patients with JAK2 V617F-positive PV and ET: update of 39 enrolled patients. *Blood, 114*, 753.

105. Pardanani, A., & Tefferi, A. (2011). Targeting myeloproliferative neoplasms with JAK inhibitors. *Curr Opin Hematol, 18*, 105–110.

106. Mitus, A. J., & Schafer, A. (1990). Thrombocytosis and thrombocythemia. *Hematol Oncol Clin North Am, 4*, 157–178.

107. Thiele, J., Kvasnicka, H. M., Orazi, A., et al. (2008). Essential thrombocythemia. In Swerdlow, S. H., Campo, E., Harris, N. L., et al. (Eds.), *WHO Classification of Tumours of Heamatopoietic and Lymphoid Tissues.* (4th ed., pp. 48–53). Lyon, France: IARC Press.

108. Passamonti, F., Mora, B., & Maffioli, M. (2016). New molecular genetics in the diagnosis and treatment of myeloproliferative neoplasms. *Curr Opin Hematol, 23*, 137–143.

109. Kuecht, H., & Streuli, R. A. (1985). Megakaryopoiesis in different forms of thrombocytosis and thrombocytopenia: identification of megakaryocyte precursors by immunostaining of intracytoplasmic factor VIII-related antigen. *Acta Haematol, 74*, 208–212.

110. Shvidel, L., Sigler, E., Haran, M., et al. (2007). Busulphan is safe and effective treatment in elderly patients with essential thrombocythemia. *Leukemia, 21*, 2071–2072.

111. Passamonti, F., Rumi, E., Arcaini, L., et al. (2008). Prognostic factors for thrombosis, myelofibrosis, and leukemia in essential thrombocythemia: a study of 605 patients. *Haematologica, 93*, 1645–1651.

112. Jacobson, R. J., Salo, A., & Fialkow, P. J. (1978). Agnogenic myeloid metaplasia: a clonal proliferation of hematopoietic stem cells with secondary myelofibrosis. *Blood, 51*, 189–194.

113. McCarthy, D. M. (1985). Fibrosis of the bone marrow, content and causes. *Br J Haematol, 59*, 1–7.

114. Lichtman, M. A., & Tefferi, A. (2016). Primary myelofibrosis. In Kaushansky, K., Lichtman, M. A., Prchal, J.T., et al. (Eds.), *Williams Hematology.* (9th ed., pp. 1319–1340). New York: McGraw-Hill.

115. Reilly, I. F. (1994). Pathogenesis of idiopathic myelofibrosis: present status and future directions. *Br J Haematol, 88*, 1–8.

116. Wang, J. C., Cheung, C. P., Fakhiuddin, A., et al. (1983). Circulating granulocyte and macrophage progenitor cells in primary and secondary myelofibrosis. *Br J Haematol, 54*, 301–307.

117. Buschle, M., Janssen, J. Y., Drexler, H., et al. (1988). Evidence for pluripotent stem cell origin of idiopathic myelofibrosis: clonal analysis of a case characterized by a N-ras gene mutation. *Leukemia, 2*, 658–660.

118. Juvonen, E. (1988). Megakaryocyte colony formation in chronic myeloid leukemia and myelofibrosis. *Leuk Res, 12*, 751–756.

119. Barosi, G., Viarengo, G., Pecci, A., et al. (2001). Diagnostic and clinical relevance of the number of circulating CD34(+) cells in myelofibrosis with myeloid metaplasia. *Blood, 98*, 3249–3255.

120. Jacobs, P., Maze, S., Tayob, F., et al. (1985). Myelofibrosis, splenomegaly, and portal hypertension. *Acta Haematol, 74*, 45–48.

121. Hobbs, G. S., & Rampal, R. K. (2015). Clinical and molecular genetic characterization of myelofibrosis. *Curr Opin Hematol, 22*, 177–183.

122. Grand, F. H., Hidalgo-Curtis, C. E., Ernst, T., et al. (2009). Frequent CBL mutations associated with 11q acquired uni-parental disomy in myeloproliferative neoplasms. *Blood, 113*, 6182–6192.

123. Mascarenhas, J., Najfield, V., Kremyanskaya, M., et. al. (2018). Primary myelofibrosis. In Hoffman, R., Benz, E. J. Jr., Silberstein, L.E., et al. (Eds.), *Hematology: Basic Principles and Practice.* (7th ed., pp. 1125–1150). Philadelphia: Elsevier.

124. Gangat, N., Caramazza, D., Vaidya, R., et al. (2011). DIPSS-Plus: a refined dynamic international prognostic indicator system (DIPSS) for primary myelofibrosis that incorporates prognostic information from karyotype, platelet count and transfusion status. *J Clin Oncol, 29*(4), 392–397.

125. Vellenga, E., Mulder, N., The, T., et al. (1982). A study of the cellular and humoral immune response in patients with myelofibrosis. *Clin Lab Haematol, 4*, 239–246.

126. Cervantes, F., Dupriez, B., Pereira, A., et al. (2009). New prognostic scoring system for primary myelofibrosis based on a study of the International Working Group for Myelofibrosis Research and Treatment. *Blood, 113*, 2895–2901.

127. Cervantes, S., Mesa, R., & Barosi, G. (2007). New and old treatment modalities in primary myelofibrosis. *Cancer J, 13*, 377–383.

128. Elliott, M. A., Mesa, R., & Barosi, G. (2002). Thalidomide treatment in myelofibrosis with myeloid metaplasia. *Br J Haematol, 117*, 288–296.

129. Thomas, D. A., Giles, F. J., Albitar, M., et al. (2006). Thalidomide therapy for myelofibrosis with myelometaplasia. *Cancer, 106*, 1974–1984.

130. Tefferi, A., Cortez, J., Verstovsek, S., et al. (2006). Lenalidomide therapy in myelofibrosis with myeloid metaplasia. *Blood, 108*, 1158–1164.

131. Tefferi, A., Lasho, T. L., Mesa, R. A., et al. (2007). Lenalidomide therapy in del(5)(q31)-associated myelofibrosis: cytogenetic and JAK2V617F molecular remissions. *Leukemia, 21*, 1827–1828.

132. Mesa, R. A., Pardanani, A. D., Hussein, K., et al. (2010). Phase 1/-2 study of pomalidomide in myelofibrosis. *Am J Hematol, 85*(2), 129–130.

133. Martinez-Trillos, A., Gaya, A., Maffioli, M., et al. (2010). Efficacy and tolerability of hydroxyuria in the treatment of the myeloproliferative manifestations of myelofibrosis: results of 40 patients. *Ann Hematol, 89*, 1233–1237.

134. Siragusa, S., Vaidya, R., & Tefferi, A. (2009). Hydroxyurea effect on marked splenomegaly associated with primary myelofibrosis: response rates and correlation with JAK2V617F allele burden. *Blood, 114*, 4971.

135. Mishchenko, E., & Tefferi, A. (2010). Treatment options for hydroxyuria-refractory disease complications in myeloproliferative neoplasms: JAK2 inhibitors, radiotherapy, splenectomy and transjugular intrahepatic portosystemic shunt. *Eur J Haematol, 85*, 192–199.

136. Mesa, R. A., Schwager, S., Radia, D., et al. (2009). The Myelofibrosis Symptom Assessment Form (MFSAF): an evidence-based brief inventory to measure quality of life and symptomatic response to treatment in myelofibrosis. *Leuk Res, 33*, 1199–1203.

137. Mesa, R. A., Niblack, J., Wadleigh, M., et al. (2007). The burden of fatigue and quality of life in myeloproliferative disorders

(MPDs): an international Internet-based survey of 1179 MPD patients. *Cancer, 109,* 68–76.

138. Verstovsek, S., Kantarjian, H., Mesa, R. A., et al. (2010). Safety and efficacy of INC018424, a JAK1 and JAK2 inhibitor, in myelofibrosis. *N Engl J Med, 363,* 1117–1127.

139. Passamonti, F., Mora, B., & Maffioli, M. (2016). New molecular genetics in the diagnosis and treatment of myeloproliferative neoplasms. *Curr Opin Hematol, 23*(2), 137–143.

140. Stein, B. L., Crispino, J. D., & Moliterno, A. R. (2011). Janus kinase inhibitors: an update on the progress and promise of targeted therapy in the myeloproliferative neoplasms. *Curr Opin Oncol, 23,* 609–616.

141. Pardanani, A., Gotlib, J. R., Jamieson, C., et al. (2011). Safety and efficacy of TG101348, a selective JAK2 inhibitor in myelofibrosis. *J Clin Oncol, 29*(7), 789–796.

142. Verstovsek, S., & Komrokji, R. S. (2015). A comprehensive review of pacritinib in myelofibrosis. *Future Oncol, 11*(20), 2819–2830.

143. Pegrum, G. D., Foadi, M., Boots, M., et al. (1981). How should we manage myelofibrosis? *J R Coll Physicians Lond, 15,* 17–18.

144. Tefferi, A., & Silverstein, M. N. (1996). Current perspective in agnogenic myeloid metaplasia. *Leuk Lymphoma, 22*(Suppl. 1), 169–171.

145. Guardiola, P., Anderson, J. E., Bandini, G., et al. (1999). Allogeneic stem cell transplantation for agnogenic myeloid metaplasia: a European Group for Blood and Marrow Transplantation, Société Française de Greffe de Moelle, Gruppo Italiano per il Trapianto del Midollo Osseo, and Fred Hutchinson Cancer Research Center Collaborative Study. *Blood, 93,* 2831–2838.

146. Pardanani, A., Gotlib, J. R., Jamieson, C., et al. (2010). Long-term follow up with TG101348 therapy in myelofibrosis confirms sustained improvement in splenomegaly, disease reolated symptoms and JAK2V617F allele burden. *Blood, 116,* 459.

147. Xu, M., Bruno, E., Chao, J., et al. (2005). The constitutive mobilization of bone marrow-repopulating cells into the peripheral blood in idiopathic myelofibrosis. *Blood, 105,* 1699–1705.

148. Ishii, T., Zhao, Y., Sozer, S., et al. (2007). Behavior of CD34+ cells isolated from patients with polycythemia vera in NOD/SCID mice. *Exp Hematol, 35,* 1633–1640.

149. James, C., Mazurier, F., Dupont, S., et al. (2008). The hematopoietic stem cell compartment of JAK2V617F-positive myeloproliferative disorders is a reflection of disease heterogeneity. *Blood, 112,* 2429–2438.

150. Pardanani, A., Fridley, B. L., Lash, T. L., et al. (2008). Host genetic variation contributes to phenotypic diversity in myeloproliferative disorders. *Blood, 111,* 2785–2789.

151. Scott, L. M., Scott, M. A., Campbell, P. J., et al. (2006). Progenitors homozygous for the V617F mutation occur in most patients with polycythemia vera but not essential thrombocythemia. *Blood, 108,* 2435–2437.

152. Xing, S., Wanting, T. H., Zhao, W., et al. (2008). Transgenic expression of JAK2V617F causes myeloproliferative disorders in mice. *Blood, 111,* 5109–5117.

153. Tiedt, R., Hao-Shin, S., Sobas, M. A., et al. (2008). Ratio of mutant JAK2-V617F to wild-type JAK2 determines the MPD phenotype in transgenic mice. *Blood, 111,* 3931–3940.

154. Kiladjian, J. J., Elkassar, N., Cassinat, B., et al. (2006). Essential thrombocythemias without V617F JAK2 mutation are clonal hematopoietic stem cell disorders. *Leukemia, 20,* 1181–1183.

155. Levine, R. L., Belisle, C., Wadleigh, M., et al. (2006). X-inactivation-based clonality analysis and quantitative JAK2V617F assessment reveal a strong association between clonality and JAK2V617F in PV but not ET/MMM, and identifies a subset of JAK2V617F-negative ET and MMM patients with clonal hematopoiesis. *Blood, 107,* 4139–4141.

156. Kralovics, R., Teo, S. S., Li, S. S., et al. (2006). Acquisition of the V617F mutation of JAK2 is a late genetic event in a subset of patients with myeloproliferative disorders. *Blood, 108,* 1377–1380.

157. Hussein, K., Bock, O., Seegers, A., et al. (2007). Myelofibrosis evolving during imatinib treatment of chronic myeloproliferative disease with coexisting BCR/ABL translocation and JAK2V617F mutation. *Blood, 109,* 4106–4107.

158. Kramer, A., Reiter, A., Kruth, J., et al. (2007). JAK2-V617F mutation in a patient with Philadelphia-chromosome positive chronic myeloid leukemia. *Lancet Oncol, 8,* 658–660.

159. Pardanani, A. D., Levine, R. L., Lasho, T., et al. (2006). MPL515 mutations in myeloproliferative and other myeloid disorders: a study of 1182 patients. *Blood, 108,* 3472–3476.

160. Li, S., Kralovics, R., De Libero, G., et al. (2008). Clonal heterogeneity in polycythemia vera patients with JAK2 exon 21 and JAK2-V617F mutations. *Blood, 111,* 3863–3866.

161. Petra, D., Li, S., Brisci, A., et al. (2008). Somatic mutations of JAK2 exon 12 in patients with JAK2 (V617F)–negative myeloproliferative disorders. *Blood, 111,* 1686–1689.

162. Kralovics, R., Stockton, D., Prchal, J., et al. (2003). Clonal hematopiesis in familial polycythemia vera suggests the involvement of multiple mutational events in the early pathogenesis of the disease. *Blood, 102,* 3793–3796.

163. Bellanne-Chantelot, C., Chaumarel, I., Labopin, M., et al. (2006). Genetic and clinical implications of the Val617Phe JAK2 mutation in 72 families with myeloproliferative disorders. *Blood, 108,* 346–352.

164. Villeval, J. L., Cohen-Solal, K., Tulliez, M., et al. (1997). High thrombopoietin production by hematopoietic cells induces a fatal myeloproliferative syndrome in mice. *Blood, 90,* 4369–4383.

165. Bain, B. J., Brunning, R. D., Vardiman, J. W., et al. (2008). Chronic neutrophilic leukemia. In Swerdlow, S. H., Campo, E., Harris, N. L., et al. (Eds.), *WHO Classification of Tumours of Haematopoietic and Lymphoid Tissues.* (4th ed., pp. 38–39). Lyon, France: IARC Press.

166. Liesveld, J. L., & Lichtman, M. A. (2016). Chronic myelogenous leukemia and related disorders. In Kaushansky, K., Lichtman, M. A., Prchal, J. T., et al. (Eds.), *Williams Hematology.* (9th ed., pp. 1437–1492). New York: McGraw-Hill.

167. Bain, B. J., Gilliland, D. G., Vardiman, J. W., et al. (2008). Chronic eosinophilic leukaemia, not otherwise specified. In Swerdlow, S. H., Campo, E., Harris, N. L., et al. (Eds.), *WHO Classification of Tumours of Haematopoietic and Lymphoid Tissues.* (4th ed., pp. 51–53). Lyon, France: IARC Press.

168. Reiter, A., & Gotlib, J. (2016). Myeloid neoplasms with eosinophilia. *Blood, 129*(6), 704–714.

169. Valent, P., Akin, C., & Metcalfe, D. D. Mastocytosis: 2016 updated WHO classification and novel emerging treatment concepts. *Blood, 129*(11), 1420–1427.

170. Horny, H. P., Metcalfe, D. D., Bennett, J. M., et al. (2008). Mastocytosis. In Swerdlow, S. H., Campo, E., Harris, N. L., et al. (Eds.), *WHO Classification of Tumours of Haematopoietic and Lymphoid Tissues.* (4th ed., pp. 54–63). Lyon, France: IARC Press.

171. Kvasnicka, H. M., Bain, B. J., Thiele, J., et al. (2008). Myeloproliferative neoplasm, unclassifiable. In Swerdlow, S. H., Campo, E., Harris, N. L., et al. (Eds.), *WHO Classification of Tumours of Haematopoietic and Lymphoid Tissues.* (4th ed., pp. 64–65). Lyon, France: IARC Press.

Myelodysplastic Syndromes

Nicholas C. Brehl*

OBJECTIVES

After completion of this chapter, the reader will be able to:

1. Define myelodysplastic syndromes (MDS).
2. Explain the etiology of MDS.
3. Recognize morphologic features of dyspoiesis in bone marrow and peripheral blood.
4. Discuss abnormal functions of granulocytes, erythrocytes, and thrombocytes in MDS.
5. Correlate peripheral blood, bone marrow, and cytogenetic and molecular findings in MDS with classification systems.
6. Compare and contrast the French-American-British and the 2016 World Health Organization classifications of MDS.
7. Discuss prognostic indicators in MDS.
8. Indicate modes of management for MDS.
9. Review the epidemiology of MDS and apply it as a contributor in differential diagnosis.
10. Suggest laboratory tests and their results that would rule out MDS in the differential diagnosis.
11. Explain the rationale for the category of myelodysplastic/myeloproliferative neoplasms (MDS/MPN).
12. Correlate peripheral blood, bone marrow, and cytogenetic findings in MDS/MPN with disease classification.
13. Review prognostic indicators in MDS.
14. Discuss treatment in MDS, including novel therapies.

OUTLINE

Etiology
Morphologic Abnormalities in Peripheral Blood and Bone Marrow
  Dyserythropoiesis
  Dysmyelopoiesis
  Dysmegakaryopoiesis
Differential Diagnosis
Abnormal Cellular Function
Classification of Myelodysplastic Syndromes
  French-American-British Classification
  World Health Organization Classification
Myelodysplastic/Myeloproliferative Neoplasms
  Chronic Myelomonocytic Leukemia

Atypical Chronic Myeloid Leukemia, BCR/ABL1 Negative
Juvenile Myelomonocytic Leukemia
Myelodysplastic/Myeloproliferative Neoplasm with Ring Sideroblasts and Thrombocytosis
Myelodysplastic/Myeloproliferative Neoplasm, Unclassifiable
Cytogenetics, Molecular Alterations, and Epigenetics
  Cytogenetics
  Molecular Alterations
  Epigenetics
Prognosis
Treatment
  Future Directions

CASE STUDY

After studying the material in this chapter, the reader should be able to respond to the following case study:

A 43-year-old man experienced fatigue and malaise. He presented with pancytopenia (white blood cell [WBC] count of 2.2×10^9/L, hemoglobin of 6.1 g/dL, platelet count of 51×10^9/L). The WBC differential was essentially normal. Mean cell volume was 132 fL (reference range, 80–100 fL), and vitamin B_{12} and folate levels were normal. The bone marrow was normocellular with a myeloid-to-erythroid ratio of 1:1 and adequate megakaryocytes. The erythroid component was dysplastic with megaloblastic features. No abnormal localization of immature precursors was noted. Chromosome analysis indicated direct duplication of

chromosome 1q. The patient was maintained with transfusions over the next 6 years. At that time his bone marrow revealed increased erythropoiesis, decreased granulopoiesis, and megakaryopoiesis, all with dysplastic changes. There were 50% to 60% ring sideroblasts.

1. What should be included in the differential diagnosis of patients with pancytopenia and elevated mean cell volume?
2. Given the normal vitamin B_{12} and folate levels, what is the patient's probable diagnosis?
3. In which World Health Organization 2016 classification does this disorder belong?

---

*The author extends appreciation to Bernadette. F. Rodak, whose work in prior editions provided the foundation for this chapter.

For decades, laboratory professionals have observed a group of morphologic abnormalities in peripheral blood films and bone marrow smears of elderly patients. The findings were heterogeneous and affected all cell lines, and the condition either remained stable for years or progressed rapidly to death.

Historically this pattern of abnormalities was referred to as *refractory anemia, smoldering leukemia, oligoblastic leukemia,* or *preleukemia.*[1,2] In 1982 the French-American-British (FAB) Cooperative Leukemia Study Group proposed terminology and a specific set of morphologic criteria to describe what are now known as *myelodysplastic syndromes* (MDS).[3] In 1997 a group from the World Health Organization (WHO) proposed a new classification that included molecular, cytogenetic, and immunologic criteria in addition to morphologic features.[4,5] The WHO classification was revised in 2008 and 2016. Emphasis in this chapter is placed on the WHO 2016 classification model.

MDS are a group of acquired clonal hematologic disorders characterized by progressive cytopenias in the peripheral blood, reflecting defects in erythroid, myeloid, and/or megakaryocytic maturation.[6,7] There is an increased risk, especially among certain subtypes, for the disease to transform into acute myeloid leukemia (AML).[6,7] The median age of diagnosis is 76 years old.[8] MDS rarely affect individuals younger than age 50 unless preceded by chemotherapy or radiation used in the treatment of another malignancy.[1,9] However, cases in young adults and children have been reported.[10,11] The incidence of MDS seems to be increasing, but this apparent increase may be attributable in part to improved techniques for identifying these diseases and to improved classification.[8] MDS are becoming a more common finding in the hematology laboratory, and familiarity with these disorders is an essential part of the body of knowledge of all medical laboratory professionals.

ETIOLOGY

As a clonal hematopoietic disorder, it was previously believed that the cell of origin for MDS was a myeloid progenitor because erythroid, myeloid, and megakaryocytic cells are most commonly affected. However, a myeloid progenitor did not explain the increased risk that MDS patients had for developing a lymphoid malignancy or the overlap of mutations that are shared between MDS and lymphoid malignancies. Recently, phenotypically normal hematopoietic stem cells (HSCs) were found to be the cell of origin for MDS.[7,12] These HSCs exist in low frequency in the bone marrow and may harbor one or more somatic mutations. The mutations in the affected HSCs make the cells more fit, leading to a clonal expansion at the expense of normal HSCs.[12,13] Otherwise healthy patients may have clonal hematopoiesis but do not develop a hematologic disorder. This condition, known as clonal hematopoiesis of indeterminate potential (CHIP), is recognized as a precursor state for many hematologic disorders, including MDS, even though the rate of transformation is low.[14,15] Approximately 10% of patients older than age 65 and nearly 20% older than age 90 have CHIP.[13,16,17] The complex interactions among additional somatic mutations, epigenetic modifications, the bone marrow

microenvironment, and environmental stimuli determine whether CHIP develops into MDS (or another hematologic disease), the severity of the subsequent disorder, and its risk for transformation into AML.[12,13,18]

The genetic mutations in the HSC that lead to MDS come from a variety of sources. De novo mutations (primary MDS) account for most of the cases. The mutations may also arise as a result of therapy (therapy-related MDS), secondary to exposure to chemicals or radiation (not associated with prior disease treatment), or they may be inherited.

Therapy-related MDS develops in patients after treatment with chemotherapy and/or radiotherapy. Although causality is impossible to determine, the effects of some leukemogenic chemotherapies and therapeutic radiation are known to cause genetic mutations and cellular disruptions.[19,20] Median onset of therapy-related MDS (t-MDS) is usually 4 to 7 years after therapy was initiated but may vary with the agents used.[21,22] In addition to inducing genetic change in hematopoietically active cells, evidence is accumulating that chemotherapies may apply a selective pressure to the bone marrow, which allows preexisting mutations to accumulate.[20,23] Patients who have received cytokines, such as G-CSF or GM-CSF, for bone marrow stimulation are also at an increased risk for developing t-MDS.[24] t-MDS is aggressive and may evolve quickly into AML.[21,22,25] The 2016 WHO classification places therapy-related MDS into the AML category of therapy-related myeloid neoplasms (Chapter 31).

The 2016 WHO classification recognizes patients who have a predisposition to develop MDS from germline mutations. Patients with inherited bone marrow failure syndromes such as Fanconi anemia, Diamond-Blackfan anemia, and Shwachman-Diamond syndrome are at a significantly increased risk for developing MDS, particularly in childhood or adolescence.[26] Other mutations, such as those commonly identified in de novo MDS, may be inheritable and confer increased risk for development of MDS.[26]

Two morphologic findings are common to all types of MDS: the presence of progressive cytopenias despite cellular bone marrow and dyspoiesis in one or more cell lines.

Disruption of apoptosis may be responsible for the ineffective hematopoiesis in MDS.[27] Apoptosis (programmed cell death) regulates cell population by decreasing cell survival. In MDS, apoptosis is increased in early disease, when peripheral blood cytopenias are evident. Later in MDS, when progression toward leukemia is apparent, apoptosis is decreased, which allows increased neoplastic cell survival and expansion of the abnormal clone.[27-29]

MORPHOLOGIC ABNORMALITIES IN PERIPHERAL BLOOD AND BONE MARROW

In MDS each of the three major myeloid cell lines has dyspoietic morphologic features. The following sections provide descriptions of common abnormal morphologic findings.[3,9,30] These descriptions are not all-inclusive because of the large number of possible cellular mutations and combinations of mutations.

Dyserythropoiesis

In peripheral blood the most common morphologic finding in dyserythropoiesis is the presence of oval macrocytes (Figure 33.1). When these cells are seen in the presence of normal vitamin B_{12} and folate values, MDS should be included in the differential diagnosis. Hypochromic microcytes in the presence of adequate iron stores also are seen in MDS. A dimorphic red blood cell (RBC) population (Figure 33.2) is another indication of the clonality of this disease. Poikilocytosis, basophilic stippling, Howell-Jolly bodies, and siderocytes also are indications that the erythrocyte has undergone abnormal development.[31]

Dyserythropoiesis in the bone marrow is evidenced by RBC precursors with more than one nucleus or abnormal nuclear shapes. The normally round nucleus may have lobes or buds. Nuclear fragments may be present in the cytoplasm (Figure 33.3). Internuclear bridging is occasionally present (Figure 33.4).[32] Abnormal cytoplasmic features may include basophilic stippling or heterogeneous staining (Figure 33.5). Ring sideroblasts are a common finding. Megaloblastoid cellular development in the presence of normal vitamin B_{12} and folate values is another indication of MDS. The bone marrows in these cases may have erythrocytic hyperplasia or hypoplasia (Box 33.1).

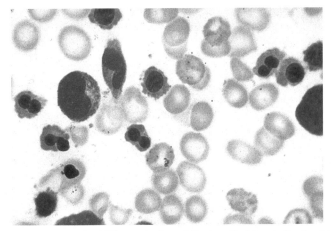

Figure 33.3 Erythroid Hyperplasia and Nuclear Budding in Erythroid Precursors. (Bone marrow, Wright-Giemsa stain, ×1000.)

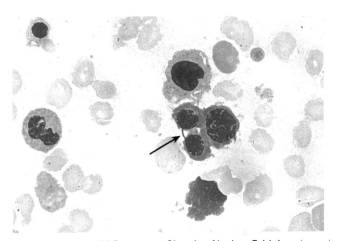

Figure 33.4 Erythroid Precursors Showing Nuclear Bridging. *(arrow)* (Bone marrow, Wright-Giemsa stain, ×1000.)

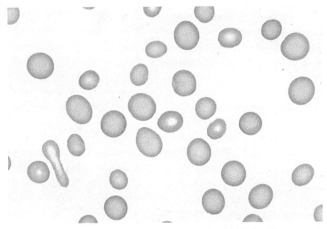

Figure 33.1 Oval Macrocytes. (Peripheral blood, Wright-Giemsa stain, ×1000.)

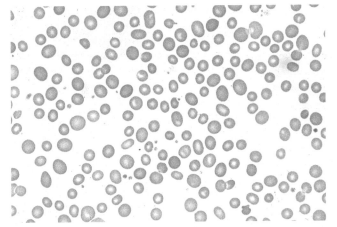

Figure 33.2 Dimorphic Erythrocyte Population. Includes macrocytic and microcytic cells. (Peripheral blood, Wright-Giemsa stain, ×500.)

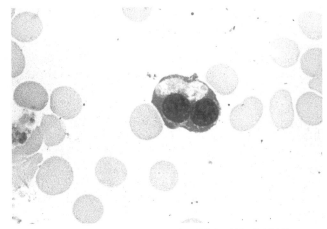

Figure 33.5 Heterogeneous Staining in a Bilobed Erythroid Precursor. (Bone marrow, Wright-Giemsa stain, ×1000.)

Dysmyelopoiesis

Dysmyelopoiesis in the peripheral blood is suspected when there is a persistence of basophilia in the cytoplasm of otherwise mature white blood cells (WBCs), indicating nuclear-cytoplasmic asynchrony (Figure 33.6). Abnormal granulation of the cytoplasm of neutrophils, in the form of larger than normal

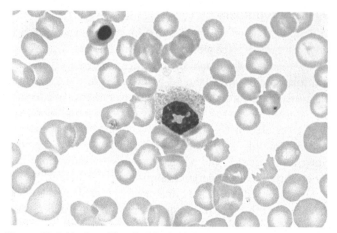

Figure 33.8 Nuclear Ring in Myeloid Cell. (Peripheral blood, Wright-Giemsa stain, ×1000.)

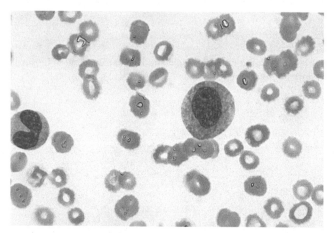

Figure 33.6 Myeloid Cells. This myelocyte *(right)* has a nucleus with clumped chromatin and a basophilic immature cytoplasm showing asynchrony. Note also the agranular myeloid cell *(left)* (Peripheral blood, Wright-Giemsa stain, ×1000.)

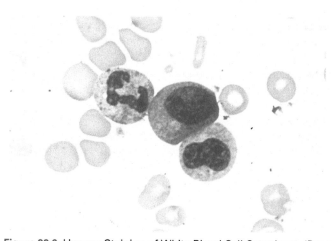

Figure 33.9 Uneven Staining of White Blood Cell Cytoplasm. (Bone marrow, Wright-Giemsa stain, ×1000.)

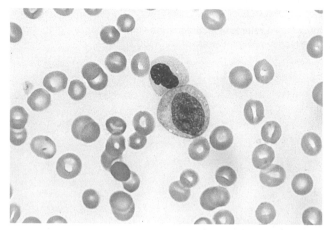

Figure 33.7 Agranular Myeloid Cells. (Peripheral blood, Wright-Giemsa stain, ×1000.)

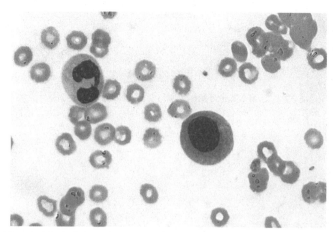

Figure 33.10 Promyelocyte or Myelocyte (right) Devoid of Granules and an Agranular Neutrophil (left). (Bone marrow, Wright-Giemsa stain, ×1000.)

granules, hypogranulation, or the absence of granules, is a common finding. Agranular bands can be easily misclassified as monocytes (Figure 33.7). Abnormal nuclear features may include hyposegmentation, hypersegmentation, or nuclear rings (Figure 33.8).[33]

In the bone marrow, dysmyelopoiesis may be represented by nuclear-cytoplasmic asynchrony. Cytoplasmic changes include uneven staining, such as a dense ring of basophilia around the periphery with a clear unstained area around the nucleus or whole sections of cytoplasm unstained, with the remainder of

the cytoplasm stained normally (Figure 33.9). There may be abnormal granulation of the cytoplasm in which promyelocytes or myelocytes or both are devoid of primary granules (Figure 33.10), primary granules may be larger than normal, or secondary granules may be reduced in number or absent, and there may be an occasional Auer rod.[34,35] Agranular promyelocytes

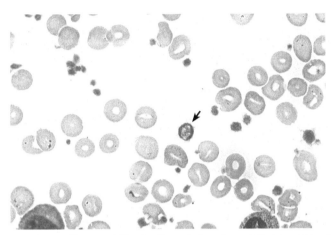

Figure 33.11 Abnormal Platelet Granulation. *(arrow)* (Peripheral blood, Wright-Giemsa stain, ×1000.)

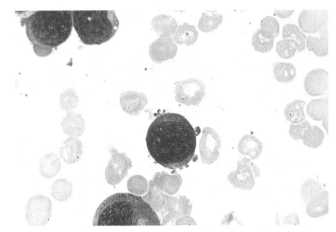

Figure 33.12 Micromegakaryocyte. (Peripheral blood, Wright-Giemsa stain, ×1000.)

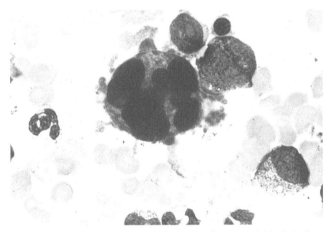

Figure 33.13 Megakaryocyte with Small Separated Nuclei. (Bone marrow, Wright-Giemsa stain, ×1000.)

may be mistaken for blasts; this could lead to misclassification of the disease in the AML scheme. Abnormal nuclear findings may include hypersegmentation or hyposegmentation and possibly ring-shaped nuclei (Box 33.2).

The bone marrow may exhibit granulocytic hypoplasia or hyperplasia. Monocytic hyperplasia is a common finding in dysplastic marrows.

Abnormal localization of immature precursors is a characteristic finding in bone marrow biopsy specimens from patients with MDS.[36] Normally, myeloblasts and promyelocytes reside along the endosteal surface of the bone marrow. In some cases of MDS these cells tend to cluster centrally in marrow sections.

Dysmegakaryopoiesis

Platelets also exhibit dyspoietic morphology in the peripheral blood. Common changes include giant platelets and abnormal platelet granulation, either hypogranulation or agranulation (Figure 33.11). Some platelets may possess large fused granules. Circulating micromegakaryocytes may be present in peripheral blood from patients with MDS (Figure 33.12).[9]

The megakaryocytic component of the bone marrow may exhibit abnormal morphology: large mononuclear megakaryocytes, micromegakaryocytes, or micromegakaryoblasts. The nuclei in these cells may be bilobed or have multiple small, separated nuclei (Figure 33.13; Box 33.3).[9]

DIFFERENTIAL DIAGNOSIS

Dysplasia by itself is not sufficient evidence for MDS, because several other conditions can cause similar morphologic features. Some examples are vitamin B$_{12}$ or folate deficiency,

which can cause pancytopenia and dysplasia, and exposure to heavy metals. Copper deficiency may cause reversible myelodysplasia.[9] Some congenital hematologic disorders, such as Fanconi anemia and congenital dyserythropoietic anemia, may also present with dysplasia. Parvovirus B19 and some chemotherapeutic agents may give rise to dysplasia similar to that in MDS. Paroxysmal nocturnal hemoglobinuria has similar features, as does human immunodeficiency virus (HIV).[37] Therefore a thorough history and physical examination, including questions about exposure to drugs and chemicals, are essential.[9]

ABNORMAL CELLULAR FUNCTION

The cells produced by abnormal maturation not only have an abnormal appearance but also have abnormal function.[9,38] The granulocytes may have decreased adhesion,[39,40] deficient phagocytosis,[40] decreased chemotaxis,[39,40] or impaired microbicidal capacity.[41] Decreased levels of myeloperoxidase and alkaline phosphatase may be found.[42] The RBCs may exhibit shortened survival,[43] and erythroid precursors may have a decreased response to erythropoietin that may contribute to anemia.[44] Patients may experience increased bleeding despite adequate platelet numbers.[9,45,46] The type and degree of dysfunction depend on the mutation present in the HSC.

CLASSIFICATION OF MYELODYSPLASTIC SYNDROMES

French-American-British Classification

In an effort to standardize the diagnosis of MDS, the FAB created five classes of MDS, each with a specific set of morphologic criteria. The categories are structured by the amount of dysplasia and the number of blasts in the bone marrow. The diagnosis of acute leukemia required at least 30% blasts in the bone marrow.[3] The FAB classification included the following:

1. Refractory anemia
2. Refractory anemia with ring sideroblasts (RARS)
3. Refractory anemia with excess blasts (RAEB)
4. Chronic myelomonocytic leukemia
5. Refractory anemia with excess blasts in transformation (RAEB-t)

The FAB classification provided a framework for discussion of a seemingly heterogeneous group of disorders; however, its reliance on morphology alone limited its usefulness as a prognostic indicator. The FAB classification did not view MDS in their totality because it did not address therapy-related MDS, hereditary forms, or childhood MDS. The WHO classification retains many of the FAB features, while incorporating advances in medical knowledge such as clinical, molecular, cytogenetic, and immunologic characteristics of these disorders.

World Health Organization Classification

The WHO classification system maintained some of the organization initiated in the FAB system but it also has undergone significant updates in pace with scientific research. The threshold for dysplasia, a requirement for the diagnosis of MDS, is defined as 10% dysplastic cells in any hematopoietic lineage.[47] The percentage of blasts required for diagnosis of an acute leukemia has decreased to 20%. The 2016 WHO classification system is outlined in Box 33.4 and detailed in Table 33.1. The classification is extensive and only the highlights are presented in this chapter.

MDS With Single Lineage Dysplasia

In 2016, WHO updated the name of refractory cytopenia with unilineage dysplasia to MDS with single lineage dysplasia (MDS-SLD).[47] The presenting symptoms of MDS-SLD are

---

> **BOX 33.4** **The 2016 World Health Organization Classification of Myelodysplastic Syndromes (MDSs)**
>
> MDS with single lineage dysplasia (MDS-SLD)
> MDS with ring sideroblasts (MDS-RS)
>   MDS-RS and single lineage dysplasia
>   MDS-RS and multilineage dysplasia
> MDS with multilineage dysplasia
> MDS with excess blasts (MDS-EB)
>   MDS-EB-1
>   MDS-EB-2
> Myelodysplastic syndrome with isolated del(5q)
> Myelodysplastic syndrome, unclassifiable
> Childhood myelodysplastic syndrome
>   Refractory cytopenia of childhood (provisional)

Adapted from Aber, D. A., Orazi, A., Hasserjian, R., et al. (2016). The 2016 revision to the World Health Organization classification of myeloid neoplasms and acute leukemia. *Blood, 127*(20), 2391–2405.

---

related to the cytopenia—namely, fatigue or shortness of breath if anemia is present; increased infections from neutropenia; and petechiae, bruising, or bleeding from thrombocytopenia. This category includes MDS cases with less than 1% blasts in the peripheral blood and less than 5% blasts in the bone marrow. Dysplasia must be present in at least one myeloid lineage. Although cytogenetic abnormalities are seen in up to 50% of cases of MDS-SLD, none is specific to the diagnosis. Median survival is 5 years, with a 2% to 12% risk of transformation to AML.[48,49]

MDS With Multilineage Dysplasia

MDS with multilineage dysplasia (MDS-MLD) (formerly known as refractory cytopenia with multilineage dysplasia) is characterized by one or more cytopenias, dysplasia in two or more myeloid cell lines, less than 1% blasts in peripheral blood, and less than 5% blasts in the bone marrow.[47] In MDS-MLD, myeloblasts do not contain Auer rods; if Auer rods are noted, the disorder is classified as MDS with excess blasts-2.[47] Median survival is about 31 to 38 months, with a 10% to 12% risk of transformation to AML within 5 years.[48,49]

MDS With Ring Sideroblasts

In 2016, WHO updated its terminology and classification of MDS with ring sideroblasts (MDS-RS) to reflect the influence of mutations in the spliceosome gene *SF3B1*. Mutations in *SF3B1* often occur early in MDS pathogenesis and precede the development of ring sideroblasts.[50] A ring sideroblast is an erythroid precursor containing at least five iron granules per cell, and these iron-containing mitochondria must circle at least one-third of the nucleus (Figure 33.14).[51] If a mutation in *SF3B1* is identified, only 5% of nucleated erythroid cells must be ring sideroblasts.[47] If a mutation in *SF3B1* is not detected, 15% of the bone marrow erythroid precursors must be ring sideroblasts to make this diagnosis.[47] Patients with MD-RS have anemia and dyserythropoiesis. The peripheral blood often demonstrates a dimorphic picture, with a mixed population of hypochromic cells and normochromic cells.

TABLE 33.1 Peripheral Blood and Bone Marrow Findings in Myelodysplastic Syndromes (MDSs)

Disease	Blood Findings	Bone Marrow Findings
MDS with single lineage dysplasia (MDS-SLD)	1–2 cytopenias No or rare blasts (<1%)	Unilineage dysplasia <5% blasts; no Auer rods <15%*/<5%† of erythroid precursors are ring sideroblasts
MDS with ring sideroblasts (MDS-RS) MDS-RS with single lineage dysplasia (MDS-RS-SLD) MDS-RS with multilineage dysplasia (MDS-RS-MLD)	No or rare blasts (<1%) 1–2 cytopenias 1–3 cytopenias	<5% blasts; no Auer rods ≥15%*/≥5%† of erythroid precursors are ring sideroblasts Unilineage dysplasia Multilineage dysplasia
MDS with multilineage dysplasia (MDS-MLD)	1–3 cytopenias No or rare blasts (<1%)	Multilineage dysplasia <5% blasts; no Auer rods <15%*/<5%† of erythroid precursors are ring sideroblasts

MDS with excess blasts (MDS-EB)
    MDS-EB-1
    MDS-EB-2
	1–3 cytopenias
	2%–4% blasts
	5%–19% blasts
		0–3 dysplastic lineages
		5%–9% blasts; no Auer rods
		10%–19% blasts; ±Auer rods‡

Myelodysplastic syndrome, unclassified (MDS-U)	0–3 cytopenias No or rare blasts (≤1%)	Unilineage or multilineage dysplasia ±MDS-defining cytogenetic abnormality <5% blasts; no Auer rods
MDS associated with isolated del(5q)	1–2 cytopenias No or rare blasts (<1%)	Unilineage or multilineage dysplasia <5% blasts; no Auer rods del(5q) cytogenetic abnormality with or without an additional cytogenetic abnormality

Dysplasia is defined as ≥10% dysplastic cells in a cell lineage.
*If a mutation in *SF3B1* is not detected.
†If a mutation in *SF3B1* is detected.
‡Patient cases with Auer rods are classified as MDS-EB-2.
Adapted from Aber, D. A., Orazi, A., Hasserjian, R., et al. (2016). The 2016 revision to the World Health Organization classification of myeloid neoplasms and acute leukemia. *Blood*, *127*(20), 2391–2405.

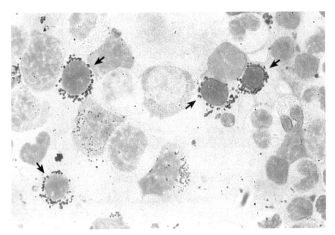

Figure 33.14 Ring Sideroblast. *(arrows)* (Bone marrow, Prussian blue stain, ×1000.)

MDS-RS is further subclassified into MDS-RS with single lineage dysplasia and MDS-RS with multilineage dysplasia. MDS-RS with single lineage dysplasia accounts for 3% to 10% of all MDS cases and has a median age of presentation of 71.[52,53] MDS-RS with multilineage dysplasia is characterized by one or more cytopenias and dysplasia in two or more myeloid cell lines.[47] MDS-RS with multilineage dysplasia has a worse prognosis than MDS with single lineage dysplasia.[52,53]

MDS With Excess Blasts

Trilineage cytopenias, as well as significant dysmyelopoiesis, dysmegakaryopoiesis, or both, are common in MDS with excess blasts (MDS-EB). WHO divided MDS-EB into two subtypes because of their respective differences in survival and rate of transformation into AML.

MDS-EB-1—5% to 9% blasts in the bone marrow or 2% to 4% blasts in the peripheral blood[47]

MDS-EB-2—10% to 19% blasts in the bone marrow and 5% to 19% blasts in the peripheral blood[47]

The presence of Auer rods, regardless of blast count, qualifies a case as MDS-EB-2. MDS-EB-2 has a more aggressive course, with a greater percentage of cases transforming to AML.[48,49]

MDS With Isolated del(5q) (5q– Syndrome)

The deletion of 5q (5q–) is the only WHO recognized MDS with a defining cytogenetic abnormality. The 2016 WHO classification now allows one additional cytogenetic abnormality to be present with del(5q).[47] MDS with isolated del(5q) is a fairly well-defined syndrome affecting predominantly women and occurring at a median age of 70.[49,54] These patients typically have anemia without other cytopenias or thrombocytosis, hypolobulated megakaryocytes, and erythroid hypoplasia.[55-57] There are less than 1% blasts in the peripheral blood.[47] Auer rods are not seen.[47] The median survival of patients ranges from 54 to 146 months.[54,56,58] The thalidomide analog lenalidomide (Revlimid) has proven to be effective in patients with isolated del(5q).[54-58]

MDS, Unclassifiable

MDS, unclassifiable (MDS-U) refers to subtypes of MDS that initially lack the specific changes necessary for classification into other MDS subtypes. If characteristics of a specific subtype develop later, the case should be reclassified into the appropriate group. The diagnosis of MDS-U is made if the patient demonstrates 1% peripheral blood blasts, single linage dysplasia and pancytopenia, or an MDS-defining cytogenetic abnormality.[47] Diagnostic criteria are described extensively in Table 33.1.

Childhood Myelodysplastic Syndromes

De novo MDS in children is very rare, and although some of the characteristics of adult MDS are present, some distinct differences exist. Investigations have revealed that the genomic landscape of childhood MDS is distinctly different than adult MDS.[59] Childhood MDS patients have an increased frequency of specific inherited gene mutations such as *RUNX1*, *SOS1*, *GATA2*, *ANKRD26*, and others.[26,59] The provisional category of *refractory cytopenia of childhood* is included in the 2008 and 2016 WHO classification systems out of concern for distinguishing these conditions from inherited bone marrow failure syndromes.[60] Refractory cytopenia of childhood presents with cytopenia and dysplasia in at least one cell line.[47]

MYELODYSPLASTIC/MYELOPROLIFERATIVE NEOPLASMS

The MDS/MPN category includes myeloid neoplasms with clinical, laboratory, and morphologic features that are characteristic of both MDS and MPN. Included in this classification are chronic myelomonocytic leukemia (CMML); atypical chronic myeloid leukemia (aCML); juvenile myelomonocytic leukemia (JMML); refractory anemia with ring sideroblasts and thrombocytosis (MDS/MPN-RS-T); and MDS/MPN, unclassifiable[47] (Box 33.5).

Chronic Myelomonocytic Leukemia

CMML is characterized by a persistent monocytosis of more than 1.0 monocyte $\times$ 10^9/L; absence of the *BCR/ABL1* fusion gene; absence of rearrangements involving *PDGFRA*, *PDGFRB*, *FGFR1*, or *PCM1-JAK2*; less than 20% blasts and promonocytes

---

BOX 33.5	**Classification of Myelodysplastic Syndromes/Myeloproliferative Neoplasms**

Chronic myelomonocytic leukemia (CMML)
Atypical chronic myeloid leukemia (aCML), *BCR/ABL1* negative
Juvenile myelomonocytic leukemia (JMML)
MDS/MPN with ring sideroblasts and thrombocytosis (MDS/MPN-RS-T)
Myelodysplastic/myeloproliferative neoplasm, unclassifiable

Adapted from Aber, D. A., Orazi, A., Hasserjian, R., et al. (2016). The 2016 revision to the World Health Organization classification of myeloid neoplasms and acute leukemia. *Blood, 127*(20), 2391–2405.

---

in the peripheral blood and bone marrow; and dysplasia in one or more myeloid cell line.[47] In the absence of dysplasia the diagnosis of CMML may still be made if unexplained monocytosis persists for more than 3 months or if a cytogenetic or a molecular mutation consistent with CMML is found.[47] The mutational landscape of CMML is complex with some patients having 8 to 14 distinct mutations in coding sequences.[61] Mutations have been found in more than 90% of CMML cases with *TET2*, *SRSF2*, *ASXL1*, and *RUNX1* being the most common.[61-64] Cytogenetic abnormalities such as trisomy 8 and loss of all or portions of chromosome 7 are also common.[61,62] Leukocytosis and dysgranulopoiesis is often evident. Splenomegaly may be present as a result of infiltration of leukemic cells. Three subgroups of CMML were recognized in the 2016 WHO classification because of the impact of blast percentages on survival. CMML-0 has less than 2% blasts in the peripheral blood and less than 5% blasts in the bone marrow.[47] CMML-1 is defined as 2% to 4% blasts in the peripheral blood and 5% to 9% blasts in the bone marrow.[47] CMML-2 has the worst prognosis with 5% to 19% blasts in the peripheral blood and 10% to 19% in the bone marrow.[47]

Atypical Chronic Myeloid Leukemia, *BCR/ABL1* Negative

Atypical CML, *BCR/ABL1* negative, is characterized by leukocytosis with morphologically dysplastic neutrophils and their precursors. Basophilia may be present, but it is not a prominent feature. Multilineage dysplasia is common. The *BCR/ABL1* fusion gene is not present, but karyotype abnormalities are seen in a third of patients, with essentially all patients demonstrating at least one gene mutation.[65] Dyspoiesis may be seen in all cell lines, but it is most remarkable in the neutrophils, which may exhibit Pelger-Huët-like cells, hypogranularity, and bizarre segmentation.[66,67] The prognosis is poor for patients with aCML because they commonly progress to AML or succumb to bone marrow failure.[62,66]

Juvenile Myelomonocytic Leukemia

JMML is a clonal disorder characterized by proliferation of the granulocytic and monocytic cell lines and affects children from 1 month to 14 years of age. Most patients have somatic or germline mutations that activate the RAS/MAPK pathway.[62] There is a strong association with congenital disorders such as Noonan syndrome and neurofibromatosis type 1.[62] Allogeneic stem cell transplantation is effective in about 50% of patients.[68]

Myelodysplastic/Myeloproliferative Neoplasm With Ring Sideroblasts and Thrombocytosis

MDS/MPN with ring sideroblasts and thrombocytosis, formerly known as MDS/MPN refractory anemia with ring sideroblasts and thrombocytosis, was proposed as a provisional category in the 2008 WHO classification.[47] The discovery that this disease is often associated with mutations in *SF3B1* and *JAK2 V617F* provided rational for the nature of the disease.[47,53] MDS/MPN-RS-T presents with anemia, 15% or more ring sideroblasts, thrombocytosis, atypical megakaryocytes, and 1% or less of blasts in the peripheral blood and 5% or less of blasts in the bone marrow.[47,53]

Myelodysplastic/Myeloproliferative Neoplasm, Unclassifiable

The designation *MDS/MPN, unclassifiable* is used for cases that meet the criteria for MDS/MPN but do not fit into one of the aforementioned subcategories. The time of diagnosis, clinical history, and the detection of molecular aberrations are important factors in properly diagnosing this condition.

CYTOGENETICS, MOLECULAR ALTERATIONS, AND EPIGENETICS

Cytogenetics

Chromosome abnormalities are found in about 50% of cases of de novo MDS and 90% to 95% of t-MDS.[19,69,70] Karyotype has a major effect on prognosis in MDS patients, and specific karyotypes can be used cautiously to predict response to treatment.[70] Balanced translocations, which are common among patients with AML, are found only rarely in cases of de novo MDS.[69,70] Except for del(5q), no cytogenetic abnormality is specific to a subtype of MDS. The most common abnormalities involve chromosomes 5, 7, 8, 18, 20, and 13.[9,69] The most common single abnormalities besides del(5q) are trisomy 8 and monosomy 7, 12p–, iso 17, –21, and loss of the Y chromosome.[69]

Molecular Alterations

Advances in molecular genetics have made testing more available for routine use, and such information is strengthening prognostic scoring models. Likewise, identification of genetic defects may allow the development of targeted therapies.[71] About 90% of patients with MDS have at least one mutation, with a median of three mutations per patient.[72,73] There are at least 47 different genes that harbor these mutations and many of them are not specific to MDS.[72,73] These mutations affect five major groups of genes: RNA splicing, DNA methylation, activated cell signaling, myeloid transcription factors, and chromatin modifiers [74] The most common mutations include *TET2*, *SF3B1*, *ASXL1*, *SRSF2*, *DNMT3A*, and *RUNX1*.[72,73] The prognostic value of these gene mutations are varied. For instance, *SF3B1*, confers a favorable prognosis, whereas others such as *TP53* confer a negative prognosis and predict a higher risk of transformation to AML.[75,76]

Epigenetics

The term *epigenetics* describes changes in gene expression that occur without altering the DNA sequence. Gene function is affected through selective activation or inactivation, rather than a change in the primary nucleotide sequence itself.[77,78] The three different ways in which epigenetics may facilitate oncogenesis are methylation of CpG islands, histone modification, and alteration of microRNA expression.[79,80] Mutations in *TET2* and *ASXL1* play important roles in altering CpG island methylation and histone methylation, respectively.[79,80] Treatment with demethylating agents may slow the progression of MDS.[81-83]

PROGNOSIS

The 2016 WHO classification system described in this chapter identifies types of MDS based on similarities in morphologic, molecular, genetic, immunologic, and clinical characteristics, but it has limited ability to provide a prognosis. The clinical phenotypes for patients with MDS are heterogeneous. Some patients are mostly asymptomatic, whereas other patients experience severe symptoms coinciding with a rapid transformation to AML and leading to shortened survival. Several prognostic scoring models have been developed to predict outcomes for patients with MDS, including the International Prognostic Scoring System (IPSS),[84] WHO classification-based Prognostic Scoring System (WPSS),[85] MD Anderson Prognostic Scoring System (MDAPSS),[86] and Revised International Prognostic Scoring System (IPSS-R).[87] Each of these systems considers cytopenias, percentage of blasts, and cytogenetics in the stratification of patients.[88,89] Each scoring system has its respective strengths, limitations, and intended uses.[89,90] As a brief example, some scoring systems were not developed or validated to be used for patients with secondary MDS, therapy-related MDS, or MDS/MPN conditions or for patients at different points in the disease course, stages of therapy, and posttherapy failure.[91-93] Additionally, scoring systems vary in their consideration of patient age and comorbidities, which may dramatically influence patient survival.[94] For brevity, IPSS and IPSS-R are the only models discussed.

IPSS and IPSS-R are the most widely used prognostic scoring models for MDS.[74,88,91,95] IPSS was introduced in 1997.[84] IPSS-R was introduced in 2012 to address growing concerns with IPSS.[87] Compared with IPSS, IPSS-R improves stratification of patients by identifying five risk categories instead of the original three.[96] IPSS-R includes additional cytogenetic abnormalities and is more sensitive to the percentage of blasts and the degree of cytopenias.[82] Other clinical features that affect survival but not transformation into AML include patient age, serum ferritin, patient performance status, and lactate dehydrogenase levels.[82] IPSS-R is not validated for all patient populations and thus needs to be applied with care.[91-93]

As our knowledge of somatic mutations in MDS increases, our understanding of their effects on prognosis becomes more refined. Mutations in at least 40 different genes have been identified in patients with MDS.[72,73,97] Some of these mutations have an independent ability to predict poor outcomes such as *TP53*, *EZH2*, *ETV6*, *RUNX1*, and *ASXL1*.[97-100] Conversely, mutations in *SF3B1* are significant for predicting positive outcomes.[98-100] The observed heterogeneity in MDS is driven by these somatic mutations, their interaction with other coexisting mutations, allele burden, karyotype abnormalities, cytokine concentrations, bone marrow microenvironment, clinical context, and numerous other factors.[90] Researchers are trying to integrate somatic mutations into existing or novel prognostic models to enhance the accuracy of prognoses for patients.[98-100]

Although many different prognostic scoring systems have been developed, it is important that users recognize limitations inherent in each one. The type of MDS or MDS/MPN, time since diagnosis, history of treatment, presence of genetic and epigenetic aberrations, age, comorbidities, and numerous other factors play an important role in deciding which prognostic system to use on a given patient.

TREATMENT

Treatment of MDS patients is challenging because many are older and have coexisting illnesses, and the heterogeneity of the disease makes the use of one standard treatment impossible. Prognostic scoring systems are often used to direct patient therapy.

Patients who are stratified into low-risk categories are usually treated less aggressively than patients with high-risk MDS. Patients with low-risk MDS are provided supportive therapy aimed at overcoming deficiencies in bone marrow production. Patient interventions may include transfusions, erythroid-stimulating agents, thrombopoietin, granulocyte colony-stimulating factor, prophylactic antibiotics, and iron chelation.[88] Immunosuppressive therapy with drugs such as antithymocyte globulin and cyclosporine has resulted in decreased risk of leukemic transformation in subsets of patients.[101-103] Lenalidomide and azanucleosides are also prescribed for patients with low-risk MDS.

Three drugs (lenalidomide, azacitidine, and decitabine) have been approved by the US Food and Drug Administration (FDA) that show promise when used either alone or in combination with other therapies.[104,105] Azacitidine and decitabine belong to a group of drugs called azanucleosides. Azanucleosides deplete intracellular methyltransferases (DMNTs) and are effective in low dose, with minimal side effects, and have improved the quality of life for patients with high-grade MDS.[104] Unfortunately, as many as 50% of patients will not respond to these agents.[106,107]

Lenalidomide a thalidomide analog that is less toxic than thalidomide, was approved by the FDA in 2005 for use in patients with low- or intermediate-risk MDS.[108,109] It has shown remarkable promise, especially in patients with del(5q), resulting in transfusion independence for many patients.[109]

Complete cytogenetic remission was seen in more than 50% of MDS patients taking lenalidomide, whereas in MDS patients taking erythropoietin, cytogenetic remission is rare.[109] Lenalidomide has also been given to patients without 5q deletions with 26% of patients becoming transfusion independent.[110] Lenalidomide has immunomodulatory and antiangiogenic effects.[108,109] The apparent efficacy of lenalidomide must be weighed against its ability to cause significant myelosuppression.[108,109]

NRAS is mutated in about 20% of MDS patients. Farnesyltransferase inhibitors interfere with this process.[101,96] Patients with high-risk MDS benefit from treatment with hypomethylating agents such as azacitidine and, to a lesser extent, decitabine.[77,78,104,105,111]

The only cure for MDS is HSC transplantation. Patients with an IPSS score of intermediate 2 or higher and patients with more than 10% blasts should be considered for allogeneic stem cell transplantation.[112,113] A patient's somatic mutations must be considered because some predict relapse and overall survival after a stem cell transplantation.[114] Stem cell transplantation is most successful in patients younger than age 70 with no comorbidity, although emerging research suggests that patients of older age should still be considered for transplantation.[9,115]

Future Directions

As research addressing the role of apoptosis in MDS continues, future therapies may be aimed at controlling apoptosis, with or without the use of chemotherapeutic agents. Additional therapies for patients that fail hypomethylating agents or relapse after stem cell transplantation should be developed.[88] Because effective treatment for MDS remains limited, it has been suggested that patients be provided with information on the prognosis for their type of MDS, available therapies, and success rates and should take part in making decisions regarding their treatment.[116,117] As more is learned about the molecular biology of MDS, it may be possible to develop customized treatment plans for individual patients.[118]

█ SUMMARY

- Myelodysplastic syndromes (MDS) are a group of clonal disorders characterized by progressive cytopenias and dyspoiesis of the myeloid, erythroid, and megakaryocytic cell lines.
- The dyspoiesis is evidenced by abnormal morphologic appearance and abnormal function of the cell lines affected.
- The World Health Organization (WHO) classification of MDS is based on morphologic, molecular, cytogenetic, and immunologic characteristics of blood cell lines.
- Prognosis in MDS depends on several factors, including percentage of bone marrow blasts, depth of cytopenias, and karyotypic abnormalities.

- Treatment of MDS depends on the prognosis. If the prognosis is favorable, patients may receive only supportive therapy.
- Other treatments that have met with limited success include chemotherapeutic agents and epigenetic modifiers.
- Currently the only cure for MDS is bone marrow or hematopoietic stem cell transplantation.
- Future treatment possibilities include the use of apoptosis-controlling drugs.

Now that you have completed this chapter, go back and read again the case study at the beginning and respond to the questions presented.

REVIEW QUESTIONS

Answers can be found in the Appendix.

1. MDS are most common in which age group?
   a. 2 to 10 years
   b. 15 to 20 years
   c. 25 to 40 years
   d. Older than 50 years

2. What is a major indication of MDS in the peripheral blood and bone marrow?
   a. Dyspoiesis
   b. Leukocytosis with left shift
   c. Normal bone marrow with abnormal peripheral blood features
   d. Thrombocytosis

3. An alert hematologist should recognize all of the following peripheral blood abnormalities as diagnostic clues in MDS EXCEPT:
   a. Oval macrocytes
   b. Target cells
   c. Agranular neutrophils
   d. Circulating micromegakaryocytes

4. For an erythroid precursor to be considered a ring sideroblast, the iron-laden mitochondria must encircle how much of the nucleus?
   a. One-quarter
   b. One-third
   c. Two-thirds
   d. Entire nucleus

5. According to the WHO classification of MDS, what percentage of blasts would constitute transformation to an acute leukemia?
   a. 5%
   b. 10%
   c. 20%
   d. 30%

6. A patient has anemia, oval macrocytes, and hypersegmented neutrophils. Which of the following tests would be most efficient in differential diagnosis of this disorder?
   a. Serum iron and ferritin levels
   b. Erythropoietin level
   c. Vitamin B_{12} and folate levels
   d. Chromosome analysis

7. A 60-year-old woman comes to the physician with fatigue and malaise. Her hemoglobin is 8 g/dL, hematocrit is 25%, RBC count is 2.00×10^{12}/L, platelet count is 550×10^9/L, and WBC count is 3.8×10^9/L. Her WBC differential is unremarkable. Bone marrow shows erythroid hypoplasia and hypolobulated megakaryocytes; granulopoiesis appears normal. Ring sideroblasts are rare. Chromosome analysis reveals the deletion of 5q only. Based on the classification of this disorder, what therapy would be most appropriate?
   a. Supportive therapy; lenalidomide if the disease progresses
   b. Aggressive chemotherapy
   c. Bone marrow transplantation
   d. Low-dose cytosine arabinoside, accompanied by *cis*-retinoic acid

8. Which of the following is LEAST likely to contribute to the death of patients with MDS?
   a. Neutropenia
   b. Thrombocytopenia
   c. Organ failure
   d. Neuropathy

9. Into what other hematologic disease does MDS often convert?
   a. Megaloblastic anemia
   b. Aplastic anemia
   c. AML
   d. Myeloproliferative disease

10. Chronic myelomonocytic leukemia is classified in the WHO system as:
   a. A myeloproliferative neoplasm
   b. Myelodysplastic syndrome, unclassified
   c. MDS/MPN
   d. Acute leukemia

REFERENCES

1. Layton, D. M., Mufti, G. J. (1986). Myelodysplastic syndromes: their history, evolution and relation to acute myeloid leukemia. *Blood, 53,* 423–436, 1986.
2. Steensma, D. P. (2012). Historical perspectives on myelodysplastic syndromes. *Leuk Res, 36,* 1441–1452.
3. Bennett, J. M., Catovsky, D., Daniel, M. T., et al. (1982). Proposals for the classification of the myelodysplastic syndromes. *Br J Haematol, 51,* 189–199.
4. Harris, N. L., Jaffe, E. S., Diebold, J., et al. (2000). The World Health Organization classification of hematological malignancies report of the Clinical Advisory Committee Meeting, Airlie House, Virginia, November 1997. *Mod Pathol, 13,* 193–207.
5. Vardiman, J. W., Harris, N. L., & Brunning, R. D. (2002). The World Health Organization (WHO) classification of the myeloid neoplasms. *Blood, 100,* 2292–2302.
6. Shastri, A., Will, B., Steidel, U., et al. (2017). Stem and progenitor cell alterations in myelodysplastic syndromes. *Blood, 129,* 1586–1594.
7. Sperling, A. S., Gibson, C. J., & Ebert, B. L. (2017). The genetics of myelodysplastic syndrome: from clonal haematopoiesis to secondary leukaemia. *Nat Rev Cancer, 17,* 5–19.
8. Ma, X., Does, M., Raza, A., et al. (2007). Myelodysplastic syndromes: incidence and survival in the United States. *Cancer, 109,* 1536–1542.

9. DeAngelo, D. J., & Stone, R. M. (2012). Myelodysplastic syndromes: biology and treatment. In Hoffman, R., Benz, E. J. Jr., Silberstein, L. E., et al., (Eds.), *Hematology: Basic Principles and Practice.* (6th ed.). Philadelphia: Saunders Elsevier, Chapter 59.

10. Hasle, H., Niemeyer, C. M., Chessells, J. M., et al. (2003). A pediatric approach to the WHO classification of myelodysplastic and myeloproliferative diseases. *Leukemia, 17,* 277–282.

11. Niemeyer, C. M., & Baumann, I. (2008). Myelodysplastic syndrome in children and adolescents. *Semin Hematol, 45*(1), 60–70.

12. Woll, P. S., Kjällquist, U., Chowdhury, O., et al. (2014). Myelodysplastic syndromes are propagated by rare and distinct human cancer stem cells in vivo. *Cancer Cell, 25,* 794–808.

13. Kennedy, J. A., & Ebert, B. L. (2017). Clinical implications of genetic mutations in myelodysplastic syndrome. *J Clin Oncol, 35,* 968–974.

14. Steensma, D. P., Bejar, R., Jaiswal, S., et al. (2015). Clonal hematopoiesis of indeterminate potential and its distinction from myelodysplastic syndromes. *Blood, 126,* 9–16.

15. Kwok, B., Hall, J. M., Witte, J. S., et al., (2015). MDS-associated somatic muttions and clonal hematopoiesis are common in idiopathic cytopenias of undetermined significance. *Blood, 126,* 2355–2361.

16. Jaiswal, S., Fontanillas, P., Flannick, J., et al. (2014). Age-related clonal hematopoiesis associated with adverse outcomes. *N Engl J Med, 371,* 2488–2498.

17. Genovese, G., Kähler, A. K., Rose, S. A., et al. (2014). Clonal hematopoiesis and blood-cancer risk inferred from blood DNA sequence. *N Engl J Med, 371,* 2477–2487.

18. Medyouf, H. (2017). The microenvironment in human myeloid malignancies: emerging concepts and therapeutic implications. *Blood, 129,* 1617–1626.

19. Zahr, A. A., Kavi, A. M., Mukherjee, S., et al. (2017). Therapy-related myelodysplastic syndromes, or are they? *Blood Rev, 31,* 119–128.

20. Ganser, A., & Heuser, M. (2017). Therapy-related myeloid neoplasms. *Curr Opin Hematol, 24,* 152–158.

21. Mufti, G. J. (2004). Pathobiology, classification, and diagnosis of myelodysplastic syndrome. *Best Pract Res Clin Haematol, 17*(4), 543–557.

22. Perkins, S. L., & McKenna, R. W. (2010). Myelodysplastic syndromes. In Kjeldsberg, C. R., Perkins, S. L., (Eds.), *Practical Diagnosis of Hematologic Disorders.* (5th ed., pp. 547–582). Chicago: ASCP Press, chap 45.

23. Mossner, M., Jann, J., Wittig, J., et al. (2016). Mutational hierarchies in myelodysplastic syndromes dynamically adapt and evolve upon therapy response and failure. *Blood, 128,* 1246–1259.

24. Hershman, D., Neugut, A. I., Jacobson, J. S., et al. (2007). Acute myeloid leukemia or myelodysplastic syndrome following use of granulocyte colony-stimulating factors during breast cancer adjuvant therapy. *J Natl Cancer Inst, 99,* 196–205.

25. Tsurusawa, M., Manabe, A., Hayashi, Y., et al. (2005). Therapy-related myelodysplastic syndrome in childhood: a retrospective study of 36 patients in Japan. *Leuk Res, 29,* 625–632.

26. Bannon, S. A., & DiNardo, C. D. (2016). Hereditary predispositions to myelodysplastic syndrome. *Int J Mol Sci, 17,* 838.

27. Yoshida, U. (2002). The role of apoptosis in the myelodysplastic syndromes. In Bennett, J. B. (Ed.), *The Myelodysplastic Syndromes: Pathobiology and Clinical Management.* (pp. 177-201). New York: Dekker.

28. Greenberg, P. L. (1998). Apoptosis and its role in the myelodysplastic syndromes: implication for disease natural history and treatment. *Leuk Res, 22,* 1123–1126.

29. Parker, J. E., & Mufti, G. J. (2001). The role of apoptosis in the pathogenesis of the myelodysplastic syndromes. *Int J Hematol, 73,* 416–428.

30. Brunning, R. D., Orazi, A., Germing, U., et al. (2008). Myelodysplastic syndromes/neoplasms, overview. In Swerdlow, S. H., Campo, E., Harris, N. L., et al., (Eds.), *WHO Classification of Tumours of Haematopoietic and Lymphoid Tissues.* (4th ed., pp. 88–93). Lyon, France: IARC Press.

31. Rodak, B. F., & Leclair, S. J. (2002). The new WHO nomenclature: introduction and myeloid neoplasms. *Clin Lab Sci, 15,* 44–54.

32. Head, D. R., Kopecky, K., Bennett, J. M., et al. (1989). Pathologic implications of internuclear bridging in myelodysplastic syndrome. An Eastern Cooperative Oncology Group/Southwest Oncology Group Cooperative Study. *Cancer, 64,* 2199–2202.

33. Langenhuijsen, M. M. (1984). Neutrophils with ring-shaped nuclei in myeloproliferative disease. *Br J Haematol, 58,* 227–230.

34. Doll, D. C., & List, A. F. (1989). Myelodysplastic syndromes. *West J Med, 151,* 161–167.

35. Seymour, J. F., & Estey, E. H. (1993). The prognostic significance of Auer rods in myelodysplasia. *Br J Haematol, 85,* 67–76.

36. Tricot, G., De Wolf-Peeters, R., Vlietinck, R., et al. (1984). Bone marrow histology in myelodysplastic syndromes. *Br J Haematol, 58,* 217–225.

37. Leguit, R. J., & van den Tweel, J. G. (2010). The pathology of bone marrow failure. *Histopathology, 57,* 655–670. Review.

38. Barbui, T., Cortelazzo, S., Viero, P., et al. (1993). Infection and hemorrhage in elderly acute myeloblastic leukemia and primary myelodysplasia. *Hematol Oncol, 11*(suppl 1), 15–18.

39. Mazzone, A., Ricevuti, G., Pasotti, D., et al. (1993). The CD11/CD18 granulocyte adhesion molecules in myelodysplastic syndromes. *Br J Haematol, 83,* 245–252.

40. Mittelman, M., Karcher, D., Kammerman, L., et al. (1993). High Ia (HLA-DR) and low CD11b (Mo1) expression may predict early conversion to leukemia in myelodysplastic syndromes. *Am J Hematol, 43,* 165–171.

41. Pomeroy, C., Oken, M. M., Rydell, R. E., et al. (1991). Infection in the myelodysplastic syndromes. *Am J Med, 90,* 338–344.

42. Boogaerts, M. A., Nelissen, V., Roelant, C., et al. (1983). Blood neutrophil function in primary myelodysplastic syndromes. *Br J Haematol, 55,* 217–227.

43. Verhoef, G. E., Zachee, P., Ferrant, A., et al. (1992). Recombinant human erythropoietin for the treatment of anemia in the myelodysplastic syndromes: a clinical and erythrokinetic assessment. *Ann Hematol, 64,* 16–21.

44. Merchav, S., Nielsen, O. J., Rosenbaum, H., et al. (1990). In vitro studies of erythropoietin-dependent regulation of erythropoiesis in myelodysplastic syndromes. *Leukemia, 4,* 771–774.

45. Lintula, R., Rasi, V., Ikkala, E., et al. (1981). Platelet function in preleukemia. *Scand J Haematol, 26,* 65–71.

46. Raman, B. K., Van Slyck, E. J., Riddle, J., et al. (1989). Platelet function and structure in myeloproliferative disease, myelodysplastic syndrome and secondary thrombocytosis. *Am J Clin Pathol, 91,* 647–655.

47. Arber, D. A., Orazi, A., Hasserjian, R., et al. (2016). The 2016 revision to the world health organization classification of myeloid neoplasms and acute leukemia. *Blood, 127,* 2391–2405.

48. Germing, U., Strupp, C., Kuemdgen, A., et al. (2006). Prospective validation of the WHO proposals for the classification of myelodysplastic syndromes. *Haematologica, 91*(12), 1596–1604.

49. Strupp, C., Nachtkamp, K., Hildebrandt, B., et al. (2017). New proposals of the WHO working group (2016) for the diagnosis of myelodysplastic syndromes (MDS): characteristics of refined MDS types. *Leuk Res, 57,* 78–84.

50. Mortera-Blanco, T., Dimitriou, M., Woll, P. S., et al. (2017). SF3B1-initiating mutations in MDS-RSs target lymphomyeloid hematopoietic stem cells. *Blood, 130,* 881–890.

51. Mufti, G. J., Bennett, J. M., Goasguen, J., et al. (2008). Diagnosis and classification of myelodysplastic syndrome: International Working Group on Morphology of myelodysplastic syndrome (IWGM-MDS) consensus proposals for the definition and enumeration of myeloblasts and ring sideroblasts. *Haematologica, 93,* 1712–1717.

52. Patnaik, M. M., Lasho, T. L., Hodnefield, J. M, et al. (2012). SF3B1 mutations are prevalent in myelodysplastic syndromes with ring sideroblasts but do not hold independent prognostic value. *Blood, 119,* 569–572.

53. Patnaik, M. M., & Tefferi, A. (2017). Refractory anemia with ring sideroblasts (RARS) and RARS with thrombocytosis (RARS-T): 2017 updated on diagnosis, risk-stratification, and management. *Am J Hematol, 92,* 297–310.

54. Gurney, M., Patnaik, M. M., Hanson, C. A., et al. (2017). The 2016 revised world health organization definition of 'myelodysplastic syndrome with isolated del(5q)': prognostic implications of single versus double cytogenetic abnormalities. *Br J Haematol, 178,* 57–60.

55. Giagounidis, A. A., Germing, U., Wainscoat, J. S., et al. (2004). The 5q– syndrome. *Hematology, 9,* 271–277.

56. Giagounidis, A. A., Germing, U., Haase, S., et al. (2004). Clinical, morphological, cytogenetic, and prognostic features of patients with myelodysplastic syndromes and del(5q) including band q31. *Leukemia, 18,* 113–119.

57. Giagounidis, A. A., Haase, S., Heinsch, M., et al. (2007). Lenalidomide in the context of complex karyotype or interrupted treatment: case reviews of del(5q) MDS patients with unexpected responses. *Ann Hematol, 86,* 133–137.

58. Fenaux, P., Giagounidis, A., Selleslag, D., et al. (2017). Clinical characteristics and outcomes according to age in lenalidomide-treated patients with RBC transfusion-dependent lower-risk MDS and del(5q). *J Hematol Oncol, 10,* 131.

59. Schwartz, J. R., Walsh, M. P., Ma, J., et al. (2016). The genomic landscape of pediatric myelodysplastic syndromes. *Blood, 128,* 956.

60. Arber, D. A., & Hasserjian, R. P. (2015). Reclassifying myelodysplastic syndromes: what's where in the new WHO and why. *Hematology Am Soc Hematol Educ Program, 2015,* 294–298.

61. Deininger, M. W. N., Tyner, J. W., & Solary, E. (2017). Turning the tide in myelodysplastic/myeloproliferative neoplasms. *Nat Rev Cancer, 17,* 425–440.

62. Mughal, T. I., Cross, N. C. P., Pardron, E., et al. (2015). An international MDS/MPN working group's perspective and recommendations on molecular pathogenesis, diagnosis and clinical characterization of myelodysplastic/myeloproliferative neoplasms. *Haematologica, 100,* 1117–1130.

63. Itzykson, R., Kosmider, O., Renneville, A., et al. (2013). Prognostic score including gene mutations in chronic myelomonocytic leukemia. *J Clin Oncol, 31,* 2428–2436.

64. Itzykson, R., Kosmider, O., Renneville, A., et al. (2013). Clonal architecture of chronic myelomonocytic leukemias. *Blood, 121,* 2186–2198.

65. Patnaik, M. M., Barraco, D., Lasho, T. L., et al. (2017). Targeted next generation sequencing and identification of risk factors in world health organization defined atypical chronic myeloid leukemia. *Am J Hematol, 92,* 542–548.

66. Vardiman, J. W., Bennett, J. M., Bain, B. J., et al. (2008). Atypical chronic myeloid leukemia, *BCR-ABL1* negative. In Swerdlow, S. H., Campo, E., Harris, N. L., et al., (Eds.), *WHO Classification of Tumours of Haematopoietic and Lymphoid Tissues.* (4th ed., pp. 80–81). Lyon, France: IARC Press.

67. Xubo, G., Xingguo, L., Xiaanguo, W., et al. (2009). The role of peripheral blood, bone marrow aspirate and especially bone marrow trephine biopsy in distinguishing atypical chronic myeloid leukemia from chronic granulocytic leukemia and chronic myelomonocytic leukemia. *Eur J Haematol, 83,* 1292–1301.

68. Locatelli, F., Nöllke, P., Zecca, M., et al. (2005). Hematopoietic stem cell transplantation (HSCT) in children with juvenile myelomonocytic leukemia (JMML): results of the EWOG-MDS/EBMT trial. *Blood, 105,* 410–419.

69. Haase, D., Germing, U., Schanz, J., et al. (2007). New insights into the prognostic impact of the karyotype in MDS and correlation with subtypes: evidence from a core dataset of 2124 patients. *Blood, 110,* 4385–4395.

70. Pedersen-Bjergaard, J., Andersen, M. T., Andersen, M. K. (2007). Genetic pathways in the pathogenesis of therapy-related myelodysplasia and acute myeloid leukemia. *Hematology Am Soc Hematol Educ Program,* 391–397.

71. Canaani, J., & Nagler, A. (2016). Established and emerging targeted therapies in the myelodysplastic syndromes. *Expert Rev Hematol, 9,* 997–1005.

72. Haferlach, T., Nagata, Y., Grossmann, V., et al. (2014). Landscape of genetic lesions in 944 patients with myelodysplastic syndromes. *Leukemia, 28,* 241–247.

73. Papaemmanuil, E., Gerstung, M., Malcovati, L., et al. (2013). Clinical and biological implications of driver mutations in myelodysplastic syndromes. *Blood, 122,* 3616–3627.

74. Haider, M., Duncavage, E. J., Afaneh, K. F., et al. (2017). New insight into the biology, risk stratification, and targeted treatment of myelodysplastic syndromes. In D. S. Dizon (Ed.), *American Society of Clinical Oncology 2017 Educational Book: Making a Difference in Cancer Care With You* (480–494). Alexandria, VA: ASCO.

75. Bejar, R., Stevenson, K., Abdel-Wahab, O., et al. (2011). Clinical effect of point mutations in myelodysplastic syndromes. *N Engl J Med, 364,* 2496–2506.

76. Malcovati, L., Karimi, M., Papaemmanuil, E., et al. (2015). SF3B1 mutation identifies a distinct subset of myelodysplastic syndrome with ring sideroblasts. *Blood, 126,* 233-241.

77. Nakao, M. (2001). Epigenetics: interaction of DNA methylation and chromatin. *Gene, 278,* 25–31.

78. Musolino, C., Sant'Antonio, E., Penna, G., et al. (2010). Epigenetic therapy in myelodysplastic syndromes. *Eur J Haematol, 84,* 463–473.

79. Milunović, V., Rogulj, I. M., Planinc-Peraica, A., et al. (2016). The role of microRNA in myelodysplastic syndromes: beyond DNA methylation and histone modification. *Eur J Haematol, 96,* 553–563.

80. Issa, J. J. (2013). The myelodysplastic syndrome as a prototypical epigenetic disease. *Blood, 121,* 3811–3817.

81. Scott, L. J. (2016). Azacitidine: a review in myelodysplastic syndromes and acute myeloid leukemia. *Drugs, 76,* 889–900.

82. Fenaux, P., Mufti, G. J., Hellstrom-Lindberg, E., et al. (2009). Efficacy of azacitidine compared with that of conventional care regimens in the treatment of higher-risk myelodysplastic syndromes: a ramdomised, open-label, phase III study. *Lancet Oncol, 10,* 223–232.

83. Kantarjian, H., Oki, Y., Garcia-Manero, G., et al. (2007). Results of a randomized study of 3 schedules of low-dose decitabine in higher-risk myelodysplastic syndrome and chronic myelomonocytic leukemia. *Blood, 109,* 52–57.

84. Greenberg, P., Cox, C., & LeBeau, M. M. (1997). International scoring system for evaluating prognosis in myelodysplastic syndromes. *Blood, 89,* 2079–2088.

85. Malcovati, L., Germing, U., Kuendgen, A., et al. (2007). Time-dependent prognostic scoring system for predicting survival and leukemic evolution in myelodysplastic syndromes. *J Clin Oncol, 25,* 3503–3510.

86. Kantarjian, H., O'Brien, S., Ravandi, F., et al. (2008). Proposal for a new risk model in myelodysplastic syndrome that accounts for events not considered in the original International Prognostic Scoring System. *Cancer, 113,* 1351–1361.

87. Greenberg, P. L., Tuechler, H., Schanz, J., et al. (2012). Revised international scoring system for myelodysplastic syndromes. *Blood, 120,* 2454–2465.

88. Garcia-Manero, G. (2015). Myelodysplastic syndromes: 2015 update on diagnosis, risk-stratification and management. *Am J Hematol, 90,* 832–841.

89. Nazha, A., & Sekeres, M. A. (2016). Improving prognostic modeling in myelodysplastic syndromes. *Curr Hematol Malig Rep, 11,* 395–401.

90. Bejar, R. (2013). Prognostic models in myelodysplastic syndromes. *Hematology Am Soc Hematol Educ Program, 504–510.*

91. Zeidan, A. M., Sekeres, M. A., Garcia-Manero, G., et al. (2016). Comparison of risk stratification tools in predicting outcomes of patients with higher-risk myelodysplastic syndromes treated with azanucleosides. *Leukemia, 30,* 649–657.

92. Cazzola, M., Della Porta, M. G., Travaglino, E., et al. (2011). Classification and prognostic evaluation of myelodysplastic syndromes. *Semin Oncol, 38,* 627–634.

93. Nazha, A., Komrokji, R. S., Garcia-Monero, G., et al. (2016). The efficacy of current prognostic models in predicting outcome of patients with myelodysplastic syndromes at the time of hypomethylating agent failiure. *Haematologica, 101,* 224–227

94. Nachtkamp, K., Stark, R., Strupp, C., et al. (2016). Causes of death in 2877 patients with myelodysplastic syndromes. *Ann Hematol, 95,* 937–944.

95. Della Porta, M. G., Tuechler, H., Malcovati, L., et al. (2015). Validation of WHO classification-based prognostic scoring system (WPSS) for myelodysplastic syndromes and comparison with the revised international prognostic scoring system (IPSS-R). A study of the international working group for prognosis in myelodysplasia (IWG-PM). *Leukemia, 29,* 1502–1513.

96. Neukirchen, J., Lauseker, M., Blum, S., et al. (2014). Validation of the revised international prognostic scoring system (IPSS-R) in patients with myelodysplastic syndrome: A multicenter study. *Leuk Res, 38,* 57–64.

97. Montalban-Bravo, G., Takahashi, K., Wang, F., et al. (2016). Clinical relevance of driver mutations and number of driver mutations in patients with myelodysplastic syndromes and chronic myelomonocytic leukemia. *Blood, 128,* 54.

98. Nazha, A., Narkhede, M., Radivoyevitch, T., et al. (2016). Incorporation of molecular data into the revised international prognostic scoring system in treated patients with myelodysplastic syndromes. *Leukemia, 30,* 2214–2220.

99. Nazha, A., Al-Issa, K., Hamilton, B. K., et al. (2017). Adding molecular data to prognostic models can improve predictive power in treated patients with myelodysplastic syndromes. *Leukemia,* Advance Online Publication.

100. Bejar, R., Papaemmanuil, E., Haferlach, T., et al. (2015). Somatic mutations in MDS patients are associated with clinical features and predict prognosis independent of the IPSS-R: analysis of combined datasets from the international working group for prognosis in MDS-molecular committee. *Blood, 126,* 907.

101. Loaiza-Bonilla, A., Gore, S., & Carraway, H. E. (2010). Novel approaches for myelodysplastic syndromes: beyond hypomethylating agents. *Curr Opin Hematol, 17,* 104–109.

102. Sloand, E. M., Wu, C. O., Greenberg, P., et al. (2008). Factors affecting response and survival in patients with myelodysplasia treated with immunosuppressive therapy. *J Clin Oncol, 26,* 2505–2511.

103. Ganán-Gómez, I., Wei, Y., Starczynowski, D. T., et al. (2015). Deregulation of innate immune and inflammatory signaling in myelodysplastic syndromes. *29, Leukemia* 1458–1469.

104. Griffiths, E. A., & Gore, S. D. (2013). Epigenetic therapies in MDS and AML. *Adv Exp Med Biol, 754,* 253–283.

105. Sekeres, M. A. (2009). Treatment of MDS; something old, something new, something borrowed. *Hematology Am Soc Hematol Educ Program, 656–663.*

106. Steensma, D. P., Baer, M. R., Slack, J. L., et al. (2009). Multicenter study of decitabine administered daily for 5 days every 4 weeks to adults with myelodysplastic syndromes: the alternative dosing for outpatient treatment (ADOPT) trial. *J Clin Oncol, 27,* 3842–3848.

107. Gore, S. D., Fenaux, P., Santini, V., et al. (2013). A multivariate analysis of the relationship between response and survival among patients with higher-risk myelodysplastic syndromes treated within azacitidine or conventional care regimens in the randomized AZA-001 trial. *Haematologica, 98,* 1067–1072.

108. Talati, C., Sallman, D., & List, A. (2017). Lenalidomide: myelodysplastic syndromes with del(5q) and beyond. *Semin Hematol, 54,* 159–166.

109. Giagounidis, A., Mufti, G. J., Germing, U., et al. (2014). Lenalidomide as a disease-modifying agent in patients with del(5q) myelodysplastic syndromes: linking mechanism of action to clinical outcomes. *Ann Hematol, 93,* 1–11.

110. Raza, A., Reeves, J. A., Feldman, E. J., et al. (2008). Phase 2 study of lenalidomide in transfusion-dependent, low-risk, and intermediate-1-risk myelodysplastic syndromes with karyotypes other than deletion 5q. *Blood, 111,* 86–93.

111. Greenberg, P. L., Stone, R. M., Al-Kali, A., et al. (2017). Myelodysplastic syndromes, version 2.2017: clinical practice guidelines in oncology. *J Natl Compr Canc Netw, 15,* 60–87.

112. Appelbaum, F. R. (2011). The role of hematopoietic cell transplantation as therapy for myelodysplasia. *Best Pract Res Clin Haematol, 24,* 541–547.

113. Gerds, A. T., & Deeg, H. J. (2012). Transplantation for myelodysplastic syndrome in the era of hypomethylating agents. *Curr Opin Hematol, 19,* 71–75.

114. Della Porta, M. G., Gallì, A., Bacigalupo, A., et al. (2016). Clinical effects of driver somatic mutations on the outcomes of patients with myelodysplastic syndromes treated with allogeneic hematopoietic stem-cell transplantation. *J Clin Oncol, 34,* 3627–3637.

115. Muffly, L., Pasquini, M. C., Martens, M., et al. (2017). Increasing use of allogeneic hematopoietic cell transplantation in patients aged 70 years and older in the United States. *Blood, 130,* 1156–1164.

116. Sekeres, M. A., Stowell, S. A., Berry, C. A., et al. (2013). Improving the diagnosis and treatment of patients with myelodysplastic syndromes through a performance improvement initiative. *Leuk Res, 37,* 422–426.

117. Besson, D., Rannou, S., Elmaaroufi, H., et al. (2012). Disclosure of myelodysplastic syndrome diagnosis: improving patients' understanding and experience. *Eur J Haematol, 90,* 151–156.

118. Scott, B. L., & Deeg, H. J. (2010). Myelodysplastic syndromes. *Annu Rev Med, 61,* 345–358.

Mature Lymphoid Neoplasms

Steven Marionneaux, Peter Maslak

OBJECTIVES

After completing this chapter, the reader will be able to:

1. Compare and contrast similarities and differences between leukemia and lymphoma with respect to clinical and laboratory findings.
2. Explain the approach to the diagnosis of lymphomas as outlined by the World Health Organization classification.
3. Describe the peripheral blood findings in chronic lymphocytic leukemia and hairy cell leukemia.
4. Recognize morphologic features of circulating malignant cells in different types of non-Hodgkin lymphoma.
5. Compare the similarities and differences between monoclonal gammopathy of unknown significance (MGUS) and monoclonal B cell lymphocytosis (MBL) with regard to laboratory findings and assessment of risk for disease progression.
6. Describe the different forms of Hodgkin lymphoma.
7. Demonstrate how clinicians use staging systems in the evaluation and management of leukemia and lymphoma.
8. Interpret diagnostic test results to identify lymphoproliferative disorders.

OUTLINE

Immunologic Diversity
Classification Schemas Based on Cell Differentiation
Approach to Diagnosis: Interface Between Clinical and
  Laboratory Medicine
  Clinical Signs and Symptoms
  Diagnostic Procedures
  Diagnostic Evaluation: Staging Systems
  Prognostic Evaluation
Leukemias
  Chronic Lymphocytic Leukemia (CLL)
  Monoclonal B Cell Lymphocytosis (MBL) and Small
    Lymphocytic Lymphoma (SLL)
  Prolymphocytic Leukemia (PLL)
  Hairy Cell Leukemia (HCL)
  Large Granular Lymphocytic (LGL) Leukemia

Lymphomas
  Adult T Cell Leukemia/Lymphoma (ATLL)
  Burkitt Lymphoma/Leukemia (BL)
  Follicular Lymphoma (FL)
  Mantle Cell Lymphoma (MCL)
  Diffuse Large B Cell Lymphoma (DLBCL)
  Marginal Zone Lymphoma (MZL)
  Nodal Marginal Zone Lymphoma
  Mycosis Fungoides (MF)/Sézary Syndrome (SS)
  Anaplastic Large Cell Lymphoma (ALCL)
  Peripheral T Cell Lymphoma-Not Otherwise Specified
    (PTCL-NOS)
  Plasma Cell Neoplasms
  Hodgkin Lymphoma (HL)

CASE STUDY

After studying the material in this chapter, the reader should be able to respond to the following case study:

A 75-year-old healthy man is seen in the emergency department for pain in his right forearm after a fall on the ice. Imaging studies reveal a fractured radius. A CBC and chemistry panel are also performed at admission.

His laboratory test results are as follows:

WBC	9.5×10^9/L
HGB	14.5 g/dL
HCT	43%
Platelets	195×10^9/L
Neutrophils	30%
Lymphocytes	60%
Monocytes	9%
Eosinophils	1%

Peripheral blood film review reveals marked smudge cells.
Lymphocytes appear mature with a dense nuclear chromatin pattern.
Chemistry tests are all within reference intervals.

1. What is the significance of the hematology test results?
2. Identify tests to be performed to aid diagnosis and predict their results.
3. Describe the diagnostic criteria required to identify and stage this condition.

Mature lymphoid neoplasms are a diverse collection of disease entities with varying clinical presentations and natural histories; however, common to all is identification with a particular lineage. Disease states in large part can be identified with a normal counterpart in the blood, bone marrow or lymph nodes. Neoplastic transformation of these cells results in abnormal changes in growth and differentiation patterns, resulting in disease.

Lymphoproliferative disorders in which the primary site of disease is the blood or bone marrow are classified as *leukemias*; disorders in which the localization of disease is in the lymph nodes and spleen are considered *lymphomas*. These categories are not mutually exclusive; there are disorders, such as chronic lymphocytic leukemia (CLL), in which the neoplastic cells are prominent in the blood yet also involve the spleen and lymph nodes. Likewise, lymphomas may have a leukemic phase in which the malignant cells are found in the peripheral blood. Plasma cell neoplasms (e.g., multiple or plasma cell myeloma) tend to be bone marrow based, although extramedullary involvement may be an important part of the clinical presentation.

In this chapter we illustrate the important role that the clinical laboratory has in the diagnosis and management of lymphoid neoplasms. The 2016 World Health Organization (WHO) classification lists over 75 different diseases spread among several different categories; therefore we highlight a few of the common or well-known disorders.[1,2]

IMMUNOLOGIC DIVERSITY

The generation of immunologic diversity is an inherently complex process with many steps. Such complexity lends itself to error, and many of the genetic abnormalities that characterize the B cell lymphomas involve the immunoglobulin genes. Mutation in individual genes sometimes results in a defective gene with an altered product that has negative implications for the cell's overall growth or function. Alternatively, chromosomal translocations cause genes to become "misplaced" and can expose them to either stimuli or suppression that results in an altered expression pattern. If such genes are involved in growth or maturation, these changes may have profound implications for the cell and result in clinical disease.[3,4] Common examples of translocated genes are *MYC*, which stimulates entry into the cell cycle; *BCL2* which suppresses apoptosis; and *BCL6*, which can suppress the transcription of other genes necessary for cell growth. These mutations are found in a number of lymphomas. Some more common chromosomal translocations and the altered genes are summarized in Table 34.1[1-4]

CLASSIFICATION SCHEMAS BASED ON CELL DIFFERENTIATION

The vast majority of the mature lymphoid neoplasms represent malignant transformation of lymphoid cells at various stages of development. Examination of the morphology is the first step in interpreting patterns of involvement; however, it is imperfect because different diseases may present with similar appearances. Flow cytometry and immunohistochemistry are important methodologies to identify disorders using the differentiation schema.

TABLE 34.1 Genetic/Molecular Changes in Mature Lymphoid Neoplasms[1-4]

Disease	Chromosomes	Genes
Chronic lymphocytic leukemia (CLL)	13q14 del	Undetermined
	Trisomy 12	Undetermined
	11q23 del	ATM
	17p13 del	TP53
Prolymphocytic leukemia (PLL)	t(8;14)	MYC
	del 17p	TP53
Hairy cell leukemia (HCL)	N/A	BRAF V(600)E
Burkitt leukemia/lymphoma (BL)	t(8;14)	MYC/IgH
	t(2;8)	MYC/Igκ
	t(8;22)	MYC/Igλ
Follicular lymphoma (FL)	t(14;18)	BCL2/IgH
	t(3;14)	BCL6/IgH
Mantle cell lymphoma (MCL)	t(11;14)	CCND1/IgH
Diffuse large B cell lymphoma (DLBCL)	3q27	BCL6
	t(14;18)	BCL2/IgH
		MYC/BCL2/BCL6 (double/triple hit)
Marginal zone lymphoma (MZL)		
Mucosa-associated lymphoid tissue lymphoma (MALT)	t(11;18)	API2/MALT1
	t(1;14)	BCL10/IgH
	t(14;18)	MALT1/IgH
	t(3;14)	FOXP1/IgH
Splenic marginal zone lymphoma (SMZL)	Trisomy 3	UD
	7q21 del	CDK6
Anaplastic large cell lymphoma (ALCL)	t(2;5)	NPM1/ALK
	t(1;2)	TPM3/ALK
	t(2;3)	TFG/ALK
	t(2;17)	CTCC/ALK
	inv(2)	ATIC/ALK
Peripheral T cell lymphoma, not otherwise specified (PTCL) (NOS)	t(5;9)	ITK/SYK (follicular variant)
Multiple (plasma cell) myeloma (MM)	Hyperdiploidy/ hypodiploidy	UD
	t(11;14)	CCND1/IgH
	t(4;14)	FGFR-3-MMSET/ IgH
	t(14;16)	CMAF/IgH
	t(14;20)	MAFB/IgH
	17p13 del	TP53
	13 del/monosomy 13	RBI/DIS3

This model fits some diseases better than others. For example, Hodgkin lymphoma and hairy cell leukemia are recognized as B cell disorders, although the normal counterpart of the transformed cells remains elusive. CLL arises in two circumstances: one version with unmutated heavy chains, representing a pregerminal center event; and one with hypermutated heavy chains, suggesting a later stage of development. The unmutated form has more clinically aggressive disease with a poorer prognosis.[5]

BOX 34.1 Clinical Behavior of Mature Lymphoid Neoplasms

BOX 34.1 Clinical Behavior of Mature Lymphoid Neoplasms

Aggressive Disease

Adult T cell leukemia/lymphoma
Prolymphocytic leukemia
Anaplastic large cell lymphoma
Mantle cell lymphoma
Sézary syndrome
Diffuse large B cell lymphoma
Peripheral T cell lymphoma
Multiple (plasma cell) myeloma
Burkitt leukemia/lymphoma

Indolent Disease

Chronic lymphocytic leukemia/small lymphocytic leukemia
Large granular lymphocytic leukemia
Hairy cell leukemia
Mycosis fungoides
Lymphoplasmacytic lymphoma (Waldentröm's)
Marginal zone lymphoma
Follicular lymphoma
Solitary plasmacytoma
Smoldering multiple myeloma

Although useful in grouping similar disease entities together, a schema based on the level of maturation is not reflective of clinical behavior. Acute lymphoid leukemia (ALL), with a stem cell or precursor phenotype, is more commonly found in the pediatric population. Although ALL is generally aggressive and has a fulminant clinical presentation, the cure rate is greater than 90%. Diseases at the terminal end of differentiation, such as plasma cell myeloma or Burkitt lymphoma, can also be clinically aggressive; however, they are more difficult to cure with currently available therapies. Therefore natural history and clinical behavior are not reflective of the phenotype of the particular disorder, but of the underlying genetic changes that determine tumor growth and response to therapy. The typical clinical behaviors of some of the more common mature lymphoid neoplasms are summarized in Box 34.1.

An appreciation of the ontogeny of B, T, and natural killer (NK) cells is helpful for understanding some of the biologic behaviors of the lymphoid neoplasms, and it forms the basis for the classification of these disorders. Neoplastic counterparts of lymphoid cells that localize to a germinal center of lymphoid tissues will likewise gravitate to and involve these areas. WHO has developed a classification system based on a multiparameter approach to diagnosis.[1,2] The 2016 schema for the mature lymphoid neoplasms is listed in Table 34.2.[1,2]

APPROACH TO DIAGNOSIS: INTERFACE BETWEEN CLINICAL AND LABORATORY MEDICINE

Clinical Signs and Symptoms

Clinical signs and symptoms for diseases discussed in this chapter range from asymptomatic disease detected on a screening complete blood count (CBC) to fulminant illness characterized by symptoms such as fever, weight loss, night sweats, and adenopathy, in addition to severe functional compromise. The history and physical exam are of utmost importance and the first step in arriving at an accurate diagnosis. Manifestations of disease can be interpreted differently, depending on the clinical context. For example, lymphadenopathy is a common presentation for non-Hodgkin lymphoma but may also be seen in reactive conditions involving infection or inflammation.

Presenting symptoms may be nonspecific; however, they are often reflective of tumor involvement of a particular organ system. Lymphadenopathy is not uncommon and is present in approximately 40% of cases of lymphoma. The pattern of involvement may be characteristic of a specific lymphoma; for example, painless cervical adenopathy in the young adult is most likely associated with Hodgkin lymphoma (HL). The presence of systematic B symptoms (Box 34.2) occurs in only 40% of cases of non-Hodgkin lymphoma (NHL), 20% of cases of early stage HL, and 50% of cases of advanced stage HL. Development of such symptoms in a patient with low-grade lymphoma or CLL who previously had been without complaints may indicate transformation to a more aggressive disease. In HL, patients can present with unique complaints of alcohol intolerance, or pruritus or skin rash upon starting ampicillin. Gastrointestinal (GI) symptoms (e.g., early satiety or nausea) often relate to direct involvement of the GI tract with tumor, but hepatosplenomegaly may be an indirect cause. Skin infiltration can occur diffusely or may be localized and appear as nodules. Although more common in T cell disorders, skin involvement also can be seen in a number of B cell diseases, such as marginal zone lymphoma (MZL).

Analysis of the cerebrospinal fluid (CSF) or pleural fluid to look for tumor involvement is important for patients presenting with central nervous system (CNS) symptoms or potential extranodal involvement or dyspnea due to pleural effusion. Cytopenias can occur when lymphoma is in the bone marrow or as a result of myelosuppressive therapy. Some forms of lymphoma have a "leukemic" phase, which can be detected with a CBC, especially when a peripheral blood film review and manual differential are included. Alternatively, abnormalities of the peripheral blood that are distinct from tumor involvement are often important for patient management.

Diagnostic Procedures

Clinical Laboratory Testing

The CBC is one of the first laboratory tests ordered to investigate a patient's symptoms in which a quantitative abnormality may be the first indication of underlying pathology. A normal lymphocyte count, automated differential, or absence of morphologic flags does not rule out the presence of abnormal cells in the peripheral blood. Therefore clinical context is crucial and communication between the clinical team and laboratory professionals is needed, particularly when a lymphoid neoplasm is suspected. Manual review of the peripheral blood film to detect abnormal lymphoid cells may be required when there is lymphadenopathy or other symptoms suggestive of a

TABLE 34.2 2016 WHO Classification of Mature Lymphoid Neoplasms[1,2]

Mature B Cell Neoplasms

Chronic lymphocytic leukemia/small lymphocytic lymphoma*
Monoclonal B cell lymphocytosis
B cell prolymphocytic leukemia
Splenic marginal zone lymphoma
Hairy cell leukemia
Splenic B cell lymphoma, unclassifiable
    Splenic diffuse red pulp small B cell lymphoma
    Hairy cell variant
Lymphoplasmacytic lymphoma*
    Waldenström's macroglobulinemia*
Monoclonal gammopathy of undetermined significance (MGUS), IgM*
μ Heavy chain disease*
γ Heavy chain disease*
α Heavy chain disease*
Monoclonal gammopathy of undetermined significance
    (MGUS), IgG/A*
Plasma cell myeloma*.**
Solitary plasmacytoma of the bone*
Extraosseous plasmacytoma*
Monoclonal immunoglobulin deposition diseases
Extranodal marginal zone lymphoma of mucosa-associated lymphoid tissue
    (MALT) lymphoma*
Nodal marginal zone*
    Pediatric nodal marginal zone lymphoma
Follicular lymphoma*
    In situ follicular neoplasm
    Duodenal-type follicular lymphoma
Pediatric-type follicular lymphoma
Large B cell lymphoma with IRF4 rearrangement
Primary cutaneous follicle center lymphoma
Mantle cell lymphoma*
    In situ mantle cell lymphoma*
Diffuse large B cell lymphoma (DLBCL), not otherwise specified —(NOS)
    Germinal center B cell type
    Activated B cell type*
    T cell/histiocyte-rich large B cell lymphoma
    Primary DLBCL of the central nervous system (NOS)
    Primary cutaneous DLBCL, leg type
    EBV+ DLBCL, NOS
    EBV+ mucocutaneous ulcer
DLBCL associated with chronic inflammation
Lymphomatoid granulomatosis
Primary mediastinal (thymic) large B cell lymphoma
Intravascular large B cell lymphoma
ALK+ Anaplastic Lymphoma Kinase + large B cell lymphoma
Plasmablastic lymphoma
Primary effusion lymphoma
Human herpesvirus 8 (HHV8+) DLBCL, NOS
Burkitt lymphoma*
    Burkitt lymphoma with 11 q aberration

High-grade B cell lymphoma with *MYC* geneand BCL2 and/or BCL6 rear-
    rangements*
High-grade B cell lymphoma
B cell lymphoma, unclassifiable with features intermediate between DLBCL
    and classic Hodgkin lymphoma

Mature T and Natural Killer (NK) Neoplasms

T cell prolymphocytic leukemia*
T cell large granular lymphocytic leukemia*
Chronic lymphoproliferative disorder of NK cells*
Aggressive NK leukemia
Systemic EBV+ T cell lymphoma of childhood
Hydroa vacciniforme-like lymphoproliferative disorder
Adult T cell leukemia/lymphoma*
Extranodal NK/T cell lymphoma, nasal type
Enteropathy-associated T cell lymphoma
Monomorphic epitheliotropic intestinal T cell lymphoma
Indolent T cell lymphoproliferative disorder of the gastrointestinal tract
Hepatosplenic T cell lymphoma
Subcutaneous panniculitis-like T cell lymphoma
Mycosis fungoides*
Sézary syndrome*
Primary cutaneous CD30+ T cell lymphoproliferative disorders
    Lymphoid papulosis
    Primary cutaneous anaplastic large cell lymphoma
Primary γδ T cell lymphoma
Primary cutaneous CD8+ aggressive epidermotropic cytotoxic T cell lymphoma
Primary cutaneous acral CD8+ T cell lymphoma
Primary cutaneous CD4+ small/medium T cell lymphoproliferative disorder
Peripheral T cell lymphoma-not otherwise specified (NOS)*
Angioimmunoblastic T cell lymphoma
Follicular T cell lymphoma
Nodal peripheral T cell lymphoma with TFH phenotype
Anaplastic large cell lymphoma , ALK+*
Anaplastic large cell lymphoma, ALK−*
Breast implant-associated anaplastic large cell lymphoma*

Hodgkin Lymphoma

Nodular lymphocyte predominant Hodgkin lymphoma
Classic Hodgkin lymphoma
    Nodular sclerosis classic Hodgkin lymphoma*
    Lymphocyte-rich classic Hodgkin lymphoma*
    Mixed cellularity classic Hodgkin lymphoma*
    Lymphocyte-depleted classic Hodgkin lymphoma*

Posttransplant Lymphoproliferative Disorders (PTLD)

Plasmacytic hyperplasia PTLD
Infectious mononucleosis PTLD
Florid follicular hyperplasia PTLD
Polymorphic PTLD
Monomorphic PTLD (B and T/NK cell types)
Classic Hodgkin lymphoma PTLD

*Discussed in the chapter text.
**Also called multiple myeloma

BOX 34.2 B Symptoms

- Unexplained weight loss (>10% body weight) in 6 months prior to staging
- Unexplained, persistent, or recurrent fever (>38° C) in prior month
- Recurrent drenching night sweats during prior month

lymphoid neoplasm. The presence of these cells may prompt further diagnostic procedures, such as flow cytometry and biopsy of the bone marrow or an enlarged lymph node. An example of a potential disparity between the automated and manual differentials is illustrated in Figure 34.1.

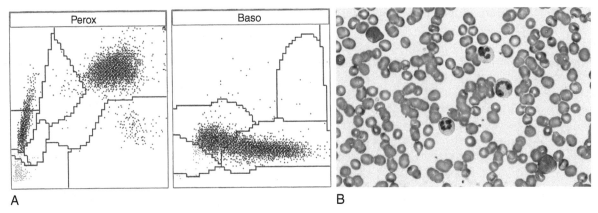

Figure 34.1 Disparity Between Automated and Manual Differentials. (A), Cytogram generated by a hematology analyzer for an 11-year-old male with a history of acute lymphoid leukemia (ALL) who was treated with hematopoietic stem cell transplantation. The cytogram shows a relatively normal pattern in which suspect/morphologic flags (e.g., "blast" or "variant lymphocyte") were not generated. **(B),** Upon manual review by the medical laboratory scientist, circulating blasts were noted, consistent with relapsed disease. This underscores the inability of modern instrumentation to always detect some lymphoid abnormalities. (Peripheral blood, Wright-Giemsa stain, ×1000.)

Flow cytometry is often used to document clonality associated with lymphoid malignancies. Immunophenotyping is undertaken with standard consensus panels, and the pattern of staining with a series of monoclonal antibodies (MoAbs) associated with lineages and degree of maturation establishes an immunologic (CD) profile[6] (Chapter 28). T and B cell disorder immunophenotypes are provided in Table 34.3. Conventional cytogenetics (karyotyping) and fluorescent in situ hybridization (FISH) detect genetic changes associated with these diseases.

Biochemical analysis may be useful for three purposes: (1) evaluating organ systems for compromise due to tumor involvement, (2) serving as an indirect measure of tumor burden, and (3) assessing prognosis. An indication of organ compromise is used to guide further diagnostic workup with a biopsy or imaging studies. Information from the biochemical panel is a good indicator of the patient's ability to tolerate chemotherapy. For example, serum creatinine levels are used to assess renal function in patients receiving treatment known to affect the kidneys. Baseline measurement of uric acid is performed in disorders with high tumor cell turnover. Patients may undergo assessment for a monoclonal protein with serum protein electrophoresis, immunofixation, and serum free light chain analysis. CLL patients presenting with sudden, unexplained anemia may require a reticulocyte count, haptoglobin,

TABLE 34.3 Common Immunophenotypes for Mature Lymphoid Neoplasms[6]

Neoplasm	Immunophenotypes
Chronic lymphocytic leukemia (CLL)	CD19+, CD20+ (CD19 > CD20), CD5+, CD23+, CD200+, surface immunoglobulin (dim), CD10−, FMC7 dim or −, CD79b dim or −
Prolymphocytic leukemia (PLL)	CD19+, CD22+ (bright), surface immunoglobulin (bright), FMC7 +, CD5 +/−, CD10 − T cell: CD4+ or CD4+/CD8+ (dual), TCL1 +, CD2+, CD3+,CD7+, CD52+,Tdt −
Hairy cell leukemia (HCL	CD20+ (bright), CD25+, CD103+, CD11c+, surface immunoglobulin (bright), CD5 + (dim) or −, CD10−
Large granular lymphocytic leukemia (LGL)	T cell type: CD8+, CD3+, CD57+, CD16+, CD2+, CD5+(dim), CD7 +(dim) or − Natural killer (NK) cell type: CD56+, CD3−, CD16+, CD2 + (dim) or −, CD7+ (dim) or −, CD57+(dim) or −
Adult T cell leukemia/lymphoma (ATLL)	CD2+, CD5+, CD3+, CD7−, CD4+, CD25+(bright), CD30+ , CCR4+, FOXP3+
Burkitt leukemia/lymphoma (BL)	CD19+, CD20+, CD22+, CD10+, surface immunoglobulin (bright), Ki67+,Tdt −
Follicular lymphoma (FL)	CD19+, CD20+ CD10+, surface immunoglobulin (bright) CD5−, CD23−
Mantle cell lymphoma (MCL)	CD19+, CD20+, CD5+, CD23−, CD200−, FMC7+, CD22+, CD79b+, CD10 +/−
Diffuse large B cell lymphoma (DLBCL)	CD19+, CD20+, CD79b+, CD22+(bright), CD10 +/−
Marginal zone lymphoma (MZL)	CD19+,CD20+, CD22+, CD79b+, surface immunoglobulin (bright), FMC7+, CD5−, CD10−, CD23−
Anaplastic large cell lymphoma (ALCL)	CD30+, ALK +/−, CD3−, CD2+, CD5+, CD4+, TIA1+
Mycosis fungoides/Sézary syndrome (MF/SS)	CD2+ , CD3+,CD5+, CD7−, CD4+, CD26−
Multiple (plasma cell) myeloma (MM)	CD45 dim or −, CD38+, CD138+, CD56+, CD117+, monotypic cytoplasmic light chains
Classic Hodgkin lymphoma (HL$_c$)	high forward scatter (large cells), CD30+, CD40+ (bright), CD95+ (bright), CD20−, CD64−

and direct antiglobulin test to rule out an associated autoimmune hemolytic anemia. Lactate dehydrogenase (LDH) and β2 microglobulin have utility as estimates of tumor burden and have been incorporated into scoring systems that have prognostic value. Measurement of the erythrocyte sedimentation rate (ESR) is indicated in Hodgkin lymphoma because elevated levels are predictive of early relapse and decreased survival. Testing for hepatitis B should be performed prior to the institution of chemoimmunotherapy. Patients who have evidence of hepatitis B surface antigen require prophylactic antiviral therapy to avoid severe complications of viral reactivation. Human immunodeficiency virus (HIV) testing should be routinely performed prior to therapy because this may significantly affect overall management.

Analyzing the peripheral blood is relatively easy; however, it may not yield sufficient information to make a diagnosis. Because lymphadenopathy is common in lymphoid neoplasms, it is logical to attempt to secure tissue from an area that is highly likely to be involved with disease. Alternatively, if suspicious cells are found in peripheral blood, bone marrow aspiration and biopsy may be indicated. In cases presenting with lymphadenopathy, it may be worthwhile to obtain a CBC prior to lymph node biopsy. Lymphadenopathy is common in CLL, but testing the peripheral blood may be sufficient to make the diagnosis, thus avoiding an invasive procedure.

Anatomic Pathology Testing

Excisional biopsy is the gold standard for lymphoma diagnosis, but fine needle aspiration (FNA) has become popular due to the ease with which specimens can be obtained. FNA coupled with advances in flow cytometry and FISH analysis make this a feasible approach for diagnosis of certain disorders and serves as a screening procedure for differentiating reactive lymphadenopathy from malignant disease

Medical Imaging Studies

Accurate staging of the tumor is fundamental for developing a treatment plan for each patient. Radiographic (medical) imaging is frequently used to assess tumor involvement. Computed tomography (CT) scans are standard for the diagnostic workup for both Hodgkin and non-Hodgkin lymphoma. Positron emission tomography (PET) with fluorodeoxyglucose (FDG) as a tracer is used to delineate areas of disease and identify sites appropriate for biopsy.

Diagnostic Evaluation: Staging Systems

Staging systems incorporate data from clinical laboratory test information, anatomic pathology analysis, and radiographic studies, along with physical exam findings. The Ann Arbor staging system was first applied to Hodgkin lymphoma to quantify nodal and extranodal sites of involvement (Table 34.4).[7-9] It was further qualified by the absence or presence of B symptoms (denoted by either the A or B suffix). The clinical utility of this system is to define limited versus extensive disease, because the treatment differs between the two.

Ann Arbor staging has also been applied to NHL but is less useful in these diseases because of biologic differences.[8] The

TABLE 34.4 Ann Arbor and Lugano Systems for Staging Hodgkin Lymphoma/Primary Nodal Non-Hodgkin Lymphoma[7-9]

Ann Arbor		Lugano
Limited		
I	1 node involved or single extranodal site (E)	1 node or group of nodes; single extranodal lesion without nodal involvement
II	2 or more nodes/groups or lymphatic structures on same side of diaphragm or involvement of limited contiguous extralymphatic organ or tissue (IIE)	2 or more nodes or nodal groups on same side of diaphragm; Stage I or II by nodal extent with limited contiguous extranodal involvement
Advanced		
III	Nodes on both sides of diaphragm (III) with involvement of spleen (IIIS) or limited contiguous extralymphatic organ or tissue involvement (IIIE) or both (IIIES)	Nodes on both sides of diaphragm / Nodes above diaphragm with spleen involvement
IV	Diffuse or disseminated foci of involvement of 1 or more extralymphatic organs or tissues with or without associated lymphatic involvement	Additional noncontiguous extralymphatic involvement

Lugano classification, a simplification of the original Ann Arbor staging, is currently used in NHL, grouping patients into limited (Stages I and II) and advanced (Stages III and IV) with a recognition that for these disorders, the intrinsic properties of the tumor have more bearing on clinical outcome than the extent of disease described by anatomic distribution.[9]

Prognostic Evaluation

The Internal Prognostic Index (IPI) has largely supplanted anatomic staging as the primary prognostic tool for NHL.[10] It was developed with data generated from over 2000 patients with aggressive histology lymphoma who were treated with standard anthracycline-containing regimens. The analysis identified five significant parameters: (1) age (greater than 60 versus less than or equal to 60 years of age); (2) serum LDH as a biochemical measure of tumor burden (less than normal versus greater than normal); (3) performance status (0/1 versus 2–4); (4) stage (limited versus advanced); and (5) extranodal involvement (less than or equal to 1 site versus greater than 1 site). Based on a scoring system assigned to the parameters, patients are categorized into four prognostic groups: low risk, low intermediate risk, high intermediate risk, and high risk. Overall survival rates vary among the different groups, with 5-year survival of 73% in the low risk group, 51% in the low intermediate group, 43% in the high intermediate group, and 26% in the high risk group. The IPI was modified after the introduction of rituximab, a CD20-targeted monoclonal antibody, because this agent improved survival across all subgroups.[11]

The IPI has been adapted to different lymphoid neoplasms. For example, the Follicular Lymphoma International

Prognostic Index (FL-IPI) has been developed to account for biologic features seen in follicular lymphoma. Disease-specific systems have been proposed for T cell lymphoma and mantle cell lymphoma.

LEUKEMIAS

Chronic Lymphocytic Leukemia (CLL)

CLL is the most common leukemia in adults in Western countries, diagnosed at an annual rate of approximately 1.1% of all new cancer cases in the United States. CLL is a disorder of B cells. Although earlier literature discussed a T cell variety, these disorders have been reclassified among mature T cell lymphoproliferative diseases.

CLL is generally a disease of the older adult; median age of diagnosis is approximately 72 years, with a slight male preponderance. The estimated incidence in the United States in 2016 was 4.6 cases per 100,000 persons. The prevalence was probably much higher because of the natural progression of the disease.[12]

Most patients are asymptomatic on presentation, and the disease is often detected by an abnormality in a routine CBC. The International Workshop on Chronic Lymphoid Leukemia (IWCLL) requires the presence of at least 5×10^9 cells/L of circulating B lymphocytes for more than 3 months to establish the diagnosis of CLL, with confirmation of clonality performed by flow cytometry.[13]

Morphology

Typical CLL presents with greater than 85% of the lymphocytes appearing small and mature with scant cytoplasm and a dense nucleus with a condensed chromatin pattern without a defined nucleolus. This characteristic chromatin pattern has been labeled as "cobblestone" or likened to a soccer ball (Figure 34.2). Prolymphocytes (PL) or atypical lymphoid cells may be seen;

however, they represent less than 10% or less than 15% of circulating lymphocytes, respectively. Typical CLL accounts for about 80% of all cases. Atypical CLL is seen in up to 20% of patients.[14] Two variant subtypes of atypical CLL exist: CLL/PLL and mixed-type/atypical CLL. Prolymphocytes represent greater than 10% but less than 55% of total lymphocytes in the CLL/PLL subtype, and greater than 15% large atypical lymphoid cells or abnormal forms that exhibit nuclear indentations/clefts are present in mixed type/atypical CLL. Atypical CLL may be identified at diagnosis or develop over time. Atypical CLL has been associated with biologic markers indicating more aggressive disease.

Smudged lymphocytes are a common finding on peripheral blood film review in CLL. Excluding or ignoring these cells during a manual differential can affect the accuracy of the results; therefore it is recommended that smudge cells be counted as lymphocytes, although only in CLL patients.[15,16] Alternately some laboratories comment in the automated differential report that smudge cells do not impact the results.

Immunophenotype

On immunophenotyping, CLL lymphocytes exhibit B cell markers CD19, CD20, and CD23 but also aberrantly co-express the T cell antigen CD5. Although CLL cells demonstrate surface immunoglobulin, the level of expression may be dim and the ability to discern light chain restriction, indicating B cell clonality, may be difficult. Antigen expression is sometimes variable; not all cases fit into a classic CLL immunophenotypic profile. To account for this variability and differentiate CLL from related B cell neoplasms, a scoring system has been developed (Box 34.3). Each criterion is given 1 point, and the total score is cumulative. A combined score greater than or equal to 4 is consistent with CLL. Low scores of 1 or 2 suggest NHL. An intermediate score of 3 remains problematic, and these cases may require biopsy of a node or molecular data to establish the diagnosis.[17]

An uncomplicated case of CLL is usually diagnosed based upon findings in the peripheral blood.[18] However, some cases require a cytospin stained for cyclin D1 or FISH for t(11;14) to rule out mantle cell lymphoma which is more clinically aggressive than CLL. Genetic and biologic biomarkers have superseded bone marrow biopsies to establish prognoses. An extensive workup that includes a full cytogenetic panel and bone marrow biopsy is often performed for patients with symptoms who require some form of therapy.[19]

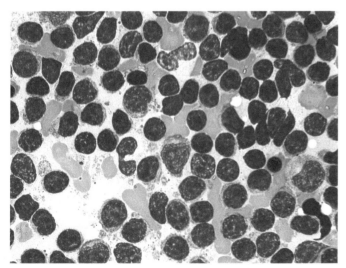

Figure 34.2 Bone Marrow Aspirate Smear from a Patient with Chronic Lymphocytic Leukemia (CLL). Bone marrow is replaced by well-differentiated lymphocytes. Leukemia cells have a high nuclear-to-cytoplasmic ratio, and the nuclear chromatin has a "cobblestone" or "soccer ball" appearance. (Tetrachrome stain, ×400.)

BOX 34.3 Catovsky-Matutes Scoring for Chronic Lymphocytic Leukemia Diagnosis[14,17]

Score 1 point for each of following:
- Weak expression of surface immunoglobulin
- Expression of CD5
- Expression of CD23
- No expression of FMC7
- Absent or weak expression of CD79b or CD22

Staging and Prognosis

Staging systems are important prognostic determinants for CLL and are used to guide clinical management. The Rai and Binet staging systems have been used for this purpose.[20,21] Both systems divide patients into risk categories reflecting the degree of organomegaly and lymphadenopathy or compromise of bone marrow function (Table 34.5) The presence of autoimmune phenomena is not an uncommon presentation in CLL; thus for patients who have evidence of rather sudden, unexplained anemia or thrombocytopenia, an underlying autoimmune process needs to be ruled out so that the patient is not inadvertently "upstaged." Therapies for autoimmune disease and CLL differ. The presence of autoimmune disease is not an indication for anti-CLL chemotherapy.

The Rai and Binet staging systems are based on clinical criteria that have prognostic implications for CLL.[5,22–24] The underlying karyotype is a strong predictor of survival and in certain cases has been associated with phenotypes of certain CLL variants. Del(17p) and *TP53* abnormalities are among the worst prognostic indicators and foretell resistance to standard chemoimmunotherapy approaches. The most powerful prognostic factor is the mutational status of the heavy chain immunoglobulin genes (*IGHv*). *IGHv* mutational status is a marker for two different subtypes of CLL – a less mature form with unmutated *IGHv* and another with a more mature phenotype associated with *IGHv* mutation. The unmutated, pregerminal center type of CLL is associated with a more aggressive clinical course and is usually accompanied by additional unfavorable genetic changes. Patients with mutated heavy chain genes do better with standard chemoimmunotherapy approaches. CD38 and ZAP70 expressions are cell markers that generally correlate with *IGHv* mutational status but also have independent prognostic value. Testing for CD38 has been incorporated into standard immunophenotyping panels for CLL. Testing for ZAP70 has been somewhat problematic because of variability in interlaboratory testing. Methylation

states of ZAP70 have been reported to be more reproducible; however, the test has not been approved by the US Food and Drug Administration (FDA) for use in the clinical laboratory. Next-generation sequencing (NGS) has identified abnormalities in *NOTCH1*, *SF3B1*, and *BIRC3* as having negative prognostic value, but these have yet to be integrated into clinical practice.

To date, no one prognostic scoring system is used for CLL. Most of these systems identify del17/*TP53* abnormalities, *IGHv* status, serum B2 microglobulin, Rai and Binet stage and age as important independent prognostic factors. These factors were however, identified in the context of standard chemo-immunotherapy approaches; evidence has not determined if they are still relevant with the newer agents used to treat CLL.

Treatment

Therapy for CLL has undergone profound changes. In the past, treatment consisted largely of oral alkylating agents such as chlorambucil or cyclophosphamide. For "fit" patients, these drugs were supplanted by the nucleoside analog fludarabine and more recently by the anti-CD20 monoclonal antibody rituximab. The emergence of targeted agents has caused a fundamental paradigm shift in CLL therapeutics. These agents include BTK inhibitors (ibrutinib), PI3k inhibitors (idelalisib), and BCL2 inhibitors (venetoclax).[25–27] New monoclonal antibodies, such as obinituzumab, designed to be more efficacious, are gradually replacing rituximab in combination regimens. With use of these newer agents, risk-adapted approaches can be explored and therapy can be individualized to the specific biology of a patient's tumor.

Monoclonal B Cell Lymphocytosis (MBL) and Small Lymphocytic Lymphoma (SLL)

Despite having a documented monoclonal B cell population in the peripheral blood, some patients fail to meet the criteria set forth by the IWCLL to establish a CLL diagnosis. Patients who are asymptomatic, without any lymphadenopathy, organomegaly, cytopenias, or systemic symptoms with less than 5×10^9/L circulating B lymphocytes are referred to as having monoclonal B cell lymphocytosis (MBL).[19] The risk for progression to CLL in these patients is 1% to 2% per year. Other individuals with less than 5×10^9/L B lymphocytes and evidence of disease elsewhere, such as adenopathy or organomegaly, are classified as having small lymphocytic lymphoma (SLL). Histologic confirmation from a bone marrow biopsy is needed to identify this disease. Clinical management of SLL is similar to that used in CLL.

Prolymphocytic Leukemia (PLL)

PLL is a rare disorder constituting about 1% to 2% of the lymphoid leukemias. It has a distinct clinical course that differs from other mature lymphoid neoplasms. PLL is a disease of the elderly, with a median age of approximately 70 years and an equal distribution between the sexes. Although both T and B forms exist as separate disorders, they share some common clinical features.

TABLE 34.5 **Staging for Chronic Lymphocytic Leukemia**[20,21]	
Rai Classification (Revised)	**Binet Classification**
Low Risk (formerly Stage 0) Lymphocytosis $> 5 \times 10^9$/L	**Stage A** Hemoglobin $\geq$ 10 g/dL and platelets $\geq 100 \times 10^9$/L and < 3 enlarged nodal areas
Intermediate Risk (formerly Stages I and II) Lymphocytes $> 5 \times 10^9$/L and (lymphadenopathy + splenomegaly) or hepatomegaly, or both	**Stage B** Hemoglobin $\geq$ 10 g/dL and platelets $\geq 100 \times 10^9$/L and ≥ 3 enlarged nodal areas
High Risk (formerly Stages III and IV) Lymphocytes $> 5 \times 10^9$/L and hemoglobin < 11 g/dL	**Stage C** Hemoglobin < 10 g/dL or platelets $< 100 \times 10^9$/L and any number of enlarged nodal areas

PLL is largely an aggressive disorder; primary manifestations are in the peripheral blood, bone marrow, and spleen. The clinical presentation is characterized by massive splenomegaly and marked absolute lymphocytosis, often more than 100×10^9/L. A rapidly rising white blood cell (WBC) count may be a clue that the diagnosis is not CLL. Lymphadenopathy is minimal, although there is a high incidence (particularly in the T cell subtype) of tissue involvement with skin as a common area of infiltration.

Morphology and Immunophenotype

Morphologically, there is a distinct appearance of the B cell subtype of PLL that accounts for 75% of cases. Cells are medium to large in size compared with a normal lymphocyte, with ample cytoplasm, a more open chromatin pattern, and a prominent nucleolus. Identifying the T cell variety is problematic because cells tend to be smaller and the nucleolus is generally less distinct (Figure 34.3). Similar to features seen in other mature T cell malignancies, the nucleus may have an irregular contour and a cerebriform appearance. Immunophenotyping and genetic studies may be useful in distinguishing T-PLL from other mature T cell neoplasms. Unlike in other post-thymic T cell disorders, CD7 is usually expressed, and the TCL-1 antigen can be detected by either flow cytometry or immunohistochemistry. FISH analysis demonstrates inv(14) in approximately 70% of patients. In PLL, hematology analyzers detect the increase in the WBC count and frequently classify the cells as lymphocytes. Because prolymphocytes are morphologically different from normal lymphocytes, the automated differential would likely have an associated atypical or variant lymphocyte flag, blast flag, or both, especially with the B cell subtype. A peripheral blood film review and manual differential should be performed. The presence of prolymphocytes is significant, and the clinician should be notified.

Treatment

Unfortunately, therapy for PLL is suboptimal. In the past, B-PLL has been treated with a standard lymphoma regimen, such as CHOP (cyclophosphamide, doxorubicin, vincristine, and prednisone). The anti-CD52 monoclonal antibody alemtuzumab has been used for the T cell subtype of PLL; however, complete responses only occur in about 20% of patients, and these are often relatively short-lived.[28] Hematopoietic stem cell transplantation is under investigation for patients who have an initial response to therapy.

Hairy Cell Leukemia (HCL)

Hairy cell leukemia (HCL) is an indolent disease of B cell lineage most commonly found in middle age (median age, 50 years), with a male preponderance. The major focus of disease is in the spleen, blood, and bone marrow. Patients typically present with splenomegaly and cytopenias. Characteristic hairy cells have round to ovoid nuclei, lack nucleoli, and have relatively abundant cytoplasm with ragged projections that extend circumferentially around the entire cell (Figure 34.4).

Morphology and Immunophenotype

Hairy cells are found in the peripheral blood and bone marrow aspirate, but they may be few in number; therefore if HCL is suspected, careful examination of the blood or bone marrow is a key step. Morphologic variants can be seen with less prominent "hairs" but exhibit the distinct kidney bean–shaped nucleus. Bone marrow aspirate can be difficult to obtain due to the presence of marrow fibrosis. Bone marrow biopsy is of the utmost importance in those instances. Patterns of bone marrow involvement may be interstitial or patchy. Immunohistochemistry with an anti-CD20 antibody may help identify clusters of hairy cells. Annexin A is specific to HCL and helps to differentiate HCL from related B cell disorders (e.g., splenic marginal zone lymphoma) that have a similar morphology.

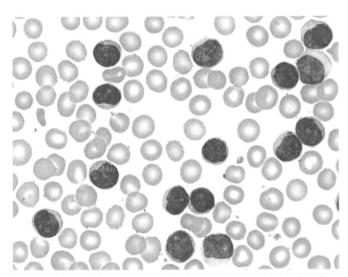

Figure 34.3 Peripheral Blood Film from a Patient with T Cell Prolymphocytic Leukemia (T-PLL). Leukemia cells have open chromatin; some with irregular nuclear contours. Nucleoli are present but are less prominent than those seen in the B cell variety of PLL. (Wright-Giemsa stain, ×1000.)

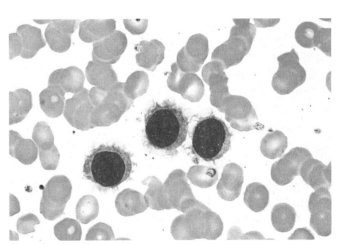

Figure 34.4 Hairy Cells. Hairy cells may be difficult to locate in the bone marrow aspirate because this disorder is often accompanied by fibrosis, which makes obtaining an adequate smear problematic. The leukemia cells have a characteristic appearance with a "shaggy" cytoplasmic border. (Peripheral blood, Wright-Giemsa stain, ×1000.)

Treatment

Historically, HCL patients have been treated with splenectomy, which removes a large reservoir of disease. Currently the nucleoside analogues cladribine and pentostatin are standard therapy.[29] Unfortunately, it is not uncommon to find evidence of minimal residual disease by flow cytometry or molecular testing in patients who have undergone therapy and have had a successful restoration of their peripheral blood counts. Recently genomic sequencing studies discovered a high frequency of the *BRAF* V600E mutation associated with this disease; subsequently the BRAF inhibitor, vemurafinib, was developed, which has proven to be highly effective in treating HCL patients refractory to other therapies.[30]

Large Granular Lymphocytic (LGL) Leukemia
Morphology

Large granular lymphocytes (LGLs) have abundant, pale blue cytoplasm with distinct medium to large azurophilic cytoplasmic granules. LGLs represent up to 15% of circulating lymphocytes, or less than 0.6×10^9/L in normal adults. LGL leukemia is a rare disease characterized by an increase in circulating LGLs in excess of 2×10^9/L. LGL leukemia is a disease of older adults (median age, 60 years), and most patients are asymptomatic at presentation. The increase in circulating LGLs may trigger a variant/atypical lymphocyte flag or blast flag on the hematology analyzer because of the size of the cells. The increased number of LGLs will be evident on peripheral blood film review and should be reported. Most patients present with neutropenia, anemia, or both. An increase in peripheral blood LGLs can also be seen in autoimmune disease and following bone marrow transplantation or administration of chemotherapy.

Immunophenotype

LGL leukemia is listed as two separate entities under the WHO classification system. T cell LGL is a clonal expansion of cytotoxic T cells,[31] expressing CD3, CD8, and CD57. Clonality can be confirmed by detection of T cell receptor (TCR) gene rearrangements. The other form of LGL leukemia is categorized as a chronic lymphoproliferative disorder of NK cells, with increased numbers of clonal NK cells in circulation. These cells are typically negative for CD3 but do express CD56. Restricted KIR expression may be used to demonstrate clonality of this population. Both types of LGL leukemia usually have an indolent course, although NK LGL leukemia can transform into a more aggressive disease.

Treatment

Most therapy for LGL leukemia is instituted in response to the cytopenias.[32] Myeloid growth factors (e.g., granulocyte colony-stimulating factor [G-CSF]) are used to treat isolated neutropenia. Although there is no standard approach to therapy, immunosuppressive agents, such as low doses of methotrexate, cyclophosphamide, or cyclosporin A, have been used to suppress the clone and improve peripheral blood counts.

LYMPHOMAS

Although centered in extramedullary areas such as the lymph nodes and spleen, many forms of lymphoma have a leukemic phase (Box 34.4). Some have a characteristic morphology or immunophenotype, but biopsy of involved tissue is often required to establish a diagnosis.

When possible lymphoma cells should be counted separately in the manual differential.[15] If the suspected lymphoma cells cannot be morphologically differentiated from normal lymphocytes with confidence, it is recommended that they be counted along with normal lymphocytes, with a comment indicating their presence.

Adult T Cell Leukemia/Lymphoma (ATLL)

Adult T cell leukemia/lymphoma (ATLL) is a post-thymic neoplastic disorder of T cells associated with retroviral infection by the human T lymphotropic virus type 1 (HTLV-1).[33,34] HTLV-1 is endemic in Japan, the Caribbean islands, Africa, South America, the Middle East, and northern Oceania. The virus is transmitted via placental circulation, breastfeeding, blood transfusion, or sex. The estimated risk of developing ATLL among HTLV-1 carriers is approximately 2.5% (women) to 5% (men) over a latency period of 55 to 70 years.

The acute form of the subtypes of ATLL is the most well-known. This disease has an aggressive clinical course marked by extensive extranodal involvement of the peripheral blood and skin. Complications of tumor involvement include osteolytic lesions, hypercalcemia, and profound immunosuppression resulting in infection. These complications represent the major source of morbidity and mortality in this disease.

Morphology and Immunophenotype

There is often marked leukocytosis in the leukemic phase of ATLL, with malignant cells exhibiting a characteristic morphology. The prototypical ATLL cells are medium to large in size and have accentuated, convoluted nuclei, coarsely clumped chromatin, and deeply basophilic cytoplasm (Figure 34.5). The term "flower cell" has been coined for this morphology. Not all ATLL cells have this distinctive appearance; malignant cells may be smaller with a pleomorphic appearance reminiscent of other peripheral T cell lymphomas, such as Sézary syndrome.

BOX 34.4 Leukemic Phase of Non-Hodgkin Lymphoma

Small lymphocytic lymphoma
Adult T cell leukemia/lymphoma
Burkitt leukemia/lymphoma (sporadic/HIV related)
Follicular lymphoma
Mantle cell lymphoma
Marginal zone lymphoma
Lymphoplasmacytic lymphoma (Waldentröm's)
Sézary syndrome/advanced mycosis fungoides
Diffuse large B cell lymphoma (rare)
Peripheral T cell lymphoma

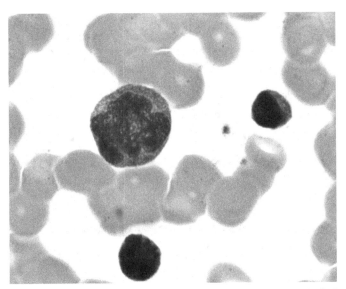

Figure 34.5 Peripheral Blood Film from a Patient with Adult T Cell Leukemia/Lymphoma (ATLL). Leukemia cells can range in size. Some have distinctive nuclear lobulation and have been termed "flower cells." (Wright-Giemsa stain, ×1000.)

The ATLL immunophenotype is generally consistent with T helper cells; CD3 and CD4 are expressed, whereas CD7 and CD8 are absent. CD25 and CCR4 are also highly expressed. The soluble form of interleukin 2 (IL-2) has prognostic significance and can be used as a tumor marker for assessing disease status.

Treatment

Despite extensive clinical trial experience (mostly undertaken by Japanese investigators), therapy for ATLL remains suboptimal. The acute form of the disease is routinely refractory to chemotherapy. The 5-year survival rate is low (less than 15%). Patients with indolent forms of ATLL tend to have a better prognosis.

A combination of interferon alpha and azidothymidine has been reported to have some efficacy against the HTLV-1 virus. Studies with experimental agents, such as the anti-CCR4 monoclonal antibody mogamulizumab, are ongoing, and these agents have shown some promise in early trials. Allogeneic stem cell transplantation has been investigated in this disease, and long-term survivors have been reported.

Burkitt Lymphoma/Leukemia (BL)

Burkitt lymphoma/leukemia (BL) is an aggressive cancer of mature B cells associated with a fulminant clinical presentation. BL has three subtypes: endemic, sporadic, and HIV associated. The endemic form is found primarily in childhood in equatorial Africa, along a geographic distribution similar to that of malaria. Extranodal involvement is common, with the orbits and mandible as typical sites of disease. Also, the EBV genome has been found to be present in the neoplastic cells.

In contrast, sporadic BL presents mostly as an abdominal disease. Extranodal involvement is not uncommon. Bone marrow and the CNS are involved in approximately 70% and 33% of cases, respectively. The HIV form has been associated with profound immunosuppression. Unlike in other subtypes, the blood and bone marrow are primary sites of disease.

Morphology and Immunophenotype

The leukemic phase develops in a subset of patients, and circulating Burkitt cells have a characteristic morphology. The cells are medium to large in size, have finely clumped chromatin, and deeply basophilic cytoplasm with distinct vacuoles. Bone marrow biopsy may show sheets of infiltrating medium-sized cells with scant cytoplasm (Figure 34.6).[6] Both bone marrow and lymph node biopsies may show a classic "starry sky" appearance, which results from the interspersed tingible body macrophages suspended in a "sea" of malignant cells.

The immunophenotypic profile of BL is that of a mature B cell in which both surface immunoglobulin and light chain restriction are present, along with the expression of CD10 and the absence of immature markers, such as CD34 or Tdt. Specimens sent for flow cytometric analysis need to be processed quickly because the high cell turnover that characterizes BL may result in poor viability, which reduces the quality of the results (Table 34.1).

Treatment

Despite its relatively fulminant presentation, BL is highly responsive to chemotherapy and is curable in greater than 90% of patients with early stage disease and in 60% to 80% of patients in more advanced stages. Intensive supportive care addressing therapy-related side effects is the key to success, because the chemotherapy regimens are of high intensity cycled over relatively short periods of time. Given the high tumor cell turnover, tumor lysis syndrome should be anticipated, and supportive efforts with aggressive intravenous (IV) hydration and antihyperuricemia medications are indicated prior to the start of cytotoxic chemotherapy.[35]

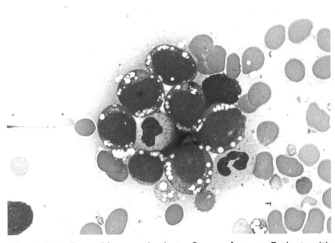

Figure 34.6 Bone Marrow Aspirate Smear from a Patient with Burkitt Leukemia/Lymphoma. Cells are of intermediate size with deeply basophilic cytoplasm and distinct cytoplasmic vacuoles. (Tetrachrome stain, ×400.)

Follicular Lymphoma (FL)

Follicular lymphomas (FLs) represent a neoplastic disorder of germinal B cells and account for approximately 12% of NHL cases. FL is generally a disease of middle to older age groups. Although FL typically has an indolent course, it is most often incurable with current therapies. The clinical pattern is one of serial responses to chemotherapy followed by recurring relapse until death.

Morphology

Most patients with FL present with painless lymphadenopathy but are otherwise asymptomatic. Peripheral blood involvement is present in about 10% of cases. Circulating FL cells have a condensed chromatin pattern and distinct nuclear clefts (Figure 34.7).[14,17] A few large cells with more pleomorphic features may also be present. Bone marrow biopsy reveals characteristic localization of tumor cells in a paratrabecular distribution. There may also be a variable degree of interstitial infiltration. The characteristic effacement of normal architecture seen in the lymph node is typically absent in the marrow. In tissue section the FL cells appear small and irregular with an angular appearance (centrocytes) or larger with round to ovoid nuclei containing one to three nucleoli located on the border within the nucleus (centroblasts). Histologically, FL is graded according to the number of larger cells. The histologic grading correlates with the clinical outcome, with grade 3 disease having the poorest outcome.

Treatment

Most FL patients are asymptomatic, therefore a "watch and wait" strategy is appropriate.[36] A separate scoring system (Fabry International Prognostic Index [FIBI]) has been developed to aid in clinical decision making. For patients who require treatment, combination chemotherapy like that used in other forms of NHL is given. More recently, specific agents targeted to unique biologic features, such as surface antigen expression (CD20, CD22, or CD37), B cell receptor signaling pathway, or genes implicated in lymphoma transformation (*BCL2, TP53*), have been investigated and, similar to the experience in CLL/SLL, have been found to be of benefit.[37] As more agents are introduced into clinical practice, treatment outcomes may improve for these patients.

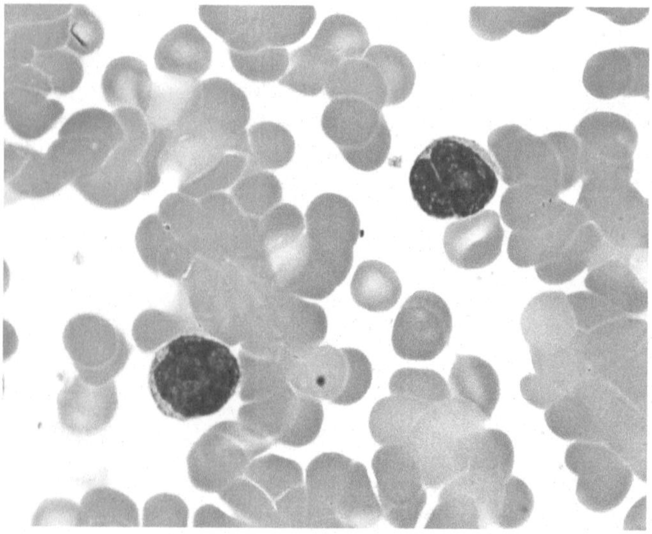

Mantle Cell Lymphoma (MCL)

Mantle cell lymphoma (MCL) constitutes approximately 3% to 6% of NHL cases.[12] The median age at diagnosis is 68 years, and males are affected more than females. MCL is considered to be a clinically aggressive disorder, although an indolent type has been described. Most patients present with extensive lymphadenopathy. Extranodal disease is not uncommon, with the GI tract acting as a primary area of involvement. Patients with the indolent form tend to have the disease restricted to the blood, bone marrow, and spleen.

Morphology

Mantle cells in peripheral blood can vary morphologically, which complicates diagnostic assessment. The small cell form of MCL can easily be mistaken for CLL/SLL or marginal zone lymphoma (Figure 34.8).[20,21] A blastoid variant of MCL with pleomorphic, immature features can be confused with acute lymphoid leukemia or diffuse large cell lymphoma. In some cases circulating mantle cells exhibit morphologic changes that can be confused with villous splenic marginal zone lymphocytes, hairy cells, or prolymphocytes. Therefore accurate diagnosis of MCL requires demonstration of either t(11,14) via FISH or overexpression of cyclin D1 by immunohistochemistry. Expression of SOX11, a transcription factor, is used to diagnose the 5% of cases that are cyclin D1 negative.

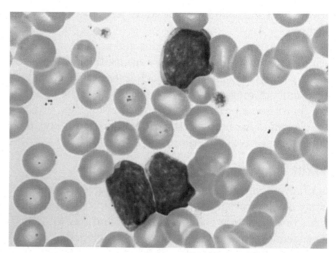

Figure 34.8 Peripheral Blood Film from a Patient with Mantle Cell Lymphoma. Cells circulating in the peripheral blood can have a variable appearance. Some cases can be confused with chronic lymphoid lymphoma/small lymphocytic lymphoma (CLL/SLL), and immunophenotyping/cytogenetic analysis is needed to differentiate between the disorders. In this case the chromatin in the lymphoma cells has a more open chromatin pattern than that typically seen with (CLL) cells. (Wright-Giemsa stain, ×1000.)

Figure 34.7 Follicular Lymphoma Cells. Follicular lymphoma cells circulating in the peripheral blood can appear as small, cleaved lymphoid cells. (Peripheral blood, Wright-Giemsa stain, ×1000.)

Treatment

A "watch and wait" strategy is appropriate for deciding when to initiate therapy for the indolent form of MCL. A separate prognostic index (Mantle Cell Lymphoma International Prognostic Index [MIPI]) may be useful in determining clinical management. Patients who develop bulky disease or B symptoms (see Box 34.2) often require therapy. Age is a major discriminator for decisions regarding therapy. Younger patients (less than 65 years old) typically are treated with high-dose chemoimmunotherapy containing cytarabine and methotrexate, followed by autologous stem cell transplantation. Older patients may not tolerate such aggressive therapy, and more standard NHL therapies, such as CHOP or bendamustine/rituximab, are used. The B-cell receptor (BCR) inhibitor, ibrutinib, has been found to be one of the most active agents for MCL patients who have relapsed, and trials investigating the incorporation of this drug into initial therapy regimens are currently underway.

Diffuse Large B Cell Lymphoma (DLBCL)

Diffuse large B cell lymphoma (DLBCL) is the most common form of NHL, representing about 25% to 30% of all cases.[12] It is generally a disease of the elderly but may occur in younger patients. DLBCL can arise de novo or result as a transformation from a more indolent form of lymphoma, such as CLL/SLL, FL, or MZL. Although DLBCL has an aggressive clinical course, it is often curable with combination chemoimmunotherapy. A number of subgroups based on morphologic or genetic criteria are recognized for this disease

The most common clinical presentation for DLBCL is rapidly expanding, painless lymphadenopathy in one or more sites. Extranodal involvement can occur in the GI tract, testis, or bone. Clinical symptoms depend on the areas of involvement. Bone marrow is affected in approximately 30% of patients, and a third of those exhibit circulating malignant cells, which often appear highly pleomorphic with large nuclei and nucleoli, resembling leukemic blasts (Figure 34.9).

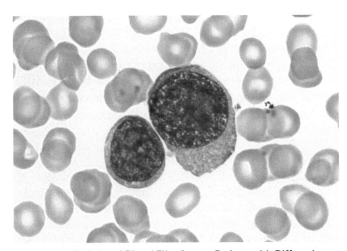

Figure 34.9 Peripheral Blood Film from a Patient with Diffuse Large B Cell Lymphoma. Peripheral blood involvement is generally rare. When present the lymphoma cells may be large with moderate amounts of cytoplasm and several nucleoli. Cells may also resemble a blast and mimic an acute leukemia. (Wright-Giemsa stain, ×1000.)

Morphology

DLBCL cells are large with a diffuse pattern in the lymph node. Morphologic variants have been described. In addition several disorders (e.g., multiple or plasma cell myeloma and anaplastic large cell lymphoma) include highly pleomorphic forms that can be confused with one of the DLBCL subtypes. Such cases require immunohistochemistry and genetic testing to rule out other lymphoid neoplasms and confirm the diagnosis.

Molecular Testing

Genetic testing reveals translocations involving the *BCL6* gene in approximately 30% of patients with DLBCL. Translocation of the *BCL2* gene, a marker associated with t(14;18) and FL, occurs in 20% to 30% of DLBCL cases and may complicate diagnosis. In addition *MYC*, a gene typically associated with Burkitt leukemia/lymphoma, is rearranged in approximately 10% of DLBCL patients. These findings demonstrate that isolated genetic differences do not define the lymphoma subtype, but instead need to be considered in the context of clinical and morphologic criteria. Up to 70% of DLBCL patients with *MYC* abnormalities have concurrent *BCL2* and/or *BCL6* abnormalities – these cases have been labeled "double (or triple) hit" lymphoma and have an exceptionally poor prognosis.[38,39] Classification of this entity has been controversial, with some considering these diseases under the WHO 2008 hybrid category B cell lymphoma; unclassifiable with features intermediate between DLBCL and Burkitt lymphoma.[1,2]

DLBCL is an example of a disease for which advances in molecular technology have had a fundamental effect on treatment. Gene expression profiling has been used to define two primary subgroups that reflect normal stages of B cell development: germinal center (GC) and activated B cell (ABC, or non-germinal center).[40] These subtypes have prognostic implications, with the GC variety having a more favorable outcome. Because gene expression profiling is not readily available in many clinical laboratories, surrogate scoring systems based on immunohistochemical algorithms have been developed to classify subtypes. However, these algorithms do not have 100% correlation with the molecular profile, and assigning therapy based on such tools does not represent the current standard of care. New molecular testing may be introduced in the near future, which will provide similar information, with better correlation and reproducibility, replacing the current immunohistochemical assays.[41]

Treatment

Although DLBCL is typically aggressive, remission can be achieved in many patients. As previously discussed, the IPI was initially developed from a cohort of DLBCL patients and remains a useful tool for clinicians. Incorporation of the anti-CD20 monoclonal antibody, rituximab, to standard combination chemotherapy has greatly improved patient outcomes. Patients with unfavorable subtypes remain a challenge, and some of the newer targeted agents are currently being tested.

Marginal Zone Lymphoma (MZL)

MZL is an indolent B cell lymphoma typically associated with chronic antigen stimulation either in the setting of infection or autoimmunity. There are three subtypes of MZL: extranodal marginal zone lymphoma of mucosa-associated lymphoid tissue (MALT), splenic marginal zone lymphoma, and nodal marginal zone lymphoma.[42]

MALT lymphomas are the most common subtype; they are usually associated with organs that seemingly lack obvious lymphoid tissue. These organs have been subjected to chronic inflammation; this in turn increases B cell proliferation, in which errors during class switching and hypermutation lead to uncontrolled growth and malignant transformation. The stomach is most often involved and is also the site most closely associated with an infection with *Helicobacter pylori* (*H. pylori*). The salivary gland, ocular adnexa, thyroid, skin, and small intestine can also be affected but are associated with different infectious stimuli. A distinct variant of MALT, immunoproliferative small intestine disease (IPSD), is seen in the Middle East, Africa, and the Mediterranean and is associated with severe malabsorption. As in the gastric-centered MALT subtype, disease spread beyond the small intestine region is uncommon, although transformation to a more aggressive histologic subtype has been described. Most therapy is centered upon relief of symptoms for MALT lymphomas. With *H. pylori*–associated disease, treatment of the underlying infection with triple antibiotic therapy may result in remission. A similar observation has been made with antibiotic therapy for IPSD. Involved field radiation has also been used for affected areas.

Morphology

Areas of involvement in splenic marginal zone lymphoma (SMZL) include the white pulp of the spleen, splenic lymph nodes, bone marrow, and very often peripheral blood. Patients typically present with massive splenomegaly and an absolute lymphocytosis in the peripheral blood often characterized by the presence of villous lymphocytes or cells similar to those seen in CLL (Figure 34.10).[43] These cells can also be confused with hairy cells; however, the cytoplasmic projections in the villous lymphocytes tend to have a polar distribution as opposed to the circumferential pattern seen in hairy cells.

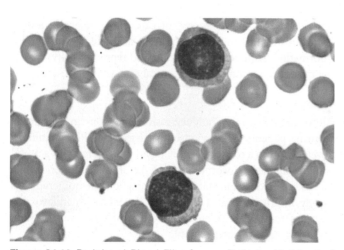

Figure 34.10 Peripheral Blood Film from a Patient with Marginal Zone Lymphoma. Cells may be intermediate in size with round nuclei. They tend to have a more open chromatin pattern compared with normal lymphocytes. (Wright-Giemsa stain, ×1000.)

In SMZL, CD103 is negative and annexin A staining is absent upon immunohistochemical staining of the lymph node biopsy. Extranodal sites of disease other than the spleen, blood, and bone marrow are rare. Approximately one third of SMZL patients also have a paraprotein present. Patients may develop severe anemia and thrombocytopenia secondary to splenic sequestration.

Treatment

Asymptomatic patients may be followed with a "watch and wait" strategy. Splenectomy is the treatment of choice when therapy is indicated. Splenectomy removes a large reservoir of disease and often corrects the cytopenias despite persistence of abnormal cells in the bone marrow and peripheral blood. Recent experience has demonstrated efficacy with the combination of bendamustine and rituximab in patients who require systemic therapy.[43]

Nodal Marginal Zone Lymphoma

Nodal marginal zone lymphoma (NMZL) is primarily localized to the lymph nodes, although bone marrow can also be involved. It is generally a disease of the elderly. NMZL cells extend from the mantle-marginal zone interface, disrupting the interfollicular region of the lymph nodes. This diagnosis represents a "waste paper basket" for disorders that morphologically resemble other low-grade B cell malignancies but lack distinguishing characteristics (i.e., cyclin D1 expression, BCL2 abnormalities), which would place NMZL among one of the other well-defined NHLs. An association with hepatitis C has been noted, and cryoglobulinemia has been identified in these patients. There is no standard therapy for NMZL. Use of targeted agents may be an approach but needs to be verified in clinical trials. Given the rare nature of this disease, evaluation of these drugs' efficacy may prove to be difficult.[44]

Mycosis Fungoides (MF)/Sézary Syndrome (SS)

Mycosis fungoides (MF)/Sézary syndrome (SS) is the most familiar form of cutaneous T cell lymphoma. Both are diseases of the elderly, with a slight male preponderance. MF is the more common disorder, making up approximately 60% to 70% of the cutaneous T cell lymphoma cases. MF is largely confined to the skin, although in the later stages of the disease, dissemination to lymph nodes, organs, and blood can be seen. MF is generally an indolent disease with a slow progressive course. SS is defined as a systemic disorder with peripheral blood involvement and a worse prognosis than MF.

Morphology and Immunophenotype

MF and SS are generally disorders of CD4+ T cells. More recently some have argued that they are distinct entities arising from separate precursors. The malignant clone in MF has been shown to have an effector memory phenotype, whereas Sézary cells are associated with central memory T cells. Malignant T cells in MF and SS have an abnormal appearance with scant cytoplasm and a cerebriform, folded nucleus, variably condensed chromatin, and inconspicuous nucleoli. In SS the malignant cells can be both large and small (Figure 34.11). A single

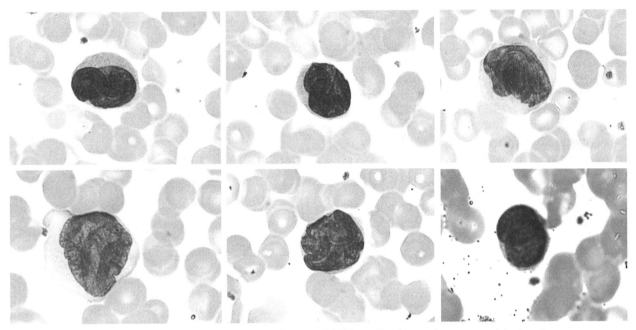

Figure 34.11 Peripheral Blood Film from a Patient with Sézary Syndrome. Appearance of the lymphoma cells can be variable. Several examples are shown here. Some cells can be small with nuclear atypia. Other cells are larger with cerebriform or folded nuclei. (Wright-Giemsa stain, ×1000.)

case may have cells of one or both types. Patients can develop a transformation from small to large cell variety.

Diagnosis of MF in the early stages can be problematic. Patients may present with psoriatic-like skin lesions requiring repeated biopsy before a definitive diagnosis is made. Longitudinal follow-up of initially nondiagnostic lesions may be required before morphologic confirmation of disease. Skin biopsy can show a characteristic localization of atypical cells in Pautrier microabscesses in the epidermis, but this occurs in only a minority of cases.

Clinically SS is characterized by erythroderma, generalized lymphadenopathy, and the presence of clonal T cells in skin, lymph nodes, and peripheral blood. An absolute Sézary cell count greater than 1×10^9/L is required to make a diagnosis of SS, underscoring the need for these abnormal lymphoid cells to be counted separately in the manual differential.[15] Pruritus can be severe for patients and difficult to control with symptomatic therapy alone. Patients have profound immunosuppression, and infection remains a major source of morbidity and mortality.

Treatment

Therapy for early-stage MF consists of agents used to treat the symptoms of the disease: topical agents such as steroids, nitrogen mustard, or phototherapy. More advanced disease is generally incurable, and allogenic stem cell transplantation has been investigated. Given the aggressive nature of advanced MF and SS, a wide variety of agents have been tested in clinical trials. Therapeutic approaches have included single-agent chemotherapy, biologic response modifiers (interferons), and monoclonal antibodies directed against CD52 (alemtuzumab), CD4 (zanolimumab), CCR4 (mogamulizumab), in addition to histone deacetylases and retinoids. Despite the wide range of investigative activity, improving outcomes in this patient population remains challenging.[45]

Anaplastic Large Cell Lymphoma (ALCL)
Morphology
Anaplastic large cell lymphoma (ALCL) is a T cell disorder that was associated with large pleomorphic cells however, there is heterogeneity in morphologic appearance, and some cells are small to medium in size (Figure 34.12). Invariably the tumor expresses CD30. The disease is divided into two subtypes,

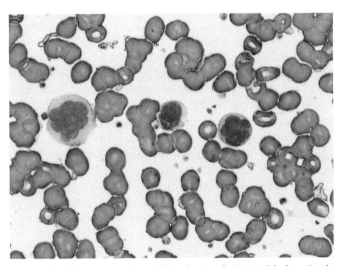

Figure 34.12 Peripheral Blood Film from a Patient with Anaplastic Large Cell Lymphoma. Lymphoma cells range in size and have irregular lobulated nuclei. In some cases the lymphoma cells resemble blasts. (Wright-Giemsa stain, ×400.)

depending on the expression of the anaplastic lymphoma kinase (ALK) protein. ALK positive (ALK+) tumors generally tend to occur in a younger cohort and have a better prognosis than most other peripheral T cell lymphomas. ALK+ ALCL constitutes approximately 10% to 30% of childhood lymphomas. The ALK negative (ALK−) form is more common in older patients, with a median age of about 57 years. A subtype of ALK− ALCL has been associated with breast implants.[46]

The clinical presentations of ALK+ and ALK- ALCL are similar. Most patients present with advanced-stage disease (Stages III and IV) and B symptoms. ALCL involves both lymph nodes and extranodal sites such as skin, bones, and soft tissue (e.g., liver and lung). There is a cutaneous variant in which the disease is localized only to the skin. Bone marrow is involved in 10% to 30% of cases, which may be subtle, and immunohistochemical stains are required to detect disease. Rare cases have been reported with a leukemic phase.

Treatment

The primary approach to treatment of ALCL is combination chemotherapy with relatively standard regimens such as CHOP. The ALK+ variety has been reported to have a 5-year survival of approximately 78% to 80% using this approach. Given several distinct disease-related features, targeted therapies have been explored, such as the anti-CD30 immunoconjugate brentuximab vedotin, approved by the FDA for use in relapsed disease. Crizotinib, an ALK inhibitor (approved for use in ALK+ non-small cell lung cancer), has shown a high response rate in a preliminary trial enrolling pediatric patients and is currently under investigation.

Peripheral T Cell Lymphoma-Not Otherwise Specified (PTCL-NOS)

Immunophenotype

Peripheral T cell lymphoma-not otherwise specified (PTCL-NOS) is a heterogeneous group of disorders. Diseases classified in this WHO category lack defining features that would place them in another category.[47] These are disorders of post-thymic T cells with rearrangement of the TCR. Immunophenotypically the abnormal cells are characterized by T cell antigen mismatch with the absence of CD7 or CD5 expression as the most common finding. More recently gene expression profiling has underscored this heterogeneity, although deregulation of genes associated with proliferation, apoptosis, and cell adhesion consistent with an activated T cell state have been noted.

Generally PTCL-NOS patients present with disseminated disease and poor performance status. Fifty percent to 70% of cases have an intermediate to high-risk IPI score. There is often diffuse nodal involvement with extranodal spread to the skin and GI tract. Bone marrow is involved in 20% to 30% of patients. Eosinophilia, in addition to anemia and thrombocytopenia, can be seen in a subset of patients (Figure 34.13).

Treatment

Given the fulminant nature of PTCL-NOS, standard treatment consists of combination chemotherapy. Approximately 30% of patients are refractory to current therapy. Patients who do

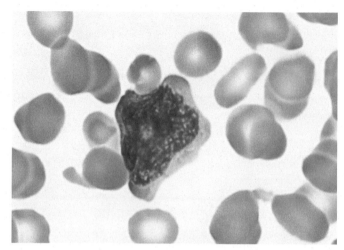

Figure 34.13 Peripheral Blood Film from a Patient with Peripheral T Cell Lymphoma. Peripheral blood involvement is uncommon. Lymphoma cells are larger, basophilic, and have a pleomorphic appearance. (Wright-Giemsa stain, ×1000.)

respond tend to relapse within a relatively short period of time. Hematopoietic stem cell transplantation has been investigated in an attempt to prolong remissions in responding patients. However, given the relatively rare nature of this disease, there is no large clinical data set to confirm the efficacy of this approach. For relapsed disease, targeted agents that are used in ALCL are currently under investigation.

Plasma Cell Neoplasms

Plasma cell neoplasms (PCNs) are malignant disorders of terminally differentiated B cells. Although they constitute approximately 1% to 2% of cancers, PCNs are the second most common hematologic malignancy. The prototypical disorder of this class, multiple (plasma cell) myeloma (MM), is generally a disease of the elderly, with a median age of 69 years. Less than 2% of patients diagnosed with this disease are younger than 40. MM is slightly more common in males than females, and in the U.S. the incidence is higher in African Americans than in Caucasians. The PCNs encompass a wide spectrum of disease states, ranging from a relatively benign condition such as MGUS, marked only by the presence of a paraprotein, to clinically aggressive plasma cell leukemia in which both tumor infiltration and paraprotein excess may produce systemic complications resulting in significant morbidity and death.

Monoclonal Gammopathy of Undetermined Significance

Monoclonal gammopathy of undetermined significance (MGUS) is a benign monoclonal proliferation of plasma cells that is usually considered with the plasma cell neoplasms because it represents a precursor state for myeloma.[48] Although the conversion to overt myeloma is relatively low overall, a subset of patients with adverse risk factors have a greater than 60% chance of progression over a 20-year period. For cases of MGUS the level of monoclonal immunoglobulin (M spike) can help predict the risk for transformation to MM or some other plasma cell neoplasm.

Multiple (Plasma Cell) Myeloma

The ability of the plasma cells to secrete monoclonal immunoglobulin (either whole or some part thereof) is an essential characteristic of the PCNs. There is a nonsecretory form of MM, but this type makes up less than 1% of cases. Monoclonal immunoglobulins in these patients can have negative effects across multiple organ systems and are responsible for most of the morbidity seen in the more advanced forms of MM.

MM is a bone marrow-based disease with extramedullary extension to bone or soft tissue. Strict criteria are followed to establish the diagnosis of MM, based on the overall tumor burden, as reflected by the percentage of plasma cells in the bone marrow, and the extent of systemic manifestations of disease, such as hypercalcemia, renal failure, anemia, and osteolytic lesions (Table 34.6).[49] Because extramedullary spread to bone is not uncommon, imaging studies of the skeleton, pelvis, or spine are a standard part of the diagnostic workup to establish the extent of disease and anticipate any potential serious complication (e.g., cord compression; fracture) that might need to be treated prophylactically.

Morphology and immunophenotype. Overt involvement of peripheral blood by circulating plasma cells is relatively rare until advanced or end-stage disease develops. Progression to plasma cell leukemia (secondary) is diagnosed when the circulating plasma cell count rises to 20% and greater than 2 × 10^9/L. Primary plasma cell leukemia is a separate entity. Both forms are associated with a dismal prognosis. The presence of rouleaux in MM is de facto evidence for a circulating paraprotein (Figure 34.14). Bone marrow involvement may be diffuse or focal (Figure 34.15). Caution should be undertaken when examining the aspirate alone, because a sampling issue may cause a relevant plasma cell population to be missed, resulting in a false negative for the presence of disease. In such instances the trephine biopsy may be more useful in detecting patchy clusters of plasma cells. Immunohistochemistry with stains for

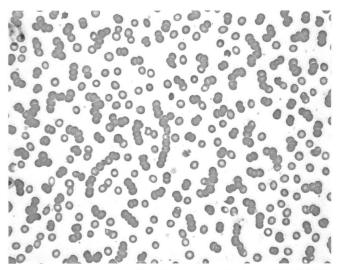

Figure 34.14 Peripheral Blood Film from a Patient with Multiple (Plasma Cell) Myeloma. Characteristic rouleaux formation of the red blood cells occurs secondary to the presence of the paraprotein. (Wright-Giemsa stain, ×100.)

TABLE 34.6	Diagnostic Criteria for Plasma Cell Neoplasms[49]	
Monoclonal gammopathy of undetermined significance (MGUS-non IgM)	Serum monoclonal protein (non-IgM) <3 g/dL Absence of end organ damage (see below)	Both criteria needed
Smoldering (asymptomatic) myeloma	Serum monoclonal protein (IgG or IgA) >3 g/dL or Urine monoclonal protein >500 mg/24 hours and/or Clonal bone marrow plasma cells 10% to 60% Absence of end organ damage or amyloidosis	Both criteria needed
Multiple (plasma cell) myeloma	Clonal bone marrow plasma cells greater than 10% or Biopsy-proven extramedullary plasmacytoma Any one of myeloma defining events (end organ damage): • Hypercalcemia • Renal insufficiency • Anemia • Bone lesions (skeletal survey/CT/ PET-CT) Clonal bone marrow plasma cells >60% or Involved/Uninvolved serum FLC ratio >100 (when involved FLC >100 mg/L) or >1 focal lesion on MRI	Three criteria needed

CT, Computed tomography; *FLC,* free light chain; *MRI,* magnetic resonance imaging; *PET,* positron emission tomography.

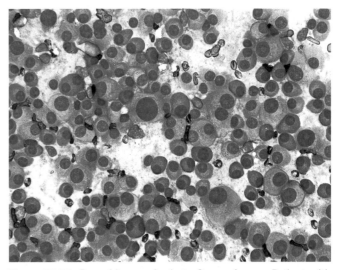

Figure 34.15 Bone Marrow Aspirate Smear from a Patient with Multiple (Plasma Cell) Myeloma. Sheets of plasma cells replace normal hematopoietic cells in the bone marrow. Plasma cells are immature and have an aberrant appearance in this aspirate specimen. (Tetrachrome stain, ×400.)

CD138 or kappa and lambda clonal excess are useful in delineating malignant plasma cells from reactive conditions. Malignant plasma cells express high levels of CD38 and CD138 and low levels of cell surface pan-leukocyte marker CD45; they also may aberrantly express the NK cell-associated marker CD56. Immunophenotyping profiles are increasingly used in myeloma diagnosis and as a measure of quantifying minimal residual disease.

Solitary plasmacytoma of bone represents a localized form of disease without an accompanying M spike in serum or urine. Definitive diagnosis of this disorder relies on testing to ensure that the plasmacytoma is localized to a single area and not a manifestation of underlying systemic disease. This distinction has therapeutic implications, because plasmacytomas may be primarily treated with radiation therapy.

Waldenström's Macroglobulinemia

Other disorders, such as Waldenström's macroglobulinemia (WM) and heavy chain disease, are, like MM, characterized by discrete secretory products. WM is a low-grade lymphoplasmacytic lymphoma associated with aberrant secretion of IgM. High levels of IgM can result in a hyperviscosity syndrome, requiring emergent plasmapheresis to alleviate symptoms. Extramedullary involvement includes nodal disease and hepatosplenomegaly. A distinct somatic mutation in the myeloid differentiation factor 88 (*MYD88*) gene, a member of the Toll-like receptor pathway, is found in over 90% of patients with WM and is a molecular marker for the disease and can differentiate it from other lymphomas that morphologically exhibit plasmacytic differentiation. Heavy chain disease is also a lymphoplasmacytic disorder. Symptoms are dependent on the heavy chain involved, but, as in MM, the paraprotein may cause significant damage to organs such as the kidney or liver.

Treatment

Patients with MGUS do not exhibit the clinical manifestations seen in MM, and given the lack of symptoms, observation alone is the standard of care. This is also true for patients with smoldering (asymptomatic) myeloma. Therapy is indicated for patients who are symptomatic. Successful treatment of MM relies not only on cytotoxic therapy to reduce the clonal plasma cell population, but also on aggressive supportive measures to reverse systemic complications.

Historically, most MM patients were treated with the alkylating agent melphalan plus the steroid prednisone. Newer therapies have included the immunomodulatory agents thalidomide and lenalidomide, in addition to the proteasome inhibitor bortezomib. Younger, "fit" patients are now often initially treated with combinations of newer drugs. These regimens have improved progression-free survival and overall survival. Despite these advances MM remains an incurable disease, with a course marked by response to therapy followed by recurrence of disease. High-dose myeloablative treatment followed by stem cell rescue has been of some benefit in patients who can endure such aggressive therapy. In this population melphalan is avoided because it has deleterious effects on stem cells used as hematopoietic rescue. Use of one of the effective agents over long periods of time to control minimal residual disease may be a more tolerable approach.

In older patients who cannot handle a high-dose approach, a melphalan-based regimen is combined with either bortezomib or lenalidomide and this has been shown to improve treatment outcomes.[50]

Relapse remains an issue in MM. Generally, repeating the prior regimen immediately prior to relapse is not efficacious. Newer drugs have been introduced and found to have a role in treating relapse disease. The second-generation proteasome inhibitor carfilzomib and the immunomodulatory agent pomalidomide have shown efficacy in patients who have relapsed. More recently the anti-CD38 antibody daratumumab has proven to be of benefit in heavily pretreated patients who have previously received combination therapy. Combinations of newer drugs continue to be explored in ongoing clinical trials in an effort to further improve outcomes in MM.[51]

Hodgkin Lymphoma (HL)

Hodgkin lymphoma (HL) is primarily a lymph node-based disease, distinct from NHL that involves the lymph nodes. HL is a relatively rare disorder, with an estimated US incidence of 2.7 cases per 100,000 persons per year. HL is associated with unique biologic and clinical features. Classic HL is generally a disease of young adults. It is one of the first tumor types cured with combination chemotherapy and therefore serves as a model for the evolution of therapeutics in modern oncology. Patients who relapse can still be cured with current therapies. This is an uncommon outcome, distinct from most cancer therapy. Approximately 86% of patients with HL are alive 5 years following diagnosis. Because this is a disease of a younger patient cohort with effective chemotherapy, survival data also provide useful information regarding long-term toxic effects of cancer therapy.

Morphology

HL has two distinct forms which differ pathologically and clinically: classic HL and lymphocyte-predominant HL. The diagnosis is established by lymph node biopsy for both types. Classic HL makes up about 95% of cases. It is characterized by the presence of Reed-Sternberg (RS) cells, which are binucleated or multinucleated and have abundant cytoplasm and distinct nuclei. RS cells are almost never found in peripheral blood. Morphologic variants of RS cells exist among the subtypes of classic HL. RS cells are of B cell origin, although they lack expression of most B cell markers. Immunophenotyping shows that RS cells primarily express CD30 and often co-express CD15 (Figure 34.16). RS and RS variants reside in lymph nodes in a "sea" of reactive cells that include lymphocytes, histiocytes, granulocytes, eosinophils, and plasma cells. There are four recognized histologic subtypes of classic HL – nodular sclerosis, mixed cellularity, lymphocyte rich, and lymphocyte depleted – which are identified based upon the background where the RS or RS-like cells are found. Previously the histologic subtype was thought to indicate prognostic significance, but this was more likely a function of disease stage; therefore all subtypes of classic HL are treated accordingly.

Lymphocyte-predominant HL (LPHL) lacks RS cells; however, the malignant cell is a lymphocytic histiocytic (L&H) cell.

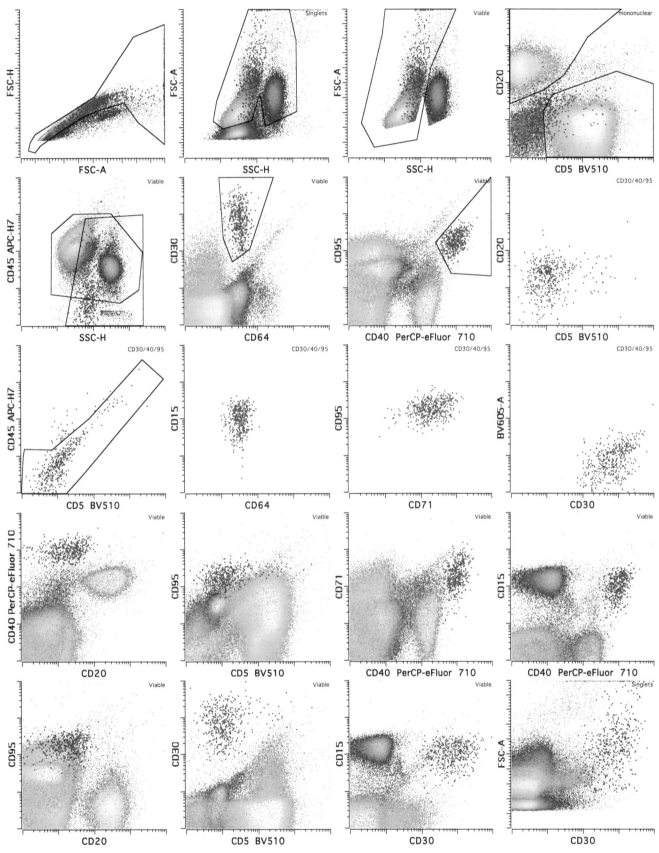

Figure 34.16 Nine-Color Flow Cytometry Assay for Classic Hodgkin Lymphoma. Reed-Sternberg cells *(red)* are large and typically have high forward and side scatter. They express CD30, CD40, CD95, and CD15 but lack CD64. T cells express CD5 *(green),* whereas B cells express CD20 *(light blue).* Flow cytometry is largely used as a confirmatory test in cases in which morphology may be problematic. (Courtesy Qi Gao, Memorial Sloan Kettering Cancer Center, NY.)

L&H cells are large with scant cytoplasm and a folded single nucleus; they are labeled "popcorn" cells because of their distinct morphology. Popcorn cells are negative for CD15 and CD30 expression, and about 50% express epithelial membrane antigen (EMA). Popcorn cells exist in a nodular background composed primarily of small lymphocytes. This disorder is also of B cell origin, although the corresponding level of neoplastic transformation from a normal counterpart is different from that in classic HL.

Classic HL has a bimodal age distribution with peaks in the 30s and again after age 50. LPHL is a disease of young adults. Clinically these patients also differ in presentation. Classic HL often presents with cervical, supraclavicular, and mediastinal adenopathy that spreads in a contiguous manner. LPHL patients have peripheral lymphadenopathy, but mediastinal adenopathy is rare. Nodal involvement is not contiguous, and extranodal involvement is rare in LPHL. Both classic HL and LPHL can be accompanied by B symptoms. Treatment decisions are based on the Ann Arbor staging criteria.

Treatment

HL is one of the initial successes associated with combination chemotherapy that established this therapeutic approach in modern oncology. The original regimen, MOPP (mechlorethamine, vincristine, procarbazine, and prednisone), was found to be effective even in advanced disease. Radiotherapy was used for patients determined to have localized disease and also to supplement chemotherapy in cases in which there was bulky lymphadenopathy. Although highly effective, treatment-related toxicity

issues began to emerge as more patients survived for longer periods of time. These complications included cardiac toxicity for those who received radiation as part of therapy to the mediastinum and also secondary malignancies. Secondary malignancies became a major concern, because patients developed solid tumors in the radiation field more than 10 years following the completion of this therapy. Patients who received high cumulative doses of alkylating agents were found to be at risk for the development of myelodysplastic syndrome or acute myeloid leukemia 3 to 5 years after completing treatment. Eventually newer regimens, such as ABVD (doxorubicin, bleomycin, vinblastine, and dacarbazine) were introduced and found to be superior and less toxic than MOPP. These therapies have largely replaced MOPP as the standard of care. As chemotherapy-based regimens with involved field radiation began to be used more frequently in limited-stage disease, approaches that limit the total dose of chemotherapy administered, and hence minimize associated adverse events, have been adopted into clinical practice.[52-55]

HL is a tumor that is highly sensitive to chemotherapy and radiation therapy. For some patients, dose attenuation designed to minimize toxicity may result in less effective disease control and result in tumor recurrence. However, such patients can still be cured. For relapse after chemotherapy, high-dose treatment followed by autologous stem cell transplant (ASCT) is effective salvage therapy, resulting in approximately 55% of patients having freedom from treatment failure at 3 year follow-up.[56] Patients with classic HL who relapse following ASCT may still achieve disease control with the CD30-directed immunoconjugate brentuximab vedotin.[57]

■ SUMMARY

- Mature lymphoid neoplasms arise from a malignant transformation at various stages of development from acquired genetic abnormalities that lead to abnormal changes in cell growth and differentiation patterns.
- Modern classification systems, such as that developed by the World Health Organization (WHO), are based on biologic features and new molecular data to refine disease models and identify prognostic markers used in identifying therapy.
- Leukemias and lymphomas are related malignancies that share cells of origin but differ in clinical presentation. Leukemias primarily involve the peripheral blood and bone marrow whereas lymphomas predominantly involve the spleen and lymph nodes. However, it is not uncommon for lymphoma cells to be found in the peripheral blood.
- Chronic lymphocytic leukemia (CLL), the most common leukemia in the western world, is characterized by an accumulation of mature appearing functionally incompetent B lymphocytes that aberrantly express CD5. Clinical behavior and outcomes in CLL are largely related to the somatic mutational status of the immunoglobulin heavy chain gene.
- Multiple (plasma cell) myeloma is a neoplasm in which proliferating malignant plasma cells in the bone marrow secrete monoclonal immunoglobulin and suppress normal

hematopoiesis. Systemic manifestations include osteolytic lesions, hypercalcemia, anemia and kidney failure. Circulating plasma cells are uncommon except in patients with end-stage disease or primary plasma cell leukemia.
- Diffuse large B cell lymphoma is the most common form of NHL. It is an aggressive disease that arises either de novo or from transformation of a more indolent form of leukemia or lymphoma. Circulating lymphoma cells can exhibit immature blast-like features.
- T cell lymphomas are less common but more aggressive than B cell lymphomas. Extranodal involvement including skin manifestations are frequently seen. Adult T cell lymphoma and Sezary cells in peripheral blood have distinctive morphology, often including irregular nuclear shapes.
- Hodgkin lymphoma is an uncommon disease of young adults characterized by painless lymphadenopathy. In the most common classical form of the disease, characteristic Reed-Sternberg cells are found in lymph node tissue. The cure rate, even in relapsed patients is greater than 85%.

Now that you have completed this chapter, go back and read again the case study at the beginning and respond to the questions presented.

REVIEW QUESTIONS

Answers can be found in the Appendix.

1. Non-Hodgkin lymphoma can be best differentiated from reactive disorders by:
   a. Genetic testing
   b. Immunophenotyping
   c. Absolute lymphocyte count
   d. Blood film review

2. Which laboratory test is most suggestive of autoimmune hemolytic anemia in a patient with CLL?
   a. Direct antiglobulin test
   b. Hemoglobin
   c. Lymphocyte count
   d. Platelet count

3. What is the best test or method for determining if a clonal population of T cells is present in a specimen?
   a. Molecular diagnostic testing
   b. Flow cytometry for CD3, CD5, and CD7
   c. Immunohistochemical stain
   d. Karyotyping

4. A rise in the lymphocyte count from 4.1×10^9/L to 5.5×10^9/L in a patient with monoclonal B lymphocytosis suggests:
   a. Acute lymphocyte leukemia
   b. Chronic lymphocytic leukemia
   c. Acute myelocytic leukemia
   d. A reactive condition

5. Which test is often used to differentiate CLL from mantle cell lymphoma?
   a. Annexin A staining
   b. Lymph node biopsy
   c. Immunohistochemistry
   d. FISH for BCL2 translocation

6. If not treated, which of the following would generally be associated with the best outcome?
   a. Peripheral T cell lymphoma
   b. Burkitt lymphoma
   c. Splenic marginal zone lymphoma
   d. Sézary syndrome

7. What do CLL and myeloma have in common?
   a. Osteolytic lesions
   b. Light chain restriction
   c. Cell of origin
   d. Immunophenotype

8. In Hodgkin lymphoma the Reed-Sternberg cell and _____ are malignant.
   a. Popcorn cells
   b. T cells
   c. B cells
   d. Histiocytes

9. In most cases the diagnosis of lymphoma relies on all of the following *except*:
   a. Microscopic examination of affected lymph nodes
   b. Immunophenotyping
   c. Molecular analysis
   d. Peripheral blood examination and complete blood count

10. Which of the following is present in monoclonal gammopathy of underdetermined significance?
    a. Hypercalcemia
    b. Serum monoclonal protein
    c. Anemia
    d. Bone lesion

REFERENCES

1. Swerdlow, S. H., Campo, E., Harris, N. L., et al. (Eds.). (2008). *WHO Classification of Tumors of Haematopoietic and Lymphoid Tissues.* (4th ed.). Lyon, France: IARC Press.

2. Swerdlow, S. H., Campo, E., Pileri, S. A., et al. (2016). The 2016 revision of the World Health Organization classification of lymphoid neoplasms. *Blood, 127*(20), 2375–2390.

3. Dave, B. J., Nelson, M., & Sanger, W. G. (2011). Lymphoma cytgenetics. *Clin Lab Med, 31*(4), 725–761.

4. Taylor, J., Xiao, W., & Abdel-Wahab, O. (2017). Diagnosis and classification of hematologic malignancies on the basis of genetics. *Blood, 130*, 410–423.

5. Hamblin, T. J., Davis, Z., Gardiner, A., et al. (1999). Unmutated Ig V(H) genes are associated with a more aggressive form of chronic lymphocytic leukemia. *Blood, 94*(6), 1848–1856.

6. Wood, B. L., Arroz, M., Barnett, D., et al. (2007). 2006 Bethesda International Consensus recommendations on the immunophenotypic analysis of hematolymphoid neoplasia by flow cytometry: optimal reagents and reporting for the flow cytometric diagnosis of hematopoietic neoplasia. *Cytometry B Clin Cytom, 72*(Suppl. 1), S14–22.

7. Lister, T. A., Crowther, D., Sutcliffe, S. B., et al. (1989). Report of a committee convened to discuss the evaluation and staging of patients with Hodgkin's disease: cotswolds meeting. *J Clin Oncol, 7*(11), 1630–1636.

8. Rosenberg, S. A. (1977). Validity of the Ann Arbor staging classification for the non-Hodgkin's lymphomas. *Cancer Treat Rep, 61*, 1923–1027.

9. Cheson, B. D., Fisher, R. I., Barrington, S. F., et al. Italian Lymphoma Foundation. (2014). Recommendations for initial evaluation, staging and response assessment of Hodgkin and non-Hodgkin lymphoma: the Lugano classification. *J Clin Oncol, 32*(27), 3059–3068.

10. International Non-Hodgkin's Lymphoma Prognostic Factors Project. (1993). A predictive model for aggressive non-Hodgkin's lymphoma. *N Engl J Med, 329*(14), 987–994

11. Sehn, H., Berry, B., Chhanabhai, M., et al. (2007). The revised International Prognostic Index (R-IPI) is a better predictor of outcome than the standard IPI for patients with diffuse large B-cell lymphoma treated with R-CHOP. *Blood, 109*(5), 1857–1861.

12. Teras, L. R., DeSantis, C. E., Cerhan, J. R., et al. (2016). 2016 US lymphoid malignancy statistics by the World Health Organization subtypes. *CA Cancer J Clin, 10.3322/caac.21357.*

13. Hallek, M., Cheson, B. D., Catovsky, D., et al. (2008). Guidelines for the diagnsosis and treatment of chronic lymphocytic leukemia: a report from the International Workshop on Chronic Lymphocytic Leukemia updating the National Cancer Institute-Working Group 1996 guidelines. *Blood*, *111*(12), 5446–5456.

14. Matutes, E., Attygalle, A., Wotherspoon, A., et al. (2010). Diagnostic issues in chronic lymphocytic leukemia (CLL). *Best Pract Res Clin Haematol*, *23*(1), 3–20.

15. Palmer, L., Briggs, C., McFadden, S., et al. (2015). ICSH recommendations for the standardization of nomenclature and grading of peripheral blood cell morphological features. *Int Jnl Lab Hem*, *37*(3), 287–303.

16. Gulati, G., Ly, V., Uppal, G., et al. (2017). Feasibility of counting smudge cells as lymphocytes in differential leukocyte counts performed on blood smears of patients with established or suspected chronic lymphocytic leukemia/small lymphocytic lymphoma. *Lab Med*, *48*(2), 137–147.

17. Matutes, E., & Polliack, A. (2000). Morphological and immunophenotypic features of chronic lymphocytic leukemia. *Rev Clin Exp Hematol*, *4*(1), 22–47.

18. Wierda, W. G., Zelenetz, A., Gordon, L. I., et al. (2017). NCCN Clinical Practice Guidelines in Oncology: chronic lymphocytic leukemia/small lymphocytic lymphoma, Version 1.2017. *J Natl Compr Canc Netw*, *15*, 293–311.

19. Rawstron, A. C., Bennett, F. L., O'Connor, S. J., et al. (2008). Monoclonal B-cell lymphocytosis and chronic lymphocytic leukemia. *N Engl J Med*, *359*(6), 575–583.

20. Rai, K. R., Sawitsky, A., Cronkite, E. P., et al. (1975). Clinical staging of chronic lymphocytic leukemia. *Blood*, *46*(2), 219–234.

21. Binet, J. L., Auquier, A. A., Dighiero, G., et al. (1981). A new prognostic classification of chronic lymphocytic leukemia derived from a multivariate survival analysis. *Cancer*, *48*(1), 198–206.

22. Dohner, H., Stilgenbauer, S., Benner, A., et al. (2000). Genomic aberrations and survival in chronic lymphocytic leukemia. *N Engl J Med*, *343*(26), 1910–1916.

23. Haferlach, C., Dicker, F., Weiss, T., et al. (2010). Toward a comprehensive prognostic scoring system in chronic lymphocytic leukemia based on a combination of genetic parameters. *Genes Chromosomes Cancer*, *49*(9), 851–859.

24. Pflug, N., Bahlo, J., Shanafelt, T. D., et al. (2014). Development of a comprehensive prognostic index for patients with chronic lymphocytic leukemia. *Blood*, *124*(1), 49–62.

25. Maddocks, K., & Jones, J. A. (2016). Bruton tyrosine kinase inhibition in chronic lymphocytic leukemia. *Semin Oncol*, *43*(2), 251–259.

26. Furman, R. R., Sharman, J. P., Coutre, S., et al. (2014). Idelalisib and rituximab in relapsed chronic lymphocytic leukemia. *N Engl J Med*, *370*(11), 997–1007.

27. Roberts, A. W., Davids, M. S., Pagel, J. M., et al. (2016). Targeting BCL2 with venetoclax in relapsed chronic lymphocytic leukemia. *N Engl J Med*, *374*(4), 311–322.

28. Dearden, C. (2015). Management of prolymphocytic leukemia. *ASH Education Book*, *2015*(1), 361–367.

29. Grever, M. R., Abdel-Wahah, O., Andritsos, L. A., et al. (2017). Consensus guidelines for the diagnosis and management of patients with classic hairy cell leukemia. *Blood*, *129*, 553–560.

30. Tiacci, E., Park, J. H., De Carolis, L. D., et al. (2015). Targeting mutant BRAF in relapsed or refractory hairy-cell leukemia. *N Engl J Med*, *373*, 1733–1747.

31. O'Malley, D. P. (2007). T-cell large granular leukemia and related proliferations. *Am J Clin Pathol*, *127*(6), 850–859.

32. Lamy, T., Moignet, A., & Loughran, T. P., Jr. (2017). LGL leukemia: from pathogenesis to treatment. *Blood*, *129*(9), 1082–1094.

33. Watanabe, T. (2017). Adult T-cell leukemia : molecular basis for clonal expansion and transformation of HTLV-1 infected T cells. *Blood*, *129*(9), 1071–1081.

34. Tsukasaki, K., Hermine, O., Bazarbachi, A., et al. (2009). Definition, prognostic factors, treatment, and response criteria of adult T-cell leukemia-lymphoma: a proposal from an international consensus meeting. *J Clin Oncol*, *27*(3), 453–459.

35. Jacobson, C., & LaCase, A. (2014). How I treat Burkitt lymphoma in adults. *Blood*, *124*, 2913–2920.

36. Nastoupil, L. J., Sinha, R., Byrtek, M., et al. (2016). Outcomes following watchful waiting for stage II-IV follicular lymphoma in the modern era. *Br J Haematol*, *172*(5), 724–734.

37. Advani, R. H., Buggy, J. J., Sharman, J. P., et al. (2013). Bruton tyrosine kinase inhibitor ibrutinib (PCI-32765) has signficant activity in patients with relapsed / refractory B-cell malignancies. *J Clin Oncol*, *31*(1), 88–94.

38. Horn, H., Ziepert, M., Becher, C., et al. (2013). MYC status in concert with BCL2 and BCL6 expression predicts outcome in diffuse large B-cell lymphoma. *Blood*, *121*(12), 2253–2263.

39. Sarkozy, C., Traverse-Glehen, A., & Coiffier, B. (2015). Double-hit and double-protein-expression lymphoma: aggressive and refractory lymphomas. *Lancet Oncol*, *16*(15), e555–e567.

40. Alizadeh, A. A., Eisen, M. B., Davis, R. E., et al. (2000). Distinct types of diffuse large B-cell lymphoma identified by gene expression profiling. *Nature*, *403*(6769), 503–511.

41. Sehn, H., Berry, B., Chhanabhai, M., et al. (2007). The revised International Prognostic Index (R-IPI) is a better predictor of outcome than the standard IPI for patients with diffuse large B-cell lymphoma treated with R-CHOP. *Blood*, *109*(5), 1857–1861.

42. Zucca, E., & Bertoni, F. (2016). The spectrum of MALT lymphoma at different sites: biological and therapeutic relevance. *Blood*, *127*, 2082–2092.

43. Arcaini, L., Rossi, D., & Paulli, M. (2016). Splenic marginal zone lymphoma: from genetics to management. *Blood*, *127*, 2072–2081.

44. Thieblemont, C., Molina, T., & Davi, F. (2016). Optimizing therapy for nodal marginal zone lymphoma. *Blood*, *127*, 2064–2071.

45. Duvic, M. (2015). Choosing a systemic treatment for advanced stage cutaneous T-cell lymphoma: mycosis fungoides and Sezary syndrome. *ASH Education Book*, *2015*(1), 529–544.

46. Hapgood, G., & Savage, K. (2015). The biology and management of systemic anaplastic large cell lymphoma. *Blood*, *126*, 17–25.

47. Broccoli, A., & Zinzani, P. L. (2017). Peripheral T cell lymphoma, not otherwise specified. *Blood*, *129*(9), 1103–1112.

48. Landgren, O. (2015). Monoclonal gammopathy of undetermined signficance and smoldering multiple myeloma: biologic insights and early treatment strategies. *ASH Education Book*, *2013*(1), 478–487.

49. Rajikumar, S. V., Dimopoulos, M. A., Palumbo, A., et al. (2014). International Myeloma Working Group updated criteria for the diagnosis of multiple myeloma. *Lancet Oncol*, *15*, e538–e548.

50. Dispenzieri, A. (2016). Myeloma: management of the newly diagnosed high-risk patient. *ASH Education Book*, *2016*, 485–494.

51. Nooka, A. K., & Lonial, S. (2016). New targets and new agents in high risk myeloma. *Am Soc Clin Oncol Educ Book*, *35*, e431–e441.

52. Johnson, P., Federico, M., Kirkwood, A. et al. (2016). Adapted treatment guided by interim PET-CT scan in advanced Hodgkin's lymphoma. *N Engl J Med*, *374*(25), 2419–2429.

53. Koontz, M. Z., Horning, S. J., Balise, R., et al. (2013). Risk of therapy-related secondary leukemia in Hodgkin lymphoma: the

Standford University experience over three generations of clinical trials *J Clin Oncol*, *31*(5), 592–598.

54. Travis, L. B., Hill, D., Dores, G. M., et al. (2005). Cumulative absolute breast cancer risk for young women treated for Hodgkin lymphoma. *J Natl Cancer Inst*, *97*(19), 1428–1437.

55. van Nimwegen, F. A., Schaapveld, M., Cutter, D. J., et al. (2016). Radiation dose-response relationship for risk of coronary heart disease in survivors of Hodgkin lymphoma. *J Clin Oncol*, *34*(3), 235–243.

56. Collins, G. P., Parker, A. N., Pocock, C., et al. (2014). British committee for standards in hematology: british society of blood and marrow transplantation. Guideline on the management of primary resistant and relapsed classical hodgkin lymphoma. *Br J Haematol*, *64*(1), 39–52.

57. Younes, A., Bartlett, N. L., Leonard, J. P., et al. (2010). Brentuximab vedotin (SGN-35) for relapsed CD30-positive lymphoma. *N Engl J Med*, *363*(1), 1812–1821.

35

Normal Hemostasis

*Jeanine M. Walenga**

OBJECTIVES

After completion of this chapter, the reader will be able to:

1. List the systems that interact to provide hemostasis.
2. Describe the properties of the vascular intima that initiate and regulate hemostasis and fibrinolysis.
3. List the hemostatic functions of tissue factor-bearing cells and blood cells, especially platelets.
4. Describe the relationships of platelets with von Willebrand factor and fibrinogen, and their impact on hemostasis.
5. Describe the nature, origin, and function of each of the tissue and plasma factors necessary for normal coagulation.
6. Explain the role of vitamin K in the production and function of the prothrombin group of plasma clotting factors.
7. Distinguish between coagulation pathway serine proteases and cofactors.
8. Describe six roles of thrombin in hemostasis.
9. Diagram fibrinogen structure, fibrin formation, fibrin polymerization, and fibrin cross-linking.
10. For each coagulation complex—extrinsic tenase, intrinsic tenase, and prothrombinase—identify the serine protease and the cofactor forming the complex, the type of cell involved, and the substrate(s) activated.
11. List the factors in order of reaction in the plasma-based extrinsic, intrinsic, and common pathways.
12. Describe the cell-based in vivo coagulation process and the role of tissue factor-bearing cells and platelets.
13. Show how tissue factor pathway inhibitor, the protein C pathway, and the serine protease inhibitor antithrombin function to regulate coagulation and prevent thrombosis.
14. Describe the fibrinolytic pathway, its regulators, and its products.

OUTLINE

Overview of Hemostasis
Vascular Intima in Hemostasis
    Anticoagulant Properties of Intact Vascular Intima
    Procoagulant Properties of Damaged Vascular Intima
    Fibrinolytic Properties of Vascular Intima
Platelets
Coagulation System
    Nomenclature of Procoagulants
    Classification and Function of Procoagulants
    The Coagulation System: Extrinsic, Intrinsic, and Common Pathways
    The Hemostatic System: Cell-Based Physiologic Coagulation

Coagulation Regulatory Mechanisms
    Tissue Factor Pathway Inhibitor
    Protein C Regulatory System
    Antithrombin
    Other Serine Protease Inhibitors
Fibrinolysis
    Plasminogen and Plasmin
    Plasminogen Activation
    Control of Fibrinolysis
    Fibrin Degradation Products and D-Dimer

---

*The author extends appreciation to Margaret G. Fritsma and George A. Fritsma, whose work in prior editions provided the foundation for this chapter.

Hemostasis is a complex physiologic process that keeps circulating blood in a fluid state and then, when an injury occurs, produces a clot to stop the bleeding, confines the clot to the site of injury, and finally dissolves the clot as the wound heals. When hemostasis systems are out of balance, hemorrhage (uncontrolled bleeding) or thrombosis (pathologic clotting) can be life threatening. The absence of a single plasma procoagulant may destine the individual to lifelong *anatomic hemorrhage,* chronic inflammation, and transfusion dependence. Conversely, absence of a control protein allows coagulation to proceed unchecked and results in *thrombosis,* stroke, pulmonary embolism, deep vein thrombosis, and cardiovascular events.

Understanding the major systems of hemostasis—blood vessels, platelets, and plasma proteins—is essential to interpreting laboratory test results and to prevent, predict, diagnose, and manage hemostatic disease.

OVERVIEW OF HEMOSTASIS

Hemostasis involves the interaction of vasoconstriction, platelet adhesion and aggregation, and coagulation enzyme activation to stop bleeding. The coagulation system, similar to other humoral amplification mechanisms, is complex because it translates a diminutive physical or chemical stimulus into a profound life-saving event.[1] The key cellular elements of hemostasis are the cells of the vascular intima, extravascular tissue factor (TF)-bearing cells, and platelets. The plasma components include the coagulation and fibrinolytic proteins and their inhibitors.

Primary hemostasis (Table 35.1) refers to the role of blood vessels and platelets in the initial response to a vascular injury or to the commonplace desquamation of dying or damaged endothelial cells. Blood vessels contract to seal the wound or reduce the blood flow (vasoconstriction). Platelets become activated, adhere to the site of injury, secrete the contents of their granules, and aggregate with other platelets to form a platelet plug. Vasoconstriction and platelet plug formation comprise the initial, rapid, short-lived response to vessel damage, but to control major bleeding in the long term, the plug must be reinforced by fibrin. Defects in primary hemostasis such as collagen abnormalities, thrombocytopenia, qualitative platelet disorders, or von Willebrand disease can cause debilitating, sometimes fatal, chronic hemorrhage.

Secondary hemostasis (Table 35.1) describes the activation of a series of coagulation proteins in the plasma, mostly serine proteases, to form a fibrin clot. These proteins circulate as inactive zymogens (proenzymes) that become activated during the process of coagulation and, in turn, form complexes that activate other zymogens to ultimately generate thrombin, an enzyme that converts fibrinogen to a localized fibrin clot. The final event of hemostasis is fibrinolysis, the gradual digestion and removal of the fibrin clot as healing occurs.[2]

Although the vascular intima and platelets are associated with primary hemostasis, and coagulation and fibrinolysis are associated with secondary hemostasis, all systems interact in early- and late-hemostatic events. For example, platelets, although a key component of primary hemostasis, also secrete coagulation factors stored in their granules and provide an essential cell membrane phospholipid on which coagulation complexes form. This chapter details vascular intima, platelets, coagulation, coagulation control, fibrinolysis, and control of fibrinolysis, and the interactions of these components, as they relate to normal hemostasis.

VASCULAR INTIMA IN HEMOSTASIS

Blood vessels, or the vasculature, carry blood throughout the body. A blood vessel is structured into three layers: an inner layer (vascular intima), a middle layer (vascular media), and an outer layer (vascular adventitia). The vascular intima provides the interface between circulating blood and the body tissues. This innermost lining of blood vessels is a monolayer of metabolically active *endothelial cells* (ECs) (Box 35.1; Figure 35.1;

TABLE 35.1 **Primary and Secondary Hemostasis**	
Primary Hemostasis	**Secondary Hemostasis**
Activated by desquamation and small injuries to blood vessels	Activated by large injuries to blood vessels and surrounding tissues
Involves vascular intima and platelets	Involves platelets and coagulation system
Rapid, short-lived response	Delayed, long-term response
Procoagulant substances exposed or released by damaged or activated endothelial cells	The activator, tissue factor, is exposed on cell membranes

BOX 35.1 **Vascular Intima of the Blood Vessel**
Innermost Vascular Lining
Endothelial cells (endothelium)
Supporting the Endothelial Cells
Internal elastic lamina composed of elastin and collagen
Subendothelial Connective Tissue
Collagen and fibroblasts in veins
Collagen, fibroblasts, and smooth muscle cells in arteries

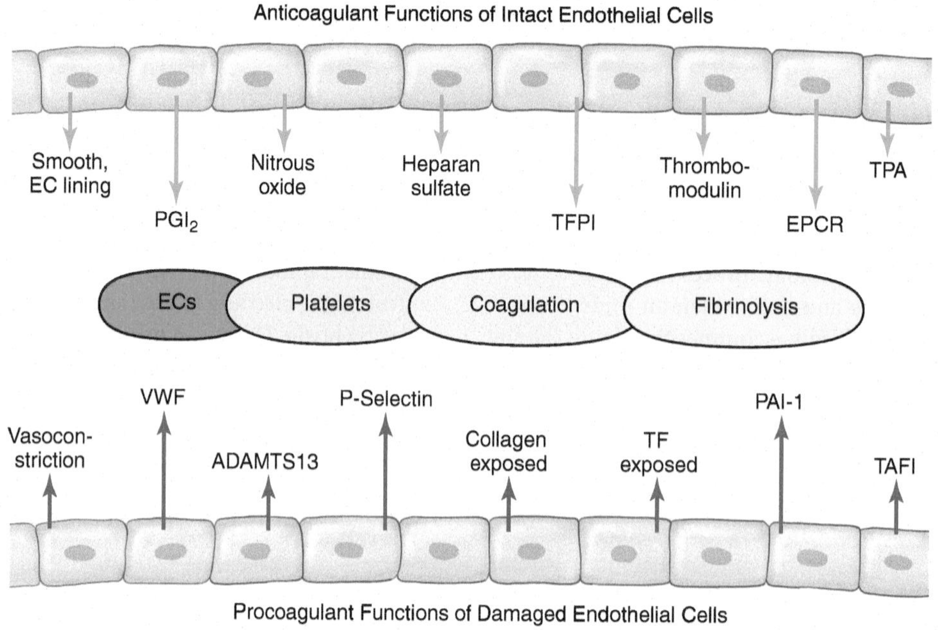

Anticoagulant Functions of Intact Endothelial Cells

Figure 35.1 Hemostatic Properties of Endothelial Cells that Line the Inner Surface of All Blood Vessels. Depicted in this cartoon are the anticoagulant properties associated with normal intact endothelial cells and the procoagulant properties associated with damaged endothelial cells as they relate to the functions of the hemostatic system listed in the center. *ADAMTS13,* A disintegrin and metalloprotease with a thrombospondin type 1 motif, member 13; *ECs,* endothelial cells; *EPCR,* endothelial cell protein C receptor; *PAI-1,* plasminogen activator inhibitor-1; *PGI₂,* prostacyclin or prostaglandin I₂; *TAFI,* thrombin activatable fibrinolysis inhibitor; *TF,* tissue factor; *TFPI,* tissue factor pathway inhibitor; *TPA,* tissue plasminogen activator; *VWF,* von Willebrand factor.

refer also to Figure 10.9A).[3] Endothelial cells are complex and heterogeneous and are distributed throughout the body. They display unique structural and functional characteristics, depending on their environment and physiologic requirements, not only in subsets of blood vessels such as arteries versus veins but also in the various tissues and organs of the body.[4,5] ECs play essential roles in immune response, vascular permeability, proliferation, and, of course, hemostasis.

ECs form a smooth, unbroken surface that eases the fluid passage of blood. A basement membrane, an elastin-rich internal elastic lamina, and its surrounding layer of connective tissues support the ECs. In all blood vessels, fibroblasts occupy the connective tissue layer and produce collagen. Smooth muscle cells in arteries and arterioles, but not in the walls of veins, venules, or capillaries, contract when an injury occurs and primary hemostasis is initiated.

Anticoagulant Properties of Intact Vascular Intima

Normally the intact vascular endothelium prevents thrombosis by inhibiting platelet aggregation, preventing coagulation activation and propagation, and enhancing fibrinolysis. Several specific anticoagulant mechanisms prevent intravascular thrombosis (Table 35.2; Figure 35.1). First, ECs are rhomboid and contiguous, providing a smooth inner surface of the blood vessel that promotes even blood flow preventing harmful turbulence that otherwise may activate platelets and coagulation enzymes. ECs form a physical barrier separating procoagulant proteins and platelets in blood from collagen in the vascular intima that promotes platelet adhesion, and TF in fibroblasts and smooth muscle cells that activates coagulation.

TABLE 35.2 Anticoagulant Properties of Intact Vascular Endothelium

Endothelial Cell Structure/Substance	Anticoagulant Property
Vascular endothelium is composed of rhomboid cells	Present a smooth, contiguous surface
ECs secrete prostacyclin	The eicosanoid platelet inhibitor
ECs secrete nitric oxide	A vascular "relaxing" factor
ECs secrete the glycosaminoglycan heparan sulfate	An anticoagulant that regulates thrombin generation
ECs secrete TFPI	A regulator of the extrinsic pathway of coagulation
ECs express the protein C receptor EPCR	An integral component of the protein C control system
ECs express cell membrane thrombomodulin	A protein C coagulation control system activator
ECs secrete TPA	Activates fibrinolysis

ECs, Endothelial cells; *EPCR,* endothelial protein C receptor; *TFPI,* tissue factor pathway inhibitor; *TPA,* tissue plasminogen activator.

ECs synthesize and secrete a variety of substances that maintain normal blood flow. Prostacyclin, a platelet inhibitor and a vasodilator, is synthesized through the eicosanoid pathway (Chapter 10) and prevents unnecessary or undesirable platelet activation in intact vessels.[6] Nitric oxide is synthesized in ECs, vascular smooth muscle cells, neutrophils, and macrophages. Nitric oxide induces smooth muscle relaxation and subsequent vasodilation, inhibits platelet activation, and promotes angiogenesis and healthy arterioles.[7,8] An important EC-produced anticoagulant is tissue factor pathway inhibitor (TFPI), which controls activation of the tissue factor pathway, also called the extrinsic coagulation pathway. TFPI limits the activation of the TF:VIIa:Xa complex.

Finally, ECs synthesize and express on their surfaces two known inhibitors of thrombin formation, thrombomodulin, facilitated by endothelial protein C receptor (EPCR), and heparan sulfate. EPCR binds protein C, and thrombomodulin catalyzes the activation of the protein C pathway. The protein C pathway downregulates coagulation by digesting activated factors V and VIII, thereby inhibiting thrombin formation. Heparan sulfate is a glycosaminoglycan that enhances the activity of antithrombin, a blood plasma serine protease inhibitor.[9] The pharmaceutical anticoagulant heparin, an important therapeutic agent used in many cardiovascular indications, resembles EC heparan sulfate in structure and its inhibitory activity when bound to antithrombin.

Procoagulant Properties of Damaged Vascular Intima

Although the intact endothelium has anticoagulant properties, when damaged, the vascular intima (ECs and the subendothelial matrix) promotes coagulation through several procoagulant properties (Table 35.3; Figure 35.1). First, any harmful local stimulus, whether mechanical or chemical, induces vasoconstriction in arteries and arterioles where blood pressure is higher than on the venous side (Figure 10.9B). Smooth muscle cells contract, the vascular lumen narrows or closes, and blood flow through the injured site is minimized. Although veins and capillaries do not have smooth muscle cells, bleeding into surrounding tissues creates extravascular pressure on the blood vessel, effectively minimizing the escape of blood.

Second, the subendothelial connective tissues of arteries and veins are rich in collagen, a flexible, elastic structural protein. Exposed with injury to the vessel, collagen binds and activates platelets (Figure 10.9B and C). This initial platelet adhesion response fills in the damaged area until new ECs grow. Some

connective tissue degeneration occurs naturally in aging, which leads to an increased bruising tendency in the elderly.

Third, ECs secrete von Willebrand factor (VWF) from storage sites called Weibel-Palade bodies when activated by vasoactive agents such as thrombin. VWF is a large multimeric glycoprotein that acts as the necessary bridge that binds platelets to exposed subendothelial collagen in arterioles and arteries where blood flows rapidly (Figure 10.9C and D).[10] VWF has been described as a "carpet" on which activated platelets assemble. ADAMTS13, also secreted from ECs, serves an important function as it cleaves large VWF multimers into shorter chains that support normal platelet adhesion.

Fourth, on activation, ECs secrete and coat themselves with P-selectin, an adhesion molecule that promotes platelet and leukocyte binding.[11] ECs also secrete immunoglobulin-like adhesion molecules called intercellular adhesion molecules (ICAMs) and platelet endothelial cell adhesion molecules (PECAMs), which further promote platelet and leukocyte binding.[12]

Finally, subendothelial smooth muscle cells and fibroblasts support the constitutive membrane protein tissue factor.[13] EC disruption exposes TF in subendothelial cells and activates the coagulation system through contact with plasma coagulation factor VII leading to fibrin formation (Figure 35.2). In pathologic conditions, TF may also be expressed on monocytes during inflammation and sepsis and by tissue factor-positive microparticles derived from membrane fragments of activated or apoptotic vascular cells and possibly on the surface of some ECs.[14] The formed fibrin surrounds the platelet plug, securing it to the damaged area, such that the blood flow does not dislodge it.

Response to pathologic conditions causes blood clot formation that occludes the vessel. In arterioles and arteries, the larger VWF multimers form a fibrillar carpet on which the platelets assemble; a white clot consisting of platelets and VWF is produced. Excess arterial occlusion causes myocardial infarction, stroke, and peripheral artery disease. In veins, a bulky red clot is produced consisting of platelets, VWF, fibrin, and red blood cells. Excess venous occlusion causes deep vein thrombosis and thromboembolic disease.

TABLE 35.3 Procoagulant Properties of Damaged Vascular Intima

Structure/Substance	Procoagulant Property
Smooth muscle cells in arterioles and arteries	Induce vasoconstriction
Exposed subendothelial collagen	Binds VWF; binds to and activates platelets
Damaged or activated ECs secrete VWF	Important for platelet binding to collagen at site of injury: platelet adhesion as a first line of defense against bleeding
Damaged or activated ECs secrete adhesion molecules: P-selectin, ICAMs, PECAMs	Promote platelet and leukocyte binding and activation at site of injury
Exposed smooth muscle cells and fibroblasts	Tissue factor exposed on cell membranes
ECs in inflammation	Tissue factor is induced by inflammation

ECs, Endothelial cells; *ICAMs,* intercellular adhesion molecules; *PECAMs,* platelet endothelial cell adhesion molecules; *VWF,* von Willebrand factor.

Fibrinolytic Properties of Vascular Intima

ECs support fibrinolysis (Table 35.2 and Figure 35.1), the removal of fibrin to restore vessel patency, with the secretion of tissue plasminogen activator (TPA). During thrombus formation, both TPA and plasminogen bind to polymerized fibrin. TPA activates fibrinolysis by converting plasminogen to plasmin, which gradually digests fibrin and restores blood flow. ECs also regulate fibrinolysis by providing inhibitors to prevent excessive plasmin generation. ECs, as well as other cells, secrete plasminogen activator inhibitor-1 (PAI-1), a TPA control protein that inhibits plasmin generation and fibrinolysis.[15] Another inhibitor of plasmin generation, thrombin activatable fibrinolysis inhibitor (TAFI), is activated by thrombin bound to EC membrane thrombomodulin.[16] Elevations in PAI-1 or TAFI can slow fibrinolysis and increase the tendency for thrombosis.

Although the significance of the vascular intima in hemostasis is well recognized, there are few valid laboratory methods to

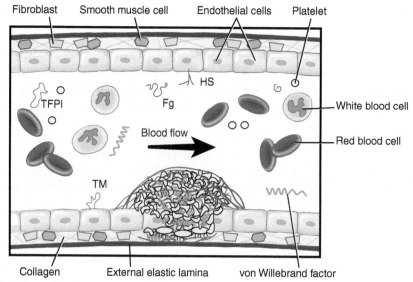

Figure 35.2 Secondary Hemostasis. Immediately after the initial response to vessel injury of platelet activation, adhesion, and aggregation (primary hemostasis) as detailed in Chapter 10 and Figure 10.9, the continued response of an injured blood vessel leads to the formation of a fibrin clot which stabilizes the initial platelet plug as shown here. Primary hemostasis requires interaction of platelets with subendothelial VWF and collagen. Secondary hemostasis requires exposure of TF from damaged endothelial cells and phospholipids from activated platelets which promotes activation of the coagulation cascade, thrombin generation, and fibrin formation that polymerizes around the platelet aggregate. *Fg*, fibrinogen; *HS*, heparan sulfate; *TF*, tissue factor, *TFPI*, tissue factor pathway inhibitor (EC bound and soluble forms exist); *TM*, thrombomodulin (EC bound and soluble forms exist).

assess the integrity of ECs, smooth muscle cells, fibroblasts, and their collagen matrix.[17] The diagnosis of blood vessel disorders is often based on clinical symptoms, family history, and laboratory tests that rule out platelet or coagulation disorders.

PLATELETS

Platelets are produced from the cytoplasm of bone marrow megakaryocytes.[18] Although platelets are only 2 to 3 μm in diameter on a fixed, stained peripheral blood film, they are complex, metabolically active cells that interact with their environment and initiate and control hemostasis.[19] Chapter 10 provides an in-depth description of platelet structure and function; an overview of the platelet functions critical in the initial stages of hemostatic control is given in this chapter.

Platelets serve as the body's first line of defense against blood loss. At the time of injury, platelets adhere, aggregate, and secrete the contents of their granules (Table 35.4; Figure 10.9).[20,21] *Adhesion* is the property by which platelets bind nonplatelet surfaces such as subendothelial collagen. Further, VWF links platelets to collagen in areas of high shear stress such as arteries and arterioles, whereas platelets may bind directly via specific receptors to collagen in damaged veins and capillaries. VWF binds platelets through their GP Ib/IX/V membrane receptor.[22] The importance of platelet adhesion is underscored by bleeding disorders such as Bernard-Soulier syndrome (Chapter 37), in which the platelet GP Ib/IX/V receptor is absent, and von Willebrand disease (Chapter 36), in which VWF is missing or defective.

Aggregation is the property by which platelets bind to one another. When platelets are activated, a change in the GP IIb/IIIa receptor allows binding of fibrinogen, as well as

TABLE 35.4	**Platelet Function**
Function	**Characteristics**
Adhesion: platelets roll and cling to nonplatelet surfaces	Reversible; seals endothelial gaps, some secretion of growth factors, in arterioles VWF is necessary for adhesion
Aggregation: platelets adhere to each other	Irreversible; platelet plugs form, platelet contents are secreted, requires fibrinogen
Secretion: platelets discharge the contents of their granules	Irreversible; occurs during aggregation, platelet contents are secreted, essential to coagulation

VWF, Von Willebrand factor.

VWF and fibronectin.[23] Fibrinogen binds to GP IIb/IIIa receptors on adjacent platelets and joins them together in the presence of ionized calcium (Ca^{2+}). Fibrinogen binding is essential for platelet aggregation, as evidenced by bleeding and compromised aggregation in patients with afibrinogenemia or in patients who lack the GP IIb/IIIa receptor (Glanzmann thrombasthenia; Chapter 37). In in vitro platelet aggregation studies, the commonly used agonists to induce aggregation are those found in vivo: thrombin (or thrombin receptor activation peptide [TRAP]), arachidonic acid, adenosine diphosphate (ADP), collagen, and epinephrine, which bind to their respective platelet membrane receptors (Chapter 41).[24]

Platelets *secrete* the contents of their granules during adhesion and aggregation, with most secretion occurring late in the platelet activation process. Platelets secrete procoagulants, such as factor V, VWF, factor VIII, and fibrinogen, as well as control proteins, Ca^{2+}, ADP, and other hemostatic molecules. See Table 35.5 for a summary of the contents of platelet α-granules and dense granules.

TABLE 35.5 Platelet Granule Contents

Platelet α-Granules (Large Molecules)	Platelet Dense Granules (Small Molecules)
β-Thromboglobulin	Adenosine diphosphate (activates neighboring platelets)
Factor V	Adenosine triphosphate
Factor XI	Calcium
Protein S	Serotonin (vasoconstrictor)
Fibrinogen	
VWF	
Platelet factor 4	
Platelet-derived growth factor	

VWF, Von Willebrand factor.

The platelet membrane consists of a phospholipid bilayer. During activation, ADP and Ca^{2+} activate phospholipase A_2. Phospholipids from the platelet membrane are converted to arachidonic acid by phospholipase A_2 (Figure 10.12). The cyclooxygenase enzyme converts arachidonic acid into the prostaglandin endoperoxides prostaglandin G_2 (PGG_2) and prostaglandin H_2 (PGH_2). In the platelet, thromboxane synthetase converts these prostaglandins into thromboxane A_2, which causes Ca^{2+} to be released from the dense tubules, thereby promoting platelet aggregation and vasoconstriction. Available Ca^{2+} (ionized calcium) is critical for normal platelet function.[25] Aspirin, a drug commonly used for its antiplatelet effect, functions via the arachidonic acid pathway to decrease platelet activity (Chapter 37).

The membrane of activated platelets is the key surface for coagulation enzyme-cofactor-substrate complex formation (Figure 35.2), which is the foundation for secondary hemostasis to occur.[26] Platelets supply Ca^{2+}, the membrane phospholipid *phosphatidylserine*, procoagulant factors, and receptors. Coagulation is initiated on tissue factor-bearing cells (such as fibroblasts) with the formation of the extrinsic tenase complex TF:VIIa:Ca^{2+}, which activates factors IX and X and produces enough thrombin to activate platelets and factors V, VIII, and XI in a feedback loop. Coagulation is then propagated on the surface of the platelet with the formation of the intrinsic tenase complex (IXa:VIIIa:phospholipid:Ca^{2+}) and the prothrombinase complex (Xa:Va:phospholipid:Ca^{2+}), ultimately generating a burst of thrombin at the site of injury. See subsequent text for more details.

Erythrocytes, monocytes, and lymphocytes also participate in hemostasis. Erythrocytes add bulk and structural integrity to the fibrin clot; there is a tendency to bleed in anemia. In inflammatory conditions, monocytes and lymphocytes, and possibly ECs, provide surface-borne TF that may trigger coagulation. Leukocytes also have a series of membrane integrins and selectins that bind adhesion molecules and help stimulate the production of inflammatory cytokines that promote the wound-healing process and combat infection.[27]

COAGULATION SYSTEM

Nomenclature of Procoagulants

Plasma transports at least 16 procoagulants, also called coagulation factors. Nearly all are glycoproteins synthesized in the liver, although monocytes, ECs, and megakaryocytes produce a few (Table 35.6; Figure 35.3). Eight are enzymes that circulate in an

TABLE 35.6 Properties of the Plasma Procoagulants

Factor	Name	Function	Molecular Weight (Daltons)	Half-Life (hr)	Mean Plasma Concentration[†]
I*	Fibrinogen	Thrombin substrate, polymerizes to form fibrin	340,000	100–150	200–400 mg/dL
II*	Prothrombin	Serine protease	71,600	60	10 mg/dL
III*	Tissue factor	Cofactor	44,000	Insoluble	None
IV*	Ionic calcium	Mineral	40	NA	8–10 mg/dL
V		Cofactor	330,000	24	1 mg/dL
VII		Serine protease	50,000	6	0.05 mg/dL
VIII	Antihemophilic factor	Cofactor	260,000	12	0.01 mg/dL
VWF	von Willebrand factor	Factor VIII carrier and platelet adhesion	600,000–20,000,000	24	1 mg/dL
IX	Christmas factor	Serine protease	57,000	24	0.3 mg/dL
X	Stuart-Prower factor	Serine protease	58,800	48–52	1 mg/dL
XI		Serine protease	143,000	48–84	0.5 mg/dL
XII	Hageman factor	Serine protease	84,000	48–70	3 mg/dL
Prekallikrein	Fletcher factor, pre-K	Serine protease	85,000	35	35–50 μg/mL
High-molecular-weight kininogen	Fitzgerald factor, HMWK	Cofactor	120,000	156	5 mg/dL
XIII	Fibrin-stabilizing factor (FSF)	Transglutaminase, transamidase	320,000	150	2 mg/dL
Platelet factor 3	Phospholipids, phosphatidyl-serine, PF3	Assembly molecule	—	Released by platelets	—

*These factors are customarily identified by name rather than Roman numeral.
†Clinically, plasma concentration of all coagulation factors, except fibrinogen, can be given as percentage of normal (%) or units/dL where the numerical value remains the same.

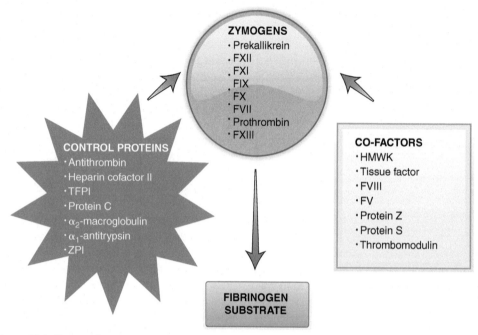

Figure 35.3 Plasma Components of the Coagulation System. Four categories of plasma-based components of the coagulation system of blood clotting include the procoagulants (zymogens), cofactors, anticoagulants (regulatory or control proteins), and final fibrinogen substrate. Throughout this chapter figures will use the above shape symbols to aid in classifying each component: zymogens as circles; activated zymogens or serine proteases as hexagons (not shown here); co-factors as rectangles; control proteins as stars; other components as ovals. *HMWK,* High-molecular-weight kininogen; *TFPI,* tissue factor pathway inhibitor; *ZPI,* protein Z-dependent protease inhibitor.

inactive form called zymogens. Others are cofactors that bind, stabilize, and enhance the activity of their respective enzymes. Fibrinogen is the substrate for the enzymatic action of thrombin, the primary enzyme of the coagulation system. In addition, there are plasma glycoproteins that act as control proteins that serve the important function of regulating the coagulation process to avoid unnecessary blood clotting. See the inside back cover of the book for the *normal clinical reference intervals* of these proteins.

In 1958 the International Committee for the Standardization of the Nomenclature of the Blood Clotting Factors officially named the plasma procoagulants using Roman numerals in the order of their initial description or discovery.[28] When a procoagulant becomes activated, a lowercase *a* appears behind the numeral; for instance, activated factor VII is VIIa. Both zymogens and cofactors become activated in the coagulation process.

We customarily call factor I fibrinogen and factor II prothrombin, although occasionally they are identified by their numerals. The numeral III was given to tissue thromboplastin, a crude mixture of TF and phospholipid. Now that the precise structure of TF has been described, the numeral designation is seldom used. The numeral IV identified the plasma cation calcium (Ca^{2+}); however, calcium is referred to by its name or chemical symbol, not by its numeral. The numeral VI was assigned to a procoagulant that later was determined to be activated factor V; VI was withdrawn from the naming system and never reassigned. Factor VIII, antihemophilic factor, is a cofactor that circulates linked to a large carrier protein, VWF.

Prekallikrein (pre-K), also called Fletcher factor, and high-molecular-weight kininogen (HMWK), also called Fitzgerald factor, have never received Roman numerals because they belong to the kallikrein and kinin systems, respectively, and their primary functions lie within these systems. Platelet phospholipids, particularly phosphatidylserine, are required for the coagulation process but were given no Roman numeral; instead they were once called collectively platelet factor 3.

Classification and Function of Procoagulants

The coagulation factors work together in a *cascade* pathway where one factor, when activated, activates the next factor in the sequence. The purpose is to generate the key thrombin enzyme and produce fibrin (a localized thrombus). The sequence of coagulation factor activation is shown in Figure 35.4.

The coagulation factors thrombin (factor IIa), factors VIIa, IXa, Xa, XIa, XIIa, and pre-K are enzymes called *serine proteases* (Table 35.7).[29] Factor XIII is an exception as it is a transglutaminase. Serine proteases are proteolytic enzymes of the trypsin family.[30] Each member has a reactive seryl amino acid residue in its active site and acts on its substrate by hydrolyzing peptide bonds, digesting the primary backbone. Small polypeptide fragments are produced from this process. Serine proteases are synthesized as inactive *zymogens* consisting of a single peptide chain. Activation occurs when the zymogen is cleaved at one or more specific sites by the action of another protease during the coagulation process.

The procoagulant cofactors that participate in complex formation are tissue factor, located on membranes of fibroblasts

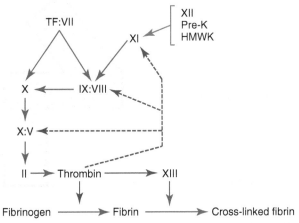

Figure 35.4 Simplified Coagulation Pathway. Exposed tissue factor *(TF)* activates factor VII, which activates factors IX and X. Factor IXa:VIIIa complex also activates X, and the factor Xa:Va complex activates prothrombin (factor II). The resulting thrombin cleaves fibrinogen to form fibrin and activates factor XIII to stabilize the clot. Thrombin also activates factors V, VIII, XI, and platelets in a positive feedback loop. Exposure to negatively charged surfaces (e.g., bacterial cell membranes) activates the contact factors XII, prekallikrein *(pre-K)* and high-molecular-weight kininogen *(HMWK)*, which activate factor XI.

TABLE 35.7 Plasma Procoagulant Serine Proteases

Inactive Zymogen	Active Protease	Cofactor	Substrate
Prothrombin (II)	Thrombin (IIa)	—	Fibrinogen, V, VIII, XI, XIII
VII	VIIa	Tissue factor	IX, X
IX	IXa	VIIIa	X
X	Xa	Va	Prothrombin
XI	XIa	—	IX
XII	XIIa	High-molecular-weight kininogen	XI
Prekallikrein	Kallikrein	High-molecular-weight kininogen	XI

BOX 35.2 Other Plasma Procoagulants

Fibrinogen
Factor XIII
Phospholipids
Calcium
Von Willebrand factor

and smooth muscle cells, and soluble plasma factors V, VIII, and HMWK.

The remaining components of the coagulation pathway are fibrinogen, factor XIII, phospholipids, calcium, and VWF (Box 35.2). Fibrinogen is the ultimate substrate of the coagulation pathway. When hydrolyzed by thrombin, soluble fibrinogen is converted to the insoluble structural protein of the fibrin clot, which is further stabilized by activated factor XIII.[31]

Ionized calcium is required for the coagulation complexes that assemble on platelet or cell membrane phospholipids. Serine proteases bind to negatively charged phospholipid surfaces, predominantly phosphatidylserine, through positively charged calcium ions. Thus coagulation activation is a localized cell-surface process, limited to the site of injury.

The molecular weights, plasma concentrations, and plasma half-lives of the procoagulant factors are given in Table 35.6.[32] These essential pieces of clinical information assist in the interpretation of laboratory tests, monitoring of anticoagulant therapy, and design of effective replacement therapies in deficiency-related hemorrhagic diseases. It is of interest to note that fibrinogen, prothrombin, and factor VIII (FVIII) are acute phase reactants and their levels increase when there is inflammation as in trauma, pregnancy, infection, and stress.

Vitamin K-Dependent Prothrombin Group

Prothrombin (factor II), factors VII, IX, and X and the regulatory proteins protein C, protein S, and protein Z are dependent on vitamin K during synthesis to produce a functional structure (Table 35.8). These are named the *prothrombin group* because of their structural resemblance to prothrombin. All seven proteins have 10 to 12 glutamic acid units near their amino terminal end. All except protein S and protein Z are serine proteases when activated; S and Z are cofactors.

Vitamin K is a quinone found in green leafy vegetables (Box 35.3) and is produced by the intestinal organisms *Bacteroides fragilis* and *Escherichia coli*. Vitamin K catalyzes an essential posttranslational modification of the prothrombin group proteins: γ-carboxylation of amino-terminal glutamic acids (Figure 35.5). Glutamic acid is modified to γ-carboxyglutamic acid when a second carboxyl group is added to the γ carbon. With two ionized carboxyl groups, the γ-carboxyglutamic acids gain a net negative charge, which enables them to bind ionic calcium (Ca^{2+}). The bound calcium enables these vitamin K-dependent coagulation factors to bind to negatively charged

TABLE 35.8 Vitamin K-Dependent Coagulation Factors

Procoagulants	Regulatory Proteins
Prothrombin (II)	Protein C
VII	Protein S
IX	Protein Z
X	

BOX 35.3 Food Sources High in Vitamin K

Kale	Asparagus
Spinach	Cabbage
Turnip greens	Green onions
Collards	Lettuce: Boston, romaine, or Bibb
Mustard greens	Avocado
Swiss chard	Cauliflower
Brussels sprouts	Parsley, fresh
Broccoli	

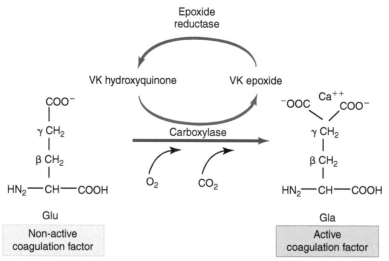

Figure 35.5 Posttranslational γ-Carboxylation of the Vitamin K-Dependent Coagulation Proteins. For coagulation factors II (prothrombin), VII, IX, and X, and control proteins C, S, and Z, vitamin K hydroxyquinone transfers a carboxyl *(COO⁻)* group to the γ carbon of glutamic acid *(Glu)*, creating γ-carboxyglutamic acid *(Gla)*. The negatively charged pocket formed by the two carboxyl groups attracts ionic calcium, which enables the molecule to bind to phosphatidylserine. Vitamin K hydroxyquinone is oxidized to vitamin K epoxide by carboxylase in the process of transferring the carboxyl group but is subsequently reduced to the hydroxyquinone form by epoxide reductase.

phospholipids to form complexes with other coagulation factors.

In vitamin K deficiency or in the presence of the anticoagulant drug Coumadin, a therapeutic inhibitor of vitamin K, the vitamin K-dependent procoagulants are released from the liver without the second carboxyl group added to the γ carbon. These are called *des-γ-carboxyl proteins* or *proteins induced by vitamin K antagonists (PIVKA) factors*. Because they lack the second carboxyl group, they cannot bind to Ca^{2+} and phospholipid, so they cannot participate in the coagulation reaction. Vitamin K antagonism is the basis for oral anticoagulant (warfarin, Coumadin) therapy (Chapter 40).

Vitamin K-dependent procoagulants are essential for the assembly of three membrane complexes leading to the generation of thrombin (Figure 35.6). Each complex is composed of a vitamin K-dependent serine protease, its nonenzyme cofactor, and Ca^{2+}, bound to the negatively charged phospholipid membranes of activated platelets or tissue factor-bearing cells. The initial complex, *extrinsic tenase,* is composed of factor VIIa and tissue factor, and it activates factors IX and X, which are components of the next two complexes, intrinsic tenase and prothrombinase, respectively (Table 35.9). *Intrinsic tenase* is composed of factor IXa and its cofactor VIIIa; it also activates factor X but much more efficiently than the TF:VIIa complex. *Prothrombinase* is composed of factor Xa and its cofactor Va; this converts prothrombin to thrombin in a multistep hydrolytic process that releases thrombin and a peptide fragment called *prothrombin fragment 1.2* (F1.2). Prothrombin fragment 1.2 in plasma is thus a marker for thrombin generation.

Cofactors in Hemostasis

Procoagulant cofactors are tissue factor, factor V, factor VIII, and HMWK. Cofactors of the coagulation control proteins are thrombomodulin, protein S, and protein Z (Table 35.10).[33] Thrombomodulin is also a cofactor in control of fibrinolysis.

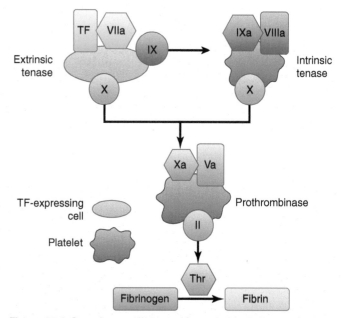

Figure 35.6 Complexes within the Coagulation Pathway. Coagulation complexes form on tissue factor *(TF)*-bearing cells (TF:VIIa) and on platelet phospholipid membranes (IXa:VIIIa and Xa:Va). Each complex consists of a vitamin K-dependent serine protease coagulation factor, a cofactor, and Ca^{2+}, bound to the cell membrane. Extrinsic tenase complex is factor VIIa and TF on the membrane of a TF-bearing cell. This complex activates both factors IX and X. Intrinsic tenase complex, which is factor IXa and its cofactor VIIIa on platelet membranes, activates factor X also. Prothrombinase complex is factor Xa and its cofactor Va, bound to the surface of platelets. Prothrombinase cleaves prothrombin to the active enzyme thrombin *(Thr)*.

Each cofactor binds its particular serine protease. When bound to their cofactors, serine proteases gain stability and increased reactivity.

Tissue factor is a transmembrane receptor for factor VIIa and is found on extravascular cells surrounding ECs such as

TABLE 35.9 Coagulation Complexes

Complex	Components	Activates
Extrinsic tenase	VIIa, tissue factor, phospholipid, and Ca²⁺	IX and X
Intrinsic tenase	IXa, VIIIa, phospholipid, and Ca²⁺	X
Prothrombinase	Xa, Va, phospholipid, and Ca²⁺	Prothrombin

TABLE 35.10 Hemostasis Cofactors

Cofactor	Function	Binds
Tissue factor	Procoagulant	VIIa
V	Procoagulant	Xa
VIII	Procoagulant	IXa
High-molecular-weight kininogen	Procoagulant	XIIa, prekallikrein
Thrombomodulin	Control (protein C)	Thrombin
	Antifibrinolytic (TAFI)	Thrombin
Protein S	Control	Protein C, TFPI
Protein Z	Control	ZPI

TAFI, Thrombin activatable fibrinolysis inhibitor; *TFPI,* tissue factor pathway inhibitor; *ZPI,* protein Z-dependent protease inhibitor.

fibroblasts and smooth muscle cells. Under normal conditions, TF is not expressed on blood vessel cells.[34] Vessel injury exposes blood to the subendothelial tissue factor-bearing cells and leads to activation of coagulation through VIIa. Thus the activation of FVII is rate limited by the injury itself. TF is expressed in high levels in cells of the brain, lung, placenta, heart, kidney, and testes. In inflammatory conditions and sepsis, leukocytes and other cells can also express TF and initiate coagulation.[35]

Factors V and VIII are soluble plasma proteins. Factor V is a glycoprotein circulating in plasma and also present in platelet α-granules. During platelet activation and secretion, platelets release partially activated factor V at the site of injury. Factor Va is a cofactor to Xa in the prothrombinase complex in coagulation. The prothrombinase complex accelerates thrombin generation more than 300,000-fold compared with Xa alone.[36] The initial small amount of thrombin generated activates the first V to Va. As described later, thrombomodulin-bound thrombin activates protein C, which inactivates Va to Vi. Therefore factor V is both activated and then ultimately inactivated by the generation of thrombin, as is factor VIII. Factor VIII is a cofactor to factor IX, which together form the intrinsic tenase complex, discussed in the next section.

HMWK is a cofactor to factor XIIa and prekallikrein in the *intrinsic contact factor complex,* a mechanism for activating coagulation in conditions where foreign objects such as mechanical heart valves, bacterial membranes, or high levels of inflammation are present.

Thrombomodulin, a transmembrane protein constitutively expressed by vascular ECs, is a thrombin cofactor in the protein C pathway. Together, thrombomodulin and thrombin activate protein C, a coagulation regulatory protein. In one of many examples of carefully regulated processes within the hemostatic system, once thrombin is bound to thrombomodulin, it loses its procoagulant ability to activate factors V and VIII, and, through activation of protein C, leads to destruction of factors V and VIII, thus suppressing further generation of thrombin—a negative feedback loop. Thrombin bound to thrombomodulin also activates TAFI, a fibrinolysis inhibitor.

Both protein S and protein Z are cofactors in the regulation and control of coagulation, discussed later in this chapter. Protein S is a cofactor to protein C, as well as TFPI. Protein Z is a cofactor to Z-dependent protease inhibitor (ZPI).

Factor VIII and von Willebrand Factor

Factor VIII and VWF are key proteins for hemostasis. These are both critically involved in all protective mechanisms to avoid blood loss (i.e., platelets, vasculature, and blood coagulation leading to fibrin formation).

Factor VIII is produced primarily by hepatocytes but also by microvascular ECs in lung and other tissues.[37] Free factor VIII is unstable in plasma; it circulates bound to VWF (Figure 35.7). During coagulation, thrombin cleaves factor VIII from VWF and activates it. Factor VIIIa binds to activated platelets and forms the intrinsic tenase complex with factor IXa and Ca²⁺. Like factor Va, factor VIIIa is also inactivated by protein C.

Factor VIII and factor IX are the two plasma procoagulants whose production is governed by genes carried on the X chromosome.[38] Factor VIII is a cofactor, but its importance in hemostasis cannot be overstated, as evidenced by the severe bleeding and symptoms associated with hemophilia A.

Factor VIII deteriorates more rapidly than the other coagulation factors in stored blood. In thawed component plasma, the factor VIII level drops to approximately 50% after 5 days.[39]

VWF is a large multimeric glycoprotein that participates in platelet adhesion and transports the procoagulant factor VIII. VWF is composed of multiple subunits of 240,000 Daltons each.[40] The subunits are produced by ECs and megakaryocytes, where they combine to form multimers that range from 500,000 to 20,000,000 Daltons.[41] VWF molecules are stored in α-granules in platelets and in Weibel-Palade bodies in ECs. ECs release ultra-large multimers of VWF into plasma, where they are normally degraded into smaller multimers by a VWF-cleaving protease, ADAMTS13 (*a d*isintegrin *a*nd *m*etalloprotease with a *t*hrombospondin type 1 motif, member *13*), in blood vessels with high shear stress.[42]

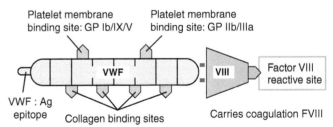

Figure 35.7 Von Willebrand Factor *(VWF)*-Factor VIII Complex. VWF molecules of various lengths from 0.5 to 20 mDaltons are in blood circulation. Factor VIII circulates covalently bound to VWF. VWF provides three other active receptor sites: VWF binds to collagen; it binds to glycoprotein *(GP)* Ib/IX/V to support platelet adhesion; and it binds to GP IIb/IIIa to facilitate platelet aggregation. VWF:Ag epitope is the target of quantitative immunoassays.

VWF has receptor sites for both platelets and collagen (Figure 35.7). This allows VWF to act as a bridge, binding platelets to exposed subendothelial collagen during platelet adhesion (Figure 10.9C), especially in arteries and arterioles where the flow of blood is faster. The primary platelet surface receptor for VWF is GP Ib/IX/V. Arginine-glycine-aspartic acid (RGD) sequences in VWF also bind a second platelet receptor, GP IIb/IIIa, during platelet aggregation (Chapter 10). A third site on the VWF molecule binds collagen. A fourth site on the VWF molecule binds the plasma procoagulant cofactor, factor VIII.

The importance of VWF in hemostasis cannot be overstated, as evidenced by the severe bleeding and symptoms associated with abnormalities in VWF molecular structure and concentration. Von Willebrand disease, an inherited disorder with several described mutations, and FVIII deficiency, which can be linked because VWF is the chaperone for FVIII, are relatively common bleeding disorders (Chapter 36).

Levels of VWF vary by ABO blood type with group O individuals having lower levels of VWF than any other blood group type.[43] VWF is an acute phase protein, as is factor VIII, and levels increase in pregnancy, trauma, infection, and stress.

Factor XI and the Contact Factors

The "contact factors" are factor XII, HMWK (Fitzgerald factor), and pre-K (Fletcher factor). They are so named because they are activated by contact with negatively charged foreign surfaces. Factor XIIa transforms pre-K, a glycoprotein that circulates bound to HMWK, into its active form kallikrein, which cleaves HMWK to form bradykinin. Factor XII and pre-K are zymogens that are activated to become serine proteases; HMWK is a nonenzymatic cofactor.

The *contact factor complex* (HMWK:pre-K:factor XIIa) activates factor XI; factor XIa is an activator of factor IX (Figure 35.4). Deficiencies of factor XII, HMWK, or pre-K do not cause clinical bleeding disorders.[44] However, deficiencies do prolong laboratory tests and necessitate investigation. Factor XII is activated in vitro by negatively charged surfaces such as non-siliconized glass, kaolin, or ellagic acid—used as test reagents for the partial thromboplastin time (PTT, APTT) assay. In vivo, foreign materials such as stents, valve prostheses, and bacterial cell membranes activate contact factors, which can lead to thrombosis.

Factor XI is activated by the contact factor complex and, more significantly, by thrombin during coagulation generated from TF activation. Factor XIa activates factor IX, and the reaction proceeds as described previously. Deficiencies of factor XI (FXI; Rosenthal syndrome) can result in mild and variable bleeeing.[44] Plasma levels of FXI do not necessarily correspond with degree of bleeding.[45]

Thrombin

Thrombin is the main enzyme of the coagulation pathway with multiple key activities. However, the primary function of thrombin is to cleave fibrinopeptides (FP) A and B from the α and β chains of the fibrinogen molecule, triggering spontaneous fibrin polymerization and the beginning of the fibrin clot (Figure 35.8). FPA and FPB are measurable in plasma and serve as a marker of thrombin activation.

Thrombin amplifies the coagulation mechanism by activating cofactors V and VIII and factor XI by a positive feedback mechanism that serves to generate more thrombin (Figure 35.4). Thrombin also activates factor XIII, which forms covalent bonds between the D domains of the fibrin polymer to cross-link and stabilize the fibrin clot (discussed in detail subsequently). Thrombin initiates aggregation of platelets. Thrombin bound to thrombomodulin activates the protein C pathway to suppress coagulation, and it activates TAFI to suppress fibrinolysis.

Thrombin therefore plays a role in coagulation (fibrin), platelet activation, regulation of coagulation activation (protein C), and controlling fibrinolysis (TAFI). Because of its multiple autocatalytic functions, thrombin is considered the key protease of the coagulation pathway.

Fibrinogen Structure and Fibrin Formation, Factor XIII

Fibrinogen is the primary substrate of thrombin, which converts soluble fibrinogen to insoluble fibrin to produce a clot. Fibrinogen is also essential for platelet aggregation because it links activated platelets through their GP IIb/IIIa platelet fibrinogen receptor. Fibrinogen is a 340,000 Dalton glycoprotein synthesized in the liver. The normal plasma concentration of fibrinogen ranges from 200 to 400 mg/dL, the most concentrated of all the plasma procoagulants. Fibrinogen is an acute phase reactant protein, whose level increases in inflammation, infection, and other stress conditions. Platelet α-granules absorb, transport, and release abundant fibrinogen.[46]

The fibrinogen molecule is a mirror-image dimer, each half consisting of three nonidentical polypeptides, designated

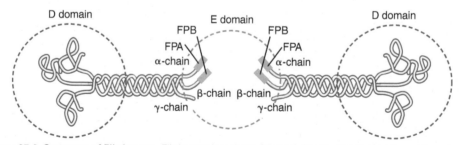

Figure 35.8 Structure of Fibrinogen. Fibrinogen has three domains. The central E domain and two terminal D domain nodules at the carboxyl ends of the molecule. The D and E domains are joined together by supercoiled α-helix regions. This trinodular structure is composed of three pairs of disulfide-bonded polypeptides, two each of the Aα, Bβ, and γ chains. *FPA,* Fibrinopeptide A; *FPB,* fibrinopeptide B.

Aα, Bβ, and γ, united by several disulfide bonds (Figure 35.8). The six N-terminals assemble to form a bulky central region called the E domain. The three carboxyl terminals on each outer end of the molecule assemble to form two D domains.[31]

Thrombin cleaves fibrinopeptides A and B from the protruding N-termini of each of the two α and β chains of fibrinogen, reducing the overall molecular weight by 10,000 Daltons. The cleaved fibrinogen is called fibrin monomer. The exposed fibrin monomer α and β chain ends (E domain) have an immediate affinity for portions of the D domain of neighboring monomers, spontaneously polymerizing to form fibrin polymer (Figure 35.9).

Factor XIII is a heterodimer whose α subunit is produced mostly by megakaryocytes and monocytes, and whose β subunit is produced in the liver.[47] After activation by thrombin, factor XIIIa covalently cross-links fibrin polymers to form a stable insoluble fibrin clot. Factor XIIIa is a transglutaminase that catalyzes the formation of covalent bonds between the carboxyl terminals of γ chains from adjacent D domains in the fibrin polymer (Figure 35.9). These bonds link the ε-amino acid of lysine moieties and the γ-amide group of glutamine units. Multiple cross-links form to provide an insoluble meshwork of fibrin polymers linked by their D domains, providing physical strength to the fibrin clot. Factor XIIIa reacts with other plasma and cellular structural proteins and is essential to wound healing and tissue integrity.

Cross-linking of fibrin polymers by factor XIIIa covalently incorporates fibronectin, a plasma protein involved in cell adhesion, and α₂-antiplasmin, rendering the fibrin mesh resistant to fibrinolysis. Plasminogen, the primary serine protease of the fibrinolytic system (discussed in detail subsequently), also becomes covalently bound via lysine moieties, as does TPA, a serine protease that ultimately hydrolyzes and activates bound plasminogen to initiate fibrinolysis, thus breaking down the clot.

The Coagulation System: Extrinsic, Intrinsic, and Common Pathways

In the past, two coagulation pathways were described, both of which activated factor X at the start of a common pathway leading to thrombin generation (Figure 35.10). The pathways were characterized as cascades in that as one enzyme became activated, it in turn activated the next enzyme in sequence.

At that time coagulation experts identified the activation of factor XII as the primary step in coagulation because this factor could be found in blood, whereas TF could not. Consequently, the reaction system that begins with factor XII and culminates in fibrin polymerization has been called the *intrinsic pathway*. The coagulation factors of the intrinsic pathway, in order of reaction, are XII, pre-K, HMWK, XI, IX, VIII, X, V, prothrombin (II), and fibrinogen. The laboratory test that detects the absence of one or more of these factors is the activated partial thromboplastin time (APTT or PTT; Chapter 41).

We now know that the contact factors XII, pre-K, and HMWK do not play a significant role in in vivo or physiologic coagulation with trauma-type injuries, although their deficiencies prolong the in vitro laboratory tests of the intrinsic pathway—in particular, the PTT. The contact system establishes a connection between inflammation and coagulation activation. However this system is complex and has only been shown in abbreviated format in this chapter.

Formation of TF:VIIa has since proven to be the primary in vivo initiation mechanism for coagulation. Because TF is not present in blood, the TF pathway has been called the *extrinsic pathway*. This pathway includes the factors VII, X, V, prothrombin, and fibrinogen. The test used to measure the integrity of the extrinsic pathway is the prothrombin time (PT; Chapter 41).

The PT and PTT are assays often used in tandem to screen for coagulation factor deficiencies. Factor VIII and factor IX are not considered to be part of the extrinsic pathway, because the

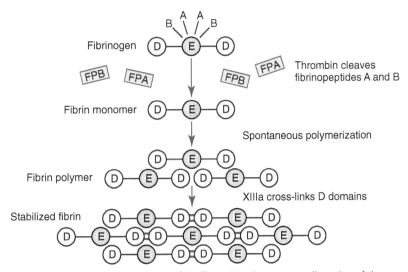

Figure 35.9 Formation of a Stabilized Fibrin Clot. Thrombin cleaves a small portion of the α and β chains in the central E domain node releasing free peptides, fibrinopeptide A *(FPA)* and fibrinopeptide B *(FPB)*. This forms fibrin monomer. Fibrin monomers spontaneously polymerize due to the affinity of thrombin-cleaved positively charged E domains for negatively charged D domains of other monomers. This forms the fibrin polymer. Factor XIIIa catalyzes the covalent cross-linking of γ chains of adjacent D domains (double red line) to form an insoluble stable fibrin clot.

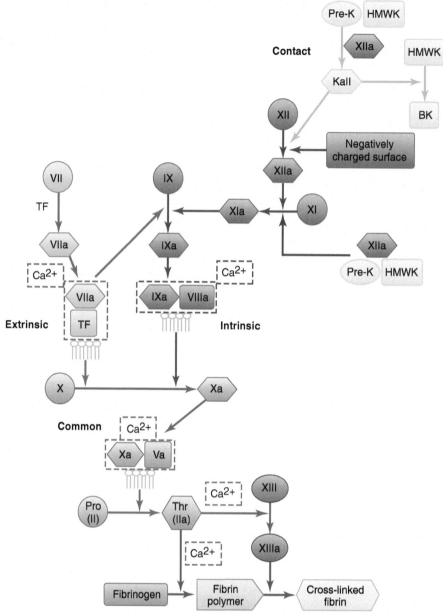

Figure 35.10 Plasma-Based Coagulation Cascade. The coagulation cascade consists of the contact system (simplified here) and the intrinsic, extrinsic, and common pathways. In the intrinsic pathway (red), the contact factors XII, prekallikrein *(pre-K)*, and high-molecular-weight kininogen *(HMWK)* are activated and proceed to activate factors XI, IX, VIII, X, and V and prothrombin, which converts fibrinogen to fibrin. In the extrinsic pathway (green), tissue factor *(TF)* activates factor VII, which activates factors X, V, and prothrombin, cleaving fibrinogen to fibrin. Both the intrinsic and extrinsic pathways converge with the activation of factor X, so factors X, V, prothrombin, and fibrinogen are called the common pathway (blue). Dashed boxes indicate the coagulation factor complexes that assemble on phospholipid (yellow symbol). These pathways are the basis of clinical coagulation laboratory tests. *Thr,* Thrombin.

PT fails to identify their absence or deficiency. But clearly the IXa:VIIIa complex in the intrinsic pathway is crucial to the activation of factor X.

The two pathways have in common factor X, factor V, prothrombin, and fibrinogen; this portion of the coagulation pathway is often called the *common pathway*. These designations—intrinsic, extrinsic, and common—are used extensively to interpret in vitro laboratory testing of blood plasma and to identify factor deficiencies; however, they do not adequately describe the complex interdependent reactions that occur in vivo.

The Hemostatic System: Cell-Based Physiologic Coagulation

An intricate combination of cellular and biochemical events function in harmony to keep blood liquid within the veins and arteries, to prevent blood loss from injuries by the formation of thrombi, and to reestablish blood flow during the healing process.[48] As noted earlier, the series of cascading proteolytic reactions in blood plasma, traditionally known as the extrinsic and intrinsic coagulation pathways, do not fully describe how coagulation occurs physiologically. These pathways are not distinct, independent, alternative mechanisms for generating thrombin but are actually *interdependent*. For example, a deficiency of factor VII in the extrinsic pathway can cause significant bleeding, even when the intrinsic pathway is intact. Similarly, deficiencies of factors VIII and IX may cause severe bleeding, regardless of the presence of a normal extrinsic pathway.[49]

In addition to procoagulant and anticoagulant plasma proteins, normal physiologic coagulation requires the presence of two cell types for formation of coagulation complexes: cells that express TF (usually extravascular) and platelets (intravascular) (Figure 35.11).[50] Operationally, coagulation can be described as occurring in two phases: *initiation*, which occurs on tissue factor-expressing cells and produces 3% to 5% of the total thrombin generated, and *propagation*, occurring on platelets, which produces 95% or more of the total thrombin.[51]

Initiation

In vivo the principle mechanism for generating thrombin is begun by formation of the extrinsic tenase complex, rather than the intrinsic pathway. The initiation phase refers to extrinsic tenase complex formation and generation of small amounts of factor Xa, factor IXa, and thrombin (Figure 35.11).

Damage to the endothelium allows blood and platelets to flow into the extravascular tissue and triggers a localized response. The magnitude of the response depends largely on the extent of the injury: how large the bleed is, how much tissue is damaged, and how many platelets are available.

About 1% to 2% of factor VIIa is present normally in blood in the activated form, but it is inert until bound to tissue factor[52] and is unaffected by TFPI and other inhibitors. Fibroblasts and other subendothelial cells provide tissue factor, a cofactor to factor VIIa. Factor VIIa binds to TF on the membrane of subendothelial cells, and the extrinsic tenase complex TF:VIIa is formed.

TF:VIIa activates low levels of both factor IX and factor X. A minute amount of thrombin is generated by membrane-bound Xa and Xa:Va prothrombinase complexes. The initial minute amount of thrombin generates feedback into the coagulation cascade to activate plasma factors V, VIII, and XI, which serves to amplify more thrombin generation.[53]

Coagulation complexes bound to cell membranes are relatively protected from inactivation by most inhibitors. However, if Xa:Va dissociates from the cell, it is rapidly inactivated by the protease inhibitors TFPI, antithrombin, and ZPI until a threshold of Xa:Va activity is reached.

Even though the amount of thrombin generated in this phase is small, platelets, cofactors, and procoagulants become activated. The low level of thrombin generated in the initiation phase (1) activates platelets through cleavage of protease activated receptors PAR-1 and PAR-4; (2) activates factor V released from platelet α-granules; (3) activates factor VIII and dissociates it from VWF; (4) activates factor XI, the intrinsic accessory procoagulant that activates more factor IX; and (5) splits fibrinogen peptides A and B from fibrinogen and forms a preliminary fibrin network. The initial platelet plug is thus formed.

Cleavage of fibrinopeptides from the fibrinogen molecule occurs at the end of the initiation phase and beginning of the propagation phase. In most clot-based coagulation assays, this is the visual endpoint of the assay.[31] It occurs with only 10 to 30 nmol/L of thrombin, or approximately 3% of the total thrombin generated.

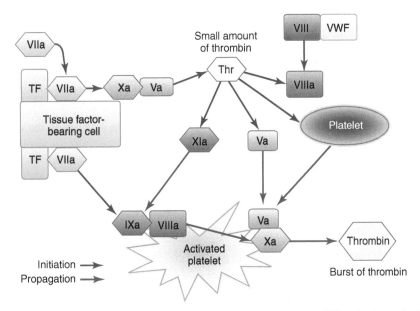

Figure 35.11 Cell-Based Coagulation. VIIa binds to cell-exposed tissue factor *(TF)* and activates both factors X and IX. Cell-bound factor Xa combines with Va and generates a small amount of thrombin *(Thr)*, which activates platelets, V, VIII, and XI and begins fibrin formation. Factor IXa, activated by both TF:VIIa and XIa, combines with factor VIIIa on the platelet surface to activate X, which binds with Va to form the prothrombinase complex (Xa:Va) and produces a burst of thrombin. *VWF,* Von Willebrand factor.

Propagation

More than 95% of thrombin generation occurs during propagation. In this phase the reactions occur on the surface of the activated platelet, which now has all the components needed for coagulation (Figure 35.11). Large numbers of platelets adhere to the site of injury, localizing the coagulation response.

Platelets are activated at the site of injury by both the low-level thrombin generated in the initiation phase and by adhering to exposed collagen. Platelets partially activated by *collagen* and *thrombin* are referred to as COAT platelets (Chapter 10).[54] These partially activated COAT platelets have a higher level of procoagulant activity than platelets exposed to collagen alone. They also provide a surface for formation and amplification of intrinsic tenase and prothrombinase complexes.

The cofactors Va and VIIIa activated by thrombin in the initiation phase bind to platelet membranes and become receptors for Xa and IXa. IXa generated in the initiation phase binds to VIIIa on the platelet membrane to form the intrinsic tenase complex IXa:VIIIa. More factor IXa is also generated by platelet-bound factor XIa. This intrinsic tenase complex activates factor X at a 50- to 100-fold higher rate than the extrinsic tenase complex.[50] Factor Xa binds to Va to form the prothrombinase complex, which activates prothrombin and generates a burst of thrombin. Thrombin cleaves fibrinogen into a fibrin clot, activates factor XIII to stabilize the clot, binds to thrombomodulin to activate the protein C control pathway, and activates TAFI to inhibit fibrinolysis.

Because coagulation depends on the presence of both tissue factor-bearing cells and activated platelets, clotting is localized to the site of injury. Protease inhibitors and intact endothelium prevent clotting from spreading to other parts of the body.

It may be helpful operationally to think of the extrinsic or TF pathway as occurring on the tissue factor-bearing cell and the intrinsic pathway (minus factors XII, HMWK, and pre-K) as occurring on the platelet surface. However, these are not separate and redundant pathways; they are interdependent and occur in parallel until blood flow has ceased and termination by control mechanisms takes place.

Both platelets and tissue factor-bearing cells are essential for physiologic coagulation. Deficiencies of any of the key proteins of coagulation complex formation and activity (VII, IX, VIII, X, V, or prothrombin) compromise thrombin generation and manifest as significant bleeding disorders.

Keep in mind that the hemostatic system described here focuses on the generation of the fibrin clot, including the role of platelets. The complete hemostatic system incorporates the regulatory control mechanisms and the fibrinolytic pathway described in the following sections, as well as the vasculature.

COAGULATION REGULATORY MECHANISMS

Inhibitors and their cofactors regulate serine proteases and cofactors in the coagulation system. They also provide feedback loops to maintain a complex and delicate balance between abnormal thrombosis and bleeding. These inhibitors, or natural anticoagulants, function to slow the activation of procoagulants and suppress thrombin production. They ensure

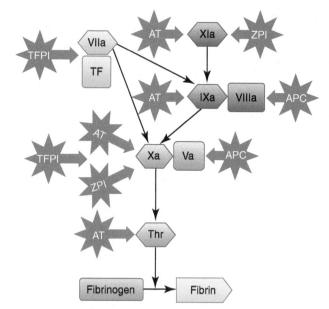

Figure 35.12 Coagulation Pathway Showing Regulatory Points. *APC,* Activated protein C; *AT,* antithrombin; *TFPI,* tissue factor pathway inhibitor; *Thr,* thrombin; *ZPI,* protein Z-dependent protease inhibitor.

that coagulation is localized and is not a systemic response, and they prevent excessive clotting or thrombosis. The principal regulators are TFPI, antithrombin (AT), and activated protein C (APC). Acquired or inherited deficiencies of these proteins may be associated with increased incidence of venous thromboembolic disease because the hemostatic balance is shifted toward increased thrombin generation and coagulation rather than normal termination of the activated pathway. Figure 35.12 illustrates coagulation mechanism regulatory points. Characteristics of these and other coagulation regulatory proteins are summarized in Table 35.11.

Tissue Factor Pathway Inhibitor

TFPI is a Kunitz-type serine protease inhibitor and is the principal regulator of the TF pathway. The Kunitz-2 domain binds to and inhibits factor Xa, and Kunitz-1 binds to and inhibits the VIIa:TF complex.[55] TFPI is synthesized primarily by ECs and is also expressed on platelets. In the initiation of coagulation, factor VIIa and TF combine to activate factors IX and X. TFPI inhibits coagulation in a two-step process by first binding and inactivating Xa. The TFPI:Xa complex then binds to TF:VIIa, forming a quaternary complex and preventing further activation of X and IX (Figure 35.13).[56,57] Alternatively, TFPI may bind to Xa in the TF:VIIa:Xa complex. TFPI provides feedback inhibition because it is not actively engaged until coagulation is initiated and factor X is activated.

Protein S, the cofactor of APC, is also a cofactor of TFPI and enhances factor Xa inhibition by TFPI tenfold.[58-60] Because of the inhibitory action of TFPI, the TF:VIIa:Xa reaction is short lived. Once TFPI shuts down the extrinsic tenase complex and Xa, additional Xa and IXa production shifts to the intrinsic pathway.[61] Propagation of coagulation occurs as factor X is activated by IXa:VIII and more factor IX is activated by factor XIa.

TABLE 35.11 Coagulation Regulatory Proteins

Name	Function	Molecular Mass (Daltons)	Half-Life (hr)	Mean Plasma Concentration
Tissue factor pathway inhibitor	With Xa, binds TF:VIIa	33,000	Unknown	60–80 ng/mL
Thrombomodulin	EC surface receptor for thrombin	450,000	Does not circulate, although soluble truncated forms can be measured	Levels of soluble thrombomodulin increase with vascular disease
Protein C	Serine protease	62,000	7–9	2–6 μg/mL
Protein S	Cofactor	75,000	Unknown	20–25 μg/mL
Antithrombin	Serpin	58,000	68	24–40 mg/dL
Heparin cofactor II	Serpin	65,000	60	30–70 μg/mL
Protein Z-dependent protease inhibitor	Serpin	72,000	Unknown	1.5 μg/mL
Protein C inhibitor	Serpin	57,000	23	2–8 μg/mL
α_1-Protease inhibitor (α_1-antitrypsin)	Serpin	60,000	Unknown	250 mg/dL
α_2-Macroglobulin	Serpin	725,000	60	150–400 mg/dL

EC, Endothelial cell; *Serpin*, Serine protease inhibitor; *TF*, tissue factor.

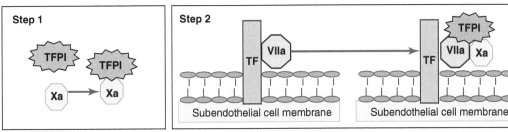

Figure 35.13 Tissue Factor Pathway Inhibitor *(TFPI)*. TFPI binds the complex of tissue factor *(TF)*:VIIa:Xa in a Xa-dependent mechanism. STEP 1, TFPI first binds to factor Xa and inactivates it. STEP 2, The TFPI:Xa complex then binds and inactivates the cell bound TF:VIIa complex, preventing more activation of Xa. Alternatively, TFPI may bind directly to Xa and VIIa in the TF:VIIa:Xa complex.

Protein C Regulatory System

During coagulation, thrombin cleaves fibrinogen generating a fibrin clot and activates factors V, VIII, XI, and XIII propagating more thrombin generation. In intact normal vessels, where coagulation would be inappropriate, thrombin avidly binds the EC membrane protein thrombomodulin and triggers an essential coagulation regulatory system called the protein C system.[62] The protein C system revises thrombin's function from a procoagulant enzyme to an anticoagulant.

EC protein C receptor (ECPR) is a transmembrane protein that binds protein C adjacent to the thrombomodulin-thrombin complex. EPCR augments the action of thrombin-thrombomodulin at least fivefold in activating protein C to the serine protease APC (Figure 35.14).[63,64] The activated form of protein C dissociates from EPCR and binds its cofactor, free plasma protein S. The stabilized APC-protein S complex hydrolyzes and inactivates factors Va and VIIIa, slowing or blocking thrombin generation and coagulation.

Protein S, the cofactor that binds and stabilizes APC, is synthesized in the liver and circulates in the plasma in two forms. About 40% of protein S is free, but 60% is covalently bound to the complement control protein C4b-binding protein (C4bBP).[65] Bound protein S cannot participate in the protein C anticoagulant pathway; only free plasma protein S can serve as the APC

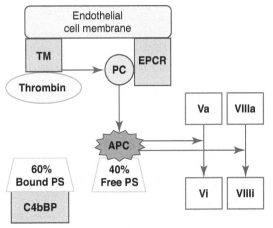

Figure 35.14 Protein C Pathway. After binding thrombomodulin *(TM)*, thrombin activates protein C *(PC)*, bound by endothelial cell protein C receptor *(EPCR)*. Free protein S *(PS;* not bound to C4b binding protein *[C4bBP])* binds and stabilizes activated protein C *(APC)*. The APC:protein S complex digests and inactivates factors Va (Vi) and VIIIa (VIIIi).

cofactor. Protein S-C4bBP binding is of particular interest in inflammatory conditions because C4bBP is an acute phase reactant. When the plasma C4bBP level increases, additional protein S is bound and free protein S levels become proportionally decreased, which may increase the risk of thrombosis.

Chronic acquired or inherited protein C or protein S deficiency or mutations of protein C, protein S, or factor V compromise the normal function of the protein C pathway to downregulate factors Va and VIIIa and are associated with venous thromboembolic disease (Chapter 39). Underscoring the importance of the protein C regulatory system, neonates who completely lack protein C have a massive thrombotic condition called purpura fulminans and die in infancy unless treated with protein C replacement and anticoagulation.[66,67]

Antithrombin

Antithrombin was the first of the coagulation regulatory proteins to be identified and the first to be assayed routinely in the clinical hemostasis laboratory.[68] AT is a serine protease inhibitor (serpin) that binds and neutralizes serine proteases, including thrombin (factor IIa) and factors IXa, Xa, XIa, XIIa, prekallikrein, and plasmin.[69]

AT requires heparin for effective anticoagulant activity.[69] *Heparin cofactor II* (HC II), an inhibitor that primarily targets thrombin, similarly requires heparin.[70] Heparin is a member of the glycosaminoglycan family of carbohydrates. It is a heterogeneous mixture of variably sulfated disaccharide units that link together to form chains of varying length and molecular weight. Physiologically, heparin is available from endothelium-associated mast cell granules or as EC heparan sulfate.

AT's activity is amplified 2000-fold by binding to heparin.[70] Heparin induces a conformational change in the AT molecule that allows binding of activated coagulation factors, which causes them to be inactivated. The inhibition of thrombin, factor X, and other serine proteases by AT is dependent on the length of the heparin chain; for thrombin, only the longer heparin chains are able to bind both molecules to produce inhibition of thrombin. Thrombin inhibition via AT binding is illustrated in Figure 35.15.

When AT covalently binds thrombin, an inactive *thrombin-antithrombin complex* (TAT) is formed, which is then released from the heparin molecule. Laboratory measurement of TAT is used as an indicator of thrombin generation.

Other Serine Protease Inhibitors

Other members of the serpin family include ZPI, protein C inhibitor, α_1-protease inhibitor (α_1-antitrypsin), α_2-macroglobulin, α_2-antiplasmin, and PAI-1.[69]

ZPI, in the presence of its cofactor protein Z, is a potent inhibitor of factor Xa.[71,72] ZPI covalently binds protein Z and factor Xa in a complex with Ca^{2+} and phospholipid. Protein Z is a vitamin K-dependent plasma glycoprotein that is synthesized in the liver. Although protein Z has a structure similar to that of the other vitamin K-dependent proteins (factors II, VII, IX, and X and protein C), it lacks an activation site and, like protein S, is nonproteolytic. Protein Z increases the ability of ZPI to inhibit factor Xa 2000-fold.[73] ZPI also inhibits factor XIa, in a separate reaction that does not require protein Z, phospholipid, and Ca^{2+}. The inhibition of factor XIa is accelerated twofold by the presence of heparin.

Protein C inhibitor is a nonspecific, heparin-binding serpin that inhibits a variety of proteases, including APC, thrombin, factor Xa, factor XIa, and urokinase.[73] It is found in plasma and also in many other body fluids and organs. Depending on its target, it can function as an anticoagulant (inhibits thrombin), as a procoagulant (inhibits thrombin-thrombomodulin and APC), or as a fibrinolytic inhibitor.

The serpins α_1-protease inhibitor and α_2-macroglobulin are able to inhibit serine proteases reversibly. See Table 35.12 and the section on fibrinolysis for further information on α_2-antiplasmin and PAI-1.

FIBRINOLYSIS

Fibrinolysis, the final stage of hemostatic activation, is the systematic, accelerating hydrolysis of fibrin by plasmin. To concentrate and localize fibrinolysis to the site of injury where the clot has formed, fibrinolytic proteins become incorporated into the fibrin clot as it is forming.

Several hours after fibrin polymerization and cross-linking (thrombus formation), and in response to inflammation and coagulation, the fibrinolytic process is activated. Two activators

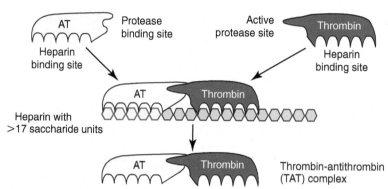

Figure 35.15 Mechanism of Antithrombin to Control Coagulation Activation. Glycosaminoglycans *(GAGs)* such as heparan sulfate and therapeutic heparin potentiate the antithrombin-thrombin reaction. When antithrombin *(AT)* binds the GAG, it is sterically modified allowing AT to covalently bind thrombin, which inactivates the active enzymatic site of thrombin. Inhibition of thrombin requires that it simultaneously binds both AT and the GAG. Thrombin and AT, covalently bound, release the GAG and form measurable plasma thrombin-antithrombin *(TAT)* complexes. Inhibition of factor Xa is accomplished on shorter GAG chains (<17 saccharide units; 5 minimum) because FXa binds only to the AT molecule when AT is in complex with the GAG.

TABLE 35.12   Proteins of the Fibrinolysis Pathway

Name	Function	Molecular Mass (Daltons)	Half-Life	Mean Plasma Concentration
Plasminogen	Active form is the plasma serine protease plasmin, digests fibrin/fibrinogen	92,000	24–26 hr	15–21 mg/dL
Tissue plasminogen activator (TPA)	Serine protease secreted by activated endothelium, activates plasminogen	68,000	Unknown	4–7 μg/dL
Urokinase plasminogen activator (UPA)	Serine protease secreted by kidney cells, activates plasminogen	54,000	Unknown	2–4 ng/mL
Plasminogen activator inhibitor-1 (PAI-1)	Serpin secreted by endothelium, inhibits tissue plasminogen activator	52,000	1 hr	14–28 mg/dL
α_2-Antiplasmin	Serpin, inhibits free plasmin	51,000	Unknown	7 mg/dL
Thrombin activatable fibrinolysis inhibitor (TAFI)	Suppresses fibrinolysis by removing fibrin C-terminal lysine binding sites blocking TPA and plasminogen binding	55,000	8–10 min	5 μg/mL

of fibrinolysis, tissue plasminogen activator (TPA) and uroki-nase plasminogen activator (UPA), are released. These convert fibrin-bound plasminogen into the principle enzyme of the fibrinolytic system, *plasmin* (Figure 35.16; Table 35.12). There is a delicate balance between the activators and inhibitors in this system.

The fibrinolytic process degrades fibrin, restoring normal blood flow during vascular repair. Fibrinolysis of the fibrinogen molecule can also occur. Excessive fibrinolysis can cause bleeding as a result of fibrinogen consumption as well as premature clot lysis before wound healing is established. On the other hand, in-adequate fibrinolysis can lead to clot extension and thrombosis.

Plasminogen and Plasmin

Plasminogen is a 92,000 Dalton plasma zymogen produced by the liver.[74,75] It is a single-chain protein possessing five glycosylated loops termed kringles. Kringles enable plasminogen, along with activators TPA and UPA, to bind the lysine moieties on the fibrin molecule during the polymerization process (Figure 35.17). This fibrin-binding step is essential to fibrinolysis.

Fibrin-bound plasminogen becomes converted into a two-chain active plasmin molecule when cleaved between arginine at position 561 and valine at position 562 by neighboring fibrin-bound TPA or UPA. Plasmin is a serine protease that systemati-cally digests fibrin polymer by the hydrolysis of arginine-related and lysine-related peptide bonds.[76] As fibrin becomes digested, the exposed carboxy-terminal lysine residues bind additional plasminogen and TPA, which further accelerates clot digestion.[77,78] There is also evidence that factors XIa, XIIa, and kallikrein pro-duce an alternative mechanism of plasminogen activation.[74]

Bound plasmin digests clots and restores blood vessel pa-tency. Its localization to fibrin through lysine binding prevents

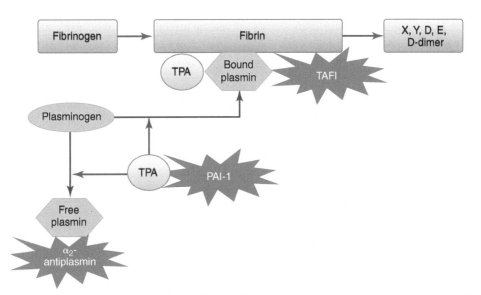

Figure 35.16 Fibrinolysis Pathway and Inhibitors. Plasminogen and tissue plasminogen activator *(TPA)* are bound to fibrin during coagulation. TPA converts bound plasminogen to plasmin, which slowly digests fibrin to form fibrin degradation products *(FDPs)* X, Y, D, E, and D-D *(D-dimer)*. D-dimer is produced from cross-linked fibrin. Free plasmin is neutralized by α_2-antiplasmin. TPA is neutralized by plasminogen activator inhibitor-1 *(PAI-1)*. Thrombin activatable fibrinolysis inhibitor *(TAFI)* inhibits fibrinolysis by cleaving lysine resi-dues on fibrin, preventing the binding of plasminogen, plasmin, and TPA.

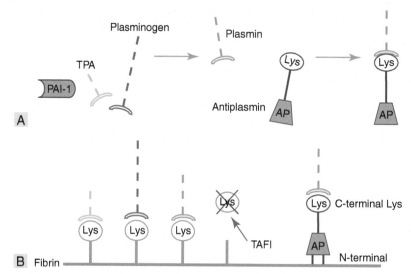

Figure 35.17 Schematic Diagram of the Action of Fibrinolytic Proteins. (A, *top*), Tissue plasminogen activator *(TPA)* activates plasminogen to the serine protease, plasmin. TPA is inhibited by plasminogen activator inhibitor-1 *(PAI-1)*. α_2-Antiplasmin *(AP)* rapidly inactivates free plasmin. **(B,** bottom), Fibrinolytic proteins TPA, plasminogen, and plasmin bind to C-terminal lysine residues *(Lys)* of fibrin during clotting. Thrombin activatable fibrinolysis inhibitor *(TAFI)* inhibits fibrinolysis by removing the C-terminal Lys from fibrin, thereby reducing binding of fibrinolytic proteins. AP N-terminus is bound to fibrin by FXIIIa cross-linking. The AP C-terminus Lys competes with fibrin C-terminus Lys to bind plasmin, which will inactivate it.

systemic activity. However, free plasmin can be found in the circulation and is capable of digesting plasma fibrinogen, factor V, factor VIII, and fibronectin. Plasma α_2-antiplasmin rapidly binds and inactivates any free plasmin. A condition known as *primary fibrinolysis* occurs when free plasmin circulates unchecked, breaking down fibrinogen and formed clots, causing a potentially fatal hemorrhagic outcome.

Plasminogen Activation

Tissue Plasminogen Activator
ECs secrete TPA, which hydrolyzes fibrin-bound plasminogen, converting it to plasmin, thus initiating fibrinolysis. TPA, with two glycosylated kringle regions, forms covalent lysine bonds with fibrin during polymerization and localizes at the surface of the thrombus with plasminogen (Figure 35.17), where it begins the digestion process by converting plasminogen to plasmin. Circulating TPA is bound to inhibitors such as PAI-1. These complexes are cleared from circulation. Synthetic recombinant TPAs, which mimic natural TPA, are a family of "clot-busting" drugs used to dissolve pathologic clots that form in venous and arterial thrombotic disease.

Urokinase Plasminogen Activator
Urinary tract epithelial cells, monocytes, and macrophages secrete another intrinsic plasminogen activator called urokinase plasminogen activator. UPA circulates in plasma at a concentration of 2 to 4 ng/mL and becomes incorporated into the mix of fibrin-bound plasminogen and TPA at the time of thrombus formation (Figure 35.17). UPA converts plasminogen to plasmin. Because it has only one kringle region, UPA does not bind firmly to fibrin and has a relatively minor physiologic effect. Like TPA, purified UPA preparations called urokinases are used therapeutically to dissolve

thrombi in patients with myocardial infarction, stroke, and deep vein thrombosis.

Control of Fibrinolysis
The regulation of fibrinolytic activity is equally important as the regulation of thrombin generation on the coagulation side of hemostasis. The control proteins of the fibrinolytic system and their function are depicted in Table 35.12 and Figure 35.16.

Plasminogen Activator Inhibitor-1
PAI-1 is the principal inhibitor of plasminogen activation, inactivating both TPA and UPA, thus preventing them from converting plasminogen to the active fibrinolytic enzyme plasmin. PAI-1 is a single-chain glycoprotein serine protease inhibitor and is produced by ECs, megakaryocytes, smooth muscle cells, fibroblasts, monocytes, adipocytes, hepatocytes, and other cell types.[79,80] Platelets store a pool of PAI-1, accounting for more than half of its availability and for its delivery to the fibrin clot. PAI-1 is present in excess of the TPA concentration in plasma, and circulating TPA normally becomes bound to PAI-1. Only at times of EC activation, such as after trauma, does the level of TPA secretion exceed that of PAI-1 to initiate fibrinolysis. Binding of TPA to fibrin protects TPA from PAI-1 inhibition.[81]

Plasma PAI-1 levels vary widely. PAI-1 deficiency has been associated with chronic mild bleeding caused by increased fibrinolysis. PAI-1 is an acute phase reactant and is increased in many conditions, including metabolic syndrome, obesity, atherosclerosis, sepsis, and stroke.[80] Increased PAI-1 levels correlate with reduced fibrinolytic activity and increased risk of thrombosis.

α_2-Antiplasmin
α_2-AP is synthesized in the liver and is the primary inhibitor of free plasmin. AP is a serine protease inhibitor with the unique

characteristic of both N- and C-terminal extensions.[82] During thrombus formation, the N-terminus of AP is covalently linked to fibrin by factor XIIIa (Figure 35.17).[83] The C-terminal contains lysine, which is capable of reacting with the lysine-binding kringles of plasmin. Free plasmin produced by activation of plasminogen can bind either to fibrin, where it is protected from AP because its lysine-binding site is occupied, or to the C-terminus of AP, which rapidly and irreversibly inactivates it. Thus AP with its C-terminal lysine slows fibrinolysis by competing with lysine residues in fibrin for plasminogen binding and also by binding directly to plasmin when in circulation and inactivating it.

The therapeutic lysine analogs, tranexamic acid and ε-aminocaproic acid, are similarly antifibrinolytic through their affinity for kringles in plasminogen and TPA. Both inhibit the proteolytic activity of plasmin, thereby reducing clinical bleeding caused by excess fibrinolysis.

Thrombin Activatable Fibrinolysis Inhibitor

TAFI is a plasma procarboxypeptidase synthesized in the liver that becomes activated by the thrombin-thrombomodulin complex. This is the same complex that activates the protein C pathway; however, the two functions are independent. Activated TAFI functions as an antifibrinolytic enzyme. It inhibits fibrinolysis by cleaving exposed carboxy-terminal lysine residues from partially degraded fibrin, thereby preventing the binding of TPA and plasminogen to fibrin and blocking the formation of plasmin (Figure 35.17).[84] In coagulation factor-deficient states, such as hemophilia, decreased thrombin production may reduce the

activation of TAFI, resulting in increased fibrinolysis that contributes to more bleeding. Conversely, in thrombotic disorders, increased thrombin generation may increase the activation of TAFI. The resulting decreased fibrinolysis may contribute further to thrombosis. TAFI also may play a role in regulating inflammation and wound healing.[85]

Fibrin Degradation Products and D-Dimer

Plasmin cleaves fibrin (and fibrinogen) producing a series of identifiable fibrin fragments: X, Y, D, E, and D-D (Figure 35.18).[86] Several of these fragments inhibit hemostasis and contribute to hemorrhage by preventing platelet activation and by hindering fibrin polymerization. Fragment X is described as the central E domain with the two D domains (D-E-D), minus some peptides cleaved by plasmin. Fragment Y is the E domain after cleavage of one D domain (D-E). Eventually these fragments are further digested to individual D and E domains.

The D-D fragment, called D-dimer, is composed of two D domains from separate fibrin molecules (not fibrinogen) cross-linked by the action of factor XIIIa. Fragments X, Y, D, and E are produced by digestion of either fibrin or fibrinogen by plasmin, but D-dimer is a specific product of digestion of cross-linked fibrin only and is therefore a marker of thrombosis and fibrinolysis.[87] In other words, D-dimer is generated via thrombin, factor XIIIa, *and* plasmin activity. Assessing D-dimer levels is an important diagnostic tool to identify disseminated intravascular coagulation and to rule out venous thromboembolism and pulmonary embolism.[88]

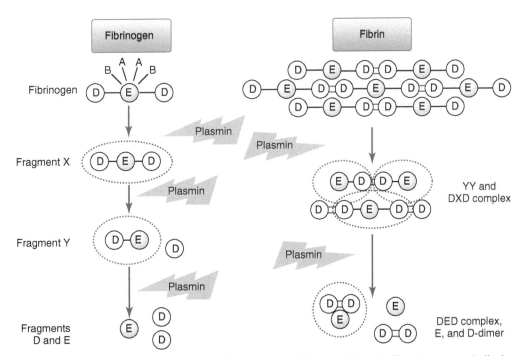

Figure 35.18 Fibrinolysis: Degradation of Fibrinogen and Fibrin by Plasmin. Plasmin systematically degrades fibrinogen and fibrin by cleaving off small peptides and digesting D-E domains. From fibrinogen, fragment X consists of a central E domain with two D domains (D-E-D); further cleavage produces fragment Y (D-E), with eventual degradation to D and E domains. From cross-linked, stabilized fibrin (note double red line on the D domains), plasmin digestion produces fragment complexes from one or more monomers. D-dimer consists of two D domains from adjacent monomers that have been cross-linked by factor XIIIa in the process of fibrin formation.

SUMMARY

- The vascular intima, platelets, tissue factor-bearing cells, and coagulation and fibrinolytic proteins interact to maintain hemostasis.
- Intact vascular intima prevents coagulation through synthesis of prostacyclin, nitric oxide, tissue factor pathway inhibitor (TFPI), thrombomodulin, and heparan sulfate.
- Damaged intima promotes coagulation by vasoconstriction, exposure of tissue factor (TF) and collagen, and secretion of von Willebrand factor (VWF) and other adhesion molecules.
- Platelets function in primary and secondary hemostasis through adhesion, aggregation, secretion of granular contents, and exposure of phosphatidylserine on activation.
- Platelets adhere to collagen through VWF and use fibrinogen to aggregate.
- Most coagulation factors are synthesized in the liver.
- The plasma factors of the prothrombin group (prothrombin; factors VII, IX, and X; protein C; protein S; and protein Z) require vitamin K in their production.
- Plasma coagulation factors include trypsin-like enzymes called serine proteases and cofactors that stabilize the proteases with the exception of factor XIIIa, which is a transamidase.
- The extrinsic pathway of coagulation consists of the membrane receptor TF and coagulation factors VII, X, V, II, and I. Prothrombin time (PT) is a screening test for these factors.
- The intrinsic pathway factors are XII, pre-kallikrein (pre-K), high-molecular-weight kininogen (HMWK), XI, IX, VIII, X, V, II, and I. Partial thromboplastin time (PTT, APTT) is a screening test for these factors.

- Activation of coagulation pathways produces thrombin, which converts fibrinogen to a fibrin polymer. Thrombin also activates platelets and factors V, VIII, XI, and XIII, and binds to thrombomodulin to activate protein C and thrombin activatable fibrinolysis inhibitor (TAFI).
- Fibrinogen is cleaved by thrombin to form first fibrin monomer, then fibrin polymer, and finally, when acted on by factor XIIIa, cross-linked fibrin.
- In vivo, coagulation is initiated on TF-bearing cells. TF:VIIa activates factors IX and X, generating enough thrombin to activate platelets and factors V, VIII, and XI. The latter step acts to amplify the generation of a larger amount of thrombin. Coagulation proceeds on activated platelet phospholipid membranes with the formation of IXa:VIIIa and Xa:Va complexes, which produces a burst of thrombin that cleaves fibrinogen to fibrin.
- The coagulation pathway is regulated by TFPI, activated protein C (APC), and the serpins, including antithrombin and protein Z-dependent protease inhibitor (ZPI). These control proteins prevent excessive thrombosis and confine clotting to the site of injury.
- The fibrinolytic pathway digests the thrombus. Plasminogen is converted to plasmin by tissue plasminogen activator (TPA). Plasmin degrades fibrin to fragments X, Y, D, and E, and D-dimer. Control proteins are plasminogen activator inhibitor (PAI)-1, α_2-antiplasmin, and TAFI.

Now that you have completed this chapter, go back and read again the case study at the beginning and respond to the questions presented.

REVIEW QUESTIONS

Answers can be found in the Appendix.

1. What intimal cell synthesizes and stores von Willebrand factor (VWF)?
   a. Smooth muscle cell
   b. Endothelial cell
   c. Fibroblast
   d. Platelet
2. What subendothelial structural protein triggers coagulation through activation of factor VII?
   a. Thrombomodulin
   b. Nitric oxide
   c. Tissue factor
   d. Thrombin
3. What coagulation plasma protein should be assayed when platelets fail to aggregate properly?
   a. Factor VIII
   b. Fibrinogen
   c. Thrombin
   d. Factor X

4. What is the primary role of vitamin K for the prothrombin group factors?
   a. Provides a surface on which the proteolytic reactions of the factors occur
   b. Protects them from inappropriate activation by compounds such as thrombin
   c. Accelerates the binding of the serine proteases and their cofactors
   d. Carboxylates the factors to allow calcium binding
5. What is the source of prothrombin fragment F1.2?
   a. Plasmin proteolysis of fibrin polymer
   b. Thrombin proteolysis of fibrinogen
   c. Proteolysis of prothrombin by factor Xa
   d. Plasmin proteolysis of cross-linked fibrin
6. What serine protease forms a complex with factor VIIIa, and what is the substrate of this complex?
   a. Factor VIIa, factor X
   b. Factor Va, prothrombin
   c. Factor Xa, prothrombin
   d. Factor IXa, factor X

7. What protein secreted by endothelial cells activates fibrinolysis?
   a. Plasminogen
   b. TPA
   c. PAI-1
   d. TAFI
8. What two regulatory proteins form a complex that digests activated factors V and VIII?
   a. TFPI and Xa
   b. Antithrombin and protein C
   c. APC and protein S
   d. Thrombomodulin and plasmin
9. What are the primary roles of VWF?
   a. Inhibit excess coagulation and activate protein C
   b. Activate plasmin and promote lysis of fibrinogen
   c. Mediate platelet adhesion and serve as a carrier molecule for factor VIII
   d. Mediate platelet aggregation via the GP IIb/IIIa receptor
10. Most coagulation factors are synthesized in:
   a. The liver
   b. Monocytes
   c. Endothelial cells
   d. Megakaryocytes

11. The events involved in secondary hemostasis:
   a. Lead to the formation of a stable fibrin clot
   b. Usually occur independently of primary hemostasis
   c. Occur in a random fashion
   d. Are the first line of defense against blood loss
12. Which of the following coagulation factors is activated by thrombin and mediates the stabilization of the fibrin clot?
   a. Tissue factor
   b. Factor VII
   c. Factor IX
   d. Factor XIII
13. Which of the following endogenous plasma inhibitors is (are) important for the control of excessive thrombin generation?
   a. AT, TFPI
   b. Platelet factor 4
   c. TAT, F1.2
   d. a and b

REFERENCES

1. Aird, W. C. (2003). Hemostasis and irreducible complexity. *J Thromb Haemost, 1,* 227–230.
2. Collen, D., & Lijnen, H. R. (2004). Tissue-type plasminogen activator: a historical perspective and personal account. *J Thromb Haemost, 2,* 541–546.
3. Ruggeri, Z. M. (2003). Von Willebrand factor, platelets and endothelial cell interactions. *J Thromb Haemost, 1,* 1335–1342.
4. Aird, W. C. (2007). Phenotypic heterogeneity of the endothelium: structure, function, and mechanisms. *Circ Res, 100,* 158–173.
5. Aird, W. C. (2007). Phenotypic heterogeneity of the endothelium: representative vascular beds. *Circ Res, 100,* 174–190.
6. Mitchell, J. A., Ferhana, A., Bailey, L., et al. (2008). Role of nitric oxide and prostacyclin as vasoactive hormones released by the endothelium. *Exp Physiol, 93,* 141–147.
7. Looft-Wilson, R. C., Billaud, M., Johnstone, S. R., et al. (2012). Interaction between nitric oxide signaling and gap junctions: effects on vascular function. *Biochim Biophys Acta, 1818*(8), 1895–1902.
8. Moncada, S. P., Palmer, R. M. J., & Higgs, A. J. (1991). Nitric oxide: physiology, pathophysiology and pharmacology. *Pharmacol Rev, 43,* 109–142.
9. Huntington, J. A. (2003). Mechanisms of glycosaminoglycan activation of the serpins in hemostasis. *J Thromb Haemost, 1,* 1535–1549.
10. Furlan, M. (1996). Von Willebrand factor: molecular size and functional activity. *Ann Hematol, 72*(6), 341–348.
11. Bevilacqua, M. P., & Nelson, R. M. (1993). Selectins. *J Clin Invest, 91,* 379–387.
12. Kansas, G. S. (1996). Selectins and their ligands: current concepts and controversies. *Blood, 88,* 3259–3287.
13. Mackman, N., Tilley, R. A., & Key, N. S. (2007). Role of the extrinsic pathway of blood coagulation in hemostasis and thrombosis. *Arterioscler Thromb Vasc Biol, 27,* 1687–1693.

14. Kretz, C. A., Vaezzadeh, N., & Gross, P. L. (2010). Tissue factor and thrombosis models. *Arterioscler Thromb Vasc Biol, 30,* 900–908.
15. Dellas, C., & Loskutoff, D. J. (2005). Historical analysis of PAI-1 from its discovery to its potential role in cell motility and disease. *Thromb Haemost, 93,* 631–640.
16. Foley, J. H., Kim, P. Y., Mutch, N. J., et al. (2013). Insights into thrombin activatable fibrinolysis inhibitor function and regulation. *J Thromb Haemost, 11*(Suppl. 1), 306–315.
17. Polgar, J., Matuskova, J., & Wagner, D. D. (2005). The P-selectin, tissue factor, coagulation triad. *J Thromb Haemost, 3,* 1590–1596.
18. Bordé, E. C., & Vainchenker, W. (2012). Platelet production: cellular and molecular regulation. In Marder, V. J., Aird, W. C., Bennett, J. S., et al. (Eds.), *Hemostasis and Thrombosis: Basic Principles and Clinical Practice.* (6th ed., pp. 349–364). Philadelphia: Lippincott Williams & Wilkins.
19. Fritsma, G. A. (1988). Platelet production and structure. In Corriveau, D. M., & Fritsma, G. A. (Eds.), *Hemostasis and Thrombosis in the Clinical Laboratory.* (pp. 206–228). Philadelphia: Lippincott.
20. Bennett, J. S. (2012). Overview of megakaryocyte and platelet biology. In Marder, V. J., Aird, W. C., Bennett, J. S., et al. (Eds.), *Hemostasis and Thrombosis: Basic Principles and Clinical Practice.* (6th ed., pp. 341–348). Philadelphia: Lippincott Williams & Wilkins.
21. Abrams, C. S., & Brass, L. F. (2012). Platelet signal transduction. In Marder, V. J., Aird, W. C., Bennett, J. S., et al. (Eds.), *Hemostasis and Thrombosis: Basic Principles and Clinical Practice.* (6th ed., pp. 449–461). Philadelphia: Lippincott Williams & Wilkins.
22. Berndt, M. C., & Andrews, R. K. (2012). Major platelet glycoproteins. GP Ib/IX/V. In Marder, V. J., Aird, W. C., Bennett, J. S., et al. (Eds.), *Hemostasis and Thrombosis: Basic Principles and Clinical Practice.* (6th ed., pp. 382–385). Philadelphia: Lippincott Williams & Wilkins.
23. Ye, F., & Ginsberg, M. H. (2012). Major platelet glycoproteins. Integrin $\alpha_{2b}\beta_3$ (GP IIb/IIIa). In Marder, V. J., Aird, W. C.,

Bennett, J. S., et al. (Eds.), *Hemostasis and Thrombosis: Basic Principles and Clinical Practice.* (6th ed., pp. 386–392). Philadelphia: Lippincott Williams & Wilkins.

24. McGlasson, D. L., & Fritsma, G. A. (2009). Whole blood platelet aggregometry and platelet function testing. *Semin Thromb Hemost, 35,* 168–180.

25. Rao, A. K. (2013). Inherited platelet function disorders: overview and disorders of granules, secretion, and signal transduction. *Hematol Oncol Clin North Am, 27,* 585–611.

26. Walsh, P. N. (2012). Role of platelets in blood coagulation. In Marder, V. J., Aird, W. C., Bennett, J. S., et al. (Eds.), *Hemostasis and Thrombosis: Basic Principles and Clinical Practice.* (6th ed., pp. 468–474). Philadelphia: Lippincott Williams & Wilkins.

27. Zarbock, A., Polanowska-Grabowska, R. K., & Ley, K. (2007). Platelet-neutrophil-interactions: linking hemostasis and inflammation. *Blood Rev, 21,* 99–111.

28. Sherry, S. (1990). The founding of the International Society on Thrombosis and Haemostasis: how it came about. *Thromb Haemost, 64,* 188–191.

29. Saito, H. (1996). Normal hemostatic mechanisms. In Ratnoff, O. D., & Forbes, C. D. (Eds.), *Disorders of Hemostasis.* (3rd ed., pp. 23–52). Philadelphia: Saunders.

30. Coughlin, S. R. (2005). Protease-activated receptors in hemostasis, thrombosis and vascular biology. *J Thromb Haemost, 3,* 1800–1814.

31. Mosesson, M. W. (2005). Fibrinogen and fibrin structure and functions. *J Thromb Haemost, 3,* 1894–1904.

32. Greenberg, D. L., & Davie, E. W. (2006). The blood coagulation factors: their complementary DNAs, genes, and expression. In: Colman, R. W., Marder, V. J., Clowes, A. M., et al. (Eds.), *Hemostasis and Thrombosis: Basic Principles and Clinical Practice.* (5th ed., pp. 21–58). Philadelphia: Lippincott Williams & Wilkins.

33. Lane, D. A., Philippou, H., & Huntington, J. A. (2005). Directing thrombin. *Blood, 106,* 2605–2612.

34. Mackman, N., Tilley, R. E., & Key, N. S. (2007). Role of the extrinsic pathway of blood coagulation in hemostasis and thrombosis. *Arterioscler Thromb Vasc Biol, 27,* 1687–1693.

35. Broze, G. J. (1995). Tissue factor pathway inhibitor and the revised theory of coagulation. *Ann Rev Med, 46,* 103–112.

36. Mann, K. G., Saulius, B., & Brummel, K. (2003). The dynamics of thrombin formation. *Arterioscler Thromb Vasc Biol, 23,* 17–25.

37. Shahani, T., Lavend'homme, R., Luttun, A., et al. (2010). Activation of human endothelial cells from specific vascular beds induces the release of a FVIII storage pool. *Blood, 115*(23), 4902–4909.

38. Jacquemin, M., De Maeyer, M., D'Oiron, R., et al. (2003). Molecular mechanisms of mild and moderate hemophilia A. *J Thromb Haemost, 1,* 456–463.

39. Scott, E., Puca, K., Heraly, J., et al. (2009). Evaluation and comparison of coagulation factor activity in fresh-frozen plasma and 24-hour plasma at thaw and after 120 hours of 1-6° C storage. *Transfusion, 49*(8), 1584–1591.

40. Sadler, J. E. (1991). Von Willebrand factor. *J Biol Chem, 266,* 22777–22780.

41. Blann, A. D. (2006). Plasma von Willebrand factor, thrombosis, and the endothelium: the first 30 years. *Thromb Haemost, 95,* 49–55.

42. Tsai, H. M. (2006). ADAMTS13 and microvascular thrombosis. *Expert Rev Cardiovasc Ther, 4,* 813–825.

43. Gill, J. C., Endres-Brooks, J., Bauer, P. J., et al. (1987). The effect of ABO group on the diagnosis of von Willebrand disease. *Blood, 69,* 1691–1695.

44. Roberts, H. R., & Escobar, M. A. (2013). Less common congenital disorders of hemostasis. In Kitchens, C. S., Konkle, B. A.,

Kessler, C. M., et al. (Eds.), *Consultative Hemostasis and Thrombosis.* (2nd ed., pp. 60–78). Philadelphia: Saunders Elsevier.

45. Santoro, C., Di Mauro, R., Baldacci, E., et al. (2015). Bleeding phenotype and correlation with factor XI (FXI) activity in congenital FXI deficiency: results of a retrospective study from a single centre. *Haemophilia, 21*(4), 496–501.

46. Harrison, P., Wilborn, B., Devilli, N., et al. (1989). Uptake of plasma fibrinogen into the alpha granules of human megakaryocytes and platelets. *J Clin Invest, 84,* 1320–1324.

47. Lorand, L. (2005). Factor XIII and the clotting of fibrinogen: from basic research to medicine. *J Thromb Haemost, 3,* 1337–1348.

48. Corriveau, D. M. (1988). Major elements of hemostasis. In Corriveau, D. M., & Fritsma, G. A. (Eds.), *Hemostasis and Thrombosis in the Clinical Laboratory.* (pp. 1–33). Philadelphia: Lippincott.

49. Monroe, D. M., & Hoffman, M. (2006). What does it take to make the perfect clot? *Arterioscler Thromb Vasc Biol, 26,* 41–48.

50. Hoffman, M. (2003). Remodeling the blood coagulation cascade. *J Thromb Thrombolysis, 16,* 17–20.

51. Mann, K. G., Brummel, K., & Butenas, S. (2003). What is all that thrombin for? *J Thromb Haemost, 1,* 1504–1514.

52. Morrissey, J. H., Macik, B. G., Neuenschwander, P. F., et al. (1993). Quantitation of activated factor VII levels in plasma using a tissue factor mutant selectively deficient in promoting factor VII activation. *Blood, 81,* 734–744.

53. Hoffman, M., & Monroe, D. M. (2007). Coagulation 2006: a modern view of hemostasis. *Hematol Oncol Clin North Am, 21,* 1–11.

54. Hoffman, M., & Cichon, L. J. H. (2013). Practical coagulation for the blood banker. *Transfusion, 53,* 1594–1602.

55. Broze, G. J. Jr., & Girard, T. J. (2013). Tissue factor pathway inhibitor: structure-function. *Front Biosci, 17,* 262–280.

56. Lwaleed, B. A., & Bass, P. S. (2006). Tissue factor pathway inhibitor: structure, biology, and involvement in disease. *J Pathol, 208,* 327–339.

57. Monroe, D. M., & Key, N. S. (2007). The tissue factor-factor VIIa complex: procoagulant activity, regulation, and multitasking. *J Thromb Haemost, 5,* 1097–1105.

58. Hakeng, T. M., Maurissen, L. F. A., Castoldi, E., et al. (2009). Regulation of TFPI function by protein S. *J Thromb Haemost, 7*(Suppl. 1), 165–168.

59. Hakeng, T. M., & Rosing, J. (2009). Protein S as cofactor for TFPI. *Arterioscler Thromb Vasc Biol, 29,* 2015–2020.

60. Hakeng, T. M., Sere, K. M., Tans, G., et al. (2006). Protein S stimulates inhibition of the tissue factor pathway by tissue factor pathway inhibitor. *Proc Natl Acad Sci USA, 103,* 3106–3111.

61. Golino, P. (2002). The inhibitors of the tissue factor: factor VII pathway. *Thromb Res, 106,* V257–V265.

62. Dahlback, B. (1995). The protein C anticoagulant system: inherited defects as basis for venous thrombosis. *Thromb Res, 77,* 1–43.

63. Taylor, F. B., Jr., Peer, G. T., Lockhart, M. S., et al. (2001). Endothelial cell protein C receptor plays an important role in protein C activation in vivo. *Blood, 97,* 1685–1688.

64. Van Hinsbergh, V. W. M. (2012). Endothelium-role in regulation of coagulation and inflammation. *Semin Immunopathol, 34,* 93–106.

65. Griffin, J. H., Gruber, A., & Fernandez, J. A. (1992). Reevaluation of total free, free, and bound protein S and C4b-binding protein levels in plasma anticoagulated with citrate or hirudin. *Blood, 79,* 3203.

66. Dreyfus, M., Magny, J. F., Bridey, F., et al. (1991). Treatment of homozygous protein C deficiency and neonatal purpura fulminans with a purified protein C concentrate. *N Engl J Med, 325,* 1565–1568.

67. Price, V. E., Ledingham, D. L., Krumpel, A., et al. (2011). Diagnosis and management of neonatal purpura fulminans. *Semin Fetal Neonatal Med, 16,* 318–322.

68. de Moerloose, P., Bounameaux, H. R., & Mannucci, P. M. (1998). Screening test for thrombophilic patients: which tests, for which patient, by whom, when, and why? *Semin Thromb Hemost, 24,* 321–327.

69. Rau, J. C., Beaulieu, L. M., Huntington, J. A., et al. (2007). Serpins in thrombosis, hemostasis and fibrinolysis. *J Thromb Haemost, 5*(Suppl. 1), 102–115.

70. Bock, S. (2013). Antithrombin and the serpin family. In Marder, V. J., Aird, W. C., Bennett, J. S., et al. (Eds.), *Hemostasis and Thrombosis: Basic Principles and Clinical Practice.* (6th ed., pp. 286–299). Philadelphia: Lippincott Williams & Wilkins.

71. Corral, J., Gonzalez-Conejero, R., Hernandez-Espinosa, D., et al. (2007). Protein Z/Z-dependent protease inhibitor (PZ/ZPI) anticoagulant system and thrombosis. *Br J Haematol, 137*(2), 99–108.

72. Broze, G. J., Jr. (2001). Protein Z-dependent regulation of coagulation. *Thromb Haemost, 86,* 8–13.

73. Chung, D. W., Xu, W., & Davie, E. W. (2013). The blood coagulation factors and inhibitors: their primary structure, complementary DNAs, genes, and expression. In Marder, V. J., Aird, W. C., Bennett, J. S., et al. (Eds.), *Hemostasis and Thrombosis: Basic Principles and Clinical Practice.* (6th ed., pp. 110–145). Philadelphia: Lippincott Williams & Wilkins.

74. Mutch, N. J., & Booth, N. A. (2013). Plasminogen activation and regulation of fibrinolysis. In Marder, V. J., Aird, W. C., Bennett, J. S., et al. (Eds.), *Hemostasis and Thrombosis: Basic Principles and Clinical Practice.* (6th ed., pp. 314–333). Philadelphia: Lippincott Williams & Wilkins.

75. Bennett, B., & Ogston, D. (1996). Fibrinolytic bleeding syndromes. In Ratnoff, O. D., & Forbes, C. D. (Eds.), *Disorders of Hemostasis.* (3rd ed., pp. 296–322). Philadelphia: Saunders.

76. Kolev, K., & Machovich, R. (2003). Molecular and cellular modulation of fibrinolysis. *Thromb Haemost, 89,* 610–621.

77. Fay, W. P., Garg, N., & Sunkar, M. (2007). Vascular functions of the plasminogen activation system. *Arterioscler Thromb Vasc Biol, 27,* 1237.

78. Esmon, C. T., & Esmon, N. L. (2013). Regulatory mechanisms in hemostasis. In Hoffman, R., Benz, E. J., Jr., Silberstein, L. E., et al. (Eds.), *Hematology: Basic Principles and Practice.* (6th ed., pp. 1842–1846). Philadelphia: Elsevier.

79. Dellas, C., & Loskutoff, D. J. (2005). Historical analysis of PAI-1 from its discovery to its potential role in cell motility and disease. *Thromb Haemost, 93,* 631–640.

80. Cesari, M., Pahor, M., & Incalzi, R. A. (2010). Plasminogen activator inhibitor-1 (PAI-1): a key factor linking fibrinolysis and age-related subclinical and clinical conditions. *Cardiovasc Ther, 28,* 72–91.

81. Weisel, J. W., & Dempfle, C. (2013). Fibrinogen structure and function. In Marder, V. J., Aird, W. C., Bennett, J. S., et al. (Eds.), *Hemostasis and Thrombosis: Basic Principles and Clinical Practice.* (6th ed., pp. 254–271). Philadelphia: Lippincott Williams & Wilkins.

82. Coughlin, P. B. (2005). Antiplasmin: the forgotten serpin? *FEBS Journal, 272,* 4852–4857.

83. Rau, J. C., Beaulieu, L. M., Huntington, J. A., et al. (2007). Serpins in thrombosis, hemostasis and fibrinolysis. *J Thromb Haemost, 5* (Suppl. 1), 102–115.

84. Bouma, B. N., & Meijers, J. C. M. (2003). Thrombin-activatable fibrinolysis inhibitor (TAFI, plasma procarboxypeptidase B, procarboxypeptidase R, procarboxypeptidase U). *J Thromb Haemost, 1,* 1566–1574.

85. Bouma, B. N., & Mosnier, L. O. (2003/2004). Thrombin activatable fibrinolysis inhibitor (TAFI) at the interface between coagulation and fibrinolysis. *Pathophysiol Haemost Thromb, 33,* 375–381.

86. Lowe, G. D. (2005). Circulating inflammatory markers and risks of cardiovascular and non-cardiovascular disease. *J Thromb Haemost, 3,* 1618–1627.

87. Adam, S. S., Key, N. S., & Greenberg, C. S. (2009). D-dimer antigen: current concepts and future prospects. *Blood, 113,* 2878–2887.

88. Geersing, G. J., Janssen, K. J. M., & Oudega, R., et al. (2009). Excluding venous thromboembolism using point of care D-dimer tests in outpatients: a diagnostic meta-analysis. *BMJ, 339,* b2990.

36

Hemorrhagic Disorders and Laboratory Assessment

George A. Fritsma

OBJECTIVES

After completion of this chapter, the reader will be able to:

1. Distinguish among the causes of localized versus generalized, anatomic versus mucocutaneous, and acquired versus congenital bleeding.
2. List and interpret laboratory tests that differentiate among acquired hemorrhagic disorders of trauma, liver disease, vitamin K deficiency, and kidney failure.
3. Discuss the laboratory monitoring of therapy for acquired hemorrhagic disorders.
4. Interpret laboratory assay results that diagnose, subtype, and monitor the treatment of von Willebrand disease.
5. Use the results of laboratory tests to identify and monitor the treatment of congenital single coagulation factor deficiencies such as deficiencies of factors VIII, IX, and XI.
6. Explain the principle and rationale for the use of each laboratory test for the detection and monitoring of hemorrhagic disorders.

OUTLINE

Bleeding Symptoms
  Localized Versus Generalized Hemorrhage
  Mucocutaneous Versus Anatomic Hemorrhage
  Acquired Versus Congenital Bleeding Disorders
Acquired Coagulopathies
  Trauma-Induced Coagulopathy
  Liver Disease Coagulopathy
  Chronic Renal Failure and Hemorrhage
  Vitamin K Deficiency and Hemorrhage

  Autoanti-Factor VIII Inhibitor and Acquired Hemophilia
  Acquired von Willebrand Disease
  Disseminated Intravascular Coagulation
Congenital Coagulopathies
  Von Willebrand Disease
  Hemophilia A (Factor VIII Deficiency)
  Hemophilia B (Factor IX Deficiency)
  Hemophilia C (Rosenthal Syndrome, Factor XI Deficiency)
  Other Congenital Single-Factor Deficiencies

CASE STUDY

After completing this chapter, the reader will be able to respond to the following case study:

A 55-year-old man comes to the emergency department with epistaxis (uncontrolled nosebleed). He reports that he has "bleeder's disease" and has had multiple episodes of inflammatory hemarthroses (joint bleeding). Physical examination reveals swollen, immobilized knees; mild jaundice; and an enlarged liver and spleen. Complete blood count results indicate that the patient is anemic and has thrombocytopenia with a platelet count of 74,400/μL (reference interval, 150,000–450,000/μL). The prothrombin time test is 18 seconds (reference interval, 12–14 seconds), and the partial thromboplastin time test is 43 seconds (reference interval, 25–35 seconds).

1. What is the most likely diagnosis?
2. What treatment does the patient need?

BLEEDING SYMPTOMS

Though most bleeding occurs as the result of an injury, bleeding may take the form of easy or spontaneous bruising, internal bleeds, or hemorrhage. *Hemorrhage* is excessive bleeding that requires medical or physical intervention. Bleeding may be *local* or *general, mucocutaneous* or *anatomic, acquired* or *congenital*. If congenital, bleeding may result from primary (platelet-related) or secondary (coagulation factor-related) hemostasis disorders or from unregulated fibrinolysis in which clots are rapidly metabolized. Congenital hemorrhage may be provoked or spontaneous. Except in emergent situations, the physician reviews the health record, conducts a comprehensive interview to document the patient's history, including a bleeding assessment test, and completes a physical examination to establish the probable cause of a bleeding event or a patient's bleeding tendency before ordering diagnostic laboratory tests.[1] In most instances, the hemostasis laboratory contributes substantially to the diagnosis, provided the physician understands the complexities of hemostasis testing and judiciously selects laboratory tests on the basis of well-defined indications.[2]

Localized Versus Generalized Hemorrhage

Bleeding from a single location usually indicates injury, infection, tumor, or an isolated blood vessel defect and is called localized bleeding or localized hemorrhage. An example of local bleeding is an inadequately cauterized or ineffectively sutured surgical site or an arteriovenous malformation (AVM). Except for AVMs, localized bleeding seldom implies a blood vessel defect. In contrast, a qualitative platelet defect, a reduced platelet count (thrombocytopenia), or a coagulation factor deficiency cause systemic and not localized bleeding.

Bleeding from multiple sites, spontaneous and recurring bleeds, or a hemorrhage that requires physical intervention is generalized bleeding. Generalized bleeding is potential evidence for a disorder of *primary hemostasis* such as a blood vessel or platelet defect (Chapters 10 and 37) or thrombocytopenia (Chapter 38); or *secondary hemostasis* characterized by single or multiple coagulation factor deficiencies or uncontrolled fibrinolysis.

Mucocutaneous Versus Anatomic Hemorrhage

Generalized bleeding may exhibit either a mucocutaneous (typically in skin or at body orifices) or anatomic (in soft tissue, muscles, joints, deep tissue) pattern. Mucocutaneous bleeding into the skin may appear as *petechiae*, red pinpoint spots (Figure 38.1A); *purpura*, purple skin lesions greater than 3 mm diameter (Figure 38.1B); or *ecchymoses* (bruises) greater than 1 cm, typically seen after trauma (Figure 38.1C).[3] The unprovoked presence of more than one such lesion may indicate a disorder of primary hemostasis. Other symptoms of a primary hemostasis defect include bleeding from the gums, epistaxis (uncontrolled nosebleed), hematemesis (vomiting of blood), blood in the urine or stool, and menorrhagia (profuse menstrual flow). Although nosebleeds are common and mostly innocent, especially in children, they suggest a primary hemostatic defect when they occur repeatedly, last longer than 10 minutes, involve both nostrils, or require physical intervention or blood products.

Mucocutaneous hemorrhage is most likely to be associated with thrombocytopenia (platelet count less than 150,000/μL; Chapter 38), qualitative platelet disorders (Chapter 37), von Willebrand disease (VWD), or vascular disorders such as scurvy or telangiectasia (Chapter 37). A thorough patient history and physical examination may distinguish between mucocutaneous and anatomic bleeding; this distinction helps direct investigative laboratory testing and subsequent treatment.

Anatomic (soft tissue) hemorrhage is seen in acquired or congenital defects in secondary hemostasis such as plasma coagulation factor deficiencies (coagulopathies).[4] Examples of anatomic bleeding include recurrent or excessive bleeding after minor trauma, dental extraction, or a surgical procedure. In such cases, hemorrhage may immediately follow a primary event, but it is often delayed or recurs minutes or hours after the event. Anatomic bleeding episodes may even be spontaneous. Most anatomic bleeds are internal, such as bleeds into joints, body cavities, muscles, or the central nervous system, and may have few initially discernible signs. Joint bleeds *(hemarthroses)*

cause swelling and acute pain. They may not be immediately perceived as hemorrhages, although experienced hemophilia patients usually recognize the symptoms at their onset. Recurrent hemarthroses cause inflammation that may culminate in permanent cartilage damage that immobilizes the joint. Bleeds into soft tissues such as muscle or fat may cause nerve compression and subsequent temporary or permanent loss of function.[5] When bleeding involves body cavities, it causes symptoms related to the organ that is affected. Bleeding into the central nervous system, for instance, may cause headaches, confusion, seizures, and coma and is managed as a medical emergency. Bleeds into the kidney may present as hematuria and may be associated with acute renal failure.

Hemostasis laboratory testing is essential whenever a generalized mucocutaneous or anatomic bleed is detected. Box 36.1 lists symptoms that suggest generalized hemorrhagic disorders. Besides a complete blood count that includes a platelet count, laboratory directors offer the prothrombin time (PT), partial thromboplastin time (PTT, activated partial thromboplastin time, APTT), thrombin time (TT, thrombin clotting time, TCT), and fibrinogen assay (FG) (Table 36.1).[6] Some laboratory practitioners add *thromboelastography*, performed

---

BOX 36.1 Generalized Bleeding Signs Heralding a Possible Hemostatic Defect

- Purpura—recurrent, chronic bruising in multiple locations; called petechiae when <3 mm, purpura when 3 mm to 1 cm, and ecchymoses when >1 cm in diameter
- Epistaxis—nosebleeds that are recurrent, bleed from both nostrils, last longer than 10 minutes, or require physical intervention
- Recurrent or excessive bleeding from trauma, surgery, or dental extraction
- Bleeding into multiple body cavities, joints, or soft tissue
- Simultaneous bleeding from several sites
- Menorrhagia (menstrual hemorrhage)
- Bleeding that is delayed or recurrent
- Bleeding that is inappropriately brisk
- Bleeding for no apparent reason
- Hematemesis (vomiting of blood)

TABLE 36.1 Primary Assays for a Generalized Hemostatic Disorder

Assay	Assesses
Hemoglobin, hematocrit; reticulocyte count	Anemia associated with chronic bleeding or a hemolytic anemia; bone marrow response
Platelet count	Thrombocytopenia
Prothrombin time (PT)	Clotting time prolonged in deficiencies of factors II (prothrombin), V, VII, or X
Partial thromboplastin time (PTT)	Clotting time prolonged in deficiencies of all factors except VII and XIII
Thrombin time (TT)	Prolonged by unfractionated heparin therapy, dysfibrinogenemia, hypofibrinogenemia, and afibrinogenemia; qualitative
Fibrinogen assay (FG)	Reduced in dysfibrinogenemia, hypofibrinogenemia, and afibrinogenemia; quantitative result

using the thromboelastograph (TEG) or *thromboelastometry* (TEM) using the rotational thromboelastometer (ROTEM) (Chapter 42). TEG and TEM are coagulometers that measure whole blood clotting, a process called global hemostasis.[7] Both report clot onset dynamics, clot strength, and fibrinolysis in 15 to 30 minutes. TEG or TEM results require interpretation by experienced laboratory practitioners.

Acquired Versus Congenital Bleeding Disorders

Liver disease, kidney failure, chronic infections, autoimmune disorders, obstetric complications, anemia, dietary deficiencies such as vitamin C or vitamin K deficiency, blunt or penetrating trauma, and inflammatory disorders may all be associated with bleeding. If a patient's bleeding episodes begin after childhood, are associated with some disease or physical trauma, and are not duplicated in relatives, they are probably acquired, not congenital. When an adult patient seeks treatment of generalized hemorrhage, the physician first looks for an underlying condition, disease, drug effect, or event and records a personal and family history (Box 36.2). The important elements of patient history are age; sex; current or past pregnancy; a systemic disorder such as diabetes or cancer; trauma; and exposure to drugs, including prescription drugs, over-the-counter nutritional supplements, alcohol abuse, and drugs of abuse. The physician determines the trigger, location, and volume of bleeding and then orders initial hemostasis laboratory assays (Table 36.1). These tests take on clinical significance when the history and physical examination have already established the existence of abnormal bleeding. Because of their propensity to generate false positive results in the absence of indications, hemostatic laboratory tests are ineffective when employed indiscriminately as population screens for healthy individuals (Chapter 2).[8]

Congenital hemorrhagic disorders are uncommon, occurring in fewer than 1 per 100 people, and are usually diagnosed in infancy or during the first years of life.[9] There may be first-degree relatives with similar symptoms. Congenital bleeding disorders lead to recurrent hemorrhages that may be spontaneous or may occur after minor injury or in unexpected locations, such as joints, body cavities, retinal veins and arteries, or the central nervous system. Patients with mild congenital hemorrhagic disorders may have no symptoms until they reach adulthood or experience some physical challenge, such as trauma, dental extraction, or a surgical procedure. The most common congenital deficiencies are VWD, factor VIII (FVIII, hemophilia A) and factor IX deficiencies (FIX, hemophilia B), and platelet function disorders (Chapters 37 and 38). Inherited deficiencies

of fibrinogen, prothrombin, and factors V, VII, X, XI, and XIII are rare.

ACQUIRED COAGULOPATHIES

We begin with the acquired coagulopathies because more patients experience acquired bleeding disorders secondary to trauma, drug exposure, or disease than possess inherited coagulopathies. Chronic disorders commonly associated with bleeding are liver disease, vitamin K deficiency, and renal failure. In all cases, laboratory test results are necessary to confirm the diagnosis and guide the management of acquired hemorrhagic events.[10]

Trauma-Induced Coagulopathy

In North America, unintentional injury is the leading cause of death among those aged 1 to 45 years. The total rises when statisticians include self-inflicted, felonious, and combat injuries. In the United States alone, trauma caused 214,000 deaths in 2015, or 63 per 100,000 residents.[11] Severe neurologic displacement accounts for 50% of trauma deaths, with most deaths occurring before the patient arrives at the hospital; however, of initial survivors, 20,000 die of hemorrhage within 48 hours.

Trauma-induced coagulopathy (TIC) accounts for most instances of fatal hemorrhage, and 3000 to 4000 hemorrhage-related deaths can be prevented through coagulopathy management.[12] *Coagulopathy* is defined as any single or multiple coagulation factor or platelet deficiency, and TIC is triggered by the combination of injury-related acute inflammation, hypothermia, acidosis, and hypoperfusion (poor distribution of blood to tissues associated with low blood pressure), all of which are elements of systemic shock. Systemic shock leads to acute reduction of ADAMTS13 (*a d*isintegrin *a*nd *m*etalloprotease with a *t*hrombo*s*pondin type 1 motif, member 13; also called VWF cleaving protease) with a related rise in ultra-large VWF multimers and VWF-triggered platelet activation.[13] Shock also leads to tissue factor release, coagulation factor activation, loss of coagulation control proteins, and hyperfibrinolysis.[14] This series of events resembles the pathophysiology of thrombotic thrombocytopenic purpura (TTP, Chapter 38), as well as conditions generated by major surgery, ruptured aortic aneurysm, gastrointestinal bleeding, esophageal varices, and postpartum hemorrhage where massive transfusion may be required.

Trauma-Induced Coagulopathy: Massive Transfusion

Trauma centers publish and maintain massive transfusion protocols (MTPs) for TIC management.[15] Massive hemorrhage is defined as blood loss exceeding total blood volume within 24 hours, loss of 50% of blood volume within a 3-hour period, blood loss exceeding 150 mL/min, or blood loss that necessitates plasma and platelet transfusion.[16] An MTP is triggered when the emergency medical team encounters an otherwise healthy trauma victim whose systolic blood pressure is less than 90 mm Hg, pulse is more rapid than 120 beats/min, pH is less than 7.25, hematocrit is less than 32%, hemoglobin is less than

---

BOX 36.2   Indications for Congenital Bleeding Disorders

- Relatives with similar bleeding symptoms
- Onset of bleeding in infancy or childhood
- Excessive bleeding from umbilical cord or circumcision wound
- Repeated hemorrhages in childhood, adulthood
- Chronic petechiae, purpura, or ecchymoses
- Bleeding into joints, central nervous system, soft tissues, peritoneum

10 g/dL, urine output is diminished, and PT is prolonged to more than 1.5 times the mean of the reference interval or generates an international normalized ratio (INR) of 1.5 or greater. These limits vary by institution, and many or all are employed in formal MTP-prediction scoring systems.[17] For example, the assessment of blood consumption (ABC) score assesses 1 point each for up to four nonlaboratory parameters: penetrating mechanism, positive focused assessment sonography for trauma (FAST), arrival systolic blood pressure of 90 mm Hg or less, and arrival heart rate of ≥120 beats/min. Any two of the four parameters activates the MTP.

Trauma center MTPs specify that unmatched thawed group AB or group A plasma be warmed and administered to the victim en route or immediately on hospital arrival.[18] Clinicians continue by administering equal amounts (1:1:1) of warmed red blood cells (RBCs), plasma, and single (random) donor platelet concentrate, approximating the makeup of whole blood.[19] Though RBCs are essential for their oxygen-carrying capacity, their administration need not exceed the volumes of the other components.[20] In most instances, clinicians administer pheresis platelet concentrate preparations that provide the equivalent of four to six random platelet concentrate preparations; consequently the practical component ratio is actually 6:6:1, with 1 representing pheresis platelet concentrate.[21]

Trauma-Induced Coagulopathy: Plasma

Plasma is a key TIC management component. Donor services separate and freeze plasma within 24 hours of collection, officially naming the product FP-24. From time-honored habit, laboratory practitioners, nurses, and physicians are inclined to call the product fresh frozen plasma (FFP), though the term no longer fits the product.[22] FP-24 may be subsequently thawed and stored at 1° C to 6° C for up to 5 days, a product officially named *thawed plasma*.[23] Trauma centers and mobile emergency services maintain an inventory of group A or AB thawed plasma ready for emergency administration. VWF and coagulation factor V and VIII activities decline to approximately 60% after 5 days of refrigerator storage, so thawed plasma may require supplementation with factor concentrates, especially in patients with VWD or hemophilia.[24,25]

Trauma-Induced Coagulopathy: Platelet Concentrate

Most trauma center MTPs now specify that platelet concentrate be administered as a standard component in equal proportion with red cells and plasma, though some stipulate platelet concentrates only be administered when the platelet count is less than, for example, 50,000/μL. Platelet concentrate inventories are limited and costly to manage, but concentrate contributes to positive outcomes because platelets halt microvascular bleeding.[26] Platelet concentrate therapy is generally ineffective when the patient has immune thrombocytopenia, thrombotic thrombocytopenic purpura, or heparin-induced thrombocytopenia (Chapter 38). In these conditions, therapeutic platelets are rapidly consumed, and their administration may therefore be contraindicated, although they may provide temporary rescue in emergent situations.[27]

Trauma-Induced Coagulopathy: Concentrates

In an effort to reduce the risk of transfusion-associated circulatory overload (TACO) and transfusion-related acute lung injury (TRALI), improve patient outcomes, and conserve resources, transfusion service directors may employ concentrates to augment or even replace component administration in TIC.[28] ADAMTS13 concentrate (SHP 665, Shire Pharmaceuticals), in clinical trials as a TTP therapeutic, shows promise in early TIC intervention and may reduce the need for MTP.[29,30] Activated prothrombin complex concentrate (APCC; FEIBA [factor eight inhibitor bypassing activity], Shire, or Autoplex T, Nabi) may be used at a dosage of 50 units/kg every 12 hours, not to exceed 200 units/kg in 24 hours.[31] The dose-response relationship of FEIBA or Autoplex T varies among recipients, and because both contain activated coagulation factors, their use, especially an overdose, may risk disseminated intravascular coagulation (DIC).[32] Nonactivated prothrombin complex concentrates (PCCs) such as four-factor concentrate Kcentra (CSL Behring) are safer and may also be employed. Kcentra was approved by the US Food and Drug Administration (FDA) in 2013 to treat hemorrhage in Coumadin overdose, but its use in TIC is off-label (not US FDA cleared for TIC).[33]

ADAMTS13 concentrate and PCCs, either activated or non-activated, may be used in conjunction with the antifibrinolytic lysine analog tranexamic acid (TXA; Cyklokapron, Pharmacia).[34,35] First US FDA cleared in 1986 to prevent bleeding in hemophilic patients about to undergo invasive procedures, TXA is effective and commonly employed for TIC, though this too is an off-label application.

Administration of *cryoprecipitate* is indicated when there is microvascular bleeding and the fibrinogen concentration is less than 100 mg/dL.[36] In postpartum hemorrhage, plunging fibrinogen levels are of particular concern because they signal the risk of major blood loss.[37] A 15 to 20 mL cryoprecipitate unit provides 150 to 250 mg of fibrinogen, and the risk of TACO is lower than the risk associated with plasma. A target fibrinogen level of 100 mg/dL should be maintained, though some recommend 200 mg/dL in postpartum hemorrhage.[38] Postpartum hemorrhage may also be managed with TXA.[39] Von Willebrand factor and FVIII concentrates are also indicated when the patient has a preexisting deficiency.[40]

Recombinant activated coagulation factor VII (rFVIIa, NovoSeven) was US FDA cleared in 1999 for treating hemophilia A or B when anti-FVIII or factor IX (FIX) inhibitors are present, respectively; its application in the treatment of TIC is off-label. A NovoSeven dosage of 30 μg/kg is rapidly effective in halting microvascular hemorrhage in nonhemophilic trauma victims, and NovoSeven does not cause DIC.[41] However, studies found a possible link between off-label NovoSeven use and arterial and venous thrombosis in patients with existing thrombotic risk factors.[42,43]

Trauma-Induced Coagulopathy: Monitoring Therapy

A skilled operator employing TEG or TEM technology may monitor the effects of plasma, platelet concentrate, PCC, activated PCC, four-factor PCC, TXA, and rFVIIa.[44,45] Cryoprecipitate efficacy may be measured using the fibrinogen assay.

Also, laboratory directors characteristically advise surgeons and emergency department physicians to monitor the effectiveness of all TIC therapy indirectly by checking for the correction of platelet count, PT, and PTT to within their respective reference intervals. Platelet aggregometry may be used to measure post-therapy platelet function, and coagulation factor assays are valuable as follow-ups to PT and PTT to determine whether the target activity of 30 units/dL has been met for each. Although PT, PTT, platelet count, and platelet function assays are accepted approaches, TEG and TEM provide immediate feedback and may be more sensitive to small physiologic improvements. ADAMTS13 assays are necessary in monitoring ADAMTS13 concentrate therapy. Once TIC has been stabilized, additional hemostasis-related therapy is seldom required.

Liver Disease Coagulopathy

The bleeding associated with liver disease may be localized or generalized, mucocutaneous or anatomic. Enlarged and collateral esophageal vessels called esophageal varices are a complication of chronic alcoholic cirrhosis; hemorrhaging from varices is localized bleeding, not a coagulopathy, though often fatal. Mucocutaneous bleeding occurs in liver disease–associated thrombocytopenia, often accompanied by decreased platelet function. Anatomic bleeding is the consequence of procoagulant dysfunction and deficiency.

Procoagulant Deficiency in Liver Disease

The liver produces nearly all of the plasma coagulation factors and regulatory proteins.[46] Hepatitis, cirrhosis, obstructive jaundice, cancer, poisoning, and congenital disorders of bilirubin metabolism may suppress the biosynthetic function of hepatocytes, reducing either the concentrations or activities of the plasma coagulation factors to less than hemostatic levels (<40 units/dL).[47]

Liver disease alters the production of the vitamin K-dependent factors II (prothrombin), VII, IX, and X and control proteins C, S, and Z. In liver disease these seven factors are produced in their *des-γ-carboxyl* forms, which cannot participate in coagulation (Chapter 35). At the onset of liver disease, factor VII, which has the shortest plasma half-life at 6 hours, is the first coagulation factor to exhibit decreased activity. Because the PT is particularly sensitive to factor VII activity, it is characteristically prolonged in mild liver disease, serving as a sensitive early marker.[48] Vitamin K may become deficient when the diet is limited. Vitamin K deficiency independent of liver disease produces a similar effect on the PT.

Declining coagulation factor V activity is a more specific marker of liver disease than deficient factors II, VII, IX, or X because factor V is non-vitamin K dependent and is not affected by dietary vitamin K deficiency. The factor V activity assay, performed in conjunction with the factor VII assay, may be used to distinguish liver disease from vitamin K deficiency.[49]

Fibrinogen is an acute phase reactant that frequently becomes elevated in early or mild liver disease. Moderately and severely diseased liver produces fibrinogen that is coated with excessive sialic acid, a condition called *dysfibrinogenemia,* in which the fibrinogen functions poorly. Dysfibrinogenemia causes generalized soft tissue bleeding associated with a prolonged TT and an exceptionally prolonged reptilase clotting time.[50] In end-stage liver disease, the fibrinogen level may fall to less than 100 mg/dL, a mark of liver failure.[51]

VWF and factors VIII and XIII are acute phase reactants that may be unaffected or elevated in mild to moderate liver disease.[52] In contrast to the other coagulation factors, VWF is produced from endothelial cells and megakaryocytes and is stored in endothelial cells and platelets.[53]

Platelet Abnormalities in Liver Disease

Moderate *thrombocytopenia* occurs in one-third of patients with liver disease.[54] Platelet counts of less than 150,000/μL may result from sequestration and shortened platelet survival associated with portal hypertension and resultant hepatosplenomegaly.[55] In alcoholism-related hepatic cirrhosis, acute alcohol toxicity also suppresses platelet production. Platelet aggregation and secretion properties are often suppressed; this is reflected in reduced platelet aggregometry and lumiaggregometry results (Chapter 41). Occasionally, platelets are hyper-reactive. Although controversial, aggregometry may be used to predict bleeding and thrombosis risk.[56,57]

Disseminated Intravascular Coagulation in Liver Disease

Chronic or compensated DIC (Chapter 39) is a significant complication of liver disease that is caused by decreased liver production of regulatory antithrombin, protein C, or protein S and by the release of activated procoagulants from degenerating liver cells. The failing liver cannot clear activated coagulation factors. In primary or metastatic liver cancer, hepatocytes may also produce nonspecific procoagulant substances that trigger chronic DIC, leading to ischemic complications.

In acute, uncompensated DIC, the PT, PTT, and TT are prolonged, the fibrinogen level is reduced to less than 100 mg/dL, and D-dimers are significantly increased.[58] If the DIC is chronic and compensated, the only elevated test result may be the D-dimer assay value, a hallmark of unregulated coagulation and fibrinolysis. Although DIC can be resolved only by removing its underlying cause, its hemostatic deficiencies may be corrected temporarily by administering RBCs, plasma, activated or nonactivated PCC, TXA, platelet concentrates, or antithrombin concentrates, which include synthetic ATryn (rEVO Biologics) and plasma-derived Thrombate III (Grifols).[59,60]

Hemostasis Laboratory Tests and Liver Disease

The PT, PTT, TT, fibrinogen concentration, platelet count, and D-dimer concentration are used to characterize the hemostatic abnormalities in liver disease (Table 36.2). Factor V and VII assays may be used in combination to differentiate liver disease from vitamin K deficiency. Both factors are decreased in liver disease, but factor V levels remain within the reference interval in simple vitamin K deficiency.

Plasminogen deficiency and an elevated D-dimer confirm systemic fibrinolysis. The *reptilase time* test occasionally may be useful to confirm dysfibrinogenemia. This test duplicates the

TABLE 36.2 Hemostasis Laboratory Tests in Liver Disease

Assay	Interpretation
Fibrinogen (FG)	>400 mg/dL (elevated) in early, mild liver disease; <200 mg/dL in moderate to severe liver disease, which causes dysfibrinogenemia and hypofibrinogenemia
Thrombin time (TT)	Prolonged in dysfibrinogenemia, hypofibrinogenemia, elevated fibrin degradation products, and unfractionated heparin therapy
Reptilase time	Prolonged in hypofibrinogenemia, significantly prolonged in dysfibrinogenemia; unaffected by heparin; assay rarely used
Prothrombin time (PT)	Prolonged, even in mild liver disease, because of des-γ-carboxyl factors replacing normal factors II (prothrombin), VII, and X
Partial thromboplastin time (PTT)	Mildly prolonged in severe liver disease because of disseminated intravascular coagulation (DIC) or des-γ-carboxyl factors II (prothrombin), IX, and X
Factor V assay	Factor V is reduced in liver disease but is unaffected by vitamin K deficiency, so the factor V level helps distinguish liver disease from vitamin K deficiency
Platelet count	Mild thrombocytopenia, platelet count <150,000/μL
Platelet aggregometry	Mild suppression of platelet aggregation and secretion in response to most agonists
Quantitative D-dimer	>240 ng/mL or >500 ng/mL fibrinogen equivalent units (FEUs)

thrombin time test except that venom of the reptile *Bothrops atrox* (common lancehead viper) is substituted for the thrombin reagent. The *Bothrops* venom triggers fibrin polymerization by cleaving fibrinopeptide A but not fibrinopeptide B from the fibrinogen molecule (Chapter 35). The subsequent polymerization is slowed by structural defects, which prolong the time interval to clot formation. The reptilase time test is unaffected by standard unfractionated heparin therapy and can be used to assess fibrinogen function even when there is heparin in the specimen.

Hemostatic Treatment to Resolve Liver Disease–Related Hemorrhage

Oral or intravenous vitamin K therapy may correct the bleeding associated with nonfunctional des-γ-carboxyl factors II (prothrombin), VII, IX, and X; however, the therapeutic effect of vitamin K is short lived compared with its effect in dietary vitamin K deficiency because of the liver's impaired biosynthetic ability. In severe liver disease, plasma transfusion provides all of the coagulation factors in hemostatic concentrations, although VWF and factors V and VIII may be reduced. Because of its small concentration and the short half-life of factor VII, plasma is unlikely to return the PT to within the reference interval.

A unit of plasma provides a volume of 200 to 280 mL. The typical adult plasma dose for liver disease is 2 units, but the dose varies widely, depending on the indication and the ability of the patient's cardiac and renal system to rapidly excrete excess fluid.

TACO is likely to occur when 30 mL/kg has been administered, but it may occur with even smaller volumes in patients with compromised cardiac or kidney function.

If the fibrinogen level is less than 50 mg/dL, spontaneous bleeding is imminent and cryoprecipitate or fibrinogen concentrate (RiaSTAP, CSL Behring) may be selected for therapy. Plasma and cryoprecipitate present a theoretical risk of virus transmission, as do other untreated single-donor biologic blood products, and allergic transfusion reactions are more common with plasma-containing products. Other therapeutic options for patients with liver disease-related bleeding are platelet concentrates, PCC, antithrombin concentrate, rFVIIa, and TXA.

Chronic Renal Failure and Hemorrhage

Chronic renal failure of any cause is often associated with platelet dysfunction and mild to moderate mucocutaneous bleeding.[61] Platelet adhesion to blood vessels and platelet aggregation are suppressed, perhaps because guanidinosuccinic acid or phenolic compounds coat the platelets.[62] Decreased RBC mass (anemia) and thrombocytopenia contribute to the bleeding. Dialysis, RBC transfusions, or erythropoietin therapy (epoetin alfa, Procrit, Janssen Pharmaceutica) may correct these disorders.[63]

Hemostasis activation syndromes that deposit fibrin in the renal microvasculature reduce glomerular function. Examples are DIC, hemolytic uremic syndrome, and thrombotic thrombocytopenic purpura. Although these are by definition thrombotic disorders, they invariably cause thrombocytopenia, which may lead to mucocutaneous bleeding. Fibrin also may be deposited in renal transplant rejection and in the glomerulonephritis syndrome of systemic lupus erythematosus.

Laboratory tests for bleeding in renal disease provide only modest information with little predictive or management value (Chapter 41). The bleeding time test may be prolonged, but it is too unreliable to provide an accurate diagnosis or to assist in monitoring treatment.[64] Platelet aggregometry is nonpredictive.[65] The PT and PTT are expected to be normal.[66]

Management of renal failure-related bleeding typically focuses on the severity of the hemorrhage without reliance on laboratory test results. Renal dialysis temporarily activates platelets and may ultimately improve platelet function, particularly when anemia is well controlled.[67,68] Desmopressin acetate may be administered intravenously (DDAVP) or intranasally (Stimate, Behring) to increase the plasma concentration of VWF high-molecular-weight multimers. The VWF aids platelet adhesion and aggregation.[69] Patients with renal failure should not take aspirin, clopidogrel, prasugrel, ticagrelor, or other platelet inhibitors, because these drugs increase the risk of hemorrhage.

Nephrotic Syndrome and Hemorrhage

Nephrotic syndrome is a state of increased glomerular permeability associated with a variety of conditions, such as chronic glomerulonephritis, diabetic glomerulosclerosis, systemic lupus erythematosus, amyloidosis, and renal vein thrombosis.[70] In nephrotic syndrome, low-molecular-weight proteins are lost through the glomerulus into the glomerular filtrate and the urine. Coagulation factors II (prothrombin), VII, IX, X, and XII have been detected in the urine, as have the coagulatory proteins antithrombin and protein C. In 25% of cases, loss of regulatory proteins takes precedence over loss of procoagulants and leads to a tendency toward venous thrombosis.

Vitamin K Deficiency and Hemorrhage

Vitamin K, required for normal function of the vitamin K–dependent prothrombin group of coagulation factors (Chapter 35; Figure 35.5), is ubiquitous in foods, especially green leafy vegetables, and the daily requirement is small, so pure dietary deficiency is rare. Body stores are limited, however, and become exhausted when the usual diet is interrupted, as when patients are fed only with parenteral (intravenous) nutrition for an extended period or when people embark upon fad diets.[71] Also, because vitamin K is fat soluble and requires bile salts for absorption, biliary duct obstruction (atresia), fat malabsorption, and chronic diarrhea may cause vitamin K deficiency. Broad-spectrum antibiotics that disrupt normal gut flora may cause a slight reduction because they destroy bacteria that produce vitamin K.[72]

Hemorrhagic Disease of the Newborn Caused by Vitamin K Deficiency

Because of their sterile intestines and the minimal concentration of vitamin K in human milk, newborns are constitutionally vitamin K deficient.[73] Hemorrhagic disease of the newborn was common in the United States before routine administration of vitamin K to infants was legislated in the 1960s, and it still occurs in developing countries. The activity levels of factors II (prothrombin), VII, IX, and X are lower in normal newborns than in adults (Chapter 43), and premature infants have even lower concentrations of these factors. Breastfeeding prolongs the deficiency because passively acquired maternal antibodies delay the establishment of gut flora.

Vitamin K Antagonists: Coumadin

The γ-carboxylation cycle of coagulation factors is interrupted by coumarin-type oral anticoagulants such as warfarin (Coumadin) that disrupt the vitamin K epoxide reductase and vitamin K quinone reductase reactions (Chapters 35 and 40; Figure 35.5).[74] In this situation the liver releases dysfunctional des-γ-carboxyl factors II (prothrombin), VII, IX, and X and proteins C, S, and Z; these inactive forms are called *proteins induced by vitamin K antagonists (PIVKA) factors*. Therapeutic overdose or the accidental or felonious administration of warfarin-containing rat poisons may result in moderate to severe hemorrhage because of the lack of functional K-dependent factors. The effect of *brodifacoum* or "superwarfarin," often used as a rodenticide, lasts for weeks to months, and treatment of poisoning with this substance requires repeated administration of vitamin K with follow-up PT monitoring.[75] Inadvertent Coumadin overdose is the single most common reason for hemorrhage-associated emergency department visits.

Detection of Vitamin K Deficiency or PIVKA Factors

A prolonged PT with or without a prolonged PTT supports the clinical suspicion of vitamin K deficiency. In PT and PTT mixing studies, if commercial platelet-free normal plasma (NP; CRYO*check* Pooled Normal Plasma, Precision BioLogic) is combined with patient plasma, the mixture yields "corrected" PT and PTT results, which indicate that factor deficiencies caused the initially prolonged PT and (perhaps) PTT. Single-factor assays will detect low factor VII (a common finding because of the short half-life of factor VII), followed in sequence by decreases in factors IX, X, and II (prothrombin), depending on the progression of the patient's abnormality.

The standard therapy for vitamin K deficiency is oral—or, in an emergency, intravenous—vitamin K. Because synthesis of functional vitamin K–dependent coagulation factors requires at least 3 hours, in the case of severe bleeding, plasma or four-factor PCC may be administered.[76] The primary assays for plasma or four-factor PCC efficacy are TEG or TEM, but the patient's recovery may be monitored indirectly using the PT/INR.

Autoanti-Factor VIII Inhibitor and Acquired Hemophilia

Acquired autoantibodies that specifically inhibit factors II (prothrombin), V, VIII, IX, and XIII and VWF have been described in nonhemophilic patients.[77] Autoanti-factor VIII is the most common. Patients who develop an autoantibody to factor VIII, which is diagnostic of acquired hemophilia, are often older than 60 and have no apparent underlying disease. Acquired hemophilia is occasionally associated with rheumatoid arthritis, inflammatory bowel disease, systemic lupus erythematosus, or lymphoproliferative disease. Pregnancy appears to trigger acquired hemophilia 2 to 5 months after delivery. Patients with inhibitor autoantibodies are prescribed immunosuppressive therapy, although autoantibodies that develop after pregnancy typically disappear spontaneously. Altogether, acquired hemophilia has an incidence of 1 per million people per year. Patients experience sudden and severe bleeding in soft tissues or bleeding in the gastrointestinal or genitourinary tract.[78] Acquired hemophilia, even when treated, remains fatal in at least 20% of cases. Autoantibodies to other procoagulants are less common but create similar symptoms.[79]

Clot-Based Assays to Detect Acquired Hemophilia

Recommended testing includes the PT, PTT, and TT for any patient with sudden onset of anatomic hemorrhage that resembles acquired hemophilia. In the presence of a factor VIII inhibitor, the PTT is likely prolonged, whereas the PT and TT are likely normal. A factor assay should reveal factor VIII activity to be less than 40 units/dL and the activity level is often undetectable.

Clot-based mixing studies confirm the presence of the inhibitor. The PTT prolongation may be corrected initially by the addition of NP to the test specimen in a 1:1 ratio, but PTT again becomes prolonged after incubation of the 1:1 NP–patient plasma mixture at 37° C for 2 hours. The return of prolongation after incubation occurs because factor VIII autoantibodies are often of the immunoglobulin G4 isotype, which are time and temperature dependent. Consequently the inhibitor effect may be evident only after the patient's inhibitor is allowed to interact with the factor VIII in the NP for 2 hours at 37° C

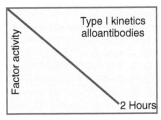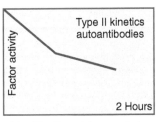

Figure 36.1 Factor Inhibitors Assayed by Clot-Based Assays. In type I linear kinetics, the inhibitor fully inactivates the coagulation factor in vitro. This is typical of alloantibodies such as factor VIII inhibitors that develop in patients with severe hemophilia A. In type II kinetics, the inhibitor and coagulation factor reach equilibrium. This is typical of autoantibodies such as the factor VIII inhibitor in acquired hemophilia A. Because of the type II kinetics, the Nijmegen-Bethesda assay is considered a semiquantitative measure in acquired hemophilia, although the results are commonly used to distinguish low-titer from high-titer autoantibodies.

before testing. Approximately 15% of inhibitors, called high-avidity inhibitors, may immediately prolong the mixture's PTT; in this case an incubated mixing study is unnecessary.

Factor VIII neutralization by an autoantibody is nonlinear. Although there is early rapid loss of factor VIII activity, residual activity remains, which indicates that the reaction has reached equilibrium. This is called type II kinetics (Figure 36.1). In contrast, alloantibodies to factor VIII, which develop in 30% of patients with severe hemophilia in response to factor VIII concentrate therapy, exhibit type I kinetics. In type I kinetics there is linear in vitro neutralization of factor VIII activity over 2 hours, which results in complete inactivation. In type I kinetics, in vitro measurement is relatively reliable, whereas in type II kinetics, the titration of inhibitor activity is semiquantitative.[80,81]

Quantitation of autoanti-VIII inhibitor is accomplished using the *Nijmegen-Bethesda assay* (Chapter 41), which is ordinarily employed to measure inhibitors in hemophilic patients with alloantibodies to factor VIII (hemophilia A with factor VIII inhibitors). Titer results help the clinician choose the proper therapy to control bleeding. Repeat titers are used to follow the response to immunosuppressive therapy but are not needed for management of the bleeding symptoms.

Factor Inhibitors Other Than Autoanti–Factor VIII

Antiprothrombin (factor II) antibodies prolong the PT. These inhibitors develop as lupus anticoagulant variants with prothrombin specificity in approximately 30% of lupus anticoagulant patients.[82,83] Like all lupus anticoagulants, antiprothrombin is typically associated with thrombosis, although a few patients experience bleeding.[84] Findings of reduced prothrombin activity by clot-based assay, antiprothrombin antibodies via enzyme immunoassay, and a positive lupus anticoagulant test result confirm the diagnosis. It is rare to detect antiprothrombin antibodies that are not associated with lupus anticoagulant.

Factor XIII inhibitors are extremely rare but cause life-threatening bleeding. They may arise spontaneously or in association with autoimmune or lymphoproliferative disorders. Autoanti-factor XIII has been documented in patients receiving isoniazid treatment for tuberculosis.[85,86]

Autoantibodies to factor V may arise spontaneously in autoimmune disorders and after exposure to bovine thrombin in

fibrin glue.[87,88] Fibrin glue-generated autoantibodies have largely disappeared since 2008 when manufacturers began to use plasma-derived human thrombin in place of bovine thrombin (Tisseel, Baxter).

Autoanti-factor X antibodies are rare; however, factor X deficiency in amyloidosis may be caused by what seems to be an absorptive mechanism.[89,90] In many cases of acquired inhibitors, mixing studies show uncorrected prolongation without incubation (immediate mixing study), and inhibitor titers may be determined by the Nijmegen-Bethesda assay.[91]

Acquired Hemophilia Management

Activated PCC or rFVIIa may bypass the coagulation factor VIII inhibitor in acquired hemophilia and thereby control acute bleeding. Patients whose inhibitor titers are less than 5 Nijmegen-Bethesda units (NBU) may respond to administration of DDAVP or factor VIII concentrates, but close monitoring of their response to therapy with serial coagulation factor VIII activity assays is warranted. Once bleeding is controlled, immune tolerance therapy may reduce the inhibitor titer. Plasma exchange may also be used in severe cases, but the response is less reliable than the response to immune tolerance therapy.[92]

Acquired von Willebrand Disease

Acquired VWF deficiency, with symptoms similar to those of congenital VWD, has been described in hypothyroidism, benign monoclonal gammopathies, Wilms tumor, intestinal angiodysplasia, congenital heart disease, pesticide exposure, uremia, lupus erythematosus, and autoimmune, lymphoproliferative, and myeloproliferative disorders.[93,94] The pathogenesis of acquired VWD may involve decreased VWF production; adsorption of VWF to abnormal cell surfaces, as seen in association with lymphoproliferative disorders and Wilms tumor; or, in less than 2% of cases, a specific VWF autoantibody.

Acquired VWD manifests with moderate to severe mucocutaneous bleeding and may be suspected in any patient with recent onset of bleeding who has no hemorrhage-related medical history.[95] Although the PT is not affected, the PTT may be moderately prolonged if the VWF reduction is severe enough to reduce factor VIII to less than 40 units/dL, because VWF serves as the factor VIII carrier molecule. As in congenital VWD, the diagnosis is based on a finding of diminished VWF activity and diminished VWF antigen by immunoassay. It may be difficult to differentiate between mild, previously asymptomatic congenital VWD and acquired VWD.[96]

If the patient requires treatment for bleeding, DDAVP or a plasma-derived factor VIII/VWF concentrate such as Humate-P (Behring), Wilate (Octapharma), or Alphanate (Grifols) is effective at controlling the symptoms. Cryoprecipitate is no longer recommended for treatment of VWD because it does not undergo viral inactivation.

Disseminated Intravascular Coagulation

DIC, although characteristically identified through its hemorrhagic symptoms, is classified as a thrombotic disorder and is described in Chapter 39.

CONGENITAL COAGULOPATHIES

Von Willebrand Disease

VWD, first described by Finnish professor Erik von Willebrand in 1926, is the most prevalent inherited mucocutaneous bleeding disorder. Any one of dozens of germline mutations may cause VWD as these mutations produce quantitative (type 1) or qualitative (functional, type 2) VWF abnormalities. Both quantitative and functional abnormalities lead to decreased platelet adhesion to injured vessel walls, impairing primary hemostasis. When solely defined by laboratory assays as VWF deficiency, VWD is reputed to afflict approximately 1% of the global population. However, when defined by the number of patients who experience bleeds serious enough to seek medical assistance, prevalence is 1 in 20,000 (0.05%).[97] The prevalence of VWD in women who report menorrhagia is 24%.[98,99] VWD inheritance is autosomal dominant and affects both sexes.[100]

Molecular Biology and Functions of von Willebrand Factor

VWF is a multimeric glycoprotein whose molecular mass ranges from 500,000 to 20,000,000 Daltons, the largest molecule in human plasma. Its plasma concentration is 0.5 to 1.0 mg/dL, but a great deal more is readily available on demand from storage organelles. VWF is synthesized in the endoplasmic reticulum of endothelial cells and stored in their cytoplasmic *Weibel-Palade bodies*. It is also synthesized in megakaryocytes and stored in the α-granules of platelets (Chapter 10). Weibel-Palade bodies and α-granules release VWF in response to a variety of hemostatic and inflammatory stimuli.[101]

The VWF gene consists of 52 exons spanning 178 kilobase pairs (kb) on chromosome 12.[102] The translated protein is a monomer of 2813 amino acids composed of four structural domains, A through D. The monomers become glycosylated, then form dimers and oligomers that migrate to the aforementioned storage organelles, where they polymerize to form ultralarge VWF (UL-VWF) multimers. At the time of storage, a propeptide, known as VWF antigen II, becomes cleaved from the end of domain D so that the mature monomers, already polymerized, consist of 2050 amino acids.[103] VWD mutations may occur anywhere on the *VWF* gene.[104]

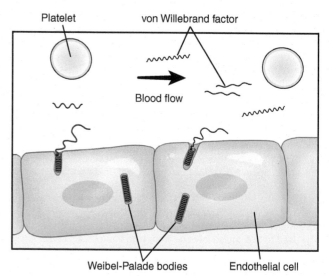

Figure 36.2 Von Willebrand Factor. Von Willebrand factor is stored in endothelial cell weibel-palade bodies and platelet α-granules. On demand, the Weibel-Palade bodies and platelet α-granules fuse with their respective plasma membranes and release VWF into the bloodstream. The ultralarge multimers of VWF are uncoiled in response to the shear forces of the blood flow where they will be cleaved by the enzyme ADAMTS13 into shorter multimers. The VWF multimers bind platelets.

As VWF is released from the Weibel-Palade bodies or platelet α-granules, blood flow shear forces cause the molecule to unfold (Figure 36.2). ADAMTS13 cleaves the now linear UL-VWF multimers, yielding multimers of various masses. ADAMTS13 deficiency results in the retention of circulating UL-VWF multimers, the basis for the devastating disorder thrombotic thrombocytopenic purpura (Chapter 38; Figure 38.6). The ADAMTS13 cleavage function also appears to modulate acute inflammation, stroke, and myocardial infarction.[105]

Epitopes of the structural domains of the VWF monomer support its various functions. Domain A supports a receptor site for collagen and a binding site (ligand) for platelet receptor glycoprotein (GP) Ib/IX/V and heparin. Domain C provides a site that binds platelet receptor GPIIb/IIIa ($\alpha_{IIb}\beta_3$), and domain D provides the carrier site for factor VIII (Figure 36.3). On release from intracellular stores, a percentage of VWF multimers complex with factor VIII. VWF protects factor VIII from proteolysis,

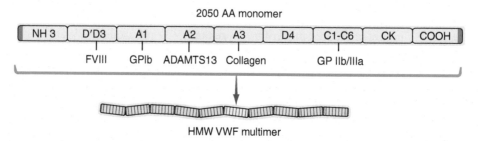

Figure 36.3 Von Willebrand Factor Monomer. The *VWF* gene, located on the p arm of chromosome 12, spans 178 kilobases, and is the template for the VWF prepropeptide of 2813 amino acids *(AA)*. Entering storage, a signal sequence of 22 AA and a propeptide of 741 AA are cleaved, leaving the mature monomer of 2050 AA, diagrammed here. The monomer consists of 12 subunits within the 4 domains (A-D) that support the active sites at the locations indicated on the diagram. The monomers polymerize to form multimers of various lengths that reach up to 20 million Daltons molecular weight.

TABLE 36.3 Nomenclature of the Factor VIII/von Willebrand Factor Complex

Term	Meaning
FVIII/VWF	Customary designation for the combination of factor VIII and VWF.
FVIII	Procoagulant factor VIII, transported on VWF. Factor VIII binds activated factor IX to form the complex of VIIIa-IXa, which digests and activates factor X. Factor VIII deficiency is called *hemophilia A*.
VWF:Ag	Epitope that is the antigenic target for the VWF immunoassay.
FVIII:C	Factor VIII coagulant activity as measured in a clot-based factor assay.

The following assays measure VWF activity, which is compared to VWF:Ag to distinguish qualitative and quantitative VWF deficiency. Most VWF activity assays measure the presence of high molecular weight VWF multimers, which are the most active multimers in platelet adhesion.

Term	Meaning
VWF:RCo	Quantitative ristocetin cofactor activity, also called VWF activity. VWF activity is measured by the ability of ristocetin to cause agglutination of reagent platelets by the patient's VWF.
VWF:CB	Collagen binding assay, a second VWF activity assay. Large VWF multimers bind immobilized target collagen, predominantly collagen III.
VWF:Immunoactivity	Automated nephelometric activity assay that employs latex microparticles and monoclonal anti-glycoprotein I–VWF receptor, a third method for assaying VWF activity.
VWF:GPIbR	Activity assay that employs ristocetin-triggered binding of recombinant glycoprotein Ib (GPIb), detected by LIA or CLIA.
VWF:GPIbM	Activity assay that employs recombinant gain-of-function GPIb that binds the VWF A1 domain without the need for ristocetin. Reaction is detected using LIA.
RIPA	Ristocetin-induced platelet aggregometry, uses ristocetin and patient's own platelets, in contrast to the VWF:RCo, which uses reagent platelets. This assay is modified by using low ristocetin concentrations to identify VWD subtype 2B in which VWF multimers exhibit increased avidity for the platelet receptor site. This method is also called the ristocetin response curve.

CLIA, Chemiluminescence immunoassay; *LIA*, latex immunoassay

prolonging its plasma half-life from a few minutes when free to 8 to 12 hours when bound to VWF. Table 36.3 lists the nomenclatures for the structural and functional components of the factor VIII/VWF molecule.

Although VWF is the factor VIII carrier molecule, its primary function is to mediate platelet adhesion to subendothelial collagen in areas of high flow rate and high shear force, as in capillaries and arterioles (Figure 35.7). VWF, released from the Weibel-Palade bodies, first unfolds and binds fibrillar intimal collagen exposed during the desquamation of endothelial cells or in a blood vessel injury (Chapter 10; Figure 10.9). Subsequently, platelets adhere through their GPIb/IX/V site to the

VWF "carpet." The high-molecular-weight (HMW-VWF) multimers are best equipped to serve the adhesion function. When VWF binds GPIb/IX/V, platelets become activated and express a second VWF binding site, GPIIb/IIIa, integrin designation $\alpha_{IIb}\beta_3$. This receptor binds arginine-glycine-aspartic acid (arginyl-glycylaspartic acid, RGD) sequences that are richly distributed in VWF and fibrinogen molecules, mediating irreversible platelet-to-platelet aggregation. The adhesion and aggregation sequences are essential to normal primary and secondary hemostasis.

Pathophysiology of von Willebrand Disease

Structural (qualitative) or quantitative VWF abnormalities reduce platelet adhesion, which leads to mucocutaneous hemorrhage of varying severity: epistaxis, ecchymosis, menorrhagia, hematemesis, gastrointestinal, and surgical bleeding. Symptoms vary over time and within kindreds because VWF production and release are susceptible to a variety of physiologic influences. In addition, severe quantitative VWF deficiency creates factor VIII deficiency as a result of the inability to protect unbound factor VIII from proteolysis. Many "low VWF" people have VWF levels in the intermediate range of 30% to 50% of normal and maintain a factor VIII level sufficient for competent coagulation. When factor VIII levels decrease to less than 30 units/dL, anatomic bleeding into joints and body cavities accompanies the typical mucocutaneous bleeding pattern of VWD.

Von Willebrand Disease Types and Subtypes

Type 1 von Willebrand disease. Type 1 VWD is a quantitative VWF deficiency caused by one of several autosomal dominant frameshifts, nonsense mutations, or deletions that may occur anywhere in the VWF gene. Type 1 comprises 40% to 70% of VWD cases.[106] The plasma concentrations of all VWF multimers and factor VIII are variably, albeit proportionally, reduced (Figure 36.4). There is mild to moderate systemic bleeding, usually after a hemostatic challenge such as dental extraction or surgery. In women, menorrhagia, which predicts postpartum hemorrhage, is a common complaint that leads to the diagnosis of VWD. However, because mucocutaneous

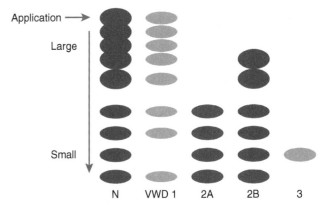

Figure 36.4 Von Willebrand Factor Multimers. Schematic of von Willebrand factor multimer analysis by polyacrylamide gel electrophoresis shows diminished concentration but normal ratios in von Willebrand disease *(VWD)* type 1 (and also subtype 2M), absence of large and intermediate multimers in subtype 2a, absence of large multimers in subtype 2b, and absence of all multimers in type 3.

(systemic) bleeding symptoms occur in normal people to varying degrees, diagnosis requires scrupulous laboratory testing.[107]

Type 2 von Willebrand disease. Type 2 VWD encompasses four qualitative VWF abnormalities. VWF levels may be normal or moderately decreased, but VWF function is consistently reduced. Laboratory testing is essential to identifying and confirming type 2 subtypes because the diagnosis affects treatment choices.

Subtype 2A von Willebrand disease. Approximately 10% to 20% of all VWD patients suffer from subtype 2A, which arises from well-characterized autosomal dominant point mutations in the A2 and D1 structural domains of the VWF molecule. These mutations render VWF susceptible to increased proteolysis by ADAMTS13, which leads to a predominance of small-molecular-weight plasma multimers (Figure 36.4). The smaller multimers support less platelet adhesion activity than the normal high- or intermediate-molecular weight multimers. Patients with subtype 2A VWD have normal or slightly reduced VWF antigen levels as measured by immunoassay, with moderate to markedly reduced VWF activity as a result of the loss of the high-molecular-weight and intermediate-molecular-weight multimers essential for platelet adhesion.

Subtype 2B von Willebrand disease. In subtype 2B VWD, identified in less than 5% of all VWD patients, mutations within the A1 domain raise the affinity of VWF for platelet GPIb/IX/V, its customary binding site; these are hence "gain-of-function" mutations. HMW-VWF multimers spontaneously bind resting platelets. The abnormal HMW-VWF multimers are consequently unavailable for normal platelet adhesion as they are cleared with the bound platelets. The electrophoretic multimer pattern is characterized by lack of HMW-VWF multimers, but intermediate-molecular-weight multimers may still be present (Figure 36.4). Subtype 2B VWD may be confirmed using a specially designed reduced-concentration, ristocetin-induced (RIPA) platelet agglutination assay. There may also exist moderate thrombocytopenia caused by chronic platelet activation because multimer-coated platelets indiscriminately bind the endothelium and become cleared.

A platelet mutation that raises GPIb affinity for normal HMW-VWF multimers creates a clinically similar disorder called *platelet-type VWD* (PT-VWD) or *pseudo-VWD*. In this instance the large multimers also are lost from the plasma, and platelets become adhesive as in subtype 2B VWD. Pseudo-VWD may be the more appropriate name, though seldom used, because this is not a true form of VWD. PT-VWD's prevalence is approximately 10% of subtype 2B VWD sufferers. Both clinically and by phenotypic laboratory assays, the two entities are indistinguishable; the diagnosis requires molecular testing. Further, platelet-type VWD is often mistaken for immune thrombocytopenia.

Subtype 2M von Willebrand disease. Subtype 2M VWD describes a qualitative VWF variant that possesses poor platelet receptor binding despite generating a normal multimeric distribution pattern in electrophoresis. The distinguishing feature of subtype 2M that separates it from type 1 is a discrepancy between the concentration of VWF:Ag and its activity as measured using the VWF ristocetin cofactor assay described later, despite a normal multimeric pattern. Subtype 2M is often incorrectly identified as type 1 or subtype 2A. It may be that the 10% to 20%

prevalence data for subtype 2A and the 40% to 70% date for type 1 are artificially elevated by misdiagnosed subtype 2M cases.

Subtype 2N von Willebrand disease (Normandy variant; autosomal hemophilia). An autosomal VWF gene missense mutation in the D9 domain impairs the protein's factor VIII binding site function. This condition, present in less than 5% of VWD patients, results in factor VIII deficiency despite a normal VWF antigen concentration assay result, normal VWF activity, and a normal multimeric pattern. The disorder is also known as autosomal hemophilia because its clinical symptoms are indistinguishable from the symptoms of hemophilia except that it affects both men and women. Subtype 2N is suspected when a girl or woman is diagnosed with hemophilia subsequent to anatomic bleeding symptoms. In boys or men, subtype 2N is suspected when a male patient misdiagnosed as a hemophilia A sufferer fails to respond to factor VIII concentrate therapy. The poor therapeutic response occurs because free factor VIII has a plasma half-life of mere minutes. The diagnosis of VWD subtype 2N is confirmed using a molecular assay that detects the specific mutation responsible for the abnormal FVIII binding function.

Type 3 von Willebrand disease. "Null allele" VWF gene translation or deletion mutations that may occur anywhere on the gene produce severe mucocutaneous and anatomic hemorrhage in compound heterozygotes or, in consanguinity, homozygotes. This is the most rare form of VWD, where the VWF concentration measured by immunoassay or by activity assay is less than 10% (Figure 36.4). Factor VIII is proportionally diminished or absent, and primary and secondary hemostasis is impaired.

Laboratory Detection and Classification of von Willebrand Disease

Definitive diagnosis of VWD depends on the combination of a personal and family history of mucocutaneous bleeding and the laboratory demonstration of decreased VWF concentration or activity (function). The physician orders a complete blood count to rule out thrombocytopenia as the cause of mucocutaneous bleeding, and a PT and PTT, which assess the coagulation cascade to rule out a coagulation factor deficiency other than VWF. No longer recommended, according to the 2009 National Heart Lung and Blood Institute (NHLBI) VWD guidelines, are the bleeding time test and the PFA-100 or other automated functional platelet assays (Chapters 2, 41, and 42). These traditional assays generate "conflicting" sensitivity and specificity data.

Owing to VWD's complexity and variability, the standard VWD test panel must incorporate at least three primary assays: VWF:Ag, VWF activity by ristocetin cofactor assay (VWF:RCo) or equivalent, and coagulation factor VIII activity.

The quantitative VWF:Ag assay is the most prominent member of the primary VWD laboratory profile. VWF:Ag may employ enzyme immunoassay (EIA) methodology, the traditional reference method, which is usually batched and performed manually; automated latex immunoassay methodology (LIA), such as the Liatest (Stago); or chemiluminescence immunoassay (CLIA) technology such as the HemosIL AcuStar VWF:Ag (Instrumentation Laboratory–Werfen). The CLIA method possesses the best sensitivity to VWF concentrations less than 10% and the best precision.[108]

Another essential primary assay is the factor VIII assay. Factor VIII assay results generally parallel VWF:Ag and VWF:RCo results in VWD types 1 and 3, and may parallel VWF:Ag in subtypes 2A, 2B, and 2M, but are markedly reduced in VWD subtype 2N.

The traditional VWF:RCo assay employs ristocetin.[109] Ristocetin, introduced in 1956 as an unsuccessful antibiotic, is added to in vitro patient plasma where it unfolds the VWF molecule and reduces repelling negative charges, enabling HMW-VWF multimers to bind reagent platelet membrane GPIb/IX/V receptors.[110] The VWF:RCo assay, typically performed using a platelet aggregometer, employs preserved reagent platelets and measures platelet agglutination, yielding a quantitative measure of VWF function.[111] The VWF:RCo has been successfully automated but has been partially replaced by automated ristocetin-triggered nonplatelet recombinant GPIb-based LIA and CLIA methods such as the HemosIL AcuStar VWF:GPIbR (Instrumentation Laboratory–Werfen), which the International Society on Thrombosis and Haemostasis Standardization Subcommittee (ISTH-SSC) for von Willebrand factor labeled VWF:GPIbR in their 2014 annual minutes.

A promising alternative to VWF:RCo and VWF:GPIbR is an assay that incorporates a gain-of-function high-affinity recombinant GPIb protein that resembles the GPIb of PT-VWD platelets. The GPIb binds the A1 domain of native VWF without the need for ristocetin. This assay has been commercialized as a LIA (Innovance VWF Ac, Siemens), and it appears to improve on ristocetin-based assays as it offers smaller VWF detection limits and less variability. The 2014 ISTH-SSC terms this assay VWF:GPIbM.[112] All VWF activity assays rely on GPIb binding avidity, a surrogate for VWF activity.

When the ratio of the VWF:RCo, VWF:GPIbR, or VWF:GPIbM assay value to the VWF:Ag concentration (VWF:GPIbR/VWF:Ag, for instance) is less than 0.5, 0.6, or 0.7 (ratio limit is generated from reference interval studies by individual laboratories), the laboratory professional infers qualitative or type 2 VWD. Secondary follow-up tests are necessary to confirm type 2 VWD and to differentiate its subtypes. Low-dose RIPA, also called the *ristocetin response curve*, identifies subtype 2B. The low-dose RIPA test is performed on platelet-rich plasma as opposed to a preserved platelet suspension used in the VWF:RCo assay. In subtype 2B the patient's platelets, because they are coated with avid VWF multimers, agglutinate in response to less than 0.5 mg/mL ristocetin; sometimes they even agglutinate in response to 0.1 mg/mL ristocetin. In comparison, normal platelets agglutinate only at ristocetin concentrations greater than 0.5 mg/mL, and platelets from a patient with subtype 2A may not agglutinate to ristocetin at all.

VWF multimer analysis by sodium dodecyl sulfate–polyacrylamide gel electrophoresis is a complex secondary confirmatory procedure that helps establish VWD type 2 and differentiates between VWD subtypes 2A, 2B, and perhaps 2M. Although both 2A and 2B lack high-molecular-weight multimers, intermediate multimers are presumed to be present in the electrophoretic pattern of subtype 2B VWD samples but are absent from the pattern of a patient with subtype 2A VWD. In type 2M the multimeric pattern appears to be normal despite the reduced function to concentration ratio. Multimer analysis is available from specialized reference laboratories for differentiation of VWD type 2 subtypes.

Table 36.4 lists the expected test results for all VWD types and subtypes. Because acquired VWD may mimic any one of the VWD types and subtypes, results of the laboratory workup seldom help to differentiate it from the inherited condition. Review of the clinical history with emphasis on age at onset of bleeding, comorbid conditions, and family history may signal acquired disease rather than the congenital form.[113]

TABLE 36.4 Detection and Classification of von Willebrand Disease: Laboratory Results*

Laboratory Test	Type 1	Subtype 2A	Subtype 2B	Subtype 2M	Subtype 2N	Type 3
VWF:RCo, VWF:CB, VWF:Immunoactivity, VWF:GPIbR, or VWF:GPIbM	Low	Low	Low	Low	Normal	Very low or absent
VWF:Ag	Low	Normal to slightly decreased	Normal to slightly decreased	Normal	Normal	Very low or absent
VWF activity to VWF:Ag ratio†	>0.5	<0.5	<0.5	<0.5	>0.5	N/A
Platelet count	Normal	Normal	Decreased	Decreased	Normal	Normal
Partial thromboplastin time (PTT)	Normal to slightly prolonged	Normal	Normal	Normal to slightly prolonged	Normal to slightly prolonged	Prolonged
RIPA	Decreased	Decreased	Increased	Decreased	Normal	Absent
Factor VIII activity	Slightly low	Normal	Normal	Normal	Low	<10 units/dL
VWF multimers	Normal pattern	Large and intermediate forms absent	Large forms absent	Normal pattern	Normal pattern	All forms absent

Ag, Antigen; *CB*, collagen binding; *GP*, glycoprotein; *N/A*, not applicable; *RCo*, ristocetin cofactor; *RIPA*, ristocetin-induced platelet aggregometry; *VWF*, von Willebrand factor.
*Results vary over time and within affected kindred.
†Limits are locally established.

Pitfalls in von Willebrand Disease Diagnosis

Varying genetic penetrance, ABO blood group, inflammation, hormones, age, and physical stress influence VWF activity.[114] Raised estrogen levels during the second and third trimesters of pregnancy nearly normalize plasma VWF activity even in women with moderate VWF deficiency. However, VWF concentration and function decrease rapidly after delivery, which may lead to acute postpartum hemorrhage in VWD, for which the obstetrician is watchful.[115] Oral contraceptives and hormone replacement therapy also raise VWF activity, and activity waxes and wanes with the menstrual cycle.

VWF activity rises substantially in acute inflammation such as occurs postoperatively, subsequent to trauma, or during an infection. Physical stress such as cold, exertion, or a child's crying or struggling during venipuncture causes VWF activity to rise. VWF activity rises when the phlebotomist allows the tourniquet to remain tied for more than 1 minute before venipuncture and descends if the specimen is stored in the refrigerator before testing. VWD patients experience fluctuation in disease severity over time, and the clinical manifestations of the disease vary from person to person within kindred, despite the assumption that everyone in the family possesses the same mutation. When the clinical presentation indicates VWD, the VWD laboratory assay panel should be repeated at least once, or until the results are conclusive.[116]

Adding to VWD diagnostic confusion is concern over the variability in the results of the VWF:RCo assay, which is based on platelet aggregometry but is performed using a variety of instruments and methods as detailed before.[117] Ristocetin avidity varies from lot to lot. In the United States proficiency surveys consistently reveal VWF:RCo assays to have an unimpressive interlaboratory coefficient of variation of 30% and a least detectable activity range of 6% to 12%.[118]

Concern over the poor reproducibility of results of the VWF:RCo assay has led to development of the *VWF collagen-binding (VWF:CB) assay*. VWF:CB employs type III collagen as its solid-phase target antigen. Developed in 1990, the VWF:CB assay produces results that more closely match those of the VWF:RCo assay than of VWF:Ag assays, because collagen type III binds predominantly HMW-VWF multimers; however, the target collagen composition requires standardization before this assay achieves routine assay status.[119] When collagen is standardized, the VWF:CB assay provides better precision than the VWF:RCo assay.[120]

Directors of specialized reference laboratories add the VWF:CB to their primary VWD assay profile. They argue that the VWF:CB assay detects abnormalities of VWF collagen binding, whereas the VWF:RCo, VWF:GPIbR, and VWF:GPIbM assays detect only abnormalities of VWF platelet GPIb binding. They cite instances in which the VWF:CB value was abnormal when the VWF:RCo value was normal, and vice versa.[121] A recently developed CLIA-based VWF:CB may improve assay sensitivity and precision when approved for clinical deployment.

In an effort to more closely reflect clinical reality and reduce false-positive type 1 VWD diagnoses, the 2009 NHLBI VWD guidelines have coined the non-disease description "*low VWF*"

for the condition in which VWF activity and antigen concentrations are between 30% and 50% of normal, the ratio of VWF:RCo to VWF:Ag is greater than 0.5, and factor VIII activity is greater than 50 units/dL. This suggested category reflects the difficulty in distinguishing mucocutaneous bleeding from self-reported "easy bruising" and recognizes that low VWF activity and bleeding often associate coincidentally. To make a definite type 1 VWD diagnosis, 30% of normal VWF activity is used as the limit. *VWF* gene mutations associate consistently with VWF levels less than 30%, whereas linkages appear in only half of instances when the VWF:Ag level is 30% to 50%.[122]

The key tendency is overdiagnosis of VWD; nevertheless, restrictive laboratory assay panels and inappropriate testing such as the bleeding time test or PFA-100 may miss documentable VWD. Rheumatoid factor and heterophile antibodies interfere to cause false positives. Occasionally, physicians may diagnose hemophilia A in patients with VWD type 3, having failed to order a VWF primary profile. Moderate VWD may fail to appear until adulthood, leading to a false diagnosis of acquired VWD. Specimen mishandling such as prolonged tourniquet application, plasma refrigeration, filtration, or ultracentrifugation lead to false positives, false negatives, or false phenotypes such as misidentifying a type 1 as a type 2 VWD.

VWF activity varies by ABO blood group, and experts have in the past recommended that laboratory directors maintain separate reference intervals for each group, as provided in Table 36.5.[123] The 2009 NHLBI VWD guidelines have recommended against this practice, noting that, "despite the ABO blood grouping and associated reference ranges, the major determinant of bleeding risk is low VWF." Therefore VWF test result reference intervals are now population based rather than ABO stratified. The internationally generalized cutoff of 50% for low VWF and 30% for VWD is clinically reasonable, although laboratory directors may choose to validate and adjust this cutoff employing internal reference interval studies.

In a well-managed tertiary care facility, laboratory professionals and physicians communicate regularly with the medical staff who are challenged with VWD diagnosis and management—nurses, pharmacists, emergency department and primary care physicians, internists, surgeons, gynecologists, and hematologists. Laboratory professionals ensure that those who manage VWD patients are aware of the effects of ABO group, estrogen levels, inflammation, and physical stress on VWF activity and that they understand the strengths and limitations of VWF laboratory assay panels, the proper interpretation of assay results, and the availability of follow-up and confirmatory assays.

TABLE 36.5   Von Willebrand Factor (VWF) Reference Intervals by Blood Group

Blood Group	Reference Interval
0	36%–157%
A	48%–234%
B	57%–241%
AB	64%–238%
Population based: "Low VWF"	<50%
Population based: von Willebrand disease	<30%

Von Willebrand Disease Treatment

Mild bleeding may resolve with the use of localized measures, such as limb elevation, pressure, and application of ice packs (the athlete's acronym is *PRICE*—for *p*rotection, *r*est, *i*ce, *c*ompression, and *e*levation).[124] Moderate bleeding may respond to estrogen and desmopressin acetate, which trigger the release of VWF from storage organelles. Therapeutic dosages are monitored using serial VWF:Ag assays. Desmopressin acetate (1-desamino-8-D arginine vasopressin) is an antidiuretic hormone analog used to control incontinence in diabetes mellitus and bedwetting; release of VWF from storage organelles is a side effect. Desmopressin acetate in its oral form, DDAVP, or oral spray form, Stimate (both from Behring), is consistently effective for type 1 and subtype 2M VWD and generally useful for subtype 2A. It is contraindicated for subtype 2B, however, because it releases abnormal VWF with increased affinity for platelet GPIb/IX/V receptors, which may intensify thrombocytopenia and lead to increased platelet activation and consumption. Because of its antidiuretic property, repeated doses may lead to hyponatremia (low serum sodium). For this reason, it is necessary to monitor and regulate electrolytes during desmopressin acetate therapy.

The lysine analogs ε-aminocaproic acid (EACA; Amicar, Akorn Pharmaceuticals) and tranexamic acid (TXA, Pfizer) inhibit fibrinolysis and may help control bleeding when used alone or in conjunction with desmopressin acetate. Therapy using nonbiologic preparations is preferred over human plasma-derived biologic therapy because nonbiologics eliminate the risk of viral disease transmission and circumvent religious objections to receipt of human blood products.

For treatment of severe VWD (type 3) and subtype 2B, three commercially prepared human plasma-derived high-purity preparations are available that provide a mixture of VWF and coagulation FVIII: Humate-P, Alphanate, and Wilate.[125] The calculation of the proper dosage follows principles identical to those used for treatment of hemophilia A provided in the next section. Laboratory monitoring by the VWF:Ag assay is essential to determine whether the given amount produced the target level of VWF and to follow its degradation between doses.[126]

Vonvendi (Shire; US FDA cleared in 2015), is a recombinant VWF that provides no accompanying factor VIII. The initial Vonvendi dose is 40 to 80 IU/kg body weight every 8 to 24 hours, adjusted to the extent of continued bleeding or the target VWF:Ag concentration. If the baseline factor VIII concentration is less than 40 IU/dL, physicians give recombinant VWF-free factor VIII within 10 minutes of completing Vonvendi infusion at a ratio of 1.3:1.

Recombinant and affinity-purified factor VIII concentrates contain no VWF and cannot be used to treat VWD. Cryoprecipitate and plasma are less desirable alternatives because of the risk of virus transmission, and the necessary plasma volume per dose may cause TACO. Therapy for bleeding secondary to acquired VWD follows the same principles as delineated previously, plus treatment of the primary disease, if applicable. Therapeutic recommendations for VWD are summarized in Table 36.6.

TABLE 36.6 Therapeutic Strategies in von Willebrand Disease

Type	Primary Approach	Other Options
1	Estrogen, DDAVP, EACA, or TXA	Factor VIII/VWF concentrate
2A	Estrogen, DDAVP, EACA, or TXA	Factor VIII/VWF concentrate
2B	Factor VIII/VWF concentrate	EACA
2M	Estrogen, DDAVP, EACA, or TXA	Factor VIII/VWF concentrate
2N	Factor VIII concentrate	EACA
3	Factor VIII/VWF concentrate	Platelet transfusions

DDAVP, Desmopressin acetate; *EACA*, ε-aminocaproic acid; *TXA*, tranexamic acid; *VWF*, von Willebrand factor.

Hemophilia A (Factor VIII Deficiency)

The hemophilias are congenital single-factor deficiencies marked by anatomic soft tissue bleeding. Second to VWD in prevalence among congenital bleeding disorders, hemophilias occur in 1 in 8000 individuals, mostly males. Of those affected, 85% are deficient in factor VIII, 14% are deficient in factor IX, and 1% are deficient in factor XI or one of the other coagulation factors, such as factors II (prothrombin), V, VII, X, or XIII. Congenital deficiency of factor VIII is called classic hemophilia or hemophilia A.[127]

Factor VIII Structure and Function

Factor VIII (FVIII) is a two-chain, 285,000-Dalton protein translated from the X chromosome.[128] When the coagulation cascade is activated, thrombin cleaves plasma FVIII and releases a large polypeptide called the *B domain* that dissociates from the molecule. This leaves behind a calcium-dependent heterodimer that detaches from its VWF carrier molecule to bind phosphatidyl serine and factor IXa. The VIIIa/IXa complex, sometimes called the *tenase complex,* cleaves and activates coagulation factor X at a rate 10,000 times faster than free factor IXa can cleave factor X (Figure 36.5). Consequently, FVIII deficiency significantly slows the coagulation pathway's production of thrombin and leads to hemorrhage. FVIII deteriorates in storage. Donor blood collected in standard citrate-dextrose-phosphate preservative provides 30 units/dL FVIII activity after 28 days' storage or approximately 50 units/dL in leukodepleted donor blood.[129]

Hemophilia A Genetics

The gene for FVIII spans 186 kilobases of the X chromosome and is the site of various deletions, stop codons, and nonsense and missense mutations. Most of these mutations result in quantitative disorders in which the FVIII coagulant activity and antigen concentration match, but in rare cases, low activity is seen despite normal antigen concentration.[130] The latter cases are due to qualitative or structural FVIII abnormalities traditionally known as cross-reacting material positive disorders.[131]

Male hemizygotes, whose sole X chromosome contains a FVIII gene mutation, experience anatomic bleeding, but female heterozygotes, who are carriers, do not. When a female carrier has children with an unaffected man, the chances of hemophilia A inheritance are a 25% chance of a normal daughter, 25% chance of a carrier daughter, 25% chance of a normal son, and

Vascular injury

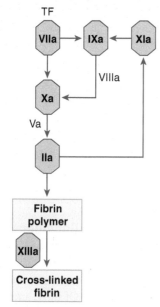

Thrombus

Figure 36.5 Factor Deficiencies that Cause Bleeding Disorders. All the coagulation factors whose absence is related to hemorrhage are depicted in this simplified diagram of the mechanism of the coagulation cascade. *TF,* tissue factor.

25% chance of a hemophilic son. All sons of men with hemophilia A and non-carrier women are normal, whereas all daughters are obligate carriers of the disease.[132] In addition, approximately 30% of newly diagnosed cases arise as a result of spontaneous germline mutations in individuals who have no family history of hemophilia A.[133] Rarely, the symptoms of hemophilia A may be seen in females. This phenomenon could be due to true homozygosity or double heterozygosity, such as in the female offspring of a hemophilic father and a carrier mother. Other possibilities include a spontaneous germline mutation in the otherwise normal allele of a heterozygous female or a disproportional inactivation of the X chromosome with the normal gene, termed extreme lyonization. Finally, VWD of the Normandy (2N) subtype may mimic hemophilia A in males and females.

Hemophilia A Clinical Manifestations

Hemophilia A causes anatomic bleeds with deep muscle and joint hemorrhages; hematomas; wound oozing after trauma or surgery; and bleeding into the central nervous system, peritoneum, gastrointestinal tract, and kidneys. Acute joint bleeds (hemarthroses) are exquisitely painful and cause temporary immobilization. Chronic joint bleeds cause inflammation and eventual permanent loss of mobility, whereas bleeding into muscles may cause nerve compression injury, with first temporary and then lasting disability. Cranial bleeds lead to severe, debilitating, and durable neurologic symptoms, such as loss of memory, paralysis, seizures, and coma, and may be rapidly fatal. Bleeding may begin immediately after a triggering event or may become manifest after a delay of several hours. Some bleeding seems to be spontaneous.

The diagnosis of hemophilia A begins with laboratory testing after the birth of an infant to a mother who has a family history of hemophilia. In the absence of a family history, abnormal bleeding in the neonatal period, which may appear as easy bruising, bleeding from the umbilical stump, postcircumcision bleeding, hematuria, or intracranial bleeding, is considered suspicious for hemophilia. Severe hemophilia usually is diagnosed in the first year of life, whereas mild hemophilia may not become apparent until a triggering event such as trauma, surgery, or dental extraction occurs in late childhood, adolescence, or adulthood.

The laboratory diagnosis of coagulopathies in the newborn or older infant is complicated by the requirement for an unhemolyzed specimen of at least 2 mL in volume from tiny veins and by the predictably low newborn levels of some coagulation factors. Medical laboratory practitioners expect the PT and PTT to be prolonged because of physiologically low levels of factors II (prothrombin), VII, IX, and X, even in full-term infants. However, normal infant FVIII levels are similar to adult levels, even in infants who are born prematurely; this allows skillful laboratory staff to provide the correct diagnosis of hemophilia A using a FVIII activity assay.

The severity of hemophilia A symptoms is inversely proportional to FVIII activity. Laboratory professionals classify an activity level of less than 1 unit/dL as severe, associated with spontaneous or exaggerated bleeding in the neonatal period. Activity levels of 1 unit/dL to 5 units/dL are seen in moderate hemophilia, which is usually diagnosed in early childhood after symptoms become apparent. In mild hemophilia, with activity levels of 5 to 40 units/dL, hemorrhage follows significant trauma and becomes a risk factor mainly in surgery or dental extractions. Patients may go for long periods without symptoms.

Hemophilia A Complications

As a result of frequent bleeds, hemophilia patients often experience debilitating and progressive musculoskeletal lesions and deformities and neurologic deficiencies subsequent to intracranial hemorrhage. In addition, other chronic disease effects, such as limited productivity, low self-esteem, poverty, drug dependency, and depression, are common problems. Before the advent of sterilized and recombinant factor concentrates, chronic hepatitis often resulted from repeated exposure to blood products. Tragically, 70% of hemophilics treated before 1984 are human immunodeficiency virus (HIV) positive or have died from acquired immunodeficiency syndrome.[134]

Hemophilia A Laboratory Diagnosis

The laboratory workup for a suspected congenital single coagulation factor deficiency starts with the PT, PTT, the fibrinogen assay, and TT and continues with specific clot-based factor assays based on the results of the initial tests. Before the physician initiates laboratory testing, however, he or she records a history of the patient's hemorrhagic symptoms and those of the patient's first-degree relatives, if available. In hemophilia A and B, the PT, fibrinogen, and TT are likely to be normal and the PTT prolonged, provided that the PTT reagent is sensitive to factor

TABLE 36.7 Results of Clot-Based Assays in Congenital Single-Factor Deficiencies*

Deficient Factor	PT	PTT	TT	Reflex Test
Fibrinogen	Prolonged	Prolonged	Prolonged	Fibrinogen assay
Prothrombin	Prolonged	Prolonged	Normal	Prothrombin, V, VII, and X assays
V	Prolonged	Prolonged	Normal	Prothrombin, V, VII, and X assays
VII	Prolonged	Normal	Normal	VII assay
VIII	Normal	Prolonged	Normal	VIII, IX, and XI assays
IX	Normal	Prolonged	Normal	VIII, IX, and XI assays
X	Prolonged	Prolonged	Normal	Prothrombin, V, VII, and X assays
XI	Normal	Prolonged	Normal	VIII, IX, and XI assays
XIII	Normal	Normal	Normal	XIII quantitative assay

PT, Prothrombin time; *PTT*, partial thromboplastin time; *TT*, thrombin clotting time.
*Results are valid when the patient is not being treated with coagulation factors or anticoagulants. Results may vary in response to reagent sensitivities.

VIII and factor IX deficiencies at or less than the 40 units/dL plasma activity level. Table 36.7 lists the expected results for each clot-based screening assay for any single-factor deficiency associated with bleeding, including deficiencies of fibrinogen and factors II (prothrombin), V, VII, VIII, IX, X, and XI. Clot-based factor VIII and factor IX assays may soon be replaced with chromogenic factor VIII and factor IX assays, which offer greater accuracy and precision. Deficiencies of contact factors (factor XII, high-molecular-weight kininogen, and prekallikrein) have no relationship to bleeding, and these factors do not appear in Table 36.7.

Hemophilia A Carrier Detection

Approximately 90% of female carriers of hemophilia A are detected by measuring the ratio of FVIII activity to VWF:Ag concentration (FVIII to VWF:Ag). This ratio is effective because VWF production is unaffected by FVIII deficiency. Using a ratio, rather than a FVIII assay value alone, normalizes for some of the physiologic variables that affect FVIII activity and VWF:Ag assays, such as estrogen levels, inflammation, physical stress, and exercise.

The laboratory professional establishes a reference interval for the FVIII to VWF:Ag ratio using plasmas from at least 30 women who are not carriers. If the ratio of the individual being tested is below the lower limit of the interval, she is likely to be a carrier. These results may be influenced by excessive lyonization, variation in VWF production, and analytical variables; consequently, if carrier status is suspected and the FVIII to VWF:Ag ratio is greater than the lower limit of the reference interval, genetic testing may be necessary to detect one of the many polymorphisms associated with FVIII deficiency.[135]

Hemophilia A Therapy

Like VWD sufferers, many mild to moderate hemophilia patients' FVIII activity rises upon on-demand self-administration of the non-biologic oral desmopressin acetate (DDAVP) or oral spray Stimate (Behring), which may be administered in combination with an antifibrinolytic such as ε-aminocaproic acid or tranexamic acid under physician supervision. If these approaches are unsuccessful, as in severe hemophilia, the patient turns to coagulation factor concentrates.

Human plasma-derived FVIII (pdFVIII) concentrates are available worldwide. Products include Alphanate (Grifols), Hemofil-M (Shire), Kogenate FS (Bayer), Humate-P (Behring), and Wilate (Octapharma). These are prepared from healthy plasma donors using chemical fractionation. They are processed using immunoaffinity columns, pasteurization, and the addition of solvent-detergent. All pdFVIII concentrates undergo viral inactivation, and since 1985, none has transmitted lipid-envelope viruses such as HIV, hepatitis B virus, or hepatitis C virus. The pdFVIIIs, however, may transmit non-lipid viruses such as parvovirus B19 and hepatitis A virus. Alphanate, Humate-P, and Wilate contain VWF, fibrinogen, and noncoagulant proteins in addition to FVIII and are used to treat VWD. The human plasma-derived factor concentrates have traditionally been employed for *on-demand* therapy.[136]

The goal of on-demand hemophilia A treatment is to raise the patient's FVIII activity to hemostatic levels whenever he experiences or suspects a bleed or anticipates a hemostatic challenge such as tooth extraction or surgery. The target activity level depends on the nature of the bleed or the bleeding risks of the procedure, but it is seldom necessary to reach activity greater than 75 units/dL. Target activity should be maintained until the threat is resolved. In the case of a bleed into soft tissue or a body cavity, the sooner the target factor level is reached, the less painful the episode, and the less likely the patient is to experience inflammation or nerve damage. Because FVIII has a half-life of 8 to 12 hours, twice-a-day infusions may be required.

In industrialized countries, 75% of hemophilia therapy relies on recombinant FVIII (rFVIII) concentrates. The first rFVIII products employed human or animal serum and albumin in their manufacturing process, thus continuing to carry the theoretical risk of viral disease transmission. These remain available as Helixate FS (Behring), Kogenate FS (Bayer), and Recombinate and Bioclate (Shire). However, manufacturers now provide rFVIII products free of all human protein, such as Advate (Shire). Additionally, deleting the large central B domain shortens rFVIII molecules, in the hope of rendering the molecule less immunogenic. The B-domain-deleted (BDD-rFVIII) preparations are ReFacto, which is produced using Chinese hamster ovary (CHO) cells grown in human albumin, and Xyntha, produced using CHO cells grown in synthetic, albumin-free culture medium.[137] Both ReFacto and Xyntha are produced by Wyeth Pharmaceuticals and distributed by Pfizer.

Because of the availability of abundant rFVIII in industrialized nations, most hemophilia patients use prophylactic regimens, administering approximately three infusions per week to maintain their FVIII activity at hemostatic levels.[138] The prophylactic approach conserves downstream resources and promotes better health by ameliorating the short- and long-term adverse effects of repeated hemorrhages.[139]

In 2014 Biogen introduced the first extended half-life rFVIII, Eloctate, a BDD-rFVIII fused with the Fc region of human immunoglobulin G1 (BDD-rFVIIIFc). The Fc fragment binds the in vivo neonatal Fc receptor, FcRn, extending the plasma half-life to nearly 20 hours and reducing the infusion frequency to once every 4 to 5 days.[140] Although the manufacturer makes no claims, Eloctate triggered no inhibitor formation during its clinical trials. Eloctate is now distributed by Sanofi.

In 2016 the US FDA approved Adynovate (Shire), a recombinant full-length rFVIII covalently conjugated with polyethylene glycol (PEG, "PEGylated" rFVIII). PEGylation is used in many drug applications; it extends the rFVIII half-life to approximately 20 hours and reduces the infusion rate to approximately twice weekly. During clinical trials, Adynovate triggered only transient inhibitors; however, the manufacturer makes no claims about inhibitor formation frequency.[141]

In 2016 the US FDA also approved Afstyla (Behring), a full-length single-chain rFVIII. Clinical trial data imply that Afstyla binds VWF with greater avidity than two-chain rFVIII formulations, resulting in extended half-life and induction of fewer inhibitors.[142] Afstyla is the third extended half-life rFVIII formulation, "rFVIII-SingleChain," that claims to closely resemble native FVIII. The one-stage clot-based FVIII assay recovers approximately 50% of Afstyla dosage, so the manufacturer recommends doubling the result, or using a chromogenic FVIII assay.

The extended half-life rFVIII formulations, be they single-chain, Fc-conjugated, or PEGylated, ultimately owe their pharmacokinetics to their "dominant partner," VWF, whose half-life of 12 to 15 hours determines their ultimate plasma life span.[143] Nevertheless, even a reduction by one infusion per week and the hint of fewer instances of inhibitor formation is attractive to hemophilic boys and their parents and caregivers.

When hematologists treat hemophilia, they base FVIII concentrate dosage calculations on the definition of an international unit (IU) of FVIII activity, which is the global mean activity present in 1 mL of normal plasma and is synonymous with 100 units/dL. They further calculate the desired increase subsequent to FVIII concentrate infusion by subtracting the patient's preinfusion factor activity from the target activity level.

The desired increase is multiplied by the patient's plasma volume to compute the dosage. The patient's plasma volume may be estimated from blood volume and hematocrit.[144] The blood volume is approximately 65 mL/kg of body weight, and the plasma volume is the "plasmacrit" (100% − hematocrit %) × blood volume. FVIII concentrate dose may be computed using the following pair of formulas:

$$\text{Plasma volume} = \text{weight in kilograms} \times 65 \text{ mL/kg} \times (1 - \text{hematocrit})$$

$$\text{FVIII concentrate dose} = \text{plasma volume} \times (\text{target FVIII level} - \text{initial FVIII level})$$

This formula may also be used to treat VWD; however, in all cases of hemophilia or VWD therapy, the product package insert formula takes precedence. There exists anecdotal evidence associating FVIII overdose with thrombosis, although the key reason for careful dosage calculation is to conserve FVIII resources.[145] No matter the formulation, FVIII pharmacokinetics vary by patient age and condition, so regardless of the dose administered, laboratory monitoring and close clinical observation are essential to predict administration frequency and therapeutic efficacy. Regrettably, the time-honored but imprecise one-stage clot-based assay does not accurately measure BDD-rFVIII or the extended half-life rFVIII formulations.[146] In vitro diagnostics manufacturers are currently developing new chromogenic factor assays to meet this clinical need.[147]

Hemophilia A and FVIII Inhibitors

Alloantibody inhibitors of FVIII arise in response to treatment in 30% of patients with severe hemophilia and 3% of those with moderate hemophilia.[148] The laboratory practitioner suspects the presence of an inhibitor when bleeding persists or when the plasma FVIII activity fails to rise to the target level after appropriately dosed concentrate administration. Most FVIII inhibitors are immunoglobulin G4, non-complement-fixing, warm-reacting antibodies. It is impossible to predict which patients are likely to develop inhibitors based on genetics, demographics, or the type of concentrate used.[148]

The first step in inhibitor detection is a one-stage clot-based FVIII assay. If the FVIII activity exceeds 30 units/dL, no inhibitor is present. If the level is less than 30 units/dL, the laboratory practitioner proceeds to perform mixing studies. Some hemostasis laboratory directors use 40 units/dL as the limit. When plasma from the bleeding patient produces a prolonged PTT, it is mixed 1:1 with NP, incubated 2 hours at 37° C, and the PTT of the mixture is measured. If no inhibitor is present, the incubated mixture should produce a PTT result within 10% of the incubated NP PTT. If an inhibitor is present, however, the FVIII from the NP is partially neutralized and the mixture's PTT remains prolonged or "uncorrected," presumptive evidence for the inhibitor.

If mixing studies and the therapeutic results suggest the presence of a FVIII inhibitor, the Nijmegen-Bethesda assay is used to quantitate the inhibitor. NP providing 100 units/dL factor activity is mixed at increasing dilutions (decreasing concentrations) in a series of tubes with the full-strength patient plasma. FVIII assays are performed on each mixture. The operator then compares the results of the various dilutions and expresses the titer as Nijmegen-Bethesda units (NBUs). One NBU is the reciprocal of the dilution that caused neutralization of 50% of the NP FVIII. The same assay is employed to measure FVIII inhibitors in acquired hemophilia. Although the complex kinetics of acquired autoantibodies diminishes the accuracy of the results in acquired hemophilia, this method adequately monitors therapy.

Hemophilia patients with inhibitors are classified as *low* or *high responders*. Low responders generate inhibitor titers of 5 NBUs or less and their inhibitor titers do not increase significantly after FVIII administration. High responders generate inhibitor titers that exceed 5 NBUs and their antibody titers further rise in response to therapy. Each laboratory director may choose to maintain a database of hemophilia patients who have inhibitors because previous titers often predict future inhibitor behavior.

Hemophilia A Treatment in Patients with Inhibitors

Every hemophilic patient with an inhibitor needs an individualized treatment plan to control bleeding episodes. Low responders often experience cessation of bleeding on administration of large doses of FVIII concentrate and may be so maintained. High responders may gain no benefit from FVIII concentrates and instead are treated with activated PCC (Autoplex T or FEIBA), or rFVIIa (NovoSeven), all of which generate thrombin despite the presence of FVIII inhibitors. The activated PCC dosage should not exceed 200 units/kg per day, distributed in two to four injections, because the activated factors may trigger DIC. NovoSeven also bypasses the physiologic FVIII requirement because it promotes thrombin formation through the tissue factor pathway. Emicizumab (HemLibra, Genentech), US FDA approved November 2017, is a "factor VIII mimetic" bispecific antibody that bypasses factor VIII by binding factor X with IXa. Hemophilic boys older than 12 with inhibitors used subcutaneous prophylactic HemLibra once a week and experienced 2.3 bleeds per year, an 80% reduction.[149] HemLibra is also available for hemophilics who have no inhibitors.

Hemophilia B (Factor IX Deficiency)

Hemophilia B, also called *Christmas disease*, totals approximately 14% of hemophilia cases in the United States, although its incidence in India nearly equals that of hemophilia A. Hemophilia B is caused by deficiency of factor IX (FIX), one of the vitamin K-dependent serine proteases. Factor IX is a substrate for both factors XIa and VIIa because it is cleaved by either to form dimeric factor IXa (Figure 36.5). Subsequently, factor IXa complexes with factor VIIIa to cleave and activate its substrate, factor X (FX). FIX deficiency reduces thrombin production and causes soft tissue anatomic bleeding that is indistinguishable from that in hemophilia A. It also is a sex-linked, markedly heterogeneous disorder involving numerous separate mutations resulting in a range of mild to severe bleeding manifestations. Determination of female carrier status is less successful in hemophilia B than in hemophilia A because of the large number of factor IX mutations and the lack of a linked molecule such as VWF that can be used as a normalization index. DNA analysis occasionally may be used to establish carrier status when hemophilia B has been diagnosed and its specific mutation identified in a relative.[150]

The laboratory is essential to the diagnosis of hemophilia B. The PTT typically is prolonged, whereas the PT, fibrinogen assay, and TT are normal. If the clinical symptoms suggest hemophilia B, the factor IX assay should be performed even if PTT is within the reference range, because the PTT reagent may be insensitive to factor IX deficiencies at the level of 30 units/dL.

Immunine (Shire) and Mononine (Behring) are plasma-derived, immunopurified FIX concentrates. When applied to on-demand therapy, dosing is calculated the same way as for FVIII concentrates in hemophilia A, except that the calculated initial dose is doubled to compensate for FIX distribution into the extravascular space. Repeat doses of FIX are given every 24 hours, reflecting the half-life of the factor. The second and subsequent doses, if needed, are half the initial dose, provided that factor assays determine that the target level of FIX was achieved. It is necessary to monitor therapy with recurring laboratory assays, because FIX pharmacokinetics are idiosyncratic.

BeneFix (Pfizer) is a recombinant FIX concentrate (rFIX) grown in CHO cells in the absence of human or animal protein. The abundance of rFIX concentrates supports prophylactic administration at a rate of 2 to 3 infusions per week. Two extended half-life preparations are the Fc-fusion Alprolix (rFIX-Fc, Sanofi) and albumin-fusion Idelvion (Behring). These preparations may extend prophylactic factor administration to as seldom as once every 2 weeks.

FIX therapy may be measured using the one-stage clot assay; however, chromogenic assays with improved accuracy, low-level sensitivity, and reproducibility are in development.[151]

FIX inhibitors arise in 3% of hemophilia B patients, bind avidly with FIX, and may be detected using the Nijmegen-Bethesda assay. Bleeding in patients with inhibitors is treated as in patients with FVIII inhibitors using activated PCC or rFVIIa and immunomodulation therapy.[152]

Hemophilia C (Rosenthal Syndrome, Factor XI Deficiency)

Factor XI (FXI) deficiency is an autosomal dominant hemophilia with mild to moderate bleeding symptoms.[153] More than half of the cases have been described in Ashkenazi Jews, but individuals of any ethnic group may be affected. The frequency and severity of bleeding episodes do not correlate with factor XI levels, and laboratory monitoring of treatment serves little purpose after the diagnosis is established. The physician treats hemophilia C with frequent plasma infusions during bleeds and times of hemostatic challenge. In the laboratory the PTT is prolonged and the PT is normal (Figure 36.5).

Other Congenital Single-Factor Deficiencies

The remaining congenital single-factor deficiencies listed in Table 36.8 are rare, are caused by autosomal recessive mutations, and are often associated with consanguinity. The PT, PTT, and TT may be employed to distinguish among these disorders, as shown in Table 36.7 (Figure 36.5). In addition, immunoassays may be performed to distinguish among the more prevalent quantitative and the less prevalent qualitative abnormalities. In qualitative disorders, often called dysproteinemias, the ratio of factor activity to antigen is less than 0.7. The bleeding symptoms in the dysproteinemias may be more severe than in quantitative deficiencies, but the risk of inhibitor formation is theoretically smaller. The clot-based measurement of factors II (prothrombin) and X may be supplemented or replaced by more reproducible chromogenic substrate assays. Fibrinogen is usually measured using the Clauss clot-based assay, a modification of the thrombin time, but it also may be measured by turbidimetry or immunoassay.

TABLE 36.8   Rare Congenital Single-Factor Deficiencies

Deficiency	Factor Levels	Symptoms	Therapy
Afibrinogenemia	No measurable fibrinogen	Severe anatomic bleeding	CRYO or FG concentrate to raise to >100 mg/dL
Hypofibrinogenemia	FG activity assay <100 mg/dL	Moderate systemic bleeding	CRYO or FG concentrate to raise to >100 mg/dL
Dysfibrinogenemia	FG activity assay <100 mg/dL	Mild systemic bleeding	CRYO or FG concentrate to control bleeding. Treat underlying cause such as liver disease
Prothrombin deficiency	Factor II < 30 units/dL	Mild systemic bleeding	PCC or plasma to raise factor II to 75 units/dL
Factor V deficiency	Factor V < 30 units/dL	Mild systemic bleeding	Platelet concentrate or plasma to raise factor V to 75 units/dL
Factor VII deficiency	Factor VII < 30 units/dL	Moderate to severe anatomic bleeding	NovoSeven, PCC, four-factor PCC, plasma to raise factor VII to 75 units/dL
Factor X deficiency	Factor X < 30 units/dL	Severe anatomic bleeding	PCC or plasma to raise factor X to 75 units/dL
Factor XI deficiency	Factor XI < 50 units/dL	Variable anatomic bleeding	Plasma to raise factor XI to 75 units/dL
Factor XIII deficiency	Factor XIII < 1 units/dL	Moderate to severe systemic bleeding, poor wound healing	Plasma or CRYO every 3 weeks

CRYO, Cryoprecipitate; *FG,* fibrinogen; *PCC,* prothrombin complex concentrate.

Because platelets transport about 20% of circulating factor V, the platelet function in *factor V deficiency* may be diminished, which is reflected in a prolonged bleeding time test but normal platelet aggregation. The PT and PTT are prolonged. Because of the concentration of factor V in platelet α-granules, platelet concentrate is an effective form of therapy for factor V deficiency. A combined factor V and VIII deficiency may be caused by a genetic defect traced to chromosome 18 that affects transport of both factors by a common protein in the Golgi apparatus.[154]

Factor VII deficiency causes moderate to severe anatomic hemorrhage.[155] The bleeding does not necessarily reflect the factor VII activity level. The half-life of factor VII is approximately 6 hours, which affects the frequency of therapy. NovoSeven at 30 μg/mL and non-activated four-factor PCC preparations are effective and may provide a target factor VII level of 10 units/dL to 30 units/dL. Many factor VII deficiencies are dysproteinemias. The PT, but not the PTT, is prolonged in factor VII deficiency.

Factor X deficiency causes moderate to severe anatomic hemorrhage that may be treated with plasma or non-activated PCC to produce therapeutic levels of 10 units/dL to 40 units/dL.[156] The half-life of factor X is 24 to 40 hours. Acquired factor X deficiency has been described in amyloidosis, in paraproteinemia, and in association with antifungal drug therapy. The hemorrhagic symptoms may be life threatening. The PT and PTT are both prolonged in factor X deficiency. In the *Russell viper venom time* test, which activates the coagulation mechanism at the level of factor X, clotting time is prolonged in deficiencies of factors X and V, prothrombin, and fibrinogen. The venom used is harvested from the Russell viper, the most dangerous snake in Asia. This test may be useful in distinguishing a factor VII deficiency, which does not prolong the Russell viper venom clotting time, from deficiencies in the common pathway, although specific factor assays are the standard approach.

Plasma *factor XIII* is a tetramer of paired α and β monomers. The intracellular form is a homodimer (two α chains) and is stored in platelets, monocytes, placenta, prostate, and uterus. The α chain contains the active enzyme site, and the β chain is a binding and stabilizing portion. Factor XIII deficiency occurs in three forms related to the affected chain, as shown in Table 36.9. Patients with factor XIII deficiency have a normal PT, PTT, and TT despite anatomic bleeds and poor wound healing. They form weak (non-cross-linked) clots that dissolve within 2 hours when suspended in a 5-molar urea solution, a traditional factor XIII screening assay. To confirm factor XIII deficiency, factor activity may be measured accurately using a chromogenic substrate assay such as the Behrichrom FXIII assay (Behring).

Finally, autosomally inherited deficiencies of the *fibrinolytic regulatory proteins* α₂-antiplasmin and plasminogen activator inhibitor-1 (PAI-1) have been reported to cause moderate to severe bleeding. Both are rare and may be diagnosed using chromogenic substrate assays.

TABLE 36.9   Factor XIII Deficiency

Type of Deficiency	Incidence	Factor XIII Activity	β-Protein	α-Protein
Type I	Rare	Absent	Absent	Absent
Type II	Infrequent	Absent	Normal	Low
Type III	Rare	Low	Absent	Low

▮ SUMMARY

- Hemorrhage is classified as localized versus generalized, acquired versus congenital, and anatomic soft tissue hemorrhage versus systemic mucocutaneous hemorrhage.

- Acquired hemorrhagic disorders that are diagnosed in the hemostasis laboratory include thrombocytopenia of various etiologies (Chapter 38), the acute coagulopathy of trauma-shock, anemia, liver and renal disease, vitamin K deficiency, acquired hemophilia or von Willebrand disease (VWD), and disseminated intravascular coagulation (DIC).

- VWD is the most common congenital bleeding disorder, and the diagnosis and classification of the type and subtypes require a series of clinical laboratory assays.
- The hemophilias are congenital single-factor deficiencies that cause moderate to severe anatomic hemorrhage. The clinical laboratory plays a key role in diagnosis, classification, and treatment monitoring in hemophilia.

Now that you have completed this chapter, go back and read again the case study at the beginning and respond to the questions presented.

REVIEW QUESTIONS

Answers can be found in the Appendix.

1. What is the most common acquired bleeding disorder?
   a. Trauma-induced coagulopathy
   b. Vitamin K deficiency
   c. Liver disease
   d. VWD
2. Which is a typical form of anatomic bleeding?
   a. Epistaxis
   b. Menorrhagia
   c. Hematemesis
   d. Central nervous system bleed
3. What factor becomes deficient early in liver disease, and what assay does its deficiency prolong?
   a. Prothrombin deficiency, the PT
   b. Factor VII deficiency, the PT
   c. FVIII deficiency, the PTT
   d. Factor IX deficiency, the PTT
4. Which of the following conditions causes a prolonged thrombin time?
   a. Antithrombin deficiency
   b. Prothrombin deficiency
   c. Hypofibrinogenemia
   d. Warfarin therapy
5. In what type or subtype of VWD is the RIPA test result positive when ristocetin is used at a concentration of less than 0.5 mg/mL?
   a. Subtype 2A
   b. Subtype 2B
   c. Subtype 2N
   d. Type 3
6. What is the typical treatment for vitamin K deficiency when the patient is bleeding?
   a. Vitamin K and plasma
   b. Vitamin K and four-factor PCC
   c. Vitamin K and platelet concentrate
   d. Vitamin K and FVIII concentrate

7. If a patient has anatomic soft tissue bleeding and poor wound healing, but the PT, PTT, TT, platelet count, and platelet functional assay results are normal, what factor deficiency is possible?
   a. Fibrinogen
   b. Prothrombin
   c. Factor XII
   d. Factor XIII
8. What therapy may be used for a hemophilic boy who is bleeding and who has a high FVIII inhibitor titer?
   a. rFVIIa
   b. Plasma
   c. Cryoprecipitate
   d. FVIII concentrate
9. What is the most prevalent form of VWD?
   a. Type 1
   b. Type 2A
   c. Type 2B
   d. Type 3
10. Which of the following assays is used to distinguish vitamin K deficiency from liver disease?
    a. PT
    b. Protein C assay
    c. Factor V assay
    d. Factor VII assay
11. Mucocutaneous hemorrhage is typical of:
    a. Acquired hemorrhagic disorders
    b. Localized hemorrhagic disorders
    c. Defects in primary hemostasis
    d. Defects in fibrinolysis

REFERENCES

1. James, P. D., Mahlangu, J., Bidlingmaier, C., et al. Global Emerging Hemostasis Experts Panel (GEHEP). (2016). Evaluation of the utility of the ISTH-BAT in haemophilia carriers: a multinational study. *Haemophilia, 22,* 912–918.
2. Kessler, C. M. (2013). A systematic approach to the bleeding patient: correlation of clinical symptoms and signs with laboratory testing. In Kitchens, C. S., Kessler, C. M., & Konkle, B. A. (Eds.), *Consultative Hemostasis and Thrombosis.* (3rd ed., pp. 16–32). St. Louis: Elsevier-Saunders.
3. Kitchens, C. S. (2013). Purpura and other hematovascular disorders. In Kitchens, C. S., Kessler, C. M., & Konkle, B. A. (Eds.), *Consultative Hemostasis and Thrombosis.* (3rd ed., pp. 150–173). St. Louis: Elsevier-Saunders.
4. Weiss, A. E. (1988). Acquired coagulation disorders. In Corriveau, D. M., & Fritsma, G. A. (Eds.), *Hemostasis and Thrombosis in the Clinical Laboratory.* (pp. 169–205). Philadelphia: Lippincott.
5. Vanderhave, K. L., Caird, M. S., Hake, M., et al. (2012). Musculoskeletal care of the hemophiliac patient. *J Am Acad Orthop Surg, 20,* 553–563.

6. Adcock, D. M. (2012). Coagulation assays and anticoagulant monitoring. *Hematology 2012, Am Soc Hematol Educ Program*, 460–465.

7. Wikkelsø, A., Wetterslev, J., Møller, A. M., et al. (2017). Thromboelastography (TEG) or rotational thromboelastometry (ROTEM) to monitor haemostatic treatment in bleeding patients: a systematic review with meta-analysis and trial sequential analysis. *Anaesthesia, 72*, 519–531.

8. Chee, Y. L., Crawford, J. C., Watson, H. G., et al. (2008). Guidelines on the assessment of bleeding risk prior to surgery or invasive procedures. British Committee for Standards in Haematology. *Br J Haematol, 140*, 496–504.

9. Fogarty, P. F., & Kessler, C. M. (2013). Hemophilia A and B. In Kitchens, C. S., Kessler, C. M., & Konkle, B. A. (Eds.), *Consultative Hemostasis and Thrombosis*. (3rd ed., pp. 45–59). St. Louis: Elsevier-Saunders.

10. Boffard, K. D., Choog, P. I. T., Kloger, Y., et al. (2009). The treatment of bleeding is to stop the bleeding! Treatment of trauma-related hemorrhage. On behalf of the NovoSeven Trauma Study Group. *Transfusion, 49*, 240S–247S.

11. Centers for Disease Control and Prevention, National Center for Injury Prevention and Control. *Web-based Injury Statistics Query and Reporting System (WISQARS)*. www.cdc.gov/injury/wisqars. Accessed March 18, 2017.

12. Balvers, K., van Dieren, S., Baksaas-Aasen, K., et al. Targeted Action for Curing Trauma-Induced Coagulopathy (TACTIC) Collaborators. (2017). Combined effect of therapeutic strategies for bleeding injury on early survival, transfusion needs and correction of coagulopathy. *Br J Surg, 104*, 222–229.

13. Kumar, M., Cao, W., McDaniel, J. K., et al. (2017). Plasma ADAMTS13 activity and von Willebrand factor antigen and activity in patients with subarachnoid haemorrhage. *Thromb Haemost, 117*, 691–699.

14. Hayakawa, M. (2017). Pathophysiology of trauma-induced coagulopathy: disseminated intravascular coagulation with the fibrinolytic phenotype. *J Intensive Care, 5*, 14. doi:10.1186/s40560-016-0200-1.

15. Frelitz, A. J. (2016). Impacts of updated transfusion guidelines on a small hospital blood bank in a Chicago suburb. *Clin Lab Sci, 29*, 16–20.

16. Savage, S. A., Sumislawski, J. J., Zarzaur, B. L., et al. (2015). The new metric to define large-volume hemorrhage: results of a prospective study of the critical administration threshold. *J Trauma Acute Care Surg, 78*, 224–229.

17. Cantle, P. M., & Cotton, B. A. (2017). Prediction of massive transfusion in trauma. *Crit Care Clin, 33*, 71–84.

18. Novak, D. J., Bai, Y., Cooke, R. K., et al. (2015). Making thawed universal donor plasma available rapidly for massively bleeding trauma patients: experience from the Pragmatic, Randomized Optimal Platelets and Plasma Ratios (PROPPR) trial. *Transfusion, 55*, 1331–1339.

19. Yonge, J. D., & Schreiber, M. A. (2016). The pragmatic randomized optimal platelet and plasma ratios trial: what does it mean for remote damage control resuscitation? *Transfusion, 56*(Suppl. 2), S149–S156.

20. Carson, J. L., Guyatt, G., Heddle, N. M., et al. (2016). Clinical practice guidelines From the AABB: red blood cell transfusion thresholds and storage. *JAMA Online*. jamanetwork.com. Accessed October 20, 2016.

21. Inaba, K., Lustenberger, T., Rhee, P., et al. (2010). The impact of platelet transfusion in massively transfused trauma patients. *J Am Coll Surg, 211*, 573–579.

22. Lu, F. Q., Kang, W., Peng, Y., et al. (2011). Characterization of blood components separated from donated whole blood after an overnight holding at room temperature with the buffy coat method. *Transfusion, 51*, 2199–2207.

23. Benjamin, R. J., & McLaughlin, L. S. (2012). Plasma components: properties, differences, and uses. *Transfusion, 52*(Suppl. 1), 9S–19S.

24. Downes, K. A., Wilson, E., Yomtovian, R., et al. (2001). Serial measurement of clotting factors in thawed plasma stored for five days. *Transfusion, 41*, 570 (letter).

25. Cardigan, R., Lawrie, A. S., Mackie, I. J., et al. (2005). The quality of fresh frozen plasma produced from whole blood stored at 4° C overnight. *Transfusion, 45*, 1342–1348.

26. Chang, R., Cardenas, J. C., Wade, C. E., et al. (2016). Advances in the understanding of trauma-induced coagulopathy. *Blood, 128*, 1043–1049.

27. American Association of Blood Banks, American Red Cross, America's Blood Centers, Armed Service Blood Program. (2013). Circular of Information for the Use of Human Blood and Blood Components. aabb.org/marketplace. Accessed March 19, 2017.

28. Narick, C., Triulzi, D. J., & Yazer, M. H. (2012). Transfusion-associated circulatory overload after plasma transfusion. *Transfusion, 52*, 160–165.

29. Zheng, X. L. (2015). ADAMTS13 and von Willebrand factor in thrombotic thrombocytopenic purpura. *Annu Rev Med, 66*, 211–225.

30. Russell, R.T., McDaniel, J.K., Cao, W., et al. (2018). Low plasma ADAMTS13 activity is associated with coagulopathy, endothelial cell damage and mortality after severe paediatric trauma. *Thromb Haemost, 118*, 676–687.

31. Wójcik, C., Schymik, M. L., & Cure, E. G. (2009). Activated prothrombin complex concentrate FVIII inhibitor bypassing activity (FEIBA) for the reversal of warfarin-induced coagulopathy. *Int J Emerg Med, 2*, 217–225.

32. Ferreira, J., & DeLosSantos, M. (2013). The clinical use of prothrombin complex concentrate. *J Emerg Med, 44*, 1201–1210.

33. Quinlan, D. J., Eikelboom, J. W., & Weitz, J. I. (2013). Four-factor prothrombin complex concentrate for urgent reversal of vitamin K antagonists in patients with major bleeding. *Circulation, 128*, 1179–1181.

34. CRASH-2 trial collaborators. (2010). Effects of tranexamic acid on death, vascular occlusive events, and blood transfusion in trauma patients with significant haemorrhage (CRASH-2): a randomised, placebo-controlled trial. *The Lancet, 376*, 23–32.

35. Maegele, M. (2016). Coagulation factor concentrate-based therapy for remote damage control resuscitation (RDCR): a reasonable alternative? *Transfusion, 56*(Suppl. 2), S157–S165.

36. Winearls, J., Campbell, D., Hurn, C., et al. (2016). Fibrinogen in traumatic haemorrhage: a narrative review. *Injury, 48*, 230–242.

37. Seto, S., Itakura, A., Okagaki, R., et al. (2017). An algorithm for the management of coagulopathy from postpartum hemorrhage, using fibrinogen concentrate as first-line therapy. *Int J Obstet Anesth. 32*, 11-16.

38. Wikkelsø, A., Lunde, J., Johansen, M., et al. (2013). Fibrinogen concentrate in bleeding patients. *Cochrane Database Syst Rev, 8*. doi:10.1002/14651858.CD008864.pub2.

39. WOMAN Trial Collaborators. (2017). Effect of early tranexamic acid administration on mortality, hysterectomy, and other morbidities in women with post-partum haemorrhage (WOMAN): an international, randomised, double-blind, placebo-controlled trial. *Lancet, 389*, 2105–2116.

40. Michiels, J. J., Berneman, Z. N., van der Planken, M., et al. (2004). Bleeding prophylaxis for major surgery in patients with type 2 von Willebrand disease with an intermediate purity FVIII-von Willebrand factor concentrate (Haemate-P). *Blood Coagul Fibrinolysis, 15*, 323–330.

41. Dutton, R. P., Parr, M., Tortella, B. J., et al, CONTROL Study Group. (2011). Recombinant activated factor VII safety in trauma patients: results from the CONTROL trial. *J Trauma, 71,* 12–19.

42. Levi, M., Peters, M., & Buller, H. R. (2005). Efficacy and safety of recombinant factor VIIa for treatment of severe bleeding: a systematic review. *Crit Care Med, 33,* 883–890.

43. Tatoulis, J., Theodore, S., Meswani, M., et al. (2009). Safe use of recombinant activated factor VIIa for recalcitrant postoperative haemorrhage in cardiac surgery. *Interact Cardiovasc Thorac Surg, 9,* 459–62.

44. da Luz, L. T., Nascimento, B., & Rizoli, S. (2013). Thrombelastography (TEG®): practical considerations on its clinical use in trauma resuscitation. *Scand J Trauma Resusc Emerg Med, 21,* 29. doi:10.1186/1757-7241-21-29.

45. Veigas, P. V., Callum, J., Rizoli, S., et al. (2016). A systematic review on the rotational thromboelastometry (ROTEM®) values for the diagnosis of coagulopathy, prediction and guidance of blood transfusion and prediction of mortality in trauma patients. *Scand J Trauma Resusc Emerg Med, 24*(1), 114-124. doi:10.1186/s13049-016-0308-2.

46. Lisman, T., & Porte, R. J. (2013). Understanding and managing the coagulopathy of liver disease. In Kitchens, C. S., Kessler, C. M., & Konkle, B. A. (Eds.), *Consultative Hemostasis and Thrombosis.* (3rd ed., pp. 688–697). St. Louis: Elsevier-Saunders.

47. Allison, M. G., Shanholtz, C. B., & Sachdeva, A. (2016). Hematological issues in liver disease. *Crit Care Clin, 32,* 385–396.

48. Robert, A., & Chazouilleres, O. (1996). Prothrombin time in liver failure: time, ratio, activity percentage, or international normalized ratio? *Hepatology, 24,* 1392–1394.

49. Lisman, T., Leebeek, F. W., & de Groot, P. G. (2002). Haemostatic abnormalities in patients with liver disease. *J Hepatol, 37,* 280–287.

50. Cunningham, M. T., Brandt, J. T., Laposata, M., et al. (2002). Laboratory diagnosis of dysfibrinogenemia. *Arch Pathol Lab Med, 126,* 499–505.

51. Shao, Z., Zhao, Y., Feng, L., et al. (2015). Association between plasma fibrinogen levels and mortality in acute-on-chronic hepatitis B liver failure. *Dis Markers, 2015,* 468596. doi:10.1155/2015/468596. Accessed March 20, 2017.

52. Hugenholtz, G. C., Adelmeijer, J., Meijers, J. C., et al. (2013). An unbalance between von Willebrand factor and ADAMTS13 in acute liver failure: implications for hemostasis and clinical outcome. *Hepatology, 58,* 752–761.

53. Ferro, D., Quintarelli, C., Lattuada, A., et al. (1996). High plasma levels of von Willebrand factor as a marker of endothelial perturbation in cirrhosis: relationship to endotoxemia. *Hepatology 23,* 1377–1383.

54. Fouad, Y. M. (2013). Chronic hepatitis C-associated thrombocytopenia: aetiology and management. *Trop Gastroenterol, 34,* 58–67.

55. Stravitz, R. T., Ellerbe, C., Durkalski, V., et al. Acute Liver Failure Study Group. (2016). Thrombocytopenia is associated with multi-organ system failure in patients with acute liver failure. *Clin Gastroenterol Hepatol, 14,* 613–620.

56. Violi, F., Basili, S., Raparelli, V., et al. (2011). Patients with liver cirrhosis suffer from primary haemostatic defects? Fact or fiction? *J Hepatol, 55,* 1415–1427.

57. Lisman, T., & Porte, R. J. (2012). Platelet function in patients with cirrhosis. *J Hepatol, 56,* 993–994; author reply 994–5.

58. Bates, S. M. (2012). D-dimer assays in diagnosis and management of thrombotic and bleeding disorders. *Semin Thromb Hemost, 38,* 673–682.

59. Cai, K., Osheroff, W. P., Buczynski, G., et al. (2014). Characterization of Thrombate III®, a pasteurized and nanofiltered therapeutic human antithrombin concentrate. *Biologicals, 42,* 133–138.

60. Wiedermann, C. J., & Kaneider, N. C. (2006). A systematic review of antithrombin concentrate use in patients with disseminated intravascular coagulation of severe sepsis. *Blood Coagul Fibrinolysis, 17,* 521–526.

61. Lambert, M. P. (2016). Platelets in liver and renal disease. *Hematology 2016, Am Soc Hematol Educ Program, (1),* 251–255.

62. Cohen, B. D. (2003). Methyl group deficiency and guanidino production in uremia. *Mol Cell Biochem, 244,* 31–36.

63. Galbusera, M., Remuzzi, G., & Boccardo, P. (2009). Treatment of bleeding in dialysis patients. *Semin Dial, 22,* 279–286.

64. Lind, S. E. (1991). The bleeding time does not predict surgical bleeding. *Blood, 77,* 2547–2552.

65. Showalter, J., Nguyen, N. D., Baba, S., et al. (2016). Platelet aggregometry cannot identify uremic platelet dysfunction in heart failure patients prior to cardiac surgery. *J Clin Lab Anal.* doi:10.1002/jcla.22084. Accessed March 24, 2017.

66. Kahan, B. D. (2008). Fifteen years of clinical studies and clinical practice in renal transplantation: reviewing outcomes with de novo use of sirolimus in combination with cyclosporine. *Transplant Proc, 40,* S17–S20.

67. Knehtl, M., Ponikvar, R., & Buturovic-Ponikvar, J. (2013). Platelet-related hemostasis before and after hemodialysis with five different anticoagulation methods. *Int J Artif Organs, 36,* 717–724.

68. Daugirdas, J. T., & Bernardo, A. A. (2012). Hemodialysis effect on platelet count and function and hemodialysis-associated thrombocytopenia. *Kidney Int, 82,* 147–157.

69. Torres, V. E. (2008). Vasopressin antagonists in polycystic kidney disease. *Semin Nephrol, 28,* 306–317.

70. Khanna, R. (2011). Clinical presentation and management of glomerular diseases: hematuria, nephritic and nephrotic syndrome. *Mo Med, 108,* 33–36.

71. DiNicolantonio, J. J., Bhutani, J., & O'Keefe, J. H. (2015). The health benefits of vitamin K. *Open Heart, 2,* e000300. doi:10.1136/openhrt-2015-000300.

72. Bolan, C. D., & Klein, H. G. (2013). Blood component and pharmacologic therapy for hemostatic disorders. In Kitchens, C. S., Kessler, C. M., & Konkle, B. A. (Eds.), *Consultative Hemostasis and Thrombosis.* (3rd ed., pp. 496–525). St. Louis: Elsevier-Saunders.

73. Burke, C. W. (2013). Vitamin K deficiency bleeding: overview and considerations. *J Pediatr Health Care, 27,* 215–221.

74. Patriquin, C., & Crowther, M. (2013). Antithrombotic agents. In Kitchens, C. S., Kessler, C. M., & Konkle, B. A. (Eds.), *Consultative Hemostasis and Thrombosis.* (3rd ed., pp. 477–495). St. Louis: Elsevier-Saunders.

75. Misra, D., Bednar, M., Cromwell, C., et al. (2010). Manifestations of superwarfarin ingestion: a plea to increase awareness. *Am J Hematol, 85,* 391–392.

76. Martin, D. T., Barton, C. A., Dodgion, C., et al. (2016). Emergent reversal of vitamin K antagonists: addressing all the factors. *Am J Surg, 211,* 919–925.

77. Kershaw, G., Jayakodi, D., & Dunkley, S. (2009). Laboratory identification of factor inhibitors: the perspective of a large tertiary hemophilia center. *Semin Thromb Hemost, 35,* 760–768.

78. Franchini, M., Vaglio, S., Marano, G., et al. (2017). Acquired hemophilia A: a review of recent data and new therapeutic options. *Hematology, 22*(9), 514-520.

79. Franchini, M., & Mannucci, P. M. (2013). Acquired haemophilia A: a 2013 update. *Thromb Haemost, 110,* 111–20.

80. Kruse-Jarres, R., Kempton, C. L., Baudo, F., et al. (2017). Acquired hemophilia A: updated review of evidence and treatment guidance. *Am J Hematol, 92*(7), 695–705.

81. Biggs, R., Austen, D. E. G., Denson, D. W. E., et al. (1972). The mode of action of antibodies which destroy FVIII: II. Antibodies which give complex concentration graphs. *Br J Haematol, 23*, 137–155.

82. Miesbach, W., Matthias, T., & Scharrer, I. (2005). Identification of thrombin antibodies in patients with antiphospholipid syndrome. *Ann NY Acad Sci, 1050*, 250–256.

83. Bertolaccini, M. L., & Sanna, G. (2016). Recent advances in understanding antiphospholipid syndrome. *F1000Res, 22, 5*, 2908. doi:10.12688/f1000research.9717.1.

84. Sreedharanunni, S., Ahluwalia, J., Kumar, N., et al. (2017) Lupus anticoagulant-hypoprothrombinemia syndrome: a rare cause of intracranial bleeding. *Blood Coagul Fibrinolysis, 28*, 416–418.

85. Franchini, M., Frattini, F., Crestani, S., et al. (2013). Acquired FXIII inhibitors: a systematic review. *J Thromb Thrombolysis, 36*, 109–114.

86. Krumdieck, R., Shaw, D. R., Huang, S. T., et al. (1991). Hemorrhagic disorder due to an isoniazid-associated acquired factor XIII inhibitor in a patient with Waldenström's macroglobulinemia. *Am J Med, 90*, 639–645.

87. Matsumoto, T., Nogami, K., & Shima, M. (2014). Coagulation function and mechanisms in various clinical phenotypes of patients with acquired factor V inhibitors. *J Thromb Haemost, 12*, 1503–1512.

88. Bowman, L. J., Anderson, C. D., & Chapman, W. C. (2010). Topical recombinant human thrombin in surgical hemostasis. *Semin Thromb Hemost, 36*, 477–484.

89. Thompson, C. A., Kyle, R., Gertz, M., et al. (2010). Systemic AL amyloidosis with acquired factor X deficiency: A study of perioperative bleeding risk and treatment outcomes in 60 patients. *Am J Hematol, 85*, 171–173.

90. Broze, G. J., Jr. (2014). An acquired, calcium-dependent, factor X inhibitor. *Blood Cells Mol Dis, 52*, 116–120.

91. Barker, B., Altuntas, F., Paranjape, G., et al. (2004). Presurgical plasma exchange is ineffective in correcting amyloid associated factor X deficiency. *J Clin Apheresis, 19*, 208–210.

92. von Depka, M. (2004). Immune tolerance therapy in patients with acquired hemophilia. *Hematology, 9*, 245–257.

93. Federici, A. B. (2011). Acquired von Willebrand syndrome associated with hypothyroidism: a mild bleeding disorder to be further investigated. *Semin Thromb Hemost, 37*, 35–40.

94. Go, A. S., Mozaffarian, D., Roger, V. L., et al. (2014). Heart disease and stroke statistics—2014 update: a report from the American Heart Association. *Circulation, 129*, 399–410.

95. Tiede, A. (2012). Diagnosis and treatment of acquired von Willebrand syndrome. *Thromb Res, 130*(Suppl. 2), S2–S6.

96. Franchini, M., & Lippi, G. (2007). Acquired von Willebrand syndrome: an update. *Am J Hematol, 82*, 368–375.

97. Favaloro, E. J., Pasalic, L., & Curnow, J. (2016). Laboratory tests used to help diagnose von Willebrand disease: an update. *Pathology, 48*, 303–318.

98. Lee, C. A., & Abdul-Kadir, R. (2005). Von Willebrand disease and women's health. *Semin Hematol, 42*, 42–8.

99. Rahbar, N., Faranoush, M., Ghorbani, R., et al. (2015). Screening of von Willebrand disease in Iranian women with menorrhagia. *Iran Red Crescent Med J, 17*, e18244. doi: 10.5812/ircmj.18244.

100. National Heart, Lung, and Blood Institute. (2009). The Diagnosis, Evaluation, and Management of Von Willebrand Disease. *NIH Publication No. 08-5832*, Bethesda, MD: US Department of Health and Human Services, National Institutes of Health.

101. James, A. H., Manco-Johnson, M. J., Yawn, B. P., et al. (2009). Von Willebrand disease: key points from the 2008 National Heart, Lung, and Blood Institute guidelines. *Obstet Gynecol, 114*, 674–678.

102. Lenting, P. J., Casari, C., Christophe, O. D., et al. (2012). Von Willebrand factor: the old, the new and the unknown. *J Thromb Haemost, 10*, 2428–2437.

103. Schneppenheim, R., & Budde, U. (2011). Von Willebrand factor: the complex molecular genetics of a multidomain and multifunctional protein. *J Thromb Haemost, 9*(Suppl. 1), 209–215.

104. Rick, M. E., & Konkle, B. A. (2013). Von Willebrand disease. In Kitchens, C. S., Kessler, C. M., & Konkle, B. A. (Eds.), *Consultative Hemostasis and Thrombosis.* (3rd ed., pp. 90–102). St. Louis: Elsevier-Saunders.

105. Cai, P., Luo, H., Xu, H., et al. (2015). Recombinant ADAMTS 13 attenuates brain injury after intracerebral hemorrhage. *Stroke, 46*, 2647–2653.

106. Favaloro, E. J. (2011). Von Willebrand disease: local diagnosis and management of a globally distributed bleeding disorder. *Semin Thromb Hemost, 37*, 425–426.

107. Ragni, M. V., Machin, N., Malec, L. M., et al. (2016). Von Willebrand factor for menorrhagia: a survey and literature review. *Haemophilia, 22*, 397–402.

108. Favaloro, E. J., & Mohammed, S. (2016). Evaluation of a von Willebrand factor three test panel and chemiluminescent-based assay system for identification of, and therapy monitoring in, von Willebrand disease. *Thromb Res, 141*, 202–211.

109. Just, S. (2017). Laboratory testing for von Willebrand disease: the past, present, and future state of play for von Willebrand factor assays that measure platelet binding activity, with or without ristocetin. *Semin Thromb Hemost, 43*, 75–91.

110. Romansky, M. J., Limson, B. M., & Hawkins, J. E. (1956–57). Ristocetin; a new antibiotic-laboratory and clinical studies; preliminary report. *Antibiot Annu, 706*, 706–715.

111. Favaloro, E. J. (2014). Diagnosing von Willebrand disease: a short history of laboratory milestones and innovations, plus current status, challenges, and solutions. *Semin Thromb Hemost, 40*, 551–570.

112. Patzke, J., Budde, U., Huber, A. et al. (2014). Performance evaluation and multicenter study of a von Willebrand factor activity assay based on GPIb binding in the absence of ristocetin. *Blood Coagul Fibrinolysis, 25*, 860–870.

113. James, A. H., Eikenboom, J., & Federici. A. B. (2016). State of the art: von Willebrand disease. *Haemophilia, 22*(Suppl. 5), 54–59.

114. Favaloro, E. J., Bonar, R., Kershaw, G., et al. (2005). Royal College of Pathologists of Australasia Quality Assurance Program in Haematology: Laboratory diagnosis of von Willebrand disorder: use of multiple functional assays reduces diagnostic error rates. *Lab Hematol, 11*, 91–97.

115. Stoof, S. C., van Steenbergen, H. W., Zwagemaker, A., et al. (2015). Primary postpartum haemorrhage in women with von Willebrand disease or carriership of haemophilia despite specialised care: a retrospective survey. *Haemophilia, 21*, 505–512.

116. Hayes, T. E., Brandt, J. T., Chandler, W. L., et al. (2006). External peer review quality assurance testing in von Willebrand disease: the recent experience of the United States College of American Pathologists proficiency-testing program. *Semin Thromb Hemost, 32*, 499–504.

117. Chandler, W. L., Peerschke, E. I. B., Castellone, D. D., et al. on behalf of the NASCOLA Proficiency Testing Committee. (2011). Von Willebrand factor assay proficiency testing. The North American Specialized Coagulation Laboratory Association Experience. *Am J Clin Pathol, 135,* 862–869.

118. Favaloro, E. J., Kershaw, G., McLachlan, A. J., et al. (2007). Time to think outside the box? Proposals for a new approach to future pharmacokinetic studies of von Willebrand factor concentrates in people with von Willebrand disease. *Semin Thromb Hemost, 33,* 745–758.

119. Favaloro, E. J. (2017). Utility of the von Willebrand factor collagen-binding assay in the diagnosis of von Willebrand disease. *Am J Hematol, 92,* 114–118.

120. Favaloro, E. J. (2007). An update on the von Willebrand factor collagen binding assay: 21 years of age and beyond adolescence but not yet a mature adult. *Semin Thromb Hemost, 33,* 727–744.

121. Ferhat-Hamida, M. Y., Boukerb, H., & Hariti, G. (2015). Contribution of the collagen binding activity (VWF:CB) in the range of tests for the diagnosis and classification of von Willebrand disease. *Ann Biol Clin (Paris), 73,* 461–468.

122. Eikenboom, J., Van Marion, V., Putter, H., et al. (2006). Linkage analysis in families diagnosed with type 1 von Willebrand disease in the European study, molecular and clinical markers for the diagnosis and management of type 1 VWD. *J Thromb Haemost, 4,* 774–782.

123. Gill, J. C., Endres-Brooks, J., Bauer, P. J., et al. (1987). The effect of ABO blood group on the diagnosis of von Willebrand disease. *Blood, 69,* 1691–1695.

124. Norton, C. (2016). How to use PRICE treatment for soft tissue injuries. *Nurs Stand, 30,* 48–52.

125. Berntorp, E., & Windyga, J. (2009). European Wilate Study Group: Treatment and prevention of acute bleedings in von Willebrand disease—efficacy and safety of Wilate, a new generation von Willebrand factor/FVIII concentrate. *Haemophilia, 15,* 122–130.

126. Batlle, J., López-Fernández, M. F., Fraga, E. L., et al. (2009). Von Willebrand factor/ FVIII concentrates in the treatment of von Willebrand disease. *Blood Coagul Fibrinolysis, 20,* 89–100.

127. Fogarty, P. F., & Kessler, C. M. (2013). Hemophilia A and B. In Kitchens, C. S., Kessler, C. M., Konkle, B. A. (Eds.), *Consultative Hemostasis and Thrombosis.* (3rd ed., pp. 45–59). St. Louis: Elsevier-Saunders.

128. Thompson, A. R. (2003). Structure and function of the FVIII gene and protein. *Semin Thromb Hemost, 29,* 11–22.

129. Kretzschmar, E., Kruse, F., Greiss, O., et al. (2004). Effects of extended storage of whole blood before leucocyte depletion on coagulation factors in plasma. *Vox Sang, 87,* 156–164.

130. Rossetti, L. C., Radic, C. P., Larripa, I. B., et al. (2005). Genotyping the hemophilia inversion hotspot by use of inverse PCR. *Clin Chem, 51,* 1154–1158.

131. Weiss, A. E. (1988). The hemophilias. In Corriveau, D. M., Fritsma, G. A. (Eds.), *Hemostasis and Thrombosis in the Clinical Laboratory.* (pp. 128–168) Philadelphia: Lippincott.

132. Lusher, J. M., & Warrier, I. (1992). Hemophilia A. *Hematol Oncol Clin North Am, 6,* 1021–1133.

133. Evatt, B. L. (2005). Demographics of hemophilia in developing countries. *Semin Thromb Hemost, 31,* 489–494.

134. Evatt, B. L. (2006). The tragic history of AIDS in the hemophilia population, 1982–1984. *J Thromb Haemost, 4,* 2295–2301.

135. Labarque, V., Perinparajah, V., Bouskill, V., et al. (2017). Utility of factor VIII and factor VIII to von Willebrand factor ratio in identifying 277 unselected carriers of hemophilia A. *Am J Hematol, 92,* E94–E96.

136. Gröner, A. (2008). Pathogen safety of plasma-derived products—Haemate P/Humate-P. *Haemophilia, 14*(Suppl. 5), 54–71.

137. Kessler, C. M., Gill, J. C., White, G. C., et al. (2005). B-domain deleted recombinant FVIII preparations are bioequivalent to a monoclonal antibody purified plasma-derived FVIII concentrate: a randomized, three-way crossover study. *Haemophilia, 11,* 84–91.

138. Gringeri, A., Lundin, V., von Mackensen, S., et al. (2009). Primary and secondary prophylaxis in children with haemophilia A reduces bleeding frequency and arthropathy development compared to on demand treatment: a 10-year, randomized clinical trial. *J Thromb Haemost, 7,* 780–786.

139. Konkle, B. A., Huston, H., & Nakaya Fletcher, S. (2017). Hemophilia A. In: Pagon, R.A., Adam, M. P., Ardinger, H. H., et al. (Eds.), *GeneReviews®* [Internet]. Seattle, WA: University of Washington, Seattle; 1993–2017. 2000 Sep 21 [updated 2017 Feb 2].

140. Sommer, J. M., Moore, N., McGuffie-Valentine, B., et al. (2014). Comparative field study evaluating the activity of recombinant factor VIII Fc fusion protein in plasma samples at clinical haemostasis laboratories. *Haemophilia, 20,* 294–300.

141. Mullins, E. S., Stasyshyn, O., Alvarez-Román, M. T., et al. (2017). Extended half-life pegylated, full-length recombinant factor VIII for prophylaxis in children with severe haemophilia A. *Haemophilia, 23,* 238–246.

142. Pabinger-Fasching, I. (2016). The story of a unique molecule in hemophilia A: recombinant single-chain factor VIII. *Thromb Res, 141*(Suppl. 3), S2–S4.

143. Pipe, S. W., Montgomery, R. R., Pratt, K. P., et al. (2016). Life in the shadow of a dominant partner: the FVIII-VWF association and its clinical implications for hemophilia A. *Blood, 128,* 2007–2016.

144. Marques, M. B., & Fritsma, G. A. (2015). *Quick Guide to Coagulation Testing.* (3rd ed., p. 89). Washington, DC: American Association for Clinical Chemistry Press.

145. Girolami, A., Cosi, E., Tasinato, V., et al. (2016). Pulmonary embolism in congenital bleeding disorders: intriguing discrepancies among different clotting factors deficiencies. *Blood Coagul Fibrinolysis, 27,* 517–525.

146. Favaloro, E. J., & Lippi, G. (2017). Emerging treatments for hemophilia: patients and their treaters spoilt for choice, but laboratories face a difficult path? *Ann Transl Med, 5,* 101–103.

147. Favaloro, E. J., Meijer, P., Jennings, I., et al. (2013). Problems and solutions in laboratory testing For hemophilia. *Semin Thromb Hemost, 39,* 816–833.

148. Franchini, M., Lippi, G., & Favaloro, E. J. (2012). Acquired inhibitors of coagulation factors: part II. *Semin Thromb Hemost, 38,* 447–453.

149. Scott, L. J., & Kim, E. S. (2018). Emicizumab-kxwh: first global approval. *Drugs, 78,* 269–274.

150. Bastida, J. M., González-Porras, J. R., Jiménez, C., et al. (2017). Application of a molecular diagnostic algorithm for haemophilia A and B using next-generation sequencing of entire F8, F9 and VWF genes. *Thromb Haemost, 117,* 66–74.

151. Kitchen, S., Tiefenbacher, S., & Gosselin, R. (2017). Factor activity assays for monitoring extended half-life FVIII and factor IX replacement therapies. *Semin Thromb Hemost, 43,* 331–337.

152. Ferreira, J., & DeLosSantos, M. (2013). The clinical use of prothrombin complex concentrate. *J Emerg Med, 44,* 1201–1210.

153. Duga, S., & Salomon, O. (2013). Congenital factor XI deficiency: an update. *Semin Thromb Hemost, 39,* 621–631.

154. Nichols, W. C., Seligsohn, U., Zivelin, A., et al. (1997). Linkage of combined factors V and VIII deficiency to chromosome 18q by homozygosity mapping. *J Clin Invest, 99,* 596–601.

155. Mariani, G., & Bernardi, F. (2009). Factor VII deficiency. *Semin Thromb Hemost, 35,* 400–406.

156. Menegatti, M., & Peyvandi, F. (2009). Factor X deficiency. *Semin Thromb Hemost, 35,* 407–415.

Qualitative Disorders of Platelets and Vasculature

Walter P. Jeske, Phillip J. DeChristopher*

OBJECTIVES

After completion of this chapter, the reader will be able to:

1. Identify the most common type of hereditary platelet defect.
2. Distinguish among the following types of inherited platelet disorders: membrane receptor abnormality, secretion disorder, and storage pool deficiency.
3. Describe the defect in each of the following hereditary disorders: storage pool disease, gray platelet syndrome, Glanzmann thrombasthenia, and Bernard-Soulier syndrome.
4. Compare and contrast Glanzmann thrombasthenia and Bernard-Soulier syndrome.
5. Discuss the mechanisms of action of antiplatelet drugs.
6. Describe the effect of aspirin on the cyclooxygenase pathway.
7. Explain the effects of paraproteins on platelet function.
8. Recognize the clinical presentation of patients with dysfunctional platelets.
9. Understand the laboratory tests used to diagnose platelet disorders.
10. Discuss the mechanism of the platelet defects associated with myeloproliferative diseases, uremia, and liver disease.
11. Recognize conditions associated with acquired vascular disorders.

OUTLINE

Qualitative Platelet Disorders
    Disorders of Platelet Aggregation (GP IIb/IIIa Function)
    Disorders of Platelet Adhesion (GP Ib/IX/V Function)
    Inherited Giant Platelet Syndromes
    Disorders of Platelet Secretion

    Other Inherited Disorders of Receptors and Signaling Pathways
    Acquired Defects of Platelet Function
Vascular Disorders
    Hereditary Vascular Disorders
    Acquired Vascular Disorders

CASE STUDY

After studying the material in this chapter, the reader should be able to respond to the following case study:

A 19-year-old woman with a chief complaint of easy bruising, occasional mild nosebleeds, and heavy menstrual periods was examined by her physician. At the time of her examination, she had a few small bruises on her arms and legs, but no other findings. Initial laboratory data revealed a normal prothrombin time and a normal partial thromboplastin time. A complete blood count (CBC), including platelet count and morphology, yielded normal results.

A detailed history revealed that the patient's bleeding problems occurred most frequently after aspirin ingestion. Her mother and one of her brothers also had some of the same symptoms. Blood was drawn for platelet function studies. Platelet aggregation tests indicated that although the response to ristocetin and adenosine diphosphate were near normal, arachidonic acid-induced aggregation

was absent, epinephrine induced only primary aggregation, and collagen-induced aggregation was decreased (although a near-normal aggregation response could be obtained with a high collagen concentration). Spontaneous aggregation was not observed.

1. What are three possible explanations for the test results?
2. Given the bleeding history in her family, which of the three explanations seems most likely?

A quantitative test for adenosine triphosphate (ATP) release was performed using the firefly luciferin-luciferase bioluminescence assay. The result of this test showed a marked decrease in the amount of ATP released when platelets were stimulated with thrombin.

3. Based on the ATP release test results, what is the likely cause of the patient's bleeding symptoms?

Clinical manifestations of bleeding disorders can be divided into two broad, rather poorly defined groups: (1) *superficial bleeding* (e.g., petechiae, epistaxis, or gingival bleeding), usually associated with a platelet defect or vascular disorder; and (2) *deep tissue bleeding* (e.g., hematomas or hemarthrosis), usually associated with plasma clotting factor deficiencies.[1] This chapter focuses on platelet and vascular disorders; thrombocytopenia specific disorders are detailed in Chapter 38. Bleeding problems resulting from defects in the coagulation mechanism are described in Chapter 36.

---

*The authors extend appreciation to Larry D. Brace, whose work in prior editions provided the foundation for this chapter.

QUALITATIVE PLATELET DISORDERS

Excessive bruising and superficial (mucocutaneous) bleeding in a patient whose platelet count is normal suggest an acquired or a congenital disorder of *platelet function*. Rapid progress in understanding these disorders began in the 1960s, following the development of instruments and test methods for measuring platelet function. Congenital disorders that result from abnormalities of each of the major phases of platelet function (adhesion, secretion, and aggregation) have been described.

Qualitative platelet disorders are summarized in Box 37.1.[2,3] This chapter discusses the individual qualitative platelet disorders, grouped by the mechanism underlying the defect. A summary of the defects associated with surface components and intracellular components of primary platelet disorders is illustrated

---

BOX 37.1   Qualitative Abnormalities: Changes in Platelet Function[3,4]

Disorders of Platelet Aggregation
Glanzmann thrombasthenia
Hereditary afibrinogenemia
Acquired defects of platelet aggregation:
  Acquired von Willebrand disease
  Acquired uremia

Disorders of Platelet Adhesion
Bernard-Soulier syndrome
Von Willebrand disease
Acquired defects of platelet adhesion:
  Myeloproliferative and lymphoproliferative disorders, dysproteinemias
  Antiplatelet antibodies
  Cardiopulmonary bypass surgery
  Chronic liver disease
  Drug-induced membrane modification

Disorders of Platelet Secretion
Storage pool diseases
Thromboxane pathway disorders
Hereditary aspirin-like defects:
  Cyclooxygenase or thromboxane synthetase deficiency
Drug inhibition of the prostaglandin pathways
Drug inhibition of platelet phosphodiesterase activity

Changes in Membrane Phospholipid Distribution
Scott syndrome
Stormorken syndrome

Hyperactive Prothrombotic Platelets

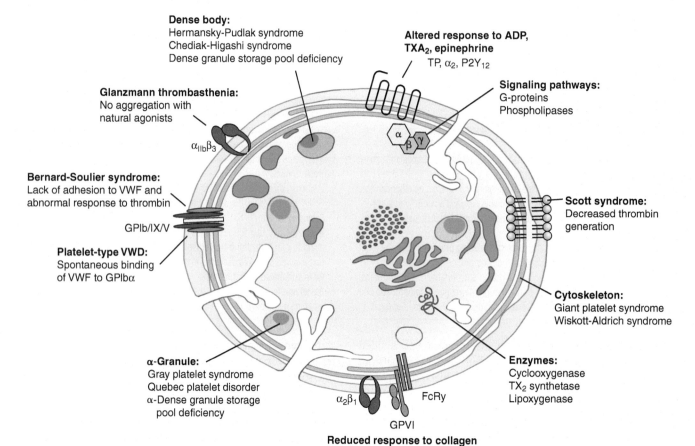

Figure 37.1 An Illustration of the Primary Disorders Associated with Defects of the Surface and Intracellular Components of Platelets.

TABLE 37.1 Genomic Defects in the Principal Inherited Platelet Function Disorders

Disorder	Gene	Chromosome Location	Autosomal Inheritance
Adhesion Defects			
• Bernard-Soulier syndrome	GP1BA	17p13.2	Recessive
	GP1BB	22q11.21	
	GP9	3q21.3	
• Platelet-type von Willebrand disease	GP1BA	17p13.2	Dominant
• GP6 deficiency	GP6	19q13.4	Recessive
Receptor and Signaling Defects			
• ADP receptor deficiency	P2RY12	3q25.1	Recessive
• Thromboxane A2 receptor deficiency	TBXA2R	19p13.3	Recessive
• PAR-4 receptor defects	F2RL3	19p13.11	Dominant
Storage Pool Disease			
• Gray platelet syndrome	NBEAL2	3p21.31	Recessive
	GF11B	9p34.13	Dominant
• Quebec platelet syndrome	PLAU	10p22.2	Dominant
• Hermansky-Pudlak syndrome	Multiple genes: HPS1, AP3B1, HPS3 to HPS9	Multiple different locations	All mutations recessive
• Chediak-Higashi syndrome	LYST	1q42.3	Recessive
Aggregation Defects			
• Glanzmann thrombasthenia	ITGA2B	17q21.31	Recessive
	ITGB3	17q21.32	
• Leukocyte adhesion deficiency-III syndrome	FERMT3	11q13.1	Recessive
Procoagulant Activity Defects			
• Scott syndrome	TMEM16F	12q12	Recessive

ADP, Adenosine diphosphate; *GP6*, glycoprotein 6; *PAR-4*, protease-activated receptor.
Adapted from Bianchi, E., Norfo, R., Pannucci, V., et al. (2016). Genomic landscape of megakaryopoiesis and platelet function defects. *Blood, 127*, 1249–1259.

in Figure 37.1.[4] Table 37.1 compiles the underlying genetic mutations associated with various inherited platelet function defects.

Disorders of Platelet Aggregation (GP IIb/IIIa Function)
Glanzmann Thrombasthenia

Glanzmann thrombasthenia (GT) originally was described as a bleeding disorder associated with abnormal in vitro clot retraction and a normal platelet count. Clot retraction is the process by which the volume of a formed clot is reduced through contraction of the intracellular actin-myosin cytoskeleton of activated platelets incorporated in the clot. GT is inherited as an autosomal recessive disorder and is seen most frequently in populations with a high degree of consanguinity. Heterozygotes

are clinically normal, whereas homozygotes have serious bleeding problems. This rare disorder manifests itself clinically in the neonatal period or infancy, occasionally with bleeding after circumcision and frequently with epistaxis and gingival bleeding. Hemorrhagic manifestations include petechiae, purpura (Figure 38.1), menorrhagia, gastrointestinal bleeding, and hematuria. Some patients may have minimal symptoms, whereas others may have frequent and serious hemorrhagic complications. The severity of the bleeding episodes seems to decrease with age.[5,6]

The biochemical lesion responsible for the disorder is a deficiency or abnormality of the platelet membrane glycoprotein (GP) IIb/IIIa (integrin $\alpha_{IIb}\beta_3$) complex, a membrane receptor capable of binding fibrinogen, von Willebrand factor (VWF), fibronectin, and other adhesive ligands (Chapter 10). Binding of fibrinogen to the GP IIb/IIIa complex mediates normal platelet aggregation responses. Failure of such binding results in a profound defect in hemostatic plug formation and the serious bleeding characteristic of thrombasthenia.[7–10]

Typically, the platelets of homozygous individuals lack surface-expressed GP IIb/IIIa, whereas the GP IIb/IIIa content of the platelets from heterozygotes has been found to be 50% to 60% of normal.[7,11] Historically, patients with GT have been designated as type 1 or type 2. Individuals with type 2 disease have more GP IIb/IIIa complexes (10% to 20% of normal) than those with type 1 disease (0% to 5% of normal), although there is considerable variability within each subdivision.[12,13] Additionally, patients with type 2 disease are less affected by abnormal clot retraction and fibrinogen binding.

Genetic mutations are distributed widely over the *ITGA2B* and *ITGB3* genes present on chromosome 17, which code for GP IIb/IIIa.[14] More than 70 mutations are known to give rise to Glanzmann thrombasthenia.[15–17] Rarely, thrombocytopenia and large platelets may be seen with some of the mutations in these genes (Table 37.1; also Table 38.1). The integrin component α_{IIb} is synthesized in megakaryocytes as pro-α_{IIb}, which complexes with the β_3 unit in the endoplasmic reticulum. This complex is transported to the Golgi body, where α_{IIb} is cleaved to heavy and light chains to form the complete complex. Uncomplexed α_{IIb} and β_3 are not processed in the Golgi body. Both proteins of the GP IIb/IIIa complex must be produced and assembled into a complex in order to be expressed on the platelet surface. Gene defects that lead to the absence of production of either protein lead to absence of the complex on the platelet surface. Defects that interfere with or prevent complex formation or affect complex stability have the same effect.

Numerous variants of GT have been described in which α_{IIb} and β_3 are produced, form a complex, and are processed normally, but one or more functions of the complex (e.g., fibrinogen binding or signal transduction) are abnormal. As expected, bleeding in these patients ranges from mild to severe.

The β_3 unit of the $\alpha_{IIb}\beta_3$ integrin is also a component of the vitronectin receptor, $\alpha_V\beta_3$, found on endothelial cells, osteoclasts, fibroblasts, monocytes, and activated B lymphocytes, where it acts as a receptor for a variety of adhesive protein ligands. Patients who have β_3 gene defects that result in the absence of $\alpha_{IIb}\beta_3$ integrin also lack the vitronectin receptor. These patients do not seem to have a more severe form of

GT.[18,19] The vitronectin receptor is thought to play a role in vascularization, but to date there is no evidence for abnormal blood vessel development in individuals lacking the vitronectin receptor. It also is unclear whether platelet vitronectin receptors play any significant role in platelet function processes.[15]

Rarely, a thrombasthenia-like state can be acquired. Such conditions include development of autoantibodies against GP IIb/IIIa, multiple myeloma in which the paraprotein is directed against GP IIIa, and afibrinogenemia. A thrombasthenia-like state also can be induced in individuals with otherwise normal platelet function by a variety of therapeutic antiplatelet drugs.[6,9]

Laboratory features. The typical laboratory features of GT include a normal platelet count, normal platelet morphology, and a lack of platelet aggregation in response to all platelet activating agents (including adenosine diphosphate [ADP], collagen, thrombin, and epinephrine).[7,9] Stimulation with strong agonists (e.g., thrombin) will induce the release/secretion reaction, even in the absence of aggregation. Ristocetin-induced binding of VWF to platelets and the resulting platelet agglutination are normal. Tests for platelet procoagulant activity, such as the platelet factor 3 test, usually show diminished activity,[11,20] for several reasons. First, when normal platelets are activated, procoagulant microvesicles are shed from the platelet surface, and coagulation factors assemble on microvesicle surfaces during activation of the coagulation cascade. In patients with GT, markedly fewer microvesicles are produced. Second, prothrombin binds directly to GP IIb/IIIa.[21] Because this complex is missing on platelets from patients with GT, significantly less thrombin is generated in response to tissue factor activation. Finally, GT platelets are activated by thrombin to a lesser degree than normal platelets.[22–25]

Treatment. Thrombasthenia is one of the few forms of platelet dysfunction in which hemorrhage is severe and disabling. Bleeding of all types, including epistaxis, ecchymosis, hemarthrosis, subcutaneous hematoma, menorrhagia, and gastrointestinal and urinary tract hemorrhage, has been reported. Treatment of bleeding episodes in patients with Glanzmann thrombasthenia requires the transfusion of normal platelets. In GT the defective platelets may interfere with the normal transfused platelets, and it may be necessary to infuse more donor platelets than expected to control bleeding.[26,27] The use of repeated transfusions in patients with GT may result in alloimmunization. Thus in GT patients who are bleeding, to minimize or prevent human leukocyte antigen (HLA) alloimmunization, it is recommended to use pre-storage, leukocyte-reduced apheresis platelets or HLA-matched donor platelets.

In general, patients with GT should avoid anticoagulants and antiplatelet agents such as aspirin and nonsteroidal antiinflammatory drugs (NSAIDs). A variety of treatments have been used successfully to control or prevent bleeding, alone or in combination with platelet transfusion. To a large extent the site of hemorrhage determines the therapeutic approach used. Hormonal therapy (norethindrone acetate) has been used to control menorrhagia. Menorrhagia at the onset of menses is uniformly severe and can be life-threatening, which has led some to suggest that birth control pills be started before menarche. Antifibrinolytic therapy (aminocaproic acid or tranexamic acid) can be used to control gingival hemorrhage or excessive bleeding after tooth extraction.[13] Recombinant factor VIIa

(rVIIa; NovoSeven, Novo) is used in surgical and nonsurgical bleeding in patients with GT who are refractory to platelet transfusions, with or without platelet antibodies. rFVIIa is thought to enhance a burst of thrombin generation after activating factor X (FX) to FXa at the wound site by stimulating tissue factor-independent thrombin generation and fibrin formation.[28] It has proved useful for treating severe bleeding in patients with isoantibodies to GP IIb/IIIa and in patients undergoing invasive procedures.[29]

Disorders of Platelet Adhesion (GP Ib/IX/V Function)
Bernard-Soulier (Giant Platelet) Syndrome

Bernard-Soulier syndrome (BSS) is a rare disorder of platelet adhesion that usually manifests in infancy or childhood with hemorrhage characteristic of defective platelet function: ecchymoses, epistaxis, and gingival bleeding. Hemarthroses and expanding hematomas are rarely seen. BSS is inherited as an autosomal recessive disorder in which the GP Ib/IX/V complex is missing from the platelet surface or exhibits abnormal function. Inability to bind to VWF accounts for the inability of platelets to adhere to exposed subendothelium and the resultant bleeding characteristic of this disorder (Chapters 10 and 36). This defect in adhesion shows the importance of initial platelet attachment for primary hemostasis. In many respects this disorder resembles the defect seen in von Willebrand disease (VWD). In contrast to VWD, however, this abnormality cannot be corrected by the addition of normal plasma or cryoprecipitate, consistent with a defect that resides in platelets.

Heterozygotes who have about 50% of normal levels of GP Ib, GP V, and GP IX have normal or near-normal platelet function. Homozygotes have enlarged platelets, thrombocytopenia, and usually decreased platelet survival, which lead to a moderate to severe bleeding disorder. Platelet counts generally range from 40,000/μL to near normal.[30] On peripheral blood films platelets typically are 5 to 8 μm in diameter (normal 2 to 3 μm), but they can be as large as 20 μm (Figure 37.2). Viewed by electron microscopy BSS platelets contain a larger number of cytoplasmic vacuoles and membrane complexes, and megakaryocytes exhibit an irregular demarcation membrane system.[2,7,31]

Four glycoproteins are required to form the GP Ib/IX/V complex: GP Ibα, GP Ibβ, GP IX, and GP V. In the complex these proteins are present in the ratio of 2:2:2:1. For surface expression of the GP Ib/IX complex it seems that synthesis of three proteins, GP Ibα, GP Ibβ, and GP IX, is required. The most frequent forms of BSS involve defects in GP Ibα synthesis or expression (Table 37.1). GP Ibα is essential to normal function because it contains binding sites for VWF and thrombin. Defects in the GP Ibβ and GP IX genes also are known to result in BSS.[32–34] Missense, frameshift, and nonsense mutations have all been reported.[35,36]

Variants. Several unusual variants of BSS have been described in which the surface expression of the GP Ib/IX/V complex is normal, but its functionality is impaired. Mutations that affect binding domains impair interactions between elements of the complex, or they result in truncation of a specific protein in the complex, resulting in complexes that fail to bind VWF or do so poorly.[33] In rare circumstances an antibody to GP Ib/V can cause a Bernard-Soulier-like syndrome (pseudo-BSS), in which the GP Ib/IX/V complex is nonfunctional.

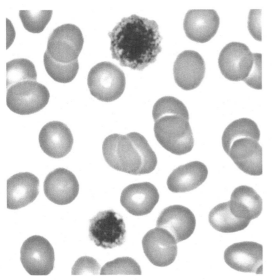

Figure 37.2 Giant Platelets in Bernard-Soulier Syndrome. (Peripheral blood, Wright-Giemsa stain, ×1000.) (Modified from Carr, J.H., & Rodak, B.F. [2009]: *Clinical Hematology Atlas.* Third Edition. Philadelphia, PA: Saunders/Elsevier.)

Several gain-of-function mutations in the GP Ib/IX/V complex can result in platelet-type VWD (pseudo-VWD).[37–39] Such mutations result in spontaneous binding of plasma VWF to the mutated GP Ib/IX/V complex. As a consequence, platelets and large VWF multimers with their associated factor VIII are removed from the circulation, resulting in thrombocytopenia and reduced factor VIII clotting activity.

Laboratory features. BSS platelets have normal aggregation responses to ADP, epinephrine, collagen, and arachidonic acid but do not respond to ristocetin and have diminished response to thrombin.[7] The lack of response to ristocetin is due to the lack of GP Ib/IX/V complexes and the inability of BSS platelets to bind VWF.

Treatment. In all cases antiplatelet therapy should be avoided. Antifibrinolytic therapy may be useful to treat mucosal bleeding. There is no specific treatment for more severe bleeding associated with BSS. Platelet transfusions are the therapy of choice, but patients invariably develop alloantibodies, limiting further platelet transfusions. BSS patients tend to do better when apheresis platelets are used for transfusion because this limits the number of donors to which the patient is exposed, and the rate of alloimmunization tends to be lower.[7] As with platelet transfusion in GT, platelets used to treat BSS should be pre-storage leukoreduced (to reduce alloimmunization). Other treatments that have been used include desmopressin acetate (DDAVP) and, more recently, recombinant factor VIIa.

Inherited Giant Platelet Syndromes

In addition to BSS there are several other inherited syndromes in which patients exhibit *large platelets and thrombocytopenia.* With few exceptions thrombocytopenia tends to be mild and bleeding tendency, if present, is also mild. In addition the platelet ultrastructure is generally normal. The exceptions include the May-Hegglin anomaly, in which there is an abnormal microtubule distribution, and Epstein syndrome, in which platelets are spherical and have a prominent surface-connected canalicular system. For most of these syndromes the cause of the large platelets and thrombocytopenia remain to be determined. See Table 37.2, Table 38.1, and Mhawech and Saleem[40] for a more complete discussion of these syndromes.

TABLE 37.2   Inherited Giant Platelet Syndromes

Disease	Inheritance	Platelet count (×10⁹/L)	Bleeding	Bleeding site	Other Clinical Characteristics
Giant platelets with velocardiofacial syndrome	Autosomal recessive	100–200	None reported		Velopharyngeal insufficiency, conotruncal heart disease
Giant platelets with abnormal surface glycoproteins and mitral valve insufficiency	Autosomal recessive	50–60	Mild	Ecchymoses, epistaxis	Mitral valve insufficiency
Familial macrothrombocytopenia with GP IV abnormality	Autosomal dominant	45–normal	Mild		Defective GP IV glycosylation
Montreal platelet syndrome		5–40		Significant bruising	Low calpain activity; defective regulation of binding sites for adhesive proteins
May-Hegglin anomaly	Autosomal dominant	60–100	Mild		Döhle body–like neutrophil inclusions
Fechtner syndrome	Autosomal dominant	30–90			Deafness, cataracts, nephritis
Sebastian syndrome	Autosomal dominant	40–120	Mild	Epistaxis, possible postoperative hemorrhage	Neutrophil inclusions
Hereditary macrothrombocytopenia	Autosomal dominant	50–120	Mild	Gingival bleeding, epistaxis, easy bruising, menorrhagia	High-frequency hearing loss
Epstein syndrome	Autosomal dominant	30–60	Mild	Epistaxis, GI bleeding, female genital tract	Nephritis, high-frequency hearing loss, proteinuria
Mediterranean macrothrombocytopenia		89–290			Stomatocytes in peripheral blood

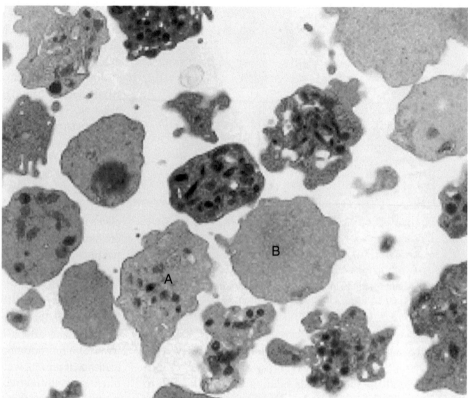

Figure 37.3 Storage Pool Disorder. Electron micrograph of platelets from a patient with storage pool disorder: The micrograph shows platelets with a normal distribution of dense granules (labeled A) and platelets with a marked decrease of dense granules (labeled B). (Barone, I., Meccariello, G, Cazzato, L., et al. [2013]: Management of platelet storage pool disease during pregnancy with recombinant factor VIIa. *Eur J Obstet Gynecol Reprod Biol, 170*, 576–577.)

Disorders of Platelet Secretion

Storage pool and *release reaction defects* are the most common of the hereditary platelet function defects. Patients with these disorders present with mucocutaneous hemorrhage and hematuria, epistaxis, and easy and spontaneous bruising. Petechiae are less common than in other qualitative platelet disorders. Hemorrhage is rarely severe but may be exacerbated by ingestion of aspirin or other antiplatelet agents. In most of these disorders the platelet count is normal. Platelet aggregation abnormalities are usually seen, but vary depending on the disorder.[7,41,42]

Storage Pool Diseases

Storage pool disorders can be related to defects of the dense granules (Figure 37.3) or defects of the α-granules. Box 37.2 lists these disorders.

Dense granule deficiencies. The dense granules are the storage site for serotonin, nucleotides (e.g., ADP and adenosine triphosphate [ATP]), calcium, and pyrophosphate (Chapter 10). The inheritance of dense granule deficiency does not follow a single mode, and it is likely that a variety of genetic abnormalities

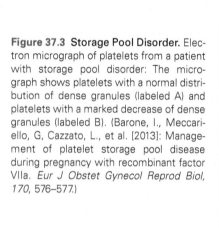

BOX 37.2 Platelet Storage Pool Diseases

Dense Granule Deficiencies
Hermansky-Pudlak syndrome
Chédiak-Higashi syndrome
Wiskott-Aldrich syndrome
Thrombocytopenia–absent radius (TAR) syndrome

α-Granule Deficiencies
Gray platelet syndrome

lead to the development of this disorder. Dense granule deficiencies can be subdivided into deficiency states associated with albinism and those in otherwise normal individuals (nonalbinos).

In the platelets of nonalbinos there is evidence for the presence of dense granule membranes in normal to near-normal numbers, which suggests that the disorder arises from an inability to package the dense granule contents.[43,44] Serotonin accumulates in normal dense granules by an active uptake mechanism in which plasma serotonin is transported by a specific carrier-mediated system across the plasma membrane into the cytoplasm, and a second carrier-mediated system in the dense granule membrane transports serotonin from the cytoplasm to the interior of the dense granules.[45] In addition to serotonin transport mechanisms a nucleotide transporter, MRP4 (ABCC4), that is highly expressed in platelets and dense granules has been identified. It would be expected that mutations in the gene for this transporter could affect nucleotide accumulation in dense granules.[46]

As an isolated abnormality, dense granule deficiency does not typically result in a serious hemorrhagic problem. Bleeding is usually mild and most often is limited to easy bruising.

The impact of dense granule deficiency can be observed in platelet aggregation tests. The contents of these granules are extruded when platelet secretion is induced, and secreted ADP plays a major role in platelet activation, recruitment, and aggregation and growth of the hemostatic plug. In the platelet function tests, addition of arachidonic acid to platelet-rich plasma fails to induce an aggregation response from platelets with dense granule deficiency (Chapter 41). Epinephrine and low-dose ADP induce a primary wave of aggregation, but a secondary wave is missing. Responses to low concentrations of collagen are decreased to absent, but a high concentration of collagen may induce a near-normal aggregation response.[42,45] This aggregation pattern, which is nearly identical to the pattern observed in patients taking aspirin (discussed later in this chapter), is caused by the lack of ADP secretion.

Hermansky-Pudlak syndrome. In addition to occurring as an isolated problem, dense granule deficiency is found in association with several disorders. Hermansky-Pudlak syndrome is an autosomal recessive disorder characterized by tyrosinase-positive oculocutaneous albinism, defective lysosomal function in a variety of cell types, ceroid-like deposition in the cells of the reticuloendothelial system, and a profound platelet dense granule deficiency.[47] Several of the mutations responsible for Hermansky-Pudlak syndrome have been mapped to chromosome 19. Mutations in at least seven genes individually can give rise to Hermansky-Pudlak syndrome. These genes encode for proteins that are involved in intracellular vesicular trafficking and are active in the biogenesis of organelles.[48]

The bleeding associated with most dense granule deficiencies is rarely severe; however, Hermansky-Pudlak syndrome can be an exception. Although most bleeding episodes in Hermansky-Pudlak syndrome are not severe, lethal hemorrhage has been reported, and in one series hemorrhage accounted for 16% of deaths in affected patients. For extensive surgery or prolonged bleeding both red blood cell (RBC) and platelet transfusions are required. Thrombin-soaked Gelfoam can be used to treat skin wounds that fail to spontaneously clot. Oral contraceptives can limit the duration of menstrual periods. A unique morphologic abnormality has been described in the platelets of four families with Hermansky-Pudlak syndrome. This abnormality consists of marked dilation and tortuosity of the surface-connecting tubular system (the so-called Swiss cheese platelet).[20,49]

Chédiak-Higashi syndrome. This is a rare autosomal recessive disorder characterized by partial oculocutaneous albinism, frequent pyogenic bacterial infections, giant lysosomal granules in cells of hematologic (Figure 26.1) and nonhematologic origin, platelet dense granule deficiency, and hemorrhage. The disorder is accompanied by severe immunologic defects and progressive neurologic dysfunction in patients who survive to adulthood.

The gene for the Chédiak-Higashi syndrome protein is located on chromosome 1 (1q42.3). A number of nonsense and frameshift mutations result in a truncated Chédiak-Higashi syndrome protein that gives rise to a disorder of generalized cellular dysfunction involving fusion of cytoplasmic granules.

In 85% of patients with Chédiak-Higashi syndrome the disorder progresses to an accelerated phase that is marked by lymphocytic proliferation in the liver, spleen, and marrow with macrophage accumulation in tissues. During this stage the pancytopenia worsens, leading to hemorrhage and ever-increasing susceptibility to infection; the result is death at an early age. Initially bleeding is increased because of dense granule deficiency and consequent defective platelet function. During the accelerated phase, however, the thrombocytopenia also contributes to a prolonged bleeding tendency. Bleeding episodes vary from mild to moderate but worsen as the platelet count decreases.[20]

Wiskott-Aldrich syndrome (WAS). This is a rare X-linked disease caused by mutations in the *WAS* gene on the short arm of the X chromosome Xp11.23 that encodes for a 502-amino acid protein – the Wiskott-Aldrich syndrome protein (WASp) – that is found exclusively in hematopoietic cells, including lymphocytes. WASp plays a crucial role in actin cytoskeleton remodeling. T cell function is defective due to abnormal cytoskeletal reorganization, leading to impaired migration, impaired adhesion, and insufficient interaction with other cells. Disease severity associated with *WAS* gene mutations ranges from the classic form of WAS with autoimmunity and/or malignancy, to a milder form with isolated microthrombocytopenia (X-linked thrombocytopenia [XLT]) (Chapter 38), to X-linked neutropenia (XLN). Approximately 50% of patients with *WAS* gene mutations have the WAS phenotype, and the other half have the XLT phenotype. WAS gene mutations causing XLN are very rare.[50] Homozygous mutations of the *WIPF1* gene on chromosome 2 that encodes WASp-interacting protein (WIP) – a cytoplasmic protein required to stabilize WASp – can also cause a WAS phenotype.[51]

The classic form of WAS, alternatively called the *eczema-thrombocytopenia immunodeficiency syndrome*, is characterized by susceptibility to infections associated with immune dysfunction, with recurrent bacterial, viral, and fungal infections, microthrombocytopenia, and severe eczema. Thrombocytopenia is present at birth, but the full expression of WAS develops over the first 2 years of life. Individuals with this disorder lack the ability to make anti-polysaccharide antibodies, which results in a propensity for pneumococcal sepsis. Patients with classic WAS tend to develop autoimmune disorders, lymphoma, or other malignancies, often leading to early death. Bleeding episodes are typically moderate to severe. In WAS a combination of ineffective thrombocytopoiesis and increased platelet sequestration and destruction accounts for the thrombocytopenia. As with all X-linked recessive disorders, it is found primarily in males.[11,20,33,52]

Wiskott-Aldrich platelets are also structurally abnormal. The number of dense granules is decreased, and the platelets are small (microthrombocytes), a feature of diagnostic importance. Other than in WAS, such small platelets are seen only in association with TORCH (toxoplasma, other agents, rubella virus, cytomegalovirus, herpesvirus) infections. Diminished levels of stored adenine nucleotides are reflected in the lack of dense granules observed on transmission electron micrographs. In laboratory testing the platelet aggregation pattern in WAS is typical of a storage pool deficiency. The platelets show a decreased aggregation response to ADP, collagen, and epinephrine and lack a secondary wave of aggregation in response to these agonists (Chapter 41). The response to thrombin is normal, however.[20]

The most effective treatment for the thrombocytopenia seems to be splenectomy, which would be consistent with a mechanism of peripheral destruction of platelets. Platelet transfusions may be needed to treat hemorrhagic episodes. Bone marrow transplantation also has been attempted, with some success.[20,53]

Thrombocytopenia with absent radii syndrome (TAR). TAR (Chapter 38) is a rare autosomal recessive disorder characterized by the congenital absence of the radial bones (the most pronounced skeletal abnormality), numerous cardiac and other skeletal abnormalities, and thrombocytopenia (90% of cases). Platelets have structural defects in dense granules, with corresponding abnormal aggregation responses. Marrow megakaryocytes may be decreased in number, immature, or normal.[54]

α-Granule deficiency: gray platelet syndrome. Platelet α-granules are the storage site for proteins (Chapter 10) produced by the megakaryocyte (e.g., platelet-derived growth factor, thrombospondin, and platelet factor 4) or present in plasma and taken up by platelets and transported to α-granules for storage (e.g., albumin, immunoglobulin G [IgG], and fibrinogen). There are 50 to 80 α-granules per platelet, which are primarily responsible for the granular appearance of platelets on stained blood films (Figure 37.4).

Gray platelet syndrome, a rare disorder first described in 1971, is characterized by the specific absence of morphologically

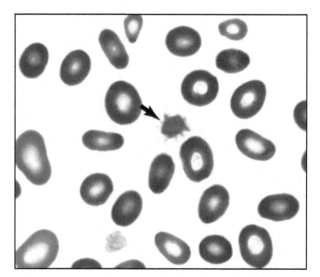

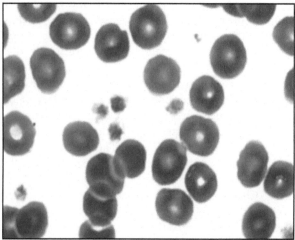

Figure 37.4 Gray Platelet Syndrome. Blood smears showing platelets from a patient with gray platelet syndrome *(top)* and, for comparison, a normal individual *(bottom)*. In gray platelet syndrome note the large pale platelet lacking the usual fine purple α granules and the large platelet with projections *(arrow)*. (Peripheral blood, Wright-Giemsa stain, ×100.) (Pozdnyakova, O. [2013]. Gray platelet syndrome. In *Hematopathology: A Volume in the High Yield Pathology Series.* Philadelphia, PA: Saunders/Elsevier.)

recognizable α-granules in platelets. The disorder is inherited in an autosomal recessive fashion. Clinically, gray platelet syndrome is characterized by lifelong mild bleeding tendencies, moderate thrombocytopenia, fibrosis of the marrow, and large platelets whose gray appearance on a Wright-stained blood film (Figure 37.4) is the source of the name of this disorder.[7,55] More recently, a mutation in region 3p21.31 involving the gene *NBEAL2* has been identified. This gene is crucial for the development of α-granules.[56,57]

In electron photomicrographs of platelets and megakaryocytes the platelets appear to have virtually no α-granules, although they do contain vacuoles and small α-granule precursors that stain positive for VWF and fibrinogen. Other types of granules are present in normal numbers. The membranes of the vacuoles and the α-granule precursors have P-selectin (CD62) and GP IIb/IIIa, which can be translocated to the cell membrane upon platelet stimulation with thrombin. This suggests that these structures are α-granules that cannot store the typical α-granule proteins. This may provide an explanation for the observation that, in gray platelet syndrome, the plasma levels of platelet factor 4 and β-thromboglobulin are increased, because although the proteins normally contained in α-granules are produced, storage in those granules is not possible. As a result the proteins are released into circulation. Most patients develop early-onset myelofibrosis, which can be attributed to the inability of megakaryocytes to store newly synthesized platelet-derived growth factors.[44]

Treatment of severe bleeding episodes may require platelet transfusions, because few other treatments are available for these patients. Cryoprecipitate has been used to control bleeding. Desmopressin acetate was found to shorten the bleeding time test (Chapter 41) and has been used as successful prophylaxis during a dental extraction procedure. Some authors believe that desmopressin acetate should be the initial therapy of choice.[7,44,58,59]

Other storage pool diseases. A rare disorder in which both α-granules and dense granules are deficient is known as α-dense storage pool deficiency. This condition seems to be inherited in an autosomal dominant manner. Other membrane abnormalities also have been described in affected patients.[33]

Quebec platelet disorder is an autosomal dominant bleeding disorder that results from a deficiency of multimerin (a multimeric protein that is stored complexed with factor V in α-granules). Even though α-granule structure is maintained, many α-granule proteins show signs of protease-related degradation. Thrombocytopenia may be present, although it is not a consistent feature.[33]

Thromboxane Pathway Disorders: Aspirin-Like Effects

Platelet secretion requires the activation of several biochemical pathways. One such pathway leads to thromboxane formation (Chapter 10). A series of phospholipases catalyze the release of arachidonic acid and several other compounds from membrane phospholipids. Arachidonic acid is converted to intermediate prostaglandins by cyclooxygenase and to thromboxane A_2 by thromboxane synthase (Figure 10.12). Thromboxane A_2 and other substances generated during platelet activation cause mobilization of ionic calcium from internal stores into the cytoplasm, initiating a cascade of events resulting in secretion and aggregation of platelets.[60]

Several acquired or congenital disorders of platelet secretion can be traced to structural and functional modifications of *arachidonic acid pathway enzymes*. Inhibition of cyclooxygenase occurs following ingestion of drugs such as aspirin and ibuprofen. As a result, the amount of thromboxane A_2 produced from arachidonic acid depends on the degree of inhibition. Thromboxane A_2 is required for storage granule secretion and maximal platelet aggregation in response to epinephrine, ADP, and low concentrations of collagen.[5,20,61]

Hereditary absence or abnormalities of the components of the thromboxane pathway are usually termed "aspirin-like defects" because the clinical and laboratory manifestations resemble those that follow aspirin ingestion. Platelet aggregation responses are similar to those in dense granule storage pool disorders (see earlier discussion). Unlike in storage pool disorders, however, ultrastructure and granular contents are normal. Deficiencies of the enzymes *cyclooxygenase* and *thromboxane synthase* are well documented, and dysfunction or deficiency of *thromboxane receptors* is known.[44]

Other Inherited Disorders of Receptors and Signaling Pathways

Collagen Receptors

The $\alpha_2\beta_1$ (GP Ia/IIa) integrin is one of the collagen receptors in the platelet membrane. A deficiency of this receptor has been reported in a patient who lacked an aggregation response to collagen, whose platelets did not adhere to collagen, and who had a lifelong mild bleeding disorder.[62] A deficiency in another collagen receptor, GP VI, also has been reported in patients with mild bleeding. The platelets of these patients failed to aggregate in response to collagen, and adhesion to collagen also was impaired.[63] A family with gray platelet syndrome and defective collagen adhesion has been described. Affected members of the family have a severe deficiency of GP VI.[64]

Adenosine Diphosphate Receptors

Platelets contain at least three receptors for ADP. $P2X_1$ is linked to an ion channel that facilitates calcium ion influx. $P2Y_1$ and $P2Y_{12}$ ($P2T_{AC}$) are members of the seven-transmembrane domain (STD) family of G protein-linked receptors (Chapter 10). $P2Y_1$ is thought to mediate calcium mobilization and shape change in response to ADP. Pathology of the $P2Y_1$ receptor has not yet been reported. $P2Y_{12}$ is thought to be responsible for macroscopic platelet aggregation and is coupled to adenylate cyclase through a G-inhibitory (G_i) protein complex.[65] Patients with an *inherited deficiency of the $P2Y_{12}$ receptor* exhibit decreased platelet aggregation in response to ADP but normal platelet shape change and calcium mobilization.[66–68] Bleeding problems seem to be relatively mild in these patients. The only treatment for severe bleeding is platelet transfusion.

Other Receptors

Congenital defects of the *α_2-adrenergic (epinephrine) receptor* associated with decreased platelet activation and aggregation in response to epinephrine are known. *PAR receptor* defects have been described in one family.[33]

Calcium Mobilization Defects

Calcium mobilization defects represent a heterogeneous group of disorders in which all elements of the thromboxane pathway are normal, but *insufficient calcium is released* from the dense tubular system, and the cytoplasmic concentration of ionic calcium in the cytoplasm never reaches levels high enough to support secretion. Such defects result from *abnormal G protein subunits and phospholipase C isoenzymes*.[20,69,70]

Scott Syndrome

Scott syndrome is a very rare autosomal recessive disorder of calcium-induced membrane phospholipid scrambling (necessary for coagulation factor assembly) and thrombin generation on platelets. Platelets secrete and aggregate normally but do not transport phosphatidylserine and phosphatidylethanolamine from the inner leaflet to the outer leaflet of the plasma membrane. This *phospholipid "flip"* normally occurs during platelet activation and is essential for the binding of vitamin K-dependent clotting factors.

In the membrane of resting platelets, phosphatidylserine and phosphatidylethanolamine are restricted to the inner leaflet of the plasma membrane, and phosphatidylcholine is expressed on the outer leaflet. This asymmetry is maintained by the enzyme aminophospholipid translocase.[71] When platelets are activated, the asymmetry is lost, and phosphatidylserine and phosphatidylethanolamine flip to the outer leaflet, providing binding sites for vitamin K-dependent clotting factors and facilitating the assembly of clotting factor complexes. The phospholipid flip is mediated by a calcium-dependent enzyme, scramblase.[72]

In Scott syndrome, platelet plug formation (including adhesion, aggregation, and secretion) occurs normally, but clotting factor complexes do not assemble on the activated platelet surface, and thrombin generation is absent or much reduced. Because lack of thrombin generation leads to inadequate fibrin formation, the platelet plug is not stabilized, and a bleeding disorder results.[73,74]

Stormorken Syndrome

Stormorken syndrome is an autosomal dominant disorder characterized by a mild bleeding tendency due to platelet dysfunction, thrombocytopenia, anemia, functional asplenia, and other constitutive disorders. Stormorken syndrome is a condition in which platelets are always in an "activated" state and *express phosphatidylserine* on the outer leaflet of the membrane without prior activation. It has been postulated that patients with this syndrome have a defective aminophospholipid translocase due to one or more mutations that result in constitutive activation of the calcium channel, with resultant inhibition of further activation.[75]

Acquired Defects of Platelet Function

Unlike inherited disorders of platelet function, which are rare, acquired disorders of platelet function are commonly encountered. The most frequent cause of acquired platelet dysfunction is drug ingestion. Therapeutic drugs have been developed with the target

TABLE 37.3   Antiplatelet Drugs

Target	Drugs
COX-1 (irreversible)	Aspirin
COX-1 (reversible)	Naproxen
	Sulfinpyrazone
	Ibuprofen (and like drugs)
ADP P2Y12 (irreversible)	Clopidogrel
	Prasugrel
ADP P2Y12 (reversible)	Ticagrelor
	Cangrelor
Thrombin PAR-1	Vorapaxar
GP IIb/IIIa	Abciximab
	Eptifibatide
	Tirofiban
Phosphodiesterase	Dipyridamole
	Aggrenox

of inhibiting platelet function. Other drugs and certain agents developed for various nonplatelet targets have an identified antiplatelet side effect. The agents that will be discussed are summarized in Table 37.3, and the actions of the main therapeutic agents are illustrated in Figure 37.5.

Drug-Induced Defects

Drugs that inhibit the prostaglandin pathway. Acetylsalicylic acid (aspirin) and other drugs that inhibit the platelet prostaglandin synthesis pathway are the most common culprits in acquired platelet dysfunction. A single 200-mg dose of aspirin can irreversibly acetylate 90% of the platelet cyclooxygenase (Figure 10.12). In platelets the acetylated cyclooxygenase (cyclooxygenase-1 [COX-1]) enzyme is completely inactive. Because platelets lack a nucleus and cannot synthesize new enzymes, the inhibitory effect is permanent for the circulatory life span of the platelet (7 to 10 days).

Endothelial cells, on the other hand, synthesize new cyclooxygenase. Endothelial cell cyclooxygenase seems to be less sensitive to aspirin than the platelet enzyme, at least at low dosages. This has led to the view that low dosages of aspirin may be better than higher dosages for cardiovascular protection – because platelet *thromboxane* production is inhibited, whereas endothelial cells recover *prostacyclin* production, with its accompanying antiplatelet effects. Others argue that inhibition of platelet function is the more important effect and that higher dosages of aspirin are better for this purpose. For these reasons there are wide-ranging opinions as to the optimal antiplatelet dosage of aspirin.

What is lost in these arguments is that endothelial cells also produce another potent platelet inhibitor, *nitric oxide* (NO), and its production is not affected by aspirin. Although aspirin may inhibit a proaggregatory mechanism (thromboxane production) and an antiaggregatory mechanism (prostacyclin production) in endothelial cells, the NO platelet inhibitory mechanism is not affected.

It may be necessary to define a test system to determine the optimal dosage of aspirin for cardiovascular protection on an

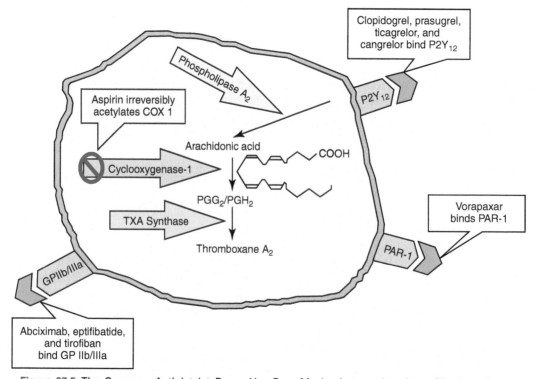

Figure 37.5 The Common Antiplatelet Drugs Use Four Mechanisms to Inactivate Platelets. Aspirin irreversibly acetylates and inactivates cyclooxygenase 1 (COX-1). Clopidogrel (irreversible), prasugrel (irreversible), ticagrelor (reversible), and cangrelor (reversible) bind the adenosine diphosphate *(ADP)* receptor P2Y$_{12}$. Abciximab (irreversible), eptifibatide (reversible) and tirofiban (reversible) block the fibrinogen binding site of the glycoprotein *(GP)* IIb/IIIa receptor. Vorapaxar blocks the thrombin binding site on the PAR-1 receptor. *PGG$_2$*, Prostaglandin G$_2$; *PGH$_2$*, prostaglandin H$_2$; *TXA*, thromboxane A$_2$.

individual basis because some patients have, or develop, *aspirin resistance*, and a dosage that previously was sufficient to inhibit platelet function effectively may no longer be able to produce that effect. In addition, unlike the practice with almost all other therapeutic agents, a single dose of aspirin is usually prescribed in a "one dose fits all" fashion (e.g., 325 mg) without regard to the patient's weight, age, health status, or other measurable parameters. Evidence is emerging, however, that there are considerable interindividual differences in the response to a single dose of aspirin.[2,20,76,77] One study has shown that patients who do not respond well to aspirin have worse cardiovascular outcomes than patients who respond well.[78] The VerifyNow (IL-Werfen) is one system that provides measurement of a patient's response to antiplatelet medication (Chapters 40, 41, and 42). Individual tests for aspirin, P2Y$_{12}$ receptor inhibitors (clopidogrel, prasugrel, ticagrelor), and GP IIb/IIIa receptor inhibitors (abciximab, eptifibatide, tirofiban) are available on the VerifyNow.

Individuals known to have a hemostatic defect, such as a storage pool deficiency, thrombocytopenia, a vascular disorder, or VWD, may experience a marked increase in bleeding tendency after aspirin ingestion, and such individuals should be advised to avoid the use of aspirin and related agents.[20]

Many drugs inhibit cyclooxygenase, but, unlike with aspirin and closely related compounds, the inhibition is *reversible*. These drugs are said to be competitive inhibitors of cyclooxygenase, and as the blood concentration of the drug decreases, platelet function is recovered. This group of drugs includes ibuprofen and related compounds, such as ketoprofen, fenoprofen, naproxen, and sulfinpyrazone. In contrast to aspirin, most of these agents have little effect on platelet function tests (Chapters 41 and 42). Except for their potential to irritate the gastric mucosa, these drugs have not been reported to cause clinically important bleeding.[5,8,20,79] Interestingly, ibuprofen appears to have a prothrombotic effect when ingested within 2 hours of aspirin because it blocks the acetylation site for aspirin on COX-1. Patients taking aspirin should be cautioned to avoid ibuprofen and related drugs near the time of aspirin ingestion.[80]

Drugs that inhibit membrane function. Many drugs interact with platelet membrane receptors and cause a clinically significant platelet function defect that may lead to hemorrhage. Some of these drugs are useful antiplatelet agents, whereas for many other drugs, their effects on the platelet membrane are an adverse side effect.[60]

P2Y$_{12}$ (ADP) receptor inhibitors. The thienopyridine derivatives clopidogrel and prasugrel; their predecessor, ticlopidine; the nucleoside ticagrelor; and the nucleotide mimetic cangrelor are antiplatelet agents that bind to the P2 Y$_{12}$ platelet receptor[66] and inhibit stimulus-response coupling between those receptors and fibrinogen binding to GP IIb/IIIa. As a consequence platelet activation and aggregation induced by ADP are markedly inhibited, and responses to other aggregating agents, such as collagen, are reduced.[66] As with aspirin inhibition of cyclooxygenase, the effect of the irreversible thienopyridines on platelet recovery of function following drug cessation is 50% of normal at 3 days, and complete at 7 to 10 days.[81] Both ticagrelor and cangrelor are reversible inhibitors of the P2Y$_{12}$ receptor.

In contrast to the immediate effect of aspirin, the effect of these agents does not reach a steady state for 3 to 5 days, although a steady state can be reached sooner with a loading dose. As prophylactic agents they have been shown to be as efficacious as aspirin. These drugs are used to prevent myocardial infarction in patients with arterial occlusive disease, to reduce the risk of thrombotic stroke in patients with cerebrovascular disease, for stroke and myocardial infarction prophylaxis, and for patients who are intolerant of aspirin. P2Y$_{12}$ inhibitors and aspirin are often used in combination to prevent arterial thrombosis, primarily based on the synergistic action of these two drugs, which inhibits platelet function by different mechanisms.

Clopidogrel (Plavix, Bristol-Myers Squibb/Sanofi; generic versions also available) is a prodrug that requires conversion to the active drug by the 2C19 (a.k.a. CYP2C19) isoform of P450 in the liver. Thus the clinical effectiveness varies from patient to patient based on the extent of metabolism to the active drug. There are numerous mutations in CYP2C19 that result in decreased activity of the enzyme and therefore inhibit the conversion of clopidogrel to the active drug. CYP2C19*1/*1 (wild type) represents two normal functioning alleles and normal metabolism of clopidogrel to the active drug. Hypofunctional alleles are CYP2C19*2 to *10, whereas CYP2C19*17 is a hyperfunctional allele. Patients with one of the mutations resulting in decreased activity (e.g., CYP2C19*1/*2) are considered intermediate metabolizers, and the usual dose of clopidogrel does not achieve the degree of platelet inhibition desired. These individuals remain at increased risk for thromboembolic events. Increasing the dose of clopidogrel may increase the degree of platelet inhibition, but it does not decrease the thromboembolic risk. Those who have two hypofunctional alleles (CYP2C19*2/*2, *2/*3, or any combination of two hypofunctional alleles) are poor metabolizers and do not derive significant benefit from clopidogrel therapy. Approximately 25% of individuals have one or two hypofunctional alleles of CYP2C19 and are considered to be clopidogrel resistant.

In contrast patients with a *17 allele are rapid metabolizers and convert clopidogrel to the active drug at a faster rate. This results in increased blood levels of the active drug following a dose of clopidogrel and an increased risk of bleeding. Those with one normal allele and one *17 allele (*1/*17) are considered to be rapid metabolizers and those who are *17/*17 are ultra-rapid metabolizers. Individuals with one hypofunctional and one hyperfunctional allele (e.g., *2/*17) have normal to intermediate clopidogrel metabolism. There are a variety of molecular methods available to test for the most common alleles of CYP2C19. Although the US Food and Drug Administration (FDA) has recommended pharmacogenetic testing for these alleles, it is not common practice due to cost.

Clopidogrel has more effect on platelet function tests than aspirin, although there is little difference in the risk of clinical bleeding.[82] Clopidogrel can occasionally produce major side effects in some patients, including long-lasting neutropenia, aplastic anemia, thrombocytopenia, gastrointestinal distress, and diarrhea.

Prasugrel (Effient, Lilly) is a third-generation thienopyridine derivative with the same mechanism of action as clopidogrel.[83]

It is also a prodrug, but its metabolism to the active form does not require CYP2C19. Instead, it is metabolized to the active drug by carboxylesterase-2 and several enzymes of the cytochrome P450 system, including CYP3A4 and CYP2B6. Because it is activated by several enzymes, mutations that result in decreased function of one or more of these enzyme have less impact, and the response is much more uniform than clopidogrel. Pharmacogenetic testing for mutations affecting prasugrel activation is not recommended.

Ticagrelor (Brilinta, AstraZeneca) is a nucleoside analog inhibitor of the P2Y$_{12}$ receptor.[83] Although its antiplatelet effect is similar, it has two important differences from prasugrel and clopidogrel. First, it is not a prodrug and therefore does not require bioactivation. Because it is rapidly absorbed, its antiplatelet effect is predictable and achieved in a short period of time. In addition, ticagrelor binds to a slightly different site on the P2Y$_{12}$ (ADP) receptor than clopidogrel or prasugrel. This difference results in reversible binding. Therefore, unlike clopidogrel and prasugrel, whose effects are irreversible, platelet function returns quite rapidly with cessation of ticagrelor. However, this shorter half-life (7 to 9 hours) necessitates twice-daily dosing and may result in compliance issues with some patients.

Cangrelor (Kengreal, The Medicines Company) is a reversible, nucleotide mimetic P2Y$_{12}$ inhibitor that, like ticagrelor, does not undergo metabolic activation.[84] Among the P2Y$_{12}$ inhibitors cangrelor is unique in that it can be administered intravenously. Cangrelor is approved for use as an adjunct treatment for reducing the risk of myocardial infarction, repeat coronary intervention, and stent thrombosis in patients undergoing percutaneous coronary intervention. Owing to its rapid onset of action (minutes) and offset of action (60 to 90 minutes), it has been suggested that cangrelor may be useful as bridge therapy in patients who need to discontinue thienopyridine therapy prior to surgery.[85]

GP IIb/IIIa ($\alpha_{IIb}\beta_3$) receptor inhibitors. Another target for antiplatelet agents to reduce cardiovascular thrombotic risk is the platelet membrane GP IIb/IIIa ($\alpha_{IIb}\beta_3$) receptor. Interference with the ability of this receptor to bind fibrinogen inhibits platelet aggregation stimulated in response to all of the usual platelet aggregating agents. Results of platelet function studies on platelets from patients receiving therapeutic doses of these drugs essentially mimic those of a mild form of Glanzmann thrombasthenia.

Two different types of agents are included in this group. The first is the mouse/human chimeric monoclonal antibody 7E3, abciximab (ReoPro, Lilly), which, by binding to the GP IIb/IIIa receptor, prevents the binding of fibrinogen and limits platelet aggregation. Numerous studies have shown the efficacy of this drug as an antiplatelet and antithrombotic agent.

The second type of agent in this group targets a site within the GP IIb/IIIa receptor that recognizes the arginine-glycine-aspartic acid (RGD) sequence found in fibrinogen and several adhesive proteins. These agents bind to the RGD recognition site, prevent the binding of fibrinogen, and consequently prevent platelet aggregation. Tirofiban (Aggrastat, Medicure) is a nonpeptide RGD mimetic, and eptifibatide (Integrilin, Merck) is a cyclic heptapeptide that is also an RGD mimetic.

The goal of therapy with these drugs is to induce a controlled thrombasthenia-like state. At present these agents are primarily used in patients undergoing percutaneous coronary intervention and are administered concurrently with heparin and other antiplatelet agents.[86–88] The use of these agents is limited by their short half-lives and the need to administer them by constant intravenous infusion. There have been attempts to make an orally active agent of this type, but none has yet been approved for use.

PAR-1 antagonists. Thrombin activates platelets via G-protein-linked receptors called *protease-activated receptors* (PARs). There are three distinct PARs on human platelets (PAR-1, PAR-2, PAR-4). Thrombin activates platelets by cleaving a portion of the N-terminus of the receptor. The newly exposed N-terminus interacts with the transmembrane domains of the receptor and acts as a tethered ligand. Vorapaxar (Zontivity, Merck) inhibits thrombin-induced platelet aggregation by blocking the ligand-binding site on PAR-1. Vorapaxar is used as secondary prevention in combination with low-dose aspirin and clopidogrel in patients with a history of myocardial infarction or peripheral artery disease. Patients with a history of stroke or transient ischemic attack should not be treated with vorapaxar due to an increased risk of bleeding.[89,90]

Other therapeutic drugs that inhibit platelet function. Dipyridamole (Aggrenox, Boehringer Ingelheim) is an inhibitor of platelet phosphodiesterase, the enzyme responsible for converting cyclic adenosine monophosphate (cAMP) to AMP. Inhibition of phosphodiesterase allows the accumulation of cAMP in the cytoplasm; elevation of cytoplasmic cAMP is inhibitory to platelet function (Figure 10.12). Dipyridamole alone does not inhibit platelet aggregation in response to the usual platelet agonists, but it promotes inhibition of agents that stimulate cAMP formation, such as prostacyclin, stable analogues of prostacyclin, and NO. Dipyridamole is most commonly used in combination with aspirin for reducing the risk of stroke in patients with a history of transient ischemic attack or thrombotic stroke.

Miscellaneous agents that inhibit platelet function. Antibiotics are well known for their ability to interfere with platelet function. Most of the drugs with this effect contain a β-lactam ring and are either a penicillin or a cephalosporin. These drugs can inhibit platelet function tests, but this effect is seen chiefly in patients receiving large parenteral doses and is thus only a problem for hospitalized patients. One postulated mechanism for the antiplatelet effect of these drugs is that they associate with the membrane via a lipophilic reaction and block receptor-agonist interactions or stimulus-response coupling between receptors and fibrinogen binding to GP IIb/IIIa. They also may inhibit calcium influx in response to thrombin stimulation, reducing the ability of thrombin to activate platelets. Although these drugs may prolong the in vitro aggregation responses to certain agonists, their association with a hemostatic defect severe enough to cause clinical hemorrhage is uncertain and is likely not predicted by laboratory test results.[2,8,61,91]

Nitrofurantoin is a non-β-lactam antibiotic that may inhibit platelet aggregation when high concentrations are present in the blood. This drug is not known to cause clinical bleeding.[91]

Dextrans are partially hydrolyzed, branched-chain polysaccharides of glucose. The two most commonly used are dextran 70 (molecular mass of 70,000 Daltons) and dextran 40 (molecular mass of 40,000 Daltons) also known as low-molecular-weight dextran. Both drugs are commonly used as plasma expanders. Although dextrans can inhibit platelet aggregation and impair platelet procoagulant activity when given as an intravenous infusion, these drugs have no effect on in vitro platelet function when added directly to platelet-rich plasma. Because of their effects on platelets, they have been extensively used as antithrombotic agents. There does not seem to be any increased risk of hemorrhage associated with the use of these agents, but their efficacy in preventing postoperative pulmonary embolism is equal to that of low-dose subcutaneous heparin.[5,52,91]

Hydroxyethyl starch, or hetastarch, is a synthetic glucose polymer with a mean molecular mass up to 450,000 Daltons that is used as a plasma expander. It has effects similar to those of the dextrans. The mechanism of action of plasma expander drugs has not been elucidated but is presumed to involve interaction with the platelet membrane.[5,52]

Several other agents of diverse chemical structure and function are known to inhibit platelet function. The mechanisms by which they induce platelet dysfunction are largely unknown. Nitroglycerin, nitroprusside, propranolol, and isosorbide dinitrate are drugs used to regulate cardiovascular function that seem to be able to cause a decrease in platelet secretion and aggregation. Patients taking phenothiazine or tricyclic antidepressants may have decreased secretion and aggregation responses, but these effects are not associated with an increased risk for hemorrhage. Local and general anesthetics may impair in vitro aggregation responses. The same is true of antihistamines. Some radiographic contrast agents are known to inhibit platelet function.[91]

Disorders that Affect Platelet Function

Myeloproliferative neoplasms. Chronic myeloproliferative neoplasms (MPNs) include polycythemia vera, chronic myelogenous leukemia (CML), essential thrombocythemia (ET), and myelofibrosis with myeloid metaplasia (Chapter 32). Platelet dysfunction is a common finding in patients with these disorders. Hemorrhagic complications occur in about one third, thrombosis occurs in another third, and, although it is uncommon, both develop in some patients. These complications are serious causes of morbidity and mortality in affected patients.

Although the occurrence of hemorrhage or thrombosis in MPN patients is largely unpredictable, certain patterns have emerged. Hemorrhage and thrombosis are less common in CML than in the other MPNs. Bleeding seems to be more common in myelofibrosis with myeloid metaplasia, but thrombosis is more common in the other MPNs.

In patients with these disorders thrombosis may occur in unusual sites, including the mesenteric, hepatic, and portal circulations. Patients with ET may develop digital artery thrombosis and ischemia of the fingers and toes, occlusions of the microvasculature of the heart, and cerebrovascular occlusions that result in neurologic symptoms.[91]

Abnormal platelet function has been postulated as a contributing cause. This hypothesis is supported by the observation that bleeding is usually mucocutaneous in nature, and thrombosis may be arterial or venous. In MPNs a variety of platelet function defects have been described, but their clinical importance is uncertain. Platelets have been reported to have abnormal shapes, decreased procoagulant activity, a decreased number of secretory granules, and shortened survival. The risk of thrombosis or hemorrhage correlates poorly with the elevation of the platelet count.

The most common functional abnormalities are decreased aggregation and secretion in response to epinephrine, ADP, and collagen.[92] Possible causes of the platelet dysfunction include loss of platelet surface membrane α-adrenergic (epinephrine) receptors, impaired release of arachidonic acid from membrane phospholipids in response to stimulation by agonists, impaired oxidation of arachidonic acid by the cyclooxygenase and lipoxygenase pathways, a decrease in the contents of dense granules and α-granules, and loss of a variety of platelet membrane receptors for adhesion and activation. There seems to be no correlation between a given MPN and the type of platelet dysfunction observed, with the exception that most patients with ET lack an in vitro platelet aggregation response to epinephrine. This observation may be helpful in the differential diagnosis.[5,8,91,93]

Multiple myeloma and Waldenström macroglobulinemia. Platelet dysfunction is observed in approximately one third of patients with IgA myeloma or Waldenström macroglobulinemia, a much smaller percentage of patients with IgG multiple myeloma, and only occasionally in patients with monoclonal gammopathy of undetermined significance.

Platelet dysfunction results from coating of the platelet membrane by paraprotein and does not depend on the type of paraprotein present. In addition to interacting with platelets, the paraprotein likely interferes with fibrin polymerization and the function of other coagulation proteins.

Almost all patients with malignant paraprotein disorders have clinically significant bleeding, but thrombocytopenia is still the most likely cause of bleeding in these patients. Other causes of bleeding include hyperviscosity syndrome, complications of amyloidosis (e.g., acquired factor X deficiency), and, in rare instances, presence of a circulating heparin-like anticoagulant or fibrinolysis.[11,91]

Cardiopulmonary bypass surgery. The use of cardiopulmonary bypass (CPB; heart-lung machine) extracorporeal blood circulation during cardiac surgery induces thrombocytopenia and a severe platelet function defect that assumes major importance in relation to postsurgical bleeding.[91] The function defect most likely results from platelet activation and fragmentation in the extracorporeal circuit. Causes of platelet activation include adherence and aggregation of platelets to fibrinogen (adsorbed onto the surfaces of the bypass circuit material), mechanical trauma and shear stresses, use of blood conservation devices (red blood cell salvage and saline suspension), bypass pump-priming solutions during surgery, hypothermia, complement activation, and exposure of platelets to the blood-air interface in bubble oxygenators.[94]

Some degree of platelet degranulation typically is found after cardiac surgery using CPB, which indicates that platelet activation and secretion have occurred during the operation. Platelet membrane fragments, or "microparticles," are found consistently in the blood of these surgical patients, providing additional evidence of the severe mechanical stress encountered by platelets during these extracorporeal procedures.

The severity of the platelet function defect closely correlates with the length of time on the bypass circuit. Normal platelet function returns in about 1 hour after an uncomplicated surgical procedure, although the platelet count does not normalize for several days. Thrombocytopenia is caused by hemodilution, accumulation of platelets on the surfaces of the bypass materials, sequestration or removal of damaged platelets by the liver and mononuclear phagocyte system, and consumption associated with normal hemostatic processes after surgery.[91]

Liver disease. Moderate to severe liver disease is associated with a variety of hemostatic abnormalities, including reduction in clotting proteins, reduction of proteins in the natural anticoagulant pathways, dysfibrinogenemia, and excessive fibrinolysis (Chapter 36). Mild to moderate thrombocytopenia is seen in approximately one third of patients with chronic liver disease in association with hypersplenism or as a result of alcohol toxicity.[7,91]

Abnormal platelet function test results seen in patients with chronic liver disease include reduced platelet adhesion, abnormal platelet aggregation (in response to ADP, epinephrine, and thrombin), abnormal phospholipid availability, and reduced procoagulant activity. An acquired storage pool deficiency also has been suggested. The abnormal platelet function in these patients may respond to infusion of desmopressin acetate. It is unclear, however, whether desmopressin acetate provides a benefit in preventing bleeding in these patients or is simply correcting an abnormal laboratory test result.

In chronic alcoholic cirrhosis, thrombocytopenia and platelet abnormalities may result from the direct toxic effects of alcohol on bone marrow megakaryocytes. Chronic, periodic, and even acute alcohol consumption may result in a transient decrease in platelet function; however, the inhibitory effect seems to be more pronounced when alcohol is consumed in excess. The impaired platelet function is thought to be related at least in part to inhibition of thromboxane synthesis. The severe bleeding diathesis associated with end-stage liver disease has many causes, such as markedly decreased or negligible coagulation factor production, excessive fibrinolysis, dysfibrinogenemia, thrombocytopenia due to acquired thrombopoietin deficiency, splenic sequestration secondary to portal hypertension, and (occasionally) disseminated intravascular coagulation. Upper gastrointestinal tract bleeding (e.g., from esophageal or gastric varices) is a relatively common complication of cirrhosis, particularly alcoholic cirrhosis, but occurs as a complication of end-stage liver disease of any etiology.[5,20,95,96]

Uremia. Uremia is commonly accompanied by bleeding caused by platelet dysfunction. Abnormal platelet function is far more common than clinically significant bleeding in uremic patients.[60,62] In uremia, guanidinosuccinic acid (GSA) is present in the circulation in higher than normal levels as a result of inhibition of the urea cycle. Because GSA is an NO donor, NO is present in the circulation at higher than normal levels in uremia. NO diffuses into platelets, activates soluble guanylate cyclase, and inhibits platelet adhesion, activation, and aggregation.[97] GSA is dialyzable, and dialysis (peritoneal dialysis or hemodialysis) is usually effective in correcting the abnormal platelet function characteristic of uremia.

Platelet aggregation pattern abnormalities are not uniform, and any combination of defects may be seen. There is evidence of a defective release reaction, such as lack of primary ADP-induced aggregation, and subnormal platelet procoagulant activity. Anemia is an independent cause of prolonged bleeding time, and the severity of anemia in uremic patients correlates with the severity of renal failure. Many uremic patients are treated with recombinant erythropoietin to increase their hematocrit.

Bleeding in uremic patients is seen more often with concurrent use of drugs that interfere with platelet function or in association with heparin use in hemodialysis. Platelet concentrates have been used to treat severe hemorrhagic episodes in patients with uremia but usually do not correct the bleeding. Other therapies that are sometimes effective in uremic bleeding include use of cryoprecipitated antihemophilic factor (to increase fibrinogen levels), DDAVP, and conjugated estrogen.

Hereditary afibrinogenemia. Congenital afibrinogenemia, a rare and inherited disorder, has been documented in more than 150 families. Although it is not truly a platelet function disorder, platelets do not exhibit normal function in the absence or near-absence of fibrinogen. Abnormal results in platelet retention and adhesion studies involving the use of glass beads also have been documented. In addition, results of all clot-based tests (including partial thromboplastin time, prothrombin time, reptilase time, thrombin time, and whole-blood clotting time) are abnormal. Addition of fibrinogen to samples or infusion of fibrinogen into the patient results in correction of the abnormal test results.[98]

A high incidence of hemorrhagic manifestations is found in patients with afibrinogenemia (or severe hypofibrinogenemia). Bleeding is the cause of death in about one third of such patients. Cryoprecipitate or fibrinogen concentrate (RiaSTAP, human fibrinogen concentrate, Behring) can be used to treat bleeding episodes. Some patients develop antibodies to fibrinogen, and this treatment then becomes ineffective.[98]

Hyperaggregable Platelets

Patients with a variety of disorders associated with thrombosis or increased risk for thrombosis, including hyperlipidemia, diabetes mellitus, peripheral arterial occlusive disease, acute arterial occlusion, myocardial infarction, and stroke, have been reported to have increased platelet reactivity. Platelets from these patients tend to aggregate at lower concentrations of aggregating agents than do platelets from individuals without these conditions.

Sticky platelet syndrome is an autosomal dominant, thrombophilic disorder that is associated with venous and arterial thromboembolic events. The disorder is characterized by hyperaggregable platelets in response to ADP, epinephrine, or both. In these patients venous and/or arterial thrombotic events are often associated with emotional stress. Prophylactic treatment of these patients with low-dose aspirin reverses clinical symptoms and normalizes hyperaggregable responses to aggregating agents in the laboratory.

Spontaneous aggregation (aggregation in response to in vitro stirring only) is an indicator of abnormally increased platelet reactivity and often accompanies increased sensitivity to platelet agonists. The presence of spontaneous aggregation by itself is considered to be consistent with the presence of a hyperaggregable state. Because participation of platelets is necessary for the development of arterial thrombosis, the presence of hyperaggregable platelets is often an indication that an antiplatelet agent should be used as part of a therapeutic or prophylactic regimen for arterial thrombosis.[99,100]

Other Causes of Platelet Function Defects

Acquired platelet function defects are seen occasionally in patients with autoimmune disorders, including systemic lupus erythematosus, rheumatoid arthritis, scleroderma, and the immune thrombocytopenias, such as immune thrombocytopenic purpura.[93]

Purified fibrin degradation products can induce platelet dysfunction in vitro. The pathophysiologic relevance of this observation is uncertain because the concentrations of fibrin degradation products required are unlikely to be reached in vivo. Patients with disseminated intravascular coagulation may have reduced platelet function, however, as a result of in vivo stimulation by thrombin and other agonists resulting in in vivo release of granule contents. This has been called *acquired storage pool disease*; the term *exhausted platelets* may be more appropriate.[101]

VASCULAR DISORDERS

The pathophysiology of disorders of vessels and their supporting tissues is obscure. Laboratory studies of platelets and blood coagulation usually yield normal results. The diagnosis is often based on medical history and is made by ruling out other sources of bleeding disorders. The usual clinical sign is the tendency to bruise easily or to bleed spontaneously, especially from mucosal surfaces. Vascular disorders are summarized in Box 37.3.

Hereditary Vascular Disorders
Hereditary Hemorrhagic Telangiectasia (Rendu-Osler-Weber Syndrome)

The mode of inheritance of hereditary hemorrhagic telangiectasia is autosomal dominant. The vascular defect of this disorder is characterized by thin-walled blood vessels with a discontinuous endothelium, inadequate smooth muscle, and inadequate or missing elastin in the surrounding stroma. Telangiectasias (dilated superficial blood vessels that create small, focal red lesions) occur throughout the body but are most obvious on the face, lips, tongue, conjunctiva, nasal mucosa, fingers, toes, and trunk and under the tongue. The lesions blanch when pressure is applied. The disorder usually manifests by puberty and progresses throughout life.

BOX 37.3 Vascular Disorders[3]

Hereditary Vascular Disorders
Hereditary hemorrhagic telangiectasia (Rendu-Osler-Weber syndrome)
Hemangioma-thrombocytopenia syndrome (Kasabach-Merritt syndrome)
Ehlers-Danlos syndrome and other genetic disorders

Acquired Vascular Disorders
Allergic purpura (Henoch-Schönlein purpura)
Paraproteinemia and amyloidosis
Senile purpura
Drug-induced vascular purpuras
Vitamin C deficiency (scurvy)

Purpuras of Unknown Origin
Purpura simplex (easy bruising)
Psychogenic purpura

Telangiectasias are fragile and prone to rupture. Epistaxis is an almost universal finding, and symptoms almost always worsen with age. The age at which nosebleeds begin is a good gauge of the severity of the disorder. Although the oral cavity, gastrointestinal tract, and urogenital tract are common sites of bleeding, bleeding can occur in virtually every organ.[102]

The diagnosis of hereditary hemorrhagic telangiectasia is based on the characteristic skin or mucous membrane lesions, a history of repeated hemorrhage, and a family history of a similar disorder.

Patients with hereditary hemorrhagic telangiectasia do well despite the lack of specific therapy and the seriousness of their hemorrhagic manifestations.[101] There are several other disorders and conditions in which telangiectasias are present, including cherry-red hemangiomas (common in older men and women), ataxia-telangiectasia (Louis-Bar syndrome), and chronic actinic telangiectasia; they also are seen in association with chronic liver disease and pregnancy.[101]

Hemangioma-Thrombocytopenia Syndrome (Kasabach-Merritt Syndrome)

Kasabach and Merritt originally described the association of a giant cavernous hemangioma (vascular tumor), thrombocytopenia, and a bleeding diathesis. The hemangiomas are visceral or subcutaneous, but rarely both. External hemangiomas may become engorged with blood and resemble hematomas. Other well-recognized complications of Kasabach-Merritt syndrome include acute or chronic disseminated intravascular coagulation (Chapter 39), sequestration of platelets in the hemangiomas, and resultant microangiopathic hemolytic anemia. A hereditary basis for this syndrome has not been established, but the condition is present at birth. Several treatment modalities are available for the angiomas and the associated coagulopathy; they range from corticosteroid therapy to surgery, but none is completely effective. The mortality rate is 30%.[103]

Ehlers-Danlos Syndrome and Other Genetic Disorders

Ehlers-Danlos syndrome may be transmitted as an autosomal dominant, recessive, or X-linked trait. It is manifested by hyperextensible skin, hypermobile joints, joint laxity, fragile tissues, and a bleeding tendency, primarily subcutaneous hematoma formation. Eleven distinct varieties of the disorder are recognized. The severity of bleeding ranges from easy bruising to arterial rupture. The disorder generally can be ascribed to defects in collagen production, structure, or cross-linking, with resulting inadequacy of the connective tissues. Platelet abnormalities have been reported in some patients.

Other inherited vascular disorders include pseudoxanthoma elasticum and homocystinuria (autosomal recessive disorders), Marfan syndrome, and osteogenesis imperfecta (autosomal dominant disorders).

Acquired Vascular Disorders

Allergic Purpura (Henoch-Schönlein Purpura)

The term *allergic purpura* or *anaphylactoid purpura* generally is applied to a group of nonthrombocytopenic purpuras characterized by apparently allergic manifestations, including skin rash and edema. Allergic purpura has been associated with certain foods and drugs, cold, insect bites, and vaccinations. The term *Henoch-Schönlein purpura* is more appropriately applied when the condition is an acute IgA-mediated disorder with widespread generalized vasculitis involving the skin, joints, kidneys, gastrointestinal tract, and, less commonly, the lungs. The purpuric skin lesions are frequently confused with the hemorrhagic rash of immune thrombocytopenic purpura.[52]

General evidence implicates autoimmune microvascular injury, but the pathophysiology of the disorder is unclear. The vasculitis is mediated by immune complexes containing IgA antibodies. It has been suggested that allergic purpura may represent autoimmunity to components of the vessel wall.

Henoch-Schönlein purpura is primarily a disease of children, occurring most commonly in children 3 to 7 years of age. It is relatively uncommon among individuals younger than age 2 or older than age 20. Twice as many boys as girls are affected. The onset of the disease is sudden, often following an upper respiratory tract infection. The infectious organism may damage the endothelial lining of blood vessels, which results in vasculitis.

Malaise, headache, fever, and rash may be the presenting symptoms. The delay in the appearance of the skin rash often poses a difficult problem in differential diagnosis. The skin lesions are urticarial and gradually become pinkish, then red, and finally hemorrhagic. The appearance of the lesions may be very rapid and accompanied by itching. The lesions have been described as "palpable purpura," in contrast to the perfectly flat lesions of thrombocytopenia and most other forms of vascular purpura. These lesions are most commonly found on the feet, elbows, knees, buttocks, and chest. Ultimately, a brownish-red eruption is seen. Petechiae also may be present.

As the disease progresses, abdominal pain, polyarthralgia, headaches, and renal disease may develop. Renal lesions are present in 60% of patients during the second to third week of the disorder. Proteinuria and hematuria are commonly present.[7] The platelet count is normal. Tests of hemostasis, including tests of blood coagulation, usually yield normal results in patients with allergic purpura. Anemia generally is not present unless the hemorrhagic manifestations have been severe. The white blood cell count and the erythrocyte sedimentation rate are usually elevated. The disease must be distinguished from other forms of nonthrombocytopenic purpura. Numerous infectious diseases that may be associated with purpura also must be considered in the differential diagnosis.

In the pediatric age group the average duration of the initial episode is about 4 weeks. Relapses are frequent, usually after a period of apparent well-being. Except for patients in whom chronic renal disease develops, the prognosis is usually good. Occasionally, death from renal failure has occurred. Management is directed primarily at symptomatic relief, because there currently is no effective treatment. Corticosteroids sometimes have been helpful in alleviating symptoms. Most patients recover without treatment.

Paraproteinemia and Amyloidosis

Platelet function can be inhibited by myeloma proteins. Abnormalities in platelet aggregation, secretion, and procoagulant activity (Chapter 41) correlate with the concentration of the plasma paraprotein and are likely due to coating of the platelet membrane with the paraprotein. Under these conditions platelet adhesion and activation receptor functions are inhibited; the paraprotein coating also inhibits assembly of clotting factors on the platelet surface. High concentrations of paraprotein can cause severe hemorrhagic manifestations as a result of a combination of hyperviscosity and platelet dysfunction. About one third of patients with IgA myeloma and Waldenström macroglobulinemia and approximately 5% of patients with IgG myeloma (usually IgG3) exhibit platelet function abnormalities. Finally, the paraprotein may contribute further to bleeding by inhibiting fibrin polymerization. In these patients there is poor correlation between abnormal results on laboratory tests (e.g., prothrombin time, activated partial thromboplastin time, thrombin time, bleeding time) and evidence of clinical bleeding. Treatment for the bleeding complications of these disorders is primarily reduction in the level of the paraprotein. This can be accomplished quickly, albeit transiently, by therapeutic plasma exchange. Longer term treatment is usually chemotherapy for the underlying plasma cell malignancy.[93,104]

Amyloid is a fibrous protein consisting of rigid, linear, nonbranching, aggregated fibrils approximately 7.5 to 10 nm wide and of indefinite length. Amyloid is deposited extracellularly and may lead to damage of normal tissues. Various proteins can serve as subunits of the fibril, including monoclonal light chains (λ more frequently than κ). Amyloidosis, the deposition of abnormal quantities of amyloid protein in tissues, may be primary or secondary, and localized or systemic. Purpura, hemorrhage, and thrombosis may be a part of the clinical presentation of patients with amyloidosis. Thrombosis and hemorrhage have been ascribed to amyloid deposition in the vascular wall and surrounding tissues. Platelet function has been shown to be abnormal in a few cases, and in rare cases patients may have thrombocytopenia. Current treatments (including chemotherapy and other targeted therapies) for most forms of amyloidosis are not effective because none reverse the buildup of amyloid proteins from tissues and organs. Chemotherapy with allogeneic stem cell transplantation has had some success treating the early stages of light-chain amyloidosis.[105]

Senile Purpura

Senile purpura occurs more commonly in elderly men than in women and is due to a lack of collagen support for small blood vessels and loss of subcutaneous fat and elastic fibers. The incidence increases with advancing age. The dark blotches are flattened, are about 1 to 10 mm in diameter, do not blanch with pressure, and resolve slowly, often leaving a brown stain in the skin (age spots) (Figure 38.1). The lesions are limited mostly to the extensor surfaces of the forearms and backs of the hands and occasionally occur on the face and neck. With the exception of increased capillary fragility, results of laboratory tests are normal, and no other bleeding manifestations are present.

Drug-Induced Vascular Purpuras

Purpura associated with drug-induced vasculitis occurs in the presence of functionally adequate platelets. A variety of drugs are known to cause vascular purpura, including aspirin, warfarin, barbiturates, diuretics, digoxin, methyldopa, and several antibiotics. Sulfonamides and iodides have been implicated most frequently. The lesions vary from a few petechiae to massive, generalized petechial eruptions. Mechanisms include development of antibodies to vessel wall components, development of immune complexes, and changes in vessel wall permeability. As soon as the disorder is recognized, the offending drug should be discontinued. No other treatment is necessary.

▌ SUMMARY

- Inherited qualitative platelet disorders can cause bleeding disorders ranging from mild to severe.
- Bernard-Soulier syndrome is caused by the lack of expression of GP Ib/IX/V complexes on the platelet surface. This receptor complex is responsible for platelet adhesion, and its absence results in a severe bleeding disorder.
- Glanzmann thrombasthenia is caused by the lack of expression of GP IIb/IIIa complexes on the platelet surface. This complex is known as the platelet aggregation receptor, and its absence is associated with a severe bleeding disorder.
- Storage pool disorders result from the absence of intraplatelet α-granules, dense granules, or both. Platelet dysfunction associated with these disorders is generally mild; bleeding symptoms also are usually mild.
- Aspirin-like effects result from defects in elements of the arachidonic acid metabolic pathway. Platelet dysfunction mimics that seen after aspirin ingestion.
- Deficiencies of several of the receptors for platelet activating substances have been documented, and bleeding symptoms of varying severity are associated with these deficiencies.

- Drugs are the most common cause of acquired platelet dysfunction, and aspirin is the most frequent culprit. New classes of antiplatelet agents with mechanisms different from aspirin, including ADP receptor antagonists, PAR-1 inhibitors, GP IIb/IIIa inhibitors, and thromboxane inhibitors, are now available.
- A variety of pathologic conditions can result in platelet dysfunction; these include hematologic malignancies, kidney disease, and liver disease.
- Vascular disorders that result in bleeding are uncommon. There are a few well-recognized inherited disorders, however, such as Ehlers-Danlos syndrome and hereditary hemorrhagic telangiectasia, that can result in substantial blood loss.
- Acquired vascular disorders are much more common than inherited disorders. Causes include the effects of aging, drug effects, and allergic reactions.

Now that you have completed this chapter, go back and read again the case study at the beginning and respond to the questions presented.

▌ REVIEW QUESTIONS

Answers can be found in the Appendix.

1. The clinical presentation of platelet-related bleeding may include all of the following *except*:
   a. Bruising
   b. Nosebleeds
   c. Gastrointestinal bleeding
   d. Bleeding into the joints (hemarthroses)
2. A defect in GP IIb/IIIa causes:
   a. Glanzmann thrombasthenia
   b. Bernard-Soulier syndrome
   c. Gray platelet syndrome
   d. Storage pool disease
3. Patients with Bernard-Soulier syndrome have which of the following laboratory test findings?
   a. Abnormal platelet response to arachidonic acid
   b. Abnormal platelet response to ristocetin
   c. Abnormal platelet response to collagen
   d. Thrombocytosis

4. Which of the following is the most common of the hereditary platelet function defects?
   a. Glanzmann thrombasthenia
   b. Bernard-Soulier syndrome
   c. Storage pool defects
   d. Multiple myeloma
5. A reduction in thrombin generation in patients with Scott syndrome results from:
   a. Defective granule secretion
   b. Altered platelet aggregation
   c. Altered expression of phospholipids on the platelet membrane
   d. Deficiency of vitamin K-dependent clotting factors
6. The impaired platelet function in myeloproliferative neoplasms results from:
   a. Abnormally shaped platelets
   b. Extended platelet life span
   c. Increased procoagulant activity
   d. Decreased numbers of α granules and dense granules

7. The platelet defect associated with increased paraproteins is:
   a. Impaired membrane activation, owing to protein coating
   b. Hypercoagulability, owing to antibody binding and membrane activation
   c. Impaired aggregation, because the hyperviscous plasma prevents platelet-endothelium interaction
   d. Hypercoagulability, because the increased proteins bring platelets closer together, which leads to inappropriate aggregation

8. In uremia, platelet function is impaired by higher than normal levels of:
   a. Urea
   b. Uric acid
   c. Creatinine
   d. NO

9. Thrombocytopenia associated with the use of cardiopulmonary bypass is *not* caused by:
   a. Anti-GP IIb/IIIa antibodies
   b. Hemodilution
   c. Platelet binding to bypass circuitry
   d. Platelet consumption associated with normal postsurgical hemostatic activity

10. Aspirin ingestion blocks the synthesis of:
    a. Thromboxane A_2
    b. Ionized calcium
    c. Collagen
    d. ADP

11. A mechanism of antiplatelet drugs targeting GP IIb/IIIa function is:
    a. Interference with platelet adhesion to the subendothelium by blocking of the collagen binding site
    b. Inhibition of transcription of the GP IIb/IIIa gene
    c. Direct binding to GP IIb/IIIa
    d. Interference with platelet secretion

12. Which is a congenital qualitative platelet disorder?
    a. Senile purpura
    b. Ehlers-Danlos syndrome
    c. Henoch-Schönlein purpura
    d. Waldenström macroglobulinemia

REFERENCES

1. Triplett, D. A. (1978). How to evaluate platelet function. *Lab Med Pract Phys*, July-Aug, 37–43.
2. Thorup, O. A. (1987). *Leavell and Thorup's Fundamentals of Clinical Hematology*. (5th ed.). Philadelphia: Saunders.
3. Thompson, A. R., & Harker, L. A. (1983). *Manual of Hemostasis and Thrombosis*. (3rd ed.). Philadelphia: FA Davis.
4. Colvin, B. T. (1985). Thrombocytopenia. *Clin Haematol, 14*, 661–681.
5. Nurden, P., & Nurden, A. T. (2008). Congenital disorders associated with platelet dysfunctions. *Thromb Haemost, 99*, 253–263.
6. George, J. N., & Shattil, S. J. (1991). The clinical importance of acquired abnormalities of platelet function. *N Engl J Med, 324*, 27–39.
7. Caen, J. P. (1989). Glanzmann's thrombasthenia. *Baillieres Clin Haematol, 2*, 609–623.
8. Coller, B. S., Mitchell, W. B., & French, D. L. (2006). Hereditary qualitative platelet disorders. In Lichtman, M. A., Beutler, E., Kipps, T. J., et al. (Eds.), *Williams Hematology*. (7th ed., pp. 1795–1832). New York: McGraw-Hill.
9. Triplett, D. A. (Ed.). (1978). *Platelet Function: Laboratory Evaluation and Clinical Application*. Chicago: American Society of Clinical Pathologists.
10. Powers, L. W. (1989). *Diagnostic Hematology: Clinical and Technical Principles*. St. Louis: Mosby.
11. Rapaport, S. I. (1987). *Introduction to Hematology*. (2nd ed.). Philadelphia: JB Lippincott.
12. Meyer, M., Kirchmaier, C. M., Schirmer, A., et al. (1991). Acquired disorder of platelet function associated with autoantibodies against membrane glycoprotein IIb-IIIa complex: 1. Glycoprotein analysis. *Thromb Haemost, 65*, 491–496.
13. Tarantino, M. D., Corrigan, J. J., Jr., Glasser, L., et al. (1991). A variant form of thrombasthenia. *Am J Dis Child, 145*, 1053–1057.
14. Friedlander, M., Brooks, P. C., Shaffer, R. W., et al. (1995). Definition of two angiogenic pathways by distinct a_v integrins. *Science, 270*, 1500–1502.

15. Nurden, A. T., & George, J. N. (2006). Inherited disorders of the platelet membrane: Glanzmann thrombasthenia, Bernard-Soulier syndrome and other disorders. In Colman, R. W., Marder, V. J., Clowes, A. W., et al. (Eds.), *Hemostasis and Thrombosis: Basic Principles and Clinical Practice*. (5th ed., pp. 987–1010). Philadelphia: Lippincott Williams & Wilkins.
16. Nurden, A. T. (2005). Qualitative disorders of platelets and megakaryocytes. *J Thromb Haemost, 3*, 1773–1782.
17. Nurden, A. T., Fiore, M., Nurden, P., et al. (2011). Glanzmann thrombasthenia: a review of *ITGA2B* and *ITGB3* defects with emphasis on variants, phenotypic variability, and mouse models. *Blood, 118*(23), 5996–6005.
18. Coller, B. S., Cheresh, D. A., Asch, E., et al. (1991). Platelet vitronectin receptor expression differentiates Iraqi-Jewish from Arab patients with Glanzmann thrombasthenia in Israel. *Blood, 77*, 75–83.
19. French, D. L. (1998). The molecular genetics of Glanzmann's thrombasthenia. *Platelets, 9*, 5–20.
20. Corriveau, D. M., & Fritsma, G. A. (1988). *Hemostasis and Thrombosis in the Clinical Laboratory*. Philadelphia: JB Lippincott.
21. Rosa, J. P., Artçanuthurry, V., Grelac, F., et al. (1997). Reassessment of protein tyrosine phosphorylation in thrombasthenic platelets: evidence that phosphorylation of cortactin and a 64 kD protein is dependent on thrombin activation and integrin $\alpha_{IIb}\beta_3$. *Thromb Haemost, 89*, 4385–4392.
22. Byzova, T. V., & Plow, E. F. (1997). Networking in the hemostatic system: integrin $\alpha_{IIb}\beta_3$ binds prothrombin and influences its activation. *J Biol Chem, 272*, 27183–27188.
23. Gemmell, C. H., Sefton, M. V., & Yeo, E. L. (1993). Platelet-derived microparticle formation involves glycoprotein IIb-IIIa: inhibition by RGDs and a Glanzmann's thrombasthenia defect. *J Biol Chem, 268*, 14586–14589.
24. Reverter, J. C., Beguin, S., Kessels, H., et al. (1996). Inhibition of platelet-mediated tissue factor-induced thrombin generation by the mouse/human chimeric 7E3 antibody: potential implications

for the effect of c7E3 Fab treatment on acute thrombosis and "clinical restenosis." *J Clin Invest, 98,* 863–874.

25. Caen, J. P. (1972). Glanzmann's thrombasthenia. *Clin Hematol, 1,* 383–392.

26. George, J. N., Caen, J. P., & Nurden, A. T. (1990). Glanzmann's thrombasthenia: the spectrum of clinical disease. *Blood, 75,* 1383–1395.

27. Jennings, L. K., Wang, W. C., Jackson, C. W., et al. (1991). Hemostasis in Glanzmann's thrombasthenia (GT): GT platelets interfere with the aggregation of normal platelets. *Am J Pediatr Hematol Oncol, 13,* 84–90.

28. Poon, M. C., d'Oiron, R., Von Depka, M., et al. (2004). International Data Collection on Recombinant Factor VIIa and Congenital Platelet Disorders Study Group: prophylactic and therapeutic recombinant factor VIIa administration to patients with Glanzmann's thrombasthenia: results of an international survey. *J Thromb Haemost, 2,* 1096–1103.

29. Lisman, T., Adelmaier, J., Heijnen, H. F. G., et al. (2004). Recombinant factor VIIa restores aggregation of $\alpha_{IIb}\beta_3$-deficient platelets via tissue factor-independent fibrin generation. *Blood, 103,* 1720–1727.

30. Geddis, A. E., & Kaushansky, K. (2004). Inherited thrombocytopenias: toward a better molecular understanding of disorders of platelet production. *Curr Opin Pediatr, 16,* 15–24.

31. Nurden, P., & Nurden, A. (1996). Giant platelets, megakaryocytes and the expression of glycoprotein Ib-IX complexes. *C R Acad Sci III, 319,* 717–726.

32. Clementson, K. J. (1997). Platelet GP Ib-V-IX complex. *Thromb Haemost, 78,* 266–270.

33. Nurden, A. T. (1998). Inherited abnormalities of platelets. *Thromb Haemost, 82,* 468–480.

34. Lopez, J. A., Andrews, R. K., Afshar-Kharghan, V., et al. (1998). Bernard-Soulier syndrome. *Blood, 91,* 4397–4418.

35. Savoia, A., Pastore, A., De Rocco, D., et al. (2011). Clinical and genetic aspects of Bernard-Soulier syndrome: searching for genotype/phenotype correlations. *Haematologica, 96*(3), 417–423.

36. Sumitha, E., Jayandharan, G. R., David, S., et al. (2011). Molecular basis of Bernard-Soulier syndrome in 27 patients from India. *J Thromb Haemost, 9*(8), 1590.

37. Takahashi, H., Murata, M., Moriki, T., et al. (1995). Substitution of Val for Met at residue 239 of platelet glycoprotein Ib alpha in Japanese patients with platelet-type von Willebrand disease. *Blood, 85,* 727–733.

38. Matsubara, Y., Murata, M., Sugita, K., et al. (2003). Identification of a novel point mutation in platelet glycoprotein Iba, Gly to Ser at residue 233, in a Japanese family with platelet-type von Willebrand disease. *J Thromb Haemost, 1,* 2198–2205.

39. Othman, M., Elbatarny, H. S., Notley, C., et al. (2004). Identification and functional characterization of a novel 27 bp deletion in the macroglycopeptide-coding region of the GPIba gene resulting in platelet-type von Willebrand disease. *Blood, 104,* Abstract 1023.

40. Mhawech, P., & Saleem, A. (2000). Inherited giant platelet disorders: classification and literature review. *Am J Clin Pathol, 113,* 176–190.

41. Pati, H., & Saraya, A. K. (1986). Platelet storage pool disease. *Indian J Med Res, 84,* 617–620.

42. Rao, A. K. (2006). Hereditary disorders of platelet secretion and signal transduction. In Colman, R. W., Marder, V. J., Clowes, A. W., et al. (Eds.), *Hemostasis and Thrombosis: Basic Principles and Clinical Practice.* (5th ed., pp. 961–974). Philadelphia: Lippincott Williams & Wilkins.

43. Weiss, H. J., Lages, B., Vicic, W., et al. (1993). Heterogeneous abnormalities of platelet dense granule ultrastructure in 20 patients with congenital storage pool deficiency. *Br J Haematol, 83,* 282–295.

44. Bennett, J. S. (2005). Hereditary disorders of platelet function. In Hoffman, R., Benz, E. J., Jr., Shattil, S. J., et al. (Eds.), *Hematology: Basic Principles and Practice.* (4th ed., pp. 2327–2345). Philadelphia: Churchill Livingstone.

45. Abrams, C. S., & Brass, L. F. (2006). Platelet signal transduction. In Colman, R. W., Marder, V. J., Clowes, A. W., et al. (Eds.), *Hemostasis and Thrombosis: Basic Principles and Clinical Practice.* (5th ed., pp. 617–630). Philadelphia: Lippincott Williams & Wilkins.

46. Jedlitschky, G., Tirwschmann, K., Lubenow, L. E., et al. (2004). The nucleotide transporter MRP4 (ABCC4) is highly expressed in human platelets and present in dense granules, indicating a role in mediator storage. *Blood, 104,* 3603–3610.

47. Spritz, R. A. (1998). Molecular genetics of the Hermansky-Pudlak and Chédiak-Higashi syndromes. *Platelets, 9,* 21–29.

48. Dell'Angellica, E. C., Aguilar, R. C., Wolins, N., et al. (2000). Molecular characterization of the protein encoded by the Hermansky-Pudlak syndrome type 1 gene. *J Biol Chem, 275,* 1300–1306.

49. White, J. G. (1987). Inherited abnormalities of the platelet membrane and secretory granules. *Hum Pathol, 18,* 123–139.

50. Villa, A., Notarangelo, L., Macchi, P., et al. (1995). X-linked thrombocytopenia and Wiskott-Aldrich syndrome are allelic diseases with mutations in the *WASP* gene. *Nat Genet, 9*(4), 414.

51. Lanzi, G., Moratto, D., Vairo, D., et al. (2012). A novel primary human immunodeficiency due to deficiency in the WASP-interacting protein WIP. *J Exp Med, 209*(1),29–34.

52. Quick, A. J. (1966). *Hemorrhagic Diseases and Thrombosis.* (2nd ed.). Philadelphia: Lea & Febiger.

53. Pai, S.-Y., & Notarangelo, L. D. (2018). Congenital disorders of lymphocytic function. In Hoffman, R., Benz, E. J., Silberstein, L. E., et al. (Eds.), *Hematology: Basic Principles and Practice.* (7th ed., pp. 710–759). Philadelphia: Elsevier.

54. de Alarcon, P. A., Graeve, J. A., Levine, R. F., et al. (1991). Thrombocytopenia and absent radii syndrome: defective megakaryocytopoiesis-thrombocytopoiesis. *Am J Pediatr Hematol Oncol, 13,* 77–83.

55. Raccuglia, G. (1971). Gray platelet syndrome: a variety of qualitative platelet disorder. *Am J Med, 51,* 818–828.

56. Gunay-Aygun, M., Zivony-Elboum, Y., Gumruk, F., et al. (2010). Gray platelet syndrome: natural history of a large patient cohort and locus assignment to chromosome 3p. *Blood, 116*(23), 4990.

57. Gunay-Aygun, M., Falik-Zaccai, T. C., Vilboux, T., et al. (2011). *NBEAL2* is mutated in gray platelet syndrome and is required for biogenesis of platelet α granules. *Nat Genet, 43*(8), 732.

58. Berrebi, A., Klepfish, A., Varon, D., et al. (1988). Gray platelet syndrome in the elderly. *Am J Hematol, 28,* 270–272.

59. Pfueller, S. L., Howard, M. A., White, J. G., et al. (1987). Shortening of the bleeding time by 1-deamino-8-arginine vasopressin (DDAVP) in the absence of platelet von Willebrand factor in gray platelet syndrome. *Thromb Haemost, 58,* 1060–1063.

60. Brace, L. D., Venton, D. L., & Le Breton, G. C. (1985). Thromboxane A_2/prostaglandin H_2 mobilizes calcium in human blood platelets. *Am J Physiol, 249,* H1–H7.

61. Moake, J. L., & Funicella, T. (1983). Common bleeding problems. *Clin Symp, 35,* 1–32.

62. Nieuwenhuis, H. K., Sakariassen, K. S., Houdijk, W. P. M., et al. (1986). Deficiency of platelet membrane glycoprotein Ia associated with a decreased platelet adhesion to subendothelium: a defect in platelet spreading. *Blood, 68,* 692–695.

63. Moroi, M., Jung, S. M., Okuma, M., et al. (1989). A patient with platelets deficient in glycoprotein VI that lack both collagen-induced aggregation and adhesion. *J Clin Invest, 84,* 1440–1445.

64. Nurden, P., Jandrot-Perrus, M., Combrie, R., et al. (2004). Severe deficiency of glycoprotein VI in a patient with gray platelet syndrome. *Blood, 104,* 107–114.

65. Cattaneo, M. (2003). Inherited platelet-based bleeding disorders. *J Thromb Haemost, 1,* 1628–1636.

66. Daniel, J. L., Dangelmaier, C., Jin, J., et al. (1998). Molecular basis for ADP-induced platelet activation: I. Evidence for three distinct ADP receptors on human platelets. *J Biol Chem, 273,* 2024–2029.

67. Nurden, P., Savi, P., Heilmann, E., et al. (1995). An inherited bleeding disorder linked to a defective interaction between ADP and its receptor on platelets. *J Clin Invest, 95,* 1612–1622.

68. Cattaneo, M., Zighetti, M. L., Lombardi, R., et al. (2003). Molecular basis of defective signal transduction in the platelet P2Y12 receptor of a patient with congenital bleeding. *Proc Natl Acad Sci U S A, 100,* 1978–1983.

69. Rao, A. K. (1998). Congenital disorders of platelet function: disorders of signal transduction and secretion. *Am J Med Sci, 316,* 69–76.

70. Rao, A. K. (2003). Inherited defects in platelet signaling mechanisms. *J Thromb Haemost, 1,* 671–681.

71. Zhou, Q., Sims, P. J., & Wiedmer, T. (1998). Expression of proteins controlling transbilayer movement of plasma membrane phospholipids in B lymphocytes from a patient with Scott syndrome. *Blood, 92,* 1707–1712.

72. Zhou, Q., Zhao, J., Stout, J. G., et al. (1997). Molecular cloning of human plasma membrane phospholipid scramblase: a protein mediating transbilayer movement of plasma membrane phospholipids. *J Biol Chem, 272,* 18240–18244.

73. Zwaal, R. F., Comfurius, P., & Bevers, E. M. (2004). Scott syndrome, a bleeding disorder caused by a defective scrambling of membrane phospholipids. *Biochim Biophys Acta, 1636,* 119–128.

74. Sims, P., & Wiedmer, T. (2001). Unraveling the mysteries of phospholipid scrambling. *Thromb Haemost, 86,* 266–275.

75. Stormorken, H., Holmsen, H., Sund, R., et al. (1995). Studies on the haemostatic defect in a complicated syndrome: an inverse Scott syndrome platelet membrane abnormality? *Thromb Haemost, 74,* 1244–1251.

76. Helgason, C. M., Bolin, K. M., Hoff, J. A., et al. (1994). Development of aspirin resistance in persons with previous ischemic stroke. *Stroke, 25,* 2331–2336.

77. Helgason, C. M., Tortorice, K. L., Winkler, S. R., et al. (1993). Aspirin response and failure in cerebral infarction. *Stroke, 24,* 345–350.

78. Eikelboom, J. W., Hirsh, J., Weitz, J., et al. (2002). Aspirin resistant thromboxane biosynthesis and the risk of myocardial infarction, stroke, or cardiovascular death in patients at high risk for cardiovascular events. *Circulation, 105,* 1650–1655.

79. Green, D. (1988). Diagnosis and management of bleeding disorders. *Compr Ther, 14,* 31–36.

80. Catella-Lawson, F., Reilly, M. P., Kapoor, S. C., et al. (2001). Cyclooxygenase inhibitors and the antiplatelet effects of aspirin. *New Eng J Med, 345,* 1809–1817.

81. Schleinitz, M. D., & Heidenreich, P. A. (2005). A cost-effectiveness analysis of combination antiplatelet therapy of high-risk acute coronary syndromes: clopidogrel plus aspirin versus aspirin alone. *Ann Intern Med, 142,* 251–259.

82. Wilhite, D. B., Comerota, A. J., Schmieder, F. A., et al. (2003). Managing PAD with multiple platelet inhibitors: the effect of combination therapy on bleeding time. *J Vasc Surg, 38,* 710–713.

83. Jacobson, K. A., & Boeynaems, J-M. (2010). P2Y nucleotide receptors: promise of therapeutic applications. *Drug Discovery Today, 15*(13–14), 570–578.

84. Sible, A. M., & Nawarskas, J. J. (2017). Cangrelor: a new route for P2Y$_{12}$ inhibition. *Cardiology in Review, 25,* 133–139

85. Angiolillo, D. J., Firstenberg, M. S., & Price M. J. (2012). Bridging antiplatelet therapy with cangrelor in patients undergoing cardiac surgery: a randomized controlled study. *JAMA, 307,* 265–274.

86. Coller, B. S. (1997). GPIIb/IIIa antagonists: pathophysiologic and therapeutic insights from studies of c7E3 Fab. *Thromb Haemost, 78,* 730–735.

87. Tcheng, J. E. (1997). Platelet glycoprotein IIb/IIIa integrin blockade: recent clinical trials in interventional cardiology. *Thromb Haemost, 78,* 205–209.

88. Van de Werf, F. (1997). Clinical trials with glycoprotein IIb/IIIa receptor antagonists in acute coronary syndromes. *Thromb Haemost, 78,* 210–213.

89. Ungar, L., Rodriguez, F., & Mahaffey, K. W. (2016). Vorapaxar: emerging evidence and clinical questions in a new era of PAR-1 inhibition. *Coron Artery Dis, 27,* 604–615

90. Gryka, R. J., Buckley, L. F., & Anderson, S. M. (2017). Vorapaxar: the current role and future directions of a novel protease-activated receptor antagonist for risk reduction in atherosclerotic disease. *Drugs R D, 17,* 65–72.

91. Diz-Küçükkaya, R., & López, J. A. (2018). Acquired disorders of platelet function (Chapter 130). In Hoffman, R., Benz, E. J., Jr., & Silberstein LE, et al. (Eds.), *Hematology: Basic Principles and Practice.* (7th ed., pp. 1932–1942). Philadelphia: Elsevier, Inc.

92. Landolfi, R., Marchioli, R., & Patrono, C. (1997). Mechanisms of bleeding and thrombosis in myeloproliferative disorders. *Thromb Haemost, 78,* 617–621.

93. Swart, S. S., Pearson, D., Wood, J. K., et al. (1984). Functional significance of the platelet alpha$_2$-adrenoreceptor: studies in patients with myeloproliferative disorders. *Thromb Res, 33,* 531–541.

94. Weerasinghe, A., & Taylor, K. M. (1998). The platelet in cardiopulmonary bypass. *Ann Thorac Surg, 66,* 2145–2152.

95. Bick, R. L., & Scates, S. M. (1992). Qualitative platelet defects. *Lab Med, 23,* 95–103.

96. Haut, M. J., & Cowan, D. H. (1974). The effect of ethanol on hemostatic properties of human blood platelets. *Am J Med, 56,* 22–33.

97. Boccardo, P., Remuzzi, G., & Galbusera, M. (2004). Platelet dysfunction in renal failure. *Semin Thromb Hemost, 30,* 579–589.

98. Gailani, D, Wheeler, A. P., & Neff, A. T. (2018). Rare coagulation factor deficiencies. In Hoffman, R., Benz, E. J., Silberstein, L. E., et al. (Eds.), *Hematology: Basic Principles and Practice.* (7th ed., pp. 2043–2050). Philadelphia: Elsevier.

99. Eldrup-Jorgensen, J., Flanigan, D. P., Brace, L. D., et al. (1989). Hypercoagulable states and lower limb ischemia in young adults. *J Vasc Surg, 9,* 334–341.

100. Helgason, C. M., Hoff, J. A., Kondos, G. T., et al. (1993). Platelet aggregation in patients with atrial fibrillation taking aspirin or warfarin. *Stroke, 24,* 1458–1461.

101. Pareti, F. I., Capitanio, A., Mannucci, L., et al. (1980). Acquired dysfunction due to circulation of "exhausted" platelets. *Am J Med, 69,* 235–240.

102. Hayward, C. P. M. (2018). Clinical approach to the patient with bleeding or bruising (Chapter 128). In Hoffman, R., Benz, E. J., Jr., Silberstein, L. E., et al. (Eds.), *Hematology: Basic Principles and Practice.* (7th ed., pp. 1912–1930). Philadelphia: Elsevier.

103. Maceyko, R. F., & Camisa, C. (1991). Kasabach-Merritt syndrome. *Pediatr Dermatol, 8,* 133–136.

104. Brace, L. D. (1981). The multiple myelomas: a review of selected aspects. *Allied Health Behav Sci, 3,* 47–61.

105. Gertz, M. A., Buadi, F. K., Lacy, M. Q., et al. (2018). Immunoglobulin light chain amyloidosis (primary amyloidosis). In Hoffman, R., Benz, E. J., Jr., Silberstein, L. E., et al. (Eds.), *Hematology: Basic Principles and Practice.* (7th ed., pp. 1432–1443). Philadelphia: Elsevier.

Thrombocytopenia and Thrombocytosis

Phillip J. DeChristopher, Walter P. Jeske*

OBJECTIVES

After completion of this chapter, the reader will be able to:

1. Define thrombocytopenia and thrombocytosis, and state their associated platelet counts.
2. Compare and contrast the clinical symptoms of platelet disorders and clotting factor deficiencies.
3. Explain the primary pathophysiologic processes of thrombocytopenia.
4. List the unique diagnostic features of at least four disorders included in congenital hypoplasia of the bone marrow and describe their inheritance patterns.
5. Differentiate between acute and chronic immune thrombocytopenia.
6. Describe the immunologic and nonimmunologic mechanisms by which drugs may induce thrombocytopenia.
7. Differentiate between neonatal alloimmune thrombocytopenia and neonatal autoimmune thrombocytopenia.
8. Explain the laboratory findings and pathophysiology associated with thrombotic thrombocytopenic purpura and hemolytic uremic syndrome.
9. Given clinical history and laboratory test results for patients with thrombocytopenia or thrombocytosis, suggest a diagnosis that is consistent with the information provided.

OUTLINE

Thrombocytopenia: Decrease in Circulating Platelets
    Decreased Platelet Production
    Increased Platelet Destruction
    Abnormalities in Distribution or Dilution

Thrombocytosis: Increase in Circulating Platelets
    Reactive Thrombocytosis
    Thrombocytosis Associated With Myeloproliferative
      Disorders

CASE STUDY

After studying the material in this chapter, the reader should be able to respond to the following case study:

  A 73-year-old Hispanic woman, who has had 4 children in the remote past, is hospitalized in the medical intensive care unit with end-stage liver disease secondary to cirrhosis as a result of chronic hepatitis B infection. Her clinical course has been complicated by recurrent massive abdominal ascites, episodes of spontaneous bacterial peritonitis, disseminated intravascular coagulation, respiratory failure (she is now intubated, on a ventilator), and worsening renal failure (thought to be secondary to hepatorenal syndrome). Her platelet counts, which average in the low 20s $\times$ 10^6/μL, have not been associated with spontaneous bleeding. She is not on any medications that affect platelet function. Wanting to start hemodialysis, her physicians have requested interventional radiology (IR) to place a central line. An IR physician insists on a preprocedure platelet count of at least 50 $\times$ 10^6/μL before line placement. Despite platelet transfusions during the last 3 days, repeat platelet counts the next day remained at baseline.

1. What is the most likely cause of her thrombocytopenia?
2. What laboratory tests should be ordered next?
3. One doctor suggested that "specialized platelets" (e.g., crossmatched or HLA-matched components) might work better. Is this suggestion true?

Bleeding disorders resulting from platelet abnormalities, whether quantitative, which will be discussed in this chapter, or qualitative (Chapter 37), usually manifest as bleeding into the skin or mucous membranes or both (mucocutaneous bleeding). Common presenting symptoms include petechiae, purpura, ecchymoses, epistaxis, and gingival bleeding. Similar findings also are seen in vascular disorders, but vascular disorders (e.g., Ehlers-Danlos syndrome, hereditary hemorrhagic telangiectasia; Chapter 37) are relatively rare. In contrast, deep tissue bleeding, such as hematoma and hemarthrosis, is associated with clotting factor deficiencies (Chapter 36).

*The authors extend appreciation to Larry D. Brace whose work in prior editions provided the foundation for this chapter.

THROMBOCYTOPENIA: DECREASE IN CIRCULATING PLATELETS

Although the reference range for the platelet count varies among laboratories, it is generally considered to be approximately 150,000 to 450,000/μL (150,000 to 450,000/mm^3 or 150 to 450 $\times$ 10^9/L). Thrombocytopenia (platelet count of fewer than 100,000/μL) is the most common cause of clinically important bleeding. True thrombocytopenia has to be differentiated from the thrombocytopenia artifact that can result from poorly prepared blood films or automated cell counts when platelet clumping or platelet satellitosis is present (Chapters 12 and 13).

Small-vessel bleeding in the skin attributed to thrombocytopenia manifests as hemorrhages of different sizes (Figure 38.1). *Petechiae* are small pinpoint hemorrhages about 1 mm in diameter, *purpura* are about 3 mm in diameter and generally round, and *ecchymoses* are 1 cm or larger and usually irregular in shape. Ecchymosis corresponds with the lay term *bruise*. Other conditions such as defective platelet function, vascular fragility, and trauma contribute to the hemorrhagic state.

Severity of clinical bleeding varies and often is not closely correlated with the platelet count. It is unusual for clinically significant bleeding to occur when the platelet count is greater than 50,000/μL, but the risk increases progressively as the platelet count decreases from 50,000/μL. In general, patients with platelet counts of fewer than 10,000/μL are considered to be at high risk for severe spontaneous bleeding. The primary pathophysiologic processes that result in thrombocytopenia are decreased platelet production, increased platelet destruction, and abnormal platelet distribution (sequestration).

Decreased Platelet Production

Abnormalities in platelet production can result from megakaryocyte hypoplasia in the bone marrow or ineffective thrombopoiesis. Factors causing decreased platelet production can be congenital or acquired. Box 38.1 categorizes these disorders.

Congenital Types of Impaired Platelet Production

It is increasingly apparent that most inherited thrombocytopenias can be linked to fairly specific chromosomal abnormalities or specific genetic defects. Table 38.1 provides a list of inherited thrombocytopenias associated with specific gene and chromosomal abnormalities, mode of inheritance, and associated features.

Lack of adequate bone marrow megakaryocytes (megakaryocytic hypoplasia) is seen in a wide variety of congenital disorders, including Fanconi anemia (pancytopenia), thrombocytopenia with absent radius (TAR) syndrome, May-Hegglin anomaly, Wiskott-Aldrich syndrome, Bernard-Soulier syndrome, and several other less common disorders. Although thrombocytopenia is a feature of Bernard-Soulier syndrome and Wiskott-Aldrich syndrome, the primary abnormality in these disorders is a qualitative defect, and these disorders are discussed in Chapter 37.

May-Hegglin anomaly is a rare autosomal dominant disorder whose exact frequency is unknown. Large platelets (20 μm in diameter) are present on the peripheral blood film, and

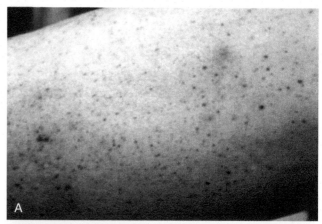
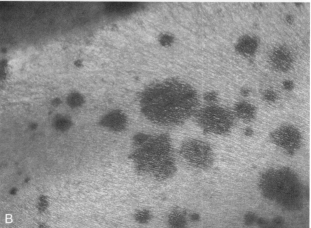
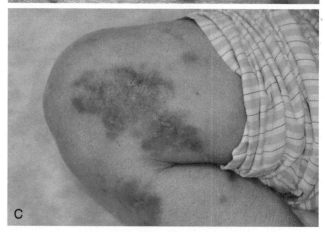

Figure 38.1 Patterns of Systemic (Mucocutaneous) Hemorrhage. The various presentations of systemic bleeding include **(A)** petechiae, **(B)** purpura, and **(C)** ecchymoses. (**A** From Abrams, C. S. [2015]. Thrombocytopenia. In Goldman L., & Schafer, A. I. (Eds.), *Goldman-Cecil Medicine* [25th ed.]. Philadelphia, PA: Elsevier; **B** From Piette, W. W. [2017]. Purpura: mechanism and differential diagnosis. In Bolognia, J. L., Schaffer, J. V., & Cerroni, L. [Eds.], *Dermatology* [4th ed., Vol. 22, pp. 357–367]. St. Louis: Elsevier; **C** From Yang, T.-H., Chen, W.-Y., & Tsai, H.-H. [2016]. Periarticular ecchymosis-like plaques and nodules. *J Am Acad Dermatol, 75*[1], e1-e2.)

Döhle-like bodies are present in neutrophils (Figure 38.2) and occasionally in monocytes. The disorder is characterized by abnormally enlarged or misshapen platelets. Thrombocytopenia of varying degrees is present in about one third to one half of affected patients. Platelet function in response to

BOX 38.1 Classification of Thrombocytopenias: Impaired or Decreased Production of Platelets

Congenital
May-Hegglin anomaly
Bernard-Soulier syndrome
Fechtner syndrome
Sebastian syndrome
Epstein syndrome
Montreal platelet syndrome
Fanconi anemia
Wiskott-Aldrich syndrome
Thrombocytopenia with absent radius (TAR) syndrome

Congenital amegakaryocytic thrombocytopenia
Autosomal dominant and X-linked thrombocytopenia

Acquired
Viral or bacterial infections
Drug induced

Neonatal

platelet-activating agents is usually normal. In some patients the number of megakaryocytes is increased and their ultrastructure is abnormal. Mutations in the *MYH9* gene that encodes for nonmuscle myosin heavy chain (a cytoskeletal protein in platelets) have been reported.[1] This mutation may be responsible for the abnormal size of platelets in this disorder. Most patients are asymptomatic unless severe thrombocytopenia is present. In severe cases with clinical bleeding, transfusion with platelets may be necessary.

Three other disorders involving mutations of the *MYH9* gene have been reported: Sebastian syndrome, Fechtner syndrome, and Epstein syndrome.[2] Sebastian syndrome is inherited as an autosomal dominant disorder characterized by large platelets, thrombocytopenia, and granulocytic

TABLE 38.1 Classification of Inherited Thrombocytopenias

Disease	Occurrence	Spontaneous Bleeding	Gene; Chromosomal Location	Platelet Size	Features
X-Linked					
Wiskott-Aldrich syndrome	****	Yes	*WAS;* Xp11.23	Small	Severe immunodeficiency; death in infancy
GATA1-related diseases	**	Yes	*GATA1;* Xp11.23	Large	Hemolytic anemia; possible congenital dyserythropoietic anemia
FLNA-related (filamin A) thrombocytopenia	*	Yes	*FLNA;* Xq28	Large	Periventricular nodular heterotopia
Autosomal Recessive					
Thrombocytopenia with absent radii	****	Yes	*RBM8A;* 1q21.1	Normal	Bilateral radial aplasia and/or other malformations; reduced megakaryocytes; platelet count normalizes into adulthood
Bernard-Soulier syndrome; biallelic	****	Yes	*GP1BA;* 17p13.2	Large	Mucosal bleeding, cutaneous bleeding, epistaxis, menorrhagia
Congenital megakaryocytic thrombocytopenia	***	Yes	*MPL;* 1p34.1	Normal	Bone marrow aplasia in infancy; defects in thrombopoietin production and reactivity
Gray platelet syndrome	**	Yes	*NBEAL2;* 3p21.31	Giant	Increased risk of developing myelofibrosis and splenomegaly
Thrombocytopenia associated with lipid accumulation	*	No	*ABCG5, ABCG8;* 2p21	Large	Anemia; tendon xanthomas; atherosclerosis
Autosomal Dominant					
MYH9-related disease	****	No	*MYH9;* 22q12–13	Large	Presenile cataracts; nephropathy; progressive hearing loss
Paris-Trousseau thrombocytopenia	****	Yes	Large deletion; 11q23.3	Large	Cardiac, facial defects, developmental delays
Bernard-Soulier syndrome; monoallelic	***	No	*GP1BB;* 22q11.21 *GP9;* 3q21.3	Large	
Familial platelet disorder/ predisposition to AML	**	No	*RUNX1;* 21q22.12	Normal	High risk of leukemia or myelodysplastic syndrome
ANKRD26-related thrombocytopenia	**	No	*ANKRD26;* 10p12.1	Normal	Risk of leukemia
ITGA2B/ITGB3-related thrombocytopenia	*	No	*ITGA2B;* 17q21.31 *ITGB3;* 17q21.32	Large	
TUBB1-related thrombocytopenia	*	No	*TUBB1;* 20q13.3	Giant	Platelet aggregation and megakaryocytes morphologically normal
CYCS-related thrombocytopenia	*	No	*CYCS;* 7p15.3	Normal	
Congenital thrombocytopenia with radioulnar bone fusion	*	Yes	*HOXA11;* 7p15.2	Normal	Possible evolution into aplastic anemia

****, ~100 Families; ***, ~50 families; **, ~10 families; *, ~10 families; *AML*, acute myelogenous leukemia.

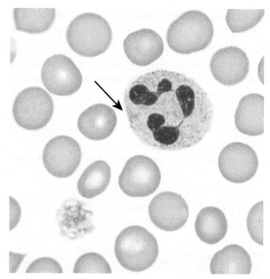

Figure 38.2 May-Hegglin Anomaly. Note the Döhle body *(arrow)* in the segmented neutrophil and the giant platelets. (Peripheral blood, Wright-Giemsa stain, ×1000.) (From Carr, J. H., & Rodak, B. F. [2013]. *Clinical Hematology Atlas* [4th ed.]. Philadelphia,: Saunders.)

inclusions. Similar abnormalities are observed in Fechtner syndrome and are accompanied by deafness, cataracts, and nephritis. In Epstein syndrome, large platelets are associated with deafness, ocular problems, and glomerular nephritis.[3] These disorders are discussed in more detail in Chapter 37.

TAR syndrome is a rare autosomal recessive disorder characterized by severe neonatal thrombocytopenia and congenital absence or extreme hypoplasia of the radial bones of the forearms with absent, short, or malformed ulnae and other orthopedic abnormalities. TAR syndrome is associated with a mutation in the *RBM8A* gene located on the long arm of chromosome 1 or a 200 kb deletion involving the *RBM8A* gene (1q21.1). In addition to bone abnormalities, up to 90% of patients may have cardiac lesions or transient leukemoid reactions with elevated white blood cell (WBC) counts (sometimes with counts >100,000/μL).[4] Platelet counts are usually 10,000 to 30,000/μL during the first 2 years of infancy. Interestingly, platelet counts usually increase over time, with normal levels usually achieved by the time these children reach school age.

Fanconi anemia is also associated with thrombocytopenia and other abnormalities, including bony abnormalities, abnormalities of visceral organs, and pancytopenia. Chapter 19 contains a more detailed description.

Congenital amegakaryocytic thrombocytopenia is an autosomal recessive disorder reflecting bone marrow failure.[5] Affected infants usually have platelet counts ≤20,000/μL at birth, petechiae and evidence of bleeding at or shortly after birth, and frequent physical anomalies. About half of the infants develop aplastic anemia in the first year of life, and there are reports of myelodysplasia and leukemia later in childhood. Allogeneic stem cell transplantation is considered curative for infants with clinically severe disease or aplasia.[6] This disorder is caused by mutations in the *MPL* gene on chromosome 1 (1p34.1), resulting in complete loss of

thrombopoietin receptor function. This loss of function results in reduced megakaryocyte progenitors and high thrombopoietin levels.[7]

Autosomal dominant thrombocytopenia has been mapped to mutations in the *ANKRD26* gene on the short arm of chromosome 10 (10p12.1). Mutations in this gene lead to incomplete megakaryocyte differentiation and resultant thrombocytopenia. Platelet morphology and size are usually normal. Until recently, autosomal dominant thrombocytopenia was considered a very rare disorder. However, *ANKRD26* mutations have recently been found in 21 of 210 thrombocytopenic pedigrees, suggesting that *ANKRD26* mutations may be a relatively common cause of autosomal dominant thrombocytopenia.[8] Bleeding in these patients is usually absent or mild, and platelet function is usually normal.[9,10]

X-linked thrombocytopenia can result from mutations in the *WAS* (Wiskott-Aldrich syndrome) gene on the X chromosome (Xp11.23) or mutations in the *GATA1* gene, also on the X chromosome at Xp11.[11-13] X-linked thrombocytopenias range from mild thrombocytopenia with small platelets and absent or mild bleeding to large platelets with severe bleeding.

Neonatal Thrombocytopenia

Neonatal thrombocytopenia (platelet count <150,000/μL) is present in 1% to 5% of infants at birth. In 75% of cases the thrombocytopenia is present at or within 72 hours of birth. The causes of neonatal thrombocytopenia are numerous as illustrated in Table 38.2. Only a minority of these patients have immunologic disorders or coagulopathy causing thrombocytopenia.

TORCH (*t*oxoplasmosis, *o*ther, (*Treponema pallidum*, varicella-zoster virus, parvovirus B19), *r*ubella, *c*ytomegalovirus [CMV], *h*erpes) syndrome infections are common causes of neonatal thrombocytopenia. Such infections cause thrombocytopenia with characteristically small platelets. CMV is the most common infectious agent causing congenital thrombocytopenia, with an overall incidence of 0.5% to 1% of all births,[14] but only 10% to 15% of infected infants have symptomatic disease,[15] which suggests that the incidence of significant neonatal thrombocytopenia caused by CMV is about 1 in 1000 infants. Although the mechanism of thrombocytopenia is not well understood, reports suggest that CMV inhibits megakaryocytes and their precursors, which results in impaired platelet production.[16] About 1 in 1000 to 1 in 3000 infants are affected by congenital toxoplasmosis. About 40% of such infants develop thrombocytopenia.[17] Although persistent thrombocytopenia is a prominent feature in infants with congenital rubella syndrome, it is now rare in countries with organized immunization programs.[18,19] Thrombocytopenia was stated to be a feature of maternal transmission of HIV to the neonate in one report,[20] but this does not generally occur.

Maternal ingestion of chlorothiazide diuretics or tolbutamide oral hypoglycemic medication (both sulfonamides) can have a direct cytotoxic effect on the fetal marrow megakaryocytes. Thrombocytopenia may be severe, with platelet counts of 70,000/μL and sometimes lower. Bone marrow examination reveals a marked decrease or absence of megakaryocytes. The thrombocytopenia develops gradually and is slow to regress when the drug is stopped. Recovery usually occurs within a few weeks after birth.[10,21,22]

Although infectious agents and certain drugs are well-known causes of neonatal thrombocytopenia, the most common cause is impaired platelet production. Most patients are preterm neonates born after pregnancies complicated by placental insufficiency or fetal hypoxia (preeclampsia and intrauterine growth restriction). These neonates have early-onset thrombocytopenia and impaired megakaryopoiesis in spite of increased levels of thrombopoietin (Table 38.2).

TABLE 38.2 Fetal and Neonatal Thrombocytopenias

		TIMING	
Cause	Fetal	Neonatal <72 hr After Birth	Neonatal >72 hrs After Birth
Alloimmune	X	X	
Autoimmune (ITP, SLE)	X		X
Aneuploidy (trisomy 13, 18, or 21 or triploidy)	X		
Bone marrow replacement (congenital leukemia)		X	
Congenital infections (TORCH)	X	X	X
Congenital inherited (Wiskott-Aldrich syndrome)			X
Congenital inherited (TAR, CAMT)		X	X
Disseminated intravascular coagulation		X	
Kasabach-Merritt syndrome		X	X
Late-onset sepsis			X
Maternal autoimmune conditions (ITP, SLE)		X	
Metabolic disease (propionic and methylmalonic acidemia)		X	X
Necrotizing enterocolitis			X
Perinatal asphyxia		X	
Perinatal infection (Escherichia coli, group B streptococcus, Haemophilus influenzae)		X	
Uteroplacental vascular insufficiency (preeclampsia, IUGR)	X	X	
Severe Rh hemolytic disease	X		
Thrombosis (aortic, renal vein)		X	

CAMT, Congenital amegakaryocytic thrombocytopenia; ITP, immune thrombocytopenic purpura; IUGR, intrauterine growth restriction; SLE, systemic lupus erythematosus; TAR, thrombocytopenia with absent radius; TORCH, toxoplasmosis, other (Treponema pallidum, varicella-zoster virus, parvovirus B19), rubella, cytomegalovirus, herpes simplex virus.

Increased platelet consumption or sequestration (discussed in detail later in this chapter) is another mechanism of neonatal thrombocytopenia, accounting for 2% to 25% of cases. Of these, 15% to 20% result from transplacental passage of maternal alloantibodies and autoantibodies. Another 10% to 15% of cases are due to disseminated intravascular coagulation (DIC), almost always in very ill infants, particularly those with perinatal asphyxia or infections. Other causes of neonatal thrombocytopenia include thrombosis, platelet activation, platelet binding at inflammatory sites such as in necrotizing enterocolitis and splenic sequestration.

Inherited thrombocytopenic syndromes are increasingly being recognized as causes of neonatal thrombocytopenia (Tables 38.1 and 38.2). Although considered to be rare, they may be more common than once believed.

Acquired Types of Impaired Platelet Production

Drug-induced hypoplasia of the bone marrow results in thrombocytopenia. Wide arrays of chemotherapeutic agents used for the treatment of hematologic and nonhematologic malignancies suppress bone marrow megakaryocyte production and the production of other hematopoietic cells. Examples include the commonly used agents methotrexate, busulfan, cytosine arabinoside, cyclophosphamide, and cisplatin. Because the resulting thrombocytopenia may lead to hemorrhage, the platelet count should be monitored closely. Drug-induced thrombocytopenia is often the dose-limiting factor for many chemotherapeutic agents. Recombinant interleukin-11 has been approved for treatment of chemotherapy-induced thrombocytopenia, and thrombopoietin or its analogs may prove to be useful for this purpose.[23-25] Zidovudine (used for the treatment of HIV infection) is also known to cause myelotoxicity and severe thrombocytopenia.[26]

Several drugs specifically affect megakaryocytopoiesis without significantly affecting other marrow elements. Anagrelide is one such agent. Although its mechanism of action is unknown, anagrelide is useful for treating thrombocytosis in patients with essential thrombocythemia and other myeloproliferative disorders.[27]

Long-term ingestion of ethanol (months to years) may result in persistent, severe thrombocytopenia. Although the mechanism is unknown, studies indicate that alcohol can inhibit megakaryocytopoiesis in some individuals. Mild thrombocytopenia is a common finding in alcoholic patients, but other causes unrelated to ethanol use, such as portal hypertension, splenomegaly, and folic acid deficiency, can also contribute. The platelet count usually returns to normal within a few weeks of alcohol withdrawal, but thrombocytopenia may persist for longer periods. A transient rebound thrombocytosis may develop when alcohol ingestion is stopped.[10]

Interferon therapy commonly causes mild to moderate thrombocytopenia, although under certain circumstances, the thrombocytopenia can be severe and life threatening. Interferon-α and interferon-γ inhibit stem cell differentiation and proliferation in the bone marrow, but the mechanism of action is unclear.[28,29]

Thrombocytopenia presumably caused by megakaryocyte suppression also has been reported to follow the administration of large doses of estrogen or estrogenic drugs such as diethylstilbestrol. Certain antibacterial agents (e.g., chloramphenicol), tranquilizers, and anticonvulsants also have been associated with thrombocytopenia caused by bone marrow suppression.[30,31]

Ineffective thrombosis can also occur. Thrombocytopenia is a usual feature of the megaloblastic anemias (pernicious anemia, folic acid deficiency, and vitamin B_{12} deficiency). Quantitative studies indicate that, as with erythrocyte production in these disorders, platelet production is ineffective. Although the bone marrow generally contains an increased number of megakaryocytes, the total number of platelets released into the circulation is decreased. Thrombocytopenia is caused by impaired DNA synthesis, and the bone marrow may contain grossly abnormal megakaryocytes with deformed, dumbbell-shaped nuclei, sometimes in large numbers. Stained peripheral blood films reveal large platelets that may have a decreased survival time and may have abnormal function. Thrombocytopenia is usually mild, and there is evidence of increased platelet destruction. Patients typically respond within 1 to 2 weeks to vitamin replacement.[22,32-34]

Infectious conditions, such as with viruses, are known to cause thrombocytopenia by acting on megakaryocytes or circulating platelets, either directly or in the form of viral antigen-antibody complexes. Live measles vaccine can cause degenerative vacuolization of megakaryocytes 6 to 8 days after vaccination. Some viruses interact readily with platelets by means of specific platelet receptors. Other viruses associated with thrombocytopenia include CMV, varicella-zoster virus, rubella virus, Epstein-Barr virus (which causes infectious mononucleosis), and some serotypes of dengue virus that cause Thai hemorrhagic fever.[10]

Certain bacterial infections are commonly associated with the development of thrombocytopenia. This may be the result of toxins of bacterial origin, direct interactions between bacteria and platelets in the circulation, or extensive damage to the endothelium, as in meningococcemia. Many cases of thrombocytopenia in childhood result from bacterial infection. Purpura may occur in many infectious diseases in the absence of thrombocytopenia, presumably because of vascular damage (Chapter 37).[10,35]

Infiltration of the bone marrow by malignant cells can cause thrombocytopenia. The result is a progressive decrease in marrow megakaryocytes as the abnormal cells replace normal marrow elements. Inhibitors of thrombopoiesis may be produced by these abnormal cells and may contribute to the thrombocytopenia associated with conditions such as myeloma, lymphoma, metastatic cancer, and myelofibrosis.[22,32,36]

Increased Platelet Destruction

Thrombocytopenia as a result of increased platelet destruction can be separated into two categories: increased platelet destruction caused by immunologic responses and increased destruction caused by mechanical damage, consumption, or sequestration. Box 38.2 categorizes these disorders. Regardless of the process,

---

> **BOX 38.2 Classification of Thrombocytopenias: Increased Platelet Destruction and Sequestration**
>
> **Immune**
> Acute and chronic immune thrombocytopenic purpura
> Drug induced: immunologic
> Heparin-induced thrombocytopenia
> Neonatal alloimmune thrombocytopenia
> Neonatal autoimmune thrombocytopenia
> Posttransfusion purpura
> Secondary autoimmune thrombocytopenia
>
> **Nonimmune**
> Gestational thrombocytopenia (in pregnancy, preeclampsia, and HELLP syndrome)
> Human immunodeficiency virus infection
> Hemolytic disease of the newborn
> Thrombotic microangiopathies (including TTP, HUS, aHUS)
> Disseminated intravascular coagulation
> Bacterial infection, other infections/sepsis
> Drug induced
>
> **Distribution or Dilution**
> Splenic sequestration (often associated with hypersplenism, chronic liver disease)
> Kasabach-Merritt syndrome
> Hypothermia
> Loss of platelets: massive blood transfusions, extracorporeal circulation

---

increased production is required to maintain a normal platelet count, and thrombocytopenia develops only when production capacity is no longer adequate to compensate for the increased rate of destruction.

Immune Mechanisms of Platelet Destruction

Immune thrombocytopenic purpura. The term idiopathic thrombocytopenic purpura (ITP) was used previously to describe cases of thrombocytopenia arising without apparent cause or underlying disease state. Although the acronym for the disorder remains the same, the word *idiopathic* has been replaced by *immune* after the realization that acute and chronic ITP are immunologically mediated.

Acute ITP is primarily a disorder of children, although a similar condition is seen occasionally in adults.[37] The incidence of acute ITP is estimated to be 4 in 100,000 children, with a peak frequency in children between 2 and 5 years of age without sex predilection.[38] The disorder is characterized by abrupt onset of bruising, petechiae, and sometimes mucosal bleeding (e.g., epistaxis) in a previously healthy child. The primary hematologic feature is thrombocytopenia, which often occurs 1 to 3 weeks after an infection.

Acute ITP is preceded by various infections or vaccinations in more than half of pediatric patients in the 4 weeks before diagnosis. When specified, the type of vaccination included MMR (measles, mumps, rubella), DTP (diphtheria, tetanus, pertussis), and other vaccines such as polio, hepatitis A, or hepatitis B. The observation that acute ITP often follows a viral illness or vaccination suggests that some children produce antibodies and immune complexes against viral antigens and that platelet destruction may result from the binding of these antibodies or immune complexes to the platelet surface.

The diagnosis of acute ITP in a child with severe thrombocytopenia almost always can be made without a bone marrow examination. If the child has recent onset of bleeding signs and symptoms, otherwise normal results on complete blood count (for all red and white blood cell parameters and cell morphology), and normal findings on physical examination (except for signs of bleeding), there is a high likelihood that the child has ITP. In addition, if the bleeding symptoms develop suddenly and there is no family history of hemorrhagic abnormalities or thrombocytopenia, the diagnosis of ITP is almost certain. There is, at present, no specific test that is diagnostic of acute or chronic ITP.

In mild cases of acute ITP, patients may have only scattered petechiae. In most cases of acute ITP, however, patients develop fairly extensive petechiae and some ecchymoses and may have hematuria or epistaxis or both. About 3% to 4% of acute ITP cases are considered severe, with platelet counts <10,000/μL and noncutaneous bleeding such as gastrointestinal bleeding, hematuria, mucous membrane bleeding, and retinal hemorrhage.[39] Of patients with severe disease, 25% to 50% are considered to be at risk for intracranial hemorrhage, which is the primary complication that contributes to the overall approximately 0.6% mortality rate for patients with acute ITP.[38]

Most patients with acute ITP recover with or without treatment in about 3 weeks, although for some, recovery may take 6 months. In about 10% to 15% of the children initially thought to have acute ITP, the thrombocytopenia persists for 6 months or longer, and these children are reclassified as having chronic ITP.[38] In a small fraction of children, recurrent episodes of acute ITP occur after complete recovery from the first episode.[40] Treatment is mandatory in children with ITP who are having active hemorrhage. In those circumstances treatment of acute ITP with corticosteroids, intravenous immunoglobulin (IVIG), or anti-D immunoglobulin is provided to treat hemorrhage. However, the value to using drugs for prevention of major bleeding in thrombocytopenic children exhibiting little or no clinical hemorrhage has not been established.

Chronic ITP can be found in patients of any age, although most cases occur in patients between the ages of 20 and 50 years. The overall incidence of chronic ITP ranges from 1 to 3 cases per 100,000 per year.[41] Females with this disorder outnumber males 2 to 3:1, with the highest incidence in women between 20 and 40 years of age. Chronic ITP usually begins insidiously, with platelet counts that are variably decreased and sometimes normal for periods. Presenting symptoms are those of mucocutaneous bleeding, with menorrhagia, recurrent epistaxis, and easy bruising (ecchymoses) being most common.

Platelet destruction in chronic ITP is the result of the binding of autoantibodies to platelets, which leads to enhanced platelet removal from the circulation by reticuloendothelial cells, primarily in the spleen. Autoantibodies that recognize platelet surface glycoproteins (GP) such as GPIIb and GPIIIa ($\alpha_{IIb}\beta_3$), GPIa/IIa, and others occur in 50% to 60% of ITP patients.[42,43] Because megakaryocytes also express GPIIb/IIIa and GPIb/IX on their membranes, these cells are also targets of the antibodies, leading to impaired megakaryocytopoiesis.[44] T cell-mediated destruction of platelets may also play a role.[45]

Platelet turnover studies have shown impaired platelet production in ITP. Overall, the life span of the platelet is shortened from the normal 7 to 10 days to a few hours. The rapidity with which platelets are removed from the circulation correlates with the degree of thrombocytopenia. If plasma from a patient with ITP is transfused into the circulation of a normal recipient, the recipient develops thrombocytopenia. The thrombocytopenia-producing factor in the plasma of the ITP patient is an immunoglobulin G (IgG) antibody that can be removed from serum by adsorption with normal human platelets.

The only abnormalities in the peripheral blood of patients with ITP are related to platelets. In most cases, platelets number between 30,000/μL and 80,000/μL. Patients with ITP undergo periods of remission and exacerbation, however, and their platelet counts may range from near normal to fewer than 20,000/μL during these periods. Morphologically, platelets appear normal, although larger in diameter than usual (Figure 38.3). This is reflected in an increased mean platelet volume as measured by electronic cell counters. The marrow typically is characterized by megakaryocytic hyperplasia. Megakaryocytes are increased in size, and young forms with a single nucleus, smooth contour, and diminished cytoplasm are common. In the absence of bleeding, infection, or other underlying disorder, erythrocyte and leukocyte precursors are normal in number and morphology. Coagulation tests showing abnormal results include tests dependent on platelet function. Although platelet-associated IgG levels are increased in most patients,[10,21,46] such testing for IgG platelet antibodies is neither sensitive or specific for ITP and therefore is not diagnostically useful for any form of ITP.[46]

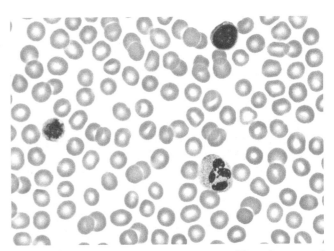

Figure 38.3 Blood Cell Morphology in Immune Thrombocytopenic Purpura. Note scarce platelets and increased platelet size but normal red blood cell and white blood cell morphology. (Peripheral blood, Wright-Giemsa stain, ×500.)

The initial treatment of chronic ITP depends on the urgency for increasing the platelet count. In ITP patients with platelet counts >30,000/μL who receive no treatment, the expected mortality rate is equal to that of the general population. In the absence of additional risk factors, ITP patients with platelet counts >30,000/μL should not be treated. If additional risk factors are present, such as old age, coagulation defects, recent surgery, trauma, or uncontrolled hypertension, the platelet count should be maintained at 50,000/μL or higher, depending on the clinical situation. In patients in whom the need is considered urgent, IVIG remains the treatment of choice. For most patients, however, the initial treatment of chronic ITP is with prednisone. About 70% to 90% of patients respond to this therapy, with an increase in platelet count and a decrease in hemorrhagic episodes. Although reported response rates vary widely, about 50% of patients have a long-term beneficial effect from corticosteroid treatment.[47]

If the response to corticosteroids is inadequate or no response is seen, steroid therapy can be supplemented with IVIG or, in some cases, anti-D immunoglobulin.[47,48] For patients in whom prednisone is ineffective, intravenous rituximab can be tried. Responses to rituximab are usually seen within 3 to 4 weeks. In patients refractory to all medical therapies, splenectomy may become necessary. Splenectomy eliminates the primary site of platelet removal and destruction, and it also removes an organ containing autoantibody-producing lymphocytes. Splenectomy is an effective treatment for adult chronic ITP, with 88% of patients showing improvement and 66% having a complete and lasting response.[49] Studies with high-dose dexamethasone, rituximab and thrombopoietin receptor agonists have suggested possible benefits to these therapies.[50] In the most severe refractory cases, immunosuppressive (chemotherapeutic) agents such as azathioprine given alone or with steroids may be necessary. In such patients, platelet transfusions may be of transient benefit in treating severe hemorrhagic episodes but should not be given routinely.[46] IVIG given alone or just before platelet transfusion also may be beneficial.[37,46]

Chronic ITP occurring in association with HIV infection, with hemophilia, or with pregnancy presents special problems in diagnosis and therapy. Unexplained thrombocytopenia in otherwise healthy members of high-risk populations may be an early manifestation of acquired immunodeficiency syndrome (AIDS).[36,46]

The differences between acute and chronic ITP are summarized in Table 38.3. Acute ITP occurs most often in children 2 to 9 years of age and in young adults, whereas chronic ITP occurs in patients of all ages, although most commonly in adults aged 20 to 50 years, and more commonly in women. Of patients with acute ITP, 60% to 80% have a history of infection, usually viral (rubella, rubeola, chickenpox, and nonspecific respiratory tract infection), occurring 2 to 21 days before ITP onset. Acute ITP also may occur after immunization with live vaccine for measles, chickenpox, mumps, and smallpox.

Acute ITP usually is self-limited, and spontaneous remissions occur in 80% to 90% of patients, although the duration of the illness may range from days to months. In chronic ITP, there is typically a fluctuating clinical course, with episodes of

---

TABLE 38.3 Differentiation of Acute and Chronic Immune Thrombocytopenic Purpura (ITP)

Characteristic	Acute ITP	Chronic ITP
Age at onset	2–6 yr	20–50 yr
Sex predilection	None	Female over male, 3:1
Prior infection	Common	Unusual
Onset of bleeding	Sudden	Gradual
Platelet count	<20,000/μL	30,000–80,000/μL
Duration	2–6 weeks	Months to years
Spontaneous remission	90% of patients	Uncommon
Seasonal pattern	Higher incidence in winter and spring	None
Therapy:		
Steroids	70% response rate	30% response rate
Splenectomy	Rarely required	<45 yr, 90% response rate >45 yr, 40% response rate

Adapted from Triplett, D. A. (Ed.). (1978). *Platelet Function: Laboratory Evaluation and Clinical Application.* Chicago: American Society of Clinical Pathologists; Quick, A. J. (1966). *Hemorrhagic Diseases and Thrombosis* (2nd ed.). Philadelphia: Lea & Febiger; and Arnold, D. M., Zeller, M. P., Smith, J. W., & Nazy, I. (2018). Diseases of platelet number: immune thrombocytopenia, neonatal alloimmune thrombocytopenia and posttransfusion purpura. In Hoffman, R., Benz, E. J., & Silberstein, L. E., et al. (Eds.), *Hematology: Basic Principles and Practice.* (7th ed., pp. 1944–1954). Philadelphia: Elsevier.

---

bleeding that last a few days or weeks. Spontaneous remissions are uncommon and usually incomplete.[46]

Symptoms of acute ITP vary, but petechial hemorrhages, purpura, and often bleeding from the gums and gastrointestinal or urinary tract typically begin suddenly, sometimes over a few hours. Hemorrhagic bullae in the oral mucosa are often prominent in patients with severe thrombocytopenia of acute onset. Usually the severity of bleeding is correlated with the degree of thrombocytopenia.[46] In contrast, presenting symptoms of chronic ITP begin with a few scattered petechiae or other minor bleeding manifestations. Occasionally a bruising tendency, menorrhagia, or recurrent epistaxis is present for months or years before diagnosis. Platelet counts range from 5000/μL to 75,000/μL and are generally higher than those in acute ITP. Giant platelets are common.

Treatment also varies for acute and chronic ITP. In chronic ITP, initial therapy often consists of glucocorticoids (corticosteroids), which interfere with splenic and hepatic macrophages to increase platelet survival time. In acute ITP, treatment for all but the most severely thrombocytopenic and hemorrhagic patients is contraindicated. When treatment is necessary, a good response to IVIG, corticosteroids, or both usually can be obtained, and splenectomy is rarely required.[37,38] Patients with chronic ITP unresponsive to all medical therapies may be candidates for splenectomy.

Immunologic drug-induced thrombocytopenia. Many drugs can induce acute thrombocytopenia (Box 38.3). Drug-dependent antibodies typically occur after 1 to 2 weeks of exposure to a new drug. Drug-induced immune-mediated thrombocytopenia can be divided into several types based on the mechanisms underlying the interaction of the antibody with the drug and platelets. The common mechanisms are depicted in Figure 38.4. and will be discussed in the following paragraphs.

Drug-dependent antibodies. One mechanism of drug-dependent antibodies recognized for more than 100 years is typified by quinidine- and quinine-induced thrombocytopenia (Figure 38.4). Antibodies induced by drugs of this type interact with platelets only in the presence of the drug. Many drugs can induce such antibodies, but quinine, quinidine, and sulfonamide derivatives do so more often than other drugs. When antibody production has begun, the platelet count falls rapidly and often may be <10,000/μL. Patients may have abrupt onset of bleeding symptoms. If this type of drug-induced thrombocytopenia develops in a pregnant woman, both she and her fetus may be affected.

The antibodies responsible for drug-dependent thrombocytopenia bind directly to platelets by their Fab regions. The Fab portion of the antibody binds to a platelet membrane constituent, usually the GPIb/IX/V complex or the GPIIb/IIIa complex, only in the presence of drug.[51,52] The mechanism by which the drug promotes binding of a drug-dependent antibody to a specific target on the platelet membrane without covalently linking to the target or the antibody remains to be determined. Because

the Fc portion of the immunoglobulin is not involved in binding to platelets, it is still available to bind the Fc receptors on phagocytic cells. This situation may contribute to the rapid onset and relatively severe nature of the thrombocytopenia. Most drug-induced platelet antibodies are of the IgG class, but in rare instances, IgM antibodies are involved.[45]

A similar pattern is seen with the antiplatelet agents abciximab, tirofiban, and eptifibatide (Figure 38.4), although with these drugs thrombocytopenia tends to occur within several hours of exposure. Such immediate reactions are due to naturally occurring antibodies to the murine structural elements of abciximab (a mouse/human monoclonal antibody fragment) or to structural changes in platelet GPIIb/IIIa induced by binding of eptifibatide or tirofiban.

Hapten-induced antibodies. A second mechanism of drug-induced thrombocytopenia is induction of hapten-dependent antibodies. Some drug molecules are too small by themselves to trigger an immune response, but they may act as a hapten and combine with a larger carrier molecule (usually a plasma protein or protein constituent of the platelet membrane) to form a complex that can act as a complete antigen.[45] Penicillin and penicillin derivatives are the primary offending agents causing drug-induced thrombocytopenia by this mechanism. Drug-induced thrombocytopenia of this type is often severe with an initial platelet count of <10,000/μL and sometimes <1000/μL. The number of bone marrow megakaryocytes is usually normal to elevated.[45] Bleeding is often severe and rapid in onset, and hemorrhagic bullae in the mouth may be prominent.

Drug-induced autoantibodies. Drug-induced autoantibodies represent a third mechanism of drug-induced thrombocytopenia. In this case the drugs stimulate the formation of an autoantibody that binds to a specific platelet membrane glycoprotein with no requirement for the presence of free drug. Gold salts, procainamide, and levodopa are examples of such drugs (Figure 38.4). The precise mechanism by which these drugs induce autoantibodies against platelets is not known with certainty.

Immune complex–induced thrombocytopenia. Heparin-induced thrombocytopenia (HIT) is a good example of immune complex–induced thrombocytopenia, the fourth mechanism of drug-induced thrombocytopenia (Figure 38.4). Binding of therapeutic heparin to platelet factor 4 (PF4), a protein released by activated platelets, or binding of PF4 to the platelet membrane causes a conformational change in PF4, resulting in the exposure of neoepitopes. The Fab portion of an IgG binds to the PF4 neoepitope. The free Fc portion of the IgG binds with the platelet FcγIIa receptor. Platelets are activated by occupancy of their FcγIIa receptor,[53,54] leading to platelet activation and aggregation. It is this activation of platelets that leads to their consumption and thrombocytopenia. Thrombocytopenia, typically beginning 5 to 14 days after heparin exposure, is usually mild to moderate, with platelet counts only rarely <15,000/μL. Paradoxically, patients with HIT rarely bleed but have a high risk of thrombosis that can be life threatening. A more detailed discussion of HIT can be found in Chapter 39.

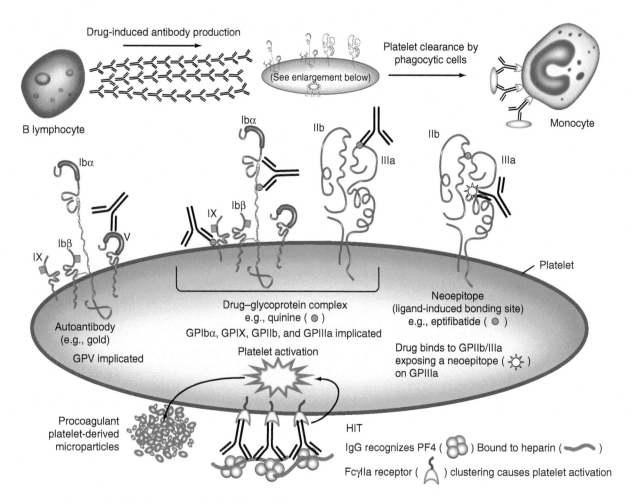

Figure 38.4 Mechanisms of Drug-Induced Thrombocytopenia. Certain drugs stimulate the production of immunoglobulins that bind a platelet membrane antigen or antigen and drug combination; monocyte/macrophage Fc receptors bind the Fc portion of the immunoglobulin bound to the platelet resulting in platelet removal *(top panel)*. Mechanisms of four specific drugs are depicted *(bottom panel)*. *GP,* Glycoprotein; *HIT,* heparin-induced thrombocytopenia; *IgG,* immunoglobulin G; *PF4,* platelet factor 4. (From Warkentin, T. E. [2018]. Thrombocytopenia caused by platelet destruction, hypersplenism, or hemodilution. In Hoffman, R., Benz, E. J., & Silberstein, L. E., et al. [Eds.], *Hematology: Basic Principles and Practice* [7th ed.]. Philadelphia: Elsevier.)

Treatment of patients with drug-induced thrombocytopenia. Treatment for any drug-induced thrombocytopenia requires identification of the offending drug, drug discontinuation, and substitution with another suitable therapeutic agent. This is often difficult to accomplish. In patients taking multiple drugs, it is not always easy to determine which of the drugs is at fault for causing thrombocytopenia. Under these conditions, identifying the causative agent may be a trial-and-error procedure in which the most likely drugs are eliminated one at a time. In addition, even if the patient is taking only one agent, there may not be a suitable replacement, or a prolonged period may be required for the alternative drug to become effective. Furthermore, laboratory testing to identify specific drugs involved is beyond the capabilities of most clinical laboratories and is usually performed by reference laboratories.

Although drugs usually are cleared from the circulation rapidly, dissociation of drug-antibody complexes may require longer periods, perhaps 1 to 2 weeks.[10] In some cases, such as those caused by gold salts, thrombocytopenia may persist for months.

Platelet transfusions may be administered to patients with life-threatening bleeds, but platelet transfusions in severe but not life-threatening bleeding should be individualized. Although the transfused platelets are destroyed rapidly, they may function to halt bleeding effectively before they are destroyed.

In addition, high-dose IVIG may be used and is generally an effective treatment for most drug-induced immune thrombocytopenias.

Neonatal Immune-Mediated Thrombocytopenias

Neonatal alloimmune thrombocytopenia. Neonatal alloimmune thrombocytopenia (NAIT) develops when the mother lacks a platelet-specific antigen that the fetus has inherited from the father. Fetal platelet antigens, which are inherited as codominant genes, may pass from the fetal to the maternal circulation as early as the 14th week of gestation.[55] If the mother is exposed to a fetal antigen she lacks, she may make antibodies to that fetal antigen. These IgG antibodies cross the placenta, attach to the antigen-bearing fetal platelets, and result in thrombocytopenia in the fetus. In this regard the pathophysiology of NAIT is similar to that of hemolytic disease of the newborn. The mother of the fetus with NAIT is usually asymptomatic.

The most common cause (~80%) of NAIT in Caucasians is the HPA-1a antigen expressed on GPIIIa of the surface membrane GPIIb/IIIa complex. HPA-5b (Br), which is found on the GPIa, accounts for 10% to 15% of cases. The antigen HPA-3a (Bak) is present on GPIIb and is an important cause of neonatal thrombocytopenia in Asians. Platelet antigen HPA-4 (Pen, Yuk) accounts for the disorder in a few affected neonates.

Clinically severe thrombocytopenia as a result of NAIT occurs in 1 in 1000 live births and, unlike hemolytic disease of the fetus and newborn, often affects the first pregnancy in an at-risk couple.[56] With the first pregnancy, about 50% of neonates born to mothers lacking a specific platelet antigen are affected, whereas with subsequent pregnancies the risk may increase to 75% to 97%.[56] The incidence of intracranial hemorrhage or death or both in affected offspring is about 25%, with about half of the intracranial hemorrhages occurring in utero in the second trimester.

Affected infants may appear normal at birth but soon manifest scattered petechiae and purpuric hemorrhages. In many infants with NAIT, serious hemorrhage does not develop, but the risks are directly associated with the degree of thrombocytopenia. Infants may recover over a 1- to 2-week period as the level of passively transferred antibody decreases.[10,38] In symptomatic cases, platelet levels are usually <30,000/μL and may decrease even further in the first few hours after birth; however, in these circumstances, affected neonates must be followed in a neonatal intensive care setting for serial assessment of platelet counts and indicated therapy.

The diagnosis of NAIT is one of exclusion of other causes of neonatal thrombocytopenia, including neonatal bacterial infection, maternal ITP and maternal ingestion of drugs known to be associated with drug-induced thrombocytopenia. The presence of thrombocytopenia in a neonate with a HPA-1a–negative mother or a history of the disorder in a sibling is strong presumptive evidence in favor of the diagnosis. Confirmation should include platelet typing of both parents and testing for evidence of a maternal antibody directed at paternal platelets.[37]

In situations in which suspicion of NAIT is high or there is a history of NAIT in a first pregnancy, it may be necessary to test or treat the fetus to prevent intracranial hemorrhage in utero. Fetal genotypes now can be determined at 15 to 16 weeks of gestation using polymerase chain reaction methods on cells obtained by chorionic villus sampling or amniocentesis.[57]

Serial cordocentesis and intrauterine platelet transfusion of fetuses has been largely abandoned because of complication rates. In cases in which the fetal postnatal platelet counts do not increase with IVIG therapy, washed maternal platelets, if available, have been infused into the fetus with good results.[58] Treatment of the mother with high-dose corticosteroids to decrease maternal antibody production is not recommended because of potential fetal toxicity.

In situations in which the diagnosis of NAIT is known or highly suspected, delivery by cesarean section at 36 to 37 weeks gestation (to ensure fetal lung maturity) is recommended to avoid fetal trauma associated with vaginal delivery. After delivery, the affected infant may be treated with transfusion of the appropriate antigen-negative platelets (usually maternal). Obtaining washed maternal platelets is always logistically difficult. In severely thrombocytopenic or bleeding neonates with NAIT, it is acceptable to transfuse random platelets. Although destined to have a suboptimal in vivo survival, such transfused platelets are hemostatically active and reduce the risk of bleeding.[59] IVIG can be used alone or in combination with platelet transfusion but should not be used as the sole treatment in a bleeding infant because response to this therapy usually takes 1 to 3 days.[56]

Neonatal autoimmune thrombocytopenia. Women commonly develop chronic ITP during pregnancy which tends to remit after delivery. Additionally, during pregnancy, relapse is relatively common for women whose ITP had been in complete or partial remission; this has been attributed to the facilitation of reticuloendothelial phagocytosis by the high estrogen levels in pregnant women.

Neonatal autoimmune thrombocytopenia results from the passive transplacental transfer of maternal ITP autoantibodies or, less commonly, from autoantibodies associated with a collagen-vascular disease such as systemic lupus erythematosus. The neonate does not have an ongoing autoimmune process per se, but rather is an incidental target of the mother's autoimmune process. Corticosteroids are the primary treatment for pregnant women with ITP, and at the dosages used, there is a low incidence of adverse fetal side effects.[60]

Neonatal autoimmune thrombocytopenia develops in about 10% of the infants of pregnant women with autoimmune thrombocytopenia, and intracranial hemorrhage occurs in 1% or less. It is no longer recommended that high-risk infants be delivered by cesarean section to avoid the trauma of vaginal delivery and accompanying risk of hemorrhage in the infant, regardless of maternal platelet count.[61]

Affected newborns may have normal to decreased platelet numbers at birth and have a progressive decrease in the platelet count for about 1 week postpartum (but could last for several months) before the platelet count begins to increase. It has been speculated that the falling platelet count is associated with maturation of the infant's reticuloendothelial system and accelerated removal of antibody-labeled platelets by cells of the reticuloendothelial system.

Although treatment is not required in most cases, severely thrombocytopenic infants generally respond quickly to IVIG treatment. If an infant develops hemorrhagic symptoms, risks should be clinically stratified and medical therapies (such as platelet transfusion, IVIG treatment, or corticosteroid therapy) should be started immediately.[37]

Posttransfusion purpura. Posttransfusion purpura (PTP) is a rare disorder that typically develops about 1 week after transfusion of platelet-containing blood products, including fresh or frozen plasma, whole blood, and packed or washed red cells. PTP is manifested by the rapid onset of severe thrombocytopenia and moderate to severe hemorrhage that may be life threatening.

The recipient's plasma is found to contain alloantibodies to antigens on the platelets or platelet membranes of the transfused blood product, directed against an antigen the recipient lacks.

The mechanism by which the recipient's own platelets are destroyed is unclear, but it requires stimulation of platelet autoantibodies, which also target recipient antigen-negative platelets. In more than 90% of cases, the primary alloantibody is directed against the HPA-1a (Pl^{A1} antigen; in most of the remaining cases, the antibodies are directed against HPA-1b (Pl^{A2}) or other epitopes on GP IIb/IIIa.[37] Involvement of other alloantigens, such as HPA-3a (Bak), HPA-4 (Pen), and HPA-5b (Br), have also been reported. Most patients with PTP are multiparous middle-aged women and almost all patients have a history of blood transfusion. PTP seems to be exceedingly rare in men who have never been transfused and in women who have never been pregnant or never been transfused.[62] PTP seems to require prior exposure to foreign platelet antigens and behaves in many respects like an anamnestic immune response.

No clinical trials have been conducted on the treatment of PTP, primarily because of the small number of cases. Therapeutic exchange transfusion has been used with some success in the past, but the treatment of choice is now IVIG. Many patients with PTP respond to a 2-day course of IVIG, generally initiated within the first 2 to 3 days of presentation, although a second course occasionally is necessary.[63] IVIG also is much easier to administer, and the response rates are higher than for therapeutic exchange transfusion. Corticosteroid therapy is not particularly efficacious when used alone but may be beneficial in combination with other, more effective treatments.[37] If PTP is untreated or treatment is ineffective, mortality rates may approach 10%.[63] In addition, untreated or unresponsive patients who happen to survive have a protracted clinical course, with thrombocytopenia typically lasting 3 weeks but in some cases up to 4 months.

Secondary thrombocytopenia, presumed to be immune mediated. Severe thrombocytopenia has been identified in patients receiving biologic response modifiers such as interferons, colony-stimulating factors, and interleukin-2.[64-66] Thrombocytopenia associated with use of these substances is reversible and, at least for interferon, may be immune mediated, because increased levels of platelet-associated IgG have been measured. Immune thrombocytopenia develops in about 5% to 10% of patients with chronic lymphocytic leukemia and in a smaller percentage of patients with other lymphoproliferative disorders.[67,68] Thrombocytopenia also is noted in 14% to 26% of patients with systemic lupus erythematosus.[69] In such secondary situations the clinical picture and the response to therapeutic interventions are similar to that of ITP in that the bone marrow has a larger than normal number of megakaryocytes, and an increased level of platelet-associated IgG often is found.[36]

Parasitic infections also are known to cause thrombocytopenia. Malaria is the most studied disease in this group and is regularly accompanied by thrombocytopenia, the onset of which corresponds to the first appearance of antimalarial antibodies, and a decrease in serum complement, and control of parasitemia. There is evidence for the adsorption of microbial antigens to the platelet surface and subsequent antibody binding via the Fab terminus.[70] Immune destruction of platelets seems to be the most likely mechanism for the thrombocytopenia.

Nonimmune Mechanisms of Platelet Destruction

Nonimmune platelet destruction may result from exposure of platelets to nonendothelial surfaces, from activation of the coagulation process, or from platelet consumption by endovascular injury without measurable depletion of coagulation factors.[36] Many of these disorders are classified as *thrombotic microangiopathies* (TMAs), a broad group of disorders characterized by the presence of thrombocytopenia, clot formation within the arterioles and capillaries, and microangiopathic hemolytic anemia. Although hemolytic uremic syndrome (HUS) and thrombotic thrombocytopenic purpura (TTP) are the most commonly known TMAs, TMA can occur secondary to a large number of clinical conditions (Box 38.4).

Thrombocytopenia in pregnancy and preeclampsia. Incidental thrombocytopenia of pregnancy, also known as pregnancy-associated thrombocytopenia and gestational thrombocytopenia, is a benign physiologic condition that is the most common cause of thrombocytopenia in pregnancy and requires no evaluation or treatment.[71] Random platelet counts in pregnant and postpartum women are slightly higher than normal, but about 5% of pregnant women develop a mild thrombocytopenia (100,000 to 150,000/μL), with 98% of such women having platelet counts >70,000/μL. These women are healthy, have no prior history of thrombocytopenia, and do not seem to be at increased risk for bleeding or for delivery of infants with neonatal thrombocytopenia. The cause of this type of thrombocytopenia is unknown. Maternal platelet counts return to normal within several weeks of delivery. Such women could experience recurrence in subsequent pregnancies.

Approximately 20% of cases of thrombocytopenia of pregnancy are associated with hypertensive disorders. These disorders include preeclampsia, preeclampsia-eclampsia, preeclampsia with chronic hypertension, chronic hypertension, and gestational hypertension. Preeclampsia complicates about 5% of pregnancies and typically occurs at about 20 weeks of gestation. The disorder is characterized by the onset of hypertension and proteinuria and may include abdominal pain, headache, blurred vision, or mental function disturbances.[72] Thrombocytopenia occurs in 15% to 20% of patients with preeclampsia, with 40% to 50% of these patients progressing to eclampsia (hypertension, proteinuria, and seizures).[73,74]

Some patients with preeclampsia have microangiopathic **h**emolysis, **e**levated **l**iver enzymes, and **l**ow **p**latelet count, termed *HELLP syndrome.* HELLP syndrome affects an estimated 4% to 12% of women with severe preeclampsia[46,75,76] and seems to be associated with higher rates of maternal and fetal complications. This disorder is difficult to differentiate from TTP, complement-mediated TMAs, HUS, and DIC. Therefore appropriate clinical differential diagnostic considerations are required (Box 38.4).

BOX 38.4 Thrombotic Microangiopathies in Association with Various Conditions

Thrombotic thrombocytopenic purpura (TTP; classical TM)
Hemolytic uremic syndrome (HUS; classical TM):
　　Shiga toxin–associated HUS (such as *Escherichia coli* O157:H7)
　　Atypical HUS (aHUS)
Drug-associated (e.g., clopidogrel, ticlopidine)
Transplant-associated (solid organ or stem cell)
Malignancy-associated
Pregnancy-associated:
　　HELLP syndrome
　　Preeclampsia/eclampsia
Disseminated intravascular coagulation (DIC)
Catastrophic antiphospholipid syndrome (CAPS)
Connective tissue/autoimmune disorders (e.g., systemic lupus erythematosus)
HIV disease
Malignant hypertension

HELLP, *h*emolysis, *e*levated *l*iver enzymes, and *l*ow *p*latelet count; *HIV*, human immunodeficiency virus; *TM*, thrombotic microangiopathy.

The development of thrombocytopenia in these patients is thought to be due to increased platelet destruction. Though the mechanism of platelet destruction remains unclear, some evidence (elevated D-dimer) suggests that these patients have an underlying low-grade DIC.[77] Elevated platelet-associated immunoglobulin is commonly found in these patients, which indicates immune involvement.[78] Early reports suggested that in vivo platelet activation may contribute to the development of preeclampsia because low-dose aspirin therapy has been shown to prevent preeclampsia in high-risk patients.[79,80] When aspirin is used to prevent preeclampsia, however, reduction in risk is only 15%.

The best treatment of preeclampsia is delivery of the infant whenever possible. After delivery, the thrombocytopenia usually resolves in a few days. In cases in which delivery is not possible (e.g., the infant would be too premature), bed rest and aggressive treatment of the hypertension may help to increase the platelet count in some patients.

As has been discussed previously, ITP is a relatively common disorder in women of childbearing age, and pregnancy does nothing to ameliorate the symptoms of this disorder. ITP should be part of the differential diagnosis of thrombocytopenia in a pregnant woman. There is little or no correlation between the level of maternal autoantibodies and the fetal platelet count. Other causes of thrombocytopenia during pregnancy include HIV infection and other comorbidities such as systemic lupus erythematosus, antiphospholipid syndromes, TTP, and HUS. Of all women who develop TTP, 10% to 25% manifest the disease during pregnancy or in the postpartum period, and TTP tends to recur in subsequent pregnancies.[81,82] Therapeutic plasma exchange is the treatment of choice to prevent maternal or fetal mortality, which can be 90% or greater without such treatment.

Hemolytic disease of the newborn. Thrombocytopenia, usually moderate in degree, occurs commonly in infants with hemolytic disease of the newborn. Although the erythrocyte destruction characteristic of this disorder is antibody mediated,

the antigens against which the antibodies are directed are not expressed on platelets. Platelets may be destroyed as a result of their interaction with products of red cell breakdown, rather than their direct participation in an immunologic reaction.[36]

Thrombotic thrombocytopenic purpura. TTP, sometimes referred to as Moschcowitz syndrome, is characterized by the triad of microangiopathic hemolytic anemia (MAHA, Chapter 22), thrombocytopenia, and neurologic abnormalities.[83] In addition, fever and renal dysfunction (forming a pentad) can be present; however, MAHA and thrombocytopenia are the most common clinical findings. Additional symptoms, including diarrhea, anorexia, nausea, weakness, and fatigue, are present in most patients at the time of diagnosis. TTP is uncommon but not rare. The prevalence of TTP has been estimated at approximately 10 cases per 1 million people with an annual incidence of approximately 1 new case per 1 million people.[84,85] About twice as many women as men are affected, and it is most common in women 30 to 40 years of age.[34,86] About half of the patients who develop TTP have a history of a viral-like illness several days before the onset of TTP, although there is no proof that such incidences are causal.

There are at least four types of TTP. In most patients, TTP occurs as a single acute episode, although a small fraction of these patients may have recurrence at seemingly random intervals. Second, recurrent TTP occurs in 11% to 28% of TTP patients.[87,88] Third, certain types of drugs can induce TTP. The primary agents involved are the thienopyridine agents ticlopidine (Ticlid) and clopidogrel (Plavix), which are used to inhibit platelet function. Ticlopidine seems to cause TTP in about 0.025% of patients, whereas the incidence of clopidogrel-induced TTP is approximately four times less.[85] These common types of TTP generally result from autoantibodies that aid in the removal of the ADAMTS13 (*a d*isintegrin *a*nd *m*etalloprotease with a *t*hrombospondin type 1 motif, member 13) enzyme or block its function.

Fourth, rarely, patients experience chronic relapsing TTP in which episodes occur at intervals of approximately 3 months starting in infancy.[89,90] This form of TTP, known as Upshaw-Shulman syndrome, is hereditary and congenital. It is associated with an autosomal recessive gene mutation that leads to ADAMTS13 dysfunction. Familial chronic relapsing TTP is characterized by recurrent episodes of thrombocytopenia with or without ischemic organ damage. TTP usually develops only when clinical conditions with increased von Willebrand factor (VWF) levels (e.g., infection) occur. In this type of TTP, ADAMTS13 activity is nearly completely deficient.[91,92]

Thrombi composed of platelets and VWF but very little fibrin or fibrinogen are found in the end arterioles and capillaries of patients with TTP.[93] As these platelet-VWF thrombi are deposited, thrombocytopenia develops (<30,000/μL). The degree of thrombocytopenia is directly related to the extent of microvascular platelet aggregation. Red blood cells (RBCs) flowing under arterial pressure are fragmented when they encounter the strands of these thrombi, which give rise to the peripheral blood findings of schistocytosis.

Hemolysis is usually quite severe, and most patients have less than 10 g/dL hemoglobin at presentation. Examination of the peripheral blood film reveals a marked decrease in platelets, RBC polychromasia, and schistocytes, a triad of features characteristic of microangiopathic hemolytic anemias (Figure 38.5). Nucleated RBC precursors also may be present, depending on the degree of hemolysis. Other laboratory evidence of intravascular hemolysis includes reduction of haptoglobin, hemoglobinuria, increased serum unconjugated bilirubin, and increased lactate dehydrogenase activity. Bone marrow examination reveals erythroid hyperplasia and a normal to increased number of megakaryocytes. The partial thromboplastin time, prothrombin time, fibrinogen, fibrin degradation products, and D-dimer test results are usually normal and may be useful in differentiating this disorder from DIC (Chapters 39 and 41).

The thrombotic lesions give rise to the other characteristic manifestations of TTP, because they are deposited in the vasculature of all organs where they occlude blood flow and lead to organ ischemia. Symptoms depend on the severity of ischemia in each organ. Neurologic manifestations range from headache

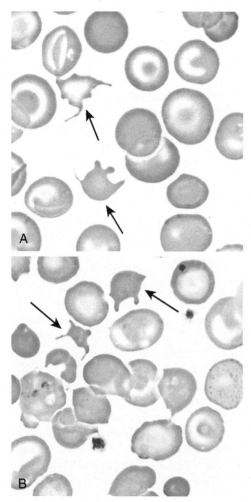

Figure 38.5 Blood Cell Morphology in Microangiopathic Hemolytic Anemia. Abundant schistocytes *(arrows)* reflect the platelet-rich clots in the microvasculature that occur with **(A)** thrombotic thrombocytopenic purpura *(TTP)* and **(B)** hemolytic uremic syndrome *(HUS)*. TTP and HUS present with similar blood morphologies. (Peripheral blood; Wright-Giemsa stain, ×1000.) (From Carr, J. H., & Rodak, B. F. [2013]. *Clinical Hematology Atlas* [4th ed.]. Philadelphia: Saunders.)

to paresthesia and coma. Visual disturbances may be of neurologic origin or may be due to thrombi in the choroid capillaries of the retina or hemorrhage into the vitreous. Renal dysfunction, present in more than half of patients,[87,88] is characterized by proteinuria and hematuria but usually does not lead to significant changes in serum creatinine or estimated glomerular filtration rate. Overwhelming renal damage with anuria and fulminant uremia usually does not occur, however, which helps distinguish TTP from HUS.[10] Gastrointestinal bleeding occurs commonly in severely thrombocytopenic patients, and abdominal pain is occasionally present as a result of occlusion of the mesenteric microcirculation.

The development of TTP is in most cases directly related to the accumulation of ultralarge von Willebrand factor (UL-VWF) multimers in the plasma. VWF multimers are made by megakaryocytes and endothelial cells, with the primary source of plasma VWF being endothelial cells. Endothelial cells store UL-VWF in Weibel-Palade bodies (endothelial cell storage granules) and secrete it into the subendothelium and plasma. In normal plasma the UL-VWF multimers are rapidly cleaved into the smaller VWF multimers, normally found in the plasma, by the VWF-cleaving protease ADAMTS13. This zinc-containing metalloprotease seems to be more effective when VWF multimers are partially unfolded by high shear stress (Figure 36.2).[94,95] Loss of ADAMTS13 activity results in an accumulation of the higher molecular weight VWF multimers. The UL-VWF multimers are more effective than the normal plasma VWF multimers at binding platelet GPIb/IX or GPIIb/IIIa complexes under fluid shear stresses[89] and will bind spontaneously to platelets to form platelet aggregates within the arterial and capillary vasculature (Figure 38.6).

Assays to measure ADAMTS13 are available[96] but commonly only performed in a reference laboratory. Functional and immuno-assays have been developed that measure ADAMTS13. Inhibitors to ADAMTS13, typically autoantibodies, can also be quantitated. Issues of assay optimization and standardization still exist. However, a recent prospective study reported that both the anti-ADAMTS13 IgG antibody level and ADAMTS13 antigen level correlate with outcome in patients with immune-mediated TTP.[97]

In patients with TTP, UL-VWF multimers tend to be present in the plasma at the beginning of the episode. These UL-VWF multimers, and usually the normal-sized plasma multimers, disappear as the TTP episode progresses and the thrombocytopenia worsens. If the patient survives an episode of TTP and does not experience a relapse, the plasma VWF multimers are usually normal after recovery. If UL-VWF multimers are found in the plasma after recovery, however, it is likely that the patient will have recurrent episodes of TTP. Because assays for UL-VWF are not readily available from clinical laboratories, recurrences of TTP are monitored based on serial hematologic testing (e.g., platelet count, hemoglobin, hematocrit).

Although ADAMTS13 levels can be measured, there is concern that a prolonged turnaround time may compromise rapid treatment of severe cases. Clinical prediction tools that use clinical and laboratory variables have been shown to be useful for determining the pretest probability of having severe

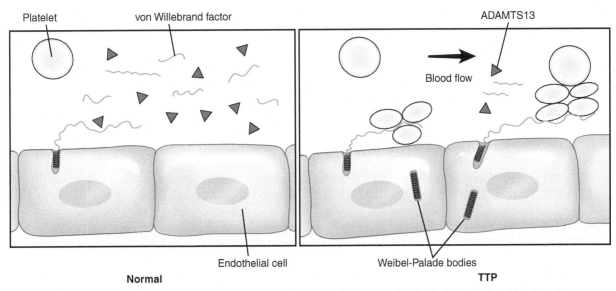

Platelet   von Willebrand factor   ADAMTS13

Blood flow

Endothelial cell   Weibel-Palade bodies

Normal   **TTP**

Figure 38.6 Mechanism for Thrombotic Thrombocytopenic Purpura *(TTP)*. Ultralarge *(UL)* von Willebrand factor *(VWF)* strands, released from endothelial cells, are normally digested by the VWF-cleaving protease ADAMTS13 into smaller multimers. In TTP the absence or dysfunction of ADAMTS13 allows the UL-VWF multimers to remain in circulation. Platelet binding to the UL-VWF multimers triggers the formation of platelet-rich thrombi.

ADAMTS13 deficiency.[98,99] The score described by Coppo, which considers creatinine levels, platelet counts and the presence of antinuclear antibodies, offers high positive predictive value and specificity but low sensitivity.

The PLASMIC score uses seven variables identified by univariate analysis to be predictive of ADAMTS13 deficiency. Patients are assigned 1 point each for platelet count <30,000/μL, hemolysis (measured in terms of reticulocyte count, haptoglobin, or indirect bilirubin), lack of active cancer, no history of solid organ or stem cell transplant, mean cell volume <90 fL, international normalized ratio <1.5, and creatinine <2 mg/dL. Patients with TTP had a median PLASMIC score of 7. In contrast, lower scores were found with rheumatologic disorders (median = 5), drug-associated TMA (median = 4), DIC (median = 4), and HUS/atypical HUS (median = 5). Three categories of risk for severe ADAMTS13 deficiency were defined: low risk for scores 0 to 4, intermediate risk for a score of 5, and high risk for scores 6 to 7. An independent external validation confirmed that a high PLASMIC score correlated with severe ADAMTS13 deficiency and predicted a high rate of response to plasma exchange therapy.[100]

Treatment decisions, based strictly on clinical criteria risk assessments, must be made immediately, often before test results are available, because TTP is a life-threatening condition.

Prophylactic plasma infusion is the most commonly used treatment of hereditary TTP caused by a mutation in ADAMTS13,[93] with higher plasma doses being administered to treat acute events. The most effective and first-line recommended treatment for acquired TTP resulting from the presence of anti-ADAMTS13 antibodies is therapeutic plasma exchange (TPE) using fresh frozen plasma.[101] Either of these plasma-replacement approaches may produce dramatic effects within a few hours. Because TPE is not available in all centers,

the patient should be given corticosteroids and infusions of fresh-frozen plasma immediately, with TPE being arranged as quickly as possible.

TPE and replacement or infusion of plasma is effective on two fronts. First, some of the UL-VWF multimers will be removed by apheresis, and plasma (simple transfusion, or exchange) supplies the deficient ADAMTS13 protease, which is able to degrade the UL-VWF multimers in the blood of the patient.

Because some patients with TTP have recovered while receiving immunosuppressive treatment (corticosteroids) alone, current recommendations are that all patients with TTP be treated with high-dose corticosteroids in addition to undergoing TPE. TPE typically is continued daily, with serial assessments of hemolysis and platelet counts. If the patient does not respond early to TPE and steroids, additional treatments need to be considered. Other agents that have been used include vincristine, azathioprine, and rituximab before consideration of splenectomy. Platelet transfusions should be avoided unless intracranial bleeding or other serious hemorrhagic problems arise.[46]

A recombinant ADAMTS13 (rADAMTS13) is being developed as a treatment for hereditary TTP. In a rat model mimicking acquired TTP, administration of rADAMTS13 prevented the full development of TTP-like symptoms (thrombocytopenia, hemolytic anemia, and VWF-rich thrombi in the kidneys and brain).[102] Analysis of plasma from treated animals confirmed the degradation of the UL-VWF multimers. A rADAMTS13 (BAX 930 or SHP 665, Shire Pharmaceuticals) has been tested in a phase I trial in patients with hereditary TTP, where it was found to be well tolerated and active in terms of cleavage of large VWF multimers.[103] The US Food and Drug Administration granted fast track designation for the development of rADAMTS13.

Before 1990, TTP was fatal in more than 90% of patients. With the means for rapid diagnosis and the advent of TPE, and new therapies on the horizon, now 80% of patients who are treated early can be expected to survive. Because patients are known to experience relapse, however, platelet counts should be monitored even after an apparent clinical remission. The detection of UL-VWF multimers in patient samples after complete remission has predicted relapse accurately in 90% of the patients tested[104]; this may prove to be useful in the long-term management of TTP.

Hemolytic uremic syndrome. HUS is another of the TMAs.[105] HUS is more common than TTP, with an annual incidence estimated at 2 to 6 per 100,000.[93] Approximately 90% of cases of HUS are caused by *Shigella dysenteriae* serotypes or enterohemorrhagic *Escherichia coli* OH serotypes, particularly O157:H7.[106] These organisms sometimes can be cultured from stool specimens. The bloody diarrhea typical of childhood HUS is caused by colonization of the large intestine with the offending organism, which causes erosive damage to the colon.

S. dysenteriae produces Shiga toxin, and enterohemorrhagic *E. coli* produces either Shiga-like toxin-1 (SLT-1) or SLT-2, which can be detected in fecal samples from patients with HUS. The toxins enter the bloodstream and attach to renal glomerular capillary endothelial cells, which become damaged and swollen and release UL-VWF multimers.[106,107] This process leads to formation of hyaline thrombi in the renal vasculature and the development of renal failure, thrombocytopenia, and microangiopathic hemolytic anemia. RBC fragmentation is usually not as severe as that seen in TTP (this is, however, not a differentiating feature).

The extent of renal involvement correlates with the rate of recovery. In more severely affected children, renal dialysis may be needed. The mortality rate associated with HUS in children is much lower than that for TTP, but there is often residual renal dysfunction that may lead to renal hypertension and severe renal failure. Because HUS in children is essentially an infectious disorder, it affects boys and girls equally and is often found in geographic clusters of cases rather than in random distribution.

The adult form of HUS is associated most often with exposure to immunosuppressive agents or chemotherapeutic agents or both, but it also may occur during the postpartum period. Usually the symptoms of HUS do not appear until weeks or months after exposure to the offending agent.[108] This disorder most likely results from direct renal arterial endothelial damage caused by the drug or one of its metabolites. The damage to endothelial cells results in release of VWF (including UL-VWF multimers), turbulent flow in the arterial system with increased shear stresses on platelets, and VWF-mediated platelet aggregation in the renal arterial system. The renal impairment in adults seems to be more severe than that in childhood HUS, and dialysis is often required. The cause of HUS associated with pregnancy or oral contraceptive use is unclear, but it may be related to development of an autoantibody to endothelial cells. In outbreaks of HUS associated with consumption of *E. coli*–contaminated water, both children and adults have developed HUS.

Clinically, HUS resembles TTP except that it is found predominantly in children 6 months to 4 years of age and is self-limiting. The cardinal signs of HUS are hemolytic anemia, renal failure, and thrombocytopenia. The thrombocytopenia is usually mild to moderate in severity. Renal failure is reflected in elevated blood urea nitrogen and creatinine levels. The urine nearly always contains RBCs, protein, and casts. The hemolytic process is shown by a hemoglobin level of less than 10 g/dL, elevated reticulocyte count, and presence of schistocytes in the peripheral blood.

Differentiating the adult form of HUS from TTP may be difficult. The lack of neurologic symptoms, the presence of renal dysfunction, and the absence of other organ involvement suggest HUS. Also, in HUS the thrombocytopenia tends to be mild to moderate (platelet consumption occurs primarily in the kidneys), whereas in TTP the thrombocytopenia is usually severe. Similarly, fragmentation of RBCs and the resultant anemia tend to be milder than that observed in TTP because RBCs are being fragmented primarily in the kidneys. In some cases of HUS, other organs become involved, and the differentiation between HUS and TTP becomes less clear. Because on initial presentation it is difficult or impossible to differentiate adult acquired TTP from adult HUS, patients are urgently started on a TPE program on a precautionary basis, until the diagnosis is better established.

Atypical hemolytic uremic syndrome. Although HUS and atypical HUS (aHUS) exhibit the same clinical signs and symptoms, each disease has a distinct mechanism of action. aHUS, like HUS, is a life-threatening disease. However, aHUS is an extremely rare, progressive disease that often has a genetic component. Unlike HUS, aHUS is not associated with an infection. Rather, aHUS is associated with a defect in the regulation of *complement activation.* A number of mutations in complement regulatory proteins have been identified. Of these, mutations in factor H that impair the control of the complement alternative pathway appear to be the most common. Although endothelial cells, RBCs, and platelets can be activated by complement, the role of each of these cell types in mediating the clinical phenotype is unclear. Eculizumab (Soliris, Alexion) is a humanized monoclonal antibody that acts as a C5 terminal complement inhibitor. Eculizumab has been approved as treatment for patients with aHUS.

Disseminated intravascular coagulation. A common cause of destructive thrombocytopenia is activation of the coagulation cascade (by a variety of agents or conditions), resulting in a consumptive coagulopathy that entraps platelets in intravascular fibrin clots. This disorder is described in more detail in Chapter 39 but is discussed here briefly for the sake of completeness. DIC has many similarities to TTP, including MAHA and deposition of thrombi in the arterial circulation of most organs. In DIC, however, the thrombi are composed primarily of platelets and fibrinogen (red clots), whereas in TTP the thrombi are composed primarily of platelets and VWF (white clots).

One form, acute DIC with rapid platelet consumption, results in severe thrombocytopenia. In addition, levels of factor V, factor VIII, and fibrinogen are decreased as a result of in vivo thrombin generation. The test for D-dimer (a breakdown product of stabilized fibrin) almost always yields positive results.

This form of DIC is life-threatening and must be treated immediately.

In chronic DIC there is an ongoing, low-grade consumptive coagulopathy. Clotting factors may be slightly reduced or normal, and compensatory thrombocytopoiesis results in a moderately low to normal platelet count.[34] D-dimer may not be elevated or may be slightly or moderately increased. Chronic DIC is not generally life-threatening, and treatment usually is not urgent. Chronic DIC, like all forms of DIC, is virtually always caused by some underlying condition, which can remain clinically elusive. If that condition can be corrected, the DIC usually resolves without further treatment. Chronic DIC should be followed closely, however, because it can convert into the life-threatening acute form.

Purpura fulminans. Purpura fulminans (PF) is a unique and devastating thrombotic disorder, often acute and fatal, that manifests as large irregular areas of blue-black cutaneous bleeding that rapidly progress to necrosis of superficial skin and deeper soft tissues. The identification of the cause of PF depends on the patient's age and context of presentation.

Occurring most commonly in neonates and children,[109] PF can be the presenting feature of acute sepsis resulting from bacterial infections with *Neisseria meningitidis*, *Streptococcus pneumoniae*, group A and B streptococci, and, less commonly, *Haemophilus influenzas* or *Staphylococcus aureus*. In sepsis there is widespread activation of the systemic inflammatory response, as well as the coagulation and complement pathways, which leads to increased bleeding. In the neonatal setting, PF may be associated with congenital or acquired deficiencies in protein C (PC) concentration or activity which promote thrombosis. The principal laboratory features of PF mirror those of DIC, including prolongation of coagulation times, thrombocytopenia, hypofibrinogenemia, and increased fibrin degradation products.

Although rare, the same clinical manifestations can occur in adults with sepsis, in whom a consistent feature is profound abnormalities in hemostasis as noted earlier.[110,111] Because of its rapid progression to multiorgan thrombotic injury, PF is a hematologic emergency requiring urgent intervention. In addition to full supportive care and urgent broad-spectrum antimicrobial therapies, PF with DIC requires plasma and platelet transfusions to replete the consumptive coagulopathy. Without effective treatment, PF causes superficial and deep soft tissues (from full-thickness skin surface down to the bone) to become gangrenous, requiring amputation. When microvascular necrosis extends to the visceral organs (lungs, kidneys, adrenals), mortality is high and morbidity is severe in survivors.

In neonates or small children with any of the heritable degrees of PC deficiency, replacement therapy with a human-derived PC concentrate (Ceprotin) is safe and effective. Intravenous dosing, however, may be required for long periods before the condition resolves. Children with more severe heritable forms of PF have ongoing risks of PF and require long-term antithrombotic therapy with PC replacement alone or in combination with Coumadin or low-molecular-weight heparin.

Nonimmune drug-induced thrombocytopenia. A few drugs directly interact with platelets to cause thrombocytopenia in a nonimmune manner. Ristocetin, an antibiotic no longer in clinical use, facilitates the interaction of VWF with platelet membrane GPIb and leads to in vivo platelet agglutination and thrombocytopenia. Hematin, used for the treatment of acute intermittent porphyria, may give rise to a transient thrombocytopenia that seems to be caused by stimulation of platelet secretion and aggregation. Protamine sulfate and bleomycin may induce thrombocytopenia by a similar mechanism.[45]

Abnormalities in Distribution or Dilution

A common clinical cause of thrombocytopenia is an abnormal distribution of platelets. The normal spleen sequesters approximately one third of the total platelet mass. Mild thrombocytopenia may be present in any of the "big spleen" syndromes, where normally produced platelets are physically sequestered. The total body platelet mass is often normal in these disorders, but numerous platelets are sequestered in the enlarged spleen, and consequently the venous blood platelet count is low. Common disorders that cause splenomegaly include end-stage liver diseases causing hepatic cirrhosis and portal hypertension. Other diseases that are associated with splenomegaly include Hodgkin lymphoma, non-Hodgkin lymphoma, sarcoidosis, leukemias (e.g., chronic myelogenous leukemia and hairy cell leukemia) and Gaucher disease.

Lowering the body temperature to less than 25° C, as is commonly done in cardiovascular surgery, results in a transient but mild thrombocytopenia secondary to platelet sequestration in the spleen and liver. An associated transient defect in function also occurs with hypothermia. Platelet count and function return to baseline values on return to normal body temperature.[32]

Thrombocytopenia often follows surgery involving extracorporeal circulatory devices (such as coronary bypass circuits, ventricular assist devices, and extracorporeal membrane oxygenation [ECMO]), as a consequence of damage and partial activation of platelets in the pump. In a few cases, severe thrombocytopenia, marked impairment of platelet function, and activation of fibrinolysis and intravascular coagulation may develop.[46]

The administration of massive amounts of stored whole blood may produce a temporary thrombocytopenia. Stored blood contains platelets whose viability is severely impaired by the effects of storage and temperature. Under these conditions, the dead or damaged platelets are rapidly sequestered by the reticuloendothelial system of the patient. This situation is only rarely encountered, however, because the practice of transfusing whole blood has been replaced virtually completely by the use of specific components. Finally, mild thrombocytopenia may be encountered in patients with chronic renal failure, severe iron deficiency, megaloblastic anemia, postcompression sickness, and chronic hypoxia.

THROMBOCYTOSIS: INCREASE IN CIRCULATING PLATELETS

Thrombocytosis is defined as an abnormally high platelet count, typically >450,000/μL.

The term *reactive thrombocytosis* is used to describe an elevation in the platelet count secondary to inflammation, trauma, or other underlying and seemingly unrelated conditions (Box 38.5). In reactive thrombocytosis the platelet count is elevated for a limited period and usually does not exceed 800,000/μL, although platelet counts greater than 1 million/μL are occasionally seen.

A marked and persistent elevation in the platelet count is a hallmark of *myeloproliferative disorders* such as polycythemia vera, chronic myelogenous leukemia, and myelofibrosis with myeloid metaplasia (or primary myelofibrosis). In these conditions the platelet count often exceeds 1 million/μL. In the myeloproliferative disorder known as essential thrombocythemia, platelet counts typically exceed 1 million/μL and may reach levels of several million.[34,112,113]

Reactive Thrombocytosis

Platelet counts between 450,000/μL and 800,000/μL with no change in platelet function can result from acute blood loss, splenectomy, childbirth, tissue necrosis secondary to surgery, chronic inflammatory disease, infection, exercise, iron deficiency anemia, hemolytic anemia, renal disorders, and various malignancies. Occasionally, patients manifest a platelet count of 1 to 2 million/μL (Figure 38.7; compare with normal platelet count in Figure 1.1).

In reactive thrombocytosis, platelet production remains responsive to normal regulatory stimuli (e.g., thrombopoietin, a glycoprotein hormone that is produced chiefly in the liver parenchyma and secondarily in the kidney) and morphologically normal platelets are produced at a moderately increased rate. This is in contrast to essential thrombocythemia (discussed later in this chapter), which is characterized by unregulated or

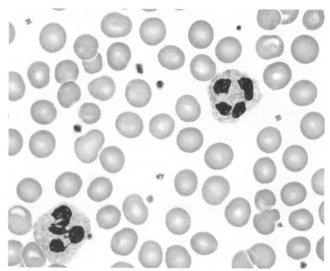

Figure 38.7 Cell Morphology in Reactive Thrombocytosis. Note the increased number of platelets but reasonably normal platelet morphology, characteristic of reactive thrombocytosis. (Peripheral blood, Wright-Giemsa stain, ×1000.)

autonomous platelet production and platelets of variable size.[112,113]

Examination of the bone marrow from patients with reactive thrombocytosis reveals a normal to increased number of megakaryocytes that are normal in morphology. Results of platelet aggregation tests induced by various agents usually reveal normal platelet function in reactive thrombocytosis.

Reactive thrombocytosis is not associated with thrombosis, hemorrhage, or abnormal thrombopoietin levels. It seldom produces symptoms per se and disappears when the underlying disorder is brought under control.[112,113]

Reactive Thrombocytosis Associated With Hemorrhage or Surgery

After acute hemorrhage, the platelet count may be low for 2 to 6 days (if no platelet transfusion) but typically rebounds to elevated levels for several days before returning to the prehemorrhage level. A similar pattern of thrombocytopenia and thrombocytosis is seen after major surgical procedures associated with significant blood loss. In both cases the platelet count typically returns to normal 10 to 16 days after blood loss.

Postsplenectomy Thrombocytosis

Removal of the spleen typically results in platelet counts that can reach or exceed 1 million/μL regardless of the reason for splenectomy. The spleen normally sequesters about one third of the circulating platelet mass. After splenectomy, one would expect an initial increase in the platelet count of approximately 30% to 50%. For unknown reasons, the platelet count, however, far exceeds levels that could result from rebalancing of the circulating platelet pool to incorporate the splenic platelet pool. Unlike after blood loss from hemorrhage or other types of surgery, the platelet count reaches a maximum 1 to 3 weeks after splenectomy and remains elevated for 1 to 3 months. In some patients who undergo splenectomy for treatment of anemias

---

BOX 38.5 Clinical States Resulting in Thrombocytosis

Conditions Associated With Reactive Thrombocytosis
Blood loss and surgery
Postsplenectomy
Iron deficiency anemia
Reactive thrombocytosis (such as infection or infection plus surgery)
Stress (including trauma and postoperative)
Rebound after myelosuppressive chemotherapy

Myeloproliferative Disorders Associated With Thrombocytosis
Polycythemia vera
Chronic myelogenous leukemia
Chronic myelomonocytic leukemia
Myelodysplastic syndrome variants (such as myelodysplasia with del[5q])
Primary myelofibrosis
Essential thrombocythemia

Adapted from Schafer, A. I. (2004). Thrombocytosis. *N Engl J Med, 350*(12), 1211–1219; and Harrison, C. N., Bareford, D., Butt, N., et al. (2010). Guideline for investigation and management of adults and children presenting with a thrombocytosis. *Br J Haematol, 149*(3), 352–375.

(e.g., autoimmune hemolytic anemia), the platelet count can remain elevated for several years.

Thrombocytosis Associated With Iron Deficiency Anemia

Mild iron deficiency anemia (IDA) secondary to chronic blood loss is associated with thrombocytosis in about 50% of cases. Thrombocytosis can be seen in severe IDA, but thrombocytopenia also has been reported. In some cases of iron deficiency, the platelet count may be 2 million/μL. After iron therapy is started, the platelet count usually returns to normal within 7 to 10 days. It is believed that iron plays some role in regulating thrombopoiesis, because treatment of the iron deficiency with iron replacement has resulted in a normalization of the platelet count in thrombocytopenic patients and has been reported to induce thrombocytopenia in patients with normal platelet counts. The mechanism underlying the role of iron in thrombopoiesis is unknown.

Thrombocytosis Associated With Inflammation and Disease

Similar to elevations in C-reactive protein, fibrinogen, VWF, and other acute phase reactants, thrombocytosis may be an indication of inflammation. Thrombocytosis may be found in association with rheumatoid arthritis, rheumatic fever, osteomyelitis, ulcerative colitis, and acute infections. In rheumatoid arthritis the presence of thrombocytosis can be correlated with activation of the inflammatory process. An elevated platelet count also may be early evidence of a tumor (e.g., Hodgkin disease) and various carcinomas. Patients with hemophilia often have platelet counts greater than normal limits, even in the absence of active bleeding.

Kawasaki disease is a disorder caused by inflammation of the walls of small and medium-sized arteries throughout the body. It is also known as mucocutaneous lymph node syndrome because it affects lymph nodes, skin, and mucous membranes in the mouth, nose, and throat. It is an acute febrile illness of infants and young children. Boys are more likely than girls to develop the disease. The highest incidence of Kawasaki disease is found in Japan and in individuals of Japanese descent, although the disease seems to occur in most, if not all, ethnic groups. It is a self-limited acute vasculitic syndrome of unknown origin, although an infectious etiology has been suspected.

Although the disease is self-limiting, there can be lifelong sequelae, including coronary artery thrombosis and aneurysms. The acute febrile stage of the disease lasts 2 weeks or longer, with a fever of 40° C or higher, and is unresponsive to antibiotic therapy. The longer the fever continues, the higher the risk of cardiovascular complications. The subacute phase lasts an additional week to 10 days. During this phase, the platelet count usually is elevated, and counts of 2 million/μL have been reported. In addition, acute phase reactants such as C-reactive protein and erythrocyte sedimentation rate are elevated, consistent with an inflammatory state. The WBC count can be moderately to markedly elevated with a left shift, and many patients develop a mild normochromic, normocytic anemia. During this phase, cardiovascular complications and aneurysms develop. The higher the platelet count, the higher the risk of

cardiovascular complications. After the subacute phase comes the convalescent phase, during which all signs of illness disappear and the acute phase reactants subside to normal.

There is no specific test for Kawasaki disease. Diagnosis is primarily by excluding other diseases that cause similar signs and symptoms (e.g., scarlet fever, juvenile rheumatoid arthritis, Stevens-Johnson syndrome, and toxic shock syndrome). The treatment for Kawasaki disease is administration of antiplatelet agents, such as aspirin and IVIG.

Exercise-Induced Thrombocytosis

Strenuous exercise is a well-known cause of relative thrombocytosis and likely is due to the release of platelets from the splenic pool or hemoconcentration by transfer of plasma water to the extravascular compartment or both. Normally the platelet count returns to its preexercise baseline level 30 minutes after completion of exercise.

Rebound Thrombocytosis

Thrombocytosis often follows the thrombocytopenia caused by marrow-suppressive therapy or other conditions. "Rebound" thrombocytosis usually peaks 10 to 17 days after withdrawal of the offending drug (e.g., alcohol or methotrexate) or after institution of therapy for the underlying condition with which thrombocytopenia is associated (e.g., vitamin B_{12} deficiency).[46]

Thrombocytosis Associated With Myeloproliferative Disorders

Primary or autonomous thrombocytosis is a typical finding in four chronic myeloproliferative disorders: polycythemia vera, chronic myelogenous leukemia, myelofibrosis with myeloid metaplasia (primary myelofibrosis), and essential thrombocythemia. Depending on the duration and stage of the myeloproliferative disorder at the time of diagnosis, it may be difficult to differentiate among these diseases. Chapter 32 provides a more complete description of these disorders. In other types of myeloproliferative disorders, the platelet count seldom reaches the extreme values characteristic of essential thrombocythemia. Diagnosis of essential thrombocythemia should not be based on the platelet count alone but should also take into account physical examination findings, history, and other laboratory data.[34,113]

Essential Thrombocythemia

Essential or primary thrombocythemia (ET), a chronic myeloproliferative neoplasm, is the most common cause of thrombocytosis and is usually diagnosed by excluding all the causes of reactive thrombocytosis. It is characterized by peripheral blood platelet counts exceeding 1 million/μL (Figure 38.8) and uncontrolled proliferation of marrow megakaryocytes. Although the platelet count may be markedly elevated in other myeloproliferative disorders (such as myelodysplastic syndromes), persistent marked elevation of the platelet count is an absolute requirement for the diagnosis of ET.

In contrast to other myeloproliferative disorders, the other marrow cell lines are not involved at the time of diagnosis of ET. There is evidence that ET is caused by a clonal proliferation of

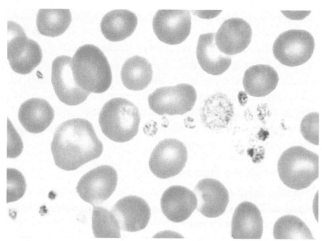

Figure 38.8 Cell Morphology in Essential Thrombocythemia *(ET).* Note the increased number of platelets and wide variation in platelet size, characteristic of ET. Red blood cell and white blood cell morphology is characteristically normal. (Peripheral blood, Wright-Giemsa stain, ×1000.) (From Carr, J. H., & Rodak, B. F. [2013]. *Clinical Hematology Atlas* [4th ed.]. Philadelphia: Saunders.)

a single abnormal pluripotent stem cell that eventually crowds out normal stem cells. As with most myeloproliferative disorders, ET is neither congenital nor hereditary, but is acquired, is prevalent in middle-aged and older patients, and affects equal numbers of men and women.

Clinical manifestations of ET. Patients with ET present with hemorrhage, platelet dysfunction, and thrombosis. The degree of thrombocytosis has not been found to reliably predict hemorrhagic or thrombotic events. There is no specific clinical sign, symptom, or laboratory test that establishes the diagnosis of ET. ET is a diagnosis of exclusion, made by ruling out the other myeloproliferative disorders and systemic illnesses that produce reactive thrombocytosis.

Thrombosis in the microvasculature is relatively common in ET, with the incidence at the time of diagnosis of 10% to 20%. This thrombosis can lead to digital pain, digital gangrene, or erythromelalgia (throbbing, aching, and burning sensation in the extremities, particularly in the palms and soles).[113] The symptoms of erythromelalgia can be explained by arteriolar inflammation and occlusive thrombosis mediated by platelets and can be relieved for several days by a single dose of aspirin.[114]

Thrombosis of large veins and arteries also may occur in ET. The arteries most commonly involved are those in the legs, the coronary arteries, and the renal arteries, but involvement of the mesenteric, subclavian, and carotid arteries is not uncommon; neurologic complications are relatively common. Venous thrombosis may involve the large veins of the legs and pelvis, hepatic veins, or splenic veins.[115] The primary cause of death of patients with ET is associated with a combination of advanced age and high incidence of cardiovascular thrombosis.[116]

Hemorrhagic episodes occur less often than thrombotic episodes in patients with ET. The hemorrhagic manifestations of ET are mucocutaneous in nature, with gastrointestinal tract bleeding occurring most often. Other sites of bleeding include the mucous membranes of the nose and mouth, the urinary tract, and the skin. Bleeding symptoms may be aggravated by aspirin use. Occasionally a patient has a paradoxical combination of thromboembolic (clotting) and hemorrhagic episodes in association with ET. A patient with ET who has had a thrombotic event may have a hemorrhagic event later.[117]

Clinical laboratory findings. Platelet size is heterogeneous, and platelets may be notably clumped on blood films. Platelets may be agranular or hypogranular and have a clear, light blue appearance on a routine Wright-stained film of the peripheral blood. The presence of giant and bizarrely shaped platelets is characteristic of myeloproliferative diseases. Megakaryocyte fragments or nuclei are commonly encountered in the peripheral blood. The number and volume of megakaryocytes are increased in the bone marrow, and they are predominantly large, show some cellular atypia, and tend to form clusters.

The platelets of some patients who have experienced thrombotic episodes are associated with increased binding affinity for fibrinogen. These patients also have elevated levels of thromboxane B_2 and β-thromboglobulin in the blood. These findings suggest enhanced in vivo platelet activation and a possible explanation for the thrombotic tendencies of patients with ET.

The bleeding manifestations may be related to a variety of qualitative abnormalities in the platelets, including deficiencies in epinephrine receptors and ultrastructural defects in granules, mitochondria, and microfilaments. Often the platelets are functionally defective when tested in vitro. Platelet aggregation is usually absent in response to epinephrine and may be decreased with adenosine diphosphate but is usually normal with collagen. Lack of an epinephrine response may help to differentiate ET from reactive thrombocytosis, because this response is usually normal in reactive thrombocytosis but absent in most cases of ET. Platelet adhesion also may be decreased.[113]

Treatment of ET. When treatment appears necessary secondary to thrombotic tendencies or splenomegaly, a variety of myelosuppressive agents (e.g., melphalan, busulfan) have been used in the past.[112] In patients with life-threatening hemorrhage or thrombosis and an extremely high platelet count, therapeutic plateletpheresis may be used to rapidly reduce, albeit only temporarily, the elevated platelet counts. In these situations, other agents are added for longer-term control of the platelet count.[118] Pegylated interferon-α has been used to treat ET and is associated with an approximately 60% rate of complete remission, but 28% of patients given the drug cannot tolerate the dosages required.[119-121] Another agent that is useful for the treatment of ET is anagrelide. This drug acts by inhibiting megakaryocyte maturation and platelet release.[122] In one large study, anagrelide decreased the platelet count in 93% of patients.[123] Many patients cannot tolerate anagrelide, however, and in these patients other, more traditional agents such as low-dose aspirin and hydroxyurea seem to be more effective.

Approximately one quarter of patients with ET have a mutation in the Janus-associated kinases (JAK1 and JAK2). The most recent medication, added to the treatment armamentarium for ET is in patients with JAK-positive mutations, is ruxolitinib (Jakafi). This drug is a kinase inhibitor and mediates the signaling of a number of cytokines and growth factors important for hematopoiesis.

The role of lowering platelet counts as a prophylactic treatment in this disease has not been established because the risks from exposure to mutagenic alkylating agents used to decrease the platelet count may be greater than the risk of thrombosis or hemorrhage. Whether a patient with ET and an elevated platelet count who is asymptomatic should or should not be treated remains controversial.

In patients with ET there is a low incidence of transformation to acute leukemia or fatal thrombotic or hemorrhagic complications. Therapy to prevent thrombotic complications seems to be effective in preventing morbidity but does not seem to improve overall survival, at least in high-risk patients.

SUMMARY

- Thrombocytopenia is the most common cause of clinically significant bleeding.
- Thrombocytopenia results from decreased platelet production, increased destruction, or abnormal distribution of platelets and manifests with small-vessel bleeding in the skin.
- Decreased production of platelets can be attributed to megakaryocyte hypoplasia, ineffective thrombopoiesis, or replacement of marrow by abnormal cells.
- An increasing number of congenital disorders, such as May-Hegglin anomaly, associated with thrombocytopenia are being identified.
- Neonatal thrombocytopenia can be caused by disorders of platelet production or increased destruction with origins in either the mother or the neonate.
- Patients experiencing increased platelet destruction become thrombocytopenic only when the rate of platelet production can no longer increase enough to compensate.
- Pathologic destruction of platelets can be caused by both immunologic and nonimmunologic mechanisms.
- Acute immune thrombocytopenic purpura (ITP) commonly occurs in children after a viral illness, and there is usually spontaneous remission. Chronic ITP is more commonly seen in women and requires treatment if the platelet count decreases to fewer than 30,000/μL.

- Treatment of drug-induced thrombocytopenia must begin with identification of the causative drug and discontinuation of its use.
- Thrombotic thrombocytopenic purpura (TTP) may present with the classic pentad of symptoms that includes microangiopathic hemolytic anemia, thrombocytopenia, and neurologic abnormalities and may be accompanied by fever and renal dysfunction. Measurements of ADAMTS13 activity or presence of an inhibitor to ADAMTS13 aid in the diagnosis of TTP.
- The hallmark signs of hemolytic uremic syndrome (HUS) of renal dysfunction, mild thrombocytopenia, mild anemia, and presentation in children, can aid in differentiating HUS from TTP.
- MAHA and thrombocytopenia are the primary laboratory abnormalities that warrant concern.
- Abnormal distribution of platelets can be caused by splenic sequestration.
- Reactive thrombocytosis is secondary to inflammation, trauma, or a variety of underlying conditions. Platelet counts are increased for a limited time. Thrombocytosis seen in myeloproliferative disorders is marked and persistent.

Now that you have completed this chapter, go back and read again the case study at the beginning and respond to the questions presented.

REVIEW QUESTIONS

Answers can be found in the Appendix.

1. The autosomal dominant disorder associated with decreased platelet production is:
   a. Fanconi anemia
   b. TAR syndrome
   c. May-Hegglin anomaly
   d. Wiskott-Aldrich anomaly
2. Which of the following is *not* a hallmark of ITP?
   a. Petechiae
   b. Thrombocytopenia
   c. Large overactive platelets
   d. Megakaryocyte hypoplasia
3. The specific antigen most commonly responsible for the development of NAIT is:
   a. Bak
   b. HPA-1a
   c. GPIb
   d. Lewis antigen a

4. A 2-year-old child with an unexpected platelet count of 15,000/μL and a recent history of a viral infection most likely has:
   a. HIT
   b. NAIT
   c. Acute ITP
   d. Chronic ITP
5. Which drug causes a reduction in platelet count by inhibiting megakaryocyte maturation?
   a. Gold salts
   b. Abciximab
   c. Anagrelide
   d. Quinidine
6. A defect in primary hemostasis (platelet response to an injury) often results in:
   a. Musculoskeletal bleeding
   b. Mucosal bleeding
   c. Hemarthroses
   d. None of the above

7. When a drug acts as a hapten to induce thrombocytopenia, an antibody forms against which of the following?
   a. Typically unexposed, new platelet antigens
   b. The combination of the drug and the platelet membrane protein to which it is bound
   c. The drug alone in the plasma, but the immune complex then binds to the platelet membrane
   d. The drug alone, but only when it is bound to the platelet membrane

8. *TAR* refers to:
   a. Abnormal platelet morphology in which the radial striations of the platelets are missing
   b. Abnormal appearance of the iris of the eye in which radial striations are absent
   c. Abnormal bone formation, including hypoplasia of the forearms
   d. Neurologic defects affecting the root (radix) of the spinal nerves

9. Neonatal autoimmune thrombocytopenia occurs when:
   a. The mother lacks a platelet antigen that the infant possesses, and she builds antibodies to that antigen, which cross the placenta
   b. The infant develops an autoimmune process such as ITP secondary to in utero infection
   c. The infant develops an autoimmune disease such as lupus erythematosus before birth
   d. The mother has an autoimmune antibody to her own platelets, which crosses the placenta and reacts with the infant's platelets

10. HUS in children is associated with:
    a. Diarrhea caused by *Shigella* species
    b. Meningitis caused by *Haemophilus* species
    c. Pneumonia caused by *Mycoplasma* species
    d. Pneumonia caused by respiratory viruses

11. Treatment with an anticomplement agent such as eculizumab is first-line therapy for:
    a. Hereditary TTP
    b. Hemolytic uremic syndrome (HUS)
    c. ITP
    d. Atypical HUS

12. Which of the following statements regarding thrombocytosis is *not* true?
    a. Thrombocytosis can be associated with hemorrhage and thrombosis
    b. Affected patients have platelet counts in excess of $450,000/\mu L$
    c. Thrombocytosis is self-correcting
    d. Thrombocytosis can be congenital or acquired

REFERENCES

1. Kelley, M. J., Jawien, W., Ortel, T. L., et al. (2000). Mutations of *MYH9*, encoding for non-muscle myosin heavy chain A, in May Hegglin anomaly. *Nat Genet, 26,* 106–108.
2. The May Hegglin/Fechtner Syndrome Consortium. (2000). Mutations in *MHY9* result in May-Hegglin anomaly, and Fechtner and Sebastian syndromes. *Nat Genet, 26,* 103–105.
3. Mhawech, P., & Saleem, A. (2000). Inherited giant platelet disorders: classification and literature review. *Am J Clin Pathol, 113,* 176–190.
4. Hall, J. G. (1987). Thrombocytopenia and absent radius (TAR) syndrome. *J Med Genet, 24,* 79–83.
5. Freedman, M. H., & Doyle, J. J. (1999). Inherited bone marrow failure syndromes. In Lilleyman, J. S., Hann, I. M., & Branchette, V. S. (Eds.), *Pediatric Hematology.* (pp. 23–49). London: Churchill Livingstone.
6. Lackner, A., Basu, M., Bierings, M., et al. (2000). Haematopoietic stem cell transplantation for amegakaryocytic thrombocytopenia. *Br J Haematol, 109,* 773–775.
7. van den Oudenrijn, S. M., Bruin, M., Folman, C. C., et al. (2000). Mutations in the thrombopoietin receptor, Mlp, in children with congenital amegakaryocytic thrombocytopenia. *Br J Haematol, 110,* 441–448.
8. Balduini, C. L., Savoia, A., & Seri, M. (2013). Inherited thrombocytopenias frequently diagnosed in adults. *J Thromb Haemost, 11,* 1006–1019.

9. Stormorken, H., Hellum, B., Egeland, T., et al. (1991). X-linked thrombocytopenia and thrombocytopathia: attenuated Wiscott-Aldrich syndrome: functional and morphological studies of platelets and lymphocytes. *Thromb Haemost, 65,* 300–305.
10. Fried, J. R., Gibbons, R. V., Kalayanarooj, S., et al. (2010) Serotype-specific differences in the risk of dengue hemorrhagic fever: an analysis of data collected in Bangkok, Thailand from 1994 to 2006. *PLOS Neglect Trop Dis, 4*(3), e617.
11. Villa, A. L., Notarangelo, P., Maachi, E., et al. (1999). X-linked thrombocytopenia and Wiskott-Aldrich syndrome are allelic diseases with mutations in the *WASP* gene. *Nat Genet, 9,* 414–417.
12. Mehaffey, M. G., Newton, A. L., Gandhi, M. J., et al. (2001). X-linked thrombocytopenia caused by a novel mutation of *GATA-1*. *Blood, 98,* 2681–2688.
13. Freson, K. K., Devriendt, G., Matthijs, G., et al. (2001). Platelet characteristics in patients with X-linked macrothrombocytopenia because of a novel *GATA-1* mutation. *Blood, 98,* 85–92.
14. Casteels, A. A., Naessens, F., Cordts, L., et al. (1999). Neonatal screening for congenital cytomegalovirus infections. *J Perinat Med, 27,* 116–121.
15. Brown, H. L., & Abernathy, M. P. (1998). Cytomegalovirus infection. *Semin Perinatol, 22,* 260–266.
16. Crapnell, K. E. D., Zanfani, A., Chaudhuri, J. L., et al. (2000). In vitro infection of megakaryocytes and their precursors by human cytomegalovirus. *Blood, 95,* 487–493.

17. McAuley, J., Boyer, D., Patel, D., et al. (1994). Early and longitudinal evaluations of treated infants and children and untreated historical patients with congenital toxoplasmosis: the Chicago Collaborative Treatment Trial. *Clin Infect Dis, 18,* 38–72.

18. Sullivan, E. M., Burgess, M. A., & Forrest, J. M. (1999). The epidemiology of rubella and congenital rubella in Australia, 1992-1997. *Commun Dis Intell, 23,* 209–214.

19. Yazigi, A., De Pecoulas, A. E., Vauloup-Fellous, C., et al. (2017) Fetal and neonatal abnormalities due to congenital rubella syndrome: a review of literature. *J Matern Fetal Neonatal Med, 30*(3), 274–278.

20. Tovo, P. A., de-Martino, M., Gabiano, C., et al. (1992). Prognostic factors and survival in children with perinatal HIV-1 infection. The Italian Register for HIV Infections in Children. *Lancet, 339,* 1249–1253.

21. Triplett, D. A. (Ed.). (1978). *Platelet Function: Laboratory Evaluation and Clinical Application.* Chicago: American Society of Clinical Pathologists.

22. Brown, B. A. (1993). *Hematology: Principles and Procedures.* (6th ed.). Philadelphia: Lea & Febiger.

23. Aster, R. (2002). Drug-induced thrombocytopenia. In Michelson, A. D. (Ed.). *Platelets.* (pp. 593–606). San Diego: Academic Press.

24. Vadhan-Raj, S. (2000). Clinical experience with recombinant human thrombopoietin in chemotherapy-induced thrombocytopenia. *Semin Hematol, 37,* 28–34.

25. Basser, R. L., Underhill, C., Davis, M. D., et al. (2000). Enhancement of platelet recovery after myelosuppressive chemotherapy by recombinant human megakaryocyte growth and development factor in patients with advanced cancer. *J Clin Oncol, 18,* 2852–2861.

26. Koch, M. A., Volberding, P. A., Lagakos, S. W., et al. (1992). Toxic effects of zidovudine in asymptomatic human immunodeficiency virus–infected individuals with CD4+cell counts of 0.5 × 10⁹/L or less: detailed and updated results from Protocol 019 of the AIDS Clinical Trials Group. *Arch Intern Med, 152,* 2286–2292.

27. Silverstein, M. N., & Tefferi, A. (1999). Treatment of essential thrombocythemia with anagrelide. *Semin Hematol, 36,* 23–25.

28. Martin, T. G., & Shuman, M. A. (1998). Interferon-induced thrombocytopenia: is it time for thrombopoietin? *Hepatology, 28,* 1430–1432.

29. Sata, M., Yano, Y., Yoshiyama, Y., et al. (1997). Mechanisms of thrombocytopenia induced by interferon therapy for chronic hepatitis B. *J Gastroenterol, 32,* 206–221.

30. Colvin, B. T. (1985). Thrombocytopenia. *Clin Haematol, 14,* 661–681.

31. Trannel, T. J., Ahmed, I., & Goebert, D. (2001). Occurrence of thrombocytopenia in psychiatric patients taking valproate. *Am J Psychiatry, 158,* 128–130.

32. Thompson, A. R., & Harker, L. A. (1983). *Manual of Hemostasis and Thrombosis.* (3rd ed.). Philadelphia: FA Davis.

33. Taghizadeh, M. (1997). Megaloblastic anemias. In Harmening, D. M. (Ed.), *Clinical Hematology and Fundamentals of Hemostasis.* (3rd ed., pp. 116–134). Philadelphia: FA Davis.

34. Corriveau, D. M., & Fritsma, G. A. (Eds.). (1988). *Hemostasis and Thrombosis in the Clinical Laboratory.* Philadelphia: JB Lippincott.

35. Quick, A. J. (1966). *Hemorrhagic Diseases and Thrombosis.* (2nd ed.). Philadelphia: Lea & Febiger.

36. Davis, G. L. (1998). Quantitative and qualitative disorders of platelets. In Steine-Martin, E. A., Lotspeich-Steininger, C., & Koepke, J. A. (Eds.), *Clinical Hematology: Principle, Procedures, Correlations.* (2nd ed., pp. 717–734). Philadelphia: Lippincott Williams & Wilkins.

37. Zeller, B., Rajantie, J., Hedlund-Treutiger, I., et al. (2005). Childhood idiopathic thrombocytopenic purpura in Nordic countries: epidemiology and predictors of chronic disease. *Acta Paediatr, 94*(2), 1708–1784.

38. Neunert, C. E., Buchanan, G. R., Imback, P., et al. (2008). Severe hemorrhage in children with newly diagnosed immune thrombocytopenic purpura. *Blood, 112*(10), 4003–4008.

39. Abrahamson, P. E., Hall, S. A., Feudjo-Tepie, M., et al. (2009). The incidence of idiopathic thrombocytopenic purpura among adults: a population-based study and literature review. *Eur J Haematol, 83,* 83–89.

40. Schulze, H., & Gaedicke, G. (2011). Immune thrombocytopenia in children and adults: what's the same, what's different? (Editorial and Perspective). *Haematologica, 96*(12), 1739–1741.

41. Stasi, R., & Provan, D. (2004). Management of immune thrombocytopenic purpura in adults. *Mayo Clin Proc, 79,* 504–522.

42. Kunicki, T. J., & Newman, P. J. (1992). The molecular immunology of human platelet proteins. *Blood, 80,* 1386–1404.

43. Beer, J. H., Rabaglio, M., Berchtold, P., et al. (1993). Autoantibodies against the platelet glycoproteins (GP) IIb/IIIa, Ia/IIa, and IV and partial deficiency in GPIV in a patient with a bleeding disorder and a defective platelet collagen interaction. *Blood, 82,* 820–829.

44. Khodadi, E., Asnafi, A. A., Shahrabi, S., et al. (2016). Bone marrow niche in immune thrombocytopenia: a focus on megakaryopoiesis. *Ann Hematol, 95*(11), 1765–1776.

45. Olsson, B., Andersson, P., Jernas, M., et al. (2003). T-cell–mediated cytotoxicity toward platelets in chronic idiopathic thrombocytopenic purpura. *Nat Med, 9,* 1123–1124.

46. George, J. N., & Kojouri, K. (2006). Immune thrombocytopenic purpura. In Colman, R. W., Marder, V. J., Clowes, A. W., et al. (Eds.), *Hemostasis and Thrombosis.* (5th ed., pp. 1085–1094). Philadelphia: Lippincott Williams & Wilkins.

47. Chong, B. H., & Ho, S-J. (2005). Autoimmune thrombocytopenia. *J Thromb Haemost, 3,* 1763–1772.

48. Jacobs, P., Wood, L., & Novitzky, N. (1994). Intravenous gammaglobulin has no advantages over oral corticosteroids as primary therapy for adults with immune thrombocytopenia: a prospective randomized clinical trial. *Am J Med, 1,* 55–59.

49. Kojouri, K., Vesely, S. K., Terrell, D. R., et al. (2004). Splenectomy for adult patients with idiopathic thrombocytopenic purpura. *Blood, 104,* 2623–2634.

50. Bussel, J. B., Cheng, G., Saleh, M. N., et al. (2007). Eltrombopag for the treatment of chronic idiopathic thrombocytopenic purpura. *N Engl J Med, 357*(22), 2237–2247.

51. Smith, M. E., Reid, D. M., Jones, C. E., et al. (1987). Binding of quinine- and quinidine-dependent drug antibodies to platelets is mediated by the Fab domain of the immunoglobulin G and is not Fc dependent. *J Clin Invest, 79,* 912–917.

52. Pfueller, S. L., Bilsont, R. A., Logan, D., et al. (1988). Heterogeneity of drug-dependent platelet antigens and their antibodies in quinine- and quinidine-induced thrombocytopenia: involvement of glycoproteins Ib, IIb, IIIa, and IX. *Blood, 11,* 190–198.

53. Chong, B. H., Fawaz, I., Chesterman, C. N., et al. (1989). Heparin-induced thrombocytopenia: mechanism of interaction of the heparin-dependent antibody with platelets. *Br J Haematol, 73,* 235–240.

54. Amiral, J., Bridley, F., Dreyfus, M., et al. (1992). Platelet factor 4 complexed to heparin is the target for antibodies generated in heparin-induced thrombocytopenia. *Thromb Haemost, 68,* 95 (letter).

55. Gruel, Y., Boizard, B., Daffos, F., et al. (1986). Determination of platelet antigens and glycoproteins in the human fetus. *Blood, 68,* 488–492.

56. Risson, D. C., Davies M. W., & Williams B. A. (2012). Review of neonatal alloimmune thrombocytopenia. *J Paediatr Child Health, 48*(9), 816–822.

57. Peterson, J. A., McFarland, J. G., Curtis, B. R., et al. (2013). Neonatal alloimmune thrombocytopenia: pathogenesis, diagnosis and management. *Br J Haematol, 116*(1), 3–14.

58. Kaplan, C., Daffos, F., Forestier, F., et al. (1988). Management of alloimmune thrombocytopenia: antenatal diagnosis and in utero transfusion of maternal platelets. *Blood, 72*, 340–343.

59. Bussel, J. B., & Pramiani, A. (2008). Fetal and neonatal alloimmune thrombocytopenia: progress and ongoing debates. *Blood Rev, 22*, 33–52.

60. Rayburn, W. F. (1992). Glucocorticoid therapy for rheumatic diseases: maternal, fetal, and breast-feeding considerations. *Am J Reprod Immunol, 28*, 138–140.

61. Clerc, J. M. (1989). Neonatal thrombocytopenia. *Clin Lab Sci, 2*, 42–47.

62. Mueller-Eckhardt, C. (1986). Post-transfusion purpura. *Br J Haematol, 64*, 419–424.

63. Vogelsang, G., Kickler, T. S., & Bell, W. R. (1986). Post-transfusion purpura: a report of five patients and a review of the pathogenesis and management. *Am J Hematol, 21*, 259–267.

64. McLaughlin, P., Talpaz, M., Quesada, J. R., et al. (1985). Immune thrombocytopenia following α-interferon therapy in patients with cancer. *JAMA, 254*, 1353–1354.

65. Yoshida, Y., Hirashima, K., Asano, S., et al. (1991). A phase II trial of recombinant human granulocyte colony-stimulating factor in the myelodysplastic syndromes. *Br J Haematol, 78*, 378–384.

66. Paciucci, P. A., Mandeli, J., Oleksowicz, L., et al. (1990). Thrombocytopenia during immunotherapy with interleukin-2 by constant infusion. *Am J Med, 89*, 308–312.

67. Fink, K., & Al-Mondhiry, H. (1976). Idiopathic thrombocytopenic purpura in lymphoma. *Cancer, 37*, 1999–2004.

68. Carey, R. W., McGinnis, A., Jacobson, B. M., et al. Idiopathic thrombocytopenic purpura complicating chronic lymphocytic leukemia: management with sequential splenectomy and chemotherapy. *Arch Intern Med, 136*, 62–66.

69. Miller, M. H., Urowitz, M. B., & Gladman, D. D. (1983). The significance of thrombocytopenia in systemic lupus erythematosus. *Arthritis Rheum, 26*, 1181–1186.

70. Kelton, J. G., Keystone, J., Moore, J., et al. (1983). Immune-mediated thrombocytopenia of malaria. *J Clin Invest, 71*, 832–836.

71. Cines, D. B., & Levine, L. D. (2017). Thrombocytopenia in pregnancy. *Blood, 130*(21), 2271–2277.

72. Barron, W. M. (1992). The syndrome of preeclampsia. *Gastroenterol Clin North Am, 21*, 851–872.

73. Schindler, M., Gatt, S., Isert, P., et al. (1990). Thrombocytopenia and platelet function defects in pre-eclampsia: implications for regional anesthesia. *Anaesth Intensive Care, 18*, 169–174.

74. Gibson, W., Hunter, D., Neame, P. B., et al. (1982). Thrombocytopenia in preeclampsia and eclampsia. *Semin Thromb Hemost, 8*, 234–247.

75. Martin, J. N. Jr., Blake, P. G., Perry, K. G. Jr., et al. (1991). The natural history of HELLP syndrome: patterns of disease progression and regression. *Am J Obstet Gynecol, 164*, 1500–1509.

76. Green, D. (1988). Diagnosis and management of bleeding disorders. *Compr Ther, 14*, 31–36.

77. Trofatter, K. F. Jr., Howell, M. L., Greenberg, C. S., et al. (1989). Use of the fibrin D-dimer in screening for coagulation abnormalities in preeclampsia. *Obstet Gynecol, 73*, 435–440.

78. Burrows, R. F., Hunter, D. J. S., Andrew, M., et al. (1987). A prospective study investigating the mechanism of thrombocytopenia in preeclampsia. *Obstet Gynecol, 70*, 334–338.

79. Benigni, A., Gregorini, G., Frusca, T., et al. (1989). Effect of low-dose aspirin on fetal and maternal generation of thromboxane by platelets in women at risk for pregnancy-induced hypertension. *N Engl J Med, 321*, 357–362.

80. Schiff, E., Peleg, E., Goldenberg, M., et al. (1989). The use of aspirin to prevent pregnancy-induced hypertension and lower the ratio of thromboxane A_2 to prostacyclin in relatively high risk pregnancies. *N Engl J Med, 321*, 351–356.

81. Ezra, Y., Rose, M., & Eldor, A. (1996). Therapy and prevention of thrombotic thrombocytopenic purpura during pregnancy: a clinical study of 16 pregnancies. *Am J Hematol, 51*, 1–6.

82. Dashe, J. S., Ramin, S. M., & Cunningham, F. G. (1998). The long-term consequences of thrombotic microangiopathy (thrombotic thrombocytopenic purpura and hemolytic uremic syndrome) in pregnancy. *Obstet Gynecol, 91*, 662–668.

83. Moschcowitz, E. (1925). An acute febrile pleiochromic anemia with hyaline thrombosis of the terminal arterioles and capillaries: a hitherto undescribed disease. *Arch Intern Med, 36*, 89–93.

84. Mariotte, E., Azoulay, E., Glaicier, L., et al. (2016). Epidemiology and pathophysiology of adulthood-onset thrombotic microangiopathy with severe ADAMTS13 deficiency (thrombotic thrombocytopenia purpura): a cross-sectional analysis of the French national registry for thrombotic microangiopathy. *Lancet Haematol, 3*(5), e237–e245.

85. Joly, B. S., Coppa, P., & Veyradier, A. (2017). Thrombotic thrombocytopenic purpura. *Blood, 129*(21), 2836–2846.

86. Moake, J. L. (2002). Thrombotic thrombocytopenic purpura and hemolytic uremic syndrome. In Michelson, A. D. (Ed.), *Platelets.* (pp. 607–620). San Diego: Academic Press.

87. Bell, W. R., Braine, H. G., Ness, P. M., et al. (1991). Improved survival in thrombotic thrombocytopenic purpura–hemolytic uremic syndrome: clinical experience in 108 patients. *N Engl J Med, 325*, 398–403.

88. Rock, G. A., Shumak, K. H., Buskard, N. A., et al. (1991). Comparison of plasma exchange with plasma infusion in the treatment of thrombotic thrombocytopenic purpura. *N Engl J Med, 325*, 393–397.

89. Moake, J. L., Turner, N. A., Stathopoulos, N. A., et al. (1986). Involvement of large plasma von Willebrand factor (VWF) multimers and unusually large VWF forms derived from endothelial cells in shear-stress induced platelet aggregation. *J Clin Invest, 78*, 1456–1461.

90. Furlan, M., Robles, R., Solenthaler, M., et al. (1997). Deficient activity of von Willebrand factor-cleaving protease in chronic relapsing thrombotic thrombocytopenic purpura. *Blood, 89*, 3097–3103.

91. Tsai, H. M., & Lian, E. C. Y. (1998). Antibodies to von Willebrand factor-cleaving protease in acute thrombotic thrombocytopenic purpura. *N Engl J Med, 339*, 1585–1594.

92. Furlan, M., & Lammle, B. (1999). von Willebrand factor in thrombotic thrombocytopenic purpura. *Thromb Haemost, 82*, 592–600.

93. Saha, M., McDaniel, J. K., & Zheng, X. L. (2017). Thrombotic thrombocytopenic purpura: pathogenesis, diagnosis and potential novel therapeutics. *J Thromb Haemost, 15*(10), 1889–1900.

94. Furlan, M., Robles, R., & Lammle, B. (1996). Partial purification and characterization of a protease from human plasma cleaving von Willebrand factor to fragments produced by in vivo proteolysis. *Blood, 87*, 4223–4234.

95. Tsai, H. M. (1996). Physiologic cleaving of von Willebrand factor by a plasma protease is dependent on its conformation and requires calcium ion. *Blood, 87*, 4235–4244.

96. Gerritsen, H. E., Turecek, P. L., Schwarz, H. P., et al. (1999). Assay of von Willebrand factor (VWF)–cleaving protease based on decreased collagen binding affinity of degraded VWF: a tool for the diagnosis of thrombotic thrombocytopenic purpura (TTP). *Thromb Haemost, 82*, 1386–1389.

97. Alwan, F., Vendramin, C., Vanhoorelbeke, K., et al. (2017). Presenting ADAMTS-13 antibody and antigen levels predict prognosis in immune-mediated thrombotic thrombocytopenic purpura. *Blood, 130*(4), 466–471.

98. Coppo, P., Schwarzinger, M., Buffet, M., et al. (2010). Predictive features of severe acquired ADAMTS13 deficiency in idiopathic thrombotic microangiopathies: the French TMA reference center experience. *PLoS One, 5,* e10208.

99. Bendapudi, P. K., Hurwitz, S., Fry, A., et al. (2017). Derivation and external validation of the PLASMIC score for rapid assessment of adults with thrombotic microangiopathies: a cohort study. *Lancet Haematol, 4*(4), e157–e164.

100. Li, A., Khalighi, P. R., Wu, Q., et al. (2018). External validation of the PLASMIC score: a clinical prediction tool for thrombotic thrombocytopenic purpura diagnosis and treatment. *J Thromb Haemost 16*(1), 164–169.

101. Byrnes, J. J., Moake, J. L., Klug, P., et al. (1990). Effectiveness of the cryosupernatant fraction of plasma in the treatment of refractory thrombotic thrombocytopenic purpura. *Am J Hematol, 34,* 169–174.

102. Tersteeg, C., Schiviz, A., De Meyer, S. F., et al. (2015). Potential for recombinant ADAMTS13 as an effective therapy for acquired thrombotic thrombocytopenic purpura. *Arterioscler Thromb Vasc Biol, 35,* 2336–2342.

103. Scully, M., Knobl, P., Kentourche, K., et al. (2017). Recombinant ADAMTS13: first-in-human pharmacokinetics and safety in congenital thrombotic thrombocytopenic purpura. *Blood, 130*(9), 2055–2063.

104. Kwaan, H. C., & Soff, G. A. (1997). Management of thrombotic thrombocytopenic purpura and hemolytic uremic syndrome. *Semin Hematol, 34,* 159–166.

105. Jokiranta, T. S. (2017), HUS and atypical HUS. *Blood, 129*(21), 2847–2856.

106. Karmali, M. A. (1992). The association of verotoxins and the classical hemolytic uremic syndrome. In Kaplan, B. S., Trompeter, R. S., & Moake, J. L. (Eds.), *Hemolytic-Uremic Syndrome and Thrombotic Thrombocytopenic Purpura.* (pp. 199–212). New York: Marcel Dekker.

107. Obrig, T. G. (1992). Pathogenesis of Shiga toxin (verotoxin)–induced endothelial cell injury. In Kaplan, B. S., Trompeter, R. S., & Moake, J. L. (Eds.), *Hemolytic-Uremic Syndrome and Thrombotic Thrombocytopenic Purpura.* (pp. 405–419). New York: Marcel Dekker.

108. Charba, D., Moake, J. L., Harris, M. A., et al. (1993). Abnormalities of von Willebrand factor multimers in drug-associated thrombotic microangiopathies. *Am J Hematol, 42,* 268–277.

109. Chalmers, E., Cooper, P., Forman, K., et al. (2011). Purpura fulminans: recognition, diagnosis and management. *Arch Dis Child, 96,* 1066–1071.

110. Francis, R. B. (1990). Acquired purpura fulminans. *Semin Thromb Hemost, 16*(4), 310–325.

111. Lerolle, N., Carlotti, A., Melican, K., et al. (2013). Assessment of the interplay between blood and skin vascular abnormalities in adult purpura fulminans. *Am J Respir Crit Care Med, 188*(6), 684–692.

112. Santhosh-Kumar, C. R., Yohannon, M. D., Higgy, K. E., et al. (1991). Thrombocytosis in adults: analysis of 777 patients. *J Intern Med, 229,* 493–495.

113. Mitus, A. J., & Schafer, A. I. (1990). Thrombocytosis and thrombocythemia. *Hematol Oncol Clin North Am, 4,* 157–178.

114. Michiels, J. J., & Ten Cate, F. J. (1992). Erythromelalgia in thrombocythemia of various myeloproliferative disorders. *Am J Hematol, 39,* 131–136.

115. Hoffman, R., Kremyanskaya, M., Nojfeld, V., et al. (2018). Essential thrombocythemia. In Hoffman, R., Benz, E. J., Silberstein, L. E., et al. (Eds.), *Hematology: Basic Principles and Practice.* (7th ed., pp 1034–1052). Philadelphia: Elsevier.

116. Lekovic, D., Gotic, M., Sefer, D., et al. (2015). Predictors of survival and cause of death in patients with essential thrombocythemia. *Eur J Haematol, 95(5),* 461–466.

117. Martin, K. (2017). Risk factors for and management of MPN-associated bleeding and thrombosis. *Curr Hematol Malig Rep, 12*(5), 389–396.

118. Panlilio, A. L., & Reiss, R. F. (1979). Therapeutic plateletpheresis in thrombocythemia. *Transfusion, 19,* 147–152.

119. Middelhoff, G., & Boll, I. (1992). A long term trial of interferon alpha-therapy in essential thrombocythemia. *Ann Hematol, 64,* 207–209.

120. Lazzarino, M., Vitale, A., Morra, E., et al. (1989). Interferon alpha-2b as treatment for Philadelphia-negative myeloproliferative disorders with excessive thrombocytosis. *Br J Haematol, 72,* 173–177.

121. Giles, F. J., Singer, C. R. J., Gray, A. G., et al. (1988). Alpha interferon for essential thrombocythemia. *Lancet, 2,* 70–72.

122. Petitt, R. M., Silverstein, M. N., & Petrone, M. E. (1997). Anagrelide for control of thrombocythemia in polycythemia and other myeloproliferative disorders. *Semin Hematol, 34,* 51–54.

123. Tefferi, A., Silverstein, M. N., Petitt, R. M., et al. (1997). Anagrelide as a new platelet-lowering agent in essential thrombocythemia: mechanism of action, efficacy, toxicity, current indications. *Semin Thromb Hemost, 23,* 379–383.

Thrombotic Disorders and Laboratory Assessment

George A. Fritsma, Jeanine M. Walenga

OBJECTIVES

After completion of this chapter, the reader will be able to:

1. List the causes and pathology of thrombosis.
2. Describe the prevalence of thrombotic disease in developed countries.
3. Define thrombophilia.
4. Differentiate among acquired thrombosis risk factors, related to lifestyle and disease, and congenital risk factors.
5. List the thrombosis risk factors that are assessed in the clinical laboratory.
6. Distinguish between venous and arterial thrombosis.
7. List the prevalence of the heritable risk factors in various people groups.
8. Offer a clot-based lupus anticoagulant test profile with diagnostic validity.
9. Perform qualitative and quantitative anticardiolipin antibody and anti-β_2-glycoprotein I antibody assays.
10. Interpret the results of lupus anticoagulant anticardiolipin antibody and anti-β_2-glycoprotein I antibody assays.
11. Diagram the protein C and protein S coagulation control pathway.
12. Describe the thrombotic relevance of antithrombin assays, protein C and protein S assays, activated protein C resistance, factor V Leiden assay, and the prothrombin G20210A assay.
13. Describe the ability of the lipoprotein (a), fibrinogen, and homocysteine assays to assess arterial thrombotic risk.
14. Describe the causes and pathophysiology of disseminated intravascular coagulation.
15. Describe the assays comprising a primary test profile for diagnosis and management of disseminated intravascular coagulation in an acute care facility.
16. Apply advanced and specialized disseminated intravascular coagulation assays.
17. Demonstrate the validity of quantitative D-dimer assays for disseminated intravascular coagulation and venous thromboembolic disease.
18. Describe the pathophysiology of heparin-induced thrombocytopenia.
19. Describe the clinical and laboratory diagnosis of heparin-induced thrombocytopenia.
20. Distinguish primary heparin-induced thrombocytopenia enzyme immunoassay assays from confirmatory platelet activation assays.

OUTLINE

CASE STUDY

After studying the material in this chapter, the reader should be able to respond to the following case study:

A 42-year-old woman with no significant medical history developed sudden onset of shortness of breath and chest pain. She was taken to an emergency department, where a pulmonary embolism was diagnosed using multislice computed tomography. The emergency department physician initiated intravenous heparin therapy. Subsequent to admission the pulmonologist ordered a thrombosis risk assay profile.

1. For what conditions can the woman be tested while she is an inpatient?
2. List potential acquired thrombosis risk factors that could account for the pulmonary embolism.
3. How does the presence of a thrombosis risk factor affect the patient's lifestyle, laboratory management, and therapy?

THROMBOSIS RISK TESTING DEVELOPMENTS

Before 1992, medical laboratory professionals performed assays to detect only three inherited venous thrombosis risk factors: deficiencies of the coagulation control factors antithrombin, protein C, and protein S.[1] Taken together, these three deficiencies accounted for approximately 7% of cases of recurrent venous thromboembolic disease and bore no apparent relationship to arterial thrombosis. Since the report by Dahlbäck and colleagues of activated protein C (APC) resistance in 1993 and the characterization by Bertina and colleagues of the factor V Leiden (FVL) mutation as its cause in 1994, efforts devoted to thrombosis risk prediction and evaluation have redefined the hemostasis laboratory.[2,3] The list of current assays includes antithrombin, protein C, protein S, APC resistance, FVL mutation, prothrombin G20210A mutation, lupus anticoagulant (LAC), and antiphospholipid antibodies, among other entities. The quantitative D-dimer assay, developed from the semiquantitative fibrin degradation products (FDP) assay, is instrumental in ruling out a venous thromboembolic event, and is also used to detect and monitor disseminated intravascular coagulation (DIC).[4]

THROMBOSIS ETIOLOGY AND PREVALENCE

Thrombosis Etiology

Thrombosis is the inappropriate formation of a platelet or fibrin clot that obstructs a blood vessel. Thrombosis is a multifaceted disorder resulting from circulatory stasis and abnormalities in the coagulation system, coagulation control mechanisms, platelet function, the blood vessel wall, or leukocyte activation molecules. Thrombotic obstructions cause *ischemia* (loss of blood supply) and *necrosis* (tissue death).[5]

Thrombophilia (once called *hypercoagulability*) is the predisposition to thrombosis secondary to a congenital or acquired condition. Known causes of thrombophilia include the following:

- Physical, chemical, or biological events such as chronic or acute inflammation that release prothrombotic mediators from damaged blood vessels or suppress blood vessel production of normal antithrombotic substances
- Uncontrolled platelet activation
- Uncontrolled blood coagulation system activation
- Blood coagulation control protein deficiencies
- Uncontrolled suppression of fibrinolysis

Thrombosis Prevalence

From 2000 to 2010 the US death rate attributable to venous and arterial thrombotic disease declined 31% and the number of thrombosis-related deaths declined by 17% per year. Yet in 2010 thrombosis accounted for one of every three deaths in the United States. Of these, 25% of initial thrombotic events were fatal, and many fatal thromboses went undiagnosed before autopsy.[6]

Prevalence of Venous Thromboembolic Disease

The annual incidence of venous thromboembolism (VTE) in the unselected US population has remained constant since before 1993 at 1 in 1000 and is more prevalent in African Americans and in women of childbearing age.[7,8] The most prevalent VTE is deep vein thrombosis (DVT), caused by clots that form in the iliac, popliteal, and femoral veins of the calves and upper legs.[9] Large occlusive thrombi may also form, although less often, in the veins of the upper extremities, liver, spleen, intestines, brain, and kidneys. Thrombosis symptoms include localized pain, the sensation of heat, erythema (redness), and edema.

Fragments of thrombi, called emboli, may separate from the proximal end of a venous thrombus, move swiftly through the right chambers of the heart, and lodge in the arterial pulmonary vasculature, causing ischemia and necrosis of lung tissue, called pulmonary emboli (PEs).[10] Nearly 95% of PEs arise from thrombi in the deep leg and calf veins. Of the 250,000 US residents per year who suffer PE, 10% to 15% die within 3 months. Many PE cases go undiagnosed because of the ambiguity of the symptoms, which may resemble those of acute coronary syndrome (ACS), pleurisy, or pneumonia. PE has been nicknamed "the great masquerader."

VTE risk factors parallel the risk factors for ACS, peripheral artery disease, and stroke. Advancing age, obesity, recent surgery or trauma, immobilization and hospitalization, hypertension, hypercholesterolemia, smoking, diabetes mellitus, and metabolic syndrome raise the risk of thrombotic disorders. The pathophysiology begins with chronic inflammation, thrombophilia, and endothelial cell injury. Coagulation system imbalances, such as inappropriate activation, gain of coagulation factor function, inadequate control of thrombin generation, or suppressed fibrinolysis, are the resulting VTE mechanisms; components of cancer, or chronic heart, lung, or renal disease are often implicated in VTE.[11] Cancers associated with VTE include gastric, pancreatic, lung, gynecologic, and testicular cancers, as well as lymphoma and acute leukemia. Predilection for DVT versus PE has a familial distribution.

Prevalence of Arterial Thrombosis

Major cardiovascular diseases, including strokes, caused 252 premature US deaths per 100,000 residents in 2014 (more than 614,000 from coronary artery disease). Approximately 80% of acute myocardial infarctions (AMIs) and 85% of strokes are caused by thrombi that block coronary arteries or carotid end arteries of the vertebrobasilar system, respectively.[12] Transient ischemic attacks and peripheral arterial occlusions are more frequent than strokes and coronary artery disease and, although not fatal, represent substantial morbidity.

One important mechanism for arterial thrombosis is the well-described vessel wall unstable atherosclerotic plaque. Activated platelets, monocytes, and macrophages embed fatty plaque within the endothelial lining, suppressing the normal release of antithrombotic molecules such as nitric oxide and exposing prothrombotic substances such as tissue factor (Chapter 35). Small plaques rupture, occluding arteries and releasing mediators that trigger thrombotic events. The mediators activate platelets, which combine with von Willebrand factor to form arterial platelet plugs—the "white thrombi" that cause arterial ischemia and necrosis of surrounding tissue (Chapter 10).

The hemostasis-related lesions we associate with arterial thrombosis are blood vessel wall destruction and platelet activation. Often these are inseparable. Researchers continue to examine new thrombosis markers that capture pathologic events in platelets and endothelial cells before a thrombotic event occurs.[13]

THROMBOSIS RISK FACTORS

Acquired Thrombosis Risk Factors

In life we acquire a legion of habits and circumstances that either help maintain or damage our hemostasis system. Their variety and interplay make it difficult to pinpoint the factors that contribute to thrombosis or to determine which have the greatest influence. These factors seem to contribute to venous and arterial thrombosis in varying degrees. Table 39.1 lists the non-disease, lifestyle risk factors implicated in thrombosis.[14]

Thrombosis Risk Factors Associated with Systemic Diseases

In addition to life events, several conditions and diseases threaten us with thrombosis. Some are listed in Table 39.2, with an indication of the laboratory's diagnostic contribution.[15]

Together, transient and chronic antiphospholipid antibodies (APLAs) such as LAC, anticardiolipin (ACL) autoantibodies, and anti-β_2-glycoprotein I (anti-β_2-GPI) autoantibodies may

be detected in 1% to 2% of the unselected population.[16] Chronic APLAs confer a risk of venous or arterial thrombosis—a condition called antiphospholipid syndrome (APS). Chronic APLAs often accompany autoimmune connective tissue disorders, such as lupus erythematosus. Some appear in patients without any apparent primary disorder.

Malignancies often are implicated in venous thrombosis. One mechanism is tumor production of tissue factor analogues that trigger chronic low-grade DIC. In addition, venous and arterial stasis and inflammatory effects raise the risk of thrombosis. Migratory thrombophlebitis, or Trousseau syndrome, is a sign of occult adenocarcinoma such as cancer of the pancreas or colon.[17]

Myeloproliferative neoplasms such as essential thrombocythemia and polycythemia vera (Chapter 32) may trigger thrombosis, probably through platelet hyperactivity. A cardinal sign of acute promyelocytic leukemia (Chapter 31) is DIC secondary to the release of procoagulant granule contents from malignant promyelocytes. DIC may intensify during therapy at the time of vigorous cell lysis.[18] Paroxysmal nocturnal hemoglobinuria (PNH) (Chapter 21) is caused by a stem cell mutation that modifies membrane-anchored platelet activation suppressors. Venous or arterial thromboses occur in at least 40% of PNH cases.[19]

Chronic inflammatory diseases cause thrombosis through a variety of mechanisms, such as elevation of fibrinogen and factor VIII, suppressed fibrinolysis, promotion of atherosclerotic plaque formation, and reduced free protein S activity secondary to raised C4b-binding protein (C4bBP) levels. Diabetes mellitus is a particularly dangerous chronic inflammatory condition,

TABLE 39.1	Non-disease (Lifestyle) Factors that Contribute to Thrombosis		
Risk Factor	**Comment**	**Contribution to Thrombosis**	**Laboratory Diagnosis**
Age	Thrombosis after age 50	Risk doubles each decade after 50	
Immobilization	Sedentary, distance driving, air travel, restriction to wheelchair or bed, obesity	Slowed blood flow raises thrombosis risk	
Diet	Fatty foods; inadequate folate, vitamin B_6, and vitamin B_{12}	Homocysteinemia associated with 2× to 7× increased risk for arterial or venous thrombosis	Plasma homocysteine, vitamin levels, and lipid profile
Lipid metabolism imbalance	Hyperlipidemia, hypercholesterolemia, dyslipidemia, elevated lipoprotein (a), elevated triglycerides, decreased HDL-C, elevated LDL-C	Moderate arterial thrombosis association with LDL-C elevation and hypercholesterolemia, may be congenital	Lipid profile: total cholesterol, HDL-C, LDL-C, triglycerides, and lipoprotein (a)
Oral contraceptive use	30 μg, formulated with progesterone	4× to 6× increased risk	
Pregnancy		3× to 5× increased risk	
Hormone replacement therapy		2× to 4× increased risk	
Femoral or tibial fracture		80% incidence of thrombosis if not treated with antithrombotic	
Hip, knee, gynecologic, prostate surgery		50% incidence of thrombosis if not treated with antithrombotic	
Smoking		Depends on degree	HSCRP
Inflammation	Chronic	Arterial thrombosis	HSCRP
Central venous catheter	Endothelial injury and activation	33% of children with central venous lines develop venous thrombosis	

HDL-C, High-density lipoprotein cholesterol; *HSCRP,* high-sensitivity C-reactive protein; *LDL-C,* low-density lipoprotein cholesterol.

TABLE 39.2	Diseases with Thrombotic Risk Components		
Disease	**Examples or Effects**	**Contribution to Thrombosis**	**Laboratory Diagnosis**
Antiphospholipid syndrome	Chronic antiphospholipid antibody often secondary to autoimmune disorders	When chronic, 1.6× to 3.2× increased risk of stroke, myocardial infarction, recurrent spontaneous abortion, venous thrombosis	PTT mixing studies, lupus anticoagulant profile, anticardiolipin antibody and anti-β_2-glycoprotein 1 immunoassays
Myeloproliferative neoplasms	Essential thrombocythemia, polycythemia vera, chronic myelogenous leukemia	Increased risk as a result of plasma viscosity, platelet activation	Platelet counts and platelet aggregometry
Hepatic disease	Diminished production of most coagulation control proteins	Increased risk as a result of deranged coagulation pathways, excess thrombin production, reduced fibrinolysis	PT, proteins C and S, and antithrombin assays, factor assays
Cancer: adenocarcinoma	Trousseau syndrome, low-grade chronic DIC	20× increased risk of thrombosis; 10%–20% of people with idiopathic venous thrombosis have cancer	DIC profile: platelet count, D-dimer, PTT, PT, fibrinogen, blood film examination
Leukemia	Acute promyelocytic leukemia, acute monocytic leukemia	Increased risk for chronic DIC	DIC profile: platelet count, D-dimer, PTT, PT, fibrinogen, blood film examination
Paroxysmal nocturnal hemoglobinuria	Platelet-related thrombosis	Increased risk for deep vein thrombosis, pulmonary embolism, DIC	Flow cytometry phenotyping for CD55 and CD59; DIC profile: platelet count, D-dimer, PTT, PT, fibrinogen, blood film examination
Chronic inflammation	Diabetes, cancer, infection, autoimmune disorder, obesity, smoking		Fibrinogen, HSCRP

DIC, Disseminated intravascular coagulation; *PT*, prothrombin time; *PTT*, partial thromboplastin time, *HSCRP*, high-sensitivity C-reactive protein.

raising the risk of cardiovascular disease six-fold.[20] Conditions associated with venous stasis, such as congestive heart failure, are also risk factors for venous thrombosis. Untreated atrial fibrillation increases the risk of ischemic strokes caused by clot formation in the right atrium and embolization to the brain.[21] Nephrotic syndrome creates protein imbalances that lead to thrombosis through loss of plasma proteins such as antithrombin. Nephrotic syndrome may also associate with hemorrhage (Chapter 36).[22]

Congenital Thrombosis Risk Factors

Clinicians suspect congenital thrombophilia when a thrombotic event occurs in young adults; occurs in unusual sites such as the mesenteric, renal, or axillary veins; is recurrent; or occurs in a patient with a family history of thrombosis (Table 39.3). Because thrombosis is multifactorial, however, even patients with congenital thrombophilia are most likely to experience thrombotic events because of a combination of constitutional and acquired conditions.[23]

The antithrombin (AT) activity assay (previously called the antithrombin III or AT III assay) has been available since 1972, and protein C (PC) and protein S (PS) activity assays became available in the mid-1980s. The 1990s brought the APC resistance assay and its confirmatory FVL mutation molecular assay, the prothrombin G20210A mutation molecular assay, and more recently tests for polymorphisms in factors VIII and XI genes, dysfibrinogenemia, plasminogen deficiency, plasma TPA, and plasma plasminogen activator inhibitor-1 (PAI-1).[24] Homocysteinemia is associated with inadequate dietary folate, vitamin B_6, or vitamin B_{12} levels and with polymorphisms affected the function of methylene tetrahydrofolate reductase (MTHFR) in the methionine metabolic pathway. Folate supplementation in

industrialized countries has reduced the incidence of homocysteinemia. Although MTHFR polymorphisms are associated with homocysteinemia, they do not correlate with incidence of arterial thrombosis. Efforts to reduce plasma homocysteine concentration do not reduce the risk of arterial thrombosis.

APC resistance is found in 3% to 8% of Caucasians worldwide. APC resistance extends to Arab and Hispanic populations, but the mutation is nearly absent from African and East Asian populations.[25] APC resistance may exist in the absence of the FVL mutation and is occasionally acquired in pregnancy or in association with oral contraceptive therapy.[26,27]

The FVL gene mutation is the most common inherited thrombosis risk factor, and the prothrombin G20210A gene mutation is the second most common inherited thrombophilia in patients with a personal and family history of deep vein thrombosis.[28] Altogether, PC, PS, and AT deficiencies are found in only 0.2% to 1.0% of the world population.

Thrombosis Double Hit

Thrombosis often is associated with a combination of genetic defect, disease, and lifestyle influences. Just because someone possesses AT, PC, or PS deficiency does not mean that thrombosis is inevitable. Many heterozygotes experience no thrombotic event during their lifetimes, whereas others experience clotting only when two or more risk factors converge. A woman who is heterozygous for the FVL mutation has a thirty-five-fold. increase in thrombosis risk when using oral contraceptives. In the Physicians' Health Study, homocysteinemia tripled the risk of idiopathic venous thrombosis, and the FVL mutation doubled it. Those with multiple congenital thrombotic risk factors coupled with homocysteinemia experience increased thrombosis risk.[29]

TABLE 39.3 Predisposing Congenital Factors and Thrombosis Risk

Risk Factor	Function	Thrombosis Relative Risk	PREVALENCE		Laboratory Assays
			Unselected Population	≥1 Thrombotic Event	
AT deficiency	AT, enhanced by heparin, inhibits serine proteases IIa, IXa, Xa, and XIa	Heterozygous: 10× to 20× Homozygous: 100%, rarely reported	1 in 2–5000	1%–1.8%	Clot-based and chromogenic AT activity assays, AT concentration by immunoassay
PC deficiency	Activated PC is a serine protease that hydrolyzes factors Va and VIIIa, requires protein S as a stabilizing cofactor	Heterozygous: 2× to 5× Homozygous: 100%; neonatal purpura fulminans	1 in 300	2.5%–5%	Clot-based and chromogenic PC activity assays, PC concentration by immunoassay
Free PS deficiency	PS is a stabilizing cofactor for activated protein C, 40% free, 60% circulates bound to C4bBP	Heterozygous: 1.6× to 11.5× Homozygous: 100% but rarely reported; neonatal purpura fulminans	Unknown	2.8%–5%	Clot-based free PS activity assays, PS concentration by free and total immunoassays
APC resistance	Factor V Leiden (R506Q) mutation gain of function renders factor V resistant to APC	Heterozygous: 3× Homozygous: 18×	3%–8% of Caucasians, rare in Asians and Africans	20%–25%	PTT-based APC resistance test and confirmatory molecular assay
Prothrombin G20210A	Mutation in prothrombin gene untranslated 3′ promoter region; moderate prothrombin activity elevation	Heterozygous: 1.6× to 11.5×	2%–3% of Caucasians, rare in Asians and Africans	4%–8%	Molecular assay only; phenotypic assay provides no specificity
Homocysteinemia	Associated with arterial thrombosis	Males: 4.3–9.9; females: 3.3–7.2 mmol/L Folate, vitamin B_6, vitamin B_{12} deficiency, MTHFR C677T and A1298C polymorphisms	Folate supplementation reduces prevalence MTHFR polymorphisms are not a risk factor for arterial thrombosis in folate supplementation		Fluorescence polarization immunoassay
Hyperfibrinogenemia	Associated with arterial thrombosis	Acute phase reactant			Clauss fibrinogen clotting assay, immunoassay, nephelometric assay

APC, Activated protein C; AT, antithrombin; C4bBP, complement component C4b-binding protein; MTHFR, methylene tetrahydrofolate reductase; PC, protein C; PS, protein S; PTT, partial thromboplastin time.

LABORATORY EVALUATION OF THROMBOPHILIA

When the physician suspects thrombophilia, it is necessary to assess all clinically significant risk factors. It is the accumulation of factors that determines the patient's risk of thrombosis.[30] Table 39.4 summarizes the clinically useful thrombosis risk assays and indicates those that can be relied on for accurate results during the acute inflammation that occurs immediately after a thrombotic event or while the patient is on anticoagulant therapy.

Experts discourage thrombosis risk testing immediately after a thrombotic event. The presence of a documented risk factor does not affect therapy for acute thrombosis. Anticoagulant therapy and ongoing or recent thrombotic events interfere with the interpretation of AT, PC, PS, factor VIII, and LAC testing results. These assays should be performed at least 14 days after anticoagulant therapy is discontinued. Connors writes, "Most patients with venous thromboembolism do not require thrombophilia testing, since the results will not affect management. Testing may be considered in younger patients with weak provoking factors, a strong family history, or recurrence at a young age."[31]

Antiphospholipid Antibodies

Antiphospholipid antibodies comprise a family of immunoglobulins that bind protein-phospholipid complexes.[32] APLAs include LACs, detected by clot-based profiles; and ACL and anti-β_2-GPI antibodies, detected by immunoassay. Chronic autoimmune APLAs are associated with antiphospholipid syndrome, which is characterized by transient ischemic attacks, strokes, coronary and peripheral artery disease, venous thromboembolism, and recurrent pregnancy complications, including spontaneous abortions.[33]

APLAs arise as immunoglobulin M (IgM) or IgG isotypes. Because they may bind a variety of protein-phospholipid complexes, they are sometimes called nonspecific inhibitors. Their name implies that they were once thought to directly bind phospholipids; however, their target antigens are actually the proteins that assemble on anionic phospholipid surfaces. The plasma protein most often bound by APLAs is β_2-GPI, although annexin V and prothrombin are sometimes implicated as APLA targets. APLAs probably develop in response to newly formed protein-phospholipid complexes, and laboratory scientists continue to investigate how they cause thrombosis.[34,35]

TABLE 39.4 Thrombophilia Laboratory Test Profile

Assay	Reference Limit or Interval	Comments
APC resistance	Ratio ≥1.8	Clot-based screen employs PTT with factor V-depleted plasma.
Factor V Leiden mutation*	Wild type	Molecular assay performed as follow-up to APC resistance ratio that is <1.8.
Prothrombin G20210A*	Wild type	Molecular assay. There is no phenotypic assay for prothrombin G20210A.
LAC profile	Negative for LAC	Minimum of two clot-based assays. Primary assays are based on DRVVT and PTT, secondary assays based on dilute PT. All include phospholipid neutralization follow-up test.
ACL antibody*	IgG: <12 GPL IgM: <10 MPL	Immunoassay for immunoglobulins of APL family. ACL depends on β_2-GPI in reaction mix.
Anti-β_2-GPI antibody*	<20 G units	Immunoassay for an immunoglobulin of APL family. β_2-GPI is key phospholipid-binding protein in family.
AT activity	78%–126%	Serine protease inhibitor suppresses IIa (thrombin), IXa, Xa, XIa. When consistently below reference limit, follow up with AT antigen assay.
PC activity	70%–140%	Digests VIIIa and Va. When consistently below reference limit, follow up with PC antigen assay.
PS activity	65%–140%	PC cofactor. When consistently below reference limit, follow up with total and free PS antigen assay, C4b-binding protein assay.
Fibrinogen	220–498 mg/dL	Clot-based assay. Chronic elevation may be associated with arterial thrombosis.
Homocysteine	Males: 4.3–9.9 Females: 3.3–7.2 mmol/L	Fluorescence polarization immunoassay. Elevation may be associated with arterial thrombosis but therapeutic reduction does not affect risk of thrombosis.

ACL, Anticardiolipin; *APC*, activated protein C; *APL*, antiphospholipid antibody; *AT*, antithrombin; β_2-GPI, β_2-glycoprotein I; *DRVVT*, dilute Russell viper venom time; *GPL*, IgG antiphospholipid antibody unit; *Ig*, immunoglobulin; *LAC*, lupus anticoagulant; *MPL*, IgM antiphospholipid antibody unit; *PC*, protein C; *PS*, protein S; *PT*, prothrombin time; *PTT*, partial thromboplastin time.
*Only measurements that are valid during active thrombosis or anticoagulant therapy. All other measurements must be performed 14 days after anticoagulant therapy is discontinued.

Clinical Consequences of Antiphospholipid Antibodies

Between 1% and 2% of unselected individuals of both sexes and all races, and 5% to 15% of individuals with recurrent venous or arterial thrombotic disease have APLAs.[36] Most APLAs arise in response to a bacterial, viral, fungal, or parasitic infection or to treatment with one of a variety of drugs (Box 39.1) and disappear within 12 weeks. These are transient alloimmune APLAs with no clinical consequences. Nevertheless, the laboratory professional must follow up any positive APLA result to determine persistence. There may exist a relationship between APLA and C-reactive protein (CRP), both of which may associate with elevated thrombotic risk, consequently many laboratory directors add the high-sensitivity CRP assay to their APLA test profile.[37,38]

Autoimmune APLAs are part of the family of autoantibodies that arise in collagen vascular diseases; 50% of patients with systemic lupus erythematosus have autoimmune APLAs. Autoimmune APLAs are also detected in patients with rheumatoid arthritis, scleroderma, and Sjögren syndrome but may arise spontaneously, a disorder called primary APS. Autoimmune APLAs may persist, and fully 30% are associated with arterial and venous thrombosis. Chronic presence of an autoimmune APLA not associated with a known underlying autoimmune disorder confers a 1.8-fold to 3.2-fold increased risk of thrombosis.[39]

Detection and Confirmation of Antiphospholipid Antibodies

Clinicians suspect APS in unexplained venous or arterial thrombosis, thrombocytopenia, or recurrent fetal loss.[40] Specialized clinical hemostasis laboratories offer APLA detection profiles that include clot-based assays for LAC and immunoassays for ACL and anti-β_2-GPI antibodies. Occasionally, an LAC is suspected because of an unexplained prolonged partial thromboplastin time (PTT) that does not correct in mixing studies (Figure 39.1).[41]

The mixing study (Chapter 41) is an important first step in the LAC laboratory workup to establish the presence of an LAC because it can differentiate an LAC from a factor deficiency. In addition to the LAC, the mixing study is sensitive to other factor inhibitors such as anti-factor VIII inhibitors.

Lupus Anticoagulant Test Profile

Clot-based assays with reduced reagent phospholipid concentrations are sensitive to LAC. There are two commonly used test systems, and both are required for an LAC profile. The need for two parallel assay systems arises from the multiplicity of LAC reaction characteristics: A confirmed positive result in one system is conclusive despite a negative result in the other. The two most commonly recommended test systems are the dilute Russell viper venom time (DRVVT) and the silica-based PTT, also called the silica clot time (SCT), both formulated with low-phospholipid concentrations designed to be LAC sensitive.[42] The time-honored dilute thromboplastin time (DTT), also named

BOX 39.1 Agents Known to Induce Antiphospholipid Antibodies

Various antibiotics	Procainamide
Phenothiazine	Phenytoin
Hydralazine	Cocaine
Quinine and quinidine	Elevated estrogens
Calcium channel blockers	

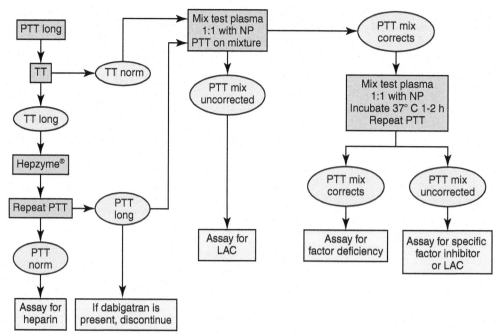

Figure 39.1 Mixing Study Employing a Partial Thromboplastin Time *(PTT)* **Reagent with Intermediate Lupus Anticoagulant** *(LAC)* **Sensitivity.** Beginning at the top left, when the PTT result exceeds the upper limit of the PTT reference interval, perform a thrombin time *(TT)* to detect unfractionated heparin (inpatient) or dabigatran (outpatient). If the TT exceeds the TT reference interval, presume that heparin or dabigatran is present. Treat an aliquot of the specimen with Hepzyme and repeat the PTT. If the new PTT is normal, assay the original sample for heparin. If the PTT remains prolonged after Hepzyme treatment, check for dabigatran. If dabigatran is present, discontinue the mixing study. If no dabigatran is present or if the TT was normal, proceed by mixing the patient plasma with normal plasma *(NP)* and perform a PTT on the mixture. If the PTT remains prolonged (uncorrected) in comparison to the NP, proceed to assay for LAC. If the PTT mixture corrects, prepare a new 1:1 mix and incubate at 37° C for 2 hours and repeat the PTT, comparing the result to incubated NP. If the incubated PTT shows a correction, assay for a factor deficiency. If the incubated PTT remains prolonged, assay for a specific inhibitor such as anti-factor VIII or LAC (Figures 39.2 and 39.3). In 15% of cases, temperature-dependent LAC may be detected after incubation.

the tissue thromboplastin inhibitor (TTI) assay, is used in many institutions and available from specialty laboratories and coagulation reagent distributors.[43] As illustrated in Figure 39.2, the PTT initiates coagulation at the level of factor XII; DRVVT at factor X; and DTT at factor VII.

The 2009 International Society on Thrombosis and Haemostasis (ISTH) update of guidelines for LAC detection requires the following sequence:

1. Prolonged phospholipid-dependent clot formation using an initial (primary) assay such as a low-phospholipid PTT or DRVVT, often called the PTT or DRVVT *screen.*
2. Failure to correct the prolonged clot time when mixing with normal platelet-poor plasma and repeating the test.[44]
3. Shortening or correction of the prolonged initial assay result by addition of a reagent formulated with excess phospholipids, often called the PTT or DRVVT *confirm.*
4. Exclusion of other coagulopathies.

Performing the clot-based lupus anticoagulant test profile.
Laboratory practitioners perform the LAC profile upon clinician request, often to find the cause for adverse thrombotic or obstetric events, or when an isolated prolonged PTT raises the presumption of an LAC. Many laboratory protocols begin with a mixing study in which the PTT is performed on

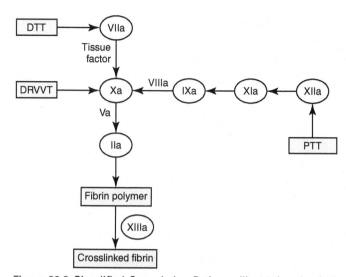

Figure 39.2 Simplified Coagulation Pathway Illustrating the Activation Points of the Lupus Anticoagulant *(LAC)* **Assays.** The dilute Russell viper venom time *(DRVVT)* assay, regarded as the most reliable LAC detection method, activates factor X. DRVVT is typically paralleled by an LAC-sensitive partial thromboplastin time assay *(PTT)* that activates factor XII. The dilute thromboplastin time test *(DTT)* activates factor VII.

patient plasma combined 1:1 with pooled normal plasma (NP) (Fig. 39.1). The mixing study includes a second 2-hour 37° C incubation step, because most specific inhibitors such as anti-factor VIII and 15% of LACs require incubation to enhance their avidity. Practitioners typically perform the initial mixing study using a PTT reagent with intermediate LAC sensitivity.[45] The mixing study includes a means for detecting unfractionated heparin (UFH), most often the thrombin clotting time (TCT, TT) or the chromogenic anti-Xa heparin assay. The practitioner may add heparinase (Hepzyme, Siemens) to the specimen to neutralize heparin, although this may be unnecessary because many LAC detection reagents provide heparin-neutralizing polybrene. Mixing studies based on a prothrombin time (PT), a DRVVT, or an LAC-sensitive PTT reagent seldom require 37° C incubation.

The NP that is mixed 1:1 with patient plasma is expected to shorten a prolonged PTT. Each laboratory director decides what degree of PTT shortening constitutes correction. Many define correction as a mixture result within 10% of the NP result; others define correction as return to a value within the PTT reference interval.

In performing mixing studies, the laboratory professional employs only platelet-poor plasma—plasma centrifuged so that it has a platelet count of less than 10,000/μL (Chapter 41). The use of platelet-poor plasma avoids LAC neutralization by platelet membrane phospholipids. Platelet membrane fragments that form during freezing and thawing can likewise neutralize LAC and lead to a false-negative LAC result.

Performing clot-based lupus anticoagulant tests. Following a mixing study whose lack of correction suggests the presence of an LAC, the practitioner performs LAC-specific testing. Most LAC protocols begin with the DRVVT, considered the more specific of the LAC assays (Figure 39.3). If the DRVVT primary (screen) reagent-patient plasma result exceeds the upper limit of the DRVVT reference interval, LAC is presumed. The practitioner then confirms LAC by mixing an aliquot of the patient specimen with the DRVVT high-phospholipid confirmatory reagent, comparing the result in seconds to the DRVVT primary reagent patient plasma result. The reagent phospholipid neutralizes LAC and shortens the DRVVT. If the primary reagent result is prolonged over the DRVVT confirm reagent result by a predetermined ratio or more, typically 1.2, LAC is confirmed.[46]

If the DRVVT primary/confirm ratio is less than 1.2, the practitioner turns to the silica-based low-phospholipid LA-sensitive PTT, using the same steps used for the DRVVT. In this instance the difference between the primary (screen) and confirmatory reagent may be expressed as a ratio or in seconds, typically a difference of 8 seconds is the threshold used to confirm an LAC.[47]

There exist numerous modifications to this algorithm. Many laboratory directors prefer to begin with the silica-based low-phospholipid PTT assay, and others include an intermediate NP mixing study step. Some incorporate the DTT. The 1.2 ratio and the 8-second difference are examples; each institution may choose to establish its own reference interval and threshold ratio or difference.

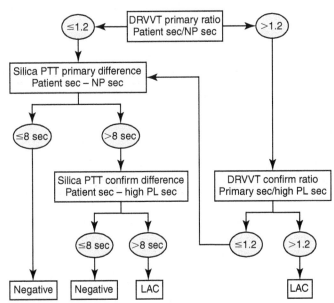

Figure 39.3 Lupus Anticoagulant *(LAC)* Algorithm. When LAC is suspected, perform the dilute Russell viper venom *(DRVVT)* primary (screen) assay, comparing the patient DRVVT result with the pooled normal plasma *(NP)* DRVVT result. If the ratio of patient to NP DRVVT in seconds is greater than 1.2, mix patient plasma 1:1 with high-phospholipid *(PL)* DRVVT *confirm* reagent and perform a new DRVVT. If the primary patient DRVVT result exceeds the DRVVT confirm patient plasma result by greater than 1.2, LAC is confirmed. If the ratio is 1.2 or less or if the primary DRVVT ratio was 1.2 or less, proceed to silica-based partial thromboplastin *(PTT)* primary and confirm assays. This step is similar to Figure 39.1, except in 39.1 the PTT reagent formulation is optional. Compare the primary patient silica-based PTT to the NP result. If the difference is 8 seconds or less, no LAC is present. If the difference is greater than 8 seconds, mix the patient plasma with high-phospholipid silica-based PTT confirm reagent and perform a new PTT. If the primary patient PTT exceeds the patient PTT confirm by more than 8 seconds, LAC is confirmed; if 8 seconds or less, LAC is not present.

Some laboratory directors choose to normalize DRVVT or PTT-based ratios using the mean of the reference interval (MRI) or the NP value. The formula for normalization using the MRI is:

$$\text{Normalized ratio} = \frac{\text{Primary mix result in seconds/MRI}}{\text{Confirm mix results in seconds/MRI}} = \frac{\text{Primary ratio}}{\text{Confirm ratio}}$$

This formula is applied to both the DRVVT and the PTT-based assays. Assays for LAC, because they are clot based, are affected by anticoagulant therapy including oral anticoagulants, current thrombosis, and factor deficiencies.

Anticardiolipin Antibody Immunoassay

LAC and ACL antibodies coexist in 60% of cases, and both may be found in APS. The ACL test is an immunoassay that is not affected by anticoagulant therapy, current thrombosis, or factor deficiencies.[48] Evidence supports that antibodies directed at cardiolipin are mainly associated with infection, whereas patients with APS have β_2-GPI bound to cardiolipin as the

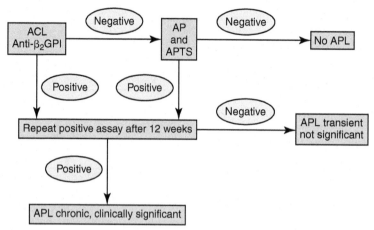

Figure 39.4 Anti-phospholipid Antibody *(APL)* Immunoassay Algorithm. If APL is suspected, perform an anti-cardiolipin *(ACL)* or anti-β$_2$-glycoprotein I *(anti-β$_2$-GPI)* immunoassay. If either is positive, confirm chronicity using a new specimen collected at least 12 weeks later. If negative, perform immunoassay to detect an anti-prothrombin *(AP)* or anti-phosphatidylserine *(APTS)* antibody. If positive, repeat after 12 weeks.

antigenic target. Better performing assays for anticardiolipin antibodies incorporate a complex of cardiolipin-β$_2$-GPI.

The manufacturer coats microplate wells with bovine heart cardiolipin and blocks (fills open receptor sites) with bovine serum. A solution containing β$_2$-GPI is then added. The laboratory practitioner pipettes test sera or plasmas to the wells alongside calibrators and controls (Figure 39.4).[49] ACL antibodies bind the solid-phase cardiolipin-β$_2$-GPI target complex and cannot be washed from the wells. The practitioner adds enzyme-labeled anti-human IgM or IgG conjugate subsequent to washing, followed by a color or fluorophore-generating substrate. A color or fluorescence change indicates the presence of ACL and intensities of the patient and control sample wells are compared with the calibrator curve wells. Results are expressed using GPL or MPL units, where 1 unit is equivalent to 1 µg/mL of an affinity-purified standard IgG or IgM sample.

Anti-β$_2$-Glycoprotein 1 Immunoassay

The practitioner performs IgM and IgG anti-β$_2$-GPI immunoassays as a part of the APS profile that includes the ACL assay. An anti-β$_2$-GPI result of greater than 20 IgG or IgM anti-β$_2$-GPI units correlates with thrombosis more closely than the presence of ACL antibodies.[50] Any positive ACL or anti-β$_2$-GPI assay repeated on a new specimen collected after 12 weeks distinguishes a transient alloantibody from a chronic autoantibody.

Antiphosphatidylserine/Antiprothrombin Immunoassay

For cases in which an APL antibody is suspected but the routine LAC, ACL, and β$_2$-GPI assay results are negative, the clinician may wish to order antiphosphatidylserine and anti-prothrombin immunoassays to detect APL antibodies specific for phosphatidylserine or prothrombin.[51] Antiphosphatidylserine and antiprothrombin assays are available from specialty reference laboratories.

Activated Protein C Resistance and Factor V Leiden Mutation

Clinical Importance of APC Resistance

When stabilized by protein S, APC hydrolyzes activated factors V and VIII (factors Va and VIIIa). A mutation in the factor V gene substitutes glutamine for arginine at position 506 of the factor V molecule (FV R506Q).[52,53] The arginine molecule is the normal cleavage site for APC, so the substitution slows or resists APC hydrolysis. The resistant factor Va remains active (a gain of function) and raises the production of thrombin, leading to thrombosis. The factor V R506Q mutation is named for the city in The Netherlands in which Bertina first described it, Leiden (factor V Leiden [FVL] mutation, also called APC resistance). Between 3% and 8% of Northern European Caucasians possess the FVL mutation (Table 39.4).[54,55] Owing to its prevalence and the associated threefold higher thrombosis risk (eighteenfold higher for homozygotes), most acute care hemostasis laboratory directors provide APC resistance detection to screen for FVL.[56]

APC Resistance Clot-Based Assay

In the APC resistance clot-based assay, patient plasma is mixed 1:4 with factor V-depleted plasma.[57] PTT reagent is added to two aliquots of the mixture and incubated for 3 minutes (Figure 39.5). A solution of calcium chloride is pipetted into one mixture, and the clot formation is timed. A solution of calcium chloride *with APC* is added to the second mixture, and clotting is timed. The interval to clot formation of the second aliquot is at least 1.8 times longer than the time to clot formation of the first, increased by the presence of APC, so the normal ratio of PTT results between the two assays is 1.8 or greater. In APC resistance the ratio is less than 1.8.

Factor V-depleted plasma compensates for potential factor deficiencies and for oral anticoagulant therapy by providing normal coagulation factors. The laboratory professional uses only platelet-poor plasma in the APC resistance test to prevent loss of sensitivity caused by the abundant release of factor V

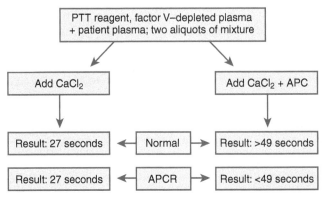

Figure 39.5 Activated Protein C Resistance Ratio *(APCR)* Measurement. Patient plasma is mixed 1:4 with factor V–depleted plasma and partial thromboplastin time *(PTT)* reagent. Two aliquots of this mixture are tested: one aliquot is mixed with calcium chloride *(CaCl₂)* alone, and the other aliquot is mixed with CaCl₂ plus activated protein C *(APC)*. The reaction in the mixture with the APC should be prolonged to at least 1.8 times longer than the mixture without APC. The results in seconds are examples. A ratio of 1.8 or less implies APC resistance.

from platelet α-granules. APC resistance reagent test kits contain polybrene or heparinase to neutralize UFH. LAC, however, affects the test system adversely.[58] If LAC is present, the molecular test for FVL is indicated.[59]

Factor V Leiden Mutation Assay

Most laboratories confirm the APC resistance diagnosis using the molecular FVL mutation test. Some laboratories omit the APC test and directly measure FVL by molecular genetic testing. The determination of zygosity is important to predict the risk for thrombosis and establish a treatment regimen.

Prothrombin G20210A

A guanine-to-adenine mutation at base 20210 of the 3′ untranslated region of the prothrombin (factor II) gene has been associated with mildly elevated plasma prothrombin levels, averaging 130%.[60] The increased risk of thrombosis in those with the mutation seems to be related to the elevated prothrombin activity.[61] The prevalence of this mutation among individuals with familial thrombosis is 5% to 18%, whereas prevalence worldwide is 0.3% to 2.4%, depending on race.[62] The risk of venous thrombosis in heterozygotes is two to three times the baseline risk.[63] Although the mutation may cause a slight prothrombin elevation, a phenotypic prothrombin activity assay is of little diagnostic value because there is considerable overlap between normal prothrombin levels and prothrombin levels in people with the mutation.[64] Diagnosis of the prothrombin G20210A mutation requires molecular genetic testing.

Antithrombin

Antithrombin (AT) is a serine protease inhibitor (SERPIN) that neutralizes factors IIa (thrombin), IXa, Xa, XIa, and XIIa, all the coagulation system serine proteases except factor VIIa (Chapter 35). AT activity is enhanced through binding to exogenous heparan sulfate found on endothelial cell surfaces. AT

activity is enhanced 1000-fold by therapeutic UFH, and 400-fold by low-molecular-weight heparin (LMWH) and synthetic pentasaccharide (fondaparinux) therapies (Fig. 35.15). AT was the first of the plasma coagulation control proteins to be identified and the first to be assayed routinely in the clinical hemostasis laboratory. Other members of the SERPIN family are heparin cofactor II, α₂-macroglobulin, α₂-antiplasmin, and α-antitrypsin. Hemostasis specialty laboratories or reference laboratories provide assays for all the SERPINs.

Antithrombin Deficiency

Adult AT levels are reached by 3 months of age, and remain steady in young adulthood, except during periods of physiologic challenge. The plasma biologic half-life is 72 hours and AT activity decreases with age.[65]

AT deficiency is defined as AT activity levels less than 70% of normal or antigen concentration less than 22 mg/dL. AT becomes depleted in pregnancy, liver disease and nephrotic syndrome, with prolonged heparin and L-asparaginase therapy, with the use of oral contraceptives, and in DIC. Hereditary AT deficiency occurs in 1 in 2000 to 1 in 5000 of the general population and accounts for 1.0% to 1.8% of recurrent venous thromboembolic disease cases.[66] About 90% of congenital AT deficiency cases are quantitative, reflected in the antigen level; the rest are caused by mutations that create structural abnormalities in the *protease-binding* site or the *heparin-binding* site. Qualitative deficiency mutations only slightly reduce AT production, but the molecules are nonfunctional, as reflected in diminished activity assay results.[67] Elevated AT levels appear to have no clinical consequence.

Severe AT deficiency causing thrombosis may be treated with an AT concentrate (Thrombate III; Grifols).[68]

Antithrombin Activity Assay

Laboratory practitioners test for AT deficiency using a clot-based or chromogenic functional assay.[69] In the chromogenic substrate method, the practitioner mixes test plasma with a solution of heparin and factor Xa (Figure 39.6) and incubates the mixture at 37° C for several minutes. During incubation, the heparin-activated plasma AT irreversibly binds a proportion of the reagent factor Xa. Residual factor Xa hydrolyzes a chromogenic substrate, added as a second reagent. The degree of hydrolysis, measurable by colored end product intensity, is inversely proportional to the activity of test plasma AT.[70] The chromogenic substrate test detects quantitative and qualitative AT deficiencies and detects mutations affecting the proteolytic site but not the heparin binding site. The clot-based assay has been available since 1972 and remains valid. Clot-based antithrombin assays are affected by, and therefore detect, mutations in both the proteolytic and heparin binding sites.

Antithrombin Antigen Assay

AT concentration is measured with a turbidometric microparticle immunoassay using a suspension of latex microbeads coated with antibody to antithrombin. In the absence of AT the wavelength of incident monochromatic light exceeds the latex

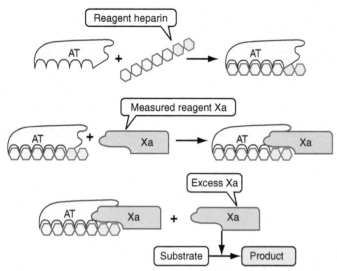

Figure 39.6 Chromogenic Antithrombin *(AT)* Functional Assay. Patient plasma is pipetted into a reagent consisting of heparin, a measured concentration of activated coagulation factor X *(Xa)*, and a chromogenic substrate specific to Xa. AT is activated by heparin and binds Xa. Excess Xa hydrolyzes the substrate and produces a yellow product, para-nitroaniline (pNA). The intensity of pNA color is inversely proportional to AT activity.

microparticle diameter, so the light passes through unabsorbed. In the presence of AT the particles form larger aggregates. The AT concentration is directly proportional to the rate of light absorption change.[71] The turbidometric immunoassay allows for a convenient application to high-throughput analyzers. Sandwich-type enzyme-linked immunosorbent assays (ELISA) are also available.

AT antigen levels are deficient in quantitative but are normal or slightly reduced in qualitative deficiencies. Coumadin therapy may raise the AT level and mask a mild deficiency. AT activity remains decreased for 10 to 14 days after a period of acute inflammation such as a thrombotic event or surgery, so the assay should not be used to establish a congenital deficiency during this period.

Heparin Resistance and the Antithrombin Assay

AT may become depleted during prolonged or intense UFH therapy, especially if the patient has a congenital deficiency. In this instance, because UFH requires AT to express its anticoagulant effect, UFH therapy at routine dosages fails to fully protect the patient. The decreased anticoagulant effect of UFH is observed in UFH monitoring assays such as the PTT, ACT, and chromogenic anti-Xa heparin assay (Chapter 40). This circumstance is known as heparin resistance. In such cases an AT assay is necessary to confirm deficiency. Patients are often managed by administering UFH at higher than therapeutic dosages until the monitoring assay provides desired results. Severe AT deficiency causing heparin resistance may be treated with plasma transfusion or an AT concentrate (Thrombate III).[68]

Protein C Control Pathway

Thrombin is an essential coagulation factor because it cleaves fibrinogen, activates platelets, and activates factors V, VIII, XI, and XIII. In the intact vessel where clotting is pathologic,

thrombin binds endothelial cell membrane thrombomodulin and becomes, paradoxically, an anticoagulant.[72] The thrombin-thrombomodulin complex cleaves and activates PC (Chapter 35). The resultant APC binds free plasma PS.[73] The stabilized APC-PS complex, simultaneously bound to the endothelial PC receptor, hydrolyzes factors Va and VIIIa to reduce thrombin production, an essential coagulation control mechanism (Figure 35.14). Recurrent venous thrombosis is the consequence of PC or PS deficiency.[74] PS, the cofactor that binds and stabilizes APC, circulates either free or covalently bound to the complement binding protein *C4bBP*. Bound PS cannot participate in the PC anticoagulant pathway; only free plasma PS is available to serve as the APC cofactor. When acute phase reactant C4bBP level rises, binding additional PS, free PS levels become proportionally decreased.

Protein C and Protein S Deficiency

PC or PS deficiency is defined as activity or concentrations levels less than 65% of normal. Heterozygous PC or PS deficiency leads to a 1.6-fold to 11.5-fold increased risk of recurrent DVTs and PEs. PS deficiency also has been implicated in transient ischemic attacks and strokes, particularly in the young.

Control proteins PC and PS (and PZ) and coagulation factors II (prothrombin), VII, IX, and X are vitamin K-dependent. Because PC's half-life is 6 hours, its level decreases as rapidly as that of factor VII at the onset of Coumadin therapy (an oral anticoagulant that reduces the vitamin K-dependent factors). In heterozygous PC deficiency, PC activity may drop to less than 65% more rapidly than the coagulation factor activities reach low therapeutic levels (less than 30%). Consequently, in early Coumadin therapy a patient may experience Coumadin-induced skin necrosis, a condition in which the anticoagulant therapy paradoxically brings on thrombosis within the dermal vessels. This complication is suspected when the patient develops painful necrotic lesions that are preceded by severe itching, called pruritus. The necrosis may require surgical debridement. To avoid this risk, hematologists recommend co-administration of UFH, LMWH, or fondaparinux with Coumadin until a satisfactory and stable international normalized ratio (INR) is reached (Chapter 40).[75]

PC and PS activity levels remain less than normal for 10 to 14 days after Coumadin therapy is discontinued. Similarly, for several days after acute inflammation caused by a thrombotic event or surgery, these proteins are diminished even if Coumadin has not been used. Their activities are depressed in pregnancy, liver or renal disease, vitamin K deficiency, DIC, and with oral contraceptive use. PC and PS assays therefore cannot be used to identify a congenital deficiency when they are employed within 14 days after an acute inflammatory event or after the cessation of Coumadin therapy, during pregnancy, or in the presence of DIC, liver disease, renal disease, vitamin K deficiency, or oral contraceptive use.[76]

Homozygous PC or PS deficiency results in neonatal purpura fulminans, a condition that is rapidly fatal when untreated (Chapter 38). Treatment includes PC concentrate and lifelong Coumadin therapy.[77]

Protein C Assays

Clot-based or chromogenic functional assays detect both quantitative and qualitative PC deficiencies.[78] For the chromogenic assay, the laboratory professional first mixes the patient's plasma with Protac (Pentapharm), derived from the venom of the Southern Copperhead serpent *Agkistrodon contortrix*, which activates PC. Subsequently a substrate is added which is hydrolyzed by the recently generated APC. The hydrolysis is reflected in the intensity of colored product, which is proportional to PC activity (Figure 39.7). The assay detects abnormalities that affect the molecule's *proteolytic* properties (active serine protease site) but misses those that affect PC's phospholipid binding site or PS binding site. In cases in which the PC chromogenic assay and immunoassay generate normal results but the clinical condition continues to indicate a possible PC deficiency, a clot-based assay may detect abnormalities at these additional sites on the molecule.

The clot-based PC assay is based on the ability of APC to prolong the PTT. The laboratory professional mixes plasma with PC-depleted NP to ensure normal levels of all coagulation factors except PC. PTT reagent mixed with Protac and a heparin neutralizer is added, followed by calcium chloride, and the interval to clot formation is measured. Prolongation is proportional to PC activity. Assay interferences include therapeutic heparin concentrations greater than 1 IU/mL, which consume the heparin neutralizer, prolong the PTT, and lead to overestimation of protein C. APC resistance (FVL mutation), LAC, and the presence of therapeutic direct thrombin inhibitors such as argatroban or dabigatran may prolong the PTT and falsely raise the PC activity level in both chromogenic and clot-based assays.

An enzyme immunoassay (EIA) may be used to measure PC antigen when the activity is low. Microtiter plates coated with rabbit anti-human protein C antibody are used to capture test plasma protein C, and the concentration of antigen is measured by color development after the sequential addition of peroxidase-conjugated anti-human protein C and orthophenylenediamine substrate. The protein C antigen concentration assay is available from specialty reference laboratories. The assay detects most acquired deficiencies and quantitative congenital deficiencies, but it may return normal or near-normal levels in qualitative congenital abnormalities.[79]

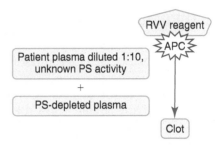

Figure 39.8 Clot-based Protein S *(PS)* Assay. Patient plasma is diluted and pipetted into PS-depleted plasma. A second reagent is composed of Russell viper venom *(RVV)*, which activates clotting at the level of factor X, and activated protein C *(APC)*. The patient PS binds the reagent APC to prolong the clotting time. Clotting time is proportional to PS activity.

Protein S Assays

PS deficiency may be detected using a clot-based functional assay. No chromogenic assay is available. In one method the laboratory practitioner mixes the patient's plasma with PS-depleted NP to ensure normal levels of all factors other than PS. APC and Russell viper venom are added in a buffer that contains a heparin neutralizer, followed by calcium chloride. The interval to clot formation is proportional to PS activity (Figure 39.8).

Assay interferences include therapeutic heparin levels greater than 1 IU/mL that consume reagent heparin neutralizer and lead to overestimation of protein S activity. APC resistance, LAC, and the presence of the therapeutic direct thrombin inhibitors argatroban or dabigatran may prolong the clot time and falsely raise the activity levels in clot-based protein S assays.[80] Coagulation factor VII activation may occur during prolonged refrigeration of plasma at 4° C to 10° C, which may cause underestimation of PS activity by the same mechanism that causes a false effect in PT-based coagulation factor assays such as factor V or factor X assays.[81]

When there is a low activity level, EIAs are employed to measure both total and free PS antigen. These assays detect most quantitative congenital deficiencies and aid in the diagnosis of qualitative congenital deficiencies characterized by normal antigen but decreased PS activity. In a third form of PS deficiency, the PS activity and the concentration of free PS antigen are reduced but not total antigen (Table 39.5). In this form the plasma C4bBP, an acute phase reactant, is elevated, proportionally reducing the concentration of free PS. The concentration of plasma C4bBP, an acute phase reactant, measured by immunoassay, helps classify this third PS deficiency type.

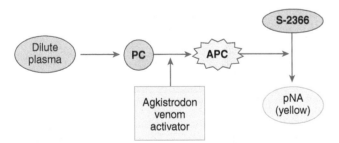

Figure 39.7 Chromogenic Protein C *(PC)* Assay. Patient plasma is pipetted into a reagent composed of *Agkistrodon contortrix* venom activator and chromogenic substrate S-2366 specific to activated protein C *(APC)*. The APC hydrolyzes the substrate to produce para-nitroaniline *(pNA)*, a yellow product. The intensity of color is proportional to APC activity.

TABLE 39.5 Anticipated Protein S Test Results in Qualitative and Quantitative Deficiencies

Type of PS Deficiency	PS Activity	PS Free Antigen	PS Total Antigen	C4bBP
I Quantitative	<65%	<65%	<65%	Normal
II Qualitative	<65%	>65%	>65%	Normal
III Inflammation	<65%	<65%	>65%	Elevated

C4bBP, C4b-binding protein; *PS,* protein S.

ARTERIAL THROMBOSIS PREDICTORS

Arterial thrombotic disease, including peripheral vascular occlusion, AMI (heart attack), and cerebrovascular ischemia (stroke), arises from atherosclerotic plaque. Eruption of unstable plaque mediates platelet-driven thrombosis formation. The traditional predictors of arterial thrombosis risk are elevated total cholesterol (TC) and low-density lipoprotein cholesterol (LDL-C), or an elevated ratio of total cholesterol to high-density lipoprotein cholesterol (TC:HDL-C) secondary to HDL-C deficiency. One third of primary cardiovascular and cerebrovascular events occur in patients whose lipid profiles are normal, however, and half of people with proven lipid risk factors never experience an arterial thrombotic event.

Researchers have sought additional arterial thrombosis predictors by performing prospective randomized studies of lipoprotein subtypes and markers of inflammation. Additional research investigations, relevant to hemostasis, encompass studies on fibrinolytic pathway components—in particular, elevated PAI-1 and thrombin activatable fibrinolysis inhibitor (TAFI); fibrinogen, factor VIII, and von Willebrand factor, which become elevated with inflammation; and activated platelets. Patients with arterial thrombosis are customarily treated with statins to reduce hyperlipidemia, with anti-inflammatories, and anti-platelet drugs.

Lipoprotein (a)

Lipoprotein "little A" (a) is low-density lipoprotein that may predict arterial thrombosis. The plasma level is measured by EIA. Although lipoprotein (a) concentrations are higher in African Americans than in European Americans, elevation is a stronger predictor of arterial thrombosis in Caucasians.[82]

Lipoprotein (a) may contribute to thrombosis by its antifibrinolytic property. The molecule competes with plasminogen for binding sites on newly formed fibrin polymer, decreasing the plasmin activity available for clot degradation. It also may contribute to the overall concentration of LDL-C. Statin drugs may reduce levels of lipoprotein (a) and LDL-C.

C-Reactive Protein

CRP is a calcium-dependent pentameric ligand-binding member of the pentraxin family. It is produced in the liver and circulates in plasma at a concentration less than 0.55 mg/L. First described in 1930, CRP is an acute phase reactant whose plasma concentration rises 1000-fold 6 to 8 hours after the onset of an inflammatory event such as an infection, trauma, or surgery. This rise remains stable over several days in vivo; the protein is resistant to in vitro degradation.[83]

Extremely high CRP levels are identified using one of several time-honored manual semiquantitative laboratory assays performed on a slide or card, all of which employ *polyclonal* anti-CRP antibodies that coat a suspension of visible latex particles. Laboratory professionals continue to use this simple and inexpensive assay in place of the erythrocyte sedimentation rate test to confirm acute inflammation and monitor the effectiveness of anti-inflammatory therapy.[84] A second CRP assay, high-sensitivity CRP (HSCRP), was developed in the late 1990s and is used to document modest but chronic CRP elevation. Various types of

immunoassays are available to quantitate HSCRP such as the automated latex microparticle immunoassay that employs *monoclonal* antibodies.

Chronic plasma CRP concentrations that remain at 1.5 mg/L or greater indicate atherosclerosis and low-grade inflammation that correlate to increased risk of myocardial infarction and stroke.[85] Consequently, HSCRP is a valid clinical measure, independent from the lipid profile, employed to predict cardiovascular or cerebrovascular disease.[86] HSCRP may also be used in relationship with TC and the TC:HDL-C ratio to establish myocardial infarction risk. Laboratory professionals may also use HSCRP to monitor the anti-inflammatory effects of statins.[87]

Fibrinogen Activity

Laboratory professionals measure fibrinogen using immunoassay, nephelometry, or the Clauss clot-based method to detect dysfibrinogenemia, hypofibrinogenemia, or afibrinogenemia (Chapter 41). The same assays may be used to detect chronic hyperfibrinogenemia, which correlates with relative risk of myocardial infarction in asymptomatic persons or patients with angina pectoris.[88] Relative risk triples from the lowest to the highest concentration of fibrinogen, and even chronic high-normal levels associate with increased risk. There also exists a correlation between fibrinogen and TC (Figure 39.9). High fibrinogen concentrations can be used to predict hypercholesterolemia and identify patients who are at high risk for new coronary events. In contrast, low normal fibrinogen levels are associated with low risk of cardiovascular events, even in people with high TC levels. Fibrinogen becomes integrated into atherothrombotic lesions and contributes to their thrombotic potential.

Although hyperfibrinogenemia predicts arterial thrombosis, the use of the fibrinogen assay for this purpose is limited. There are no independent therapeutic regimens that specifically lower fibrinogen, and no clinical trials suggest that fibrinogen reduction reverses the odds of thrombosis. Further, the various

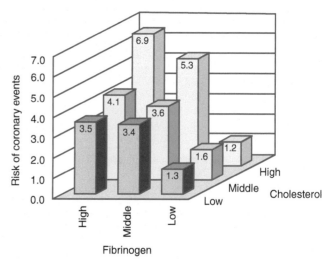

Figure 39.9 Coronary Thrombosis Risk Prediction By Fibrinogen and Cholesterol Concentrations. Fibrinogen and total cholesterol synergistically predict coronary risk. Tertiles of fibrinogen concentration are shown in relation to tertiles of total cholesterol concentration with the relative risk of coronary events indicated for each combination.

fibrinogen assay methods await harmonization. Nevertheless, statin therapy, smoking cessation, and exercise lower fibrinogen levels alongside LDL-C and TC levels, and the assay results parallel those for the other members of the risk prediction profile.

Plasma Homocysteine

Homocysteine is a naturally occurring sulfur-containing amino acid intermediate in the metabolism of dietary methionine. Fasting homocysteinemia is an independent risk factor for arterial thrombosis, with relative risk ratios of 1.7 for coronary artery disease, 2.5 for cerebrovascular disease, and 6.8 for peripheral artery disease.[89] Several theories link homocysteinemia with coronary artery disease, most citing damage to the endothelial cell.[90]

The enzyme 5,10-methylenetetrahydrofolate reductase (MTHFR) is required for the remethylation of homocysteine to methionine in the folic acid cycle. Common functional polymorphisms of the MTHFR gene raise plasma homocysteine; thus some thrombosis risk testing profiles include molecular assays for MTHFR, though MTHFR polymorphisms have not been empirically linked directly to thrombosis.

The reference intervals for homocysteine appear on the inside back cover of this text. Intervals differ for men and women, and they rise with age. Homocysteine levels are affected by dietary folate, vitamin B_6, and vitamin B_{12}. In industrialized countries, grains are supplemented with folate, primarily to reduce the risk of fetal neural tube closure (spina bifida) defects, reducing the overall prevalence of hyperhomocysteinemia.

Factor VIII

Factor VIII assays are designed to detect factor VIII deficiency and may lack accuracy at levels greater than the upper limit of the reference interval, typically 150 U/dL. Like fibrinogen, coagulation factor VIII is an acute phase reactant; consequently, an isolated case of elevated factor VIII may relate to acute inflammation and provide little thrombosis risk predictive value. However, chronically elevate factor VIII, like chronic hyperfibrinogenemia, may predict both arterial and venous thrombosis.

VENOUS THROMBOEMBOLIC DISEASE DIAGNOSIS

VTE, which comprises DVT and PE, is the third most common thrombotic disease, just after ACS and stroke. PE causes 100,000 to 180,000 US deaths per year, many of which occur within minutes of initial symptoms.[91] DVT and PE present specific diagnostic challenges that are addressed through the D-dimer assay.[92]

Deep Venous Thrombosis Symptoms

The cardinal symptoms for DVT are edema, erythema, pain, and the sensation of heat. Depending on clot location, symptoms may involve the entire leg, calf, or ankle and foot. Often the sufferer first misidentifies DVT as muscle strain or a "charley horse"; however, the symptoms persist and grow over several days.

When symptoms are ambiguous, the clinician may apply the Wells DVT scoring system.[93] One point each is scored for cancer, paralysis or recent plaster cast of lower extremities, bed rest for longer than 3 days or surgery within the previous 4 weeks, pain upon palpation of deep veins, swelling of the entire leg, diameter of the affected calf exceeding that of the unaffected calf by 3 cm or more, pitting edema, and dilated superficial veins. Two points are deducted for a compelling alternate diagnosis. A score of zero eliminates the diagnosis of DVT, 1 or 2 points signals intermediate or equivocal pre-test probability, 3 or more signal a high probability. The differential diagnosis for DVT includes superficial thrombophlebitis, ruptured Baker cyst, cellulitis, venous insufficiency, varicose veins, erythema nodosum, or postphlebitic syndrome.

Pulmonary Embolism Symptoms

Owing to the diagnostic predisposition toward acute coronary syndrome, clinicians attempt to maintain a heightened PE suspicion. PE symptoms include dyspnea, shortness of breath, syncope, transient cyanosis, tachycardia, pleuritic pain, and distended neck veins. Physicians apply the Wells PE scoring system (separate from the Wells DVT scoring system).[94] Wells criteria include current signs and symptoms of DVT, pulse greater than 100, immobilization or surgery within previous 4 weeks, prior PE or DVT, hemoptysis, or cancer. Other clinical scoring systems exist; all report one of two categories: PE likely, PE unlikely.

Deep Venous Thrombosis and Pulmonary Embolism Diagnostic Tests: D-Dimer

Using a clinical scoring system, high DVT or PE pre-test probability triggers non-invasive imaging tests. Ultrasonography is effective for most DVT cases, whereas "multislice" or spiral chest computed tomography (CT) angiography is the reference method for PE. The CT scan readily distinguishes PE from pneumonia, pleurisy, and ACS, supporting the differential diagnosis.

For low or intermediate pre-test probability scores, the plasma *D-dimer* assay is chosen over imaging for its robust sensitivity and negative predictive index. The D-dimer is "promiscuous," rising in response to all acute inflammatory conditions, especially ACS, congestive heart failure, pneumonia, sepsis, cancer, surgery, or pregnancy. For this reason, the D-dimer cannot be employed to "rule in" DVT or PE; however, a normal D-dimer reliably rules out either condition without the need for imaging when the pre-test probability score is low. If the D-dimer is negative, the clinician considers alternative diagnoses.

The plasma D-dimer assay is reported in *D-dimer units* (DDUs) or *fibrinogen equivalent units* (FEUs), depending on the nature of the monoclonal antibody (MAB) employed in the selected kit. One manufacturer's automated D-dimer MAB binds a form of D-dimer that is crosslinked through FDP "E" fragments (the D-E-D unit), yielding a molecular weight of 340,000 Daltons. The automated D-dimer assays of competing manufacturers' MABs detect D-D fragments of 170,000 Daltons (Figure 35.18). Consequently the typical FEU decision limit is 500 ng/mL, whereas the DDU "cutoff" is often 240 ng/mL. In general, FEU results are about 1.7 times greater than DDU results; however, small differences exist in MAB specificity, and thus laboratory directors establish local limits and discourage a simple multiplying conversion between reporting methods. While maintaining DDU and FEU distinctions, individual laboratory directors may choose to express results in milligrams per milliliter, milligrams per deciliter, or other units, a historical circumstance that demands ongoing laboratory-clinician communication and establishes a need for harmonization.

Further, D-dimer levels rise with advancing age, moving physicians to request that the laboratory provide age-adjusted limits for people older than 50. When reporting in FEUs, age adjustment relies on multiplication of age by 10 FEUs in nanograms per milliliter; thus the limit at age 60 would be 600 ng/mL FEUs, 700 ng/mL at age 70, and so on.[95] Those who use a kit that reports in DDUs may choose to use age times 5 DDUs in ng/mL, thus 300 and 350 DDUs in ng/mL for ages 60 and 70, respectively. This approach is discouraged because age-related limit studies were performed using FEUs and there doesn't exist a precise doubling relationship.

DISSEMINATED INTRAVASCULAR COAGULATION

DIC, also named defibrination syndrome or consumption coagulopathy, is generalized and uncontrolled hemostasis activation secondary to a systemic disorder. DIC is the "Black Death" of the Middle Ages, and it involves all hemostatic systems: vascular intima, platelets, leukocytes, coagulation pathways, coagulation control pathways, and fibrinolysis.[96] DIC is microangiopathic, a condition in which fibrin microthrombi form in and occlude small vessels where they consume platelets, coagulation factors, coagulation control proteins, and fibrinolytic enzymes. Microangiopathic pathology produces schistocytes (Figure 16.1) visible on peripheral blood films. Fibrin/fibrinogen degradation products (FDPs), including D-dimer, become elevated and interfere with normal fibrin formation as they coat platelets and fibrin.[97] This combination of events sets loose a series of toxic and inflammatory processes with secretion of the proinflammatory cytokines tumor necrosis factor-α (TNF-α), interleukin-1β (IL-1β), and IL-6.[98]

DIC may be *acute and uncompensated*, with deficiencies of multiple hemostasis components, or *chronic*, with slightly reduced, normal, or even elevated clotting factor levels. In chronic DIC, liver coagulation factor production and bone marrow platelet production incompletely compensate for consumption. Although DIC is a thrombotic process, the thrombi that form are small and ineffective, so systemic hemorrhage is often the first or most apparent symptom. Acute DIC is fatal in 25% to 50% of cases, depending on cause, and requires immediate medical intervention. DIC diagnosis relies heavily on the hemostasis laboratory, and medical laboratory professionals often perform a DIC profile under emergent circumstances.

Causes of DIC

Any disorder that contributes hemostatic molecules or promotes their endogenous secretion may cause DIC. Listing and classifying all the causes of DIC is impractical, but the major triggering mechanisms and examples of each are listed in Table 39.6.

TABLE 39.6   Disseminated Intravascular Coagulation-Associated Conditions by Mechanism

Mechanism That Induces DIC	Examples of Conditions
Tissue factor is released into circulation through endothelial cell damage or monocyte activation	Physical trauma: crush or brain injuries, surgery Degradation of muscle; rhabdomyolysis Tissue ischemia; myocardial infarction Thermal injuries: burns or cold Adenocarcinoma Acute inflammation
Exposure of subendothelial tissue factor during vasodilatation	Hypovolemic and hemorrhagic shock Malignant hypertension Asphyxia and hypoxia Heat stroke Vasculitis
Endotoxins that activate cytokines	Bacterial, protozoal, fungal, and viral infections, septicemia Toxic shock syndrome
Circulating immune complexes	Heparin-induced thrombocytopenia with thrombosis Drugs that trigger an immune response Acute hemolytic transfusion reactions Allergic reactions and anaphylaxis Bacterial and viral infections Graft rejection
Particulate matter from tissue injury	Eclampsia, preeclampsia, HELLP syndrome Retained dead fetus or missed abortion Amniotic fluid embolism Abruptio placentae Rupture of uterus Tubal pregnancy Fat embolism Heatstroke
Infusion of activated clotting factors	Activated prothrombin complex concentrate therapy
Secretion of proteolytic enzymes	Acute promyelocytic or myelomonocytic leukemia Bacterial, protozoal, fungal, and viral infections Pancreatitis
Toxins that trigger coagulation	Snake or spider envenomation Pancreatitis
Thrombotic disease or thrombogenic conditions	Thrombotic thrombocytopenic purpura, hemolytic uremic syndrome Pregnancy, postpartum period, estrogen therapy Deep vein thrombosis, pulmonary embolus Coagulation control system deficiencies Purpura fulminans, skin necrosis
Severe hypoxia or acidosis	Trauma-induced coagulopathy Chronic inflammation Diabetes mellitus
Platelet activation	Vascular surgery, coronary artery bypass surgery Thrombocytosis, thrombocythemia, polycythemia Vascular tumors Vascular prostheses Aortic aneurysm

HELLP, **H**emolysis, **e**levated **l**iver enzymes, and **l**ow **p**latelet count.

Chronic DIC may be associated with tissue necrosis, liver disease, renal disease, chronic inflammation, vascular prostheses, vascular tumors, and adenocarcinoma. The malignancies most associated with DIC are pancreatic, prostatic, ovarian, and lung cancers; multiple myeloma; acute promyelocytic leukemia, and myeloproliferative neoplasms. Trousseau syndrome, first described in 1865, is a term for tumor-induced chronic DIC that generates DVT and migrating sub-epithelial thromboses causing ecchymosis and purpura fulminans.[99] Trousseau syndrome is difficult to manage and may be the first symptom of previously undocumented adenocarcinoma.

The more acutely ill the patient, the more dangerous the DIC's pathology. Acute DIC is seen in association with obstetric emergencies, intravascular hemolysis, septicemia, viremia, burns, acute inflammation, crush injuries, dissecting aortic aneurysms, and cardiac disorders.

Pathophysiology of DIC

Tissue damage, endothelial damage, endothelial exposure to bacterial products, and exposure of blood to the subendothelium releases tissue factor, triggering the extrinsic pathway at the level of factor VII and activating platelets. Exposure to TNF-α, IL-1β, hemolysis, and cell necrosis triggers activation of factor XII and the intrinsic pathway. The osmotic imbalance of shock and endothelial exposure to TNF-α and IL-6 trigger the release of tissue plasminogen activator (TPA), activating plasminogen. Although extrinsic coagulation pathway activation dominates, these events occur simultaneously, and once triggered, DIC proceeds in a predictable sequence. Circulating thrombin becomes the primary culprit because it further activates platelets and coagulation factors, leading to fibrin formation (Chapter 35). Thrombin further activates fibrinolysis, resulting in expression of free plasmin.

Thrombin cleaves fibrinogen, producing fibrin monomers. In normal hemostasis, fibrin monomers spontaneously polymerize to form an insoluble gel that binds plasmin during its formation (Figure 35.9). The polymer becomes strengthened through factor XIII-mediated cross-linking. In DIC a percentage of fibrin monomers fail to polymerize and circulate in plasma as soluble fibrin monomers. The monomers coat platelets and coagulation proteins, creating an anticoagulant effect that prolongs the thrombin clotting time (TCT, TT), PT, and PTT assays.

Thrombin, soluble fibrin monomers, fibrin polymer, and cross-linked fibrin all activate plasminogen to form active *plasmin.* Normally, plasmin functions locally to digest only the solid fibrin clot to which it is bound (Chapter 35). In DIC, as a result of antiplasmin consumption, plasmin circulates in the plasma and digests all forms of fibrinogen and fibrin (Figure 35.18).[100] Consequently, FDPs labeled X, Y, D, E, and D-dimer are detectable in the plasma in concentrations exceeding 20,000 ng/mL. D-dimer arises from cross-linked fibrin polymer, whereas the other FDPs may be produced from fibrinogen or fibrin monomers or polymers.[101]

Platelets become enmeshed in the fibrin polymer or are exposed to thrombin; both events trigger platelet activation, which further drives coagulation and is reflected in moderate thrombocytopenia. Concurrently, coagulation pathway control is lost as PC, PS, and AT are consumed. The combination of thrombin activation, circulating plasmin, loss of control, and thrombocytopenia contributes to the overall hemorrhagic outcome.

Free plasmin digests factors V, VIII, IX, and XI, as well as other plasma proteins. Thrombin and plasmin also may trigger the complement pathway, which leads to hemolysis, and the kinin system, which results in inflammation, hypotension, and shock.

During fibrinolytic therapy, in late-phase cardiopulmonary bypass surgery, liver disease and transplant surgery, trauma, and amyloidosis, plasminogen sometimes becomes activated independent of the coagulation pathway. This rare condition, called systemic fibrinolysis or primary fibrinolysis, produces laboratory-measurable fibrinogen and FDPs, including D-dimer, and prolongs the PT and PTT with a normal platelet count.[102]

Symptoms of DIC

The symptoms signaling DIC often are masked by the symptoms of the underlying disorder and may be chronic, acute, or even fulminant. Ischemia of major organ microvasculature produces symptoms of organ dysfunction such as renal function impairment, acute respiratory distress syndrome, and central nervous system manifestations such as sudden vision loss or seizures. Skin, bone, and bone marrow necrosis may be seen. Purpura and ecchymoses leading to purpura fulminans (Chapter 38) are seen in meningococcemia, chickenpox, and spirochete infections.

Laboratory Diagnosis of DIC

DIC is foremost a clinical diagnosis that requires speedy laboratory confirmation (Chapter 41). The initial laboratory profile includes a platelet count, blood film examination (Chapters 12 and 13), PT, PTT, TT, fibrinogen assay, and D-dimer. Table 39.7 lists anticipated DIC laboratory results. Prolonged PT and PTT reflect coagulation factor consumption in 50% to 75% of cases. Fibrinogen may decrease in DIC, but because fibrinogen levels rise in inflammation, the fibrinogen concentration alone provides little reliable diagnostic information. The platelet count and peripheral blood film platelet estimate confirm thrombocytopenia in 90% of cases, though the platelet count remains greater than 30,000 to 40,000/μL, and the presence of schistocytes, denoting microangiopathic hemolytic anemia (MAHA), helps establish the diagnosis of DIC in 50% of cases.[103]

The D-dimer reference limit is typically 240 DDU ng/mL or 500 FEU ng/mL. In 85% of DIC cases, D-dimer levels reach 10,000 to 20,000 ng/mL. A normal D-dimer assay result rules out DIC.[104] D-dimer concentrations are typically elevated in VTE, inflammation, sickle cell crisis, pregnancy, and renal disease, so an abnormal result alone cannot be used to definitively diagnose DIC.[105] The PT, PTT, TT, fibrinogen assay, platelet count, and blood film examination must be performed alongside the D-dimer to rule out other disorders.

The time-honored semiquantitative FDP assay may be used in acute care settings or in under-resourced locations. FDP results reflect D-dimer results.

TABLE 39.7   Anticipated Results of Disseminated Intravascular Coagulation (DIC) Primary Laboratory Profile

Test	Reference Interval	Typical Value in DIC
Platelet count	150,000–450,000/μL	<150,000/μL
Peripheral blood film exam	Anemia with schistocytes	Schistocytes (MAHA) are present in 50% of DIC cases; leukocytosis is common.
PT	11–14 sec	>14 sec
PTT	25–35 sec	>35 sec
Thrombin time, reptilase time	Prolonged	Fibrinogen levels <80 mg/dL, elevated FDPs, and soluble fibrin monomer all prolong thrombin time and reptilase time.
D-dimer	0–240 ng/mL DDU or 0–500 ng/mL FEU	>240 ng/mL DDU or >500 ng/mL FEU, often 10,000–20,000 ng/mL
Fibrinogen	220–498 mg/dL	<220 mg/dL, often higher, because fibrinogen is an acute phase reactant

DDU, D-dimer units; *FDP*, fibrin degradation products; *FEU*, fibrinogen equivalent units; *MAHA*, microangiopathic hemolytic anemia; *PT*, prothrombin time; *PTT*, partial thromboplastin time

Specialized Laboratory Tests for DIC

Table 39.8 lists specialized laboratory tests that may be used to further diagnose and classify DIC.[106] Results consistent with DIC and clinical comments are included. Many of these tests are available in acute care facilities, but they are not routinely applied to the diagnosis of DIC. Others are available only in tertiary care facilities and specialized hemostasis reference laboratories.[107]

PC, PS, and AT are consumed in DIC, and their assay may contribute to the diagnosis. When plasma or AT concentrate

TABLE 39.8   Specialized Laboratory Assays to Assist in the Diagnosis of Disseminated Intravascular Coagulation (DIC)

Assay	Value in DIC	Comments
Protein C, protein S, and AT activity assays	<50%	Use to monitor plasma, AT concentrate
Serum FDP	>10 μg/mL	Largely replaced by quantitative D-dimer
Plasminogen, tissue plasminogen activator, plasminogen activator inhibitior-1	Decreased	May be useful for analyzing systemic fibrinolysis; specimen management protocol must be strictly observed
Soluble fibrin monomer	Positive	Hemagglutination assay
Factor assays: II (prothrombin), V, VIII, X	<30%	Factors V and VIII rise in inflammation; assays may give misleading results

AT, Antithrombin; *FDP*, fibrin degradation products; *MAHA*, microangiopathic hemolytic anemia.

(Thrombate III) is used to treat DIC, the AT assay is used to establish the necessity for therapy and monitor its effect.[108] Factor assays may clarify PT and PTT results.

Tests of the fibrinolytic pathway include chromogenic plasminogen activity assay and TPA and PAI-1 immunoassays.[109] These tests are seldom offered in the acute care hemostasis laboratory because they require meticulous specimen management, but they may help in the diagnosis of primary fibrinolysis.

Differential Diagnosis of DIC

Hemostasis laboratory assays cannot distinguish DIC from severe liver disease. Whereas in DIC, coagulation factors and controls, platelets, and the components of fibrinolysis are consumed, in advanced liver disease their production is diminished. In liver disease, D-dimers rise in response to inflammation and diminished hepatic clearance. The clinician must base the diagnosis and management on history, symptoms, and liver enzyme assays.[110]

Dilutional coagulopathy may occasionally resemble DIC, prolonging the PT, PTT, and TT, and reducing the platelet count. Treatment of severe hemorrhage with plasma, cryoprecipitate, red blood cells, and platelet concentrate causes dilutional coagulopathy. The clinician distinguishes DIC from dilutional coagulopathy on the basis of recent history. In shock secondary to trauma, hypotension, acidosis, and hypothermia lead to DIC, which may coexist with dilutional coagulopathy.[111]

Obstetric complications pre-eclampsia, eclampsia, acute fatty liver of pregnancy, and HELLP syndrome (**h**emolysis, **e**levated **l**iver function tests, and **l**ow **p**latelets) may all mimic DIC laboratory results and must be resolved on the basis of history and symptoms. Resolution in all these cases calls for early delivery of the fetus and placenta.[112]

Thrombotic thrombocytopenic purpura (TTP) and its sibling, hemolytic-uremic syndrome (HUS) (Chapter 38), both platelet activation-based microangiopathic thrombosis disorders, may resemble DIC in symptoms and laboratory results. In both disorders, however, the PT, PTT, and TT remain relatively normal while the platelet count drops to as low as 40,000 to 50,000/μL. Clinically, DIC arises from an existing condition, whereas TTP arises in individuals with no identifiable primary disorder.

Treatment of DIC

To arrest DIC the physician must diagnose and treat the underlying disorder. Surgery, antiinflammatory agents, antibiotics, or obstetric procedures as appropriate may normalize hemostasis without requiring efforts to directly correct the coagulopathy. Supportive therapy, such as maintenance of fluid and electrolyte balance, always accompanies medical and surgical management.

In acute DIC, where ischemic multiorgan dysfunction and bleeding threaten the life of the patient, heroic measures are necessary. Treatment involves therapies that slow the clotting process and therapies that replace missing platelets and coagulation factors.

UFH may be used for its anti-thrombotic properties to stop the uncontrolled activation of the coagulation cascade. Because

UFH aggravates bleeding, careful dosing, observation, and support are required. Periodic chromogenic anti-factor Xa heparin assays are necessary to control UFH dosage because in DIC the PTT is ineffective (non-specific) for monitoring heparin therapy.

Plasma provides all the necessary coagulation factors and replaces blood volume lost during acute DIC hemorrhage. Prothrombin complex concentrate (Proplex T complex, Baxter; or Kcentra, Behring), fibrinogen concentrate (RiaSTAP, Behring), and factor VIII concentrate (ADVATE, Baxter) may be used in place of plasma, particularly if there is concern for transfusion-associated circulatory overload. Periodic fibrinogen, PT, PTT, and TT assays are necessary to confirm the effectiveness of these therapeutics.[113] Platelet transfusions are necessary when thrombocytopenia is severe. Platelet counts are used to monitor the effectiveness of platelet concentrate and platelet consumption (Chapters 12 and 13). Red blood cells are administered as necessary to treat the resulting anemia. Antifibrinolytic therapy is contraindicated, except in proven systemic fibrinolysis.[114]

HEPARIN-INDUCED THROMBOCYTOPENIA

Heparin-induced thrombocytopenia (HIT) is the consequence of an immune response to UFH (standard intravenous heparin) and LMWH that is reflected in a reduced platelet count.[115] HIT may progress to venous and arterial thrombosis. The incidence of HIT as a response to UFH therapy is 0.5% to 5%. The risk for HIT in LMWH therapy in patients with major surgery is 1% to 10% the risk of its occurrence in response to UFH.[116] Risk

levels depend on the diagnosis, medical or surgical history, obstetric events, and the patient's general health. The incidence of HIT also relates to duration and dosage of heparin therapy, though there are published cases in which HIT follows a single dose or even the incidental use of heparin to flush a line.[117] Arterial and venous thromboembolic complications include deep vein thrombosis, PE, myocardial infarction, thrombotic stroke, limb ischemia, vein graft occlusion, and injection site skin lesions.[118] Mortality among patients with thrombosis rises to 30%, and up to 20% of those who survive require amputation.[119] HIT diagnosis and treatment is complex, as 30% of patients who are receiving heparin develop mild thrombocytopenia with no additional consequence. Nevertheless, HIT must be considered with a high index of suspicion in the clinical management of patients exposed to UFH and LMWH because of its grave outcomes.[120]

Pathophysiology of HIT

HIT involves platelet activation, inflammation, and thrombosis.[121] HIT antibodies are specific for *platelet factor 4 (PF4) complexed with heparin* (UFH or LMWH).[122] PF4 is a positively charged tetrameric protein stored in alpha granules. When exposed, the charged amino acids on the PF4 protein bind negatively charged heparin to form H:PF4.[123] H:PF4 is a hapten that triggers immune production of IgG isotype anti-H:PF4 antibodies that now bind the H:PF4, targeting a neoepitope on PF4 that is expressed with heparin binding. The Fc portion of the resultant IgG:H:PF4 immune complex binds platelet FcγIIa receptors, activating platelets and releasing additional

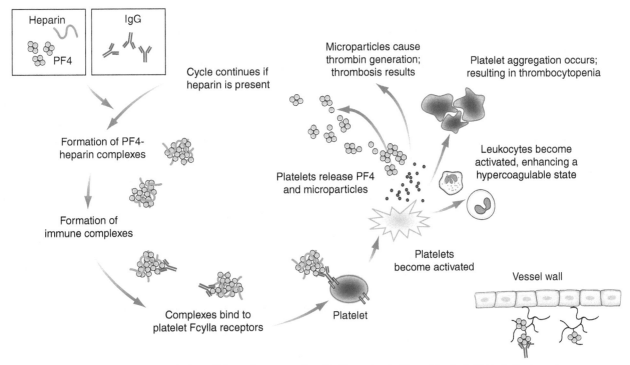

Figure 39.10 Heparin-induced Thrombocytopenia with Thrombosis. The antibody *(IgG)* binds the heparin-platelet factor 4 complex in plasma or on the platelet membrane. The Fc portion of the antibody binds monocyte or platelet Fc receptors causing cellular activation. The activated platelets release procoagulant microparticles and aggregate to form platelet thrombi in the arterial or venous circulation. Platelet activation releases additional PF4 from granular stores contributing to continuation of the cycle if heparin is present.

PF4, initiating a cycle of platelet activation that generates pro-coagulant platelet microparticles (Figure 39.10).[124] Sustained platelet activation contributes to platelet clearance, and platelet microparticles generate thrombin, resulting in thrombocytopenia and HIT-associated thrombosis.[125]

HIT antibodies also recognize PF4 bound to cell membranes.[126] For instance, the endothelial cell glycosaminoglycan heparan sulfate binds PF4, forming an H:PF4-like complex recognized by HIT antibodies.[127] The reaction triggers an inflammatory state in which endothelial cells, macrophages, monocytes, and neutrophils release tissue factor, PAI-1, and cytokines.[128] Inflammatory adhesion molecules promote additional platelet and monocyte binding.[129] The interrelationships of platelets, leukocytes, the endothelium, and inflammatory cytokines determine the clinical expression of HIT and may provide loci for thrombus formation.[130-132]

Platelet Counts and Clinical Scoring for HIT

Early diagnosis demands a comprehensive interpretation of clinical and laboratory information. Surveillance begins with consecutive platelet counts, at least once every 48 hours during and after therapy.[133] Hematologists customarily define HIT-related thrombocytopenia as a 30% to 50% drop in platelet count from the pre-heparin level.[134] The resultant platelet count may remain within the reference interval, though in most cases the count falls to less than 150,000/μL, the lower limit of the reference interval, or even less than 100,000/μL. HIT patients rarely experience bleeding. In de novo HIT, the count begins to fall 5 to 10 days after heparin therapy is initiated, but if the patient has had heparin less than 120 days prior to the current therapy, thrombocytopenia may appear within hours. Delayed HIT may appear up to 30 days subsequent to discontinuation of therapy.

Thrombosis, which occurs in 30% of heparin-treated patients with thrombocytopenia, is a significant HIT signal. Patients with thrombocytopenia but without thrombosis at discharge continue with a 50% risk of thrombosis within 30 days subsequent to the initial platelet count fall.

Clinicians employ platelet counts and thrombosis in the 4Ts scoring system to evaluate the initial likelihood of HIT (Table 39.9).[135] Best practices dictate that scoring is essential prior to specialized HIT testing. There are many causes of thrombocytopenia in hospitalized patients; scoring improves diagnosis and management while preserving resources and reducing patient risk. The 4Ts system generates low, intermediate, and high probability scores.[136] Low scores provide reliable negative predictive value, whereas intermediate or high 4T scores make it necessary to employ advanced laboratory methods.

The HIT Expert Probability (HEP) score is an alternative that further evaluates thrombosis and other causes of thrombocytopenia.[137] A separate scoring system for cardiopulmonary bypass patients assesses the timing and extent of platelet count decline and duration of extra-corporeal circulation.[138]

Enzyme Immunoassays for HIT

Clinicians assess specialized HIT assay results with reference to the clinical context to avoid false positive conclusions that lead to expensive alternative anticoagulants with increased bleeding risk.[139] Clinicians, laboratorians, and pharmacists meet to develop comprehensive diagnostic and treatment algorithms that rely on scoring systems to enhance diagnostic accuracy and effective therapy.[140] Subsequent to scoring, HIT testing begins with manual EIA methods, available within many acute care facility laboratories, to determine whether antibodies to the H:PF4 complex are present.[141] Though unnecessary when the pre-test score is low, the combination of a low pre-test score and negative EIA HIT assay rules out HIT.

TABLE 39.9 The 4Ts Scoring System: Laboratory and Clinical Pretest Probability of Heparin-Induced Thrombocytopenia (HIT)

Indicator	SCORE		
	2	1	0
Acute thrombocytopenia	>50% decrease in platelet count to nadir of ≥20,000/μL	30%–50% decrease in platelet count, >50% if directly resulting from surgery, or to nadir of 10,000–19,000/μL	<30% decrease in platelet count, or to nadir of <10,000/μL
Timing of platelet count decrease, thrombosis, or other sequelae of HIT (first day of heparin therapy is day 0)	Onset of decrease on days 5–10, or onset of decrease on day 1 if previous heparin exposure within past 5–30 days	Apparent decrease on days 5–10, but unclear due to missing platelet counts; or decrease after day 10; or decrease on day 1 if previous heparin exposure within past 31–100 days	Decrease at ≤4 days without recent heparin exposure
Thrombosis, skin lesions, acute system reaction	Proven new thrombosis or skin necrosis; acute systemic reaction after heparin exposure	Progressive, recurrent, or suspected thrombosis; erythematous skin lesions	None
Other causes for thrombocytopenia	No explanation for platelet count decrease is evident	Possible other cause is evident	Probable other cause is evident

Maximum pretest probability score is 8; a score of 6 to 8 indicates high probability of HIT; 4 to 5, intermediate probability; 0 to 3, low probability. The most immunizing heparin exposure is considered first; unfractionated heparin (UFH) received during cardiac surgery is more immunogenic than UFH or low-molecular-weight heparin received for acute coronary syndrome. The day the platelet count begins to fall is considered the day of onset of thrombocytopenia. It generally takes 1 to 3 days before an arbitrary threshold that defines thrombocytopenia, such as 150,000 platelets/μL, is passed. From Crowther, M. A., Cook, D. J., Albert, M., et al. (2010). Canadian Critical Care Trials Group: The 4Ts scoring system for heparin-induced thrombocytopenia in medical-surgical intensive care unit patients. *J Crit Care, 25,* 287–293.

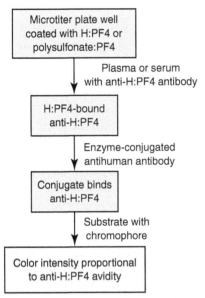

Figure 39.11 Enzyme Immunoassay for Heparin-Induced Thrombo-cytopenia *(HIT)*. The solid-phase target antigen is a complex of platelet factor 4 *(PF4)* and heparin or a heparin surrogate *(H)*. Anti-heparin/platelet factor 4 *(anti-H:PF4)* antibody in the patient plasma or serum binds the H:PF4 target and is bound in turn by enzyme-labeled anti-human antibody. The bound enzyme catalyzes the release of a chromophore from the anti-human antibody substrate; intensity of the chromophore color is proportional to the level of anti-H:PF4 antibody.

HIT EIAs employ solid phase antigen targets surrogate to the H:PF4 complex.[142] EIAs are sensitive and prone to a high false-positive rate and must be confirmed using more specific follow-up platelet-based functional assays (see Confirmatory Platelet Activation Assays for HIT). Though the anti-H:PF4 antibodies detectable by EIA are a critical part of the HIT mechanism, without platelet interaction they fail to trigger thrombosis. Non-thrombotic anti-H:PF4 antibodies are the source for EIA false-positive results.

The Lifecodes PF4 IgG (Immucor GTI) kit illustrates EIA technology. Patient plasma or serum is incubated in microtiter plate wells coated with a solid-phase complex of purified PF4 and polysulfonate, a heparin surrogate (Figure 39.11).

Anti-H:PF4 antibodies bind the polysulfonate:PF4 complex. Enzyme-conjugated anti-human IgG antibodies attach to the bound antibodies and a substrate chromophore is added. Manual EIA technology requires two intermediate washing phases and two one-hour incubation phases. The operator employs a plate reader to record the resultant color intensity of each well as semiquantitative absorbance or optical density units that are proportional to HIT antibody concentration and avidity. Manufacturers may provide a positive decision point in absorbance or optical density units, or local operators may establish their own. Besides initial testing subsequent to scoring, EIA methodology is used to monitor HIT patient progress during therapy.

Operators may follow up positive EIA results with a confirmatory step. They add high heparin buffers, typically 100 units/mL, displacing or blocking solid-phase PF4. They repeat the EIA from the beginning where a negative outcome confirms the heparin-dependent nature of the HIT antibody. It remains necessary to reflex to a functional assay.

Confirmatory Platelet Activation Assays for HIT

Positive EIA results are confirmed in a reflex-testing algorithm using a platelet function test, typically the washed platelet ^{14}C-serotonin release assay (SRA), available from a handful of high-quality specialized laboratories that possess isotope licenses.[143] Light transmittance platelet aggregometry using washed donor platelet-rich plasma was once an alternative that avoided radioactive labeling; however, the SRA offers superior sensitivity and is universally considered the reference assay (Figure 39.12).[144,145]

The SRA demonstrates the ability of the anti-H:PF4 HIT antibody to activate platelets in the presence of heparin. The operator obtains fresh platelet concentrate from a donor whose platelets demonstrated consistent reactivity in this assay. The platelets are washed in two special Tyrode buffers and labeled with ^{14}C-serotonin. Heparin and patient serum are added to the suspension, and platelet activation is reported by measurable ^{14}C-serotonin release, confirming HIT.

The operator continues to a high-concentration heparin confirmatory step similar to the EIA confirmatory step. Excess

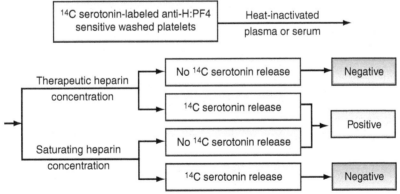

Figure 39.12 The Serotonin Release Assay *(SRA)* for Heparin-Induced Thrombocytopenia *(HIT)*. Donor platelets proven to be antiheparin/platelet factor 4 *(anti-H:PF4)* antibody sensitive are washed and labeled with ^{14}C-serotonin, then suspended in albumin-free Tyrode buffer. Heat-inactivated patient plasma or serum is added. Heparin is added to two aliquots in therapeutic (0.1 to 0.4 U/dL) and saturating concentrations (100 U/dL), respectively. Release of radioactive serotonin in the therapeutic aliquot compared to no release from the saturating aliquot confirms HIT. This pattern demonstrates H:PF4 antibody binding to and activating platelets in a heparin-dependent manner. Any platelet activation with saturating concentrations of heparin likely is due to nonspecific anti-platelet antibodies.

heparin does not allow for the conformation of the H:PF4 complexes that are recognized as an antigenic target by the HIT antibody. Thus there is no binding of the antibody to the platelet and no platelet activation. A negative response confirms the heparin-dependent nature of the HIT antibody.

Rapid Turnaround Assays for HIT

Because of their manual format and lengthy incubations, EIAs are batched and performed once a day, necessitating a 24-hour turnaround time.[146] The SRA is a send-out whose turnaround time may be 2 to 3 days. As HIT is an emergent diagnosis, clinicians make initial decisions to replace heparin therapy based solely on platelet count and the 4Ts (or other) scoring system, relying on advanced laboratory assays for subsequent confirmation.[147] Manufacturers have developed rapid turnaround HIT assays to alleviate the diagnostic stress.

In Europe, BioRad Laboratories offers a 20-minute gel-agglutination immunoassay that employs a suspension of colored polystyrene particles coated with heparin and human PF4. Patient serum is incubated with the particles. After centrifugation through a gel matrix, particles bound to anti-H:PF4 remain on top of or within the gel, visibly confirming the antibody.

Instrumentation Laboratory (IL) offers a 30-minute turn-around latex-based HemosIL HIT-Ab chemiluminescent assay approved for North American and European markets. HemosIL HIT-Ab is adapted to IL's automated coagulometers.

These and other rapid turnaround assays generate clinical efficacy statistics similar to or somewhat more favorable than manual EIA methods and may be used in conjunction with a scoring system to rule out HIT.[148] Positive results are confirmed by SRA. Developers continue to search for rapid turnaround methods with reliable false-negative and false-positive rates that can reduce reliance on the SRA assay.

Therapy for HIT

When the clinician is convinced of HIT, heparin therapy is stopped immediately. Effective alternatives are fondaparinux (Arixtra), argatroban, and bivalirudin (Angiomax), discussed in Chapter 40.[149] Though considered safe, these alternatives have a higher rate of serious bleeding that should be considered as part of the HIT therapeutic decision. Direct oral anticoagulant therapy portends new and potentially safer alternatives.[150,151]

THROMBOSIS RISK TESTING FUTURE

Before Dr. Dahlbäck described activated protein C resistance in 1993, the typical hemostasis laboratory existed only to monitor Coumadin and heparin and to diagnose and treat the occasional hemophilia or thrombocytopenia patient. Suddenly in 1994, with the advent of thrombosis risk testing for acquired and congenital clotting disorders in veins and arteries, hemostasis moved to center stage. Coagulationists could now assess risk, diagnose, and monitor treatment for a variety of thrombotic disorders whose resolution required a combination of laboratory and clinical science in close communication. Antithrombin, protein C, protein S, activated protein C resistance, factor V Leiden mutation, prothrombin 20210 mutation, HIT, and DIC, lost causes in 1992, are now managed successfully through precise laboratory assays directing pinpoint therapies. The near future will connect thrombophilia and thrombosis risk testing with chronic and acute inflammation, endothelial cell analyses, molecular diagnostics, high-throughput human genome studies, and cytokine libraries. The laboratory contribution will continue to make inroads into arterial disease and platelet hyperactivity and reduce the burden of chronic disease.

SUMMARY

- Thrombosis is the most prevalent condition in developed countries and accounts for most illnesses and premature death.
- Thrombosis may be arterial, causing peripheral artery disease, heart disease, and stroke, or venous, causing deep vein thrombosis and pulmonary emboli.
- Most thrombosis occurs as a result of disease, lifestyle habits and aging, but many thrombotic disorders are related to congenital risk factors.
- Thrombosis risk profiles may be offered to clinicians for screening purposes in high-risk populations.
- The main hemostasis predictors of arterial thrombotic disease are elevated levels of C-reactive protein (CRP, measured by high-sensitivity assay), homocysteine, fibrinogen, lipoprotein (a), and coagulation factors.
- The main hemostasis predictors of venous thromboembolic disease are antiphospholipid antibodies; antithrombin, protein C and protein S deficiencies; factor V Leiden mutation; and prothrombin G20210A.
- Antiphospholipid antibody testing requires a series of essential hemostasis laboratory assays—clot-based tests and immunoassays.

- Antithrombin may be assayed using chromogenic substrate and enzyme immunoassay analyses.
- The tests for evaluating the protein C pathway include protein C and protein S activity and concentration, activated protein C (APC) resistance, factor V Leiden (FVL) assay, and C4b-binding protein (C4bBP) assay.
- The molecular test for the prothrombin G20210A mutation predicts the risk of venous thrombosis.
- Disseminated intravascular coagulation (DIC) is a clinical diagnosis that requires laboratory confirmation using a series of assays in the acute care facility.
- The quantitative D-dimer assay may be used to rule out venous thromboembolic disease and to diagnose and monitor disseminated intravascular coagulation.
- Heparin-induced thrombocytopenia is often associated with thrombosis; its diagnosis requires high-complexity laboratory assays.

Now that you have completed this chapter, go back and read again the case study at the beginning and respond to the questions presented.

REVIEW QUESTIONS

Answers are found in the Appendix.

1. What is the prevalence of venous thrombosis in the United States?
   a. 0.01
   b. 1 in 1000
   c. 10% to 15%
   d. 500,000 cases per year

2. What is thrombophilia?
   a. Predisposition to thrombosis secondary to a congenital or acquired disorder
   b. Inappropriate triggering of the plasma coagulation system
   c. A condition in which clots form uncontrollably
   d. Inadequate fibrinolysis

3. What acquired thrombosis risk factor is assessed in the hemostasis laboratory?
   a. Smoking
   b. Immobilization
   c. Obesity
   d. Lupus anticoagulant

4. Trousseau syndrome, a low-grade chronic DIC, is often associated with what type of disorder?
   a. Renal disease
   b. Hepatic disease
   c. Adenocarcinoma
   d. Chronic inflammation

5. What is the most common heritable thrombosis risk factor in Caucasians?
   a. APC resistance (factor V Leiden mutation)
   b. Prothrombin G20210A mutation
   c. Antithrombin deficiency
   d. Protein S deficiency

6. In most LAC profiles, what test is primary (performed first) because it detects LAC with the least interference?
   a. Low-phospholipid PTT
   b. DRVVT
   c. KCT
   d. PT

7. A patient with venous thrombosis is tested for protein S deficiency. The protein S activity, antigen, and free antigen are all less than 65%, and the C4bBP level is normal. What type of deficiency is likely?
   a. Type I
   b. Type II
   c. Type III
   d. No deficiency is indicated, because the reference range includes 65%

8. An elevated level of what fibrinolytic system assay is associated with arterial thrombotic risk?
   a. PAI-1
   b. TPA
   c. Factor VIIa
   d. Factor XII

9. How does lipoprotein (a) cause thrombosis?
   a. It causes elevated factor VIII levels
   b. It coats the endothelial lining of arteries
   c. It substitutes for plasminogen or TPA in the forming clot
   d. It contributes additional phospholipid in vivo for formation of the tenase complex

10. What test may be used to *confirm* the presence of LAC?
    a. PT
    b. Bethesda titer
    c. Antinuclear antibody
    d. DRVVT using high-phospholipid reagent

11. What molecular test may be used to *confirm* APC resistance?
    a. Prothrombin G20210A
    b. MTHFR 1298
    c. MTHFR 677
    d. Factor V Leiden

12. What therapeutic agent may occasionally cause DIC?
    a. Factor VIII
    b. Factor VIIa
    c. Antithrombin concentrate
    d. Activated prothrombin complex concentrate

13. Which is *not* a fibrinolysis control protein?
    a. Thrombin-activatable fibrinolysis inhibitor
    b. Plasminogen activator inhibitor-1
    c. α_2-Antiplasmin
    d. D-dimer

14. What is the most important application of the quantitative D-dimer test?
    a. Diagnose primary fibrinolysis
    b. Diagnose liver and renal disease
    c. Rule out deep venous thrombosis
    d. Diagnose acute myocardial infarction

15. What is the first laboratory assay necessary to detect heparin-induced thrombocytopenia?
    a. Platelet count
    b. H:PF4 immunoassay
    c. Quick turnaround test
    d. Serotonin release assay

REFERENCES

1. Francis, J. L. (1998). Laboratory investigation of hypercoagulability. *Semin Thromb Hemost, 24,* 111–126.
2. Dahlback, B., Carlsson, M., & Svensson, P. J. (1993). Familial thrombophilia due to a previously unrecognized mechanism characterized by poor anticoagulant response to activated protein C: prediction of a cofactor to activated protein C. *Proc Natl Acad Sci U S A, 90,* 1004–1008.
3. Bertina, R. M., Koeleman, B. P. C., Koster, T., et al. (1994). Mutation in blood coagulation factor V associated with resistance to activated protein C. *Nature, 369,* 64–67.
4. Yamaguchi, T., Wada, H., Miyazaki, S., et al. (2016). Fibrin-related markers for diagnosing acute-, subclinical-, and pre-venous

thromboembolism in patients with major orthopedic surgery. *Int J Hematol, 103,* 560–566.

5. Heit, J. A. (2013). Thrombophilia: clinical and laboratory assessment and management. In Kitchens, C. S., Kessler, C. M., & Konkle, B. A. (Eds.), *Consultative Hemostasis and Thrombosis* (3rd ed., pp. 205–239). Philadelphia: Saunders.

6. Mozaffarian, D., Benjamin, E. J., Go, A. S., et al. (2015). Heart disease and stroke statistics—2015 update: a report from the American Heart Association. *Circulation, 131,* e29-e322.

7. Heit, J. A. (2008). The epidemiology of venous thromboembolism in the community. *Arterioscler Thromb Vasc Biol, 28,* 370–372.

8. Zöller, B., Li, X., Sundquist, J., et al. (2012). Shared familial aggregation of susceptibility to different manifestations of venous thromboembolism: a nationwide family study in Sweden. *Br J Haematol, 157,* 146–148.

9. Olaf, M., & Cooney, R. (2017). Deep venous thrombosis. *Emerg Med Clin North Am, 35,* 743–770.

10. Giordano, N. J., Jansson, P. S., Young, M. N., et al. (2017). Epidemiology, pathophysiology, stratification, and natural history of pulmonary embolism. *Tech Vasc Interv Radiol, 20,* 135–140.

11. Rosendaal, F. R., & Reitsma, P. H. (2009). Genetics of venous thrombosis. *J Thromb Haemost, 7*(Suppl. 1), 301–304.

12. Kochanek, K. D., Murphy, S. L., & Xu, J. (2016). National vital statistics report. Deaths: final data for 2014. *National Vital Statistics System, 54*(4), 1–22.

13. Vemulapalli, S., & Becker, R. C. (2013). Hemostatic aspects of cardiovascular medicine. In Kitchens, C. S., Kessler, C. M., & Konkle, B. A. (Eds.), *Consultative Hemostasis and Thrombosis* (3rd ed., pp. 342–394). Philadelphia: Saunders.

14. Office of the Surgeon General. (2008). *The Surgeon General's Call to Action to Prevent Deep Vein Thrombosis and Pulmonary Embolism.* Rockville, MD: Office of the Surgeon General. http://www.ncbi.nlm.nih.gov/books/NBK44178/. Accessed December 11, 2017.

15. Piazza, G., & Goldhaber, S. Z. (2010). Venous thromboembolism and atherothrombosis: an integrated approach. *Circulation, 121,* 2146–2150.

16. Rand, J. H., & Wolgast, L. R. (2013). Antiphospholipid syndrome: pathogenesis, clinical presentation, diagnosis, and patient management. In Kitchens, C. S., Kessler, C. M., Konkle, B. A. (Eds.), *Consultative Hemostasis and Thrombosis* (3rd ed., pp. 321–341). Philadelphia: Saunders.

17. Rak, J., Milsom, C., May, L., et al. (2006). Tissue factor in cancer and angiogenesis: the molecular link between genetic tumor progression, tumor neovascularization, and cancer coagulopathy. *Semin Thromb Hemost, 32,* 54–70.

18. Sanz, M. A., Grimwade, D., & Tallman, M. S. (2009). Management of acute promyelocytic leukemia: recommendations from an expert panel on behalf of the European Leukemia Net. *Blood, 13,* 1875–1891.

19. Nishimura, J., Ware, R. E., Burnette, A., et al. (2002). The hematopoietic defect in PNH is not due to defective stroma, but is due to defective progenitor cells. *Blood Cells Mol Dis, 29,* 159–167.

20. Lontchi-Yimagou, E., Sobngwi, E., Matsha, T. E., et al. (2013). Diabetes mellitus and inflammation. *Curr Diab Rep, 13,* 435–444.

21. Melgaard, L., Rasmussen, L. H., Skjøth, F., et al. (2014). Age dependence of risk factors for stroke and death in young patients with atrial fibrillation: a nationwide study. *Stroke, 45,* 1331–1337.

22. Bramham, K., Hunt, B. J., & Goldsmith, D. (2009). Thrombophilia of nephrotic syndrome in adults. *Clin Adv Hematol Oncol, 7,* 368–372.

23. Middeldorp, S. (2016). Inherited thrombophilia: a double-edged sword. *Hematology Am Soc Hematol Educ Program, 2016,* 1–9.

24. Martin-Fernandez, L., Gavidia-Bovadilla, G., Corrales, I., et al. (2017). Next generation sequencing to dissect the genetic architecture of *KNG1* and *F11* loci using factor XI levels as an intermediate phenotype of thrombosis. *PLoS One, 12,* e0176301. doi:10.1371/journal.pone.0176301.

25. Itakura, H. (2005). Racial disparities in risk factors for thrombosis. *Curr Opin Hematol, 12,* 364–369.

26. Mohammed, S., & Favaloro, E. J. (2017). Laboratory testing for activated protein C resistance (APCR). *Methods Mol Biol, 1646,* 137–143.

27. Sedano-Balbás, S., Lyons, M., Cleary, B., et al. (2011). Acquired activated protein C resistance, thrombophilia and adverse pregnancy outcomes: a study performed in an Irish cohort of pregnant women. *J Pregnancy, 2011,* 1–9.

28. Berg, A. O., Botkin, J., Calonge, N., et al. Evaluation of Genomic Applications in Practice and Prevention (EGAPP) Working Group. (2011). Recommendations from the EGAPP Working Group: routine testing for Factor V Leiden (R506Q) and prothrombin (20210G.A) mutations in adults with a history of idiopathic venous thromboembolism and their adult family members. *Genet Med, 13,* 67–76.

29. Glueck, C. J., Smith, D., Gandhi, N., et al. (2015). Treatable high homocysteine alone or in concert with five other thrombophilias in 1014 patients with thrombotic events. *Blood Coagul Fibrinolysis, 26,* 736–742.

30. Reitsma, P. H., Versteeg, H. H., & Middeldorp, S. (2012). Mechanistic view of risk factors for venous thromboembolism. *Arterioscler Thromb Vasc Biol, 32,* 563–568.

31. Connors, J. M. (2017). Thrombophilia testing and venous thrombosis. *N Engl J Med, 377,* 1177–1187.

32. Favaloro, E. J., & Wong, R. C. (2014). Antiphospholipid antibody testing for the antiphospholipid syndrome: a comprehensive practical review including a synopsis of challenges and recent guidelines. *Pathology, 46,* 481–495.

33. Chaturvedi, S., & McCrae, K. R. (2017). Diagnosis and management of the antiphospholipid syndrome. *Blood Rev, 31,* 406–417.

34. Negrini, S., Pappalardo, F., Murdaca, G., et al. (2017). The antiphospholipid syndrome: from pathophysiology to treatment. *Clin Exp Med, 17,* 257–267.

35. López-Pedrera, C., Buendía, P., Barbarroja, N., et al. (2006). Antiphospholipid-mediated thrombosis: interplay between anticardiolipin antibodies and vascular cells. *Clin Appl Thromb Hemost, 12,* 41–45.

36. Chaturvedi, S., & McCrae, K. R. (2015). The antiphospholipid syndrome: still an enigma. *Hematology Am Soc Hematol Educ Program, 2015,* 53–60.

37. Miesbach, W., Gökpinar, B., Gilzinger, A., et al. (2005). Predictive role of hs-C-reactive protein in patients with antiphospholipid syndrome. *Immunobiology, 210,* 755–760.

38. Schouwers, S. M., Delanghe, J. R., & Devreese, K. M. J. (2010). Lupus anticoagulant (LAC) testing in patients with inflammatory status: does C-reactive protein interfere with LAC test results? *Thromb Res, 125,* 102–104.

39. Marques, M. B., & Fritsma, G. A. (2015). *Quick Guide to Hemostasis* (3rd ed.). Washington, DC: AACC Press.

40. Devreese, K., & Hoylaerts, M. F. (2010). Challenges in the diagnosis of the antiphospholipid syndrome. *Clin Chem, 56,* 930–940.

41. Fritsma, G. A., Dembitzer, F. R., Randhawa, A., et al. (2012). Recommendations for appropriate activated partial thromboplastin time reagent selection and utilization. *Am J Clin Pathol, 137,* 904–908.

42. Pengo, V., Tripodi, A., Reber, G., et al. (2009). Update of the guidelines for lupus anticoagulant detection. Subcommittee on Lupus Anticoagulant/Antiphospholipid Antibody of the Scientific and Standardisation Committee of the International Society on Thrombosis and Haemostasis. *J Thromb Haemost, 7,* 1737–1740.

43. Yao, K., Zhang, L., Zhou, H., et al. (2017). Plasma antiphospholipid antibodies effects on activated partial thromboplastin time assays. *Am J Med Sci, 354,* 22–26.

44. Devreese, K. M., & de Laat, B. (2015). Mixing studies in lupus anticoagulant testing are required at least in some type of samples. *J Thromb Haemost, 13,* 1475–1478.

45. Moore, G. W., Culhane, A. P., Daw, C. R., et al. (2016). Mixing test specific cut-off is more sensitive at detecting lupus anticoagulants than index of circulating anticoagulant. *Thromb Res, 139,* 98–101.

46. Froom, P., Saffuri-Elias, E., Rozenberg, O., et al. (2014). The association of serum antiphospholipid antibodies and dilute Russell's viper venom times. *J Clin Pathol, 67,* 441–444.

47. Tripodi, A., & Chantarangkul, V. (2017). Lupus anticoagulant testing: activated partial thromboplastin time (APTT) and silica clotting time (SCT). *Methods Mol Biol, 1646,* 177–183.

48. Willis, R., Papalardo, E., & Nigel Harris, E. (2017). Solid phase immunoassay for the detection of anticardiolipin antibodies. *Methods Mol Biol, 1646,* 185–199.

49. Cohen, D., Berger, S. P., Steup-Beekman, G. M., et al. (2010). Diagnosis and management of the antiphospholipid syndrome. *BMJ, 340,* c2541.

50. Willis, R., Papalardo, E., & Nigel Harris, E. (2017). Solid phase immunoassay for the detection of anti-β_2 glycoprotein I antibodies. *Methods Mol Biol, 1646,* 201–215.

51. Shi, H., Zheng, H., Yin, Y. F., et al. (2018). Antiphosphatidylserine/prothrombin antibodies (aPS/PT) as potential diagnostic markers and risk predictors of venous thrombosis and obstetric complications in antiphospholipid syndrome. *Clin Chem Lab Med, 56,* 614–624.

52. Dahlbäck, B., & Hildebrand, B. (1994). Inherited resistance to activated protein C is corrected by anticoagulant cofactor activity found to be a property of factor V. *Proc Natl Acad Sci U S A, 91,* 1396–1400.

53. De Ronde, H., & Bertina, R. M. (1994). Laboratory diagnosis of APC-resistance: a critical evaluation of the test and the development of diagnostic criteria. *Thromb Haemost, 72,* 880–886.

54. Segers, K., Dahlbäck, B., & Nicolaes, G. A. (2007). Coagulation factor V and thrombophilia: background and mechanisms. *Thromb Haemost, 98,* 530–542.

55. Bouaziz-Borgi, L., Nguyen, P., Hezard, N., et al. (2007). A case control study of deep venous thrombosis in relation to factor V G1691A (Leiden) and A4070G (HR2 haplotype) polymorphisms. *Exp Mol Pathol, 83,* 480–483.

56. Favaloro, E. J., McDonald, D., & Lippi, G. (2009). Laboratory investigation of thrombophilia: the good, the bad, and the ugly. *Semin Thromb Hemost, 35,* 695–710.

57. Johnson, N. V., Khor, B., & Van Cott, E. M. (2012). Advances in laboratory testing for thrombophilia. *Am J Hematol, 87*(Suppl. 1), S108–S112.

58. Ragland, B. D., Reed, C. E., Eiland, B. M., et al. (2003). The effect of lupus anticoagulant in the second-generation assay for activated protein C resistance. *Am J Clin Pathol, 119,* 66–71.

59. Emadi, A., Crim, M. T., Brotman, D. J., et al. (2010). Analytic validity of genetic tests to identify factor V Leiden and prothrombin G20210A. *Am J Hematol, 85,* 264–270.

60. Poort, S. R., Rosendaal, F. R., Reitsma, P. Y., et al. (1996). A common genetic variation in the 3'-untranslated region of the prothrombin gene is associated with elevated plasma prothrombin levels and an increase in venous thrombosis. *Blood, 88,* 3698–3703.

61. Dziadosz, M., & Baxi, L. V. (2016). Global prevalence of prothrombin gene mutation G20210A and implications in women's health: a systematic review. *Blood Coagul Fibrinolysis, 27,* 481–489.

62. Naeem, M. A., Anwar, M., Ali, W., et al. (2006). Prevalence of prothrombin gene mutation (G-A 20210 A) in general population: a pilot study. *Clin Appl Thromb Hemost, 12,* 223–226.

63. Gao, H., & Tao, F. B. (2015). Prothrombin G20210A mutation is associated with recurrent pregnancy loss: a systematic review and meta-analysis update. *Thromb Res, 135,* 339–446.

64. Danckwardt, S., Hartmann, K., Gehring, N. H., et al. (2006). 3' end processing of the prothrombin mRNA in thrombophilia. *Acta Haematol, 115,* 192–197.

65. Cooper, P. C., Coath, F., Daly, M. E., et al. (2011). The phenotypic and genetic assessment of antithrombin deficiency. *Int J Lab Hematol, 33,* 227–237.

66. Di Minno, M. N., Dentali, F., Lupoli, R., et al. (2014). Mild antithrombin deficiency and risk of recurrent venous thromboembolism: a prospective cohort study. *Circulation, 129,* 497–503.

67. De Stefano, V., & Rossi, E. (2013). Testing for inherited thrombophilia and consequences for antithrombotic prophylaxis in patients with venous thromboembolism and their relatives. A review of the Guidelines from Scientific Societies and Working Groups. *Thromb Haemost, 110,* 697–705.

68. Cai, K., Osheroff, W. P., Buczynski, G., et al. (2014). Characterization of Thrombate III®, a pasteurized and nanofiltered therapeutic human antithrombin concentrate. *Biologicals, 42,* 133–138.

69. Cooper, P. C., Coath, F., Daly, M. E., et al. (2011). The phenotypic and genetic assessment of antithrombin deficiency. *Int J Lab Hematol, 33,* 227–237.

70. Gausman, J. N., & Marlar, R. A. (2017). Assessment of hereditary thrombophilia: performance of antithrombin (AT) testing. *Methods Mol Biol, 1646,* 161–167.

71. Antovic, J., Söderström, J., Karlman, B., et al. (2001). Evaluation of a new immunoturbidimetric test (Liatest antithrombin III) for determination of antithrombin antigen. *Clin Lab Haematol, 23,* 313–316.

72. Dahlbäck, B. (1995). The protein C anticoagulant system: inherited defects as basis for venous thrombosis. *Thromb Res, 77,* 1–43.

73. Gausman, J. M., & Marlar, R. A. (2017). Assessment of hereditary thrombophilia: performance of protein C (PC) testing. *Methods Mol Biol, 1646,* 145–151.

74. Mann, H. J., Short, M. A., & Schlichting, D. E. (2009). Protein C in critical illness. *Am J Health Syst Pharm, 15,* 1089–1096.

75. Weeda, E. R., Kohn, C. G., Peacock, W. F., et al. (2016). Rivaroxaban versus heparin bridging to warfarin therapy: impact on hospital length of stay and treatment costs for low-risk patients with pulmonary embolism. *Pharmacotherapy, 36,* 1109–1115.

76. Khor, B., & Van Cott, E. M. (2010). Laboratory tests for protein C deficiency. *Am J Hematol, 85,* 440–442.

77. Manco-Johnson, M. J., Bomgaars, L., Palascak, J., et al. (2016). Efficacy and safety of protein C concentrate to treat purpura fulminans and thromboembolic events in severe congenital protein C deficiency. *Thromb Haemost, 116,* 58–68.

78. Martos, L., Bonanad, S., Ramón, L. A., et al. (2016). A simplified assay for the quantification of circulating activated protein C. *Clin Chim Acta, 459*, 101–104.

79. Espana, F., Zuazu, I., Vicente, V., et al. (1996). Quantification of circulating activated protein C in human plasma by immunoassays—enzyme levels are proportional to total protein C levels. *Thromb Haemost, 75*, 56–61.

80. Van Cott, E. M., Ledford-Kraemer, M., Meijer, P., et al., NASCOLA Proficiency Testing Committee. (2005). Protein S assays: an analysis of North American Specialized Coagulation Laboratory Association proficiency testing. *Am J Clin Pathol, 123*, 778–785.

81. Ens, G. E., & Newlin, F. (1995). Spurious protein S deficiency as a result of elevated factor VII levels. *Clin Hemost Rev, 9*, 18.

82. Rigamonti, F., Carbone, F., Montecucco, F., et al. (2018). Serum lipoprotein (a) predicts acute coronary syndromes in patients with severe carotid stenosis. *Eur J Clin Invest, 48*. doi:10.1111/eci.12888.

83. Yousuf, O., Mohanty, B. D., Martin, S. S., et al. (2013). High-sensitivity C-reactive protein and cardiovascular disease: a resolute belief or an elusive link? *J Am Coll Cardiol, 62*, 397–408.

84. Turner, D., Mack, D. R., Hyams, J., et al. (2011). C-reactive protein (CRP), erythrocyte sedimentation rate (ESR) or both? A systematic evaluation in pediatric ulcerative colitis. *J Crohns Colitis, 5*, 423–429.

85. Lelubre, C., Anselin, S., Zouaoui Boudjeltia, K., et al. (2013). Interpretation of C-reactive protein concentrations in critically ill patients. *Biomed Res Int, 2013*, 124021.

86. Ridker, P. M. (1999). Evaluating novel cardiovascular risk factors: can we better predict heart attacks? *Ann Intern Med, 130*, 933–937.

87. Jellinger, P. S., Handelsman, Y., Rosenblit, P. D., et al. (2017). American Association of Clinical Endocrinologists and American College of Endocrinology guidelines for management of dyslipidemia and prevention of cardiovascular disease—executive summary. *Endocr Pract, 23*, 479–497.

88. Franchini, M., & Veneri, D. (2005). Inherited thrombophilia: an update. *Clin Lab, 51*, 357–365.

89. Ciaccio, M., & Bellia, C. (2010). Hyperhomocysteinemia and cardiovascular risk: effect of vitamin supplementation in risk reduction. *Curr Clin Pharmacol, 5*, 30–36.

90. Ganguly, P., & Alam, S. F. (2015). Role of homocysteine in the development of cardiovascular disease. *Nutr J, 14*, 6. doi:10.1186/1475-2891-14-6.

91. Guanella, R., Ducruet, T., Johri, M., et al. (2011). Economic burden and cost determinants of deep vein thrombosis during 2 years following diagnosis: a prospective evaluation. *J Thromb Haemost, 9*, 2397–2405.

92. Huisman, M. V., & Klok, F. A. (2013). Diagnostic management of acute deep vein thrombosis and pulmonary embolism. *J Thromb Haemost, 11*, 412–422.

93. Wells, P. S., Anderson, D. R., Bormanis, J., et al. (1997). Value of assessment of pretest probability of deep-vein thrombosis in clinical management. *Lancet, 350*, 1795–1798.

94. Wells, P. S., Anderson, D. R., Rodger, M., et al. (2000). Derivation of a simple clinical model to categorize patients probability of pulmonary embolism: increasing the models utility with the Simplired D-dimer. *Thromb Haemost, 83*, 416–420.

95. Righini, M., Van Es, J., Den Exter, P. L., et al. (2014). Age-adjusted D-dimer cutoff levels to rule out pulmonary embolism: the ADJUST-PE study. *JAMA, 311*, 1117–1124.

96. Mandernach, M. W., & Kitchens, C. S. (2013). Disseminated intravascular coagulation. In Kitchens, C. S., Kessler, C. M., & Konkle, B. A. (Eds.), *Consultative Hemostasis and Thrombosis* (3rd ed., pp. 174–189). Philadelphia: Elsevier Saunders.

97. Madoiwa, S., Kitajima, I., Ohmori, T., et al. (2013). Distinct reactivity of the commercially available monoclonal antibodies of D-dimer and plasma FDP testing to the molecular variants of fibrin degradation products. *Thromb Res, 132*, 457–464.

98. Levi, M., Feinstein, D. I., Colman, R. W., et al. (2013). Consumptive thrombohemorrhagic disorders. In Marder, V. J., Aird, W. C., Bennett, J. S., et al. (Eds.), *Hemostasis and Thrombosis: Basic Principles and Clinical Practice.* (6th ed., pp. 1178–1196). Philadelphia: Lippincott Williams & Wilkins.

99. Trousseau, A. (1865). Phlegmasia alba dolens: Clinique Medicale de L'Hotel Dieu de Paris. *The New Sydenham Society, 3*, 94.

100. Longstaff, C., & Kolev, K. (2015). Basic mechanisms and regulation of fibrinolysis. *J Thromb Haemost, 13*(Suppl. 1), S98–S105.

101. Linkins, L. A., & Takach Lapner, S. (2017). Review of D-dimer testing: good, bad, and ugly. *Int J Lab Hematol, 39*(Suppl. 1), 98–103.

102. Kashuk, J. L., Moore, E. E., Sawyer, M., et al. (2010). Primary fibrinolysis is integral in the pathogenesis of the acute coagulopathy of trauma. *Ann Surg, 252*, 434–442.

103. Kappler, S., Ronan-Bentle, S., & Graham, A. (2017). Thrombotic microangiopathies (TTP, HUS, HELLP). *Hematol Oncol Clin North Am, 31*, 1081–1103.

104. Khoury, J. D., Adcock, D. M., Chan, F., et al. (2010). Increases in quantitative D-dimer levels correlate with progressive disease better than circulating tumor cell counts in patients with refractory prostate cancer. *Am J Clin Pathol, 134*, 964–969.

105. Tripodi, A. (2011). D-dimer testing in laboratory practice. *Clin Chem, 57*, 1256–1262.

106. Sawamura, A., Hayakawa, M., Gando, S., et al. (2009). Disseminated intravascular coagulation with a fibrinolytic phenotype at an early phase of trauma predicts mortality. *Thromb Res, 124*, 608–613.

107. Singh, N., Pati, H. P., Tyagi, S., et al. (2017). Evaluation of the diagnostic performance of fibrin monomer in comparison to D-dimer in patients with overt and nonovert disseminated intravascular coagulation. *Clin Appl Thromb Hemost, 23*, 460–465.

108. Gando, S., Saitoh, D., Ishikura, H., et al. (2013). A randomized, controlled, multicenter trial of the effects of antithrombin on disseminated intravascular coagulation in patients with sepsis. *Crit Care, 17*, R297.

109. Favaloro, E. J. (2010). Laboratory testing in disseminated intravascular coagulation. *Semin Thromb Hemost, 36*, 458–467.

110. Ben-Ari, Z., Osman, E., Hutton, R. A., et al. (1999). Disseminated intravascular coagulation in liver cirrhosis: fact or fiction? *AM J Gastroenterol, 94*, 2977–2982.

111. Cosgriff, N., Moore, E. E., Sauaia, A., et al. (1997). Predicting life-threatening coagulopathy in the massively transfused trauma patient: hypothermia and acidoses revisited. *J Trauma, 41*, 857–861.

112. Haram, K., Mortensen, J. H., Mastrolia, S. A., et al. (2017). Disseminated intravascular coagulation in the HELLP syndrome: how much do we really know? *J Matern Fetal Neonatal Med, 30*, 779–788.

113. Levi, M., de Jonge, E., & van der Poll, T. (2006). Plasma and plasma components in the management of disseminated intravascular coagulation. *Best Pract Res Clin Haematol, 19*, 127–142.

114. Gorog, D. A. (2010). Prognostic value of plasma fibrinolysis activation markers in cardiovascular disease. *J Am Coll Cardiol*, *15*, 2701–2709.

115. Salter, B. S., Weiner, M. M., Trinh, M. A., et al. (2016). Heparin-induced thrombocytopenia: a comprehensive clinical review. *J Am Coll Cardiol*, *67*, 2519–2532.

116. Junqueira, D. R., Zorzela, L. M., & Perini, E. (2017). Unfractionated heparin versus low molecular weight heparins for avoiding heparin-induced thrombocytopenia in postoperative patients. *Cochrane Database Syst Rev*, *4*, CD007557. doi:10.1002/14651858.CD007557.pub3.

117. Lovecchio, F. (2014). Heparin-induced thrombocytopenia. *Clin Toxicol (Phila)*, *52*, 579–583.

118. Ban-Hoefen, M., & Francis, C. (2009). Heparin induced thrombocytopenia and thrombosis in a tertiary care hospital. *Thromb Res*, *124*, 189–192.

119. Levy, J. H., & Hursting, M. J. (2007). Heparin-induced thrombocytopenia, a prothrombotic disease. *Hematol Oncol Clin North Am*, *21*, 65–88.

120. Smith, B. W., Joseph, J. R., & Park, P. (2017). Heparin-induced thrombocytopenia presenting as unilateral lower limb paralysis following lumbar spine surgery: case report. *J Neurosurg Spine*, *26*, 594–597.

121. Warkentin, T. E. (2003). Heparin-induced thrombocytopenia: pathogenesis and management. *Br J Haematol*, *121*, 535–555.

122. Staibano, P., Arnold, D. M., Bowdish, D. M., et al. (2017). The unique immunological features of heparin-induced thrombocytopenia. *Br J Haematol*, *177*, 198–207.

123. Warkentin, T. E., & Greinacher, A. (2013). Heparin-induced thrombocytopenia. In Marder, V. J., Aird, W. C., Bennett, J. S., et al. (Eds.), *Hemostasis and Thrombosis: Basic Principles and Clinical Practice.* (6th ed., pp. 1293–1307). Philadelphia: Lippincott Williams & Wilkins.

124. Warkentin, T. E., Hayward, C. P., Boshkov, L. K., et al. (1994). Sera from patients with heparin-induced thrombocytopenia generate platelet-derived microparticles with procoagulant activity: an explanation for the thrombotic complications of heparin-induced thrombocytopenia. *Blood*, *84*, 3691–3699.

125. Rauova, L., Hirsch, J. D., Greene, T. K., et al. (2010). Monocyte-bound PF4 in the pathogenesis of heparin-induced thrombocytopenia. *Blood*, *116*, 5021–5031.

126. Visentin, G. P., Ford, S. E., Scott, J. P., et al. (1994). Antibodies from patients with heparin-induced thrombocytopenia/thrombosis are specific for platelet factor 4 complexed with heparin or bound to endothelial cells. *J Clin Invest*, *93*, 81–88.

127. Blank, M., Shoenfeld, Y., Tavor, S., et al. (2002). Anti-platelet factor 4/heparin antibodies from patients with heparin-induced thrombocytopenia provoke direct activation of microvascular endothelial cells. *Int Immunol*, *14*, 121–129.

128. Arepally, G. M., & Mayer, I. M. (2001). Antibodies from patients with heparin-induced thrombocytopenia stimulate monocytic cells to express tissue factor and secrete interleukin-8. *Blood*, *98*, 1252–1254.

129. Fareed, J., Walenga, J. M., Hoppensteadt, D. A., et al. (1999). Selectins in the HIT syndrome: pathophysiologic role and therapeutic modulation. *Semin Thromb Hemost*, *25*(Suppl. 1), 37–42.

130. Walenga, J. M., Jeske, W. P., & Messmore, H. L. (2000). Mechanisms of venous and arterial thrombosis in heparin-induced thrombocytopenia. *J Thromb Thrombolysis*, *10*, S13–S20.

131. Walenga, J. M., Jeske, W. P., Prechel, M. M., et al. (2004). Newer insights on the mechanism of heparin-induced thrombocytopenia. *Semin Thromb Hemost*, *30*(Suppl. 1), 57–67.

132. Poncz, M. (2005). Mechanistic basis of heparin-induced thrombocytopenia. *Semin Thorac Cardiovasc Surg*, *17*, 73–79.

133. Kuter, D. J., Konkle, B. A., Hamza, T. H., et al. (2017). Clinical outcomes in a cohort of patients with heparin-induced thrombocytopenia. *Am J Hematol*, *92*, 730–738.

134. Warkentin, T. E., & Sheppard, J. A. (2006). Testing for heparin-induced thrombocytopenia antibodies. *Transfus Med Rev*, *20*, 259–272.

135. Vatanparast, R., Lantz, S., Ward, K., et al. (2012). Evaluation of a pretest scoring system (4Ts) for the diagnosis of heparin-induced thrombocytopenia in a university hospital setting. *Postgrad Med*, *124*, 36–42.

136. Crowther, M., Cook, D., Guyatt, G., et al. (2014). Heparin-induced thrombocytopenia in the critically ill: interpreting the 4Ts test in a randomized trial. *J Crit Care*, *29*, 470.e7–e15.

137. Cuker, A., Arepally, G., Crowther, M. A., et al. (2010). The HIT expert probability (HEP) score: a novel pre-test probability model for heparin-induced thrombocytopenia based on broad expert opinion. *J Thromb Haemost*, *8*, 2642–2650.

138. Demma, L. J., Winkler, A. M., & Levy, J. H. (2011). A diagnosis of heparin-induced thrombocytopenia with combined clinical and laboratory methods in cardiothoracic surgical intensive care unit patients. *Anesth Analg*, *113*, 697–702.

139. Prechel, M., & Walenga, J. M. (2012). Heparin-induced thrombocytopenia: an update. *Semin Thromb Hemost*, *38*, 483–496.

140. Minet, V., Dogné, J. M., & Mullier, F. (2017). Functional assays in the diagnosis of heparin-induced thrombocytopenia: a review. *Molecules*, *22*, E617. doi:10.3390/molecules22040617.

141. Sylvester, K. W., Fanikos, J., & Anger, K. E. (2013). Impact of an immunoglobulin G-specific enzyme-linked immunosorbent assay on the management of heparin-induced thrombocytopenia. *Pharmacotherapy*, *33*, 1191–1198.

142. Vianello, F., Sambado, L., Scarparo, P., et al. (2015). Comparison of three different immunoassays in the diagnosis of heparin-induced thrombocytopenia. *Clin Chem Lab Med*, *53*, 257–263.

143. Warkentin, T. E., Arnold, D. M., Nazi, I., et al. (2015). The platelet serotonin-release assay. *Am J Hematol*, *90*, 564–572.

144. Vitale, M., Tazzari, P., Ricci, F., et al. (2001). Comparison between different laboratory tests for the detection and prevention of heparin-induced thrombocytopenia. *Cytometry*, *46*, 290–295.

145. Brace, L. D. (1992). Testing for heparin-induced thrombocytopenia by platelet aggregometry. *Clin Lab Sci*, *5*, 80–81.

146. Tan, C. W., Ward, C. M., & Morel-Kopp, M. C. (2012). Evaluating heparin-induced thrombocytopenia: the old and the new. *Semin Thromb Hemost*, *38*, 135–143.

147. Crowther, M. A., Cook, D. J., Albert, M., et al. (2010). The 4Ts scoring system for heparin-induced thrombocytopenia in medical-surgical intensive care unit patients. *J Crit Care*, *25*, 287–293.

148. Sun, L., Gimotty, P. A., Lakshmanan, S., et al. (2016). Diagnostic accuracy of rapid immunoassays for heparin-induced thrombocytopenia. A systematic review and meta-analysis. *Thromb Haemost*, *115*, 1044–1055.

149. Warkentin, T. E., Pai, M., Sheppard, J. I., et al. (2011). Fondaparinux treatment of acute heparin-induced thrombocytopenia confirmed by the serotonin-release assay: a 30-month, 16-patient case series. *J Thromb Haemost*, *9*, 2389–2396.

150. Skelley, J. W., Kyle, J. A., & Roberts, R. A. (2016). Novel oral anticoagulants for heparin-induced thrombocytopenia. *J Thromb Thrombolysis*, *42*, 172–178.

151. Warkentin, T. E., Pai, M., & Linkins, L. A. (2017). Direct oral anticoagulants for treatment of HIT: update of Hamilton experience and literature review. *Blood*, *130*, 1104–1113.

Antithrombotic Therapies and Their Laboratory Assessment

George A. Fritsma

OBJECTIVES

After completion of this chapter, the reader will be able to:

1. Describe the purpose of antithrombotic drug administration and distinguish between anticoagulants and antiplatelet therapy.
2. Diagram the mechanism of action of each of the antithrombotic drugs.
3. Describe the indications for, dosage of, and management of Coumadin therapy, including how to detect and manage Coumadin overdose.
4. Monitor Coumadin therapy using the prothrombin time (PT) and international normalized ratio (INR), and compare these tests with the chromogenic factor X assay.
5. Describe conditions that affect PT/INR and the relevance of the results to patient management.
6. Describe the indications for, dosage of, and laboratory monitoring of unfractionated heparin therapy, including how to establish the unfractionated heparin partial thromboplastin time therapeutic range.
7. Perform and interpret the results of the partial thromboplastin time and activated clotting time assays for monitoring unfractionated heparin therapy, and compare these tests with the chromogenic anti-factor Xa heparin assay.

8. Describe the indications, dosages, and laboratory measurement of low-molecular-weight heparin therapy, fondaparinux therapy, and oral factor Xa inhibitors.
9. Perform and interpret the results of the chromogenic anti-Xa assay for measuring unfractionated heparin, low-molecular-weight heparin, fondaparinux, rivaroxaban, apixaban, and edoxaban therapy.
10. Describe the indications for oral direct thrombin inhibitor therapy with dabigatran and the indications for intravenous thrombin inhibitor therapy with argatroban and bivalirudin.
11. Measure the direct thrombin inhibitors using the partial thromboplastin time, ecarin clotting time, ecarin chromogenic assay, plasma-diluted thrombin time, and the activated clotting time where indicated.
12. Describe the indications for intravenous platelet glycoprotein IIb/IIIa inhibitors abciximab, eptifibatide, and tirofiban, and describe how their effects are measured.
13. Describe the indications for oral platelet inhibitors aspirin, clopidogrel, prasugrel, and ticagrelor, and describe how their effects are measured.

OUTLINE

THROMBOSIS AND ANTICOAGULATION

Thrombosis, described in Chapter 39, is the pathologic development of blood clots in veins or arteries that obstruct flow and cause tissue ischemia and necrosis. Antithrombotic drugs have been employed to prevent and treat thrombosis since intravenous heparin was first described in 1914.[1] Antithrombotics include anticoagulants, which suppress coagulation and reduce thrombin formation, and antiplatelet drugs, which suppress platelet activation. Fibrinolytics are also employed to disperse or reduce existing clots clogging veins and arteries.

Antithrombotic drugs can be categorized into three groups: the original drugs heparin, Coumadin, and aspirin; drugs that entered clinical use in the 1990s, including heparin derivatives and antiplatelet drugs; and the newest drugs, the direct-acting oral and intravenous anticoagulants. Table 40.1 provides a list of pre-2010 antithrombotics with their indications. The direct-acting oral anticoagulants (DOACs; once called novel oral anticoagulants or NOACs) are detailed separately in this chapter.

Venous thromboembolic disease (VTE, venous thromboembolism) includes superficial and deep vein thrombosis (DVT) and pulmonary embolism (PE). Physicians and surgeons treat VTE with intravenous standard unfractionated heparin (UFH), subcutaneous low-molecular-weight heparin (LMWH), subcutaneous synthetic pentasaccharide (fondaparinux), or one of the DOACs. VTE is also managed using the oral vitamin K antagonist warfarin sodium (Coumadin). Clinicians can employ these anticoagulants prophylactically to prevent strokes in non-valvular atrial fibrillation and to prevent VTE subsequent to total hip and total knee replacement surgery, orthopedic repair surgery, immobilization, and in several medical conditions. For thrombosis prevention, lower prophylactic drug dosages may be employed in an effort to reduce adverse events such as bleeding, whereas for established thrombosis, higher treatment dosages are used for a more potent effect.

One of two intravenous direct thrombin inhibitors (DTIs), argatroban or bivalirudin, is substituted for UFH in patients

TABLE 40.1 Antithrombotic Drugs Before 2010

Antithrombotic	Indication	Mode of Action	Half-Life	Measurement	Reversal	FDA Approval
Coumadin	Prevent post-VTE rethrombosis, ischemic stroke in NVAF	Oral VK antagonist	5 d	Monitor: PT/INR; CFX	Vitamin K, 4-factor PCC, rFVIIa	1954
UFH	Prevent post-VTE and ACS rethrombosis; intraoperative anticoagulation	IV antithrombin activation, suppresses IIa & Xa	1–2 hr	Monitor: PTT, ACT, anti-Xa	Protamine	1936
LMWH	Prevent thrombosis after surgery, in medical conditions or in ACS; DVT/PE treatment	SC antithrombin activation, anti-Xa	3–5 hr	Anti-Xa	Protamine (partial)	1993
Fondaparinux			12–17 hr	Anti-Xa		2001
Argatroban	Anticoagulation in HIT	IV DTI	50 min	PTT	Discontinue therapy	1997
Bivalirudin		IV DTI	25 min			2000
Aspirin		Oral antiplatelet COX inhibitor		VerifyNow Aspirin, Aspirin-Works, platelet aggregation		1900
Clopidogrel	Prevent acute coronary syndrome recurrence	Oral, bind platelet P2Y$_{12}$		VerifyNow P2Y		2000
Prasugrel						2009
Ticagrelor						2011
Eptifibatide	Maintain vascular patency during PCI and medical therapy for ACS	IV, bind platelet GPIIb/IIIa	2.5 hr	VerifyNow GPI		1998
Abciximab			1030 min			1993
Tirofiban			2.5 hr			1998

ACS, Acute coronary syndrome; *CFX,* chromogenic factor X activity; *COX,* cyclooxygenase; *DTI,* direct thrombin inhibitor; *US FDA,* Food and Drug Administration; *DVT,* deep vein thrombosis; *FEIBA,* factor VIII inhibitor bypassing activity; *GPI,* glycoprotein inhibitor; *HIT,* heparin-induced thrombocytopenia with thrombosis; *INR,* international normalized ratio; *IV,* intravenous; *LMWH,* low-molecular-weight heparin; *NVAF,* nonvalvular atrial fibrillation; *PCC,* prothrombin complex concentrate; *PCI,* percutaneous coronary intervention; *PE,* pulmonary embolism; *PTT,* partial thromboplastin time; *PT,* prothrombin time; *rFVIIa,* recombinant activated factor VII; *UFH,* unfractionated heparin; *VK,* vitamin K; *VTE,* venous thromboembolism.

who have developed heparin-induced thrombocytopenia with thrombosis (HIT), a devastating arterial and venous thrombotic side effect of UFH therapy (Chapter 39).

Arterial thrombosis includes acute myocardial infarction (AMI), ischemic cerebrovascular accident (CVA, stroke), transient ischemic attack (TIA), and peripheral arterial occlusion (PAO or peripheral artery disease, PAD). These disorders are managed with UFH, LMWH, fondaparinux, Coumadin, and the antiplatelet drugs aspirin, clopidogrel, prasugrel, and ticagrelor. Aspirin is taken prophylactically by many healthy people at less than 100 mg/day and is particularly effective in reducing mortality when taken within minutes of the acute onset of stroke or cardiac symptoms. The intravenous platelet glycoprotein IIb/IIIa inhibitor (GPI) drugs eptifibatide, abciximab, and tirofiban are used to prevent thrombosis during percutaneous coronary intervention (PCI, cardiac catheterization).

Fibrinolytics or thrombolytic therapy may be used to resolve DVT, PE, PAO, AMI, and stroke, particularly when used 3 to 4 hours after the onset of symptoms.[2] Thrombolytic therapy employs recombinant forms of tissue plasminogen activator (reteplase, alteplase, and tenecteplase). Thrombolytic therapy raises the risk of hemorrhage, particularly intracranial hemorrhage. The effects of thrombolytic therapy are seldom measured, though laboratory testing for a disseminated intravascular coagulation (DIC) profile may be used to rule out primary fibrinolysis (Chapter 39).[3]

Many lives have been saved through the judicious use of antithrombotic therapy, and countless more healthy individuals have been spared thrombotic disease through long-term antithrombotic prophylaxis in moderate-risk circumstances and conditions. However, antithrombotics are dangerous because their effective dosage ranges are narrow.[4] Overdose is critical and leads to emergency department visits for uncontrolled bleeding; inadequate dosages lead to secondary (repeat), often fatal, thrombotic events. Dosages and half-lives differ among the antithrombotics because of variations in formulation and metabolism.[5]

Because of these risks, laboratory monitoring or measurement of anticoagulant therapy is essential. Coagulation laboratory scientists and technicians perform countless prothrombin time (PT) assays, partial thromboplastin time (PTT, activated partial thromboplastin time, APTT), and chromogenic anti-Xa heparin assays to measure or monitor anticoagulant therapy; meanwhile, physicians and nurses regularly modify Coumadin and UFH dosages in response to laboratory outcomes. Although anticoagulant therapy measurement or monitoring may seem routine, vigilance is essential to provide consistently valid results.[6]

The antiplatelet drugs aspirin, clopidogrel, prasugrel, and ticagrelor, as well as LMWH, fondaparinux, and the DOACs, have fixed dose-response characteristics and require only on-demand assays or laboratory-directed dose adjustment. However, these antiplatelet drugs and all antithrombotics require measurement in the conditions listed in Box 40.1.

COUMADIN AND THE PT/INR

Coumadin: A Vitamin K Antagonist

As detailed in Chapter 35, the coagulation factors II (prothrombin), VII, IX, and X depend on vitamin K for normal

> **BOX 40.1   Clinical Conditions That Require Anticoagulant and Antiplatelet Drug Measurement**
>
> - Renal disease: inadequate excretion, CrCl <30 mL/min
> - Concern for noncompliance and underdosing
> - Detection of comedication interference
> - Overdose, effects of comedication
> - Acute hemorrhage
> - Detection and identification; what anticoagulant is it?
> - Determine whether reversal is effective
> - Bridging from one anticoagulant to another before surgery
> - Discontinuing anticoagulant before surgery
> - Resuming anticoagulant after surgery
> - Unstable coagulation: pregnancy, liver disease, malignancy, chronic DIC
> - >75 years old (excluded from clinical trials)
> - Extremes of body weight (creates marginal fluid compartment [excluded from clinical trials])
>   - >150 kg: proportionally reduced fluid compartment
>   - <50 kg or pediatric: proportionally increased fluid compartment

CrCl, Creatinine clearance; *DIC,* disseminated intravascular coagulation.

production, as do coagulation control proteins C, S, and Z. Vitamin K is responsible for the γ-carboxylation of a series of 12 to 18 glutamic acids near each molecule's N-terminus (amino terminus), a posttranslational modification that enables these coagulation factors and coagulation control proteins to bind ionic calcium (Ca^{2+}) and cell membrane phospholipids, especially phosphatidylserine (Figure 35.5). Vitamin K is concentrated in green tea, avocados, and green leafy vegetables and is produced by gut flora; its absence results in the production of nonfunctional *des-γ carboxyl* forms of factors II, VII, IX, and X and proteins C, S, and Z.

Warfarin sodium (4-hydroxycoumarin, Coumadin) is a member of the coumarin drug family and is the formulation of coumarin most often used in North America.[7] Another coumarin is dicoumarol (3,3′-methylenebis-[4-hydroxycoumarin]), the original anticoagulant extracted from moldy sweet clover, described in 1940, and used for many years as a rodenticide.[8] Coumadin is a vitamin K antagonist that suppresses γ-carboxylation of glutamic acid by slowing the activity of the enzyme vitamin K epoxide reductase. During Coumadin therapy, the activities of factors II, VII, IX, and X and proteins C, S, and Z become reduced as the nonfunctional des-carboxyl proteins are produced in their place. These are sometimes called proteins induced by vitamin K antagonists (PIVKA); they bind few calcium ions, do not assemble on phospholipid surfaces with their substrates, and therefore do not participate in coagulation. PIVKA factor concentration assays are available from hemostasis reference laboratories.

Coumadin Prophylaxis and Therapy

Coumadin is a widely used, often prescribed oral anticoagulant. Until 2010 it was the only oral anticoagulant available for long-term outpatient management. The goal of Coumadin therapy is to reduce but not eradicate thrombin generation. Physicians prescribe Coumadin prophylactically to prevent TIAs and strokes in patients with nonvalvular atrial fibrillation and to

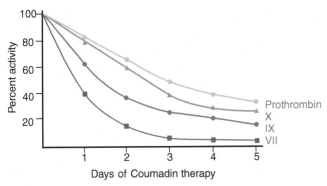

Figure 40.1 The Anticoagulant Effect of Coumadin at Initiation of Therapy. Factor VII activity decreases to 50% of normal 6 hours after Coumadin therapy is begun, prolonging the factor VIIa-sensitive prothrombin time *(PT)* to near the therapeutic international normalized ratio (INR) of 2 to 3. The half-lives of factors II (prothrombin), IX, and X are longer than that of VII; factor II activity requires at least 3 days to decline by 50%. The patient gains full anticoagulation effects approximately 5 days after the start of Coumadin therapy.

TABLE 40.2 Functional Properties of the Coagulation Factors

Factor	Half-Life	Plasma Level	Hemostatic Level*
Fibrinogen	4 days	280 mg/dL	50 mg/dL
Prothrombin	60 hr	1300 μg/mL	20%
V	16 hr	680 μg/mL	25%
VII	6 hr	120 μg/mL	20%
VIII	12 hr	0.24 μg/mL	30%
IX	24 hr	5 μg/mL	30%
X	30 hr	1 mg/dL	25%
XI	2–3 days	6 μg/mL	25%
XIII	7–10 days	290 μg/mL	2%–3%
Von Willebrand factor	30 hr	6 μg/mL	50%

*Minimum effective hemostatic level as a percentage of normal level.

prevent VTE after trauma, orthopedic surgery, and general surgery and in a number of chronic medical conditions. They also prescribe Coumadin therapeutically to prevent DVT or PE recurrence. Coumadin is also used therapeutically after an AMI if the event is complicated by congestive heart failure or coronary insufficiency and to control clotting in patients with mechanical heart valves.

Whether prescribed prophylactically or therapeutically, the standard Coumadin regimen begins with a 5-mg daily oral dose. The starting dosage for people older than 70 and people who are debilitated, malnourished, or have congestive heart failure is 2 mg/day. Coumadin is packaged in dosages from 1 to 10 mg. For people simultaneously taking drugs that are known to raise Coumadin sensitivity, the starting dosage is 2 mg/day, and 2 mg/day is also the dosage used for those with inherited Coumadin sensitivity. There is no loading dose, and subsequent dosing is based on patient response as measured by the PT/INR.

The activity of each of the vitamin K–dependent coagulation factors begins to decline immediately but at different rates (Figure 40.1), and it takes about 5 days for all the factors to reach therapeutic levels. Table 40.2 lists the plasma half-life, plasma concentration, and minimum effective percentage of normal factor activity for the coagulation factors. Knowing the functional properties of the vitamin K–dependent coagulation factors explains the anticoagulant action of Coumadin.

Control protein activities also become reduced on Coumadin onset, especially the activity of protein C, which has a 6-hour half-life. So for the first 2 or 3 days of Coumadin therapy the patient actually incurs the risk of thrombosis. For this reason, Coumadin therapy is "covered" by UFH, LMWH, or fondaparinux therapy for up to 5 days. Failure to provide anticoagulant therapy during this period may result in Coumadin-induced skin necrosis, a severe thrombotic reaction requiring debridement of dead tissue.[9]

Coumadin is contraindicated during pregnancy because it causes birth defects. When anticoagulation is desired during pregnancy—for instance, in women who possess a thrombosis risk factor—LMWH or fondaparinux is prescribed.

Monitoring Coumadin Therapy
The PT/INR

The PT effectively monitors Coumadin therapy because it is sensitive to reductions of factors II, VII, and X (Figure 40.2) (Chapter 35). The PT reagent consists of tissue factor, phospholipid, and ionic calcium, so it triggers the coagulation pathway at the level of factor VII (Chapter 41). Owing to the 6-hour half-life of factor VII, the PT begins to prolong within 6 to 8 hours of Coumadin dosing; however, anticoagulation becomes therapeutic only when the activities of factors II and X decrease to less than 50% of normal, after approximately 5 days.

The first specimen for PT testing is collected and performed 24 hours after Coumadin therapy is initiated; subsequent PTs are performed daily until at least two consecutive results are within the target therapeutic range. Monitoring continues every 4 to 6 weeks until the completion of therapy, which often lasts for 6 months after a thrombotic event.[10] Monitoring is performed more frequently if there is a dose change, when another medication is being started or stopped, or when the medical condition of the patient changes. The duration of Coumadin therapy for stroke prevention in atrial fibrillation is indefinite, possibly lifelong. Because the therapeutic range is narrow, diligent monitoring is essential for successful Coumadin therapy. Underanticoagulation signals the danger of thrombosis or secondary thrombosis (rethrombosis); overdose carries the danger of hemorrhage.

PT results and the INR. The medical laboratory technician or scientist reports PT results to the nearest tenth of a second and provides the PT reference interval in seconds for comparison. In view of the inherent variations among thromboplastin reagents and to accomplish interlaboratory normalization, all laboratories report the international normalized ratio (INR) for patients who have reached a stable response to Coumadin therapy. The INR has been validated only for use

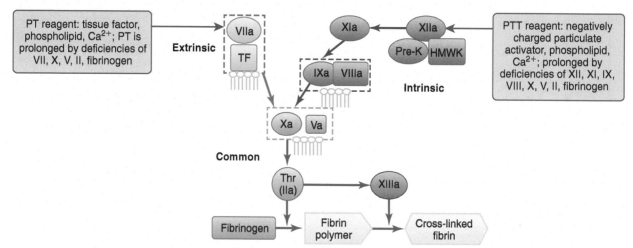

Figure 40.2 The Prothrombin Time (PT) and Partial Thromboplastin Time (PTT) Tests. The PT reagent activates the extrinsic coagulation pathway beginning with factor VII. The PT is prolonged by deficiencies of factors VII, X, V, and II (prothrombin); and fibrinogen when the fibrinogen concentration is less than 100 mg/dL. The PT is prolonged in Coumadin therapy because it responds to the reduced VII, X, and prothrombin activity. The PTT reagent activates the intrinsic coagulation pathway through factor XII, in association with prekallikrein (pre-K) and high-molecular-weight kininogen (HMWK). The PTT is prolonged by deficiencies of pre-K; HMWK; factors XII, XI, IX, VIII, and X; prothrombin; and fibrinogen when the fibrinogen concentration is less than 100 mg/dL. The PTT is prolonged in unfractionated heparin (UFH) therapy because UFH activates the plasma control protein antithrombin, which neutralizes the serine proteases XIIa, XIa, Xa, IXa, and IIa (thrombin [Thr]). The PTT is also prolonged by lupus anticoagulant. TF, Tissue factor.

with Coumadin monitoring. Laboratory practitioners use the following formula:[11]

$$INR = (PT_{patient}/PT_{normal})^{ISI}$$

where $PT_{patient}$ is the PT of the patient in seconds, PT_{normal} is the geometric mean of the PT reference interval in seconds, and ISI is the international sensitivity index applied as an exponent.

Thromboplastin producers generate the ISI by performing a regression analysis comparing the results of their PT reagents for 50 or more Coumadin plasma specimens and 10 or more normal specimens with the results of the international reference thromboplastin (World Health Organization human brain thromboplastin) on the same plasmas specimens.[12] Most manufacturers provide ISIs for a variety of coagulation instruments because each coagulometer may respond differently to their thromboplastins; for instance, some coagulometers rely on photometric plasma changes, whereas others use an electromechanical system (Chapter 42). Most thromboplastin reagents have ISIs near 1.0, matching the ISI of the World Health Organization's international reference thromboplastin. Automated coagulometers "request" the reagent ISI from the operator or obtain it electronically from a reagent vial label bar code, and compute the INR for each assay result. Although INRs are meant to be computed only for patients in whom the response to Coumadin has stabilized, they typically are reported for all patients, even those who are not taking Coumadin. During the first 5 days of Coumadin therapy, the astute physician and medical laboratory practitioner ignore the INR as unreliable and interpret the PT results in seconds, comparing it with the reference interval.

Coumadin INR therapeutic range. The physician adjusts the Coumadin dosage to achieve the desired INR of 2 to 3, or 2.5 to 3.5 if the patient has a mechanical heart valve. INRs greater than 5 are associated with increased risk of hemorrhage and require immediate communication with the clinician who is managing the patient's case.[13,14] Dosage adjustments are made conservatively because the INR requires 4 to 7 days to stabilize, but an elevated INR accompanied by the symptoms of anatomic bleeding is a medical emergency.

Chromogenic Factor X Assay

The chromogenic coagulation factor X assay (not to be confused with the chromogenic anti-Xa heparin assay) may be used as an alternative to the PT/INR system, eliminating the necessity for normalization of test results using the INR.[15] The therapeutic range is typically about 20% to 40% of normal factor X activity, determined locally by comparison with the INR.[16] The chromogenic factor X assay is useful when the PT is compromised by a lupus anticoagulant, a factor inhibitor, or a coagulation factor deficiency.[17]

Diet and Drug Interference on Coumadin Activity

Dietary vitamin K decreases Coumadin's effectiveness and reduces the INR. Green vegetables are an important source of vitamin K, but vitamin K also is concentrated in green tea, cauliflower, liver, avocados, parenteral nutrition formulations, multivitamins, red wine, over-the-counter nutrition drinks, and over-the-counter dietary supplements. A patient who is taking Coumadin is counseled to maintain a regular balanced diet, avoid supplements, and follow up dietary changes or dietary supplement changes with additional PT assays and dosage adjustments, if indicated.

Coumadin is metabolized in the mitochondrial cytochrome P450 (CYP2C9) pathway of hepatocytes—the "disposal system" for at least 80 drugs. Theoretically, parallel therapy with any drug metabolized through the CYP2C9 pathway may unpredictably suppress or enhance the effects of Coumadin due to competition for sites within the pathway. Amiodarone, metronidazole, and cimetidine suppress the pathway and typically double or triple the INR. Any change in drug therapy must be followed up with additional PT assays and dosage adjustments.

Sensitivity to Coumadin

Two genetic polymorphisms generate variations in enzymes of the cytochrome P450 pathway. These are *CYP2C9*2* and *CYP2C9*3*, which reduce enzyme pathway activity and slow the metabolic breakdown of Coumadin. Likewise, there is a genetic polymorphism located at 16p11.2 that affects the key enzyme of vitamin K metabolism, vitamin K epoxide reductase.[18] This polymorphism, named *VKORC1*, slows vitamin K reduction, which makes the patient more sensitive to Coumadin. In patients possessing one, two, or all three of these polymorphisms, Coumadin therapy should begin at 2 mg/day and should be adjusted and monitored daily until the INR remains consistently in the therapeutic range. The standard 5 mg/day regimen risks hemorrhage in patients who possess these polymorphisms. In 2007 the US Food and Drug Administration (FDA) required that drug manufacturers add a statement on all vials of Coumadin recommending that physicians screen patients for these common dosage-affecting polymorphisms. Numerous molecular diagnostics manufacturers have developed short turnaround assays for these three polymorphisms.[19]

Conversely, Coumadin receptor insufficiency ("Coumadin resistance") may render the patient unresponsive to typical Coumadin dosages. Some patients require dosages of 20 mg/day or higher to achieve a therapeutic INR. Coumadin resistance has been traced to up to 26 mutations also of the VKORC1 gene. These mutations parallel polymorphisms that render rodents resistant to warfarin poisoning.[20]

Switching Anticoagulants and the PT/INR

Physicians switch from an intravenous anticoagulant to an oral anticoagulant, often Coumadin, once the patient is recovering. The crossover period is necessary because of the 5 days required to achieve full Coumadin anticoagulation. When UFH, monitored by the PTT, is the intravenous drug, the transition to Coumadin, monitored by the PT/INR, is without issue. However, in switching from the intravenous DTI argatroban or bivalirudin to Coumadin, the combination nearly doubles

the PT.[21] The chromogenic factor X assay is an effective means for monitoring Coumadin dosage during the crossover period.

Reversing Coumadin

Table 40.3 provides recommendations for Coumadin overdose reversal based on the INR and evidence of bleeding. Reversal requires oral or intravenous vitamin K and, if bleeding is severe, a means for substituting active coagulation factors such as plasma, recombinant activated factor VII (rVIIa, NovoSeven), activated prothrombin complex concentrate (FEIBA), three-factor nonactivated prothrombin complex concentrate (Profilnine), or four-factor prothrombin complex concentrate (Kcentra). The effects of reversal are assessed through clinical observation and repeated PT/INR assays.[22]

UNFRACTIONATED HEPARIN

Heparin Activates Antithrombin to Neutralize Serine Proteases

Standard UFH, often simply called heparin, was first used clinically in 1935. It is a mixture of sulfated glycosaminoglycans (polysaccharides) extracted from porcine mucosa. The molecular weight of UFH ranges from 3000 to 30,000 Daltons (average 15,000 Daltons). Approximately one-third of its molecules support somewhere on their length a series of 5 specific sugar units, a pentasaccharide, which binds plasma antithrombin with high affinity. The mixture of polysaccharide chains provides additional binding sites for antithrombin, but none that produce the high affinity binding as this specific pentasaccharide sequence.

The anticoagulant action of UFH is indirect and catalytic, relying on antithrombin. Pentasaccharide-bound antithrombin undergoes a steric change (allostery), exposing an anticoagulant site that covalently binds and inactivates the coagulation pathway serine proteases, factors IIa (thrombin), IXa, Xa, XIa, and XIIa (Chapter 35). Principal among these are heparin's inhibition of thrombin and factor Xa. Laboratory practitioners call activated antithrombin a *serine protease inhibitor* (SERPIN), and the protease-binding reaction yields, among other products, the measurable inactive plasma complex thrombin-antithrombin (TAT) (Figure 35.15). When UFH binds antithrombin the combination increases the rate of antithrombin inhibition of thrombin 1000-fold.

TABLE 40.3 Recommendations for Reversal of Coumadin Overdose Based on INR and Bleeding		
Bleeding	**INR**	**Intervention**
No significant bleeding	3–5	Reduce dosage or omit one dose, monitor INR frequently
	5–9	Omit Coumadin, monitor INR frequently, consider oral vitamin K ($\leq$5 mg) if high risk for bleeding (surgery)
	>9	Stop Coumadin, give 5–10 mg oral vitamin K, monitor INR frequently
Serious bleeding	Any INR	Stop Coumadin, give 10 mg vitamin K by intravenous push (may repeat every 12 hr); give thawed fresh-frozen plasma, prothrombin complex concentrate, or recombinant factor VIIa
Life-threatening bleeding	Any INR	Same as for serious bleeding, except stronger indication for recombinant factor VIIa

INR, International normalized ratio.

UFH supports the thrombin-antithrombin reaction through a "bridging" mechanism. If the UFH molecule exceeds approximately 17 linear saccharide units, thrombin assembles on the UFH molecule near the bound, activated antithrombin. Bridging drives the thrombin-antithrombin reaction at a rate four times that of the factor Xa-antithrombin reaction, because factor Xa becomes inactivated only through binding to the sterically modified antithrombin; factor Xa itself does not bind UFH.

UFH preparations vary in average molecular weight, the chain length and chemical structure, and in particular the saccharide unit sulfation patterns. These variations affect UFH's efficacy among manufacturers and between lots. Further, individual patient UFH dose responses diverge markedly because numerous plasma and cellular proteins bind UFH at varying rates. Consequently, laboratory monitoring is essential.[23]

Heparin Therapy

Physicians administer UFH intravenously to treat VTE, to provide initial treatment of AMI, to prevent reocclusion after stent placement, and to maintain vascular patency during cardiac surgery using cardiopulmonary bypass (CPB) with extracorporeal circulation. For VTE treatment, therapy begins with a bolus of 5000 to 10,000 units, followed by continuous infusion at approximately 1300 units/hour, adjusted to patient weight. Cardiac surgeons use much higher dosages during bypass surgery. UFH therapy is discontinued when the acute clinical state has resolved or after the procedure or surgery. If necessary, the patient will be switched to an oral anticoagulant to reduce the risk of future thrombotic events.[24]

Monitoring Heparin Therapy

Because of its inherent pharmacologic variations and narrow therapeutic range, laboratory professionals diligently monitor UFH therapy using the PTT or the chromogenic anti-Xa heparin assay. For PTT monitoring, blood is collected and assayed before therapy is begun to ensure that the baseline PTT is normal.[25] A prolonged baseline PTT may indicate an underlying coagulopathy or the presence of lupus anticoagulant. In this case the chromogenic anti-Xa assay is employed.

A second PTT specimen is collected a minimum of 4 to 6 hours but not longer than 24 hours after the initial UFH bolus. The PTT becomes prolonged within minutes of UFH administration, reflecting the immediate anticoagulation effect of UFH. The result for the second specimen should fall within the target therapeutic range (discussed in the following section), which is established by the laboratory practitioner and reported with the result. The physician or nurse adjusts the infusion rate to ensure that the PTT result remains within the target range. PTT measurement is subsequently repeated every 24 hours, and the dosage is continually readjusted until UFH anticoagulation is complete. The physician also requests that the laboratory monitors the platelet count daily. A 40% or greater reduction in the platelet count, even within the reference interval, is presumptive evidence for HIT. (See the discussion of the "4Ts" HIT diagnosis system in Chapter 39.) If HIT is suspected and thrombosis is present, UFH therapy is immediately discontinued and replaced with intravenous DTI therapy. If thrombosis has not developed, fondaparinux or a DOAC can be administered.

Determining the PTT Therapeutic Range for Heparin Therapy

The hemostasis laboratory establishes and communicates a PTT therapeutic range to monitor and manage UFH therapy. The practitioner collects 20 to 30 plasma specimens from patients being infused with UFH at all levels of anticoagulation, ensuring that fewer than 10% of the specimens are collected from the same patient, and measures PTT for all.[26] The specimens must be from patients who are not receiving simultaneous Coumadin therapy; that is, their PT results must be normal. The practitioner also performs PTTs on specimens from 10 normal healthy non-anticoagulated subjects. A chromogenic anti-Xa heparin assay is performed on aliquots of all specimens and the paired results are displayed on a linear graph (Figure 40.3). The range in seconds of PTT results that corresponds to 0.3 to 0.7 chromogenic anti-Xa heparin units/mL is the therapeutic range.[27] This therapeutic range method, known as the ex vivo or Brill-Edwards method, is required by laboratory certification and licensing agencies. The UFH therapeutic range is communicated to the pharmacy and all inpatient facility units.

Other therapeutic range approaches are discouraged. For instance, experts once recommended a PTT therapeutic range of 1.5 to 2.5 times the mean of the reference interval. This approach, however, consistently results in underanticoagulation, which raises the risk of a secondary thrombotic event. The practice of developing a therapeutic range by "spiking" normal plasma with measured volumes of heparin is prohibited because the curve that is generated tends to flatten at higher concentrations and does not represent the clinical condition.[28]

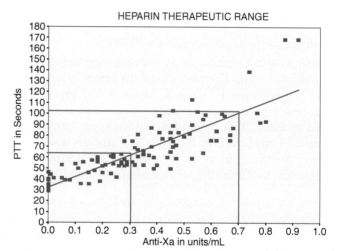

Figure 40.3 Heparin Therapeutic Range. Laboratory practitioners establish the partial thromboplastin time *(PTT)* therapeutic range for unfractionated heparin *(UFH)* by collecting specimens from 20 to 30 patients receiving UFH at representative dosages who have normal prothrombin times and at least 10 individuals not receiving heparin. PTT and chromogenic anti-factor Xa heparin assays are performed on all specimens, and a linear graph of paired results is prepared with PTT on the vertical scale. The PTT range in seconds is correlated with the chromogenic anti-factor Xa therapeutic range of 0.3 to 0.7 units/mL or the prophylactic range of 0.1 to 0.4 units/mL.

Clinical Practice of Heparin Therapy Monitoring Using the PTT

The medical laboratory practitioner reports the PTT results, the reference interval, and the UFH therapeutic range to the clinician who is managing the patient's UFH dosage. Because reagent sensitivity varies among producers and among individual producers' reagent lots, the clinician must evaluate PTT results in relationship to the institution's published therapeutic range and reference interval.[29] No system analogous to the INR exists for normalizing PTT results because reagents and patient responses are inconsistent.

Limitations of Heparin Therapy Monitoring Using the PTT

Several conditions render the patient unresponsive to UFH therapy, a circumstance called heparin resistance.[30] These conditions may affect heparin's anticoagulation efficacy and may interfere with the PTT. Inflammation is typically accompanied by fibrinogen levels raised to greater than 500 mg/dL and factor VIII activities of greater than 190 U/dL. Both elevations render the PTT less sensitive to heparin's effects, though the therapeutic effect is unchanged. Further, in many patients, antithrombin activity becomes depleted as a result of prolonged UFH therapy or an underlying deficiency secondary to chronic inflammation. In this instance the PTT result remains below the therapeutic range, becoming only modestly prolonged despite ever-increasing UFH dosages.

The physician may reduce inflammation with steroids, aspirin, or other nonsteroidal antiinflammatory drugs and may administer antithrombin concentrate. In the interim, however, it is necessary to use an alternative assay for UFH monitoring such as the chromogenic anti-Xa heparin assay. In this case the laboratory director needs to consider the type of anti-Xa heparin assay. One type is designed with reagent antithrombin, which will provide the concentration or amount of heparin in the blood; the other type, more often used, depends on the patient's own antithrombin and is thus affected in the same way as the PTT.

Platelets in whole-blood specimens release platelet factor 4 (PF4), a heparin-neutralizing protein (Chapter 10). In specimens from patients receiving UFH therapy, the PTT begins to shorten, masking the effect of UFH, as early as 1 hour after collection because of in vitro PF4 release. For all UFH assays, it is imperative that patient specimens are centrifuged and the platelet-poor plasma is removed from the cells within 1 hour of collection (Chapter 41).[31]

Hypofibrinogenemia, factor deficiencies, and the presence of lupus anticoagulant, fibrin degradation products, or paraproteins falsely prolong the PTT independent of UFH levels. Here too the chromogenic anti-Xa assay is preferred for UFH monitoring.

Monitoring Heparin Using the Chromogenic Anti-Xa Assay

Owing to fewer interferences and improved assay stability, the chromogenic anti-Xa heparin assay is rapidly replacing the PTT in routine clinical use. Its stability leads to fewer dosage drip-rate adjustments and significant reductions in red cell transfusions.[32]

Conversely, the PTT provides a global impression of anticoagulation status, which some physicians prefer, particularly for high-risk patients. Further, the chromogenic anti-Xa heparin assay reflects only the changes in antithrombin-Xa binding, whereas the PTT responds to all plasma-based heparin activities. Some facilities offer the anti-Xa heparin assay for routine UFH monitoring but offer the PTT on physician request. Refer to Measuring LMWH further in this chapter for a description of the chromogenic anti-Xa heparin assay mechanism.

Monitoring Heparin Therapy Using The ACT

Activated clotting time (ACT) is a 1966 modification of the time-honored but obsolete Lee-White whole blood clotting time assay.[33] The ACT is a popular point-of-care test employed to monitor UFH dosages that yield plasma levels of 1 to 2 units/mL, exceeding PTT and anti-Xa analytical range limits. Surgeons employ these high UFH dosages during extracorporeal membrane oxygenation (ECMO) life support for patients with heart-lung disorders, with PCI, and in cardiac surgeries where the caradioplumonary bypass (CPB) unit is used for extracorporeal blood circulation, such as in coronary artery bypass graft (CABG) surgery.[34]

ACT assay distributors such as the makers of the Hemochron Response (Chapter 42) provide evacuated blood specimen collection tubes with no anticoagulant but with a particulate clot activator and a small magnet. The negative tube pressure collects 2 mL of blood. Immediately on collection, the tube is placed in the angled cuvette well, where it is continuously rotated. When a clot forms, the magnet pulls away from a sensing device, stopping the timer, and the time interval to clot formation is recorded.

ACT results are comparable to those of the PTT within the PTT analytical range. The median of the ACT reference interval is 98 seconds. Heparin is administered to yield results of 200 to 240 seconds in PCI or 480 to 600 seconds during CABG.[35]

Reversing Heparin

When CPB is discontinued, UFH anticoagulation must be quickly reversed. Protamine sulfate, (in Europe, protamine chloride) a cationic protein extracted from salmon sperm, binds UFH and neutralizes it at a ratio of 100 units of UFH per milligram protamine. The surgeon or anesthetist administers protamine sulfate slowly by intravenous push, targeting median ACT results, approximately 98 seconds, as their indication of reversal. Protamine sulfate may also be employed to reverse bleeding in UFH-aspirin coadministration, UFH overdose, or fibrinolytic therapy.

Protamine sulfate may cause a delayed form of HIT; consequently, platelet counts for patients who have received protamine sulfate are routinely monitored.[36]

LOW-MOLECULAR-WEIGHT HEPARIN AND THE ANTI-FACTOR Xa ASSAY

LMWH Produced From UFH

Uncertainty about UFH dose response and the ever-present threat of HIT led to the development of LMWH (enoxaparin, tinzaparin, dalteparin), first cleared for anticoagulant prophylaxis in the United States and Canada in 1993.[37] LMWH is

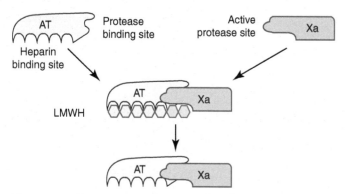

Figure 40.4 The Anti-Factor Xa Mechanism of Action of Low-Molecular-Weight Heparin *(LMWH).* Antithrombin *(AT)* molecules bind a pentasaccharide region on heparin polysaccharide chains, producing an allosteric change that activates AT, facilitating FXa binding. The LMWH molecule is too short to support a factor IIa (thrombin)-AT reaction (Figure 35.15 shows the mechanism for the longer chains of unfractionated heparin). The activated AT binds factor Xa independently of the bridging phenomenon required for thrombin, producing an AT-factor Xa complex.

prepared from UFH using chemical or enzymatic fractionation, which cleaves the long polysaccharide chains to yield a product with a mean molecular weight of 4500 to 5000 Daltons, about one third the mass of UFH.

LMWH possesses the same antithrombin-binding pentasaccharide sequence as UFH; however, the overall shorter polysaccharide chains support less thrombin-antithrombin bridging. The factor Xa neutralization response is unchanged, however, because this reaction does not rely on factor Xa binding to heparin's polysaccharide chain (Figure 40.4). LMWH provides similar anticoagulant efficacy as UFH, although predominantly through factor Xa inhibition.

LMWH Therapy

LMWH is administered by subcutaneous injection once or twice a day using premeasured syringes at selected dosages—for instance, 30 mg subcutaneously every 12 hours or 40 mg subcutaneously once daily. Prophylactic applications provide coverage during or after general and orthopedic surgery and trauma, typically for 14 days from the time of the event. LMWH also is used to treat VTE. LMWH is indicated during pregnancy for women at risk of VTE, because Coumadin causes birth defects. When patients who are taking Coumadin require surgery, it is discontinued for up to a week before the procedure and replaced with an LMWH because of its shorter half-life, a process called "bridging."[38]

The advantages of LMWH over UFH include home therapy, a half-life of 3 to 5 hours compared with 60 to 90 minutes for UFH, increased bioavailability after subcutaneous injection, less plasma protein binding resulting in a more predictable dose response, and lower bleeding risk. The predictable dose response and safety of LMWH treatment eliminates the need for periodic laboratory monitoring, although laboratory measurement is still required for the conditions listed in Box 40.1.

Protamine sulfate may be used to reverse LMWH-associated bleeding, an uncommon event. In contrast to its effect on UFH, LMWH reversal is only partially effective. The incomplete

neutralization is reflected in the results of the chromogenic anti-Xa heparin assay.

To avoid HIT (Chapter 39), LMWH or other anticoagulants are used in place of UFH where possible.[39] LMWH reduces the risk of HIT by 90% compared with UFH in patients who have never received UFH. However, LMWH may cross-react with previously formed antibodies against the heparin-PF4 epitope. Consequently, LMWH is contraindicated in patients who developed HIT after UFH therapy.

Measuring LMWH

The kidneys alone clear LMWH, so it accumulates in patients with renal insufficiency. Laboratory measurement of LMWH therapy is necessary when the creatinine clearance is less than 30 mL/min or the serum creatinine is greater than 4 mg/dL. During LMWH therapy, creatinine assays are performed periodically to document kidney function and avoid the risk of LMWH accumulation in plasma. LMWH therapy in children and adults weighing less than 50 kg, in adults weighing more than 150 kg, and during pregnancy also require measurement because of fluid compartment imbalances or unstable coagulation (Box 40.1).

LMWH selectively catalyzes the neutralization of factor Xa more avidly than the neutralization of thrombin; thus its effects cannot be measured using the PTT. For LMWH the chromogenic anti-Xa assay is the assay of choice.

The phlebotomist collects a blood specimen 4 hours after subcutaneous injection. The chromogenic anti-Xa heparin assay employs a reagent that provides a fixed concentration of factor Xa and a substrate specific to factor Xa (Figure 40.5).

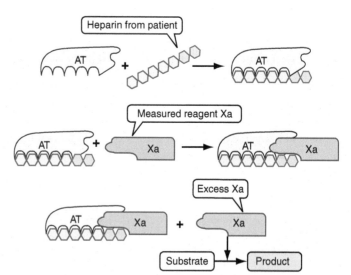

Figure 40.5 The Chromogenic Anti-Xa Heparin Assay. Patient heparin (plasma specimen) binds antithrombin (AT, either from patient plasma or kit reagent), and this complex binds reagent factor Xa. The assay kit provides a measured excess of reagent factor Xa. Factor Xa not bound to the complex digests its substrate to produce a colored end product. The intensity of the product is inversely proportional to plasma heparin. This assay is used for unfractionated heparin *(UFH),* low-molecular-weight heparin *(LMWH),* fondaparinux, and the anti-Xa direct-acting oral anticoagulants *(DOACs).* Standard curves for UFH/LMWH combination, fondaparinux, or the individual DOACs are prepared using calibrators specific to the patient's therapy.

Some distributors add fixed concentrations of antithrombin, and others none; the latter rely on the patient's plasma antithrombin and provide sensitivity to antithrombin depletion or deficiency. Heparin forms a complex with reagent factor Xa and antithrombin; a measured excess of factor Xa digests the substrate, yielding a colored product whose intensity is inversely proportional to heparin concentration.

To prepare a calibration curve, the laboratory practitioner obtains LMWH calibrators from the assay manufacturer, then computes and prepares dilutions that "bracket" the reference and the therapeutic range. If the chromogenic anti-factor Xa heparin assay is to be used to monitor UFH and LMWH, a single hybrid standard curve may be prepared.[40] The prophylactic range for LMWH is 0.2 to 0.5 unit/mL, and the therapeutic range is 0.5 to 1.2 units/mL.[41]

Other anti-Xa anticoagulants, such as fondaparinux and the DOACs, are measured by the chromogenic anti-Xa assay. It is necessary to prepare separate curves using calibrators of the target drug.

FONDAPARINUX AND THE ANTI-FACTOR Xa ASSAY

Fondaparinux sodium (Arixtra) is a synthetic formulation of the active pentasaccharide sequence in UFH and LMWH (Figure 40.6). This is the only synthetic heparin; all other heparin products are from a biologic source. Fondaparinux is composed of only one molecular structure; it is not a mixture of polysaccharide units, unlike UFH or LMWH. The pentasaccharide sequence is specific in the type, number, and placement of saccharide units, in particular the placement and number of sulfate groups, producing the highest antithrombin affinity. Other saccharide sequences by which heparin binds antithrombin are found within UFH and LMWH, but none provide the avidity of fondaparinux.

Fondaparinux, because of its short chain length, inhibits only factor Xa through antithrombin. It has no inhibitory effect on thrombin or other serine proteases. Fondaparinux raises antithrombin activity 400-fold.[42] It is equivalent in clinical efficacy and reproducible dose response to LMWH. Compared with LMWH, fondaparinux has a reduced major bleeding effect

and a longer half-life of 17 to 21 hours, and consequently it is administered in once-a-day subcutaneous injections of 2.5 to 7.5 mg.[43] Fondaparinux is FDA cleared for prevention of VTE after orthopedic and abdominal surgery and for treatment of acute VTE events, but its use is contraindicated in patients with creatinine clearance values of less than 30 mL/min.[44]

Owing to its favorable safety and efficacy profile, physicians seldom order fondaparinux assays. The chromogenic anti-Xa heparin assay is used, however, to measure fondaparinux therapy in children, adults weighing less than 50 kg or more than 150 kg, patients receiving treatment for more than 7 to 8 days, and pregnant women and whenever there is a question related to therapy.[45-47]

Blood is collected 4 hours after injection, and the target range is 0.2 to 0.4 mg/mL for a 2.5-mg dose and 0.5 to 1.5 mg/mL for a 7.5-mg dose. The operator prepares a calibration curve using fondaparinux—not UFH, LMWH, or a hybrid calibrator—because concentrations are expressed in milligrams per milliliter, not units per milliliter. The PTT is not sensitive to the effect of fondaparinux because, although fondaparinux reacts with antithrombin to inhibit factor Xa, it does not inhibit thrombin or factors IXa, XIa, or XIIa.

In the event of bleeding associated with fondaparinux overdose, protamine sulfate is ineffective. Recombinant factor VIIa (NovoSeven) may partially reverse the anticoagulant effect of fondaparinux.[48,49]

ORAL FACTOR Xa INHIBITORS AND THEIR ASSESSMENT

Anticoagulant Activity

Four DOACs directly and stoichiometrically inhibit coagulation factor Xa whether it is free, clot-bound, or bound to coagulation factor IXa (Table 40.4).[50] These are rivaroxaban (Xarelto), apixaban (Eliquis), edoxaban (Savaysa), and the newest, betrixaban (Bevyxxa).[51] These drugs do not require antithrombin to express their anticoagulant activity. Because these drugs are oral, they are replacing Coumadin.

As established by results of several clinical trials, the direct anti-Xa DOACs possess efficacy and safety characteristics equivalent to or better than UFH, enoxaparin, or Coumadin.[52]

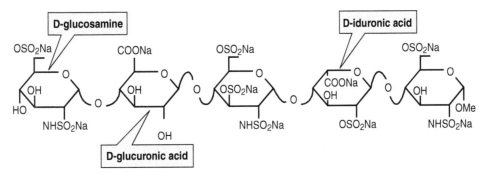

Figure 40.6 The Specific Pentasaccharide Sequence Synthesized to Produce Fondaparinux. The illustrated pentasaccharide sequence of heparin (glucosamine, glucuronic acid, glucosamine, iduronic acid, and glucosamine with associated sulfate groups at the defined positions) allows for the highest affinity binding of antithrombin *(AT)* to heparin. This is the minimum sequence of saccharide units, necessarily composed of the illustrated saccharide units of the shown specific chemical structures, that binds to AT with highest affinity and also produces an anti-factor Xa activity. (From Turpie, A. G. G. [2002]. Pentasaccharides. *Semin Hematol, 39,* 159–171.)

TABLE 40.4   Comparison of the Direct Oral Anticoagulants (DOACs)

Generic Name	Dabigatran	Rivaroxaban	Apixaban	Edoxaban	Betrixaban
Trade Name	Pradaxa	Xarelto	Eliquis	Savaysa	Bevyxxa
Manufacturer	Boehringer Ingelheim	Janssen Pharmaceutical	Pfizer, Bristol-Myers-Squibb	Daiichi-Sankyo	Portola
Indication	Prophylaxis for stroke in NVAF, VTE[1]; treatment of VTE				VTE[2] prophylaxis
US FDA Approval	10/2010	7/2011	12/2012	1/2015	6/2017
Function	DTI	Direct factor Xa inhibitor			
Dosage	75 or 150 mg capsule	15 or 20 mg	10, then 2.5 or 5 mg[3]	15, 30, 60 mg	160 then 80 mg[4]
Daily schedule	Twice	Once[5]	Twice	Once	Once
Half-life	Half-life for DOACS is 10–18 hr when kidney function is normal				
Laboratory assay: peak	Dilute TT, ECA (RUO)	Chromogenic anti-Xa (RUO)			
Kidney function	Normal function required				
Food effect	No	Take with food	No	No	Take with food
Drug interactions	Few				
Reversal	Praxbind	Andexanet Alpha		None	None

1. VTE prophylaxis indication for dabigatran, rivaroxaban, and apixaban is subsequent to orthopedic surgery.
2. VTE prophylaxis for betrixaban is indicated for medical conditions and immobilization.
3. Seven days' loading dose of 10 mg twice a day, then 2.5 or 5 mg.
4. One loading dose at 160 mg followed by daily doses of 80 mg.
5. For VTE, use 3-week loading period of twice daily.

DTI, Direct thrombin inhibitor; *DOAC,* direct oral anticoagulant; *ECA,* ecarin chromogenic assay; *FDA,* US Food and Drug Administration; *NVAF,* nonvalvular atrial fibrillation; *VTE,* venous thromboembolic disease including deep venous thrombosis (DVT) and pulmonary embolism (PE); *TT,* thrombin time; *RUO,* research use only, not approved by US FDA.

Rivaroxaban, apixaban, and edoxaban are approved by the US FDA, Health Canada, and the European Medicines Agency for prevention of secondary thrombosis subsequent to VTE, VTE prophylaxis in patients who are undergoing total knee or total hip replacement surgery, and prevention of ischemic stroke in patients with chronic nonvalvular atrial fibrillation.[53] Betrixaban was approved in 2017 for VTE prophylaxis in patients with chronic medical conditions or immobilization. None of the DOACs have been approved for post-AMI therapy, for use in pregnant women, or for use in patients with HIT.[54]

The anti-factor Xa DOACs possess half-lives of 10 to 18 hours and are cleared through the kidney, except for apixaban—70% of active apixaban is cleared by the liver. When DOACs are prescribed, frequent kidney function tests are necessary. For overdose-related hemorrhages, some clinicians report normalization of laboratory test results by the use of FEIBA, Kcentra, or NovoSeven.[55] A specific reversal agent, andexanet alfa (AndexXa) was cleared for clinical use by the FDA in May 2018.[56,57]

Laboratory Assessment

All anti-factor Xa DOACs are prescribed without laboratory monitoring, however, the clinical conditions listed in Box 40.1 dictate the need to assess DOAC levels at indicated times.[58] There is minimal effect on the PTT.[58,59] The relationship of Coumadin dosing and bleeding risk to PT/INR, the mainstay of oral anticoagulation monitoring since 1960, does not exist with the anti-Xa DOACs. However, the tendency to bleed increases with increasing DOAC doses.

Rivaroxaban prolongs the PT in a reagent-dependent manner, edoxaban to a lesser degree, and apixaban has no effect on the PT. Attempts to correlate PT results with dosage have revealed variability among DOAC responses and among PT reagents, rendering the PT only partially valid.[60] The PT shortcomings include a lack of low-end sensitivity and linearity over the therapeutic range. DOAC overdose may be reflected with prolonged PT results; however, the PT cannot be used to quantitate their activity.

Anti-Xa DOACs may be measured using drug-specific versions of the chromogenic anti-Xa heparin assay.[61] The assay is calibrated using the respective DOAC in place of UFH, LMWH, or fondaparinux.[62] Manufacturers have produced calibrators and controls dedicated to chromogenic anti-factor Xa assays for rivaroxaban, apixaban, and edoxaban and soon for betrixaban. These await FDA approval and thus are labeled for research use only (RUO). Laboratory practitioners are working to correlate laboratory results with clinical outcomes in an effort to provide a therapeutic range.

One other test option is liquid chromatography used in tandem with mass spectrometry (LC-MS/MS), similar to high performance liquid chromatography (HPLC). This assay served as the reference assay in clinical trials. LC-MS/MS quantitates the drug level, but does not provide functional anticoagulation information. This technique is sensitive and specific but requires trained staff and instrumentation is in few clinical laboratories.

Anti-Xa DOACs interfere with PT and PTT-based coagulation assays. Factor assay results are falsely decreased. Tests for lupus anticoagulant, protein C, protein S, and antithrombin are falsely prolonged leading to false positive lupus anticoagulant tests and falsely increased antithrombin, protein C, and protein S. Immunoassays are unaffected.

A tablet-form RUO product, DOAC-Stop (Haematex, Dia-Pharma) depletes dabigatran, rivaroxaban, apixaban, edoxaban at 1 tablet per mL test plasma, so that the treated specimen yields PT, PTT, and dilute Russell viper venom time (DRVVT) results equivalent to the same specimen without DOACs. DOAC-Stop absorbs up to an estimated 2000 ng/mL of any DOAC in less than 5 minutes and does not appear to interfere with Coumadin or heparin-based anticoagulants.[63] As well as providing DOAC-free plasma for testing, DOAC-Stop may be used to identify the presence of a DOAC.

DIRECT THROMBIN INHIBITORS AND THEIR ASSESSMENT

Oral Dabigatran
Anticoagulant Activity

Oral dabigatran etexilate (Pradaxa) is a DOAC prodrug that converts upon digestion to active dabigatran, a DTI that binds both free and clot-bound thrombin (Table 40.4). Dabigatran does not require antithrombin as a cofactor to inhibit thrombin for its anticoagulant effect; thus, like the anti-factor Xa DOACs, dabigatran is a direct acting inhibitor.

Dabigatran's efficacy and safety match those of enoxaparin and Coumadin, and it has shown no food interactions. It is cleared by the kidneys, has a half-life of 10 to 18 hours, and is not metabolized by liver cytochrome enzymes. However, it relies on the P-glycoprotein transport system, which leads to drug-drug interactions that may raise or lower the plasma concentration.[64]

Like the anti-Xa DOACS, dabigatran is approved for VTE prophylaxis and therapy and for stroke prevention in nonvalvular atrial fibrillation. In renal disease the half-life may be prolonged to as much as 60 hours. Dabigatran activity is rapidly reversed using idarucizumab (Praxbind), a monoclonal antibody.[65]

Laboratory Assessment

Dabigatran, like all DOACs, is prescribed without periodic monitoring. Measurement becomes necessary when one of the clinical situations listed in Box 40.1 apply. Dabigatran prolongs the thrombin time (TT), PTT, and ecarin clotting time (ECT). The standard TT is exceptionally sensitive and is convenient for ruling out the presence of dabigatran; a normal TT indicates definitively that no drug is present. A prolonged TT may indicate that dabigatran is present, but the concentration cannot be determined. The PTT generates a "curvilinear" response to dabigatran and is unreliable at low levels, but a normal PTT can be used to rule out a dabigatran overdose. There is considerable variability in sensitivity to dabigatran among PTT reagents.[66]

The ecarin chromogenic assay (ECA) provides a precise, accurate linear response to dabigatran, with an analytical range of 18 to 470 ng/mL. Ecarin is a snake venom that activates prothrombin to form meizothrombin, an intermediate form of thrombin. Meizothrombin acts on its substrate, producing a

color whose intensity is proportional to the dabigatran plasma concentration.[67] The ECA can be adapted to all coagulometers.

Further, a modification of the TT called the plasma-diluted thrombin time (Hemoclot Direct Thrombin Inhibitor Assay) is available.[68] Patient plasma is diluted with normal human plasma and the TT is performed using standard assay technique. The assay provides linearity and analytical sensitivity data similar to the ECA. The ECA and the plasma-diluted thrombin time, both of which require a sodium citrate plasma specimen, await FDA approval and are available in the RUO category.[69] The ECA and plasma-diluted TT, when combined with dabigatran calibrators, may become the assays of choice for determining plasma concentration of dabigatran. The LC-MS/MS, as described for the anti-Xa DOACs, can also be used for dabigatran assessment.

Any clot-based coagulation assay, such as PT, PTT, factor assay, or lupus anticoagulant profile, is prolonged by dabigatran, leading to invalid test results.

Intravenous Direct Thrombin Inhibitors

For patients with HIT, anticoagulation is a necessity. However, they cannot be administered any heparin product that cross-reacts with the HIT antibody. Coumadin is also contraindicated for its slow startup. The intravenous DTIs argatroban or bivalirudin offer rapid onset and efficacy, and their chemical structure avoids generating or cross-reacting with heparin-PF4 antibodies.

The DTIs bind and inactivate free and clot-bound thrombin (Figure 40.7). DTIs substitute for UFH or LMWH when HIT is suspected or confirmed using the 4Ts assessment system (Chapter 39).[70] Without argatroban or bivalirudin, the risk of thrombosis is 50% for 30 days after heparin is discontinued.[71] Because of their cost and increased bleeding risk, argatroban and bivalirudin are limited to patients with HIT.

Argatroban

Argatroban (Novastan) is a non-protein L-arginine derivative with a molecular weight of 527 Daltons.[72] Argatroban was

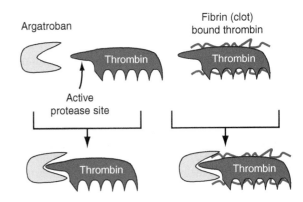

Figure 40.7 The Mechanism of Action of Direct Thrombin Inhibitors *(DTIs).* The thrombin inhibitor argatroban binds directly to and inhibits the active site of free and fibrin/clot-bound thrombin *(factor IIa).* Antithrombin is not involved in this reaction. Bivalirudin and dabigatran directly inhibit thrombin by interacting at the same site but with their own specific binding characteristics.

FDA approved in 1997 for thrombosis prophylaxis and treatment and for anticoagulation during PCI for patients with HIT.[73]

Due to its 50-minute half-life, argatroban is administered by continuous infusion. The physician initiates infusion at 2 μg/kg per minute or in hepatic disease at 0.5 μg/kg per minute. During PCI, a bolus of 350 μg/kg is given over 3 to 5 minutes, followed by infusion at 25 μg/kg per minute. Argatroban is cleared by the liver and excreted in stool. There is a remarkable 5% general bleeding risk and no direct reversal agent; however, on discontinuance, argatroban clears completely in 2 to 4 hours.

Bivalirudin

Bivalirudin (Angiomax) is a synthetic 20-amino acid, 2180 Dalton molecular weight peptide analogue of the active site of hirudin, an anticoagulant produced in trace amounts in the saliva of the medicinal leech *Hirudo medicinalis*. The FDA cleared bivalirudin in 2000 for use as an anticoagulant in patients with unstable angina at risk for HIT who are undergoing PCI.[74] Bivalirudin is used as an anticoagulant in any patient with HIT, including emergency cardiac surgery.

Bivalirudin is intended for use with concurrent 325 mg/day aspirin because it has been studied only in patients receiving aspirin.[75] For PCI, surgeons provide an intravenous bolus dose of 0.75 mg/kg bivalirudin, followed by an infusion of 1.75 mg/kg per hour for the duration of the procedure. After 4 hours, an additional intravenous infusion may be given at a rate of 0.2 mg/kg per hour for up to 20 hours. The manufacturer provides specialized dosing and monitoring recommendations.

The rate of major hemorrhage with bivalirudin is a striking 4%. There is no reversal agent; however, in patients with normal renal function, the half-life is 25 minutes. Anticoagulation reversal is accomplished by discontinuing the infusion. The dosage is decreased in patients with reduced creatinine clearance or elevated serum creatinine.[76]

Monitoring Argatroban and Bivalirudin

Argatroban and bivalirudin are monitored to ensure that patients are maintained within the therapeutic range. Both prolong the thrombin time, PT, PTT, and ACT.[77] For nonsurgical therapy, distributors recommend assaying with the PTT using the target therapeutic range of 1.5 to 3 times the mean of the laboratory reference interval, but not more than 90 seconds. Blood is collected 2 hours after initiation of intravenous therapy for argatroban and 4 hours after therapy initiation for bivalirudin, and the dosage is adjusted to achieve a PTT within the therapeutic range.

The point-of-care ACT offers immediate turnaround during PCI because it detects the higher dosages required for interventional cardiology procedures. The target ACT for bivalirudin therapy is 320 to 400 seconds with a median normal value of 98 seconds.[78]

When the baseline PTT is prolonged by lupus anticoagulant, factor inhibitors, or factor deficiencies, the ECT provides an alternative. Argatroban and bivalirudin bind meizothrombin and generate a linear, dose-dependent prolongation of the ECT.

Aside from DTIs, the ECT is prolonged only by reduced prothrombin or fibrinogen activity.

Intravenous DTI Interference in Coagulation Assays

Transition from argatroban or bivalirudin to Coumadin requires monitoring of both anticoagulants using PTT and PT/INR, respectively. This is challenging because the DTIs prolong the PT and raise the INR. It is possible to see INR values of 6 or higher during combined treatment.[21,79] Studies have found, however, that the PT/INR elevation is an artifact that does not signal increased bleeding risk. Physicians ensure that the INR reaches the therapeutic range of 2 to 3 when DTIs are discontinued.[80]

Clot-based coagulation assays such as the PT and PTT are prolonged by argatroban or bivalirudin, leading to invalid results. As a consequence, factor assays and fibrinogen levels are falsely low and protein C and S levels are falsely elevated.

ANTIPLATELET THERAPY AND PLATELET FUNCTION ASSAYS

Although aspirin has been used medicinally for more than 100 years, its antiplatelet effect and role in reducing the risk of arterial thrombosis were first appreciated in the 1990s when the cardiology community undertook clinical trials that established aspirin's property of reducing heart disease.[81] Chapter 37 provides a detailed description of aspirin, other antiplatelet drugs, and their effect on platelet function.

Intravenous Antiplatelet Drugs for PCI

The intravenous glycoprotein IIb/IIIa inhibitors fill $\alpha_{IIb}\beta_3$ receptor sites and block fibrinogen or von Willebrand factor binding, reducing platelet aggregation (Figure 37.5).[82]

Cardiologists infuse GPIs to maintain vascular patency during PCI for intracoronary stent placement and angioplasty.[83] Before GPI infusion, the PT, PTT, ACT, hemoglobin, hematocrit, and platelet count are determined to detect any hemostatic or hematologic abnormality. During infusion, the ACT is maintained within the specified UFH therapeutic range. Platelet counts are performed at 2 hours, 4 hours, and 24 hours after the initial bolus. If the platelet count drops by 25% or more, UFH and GPI are discontinued and the platelet count is monitored daily until it returns to within the reference interval.[84] GPI efficacy may be measured using the Multiplate analyzer or VerifyNow IIb/IIIa assay.[85]

Abciximab (ReoPro) is the 47,615 Dalton Fab fragment of a mouse monoclonal antibody specific for $\alpha_{IIb}\beta_3$ that effectively fills the receptor site. The dose is 0.25 mg/kg given by intravenous bolus administered 10 to 60 minutes before the start of cardiac catheterization, followed by continuous infusion of 0.125 μg/kg per minute for up to 12 hours. Abciximab is always coadministered with UFH and aspirin.

Eptifibatide (Integrilin) is an 832 Dalton heptapeptide GPI. It is coadministered with aspirin and UFH. An intravenous bolus of 180 μg/kg is given as soon as possible after initial diagnosis, and a continuous intravenous drip of 2 μg/kg per minute is continued for up to 96 hours after the initial bolus, including throughout cardiac catheterization.

Tirofiban hydrochloride (Aggrastat) is a 495 Dalton non-protein GPI that is coadministered with aspirin and UFH. It is administered intravenously at an initial rate of 0.4 μg/kg per minute for 30 minutes and then continued at 0.1 μg/kg per minute throughout cardiac catheterization and for 12 to 24 hours after catheterization. Tirofiban is excreted through the kidney, so the dosage is halved when the creatinine clearance is less than 30 mL/min.

Oral Antiplatelet Drugs to Reduce the Incidence of Arterial Thrombosis

The most commonly prescribed oral antiplatelet drugs are aspirin, clopidogrel (Plavix), prasugrel (Effient), and ticagrelor (Brilinta) (Figure 37.5).[86,87] The thienopyridines clopidogrel, and prasugrel, and the purine analogue ticagrelor occupy the platelet membrane adenosine diphosphate (ADP) receptor $P2Y_{12}$, suppressing the normal platelet aggregation and secretion response to ADP.[88]

Aspirin, alone or in combination with clopidogrel, prasugrel, or ticagrelor, called dual antiplatelet therapy, is prescribed at 81 or 325 mg/day to prevent secondary thrombotic events in patients with stable or unstable angina, AMI, transient cerebral ischemia, peripheral vascular disease, or stroke.[89] Many primary care practitioners recommend that healthy people older than 55 take one aspirin tablet per day. This regimen carries a risk of gastrointestinal bleeding but prevents four thrombotic events per 1000 individuals per year.[90]

Clopidogrel is prescribed at 75 mg/day together with aspirin. Clopidogrel is a prodrug, and patients have varying dose responses. Patients who possess a variant of the CYP2C19 liver enzyme responsible for activating clopidogrel, detected through molecular diagnostic techniques, may not get the full therapeutic effect. This raises the need for platelet function assays and dosage adjustment.[91]

Prasugrel, administered with aspirin, is an oral prodrug that is converted in the liver via several cytochrome P450 pathways to an active metabolite whose elimination half-life is about 7 hours. Treatment begins with a single 60-mg oral loading dose and continues at 10 mg daily, or 5 mg daily for patients who weigh less than 60 kg. Prasugrel is to be taken with aspirin at 81 mg or 325 mg daily. Up to 14% of patients may not achieve the full effect of prasugrel because of a genetic variant of the CYP2C19 liver activation enzyme. In addition, prasugrel dosage is affected by drug interactions. Prasugrel carries a higher risk of bleeding than clopidogrel and may be associated with an increased risk of solid tumors. Platelet function assays, though optional, may be used to assess the antiplatelet effect of prasugrel.[92]

Ticagrelor is coadministered with aspirin. Ticagrelor is a prodrug whose main active metabolite is formed via the CYP3A4 liver enzyme. It is provided in 90-mg tablets. Therapy is begun with 180 mg, taken with 325 mg of aspirin, followed by 90 mg of ticagrelor twice a day and aspirin once a day. Ticagrelor reaches full effectiveness in 1.5 hours and maintains a steady state for at least 8 hours. Ticagrelor is susceptible to drug interactions and platelet function assays may be used to assess the antiplatelet effect of ticagrelor.

Laboratory Assessment of Antiplatelet Drugs

Several investigations confirm that 10% to 20% of people who are taking aspirin generate an inadequate response as measured by arachidonic acid-triggered platelet aggregometry. Inadequate response has been termed *aspirin resistance*.[93,94] Likewise, the response to clopidogrel, prasugrel, or ticagrelor, as measured by ADP-triggered aggregometry, varies markedly among patients. Aggregometry results may be used to adjust dosage.[95] Prasugrel and ticagrelor generate less interpatient variation than aspirin or clopidogrel. Aggregometry (Chapter 41) is the reference method; however, several rapid assays are available.[95,96]

The point-of-care VerifyNow system uses light transmittance aggregometry to test for responses to aspirin, clopidogrel, prasugrel, ticagrelor, and the GPIs. For each assay a cartridge provides the desired agonist and a suspension of fibrinogen-coated beads. VerifyNow Aspirin uses arachidonic acid as its agonist. VerifyNow $P2Y_{12}$ uses ADP, and VerifyNow IIb/IIIa uses thrombin receptor-activating peptide (TRAP), which activates platelets by binding the thrombin receptor protease-activated receptor 1 (PAR1; Chapter 10; Figure 37.5). The laboratory establishes reference interval and therapeutic target limits for each assay. Results that are outside the therapeutic target range indicate possible treatment failure and the need to revise dosage or change to a new antiplatelet drug. All three Accumetrics VerifyNow assays are US FDA approved.

The semiautomated point-of-care Multiplate analyzer, available in Europe, employs impedance aggregometry (Chapters 41 and 42) to simultaneously or individually test for responses to aspirin, clopidogrel, and GPIs. The Multiplate requires a total of 300 μL of whole blood. The aspirin resistance assay uses arachidonic acid as its agonist, the clopidogrel response assay uses ADP, and the GPI response uses TRAP. The instrument integrates three aggregometry parameters—aggregation velocity, maximum aggregation, and area under the aggregation curve—to produce measurement units. The local laboratory establishes reference interval limits and expected therapeutic target ranges. Results that are outside the therapeutic target range indicate possible treatment failure and the need to revise dosage or change to a new antiplatelet drug.

The PlateletWorks assay determines the percent platelet aggregation in whole blood. Fresh whole blood is transferred to EDTA tubes coated with the agonists ADP or collagen, plus plain EDTA tubes. The practitioner performs platelet counts on the EDTA-only tube (baseline) and the agonist-treated EDTA tubes using an electronic cell counter. The differences, expressed as percentages, indicate the degree of platelet aggregation triggered by each agonist. An expected response is 40% to 60% reduction from normal.

The PFA-100 system uses two cartridges. The first provides an aperture impregnated with collagen and epinephrine, and the second impregnated with collagen and ADP. The operator pipettes 800 μL whole blood per cartridge and places each cartridge in turn on the instrument. The specimen passes through the aperture until activation by the agonist causes occlusion, generating a parameter called closure time. The PFA-100 tests for aspirin resistance but not for clopidogrel or the GPIs.

A closure time that is shorter than the anticipated therapeutic range for aspirin indicates resistance. The PFA-100 is also used to reach a presumptive diagnosis for platelet function deficiency or von Willebrand disease.

The AspirinWorks immunoassay measures a urine metabolite of platelet eicosanoid synthesis, 11-dehydrothromboxane B_2 (Chapter 10). Hepatocyte 11-hydroxythromboxane dehydrogenase acts upon platelet-derived plasma thromboxane B_2, the end product of eicosanoid synthesis and the stable analogue of thromboxane A_2, to produce water-soluble 11-dehydrothromboxane B_2.[97] The urine concentration of the metabolite is sufficient for measurement without extraction and, because platelets seem to be its primary source, reflects platelet activity within the previous 12 hours. Urine levels of 11-dehydrothromboxane B_2 are frequently elevated in atherosclerosis; after stroke, transient ischemic attack, or intracerebral hemorrhage; and in atrial fibrillation. Levels of the metabolite are decreased in patients receiving aspirin therapy, even in those with atherosclerosis, AMI, and atrial fibrillation, but appear to remain normal in patients who have aspirin resistance. Aspirin resistance is associated with increased risk of stroke and AMI.

FUTURE OF ANTITHROMBOTIC THERAPY

Antithrombotic therapy, unchanged for more than 50 years, is likely to see further changes between 2020 and 2025. Several DOACs in development or awaiting clearance are likely to replace Coumadin, LMWH, and fondaparinux. Some of the newest antithrombotics inhibit factors other than thrombin or Xa. Particular interest is being directed at the inhibition of factor XI. Likewise, a series of new and emerging antiplatelet drugs will augment the time-honored aspirin tablet. The work of the clinical laboratory will reflect these changes, moving from the PT and PTT to the chromogenic anti-Xa heparin assay, modifications of the thrombin time, the ecarin clotting time, chromogenic assays, and new molecular assays. Antiplatelet response measuring will grow in convenience and take advantage of flow cytometry, immunoassays, mass spectrometry, and rapid molecular assays.

▌ S U M M A R Y

- Warfarin was first used as an anticoagulant in 1952. It protects against venous thromboembolic disease (VTE), but it has a narrow therapeutic range, and an overdose causes hemorrhage. Coumadin therapy is monitored by the prothrombin time (PT) assay and reported as an international normalized ratio (INR). PT measurement is available on portable point-of-care instrumentation. Anticoagulation clinics are available to facilitate Coumadin monitoring and provide patient education and support.
- Unfractionated heparin (UFH) is administered intravenously to provide immediate coagulation control. Its therapeutic effect is monitored using the partial thromboplastin time (PTT), which requires the laboratory practitioner to develop a therapeutic range in seconds calibrated to the chromogenic anti-Xa heparin assay. PTT results are subject to several interferences. Heparin is also used during percutaneous coronary intervention (PCI) or cardiac surgery that requires extracorporeal circulation. In these acute settings it is monitored by the activated clotting time (ACT) for its point-of-care capabilities and sensitivity to high heparin doses.
- Low-molecular-weight heparin (LMWH) and fondaparinux are used as substitutes for UFH and are administered subcutaneously for both prophylaxis and therapy. Both provide near-complete bioavailability, predictable dose response, longer half-lives than UFH, and low risk of bleeding. LMWH and fondaparinux therapy require laboratory measurement only in patients with renal insufficiency, pregnant women, obese patients, children, and underweight adults using the chromogenic anti-Xa heparin assay.
- Rivaroxaban, apixaban, edoxaban, and betrixaban are direct oral anticoagulants (DOACs) that function by inhibiting factor Xa and require little laboratory measurement. New measurement techniques include the chromogenic anti-Xa assays using rivaroxaban, apixaban, edoxaban, and betrixaban calibrators and controls.
- Dabigatran is another DOAC that functions by inhibiting thrombin and requires laboratory measurement for specific indications. Dabigatran may be measured using the ecarin chromogenic assay (ECA) or the plasma-diluted thrombin time.
- The intravenous direct thrombin inhibitors (DTIs) argatroban and bivalirudin directly bind thrombin and are substituted for heparin in patients with heparin-induced thrombocytopenia with thrombosis (HIT). Intravenous DTI therapy is monitored using the PTT or ECT. These drugs affect the PT results when bridging to Coumadin therapy and other clot-based assays. At higher doses, as used during coronary intervention or cardiac surgery, argatroban and bivalirudin are monitored by the ACT.
- The intravenous antiplatelet drugs abciximab, eptifibatide, and tirofiban are used during coronary interventional procedures to maintain vascular patency. Because they may cause thrombocytopenia, the platelet count is monitored carefully. Their efficacy may be monitored using the VerifyNow system, PlateletWorks, or the Multiplate system.
- The oral antiplatelet drugs aspirin, clopidogrel, prasugrel, and ticagrelor are used after arterial thrombotic events to prevent secondary acute myocardial infarction, stroke, and peripheral arterial occlusion. Patient responses to aspirin and clopidogrel therapy vary. Response variation is detected using platelet aggregometry, the VerifyNow system, the Multiplate system, PlateletWorks, the PFA-100, or the AspirinWorks assay; the latter two measure aspirin only.

Now that you have completed this chapter, go back and read again the case study at the beginning and respond to the questions presented.

REVIEW QUESTIONS

Answers can be found in the Appendix.

1. What is the PT/INR therapeutic range for Coumadin therapy when a patient has a mechanical heart valve?
   a. 1 to 2
   b. 2 to 3
   c. 2.5 to 3.5
   d. Coumadin is not indicated for patients with mechanical heart valves

2. Monitoring of a patient taking Coumadin showed that her anticoagulation results remained stable over a period of about 7 months. The frequency of her visits to the laboratory began to decrease, so the period between testing averaged 6 weeks. This new testing interval is:
   a. Acceptable for a patient with stable anticoagulation results after 6 months
   b. Unnecessary, because monitoring for patients taking oral anticoagulants can be discontinued entirely after 4 months of stable test results
   c. Too long even for a patient with previously stable test results; 4 weeks is the standard
   d. Acceptable as long as the patient performs self-monitoring daily using an approved home testing instrument and reports unacceptable results promptly to her physician

3. What is the greatest advantage of point-of-care PT testing?
   a. It permits self-dosing of Coumadin
   b. It is inexpensive
   c. It is convenient
   d. It is precise

4. You collect a citrated whole-blood specimen to monitor UFH therapy. What is the longest it may stand before the plasma must be separated from the cells?
   a. 1 hour
   b. 4 hours
   c. 24 hours
   d. Indefinitely

5. What test is used to monitor high-dose UFH therapy during an interventional cardiology procedure?
   a. PT
   b. PTT
   c. Bleeding time
   d. ACT

6. What test is used most often to monitor UFH therapy in the central laboratory?
   a. PT
   b. PTT
   c. ACT
   d. Chromogenic anti-factor Xa heparin assay

7. What test is used most often to monitor LMWH therapy in the central laboratory?
   a. PT
   b. PTT
   c. ACT
   d. Chromogenic anti-factor Xa heparin assay

8. What is an advantage of LMWH therapy over UFH therapy?
   a. It is cheaper
   b. It causes no bleeding
   c. It has a predictable dose response
   d. There is no risk of HIT

9. In what situation is an intravenous DTI used?
   a. DVT
   b. HIT
   c. Any situation in which Coumadin could be used
   d. Uncomplicated AMI

10. What laboratory test may be used to monitor intravenous DTI therapy when PTT results are unreliable?
   a. PT
   b. ECT
   c. Reptilase clotting time
   d. Chromogenic anti-factor Xa heparin assay

11. What is the reference method for detecting aspirin or clopidogrel resistance?
   a. Platelet aggregometry
   b. AspirinWorks
   c. VerifyNow
   d. PFA-100

12. What is the name of the measurable platelet activation metabolite used in the AspirinWorks assay to monitor aspirin resistance?
   a. 11-dehydrothromboxane B_2
   b. Arachidonic acid
   c. Thromboxane A_2
   d. Cyclooxygenase

13. Which is an intravenous antiplatelet drug used during an interventional cardiology procedure?
   a. Abciximab
   b. Ticagrelor
   c. Prasugrel
   d. Clopidogrel

14. Which of the following is a DOAC?
   a. Argatroban
   b. Fondaparinux
   c. Bivalirudin
   d. Rivaroxaban

REFERENCES

1. Galanaud, J. P., Laroche, J. P., & Righini, M. (2013). The history and historical treatments of deep vein thrombosis. *J Thromb Haemost, 11,* 402–411.

2. Mair, G., von Kummer, R., Adami, A., et al. (2017). Arterial obstruction on computed tomographic or magnetic resonance angiography and response to intravenous thrombolytics in ischemic stroke. *Stroke, 48,* 353–360.

3. Marder, V. J. (2013). Thrombolytic therapy. In Kitchens, C. S., Kessler, C. M., Konkle, B. A. (Eds.), *Consultative Hemostasis and Thrombosis.* (3rd ed., pp. 526–537). Philadelphia: Saunders.

4. Whitlock, R. P., Sun, J. C., Fremes, S. E., et al. (2012). Antithrombotic and thrombolytic therapy for valvular disease: antithrombotic therapy and prevention of thrombosis, 9th ed. American College of Chest Physicians Evidence-Based Clinical Practice Guidelines. *Chest, 141*(Suppl. 2), e576–e600s.

5. Patriquin, C., & Crowther, M. (2013). Antithrombotic agents. In Kitchens, C. S., Kessler, C. M., Konkle, B. A. (Eds.), *Consultative Hemostasis and Thrombosis.* (3rd ed., pp. 477–495). Philadelphia: Saunders.

6. Adverse events and deaths associated with laboratory errors at a hospital—Pennsylvania. (2001). *MMWR Morb Mortal Wkly Rep, 50*, 710–711.

7. Ageno, W., Gallus, A. S., Wittkowsky, A., et al. (2012). Oral anticoagulant therapy: antithrombotic therapy and prevention of thrombosis: American College of Chest Physicians Evidence-Based Clinical Practice Guidelines (9th edition). *Chest, 141*, e44S–e88S.

8. Duxbury, B. M., & Poller, L. (2001). The oral anticoagulant saga: past, present, and future. *Clin Appl Thromb Hemost, 7*, 269–275.

9. Nazarian, R. M., Van Cott, E. M., Zembowicz, A., et al. (2009). Warfarin-induced skin necrosis. *J Am Acad Dermatol, 61*, 325–332.

10. Witt, D. M. (2012). Approaches to optimal dosing of vitamin K antagonists. *Semin Thromb Hemost, 38*, 667–672.

11. Ng, V. L. (2009). Anticoagulation monitoring. *Clin Lab Med, 29*, 283–304.

12. Poller, L., Keown, M., Chauhan, N., et al. (2005). European Concerted Action on Anticoagulation. A multicentre calibration study of WHO international reference preparations for thromboplastin, rabbit (RBT/90) and human (rTF/95). *J Clin Pathol, 58*, 667–669.

13. Korn, D., Sean McMurtry, M., George-Phillips, K., et al. (2017). Critical international normalized ratio results after hours: to call or not to call? *Can Fam Physician, 63*, e170–e176.

14. Lippi, G., Adcock, D., Simundic, A., et al. (2017). Critical laboratory values in hemostasis: toward consensus. *Ann Med, 49*(6), 455–461.

15. Rosborough, T. K., Jacobsen, J. M., & Shepherd, M. F. (2009). Relationship between chromogenic factor X and INR differs during early Coumadin initiation compared with chronic warfarin administration. *Blood Coagul Fibrinolysis, 20*, 433–435.

16. Rosborough, T. K., & Shepherd, M. F. (2004). Unreliability of international normalized ratio for monitoring warfarin therapy in patients with lupus anticoagulant. *Pharmacotherapy, 24*, 838–842.

17. McGlasson, D. L., Romick, B. G., & Rubal, B. J. (2008). Comparison of a chromogenic factor X assay with INR for monitoring oral anticoagulation therapy. *Blood Coagul Fibrinolysis, 19*, 513–517.

18. Caldwell, M. D., Awad, T., & Johnson, J. A. (2008). CYP4F2 genetic variant alters required warfarin dose. *Blood, 111*, 4106–4112.

19. Cavallari, L. H., & Limdi, N. A. (2009). Warfarin pharmacogenomics. *Curr Opin Mol Ther, 11*, 243–251.

20. Oldenburg, J., Müller, C. R., Rost, S., et al. (2014). Comparative genetics of warfarin resistance. *Hamostaseologie, 34*, 143–159.

21. Linkins, L. A., Dans, A. L., Moores, L. K., et al. (2012). Treatment and prevention of heparin-induced thrombocytopenia: antithrombotic therapy and prevention of thrombosis: American College of Chest Physicians Evidence-Based Clinical Practice Guidelines (9th ed.). *Chest, 141*, e495S–e530S.

22. Pabinger-Fasching, I. (2008). Warfarin-reversal: results of a phase III study with pasteurized, nanofiltrated prothrombin complex concentrate. *Thromb Res, 122*(Suppl. 2), S19–S22.

23. Garcia, D. A., Baglin, T. P., Weitz, J. I., et al. (2012). Parenteral anticoagulants: antithrombotic therapy and prevention of thrombosis: American College of Chest Physicians Evidence-Based Clinical Practice Guidelines (9th ed.). *Chest, 141*, e24S–e43S.

24. Cuker, A. (2012). Unfractionated heparin for the treatment of venous thromboembolism: best practices and areas of uncertainty. *Semin Thromb Hemost, 38*, 593–599.

25. Olson, J. D., Arkin, C. F., Brandt, J. T., et al. (1998). College of American Pathologists Conference XXXI on laboratory monitoring of anticoagulant therapy: laboratory monitoring of unfractionated heparin therapy. *Arch Pathol Lab Med, 122*, 782–798.

26. Marlar, R. A., & Gausman, J. (2013). The optimum number and type of plasma samples necessary for an accurate activated partial thromboplastin time-based heparin therapeutic range. *Arch Pathol Lab Med, 137*, 77–82.

27. Brill-Edwards, P., Ginsberg, J. S., Johnston, M., et al. (1993). Establishing a therapeutic interval for heparin therapy. *Ann Intern Med, 119*, 104–109.

28. Eikelboom, J. W., & Hirsh, J. (2006). Monitoring unfractionated heparin with the aPTT: time for a fresh look. *Thromb Haemost, 96*, 547–552.

29. Tripodi, A., & van den Besselaar, A. (2009). Laboratory monitoring of anticoagulation: where do we stand? *Semin Thromb Hemost, 35*, 34–41.

30. Knapik, P., Cieśla, D., Przybylski, R., et al. (2012). The influence of heparin resistance on postoperative complications in patients undergoing coronary surgery. *Med Sci Monit, 18*, 105–111.

31. Adcock, D. M., Kressin, D. C., & Marlar, R. A. (1998). The effect of time and temperature variables on routine coagulation tests. *Blood Coagul Fibrinolysis, 9*, 463–470.

32. Belk, K. W., Laposata, M., & Craver, C. (2016). A comparison of red blood cell transfusion utilization between anti-activated factor X and activated partial thromboplastin monitoring in patients receiving unfractionated heparin. *J Thromb Haemost, 14*, 2148–2157.

33. Lenahan, J. G., Frye, S., Jr., & Phillips, G. E. (1966). Use of the activated partial thromboplastin time in the control of heparin administration. *Clin Chem, 12*, 263–268.

34. Slight, R. D., Buell, R., Nzewi, O. C., et al. (2008). A comparison of activated coagulation time–based techniques for anticoagulation during cardiac surgery with cardiopulmonary bypass. *J Cardiothorac Vasc Anesth, 22*, 47–52.

35. Horton, S., & Augustin, S. (2013). Activated clotting time (ACT). *Methods Mol Biol, 992*, 155–167.

36. Bakchoul, T., Zoliner, H., Amiral, J., et al. (2013). Anti-protamine-heparin antibodies: incidence, clinical relevance, and pathogenesis. *Blood, 121*, 2821–2827.

37. Hull, R. D., Raskob, G. E., Pineo, G. F., et al. (1992). Subcutaneous low molecular weight heparin compared with continuous intravenous heparin in the treatment of proximal-vein thrombosis. *N Engl J Med, 326*, 975–982.

38. Douketis, J. D., Spyropoulos, A. C., Spencer, F. A., et al. (2012). Perioperative management of antithrombotic therapy: antithrombotic therapy and prevention of thrombosis: American

College of Chest Physicians Evidence-Based Clinical Practice Guidelines (9th ed.). *Chest, 141,* e326S–e350S.

39. Cuker, A. (2012). Current and emerging therapeutics for heparin-induced thrombocytopenia. *Semin Thromb Hemost, 38,* 31–37.

40. McGlasson, D. L., Kaczor, D. A., Krasuski, R. A., et al. (2005). Effects of pre-analytical variables on the anti-activated factor X chromogenic assay when monitoring unfractionated heparin and low molecular weight heparin anticoagulation. *Blood Coagul Fibrinolysis, 16,* 173–176.

41. McGlasson, D. L. (2005).Using a single calibration curve with the anti-Xa chromogenic assay for monitoring heparin anticoagulation. *Lab Med, 36,* 297–299.

42. Turpie, A. G. G. (2002). Pentasaccharides. *Semin Hematol, 39,* 158–171.

43. Heit, J. A. (2002). The potential role of fondaparinux as venous thromboembolism prophylaxis after total hip or knee replacement of hip fracture surgery. *Arch Intern Med, 162,* 1806–1808.

44. Samama, M. M., & Gerotziafas, G. T. (2010). Newer anticoagulants in 2009. *J Thromb Thrombolysis, 29,* 92–104.

45. Turpie, A. G. G., Bauer, K. A., Eriksson, B. I., et al. (2002). Fondaparinux vs. enoxaparin for the prevention of venous thromboembolism in major orthopedic surgery: a meta-analysis of 4 randomized double-blind studies. *Arch Intern Med, 162,* 1833–1840.

46. Fuji, T., Fujita, S., Tachibana, S., et al. (2008). Randomized, double-blind, multi-dose efficacy, safety and biomarker study of the oral factor Xa inhibitor DU-176b compared with placebo for prevention of venous thromboembolism in patients after total knee arthroplasty. *Blood, 112,* Abstract 34.

47. Bauer, K. A., Homering, M., & Berkowitz, S. D. (2008). Effects of age, weight, gender and renal function in a pooled analysis of four phase III studies of rivaroxaban for prevention of venous thromboembolism after major orthopedic surgery. *Blood, 112,* Abstract 436.

48. Bijsterveld, N. R., Moons, A. H., Boekholdt, S. M., et al. (2002). Ability of recombinant factor VIIa to reverse the anticoagulant effect of the pentasaccharide fondaparinux in healthy volunteers. *Circulation, 106,* 2550–2554.

49. Desmurs-Clavel, H., Huchon, C., Chatard, B., et al. (2009). Reversal of the inhibitory effect of fondaparinux on thrombin generation by rFVIIa, aPCC and PCC. *Thromb Res, 123,* 796–798.

50. Quinlan, D. J., & Eriksson, B. I. (2013). Novel oral anticoagulants for thromboprophylaxis after orthopaedic surgery. *Best Pract Res Clin Haematol, 26,* 171–182.

51. Cohen, A. T., Hamilton, M., Mitchell, S. A., et al. (2015). Comparison of the novel oral anticoagulants apixaban, dabigatran, edoxaban, and rivaroxaban in the initial and long-term treatment and prevention of venous thromboembolism: systematic review and network meta-analysis. *PLoS One, 10,* e0144856. doi:10.1371/journal.pone.0144856.

52. US Dept of HHS Agency for Healthcare Research and Quality. (2008). http://www.ahrq.gov/qual/vtguide/vtguideapa.htm. Accessed July 5, 2013.

53. Shirasaki, Y., Morishima, Y., & Shibano, T. (2014). Comparison of the effect of edoxaban, a direct factor Xa inhibitor, with a direct thrombin inhibitor, melagatran, and heparin on intracerebral hemorrhage induced by collagenase in rats. *Thromb Res, 133,* 622–628.

54. Schulman, S., & Spencer, F. A. (2010). Antithrombotic drugs in coronary artery disease: risk benefit ratio and bleeding. *J Thromb Haemost, 8,* 641–650.

55. Levi, M., Moore, T., Castillejos, C. F., et al. (2013). Effects of 3-factor and 4-factor prothrombin complex concentrates on the pharmacodynamics of rivaroxaban. *J Thromb Haemost, 11* (Suppl. 2), Abstract OC 36.5.

56. Laulicht, B., Bakhru, S., Jiang, X., et al. (2013). Antidote for new oral anticoagulants: mechanism of action and binding specificity of PER977. *J Thromb Haemost, 11*(Suppl. 2), Abstract AS 47.1.

57. Crowther, M., Kitt, M., Lorenz, T., et al. (2013). A phase 2 randomized, double-blind, placebo controlled trial of PRT064445, a novel, universal antidote for direct and indirect factor Xa inhibitors. *J Thromb Haemost, 11*(Suppl. 2), Abstract OC 20.1.

58. Baglin, T., Hillarp, A., Tripodi, A., et al. (2013). Measuring oral direct inhibitors of thrombin and factor Xa: a recommendation from the Subcommittee on Control of Anticoagulation of the Scientific and Standardization Committee of the International Society on Thrombosis and Haemostasis. *J Thromb Haemost, 11,* 756–760.

59. ten Cate, H., Henskens, Y. M. C., & Lance, M. D. (2017). Practical guidance on the use of laboratory testing in the management of bleeding inpatients receiving direct oral anticoagulants. *Vasc Health Risk Manag, 13,* 457–467.

60. Tripodi, A. (2013). Which test to use to measure the anticoagulant effect of rivaroxaban: the prothrombin time test. *J Thromb Haemost, 11,* 576–578.

61. Samama, M. M. (2013). Which test to use to measure the anticoagulant effect of rivaroxaban: the anti-factor Xa assay. *J Thromb Haemost, 11,* 579–580.

62. Favaloro, E. J., & Lippi, G. (2012). The new oral anticoagulants and the future of haemostasis laboratory testing. *Biochemia Medica, 22,* 329–341.

63. Exner, T., Michalopoulos, N., Pearce, J., et al. (2018). Simple method for removing DOACs from plasma samples. *Thromb Res, 163,* 117–122.

64. Celikyurt, I., Meier, C. R., Kühne, M., et al. (2017). Safety and interactions of direct oral anticoagulants with antiarrhythmic drugs. *Drug Saf, 40,* 1091–1098.

65. Khadzhynov, D., Wagner, F., Formella, S., et al. (2013). Effective elimination of dabigatran by haemodialysis. A phase I single-centre study in patients with end-stage renal disease. *Thromb Haemost, 109,* 596–605.

66. Harenberg, J., Giese, C., Marx, S., et al. (2012). Determination of dabigatran in human plasma samples. *Semin Thromb Hemost, 38,* 16–22.

67. Gosselin, R. C., Dwyre, D. M., & Dager, W. E. (2013). Measuring dabigatran concentrations using a chromogenic ecarin clotting time assay. *Ann Pharmacother, 47,* 1635-1640.

68. Avecilla, S. T., Ferrell, C., Chandler, W. L., et al. (2012). Plasma-diluted thrombin time to measure dabigatran concentrations during dabigatran etexilate therapy. *Am J Clin Pathol, 137,* 572–574.

69. Antovic, J. P., Skeppholm, M., Eintrei, J., et al. (2013). How to monitor dabigatran when needed: comparison of coagulation laboratory methods and dabigatran concentrations in plasma. *J Thromb Haemostas, 11*(Suppl. 2), Abstract AS 02-3.

70. Sun, Z., Lan, X., Li, S., et al. (2017). Comparisons of argatroban to lepirudin and bivalirudin in the treatment of heparin-induced thrombocytopenia: a systematic review and meta-analysis. *Int J Hematol, 106,* 476–483.

71. Grouzi, E. (2014). Update on argatroban for the prophylaxis and treatment of heparin-induced thrombocytopenia type II. *J Blood Med, 5,* 131–141.

72. Shantsila, E., Lip, G. Y., & Chong, B. H. (2009). Heparin-induced thrombocytopenia. A contemporary clinical approach to diagnosis and management. *Chest, 135*, 1651–1654.

73. Prechel, M., & Walenga, J. M. (2008). The laboratory diagnosis and clinical management of patients with heparin-induced thrombocytopenia: an update. *Semin Thromb Hemost, 34*, 86–96.

74. Joseph, L., Casanegra, A. I., Dhariwal, M., et al. (2014). Bivalirudin for the treatment of patients with confirmed or suspected heparin-induced thrombocytopenia. *J Thromb Haemost, 12*, 1044–1053.

75. Curran, M. P. (2010). Bivalirudin: in patients with ST-segment elevation myocardial infarction. *Drugs, 70*, 909–918.

76. Zeng, X., Lincoff, A. M., Schulz-Schüpke, S., et al. (2018). Efficacy and safety of bivalirudin in coronary artery disease patients with mild to moderate chronic kidney disease: meta-analysis. *J Cardiol, 71*, 494–504.

77. Chia, S., Van Cott, E. M., Raffel, O. C., et al, (2009). Comparison of activated clotting times obtained using Hemochron and Medtronic analyzers in patients receiving anti-thrombin therapy during cardiac catheterization. *Thromb Haemost, 101*, 535–540.

78. Qaderdan, K., Vos, G. A., McAndrew, T., et al. (2017). Outcomes in elderly and young patients with ST-segment elevation myocardial infarction undergoing primary percutaneous coronary intervention with bivalirudin versus heparin: pooled analysis from the EUROMAX and HORIZONS-AMI trials. *Am Heart J, 194*, 73–82.

79. Walenga J. M., Fasanella A. R., Iqbal O., et al. (1999). Coagulation laboratory testing in patients treated with argatroban. *Semin Thromb Hemost, 25*(Suppl 1), 61–66.

80. Bartholomew, J. R., & Hursting, M. J. (2005). Transitioning from argatroban to warfarin in heparin-induced thrombocytopenia: an analysis of outcomes in patients with elevated international normalized ratio (INR). *J Thromb Thrombolysis, 19*, 183–188.

81. Muhlestein, J. B. (2010). Effect of antiplatelet therapy on inflammatory markers in atherothrombotic patients. *Thromb Haemost, 103*, 71–82.

82. van't Hof, A. W., & Valgimigli, M. (2009). Defining the role of platelet glycoprotein receptor inhibitors in STEMI: focus on tirofiban. *Drugs, 69*, 85–100.

83. Rubboli, A., & Patti, G. (2018). What is the role for glycoprotein IIb/IIIa inhibitor use in the catheterisation laboratory in the current era? *Curr Vasc Pharmacol, 16*, 451–458.

84. Dézsi, D. A., Bokori, G., Faluközy, J., et al. (2016). Eptifibatide-induced thrombocytopenia leading to acute stent thrombosis. *J Thromb Thrombolysis, 41*, 522–524.

85. Gibbs, N. M. (2009). Point-of-care assessment of antiplatelet agents in the perioperative period: a review. *Anaesth Intensive Care, 37*, 354–369.

86. Freeman, M. K. (2010). Thienopyridine antiplatelet agents: focus on prasugrel. *Consult Pharm, 25*, 241–257.

87. Gilroy, D. W. (2010). Eicosanoids and the endogenous control of acute inflammatory resolution. *Int J Biochem Cell Biol, 42*, 524–528.

88. Winter, M. P., Grove, E. L., De Caterina, R., et al. (2017). Advocating cardiovascular precision medicine with P2Y12 receptor inhibitors. *Eur Heart J Cardiovasc Pharmacother, 3*, 221–234.

89. Giustino, G., Baber, U., Sartori, S., et al. (2015). Duration of dual antiplatelet therapy after drug-eluting stent implantation: a systematic review and meta-analysis of randomized controlled trials. *J Am Coll Cardiol, 65*, 1298–1310.

90. Eikelboom, J. W., Hirsh, J., Weitz, J. I., et al. (2002). Aspirin-resistant thromboxane biosynthesis and the risk of myocardial infarction, stroke, or cardiovascular death in patients at high risk for cardiovascular events. *Circulation, 105*, 1650–1655.

91. Flechtenmacher, N., Kämmerer, F., Dittmer, R., et al. (2015). Clopidogrel resistance in neurovascular stenting: correlations between light transmission aggregometry, VerifyNow, and the Multiplate. *Am J Neuroradiol, 36*, 1953–1958.

92. Alexopoulos, D., Xanthopoulou, I., Perperis, A., et al. (2013). Factors affecting residual platelet aggregation in prasugrel treated patients. *Curr Pharm Des, 19*, 5121–5126.

93. Gum, P. A., Kottke-Marchant, K., Welsh, P. A., et al. (2003). A prospective, blinded determination of the natural history of aspirin resistance among stable patients with cardiovascular disease. *J Am Coll Cardiol, 41*, 961–965.

94. Knoepp, S. M., & Laposata, M. (2005). Aspirin resistance: moving forward with multiple definitions, different assays, and a clinical imperative. *Am J Clin Pathol, 123*, S125–S132.

95. van Werkum, J. W., Harmsze, A. M., Elsenberg, E. H., et al. (2008). The use of the VerifyNow system to monitor antiplatelet therapy: a review of the current evidence. *Platelets, 19*, 479–488.

96. Mueller, T., Dieplinger, B., Poelz, W., et al. (2009). Utility of the PFA-100 instrument and the novel Multiplate analyzer for the assessment of aspirin and clopidogel effects on platelet function in patients with cardiovascular disease. *Clin Appl Thromb Hemost, 15*, 652–659.

97. McGlasson, D. L., Chen, M., & Fritsma, G. A. (2005). Urinary 11-dehydrothromboxane B_2 levels in healthy individuals following a single dose response to two concentrations of aspirin. *J Clin Ligand Assay, 28*, 147–150.

Laboratory Evaluation of Hemostasis

George A. Fritsma

OBJECTIVES

After completion of this chapter, the reader will be able to:

1. Properly collect and transport hemostasis blood specimens.
2. Reject hemostasis blood specimens due to clots, short draws, or hemolysis.
3. Prepare hemostasis blood specimens for analysis.
4. Describe the principles of light transmittance and impedance platelet aggregometry.
5. Apply appropriate platelet function tests in a variety of conditions and interpret their results.
6. Analyze the plasma markers of platelet activation.
7. Describe the principle of, appropriately select, and correctly interpret the results of clot-based coagulation tests, including prothrombin time, partial thromboplastin time, and thrombin clotting time.
8. Interpret clot-based assay results collectively to reach presumptive diagnoses, and then recommend and perform confirmatory tests.
9. Perform partial thromboplastin time mixing studies to detect factor deficiencies, lupus anticoagulants, and specific factor inhibitors.
10. Describe the principle of, select, and correctly interpret coagulation factor assays.
11. Describe the principle of and correctly interpret Nijmegen-Bethesda assays for coagulation factor inhibitors.
12. Describe the principle of, select, and correctly interpret tests of fibrinolysis, including D-dimer, plasminogen, plasminogen activator, and plasminogen activator inhibitor.
13. Interpret global coagulation assays: thromboelastography, thromboelastometry, and thrombin generation assays.
14. Employ high-throughput genomic sequencing to detect coagulopathies and platelet abnormalities.

OUTLINE

CASE STUDY

After studying the material in this chapter, the reader should be able to respond to the following case study:

A 54-year-old woman experienced a pulmonary embolism on September 26 and began oral anticoagulant therapy. Monthly prothrombin time (PT) values were collected to monitor therapy. From October through January, her international normalized ratio (INR) was stable at 2.4, but on February 1, her INR was 1.3. The reduced INR was reported to her physician.

On questioning, the patient reported that there had been no change in her warfarin (Coumadin) dosage or in her diet. She recalled, however, that the phlebotomist had used a tube with a red and black ("tiger-top") closure. She had thought this to be out of the ordinary and had remarked about it to the phlebotomist, who made no response. The medical laboratory practitioner who had performed the PT assay reexamined the blood specimen and saw that it was in a blue-closure tube.

1. What did the phlebotomist do?
2. What was the consequence of this action?
3. What else could cause an unexpectedly short PT?

HEMOSTASIS LABORATORY TESTING

This chapter describes the techniques that underlie clinical hemostasis laboratory testing. Included are the techniques for specimen collection and management, platelet function tests, routine clot-based assays, factor assays, and assays to identify defects in coagulation control and fibrinolysis. For assays specific to bleeding disorders (Chapter 36), platelet defects (Chapters 37 and 38), thrombotic disorders (Chapter 39), and antithrombotic drug monitoring (Chapter 40), refer to the respective chapters devoted to these topics.

For diagnostic purposes, it is important to obtain results from assays that provide information on the function of platelets, coagulation factors, control proteins, and fibrinolytic components. Quantitative assays such as immunoassays are often essential but may not provide functional information.

HEMOSTASIS SPECIMEN COLLECTION

Blood collectors, including medical laboratory practitioners, phlebotomists, patient care technicians, nurses, and physicians who collect and manage hemostasis blood specimens must adhere closely to published protocols (see the Evolve website) to ensure assay validity. Blood specimen collection and management are the most vulnerable stages of the hemostasis blood testing process because every stage is manual and thus error-fraught. The laboratory or nursing supervisor is responsible for the up-to-date validity of specimen collection and management protocols and ensures that personnel employ approved techniques.[1]

Most hemostasis procedures are performed on platelet-poor plasma (PPP, plasma whose platelet count is less than 10,000/μL) prepared from venous whole blood collected by venipuncture. At the moment of collection, blood is mixed with sodium citrate anticoagulant and is maintained as well-mixed whole blood for assays that require whole blood such as platelet function tests, or centrifuged to provide platelet-rich plasma (PRP, plasma whose platelet count is approximately 200,000/μL) for light transmittance platelet aggregometry, or PPP for clot-based assays.

Patient Management

The medical laboratory practitioner, pharmacist, nurse, and physician shoulder substantial responsibility for preparing a patient for hemostasis testing, starting with a diligent bleeding and thrombosis risk assessment. The clinician asks about family clotting and bleeding history, blood group (group O people have a higher von Willebrand disease prevalence), pregnancy (prothrombotic), liver or kidney disease, leukemia, anemia, and malnutrition. Bleeding and clotting characteristics come next, including location, frequency, volume, and whether events are spontaneous or follow an injury or a surgical or dental procedure. Of equal importance is a 2-week drug history, including anticoagulants (blood thinners), antiplatelet drugs, especially aspirin (ASA) and nonsteroidal antiinflammatory drugs (NSAIDS), contraceptives, and hormone replacement therapy, which are prothrombotic.[2] The patient is also asked about over-the-counter remedies and dietary supplements, such as garlic, vitamin K, ginger, and St. John's wort, and is instructed to discontinue nonprescription drugs at least a week prior to blood collection. Anticoagulants such as Coumadin or direct oral anticoagulants (DOACs) and antiplatelet drugs such as ASA or clopidogrel are continued when the purpose is to assess their efficacy. Lastly, the clinician examines the patient for evidence of bleeding; bruises and swelling. Standardized bleeding assessment tools (BAT) may be employed to enhance bleeding history accuracy.[3] Patients need only fast under arranged circumstances but are advised to avoid caffeine and exercise for 2 hours and smoking for 30 minutes before collection. Patients should be inactive for 5 minutes before collection.[4]

Blood collectors manage patients using standard protocols for identification, cleansing, tourniquet use, and venipuncture (see the Evolve website).[5] If there is a reason to anticipate excessive bleeding—for instance, if the patient has multiple bruises, mentions a tendency to bleed, or possesses a high-risk BAT score—the phlebotomist should extend the time for observing the venipuncture site from the usual 1 minute to 5 minutes and should apply a pressure bandage before dismissing the patient.[6]

Materials for Hemostasis Blood Specimen Collection

Needle Selection

The blood collector fits a 20-gauge or 21-gauge, thin-walled, double-point needle to an adapter for standard evacuated tube collection. In the case of small, scarred, or fragile veins, the collector may fit a 23-gauge Luer-adapter needle or 23-gauge "butterfly" needle infusion tube to a syringe, which enables the collector to reduce and control the negative collection pressure.[7] The needle bore should be sufficient to prevent hemolysis and to prevent the activation of platelets and procoagulants (Table 41.1). Needles are equipped with safety devices that prevent accidental needle-stick injury subsequent to specimen collection.

TABLE 41.1 Hemostasis Specimen Collection Needle Selection

Application	Preferred Needle Gauge and Length
Adult with good veins	20 or 21 gauge, thin-walled, 1.0 or 1.25 inches long
Child or adult with small, fragile, or hardened veins	23-gauge, winged-needle set; collect with small evacuated tubes or syringe
Transfer of blood from syringe to tube	19-gauge safety transfer unit; slowly inject through tube closure

Hemostasis Specimen Collection Tubes

Most hemostasis specimens are collected in plastic blue-closure (blue-top, blue-stopper) sterile evacuated blood collection tubes containing a measured volume of buffered sodium citrate anticoagulant.[8] Siliconized (plastic-coated) glass tubes are available, but their use is declining because of concern for potential breakage, with consequent risk of exposure to bloodborne pathogens. Tubes of uncoated soda-lime glass are unsuitable.[9]

Anticoagulants for Hemostasis Specimens

Sodium citrate. The anticoagulant used for most hemostasis testing is buffered 0.105 to 0.109 M (3.2%) sodium citrate, $Na_3C_6H_5O_7 \cdot 2H_2O$, molecular weight 294.1 Daltons. Sodium citrate binds calcium ions to prevent coagulation, and the buffer stabilizes specimen pH as long as the tube closure remains in place.[10]

Upon collection, the anticoagulant solution mixes with blood to produce a 9:1 ratio—9 parts whole blood to 1 part anticoagulant. In most cases, 0.3 mL of anticoagulant mixes with 2.7 mL of whole blood, the volumes in the most commonly used evacuated plastic collection tubes, but any volume is valid, provided that the 9:1 ratio is maintained. The ratio yields a final citrate concentration of 10.5 to 10.9 mM of anticoagulant in whole blood.[11]

Sodium citrate volume adjustment for elevated hematocrits. The 9:1 blood-to-anticoagulant ratio is effective, provided the patient's hematocrit is 55% or below. In polycythemia the decrease in plasma volume relative to whole blood unacceptably raises the anticoagulant-to-plasma ratio, which causes falsely prolonged results for clot-based coagulation tests. The phlebotomist must prepare specially marked tubes with relatively reduced anticoagulant volumes for collection of blood from a patient whose hematocrit is known to be 55% or higher. The amount of anticoagulant may be computed by using this formula:

$$C = (1.85 \times 10^{-3})(100 - HCT)V$$

where C is the volume of sodium citrate in milliliters, V is volume of whole blood-sodium citrate solution in milliliters, and HCT is the hematocrit in percent.

For example, to collect 3 mL of blood/anticoagulant mixture from a patient who has a hematocrit of 65%, calculate the sodium citrate volume as follows:

$$C = (1.85 \times 10^{-3})(100 - 65) \times 3.0 \, mL$$
$$C = (1.85 \times 10^{-3})(35) \times 3.0 \, mL$$
$$C = 0.19 \, mL \text{ of sodium citrate}$$

Remove the stopper from a 3-mL blue closure collection tube, pipette and discard 0.11 mL from the 0.3 mL of anticoagulant, leaving 0.19 mL. Collect blood in a syringe and transfer 2.81 (2.8) mL of blood to the tube, replace the stopper, and immediately mix by gently inverting at least three times. Alternatively the laboratory practitioner can prepare for collection of 10 mL of blood and anticoagulant solution in a 12-mL centrifuge tube as follows:

$$C = (1.85 \times 10^{-3})(100 - 65) \times 10.0 \, mL$$
$$C = (1.85 \times 10^{-3})(35) \times 10.0 \, mL$$
$$C = 0.64 \, mL \text{ of sodium citrate}$$

In this instance 0.64 mL of sodium citrate is pipetted into the tube, and 9.36 (9.4) mL of whole blood is transferred from the collection syringe.

This formula may be expressed as a nomogram as shown in Figure 41.1. A complete nomogram appears in Clinical and Laboratory Standards Institute (CLSI) Standard GP41. There exists no evidence suggesting a need for increasing the volume of anticoagulant for specimens from patients with anemia, even when the hematocrit is less than 20%.

Other anticoagulants for hemostasis specimens. Laboratory practitioners do not use ethylenediaminetetraacetic acid (EDTA, lavender closure) anticoagulated specimens for clot-based coagulation testing because EDTA irreversibly chelates calcium ions.[12] Calcium ion chelation with citrate, on the other hand, is reversed with the addition of calcium chloride.

EDTA is the anticoagulant used to collect specimens for complete blood counts, including platelet counts. Heparinized (green closure) specimens have never been validated for plasma coagulation testing but may be necessary to produce accurate platelet counts in cases of platelet satellitosis (satellitism) as a substitute for specimens collected in EDTA.

EDTA may be required for specimens used for molecular diagnostic testing, such as testing for the factor V Leiden mutation. Likewise, acid citrate dextrose (ACD, yellow closure) and dipotassium EDTA (K_2EDTA, white closure) gel tubes may be used for molecular diagnosis, as specified by institutional protocol.

Citrate theophylline adenosine dipyridamole (CTAD, blue closure) tubes suppress in vitro platelet or coagulation activation for specialty assays such as the platelet activation marker platelet factor 4 (PF4) or the coagulation activation marker thrombin-antithrombin complex (TAT).

Specimen Collection Procedures
Venipuncture

The blood collector adheres strictly to standard venipuncture procedures for evacuated tube or syringe collection. Specialized hemostasis laboratories may employ trained collectors to ensure specimen integrity.[13] Table 41.2 lists collection errors to avoid.

The blood collector consults the manufacturer's "order of draw" chart. If a series of evacuated tubes is to be filled from a single venipuncture site, the hemostasis specimen must be collected first or immediately after a *nonadditive* tube. The hemostasis tube may not immediately follow a tube that contains heparin, EDTA, sodium fluoride (gray closure), or clot-promoting silica particles that are contained in plastic

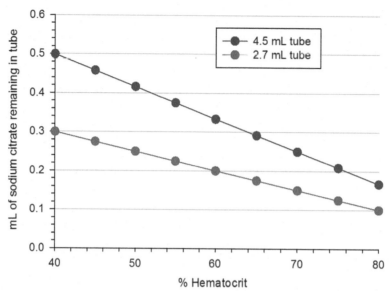

Figure 41.1 Adjusted Citrate Volume for High Hematocrit Specimens. This graph is used for determining the volume of sodium citrate anticoagulant to add to the hemostasis blood collection tube when the patient's hematocrit is 55% or more. Illustration is provided for the typical blood collection tubes: 2.7 mL blood with 0.3 mL citrate for a normal hematocrit and 4.5 mL blood with 0.5 mL citrate for a normal hematocrit.

TABLE 41.2 Hemostasis Specimen Collection and Management Errors That Require Specimen Rejection

Error	Comments
Short draw	Whole-blood volume less than 90% of required volume or less than manufacturer specified minimum. PT and PTT are falsely prolonged.
Specimen clot	Each specimen is inspected visually before centrifugation or during analysis; even a small clot interferes with hemostasis test results.
Visible hemolysis	Pink or red plasma indicates in vitro activation of platelets and coagulation; unpredictable hemostasis test interference. Further, hemolysis interferes with optical endpoint coagulometer results.
Lipemia or icterus	Optical instruments may fail to measure clots in cloudy or highly colored specimens. Interferes with chromogenic substrate methods. The practitioner must employ an electro-mechanical detection method instrument.
Tourniquet application >1 minute	Blood stasis activates endothelial cells and elevates the concentration of von Willebrand factor and fibrinogen, falsely shortening clot-based test results.
Specimen storage at 1–6° C	Storage at refrigerator temperatures causes precipitation of large von Willebrand factor multimers, activation of coagulation factor VII, activation of platelets, and destruction of platelet integrity.
Specimen storage at >25° C	Storage at above standard room temperature causes coagulation factors V and VIII to deteriorate.

PT, Prothrombin time; *PTT*, partial thromboplastin time.

red-closure or serum separator (gold or red-gray closure with gel, SST) tubes. These additives may transfer to the hemostasis specimen and invalidate hemostasis test results. Nonadditive tubes include red-closure glass (but not plastic) tubes and clear-closure plastic tubes. If nonadditive tubes are unavailable, the phlebotomist may use and discard a preliminary blue-closure tube when following an additive tube.[14]

Evacuated tubes are designed so that the negative internal pressure collects the correct volume of blood. Collection tube manufacturers indicate the allowable range of collection volume error in package inserts and provide a minimum volume indication on each tube. In most cases the volume of blood collected must be within 90% of the calibrated volume. A *short draw*—that is, a specimen with a smaller volume than the minimum specified by the manufacturer—generates erroneously prolonged clot-based coagulation test results because the excess

anticoagulant relative to blood volume adversely neutralizes test reagent calcium.[15] Short-draw specimens are discarded, and a fresh specimen is collected. The smaller the collection tube, the narrower the tolerance for short draws.

When collecting a specimen using a butterfly set, the blood collector compensates for the internal volume of the tubing, which is typically 12 inches long and contains approximately 0.5 mL of air, by collecting and discarding a nonadditive tube or a blue-closure tube. This step ensures that the needle set tubing is filled with fresh patient blood before the hemostasis specimen is collected and avoids an inadvertent short draw.[16]

When collecting by syringe, the collector replaces the Luer adaptor needle or butterfly needle with a Luer adaptor-equipped large-bore safe transfer device and gently transfers the specimen from the syringe into evacuated tubes, using the same order of tube selection as for standard evacuated tube collection.

Clotted specimens are useless for hemostasis testing, even if the clot is small. A few seconds after collection, the blood collector must gently invert the specimen end over end at least three times to mix the blood with the anticoagulant and prevent clot formation. Excessive specimen agitation, called "cocktail shaking," causes hemolysis (RBC rupture), procoagulant activation, and platelet activation. Later the medical laboratory practitioner visually examines the specimen for clots just before centrifugation and testing. Many coagulometers are equipped to detect the presence of clots. Clotted specimens are discarded, and a new specimen is collected.

Blood specimens for hemostatic testing must be collected using atraumatic technique. Excess needle manipulation may promote the release of connective tissue procoagulants that contaminate the specimen by activating clotting factors. Consequently, time to clot test results from specimens collected during a traumatic venipuncture may be falsely shortened and unreliable.[17]

During blood collection, the phlebotomist must remove the tourniquet within 1 minute of its application to avoid stasis, which slows venous flow.[18] Stasis results in endothelial cell activation and hemoconcentration with the local accumulation of coagulation factors V, VII, VIII, XII, and von Willebrand factor (VWF), which may falsely shorten clot-based coagulation test results.

Specimen Collection From Vascular Access Devices

Although CLSI Standard GP41 discourages the practice, specimens may of necessity be collected from heparin or saline locks, ports in intravenous (IV) lines, peripherally inserted central catheters (PICC tubes), central venous catheters, or dialysis catheters. Vascular access device management requires strict adherence to protocol to ensure sterility, prevent emboli, and prevent damage to the device. Blood collectors must be proficient and must recognize the signs of complications and take appropriate action. Institutional protocol may limit vascular access device blood collection to physicians and nurses. Before blood is collected for hemostasis testing, the line must be flushed with 5 mL of saline, and the first 5 mL of blood, or six times the volume of the blood collection tube, must be collected and discarded. The blood collector *must not flush with heparin*. Blood is collected into a syringe and transferred to an evacuated tube using a safety transfer device.[19]

Though the practice is discouraged, often nurses and phlebotomists collect blood specimens while starting IV lines. Although a necessary convenience for the patient, IV cannulas are notorious for causing hemolysis. Once the site is flushed, and before the IV drip is started, the phlebotomist or nurse collects the specimen via syringe, exerting minimal negative pressure. The test results from visibly hemolyzed specimens are unreliable, and the specimen must be recollected.[20]

Specimen Collection Using Capillary Puncture

Point-of-care coagulometers generate PT/international normalized ratio (INR) results from a specimen consisting of 10 to 50 μL of whole blood. These instruments are designed to test either anticoagulated venous whole blood or capillary (fingerstick) blood. They are a significant convenience to patients and to anticoagulation clinics,[21] and some are designed for patient self-testing and pediatric or neonatal testing. Laboratory

practitioners are often charged with training nurses, pharmacists, and patients in proper capillary puncture technique.[22]

Capillary specimen skin punctures are made using sterile spring-loaded lancets designed to produce an incision of standard depth and width, while avoiding injury. The collector or patient cleanses the third (middle) finger or fourth (ring) finger and activates the device so that it produces a puncture that is just off center of the fingertip and perpendicular to the fingerprint lines. After wiping away the first drop of blood, which is likely to be contaminated by connective tissue procoagulants, the blood collector places the collection device adjacent to the free-flowing blood and allows the device to fill by capillary action and gravity. The collector then presses a gauze pad to the wound and instructs the patient to maintain pressure until bleeding ceases. Next the collector wipes excess blood from the outside of the device and introduces it to the coagulometer to complete the assay.

The key to accurate capillary PT/INR measurement is a free-flowing puncture. Often it is necessary for the collector to warm the patient's hand to increase blood flow to the fingertips. Blood collection device distributors provide dry, disposable warming devices for this purpose. The collector avoids squeezing ("milking") the finger, because this raises the concentration of tissue fluid relative to plasma and blood cells.[23]

HEMOSTASIS SPECIMEN MANAGEMENT

Hemostasis Specimen Transport and Storage

Table 41.3 provides information for proper specimen transport and storage, including time interval and temperature.

Sodium citrate-anticoagulated whole blood specimens are placed in a rack and allowed to stand in a vertical position with the closure intact and uppermost. Maintaining the blood collection tube seal minimizes CO_2 diffusion, which otherwise allows the pH to rise, falsely prolonging the PT and PTT.[24] Specimens are maintained at ambient temperature, 15° C to 25° C, never at refrigerator temperatures or on ice. Storage at 1° C to 6° C activates factor VII, activates platelets, and precipitates large VWF multimers.[25,26] Specimens are never stored or transported at temperatures greater than 25° C because heat deteriorates coagulation factors V and VIII.

Specimens collected for PTs may be held uncentrifuged or centrifuged at 15° C to 25° C and tested within 24 hours of the time of collection.[27] Specimens collected for PTTs and most other clot-based assays are also held uncentrifuged or centrifuged at 15° C to 25° C, but they must be tested within 4 hours of time of collection. If a patient is receiving unfractionated heparin (UFH) therapy, PTT specimens must be centrifuged within 1 hour of the time of collection to avoid depletion of the heparin. Centrifuges that are used to prepare hemostasis specimens must maintain a temperature of 15° C to 25° C.[28]

If any plasma-based hemostasis assay cannot be completed within the prescribed interval, the practitioner must centrifuge the specimen within 1 hour of collection. The practitioner immediately transfers the plasma by plastic pipette to a plastic freezer tube, taking care to avoid stirring up the buffy coat. Never use glass containers because glass stimulates the intrinsic coagulation pathway. The freezer tube is labeled, sealed, and frozen. It may be stored at −20° C for up to 2 weeks or at −70° C for long-term

TABLE 41.3 **Hemostasis Specimen Storage Times and Temperatures**

Application	Temperature	Specimen Stability
PT with no UFH	15° C–25° C	Test within 24 hr, maintain upright and sealed
PTT with no UFH		Test within 4 hr, maintain upright and sealed
PTT for monitoring UFH		Centrifuge to separate plasma within 1 hour, test within 4 hr
PT when UFH is present		Centrifuge to separate plasma within 1 hour, test within 4 hr
Factor assays		Test within 4 hr, maintain upright and sealed
Optical platelet aggregometry using PRP		Wait 30 min after centrifugation, test within 4 hr of collection
Whole-blood aggregometry		Test within 4 hours of collection, maintain upright and sealed
Storage in household freezer	−20° C	2 weeks
Storage for 6 months	−70° C	6 months or indefinite

PRP, Platelet-rich plasma; *PT,* prothrombin time; *PTT,* partial thromboplastin time, *UFH,* unfractionated heparin.

storage.[29,30] At the time the test is performed, the frozen specimen is thawed rapidly at 37° C, mixed, and tested within 1 hour of the time it is removed from the freezer. If it cannot be tested immediately, the specimen may be stored at 1° C to 6° C for up to 2 hours after thawing.[31] To avoid cryoprecipitation of VWF, specimens may not be frozen and thawed more than once.

Preparation of Hemostasis Specimens

Whole-Blood Specimens for Platelet Aggregometry

Blood for whole-blood platelet aggregometry, lumiaggregometry, thromboelastography (TEG), or thromboelastometry (ROTEM) is collected with 3.2% sodium citrate and held at 15° C to 25° C until testing. Chilling destroys platelet activity and is to be avoided. Aggregometry should be started immediately and must be completed within 4 hours of specimen collection (for undiminished ex vivo platelet activity). The practitioner mixes the specimen by gentle inversion, checks for clots just before testing, and rejects specimens with clots. Most specimens for whole-blood aggregometry are mixed 1:1 with normal saline before testing, although if the platelet count is less than 100,000/μL the specimen is tested undiluted.[32]

Platelet-Rich Plasma for Light Transmittance Platelet Aggregometry

Light-transmittance (optical) platelet aggregometers are designed to test PRP, plasma with a platelet count of 200,000 to 300,000/μL. Sodium citrate-anticoagulated blood is first checked visually for clots and then centrifuged at a relative centrifugal force (RCF) of 50 × g for 30 minutes with the closure in place to maintain the pH. The supernatant PRP is transferred by plastic pipette to a clean plastic tube (never glass), and the tube is sealed and stored at 15° C to 25° C (ambient temperature) until the test is begun. Specimens for PRP-based light-transmittance aggregometry must stand undisturbed for 30 minutes after centrifugation while the platelets regain responsiveness. Specimens must be tested within 4 hours of collection to avoid spontaneous in vitro platelet activation and loss of normal activity. To produce sufficient PRP, the original specimen must measure 9 to 12 mL of whole blood.

Light-transmittance aggregometry is unreliable when the patient's whole-blood platelet count is less than 100,000/μL.

Platelet-Poor Plasma for Clot-Based Testing

Clot-based plasma coagulation tests require PPP with a platelet count of less than 10,000/μL.[33] Sodium citrate-anticoagulated whole blood is centrifuged at 1500 × g RCF for 15 minutes in a horizontal-head centrifuge to produce supernatant PPP. Alternatively, a HemoCue StatSpin type of centrifuge that generates 4400 × g RCF can produce PPP within 3 minutes. The advantage of the horizontal centrifuge head is that it produces a straight, level plasma-blood cell interface, making it possible for automated coagulometers to sample from the supernatant plasma of the blood collection tube (the "primary" tube). Angled centrifuge heads cause platelets to adhere to the side of the tube. If the "angle-spun" tube is allowed to stand, the adherent platelets drift back into the plasma and release granule contents. Each hemostasis laboratory manager establishes the correct centrifugation speed and times locally.

In the special hemostasis laboratory the manager may choose a double-spin approach. The primary tube is centrifuged and the plasma is transferred to a secondary plastic tube, which is labeled and centrifuged again. The double-spin approach may be used to produce PPP with a plasma platelet count of less than 5000/μL, which some laboratory directors prefer for lupus anticoagulant (LAC) testing and for freezing.

A plasma platelet count greater than 10,000/μL affects clot-based test results. Platelets become activated in vitro and release microparticles and the membrane phospholipid phosphatidylserine, which trigger plasma coagulation and interfere with LAC testing. Platelets also secrete fibrinogen, factors V and VIII, and VWF (Chapter 10). These may desensitize PT and PTT assays and interfere with clot-based coagulation assays. In addition, platelets release PF4, a protein that binds and neutralizes therapeutic heparin in vitro, falsely shortening the PTT and interfering with heparin management.

The hemostasis laboratory manager arranges to perform PPP platelet counts on coagulation plasmas at regular intervals to ensure that they are consistently platelet poor. Many managers select 10 to 12 specimens from each centrifuge every 6 months, perform plasma platelet counts, and document that their samples remain appropriately platelet poor, even if the initial platelet count is elevated.

Laboratory practitioners inspect hemostasis plasmas for hemolysis, lipemia (cloudy, milky), and icterus (golden yellow from bilirubin). Visible hemolysis implies platelet or coagulation pathway activation. Visibly hemolyzed specimens are rejected, and new specimens must be obtained. Lipemia and icterus may affect the end-point results of optical coagulation instruments. The hemostasis laboratory manager may choose to maintain a separate mechanical end-point coagulometer to substitute for the optical instrument if the specimen is too cloudy for optical determinations. Conversely, some optical instruments detect and compensate for lipemia and icterus via spectrophotometric analysis.[34]

PLATELET FUNCTION TESTS

Platelet function tests are designed to detect qualitative (functional) platelet abnormalities in patients who are experiencing the symptoms of mucocutaneous bleeding (Chapters 36, 37, and 38). A platelet count is performed, and the blood film is reviewed before platelet function tests are begun, because thrombocytopenia is a common cause of hemorrhage.[35] Qualitative platelet abnormalities are suspected only when bleeding symptoms are present and the platelet count exceeds 50,000/μL.

Bleeding Time Test

The bleeding time test, now obsolete, was the original test of platelet function. The phlebotomist used a lancet to make a small, controlled puncture wound and recorded the duration of bleeding, comparing the results with the reference interval of 2 to 9 minutes. The bleeding time test was first described by Duke in 1912 and modified by Ivy in 1941.[36,37] In 1969, Mielke attempted to standardize the bleeding time by specifying a lancet that used a template to establish incision depth and applying a blood pressure cuff inflated to 40 mm Hg to the upper arm. In 1976 a calibrated spring-loaded lancet (Surgicutt Bleeding Time Device) was developed. The device was triggered on the volar surface of the forearm a few inches distal to the antecubital crease, and the resulting wound was blotted every 30 seconds with filter paper until bleeding stopped.[38,39]

A prolonged bleeding time could theoretically signal von Willebrand disease (VWD), a functional platelet disorder such as Glanzmann thrombasthenia, or a vascular disorder such as scurvy or vasculitis, and was thought to have a predictable result in therapy using aspirin and other NSAIDs. Surgeons routinely requested bleeding time screens in a futile attempt to predict surgical bleeding, but a series of studies in the 1990s revealed that the test has inadequate predictive value.[40] The bleeding time is affected by the nonplatelet variables of intracapillary pressure, skin thickness at the puncture site, and size and depth of the wound, all of which interfere with accurate interpretation of the test results.[41]

Platelet Aggregometry

Functional platelets adhere to subendothelial collagen, aggregate with one another, and secrete the contents of their α-granules

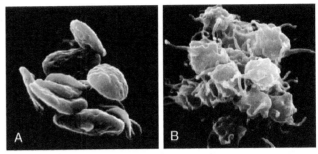

Figure 41.2 Scanning Electron Micrograph of Resting (**A**) and Activated (**B**) Platelets.

and dense granules (Figure 41.2; Chapter 10). Normal adhesion requires intact platelet membranes and functional plasma VWF. Normal aggregation requires that platelet membranes and platelet activation pathways are intact, that the plasma fibrinogen concentration is normal, and that normal secretions are released from platelet granules. Platelet adhesion, aggregation, and secretion are assessed using platelet aggregometry that can be detected by one of three different types of instruments, described later and depicted in Chapter 42. Platelet aggregometry is a high-complexity laboratory test requiring a skilled, experienced operator.

Platelet Aggregometry Using Platelet-Rich Plasma

PRP aggregometry is performed using a specialized photometer called a *light-transmittance aggregometer* distributed by Chrono-Log or BioData.[42] After calibrating the instrument in accordance with manufacturer instructions, the operator pipettes the PRP to instrument-compatible cuvettes, usually 500 μL; drops in one clean plasticized stir bar per sample; places the cuvettes in incubation wells; and allows the samples to warm to 37° C for 5 minutes. The operator then transfers the first cuvette, containing specimen and stir bar, to the instrument's reaction well and starts the stirring device and the recording computer. The stirring device turns the stir bar at

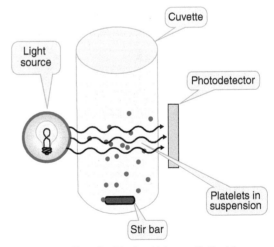

Figure 41.3 Platelet Function Testing Using an Optical Aggregometer. Platelets, in a platelet-rich plasma specimen, are maintained in suspension by a magnetic stir bar turning at 800 to 1200 rpm. As platelet aggregation proceeds, the platelets form large clumps that allow more light transmission through the specimen. (Courtesy Kathy Jacobs, Chrono-Log Corp., Havertown, PA.)

TABLE 41.4   Platelet Aggregometry Agonists and Their Target Mechanism

Agonist	Typical Final Concentration	Platelet Membrane Receptors Targeted by the Agonist
Thrombin	1 unit/mL	PAR1 and PAR4; GPIbα and GPV
TRAP	10, 50, 100 μM	PAR1 and PAR4; GPIbα and GPV
ADP	1–10 μM	P2Y₁, P2Y₁₂
Epinephrine	2–10 μg/mL	α₂-adrenergic receptor
Collagen	5 μg/mL	GP Ia/IIa, GP VI
Arachidonic acid	500 μM	TPα, TPβ
Ristocetin	1 mg/mL	GPIb/IX/V in association with von Willebrand factor

ADP, Adenosine diphosphate; *GP*, glycoprotein; *PAR*, protease-activatable receptor; *P2Y*, platelet membrane ADP receptor; *TP*, thromboxane receptor; *TRAP*, thrombin receptor-activating peptide.

800 to 1200 rpm, a gentle speed that keeps the platelets in suspension. The instrument directs focused light through the sample cuvette to a photodetector (Figure 41.3). As the PRP is stirred, the recorder tracing stabilizes to generate a baseline, near 0% light transmittance. After a few seconds, the operator pipettes an agonist (platelet activator) (Table 41.4) directly into the sample to trigger aggregation. In a normal specimen, after

the agonist is added, the shape of the suspended platelets changes from discoid to spherical followed by pseudopod extension (Figure 41.2), and the intensity of light transmittance initially (and briefly) decreases, then increases in proportion to the degree of shape change. Percent light transmittance is monitored continuously and recorded (Figure 41.4). As platelet aggregates form, more light passes through the PRP, and the tracing begins to move toward 100% light transmittance. Platelet function deficiencies are reflected in diminished or absent aggregation; many laboratory directors choose 40% aggregation as the lower limit of normal.

Whole-Blood Platelet Aggregometry

In whole-blood platelet aggregometry, platelet aggregation is measured by *electrical impedance*. Specimens are diluted 1:1 with normal saline and tested immediately.[43] The operator pipettes aliquots of properly mixed whole blood suspension to cuvettes and adds equal volumes of physiologic saline. Suspension volume may be 300 to 500 μL. The operator drops in one stir bar per cuvette and places the cuvettes in 37° C incubation wells for 5 minutes. The operator transfers the first cuvette to a reaction well, pipettes an agonist directly into the specimen, and suspends a pair of low-voltage cartridge-mounted disposable direct current electrodes in the mixture. As aggregation occurs, platelets adhere to the electrodes and one another, impeding the current (Figure 41.5). The rise in impedance, which is directly proportional to platelet aggregation, is amplified and

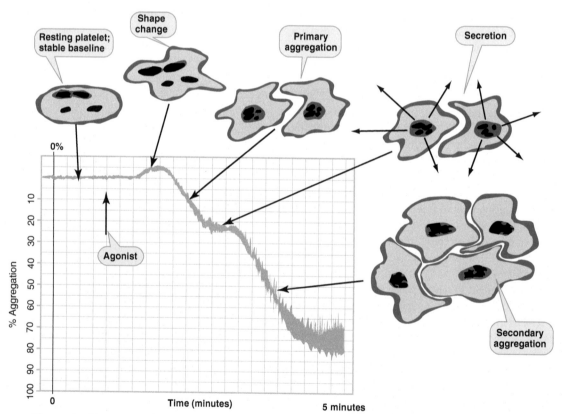

Figure 41.4 Platelet Aggregation Response. This optical aggregometry tracing shows the five phases of platelet aggregation: baseline at 0% aggregation, shape change after the addition of the agonist, primary aggregation, release of adenosine diphosphate *(ADP)* and adenosine triphosphate *(ATP)* from platelet granules, and second-wave aggregation that forms large clumps. The percentage of aggregation is measured by intensity of light transmittance through the test specimen. (Courtesy Kathy Jacobs, Chrono-Log Corp., Havertown, PA.)

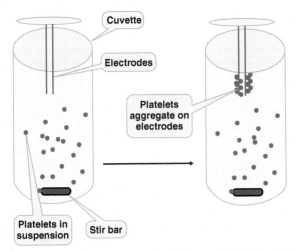

Figure 41.5 Platelet Function Testing Using a Whole-Blood Platelet Aggregometer. Aggregating platelets form a layer on the electrodes. As the platelet layer grows with aggregated platelets, the electrical current is impeded. Impedance (in ohms) is proportional to aggregation, and a tracing is provided that resembles the tracing obtained using optical aggregometry. (Courtesy Kathy Jacobs, Chrono-Log Corp., Havertown, PA.)

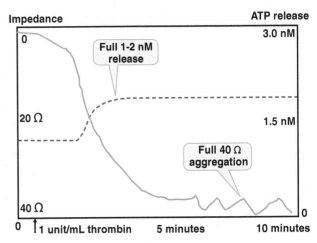

Figure 41.6 Lumiaggregometry Tracing of Normal Platelet Function. This tracing of platelet activity illustrates a monophasic aggregation curve with superimposed secretion (release) reaction curve. Aggregation is measured in ohms (Ω) using the left *y*-axis scale; release is measured in nM of adenosine triphosphate *(ATP)* based on luminescence using the right *y*-axis scale. Curve illustrates full aggregation and secretion response to 1 unit/mL of thrombin.

recorded by instrument circuitry. A whole-blood aggregometry tracing closely resembles a PRP-based light-transmittance aggregometry tracing (Figure 41.4).

Platelet Lumiaggregometry

The Chrono-Log Model 700 Whole Blood/Optical Lumi-Aggregometer is used for the simultaneous measurement of platelet aggregation and the *secretion of adenosine triphosphate* (ATP) from activated platelet dense granules.[44] The procedure for lumiaggregometry differs little from that for light-transmittance or whole blood aggregometry, but because of its detection properties lumiaggregometry simplifies the diagnosis of platelet dysfunction.[45,46] As ATP is released, it oxidizes a firefly derived luciferin-luciferase reagent (Chrono-Lume from Chrono-Log) to generate cold chemiluminescence proportional to the ATP concentration.[47] A photodetector amplifies the luminescence, which is recorded as a second tracing on the aggregation report (Figure 41.6).[48]

To perform lumiaggregometry, the operator adds an ATP standard to the first sample and then adds luciferin-luciferase and tests for full luminescence. The operator then adds luciferin-luciferase and an agonist to the second sample; the instrument monitors for aggregation and secretion simultaneously. Thrombin (or thrombin receptor-activating peptide, TRAP) is typically the first agonist used because thrombin induces full secretion. The operator ordinarily begins with 1 unit/mL of thrombin to induce the release of 1 to 2 nM of ATP, detected by luminescence of the firefly luciferin-luciferase. The luminescence induced by thrombin is measured, recorded, and used for comparison with the luminescence produced by the additional agonists (Table 41.5). Normal secretion induced by agonists other than thrombin produces luminescence at a level of about 50% of that resulting from thrombin. Thrombin-induced secretion may be diminished to less than 1 nM in storage pool deficiencies (Chapter 37), but it is relatively unaffected by membrane disorders or pathway enzyme deficiencies.

TABLE 41.5 Typical Platelet Impedance Lumiaggregometry Reference Intervals

Agonist	Final Concentration	Aggregation RI	ATP Secretion
Thrombin	1 unit/mL	Often causes clotting	1.0–2.0 nM
TRAP	10, 50, 100 μM	15–27 Ω	1.0–2.0 nM
Collagen	1 μg/mL	15–27 Ω	0.5–1.7 nM
	5 μg/mL	15–31 Ω	0.9–1.7 nM
ADP	5 μM	1–17 Ω	0.0–0.7 nM
	10 μM	6–24 Ω	0.4–1.7 nM
Arachidonic acid	500 μM	5–17 Ω	0.6–1.4 nM
Ristocetin	1 mg/mL	>10 Ω	Not recorded

ADP, Adenosine diphosphate; *ATP,* adenosine triphosphate; *RI,* reference interval; *TRAP,* thrombin receptor-activating peptide.

Figure 41.6 depicts simultaneous aggregation and secretion responses to thrombin.

Platelet Agonists in Aggregometry

The agonists used to activate platelets are thrombin or synthetic TRAP, adenosine diphosphate (ADP), epinephrine, collagen, arachidonic acid, and ristocetin. Tables 41.4 and 41.5 list representative agonists and the final reaction mixture concentrations used in light-transmittance, whole blood, and lumiaggregometry. Small volumes (2 to 5 μL) of concentrated agonist are used so that they have little dilutional effect in the reaction system.[49]

Laboratory practitioners use these platelet agonists to test for abnormalities of specific membrane binding sites. Arachidonic acid is the agonist used to check for deficiencies in the eicosanoid synthesis pathway. Ristocetin is used to check for abnormalities of plasma VWF in VWD. Lumiaggregometry provides more definitive information for conditions where recording platelet secretion, in addition to platelet aggregation, is an important diagnostic factor.

Thrombin (or TRAP) cleaves two platelet membrane protease activatable receptors (PARs), PAR-1 and PAR-2, both members of the seven-transmembrane repeat receptor family. Thrombin or TRAP also cleaves glycoprotein (GP) 1bα and GPV. Membrane-associated G proteins and both the eicosanoid and the diacylglycerol pathways trigger internal platelet activation. Thrombin-induced activation results in full secretion and aggregation. Thrombin has the disadvantage that it often triggers coagulation (fibrin formation) simultaneously with aggregation, abolishing the value of the aggregation tracing. The use of TRAP avoids this pitfall. Reagent thrombin is stored dry at –20° C or –70° C and is reconstituted with physiologic saline immediately before use. Leftover reconstituted thrombin may be divided into aliquots, frozen, and thawed for later use.

ADP binds platelet membrane receptors $P2Y_1$ and $P2Y_{12}$, also members of the seven-transmembrane repeat receptor family. ADP-induced platelet activation relies on the physiologic response of membrane-associated G protein and the eicosanoid synthesis pathway. The end product of eicosanoid synthesis, thromboxane A_2, raises cytosolic free calcium, which mediates platelet activation and induces secretion of the ADP stored in dense granules. The secreted ADP activates neighboring platelets.

ADP is the most commonly used agonist, particularly in aggregometry systems that measure only aggregation and not luminescence. The operator adjusts the ADP concentration to between 1 and 10 μM to induce "biphasic" aggregation (Figure 41.4). At ADP concentrations near 1 μM, platelets achieve only primary aggregation, followed by disaggregation: The aggregometry recording line deflects from the baseline for 1 to 2 minutes and then returns to baseline. Primary aggregation involves shape change with formation of microaggregates; both are reversible processes. Secondary aggregation is full platelet aggregation after release of platelet dense granule ADP. At agonist ADP concentrations near 10 μM, there is simultaneous irreversible shape change, secretion, and formation of aggregates, resulting in a monophasic curve and full deflection of the aggregometry tracing. ADP concentrations between 1 and 10 μM may induce a biphasic curve: primary aggregation followed by a brief flattening of the curve called the lag phase and then secondary aggregation.

Operators expend considerable effort to discover the ADP concentration that generates a biphasic curve with a visible lag phase because the appropriate concentration varies among patients. This enables operators to use aggregometry alone to distinguish between membrane-associated platelet defects and storage pool or release defects.

Lumiaggregometry provides a clearer and more reproducible measure of platelet secretion, rendering the quest for the biphasic curve unnecessary. Secretion in response to ADP at 5 μM is diminished in platelet membrane disorders, eicosanoid synthesis pathway enzyme deficiencies, or ASA therapy, NSAIDs, or clopidogrel. Secretion is absent in storage pool deficiency when thrombin or TRAP is used as the agonist.

Reagent ADP is stored at –20° C or –70° C, reconstituted with physiologic saline, and used immediately after reconstitution. Leftover reconstituted ADP may be aliquoted and frozen for later use.

The thienopyridine antiplatelet drugs clopidogrel and prasugrel irreversibly occupy the ADP receptor $P2Y_{12}$, whereas the nucleoside ticagrelor is reversibly bound (Chapter 37). The $P2Y_{12}$ inhibitors suppress aggregation and secretion responses to ADP.[50] Platelet aggregometry is employed to monitor response to these antiplatelet drugs.[51] The VerifyNow system (Accriva) offers specific assays for monitoring the effect of the $P2Y_{12}$ inhibitors (Chapter 40) and is available in point-of-care settings (Chapter 42).

Epinephrine binds platelet α-adrenergic receptors, identical to muscle receptors, and activates the platelets through the same metabolic pathways as reagent ADP. The results of epinephrine-induced aggregation match those of ADP, except that epinephrine cannot induce aggregation in storage pool disorder or eicosanoid synthesis pathway defects no matter how high its concentration. Epinephrine does not work in whole-blood aggregometry. Epinephrine is stored at 1° C to 6° C and reconstituted with distilled water immediately before it is used. Leftover reconstituted epinephrine may be aliquoted and frozen for later use.

Collagen binds GPIa/IIa and GPVI, but it induces no primary aggregation. After a lag of 30 to 60 seconds, aggregation begins and a monophasic curve develops. Aggregation induced by collagen at 5 μg/mL requires intact membrane receptors, functional membrane G proteins, and normal eicosanoid pathway function. Loss of collagen-induced aggregation may indicate a membrane abnormality, storage pool disorder, release defect, or the presence of aspirin. Most laboratory managers purchase lyophilized fibrillar collagen preparations such as Chrono-Par Collagen (Chrono-Log). Collagen is stored at 1° C to 6° C and used without further dilution. Collagen may not be frozen.

Arachidonic acid assesses the viability of the eicosanoid synthesis pathway. Free arachidonic acid agonist is added to induce a monophasic aggregometry curve with virtually no lag phase. Aggregation is independent of membrane integrity. Deficiencies in eicosanoid pathway enzymes, including deficient or aspirin-suppressed cyclooxygenase, result in reduced aggregation and secretion. Arachidonic acid is readily oxidized and must be stored at –20° C or –70° C in the dark. The operator dilutes arachidonic acid with a solution of bovine albumin for immediate use. Aliquots of bovine albumin-dissolved arachidonic acid may be frozen for later use.

NSAIDs such as aspirin, ibuprofen, indomethacin, and sulfinpyrazone permanently inactivate or temporarily inhibit cyclooxygenase.[52] The NSAIDs limit or eliminate the aggregation and secretion responses to arachidonic acid and collagen. Platelet aggregometry is employed to monitor response to these antiplatelet drugs.[53] The VerifyNow system (Accriva) offers specific assays for monitoring the effect of aspirin (Chapter 40) and is available in point-of-care settings (Chapter 42).

Von Willebrand Factor Activity Assays

VWF analysis requires a panel of quantitative and functional assays. These include the VWF antigen (VWF:Ag) immunoassay, the clot-based coagulation factor VIII assay, the functional VWF ristocetin cofactor assay (VWF:RCo), and the dilute ristocetin-induced platelet aggregation assay (RIPA), also called the ristocetin response curve, which is employed to diagnose VWD subtype 2B. These assays and several current refinements are described in Chapter 36.

Two manual enzyme-linked immunosorbant assays (ELISAs), the VWF Activity Immunoassay (REAADS von Willebrand Factor Activity enzyme immunoassay) and the VWF Collagen Binding Assay (Technozyme VWF:CBA ELISA Collagen Type I) are available. The former employs a monoclonal antibody specific for an active VWF epitope, and the latter mimics VWF's in vivo collagen adhesion property. Both reflect VWF activity rather than concentration and offer improved precision when compared to the VWF:RCo.

Heparin-Induced Thrombocytopenia Assays

A description of the clinical manifestations and mechanism of heparin-induced thrombocytopenia (HIT) is provided in Chapters 38 and 39. Although a number of enzyme immunoassay and rapid tests are available (Chapter 39), aggregation-based assays remain available to assess the functional platelet response to the HIT antibodies.[54,55] The aggregation-based tests for HIT include light-transmittance aggregometry, washed platelet light-transmittance aggregometry, washed platelet lumiaggregometry, and whole-blood lumiaggregometry.[56,57] The washed platelet carbon-14 (^{14}C) serotonin release assay (SRA, not to be confused with the assay for serotonin) is an aggregation assay that measures platelet activation and secretion induced by HIT antibodies in the presence of heparin.[58] All these tests employ UFH as their agonist. The ^{14}C-SRA is available from specialized reference laboratories and is regarded as both the reference and the confirmatory method for a diagnosis of HIT. Few local institutions provide the ^{14}C-SRA because a radioisotope license is required. Compared with the ^{14}C-SRA, aggregometry and lumiaggregometry tests for HIT have proven to be less sensitive and have been largely discontinued.[59]

PLATELET ACTIVATION MARKERS

Elevated plasma levels of PF4 (not to be confused with the HIT antibody) may accompany thrombotic stroke or coronary thrombosis, reflecting raised platelet activation.[60] A PF4 immunoassay is available from Hyphen BioMed and its measurement may be of diagnostic or prognostic significance.[61] Blood collectors employ CTAD tubes to prevent in vitro platelet activation.[62]

Thromboxane A_2, the active product of the eicosanoid pathway, has a half-life of 30 seconds, diffuses from the platelet, and spontaneously reduces to thromboxane B_2, a stable, measurable plasma metabolite (Chapter 10). Efforts to produce a clinical assay for plasma thromboxane B_2 have been unsuccessful because specimens must be collected in CTAD tubes to prevent in vitro platelet activation and must undergo a cumbersome extraction step before the assay is performed.

Liver enzymes act on thromboxane B_2 to produce an array of soluble urine metabolites, including 11-dehydrothromboxane B_2, which is stable and measurable.[63] Immunoassays of urine 11-dehydrothromboxane B_2, available from specialized reference laboratories, are employed to characterize in vivo platelet activation.[64] These assays require no special specimen management and can be performed on random urine specimens. The urinary 11-dehydrothromboxane B_2 assay also may be used to monitor aspirin therapy and to identify cases of aspirin therapy failure.[65,66]

CLOT-BASED SCREENING TESTS FOR COAGULATION DISORDERS

The Lee-White whole-blood coagulation time test, described in 1913, was the first laboratory procedure designed to assess coagulation.[67] The Lee-White test is no longer used, but it was the first in vitro clot procedure that employed the principle that the time interval from the initiation of clotting to visible clot formation reflects the condition of the coagulation mechanism. A prolonged clotting time indicates a *coagulopathy,* a coagulation deficiency. A 1953 modification, the activated clotting time (ACT) test, uses a particulate clot activator in the test tube, which speeds the clotting process (Chapter 40). The ACT is still widely used as a point-of-care assay to monitor UFH therapy in high-dose applications, cardiac catheterization and coronary artery bypass graft surgery.

The standard clot-based coagulation screening tests—PT, PTT, fibrinogen assay, and thrombin clotting time (TCT)—use the clotting time principle of the Lee-White test. Many specialized tests, such as coagulation factor assays, tests of fibrinolysis, inhibitor assays, reptilase time, Russell viper venom time, and dilute Russell viper venom time, are also based on the relationship between time to clot formation and coagulation system function. Typical reference intervals are provided on the inside back cover.

Prothrombin Time
Prothrombin Time Principle
PT reagents, often called thromboplastin or tissue thromboplastin, consist of recombinant or affinity-purified *tissue factor* suspended in *phospholipids* mixed with a buffered 0.025 M solution of *calcium chloride.*[68] A few thromboplastins are organic extracts of emulsified rabbit brain or lung suspended in calcium chloride. When mixed with citrated PPP, the PT reagent triggers fibrin polymerization by adding calcium ions and activating plasma factor VII (Figure 41.7). Calcium and phospholipids participate in the formation of the tissue factor-factor VIIa complex, the factor VIIIa-factor IXa complex, and the factor Va-factor Xa complex. The clot is detectable by optical or electromechanical sensors (Chapter 42). Although analysis of the coagulation pathway would seem to imply that the PT would prolong in deficiencies of fibrinogen, prothrombin, and factors V, VII, and X, the procedure is most sensitive to factor VII deficiencies, moderately sensitive to factor V and X deficiencies, sensitive to severe fibrinogen and prothrombin deficiencies, and insensitive to deficiencies of factors VIII, IX, and XIII.[69] The PT is prolonged in multiple factor deficiency disorders that include deficiencies of factors VII and X and is

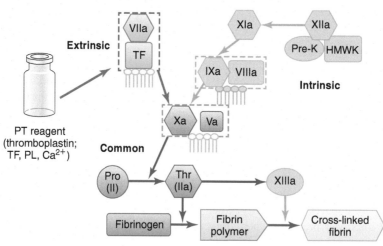

Figure 41.7 Prothrombin time *(PT)* Assay. The PT reagent (thromboplastin) consists of tissue factor *(TF)*, phospholipid *(PL)*, and ionized calcium *(Ca²⁺)*. The reagent activates the extrinsic and common pathways of the coagulation mechanism beginning with factor VII (colored area in figure). The PT is prolonged by deficiencies of factors VII, X, and V; prothrombin; and fibrinogen when fibrinogen is less than 100 mg/dL. The PT is prolonged in Coumadin therapy because production of factor VII, factor X, and prothrombin is suppressed. *a,* Activated form of each factor *HMWK,* high-molecular-weight kininogen; *Pre-K,* prekallikrein; *Pro,* prothrombin (II); *Thr,* thrombin.

used most often to monitor the effects of therapy with the oral anticoagulant Coumadin (Chapter 40).

Prothrombin Time Procedure

The tissue factor-phospholipid-calcium chloride reagent is warmed to 37° C. An aliquot of test PPP, 50 or 100 µL, is transferred to the reaction vessel, which also is maintained at 37° C. The PPP aliquot is incubated at 37° C for at least 3 and for no more than 10 minutes. Aliquots that are incubated longer than 10 minutes become prolonged as coagulation factors begin to deteriorate or are affected by evaporation and pH change. A premeasured volume of reagent, 100 or 200 µL, respectively, is speedily and directly added to the PPP aliquot, and a timer is started. As the clot forms, the timer stops, and the elapsed time is recorded. Most laboratory practitioners perform PTs using semiautomated or automated instruments that strictly control temperature, pipetting, and interval timing (Chapter 42).

Prothrombin Time Quality Control

The medical laboratory practitioner tests commercially prepared normal and prolonged control PPP specimens at the beginning of each 8-hour shift or with each change of reagent. Controls may be shipped frozen or lyophilized, but in either case are tested alongside patient specimens using the same protocol as for patient PPP testing. Frozen controls must be rapidly thawed at 37° C and mixed well. Lyophilized control materials are reconstituted with the supplied buffer, using caution to ensure no material is expelled during reconstitution, mixed well, and allowed to stand for 20 to 30 minutes following manufacturer specifications. Once prepared, controls are placed in temperature-controlled wells.

The normal control result should be within the reference interval, and the prolonged control result should be within the therapeutic range for Coumadin. If the control results fall within the stated limits provided in the laboratory protocol, the test results are considered valid. If the results fall outside the control limits, the reagents, control, and equipment are checked; the problem is corrected; and the control and patient specimens are retested. The operator records all the actions taken. Control results are recorded and analyzed at regular intervals to determine the long-term validity of results.

Reporting Prothrombin Time Results and the International Normalized Ratio

The medical laboratory practitioner reports PT results to the nearest tenth of a second, along with the PT reference interval.

When the PT is used for Coumadin monitoring, the INR, detailed in Chapter 40, is employed to normalize results from laboratories around the world.[70] Laboratories typically report a combination of the PT in seconds and the INR together as the PT/INR, though clinicians are encouraged to use the PT in seconds for all non-Coumadin applications.

Prothrombin Time Reference Interval

The PT reference interval, computed from PT values of healthy individuals, varies from site to site, depending on the patient population, type of thromboplastin used, type of instrument used, and pH and purity of the reagent diluent. Each center must establish its own interval for each new lot of reagents, or at least once a year. This may be done by testing a sample of at least 30 specimens from healthy donors of both sexes spanning the adult age range over several days and computing the 95% confidence interval of the results. A typical PT reference interval is 12.6 to 14.6 seconds, though the interval varies among facilities.

The Prothrombin Time as a Diagnostic Assay

The PT is performed diagnostically when any coagulopathy is suspected. Acquired multiple deficiencies such as disseminated intravascular coagulation (DIC), liver disease, and vitamin K deficiency all affect factor VII activity and are detected through prolonged PT results. The PT is particularly sensitive to liver disease, in which factor VII levels rapidly diminish because the half-life of factor VII is only 6 hours (Chapter 36).

Vitamin K deficiency is seen in severe malnutrition, during use of broad-spectrum antibiotics that destroy gut flora, with parenteral nutrition, and in malabsorption syndromes. Vitamin K levels are low in newborns, in which bacterial colonization of the gut has not begun. Hemorrhage is likely in vitamin K deficiency, and the PT is the best indicator. To distinguish between vitamin K deficiency and liver disease, the laboratory practitioner determines factor V and factor VII levels. Both factor V and factor VII are reduced in liver disease; only factor VII is reduced in vitamin K deficiency. Chapter 36 provides details regarding liver disease and vitamin K deficiency.

The PT is prolonged in congenital single-factor deficiencies of factor X, VII, or V, profound prothrombin deficiency, and fibrinogen deficiency when the fibrinogen level is 100 mg/dL or less. When the PT is prolonged, but the PTT and TCT test results are normal, factor VII activity may be deficient. Any suspected single-factor deficiency is confirmed with a factor assay. The PT is not affected by factor VIII or IX deficiency, because the concentration of tissue factor in the reagent is high, and those factors are bypassed in thrombin generation.

Minimal Effectiveness of Prothrombin Time as a Screening Tool

Preoperative PT screening of asymptomatic surgical patients to predict intraoperative hemorrhage is not supported by prevalence studies.[71] No clinical data support the use of the PT as a general screening test for individuals at low risk of bleeding, and the PT is not useful for establishing baseline values in Coumadin therapy.[72] The PT's diagnostic efficacy rises when used in the context of a bleeding indication.

Prothrombin Time Limitations

Specimen variations profoundly affect PT results (Table 41.6). The ratio of whole blood to anticoagulant is crucial, so collection tubes must be filled to within tube manufacturers' specifications and not underfilled or overfilled. Anticoagulant volume must be adjusted when the hematocrit is greater than 55% to avoid false prolongation of the results. Specimens must be inverted at least three times immediately after collection to ensure good anticoagulation, but the mixing must be gentle. Practitioners must reject clotted and visibly hemolyzed specimens because they give unreliable results. Plasma lipemia or icterus may affect the results obtained with optical instrumentation.

Heparin may prolong the PT. If the patient is receiving therapeutic heparin, it should be noted on the order and commented on when the results are reported. The laboratory manager selects thromboplastin reagents that are maximally sensitive to Coumadin and relatively insensitive to heparin. Many reagent manufacturers incorporate polybrene (5-dimethyl-1,5-diazaundecamethylene polymethobromide, or hexadimethrine bromide, Millipore Sigma) in their thromboplastin reagent to neutralize heparin. The medical laboratory practitioner may detect unexpected heparin by using the TCT test.

TABLE 41.6	Factors That Interfere with the Validity of Clot-Based Test Results
Specimen Variation	**Solution**
Blood collection volume less than specified minimum	PT and PTT falsely prolonged; recollect specimen.
Hematocrit ≥ 55%	Adjust anticoagulant volume using formula or nomogram and recollect specimen using new anticoagulant volume.
Specimen clot	All results are affected unpredictably; recollect specimen.
Visible hemolysis	PT and PTT falsely shortened; recollect specimen.
Icterus or lipemia	Measure PT and PTT using a mechanical coagulometer.
UFH therapy	Use reagent known to be insensitive to UFH or one that includes a UFH neutralizer such as polybrene.
Lupus anticoagulant	PT and PTT results invalid; use alternative methods, for instance, chromogenic assays.
Incorrect calibration, incorrect dilution of reagents	Correct analytical error and repeat assay.

PT, Prothrombin time; *PTT*, partial thromboplastin time; *UFH*, unfractionated heparin.

LACs prolong some thromboplastins. LACs are members of the antiphospholipid antibody family and may partially neutralize PT reagent phospholipids. Coumadin often is prescribed to prevent thrombosis in patients with LACs, but the PT may be an unreliable monitor of therapy in such cases. Patients who have an LAC and are taking Coumadin should be monitored using an alternative system, such as the chromogenic factor X assay.[73-75]

Reagents must be reconstituted with the correct diluents and volumes following manufacturer instructions. Reagents must be stored and shipped according to manufacturer instructions and never used after the expiration date.

Partial Thromboplastin Time
Partial Thromboplastin Time Principle

The PTT (also called the activated partial thromboplastin time, or APTT) is employed to monitor the effects of UFH and to detect LAC and specific coagulation factor antibodies such as antifactor VIII antibody.[76] The PTT is also prolonged in all congenital and acquired procoagulant deficiencies, except for deficiencies of factor VII or XIII.[77]

The PTT reagent contains *phospholipid* (previously called partial thromboplastin or cephalin) and a *negatively charged particulate activator* such as silica, kaolin, ellagic acid, or celite in suspension. The phospholipid mixture, which was historically extracted from rabbit brain, is now produced synthetically. The activator provides a surface that mediates a conformational change in plasma factor XII that results in its activation (Figure 41.8). Factor XIIa forms a complex with two other plasma components: high-molecular-weight kininogen

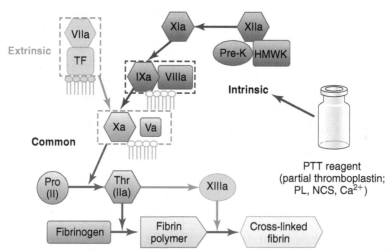

Figure 41.8 Partial Thromboplastin Time *(PTT)* Assay. The PTT reagent (partial thromboplastin) consists of phospholipid *(PL)*, a negatively charged particulate activator *(NCS)*, and ionized calcium *(Ca²⁺)*. The reagent activates the intrinsic and common pathways of the coagulation mechanism through the contact factors XII, prekallikrein *(pre-K)*, and high-molecular-weight kininogen *(HMWK)* (colored area in figure). The PTT is prolonged by deficiencies in pre-K; HMWK; factors XII, XI, IX, VIII, and X and prothrombin; and fibrinogen when less than 100 mg/dL. The PTT is prolonged in unfractionated heparin *(UFH)* therapy because UFH bound to antithrombin neutralizes thrombin (IIa), factor Xa, and other coagulation serine proteases. The PTT is prolonged in the presence of lupus anticoagulant *(LAC)* because LAC neutralizes reagent phospholipids. *a*, Activated form of each factor; *Pro*, prothrombin (factor II); *TF*, tissue factor; *Thr*, thrombin.

(Fitzgerald factor) and prekallikrein (Fletcher factor). These three plasma glycoproteins, termed the contact activation factors, initiate in vitro clot formation through the intrinsic pathway but are not part of in vivo coagulation. The complexed factor XIIa, a serine protease, activates factor XI (XIa), which activates factor IX (IXa) (Chapter 35).

Factor IXa forms a complex with factor VIIIa, reagent calcium, and reagent phospholipid. This complex catalyzes factor X. The resultant factor Xa forms a second complex with calcium, phospholipid, and factor Va, catalyzing the conversion of prothrombin to thrombin. Thrombin catalyzes the polymerization of fibrinogen and the formation of the fibrin clot, which is the endpoint of the PTT.

Most PTT reagents are designed so that the PTT is prolonged when the specimen has less than approximately 30 units/mL of factors VIII, IX, or XI.[78]

Partial Thromboplastin Time Procedure

To initiate contact activation, 50 or 100 μL of warmed (37° C) reagent consisting of phospholipid and particulate activator is mixed with an equal volume of warmed PPP. The mixture is allowed to incubate for the exact manufacturer-specified time, usually 3 minutes. Next, 50 or 100 μL of warmed 0.025 M calcium chloride is forcibly added to the mixture, and a timer is started. When a fibrin clot forms, the timer stops, and the interval is recorded. Timing may be done with an automatic electromechanical or photo-optical device. Results are reported to the nearest tenth of a second, along with the PTT reference interval.

Partial Thromboplastin Time Quality Control

The medical laboratory practitioner tests normal and prolonged control plasma specimens at the beginning of each 8-hour shift or with each new batch of reagent. The laboratory director may require more frequent use of controls. Controls are tested using the protocol for patient plasma testing.

The normal control result should be within the reference interval, and the abnormal control result should be within the UFH therapeutic range (Chapter 40). If the control results fall within the stated limits in the laboratory protocol, the test results are considered valid. If the results fall outside the control limits, the reagents, control, and equipment are checked; the problem is corrected; and the control and patient specimens are retested. The operator records each control run and all the actions taken. Control results are recorded and analyzed at regular intervals to determine the long-term validity of results.

Reagents and controls must be reconstituted with the correct diluents and volumes or thawed following manufacturer instructions. Reagents must be stored and shipped according to manufacturer instructions and never used after the expiration date. Specimen errors that affect the PT similarly affect the PTT (Table 41.6).

Partial Thromboplastin Time Reference Interval

The PTT reference interval varies from site to site, depending on the patient population, type of reagent, type of instrument, and pH and purity of the diluent. One medical center laboratory has established 26 to 38 seconds as its reference interval. This is typical, but each center must establish its own interval for each new lot of reagent, or at least once a year. This may be done by testing a sample of 30 or more specimens from healthy donors of both sexes spanning the adult age range over several days and computing the 95% confidence interval of the results.

Monitoring Heparin Therapy with the Partial Thromboplastin Time

Since the early 1970s, the PTT has been the standard method for monitoring UFH, which is used to treat patients with venous thrombosis, pulmonary embolism, myocardial infarction, and a variety of thrombotic events.[79] The laboratory practitioner establishes a therapeutic range using the ex vivo Brill-Edwards curve, and publishes it to all units. A typical therapeutic range is 60 to 100 seconds; however, the range varies widely and must be established locally.[80] The range must be reestablished with each change of PTT reagent, including each lot change, and on instrument recalibration. Details on UFH monitoring and establishment of the PTT therapeutic range are provided in Chapter 40.

The Partial Thromboplastin Time as a Diagnostic Assay

The physician orders a PTT when a hemorrhagic disorder is suspected or when recurrent thrombosis or the presence of an autoimmune disorder points to the possibility of LAC.[81] The PTT result is prolonged when there is a deficiency of one or more of the following coagulation factors: prothrombin; factors V, VIII, IX, X, XI, or XII; or fibrinogen when the fibrinogen level is 100 mg/dL or less. The most common deficiencies that are reflected in an isolated prolonged PTT are deficiencies of factors VIII, IX, or XI; hemophilia A, hemophilia B, and Rosenthal syndrome, respectively. Factor VII and factor XIII deficiencies have no effect on the PTT. Deficiencies of factor XII, prekallikrein, or high-molecular-weight kininogen prolong the PTT but do not associate with bleeding.

The PTT also is prolonged in the presence of a specific inhibitor, such as anti-factor VIII or anti-factor IX; a nonspecific inhibitor, such as LAC, an immunoglobulin with affinity for phospholipid-bound proteins; and interfering substances, such as fibrin degradation products (FDPs) or paraproteins, which are present in myeloma.

DIC prolongs PTT results because of consumption of multiple procoagulants, but the PTT results must be confirmed using the D-dimer, platelet count, and erythrocyte morphology. Vitamin K deficiency results in diminished activities of procoagulant factors II (prothrombin), VII, IX, and X, and the PTT is eventually prolonged. Because factor VII deficiency does not affect the PTT, however, and because it is the first coagulation factor whose activity becomes deficient, the PTT is less sensitive to vitamin K deficiency or Coumadin therapy than the PT.

PTT Mixing Studies
Lupus Anticoagulants

LACs are IgG immunoglobulins directed against a number of phospholipid-protein complexes.[82] LACs prolong the phospholipid-dependent PTT reaction. Most laboratories employ a moderate-phospholipid or high-phospholipid PTT reagent in their routine PTT assay, which is designed to monitor UFH therapy and detect coagulopathies. Laboratories use a second low-phospholipid PTT reagent such as PTT-LA (Diagnostica Stago), which is more sensitive to LAC, for LAC detection (Chapter 39). Because they have a variety of target antigens, LACs are called nonspecific inhibitors. Every acute care laboratory provides a means for their initial detection as their presence signals a potential thrombotic risk.[83] Laboratory directors employ repeated LAC assays separated by a minimum 12-week interval to distinguish chronic from acute LACs as thrombotic risk has been traditionally associated with chronic LAC presence, although additional evidence implicates transient LACs with thrombosis as well. Together, chronic and transient LACs are found in 1% to 2% of randomly selected individuals.

Specific Factor Inhibitors

Specific factor inhibitors are IgG immunoglobulins directed against coagulation factors. Specific inhibitors arise in severe congenital factor deficiencies in response to factor concentrate treatment. Anti-factor VIII, the most common of the specific inhibitors, is detected in 10% to 20% of patients with severe hemophilia and anti-factor IX is detected in 1% to 3% of factor IX-deficient patients. Autoantibodies to factor VIII occasionally arise in individuals without hemophilia, usually in young women, where they are associated with a postpartum bleeding syndrome or in patients over 60 with autoimmune disorders. The presence of these types of antibodies is called acquired hemophilia (Chapter 36). Alloantibodies and autoantibodies to factor VIII are associated with severe anatomic hemorrhage.

Detection of Lupus Anticoagulants, Other Inhibitors, and Factor Deficiencies

LAC testing is part of every thrombophilia profile and may be ordered when a physician confirms a primary thrombotic patient event (Chapter 39). An unexpectedly prolonged initial PTT may also trigger an LAC investigation. PTT mixing studies are necessary for the presumptive detection of LACs.[84] Mixing studies also distinguish LACs from specific inhibitors and factor deficiencies and should be available from all coagulation laboratories.[85]

When the PTT is prolonged beyond the upper limit of the reference interval, the laboratory practitioner first tests for UFH using the TCT. A TCT result that exceeds the upper limit of the TCT reference interval is evidence for UFH. In fact, UFH often prolongs the TCT to 30 to 40 seconds. UFH may be neutralized using polybrene or heparinase (Hepzyme; Siemens), and the treated sample may be used for PTT mixing studies.

The UFH-free or UFH-neutralized patient plasma is then mixed 1:1 with reagent *platelet-poor normal plasma* (PNP; Figure 39.1). Several manufacturers prepare and distribute PNP—for example, frozen CRYO*Check* Normal Reference Plasma (Precision BioLogic). A repeat PTT is performed immediately on the 1:1 patient plasma-PNP mixture. If the mixture PTT corrects to within 10% of the PNP PTT (or to within the reference interval) and the patient is experiencing bleeding, the operator presumes there is a coagulation factor deficiency (coagulopathy).[86]

About 15% of LACs appear to be temperature-dependent and 85% of anti-factor VIII inhibitors are temperature-dependent IgG4-class antibodies, so an incubated mix becomes necessary. If the immediate mix PTT corrects, a new 1:1 mixture is prepared and incubated 2 hours at 37° C. If the incubated mixture's PTT fails to correct to within 10% of the incubated PNP PTT, an inhibitor may be present. The inhibitor could be an LAC, but if the patient is bleeding, a specific inhibitor such as anti-factor VIII is suspected and a factor VIII activity assay is performed. Although anti-factor IX and other inhibitors have been documented, anti-factor VIII is the most common. The Nijmegen-Bethesda assay, discussed later in this chapter, is used to confirm the presence of specific anticoagulation factor antibodies.

If the PTT of the initial or incubated mixture fails to correct and the patient is not bleeding, the laboratory practitioner suspects LAC and automatically orders an LAC profile, as described in Chapter 39. LAC profiles are available from tertiary care facilities and specialty reference laboratories.

Thrombin Clotting Time

Thrombin Clotting Time Reagent and Principle

Commercially prepared bovine thrombin reagent at 5 National Institutes of Health (NIH) units/mL cleaves fibrinopeptides A and B from plasma fibrinogen to form a detectable fibrin polymer (Figure 41.9).[87]

Thrombin Clotting Time Procedure

Reagent thrombin is warmed to 37° C for a minimum of 3 and a maximum of 10 minutes. Thrombin deteriorates during incubation and must be used within 10 minutes of the time incubation is begun. An aliquot of patient plasma, usually 100 μL, is also incubated at 37° C for a minimum of 3 and a maximum of 10 minutes. The operator pipettes 200 μL of thrombin into the PPP aliquot, starts a timer, and records the interval to clot formation. Automated TCT assays are available on all coagulometers.

Thrombin Clotting Time Quality Control

The medical laboratory practitioner tests a normal control sample and an abnormal control sample with each batch of TCT assays and records the results. The normal control results should fall within the laboratory's reference interval. The abnormal control results should be prolonged to the range reached by the TCT in moderate hypofibrinogenemia. If the results fall outside the laboratory protocol's control limits, the reagents, control, and equipment are checked; the problem is corrected; and the control is retested. The actions taken to correct out-of-limit tests are recorded. Control results are analyzed at regular intervals (weekly is typical) to determine the longitudinal validity of the procedure. Specimen errors that affect the PT and PTT likewise affect the TCT (Table 41.6).

Reporting of Thrombin Clotting Time Results and Clinical Utility

Although the TCT reference interval is established locally, a typical TCT reference interval is 15 to 20 seconds. The TCT is prolonged when the fibrinogen level is less than 100 mg/dL (*hypofibrinogenemia*) or in the presence of antithrombotic materials such as FDPs, paraproteins, or UFH. *Afibrinogenemia* (absence of fibrinogen) and *dysfibrinogenemia* (presence of fibrinogen that is biochemically abnormal and nonfunctional) also prolong the TCT. Before a prolonged TCT may be considered as evidence of diminished or abnormal fibrinogen, the presence of antithrombotic substances, such as UFH, FDPs, or paraproteins, must be ruled out. The TCT is part of the PTT mixing study protocol (Figure 39.1) and is used to determine whether UFH is present whenever the PTT is prolonged. The TCT is not sensitive to factor XIII (FXIII) deficiency.

The TCT may also assess the presence of the oral direct thrombin inhibitor dabigatran. The TCT provides binary (qualitative) evidence for dabigatran; if drug is present, the TCT is markedly prolonged. A normal TCT rules out dabigatran. A TCT modification, the plasma-diluted TCT, provides a quantitative measure of dabigatran when used with calibrators of specific drug concentrations.[88]

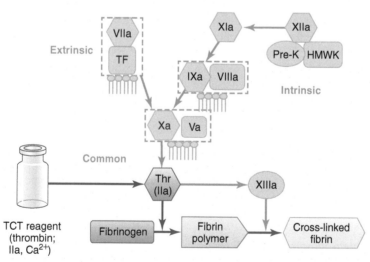

Figure 41.9 Thrombin Clotting Time *(TCT)* Assay. The portion of the coagulation pathway evaluated in the TCT is the same as the pathway evaluated in the reptilase time assay. The reagent activates the coagulation pathway at the level of thrombin and tests for the polymerization of fibrinogen (colored area in figure). The TCT is prolonged by unfractionated heparin *(UFH)*, direct thrombin inhibitors; fibrin degradation products; and dysfibrinogenemia, hypofibrinogenemia, and afibrinogenemia. The reptilase time is unaffected by heparin. *a,* Activated form of each factor; *HMWK,* high-molecular-weight kininogen; *Pre-K,* prekallikrein; *TF,* tissue factor; *Thr,* thrombin.

Venom Activated Assays

Reptilase Time

Reptilase is a thrombin-like enzyme, batroxobin, isolated from the venom of *Bothrops atrox* that catalyzes the conversion of fibrinogen to fibrin (Pefakit Reptilase Time; Pentapharm). In contrast to thrombin, this enzyme cleaves only fibrinopeptide A from the ends of the fibrinogen molecule, whereas thrombin cleaves both fibrinopeptides A and B.[89]

The specimen requirements, procedure, and quality assurance protocol are the same as those for the TCT. The reagent is reconstituted with distilled water and is stable for 1 month when stored at 1° C to 6° C. Reptilase time reagent may be fatal if it enters the bloodstream.

The reptilase time assay is insensitive to UFH and FXIII deficiency but is markedly prolonged in dysfibrinogenemia, so it is occasionally employed to rule out UFH in a patient who has a prolonged PTT. This renders the reptilase time test useful for detecting hypofibrinogenemia or dysfibrinogenemia in patients receiving UFH therapy, and it may be used to work up a bleeding patient whose factors VIII, IX, and XI are normal. The reptilase time is prolonged in the presence of FDPs and paraproteins.

Russell Viper Venom Test

Russell viper venom (RVV) from the *Daboia russelii* viper, which triggers coagulation at the level of factor X, was once used as an alternative to the PT. The assay was named the Stypven time, but is now obsolete. However, buffer-diluted RVV is prolonged by the LAC, and the dilute RVV time is routinely employed to detect LAC, as described in Chapter 39.

COAGULATION FACTOR ASSAYS

Fibrinogen Assay

The clot-based method of Clauss, a modification of the TCT, is the recommended procedure for estimating fibrinogen function.[90] Patient PPP is diluted 1:10 with Owren buffer. The operator adds reagent bovine thrombin at 50 to 100 NIH units/mL to the diluted patient specimen, converting fibrinogen to fibrin polymer. There is an inverse relationship between the interval to clot formation and the concentration of functional fibrinogen. When the thrombin reagent is concentrated and the PPP is diluted, the relationship is linear provided the fibrinogen concentration is 100 to 500 mg/dL. Diluting the PPP minimizes the antithrombotic effects of UFH, FDPs, and paraproteins; UFH levels less than 0.6 units/mL and FDP levels less than 100 μg/dL do not affect the results of the assay provided the fibrinogen concentration is 150 mg/dL or greater. A calibration curve is prepared in each laboratory and updated regularly; for patient PPP the interval to clot formation is read from the curve.[91]

An attractive alternative to the Clauss method is the automated PT-derived fibrinogen assay. Optical coagulometers (ACL TOP, Instrumentation Laboratory [IL]-Werfen) estimate fibrinogen by assessing reaction mixture turbidity while performing the PT.[92] These offer the convenience of a fibrinogen result with each PT.

Fibrinogen Assay Procedure

Clauss fibrinogen assay thrombin reagent. Laboratory managers choose commercially manufactured lyophilized bovine thrombin reagent such as HemosIL QFA, 100 NIH units/mL (IL-Werfen).[93] The reagent is reconstituted according to manufacturer instructions and placed on the coagulometer.

Clauss fibrinogen assay calibration curve. The laboratory practitioner orders the coagulometer to generate a calibration curve at 6-month or shorter intervals, with each change of reagent lot numbers, shift in control results, and subsequent to instrument maintenance. The instrument prepares 1:5, 1:10, 1:15, 1:20, and 1:40 dilutions using reconstituted fibrinogen calibration plasma (Helena Laboratories). An aliquot of each dilution, for instance, 200 μL, is transferred to reaction cuvettes, warmed to 37° C, and tested by adding 100 μL of thrombin reagent. Time from addition of thrombin to clot formation is recorded and the values in seconds are graphed against computed fibrinogen concentration (Figure 41.10). Because patient PPPs are diluted 1:10 before testing, the 1:10 calibration plasma dilution is assigned the same fibrinogen value as that of the undiluted reconstituted calibration plasma.

Clauss fibrinogen assay test protocol. The coagulometer prepares a 1:10 dilution of each patient and control PPP with Owren buffer. An aliquot of each of the diluted samples is warmed to 37° C in a cuvette for 3 minutes. After incubation, thrombin reagent is added; the timer starts and then stops when a clot forms. The interval in seconds is compared with the calibration curve and results are reported in mg/dL.

If the clotting time of the patient PPP dilution is short, indicating a fibrinogen level greater than 480 mg/dL, the instrument prepares and assays a 1:20 Owren buffer dilution, then multiplies the initial result by the dilution factor. If the clotting time is prolonged, indicating less than 200 mg/dL of fibrinogen, the instrument employs a low concentration curve.

Fibrinogen Assay Quality Control

Normal and abnormal control samples are assayed with each batch of patient samples. The normal control results should fall

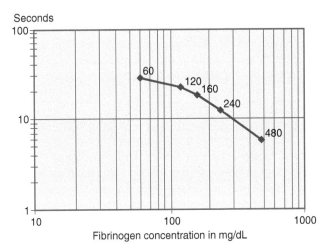

Figure 41.10 Fibrinogen Assay Calibration. This graph illustrates a calibration curve of fibrinogen concentration plotted against the clot times obtained from the fibrinogen assay, using log-log axes.

within the laboratory's reference interval and the abnormal control results should be near or less than 100 mg/dL. If either control result falls outside the control limits, the reagents, control, and equipment are checked; the problem is corrected; and the control is retested. The actions taken to correct out-of-limit tests are recorded. Specimen errors that affect the PTT likewise affect the fibrinogen assay and all factor assays (Table 41.6).

Fibrinogen Assay Results and Clinical Utility

One institution's reference interval for fibrinogen concentration is 220 to 498 mg/dL, although each local institution prepares its own interval. Hypofibrinogenemia, a fibrinogen level of less than 220 mg/dL, may be congenital or may be associated with DIC or severe liver disease. Conversely, early or moderate liver disease, pregnancy, and chronic inflammation may raise the fibrinogen level to greater than 498 mg/dL. Congenital afibrinogenemia is reflected in prolonged clotting times and is associated with variable anatomic hemorrhage. Dysfibrinogenemia may resemble hypofibrinogenemia by the Clauss method, as abnormal fibrinogen species are hydrolyzed more slowly by thrombin than is normal fibrinogen. Conversely, the PT-derived fibrinogen assay, though able to estimate hypofibrinogenemia and dysfibrinogenemia, usually returns normal results for dysfibrinogenemia.[94]

Fibrinogen Assay Limitations

Although antithrombotic effects are minimized by the dilution of PPP specimens, UFH levels greater than 0.6 units/mL and FDP levels greater than 100 μg/mL prolong the clotting time and give falsely lowered fibrinogen results. The operator ensures that the thrombin reagent is pure and has not degenerated. Exposure to sunlight or oxidation results in rapid thrombin breakdown.

Single-Factor Assays Using the PTT

Principle of Single-Factor Assays Based on Partial Thromboplastin Time

If the PTT is prolonged and the PT is normal, and a normal TCT indicates there is no heparin therapy, a mixing study is the next step. If there is correction after the immediate and incubated mix, the operator suspects a congenital single-factor deficiency (Table 41.7).[95] Three factor deficiencies that give this reaction pattern and accompany anatomic hemorrhage are factor VIII deficiency (hemophilia A), factor IX deficiency (hemophilia B), and factor XI deficiency (Rosenthal syndrome).[96] These deficiencies are most often diagnosed in childhood using PTT-based single-factor assays; however, factor assays are more often performed on specimens from patients with previously identified single-factor deficiencies. Their purpose is to regularly monitor prophylactic therapy or to document the efficacy of on-demand therapy during bleeds or invasive procedures. Because hemophilia A is the most common single-factor deficiency disorder, the following discussion is confined to the factor VIII assay.

The medical laboratory practitioner uses the PTT system to estimate the activity of functional factor VIII by incorporating commercially prepared factor VIII-depleted PPP in the test

system (CRYO*Check* Factor VIII Deficient Plasma; Precision BioLogic). Distributors collect plasma from normal donors and employ immunodepletion, relying on an anti-factor VIII antibody bound to a separatory column, to prepare factor VIII-depleted plasma.[97] Because immunodepletion may reduce VWF activity, some laboratory managers prefer plasma collected from congenitally factor VIII-deficient donors, whose VWF levels are normal (George King Bio-Medical).

In the PTT-based factor assay system, factor VIII-depleted or -deficient PPP provides normal activity of all procoagulants except factor VIII. Tested alone, factor VIII-depleted or -deficient PPP has a prolonged PTT, but when normal PPP is added, the PTT reverts to normal. In contrast, a prolonged result for a mixture of patient PPP and factor VIII-depleted PPP implies that the patient PPP is factor VIII deficient. The clotting time interval for the mixture of patient PPP and factor VIII-depleted PPP is compared with a calibrated reference curve to estimate the level of factor VIII activity in the patient PPP. The factor assay is typically performed on an automated coagulometer.[98]

Factor VIII Assay Reference Curve

To prepare a reference curve for the factor VIII assay, the laboratory practitioner obtains reference plasma such as CRYO*Check* Normal Reference Plasma (Precision BioLogic) and programs the coagulometer to prepare a series of dilutions with buffered saline.[99] Although laboratory protocols vary, most laboratory practitioners prepare a series of five dilutions, from 1:5 to 1:500. Each dilution is mixed with reagent factor VIII-depleted or -deficient plasma and tested using the PTT reagent system, generating a linear-log graph (Figure 41.11). The 1:10 dilution is assigned the factor VIII assay activity value found on the package insert. When patient PPP is tested, the time interval obtained is automatically entered on the vertical coordinate and converted to a percentage of activity or units per deciliter.

Factor VIII Assay Procedure

The coagulometer is programmed to prepare 1:10, 1:20, 1:40, and 1:80 or similar dilutions of each patient PPP and control specimen and then mixes each dilution with equal volumes of factor VIII-depleted or -deficient plasma and PTT reagent. In

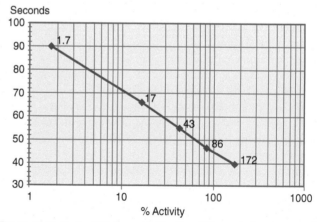

Figure 41.11 Factor VIII Assay Calibration. This graph illustrates a calibration curve of factor VIII concentration plotted against the clot times obtained from the factor VIII assay, using linear-log axes.

most cases, 100 μL of PTT reagent is mixed with 100 μL each of patient PPP dilution and factor VIII-depleted (-deficient) plasma mixture. After incubation at 37° C for the manufacturer-specified time, typically 3 minutes, 100 μL of 0.025 M calcium chloride is dispensed, and a timer starts. The interval in seconds for each dilution is entered into the curve and factor VIII in percentages or units per deciliter is reported for each. Factor activity results for the 1:20, 1:40, and 1:80 dilutions are multiplied by 2, 4, and 8, respectively, to compensate for the dilutions. The results should match the results of the 1:10 dilution within 10%. If the results of the higher dilutions do not match the 1:10 dilution within 10%, they are considered *nonparallel*. A factor VIII inhibitor or LAC may be present, and the assay cannot provide a reliable estimate of factor VIII activity.

Tests for factors IX and XI are performed using the same approach, except that the appropriate factor-depleted (-deficient) plasma is substituted for factor VIII-depleted (-deficient) plasma. Tests for the contact factors XII, prekallikrein, and high-molecular-weight kininogen are seldom requested because deficiencies are not associated with bleeding disorders. Acquired and congenital contact factor deficiencies are relatively common, however, and cause PTT prolongation. Factor XII, prekallikrein, and high-molecular-weight kininogen assays are available from hemostasis reference laboratories, and they may be necessary to account for an unexplained prolonged PTT.

Expected Results and Clinical Utility of Single-Factor Assays

One facility's reference interval for factor VIII activity is 50 to 186 units/dL. The test is used most often to estimate the plasma level of factor VIII activity during therapy (Chapter 36). Spontaneous hemophilia A and B bleeds occur at activity levels of 10 units/dL or less, and regrettably, the factor assay offers poor accuracy at less than 10 units/dL.[100] Chronically elevated factor VIII implies a risk of venous thrombotic disease (Chapter 39).[101]

Single-Factor Assay Quality Control

The laboratory practitioner tests a normal and a deficient control specimen with each assay and records the results. The normal control results should fall within the reference interval. The deficient control results should be in the range of 10 units/dL factor VIII activity or below. If either control result falls outside the control limits, the reagents, control, and equipment are checked; the problem is corrected; and the control is retested. The practitioner records all actions taken to correct out-of-limit tests. Control results are analyzed at regular intervals (weekly is typical) to determine the longitudinal validity of the procedure.

Limitations of Clot-Based Single-Factor Assays

Interlaboratory coefficients of variation for factor VIII assay proficiency testing surveys reach 80%, implying undesirable imprecision in the interpretation of therapeutic monitoring results from separate institutions. To reduce inherent variation, the medical laboratory practitioner uses commercial calibrated plasma to prepare the reference curve and selects reference dilutions that correspond to only the linear portion of the curve. In many facilities the curve is included in each test run, despite the expense.[102] The laboratory must assay three or more dilutions of patient PPP to check for inhibitors. The practitioner also selects a matching reagent-instrument system with a demonstrated internal day-to-day coefficient of variation of less than 5%. As with the PT, PTT, and TCT, good specimen management is essential. Clotted, hemolyzed, icteric, or lipemic specimens are rejected because they give unreliable results. Reagents must be reconstituted with the correct diluents and volumes following manufacturer instructions. Reagents must be stored and shipped in accordance with manufacturer instructions and never used after the expiration date.

Regrettably, clot-based assays do not accurately measure B-domain-deleted rFVIII or the extended half-life rFVIII formulations that have been available for therapy since 2014.[103] In vitro diagnostics manufacturers are currently developing new approaches to factor estimation, of which chromogenic substrate factor assays appear to be the most likely successors.[104]

Nijmegen-Bethesda Assay for Anti-Factor VIII Inhibitor

The Nijmegen-Bethesda assay (NBA) confirms and quantifies anti-factor VIII inhibitors, which are typically IgG4-class immunoglobulins.[105] Using the traditional Bethesda titer, prior to the Nijmegen upgrade, 200 μL of patient PPP is incubated with 200 μL of PNP for 2 hours at 37° C. A so-called "control" consisting of 200 μL of imidazole buffer at pH 7.4 mixed with 200 μL of PNP is incubated simultaneously. During incubation, anti-factor VIII inhibitor from the patient PPP neutralizes a percentage of the PNP factor VIII activity, originally 100 units/dL. The percentage of factor VIII activity neutralized is proportional to the level of inhibitor activity. After incubation, residual factor VIII activity in the patient PPP-PNP mixture is measured using the factor VIII factor activity assay as described in the section on factor assays using the PTT.

The traditional Bethesda titer is expressed as a percentage of the control. If the patient PPP-PNP mixture retains 75% of the residual factor VIII activity of the control, presumably 75 units/dL, no factor VIII inhibitor is present. If the residual factor VIII level is 25% that of the control, 25 units/dL, the patient PPP factor VIII inhibitor level is titered using several dilutions of the patient specimen in reagent normal PPP. One Bethesda unit of activity is the amount of antibody that leaves 50% residual factor VIII activity in the mixture.

A median 40% of severe hemophilia patients are tested for inhibitors at US hemophilia centers using the Bethesda titer. Regrettably, the traditional method is characterized by a 32% false-positive rate, a 5% false-negative rate, and an interlaboratory coefficient of variation that exceeds 50%.[106] Patients must become cleared of therapeutic factor concentrate before the specimen is collected, exposing them to bleeding risk. The Bethesda titer is affected by residual patient plasma coagulation factor, dabigatran, UFH, coexistence of LAC, differences in inhibitor epitope specificity, and neutralizing versus nonneutralizing inhibitor kinetics.[107]

Refinements to the Bethesda titer were offered in 1995, whereupon the procedure was renamed the *Nijmegen-Bethesda assay* (NBA).[108] In 2012 the US Centers for Disease Control and Prevention expanded on these modifications to reduce NBA variability and improve specificity.[109] The 1995 and 2012 refinements combined are the following:

- Include an inhibitor positive control in all NBA runs.
- Heat patient plasma at 56° C for 30 minutes and centrifuge to eliminate residual factor VIII.
- Serially dilute heated patient plasma in FVIII-depleted (-deficient) plasma, not imidazole buffer, or alternatively dilute in bovine serum albumin (BSA).
- Serially dilute unheated commercial 100 Nijmegen-Bethesda unit (NBU)/dL-positive PNP in FVIII-deficient plasma or BSA.
- Incubate at 37° C for 2 hours, then perform the PTT-based FVIII assay.
- Convert residual FVIII activity to NBU per milliliter.

Few laboratories have made this full conversion; however, 70% of US laboratories use a "hybrid" NBA that substitutes imidazole buffered saline diluent, pH 7.4, for factor VIII-deficient plasma to reduce expense. For these laboratory managers, BSA may become an acceptable alternative.

Promising additional approaches are the fluorogenic and chromogenic NBA. Instead of employing the PTT, the operator adds FXa fluorogenic or chromogenic substrate with thrombin inhibitor and stopping buffer to measure FXa production as a surrogate to FVIII activity. One fluorogenic or chromogenic Bethesda unit (CBU) equals the level of inhibitor per milliliter of patient PPP that inactivates 50% of FVIII in 1 mL of PNP.[110]

Single-Factor Assays Using the PT

If the PTT and the PT are both prolonged, the TCT is normal, and there is no ready explanation for the prolonged test results, such as liver disease, vitamin K deficiency, DIC, or Coumadin therapy, the medical laboratory practitioner may suspect a congenital single-factor deficiency of the common pathway (Chapter 35). Three relatively rare factor deficiencies that give this reaction pattern and cause hemorrhage are prothrombin deficiency, factor V deficiency, and factor X deficiency. If the PT is prolonged and all other test results are normal, factor VII deficiency is suspected. The next step is the performance of a one-stage single-factor assay based on the PT. The principles and procedure described in the section on single-factor assay using the PTT system may be applied except that PT reagent replaces the PTT reagent in the test system, and the PT protocol is followed. Factor II (prothrombin)-depleted, factor V-depleted, factor VII-depleted, and factor X-depleted plasmas are available (Table 41.7).

Factor XIII Assay

Coagulation factor XIII is a transglutaminase that catalyzes covalent cross-linking bonds between the α and γ chains of fibrin polymer.[111] Cross-linking strengthens the fibrin clot and renders it resistant to proteases. This is the final event in coagulation, and it is essential for normal hemostasis and normal wound healing, but neither the PT nor the PTT is prolonged by factor XIII deficiency.

TABLE 41.7 Factor Assays Using the TCT, PT, and PTT Test Systems

Factor	System
Fibrinogen (I)	Clauss method; modified TCT
Prothrombin (II)	PT
Factor V	PT
Factor VII	PT
Factor VIII	PTT
Factor IX	PTT
Factor X	PT
Factor XI	PTT
Factor XIII	Chromogenic assay

PT, Prothrombin time; *PTT,* partial thromboplastin time; *TCT,* thrombin clotting time.

Inherited factor XIII deficiency, an autosomal recessive disorder, affects both sexes in all races. The first report of the deficiency appeared in 1960, and the frequency is estimated at 0.5 in a million. Factor XIII levels also may be low in chronic DIC secondary to Crohn disease, leukemias, ulcerative colitis, sepsis, inflammatory bowel disease, surgery, and Henoch-Schönlein purpura. In these cases the factor XIII level decreases to 50% of normal, not low enough to create symptoms, although occasionally acquired factor XIII deficiencies produce low enough levels to cause mild bleeding. Acquired factor XIII inhibitors have been described in patients treated with isoniazid, penicillin, valproate, and phenytoin.[112] These drugs may cause complete absence of factor XIII.

Factor XIII activity levels lower than 5% result in hemorrhage. In congenital factor XIII deficiency, bleeding is evident in infants, with seepage at the umbilical stump.[113] In adults bleeding is slow but progressive, accompanied by poor wound healing and slowly resolving hematomas. Recurrent spontaneous abortion and posttraumatic hemorrhage are common. Acquired factor XIII inhibitors cause severe bleeding that does not respond to therapy.

When a patient comes for treatment of bleeding and poor wound healing and the PTT, PT, platelet count, and fibrinogen level are normal, the laboratory practiter may recommend a chromogenic factor XIII assay such as the Technochrom Factor XIII (DiaPharma).[114] In this representative assay, quantitation of factor XIII activity is based on the measurement of ammonia released during an in vitro transglutaminase reaction. Plasma factor XIII is first activated by reagent thrombin. The resultant factor XIIIa then cross-links the fibrin amine substrate glycine ethyl ester to the glutamine residue of a peptide substrate, releasing ammonia. The concentration of ammonia is monitored in a glutamate dehydrogenase-catalyzed reaction that depends on NADPH, the reduced form of nicotinamide adenine dinucleotide phosphate. NADPH consumption is measured by the decrease of absorbance at 340 nm. The absorbance is inversely proportional to factor XIII activity. Several manufacturers also market immunoassays for factor XIII, which provide factor XIII concentration values but do not identify functional factor XIII abnormalities.

FIBRINOLYSIS ASSAYS

D-Dimer Immunoassay

During coagulation, fibrin polymers become cross-linked by factor XIIIa and simultaneously bind plasma plasminogen and tissue plasminogen activator (TPA) (Chapter 35). Over several hours, bound TPA activates nearby plasminogen to form plasmin. The bound plasmin cleaves fibrin and yields FDPs D, E, X, and Y and D-dimer. The FDPs are fragments of the original *fibrinogen* domains, and D-dimers are a subset of covalently linked D domains reflecting the cross-linking effects of factor XIIIa in the production of *fibrin*.[115] FDP assays, including D-dimer, are convenient for detecting active fibrinolysis, which indirectly implies thrombosis. Normally, FDPs, including D-dimer, circulate at concentrations of less than 2 ng/mL. Fibrinolysis generates FDPs and D-dimer at concentrations greater than 200 ng/mL. Increased FDP and D-dimer concentrations are characteristic of acute and chronic DIC, systemic fibrinolysis, deep vein thrombosis, and pulmonary embolism, and may predict stroke.[116,117] FDPs, including D-dimer, also are detected in plasma after thrombolytic therapy.[118]

Principle of the Quantitative D-Dimer Assay

Plasma D-dimer immunoassays abound, and several diagnostics distributors offer automated quantitative immunoassays for plasma D-dimers that generate results within 30 minutes.[119] Microlatex particles in buffered saline are coated with monoclonal anti-D-dimer antibodies. The coated particles are agglutinated by patient plasma D-dimer; the resultant turbidity is measured by turbidometric or nephelometric technology (Chapter 42). Sensitivity varies, depending on the avidity of the monoclonal anti-D-dimer antibody and the detection method; however, most methods detect concentrations as low as 10 ng/mL. D-dimer results may be reported in D-dimer units (DDU) or fibrinogen equivalent units (FEU) depending on the monoclonal antibody target. See Chapter 39 for a discussion of D-dimer results and interpretation.

Fibrin Degradation Product Immunoassay

Although the FDP assay has largely been replaced by the automated quantitative D-dimer assay, FDPs may be detected using a qualitative visible agglutination immunoassay that detects FDPs in serum and urine.[120] One such method is the Thrombo-Wellcotest (Thermo-Fisher).[121] Thrombo-Wellcotest is a slide agglutination method in which the practitioner mixes one drop of sample with one drop of latex suspension. The polystyrene latex particles in buffered saline are coated with polyclonal antibodies specific for D and E fragments (Figure 35.18) calibrated to detect FDPs at a concentration of 2 μg/mL or greater by the appearance of visible agglutination. The assay usually is performed on urine or serum collected in special tubes that promote clotting and prevent in vitro fibrinolysis. Owing to inadequate sensitivity at low concentrations, qualitative FDP assays are confined to diagnosis and monitoring of DIC.

Plasminogen Assay

Plasminogen, the inactive precursor of the trypsin-like proteolytic enzyme plasmin, is produced in the liver and circulates as a single-chain glycoprotein (Chapter 35). When bound to fibrin, plasminogen is converted to plasmin by the action of nearby TPA. Bound plasmin degrades fibrin, whereas a circulating inhibitor, α_2-antiplasmin, rapidly inactivates free plasmin. Plasmin is the central enzyme of the fibrinolytic pathway.

Excessive fibrinolysis occurs in trauma and inflammation, reflected in a radical increase in circulating plasmin that may associate with hemorrhage. Bone trauma, fractures, and surgical dissection of bone, as in cardiac surgery, also increase fibrinolysis. *Hyperfibrinolysis* may be documented using a global assay such as ROTEM or TEG, discussed later in this chapter.

Conversely, *hypofibrinolysis* occurs when TPA or plasminogen levels become depleted or when excess secretion of plasminogen activator inhibitor-1 (PAI-1) suppresses TPA activity. Congenital plasminogen deficiencies are associated with thrombosis in some families.[122] Acquired plasminogen deficiencies are seen in DIC and acute promyelocytic leukemia.[123] Further, thrombolytic therapy is ineffective when plasminogen activity is low.

Principle of the Plasminogen Chromogenic Substrate Assay

The chromogenic substrate assay mimics the natural enzymatic process whereby plasminogen is converted to active plasmin which cleaves its substrate fibrinogen. For the assay streptokinase, derived from cultures of β-hemolytic streptococci, is used as the plasminogen activator. To detect plasmin, its natural substrate fibrinogen is mirrored in the synthetic chromogenic substrate S-2251, composed of H-D-Val-Leu-Lys-pNA. Streptokinase is added to patient PPP, where it binds and activates plasminogen to form plasmin. The resulting streptokinase-plasmin complex hydrolyzes a bond in the S-2251 valine-leucine-lysine (Val-Leu-Lys) sequence. Para-nitroaniline (pNA), which is covalently bound to the carboxyl terminus of the oligopeptide substrate, is released on digestion producing a color (Figure 41.12). Color intensity is proportional to the plasminogen concentration. Results of patient specimens and controls read from a calibration curve are recorded. Several analogous chromogenic and fluorogenic substrates are suitable for plasminogen measurement.

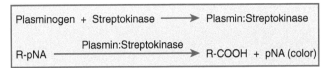

Figure 41.12 Plasminogen Assay. Plasma levels of plasminogen are quantitated using a chromogenic substrate method. Reagent streptokinase activates plasminogen to form plasmin. R-pNA designates a chromogenic substrate, where R indicates a peptide sequence specific to the enzyme being measured and pNA (para-nitroaniline) is the chromophore. In the case of plasminogen, the R represents the peptide sequence valine-leucine-lysine (Val-Leu-Lys). Plasmin recognizes the Val-Leu-Lys amide sequence as its enzymatic cleavage site, releasing the pNA, which generates a yellow color.

Clinical Significance of Plasminogen

A typical plasminogen reference interval is 5 to 13.5 mg/dL. Plasminogen levels are decreased in thrombolytic therapy, DIC, hepatitis, and cancer, or may be hereditary. Decreased plasminogen is associated with thrombosis. Plasminogen rises in systemic fibrinolysis, acute inflammation, and during pregnancy, and high levels may be associated with hemorrhage. Plasminogen assays are available from specialty reference laboratories.

Tissue Plasminogen Activator Assay

The two physiologic human plasminogen activators are TPA and urokinase.[124,125] TPA is synthesized in vascular endothelial cells and released into the circulation, where its half-life is approximately 3 minutes and its plasma concentration averages 5 ng/mL. Urokinase is produced in the kidney and vascular endothelial cells and has a half-life of approximately 7 minutes and a concentration of 2 to 4 ng/mL. Both activators are serine proteases that form ternary complexes with bound plasminogen at the surface of fibrin, activating plasminogen to form plasmin and initiating thrombus degradation. The endothelial-secreted PAI-1 covalently inactivates both.

Specimen Collection for the TPA Assay

TPA activity exhibits diurnal variation and rises upon exercise. Further, TPA is unstable in vitro because it rapidly binds PAI-1 after collection. For specimen collection, patients should be at rest, tourniquet application should be minimal, the phlebotomist should record the collection time, and immediate acidification of the specimen in acetate buffer is necessary.[126] Acidification may be accomplished using the Biopool Stabilyte acidified citrate tube (DiaPharma). Supernatant PPP may be frozen at –70° C until the assay is performed.

Principle of the TPA Assay

Plasma concentration of TPA antigen may be estimated by enzyme immunoassay. To measure TPA activity, a specified concentration of reagent plasminogen is added to the patient plasma (Chromolyse TPA Activity; Diagnostica Stago). Plasma TPA activates the plasminogen, and the resultant plasmin activity is measured using a chromogenic substrate. The resulting color intensity is proportional to TPA activity (Figure 41.13). The system may incorporate soluble fibrin to increase TPA activity.

Clinical Significance of TPA

The reference interval upper limit for TPA activity is 1.1 units/mL, and the upper limit for TPA antigen concentration is 14 ng/mL.

TPA is the primary mediator of fibrinolysis and is the model for therapeutic, synthetic TPA (Activase, alteplase; Genentech). Decreased TPA levels may correlate with increased risk of myocardial infarction, stroke, or deep vein thrombosis.[127] Impaired fibrinolysis in the form of TPA deficiency or PAI-1 excess also is associated with deep vein thrombosis and myocardial infarction.

Plasminogen Activator Inhibitor-1 Assay

PAI-1 is produced by vascular endothelial cells and hepatocytes and circulates in plasma bound to vitronectin at an average concentration of 10 ng/mL with diurnal variations.[128] An inactive form of PAI-1 is stored in high concentrations in platelets. PAI-1 inactivates free TPA by covalent binding. Elevated PAI-1 is associated with venous thrombosis and may be a cardiovascular risk factor and a marker of senescence.[129,130] A few cases of PAI-1 deficiency have been reported; however, hemorrhage apparently occurs only when homozygous or compound heterozygous *SERPINE1* mutation is detected, causing complete PAI-1 deficiency.[131] Because the reference interval of PAI-1 activity starts at zero in most laboratories, the ability to discriminate between normal and low levels by phenotype alone is limited. The incidence of complete PAI-1 deficiency is elevated in the Old Order Amish population of eastern and southern Indiana implying a pathogenic founder variant. Confirmation of total PAI-1 deficiency may be accomplished using the serum PAI-1 assay. In serum, platelet PAI-1 is expressed in excess. In true PAI-1 absence, no PAI-1 is detectable in serum.

Principle of PAI-1 Assays

Blood is collected from patients at rest into an acidified citrate tube (Stabilyte) and centrifuged immediately to make PPP; this avoids in vitro release of platelet PAI-1.[132] Several immunologic and chromogenic substrate methods are available for estimation of PAI-1 antigen and PAI-1 activity, respectively. One enzyme immunoassay for functional PAI-1 uses urokinase to bind PAI-1. The urokinase-PAI-1 complex is immobilized with solid-phase monoclonal anti-PAI-1 and is measured using monoclonal antiurokinase immunoglobulin as the detecting antibody.

Most chromogenic substrate kits for PAI-1 use an indirect measurement approach (Spectrolyse PAI-1 Activity Assay, Bio-Medica Diagnostics). Patient PPP is mixed with a measured amount of reagent TPA. Residual TPA is assayed in the plasminogen system as shown in Figure 41.14. The resulting color intensity is inversely proportional to plasma PAI-1 activity.

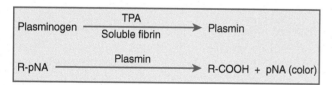

Figure 41.13 Tissue Plasminogen Activator (TPA) Assay. Plasma levels of TPA are quantitated using a chromogenic substrate method. To assay, plasma that contains TPA is added to plasminogen to produce plasmin. Plasmin activity is measured using the same chromogenic substrate as in the plasminogen assay illustrated in Fig. 41.12. The intensity of color is proportional to TPA activity. *pNA,* Para-nitroaniline; *R,* variable peptide sequence.

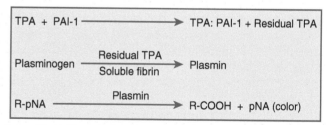

Figure 41.14 Plasminogen Activator Inhibitor-1 (PAI-1) Assay. Activity of PAI-1 is measured using a chromogenic substrate method. Plasma containing PAI-1 is added to reagent tissue plasminogen activator *(TPA)* of known concentration. The residual TPA is assayed, as shown in Figure 41.13. The intensity of color is inversely proportional to PAI-1 level. *pNA,* Para-nitroaniline; *R,* variable peptide sequence.

GLOBAL COAGULATION ASSAYS

TEG and ROTEM

Thromboelastography and its more recent modification rotational thromboelastometry have their beginning in the 1940s as one of the original assays to assess the hemostatic status of patients. The TEG 5000 and TEG 6S Thromboelastograph Hemostasis Analyzers (Haemonetics) and the ROTEM (IL-Werfen) are global *whole-blood* analyzers that measure clotting time and the dynamics of clot formation and dissolution as effected by the kinetics of thrombin generation, platelet activation, fibrin generation, clot strength, clot stability, and inhibitory effects on any aspect.[133] These manual coagulometers used mainly in liver surgery, cardiac surgery, and trauma are described in detail in Chapter 42.

Thrombin Generation Assays

Although the endpoint of clotting assays is based on thrombin generation followed by thrombin conversion of soluble fibrinogen to insoluble fibrin, the clotting time result of the PT and PTT may differ from the amount of thrombin formed. Assay systems that assess thrombin generation, such as the Calibrated Automated Thrombogram (CAT, Diagnostica Stago) and the Technothrombin TGA (DiaPharma), have been developed and are under investigation for their clinical utility. These systems measure the phased kinetics of thrombin generation from initiation and peak generation through downregulation and inactivation. Thrombin generation assays may help to better categorize the physiologic mechanisms of hemostasis and to better assess bleeding risk, thrombotic risk, and their modification by hemostatic or antithrombotic agents.

GENETIC TESTING FOR HEMOSTATIC DISORDERS

High-throughput genetic sequencing (HTS) has, since 2007, become the reference approach to identifying the genetic variants that underlie platelet-related and coagulopathy-related bleeding disorders, having replaced the pioneering but less precise Sanger sequencing. Table 41.8 illustrates the genetic variants whose presence has been definitively identified with the listed coagulation disorders. Table 37.1 and Table 38.1 list the identified genetic variants associated with platelet disorders. HTS is being developed as a clinical assay and may include whole-genome sequencing, whole-exome sequencing, or gene-targeted methods. Sequencing costs continually decline, and it is likely that whole-genome HTS will become the clinical

TABLE 41.8 Clinically Detectable Genetic Variants That Have Been Associated with Coagulopathies

Variant	Coagulopathy	MOI
F2	Prothrombin deficiency	AR
F5	Factor V deficiency	AR
F7	Factor VII deficiency	AR
F8	Hemophilia A	XR
F9	Hemophilia B	XR
F10	Factor X deficiency	AR
F11	Factor XI deficiency	AR
F13A1. F13B	Factor XIII deficiency	AR
FG4, FGB, FGG	Fibrinogen deficiency	AD, AR, AR
LMAN1, MCFD2	Combined V and VIII deficiency	AR, AR
KLKB1	Prekallikrein (Fletcher factor) deficiency	AR
KNG1	Kininogen (Fitzgerald factor) deficiency	AR
VWF	Von Willebrand disease	AD
PLG	Plasminogen deficiency	AR
SERPINE1	Plasminogen activator inhibitor 1 deficiency	AR
GGCX	Multiple coagulation factor deficiency type 1	AR
VKORC1	Multiple coagulation factor deficiency type 2	AR

AD, Autosomal dominant; *AR*, autosomal recessive; *XR*, X-linked recessive; *MOI*, mode of inheritance.

standard, gradually replacing inherently imprecise phenotypic assays, such as the time-honored platelet function testing, quantitative platelet activation immunoassays, and clot-based coagulation factor assays.

Besides the currently known hemostatic variants, HTS's extreme precision enables the detection of many additional variants whose provenance requires statistical comparison with the current phenotypic methodology and clinical outcomes for disorders currently unnamed or identified by trivial nomenclature. This effort has produced phenotypic ontologies (formal naming systems) more precise than the *International Classification of Diseases, Tenth Revision* (ICD-10) such as the Human Phenotypic Ontology, leading to further platelet and coagulopathy disorder associations and to consolidation of terminology.[134]

SUMMARY

- Proper specimen collection, transport, storage, and centrifugation ensure a valid hemostasis test result.
- Specimens that are short draws, clotted, or hemolyzed are rejected.
- Platelet function testing, including aggregometry, helps determine the cause of nonthrombocytopenic mucocutaneous bleeding.

- Von Willebrand disease (VWD) is diagnosed and monitored through the judicious selection and performance of plasma and platelet function-based laboratory tests.
- Plasma platelet factor 4 (PF4) and urinary 11-dehydrothromboxane B_2 are used to assess platelet activation.
- Clot-based routine coagulation tests include the prothrombin time (PT), partial thromboplastin time (PTT), and thrombin clotting time (TCT).

- Mixing studies are employed in acute care facilities to differentiate factor deficiencies, lupus anticoagulants (LACs), and specific factor inhibitors.
- Clot-based coagulation factor assays detect and measure coagulation factor deficiencies.
- Nijmegen-Bethesda assays detect and measure coagulation factor inhibitors.
- Tests of fibrinolysis include assays for fibrin degradation products (FDPs), D-dimer, plasminogen, tissue plasminogen activator (TPA), and plasminogen activator inhibitor-1 (PAI-1).
- Thromboelastography and thromboelastometry are global whole blood hemostasis methods that assess the spectrum of hemostatic components required for thrombus formation and fibrinolysis.
- Thrombin generation assays may become common in future hemostasis laboratory testing.
- High-throughput genomic sequencing is beginning to replace less precise phenotypic methods to identify platelet function disorders and coagulopathies.

Now that you have completed this chapter, go back and read again the case study at the beginning and respond to the questions presented.

REVIEW QUESTIONS

Answers can be found in the Appendix.

1. What happens if a coagulation specimen collection tube is underfilled?
   a. The specimen clots and is useless
   b. The specimen is hemolyzed and is useless
   c. Clot-based test results are falsely prolonged
   d. Chromogenic test results are falsely decreased

2. If you collect blood into a series of tubes, when in the sequence should the hemostasis (blue stopper) tube be filled?
   a. After a lavender-topped or green-topped tube
   b. First, or after a nonadditive tube
   c. After a serum separator tube
   d. Last

3. What is the effect of hemolysis on a hemostasis specimen?
   a. In vitro platelet and coagulation activation
   b. The specimen is icteric or lipemic
   c. Hemolysis has no effect
   d. The specimen is clotted

4. Except for platelet aggregometry, most coagulation testing must be performed on PPP, which is plasma with a platelet count less than:
   a. 1000/μL
   b. 10,000/μL
   c. 100,000/μL
   d. 1,000,000/μL

5. You wish to obtain a 5-mL specimen of whole-blood/anticoagulant mixture. The patient's hematocrit is 65%. What volume of anticoagulant should you use?
   a. 0.32 mL
   b. 0.5 mL
   c. 0.64 mL
   d. 0.68 mL

6. You perform whole-blood lumiaggregometry on a specimen from a patient who complains of easy bruising. Aggregation and secretion are diminished when the agonists thrombin, ADP, arachidonic acid, and collagen are used. What is the most likely platelet abnormality?
   a. Storage pool disorder
   b. Aspirin-like syndrome
   c. ADP receptor anomaly
   d. Glanzmann thrombasthenia

7. What is the reference assay for HIT?
   a. Enzyme immunoassay
   b. Serotonin release assay
   c. Platelet lumiaggregometry
   d. Washed platelet aggregation

8. What agonist is used in platelet aggregometry to detect VWD?
   a. Arachidonic acid
   b. Ristocetin
   c. Collagen
   d. ADP

9. Deficiency of which congenital single factor is likely when the PT result is prolonged and the PTT result is normal?
   a. Factor V
   b. Factor VII
   c. Factor VIII
   d. Prothrombin

10. A prolonged PT, a low factor VII level, but a normal factor V level are characteristic of an acquired coagulopathy associated with which of the following?
    a. Vitamin K deficiency
    b. Thrombocytopenia
    c. Liver disease
    d. Hemophilia

11. The patient has deep vein thrombosis. The PTT is prolonged and is not corrected in an immediate mix of patient PPP with an equal part of PNP. What is the presumed condition?
    a. Factor VIII inhibitor
    b. Lupus anticoagulant
    c. Factor VIII deficiency
    d. Factor V Leiden mutation

12. What condition causes the most pronounced elevation in the result of the quantitative D-dimer assay?
    a. Deep vein thrombosis
    b. Fibrinogen deficiency
    c. Paraproteinemia
    d. DIC

13. What is the name given to the type of assay that uses a synthetic polypeptide substrate that releases a chromophore on digestion by its serine protease?
    a. Clot-based assay
    b. Molecular diagnostic assay
    c. Fluorescence immunoassay
    d. Chromogenic substrate assay

14. What component of the fibrinolytic process binds and neutralizes free plasmin?
    a. TPA
    b. PAI-1
    c. Urokinase
    d. α_2-antiplasmin

15. What type of high-throughput genomic sequencing is likely to become a standard clinical assay?
    a. Human genotypic ontogeny
    b. Whole-genome sequencing
    c. Whole-exome sequencing
    d. Gene-targeted sequencing

REFERENCES

1. Clinical and Laboratory Standards Institute. (2008). *Collection, Transport, and Processing of Blood Specimens for Testing Plasma-Based Coagulation Assays: Approved Guideline.* (5th ed.). CLSI Document H21-A5, Wayne, PA: Clinical and Laboratory Standards Institute.

2. Magnette, A., Chatelain, M., Chatelain, B., et al. (2016). Pre-analytical issues in the haemostasis laboratory: guidance for the clinical laboratories. *Thrombosis Journal, 14,* 49–63.

3. Rodeghiero, F., Tosetto, A., Abshire, T., et al. (2010). Perinatal/pediatric hemostasis subcommittees working group, ISTH SSC. Bleeding assessment tool, a standardized questionnaire and a new bleeding score for inherited bleeding disorders. *J Thromb Haemost, 8,* 2063–2065.

4. Guder, W. G., & Narayanan, S. (2015). *Pre-examination Procedures in Laboratory Diagnostics: Preanalytical Aspects and Their Impact on the Quality of Medical Laboratory Results.* Berlin, Germany: DeGruyter.

5. Bennett, A., Fritsma, G. A., & Ernst, D. J. (2016). *Quick Guide to Blood Collection.* (2nd ed.). Washington, DC: AACC Press.

6. Tosetto, A., Castaman, G., & Rodeghiero, F. (2013). Bleeders, bleeding rates, and bleeding score. *J Thromb Haemost, 11* (Suppl 1), 142–150.

7. Lippi, G., Becan-McBride, F., Behulova, D., et al. (2012). Preanalytical quality improvement; in quality we trust. *Clin Chem Lab Med, 51,* 229–241.

8. Ernst, D. J. (2017). *Procedures for the Collection of Diagnostic Blood Specimens by Venipuncture: Approved Standard.* (7th ed.). CLSI Document GP41, Wayne, PA: Clinical and Laboratory Standards Institute.

9. Dubrovny, N. (2010). *Tubes and Additives for Venous Blood Specimen Collection: Approved Standard.* (6th ed.). CLSI Document. GP39, Wayne, PA: Clinical and Laboratory Standards Institute.

10. Adcock-Funk, D. M., Lippi, G., & Favaloro, E. J. (2012). Quality standards for sample processing, transportation, and storage in hemostasis testing. *Semin Thromb Hemost, 38,* 576–585.

11. van den Besselaar, A. M., Meeuwisse-Braun, J., Schaefer-van Mansfeld, H., et al. (1997). Influence of plasma volumetric errors on the prothrombin time ratio and international sensitivity index. *Blood Coagul Fibrinolysis, 8,* 431–435.

12. Horsti, J. (2001). Use of EDTA samples for prothrombin time measurement in patients receiving oral anticoagulants. *Haematologica, 86,* 851–855.

13. McCall, R., & Tankersley, C. (2012). *Phlebotomy Essentials.* (5th ed.). Philadelphia: Lippincott Williams & Wilkins.

14. McGlasson, D. L., More, L., Best, H. A., et al. (1999). Drawing specimens for coagulation testing: is a second tube necessary? *Clin Lab Sci, 12,* 137–139.

15. Lippi, G., Salvagno, G. L., Montagnara, M., et al. (2012). Quality standards for sample collection in coagulation testing. *Semin Thromb Hemost, 38,* 565–575.

16. Ernst, D. J. (2008). *Blood Specimen Collection FAQs.* Ramsey, IN: Center for Phlebotomy Education.

17. Marques, M., & Fritsma, G. A. (2015). *Quick Guide to Coagulation Testing.* (3rd ed.). Washington, DC: AACC Press.

18. Lima-Oliveira, G., Lippi, G., Salvango, G. L., et al. (2013). The effective reduction of tourniquet application time after minor modification of the CLSI H03-A6 blood collection procedure. *Biochem Med (Zagreb), 23,* 308–315.

19. Ernst, C., & Ernst, D. J. (2001). *Phlebotomy for Nurses and Nursing Personnel.* Ramsey, IN: Center for Phlebotomy Education.

20. Marcus, N. (2010). Coagulation testing in the context of the automated hospital lab and optimizing for the effects of common interferences. *Clin Chem, 56*(Suppl.), Abstract A172.

21. Sunderji, R., Gin, K., Shalansky, K., et al. (2005). Clinical impact of point-of-care vs. laboratory measurement of anticoagulation. *Am J Clin Pathol, 123,* 184–188.

22. McGlasson, D. L., Paul, J., & Shaffer, K. M. (1993). Whole blood coagulation testing in neonates. *Clin Lab Sci, 6,* 76–77.

23. Clinical and Laboratory Standards Institute. (2008). *Procedures and Devices for the Collection of Diagnostic Capillary Blood Specimens. Approved Standard.* CLSI Document GP42, Wayne, PA: Clinical and Laboratory Standards Institute.

24. McGraw, A., Hillarp, A., & Echenegucia, M. (2010). Considerations in the laboratory assessment of haemostasis. *Haemophilia, 16*(Suppl 5), 74–78.

25. Ens, G. E., & Newlin, F. (1995). Spurious protein S deficiency as a result of elevated factor VII levels. *Clin Hemost Rev, 9,* 18.

26. National Heart, Lung, and Blood Institute. (2007). *The Diagnosis, Evaluation, and Management of Von Willebrand Disease.* NIH Publication No. 08-5832, Bethesda, MD: US Department of Health and Human Services, National Institutes of Health.

27. Toulon, P., Metge, S., & Hangard, M. (2017). Impact of different storage times at room temperature of unspun citrated blood samples on routine coagulation tests results. Results of a bicenter study and review of the literature. *Int J Lab Hem, 39,* 1–11.

28. Polack, B., Schved, J. F., & Boneu, B. (2001). Preanalytical recommendations of the 'Groupe d'Etude sur l'Hémostase et la Thrombose' (GEHT) for venous blood testing in hemostasis laboratories. *Haemostasis, 31,* 61–68.

29. Foshat, M., Bates, S., Russo, W., et al. (2015). Effect of freezing plasma at −20° C for 2 weeks on prothrombin time, activated partial thromboplastin time, dilute Russell viper venom time, activated protein C resistance, and D-dimer levels. *Clin Appl Thromb Hemost, 21,* 41–47.

30. Gosselin, R. C., Honeychurch, K., Kang, H. J., et al. (2015), Effects of storage and thawing conditions on coagulation testing. *Int J Lab Hem, 37,* 551–559.

31. Rimac, V., & Herak, D. C. (2017). Is it acceptable to use coagulation plasma samples stored at room temperature and 4° C for 24 hours for additional prothrombin time, activated partial thromboplastin time, fibrinogen, antithrombin, and D-dimer testing? *Int J Lab Hem, 39,* 1–7.

32. Dyszkiewicz-Korpanty, A. M., Frenkel, E. P., & Sarode, R. (2005). Approach to the assessment of platelet function: comparison between optical-based platelet-rich plasma and impedance-based whole blood platelet aggregation methods. *Clin Appl Thromb Hemost, 11,* 25–35.

33. Pierangeli, S. S., & Harris, E. N. (2005). Clinical laboratory testing for the antiphospholipid syndrome. *Clin Chim Acta, 357,* 17–33.

34. Lippi, G., Plebani, M., & Favaloro, E. J. (2013). Interference in coagulation testing: focus on spurious hemolysis, icterus, and lipemia. *Semin Thromb Hemost, 39,* 258–266.

35. Matthews, D. C. (2013). Inherited disorders of platelet function. *Pediatr Clin North Am, 60,* 1475–1478.

36. Duke, W. W. (1912). The pathogenesis of purpura haemorrhagica with especial reference to the part played by the blood platelets. *Arch Intern Med, 10,* 445.

37. Ivy, A. C., Nelson, D., & Bucher, G. (1941). The standardization of certain factors in the cutaneous "venostasis" bleeding time technique. *J Lab Clin Med, 26,* 1812.

38. Kumar, R., Ansell, J. E., Canoso, R. T., et al. (1978). Clinical trial of a new bleeding device. *Am J Clin Pathol, 70,* 642–645.

39. Mielke, C. H., Jr., Kaneshiro, M. M., Maher, I. A., et al. (1969). The standardized normal Ivy bleeding time and its prolongation by aspirin. *Blood, 34,* 204–215.

40. Lind, S. E. (1991). The bleeding time does not predict surgical bleeding. *Blood, 77,* 2547–2552.

41. Finazzi, G., Budde, U., & Michiels, J. J. (1996). Bleeding time and platelet function in essential thrombocythemia and other myeloproliferative syndromes. *Leuk Lymphoma, 22*(Suppl 1), 71–78.

42. Cattaneo, M. (2009). Light transmission aggregometry and ATP release for the diagnostic assessment of platelet function. *Semin Thromb Hemost, 35,* 158–167.

43. McGlasson, D. L., & Fritsma, G. A. (2009). Whole blood platelet aggregometry and platelet function testing. *Semin Thromb Hemost, 35,* 168–180.

44. Fritsma, G. A. (2007). Platelet function testing: aggregometry and lumiaggregometry. *Clin Lab Sci, 20,* 32–37.

45. Vucenik, I., & Podczasy, J. J. (1998). Whole blood lumi-aggregation: evaluation of reagents. *Clin Appl Thromb Hemost, 4,* 253–256.

46. White, M. M., Foust, J. T., Mauer, A. M., et al. (1992). Assessment of lumiaggregometry for research and clinical laboratories. *Thromb Haemost, 67,* 572–577.

47. Goldenberg, S. J., Veriabo, N. J., & Soslau, G. (2001). A micromethod to measure platelet aggregation and ATP release by impedance. *Thromb Res, 103,* 57–61.

48. Podczasy, J. J., Lee, J., & Vucenik, I. (1997). Evaluation of whole blood lumi-aggregation. *Clin Appl Thromb Hemost, 3,* 190–195.

49. Ren, Q., Ye, S., & Whiteheart, S. W. (2008). The platelet release reaction: just when you thought platelet secretion was simple. *Curr Opin Hematol, 15,* 537–541.

50. Sharma, R. K., Reddy, H. K., Singh, V. N., et al. (2009). Aspirin and clopidogrel hyporesponsiveness and nonresponsiveness in patients with coronary artery stenting. *Vasc Health Risk Manag, 5,* 965–972.

51. Legrand, D., Barbato, E., Chenu, P., et al. (2015). The STIB score: a simple clinical test to predict clopidogrel resistance. *Acta Cardiol, 70,* 516–521.

52. Guirgis, M., Thompson, P., & Jansen, S. (2017). Review of aspirin and clopidogrel resistance in peripheral arterial disease. *J Vasc Surg, 66,* 1576–1586.

53. Raichand, S., Moore, D., Riley, R. D., et al. (2013). Protocol for a systematic review of the diagnostic and prognostic utility of tests currently available for the detection of aspirin resistance in patients with established cardiovascular or cerebrovascular disease. *Syst Rev, 26,* 2–16.

54. Nagler, M., & Cuker, A. (2017). Profile of Instrumentation Laboratory's HemosIL® AcuStar HIT-Ab(PF4-H) assay for diagnosis of heparin-induced thrombocytopenia. *Expert Rev Mol Diagn, 17,* 419–426.

55. Nazi, I., Arnold, D. M., Moore, J. C., et al. (2015). Pitfalls in the diagnosis of heparin-induced thrombocytopenia: a 6-year experience from a reference laboratory. *Am J Hematol, 90,* 629–633.

56. Warkentin, T. (2013). Heparin-induced thrombocytopenia. In Kitchens, C. S., Kessler, C. M., & Konkle, B. A. (Eds.), *Consultative Hemostasis and Thrombosis.* (3rd ed., pp. 442–476). Elsevier, St. Louis.

57. Warkentin, T. E., Pai, M., Sheppard, J. I., et al. (2011). Fondaparinux treatment of acute heparin-induced thrombocytopenia confirmed by the serotonin-release assay: a 30-month, 16-patient case series. *J Thromb Hemost, 9,* 2389–2396.

58. Warkentin, T. E., Arnold, D. M., Nazi, I., et al. (2015). The platelet serotonin-release assay. *Am J Hematol, 90,* 564–572.

59. Morel-Kopp, M. C., Aboud, M., Tan, C. W., et al. (2010). Whole blood impedance aggregometry detects heparin-induced thrombocytopenia antibodies. *Thromb Res, 125,* e234–e239.

60. Ferroni, P., Riondino, S., Vazzana, N., et al. (2012). Biomarkers of platelet activation in acute coronary syndromes. *Thromb Haemost, 108,* 1109–1123.

61. Kubota, Y., Alonso, A., & Folsom. A. R. (2017). β-thromboglobulin and incident cardiovascular disease risk: the Atherosclerosis Risk in Communities study. *Thromb Res, 155,* 116–120.

62. Rand, M. L., Leung, R., & Packham, M. A. (2003). Platelet function assays. *Transfus Apher Sci, 28,* 307–317.

63. Fritsma, G. A., Ens, G. E., Alvord, M. A., et al. (2001). Monitoring the antiplatelet action of aspirin. *JAAPA, 14,* 57–62.

64. Eikelboom, J. W., & Hankey, G. J. (2004). Failure of aspirin to prevent atherothrombosis: potential mechanisms and implications for clinical practice. *Am J Cardiovasc Drugs, 4,* 57–67.

65. Eikelboom, J. W., Hankey, G. J., Thom, J., et al. (2008). Incomplete inhibition of thromboxane biosynthesis by acetylsalicylic acid: determinants and effect on cardiovascular risk. *Circulation, 118,* 1705–1712.

66. Tran, H. A., Anand, S. S., Hankey, G. J., et al. (2007). Aspirin resistance. *Thromb Res, 120,* 337–346.

67. Lee, R. I., & White, P. D. (1913). A clinical study of the coagulation time of blood. *Am J Med Sci, 243,* 279–285.

68. Clinical and Laboratory Standards Institute. (2008). *One-Stage Prothrombin Time (PT) Test and Activated Partial Thromboplastin Time (APTT) Test; Approved Guideline*. (2nd ed.). CLSI Document H47-A2, Wayne, PA: Clinical and Laboratory Standards Institute.

69. Mannucci, P. M., & Tripodi, A. (2012). Hemostatic defects in liver and renal dysfunction. *Am Soc Hematol Educ Program, 2012*, 168–173.

70. Poller, L. (1986). Laboratory control of anticoagulant therapy. *Semin Thromb Hemost, 12*, 13–19.

71. Capoor, M. N., Stonemetz, J. L., Baird, J. C., et al. (2015). Prothrombin time and activated partial thromboplastin time testing: a comparative effectiveness study in a million-patient sample. *PLoS ONE, 10*(8), e0133317. doi:10.1371/journal.

72. McKinly, L., & Wrenn, K. (1993). Are baseline prothrombin time/partial thromboplastin time values necessary before instituting anticoagulation? *Ann Emerg Med, 22*, 697–702.

73. Baumann Kreuziger, L. M., Datta, Y. H., Johnson, A. D., et al. (2014). Monitoring anticoagulation in patients with an unreliable prothrombin time/international normalized ratio: factor II versus chromogenic factor X testing. *Blood Coagul Fibrinolysis, 25*, 232–236.

74. Rosborough, T. K., Jacobsen, J. M., & Shepherd, M. F. (2009). Relationship between chromogenic factor X and international normalized ratio differs during early warfarin initiation compared with chronic warfarin administration. *Blood Coagul Fibrinolysis, 20*, 433–435.

75. McGlasson, D. L., Romick, B. G., & Rubal, B. J. (2008). Comparison of a chromogenic factor X assay with international normalized ratio for monitoring oral anticoagulation therapy. *Blood Coagul Fibrinolysis, 19*, 513–517.

76. Marlar, R. A., Clement, B., & Gausman, J. (2017). Activated partial thromboplastin time monitoring of unfractionated heparin therapy: issues and recommendations. *Semin Thromb Hemost, 43*, 253–260.

77. Tripodi, A., Lippi, G., & Plebani, M. (2016). How to report results of prothrombin and activated partial thromboplastin times. *Clin Chem Lab Med, 54*, 215–222.

78. Lawrie, A. S., Kitchen, S., Efthymiou, M., et al. (2013). Determination of APTT factor sensitivity—the misguiding guideline. *Int J Lab Hematol, 35*, 652–657.

79. Alsulaiman, D., Sylvester, K., Stevens, C., et al. (2016). Comparison of time to therapeutic aPTT in patients who received continuous unfractionated heparin after implementation of pharmacy-wide intervention alerts. *Hosp Pharm, 51*, 656–661.

80. Marlar, R. A., & Gausman, J. (2013). The optimum number and types of plasma samples necessary for an accurate activated partial thromboplastin time-based heparin therapeutic range. *Arch Pathol Lab Med, 137*, 77–82.

81. Hayward, C. P., Moffat, K. A., & Liu, Y. (2012). Laboratory investigations for bleeding disorders. *Semin Thromb Hemost, 38*, 742–752.

82. Moore, G. W. (2014). Commonalities and contrasts in recent guidelines for lupus anticoagulant detection. *Int J Lab Hematol, 36*, 364–373.

83. Medina, G., Briones-García, E., Cruz-Domínguez, M. P., et al. (2017). Antiphospholipid antibodies disappearance in primary antiphospholipid syndrome: thrombosis recurrence. *Autoimmun Rev, 16*:352–354.

84. Kershaw, G. K., & Orellana, D. (2013). Mixing tests: diagnostic aides in the investigation of prolonged prothrombin times and activated partial thromboplastin times. *Semin Thromb Hemost, 39*, 283–290.

85. Ledford-Kraemer, M. R. (2008). Laboratory testing for lupus anticoagulants: pre-examination variables, mixing studies, and diagnostic criteria. *Semin Thromb Hemost, 34*, 380–388.

86. Pengo, V., Tripodi, A., & Reber, G. (2009). Update of the guidelines for lupus anticoagulant detection. Subcommittee on Lupus Anticoagulant/Antiphospholipid Antibody of the Scientific and Standardisation Committee of the International Society on Thrombosis and Haemostasis. *J Thromb Haemost, 7*, 1737–1740.

87. Ignjatovic, V. (2013). Thrombin clotting time. *Methods Mol Biol, 992*, 131–138.

88. Winkler, A. M., & Tormey, C. A. (2013). Education Committee of the Academy of Clinical Laboratory Physicians and Scientists. Pathology consultation on monitoring direct thrombin inhibitors and overcoming their effects in bleeding patients. *Am J Clin Pathol, 40*, 610–662.

89. Karapetian, H. (2013). Reptilase time (RT). *Methods Mol Biol, 992*, 273–277.

90. Clinical and Laboratory Standards Institute. (2001). *Procedure for the Determination of Fibrinogen in Plasma: Approved Guideline*. (2nd ed.). CLSI Document H30-A2, Wayne, PA: Clinical and Laboratory Standards Institute.

91. Stang, L. J., & Mitchell, L. G. (2013). Fibrinogen. *Methods Mol Biol, 992*, 181–192.

92. van den Besselaar, A. M., Haas, F. J., van der Graaf, F., et al. (2009). Harmonization of fibrinogen assay results: study within the framework of the Dutch project 'Calibration 2000'. *Int J Lab Hematol, 31*, 513–520.

93. Lew, W. K., & Weaver, F. A. (2008). Clinical use of topical thrombin as a surgical hemostat. *Biologics, 2*, 593–599.

94. Miesbach, W., Schenk, J., Alesci, S., et al. (2010). Comparison of the fibrinogen Clauss assay and the fibrinogen PT derived method in patients with dysfibrinogenemia. *Thromb Res, 126*, e428–e433.

95. Kershaw, G. K., & Orellana, D. (2013). Mixing tests: diagnostic aides in the investigation of prolonged prothrombin times and activated partial thromboplastin times. *Semin Thromb Hemost, 39*, 283–290.

96. James, P., Salomon, O., Mikovic, D., et al. (2014). Rare bleeding disorders—bleeding assessment tools, laboratory aspects and phenotype and therapy of FXI deficiency. *Haemophilia, 20*(Suppl. 4), 71–75.

97. Takeyama, M., Nogami, K., Okuda, M., et al. (2008). Selective factor VIII and V inactivation by iminodiacetate ion exchange resin through metal ion adsorption. *Br J Haematol, 142*, 962–970.

98. Fritsma G. A. (2002). Factor assays—intrinsic pathway. In Adcock, D. M., Jensen, R., Johns C. S., et al. (Eds.), *Esoterix Coagulation Handbook*, Denver, CO: Colorado Coagulation Consultants.

99. Lattes, S., Appert-Flory, A., Fischer, F., et al. (2011). Measurement of factor VIII activity using one-stage clotting assay: a calibration curve has not to be systematically included in each run. *Haemophilia, 17*, 139–142.

100. Castellone, D. D., & Adcock, D. M. (2017). Factor VIII activity and inhibitor assays in the diagnosis and treatment of hemophilia A. *Semin Thromb Hemost, 43*, 320–330.

101. Yap, E. S., Timp, J. F., Flinterman, L. E., et al. (2015). Elevated levels of factor VIII and subsequent risk of all-cause mortality: results from the MEGA follow-up study. *J Thromb Haemost, 13*, 1833–1842.

102. Lattes, S., Appert-Flory, A., Fischer, F., et al. (2011). Measurement of factor VIII activity using one-stage clotting assay: a calibration curve has not to be systematically included in each run. *Haemophilia, 17*, 139–142.

103. Favaloro, E. J., & Lippi, G. (2017). Emerging treatments for hemophilia: patients and their treaters spoilt for choice, but laboratories face a difficult path? *Ann Transl Med, 5,* 101–103.

104. Favaloro, E. J., Meijer, P., Jennings, I., et al. (2013). Problems and solutions in laboratory testing for hemophilia. *Semin Thromb Hemost, 39,* 816–833.

105. Kershaw, G., Jayakodi, D., & Dunkley, S. (2009). Laboratory identification of factor inhibitors: the perspective of a large tertiary hemophilia center. *Semin Thromb Hemost, 35,* 760–768.

106. Soucie, J. M., Miller, C. H., Kelly, F. M., et al. (2014). National surveillance for hemophilia inhibitors in the United States: summary report of an expert meeting. *Am J Hematol, 89,* 621–625.

107. Favaloro, E. J., Verbruggen, B., & Miller, C. H. (2014). Laboratory testing for factor inhibitors. *Haemophilia, 20*(Suppl 4), 94–98.

108. Verbruggen, B., Novakova, I., Wessels, H., et al. (1995). The Nijmegen modification of the Bethesda assay for factor VIII:C inhibitors: improved specificity and reliability. *Thromb Haemost, 73,* 247–251.

109. Miller, C. J., Platt, S. J., Rice, A. S., et al. (2012). Validation of Nijmegen-Bethesda assay modifications to allow inhibitor measurement during replacement therapy and facilitate inhibitor surveillance. *J Thromb Haemost, 10,* 1055–1061.

110. Miller, C. H., Rice, A. S., Boylan, B., et al. (2013). Hemophilia Inhibitor Research Study Investigators. Comparison of clot-based, chromogenic and fluorescence assays for measurement of factor VIII inhibitors in the US Hemophilia Inhibitor Research Study. *J Thromb Haemost, 11,* 1300–1309.

111. Duval, C., Philippou, H., & Ariens, R. A. S. (2013). Factor XIII. In Marder, V. J., Aird, W. C., Bennett, J. S., et al. (Eds.), *Hemostasis and Thrombosis: Basic Principles and Clinical Practice.* (6th ed., pp. 272–285). Philadelphia: Lippincott Williams & Wilkins.

112. Krumdieck, R., Shaw, D. R., Huang, S. T., et al. (1991). Hemorrhagic disorder due to an isoniazid-associated acquired factor XIII inhibitor in a patient with Waldenström's macroglobulinemia. *Am J Med, 90,* 639–645.

113. Karimi, M., Bereczky, Z., Cohan, N., et al. (2009). Factor XIII deficiency. *Semin Thromb Hemost, 35,* 426–438.

114. Schroeder, V., & Kohler, H. P. (2013). Factor XIII deficiency: an update. *Semin Thromb Hemost, 39,* 632–641.

115. Linkins, L. A., & Takach Lapner, S. (2017). Review of D-dimer testing: good, bad, and ugly. *Int J Lab Hematol, 39*(Suppl 1), 98–103.

116. Wannamethee, S. G., Whincup, P. H., Lennon, L., et al. (2012). Fibrin D-dimer, tissue-type plasminogen activator, von Willebrand factor, and risk of incident stroke in older men. *Stroke, 43,* 1206–1211.

117. Southern, D. K. (1992). Serum FDP and plasma D-dimer testing: what are they measuring? *Clin Lab Sci, 5,* 332–333.

118. Lawler, C. M., Bovill, E. G., Stump, D. C., et al. (1990). Fibrin fragment D-dimer and fibrinogen B beta peptides in plasma as markers of clot lysis during thrombolytic therapy in acute myocardial infarction. *Blood, 76,* 1341–1348.

119. Pernod, G., Wu, H., de Maistre, E., et al. (2017). Validation of STA-Liatest D-Di assay for exclusion of pulmonary embolism according to the latest Clinical and Laboratory Standard Institute/Food and Drug Administration guideline. Results of a multicenter management study. *Blood Coagul Fibrinolysis, 28,* 254–260.

120. Drewinko, B., Surgeon, J., Cobb, P., et al. (1985). Comparative sensitivity of different methods to detect and quantify circulating fibrinogen/fibrin split products. *Am J Clin Pathol, 84,* 58–66.

121. Garvey, M. B., & Black, J. M. (1972). The detection of fibrinogen-fibrin degradation products by means of a new antibody-coated latex particle. *J Clin Pathol, 25,* 680–682.

122. Schuster, V., Hügle, B., & Tefs, K. (2007). Plasminogen deficiency. *J Thromb Haemost, 5,* 2315–2322.

123. Mehta, R., & Shapiro, A. D. (2008). Plasminogen deficiency. *Haemophilia, 14,* 1261–1268.

124. Mutch, N. J., & Booth, N. A. (2013). Plasminogen activation and regulation of fibrinolysis. In Marder, V. J., Aird, W. C., Bennett, J. S., et al. (Eds.), *Hemostasis and Thrombosis: Basic Principles and Clinical Practice.* (6th ed., pp. 314–333). Philadelphia: Lippincott Williams & Wilkins.

125. Gebbink, M. F. (2011). Tissue-type plasminogen activator-mediated plasminogen activation and contact activation, implications in and beyond haemostasis. *J Thromb Haemost, 9* (Suppl. 1), 174–181.

126. Chandler, W. L., Schmer, G., & Stratton, J. R. (1989). Optimum conditions for the stabilization and measurement of tissue plasminogen activator activity in human plasma. *J Lab Clin Med, 113,* 362–371.

127. Prabhudesai, A., Shetty, S., Ghosh, K., et al. (2017). Dysfunctional fibrinolysis and cerebral venous thrombosis. *Blood Cells Mol Dis, 65,* 51–55.

128. Oishi, K. (2009). Plasminogen activator inhibitor-1 and the circadian clock in metabolic disorders. *Clin Exp Hypertens, 31,* 208–219.

129. D'Elia, J. A., Bayliss, G., Gleason, R. E., et al. (2016). Cardiovascular-renal complications and the possible role of plasminogen activator inhibitor: a review. *Clin Kidney J, 9,* 705–712.

130. Vaughan, D. E., Rai, R., Khan, S. S., et al. (2017). Plasminogen activator inhibitor-1 is a marker and a mediator of senescence. *Arterioscler Thromb Vasc Biol, 37,* 1446–1452.

131. Heiman, M., Gupta, S., Khan, S. S., et al. (2017). Complete plasminogen activator inhibitor 1 deficiency. In Pagon, R. A., Adam, M. P., Ardinger, H. H., et al. (Eds.), *GeneReviews®* [Internet]. Seattle, WA: University of Washington, Seattle; 1993–2017.

132. Macy, E. M., Meilahn, E. N., Declerck, P. J., et al. (1993). Sample preparation for plasma measurement of plasminogen activator inhibitor-1 antigen in large population studies. *Arch Pathol Lab Med, 117,* 67–70.

133. Whiting, D., & DiNardo, J. A. (2014). TEG and ROTEM: technology and clinical applications. *Am J Hematol, 89,* 228–232.

134. Freson, K., & Turrot, E. (2017). High-throughput sequencing approaches for diagnosing hereditary bleeding and platelet disorders. *J Thromb Haemost, 15,* 1262–1272.

Hemostasis and Coagulation Instrumentation

Debra A. Hoppensteadt, Jo Ann Molnar

OBJECTIVES

After completion of this chapter, the reader will be able to:

1. Describe methodologies in the hemostasis laboratory that were previously considered as specialized but are now routinely available on clinical analyzers.
2. Identify assay endpoints for various coagulation analyzers.
3. Identify the methods of end-point detection used in coagulation analyzers.
4. List common coagulation instrument flags that alert operators to specimen and instrument problems.
5. Describe the advantages and disadvantages of each method of clot detection.
6. Describe the differences between manual, semiautomated, and automated coagulation analyzers.
7. Identify characteristics that should be evaluated when selecting the appropriate coagulation analyzer for an individual laboratory setting.
8. Define the similarities and differences between TEG and ROTEM.
9. Describe the different assays available for point-of-care coagulation testing.
10. Know the advantage of using platelet function testing analyzers in the hemostasis laboratory.
11. Identify the role of flow cytometry in the hemostasis laboratory.
12. Describe the methods available for molecular testing in the clinical hemostasis laboratory and the analytes that can be measured using these techniques.
13. Develop a plan of action for the evaluation of a new hemostasis analyzer.
14. Describe the newer technologies that will be helpful in the future for diagnosing hemostatic disorders.

OUTLINE

The Clinical Coagulation Laboratory
  Historical Perspective of Blood Clot Assessment
Assay End-Point Detection Principles
  Mechanical Clot End-Point Detection
  Photo-Optical Clot End-Point Detection
  Viscoelastic Clot Detection
  Chromogenic End-Point Detection
  Nephelometric End-Point Detection
  Immunologic Light Absorbance End-Point Detection
Advantages and Disadvantages of Detection Methods
Coagulation Instrumentation and Technology Advancements
  Improved Accuracy and Precision
  Random Access Testing
  Improved Reagent Handling

Improved Specimen Management
Expanded Computer Capabilities
Quality Features of Automated Assay Performance
Specimen Quality Set Points
Selection of Coagulation Instrumentation
Point-of-Care Coagulation Testing
Global Hemostasis Assessment
Platelet Function Testing
  Platelet Aggregometers
  Platelet Function Analyzers
  Flow Cytometry
Molecular Coagulation Testing
Future Technologies for the Coagulation Laboratory
Currently Available Coagulation Instruments

CASE STUDY

After studying the material in this chapter, the reader should be able to respond to the following case study:

A 65-year-old woman came to the ED with swollen legs and shortness of breath. A chest x-ray and venogram where ordered. After reviewing the results the physician made a diagnosis of deep vein thrombosis and pulmonary embolism. The woman was hospitalized and started on heparin. The following day she was also given Coumadin at 10 mg/day. On days 3 and 5 after starting Coumadin, her blood was drawn for PT/INR. The specimen arrived in the laboratory, it was centrifuged, and it was processed by an automated analyzer using photo-optical end-point detection methodology, and the following results were obtained:

Test	Results – Day 3	Results – Day 5	Reference Interval
Prothrombin time/INR	16.7 sec/2.6	7.3 sec/0.4 (Flag)	10.9–13.0 sec

The laboratory's policy is to investigate all flagged results and to retest all unusual coagulation results. The day 5 prothrombin time assay was repeated; similar values were obtained.

1. Should the operator report the test results as shown for day 5?
2. What action should the operator take to address the results of the specimen on day 5?
3. On day 5 would you expect this patient to be at risk for bleeding based on these test results?

THE CLINICAL COAGULATION LABORATORY

The clinical coagulation laboratory is an ever-changing environment populated by automated analyzers that offer advances in both volume and variety of tests.[1] For many years, the routine coagulation test menu consisted of only prothrombin time (PT) with the international normalized ratio (INR), partial thromboplastin time (PTT; also referred to as the activated partial thromboplastin time [APTT]), fibrinogen, and thrombin time assays (Chapter 41). More specialized testing was performed in tertiary care institutions or reference laboratories employing medical laboratory scientists with specialized training.

With the introduction of new instrumentation and test methodologies, coagulation testing capabilities have expanded significantly, so many formerly "specialized" tests now can be performed easily by general medical laboratory staff. New instrumentation has also made coagulation and expanded hemostasis testing more standardized, consistent, and cost-effective.

Automation has not advanced, however, to the point of making coagulation testing foolproof or an exact science. Operators must develop expertise in correlating critical test results with the patient's diagnosis and when monitoring antithrombotic therapy. Good method validation of procedures, cognitive ability, and theoretical understanding of the hemostatic mechanisms are still required to ensure the accuracy and validity of test results so that the physician can make an informed decision about patient care.

Historical Perspective of Blood Clot Assessment

Visual clot-based testing began in the 18th century. The first observation of blood clotting was from blood taken from the vein of a dog; the sample was completely "jellied" in about 7 minutes. In 1780 Hewson measured that human blood clotted in 7 minutes, using a basin to collect the blood. With the discovery of the microscope, scientists were able to observe visible clot formation and turbidity.[1,2]

Many advances in the assessment of blood clotting took place from 1822 to 1921. These included temperature control during clot formation, passing objects such as a fine needle through the blood to detect resistance, and using different sizes and shapes of glass tubes to view clot formation. In the early 1900s researchers monitored the length of time it took whole blood to clot in a glass tube while it was being tilted, a precursor to the Lee-White clotting time (1913). These early clotting time tests depended on observation of the clot directly (visually) or microscopically.

In 1910 the first clot detection instrument, the "Koaguloviskosimeter," was developed by Kottman. This apparatus measured the change in the viscosity of blood as it clotted. This process generated a voltage change that was recorded by a direct readout system. Voltage changes were plotted against time to measure clot formation. Using the principle of a change in viscosity as blood clots, Hartert developed the thromboelastograph (TEG; detailed later in this chapter) in 1948, and a related clot detection device based on sonar clot detection followed. Both devices are still in use today.[2]

Citrated plasma (usually platelet-poor plasma, or plasma with a platelet count of less than 10,000/μL) came to replace whole blood in coagulation testing. Except for a few specific coagulation tests (e.g., point-of-care testing, for which whole blood is still used), citrated plasma remains the specimen of choice for the largest volume of coagulation testing. However, the principle of interval to clot formation lives on.[1,2]

Plasma coagulation testing began in 1920 when Gram added calcium chloride to anticoagulated plasma at 37° C. He measured the increasing viscosity of the plasma during fibrin monomer polymerization, laying the groundwork for the PT and PTT assays.[3]

In these early days and for many years hence coagulation testing, largely via only the PT and PTT assays, was typically performed by adding plasma and reagents to a glass tube held in a 37° C water bath. Clot formation was determined by visual inspection of the plasma as the tube was tilted, and a stopwatch was used to determine the time to clot formation. This was referred to as the *tilt-tube technique.*

The first instruments dedicated to coagulation testing were nephelometers, developed in 1920. These devices measure 90-degree light dispersion of a colloidal suspension. As plasma clots, a change in light scatter can be measured over time, a principle still in use today.

The 1950s witnessed the dawn of the modern era of instrumentation in coagulation testing with the development of the first coagulometer, the BBL Fibrometer. This instrument used a movable electrode that detected a plasma clot via electromechanical methodology. This advancement allowed laboratories to transition from the manual tilt tube or the manual wire loop method to a more accurate semiautomated testing process. The Fibrometer became the mainstay instrument for clinical coagulation testing and remained so for many years. It can still be found in some coagulation laboratories, although it is no longer manufactured.

Subsequent 20th century developments in clot detectors included a rolling steel ball and photo-optical measurements that are commonly in use today. The technologies used in current instrumentation, along with computerization and software innovations, have created many further enhancements, as will be detailed in this chapter.

Finally, hemostasis laboratory test menus today consist not only of clot-based assays, which still make up the highest volume of the clinical workload, but also new methodologies using synthetic substrates and monoclonal antibodies for measurements of single proteins. These advances have increased our ability to identify specific causes of thrombotic and bleeding disorders.[4,5] Modern instrumentation has the capability to measure these multiple different end-points on one device. Thus the clinical laboratory has moved from the simple assessment of time for whole blood to clot, to assessment of the coagulation cascade using a clot-based assay, to assessment of singular enzymes, inhibitors, and platelet function in the modern hemostasis laboratory with advanced testing capabilities.

ASSAY END-POINT DETECTION PRINCIPLES

Instrument methodologies used for high-volume coagulation and hemostasis testing are classified into six groups based on the type of end-point detection principle (Box 42.1). Instrumentation for specialized (low volume) hemostatic testing beyond coagulation factors will be discussed later in this chapter.

Coagulation instruments apply clot detection principles that either "observe" the clot formation (optical and nephelometric devices) or detect the clot by "feel" (mechanical and viscosity-based devices). The original instruments for coagulation testing typically had a single end-point detection system based on the mechanical principle. The most commonly used end-point in today's clinical coagulation instruments, however, has become photo-optical detection that reads at a fixed wavelength

---

BOX 42.1 End-Point Detection Principles Used in Coagulation Analyzers

Mechanical
Photo-optical (turbidometric)
Nephelometric
Chromogenic (amidolytic)
Immunologic
Viscoelastic

---

between 500 and 600 nm. Dedicated instrumentation with viscoelastic end-point detection can still be found in today's laboratories for specialty testing.

With the growth in understanding of the physiologic mechanisms of coagulation and hemostasis (Chapter 35), laboratory testing also expanded. The newly identified analytes were evaluated by clot-based tests and also by a novel, at the time, test methodology using a color end-point. Thus a second type of instrument was designed to read optical densities at 405 nm to perform the chromogenic (colorimetric, amidolytic) assays. The next step was the development of immunoassays for specific hemostatic analyte measurements. The end-point detection for these assays used nephelometry or other means of detection. Early on, laboratories were required to purchase multiple analyzers in order to offer clot-based, chromogenic-based, and immunoassay-based testing methods.

Instrumentation for today's modern hemostasis clinical laboratory now incorporates all three end-point mechanisms into one platform. Since 1990 instrument manufacturers have successfully incorporated multiple detection methods into single analyzers, which allows a laboratory to purchase and train on only one instrument providing routine and specialized testing capabilities.[4]

Mechanical Clot End-Point Detection

Electromechanical clot detection systems measure a change in conductivity between two metal electrodes in plasma. The BBL Fibrometer was the first semiautomated instrument to be used routinely in the coagulation laboratory. The probe of this instrument has one stationary and one moving electrode. During clotting, the moving electrode enters and leaves the plasma at regular intervals. The current between the electrodes is broken as the moving electrode leaves the plasma. When a clot forms, the fibrin strand conducts current between the electrodes even when the moving electrode exits the solution. The current completes a circuit that stops the timer.[6]

Another mechanical clot detection method uses a magnetic sensor that monitors the movement of a steel ball within the test plasma. Two principles are used for this type of mechanical clot detection in routinely used coagulation instruments. In one system, an electromagnetic field detects the oscillation of a steel ball within the plasma-reagent solution.[3] As fibrin strands form, the viscosity starts to increase, slowing the movement (Figure 42.1). When the oscillation decreases to a predefined rate, the timer stops, indicating the clotting time of the plasma. This methodology is found on all Diagnostica Stago analyzers.

In the second system, a steel ball is positioned in an inclined well. The position of the ball is detected by a magnetic sensor. As the well rotates, the ball remains positioned on the incline. When fibrin forms, the ball is swept out of position. As it moves away from the sensor, there is a break in the circuit, which stops the timer. This technology can be found on AMAX and Destiny instruments distributed by Tcoag and on the original Hemochron ACT instruments.

Photo-Optical Clot End-Point Detection

Photo-optical (turbidometric) coagulometers detect a change in plasma optical density (OD; light transmittance) during the clotting process. Light of a specified wavelength passes through

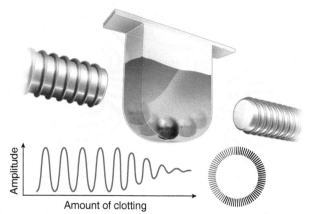

Figure 42.1 Viscosimetric (Electromechanical) Clot Detection. A steel ball oscillates in an arc from one side of the cuvette holding patient plasma to the other. Movement is monitored continuously within a magnetic field. As the specimen clots, viscosity rises and movement of the steel ball is impeded. Variation in amplitude stops the timer, and the interval is the clotting time.

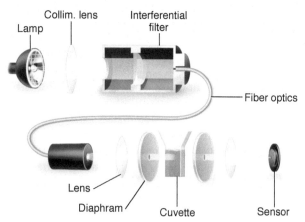

Figure 42.2 Photo-Optical (Turbidometric) Clot Detection. Polychromatic light is focused by a collimator and filtered to transmit a selected wavelength. Monochromatic light is transmitted by fiber optics and focused on the reaction cuvette where the plasma specimen is held. As fibrin forms, opacity increases and the intensity of light reaching the sensor decreases. *Collim.,* Collimator.

plasma, and its intensity (OD) is recorded by a photodetector over the period of clot formation (Figure 42.2). The OD depends on the color and clarity of the specimen, which is used to establish a baseline. Formation of fibrin strands causes light to scatter, allowing less light to fall on the photodetector, thus generating an increase in OD, which becomes greater as the clot becomes denser. When the OD rises to a predetermined variance from baseline, the timer stops, indicating clot formation. Because the baseline OD is subtracted from the final OD, effects of lipemia and icterus are minimized. Many optical systems use multiple wavelengths that discriminate and filter out the effects of icterus and lipemia. Most of the automated and semiautomated coagulation instruments developed since 1970 use photo-optical clot detection.

Viscoelastic Clot Detection

The viscoelastic technique used to detect clot formation in the past is still used today in particular instruments for whole blood clotting. These assays are not high volume, but their

design provides much information about the entire blood clotting process. Depending on the instrument and assay, information can be obtained on the time to clot, kinetics of whole blood clot formation, clot strength, and fibrinolytic activity. Viscoelastic instrumentation is detailed in the Global Hemostasis Assessment section below.

Chromogenic End-Point Detection

Chromogenic (synthetic substrate, amidolytic) methodology uses a synthetic small peptide substrate conjugated to a chromophore, usually para-nitroaniline (pNA). Chromogenic analysis is a means for measuring the activity of a specific coagulation factor because it exploits the factor's enzymatic (protease) properties. The oligopeptide substrate is a series of usually three amino acids whose sequence matches the natural substrate of the factor being measured.[7–10] The hemostatic factor cleaves the chromogenic substrate at the site binding the oligopeptide to the pNA, freeing the pNA. Free pNA is yellow (bound pNA is clear). The OD of the solution is proportional to protease activity and is measured by a photodetector at 405 nm. Simple spectrophotometers can be used for end-point detection.

For examples of chromogenic assays, see Figures 39.6, 39.7, 41.12, 41.13, and 41.14. The activity of coagulation enzymes is measured by direct or indirect chromogenic methods:

- *Direct chromogenic assay:* OD is proportional to the activity of the analyte being measured. For instance, protein C activity is measured by a chromogenic substrate specific for protein C.
- *Indirect chromogenic assay:* The protein or analyte being measured inhibits a target enzyme. It is the target enzyme that has activity directed toward the chromogenic substrate. The greater the inhibition of the target enzyme, the less target enzyme that is available to react with the substrate. The change in OD is thus inversely proportional to the concentration or activity of the substance being measured. This principle is illustrated by heparin quantitation using the anti-factor Xa assay.

Nephelometric End-Point Detection

Nephelometry is a modification of photo-optical end-point detection in which 90-degree or forward-angle light scatter, rather than OD, is measured. A light-emitting diode produces incident light at approximately 600 nm, and a photodetector detects variations in light scatter at 90 degrees (side scatter) and 180 degrees (forward-angle scatter) (Figure 42.3). As fibrin polymers form, side scatter and forward-angle scatter rise.[4,11,12] The timer stops when scatter reaches a predetermined intensity, and the time to clot interval is recorded.

Nephelometry can be adapted to measure the dynamics or kinetics of clot formation. When continuous readings are taken throughout the clotting period, the entire clotting sequence is measured to completion, and a clot curve or "signature" is produced.

Nephelometry was first applied to immunoassays, an application that can still be found today. As antigen-antibody complexes (immune complexes) are formed, they precipitate, and the resulting turbidity scatters the incident light.[13] In reactions in which the immune complexes are known to be too small for detection, the antibodies are first attached to microlatex

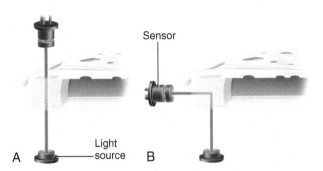

Figure 42.3 Nephelometric Clot Detection. (A), For forward-angle light scatter detection, light from below passes through the patient plasma specimen in a cuvette (yellow area) to the detector above. **(B),** For side scatter light detection, as fibrin polymerizes, light is deflected and is detected at an angle from the original path.

particles. Nephelometry provides a quantitative, not a functional, assay of coagulation factors. Nephelometry is often used in today's high-volume, complex, automated coagulometers that allow for multiple-assay coagulation profiles using both clot-based assays and immunoassays on one platform.

Immunologic Light Absorbance End-Point Detection

Immunologic assays are the newest assays available for routine coagulation testing. These assays are based on antigen-antibody reactions. In slight contrast to the nephelometry principle described previously, which uses a light scatter end-point, another common means to detect an end-point in an immunoassay is to use light absorbance. Latex microparticles are coated with

antibodies directed against the selected analyte (antigen). Monochromatic light passes through the suspension of latex microparticles. When the wavelength is greater than the diameter of the particles, only a small amount of light is absorbed.[7] When the coated latex microparticles come into contact with their antigen, however, the antigen attaches to the antibody and "bridges" are formed, which causes the particles to agglutinate. As the diameter of the agglutinates increases relative to the wavelength of the monochromatic light beam, light is absorbed. The increase in light absorbance is proportional to the size of the agglutinates, which in turn is proportional to the antigen level.

Immunoassay technology became available on coagulometers in the 1990s and is used to measure a growing number of coagulation factors and proteins, such as D-dimer. These assays, which used to take hours or days to perform using traditional antigen-antibody detection methodologies (e.g., enzyme-linked immunosorbent assay [ELISA] or electrophoresis), now can be done in minutes on an automated analyzer.

ADVANTAGES AND DISADVANTAGES OF DETECTION METHODS

As stated, coagulation testing is not foolproof or an exact science. Operator expertise in performing quality testing and interpreting results is a key component of a professional hemostasis laboratory. Some basic technical issues are an important consideration in quality coagulation laboratory testing. Table 42.1 summarizes advantages and disadvantages of the different detection methodologies.

TABLE 42.1 Advantages and Disadvantages of Detection Systems of Hemostatic Analyzers

End-Point Detection Method	Advantages	Disadvantages
Mechanical	• No interference from specimen lipemia or bilirubinemia (icterus) • Ability to use specimen and reagent volumes as small as 25 μL in some instruments • Able to detect weak clots	• Reliance on the integrity of the entire coagulation cascade • Inability to observe graph of clot formation
Photo-optical	• Good precision • Increased test menu flexibility and specimen quality information when multiple wavelengths are used • Ability to observe graph of clot formation with some instrumentation	• Interference from lipemia, hemolysis, bilirubinemia, and increased plasma proteins; this issue has been addressed by some manufacturers with readings from multiple wavelengths • May not detect short clotting times owing to long lag phase • May not detect small friable clots that are translucent
Chromogenic	• Ability to measure proteins that do not clot • More specific than clot-based assays • Expanded menu options to replace clottable assays affected by preanalytical variables, such as heparin, thrombin inhibitors (e.g., argatroban, dabigatran) or FXa inhibitors (e.g., rivaroxaban) • Most automated systems now have cost-effective chromogenic capabilities	• Limited by wavelength capabilities of some instruments • May need large test volume to be cost effective
Immunologic	• Ability to automate tests previously available only with manual, time-consuming methods, such as enzyme-linked immunosorbent assays • Expanded test menu capabilities	• Limited number of automated tests available • Higher cost of instruments and reagents • May need to have additional instruments available to run routine tests in laboratories without automated coagulation analyzers that have random access capability
Nephelometric	• Ability to measure antigen-antibody reactions for proteins present in small concentrations	• Limited number of tests available • Higher cost of reagents • Need for special staff training

All coagulation tests that use clot-based end-points need special considerations when results are interpreted. There are many variables that affect coagulation function. It is important to always keep in mind that the integrity of the entire coagulation cascade is relevant to the final test result. Thus these assays are not highly specific. This would not be true for chromogenic or immunologic end-point assays that do not rely on the coagulation cascade, but rather are single analyte specific.

Assays based on a chromogenic end-point (rather than a clot-based assay) are useful to evaluate specimens from patients who have circulating inhibitors or who are on anticoagulant treatment because the inhibitors do not interfere in the chromogenic assay. For clot-based assays the entire coagulation cascade is part of the test system, whereas for chromogenic assays the test is isolated to the specific chemical (enzymatic) reaction in question. Chromogenic substrate assays are thus more specific than clot-based assays.

Some other common issues include the following. Photo-optical clot end-point detection may be confounded by icterus or lipemia, which erroneously prolongs the clotting time because the change in OD is masked by the color or turbidity of the specimen. Some coagulation instruments may be unable to use PT and PTT reagents manufactured with synthetic material because their greater translucency compared to other reagents can generate a plasma clot that is not detected by certain instruments.[14]

Other important advantages of mechanical clot-based methods (as opposed to photo-optical clot-based methods) are that they are not affected by icteric or lipemic plasma. Mechanical methods also provide a sensitive end-point able to detect weak clots, such as those formed in plasmas with low fibrinogen or a factor XIII deficiency, in which clots are not stable.

COAGULATION INSTRUMENTATION AND TECHNOLOGY ADVANCEMENTS

Coagulometers are manual, semiautomated, or automated (Table 42.2). Manual and semiautomated coagulometers require the operator to deliver test plasma and reagents manually to the reaction cuvette and limit testing to one or two specimens at a time. Manual result recording and calculation of the results are also done. The use of manual and semiautomated coagulometers requires considerable operator time and expertise. These are relatively inexpensive instruments, and they are useful for low-volume clinical laboratories and for research laboratories.

Significant advances have been made in the capability and flexibility of coagulation instrumentation. Current technology in automated instrumentation allows a "walkaway" environment. After specimens and reagents are loaded and the testing sequence is initiated, the operator can move on to perform other tasks. Fully automated analyzers provide pipetting systems that automatically transfer reagents and test plasma to reaction vessels and measure the end-point without operator intervention. Multiple specimens can be tested simultaneously. Automated coagulometers are expensive, and laboratory staff require specialized training to operate and maintain them.

Regardless of technology all automated and semiautomated analyzers offer better coagulation testing accuracy and precision than the manual methods. Clot end-point detection methods have remained consistent through the years, but with the advent of chromogenic- and immunologic-based assays, other instrumentation needed to be brought into the coagulation laboratory. Multiple methodologies are now incorporated into single analyzers. From instruments that performed only clot-based assays, clinical laboratory instruments have been developed that perform both clot-based and chromogenic-based assays.[8–10] The most recent advancement has been the development of a single instrument that performs clot-based, chromogenic, and immunologic assays on one platform.

Many technical advances have greatly improved specimen, reagent, and data management, improved test performance, and increased throughput as will be detailed below.

Improved Accuracy and Precision

In the days of visual methods, coagulation assays were performed in duplicate to reduce the coefficient of variation, which generally exceeded 20%. Semiautomated instruments

TABLE 42.2	Levels of Coagulation Instrumentation Automation	
Level	**Description**	**Examples**
Manual	All reagents and specimens are transferred manually by the operator. Temperature is maintained by a water bath or heat block; external measurement by operator may be required. End-point is determined visually by the operator. Timer is initiated and stopped by the operator.	Tilt tube Wire loop
Semiautomated	All reagents and specimens are transferred manually by the operator. Instrument usually contains a device for maintaining constant 37° C temperature. Analyzer may internally monitor temperature. Instrument has a mechanism to initiate a timing device automatically on addition of final reagent and a mechanism for detecting clot formation and stopping the timer.	Fibrometer STart 4 Cascade M and M-4 BFT-II KC1 and KC4
Automated	All reagents are automatically pipetted by the instrument. Specimens may or may not be automatically pipetted. Analyzer contains monitoring devices and an internal mechanism to maintain and monitor constant 37° C temperature throughout the testing sequence. Timers are initiated and clot formation is detected automatically.	ACL TOP STA-R Evolution STA Compact and Compact CT Sysmex CA-series BCS XP CoaLAB

improved upon precision, but the requirement for manual pipetting of plasma and reagents continued to necessitate duplicate testing. With the advent of fully automated instruments, precision improved to the extent that duplicate testing is no longer necessary, halving material and reagent costs. Assays are performed with confidence as coefficients of variation of less than 5% are typically achieved, and even less than 1% for some tests.

Random Access Testing

Automated coagulometers provide random access testing. Through simple programming, a variety of tests can be run in any order on single or multiple specimens within a testing sequence. Previous automated analyzers were capable of running only one or two assays at a time, so batching was necessary. The disadvantage was that specimens with multiple orders had to be handled multiple times and stat testing could be challenging. For current automated analyzers, the ability to run multiple tests is limited only by the number of reagents that can be stored in the analyzer and the instrument's ability to simultaneously interweave tests that require different end-point detection methodologies (clot-based, chromogenic, and/or immunologic). Random access benefits include improved turnaround times, reduced errors, and reduced labor costs.

Improved Reagent Handling
Reduced Reagent and Specimen Volumes

Automated and semiautomated coagulometers now have the capability to perform tests on smaller specimen volumes. Traditionally, PT assays required 100 μL of patient plasma and 200 μL of thromboplastin/calcium chloride reagent. PTT was measured using 100 μL of plasma, 100 μL of activated partial thromboplastin, and 100 μL of calcium chloride. Current analyzers can perform the same tests using one half or even one quarter the traditional volumes of reagents and patient specimens. This promotes the use of smaller specimen volumes, especially from pediatric patients or those from whom specimens are difficult to draw, thus further reducing reagent costs.

Open Reagent Systems

Laboratory directors want the flexibility of selecting reagents that best suit their needs, and prefer not to be restricted in their choices by the analyzer being used. Recognizing that the ability to select reagents independently of the analyzer is a high priority, instrument manufacturers have responded by developing systems that provide optimal performance with the variety of coagulation test reagents available from alternative manufacturers, provided that the reagents are compatible with the instrument's methodology.

Reagent Tracking

Many automated instruments keep records of reagent lot numbers and expiration dates, which makes it easier for the laboratory to maintain reagent integrity and comply with regulatory requirements. An additional feature on current instrumentation includes on-board monitoring of reagent volumes with flagging systems to alert the operator when an insufficient volume of reagent is present in relation to the number of specimens programmed to be run. Reagent bar coding supports record keeping by tracking reagent properties and enabling the operator to load reagents onto the coagulometer without stopping specimen analysis.

Improved Specimen Management
Primary Tube Sampling

The design of many coagulometers encourages the operator to place the primary specimen collection tube on the instrument after centrifugation, which eliminates the need to separate the plasma into a secondary tube. In addition, instruments often accommodate multiple tube sizes. Significant time savings occur as a result of elimination of the extra specimen preparation steps, and errors resulting from mislabeling of the aliquot tube are reduced.

Closed-Tube Sampling

Closed-tube sampling of specimens has improved the safety and efficiency of coagulation testing. After centrifugation the operator places the primary blood collection tube on the analyzer without removing the blue stopper. The cap is pierced by a needle in the instrument that aspirates plasma. The probe is incorporated with a sensor that recognizes the presence of liquid and stops at the optimized liquid level, between 4 and 250 μL. This allows aspiration of the specimen to occur without disturbing the red blood cell layer. Cross-over between specimens is eliminated by washing the needle between specimens with a rinse solution.

Not only does closed-tube sampling save staff time, it also reduces the risk to the staff of specimen exposure through aerosols or spillage and promotes plasma pH stabilization. When closed-tube sampling is used, as a measure of quality assurance, specimens are visually checked for clots after centrifugation by looking for the presence of fibrin strands. For example, if the assay result is a short clotting time or the corresponding coagulation tracing (available on some instruments) is abnormal, then the staff rims the specimen with wooden sticks to determine if a clot is present.

Automatic Dilutions

Many instruments perform multiple dilutions on patient specimens, calibrators, or controls, eliminating the need for the operator to perform this task manually and reducing the potential for dilution errors. These conditions can be automatically programmed into the individual test setups on the analyzer.

Expanded Computer Capabilities

The computer circuitry of coagulation analyzers now incorporates internal data storage and retrieval systems. Hundreds of results can be stored, retrieved, and compiled into cumulative reports. Multiple calibration curves can be stored and accessed. Quality control files can be stored, which eliminates the time-consuming task of manually logging and graphing quality control values. Westgard rules can be applied, and failures are automatically flagged. Some analyzers feature automatic repeat testing when failures occur on the initial run. The quality control files can be reviewed or printed on a regular basis to meet regulatory requirements.

The programming flexibility of modern analyzers has enhanced the laboratory's opportunities to provide expanded test menus. Most advanced analyzers are preprogrammed with several routine test protocols ready for use. Specimen and reagent volumes, incubation times, and other testing parameters do not need to be determined by the operator but can be changed easily when necessary. Additional tests can be programmed into the analyzer by the user whenever needed, which allows for enhanced flexibility of the analyzer and reduces the need for laboratories to have multiple instruments.

Instrument interfacing to laboratory information systems and specimen bar coding capabilities have become a priority as facilities of all sizes endeavor to reduce dependence on manual record keeping. Bidirectional interfaces improve efficiency through the ability of the instrument to send specimen bar code information to the laboratory information systems and receive a response listing the tests that have been ordered. This eliminates the need for the operator to program each specimen and test.

Quality Features of Automated Assay Performance
Flagging

Improved flagging capabilities alert the operator when preset criteria have been exceeded for instrument performance and specimen quality. A selection of common instruments flags are given in Box 42.2.

Reflex Testing

Reflex testing is the automatic ordering of tests based on preset parameters or the results of prior tests. Instruments may make additional dilutions if the initial result is outside the linearity limits, or supplementary tests can be run automatically if clinically indicated by the initial test result. The first result does not need to wait for review by the operator before follow-up action is initiated by the instrument.

Kinetics of Clot Formation

Graphing of the kinetics of clot formation is provided on some analyzers, such as the ACL TOP from Instrumentation Laboratory. The graph is generated by an algorithm used to convert multiple raw optical measurements collected over the course of

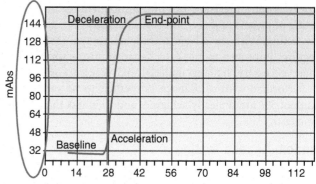

Figure 42.4 Clot Signature from the ACL TOP Coagulation Analyzer (Instrumentation Laboratory). As the fibrinogen in the patient plasma specimen converts to fibrin and a solid clot, the change in light transmission through the specimen is recorded. The clot curve consists of baseline, acceleration phase, deceleration phase, and end-point. The baseline is recorded before clotting occurs. Acceleration reflects clotting and is normally steep because clotting is rapid. The deceleration phase represents the decreasing rate of clot formation as all available fibrinogen converts to fibrin. The end-point is flat and stable, reflecting consumption of all fibrinogen. A key component in evaluating the clot curve is the y-axis, absorbance, which provides the time interval at a defined minimum that identifies that a clot has developed. Absorbance adjusts to compensate for baseline fibrinogen and interferences such as lipemia or icterus. (Image courtesy of Beckman-Coulter, Brea, CA.)

the assay into a final result. In addition to determining the time to clot, this instrument smooths the raw data into a visible curve and uses the curve to check for clot formation integrity. Multiple checks are performed to ensure an accurate and reproducible result. Should the data not meet all of the acceptable criteria, an error flag is generated. The clot curve is examined to troubleshoot potential technical aberrations. The clot formation graph may also be used as a clot "signature" of the patient specimen that correlates with the disease state. Figure 42.4 shows an example of a typical clot curve.

Specimen Quality Set Points

Specimen quality flags, such as the following, are included on some coagulation instrumentation:

- *Clotted:* Will cause falsely shortened clotting times because of premature activation of coagulation factors and platelets that generate FVIIa and thrombin.
- *Lipemia:* May cause falsely prolonged clotting times on OD-sensing instruments because of interference with light transmittance.
- *Hemolysis:* May cause falsely shortened clotting times because of premature activation of coagulation factors and platelets that generate FVIIa and thrombin.[15]
- *Icterus (bilirubinemia):* Indicates liver dysfunction that may lead to prolonged clotting times because of inadequate clotting factor production; also may interfere with OD-sensing instruments.
- *Abnormal clot formation:* May lead to falsely elevated clotting times because of instrument inability to detect an end-point.
- *No end-point detected:* Indicates that the instrument was unable to detect clot formation; the specimen may need to be tested using an alternative type of instrument.

BOX 42.2   Some Types of Warning Flags Available on Coagulometers

Instrument Malfunction Flags
Temperature error
Photo-optics error
Mechanical movement error
Probe not aspirating

Sample Quality Flags
Lipemia
Hemolysis
Icterus
Abnormal clot formation
No end-point detected

SELECTION OF COAGULATION INSTRUMENTATION

In today's clinical laboratory, more than ever before, cost effectiveness, testing capabilities, and standardization are top priorities. As an increasing number of tests become available, laboratories must determine what tests to incorporate to provide guidance to physicians in diagnosis and treatment. Identification of testing needs based on patient population should be the first step in the process. The decisions regarding which tests are the most appropriate for the clinical situations encountered by each laboratory should be made in conjunction with the medical staff. When that input has been obtained, the laboratory can determine the availability and cost of instruments that would meet those requirements.

An instrument should be matched to the anticipated workload. It may not be necessary to purchase a highly sophisticated analyzer capable of performing a large menu of tests if the setting is a small hospital laboratory ordering very few of the more "esoteric" test options. A batch analyzer with high throughput of the routine coagulation tests may be more appropriate for this situation. The option to send out esoteric tests and/or low-volume tests to a reference laboratory is always available.

Instrument selection criteria may include, but are not limited to, the items listed in Box 42.3. When the choices have been narrowed based on the most desirable criteria, consideration

should be given to additional features. Because no instrument has all the desired features, prioritizing helps the laboratory focus on the capabilities that would be the most advantageous for them. Table 42.3 summarizes several of these specialized features. The final section, Currently Available Coagulation Instruments, provides a comparison of instrumentation.

BOX 42.3 Selection Criteria for Hemostasis Instrumentation

- Instrument cost
- Consumables cost
- Service response time
- Reliability and downtime
- Maintenance requirements and time
- Operator ease of use
- Breadth of testing menu
- Ability to add new testing protocols
- Reagent lot to lot variation
- Throughput for high-volume testing
- Laboratory information systems (LIS) interface capabilities
- Footprint (the space the instrument occupies; benchtop or floor model)
- Special requirements (water, power, waste drain)
- Flexibility in using other manufacturers' reagents
- Availability of a training program and continued training support

---

TABLE 42.3 Specialized Features on Current Coagulometers

Instrument Feature	Comment
Random access	A variety of tests can be performed on a single specimen or multiple specimens in any order as determined by the operator.
Primary tube sampling	Plasma is directly aspirated from an open or a capped centrifuged primary collection tube on the analyzer.
Cap piercing	Analyzer aspirates plasma from the closed centrifuged primary collection tube.
Bar coding	Reagents and specimens are identified with a bar code; eliminates manual information entry.
Bidirectional laboratory information system (LIS) interface	Analyzer queries the host computer (LIS) to determine which tests have been ordered. Results are returned to the LIS after verification.
Specimen and instrument flagging	Automated alerts indicate problems with specimen integrity or instrument malfunction.
Liquid level sensing	Operator is alerted when there is inadequate specimen or reagent volume. An alert is also given when the instrument fails to aspirate the required specimen volume. Volume is verified each time a specimen or reagent is aspirated.
On-board quality control	Instrument stores and organizes quality control data; may include application of Westgard rules for flagging out-of-range results; instrument may transmit quality control data to the LIS.
Stat capabilities	Operator can interrupt a testing sequence to place a stat specimen next in line for testing.
On-board refrigeration of specimens and reagents	Refrigeration maintains the integrity of specimens and reagents throughout testing and allows reagents to be kept in the analyzer for extended periods, which reduces setup time for less frequently performed tests.
On-board specimen storage capacity	Indicates the number of specimens that can be loaded at a time.
Reflex testing	Instrument can be programmed to perform repeat or additional testing under operator-defined circumstances.
Patient data storage	Test results can be stored for future retrieval; clot formation graphs may be included.
Throughput	Number of tests that can be processed within a specified interval, usually the number of tests per hour; depends on test mix and methodologies.
Total testing (dwell) time	Length of time from specimen placement in the analyzer until testing is completed; depends on the type and complexity of the procedure.
Graph of clot formation	Operator can visualize how the clot is formed over time.

TABLE 42.4   Comparison of Point-of-Care Instruments for Coagulation Testing

Manufacturer/ Instrument	First Year Marketed	Test	Specimen	Clot Detection Principle	Includes QC
Abbott iSTAT	2000	PT/INR, PTT, ACT	Whole blood	Electrogenic	Yes
Alere INRatio/INRatio2	2003/2008	PT/INR	Fingerstick	Electrochemical, impedance	Yes
Helena Cascade POC	2000	PT/INR, PTT, ACT, low molecular weight heparin	Whole blood/fingerstick	Photo-mechanical	Yes
Helena Actalyke Mini II	2004	ACT	Whole blood	2-point electromechanical	Yes
Helena Actalyke XL	2002	ACT	Whole blood	2-point electromechanical	Yes
Instrumentation Laboratory Gem PCL Plus	2003	PT/INR, PTT, ACT	Whole blood/fingerstick	Mechanical end-point monitored optically	Yes
Accriva ProTime Micro Coagulation System	1995/2003/2006	PT/INR	Fingerstick	Mechanical clot	Yes
Accriva Hemochron Signature Elite	2005	PT/INR, PTT, ACT	Whole blood/fingerstick	Mechanical clot	Yes
Accriva Hemochron Signature +	2002	PT/INR, PTT, ACT	Whole blood/fingerstick	Mechanical clot	Yes
Accriva Hemochron Response	2000	PT/INR, PTT, ACT, TT	Whole blood/fingerstick	Mechanical clot	Yes
Medtronic HMS Plus	1999	ACT, protamine titration	Whole blood	Mechanical clot	Yes
Medtronic ACT Plus	2003	ACT	Whole blood	Mechanical clot	Yes
Roche CoaguCheck XS	2007	PT/INR	Whole blood/fingerstick	Amperometric	No
Roche CoaguCheck XS Plus	2007	PT/INR	Whole blood/fingerstick	Amperometric	Yes
Roche CoaguCheck XS Pro	2010	PT/INR	Whole blood/fingerstick	Amperometric	Yes
CoaguSense PT/INR Monitoring System	2010	PT/INR	Fingerstick	Mechanical	Yes
Siemens Xprecia Stride	2015	PT/INR	Fingerstick	Electrochemical with amperometric	Yes

POINT-OF-CARE COAGULATION TESTING

Point-of-care (POC) instruments are handheld devices that permit near-patient testing during clinical procedures or surgeries, bedside testing for hospitalized patients, and self-testing for outpatients. In addition, the small specimen volume is an advantage for testing in infants. The instantaneous turnaround time of results, portability of the devices, and small specimen volume are conveniences appreciated by both physicians and patients. Table 42.4 summarizes the variety of US Food and Drug Administration (FDA)-cleared POC devices and assays currently available.[16]

Various end-point detection techniques are used in the POC devices. Each device uses an individual patented technology. The newer versions of POC devices include touch screen, wireless transmission of results in real-time, and micro-blood volumes.

POC coagulation analyzers often use capillary (fingerstick) whole blood, but some will require anticoagulated whole blood (venipuncture). Typically a 10 to 50 μL whole blood specimen is transferred to a test cartridge that contains the test reagents, which is immediately inserted into the test module. Other instruments will require nonanticoagulated whole blood with higher volumes of blood.

POC coagulation testing has been in practice since 1966 with the introduction of the whole blood activated clotting time (ACT) for heparin monitoring during cardiac surgery (Chapter 40). The fast turnaround time of the ACT is necessary to allow for immediate heparin dosage changes, avoiding both bleeding and clotting in the patient and clotting of the cardiopulmonary bypass pump. At the conclusion of surgery the high dose of heparin used during the procedure is reversed with protamine. This practice is also monitored with the ACT to assure there is no residual heparin in the patient that can cause postoperative bleeding.

A second common POC test is the prothrombin time/ international normalized ratio (PT/INR) for monitoring the oral anticoagulant Coumadin (Chapter 40). Anticoagulation clinics can be high-volume users of POC testing. Patients on oral anticoagulant therapy with Coumadin are required to be monitored monthly. Anticoagulation clinics provide this service in the outpatient setting using the PT/INR test on a POC device. Having test results quickly available allows for dose adjustments at the same clinic visit, eliminating patient waiting time.

Other POC coagulation tests, including the PTT and thrombin clotting time, are available but not widely accepted as yet. Another assay that would be beneficial as a near-patient test for trauma or surgical patient care is a test to determine the level of fibrinogen. This is a clinical need, and POC assays are already in development.

Before POC devices are placed in service, laboratory scientists validate the results against the plasma-based assay performed in the central laboratory, which is considered the primary coagulometer and reference method (Chapter 2). The whole blood ACT (never designed as a plasma-based assay) is validated in a different manner. Because POC assays and the plasma-based central laboratory assays can show a weak correlation due to differences in instrumentation, reagents, and specimens, care must be taken to understand the differences between POC and central laboratory results to ensure that clinical decisions are accurate. In the case of the anticoagulation clinic, an INR that exceeds 6.0 or any unexpected INR change is confirmed with a venipuncture blood specimen tested by the plasma-based assay in the central laboratory.

GLOBAL HEMOSTASIS ASSESSMENT

Thromboelastography was developed in 1948 and to this day follows the same general format. This technique uses the viscoelastic property of blood clotting described previously. The assay provides information on the entire kinetic process of whole blood clot formation. An advantage is that whole blood, not plasma, is used as the specimen; this allows evaluation of the interactions of platelets, erythrocytes, leukocytes, plasma coagulation factors, and plasma proteins, in addition to their individual contribution to the clotting process. This technique assesses both bleeding and thrombosis risk, and it also provides an evaluation of fibrinolysis and a hypercoagulable state. For example, thromboelastography is useful for defining the global (or entire) hemostatic status of patients with hepatic disease, obstetrical disorders, or trauma, and that of patients undergoing liver transplantation or cardiac surgery. This assay helps determine specific patient management needs for clotting factor and/or platelet replacement, in addition to anticoagulant, fibrinolytic, or antiplatelet therapy. Algorithms have been developed to aid in diagnosis.

The TEG Thromboelastograph Hemostasis Analyzer System from Haemonetics is based on the original instrument design. Nonanticoagulated or citrated whole blood is pipetted into a cylindrical cup that oscillates by 4.75 degrees. A stationary pin with a diameter 1 mm smaller than the cup's diameter is suspended by a torsion wire into the cup. Kaolin (or another activator) is added to trigger clotting. As the blood clots, fibrin links the pin to the cup, and viscoelasticity changes are transmitted to the pin. The resulting pin torque generates an electrical signal from the torsion wire. The signal is plotted as a function of time to produce a

TEG tracing. The tracing is analyzed to determine the speed, strength, and stability of clot formation and the downstream effect of fibrinolysis (Figure 42.5). Through computerization the trace furnishes real-time information about the evolving clot from platelet activation and initial fibrin formation through fibrin cross-linkage and fibrinolysis.[17] Two test channels are available on each instrument; manual pipetting is required. Assay kits are available for specific platelet function and other testing.

A new version of thromboelastography is the ROTEM, or rotational thromboelastometry, from Instrumentation Laboratory. The enhancements of the ROTEM are that the instrument is not sensitive to vibrations, it has four test channels, a touch screen, and an automated pipettor. In this system a whole blood specimen is placed in a cuvette, with one of various coagulation activators, and a suspended pin is immersed into the blood. The pin rotates (the cup is stationary), and upon clot formation, the increased tension from fibrin binding the cup to the pin is detected by sensors. The tracing is recorded as the clot evolves over time. The clot signature of the ROTEM is the same as that for the TEG.[18] The TEG and ROTEM clot signatures and their parameters are directly compared in Figure 42.5. For both devices reagents are available for several coagulation assays that assess factor and fibrinogen deficiency, platelet function, fibrinolysis, and anticoagulant influence on hemostasis. Reagent-dependent differences will determine appropriate result interpretation. Differences between TEG and ROTEM can also be found in the quality control (QC) and instrument maintenance schedules.

The TEG and ROTEM devices are often placed in the operating room and emergency department in addition to the central laboratory. Results are available within 10 to 20 minutes. Certain disadvantages of both the TEG and ROTEM are that the assay results are operator dependent, require training, and demand a certain level of skill to perform a quality assay. Result interpretation also requires skill, knowledge, and experience.

PLATELET FUNCTION TESTING

In addition to coagulation factor testing, clinical hemostasis laboratories have expanded their test menu to include assays that evaluate platelet function. This section will detail the instrumentation available for platelet function assays.

The demand for rapid, cost-effective methods for the evaluation of platelet function has increased due to the need to monitor the efficacy of antiplatelet therapy, such as aspirin, clopidogrel, and glycoprotein IIb/IIIa inhibitors used in cardiovascular patients (Chapters 37 and 40). In addition, preoperative evaluation of platelet function is important in hemostatic management, particularly if the patient has a history of bleeding or if the patient is on antiplatelet medication.[19]

Platelet function testing has been a challenge for the clinical laboratory because of the lack of reliable, accurate, and easy to perform assays. In addition, proper specimen procurement and handling for platelet function testing plays an important role in the reliability and accuracy of the test. Platelet function historically has been assessed by the bleeding time test and platelet aggregation assays (Chapter 41). The bleeding time is technically demanding and highly dependent on the individual

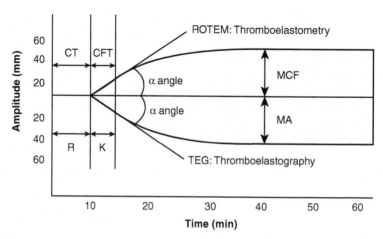

Parameter	TEG	ROTEM	Comment
Clot initiation or clotting time	R (reaction time)	CT (clotting time)	Time of initial fibrin formation
Clot kinetics	K	CFT (clot formation time)	A measure of the speed to reach a specific level of clot strength
Angle	α (angle in degrees)	α	Measure of the rate of clot formation, reflects the rate of fibrin formation and cross linking
Clot strength	MA (maximum amplitutde)	MCF (maximum clot firmness)	Measure of the strength of the clot
Clot stability	Ly30 (lysis at 30 minutes as a ratio of MA)	CLI (clot lysis index)	Measure of the rate of amplitude reduction

Figure 42.5 Comparison of the Clot Signatures of the TEG and ROTEM. The thromboelastograph *(TEG)* and the rotational thromboelastometry *(ROTEM)* instruments produce the same pattern of the dynamics of clot formation. The parameters measured from the kinetic reaction of clot formation are also the same but are labeled differently.

performing the test; also, results fail to correlate with intraoperative bleeding risk.[20–23] Thus the bleeding time test has been discontinued in most institutions. New platelet aggregometers and several new devices are making it easier to assess platelet function.

Platelet Aggregometers

Classic platelet aggregometry using the light transmission principle was developed in 1962 by Born. This test system measures the increase in light transmission that occurs in direct proportion to platelet aggregation (Figure 41.4) induced by various agonists (e.g., collagen, adenosine diphosphate [ADP], epinephrine). The reduced amount of light able to be transmitted through a platelet-rich plasma (PRP) specimen is compared to the increased light that can be transmitted through a specimen in which the aggregated platelet clumps have cleared the plasma. Since its inception, platelet aggregation using PRP assays and light transmission aggregation (LTA) detection has been the primary means to assess platelet function.

Table 42.5 compares commonly used US FDA-cleared platelet aggregometers. Three parameters are calculated from each specimen: maximum percentage aggregation, area under the curve, and velocity. In addition to LTA several new devices to detect platelet aggregation based on whole blood impedance, luminescence, and light scatter have been developed. Whole blood platelet aggregation by impedance is based on the principle that upon activation, platelets become sticky and adhere to metal sensor wires (electrodes) (Figure 41.5).[24] The theoretical advantage of whole blood aggregometry is that it is a more physiologic test due to the ability to measure platelet aggregation in the presence of erythrocytes and leukocytes. The advantage of lumi-aggregation, described in Chapter 41, is that the properties of platelet secretion and platelet aggregation are simultaneously evaluated.

The PAP-8E from BioData is an eight-channel platelet aggregometer with a touch screen and on-screen procedure templates (Figure 42.6). It has a programmable pipette and an optional bar code scanner. The PAP-8E uses LTA and a low sample volume (225 μL). BioData also has a dedicated centrifuge for preparing the PRP specimen (Figure 42.7).[25] PRP can be prepared in 3 minutes, platelet-poor plasma can be prepared in 120 seconds, and platelet-free plasma can be prepared in 180 seconds, a tremendous time-saving improvement over the traditional centrifugation procedure.

TABLE 42.5 Comparison of Platelet Aggregometers

Parameter	BioData Corp.	Chrono-Log Corp.	Helena Laboratories	DiaPharma Group/ Roche Diagnostics
Instrument name (first year sold)	Platelet Aggregation Profiler, Model PAP-8E (2005)	Whole Blood/Optical Lumi-Aggregation System Model 700-2/700-4 (2006)	AggRAM (2005)	Multiplate Analyzer
Operational type	Batch, random access	Batch, random access	Batch, random access	Batch, random access
Reagent type	Open reagent system, assay kits, reagents, controls, diluents, buffers	Open reagent system, assay kits, reference plasma, controls	Open reagent system	Open reagent
Operates on whole blood or spun plasma	Spun plasma, optional centrifugation with PDQ to obtain PRP in 3 minutes	Whole blood, spun plasma	Spun plasma	Whole blood
Plasma volume/test	225 μL	225 μL	225 μL	175 μL/300 μL
Model type	Benchtop	Benchtop	Benchtop	Benchtop
Number of channels	8	2–4	4–8	5
Time required for maintenance by lab staff	Weekly:15 minutes; monthly: 30 minutes	30 minutes when optical calibration required	Daily: 15 minutes; weekly: 15 minutes; monthly: 1 hour	Daily: Clean and disinfect the analyzer and pipette. Periodically: Replace sensor cables.

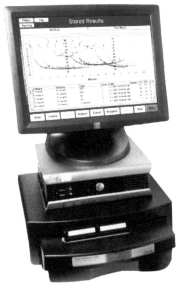

Figure 42.6 The PAP-8E Platelet Aggregometer (BioData). The PAP-8E is an eight-channel platelet aggregometer that detects platelet aggregation by changes in light transmission through the platelet rich plasma specimen; as platelets clump together more light is able to pass thought the cleared plasma. This instrument allows for the analysis of platelet function, measurement of ristocetin cofactor activity for detecting von Willebrand disease, identifying platelet function abnormalities such as heparin-induced thrombocytopenia, and monitoring antiplatelet therapy. (Photo courtesy of BioData Corp, Horsham, PA.)

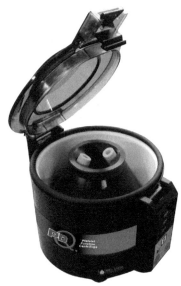

Figure 42.7 The PDQ Platelet Function Centrifuge (BioData). This is an optional unit to the PAP-8E platelet aggregometer. This centrifuge is dedicated to preparing standardized specimens for platelet function testing. The PDQ produces platelet-rich plasma, platelet-poor plasma, and platelet-free plasma within 5 minutes. (Photo courtesy of BioData Corp, Horsham, PA.)

Chrono-Log has a Whole Blood/Optical Lumi-Aggregation System. The Model 700 aggregometer provides for platelet aggregation in whole blood or PRP, while simultaneously measuring the platelet secretion response using the luciferase reagent (Figure 41.6). Electrical impedance is used to detect aggregation, and optical density to detect luminescence identifies platelet secretion. The instrument can be configured as either a two- or four-channel aggregometer.[26] Either disposable or reusable electrodes can be used for impedance measurements. Chrono-Log has several other optical and impedance-based instruments for evaluating platelet function.

The Multiplate Analyzer from Diapharma, also called the Whole-Blood Multiple Electrode Platelet Aggregometer (MEA), which monitors platelet function by impedance, is the latest development.[24] Multiplate results correlate well with LTA in testing the therapeutic efficacy of clopidogrel and glycoprotein

IIb/IIIa inhibitors. Further studies to determine correlations between Multiplate and LTA, and the clinical predictive value of Multiplate results, are in progress. The hematocrit and platelet count may limit assay sensitivity. US FDA approval is pending.

The AggRAM from Helena is a modular system for platelet aggregation and ristocetin cofactor testing. Its advanced optics use a laser diode measuring at a wavelength of 650 nm to enhance precision of the aggregation tracing.[27] The AggRAM has four channels capable of microvolume testing, customized result reporting, and internal quality control programs.

Platelet Function Analyzers

The Siemens PFA-100 Platelet Function Analyzer is an automated instrument that provides rapid results on quantitative and qualitative platelet abnormalities. Test cartridges contain membranes coated with collagen/epinephrine or collagen/ADP to stimulate platelet aggregation. Whole blood is aspirated under controlled flow conditions through a microscopic aperture in the membrane. The time required for a platelet plug to occlude the aperture is an indication of platelet function.[28] The PFA-100 system is successful at detecting von Willebrand disease and the efficacy of aspirin therapy.[29,30]

The Verify Now from Accriva Diagnostics is an optical detection system that measures platelet aggregation by microbead agglutination. The system uses a disposable cartridge that contains lyophilized fibrinogen-coated beads and a platelet agonist specific for the test. Whole blood is dispensed from a special blood collection tube into the assay device, with no blood handling or pipetting required by the operator. The instrument provides an aspirin assay using arachidonic acid as the test reagent, a glycoprotein IIb/IIIa inhibitor (abciximab, tirofiban, eptifibatide) assay using thrombin receptor activation peptide (TRAP) as the test reagent, and a P2Y₁₂ inhibitor (clopidogrel, prasugrel, ticagrelor) assay using ADP as the test reagent.[31–34] Results, available in about 10 minutes, can be used to modify drug dosing. This device can be found in clinical laboratories or in surgical/procedure rooms for near-patient testing.

The Plateletworks platelet function assay is available from Helena. This assay kit can be run on any standard impedance cell counter found in the hematology laboratory. Aggregation results are based on a platelet count before (high count) and after (lower count) platelet activation. Blood specimens are collected via venipuncture directly into tubes provided in the kit: an ethylenediaminetetraacetic acid (EDTA) tube for the baseline specimen and tubes with different agonists to aggregate platelets. Testing requires 1 mL of whole blood for the baseline count and 1 mL whole blood for each additional agonist-containing reagent tube. Results can be obtained in 2 minutes. The Plateletworks platelet function kit can be used for presurgical screening and to monitor antiplatelet therapy.[35]

Flow Cytometry

Flow cytometric assays are being developed for platelet function analysis. Flow cytometry offers several advantages over conventional platelet aggregation studies. Whole blood testing is performed, making for a more physiologic evaluation. Minimal specimen volumes are required (about 5 µL/test), allowing for ease of testing of pediatric and difficult-to-draw patients. The method is highly sensitive and able to capture platelet activity in patients with thrombocytopenia. Flow cytometry can measure multiple cellular activation-dependent changes related to platelet surface receptor upregulation and activation, generation of platelet microparticles, and binding of platelets to leukocytes, in addition to the traditional platelet secretion and aggregation markers. Flow cytometry assays are also available for the diagnosis of heparin-induced thrombocytopenia (HIT). At this time all platelet assays using flow cytometry analysis are laboratory developed tests (LDTs).

MOLECULAR COAGULATION TESTING

Molecular testing in the coagulation laboratory is available for patients with thrombophilia. Molecular testing is now readily available for gene mutations of factor V (FV Leiden) and prothrombin (prothrombin G20210A) for thrombophilia testing (Chapter 39). Testing for mutations of the methylene-tetrahydrofolate reductase (MTHFR) gene, a cause of thrombosis, are also performed to aid in the diagnosis. However, the clinical utility of MTHFR testing is not clear, and the American College of Medical Genetics and Genomics (ACMG) has recommended that MTHFR testing should not be routinely performed for the workup of patients with thrombophilia.[36]

There are several testing methods available for the clinical laboratory for the more commonly occurring, clinically relevant genetic mutations (Table 42.6). Cost and labor are considered when evaluating which test system to choose. The most

TABLE 42.6 Molecular Techniques for the Evaluation of a Hypercoagulable State

Assay	Accuracy	Throughput	Clinical Applications: Genetic Mutations Detected
PCR/RFLP	Good	Limited	Factor V Leiden, prothrombin G20210A, MTHFR
PCR/ARMS	Excellent	Intermediate	Factor V Leiden, prothrombin G20210A, MTHFR
Light cycler	Excellent	Intermediate	Factor V Leiden, prothrombin G20210A, MTHFR
Array technology	Excellent	Very high	Factor V Leiden, prothrombin G20210A, MTHFR
Invader assays	Excellent	Limited	Factor V Leiden, prothrombin G20210A, MTHFR
Ligand-based technologies	Excellent	Very high	Factor V Leiden, prothrombin G20210A, MTHFR

ARMS, Amplification refractory mutation system; *MTHFR,* methylene-tetrahydrofolate reductase; *PCR,* polymerase chain reaction; *RFLP,* restriction fragment length polymorphism.

common methods used are polymerase chain reaction (PCR)-based assays. PCR is accurate for the detection of both point mutations and single-nucleotide polymorphisms. FV Leiden, prothrombin G20210A, and *MTHFR* mutations are detectable by this method. A common method to analyze PCR products is restriction fragment-length polymorphism (RFLP) analysis. However, RFLP analysis is not a high-throughput method and is not suitable for high-volume laboratories.

Other methods for molecular testing in the clinical laboratory that are PCR based or not PCR based, that no longer require restriction digestion, are also available.[37–39] A popular non-PCR-based method is the Invader assay, which uses allele-specific hybridization in a high-throughput format.

In an effort to obtain rapid and reliable results, several new molecular methods have been developed. Sequence-specific primers, allele-specific oligonucleotides, hybridization, rapid-cycle PCR using LightCycler instrumentation, and nanochips are now available.

Major advantages of molecular testing for hemostatic biomarkers are the high sensitivity and specificity, and the lack of interference by anticoagulants or inhibitors in these assays.[38,39]

Molecular diagnostics in hemophilia and von Willebrand disease are available but currently limited. There is a strong potential for use of these assays in the diagnosis and classification of the subgroups of von Willebrand disease. Molecular diagnostics also may have a role in the diagnosis of hemophilia, mutations involved in factor VIII and factor IX genes, and potentially other coagulopathy associated mutations (Table 41.8) in the future.[39] Testing for these disorders is becoming more accessible with the decrease in cost of sequencing and availability of high-throughput next generation sequencing technologies. These newer sequencing technologies allow for simultaneous investigation of several genes, even though they may span a very extensive region. Genetic mutations associated with inherited platelet-dependent bleeding disorders are increasingly being identified. Currently known mutations are described in Chapters 37 and 38. As these mutations tend to be rare, reference laboratories that specialize in molecular testing aid in patient diagnosis and in discovering new clinically relevant genetic mutations.

More recently high-throughput sequencing (HTS) has become available for the diagnosis of hereditary bleeding and platelet disorders. The traditional sequencing information used a low-throughput technique called Sanger sequencing. This technique was slow, expensive, and had a low sensitivity. HTS allows for the sequencing of multiple DNAs in parallel, resulting in the sequencing of millions of DNA molecules at the same time. HTS can sequence an entire exome that can be used to identify variants or mutations in DNA and RNA responsible for different diseases. HTS has become the primary means of identifying genetic variants.[40] The complexity and size of the sequencing data require changes in the diagnostic process such that teams composed of clinicians, geneticists, and bioinformaticians are needed.

The role of molecular diagnostics in thrombophilia and bleeding disorders will continue to grow due to the identification of associated genetic mutations and polymorphisms.

The challenge for the laboratory is to determine which tests to offer and their relevance to patient management.

FUTURE TECHNOLOGIES FOR THE COAGULATION LABORATORY

With advances in technology, novel techniques that can potentially be used for coagulation testing are being developed. Lateral flow assays are a paper-based platform for the detection and quantitation of analytes in a complex mixture using antibody detection. This technology provides rapid results at a low cost. The principle is that a specimen containing the target analyte moves by capillary action through zones of a polymeric strip in which reagents are embedded. A typical test strip consists of overlapping membranes that are mounted on a backing card. The specimen is applied to one end of the strip; it travels through the sample pad, where it is buffered and then bound. The specimen then migrates through the conjugate release pad and is bound to a conjugated antibody that contains colored or fluorescent particles. In a final step, the target analyte-conjugated antibody migrates into the detection zone. A control line indicates the proper flow of the liquid through the strip. The difference between the intensities of the test line and the control line is the readout of the test result.[41]

The multifluidic chips using photolithography (semiconductors) can also be used for the application of multiple protein assays using a drop of blood. This technique integrates fluid handling with silver reduction in microelectronic chips. It allows for the measurement of several proteins at one time, with increased sensitivity for a more accurate diagnosis – this has been termed "lab on a chip (LOC)."[42]

These novel diagnostic technologies will no doubt become increasingly important for the prevention and diagnosis of diseases. As additional biomarkers are discovered, the diagnosis of diseases by determining levels of proteins, nucleic acids, and small molecules in blood will be an important tool in modern medicine. The new techniques should provide a low-cost, sensitive, and user friendly way to assist the health care team.

CURRENTLY AVAILABLE COAGULATION INSTRUMENTS

The heart of any clinical coagulation laboratory is the instrumentation that performs the high-volume tests of PT, PTT, and related clot-based assays, with the option of integrated chromogenic and immunoassays on the same platform. A variety of coagulometers address the increasing demand for test volume, random access testing, and test variety. All analyzers perform routine testing quickly and efficiently. The challenges lie in determining which instruments should be considered for a particular laboratory setting and in developing an organized approach for instrument evaluation. Table 42.7 lists several of the coagulation analyzers currently available, the type of end-point detection offered, and selected specialized features highlighted by the manufacturers in their product information.[43,44]

TABLE 42.7   Comparison of Available Coagulation Analyzers

Instrument Name/ Manufacturer	Sample Handling System	FDA-Cleared Clot-Based Tests	FDA-Cleared Chromogenic Tests	FDA-Cleared Immunologic Tests	Methodologies Supported	Standard Specimen Volume PT/PTT	Detection of Hemolysis/ Turbidity
Diagnostica Stago STA Satellite	Carousel—primary tube	PT, PTT, fibrinogen	Heparin (UFH, LMWH), AT	D-dimer	Clot detection, mechanical; chromogenic; immunologic	5 µL	No/no (mechanical method)
Diagnostica Stago STA-R Evolution	Rack with continuous access	PT, PTT, TT, fibrinogen, reptilase, factors, protein C, protein S, lupus anticoagulant, DRVVT screen and confirm	Heparin (UFH, LMWH), protein C, AT, plasminogen, antiplasmin	D-dimer, VWF, total and free protein S, AT antigen	Clot detection, mechanical; chromogenic; immunologic	5 µL	No/no (mechanical method)
Diagnostica Stago STA Compact, Max	Continuous specimen access—primary tube	PT, PTT, TT, fibrinogen, reptilase, factors, protein C, protein S, lupus anticoagulant, DRVVT	Heparin (UFH, LMWH), protein C, AT, plasminogen, antiplasmin	D-dimer, VWF, total and free protein S, AT antigen	Clot detection, mechanical	5 µL	No/no (mechanical method)
Helena Laboratories Cascade M-4	Manual	PT, PTT, fibrinogen, TT, factors II, V, VII to XII	None	None	Clot detection, optical, turbidometric	100 µL	No/no
Instrumentation Laboratory ACL 300/350	Continuous rack loading	PT, PTT, fibrinogen, TT, factors, FVIII (with VWF)	Anti-Xa, AT	D-dimer, D-dimer HS, HIT	Clot detection, LED optical; chromogenic; immunologic (turbidometric)	PT, PTT: 50 µL	Optional
Instrumentation Laboratory ACL 500/500	Continuous rack loading	PT, PTT, fibrinogen, TT, factors, lupus (SCT and DRVVT), protein C, protein S, aPCR-V, FVIII (with VWF)	Heparin anti-FXa, protein C, AT, plasminogen, plasmin inhibitor	D-dimer, D-dimer HS, VWF (activity and antigen), free protein S, FXIII antigen, homocysteine, HIT	Clot detection, LED optical; chromogenic; immunologic (turbidometric)	PT and PTT: 50 µL; FVIII: 25 µL	Optional
Instrumentation Laboratory ACL 700/750	Continuous rack loading	PT, PTT, fibrinogen, TT, factors, lupus (SCT and DRVVT), aPCR-V, protein C, protein S, FVIII (with VWF)	Heparin anti-FXa, protein C, AT, plasminogen, plasmin inhibitor	D-dimer, D-dimer HS, VWF (activity and antigen), free protein S, FXIII antigen, homocysteine, HIT	Clot detection, LED optical; chromogenic; immunologic	PT and PTT: 50 µL; FVIII: 25 µL	Optional
Instrumentation Laboratory ACL Elite Series	Tray-primary tubes	PT, PTT, fibrinogen, TT, factors, protein C, protein S, lupus (SCT and DRVVT), aPCR-V	Heparin anti-FXa, protein C, AT, plasminogen, antiplasmin, FVIII	D-dimer, VWF (activity and antigen), free protein S, FXIII antigen, homocysteine	Clot detection, LED optical (nephelometric); chromogenic; immunologic	PT and PTT: 60 µL; FVIII: 18 µL	No/no

Continued

Instrument	Sample handling	Clot-based assays	Chromogenic/immunologic assays	D-dimer	Detection	Sample volume	
Siemens CA-2500	10-Tube position sample rack × 5	PT, PTT, fibrinogen, TT, reptilase time, factors, DRVVT screen and confirm, FV Leiden, protein C clot, protein S activity	Innovance AT, Berichrom AT, plasminogen, FVIII chromogenic, antiplasmin, protein C chromogenic, heparin	Innovance D-dimer	Clot detection, optical, turbidometric; chromogenic; immunologic	50 µL/5 µL	No/yes
Siemens CA-5100	Rack	PT, PTT, fibrinogen, TT, reptilase time, factors, DRVVT screen and confirm, FV Leiden, protein C clot, protein S activity	Innovance AT, Berichrom AT, plasminogen, FVIII chromogenic, antiplasmin, protein C chromogenic, heparin	Innovance D-dimer	Clot detection, optical, turbidometric; chromogenic; immunologic	50 µL/5 µL	No/yes
Siemens BCS XP	10-Tube position specimen rack	PT, PTT, fibrinogen, TT, reptilase time, factors, DRVVT screen and confirm, FV Leiden, protein C clot, protein S activity	Innovance AT, Berichrom AT, plasminogen, FVIII chromogenic, antiplasmin, protein C chromogenic, heparin	Innovance D-dimer	Clot detection, optical (xenon flasher lamp); chromogenic; immunologic	50 µL/20 µL min. 100 µL (includes dead volume)/50 µL	Yes/no
Siemens CA-600	10-Tube position specimen rack	PT, PTT, fibrinogen, TT, reptilase time, protein C clot, factor assays	Innovance AT, Berichrom AT, protein C chromogenic, heparin	Innovance D-dimer	Clot detection, optical; turbidometric; chromogenic; immunologic	50 µL/5 µL	No/yes
LABiTech GmbH CoaData 2004 and 4004	Semiautomated manual pipette—auto start	PT, PTT	None	None	Clot detection, optical; turbodensitometric	50 µL	No/no

aPCR, Activated protein C resistance; *AT,* antithrombin; *DRVVT,* dilute Russell viper venom test; *F,* factor; *FDA,* US Food and Drug Administration; *LMWH,* low molecular weight heparin; *HS,* high sensitivity; *PT,* prothrombin time; *PTT,* partial thromboplastin time; *SCT,* silica clotting test; *TT,* thrombin clotting time; *UFH,* unfractionated heparin; *VWF,* von Willebrand factor.

SUMMARY

- Advanced technology used in semiautomated and automated analyzers has greatly improved coagulation testing accuracy and precision.
- End-point detection methodologies used by modern coagulation analyzers include mechanical, photo-optical, nephelometric, chromogenic, and immunologic methods.
- Advances in end-point detection methodologies have greatly expanded the testing capabilities available in the routine coagulation laboratory.
- Markedly improved instrument precision and reduced reagent volume requirements have led to substantial cost savings in coagulation testing.
- Instrument manufacturers have incorporated many features that have enhanced efficiency, safety, and diagnostic capabilities in hemostasis testing.
- Coagulation analyzer flagging alert functions warn the operator when specimen or instrument conditions exist that might lead to invalid test results, so that appropriate actions can be taken to ensure test accuracy.

- Each method of end-point detection has advantages and disadvantages that must be recognized and understood to ensure the validity of test results.
- Coagulation testing has been incorporated into the arena of point-of-care testing primarily to enhance the patient's and physician's ability to monitor oral anticoagulant therapy.
- Several methods to evaluate platelet function are available for both general platelet function testing and antiplatelet drug monitoring.
- The role of molecular diagnostics will continue to grow to identify new mutations and polymorphisms associated with bleeding and clotting disorders.
- A systematic approach to the evaluation and selection of a new coagulation analyzer should be developed and followed to determine the best instrument for a specific laboratory setting.

Now that you have completed this chapter, go back and read again the case study at the beginning and respond to the questions presented.

REVIEW QUESTIONS

Answers can be found in the Appendix.

1. Which of the following includes the advances made in technology in the coagulation lab?
   a. Primary tube sampling
   b. Random access testing
   c. Reduced specimen and reagent volumes
   d. All of the above

2. Which of the following is considered to be an advantage of the mechanical end-point detection methodology?
   a. It is not affected by lipemia in the test specimen
   b. It has the ability to provide a graph of clot formation
   c. It can incorporate multiple wavelengths into a single testing sequence
   d. It can measure proteins that do not have fibrin formation as the end-point

3. What method of detection is used in both the TEG and ROTEM?
   a. Photo-optical
   b. Chromogenic end-point
   c. Viscoelastic
   d. Immunologic

4. Which of the following is a feature of semiautomated coagulation testing analyzers?
   a. The temperature is maintained externally by a heat block or water bath
   b. Reagents and specimens usually are added manually by the operator
   c. Timers are automatically started as soon as the analyzer adds reagents to the test cuvette
   d. The end-point must be detected by the operator

5. When a specimen has been flagged as being icteric by an automated coagulation analyzer, which method would be most susceptible to erroneous results because of the interfering substance?
   a. Mechanical clot detection
   b. Immunologic antigen-antibody reaction detection
   c. Photo-optical clot detection
   d. Chromogenic end-point detection

6. Which of the following newer techniques can be used for the measurement of platelet function testing in patients with thrombocytopenia and in pediatrics?
   a. PFA-100
   b. Flow cytometry
   c. Lumi-aggregation
   d. PAP-8E

7. All of the following are performance characteristics to consider in the selection of a coagulation analyzer *except:*
   a. Location of the manufacturer's home office
   b. Instrument footprint
   c. Ease of use for the operator
   d. Variety of tests the instrument can perform

8. Platelet function is measured by the PFA-100 using which of the following methods?
   a. Detecting the change in blood flow pressure along a small tube when a clot impairs blood flow
   b. Detecting the aggregation of latex beads coated with platelet activators
   c. Graphing the transmittance of light through platelet-rich plasma over time after addition of platelet activators
   d. Detecting the time it takes for a clot to form as blood flows through a small aperture in a tube coated with platelet activators

9. A clinical setting where point-of-care testing is used in high volume is:
   a. To monitor patients receiving oral anticoagulant therapy
   b. To monitor patients taking platelet inhibitors such as aspirin
   c. To provide a baseline for all subsequent patient test result comparisons when the patient starts any kind of anticoagulant therapy
   d. To monitor obstetric patients at risk of fetal loss

10. Molecular testing can be used to diagnose patients with:
    a. Thrombocytopenia
    b. Factor V Leiden
    c. Prothrombin 20210A
    d. Both b and c

REFERENCES

1. McGlinchey, K. (2009). Sophistication in coagulation platforms. *Adv Med Lab Prof, 20,* 20–21.
2. Owen, C. A. (2002). History of blood coagulation. *JAMA, 87,* 1051–1052.
3. Bender, G. T. (1998). *Principles of Chemical Instrumentation: STA-R Operator's Manual.* (pp.119-124). Parsippany, NJ: Diagnostica Stago.
4. Johns, C. S. (2007). Coagulation instrumentation. In Rodak, B. G., Fritsma, G. A., & Doig, K. (Eds.), *Hematology: Clinical Principles and Applications.* (3rd ed., pp. 714–728). St. Louis, Elsevier.
5. Gram, J., & Jespersen, J. (1999). Introduction to laboratory assays in haemostasis and thrombosis. In Jepersen, J., Bertina, R. M., & Haverkate, F. (Eds.), *Laboratory Techniques in Thrombosis—A Manual.* (2nd ed., pp. 1–7). Boston: Kluwer Academic Publishers.
6. *BBL FibroSystem Manual.* (1992). Sparks, MD: BD Diagnostics Systems.
7. *STA Liatest D-Di.* (2005). Parsippany, NJ: Diagnostica Stago.
8. Fareed, J., Bermes, E. W. Jr., & Walenga, J. (1984). Automation in coagulation testing. *J Clin Lab Auto, 4,* 415–425.
9. Fareed, J., & Walenga, J. (1983). Current trends in hemostatic testing. *Semin Thromb Hemost, 9,* 379–391.
10. Fareed, J., Bick, R. L., Squillaci, G., et al. (1983). Molecular markers of hemostatic disorders: implications in the diagnosis and therapeutic management of thrombotic and bleeding disorders. *Clin Chem, 29,* 1641–1658.
11. Thomas, L. C., & Sochynsky, C. L. (1999). Multiple measuring modes of coagulation instruments. *Clin Hemost Rev, 13,* 8.
12. *Behring Nephelometer 100 Operator's Manual.* (1995). Deerfield, IL: Dade Behring, Inc.
13. Schueter, A., & Olson, J. D. (2002). Coagulation instrumentation: the hospital laboratory to the home. *Adv Lab Methods Haematol,* 316–336.
14. Allen, R., & Sheridan, B. (1999, Jan). Service above all. *CAP Today.* (pp. 39–60).
15. Laga, A. C., Cheves, T. A., & Sweeney, J. D. (2006). The effect of specimen hemolysis on coagulation test results. *Am J Clin Pathol, 126,* 748–756.
16. Dabkowski, B. (2012, May). Coagulation analyzers—point of care, self monitoring. *CAP Today.* (pp. 20–30).
17. Hobson, A. R., Agarwala, R. A., Swallow, K. D., et al. (2006). Thromboelastography: current clinical applications and its potential role in interventional cardiology. *Platelets, 17,* 509–518.
18. *ROTEM delta Manual.* (2011). Munich, Germany: Tem Innovations GmbH.
19. Harrison, P., & Mumford, A. (2009). Screening tests of platelet function: update on their appropriate uses for diagnostic testing. *Semin Thromb Hemost, 35,* 150–157.
20. Rodgers, R. P. C., & Levin, J. (1990). A critical reappraisal of the bleeding time. *Semin Thromb Hemost, 16,* 1–20.
21. Lind, D. E. (1991). The bleeding time does not predict surgical bleeding. *Blood, 77,* 2547–2552.
22. Gerwitz, A. S., Miller, M. L., & Keys, T. F. (1996). The clinical usefulness of the preoperative bleeding time. *Arch Pathol Lab Med, 120,* 353–356.
23. Peterson, P., Hayes, T. C., Arkin, C. F., et al. (1998). The preoperative bleeding time test lacks clinical benefit: College of American Pathologists' and American Society of Clinical Pathologists' position article. *Arch Surg, 133,* 134–139.
24. *Multiplate 5.0 Analyzer Product Information.* (2013). West Chester, OH: DiaPharma Corporation.
25. *PAP-8E Product Information.* (2005). Horsham, PA: BioData Corporation.
26. *Model 700 Aggregometer Product Information.* (2006). Havertown, PA: Chrono-Log Corporation.
27. *AggRAM Product Information.* (2005). Beaumont, TX: Helena Laboratories.
28. Kundu, S. K., Heilmann, E. F., Sio, R., et al. (1996). Characterization of an in vitro platelet function analyzer, PFA-100. *Clin Appl Thromb Hemost, 2,* 241–249.
29. Franchini, M. (2005). The platelet function analyzer (PFA-100): an update on its clinical use. *Clin Lab, 51,* 367–372.
30. Favaloro, E. J. (2008). Clinical utility of the PFA-100. *Semin Thromb Hemost, 34,* 709–733.
31. McKee, S. A., Sane, D. C., & Deliargyris, E. N. (2002). Aspirin resistance in cardiovascular disease: a review of prevalence, mechanisms, and clinical significance. *Thromb Haemost, 88,* 711–715.
32. Lordkipanidze, M., Pharand, C., Schampaert, E., et al. (2007). A comparison of six major platelet function tests to determine the prevalence of aspirin resistance in patients with stable coronary artery disease. *Eur Heart J, 28,* 1702–1708.
33. Dyskiewicz-Korpanty, D. M., Kim, A., Durner, J. D., et al. (2007). Comparison of a rapid platelet function assay—VerifyNow Aspirin—for the detection of aspirin resistance. *Thromb Res, 120,* 485–488.
34. McGlasson, D. L., & Fritsma, G. A. (2008). Comparison of four laboratory methods to assess aspirin sensitivity. *Blood Coagul Fibrinolysis, 19,* 120–123.
35. Hussein, H. M., Emiru, T., Georgiadis, A. L., et al. (2013). Assessment of platelet inhibition by point-of-care testing in neuroendovascular procedures. *Am J Neuroradiol, 34,* 700–706.
36. Hickey, S. E., Curry, C. J., & Toriello, H. V. (2013). ACMG Practice Guideline: lack of evidence for MTHFR polymorphism testing. *Genet Med, 15,* 153–156.
37. Nagy, P. L., Schrijver, I., & Zehnder, J. L. (2004). Molecular diagnosis of hypercoagulable states. *Lab Med, 35,* 214–221.

38. Ballestros, E. (2006). Molecular diagnostics in coagulation. In Coleman, W. B., & Tsongalis, J. (Eds.), *Molecular Diagnostics For the Clinical Laboratorian.* (2nd ed., pp. 311–320). New York: Humana Press.

39. Perrotta, P. L., & Svensson, A. M. (2009). Molecular diagnostics in hemostatic disorders. *Clin Lab Med, 29,* 367–90.

40. Freson, K., & Turro, E. (2017). High-throughput sequencing approaches for diagnosing hereditary bleeding and platelet disorders. *J Thromb Haemost, 15,* 1262–1272.

41. Koczula, K. M., & Gallotta, A. (2016). Lateral flow assays. *Essays Biochem, 60,* 111–120.

42. Song, Y., Huang, Y., Liu, X., et al. (2014). Point-of-care technologies for molecular diagnostics using a drop of blood. *Trends Biotechnol, 32,* 132–139.

43. Dabkowski, B. (2013, Jan). Coagulation analyzers. *CAP Today.* (pp. 14–24).

44. Dabkowski, B. (2009, Jan). Coagulation analyzers offering speed, full menus and more. *CAP Today.* (pp. 19–29).

43

Hematology and Hemostasis in the Pediatric, Geriatric, and Pregnant Populations

Linda H. Goossen

OBJECTIVES

After completion of this chapter, the reader will be able to:

1. Describe the major differences in reference intervals for the complete blood count, reticulocyte count, and nucleated red blood cells in preterm newborns, full-term newborns, infants, children, adults, and elderly adults.
2. Explain the cause of physiologic anemia of infancy and the time frame in which it is expected.
3. Describe normal red blood cell (RBC) morphology in neonates.
4. Compare RBC survival in preterm and full-term infants with that in adults.
5. Recognize and list factors affecting specimen collection that can have an impact on the interpretation of hematology values in newborns.
6. Compare and contrast the morphology of lymphocytes in children and in adults, and indicate reasons for differences.
7. Describe the general association between age and hemoglobin levels in elderly adults.
8. Explain the clinical significance of anemia in elderly adults.
9. Name the two most common anemias in elderly adults and their common causes in this age group.
10. List other anemias affecting elderly individuals.
11. Compare the frequency of acute lymphoblastic leukemias and chronic lymphocytic leukemias in children and elderly adults.
12. Name hematologic malignancies that are more common in elderly adults than in other age groups.
13. Define and describe the physiologic anemia of pregnancy.
14. Compare the hemostatic systems of newborns, children, adults, pregnant women, and elderly adults, including the risk of bleeding and thrombosis.

OUTLINE

Pediatric Hematology and Hemostasis
Hematopoiesis
Pediatric Developmental Stages
Gestational Age and Birth Weight
Specimen Collection for the Neonate
Red Blood Cell Values in the Neonate
White Blood Cell Values in the Neonate
Platelet Values in the Neonate
Neonatal Hemostasis

Geriatric Hematology and Hemostasis
Aging and Hematopoiesis
Hematologic Parameters in Elderly Adults
Anemia and Elderly Adults
Hematologic Neoplasia in Elderly Adults
Geriatric Hemostasis
Gestational Hematology and Hemostasis
Anemia and the Pregnant Woman
Gestational Hemostasis

Hematology and hemostasis values are fairly stable throughout adult life, but significant differences exist in the pediatric and, to some extent, the geriatric and pregnant populations. This chapter focuses on the more significant differences.

PEDIATRIC HEMATOLOGY AND HEMOSTASIS

Children are not merely "small adults." The newborn infant, older child, and adult exhibit profound hematologic differences from one another; thus it is inappropriate to use adult reference intervals for the assessment of pediatric blood values. Historically, pediatric reference intervals were inferentially established from adult data because of the limitations in attaining analyzable data. Pediatric procedures required large blood draws and tedious methodologies and lacked standardization. The implementation of child-friendly phlebotomy techniques and micropediatric procedures has revolutionized laboratory testing. Pediatric hematology has emerged as a specialized science with age-specific reference intervals that correlate with the hematopoietic, immunologic, and chemical changes in a developing child.

Dramatic changes occur in the blood and bone marrow of the newborn infant during the first hours and days after birth, and there are rapid fluctuations in the quantities of all hematologic elements. Significant hematologic differences are seen between term and preterm infants and among newborns, infants, young children, and older children. This chapter reviews neonatal hematopoiesis, discussed in detail in Chapter 4, as a prerequisite to understanding the changes in pediatric hematologic reference intervals, morphologic features, and age-specific physiology that will be covered.

Hematopoiesis
Prenatal Hematopoiesis

Hematopoiesis, the formation and development of blood cells from hematopoietic stem cells, begins in the first weeks of embryonic development and proceeds systematically through three phases of development: mesoblastic (yolk sac), hepatic (liver), and myeloid (bone marrow). The first cells produced in the developing embryo are primitive erythroblasts formed in the yolk sac. These cells appear megaloblastic and circulate as large nucleated cells, synthesizing embryonic hemoglobins. A second wave of yolk-sac-derived erythroid progenitor cells, termed burst forming units-erythroid (BFU-E), appear around 4 weeks and are thought to seed the fetal liver.[1-3]

By the second month of gestation, hematopoiesis ceases in the yolk sac, and the liver becomes the center for hematopoiesis, reaching its peak activity during the third and fourth gestational months. Megakaryocytes and leukocytes of each cell type systematically make their appearance. In week 9 of gestation, lymphocytes can be detected in the region of the thymus. They are subsequently found in the spleen and lymph nodes. During the fourth and fifth gestational months, the bone marrow emerges as a major site of blood cell production, and it becomes the primary site by birth (Chapter 4).[1-3]

Hematopoiesis of the Neonate

Hematopoietically active bone marrow is referred to as red marrow, as opposed to inactive yellow (fatty) marrow. At the time of birth, the bone marrow is fully active and almost completely cellular, with all hematopoietic cell lineages undergoing cellular differentiation and amplification. In addition to the mature cells in fetal blood, there are significant numbers of circulating progenitor cells in cord blood.[2]

In a full-term infant, hepatic hematopoiesis has ceased except in widely scattered small foci that become inactive soon after birth.[1-3] Extramedullary hematopoiesis may be seen in times of stress, most commonly in the liver, spleen, lymph nodes, and paravertebral regions.[4]

Pediatric Developmental Stages

Pediatric hematologic values change markedly in the first weeks and months of life, and many variables influence the interpretation of what might be considered healthy at the time of birth. Thus it is important to provide age-appropriate pediatric hematology reference intervals that extend from neonatal life through adolescence. The pediatric population can be categorized with reference to three different developmental stages: the neonatal period, which represents the first 4 weeks of life; infancy, which incorporates the first year of life; and childhood, which spans age 1 to puberty (ages 8 to 12 years). Refer to the inside front cover for pediatric hematology reference ranges.

Gestational Age and Birth Weight

Hematologic values obtained from full-term infants generally do not apply to preterm infants, and laboratory values for low-birth-weight preterm infants differ from values for extremely low-birth-weight infants. A *full-term infant* is defined as an infant who has completed 37 to 42 weeks of gestation. Infants born before 37 weeks' gestation are referred to as *premature* or *preterm*, whereas infants delivered after 42 weeks are considered *postterm*.[5-7] Infants can be subcategorized further by birth weight as (1) appropriate size for gestational age; (2) small for gestational age, including low-birth-weight infants (2500 g or less); (3) very low-birth-weight infants (1500 g or less); (4) extremely low-birth-weight micropreemies (1000 g or less); and (5) large for gestational age (more than 4000 g).[6,7]

Specimen Collection for the Neonate

Neonatal hematologic values are affected by the gestational age of the infant, birth weight, the age in hours after delivery, the presence of illness, and the level of support required. Other important variables to be considered when evaluating laboratory data include site of sampling and technique (capillary vs. venous puncture, warm or unwarmed extremity), timing of sampling, and conditions such as the course of labor and the treatment of the umbilical vessels, and maternal drug use.[1,2] The presence of fetal hemoglobin (Hb F), bilirubin, and lipids in newborns can also interfere with hematology laboratory testing.[8] As with all laboratory testing, each laboratory should establish reference intervals based on its instrumentation, methods, and patient population (Chapter 2).

Red Blood Cell Values in the Neonate

Refer to the inside front cover of this book for red blood cell (RBC) reference intervals. The RBC count increases during the first 24 hours of life, remains at this plateau for about 2 weeks, and then slowly declines. This *"polycythemia" of the newborn*[9] may be explained by in utero hypoxia, which becomes more pronounced as the fetus grows. Hypoxia, the trigger for increased secretion of erythropoietin, stimulates erythropoiesis. At birth, the physiologic environment changes, and the fetus makes the transition from its placenta-dependent oxygenation to the increased tissue oxygenation by the lungs. This increased oxygen tension suppresses erythropoietin production, which is followed by a decrease in RBC and hemoglobin production. Studies show that erythropoietin levels before birth are equal to or greater than adult levels with a gradual drop to near zero a few weeks after birth.[10-12] This decline corresponds to the physiologic anemia seen at 5 to 8 weeks of life, with the RBCs reaching their lowest count at 7 weeks of age and hemoglobin reaching its lowest concentration at 9 weeks of age.

Erythrocyte morphology of the neonate. Early normoblasts are megaloblastic, hypochromic, and irregularly shaped. During hepatic hematopoiesis, normoblasts are smaller than the megaloblasts of the yolk sac but are still macrocytic. Erythrocytes remain macrocytic from the first 11 weeks of gestation until day 5 of postnatal life (Figure 43.1).[1,2,10,12,13]

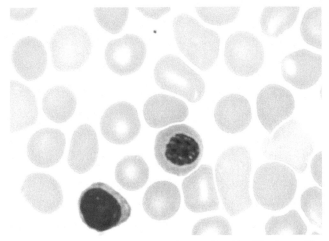

Figure 43.1 Peripheral Blood Film from a Healthy Newborn. Note the normal lymphocyte, macrocytes, polychromasia, and one nucleated red blood cell. (Peripheral blood, Wright-Giemsa stain, ×1000.)

The macrocytic RBC morphology gradually changes to the characteristic normocytic, normochromic morphology. Orthochromic normoblasts often are identified in the full-term infant on the first day of life but disappear within postnatal days 3 to 5. These nucleated RBCs (NRBCs) may persist longer than a week in immature infants. The average number of NRBCs ranges from 3 to 10 per 100 white blood cells (WBCs) in a healthy full-term infant to 25 NRBCs per 100 WBCs in a premature infant. The presence of NRBCs for more than 5 days suggests hemolysis, hypoxic stress, or acute infection.[1,2,10-12]

The erythrocytes of newborns show additional morphologic differences. The number of biconcave discs relative to stomatocytes is reduced in neonates (43% discs, 40% stomatocytes) compared with adults (78% discs, 18% stomatocytes).[14] In addition, increased numbers of pitted cells, burr cells, spherocytes, and other abnormally shaped erythrocytes are seen in neonates. The number of these "dysmorphic" cells is even higher in premature infants. Zipursky and colleagues found 40% discs, 30% stomatocytes, and 27% additional poikilocytes in premature infants.[1,14]

Reticulocyte Count

An apparent reticulocytosis exists during gestation, decreasing from 90% reticulocytes at 12 weeks' gestation to 15% at 6 months' gestation and ultimately to 4% to 6% at birth. Reticulocytosis persists for about 3 days after birth and then declines abruptly to 0.8% reticulocytes on postnatal days 4 to 7. At 2 months the number of reticulocytes increases slightly, followed by a slight decline from 3 months to 2 years, when adult levels of 0.5% to 2.5% are attained.[1,2,10-12] The reticulocyte count of premature infants is typically higher than that of term infants; however, the count can vary dramatically, depending on the extent of illness in the newborn. Significant polychromasia seen on a Wright-stained blood film is indicative of postnatal reticulocytosis (Figure 43.2).

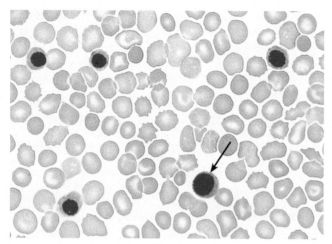

Figure 43.2 Peripheral Blood Film from a Premature Infant. Note the normal lymphocyte *(arrow)*, four nucleated red blood cells, and increased polychromasia. (Peripheral blood, Wright-Giemsa stain, ×500.)

Hemoglobin

Hemoglobin synthesis results from an orderly evolution of a series of embryonic, fetal, and adult hemoglobins. At birth Hb F constitutes 53% to 95% of the total hemoglobin.[2] Hb F declines from 90% to 95% at 30 weeks' gestation to approximately 7% at 12 weeks after birth and stabilizes at 2% to 3% by 6 months of age.[2] The switch from Hb F to Hb A is genetically controlled and determined by gestational age; it does not appear to be influenced by the age at which birth occurs.[2,12] Chapter 7 provides an in-depth discussion of the ontogeny, structure, and types of hemoglobin.

The concentration of hemoglobin fluctuates dramatically in the weeks and months after birth as a result of physiologic changes, and various factors must be considered when analyzing pediatric hematologic values. The site of sampling, gestational age, and time interval between delivery and clamping of the umbilical cord can influence the hemoglobin level in newborn infants.[1,2,5,6] In addition, there are significant differences between capillary and venous blood hemoglobin levels. Capillary specimens in newborns generally have a higher hemoglobin concentration than venous specimens, which can be attributed to circulatory factors.[10,12,13] Racial differences must also be considered when evaluating hemoglobin levels in children. Black children have hemoglobin levels averaging 0.5 g/dL lower than those in white children.[15,16]

The reference interval for hemoglobin for a full-term infant at birth is 16.5 to 21.5 g/dL; levels less than 14 g/dL are considered abnormal.[2,10] The average hemoglobin value for a preterm infant who is small for gestational age is 17.1 g/dL, lower than that for a full-term infant; hemoglobin values less than 13.7 g/dL are considered abnormal in preterm infants.[10]

Physiologic anemia of the neonate. The hemoglobin concentration of term infants decreases during the first 5 to 8 weeks of life, a condition known as physiologic anemia of infancy. Infants born prematurely also experience a decrease in hemoglobin concentration, which is termed *physiologic anemia of*

prematurity.[2,12] Along with a decrease in hemoglobin, there is a reduction in the number of RBCs, a decrease in the reticulocyte percentages (Table 43.1), and undetectable levels of erythropoietin associated with the transition from the placenta to the lungs as a source of oxygen. When the hemoglobin concentration decreases to approximately 11 g/dL, erythropoietic activity increases until it reaches its adult levels by age 14 years.[2,9,17,18] Also contributing to the physiologic anemia is the shortened life span of the fetal RBC. The lifespan of erythrocytes in term neonates is 60 to 70 days, compared with 35 to 50 days for premature neonates.[4] The more immature the infant, the shorter the lifespan.[1,12]

This physiologic anemia is not known to be associated with any abnormalities in the infant. The hemoglobin levels of premature infants are typically 1 g/dL or more below the values of full-term infants. Thereafter, a gradual recovery occurs, which results in values approximating those of healthy full-term infants by about 1 year of age.[9,11] Very low-birth-weight infants (less than 1500 g) show a progressive decline in hemoglobin, RBC count, mean cell volume (MCV), mean cell hemoglobin (MCH), and mean cell hemoglobin concentration (MCHC) and have a slower recovery than other preterm and term infants.

Hematocrit

The average capillary hematocrit (HCT) at birth for healthy full-term infants is 61% (reference interval, 48% to 68%).[1,2,12] Often newborns with increased HCTs, especially values greater than 65%, experience hyperviscosity of the blood. This can cause problems in producing a high-quality peripheral blood film.

The HCT usually increases approximately 5% during the first 48 postnatal hours; this is followed by a slow linear decline to 46% to 62% at 2 weeks and 32% to 40% between the second and fourth months.[1,2,13] Adult values of 47% for males and 42% for females are achieved during adolescence. Very low-birth-weight preterm infants are often anemic at birth (Table 43.1). Many require transfusions or erythropoietin injections or both.

Red Blood Cell Indices

The RBC indices and RBC distribution width provide one means for assessing the type of anemia (Chapter 16) described later.

TABLE 43.1 Hematologic Values for Very Low-Birth-Weight Infants During the First 6 Weeks of Life[18]

	AGE OF INFANT (DAYS)			
Hematologic Value	**3**	**12–14**	**24–26**	**40–42**
Hemoglobin (g/dL)	15.6	14.4	12.4	10.6
Hematocrit (%)	47	44	39	33
Red blood cells (×10^{12}/L)	4.2	4.1	3.8	3.4
Reticulocytes (%)	7.1	1.7	1.5	1.8
Platelets (×10^{9}/L)	203.5	318	338	357
White blood cells (×10^{9}/L)	9.5	12.3	10.4	9.1

Mean cell volume. The erythrocytes of newborn infants are markedly macrocytic at birth. The average MCV for full-term infants is 119 ± 9.4 fL; however, a sharp decrease occurs during the first 24 hours of life.[1,2] The MCV continues to decrease to 90 ± 12 fL in 3 to 4 months.[2,9,17] The more premature the infant, the higher the MCV. A newborn with an MCV of less than 94 fL should be evaluated for α-thalassemia or iron deficiency.[1,19]

Mean cell hemoglobin. MCH is 30 to 42 pg in healthy neonates and 27 to 41 pg in premature infants.[9,17]

Mean cell hemoglobin concentration. The average MCHC is the same for full-term infants, premature infants, and adults: approximately 33 g/dL.

Red blood cell distribution width. The red blood cell distribution width (RDW) is elevated in newborns, with a reference interval of 14.2% to 17.8% the first 30 days of life. After that it gradually decreases and reaches the adult reference interval by 6 months of age.[13]

Anemia in Infants and Children

Nutritional deficiencies in infants and children can result in iron deficiency anemia and, rarely, in megaloblastic anemia (Chapters 17 and 18), particularly in low-birth-weight and premature infants. These anemias are associated with abnormal psychomotor development; however, they can easily be treated with dietary fortification.[20,21]

Iron deficiency anemia. Iron deficiency anemia is the most common pediatric hematologic disorder and the most common cause of anemia in childhood.[22,23] Iron deficiency anemia is more prevalent in premature infant because the majority of the placental transfer of maternal iron occurs late in the third trimester.[4] The occurrence of iron deficiency anemia in infants has decreased in the United States because of iron fortification of infant formula and increased rates of breastfeeding.[24] However, the prevalence is still 2% in toddlers 1 to 2 years of age and 3% in children 3 to 5 years of age[25] and is related to early introduction and excessive intake of whole cow's milk.[20,25] Chapter 17 provides an in-depth discussion of iron deficiency anemia.

Ancillary tests for anemia in infants and children. The differential diagnosis of anemia in infants and children relies on a variety of ancillary tests. The reference intervals for a number of these tests differ from those for adults. Haptoglobin levels are so low as to be undetectable in neonates, which makes it unreliable as a marker of infant hemolysis.[26] Transferrin levels are also lower in neonates, increasing rapidly after birth and reaching adult levels at 6 months.[26] Both serum ferritin and serum iron are high at birth, rise during the first month, drop to their lowest level between 6 months and 4 years of age, and remain low throughout childhood.[27,28] Consideration of these differences is important when interpreting hematology laboratory results for infants and children.

White Blood Cell Values in the Neonate

Fluctuations in the number of WBCs are common at all ages but are greatest in infants (references ranges on inside front cover of the book). *Leukocytosis* is typical at birth for full-term and preterm infants, with a wide reference interval.[9] There is an excess of segmented neutrophils and bands and an occasional metamyelocyte, with no evidence of disease. The absolute neutrophil count rises within the first 8 to 12 hours after birth and then declines by 12 hours to a constant level.[2,9,29,30]

Neutrophilic Leukocytes

Term and premature infants have a greater absolute neutrophil count than that found in older children, who characteristically maintain a predominance of lymphocytes. Band forms are also higher for the first 3 to 4 days after birth (Table 43.2). Newborn girls have absolute neutrophil counts averaging 2000 cells/μL higher than those of boys; neonates whose mothers have undergone labor have higher counts than neonates delivered by cesarean section with no preceding maternal labor.[29,30] There is some evidence that absolute neutrophil counts are lower in healthy black children than in white children.[31]

Premature infants. At birth, preterm infants exhibit a left shift, with promyelocytes and myelocytes commonly observed. The trend to lymphocyte predominance occurs later than in full-term infants. The neutrophil counts in premature infants are similar to or slightly lower than the neutrophil counts in full-term infants during the first 5 days of life; however, the count gradually declines to 2.5×10^9/L (1.1 to 6.0×10^9/L) at 4 weeks.[32] There is no significant difference in the absolute neutrophil count of infants by birth weight or gestational age; however, very low-birth-weight infants have a significantly lower limit (1.0×10^9/L) compared with larger infants.[32,33]

Neutropenia. Neutropenia is defined as a reduction in the number of circulating neutrophils to less than 1.5×10^9/L. Neutropenia accompanied by bands and metamyelocytes is often associated with infection, particularly in preterm neonates. Neutropenia represents a decrease in neutrophil production or an increase in consumption.[34]

TABLE 43.2 Neutrophil and Band Counts for Newborns During the First 2 Days of Life

Age	Absolute Neutrophil Count ($\times 10^9$/L)	Absolute Band Count ($\times 10^9$/L)
Birth	3.5–6.0	1.3
12 hr	8.0–15.0	1.3
24 hr	7.0–13.0	1.3
36 hr	5.0–9.0	0.7
48 hr	3.5–5.2	0.7

Reference intervals were obtained from the assessment of 3100 separate white blood cell counts obtained from 965 infants; 513 counts were from infants considered to be completely healthy at the time the count was obtained and for the preceding and subsequent 48 hours. There was no difference in the reference intervals when values were stratified by infant birth weight or gestational age.

Modified from Luchtman-Jones, L., & Wilson, D. B. (2011). The blood and hematopoietic system. In Martin, R. J., Fanaroff, A. A., & Walsh, M. C. (Eds.), *Fanaroff and Martin's Neonatal-Perinatal Medicine* (9th ed., p. 1325). Philadelphia: Mosby.

Neutrophilia. *Neutrophilia* refers to an increase in the absolute number of neutrophils to greater than 8.0×10^9/L. Morphologic changes associated with infection include Döhle bodies, vacuoles, and toxic granulation.[35]

Eosinophils and Basophils

The percentages of eosinophils and basophils remain consistent throughout infancy and childhood. Refer to the inside front cover of this book for reference intervals.

Lymphocytes

Lymphocytes constitute about 30% of the leukocytes at birth and increase to 60% at 4 to 6 months. They decrease to 50% by 4 years, to 40% by 6 years, and to 30% by 8 years.[10] *Benign immature B cells* (hematogones), although predominantly found in the bone marrow, can sometimes be seen in the peripheral blood of newborns. These lymphocytes are primarily midstage B cells.[36,37] They vary in diameter from 10 to 20 μm, have scant cytoplasm and condensed but homogeneous nuclear chromatin, and may have small, indistinct nucleoli (Figures 43.3 and 43.4).[38] Although these lymphocytes may be similar in appearance to the malignant cells seen in childhood acute lymphoblastic leukemia (ALL), these benign cells lack the asynchronous or aberrant antigen expression seen in ALL and thus can be differentiated from the lymphocytes of infant ALL by immunophenotyping (Chapter 28).[39,40]

Monocytes

The mean monocyte count of neonates is higher than adult values. At birth the average proportion of monocytes is 6%. During infancy and childhood, an average of 5% is maintained, except in the second and third weeks, when the proportion increases to around 9%. The count reaches adult levels at 3 to 5 months.[13]

Neonatal hematologic response to infection. The immune response of newborns is considered "immature," with decreased responsiveness to agonists. This distinct immune response is postulated to be related to the demands of the fetal environment

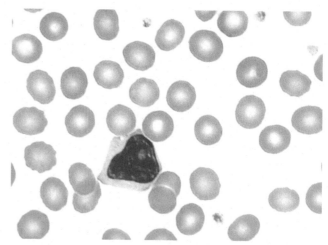

Figure 43.4 Peripheral Blood Film from a Healthy Newborn. Note the benign lymphocyte with visible nucleoli. (Peripheral blood, Wright-Giemsa stain, ×1000.)

and the need to avoid response to maternal antigens.[41] Sepsis in neonates is a common cause of morbidity, particularly in premature and low-birth-weight infants.[2,42,43] Defective B cell response against polysaccharide agents, as well as abnormal cytokine release by neutrophils and monocytes, has been implicated.[44-46] Because of the transient neutrophilia that occurs during the first 24 hours after birth, followed by a rapid decline, the neutrophil count is not a satisfactory index of infection in the newborn. Newborns with bacterial infections often have neutrophil counts within or less than the reference interval with a shift to the left. Thus many practitioners depend on the band count and its derived immature-to-total neutrophil ratio as an indicator of sepsis in neonates,[47] although CD64 index, C-reactive protein (CRP), and procalcitonin levels have been suggested as more sensitive markers of sepsis in infants and children.[47-49]

Platelet Values in the Neonate

The platelet count ranges from 150 to 400×10^9/L for full-term and preterm infants, comparable to adult values (Table 43.3).[2] Thrombocytopenia of fewer than 100×10^9/L may be seen in high-risk infants with sepsis or respiratory distress and neonates with trisomy syndromes.[2] Platelets of a newborn infant

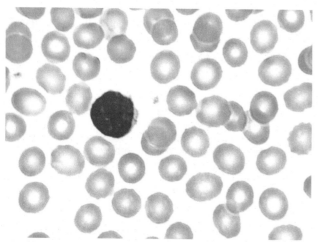

Figure 43.3 Peripheral Blood Film from a Healthy Newborn. Note the benign lymphocyte. (Peripheral blood, Wright-Giemsa stain, ×1000.)

TABLE 43.3	**Platelet Count Reference Intervals for Full-Term and Preterm Infants**	
Age	**Platelet Count** **($\times 10^9$/L; mean ± 1 SD)**
Preterm infants, 27–31 wk	275 ± 60
Preterm infants, 32–36 wk	290 ± 70
Term infants	310 ± 68
Healthy child/adult	300 ± 50

SD, Standard deviation.
Adapted from Oski, F. A., & Naiman, J. L. (1982). Normal blood values in the newborn period. In *Hematologic Problems in the Newborn*, Philadelphia: WB Saunders.

have great variation in size and shape and are characterized as hypofunctional compared with adult platelets. Cord-blood–derived platelets have impaired calcium mobilization, glycoprotein IIb/IIIa (GPIIb/IIIa) activation, dense granule secretion, and α-granule release compared with adult platelets. However, bleeding times, PFA-100 closure times, and thromboelastography have superior functionality (tests described in Chapters 41 and 42). Although neonatal platelets function differently than adult platelets, they are effective in their role of primary hemostasis.[50] Neonatal thrombocytopenia is discussed in Chapter 38.

Neonatal Hemostasis
Specimen Collection and Management
Specimen collection and handling for hemostatic testing in neonates follows the principles described in Chapter 41. However, for this population attention should be given to the collection procedure guidelines established for patients with small vessels, capillary specimen collection by skin puncture, and procedures for heel stick specimen collection described on the Evolve website.

Hemostatic Components
The physiology of the hemostatic system in infants and children is different from that in adults (Chapter 35) (reference ranges are on the inside back cover of the book). The vitamin K-dependent coagulation factors (factors II, VII, IX, and X) are about 30% of adult values at birth; they reach adult values after 2 to 6 months, although the mean values remain lower in children than in adults. Levels of factor XI, factor XII, prekallikrein, and high-molecular-weight kininogen are between 35% and 55% of adult values at birth, reaching adult values after 4 to 6 months.

In contrast, the levels of fibrinogen, factor VIII, and von Willebrand factor (VWF) are similar to adult values throughout childhood.[51,52] Factor V decreases during childhood, with lower levels during the teen years compared with adults.

The physiologic anticoagulants and inhibitors of coagulation (protein C, protein S, and antithrombin) and a disintegrin and metalloprotease with a thrombospondin type 1 motif, member 13 (ADAMTS13) that cleaves ultralong VWF multimers are reduced at about 30% to 40% at birth. Antithrombin and protein S reach adult values by 3 months, whereas protein C does not reach adult levels until after 6 months.[51]

In the fibrinolytic system, plasminogen has both lower levels and decreased activity in neonates compared with adults; α2-antiplasmin is lower than adult levels at birth (Table 43.4).

Tissue plasminogen activator (TPA) and plasminogen activator inhibitor-1 (PAI-1) levels are increased; however, 5 times the amount of TPA is required to activate plasminogen compared with activation of plasminogen in adults.[53]

The hemostatic components are not only changing in concentration over the first few weeks to months of life, but their values are also dependent on the gestational age of the child. Premature infants have different values at birth than term infants. Prothrombin time (PT) and partial thromboplastin time (PTT) tests are longer, most coagulation factor assays measure lower values, and control proteins levels are lower in healthy preterm infants than in term infants, whereas plasminogen level is lower and TPA is the same.[53]

Bleeding and Thrombosis
The risk of bleeding is not increased in a healthy newborn despite the decreased levels of the vitamin K-dependent coagulation factors. This is primarily related to the reduced levels of the physiologic anticoagulants protein C and protein S.[54]

The risk of thrombosis is considerably less in neonates and children than in adults. However, two age-related peaks in frequency occur: the first in the neonatal period and the second in postpuberty adolescence.[55] Central venous catheters, cancer, and chemotherapy are the most common risk factors in both of these groups.[56,57] Hemorrhagic and thrombotic disorders are discussed in Chapters 36 and 39, respectively.

GERIATRIC HEMATOLOGY AND HEMOSTASIS

In 2014 there were 46 million people in the United States aged 65 and older, accounting for 15% of the population. The older population in 2030 is projected to be twice as large as in 2000, growing from 35 million to 74 million and representing 21% of the total US population.[58] The life expectancy and quality of life of elderly adults have improved dramatically in recent decades. Life expectancies at both age 65 and age 85 have increased. Under current conditions, people who survive to age 65 can expect to live an average of 19.4 more years—almost 5 years longer than people aged 65 in 1960.[59] In 2015 the life expectancy of people who survived to age 85 was 13 years for women and 11.2 years for men.[60]

Elderly adults can be roughly divided into three age categories: the *young-old*, aged 65 to 74; the *old-old*, aged 74 to 84; and the *very old*, aged 85 and older.[61] Although disease and disabilities are not a function of age, age is a risk factor for

TABLE 43.4 Reference Intervals for Fibrinolytic Proteins in the Healthy Full-Term Infant During the First 6 Months of Life

Fibrinolytic Proteins	Day 1	Day 5	Day 30	Day 90	Day 180	Adult
Plasminogen (%)	125–265	141–293	126–270	174–322	221–381	248–424
Tissue plasminogen activator (ng/mL)	5.0–18.9	4.0–10.0	1.0–6.0	1.0–5.0	1.0–6.0	1.4–8.4
α2-Antiplasmin (%)	55–115	70–130	76–124	76–140	83–139	68–136
Plasminogen activator inhibitor-1 (%)	20–151	0–81	0–88	10–153	60–130	0–110

From Andrew, M., Paes, B., & Johnston, M. (1990). Development of the hemostatic system in the neonate and young infant. *Am J Pediatr Hematol Oncol, 12*(1), 95–104.

many diseases. With the increase in the aging population, the incidence of age-related health conditions also is likely to increase.

Aging and Hematopoiesis

The aging process is associated with the functional decline of several organ systems, such as cardiovascular, renal, musculoskeletal, and pulmonary, and bone marrow reserve. Certain cells lose their ability to divide (e.g., nervous tissue, muscles), whereas others, such as bone marrow and the gastrointestinal mucosa, remain mitotic. Marrow cellularity begins at 80% to 100% in infancy and decreases to about 50% after 30 years, followed by a decline to 30% after age 65.[62,63] These changes may be due to a reduction in the volume of cancellous (trabecular or spongy) bone, along with an increase in fat, rather than to a decrease in hematopoietic tissue.[63] Telomere shortening, which determines the number of divisions a cell undergoes, has not been definitively correlated to age-related hematopoietic stem cell exhaustion in humans[64]; however, it is speculated to be associated with hematopoietic stem cell differentiation.[65]

Hematologic Parameters in Elderly Adults

In 1930 Wintrobe published hematologic reference ranges that are still in use today. These were derived from healthy young adults, yet what constitutes "normal" for elderly patients is a matter of considerable debate. There is controversy concerning the assignment of geriatric age-specific reference intervals, especially because aging is often accompanied by physiologic changes and the prevalence of disease increases markedly.

The baseline values for elderly adults are the same reference intervals used for healthy adults; however, the heterogeneity in the aging process and difficulty in separating the effects of age from the effects of occult diseases that accompany aging emphasize the importance of proper interpretation of hematologic data and requires a complete understanding of the association between disease and older age. This section focuses on hematologic changes in elderly adults and discusses hematologic reference intervals for various geriatric age groups as well as hematopathologic conditions seen in the geriatric population.

Red Blood Cells

Most RBC parameters (e.g., RBC count, indices, and RDW) for healthy elderly adults do not show significant deviations from those for younger adults. There is a gradual decline in hemoglobin starting at middle age, with the mean level decreasing by about 1 g/dL during the sixth through eighth decades.[66] Men older than 60 years have average hemoglobin levels of 12.4 to 15.3 g/dL. The hemoglobin levels in women may increase slightly with age or remain unchanged. Elderly women have hemoglobin concentrations ranging from 11.7 to 13.8 g/dL. Men normally have higher hemoglobin levels than women because of the stimulating effect of androgens on erythropoiesis; however, the difference narrows as androgen levels decrease in elderly men and estrogen levels decrease in older women. Typically the lowest hemoglobin levels are found in the oldest patients (Table 43.5).

TABLE 43.5 Hematologic Values in Ambulatory Healthy Adults

	84–98 yr	30–50 yr
Red Blood Cells (×10^{12}/L)		
Males	4.8 ± 0.4	5.1 ± 0.2
Females	4.5 ± 0.3	4.6 ± 0.3
Hemoglobin (g/dL)		
Males	14.8 ± 1.1	15.6 ± 0.7
Females	13.6 ± 1.0	14.0 ± 0.8
Hematocrit (%)		
Males	43.8 ± 3.3	45.3 ± 2.2
Females	40.7 ± 2.9	41.6 ± 2.3
Mean Cell Volume (fL)		
Males	91.3 ± 5.4	87.8 ± 2.8
Females	90.5 ± 4.1	90.5 ± 5.0
Mean Cell Hemoglobin (pg)		
Males	31.0 ± 2.0	30.1 ± 1.6
Females	30.2 ± 1.2	30.3 ± 2.1
Mean Cell Hemoglobin Concentration (g/dL)		
Males	33.7 ± 1.5	34.2 ± 1.5
Females	33.4 ± 1.2	33.5 ± 1.5
White Blood Cells (×10^9/L)		
	7.6 ± 0.5	8.8 ± 0.4
Platelets (×10^9/L)		
	277 ± 21	361 ± 38
Neutrophils (×10^9/L)		
	4.5 ± 0.3	5.9 ± 0.3
Lymphocytes (×10^9/L)		
	1.9 ± 0.3	1.9 ± 0.8

Mean values ± 1 standard deviation.
Adapted from Zauber, N. P., & Zauber, A. G. (1987). Hematologic data of healthy very old people. *JAMA, 257,* 2181–2184; and Chatta, G. S., & Lipschitz, D. A. (2003). Aging of the hematopoietic system. In Hazzard, W. R., Blass, J. P., Halter, J. B., et al. (2003). *Principles of Geriatric Medicine and Gerontology,* (5th ed., p. 767). New York: McGraw-Hill.

Leukocytes

In the absence of any underlying pathologic condition, there are no statistically significant differences between the total leukocyte count and WBC differential for the young-old and old-old and those for middle-aged adults. Some investigators, however, have reported a lower leukocyte count in elderly adults, owing primarily to a decrease in the lymphocyte count.[67] Other studies have found no change in WBC with age.[68]

Immune response in elderly adults. Infectious diseases are an important cause of morbidity and mortality in elderly adults. Aged adults are more susceptible to infection, take longer to recover from infection, and are often less responsive to vaccination.[69] The adverse changes that occur in the function of the immune system with age are called immunosenescence.[70] Although all components of immunity are affected, T cells appear to be the most susceptible.[71,72] The thymus disappears by early middle age, and adults must then depend on their T-lymphocyte pool in the secondary tissues to mediate T cell–dependent immune responses. The number of naive T cells decreases in elderly adults, which increases the dependence on memory T cells. T cells of elderly adults have impaired responsiveness to mitogens and antigens as a result of decreased expression of costimulator receptor ligand molecules CD80 and CD86.[72] T cells are turned off as a result of increased expression of PD-L1 ligand that binds to PD-1, a negative costimulatory receptor.[72] There is also an alteration of T cell signaling with aging.[73-75] B-lymphocyte function depends on T cell interaction. Thus the decreased ability to generate antibody responses, especially to primary antigens, may be the result of T cell changes rather than intrinsic defects in B lymphocytes.

Many neutrophil functions are decreased in elderly adults, including chemotaxis, phagocytosis of microorganisms, and generation of superoxide. Studies indicate that these defects may be associated with changes to the cell membrane or to receptor signaling.[69]

Monocytes and Macrophages

The aging process does not significantly affect the number of monocytes. Information on the effects of aging on monocyte and macrophage function is limited and often conflicting.[69] Recent studies provide evidence for defects in the Toll-like receptor (TLR) function in monocytes and macrophages in older individuals.[69] The TLRs play a crucial role in the immune response.[76]

Platelets

The platelet count does not significantly change with age. There have been reports of increased levels of β-thromboglobulin and platelet factor 4 in the α-granules of platelets and increased platelet phospholipid content.[77] Thrombocytopenia may be drug induced or secondary to marrow infiltration of metastatic cancer, lymphoma, or leukemia (Chapter 38). Essential thrombocythemia is a myeloproliferative neoplasm characterized by sustained proliferation of megakaryocytes, resulting in platelet counts of 450×10^9/L or greater (Chapter 32).[78] Primary thrombocytosis can also be seen in chronic myeloid leukemia.

Anemia and Elderly Adults

Anemia is common in elderly adults and its prevalence increases with age; however, anemia should not be viewed as an inevitable consequence of aging.[79,80] Although anemia in elderly adults is typically mild, it has been associated with substantial morbidity and mortality.[81] The World Health Organization (WHO) defines anemia as hemoglobin less than 13 g/dL in men and less than 12 g/dL in women. Using the WHO definition of anemia, the Third National Health and Nutrition Examination Survey (NHANES III), a national study that samples clinical specimens, found the prevalence of anemia in the United States in individuals older than 65 years to be 11% in men and 10.2% in women. This prevalence increases rapidly with age, and exceeds 20% in individuals aged 85 or older.[82]

The factors contributing to anemia include a decrease in bone marrow function, a decline in physical activity, nutritional deficiencies, cardiovascular disease, and chronic inflammatory disorders. Unexplained anemia, anemia of inflammation, iron deficiency anemia, and anemia as a result of hematologic malignancies are the most common causes of anemia in elderly adults.[83]

Ineffective erythropoiesis and hypoproliferation are also seen in elderly adults. Ineffective erythropoiesis is associated with vitamin B_{12} or folate deficiency, myelodysplastic syndrome, sideroblastic anemia, and thalassemia. Hypoproliferative anemia often occurs secondary to iron deficiency, vitamin B_{12} or folate deficiency, renal failure, hypothyroidism, chronic inflammation, or endocrine disease.[83] To a lesser extent, elderly adults are at risk for anemias such as aplastic anemia, hemolytic anemia, myelophthisic anemia, and anemia caused by protein-calorie malnutrition.

The initial laboratory evaluation of anemia should include a complete blood count (CBC), reticulocyte count, peripheral blood film review, and chemistry panel, along with other diagnostic tools, including iron studies (with ferritin), vitamin B_{12}, and folate levels. Table 43.6 indicates the types of anemia suggested by MCV and RDW results. In addition, assessment for signs of gastrointestinal blood loss, hemolysis, nutritional deficiencies, malignancy, chronic infection, renal or hepatic disease, or other chronic disease can provide important information for the evaluation of anemia in elderly adults.

TABLE 43.6 Classification of Geriatric Anemia Based on Typical Mean Cell Volume (MCV) and Red Cell Distribution Width (RDW)

MCV	RDW	Anemia
Normal	Normal	Anemia of chronic inflammation (some) Hemorrhagic anemia Leukemia-associated anemia
	High	Early iron deficiency anemia Mixed deficiency anemia (e.g., vitamin B_{12} and iron) Sideroblastic anemia
Low	Normal	Anemia of chronic inflammation (some)
	High	Iron deficiency anemia
High	Normal	Anemia associated with myelodysplastic syndrome
	High	Vitamin B_{12} deficiency anemia Folate deficiency anemia Hemolytic anemia

Note that this classification is not absolute because there can be an overlap of RDW values among some of the conditions in each MCV category.

Anemia of Chronic Inflammation

Anemia of inflammation, also known as *anemia of chronic disease,* often occurs with chronic inflammatory disorders (e.g., rheumatoid arthritis, vasculitis, liver disease), chronic infections, congestive heart failure, and malignant diseases (e.g., Hodgkin lymphoma, leukemia, plasma cell myeloma).[84] This hypoproliferative anemia is the most common form of anemia in the hospitalized geriatric population.[85] Hepcidin-induced inhibition of iron absorption in the intestines and iron mobilization from macrophages and hepatocytes and impaired erythropoietin-dependent erythropoiesis triggered by inflammatory cytokines are involved in the pathogenesis of anemia of chronic inflammation (Chapter 17).[86]

Iron Deficiency Anemia

Iron deficiency anemia is common cause of anemia in elderly adults, with a prevalence of 25%.[82] Iron deficiency affects not only erythrocytes but also the metabolic pathways of iron-dependent tissue enzymes. Hemoglobin synthesis is reduced, and even a minimal decrease can cause profound functional disabilities in an elderly patient. The serum iron level decreases progressively with each decade of life, particularly in women. Nevertheless, healthy elderly adults usually have serum iron levels within the adult reference interval.

Iron deficiency anemia in elderly adults rarely is due to dietary deficiency in industrialized nations because of the prevalence of iron fortification of grains, as well as a diet that includes meats containing heme iron. Iron deficiency in elderly adults most often results from conditions leading to chronic gastrointestinal blood loss, including long-term use of nonsteroidal antiinflammatory medications, gastritis, peptic ulcer disease, gastroesophageal reflux disease with esophagitis, colon cancer, and angiodysplasia.[87,88] It also may be due to poor diet in an elderly individual who has lost the taste or desire for food or is unable to prepare nutritious meals. Chapter 17 discusses iron disorders in detail.

Unexplained Anemia of the Elderly

Unexplained anemia of the elderly (UAE) is responsible for approximately 30% of anemias in elderly adults.[82,89] UAE is a hypoproliferative anemia that is not caused by nutritional deficiency, chronic kidney disease, or inflammatory disease. The anemia is typically mild and normocytic, with hemoglobin levels between 10 to 12 g/dL. Data suggest that UAE occurs as result of a failure of a normal erythropoietin response to anemia.[82,85] It is hypothesized that UAE is related to a declining testosterone level, underlying stem cell disorder, or increased proinflammatory cytokines that are expressed in the aging population.[82,86,89]

Ineffective Erythropoiesis

Ineffective erythropoiesis has been attributed not only to maturation disorders such as vitamin B_{12} and folic acid deficiency but also to sideroblastic anemia, thalassemia, and myelodysplastic syndrome. Sideroblastic anemias are characterized by impaired heme synthesis, and abnormal globin synthesis occurs in the thalassemias (Chapters 17 and 25). Megaloblastic anemia results from defective synthesis of DNA with compromised cell division but normal cytoplasmic development (i.e., asynchrony) (Chapter 18).[90] These megaloblastic cells are more prone to destruction in the bone marrow, which results in ineffective erythropoiesis. Two causes of megaloblastic anemia are vitamin B_{12} deficiency and folate deficiency. Myelodysplastic syndrome results in ineffective hematopoiesis as a result of mutations in hematopoietic stem cells and progenitor cells. It is more common in elderly adults and is discussed later.

Vitamin B_{12} deficiency. Vitamin B_{12} (cobalamin) deficiency has been reported in 10% to 20% of elderly patients; however, clinically significant vitamin B_{12} deficiency is identified in less than 1% of the elderly population.[82] Neurologic complications are found in 75% to 90% of individuals with clinically apparent vitamin B_{12} deficiency.[91] In the absence of anemia, neurologic symptoms may be the only indication. Even when anemia is present, it does not always manifest with the classic macrocytic and megaloblastic picture but may be normocytic.

Vitamin B_{12} deficiency in elderly adults has been attributed to inadequate intestinal absorption of food-bound vitamin B_{12} rather than pernicious anemia or inadequate intake.[92,93] Many elderly individuals have atrophic gastritis resulting in decreased gastric production of acid. In this condition there is low vitamin B_{12} absorption because protein-bound vitamin B_{12} is not dissociated from food proteins and therefore cannot bind to intrinsic factor for absorption.[94] In addition, the loss of gastric acid can result in bacterial overgrowth, particularly with *Helicobacter pylori*, which also interferes with vitamin B_{12} absorption. Inadequate vitamin B_{12} absorption in elderly adults has also been reported in other uncommon conditions such as small bowel disorder, gastric resection, pancreatic insufficiency, resection of the terminal ileum, blind loop syndrome, and tropical sprue.[95] Pernicious anemia develops slowly and insidiously in patients when autoimmune antibodies to intrinsic factor or to parietal cells destroy their parietal cells so that they are left without intrinsic factor.[96] Given the risk of vitamin B_{12} deficiency in the aged and the risks of the condition, some authors have proposed that all elderly adults be screened periodically for vitamin B_{12} deficiency.[97] Chapter 18 discusses megaloblastic anemias.

Folate deficiency. A second megaloblastic anemia that may be seen in elderly adults results from folate deficiency. In contrast to vitamin B_{12} deficiency, folic acid deficiency usually develops from inadequate dietary intake because the body stores little folate.[98] However, the incidence of low serum and RBC folate levels has declined in all age groups, including elderly adults, since countries began to fortify their grains with folic acid in the 1990s.[99] Alcoholic elderly patients are particularly at risk for folic acid deficiency, mainly as a consequence of a poor diet. Alcohol may also interfere with folate absorption and the induction of enzymes involved in folate catabolism (Chapter 18).[98]

Hematologic Neoplasia in Elderly Adults

Although hematologic malignancies may occur at any age, certain disorders are common in those older than 50 years. A brief overview of these disorders is included in this chapter, with references to more detailed discussions.

Chronic Myeloid Neoplasms

The 2016 WHO classification of myeloid neoplasms and acute leukemia revises the 2008 classification based on recently identified molecular diagnostic markers, improved characterization and standardization of morphologic features that aid in the differentiation of the disease groups, and an integration of hematologic, morphologic, cytogenetic, and molecular knowledge. Box 43.1 lists the major subtypes of myeloid neoplasms and acute leukemias according to the 2016 WHO classification.[100] The myeloid neoplasms and acute leukemias have increased incidence in elderly adults, peaking at 75 to 99 years.[101]

Myelodysplastic syndrome. Myelodysplastic syndrome (MDS) represents a heterogeneous group of clonal bone marrow disorders that may affect multiple cell lineages. Myelodysplastic syndrome is the most common hematologic malignancy in elderly adults, with a median age at diagnosis of 68 to 75 years.[83,102] The incidence of myelodysplastic syndrome increases from a total annual incidence of 4 cases per 100,000 to approximately 40 per 100,000 at age 70 years or older and 50 per 100,000 at 80 years or older.[102] Typical features include progressive cytopenias, dyspoiesis in one or more cell lines, and an increase in blasts in the peripheral blood and bone marrow. With the aging of the population, the incidence of MDS will increase in the future. Chapter 33 provides a complete discussion of myelodysplastic syndrome.

Myeloproliferative neoplasms. Myeloproliferative neoplasms are monoclonal proliferations of hematopoietic stem cells with overaccumulation of RBCs, WBCs, or platelets in various combinations. Myeloproliferative disorders include chronic myeloid leukemia; polycythemia vera; essential thrombocythemia; primary myelofibrosis; chronic eosinophilic leukemia, not otherwise specified; mastocytosis; chronic neutrophilic leukemia; and unclassifiable myeloproliferative neoplasms. The incidence of myeloproliferative neoplasms increases from 6.8 per 100,000 for individuals aged 60 to 69, to 12.0 per 100,000 for those aged 70 to 79, and to 15.9 per 100,000 for those aged 80 years and older.[103] Chapter 32 discusses the myeloproliferative neoplasms.

Leukemia

Leukemia is a neoplastic disease characterized by a malignant proliferation of hematopoietic stem cells in the bone marrow, peripheral blood, and often other organs. Leukemia is broadly classified on the basis of the cell type involved (lymphoid or myeloid) and the stage of maturity of the leukemic cells (acute or chronic). Although the overall incidence of leukemia has decreased in the past 5 decades, there is a disproportionately greater incidence of leukemia in elderly adults (Table 43.7). The incidence of acute myeloid leukemia (Chapter 31) increases from 2.0 per 100,000 for those young than 65 years to 20.1 per 100,000 for those 65 and older and peaks at 28.5 per 100,000 for the group aged 80 to 84 years. Chronic lymphocytic leukemia (Chapter 34) has the most dramatic age-related increase in incidence, increasing in incidence from 1.5 per 100,000 for those younger than 65 years to 26.7 per 100,000 for those 65 and older, reaching a peak at 36.9 per 100,000 for those 85 and older.[103]

Geriatric Hemostasis

Age-related changes occur in the vascular and hemostatic systems, including alterations in platelets, coagulation, and fibrinolytic factors. These changes contribute to the *increased incidence of thrombosis in elderly adults.* The rate of venous thromboembolism, for example, increases from 1 per 10,000 in the young (25 to 30 years) to 8 per 1000 in elderly adults (85 years and older).[104] Approximately 60% of venous thrombosis events occur in those aged 70 years and older (Chapter 39).[105] Overall, elderly adults demonstrate a shift of the hemostatic balance toward increased coagulation and decreased fibrinolysis.

TABLE 43.7 SEER Incidence of Leukemia in the Elderly in the United States per 100,000 (2000–2010)[103]

Age at Diagnosis	All Leukemias	ALL	CLL	AML	CML	AMoL
65–69 yr	36.8	1.3	16.7	10.4	4.4	0.7
70–74 yr	49.4	1.4	21.9	14.9	5.7	0.9
75–79 yr	65.7	1.5	28.5	19.7	7.9	1.2
80–84 yr	77.8	1.6	32.4	23.2	9.7	1.4
≥85 yr	88.5	1.8	37.5	22.7	10.1	1.5

ALL, Acute lymphoblastic leukemia; *AML*, acute myeloid leukemia; *AMoL*, acute monocytic leukemia; *CLL*, chronic lymphocytic leukemia; *CML*, chronic myeloid leukemia; *SEER*, Surveillance, Epidemiology, and End Results.

Fibrinogen, factors V, VII, VIII, IX, and XIII, VWF, high-molecular-weight kininogen, and prekallikrein increase in healthy individuals as they age.[106] Fibrinogen, which has been implicated as a primary risk factor for thrombotic disorders, including ischemic heart disease, increases approximately 10 mg/dL per decade in elderly adults (65 to 79 years), from 280 mg/dL to more than 300 mg/dL.[107] In addition, there are seasonal variations in fibrinogen in elderly adults, with the highest plasma levels occurring during the coldest months.[108] Elevated levels of factor VIII also have been associated with increased risk of venous thrombosis, and a positive relationship has been found between plasma VWF and atherosclerosis in the elderly population. Studies of the association between factor VII and thrombotic disorders have yielded conflicting findings.[106,108] Fibrinolysis is impaired in elderly adults, especially as a result of an increase in PAI-1. PAI-1 has been found to promote age-dependent thrombosis in animal models and could play an important role in causing hypercoagulability in elderly adults.[109,110] D-dimer levels trend upward in adults 50 years and older.

Platelets increase in activity with age, as evidenced by a decrease in bleeding time in elderly adults and an increase in markers of platelet activation such as β-thromboglobulin and platelet factor 4.[111] Increased platelet activity with aging is also associated with increased platelet phospholipids, which suggests an age-related increase in platelet transmembrane signaling.[112]

Many conventional risk factors associated with venous thrombosis are likely to also increase the risk of thrombosis in elderly adults. These factors include immobility, malignant disease, comorbidities, and prescription drugs that influence coagulation or platelet function.[92,104]

GESTATIONAL HEMATOLOGY AND HEMOSTASIS

Pregnancy brings about numerous physiologic changes in women to meet the needs of the developing fetus. These physiologic changes are largely beneficial to the mother and the baby but can sometimes cause problems. Expansion of the RBC mass and plasma volume are necessary to maintain the blood supply for the developing fetus. These changes can lead to a physiologic anemia as well as iron deficiency anemia. The increase in uterine blood flow can also lead to hemorrhage at the time of delivery. Changes in coagulation factors help to combat this but result in a hypercoagulable state and increase the risk for thromboembolic events. Recognizing and treating the hematologic and hemostatic disorders that occur during pregnancy can be difficult because of the scarcity of data available that are specific to the hematology and hemostasis of pregnancy. This section discusses the physiologic changes and related disorders that occur in the hematologic system during pregnancy (Table 43.8).

Anemia and the Pregnant Woman

The most common hematologic complication during pregnancy is anemia. Several normal physiologic changes occur

TABLE 43.8 Hematologic and Hemostatic Changes during Pregnancy

Anemia	Disorders of Hemostasis
Deficiency	Venous thromboembolism (VTE)
Iron	Antiphospholipid syndrome
Folic acid	Thrombocytopenia
Vitamin B$_{12}$	Gestational thrombocytopenia
Hemoglobinopathies	Thrombotic thrombocytopenia purpura
Thalassemias	(TTP)
Sickle cell anemia	Immune thrombocytopenia (ITP)
Parasitic infections	Preeclampsia & HELLP syndrome
Ancylostoma	
Trichuris trichiura	
Ascaris lumbricoides	

HELLP, hemolysis, elevated liver enzymes, and low platelet count

during pregnancy that lead to the term *physiologic anemia of pregnancy*. The plasma volume expands 40% to 50%, compared with the proportionally smaller increase in RBC mass of 20% to 30%, accounting for the anemia, which is maximal at 32 weeks.[113-115] The increase in plasma volume and red cell mass supports amniotic fluid production, diminishes hemodynamic insults such as hemorrhage, improves oxygen binding capacity, and facilitates tissue oxygen delivery. The physiologic anemia of pregnancy is generally normochromic and normocytic; therefore, if a pregnant woman has a microcytic hypochromic anemia, nonphysiologic causes must be considered. Iron deficiency is the most common cause of nonphysiologic anemia during pregnancy.[116]

Iron Deficiency Anemia

Anemia of pregnancy is identified in the first and third trimesters if the hemoglobin is less than 11 g/dL or the HCT is less than 33% and in the second trimester if the hemoglobin is less than 10.5 g/dL or the HCT is less than 32%.[117,118] If hemoglobin concentration falls to less than 11 g/dL, testing for iron deficiency anemia should be initiated, because iron deficiency is the most common cause of anemia diagnosed during pregnancy. Under normal circumstances there is an increased requirement for total iron during pregnancy of approximately 1200 mg, an increase in daily iron intake between 15 mg/day to 30 mg/day.[113,118,119] Iron is used primarily for the increase in maternal red blood cells, the placenta, the fetus, general losses, and blood loss at delivery.[118,119]

Most women do not have adequate iron stores to maintain iron needs during pregnancy, even under optimal circumstances. Fifty two percent of pregnant women from underdeveloped or developing countries and 20% from industrialized nations are anemic.[118] The risk of anemia increases with progression of the pregnancy. According to criteria established by the Centers for Disease Control and Prevention, among low-income pregnant women in the United States, 8% are anemic during the first trimester, 12% in the second trimester, and 34% in the third trimester.[117,118] Iron deficiency has been associated with low birth weight, intrauterine growth retardation

(IUGR), increased neonatal mortality, anemia, and impaired cognitive development in the infant.[115,118] Fatigue, pallor, lightheadedness, tachycardia, and preterm labor, as well as postpartum depression, poor maternal-infant interactions, and impaired lactation, are associated with iron deficiency in the pregnant or postpartum woman.[118,120]

Diagnosis of iron deficiency anemia in pregnancy. Diagnosis of iron deficiency anemia can be difficult because serum ferritin increases during the third trimester of pregnancy and microcytosis can be masked by the physiologic increase of 5 to 10 fL in MCV.[114,118] Serum ferritin is an acute phase reactant and as such increases 1 month before delivery. If the ferritin level is normal or elevated and there is evidence of a microcytic, hypochromic anemia, iron deficiency anemia should be considered.[118] Serum ferritin is primarily influenced by obstetric delivery, experiencing a postpartum increase similar to that of CRP or interleukin-6, which does not reflect iron stores.[120] Refer to Chapter 17 for additional information about the diagnosis of iron deficiency anemia.

Treatment of iron deficiency anemia in the pregnant woman. There is disagreement about iron requirements and whether routine supplementation is appropriate in pregnancy. However, it is safer and less expensive to prescribe daily iron supplements to all pregnant women because it appears to do no harm to either the mother or the developing fetus. Most guidelines recommend an increase in iron consumption of 15 to 30 mg/day from the beginning of gestation to 3 months postpartum. This amount readily is met by most prenatal vitamin formulations.

Megaloblastic Anemia

Megaloblastic anemia is the second most common nutritional anemia in pregnancy.[119] Folate and vitamin B_{12} requirements increase during pregnancy because both are involved in nucleic acid formation in the developing fetus.[114] Because of the increased risk of neural tube defects in women who are deficient in folate (Chapter 18), prenatal vitamins are routinely fortified with oral folic acid at a dose of 0.4 mg.[113,115,118] Supplementation must begin during the first trimester to reduce the risk of neural tube defects in the fetus.

Serum vitamin B_{12} levels can decrease to as low as 100 ng/mL during pregnancy, primarily because of a dilutional effect rather than a true deficiency.[114] The decrease does not result in an anemia of pregnancy or produce megaloblastic changes in the bone marrow.[115] Most prenatal vitamins are fortified with 6 μg vitamin B_{12}. Chapter 18 provides an in-depth discussion of folate and vitamin B_{12} and their role in megaloblastic anemia.

Hemoglobinopathies

Early screening for sickle cell anemia, thalassemia, and other hemoglobinopathies is critical for prenatal diagnosis and use of genetic counseling.[114] Individuals with these conditions require additional medical care to address sequelae associated with hemoglobinopathies and decrease risks to the fetus and the mother during pregnancy. For example, all women with chronic hemolysis during pregnancy need extra folic acid supplementation.[115] Since 2006, all US states have instituted universal newborn screening for sickle cell disease.[118] Refer to Chapters

24 and 25 for in-depth discussions of sickle cell anemia and the thalassemias.

Parasitic Infections

Organisms such as *Ancylostoma* (hookworm), *Trichuris trichiura* (whipworm), and *Ascaris lumbricoides* (roundworm), and *Plasmodium* (malaria) are common causes of infections in less developed countries.[118] These infections often result in an anemia as a result of nutritional depletion, gastrointestinal bleeding, and hemolysis.[116,118] Coinfection with these organisms is common and lead to complex problems for pregnant women.

Gestational Hemostasis

Profound hemostatic changes occur during pregnancy. Normal pregnancy is considered to be a *hypercoagulable state* associated with significantly increased concentrations of coagulation factors and decreasing levels of anticoagulation proteins. The hemostatic balance shifts toward enhanced coagulation—which, on the one hand, protects pregnant women from excessive bleeding and hemorrhage during delivery and the postpartum period (puerperium), but, on the other hand, predisposes them to thromboembolism. See Chapter 39 for a detailed discussion on thrombosis.

Thrombophilia and Thrombosis in Pregnancy

Thrombotic processes have been described as an important pathogenic factor of several severe obstetric conditions such as preeclampsia, intrauterine growth restriction (IUGR), and placental abruption by influencing the placental perfusion. Preeclampsia, placental abruption, IUGR, and intrauterine fetal death (IUFD) contribute to maternal morbidity and mortality.

Venous thromboembolism. Overall there is a 4- to 10-fold *increased risk of thrombosis* throughout gestation and the postpartum period.[121] Venous thromboembolism (VTE) is a major cause of maternal mortality. The risk of thrombosis increases as pregnancy progresses and peaks during the puerperium. Virchow's triad of hypercoagulability, stasis, and endothelial damage underlie the pathogenesis of VTE in pregnancy. The hypercoagulable state is created by an increase in coagulation factors, including factors V, VII, VIII, IX, X, and XII, fibrinogen, and VWF; acquired resistance to activated protein C (found with multiple myeloma); decreased free protein S; and impaired fibrinolysis.[113,121] Diminished blood flow to the lower extremities creates stasis, and endothelial damage occurs during vaginal delivery or cesarean section.

Both inherited and acquired thrombophilia are implicated in pathophysiologic processes associated with thrombotic damage of the placenta and are associated with increased risk of VTE. The prevalence of VTE during gestation and puerperium is increased in women with inherited thrombophilic states such as deficiencies of antithrombin, protein C, and protein S. Activated protein C resistance caused by the factor V Leiden mutation (c.1619G>A) is the most common inherited thrombophilia, accounting for up to 44% of cases.[114,122] As an inherited condition, the hypercoagulable state related to factor V Leiden mutation is a lifelong risk factor for VTE, and the risk rises during pregnancy. The factor II mutation (prothrombin G20210A allele variation, c.*97G>A) is also an important inherited risk factor for VTE in pregnant women. There is inconsistent evidence as to whether the factor V Leiden and the prothrombin gene mutations are associated with increased incidence of pregnancy loss.[123]

Screening for thrombophilia is not routine; however, it may be indicated if the result would justify prophylactic treatment. If required, testing should include antithrombin level, protein C level, and polymerase chain reaction for factor V Leiden and prothrombin G20210A.[114]

Treatment of venous thromboembolism in the pregnant woman. Women with previous recurrent VTE should receive prophylactic low-molecular-weight heparin (LMWH; Chapter 40) during gestation. Women who have had a single previous thromboembolic episode are commonly given prophylactic low-dose aspirin during their pregnancy. Women with thrombophilia with no previous VTE and with no placental vascular complications should receive postpartum prophylaxis for 6 weeks with heparin or Coumadin.[113,115]

The use of Coumadin for treatment of VTE during pregnancy is avoided because of the risk of maternal and fetal hemorrhage and fetal *embryopathy* early in the pregnancy. Vitamin K antagonists cross the placenta and are teratogenic. Unfractionated heparin (UFH) and LMWH do not cross the placenta and thus do not have the potential to cause fetal bleeding or teratogenicity. LMWH is thought to have advantages over UFH such as less bleeding risk, longer half-life, less osteoporosis, and less heparin-induced thrombocytopenia.[121] Coumadin, UFH, LMWH, and aspirin are all safe to use when breastfeeding.

Antiphospholipid syndrome. Antiphospholipid syndrome (APS) is an autoimmune disorder and an acquired thrombophilic state that is characterized by the presence of specific antibodies, including lupus anticoagulant (LAC), anticardiolipin antibodies (ACLs), and anti-β_2-glycoprotein I (anti-β_2-GPI). Antiphospholipid antibodies (APLAs) have been found to inhibit trophoblast proliferation and implantation as well as embryo implantation. The presence of APLAs is associated with increased risk of *recurrent pregnancy loss.*[124]

Laboratory testing for APS includes detection of ACLs, a LAC, or anti-β_2-GPI antibodies (Chapter 39). Repeat testing on a new specimen collected more than 12 weeks later will distinguish a chronic autoantibody from a transient alloantibody. Treatment with low-dose aspirin and prophylactic UFH/LMWH has increased the rates of live births from 10% to 70%.[114]

Thrombocytopenia and Bleeding Disorders

Thrombocytopenia in pregnancy is defined as a platelet count of less than 150,000/μL and can be caused by either decreased production or increased destruction of platelets. Thrombocytopenia is common in pregnancy (6% to 10%), with *gestational thrombocytopenia* occurring in 75% of all cases.[125,126] The thrombocytopenia seen in pregnant women is usually secondary to the physiologic changes that occur in pregnancy, such as the increase in blood volume, platelet activation, and increased platelet clearing. Most cases are mild, with platelet counts of 100,000 to 150,000/μL, and are not associated with any adverse events for the mother or baby. The decrease is most pronounced during the third trimester but rarely drops to less than 70,000 to 80,000/μL, and counts typically return to normal by 6 weeks postpartum.[113,114]

The differential diagnosis of maternal thrombocytopenia includes thrombotic thrombocytopenia purpura (TTP), immune thrombocytopenic purpura (ITP), HELLP (**h**emolysis, **e**levated **l**iver enzymes, and **l**ow **p**latelet count) syndrome, hemolytic uremic syndrome (HUS), and conditions resulting in disseminated intravascular coagulation (DIC). Each is described in detail in Chapter 38.

Immune thrombocytopenia. ITP is the second most common cause of thrombocytopenia after gestational thrombocytopenia and should be considered if the platelet count drops to less than 80,000/μL during the first trimester. Two thirds of pregnant women with ITP will require observation only; treatment is indicated if there is maternal hemorrhage, if the platelet count is less than 20,000 to 30,000/μL, or if delivery is imminent when a count of more than 50,000 to 75,000/μL is required.[113,114]

Treatment of ITP during pregnancy is similar to treatment of ITP in the nonpregnant patient. During the first and second trimesters, corticosteroids or intravenous immunoglobulin (IVIG) are typically administered if the platelet count falls to less than 20,000 to 30,000/μL. Corticosteroids have side effects that should be considered before treatment. For example, corticosteroids may exacerbate gestational diabetes mellitus or maternal hypertension. It is important to note that maternal antiplatelet antibodies can cross the placenta and induce thrombocytopenia in the fetus.[125,126]

Thrombotic thrombocytopenia. TTP is a systemic disorder of microvascular thrombosis associated with a severe deficiency of ADAMTS13 and is most often an acquired autoimmune disorder. An association between pregnancy and onset of TTP has been suspected but not confirmed. Because TTP affects women in their reproductive years, it may be a coincidental occurrence during pregnancy. TTP does not cause fetal thrombocytopenia but may result in IUGR and loss of the fetus. Patients with TTP during pregnancy should be treated as other patients with plasma exchange, guided by ADAMTS13 levels and urgent delivery of the fetus when possible. Untreated TTP is associated with a 90% maternal mortality.[114,127]

Preeclampsia and HELLP syndrome. Preeclampsia is the most common cause of pregnancy-related mortality worldwide, affecting up to 6% of all first pregnancies.[125] Preeclampsia is characterized by gestational hypertension and proteinuria after 20 weeks gestation and is commonly responsible for thrombocytopenia in the second and third trimesters. Hematologic complications include microangiopathic hemolytic anemia with fragmented red blood cells in the peripheral blood, and coagulation abnormalities. Inadequate placentation and endothelial damage are thought to be responsible for the pathogenesis of preeclampsia.[113,116] Multiple organ systems are affected in preeclampsia, reflecting systemic endothelial dysfunction, with the kidneys being the most seriously affected.

HELLP syndrome occurs in 10% to 20% of women with preeclampsia. Laboratory results include elevated lactate dehydrogenase (>600 U/mL), increased aspartate aminotransferase (≥70 U/mL), and thrombocytopenia (<100,000/μL).[113,116]

Approximately 70% of the cases occur during the third trimester, with the remaining 30% occurring during the postpartum period. Prompt delivery of the fetus if the gestational age is 34 weeks or more is the mainstay of treatment for HELLP syndrome.[113,116,128]

SUMMARY

- The newborn infant, preadolescent child, elderly adult, and pregnant woman exhibit profound hematologic differences from one another.
- Newborn hematologic parameters continue to change and evolve over the first few days, weeks, and months of life. Laboratory results must be assessed in light of gestational age, birth weight, and developmental differences between newborns and older infants.
- The erythrocytes of newborn infants are markedly macrocytic at birth. A condition known as physiologic anemia of infancy occurs after the first few weeks of life. Infants born prematurely also experience a decrease in hemoglobin concentration, which is termed physiologic anemia of prematurity.
- Iron deficiency is the most common cause of anemia in children.
- Fluctuations in the number of white blood cells are common at all ages but are greatest in infants. Leukocytosis is typical at birth for healthy full-term and preterm infants, with a mean of 22×10^9 cells/L (range 9 to 30×10^9 cells/L) at 12 hours of life. There is an increase in segmented neutrophils, bands, and occasional metamyelocytes with no evidence of disease.
- Sepsis in neonates is a common cause of morbidity, particularly in premature and low-birth-weight infants. Defective B cell response against polysaccharide agents and abnormal cytokine release by neutrophils and monocytes have been implicated.
- Although hemostatic values are different in infants and children from those in adults, this population is not at increased risk of bleeding or thrombosis.
- There is a gradual decline in hemoglobin starting at middle age, and the mean level decreases by about 1 g/dL during the sixth through eighth decades.
- Although anemia is common in elderly patients, it is not a normal occurrence in the aging process. The cause of anemia may be multifactorial in elderly patients.

- Unexplained anemia of the elderly, iron deficiency anemia, and anemia of chronic inflammation are the most common anemias seen in elderly adults.
- Immunosenescence refers to the adverse changes in the immune system associated with aging.
- Elderly adults experience an increased frequency of many neoplastic and malignant disorders, such as acute and chronic leukemias, myelodysplastic syndromes, and myeloproliferative neoplasms, which are associated with hematologic disorders.
- Elderly adults are at an increased risk of thrombosis associated with age-related changes in the vascular and hemostatic systems.
- The most common hematologic complication during pregnancy is anemia.
- Physiologic anemia of pregnancy is caused by an expansion of the plasma volume of 40% to 50% while the red blood cell (RBC) mass expands only by 20% to 30%.
- The increased need for iron during pregnancy—for maternal RBC production, for the placenta and the fetus, and to recover from blood loss—often results in iron deficiency anemia in the mother.
- Megaloblastic anemia is the second most common nutritional anemia in pregnancy and is caused by the increased need for folate and vitamin B_{12} for nucleic acid formation in the developing fetus.
- Normal pregnancy is considered to be a hypercoagulable state with significantly increased concentrations of coagulation proteins and decreased levels of anticoagulant proteins.
- There is a 4- to 10-fold increased risk of thrombosis throughout gestation and the postpartum period.
- Thrombocytopenia is common in pregnancy, occurring in approximately 6% of all pregnancies.

Now that you have completed this chapter, go back and read again the case study at the beginning and respond to the questions presented.

REVIEW QUESTIONS

Answers can be found in the Appendix.

1. The CBC results for children (aged 3 to 12 years) differ from those of adults chiefly in what respect?
   a. NRBCs are present
   b. Notable polychromasia is seen, indicating increased reticulocytosis
   c. Platelet count is lower
   d. The percentage of lymphocytes is higher

2. Physiologic anemia of infancy results from:
   a. Iron deficiency caused by a milk-only diet during the early neonatal period
   b. Increased oxygenation of blood and decreased erythropoietin
   c. Replacement of active marrow with fat soon after birth
   d. Hb F and its diminished oxygen delivery to tissues

3. Morphologically, the hematogones in newborns are:
   a. Similar to those seen in megaloblastic anemia
   b. Easily confused with leukemic blasts
   c. Monocytoid in appearance
   d. Similar to adult lymphocytes

4. The most common cause of anemia in childhood is:
   a. Vitamin B_{12} deficiency
   b. Drug-related hemolysis
   c. Iron deficiency
   d. Folate deficiency

5. Which of the following are the most common anemias in the elderly population?
   a. Megaloblastic anemia and iron deficiency anemia
   b. Sideroblastic anemia and megaloblastic anemia
   c. Myelophthisic anemia and anemia of chronic inflammation
   d. Iron deficiency anemia and anemia of chronic inflammation

6. When iron deficiency is recognized in an elderly individual, the cause is usually:
   a. An iron-deficient diet
   b. Gastrointestinal bleeding
   c. Diminished absorption
   d. Impaired incorporation of iron into heme as a result of telomere loss

7. Which of the following conditions is least likely in an elderly individual?
   a. Acute lymphoblastic leukemia
   b. Multiple myeloma
   c. Myelodysplasia
   d. Chronic lymphocytic leukemia

8. The physiologic anemia of pregnancy is a result of:
   a. A decrease of EPO response during pregnancy
   b. Inability of the pregnant woman to absorb dietary iron
   c. Increased hepcidin synthesis during gestation
   d. Increased plasma volume proportionally greater than the increase in RBC mass

9. Which of the following is recommended as treatment for venous thromboembolism in pregnant women?
   a. Coumadin
   b. Unfractionated heparin (UFH)
   c. Low-molecular-weight heparin (LMWH)
   d. Aspirin

10. A pregnant woman was seen in the emergency department with the following: decreased platelet count, proteinuria, fragmented RBCs, and increased liver enzymes. What is the most likely cause of these abnormalities?
    a. HELLP syndrome
    b. ITP
    c. Antiphospholipid syndrome (APS)
    d. DIC

REFERENCES

1. Brugnara, C., & Platt, O. S. (2009). The neonatal erythrocyte and its disorders. In Orkin, S. H., Nathan, D. G., Ginsburg, D., et al. (Eds.), *Nathan and Oski's Hematology of Infancy and Childhood.* (7th ed., pp. 21–66). Philadelphia: Saunders.

2. Palis, J., & Segal, G. B. (2016). Hematology of the fetus and newborn. In Kaushansky, K., Lichtman, M. A., Prchal JT., et al. (Eds.), *Williams Hematology.* (9th ed., pp. 99–118). New York: McGraw-Hill.

3. Christensen, R. D., & Ohls, R. K. (2016). Development of the hematopoietic system. In Kliegman, R., Stanton, B. F., Geme J. W., III, et al. (Eds.), *Nelson Textbook of Pediatrics.* (20th ed., pp. 2304–2309). Philadelphia: Elsevier.

4. Diaz-Miron, J., Miller, J., & Vogel, A. M. (2013). Neonatal hematology. *Semin Pediat Surg, 22,* 199–204.

5. Stavis, R. L. Postmature (postterm) infant. Merck Manual Professional Version. https://www.merckmanuals.com/professional/pediatrics/perinatal-problems/postmature-postterm-infant. Accessed May 27, 2018.

6. Waldemar, A. C. (2016). The high risk infant. In Kliegman, R., Stanton, B. F., Geme J. W., III, et al. (Eds.), *Nelson Textbook of Pediatrics.* (20th ed., pp. 818–831). Philadelphia: Elsevier.

7. Peterec, S. M., & Warshaw, J. B. (2006). The premature newborn. In McMillan, J. A. (Ed.), *Oski's Pediatrics.* (4th ed., pp. 220–235). Philadelphia: Lippincott Williams & Wilkins.

8. Puukka, R., & Puukka, M. (1994). Effect of hemoglobin F on measurements of hemoglobin A_{1c} with physicians' office analyzers. *Clin Chem, 40,* 342–343.

9. Geaghan, S. M. (1999). Hematologic values and appearances in the healthy fetus, neonate, and child. *Clin Lab Med, 19,* 1–37.

10. Christensen, R. D., & Ohls, R. K. (2012). Anemia in the neonatal period. In Buonocore, G., Bracci, R., & Weingling, M. (Eds.), *Neonatology a Practical Approach to Neonatal Diseases.* (pp. 784–798). Milan: Springer.

11. Pahal, G. S., Jauniaux, E., Kinnon, C., et al. (2000). Normal development of human fetal hematopoiesis between eight and seventeen weeks' gestation. *Am J Obstet Gynecol, 183,* 1029–1034.

12. Diab Y., & Luchtman-Jones, L. (2015). Hematologic and oncologic problems in the fetus and neonate. In Martin, R. J., Fanaroff, A. A., & Walsh, M. C. (Eds.), *Neonatal-Perinatal Medicine; Diseases of the Fetus and Infant.* (10th ed., pp. 1294–1343). St. Louis: Saunders Elsevier.

13. Soldin, S., Wong, E. C., Brugnara, C., et al. (Eds.). (2011). *Pediatric Reference Intervals.* (7th ed.). Washington, DC: AACC Press.

14. Zipursky, M. D., Brown, E., Palko, J., et al. (1983). The erythrocyte differential count in newborn infants. *Am J Pediatr Hematol Oncol, 3,* 45–51.

15. Dallman, P. R., George, D. B., Allen, C. M., et al. (1978). Hemoglobin concentration in white, black, and oriental children: is there a need for separate criteria in screening for anemia? *Am J Clin Nutr, 31,* 377–380.

16. Alur, P., Satish, S., Super, D. M., et al. (2000). Impact of race and gestational age on red blood cell indices in very low birth weight infants. *Pediatrics, 106,* 306–310.

17. Cavaliere, T. A. (2004). Red blood cell indices: implications for practice. *Newborn Infant Nurs Rev, 4,* 231–239.

18. Obladen, M., Diepold, K., & Maier, R. F. (2000). Venous and arterial hematologic profiles of very low birth weight infants. *Pediatrics, 106,* 707–711.

19. Christensen, R. D. & Ohls, R. K. (2014). Anemias unique to the fetus and neonate. In Greer, J. P., Arber, D. A., Glader, B., et al. (Eds.), *Wintrobe's Clinical Hematology.* (13th ed., pp 1018–1031). Philadelphia: Wolters Kluwer/Lippincott Williams & Wilkins.

20. Nickerson, H. J., Silberman, T., Park, R. W., et al. (2000). Treatment of iron deficiency anemia and associated protein-losing enteropathy in children. *J Pediatr Hematol Oncol, 22,* 50–54.

21. Bridges, K. R., & Pearson, H. A. (2008). *Anemias and Other Red Cell Disorders.* (pp. 99–100). New York: McGraw-Hill.

22. Will, A. M. (2006). Disorders of iron metabolism: iron deficiency, iron overload and the sideroblastic anemias. In Arceci, R. J., Hann, I. M., & Smith, O. P. (Eds.), *Pediatric Hematology.* (3rd ed., pp. 79–104). Malden, Mass: Blackwell.

23. Baker, R. D., Greer, F. R., and The Committee on Nutrition. (2010). Diagnosis and prevention of iron deficiency and iron deficiency anemia in infants and young children (0-3 years of age). *Pediatrics, 126,* 1040–1050.

24. Fleming, M. D. (2015). Disorders of iron and copper metabolism and sideroblastic anemias, and lead toxicity. In Orkin S. H., Fisher D. E., Ginsberg D., et al. (Eds.), *Nathan and Oski's Hematology and Oncology of Infancy and Childhood.* (8th ed., pp. 344–381). Philadelphia: Elsevier Saunders.

25. Looker, A. (2002). Iron deficiency—United States, 1999–2000. *MMWR Morb Mortal Wkly Rep, 51,* 897–899.

26. Kanakoudi, F., Drossou, V., Tzimouli, V., et al. (1995). Serum concentrations of 10 acute-phase proteins in healthy term and preterm infants from birth to age 6 months. *Clin Chem, 41,* 605–608.

27. Minder, N., & Cohn, J. (1984). Serum iron, serum transferrin and transferrin saturation in healthy children without iron deficiency. *Eur J Pediatr, 143,* 96–98.

28. Saarinen, U. M., & Siimes, M. A. (1978). Serum ferritin in assessment of iron nutrition in healthy infants. *Acta Paediatr Scand, 67,* 745–751.

29. Schmutz, N., Henry, E., Jopling, J., et al. (2008). Expected ranges for blood neutrophil concentrations of neonates: the Manroe and Mouzinho charts revisited. *J Perinatol, 28,* 275–281.

30. Christensen, R. D., Henry, E., Jopling, J., et al. (2009). The CBC: reference ranges for neonates. *Semin Perinatol, 33,* 3–11.

31. Reich, D., Nalls, M. A., Kao, W. H., et al. (2009). Reduced neutrophil count in people of African descent is due to a regulatory variant in the duffy antigen receptor for chemokines gene. *Plos Genet, 5(1),* 1–14.

32. Mouzinho, A., Rosenfeld, C. R., Sanchez, P. J., et al. (1994). Revised reference ranges for circulating neutrophils in very-low-birth-weight neonates. *Pediatrics, 94,* 76–82.

33. Alexander, G. R., Kogan, M., Bader, G., et al. (2003). US birth weight/gestational age–specific neonatal mortality: 1995–1997 rates for whites, hispanics and blacks. *Pediatrics, 111,* e61–e66.

34. Dinauer, M. C., Newburger, P. E. & Borregaard N. (2015). The phagocyte system and disorders of granulopoiesis and granulocyte function. In Orkin S.H., Fisher D.E., Ginsberg D., et al. (Eds.), *Nathan and Oski's Hematology and Oncology of Infancy and Childhood.* (8th ed., pp. 773–847). Philadelphia: Elsevier Saunders.

35. Grace R. F. (2015). Hematologic manifestations of systemic diseases. In Orkin S.H., Fisher D.E., Ginsberg D., et al. (Eds.), *Nathan and Oski's Hematology and Oncology of Infancy and Childhood.* (8th ed., pp. 1167–1202). Philadelphia: Elsevier Saunders.

36. Wright, B., McKenna, R. W., Asplund, S. L., et al. (2002). Maturing B-cell precursors in bone marrow: a detailed subset analysis of 141 cases by 4-color flow cytometry. *Mod Pathol, 15,* 270A.

37. Rimsza, L. M., Douglas, V. K., Tighe, P., et al. (2004). Benign B-cell precursors (hematogones) are the predominant lymphoid population in the bone marrow of preterm infants. *Biol Neonate, 86,* 247–253.

38. Muehleck, S. D., McKenna, R. W., Gale, P. F., et al. (1983). Terminal deoxynucleotidyl transferase (TdT)–positive cells in bone marrow in the absence of hematologic malignancy. *Am J Clin Pathol, 79,* 277–284.

39. McKenna, R. W., Washington, L. T., Aquino, D. B., et al. (2001). Immunophenotypic analysis of hematogones (B-lymphocyte precursors) in 662 consecutive bone marrow specimens by 4-color flow cytometry. *Blood, 98,* 2498–2507.

40. Intermesoli, T., Mangili, G., Salvi, A., et al. (2007). Abnormally expanded pro-B hematogones associated with congenital cytomegalovirus infection. *Am J Hematol, 82,* 934–936.

41. Cuenca, A. G., Wynn, J. J., Moldawer, I. L., et al. (2013). Role of innate immunity in neonatal infection. *Am J Perinat, 30,* 105–112.

42. Garra, G., Cunningham, S. J., & Crain, E. F. (2005). Reappraisal of criteria used to predict serious bacterial illness in febrile infants less than 8 weeks of age. *Acad Emerg Med, 12,* 921–925.

43. Lukacs, S. L. & Schrag, S. J. (2012).Clinical sepsis in neonates and young infants, United States, 1988–2006. *J Pediatr, 160(6),* 960–965.

44. Davidson, D., Miskolci, V., Clark, D. C., et al. (2007). Interleukin-10 production after pro-inflammatory stimulation of neutrophils and monocytic cells of the newborn. *Neonatology, 92,* 127–133.

45. Rondini, G., & Chirico, G. (1999). Hematopoietic growth factor levels in term and preterm infants. *Curr Opin Hematol, 6,* 192–197.

46. Kotiranta-Ainamo, A., Rautonen, J., & Rautonen, N. (2004). Imbalanced cytokine secretion in newborns. *Biol Neonate, 85,* 55–60.

47. Bhandari, V., Wang, C., Rinder, C., et al. (2008). Hematologic profile of sepsis in neonates: neutrophil CD64 as a diagnostic marker. *Pediatrics, 121,* 129–134.

48. Rey, C., Los Arcos, M., Concha, A., et al. (2007). Procalcitonin and C-reactive protein as markers of systemic inflammatory response syndrome severity in critically ill children. *Intensive Care Med, 33,* 477–484.

49. Elawady, S., Botros, S. K., Sorour, A. E., et al. (2014). Neutrophil CG64 as a diagnostic marker of sepsis in neonates. *J Invest Med, 62(3),* 644–649.

50. Haley, K. M., Recht, M., & McCarty, O. J. T. (2014). Neonatal platelets: mediators of primary hemostasis in the developing hemostatic system. *Pediatr Res, 76(3),* 230–237.

51. Andrew, M., Paes, B., Milner, R., et al. (1987). Development of the human coagulation system in the full-term infant. *Blood, 70,* 165–172.

52. Andrew, M., Vegh, P., Johnston, M., et al. (1992). Maturation of the hemostatic system during childhood. *Blood, 80,* 1998–2005.

53. Revel-Vilk, S. (2012). The conundrum of neonatal coagulopathy. *ASH Education Program Book,* 450–454.

54. Manno, C. S. (2005). Management of bleeding disorders in children. *ASH Education Program Book,* 416–422.

55. Pabinger, I., & Schneider, B. (1996). Thrombotic risk in hereditary antithrombin III, protein C, or protein S deficiency. A cooperative, retrospective study. Gesellschaft für Thrombose- und Hamostaseforschung (GTH) Study Group on Natural Inhibitors. *Arterioscler Thromb Vasc Biol, 12,* 742–748.

56. Will, A. (2015). Neonatal haemostasis and the management of neonatal thrombosis. *Brit J Haematol, 169,* 324–332.

57. Parasuraman, S., & Goldhaber, S. Z. (2006). Venous thromboembolism in children. *Circulation, 113,* e12–e16.

58. Federal Interagency Forum on Aging Related Statistics. (2016). *Older Americans 2016: key indicators of well-being.* http://www.AgingStats.gov. Accessed September 25, 2017.

59. Centers for Disease Control and Prevention National Center for Health Statistics. *Mortality in the United States, 2015.* https://www.cdc.gov/nchs/products/databriefs/db267.htm. Accessed September 25, 2017.

60. Centers for Disease Control and Prevention National Center for Health Statistics. *Health, United States 2016, table 15.* https://www.cdc.gov/nchs/fastats/life-expectancy.htm. Accessed September 25, 2017.

61. Zauber, N. P., & Zauber, A. G. (1987). Hematologic data of healthy old people. *JAMA, 257,* 2181–2184.

62. Lansdorp, P. M. (1997). Self-renewal of stem cells. *Biol Blood Marrow Transplant, 3,* 171–178.

63. Ricci, C., Cova, M., Kang, Y., et al. (1990). Normal age-related pattern of cellular and fatty bone marrow distribution in the axial skeleton: MR imaging study. *Radiology, 177,* 83–88.

64. Frenck, R. W., Jr., Blackburn, E. H., & Shannon, K. M. (1998). The rate of telomere sequence loss in human leukocyte varies with age. *Proc Natl Acad Sci U S A, 95,* 5607–5610.

65. Sahin, E., & DePinho, R. A. (2010). Linking functional decline of telomeres, mitochondria and stem cells during ageing. *Nature, 464,* 520–528.

66. Nilsson-Ehle, H., Jagenburg, R., Landahl, S., et al. (2000). Blood haemoglobin values in the elderly: implications for reference intervals from age 70 to 88. *Eur J Haematol, 65,* 296–305.

67. Tatar, E., Mirili, C., Isikyakar, T., et al. (2016). The association of neutrophil/lymphocyte ratio and platelet/lymphocyte ratio with clinical outcomes in geriatric patients with stage 3-5 chronic kidney disease. *Acta Clinica Belgica, 71(4),* 221–226.

68. Compte, N., Bailly, B., DeBreucker, S., et al. (2015). Study of the association of total and differential white blood cell counts with geriatric conditions, cardio-vascular diseases, seric IL-6 levels and telomere length. *Exp Gerintol, 61,* 105–112.

69. Panda, A., Arjona, A., Sapey, E., et al. (2009). Human innate immunosenescence: causes and consequences for immunity in old age. *Trends Immunol, 30,* 325–333.

70. Fulop, T., Pawalec, G., Castle, S., et al. (2009). Immunosenescence and vaccination in nursing home residents. *Clin Infect Dis, 48,* 443–448.

71. Fulop, T., Larbi, A., Wikby, A., et al. (2005). Dysregulation of T cell function in the elderly: scientific basis and clinical implications. *Drugs Aging, 22,* 589–603.

72. Pawelec, G., Derhovanessian, E., & Larbi, A. (2010). Immunosenescence and cancer. *Crit Rev Oncol Hemat, 75,* 165–172.

73. Nel, A. E., & Slaughter, N. (2002). T-cell activation through the antigen receptor, part 2: role of signaling cascades in T-cell differentiation, anergy, immune senescence, and development of immunotherapy. *J Allergy Clin Immunol, 109,* 901–915.

74. Larbi, A., Douziech, N., Dupuis, G., et al. (2004). Age-associated alterations in the recruitment of signal transduction proteins to lipid rafts in human T lymphocytes. *J Leukoc Biol, 75,* 373–381.

75. Larbi, A., Dupuis, G., Khalil, A., et al. (2006). Differential role of lipid rafts in the functions of CD41 and CD81 human T lymphocytes with aging. *Cell Signal, 18,* 1017–1030.

76. Kawai, T., & Akira, S. (2007). TLR signaling. *Semin Immunol, 19,* 24–32.

77. Grubeck-Lobenstein, B. (1997). Changes in the aging immune system. *Biologicals, 25,* 205–208.

78. Tefferi, A., Thiele, J., Orazi, A., et al. (2007). Proposals and rationale for revision of the World Health Organization diagnostic criteria for polycythemia vera, essential thrombocythemia, and primary myelofibrosis: recommendation from an ad hoc international expert panel. *Blood, 110,* 1092–1097.

79. Balducci, L. (2003). Anemia, cancer, and aging. *Cancer Control, 10,* 478–486.

80. Guralnik, J., Eisenstaedt, R., Ferrucci, L., et al. (2004). Prevalence of anemia in persons 65 years and older in the United States: evidence for a high rate of unexplained anemia. *Blood, 104,* 2263–2268.

81. Lipschitz, D. (2003). Medical and functional consequences of anemia in the elderly. *J Am Geriatr Soc, 51*(Suppl),10–13.

82. Goodnough, L. T. & Schrier, S. (2013). Evaluation and management of anemia in the elderly. *Am J Hematol, 89(1),* 88–96.

83. Price, E. A., Mehra, R., Holmes, T. H., et al. (2011). Anemia in older persons: etiology and evaluation. *Blood Cell Mol Dis, 46,* 159–165.

84. Means, R. T. (2014). Anemia secondary to chronic disease and systemic disorders. In Greer, J. P., Arber, D. A., Glader, B., et al. (Eds.), *Wintrobe's Clinical Hematology.* (13th ed., pp. 998–1011). Philadelphia: Wolters Kluer/Lippincott Williams & Wilkins.

85. Joosten, E. (2004). Strategies for the laboratory diagnosis of some common causes of anaemia in elderly patients. *Gerontology, 50,* 49–56.

86. Berliner, N. (2013). Anemia in the elderly. *Trans Am Clin Climatol Assoc, 124,* 230–237.

87. Smith, D. I. (2000). Anemia in the elderly. *Am Fam Physician, 62,* 1565–1572.

88. Chiari, M. M., Bagnoli, R., DeLuca, P., et al. (1995). Influence of acute inflammation on iron and nutritional status indexes in older inpatients. *J Am Geriatr Soc, 43,* 767–771.

89. Ersher, W. B., Artz, A. S., & Kanapuru, B. (2015). Hematology in older persons. In Kaushansky, K., Lichtman, M. A., Prchal, J. T., et al. (Eds.), *Williams Hematology.* (9th ed., pp. 129–144). New York: McGraw-Hill.

90. Stabler, S. P. (2013). Vitamin B_{12} Deficiency. *N Engl J Med, 368(2),* 149–160.

91. Savage, D. G., & Lindenbaun, J. (1995). Neurological complications of acquired cobalamin deficiency: clinical aspects. *Baillieres Clin Haematol, 8,* 657–678.

92. Ershler, W. B. (2010) Blood disorders in older adults. In Fillit, H. M., Rockwood, K., & Young, J. (Eds.), *Brocklehurst's Textbook of Geriatric Medicine and Gerontology.* (8th ed., pp 757–771). Philadelphia, Elsevier.

93. Matthews, J. H. (1999). Cobalamin and folate deficiency in the elderly. *Baillieres Clin Haematol, 54,* 245–253.

94. Kozyraki, R. & Cases, O. (2013). Vitamin B_{12} absorption: mammalian physiology and acquired and inherited disorders. *Biochimie, 95,* 1002–1007.

95. Baik, H. W., & Russell, R. M. (1999). Vitamin B_{12} deficiency in the elderly. *Annu Rev Nutr, 19,* 357–377.

96. Carmel, R. (1996). Prevalence of undiagnosed pernicious anemia in the elderly. *Arch Intern Med, 156,* 1097–1100.

97. Loikas, S., Koskinen, P., Irjala, K., et al. (2007). Vitamin B_{12} deficiency in the aged: a population-based study. *Age Ageing, 36,* 177–183.

98. Wickramasinghe, S. N. (2006). Diagnosis of megaloblastic anemia. *Blood Rev, 20,* 299–318.

99. Pfeiffer, C. M., Johnson, C. L., Jain, R. B., et al. (2007). Trends in blood folate and vitamin B-12 concentrations in the United States, 1988–2004. *Am J Clin Nutr, 86,* 718–727.

100. Arber, D. A., Orazi, A., Hasserjian, R., et al. (2016). The 2016 revision to the World Health Organization classification of myeloid neoplasms and acute leukemia. *Blood, 127*(20), 2391–2405.

101. Hassan, M., & Abedi-Valugerdi, M. (2014). Hematologic malignancies in elderly patients. *Haematologica, 99*(7), 1124–1127.

102. Burgstaller, S., Wiesinger, P., & Stauder, R. (2015). Myelodysplastic syndromes in the elderly: treatment options and personalized management. *Drug Aging, 32,* 891–905.

103. Howlader, N., Noone, A. M., Krapcho, M., et al. (Eds.), *SEER Cancer Statistics Review, 1975–2014.* Bethesda, MD: National Cancer Institute. https://seer.cancer.gov/csr/1975_2014/, based on November 2016 SEER data subsion, posted to the SEER web site, April 2017. Accessed September 29, 2017.

104. Engbers, M. J., Van Hylckama Vlieg, A., & Rosendall, F. R. (2010). Venous thrombosis in the elderly: incidence, risk factors and risk groups. *J Thromb Haemost, 8,* 2105–2112.

105. Naess, I. A., Christiansen, S. C., Romendstad, P., et al. (2007). Incidence and mortality of venous thrombosis: a population-based study. *J Thromb Haemost, 5,* 692–699.

106. Franchini, M. (2006). Hemostasis and aging. *Crit Rev Oncol Hematol, 60,* 144–151.

107. Kannel, W. B., Wolf, P. A., Castelli, W. P., et al. (1987). Fibrinogen and risk of cardiovascular disease. The Framingham Study. *JAMA, 258, 1183*–1186.

108. Mari, D., Coppola, R., & Provensano, R. (2008). Hemostasis factors and aging. *Exp Gerontol, 43,* 66–73.

109. Yamamoto, K., Takeshita, K., Shimokawa, T., et al. (2002). Plasminogen activator inhibitor-1 is a major stress-regulated gene: implications for stress-induced thrombosis in aged individuals. *Proc Natl Acad Sci USA, 99,* 890–895.

110. Yamamoto, K., Takeshita, K., Kojima, T., et al. (2005). Aging and plasminogen activator inhibitor-1 (PAI-1) regulation: implication in the pathogenesis of thrombotic disorders in the elderly. *Cardiovasc Res, 66,* 276–285.

111. Zahavi, J., Jones, N. A., Leyton, J., et al. (1980). Enhanced in vivo platelet "release reaction" in old healthy individuals. *Thromb Res, 17,* 329–336.

112. Bastyr, E. J., 3rd., Kadrofske, M. M., & Vinik, A. I. (1990). Platelet activity and phosphoinositide turnover increase with advancing age. *Am J Med, 88,* 601–606.

113. Townsley, D. M. (2013). Hematologic complications of pregnancy. *Semin Hematol, 50*(3), 222–231.

114. Robinson, S., Longmuir, K., & Pavord, S. (2017). Haematology of pregnancy. *Medicine, 45*(4), 251–255.

115. Letsky, E. A. (2004). Haematology of pregnancy. *Medicine, 32*(5), 42–45.

116. Means, R. T. (2014). Anemias during pregnancy and the postpartum period. In Greer, J. P., Arber, D. A., Glader, B., et al. (Eds.), *Wintrobe's Clinical Hematology.* (13th ed., pp. 1012–1017). Philadelphia: Lippincott Williams & Wilkins.

117. Current trends CDC criteria for anemia in children and childbearing-aged women. (1989). *Morbidity Mortality Weekly Report (MMWR). 38*(22), 400–404.

118. Lee, A. I., & Okam M. M. (2011). Anemia in pregnancy. *Hematol Oncol Clin N Am, 25,* 241–259.

119. Horowitz, K. M., Ingardia, C. J., & Borgida, A. F. (2013). Anemia in pregnancy. *Clin Lab Med, 33,* 281–291.

120. Breymann, C. (2015). Iron deficiency anemia in pregnancy. *Semin Hematol, 52*(4), 339–347.

121. Brenner, B., Aharon, A., & Lanir, N. (2005). Hemostasis in normal pregnancy. *Thromb Res, 115S,* 6–10.

122. Hammerova, L., Chabada, J., Drobny, J., et al. (2014). Longitudinal evaluation of markers of hemostasis in pregnancy. *Bratisl Lek Listy, 115*(3), 140–144.

123. Bates, S. M. (2010). Consultative hematology: the pregnant patient pregnancy loss. *ASH Education Program Book,* 166–172.

124. Brenner, B. (2005). Thrombophilia and pregnancy. *Hematology, 10*(Suppl. 1), 186–189.

125. McCrae, K. R. (2010). Thrombocytopenia in pregnancy. *ASH Education Program Book,* 397–402.

126. Adams, T. M. (2013). Maternal thrombocytopenia in pregnancy: diagnosis and management. *Clin Lab Med, 33,* 327–341.

127. Tsai, H-M. (2014). Thrombotic thrombocytopenic purpura, hemolytic-uremic syndrome, and related disorders. In Greer, J. P., Arber, D. A., Glader, B., et al. (Eds.), *Wintrobe's Clinical Hematology.* (13th ed., pp. 1077–1096). Philadelphia: Lippincott Williams & Wilkins.

128. Levi, M., & Seligsohn, U. (2015). Disseminated intravascular coagulation. In Kaushansky, K., Lichtman, M. A., Prchal, J. T., et al. (Eds.), *Williams Hematology.* (9th ed., pp. 2199–2220). New York: McGraw-Hill.

APPENDIX A: ABBREVIATIONS

ACA	anticardiolipin antibody
ACL	anticardiolipin
ACT	activated clotting time
ADAMTS13	a disintegrin and metalloprotease with a thrombospondin type 1 motif, member 13
AFIB	atrial fibrillation
Ag	antigen
AHF	antihemophilic factor
AHG	antihuman globulin
AHTR	acute hemolytic transfusion reaction
AIDS	acquired immunodeficiency syndrome
AIHA	autoimmune hemolytic anemia
ALL	acute lymphoblastic leukemia
AML	acute myeloid leukemia
AMoL	acute monocytic leukemia
ANC	absolute neutrophil count
AOI	anemia of inflammation; also ACD, anemia of chronic disease
APC	activated protein C
APCC	activated prothrombin complex concentrate
APCR	activated protein C resistance
APL	acute promyelocytic leukemia; also antiphospholipid antibody
APS	antiphospholipid syndrome
APTT	activated partial thromboplastin time; also PTT
ARC	absolute reticulocyte count
ASA	aspirin; acetylsalicylic acid
AT	antithrombin
ATRA	all-trans-retinoic acid
BAL	bronchoalveolar lavage
BAND	band neutrophil
BASO	basophil
β_2-GPI	beta$_2$-glycoprotein 1
BFU	burst-forming unit
BSS	Bernard-Soulier syndrome
BT	bleeding time
CABG	coronary artery bypass graft
CAD	cold agglutinin disease; also coronary artery disease
CBC	complete blood count
CD	cluster of differentiation
CDA	congenital dyserythropoietic anemia
CEL	chronic eosinophilic leukemia
CFU	colony-forming unit
CGH	comparative genomic hybridization
CHr	reticulocyte hemoglobin; also Ret-He
CI	confidence interval
CKD	chronic kidney disease
CLIA	Clinical Laboratory Improvement Amendments of 1988
CLL	chronic lymphocytic leukemia
CLP	common lymphoid progenitor
CLSI	Clinical and Laboratory Standards Institute
CMA	chromosomal microarray
CML	chronic myeloid (myelogenous) leukemia
CMML	chronic myelomonocytic leukemia

CMP	common myeloid progenitor
CMV	cytomegalovirus
CNL	chronic neutrophilic leukemia
CNP	circulating neutrophil pool
COAT	collagen and thrombin (refers to platelet activation)
COX	cyclooxygenase
CPB	cardiopulmonary bypass
CRYO	cryoprecipitate
CSF	cerebrospinal fluid; colony-stimulating factor
CV	coefficient of variation (%)
CVA	cerebrovascular accident
DAPT	dual antiplatelet therapy
DAT	direct antiglobulin test; formerly direct Coombs test
DBA	Diamond-Blackfan anemia
DDAVP	desamino-8-D-arginine vasopressin, desmopressin
DHS	dehydrated hereditary stomatocytosis; also HX, hereditary xerocytosis
DHTR	delayed hemolytic transfusion reaction
DIC	disseminated intravascular coagulation
DIIHA	drug-induced immune hemolytic anemia
DLBCL	diffuse large B cell lymphoma
DOAC	direct acting oral anticoagulant
DRVVT	dilute Russell viper venom time
DTI	direct thrombin inhibitor
DTS	dense tubular system
DVT	deep venous thrombosis
EBV	Epstein-Barr virus
EC	endothelial cell
ECM	extracellular matrix
ECT	ecarin clotting time
EDTA	ethylenediaminetetraacetic acid
EIA	enzyme immunoassay
ELISA	enzyme-linked immunosorbent assay
EMA	eosin-5'-maleimide binding test
EO	eosinophil
EPCR	endothelial cell protein C receptor
EPO	erythropoietin
ER	endoplasmic reticulum
ESA	erythropoiesis-stimulating agent
ESR	erythrocyte sedimentation rate
ET	essential thrombocythemia
F1+2	prothrombin fragment 1+2
FA	Fanconi anemia
FAB	French-American-British classification
FB	fibroblast
FDA	US Food and Drug Administration
FDP	fibrin degradation products; also FSP, fibrin split products
FEIBA	factor VIII inhibitor bypassing activity
FEP	free erythrocyte protoporphyrin
FFP	fresh frozen plasma
Fg, FG	fibrinogen
FID	functional iron deficiency
FISH	fluorescence in situ hybridization
FP24	24-hour frozen plasma
FPA, FPB	fibrinopeptide A, fibrinopeptide B

FVIII	factor VIII		MPV	mean platelet volume
FVIII:Ag	factor VIII related antigen		N:C	nucleus-to-cytoplasm ratio
FVIII:C	factor VIII coagulant activity		NEUT	neutrophil; also seg, segmented neutrophil; formerly PMN, polymorphonuclear neutrophil
FVL	factor V Leiden mutation		NHL	non-Hodgkin lymphoma
G6PD	glucose-6-phosphate dehydrogenase		NO	nitric oxide
GP	glycoprotein		NOAC	new, novel, non-VKA oral anticoagulant
GPI	glycosylphosphatidylinositol; also glycoprotein inhibitor		NP	normal plasma
GT	Glanzmann thrombasthenia		NRBC	nucleated red blood cell
GVHD	graft-versus-host disease		NSAID	nonsteroidal antiinflammatory drug
Hb	hemoglobin		NVAF	non-valvular atrial fibrillation
HBV	hepatitis B virus		OC	oral contraceptive
HCL	hairy cell leukemia		OHS	overhydrated hereditary stomatocytosis; also hereditary hydrocytosis
HCT	hematocrit; also PCV, packed cell volume		PAD	peripheral artery disease
HDFN	hemolytic disease of the fetus and newborn; also erythroblastosis fetalis		PAI-1	plasminogen activator inhibitor-1
HE	hereditary elliptocytosis		PAO	peripheral artery occlusion
HGB	hemoglobin concentration		PAP	plasmin-antiplasmin complex
HIT	heparin-induced thrombocytopenia		PAR	protease activated receptor
HL	Hodgkin lymphoma		PAS	periodic acid-Schiff
HLA	human leukocyte antigen		PC	protein C
HMWK	high-molecular-weight kininogen (Fitzgerald factor)		PCC	prothrombin complex concentrate
HNSHA	hereditary nonspherocytic hemolytic anemia		PCH	paroxysmal cold hemoglobinuria
HPA	human platelet antigen		PCI	percutaneous coronary intervention
HPFH	hereditary persistence of fetal hemoglobin		PCR	polymerase chain reaction
HPLC	high-performance liquid chromatography		PE	pulmonary embolism
HPP	hereditary pyropoikilocytosis		PECAM	platelet-endothelial cell adhesion molecule
HS	hereditary spherocytosis; also heparan sulfate		PF4	platelet factor 4
HSC	hematopoietic stem cell		PFA	platelet function analyzer
HSCT	hematopoietic stem cell transplantion		PFP	platelet-free plasma
HUS	hemolytic uremic syndrome		PG	prostaglandin
IAT	indirect antiglobulin test		PIVKA	proteins induced by vitamin K antagonists
ID, IDA	iron deficiency, iron deficiency anemia		PK	prekallikrein (Fletcher factor); also pyruvate kinase
Ig	immunoglobulin		PLA2	phospholipase A_2
IL	interleukin		PLC	phospholipase C
INR	international normalized ratio		PLL	prolymphocytic leukemia
IRF	immature reticulocyte fraction		PLT	platelet; also thrombocyte
IRP	international reference preparation		PMF	primary myelofibrosis
ISI	international sensitivity index		PNH	paroxysmal nocturnal hemoglobinuria
ITP	immune thrombocytopenic purpura		POCT	point-of-care testing
IU	international unit		PPP	platelet-poor plasma
LAC	lupus anticoagulant; also LA		PRP	platelet-rich plasma
LAP	leukocyte alkaline phosphatase		PS	protein S
LD	lactate dehydrogenase; formerly LDH		PT	prothrombin time
LIA	latex immunoassay		PTT	partial thromboplastin time; also APTT
LMWH	low-molecular-weight heparin		PV	polycythemia vera
LYMPH	lymphocyte		RAEB	refractory anemia with excess blasts
MAHA	microangiopathic hemolytic anemia		RARS	refractory anemia with ring sideroblasts
MALDI-TOF	matrix-assisted laser desorption/ionization-time of flight		RBC	red blood cell; also erythrocyte
MCH	mean cell hemoglobin		RDW	red cell distribution width
MCHC	mean cell hemoglobin concentration		Ret-He	reticulocyte hemoglobin; also CHr
MCV	mean cell volume		RETIC	reticulocyte count
MDS	myelodysplastic syndromes		RhIg	Rh immune globulin
M:E	myeloid-to-erythroid ratio		RI	reference interval
MHC	major histocompatibility complex		RIPA	ristocetin-induced platelet aggregation
MK	megakaryocyte		ROTEM	rotational thromboelastometry; also TEM
MMA	methylmalonic acid		RPI	reticulocyte production index
MNP	marginal neutrophil pool		RT-PCR	reverse transcriptase polymerase chain reaction
MONO	monocyte		RUO	research use only
MPO	myeloperoxidase		SAO	Southeast Asian ovalocytosis; also hereditary ovalocytosis
MPN	myeloproliferative neoplasm		SCA, SCD	sickle cell anemia, sickle cell disease

SCCS	surface connected canalicular system	TPO	thrombopoietin
SD	standard deviation	TRAP	tartrate resistant acid phosphatase; also thrombin receptor activating peptide
SERPIN	serine protease inhibitor		
SLE	systemic lupus erythematosus	TTP	thrombotic thrombocytopenic purpura
SMC	smooth muscle cell	TXA2, TXB2	thromboxane A_2, thromboxane B_2
SNP	single nucleotide polymorphism	UFH	unfractionated heparin
STR	seven-transmembrane receptor	ULVWF	ultra-long von Willebrand factor
sTfR	soluble transferrin receptor	VKA	vitamin K antagonist
TAFI	thrombin activated fibrinolysis inhibitor	VTE	venous thromboembolism
TAT	thrombin-antithrombin complex	VWD	von Willebrand disease
TCR	T cell receptor	VWF	von Willebrand factor
TCT, TT	thrombin clotting time; also thrombin time	VWF:Ag	von Willebrand factor antigen
TEG	thromboelastography	VWF:CBA	von Willebrand factor collagen binding activity
TEM	thromboelastometry	VWF:RCo	von Willebrand factor ristocetin cofactor activity
TF	tissue factor		
TIA	transient ischemic attack	WAIHA	warm autoimmune hemolytic anemia
TFPI	tissue factor pathway inhibitor	WBC	white blood cell; also leukocyte
TIBC	total iron-binding capacity	WHO	World Health Organization
TM	thrombomodulin	ZPI	Z-dependent protease inhibitor
TNF	tumor necrosis factor	ZPP	zinc protoporphyrin
TPA	tissue plasminogen activator		

Cell Counts (Hemacytometer)

$$\text{Count/L} = \frac{\text{cells counted} \times \text{dilution factor} \times 10^6}{\text{area counted (mm}^2) \times \text{depth (0.1)}}$$

$$\text{Count/}\mu\text{L} = \frac{\text{cells counted} \times \text{dilution factor}}{\text{area counted (mm}^2) \times \text{depth (0.1)}}$$

Correction for NRBCs if NRBCs > 5/100 WBCs

$$\text{Corrected WBC count} = \frac{\text{uncorrected WBC count} \times 100}{\text{number of NRBCs per 100 WBCs} + 100}$$

Absolute WBC Count

$$\text{Absolute count} = \frac{\text{relative count (\%)}}{100} \times \text{total WBC count}$$

$$\text{Absolute neutrophil count or ANC} = \frac{\text{bands} + \text{neutrophils (\%)}}{100} \times \text{total WBC count}$$

Cell Count Estimates from Peripheral Blood Film

Estimated WBC per μL = average number WBC per field with 40 × objective × 2000
Estimated WBC per μL = average number WBC per field with 50 × objective × 3000
Estimated PLT per μL = average number PLT per field with 100 × objective × 20,000
Estimated PLT per μL (in anemia or polycythemia) =

$$\frac{\text{average number PLT per field with 100} \times \text{objective} \times \text{RBC count}}{\text{200 RBCs per field}}$$

Estimation factors provided are general guidelines; the estimated factor should be determined and validated for each microscope in use.

Rule of Three

RBC × 3 = HGB ± 3
HGB × 3 = HCT ± 3
RBC × 9 = HCT ± 3
Only applies when cells are normocytic and normochromic

Mean Cell Volume (MCV), fL

$$\text{MCV} = \frac{\text{HCT (\%)} \times 10}{\text{RBC (}\times 10^{12}\text{/L)}}$$

Mean Cell Hemoglobin (MCH), pg

$$\text{MCH} = \frac{\text{HGB (g/dL)} \times 10}{\text{RBC (}\times 10^{12}\text{/L)}}$$

Mean Cell Hemoglobin Concentration (MCHC), g/dL

$$\text{MCHC} = \frac{\text{HGB (g/dL)} \times 100}{\text{HCT (\%)}}$$

Reticulocyte Count, % (Miller Disc)

$$\text{Reticulocyte count (\%)} = \frac{\text{number reticulocytes in large square} \times 100}{\text{number RBCs in small square} \times 9}$$

Absolute Reticulocyte Count (ARC), × 10⁹/L

$$\text{ARC} = \frac{\text{reticulocyte (\%)} \times \text{RBC count (}\times 10^{12}\text{/L)} \times 1000}{100}$$

Corrected Reticulocyte Count, %

$$\text{Corrected reticulocyte count (\%)} = \text{reticulocyte (\%)} \times \frac{\text{patient HCT (\%)}}{45}$$

Reticulocyte Production Index (RPI)

$$\text{RPI} = \frac{\text{corrected reticulocyte count}}{\text{maturation time}}$$

International Normalized Ratio (INR)

$$\text{INR} = (\text{PT}_{patient}/\text{PT}_{normal})^{ISI}$$

Sodium Citrate Blood Collection Anticoagulant Adjustment for Hematocrit >55%

$$C = (1.85 \times 10^{-3})(100 - \text{HCT})\,V$$

where C is the volume of sodium citrate in milliliters, V is volume of whole blood-sodium citrate solution in milliliters, and HCT is the hematocrit in percent.

CHAPTER 2: QUALITY ASSURANCE IN HEMATOLOGY AND HEMOSTASIS TESTING

Case Study

1. This is a systematic error because the magnitude of error remains constant at three ranges of test results.
2. It is not acceptable to continue using the instrument or to simply subtract the systematic error from test specimen results. All the specimens in a two out-of-control test run must be reassayed after the error is corrected.
3. Determine from the quality control charts at what moment the error occurred. Investigate potential changes in instrument settings, calibration, reagent changes, or instrument malfunction that may have occurred at the time the error was recorded.

Review Questions

1. d; 2. c; 3. b; 4. b; 5. b; 6. a; 7. d; 8. a; 9. d; 10. c; 11. d; 12. c; 13. b; 14. b; 15. a; 16. a; 17. b

CHAPTER 3: CELLULAR STRUCTURE AND FUNCTION

Review Questions

1. b; 2. b; 3. a; 4. b; 5. c; 6. a; 7. d; 8. d; 9. c; 10. b; 11. a; 12. d; 13. b; 14. a; 15. d

CHAPTER 4: HEMATOPOIESIS

Case Study

1. Specimens from the bone marrow are typically collected from the posterior superior iliac crest. The pelvic bones are both easier and safer to access to obtain both aspirate and biopsy specimens. More detail on bone marrow specimen collection is found in Chapter 14.
2. Hematopoiesis in a fetus begins in the yolk sac, followed by production in the liver, peaking at 4.5 months gestation, with additional production in the spleen from the second to seventh month of gestation. The bone marrow begins hematopoeisis in the fourth month and takes over completely by 9 months. Lymph nodes are also involved in the maturation of lymphocytes beginning in the fourth month of gestation and continuing throughout the life span.

   At birth the bone marrow is the primary source of hematopoiesis. More bones are sources for hematopoiesis in the infant (and child) than in the adult (Figures 4.1 and 4.2). As the individual ages the femur and tibia no longer produce hematopoietic cells. The primary sites for hematopoiesis occur in the iliac crest, vertebrae, sternum, skull and proximal ends of the large bones (femur and humerus).
3. The bone marrow is expected to be hypocellular, with more fat cells than hematopoietic cells, given that all three cell lineages, leukocyte, erythrocytes and platelets, are less than the reference intervals. Her clinical signs and symptoms support the decrease in all cell lineages and a hypocellular bone marrow.

Review Questions

1. a; 2. d; 3. c; 4. a; 5. b; 6. c; 7. c; 8. b; 9. a; 10. d; 11. a; 12. b

CHAPTER 5: ERYTHROCYTE PRODUCTION AND DESTRUCTION

Case Study

1. When the blood is not well oxygenated, the bone marrow responds by producing more red blood cells to carry more oxygen.
2. The hormone that stimulates red blood cell (RBC) production is erythropoietin (EPO). The peritubular cells of the kidney detect hypoxia. A hypoxia-sensitive transcription factor is produced that moves to the peritubular cell nucleus and upregulates transcription of the EPO gene. EPO acts by preventing apoptosis of the erythroid colony-forming unit. In RBC precursors, it also shortens the cell cycle time between mitoses and reduces the number of mitotic divisions; and it promotes early release of reticulocytes from the bone marrow.
3. Once the patient was receiving oxygen therapy, hypoxia diminished and EPO production also declined. Thus, production of new RBCs slowed. At the same time, RBCs reaching 120 days of age were removed from the circulation. Thus the total number of circulating RBCs decreased.

Review Questions

1. c; 2. a; 3. d; 4. b; 5. b; 6. d; 7. a; 8. d; 9. a; 10. c

CHAPTER 6: ERYTHROCYTE METABOLISM AND MEMBRANE STRUCTURE AND FUNCTION

Case Study

1. A reducing agent is able to donate an electron to an oxidized compound so that the oxidized compound has one fewer unpaired proton. The compound receiving the electron becomes reduced and the donating compound becomes oxidized.
2. When heme iron is oxidized, the molecule cannot carry oxygen and patients become cyanotic. Because vitamin C eliminated the cyanosis, it must be able to reduce methemoglobin and restore the oxygen-carrying capacity of the blood.
3. Because this condition affected brothers, a hereditary condition was suggested in which hemoglobin became oxidized more than is usual. The condition affecting these brothers was later identified as familial idiopathic methemoglobinemia.

Review Questions

1. c; 2. b; 3. a; 4. c; 5. a; 6. b; 7. d; 8. c; 9. d; 10. b; 11. c; 12. d

CHAPTER 7: HEMOGLOBIN METABOLISM

Case study

1. The mother's and infant's hemoglobin results were within the reference intervals. (Reference intervals: adult women, 12.0 to 15.0 g/dL; newborns, 16.5 to 21.5 g/dL.)

2. The major hemoglobin (Hb) at birth is Hb F. It has a high oxygen affinity because it weakly binds 2,3-bisphosphoglycerate (2,3-BPG), resulting in decreased delivery of oxygen to the tissues. The hypoxia triggers an increase in synthesis of erythropoietin by the fetal kidney, which results in an increase in the production and release of red blood cells from the fetal bone marrow. The resultant increase in red blood cell count, hemoglobin concentration, and hematocrit compensates for the high Hb F oxygen affinity and reduced oxygen transfer to tissues. The Hb F concentration gradually decreases to adult physiologic levels by 1 to 2 years of age as most of the Hb F is replaced by Hb A.

3. The hemoglobin assay measures concentration; high-performance liquid chromatography (and hemoglobin electrophoresis) identifies and quantifies hemoglobin types.

4. These are the expected results for hemoglobin fractions for a healthy mother and infant. In the second and third trimesters of fetal life, the α- and γ-globin genes are activated, producing α- and γ-globin chains that combine to form Hb F. In late fetal life, γ-β switching begins in which transcription of the β-globin gene begins to be upregulated and the γ-globin gene begins to be repressed. With the increase in transcription of the β-globin gene, the β chains combine with the α chains to form Hb A. The Hb F level decreases from 60% to 90% at birth to 1% to 2% by 1 to 2 years of age, and the Hb A increases from 10% to 40% at birth to greater than 95% at 1 to 2 years of age and throughout life. The synthesis of Hb A_2 begins shortly before birth and remains at less than 3.5% throughout life.

Review Questions

1. d; 2. a; 3. a; 4. a; 5. a; 6. d; 7. c; 8. b; 9. d; 10. b; 11. c

CHAPTER 8: IRON KINETICS AND LABORATORY ASSESSMENT

Case Study

1. Iron loss via blood donations and normal physiologic loss was not compensated by diet or supplementation.

2. Adaptation to the low iron levels. Iron stores of ferritin were mobilized first. But when storage iron declined, hepcidin levels declined, and as a result, duodenal iron absorption increased.

3. Ferritin

4. Transferrin saturation is a calculation that relies on the serum iron value and the total iron-binding capacity (TIBC). The serum iron reflects iron in transit in the blood, whereas the TIBC reflects the number of transferrin binding sites available for iron; an indirect assessment of transferrin. The diagnostic value of the % transferrin saturation is not as great as ferritin in assessing iron stores, though the % transferrin saturation would be expected to decline as iron stores decline.

Review Questions

1. c; 2. b; 3. c; 4. c; 5. a; 6. b; 7. d; 8. b; 9. d; 10. c; 11. b; 12. d; 13. b; 14. a; 15. b

CHAPTER 9: LEUKOCYTE DEVELOPMENT, KINETICS, AND FUNCTIONS

Case Study

1. The patient had an asthmatic attack. Eosinophils play an important role in the initiation and maintenance of symptoms. Eosinophils release basic proteins, lipid mediators, and reactive oxygen species that cause inflammation and damage to the mucosal cells lining the airway.

2. Eosinophils are typically elevated in the peripheral blood and also in the sputum of asthmatic patients. The number of eosinophils in the blood correlates with the severity of the case.

3. Interleukin-5 (IL-5) plays an important role in the differentiation and proliferation of eosinophils. Monoclonal antibodies to IL-5 block eosinophil development. Because eosinophils are reduced, the symptoms of asthma are controlled.

Review Questions

1. b; 2. d; 3. a; 4. c; 5. b; 6. c; 7. c; 8. a; 9. b; 10. d

CHAPTER 10: PLATELET PRODUCTION, STRUCTURE, AND FUNCTION

Case study

1. Bleeding characterized by petechiae, purpura, and ecchymoses is known as mucocutaneous bleeding, also called systemic bleeding. By contrast, anatomic bleeding is bleeding into soft tissue, muscles, joints, or body cavities.

2. Thrombocytopenia, or low platelet count, is a common cause of mucocutaneous bleeding. Another is diseases that weaken vascular collagen such as scurvy.

3. No, the bone marrow megakaryocyte estimate is high, indicating an increase in platelet production.

4. Thrombopoietin and interleukin-11 have the greatest effect on recruitment and proliferation of megakaryocytes and their progenitors. Also involved in early progenitor recruitment are interleukin-3 and interleukin-6. Other cytokines and hormones that participate synergistically with thrombopoietin and the interleukins are KIT ligand, also called stem cell factor or mast cell growth factor; granulocyte-macrophage colony-stimulating factor; granulocyte colony-stimulating factor; and erythropoietin.

Review Questions

1. d; 2. d; 3. c; 4. b; 5. d; 6. d; 7. a; 8. a; 9. c; 10. c; 11. b; 12. c

CHAPTER 11: MANUAL, SEMIAUTOMATED, AND POINT-OF-CARE TESTING IN HEMATOLOGY

Case Studies

Case 1

1. HGB × 3 = HCT ± 3
   15 × 3 = 45 ± 3 (42−48)

2. Hemoglobin can be falsely elevated by lipemia, increased white blood cell (WBC) count, or presence of hemoglobin (Hb) S or Hb C. Hematocrit can be falsely decreased by a short draw in an EDTA-anticoagulated tube causing red blood cell (RBC) shrinkage, or contamination of the specimen with intravenous fluids. In the microhematocrit method, false decreases can be caused by improper sealing of the capillary tube, errors in reading the microhematocrit reader, excessive centrifugation, and improper mixing of the specimen.

3. For lipemia, replace lipemic plasma with an equal amount of saline and retest; or use a plasma blank. For increased WBC count, centrifuge the hemoglobin/reagent solution and read the % T of the supernatant (manual procedure). For specimens with Hb S or Hb C, make a 1:2 dilution of blood with distilled water and multiply the result by 2. For the microhematocrit, check if the specimen tube was filled to the proper level, and ensure the procedure is performed correctly.

Case 2

1. Mean cell volume (MCV)=59 fL; mean cell hemoglobin (MCH)=18.1 pg; mean cell hemoglobin concentration (MCHC)=30.7 g/dL.

2. Microcytic, hypochromic red blood cells.

3. Examine the patient's peripheral blood film.

Case 3

1. The sodium concentration could affect the hematocrit. The specimen electrolyte concentration is used to correct the measured conductivity before reporting hematocrit results. Factors that affect sodium concentration will therefore also affect the hematocrit.

2. A high sodium concentration would falsely decrease the hematocrit.

3. Factors that decrease the hematocrit by this method are low total protein, settling of red blood cells in the collection device, presence of cold agglutinins, and specimen contamination by intravenous solutions.

Review Questions

1. b; 2. c; 3. c; 4. d; 5. d; 6. b; 7. c; 8. c; 9. a; 10. d

CHAPTER 12: AUTOMATED BLOOD CELL ANALYSIS

Case Study

1. RBC, HCT, MCV, MCH, MCHC, RDW.

2. Due to the elevated MCV and impossibly high MCHC in combination with a very low RBC count, a cold agglutinin should be considered. The cold agglutinin will cause the RBC to agglutinate at room temperature in the specimen. Automated blood cell analyzers will measure each agglutinate (consisting of multiple RBCs) as one large cell. The RDW will also be elevated because of the variation in volume of the agglutinates and single RBCs.

3. Check the blood film for RBC agglutination. Incubate the specimen for 15 to 30 minutes at 37° C and reanalyze. If the cold agglutinin caused the spurious CBC results, the post-incubation results will show an increase in RBC count and a decrease in MCV, MCHC, and RDW. A CBC was repeated after incubation with the following results, thus confirming the cold agglutinin: WBC = 9.3 × 10^9/L, RBC = 4.22 × 10^{12}/L, HGB = 12.2 g/dL, HCT = 36.8%, MCV = 87.2 fL, MCH = 28.9 pg, MCHC = 33.2 g/dL, RDW = 15%, and PLT = 201 × 10^9/L.

Review Questions

1. d; 2. a; 3. d; 4. c; 5. c; 6. Impedance, c; RF, b; optical scatter, a; 7. b; 8. b; 9. c; 10. Abbott CELL-DYN Sapphire, b; Siemens ADVIA 2120i, c; Sysmex XN-1000, d; Beckman Coulter UniCel DxH 800, a.

CHAPTER 13: EXAMINATION OF THE PERIPHERAL BLOOD FILM AND CORRELATION WITH COMPLETE BLOOD CELL COUNT

Case Study

1. The patient's hemoglobin shows neither anemia or polycythemia; hence it is normal. Red blood cells are normocytic and normochromic with no anisocytosis. The blood picture shows leukocytosis and thrombocytopenia. The mean platelet volume is slightly low, which suggests small average platelet volume. There is no white blood cell (WBC) differential.

2. The platelet count and WBC count should be questioned because of platelet clumping. EDTA-induced pseudothrombocytopenia and pseudoleukocytosis most likely occurred.

3. The specimen should be recollected in sodium citrate and processed through the automated analyzer. The new WBC and platelet counts should then be adjusted for the sodium citrate dilution by multiplying the results by the dilution factor 10/9 or 1.1. The following are the new results:
   a. WBCs for specimen drawn in sodium citrate: (8.4 × 10^9 /L) × 1.1 = 9.2 × 10^9 /L (the corrected WBC count)
   b. Platelets for specimen drawn in sodium citrate: (231 × 10^9 /L) × 1.1 = 254 × 10^9 /L (the corrected platelet count)

Review Questions

1. d; 2. c; 3. a; 4. c; 5. b; 6. c; 7. a; 8. b; 9. b; 10. a

CHAPTER 14: BONE MARROW EXAMINATION

Case Study

1. Bone marrow cellularity, estimated from the core biopsy specimen, or the aspirate if a biopsy specimen is unavailable, provides information on blood cell production.

2. The ratio is 9:1, which indicates myeloid hyperplasia.

3. When a bone marrow aspirate or core biopsy specimen is reviewed, the normal megakaryocyte distribution is 2 to 10 per low-power field. Counts outside these limits are characterized as decreased or increased megakaryocytes. Megakaryocyte morphology is also reviewed for diameter, granularity, and nuclear lobularity.

Review Questions

1. d; 2. b; 3. c; 4. a; 5. d; 6. c; 7. d; 8. b; 9. b; 10. b; 11. b; 12. a; 13. d

CHAPTER 15: BODY FLUID ANALYSIS IN THE HEMATOLOGY LABORATORY

Case Study

1. Tube 3 or the least bloody tube.
2. A 1:53 dilution with saline is necessary for a satisfactory cytocentrifuge slide.
3. Bacteria.
4. The most likely diagnosis is bacterial meningitis.

Review Questions

1. b; 2. a; 3. c; 4. b; 5. a; 6. b; 7. c; 8. d; 9. c; 10. a

CHAPTER 16: ANEMIAS: RED BLOOD CELL MORPHOLOGY AND APPROACH TO DIAGNOSIS

Case Study

1. Anemia is not a disease or diagnosis in itself but is the symptom of an underlying disorder. A complete history and physical examination are necessary to help identify the cause(s) of the anemia. If the underlying cause is not determined and corrected, the patient will continue to be anemic. Questions regarding lifestyle, medications, and bleeding history are only some of the questions that should be asked.
2. The reticulocyte count differentiates anemias into those involving impaired production (decreased reticulocyte count) and increased destruction (increased reticulocyte count). Anemia can also be classified on the basis of mean cell volume into normocytic, microcytic, or macrocytic. With that knowledge, appropriate laboratory testing can be ordered to determine the cause.
3. The peripheral blood film yields valuable information about the volume and hemoglobin content of the erythrocytes as well as any abnormal shapes, which may be correlated with specific causes. Some anemias are also associated with white blood cell and/or platelet abnormalities, which may be noted on the blood film.

Review Questions

1. c; 2. b; 3. d; 4. c; 5. c; 6. b; 7. c; 8. d; 9. b; 10. c; 11. d

CHAPTER 17: DISORDERS OF IRON KINETICS AND HEME METABOLISM

Case Study

1. The patient's results demonstrate a severe hypochromic, microcytic anemia with anisocytosis. There is no evidence of a bone marrow response because there is no polychromasia mentioned in the morphology report. However, there is mention of unspecified poikilocytosis, anisocytosis, hypochromia, and microcytosis, all of which are consistent with the numerical values. The white blood cells are unremarkable in number, distribution, and morphology as are the platelets.
2. Hypochromic, microcytic anemias to be considered include iron deficiency anemia, thalassemia, hemoglobin E disease, sideroblastic anemias, and possibly anemia of chronic inflammation.
3. Thalassemia and hemoglobin E disease can be eliminated because they are not conditions that would be acquired late in life.
4. Anemia of chronic inflammation could be eliminated in this case because the woman is otherwise healthy. Although iron deficiency anemia is not common in women after menopause, it is probably the most likely of the remaining possibilities for an anemia that is this severe.
5. Iron studies, including ferritin, would be useful in clarifying the patient's diagnosis. Assuming that she is iron deficient, the serum ferritin, total serum iron, and percent transferrin saturation should all be decreased, whereas total iron-binding capacity (TIBC) would be expected to be increased. On hospitalization, the patient was immediately placed on oxygen while laboratory tests were ordered. With the confirmation by the hospital laboratory of a dangerously low hemoglobin concentration, transfusions were ordered, and the patient received 3 units of packed cells over the first 2 days of hospitalization. The transfusions were administered very slowly so as not to stress her cardiovascular system with added volume. Noting the hypochromic, microcytic blood picture, the physician ordered iron studies on blood specimens drawn before the transfusions were initiated. The results were as follows: serum iron decreased, TIBC increased, percent transferrin saturation decreased, and serum ferritin decreased. The possibility of gastrointestinal bleeding as a cause for iron deficiency was investigated. Results of tests for occult blood in the stool were negative. The hospital dietitian assessed the patient's usual diet of tea, toast, canned soup, and crackers and determined that it was quite inadequate not only in iron, but also in other important nutrients. The physician concluded that the patient's dietary iron deficiency had developed slowly, which had allowed her to adapt to the exceedingly low hemoglobin level. Furthermore, her low level of activity meant that she rarely experienced the effects of the anemia. She was started on a course of oral iron supplementation and arrangements were made for her to receive one balanced meal daily from the Meals on Wheels program sponsored through a community service organization for senior citizens. She was quite responsible about taking her iron supplements, and her hemoglobin concentration was within the reference interval within 3 months.

Review Questions

1. b; 2. a; 3. d; 4. a; 5. c; 6. a; 7. d; 8. c; 9. b; 10. d; 11. b; 12. d

CHAPTER 18: ANEMIAS CAUSED BY DEFECTS OF DNA METABOLISM

Case Study

1. The complete blood cell count findings for this patient (notably macrocytic, normochromic anemia; pancytopenia; hypersegmentation of neutrophils; and oval macrocytes) were consistent with the physician's suspicion of megaloblastic anemia as suggested by the clinical findings.

2. Although the relative reticulocyte count was within the reference interval of 0.5% to 2.5%, and the calculated absolute reticulocyte count (approximately 40×10^9/L) was within the reference interval of 20 to 115×10^9/L, the calculated reticulocyte production index was 0.5, which was clearly inadequate to compensate for a substantial anemia (Chapter 11).

3. The patient's vitamin assays point to a deficiency of vitamin B_{12} substantiated by an increase in serum methylmalonic acid.

4. Based on these results, a test for intrinsic factor blocking antibodies would be appropriate. However, the physician also inquired further about the patient's dietary habits and learned that he enjoyed dishes of raw fish obtained from the surrounding lakes. Therefore the physician ordered a stool analysis for ova and parasites. The study indicated the presence in the stool of both eggs and proglottids of the fish tapeworm *Diphyllobothrium latum*. The patient was treated with a suitable purgative, and the scolex of the tapeworm was discovered in a stool specimen after a single treatment. The patient was counseled on the proper preparation of fresh fish to avoid reinfection. He received injections of cyanocobalamin to replenish his vitamin B_{12} stores. His hemoglobin concentration returned to normal over the next month, and his neurologic symptoms subsided.

Review Questions

1. d; 2. c; 3. c; 4. b; 5. a; 6. b; 7. c; 8. d; 9. a; 10. c

CHAPTER 19: BONE MARROW FAILURE

Case Study

1. The term used to describe a decrease in all cell lines is *pancytopenia*.

2. Acquired aplastic anemia should be considered because of the pancytopenia, reticulocytopenia, bone marrow hypocellularity, normal vitamin B_{12} and folate levels, absence of blasts and abnormal cells in the bone marrow and peripheral blood, normal myelopoiesis and megakaryopoiesis, and history of autoimmune hepatitis.

3. An increase in blasts or reticulin in the bone marrow suggests a diagnosis of myelodysplasia or leukemia.

4. The extent of the patient's bone marrow hypocellularity and her hemoglobin concentration and neutrophil and platelet counts place her disorder in the severe aplastic anemia category.

5. Because of her age and the severity of her aplastic anemia, hematopoietic stem cell transplant is the treatment of choice if she has an HLA-identical sibling. If an HLA-identical sibling is not available, an HLA-matched unrelated donor or immunosuppressive therapy (anthymocyte globulin and cyclosporine) may be considered. Blood product replacement should be given judiciously to avoid alloimmunization. In general, red blood cells would be transfused if the patient had symptoms of anemia, whereas platelet transfusions would be given if her platelet count fell to less than 10×10^9/L.

Review Questions

1. c; 2. d; 3. b; 4. d; 5. b; 6. d; 7. c; 8. d; 9. c; 10. d; 11. a; 12. a

CHAPTER 20: INTRODUCTION TO INCREASED DESTRUCTION OF ERYTHROCYTES

Case Study

1. Intravascular hemolysis is suspected in the patient because the color of the urine suggests oxidized hemoglobin.

2. Tests for serum haptoglobin, serum lactate dehydrogenase, plasma hemoglobin, urine hemoglobin, and examination of a peripheral blood film can differentiate the mechanism of hemolysis as fragmentation or macrophage mediated. Bilirubin assays, urinary urobilinogen, and reticulocyte counts will be similar in both types of hemolysis.

3. Because of the likelihood that the patient had hemoglobinuria, fragmentation hemolysis was suspected. Therefore the serum haptoglobin would be markedly decreased, whereas the serum lactate dehydrogenase and plasma hemoglobin levels would be increased, if measured. Routine urinalysis should yield positive results for blood on the test strip with no intact red blood cells in the urine sediment. The serum indirect bilirubin does not increase immediately after an episode of intravascular hemolysis but should begin to increase within several days. Urinary urobilinogen may rise a little sooner. The peripheral blood film may demonstrate schistocytes immediately, with reticulocytosis occurring several days later.

Review Questions

1. a; 2. b; 3. d; 4. b; 5. c; 6. a; 7. d; 8. c; 9. c; 10. c

CHAPTER 21: INTRINSIC DEFECTS LEADING TO INCREASED ERYTHROCYTE DESTRUCTION

Case Study

1. On the basis of the patient's jaundice and splenomegaly, history of gallstones, family history of anemia, low hemoglobin concentration, increased mean cell hemoglobin concentration and red cell distribution width, and spherocytes and polychromasia on the peripheral blood film, hereditary spherocytosis (HS) is suspected.

2. Additional laboratory tests to confirm HS should demonstrate increased hemolysis (increased serum indirect bilirubin level and lactate dehydrogenase activity, decreased serum haptoglobin level), increased erythropoiesis to compensate for the premature hemolysis (increased reticulocyte count), and the nonimmune nature of the hemolysis (negative result on the direct antiglobulin test). Testing family members to establish a mode of inheritance is desirable. The osmotic fragility test is expected to show increased fragility and the eosin-5'-maleimide (EMA) binding test is expected to show

low mean fluorescence intensity of the red blood cells when measured in a flow cytometer. However, special tests are not required for diagnosis of HS in a patient with a familial inheritance pattern and the typical clinical and laboratory findings.

3. HS is an inherited intrinsic hemolytic anemia caused by a mutation that disrupts the vertical protein interactions in the red blood cell (RBC) membrane. Various mutations in five known genes can result in the HS phenotype. The defective membrane protein causes the RBCs to lose unsupported lipid membrane over time as a result of local disconnections between transmembrane proteins and the cytoskeleton. The loss of membrane with minimal loss of cell volume results in a decreased surface area-to-volume ratio and the formation of spherocytes. Spherocytes do not have the deformability of normal biconcave discoid RBCs. As the cells repeatedly go through the spleen, they lose more membrane due to splenic conditioning and eventually become trapped in the spleen and removed by the splenic macrophages. The RBC membrane also has abnormal permeability to cations, particularly sodium and potassium, likely because of the disruption of the cytoskeleton by the mutated protein.

Review Questions

1. c; 2. b; 3. c; 4. a; 5. b; 6. a; 7. a; 8. a; 9. c; 10. d; 11. c; 12. c

CHAPTER 22: EXTRINSIC DEFECTS LEADING TO INCREASED ERYTHROCYTE DESTRUCTION—NONIMMUNE CAUSES

Case Study

1. Many ring forms, with multiple ring forms in individual red blood cells (RBCs), are present in the thin peripheral blood film. Many ring forms and a crescent-shaped gametocyte are also present in the thick peripheral blood film.

2. A diagnosis of malaria is suspected. Note that the high parasitemia, the presence of multiple ring forms in individual RBCs, the crescent-shaped gametocyte on the thick film, and the absence of other parasite stages in the thin and thick peripheral blood films suggest *Plasmodium falciparum*.

3. The patient had typical symptoms of malaria after a recent 3-week trip to Ghana in West Africa where malaria is endemic.

4. Anemia in malaria is due to direct lysis of infected RBCs during schizogony; immune destruction of infected and noninfected RBCs by macrophages in the spleen; and inhibition of erythropoiesis and ineffective erythropoiesis.

Review Questions

1. c; 2. a; 3. b; 4. b; 5. c; 6. c; 7. c; 8. d; 9. c; 10. a

CHAPTER 23: EXTRINSIC DEFECTS LEADING TO INCREASED ERYTHROCYTE DESTRUCTION—IMMUNE CAUSES

Case Study

1. The white blood cells (WBCs) can be elevated because of an underlying infection or the autoimmune response itself (inflammation). The mean cell volume (MCV) is elevated because of the reticulocytosis; the red cell distribution width (RDW) is slightly elevated because of the anisocytosis and occasional schistocytes. The reticulocyte count is increased as a result of a surge in red blood cell (RBC) production in the bone marrow in response to the anemia.

2. In this immune process, spherocytes develop from immunoglobulin G (IgG)-sensitized RBCs that have had the membranes seal and the cells become spherocytic. The red pulp of the spleen eventually entraps the spherocytes, which are less deformable, and macrophages engulf and digest them, thus shortening their life span.

3. The direct antiglobulin test detected an IgG autoantibody that attached to the patient's RBCs in vivo, which is a hallmark of warm autoimmune hemolytic anemia (WAIHA). The IgG autoantibody was also detected in the serum with the antibody screen using the indirect antiglobulin test. The patient's RBCs, sensitized with IgG autoantibody, were prematurely ingested and destroyed by macrophages (extravascular or macrophage-mediated hemolysis); within the macrophages hemoglobin is degraded to polypeptide chains, iron, and the protoporphyrin ring (Chapter 20). The protoporphyrin is converted to unconjugated bilirubin and is transported to the liver, where it is conjugated with glucuronic acid to form conjugated bilirubin. When there is excessive hemolysis, the liver cannot process all the excess unconjugated bilirubin that is being formed, so it accumulates in the serum. The excess conjugated bilirubin formed in the liver is excreted through the bile duct to the intestines where it is converted to urobilinogen. Because of the increased urobilinogen produced in the intestines, an increased amount is reabsorbed into the blood, and an increased amount is excreted in the urine. There is also an increase in intravascular hemolysis, which liberates lactate dehydrogenase and elevates the level in serum. Free hemoglobin is also liberated and is bound by haptoglobin. The hemoglobin-haptoglobin complex is taken up and degraded by macrophages, resulting in a decrease in serum haptoglobin. When the serum haptoglobin is depleted, the excess hemoglobin accumulates in the plasma. Some is salvaged by hemopexin, but the excess is filtered by the kidney. Some hemoglobin is absorbed by the proximal tubular cells; the iron is removed and converted to hemosiderin. When the tubular cells slough off into the urine, the hemosiderin can be detected. The excess hemoglobin that is not absorbed by the tubular cells flows into the urine resulting in hemoglobinuria.

4. Prednisone is a glucocorticosteroid with immunosuppressive properties, such as reducing WBC response to inflammation. When a patient with an autoimmune disorder is given prednisone, most of these inflammatory mechanisms are switched off or slowed down, which in turn reduces the body's autoimmune response. The patient probably had an acute form of WAIHA because the symptoms and severe anemia developed suddenly and there was no evidence of an underlying condition.

Review Questions

1. b; 2. a; 3. a; 4. d; 5. d; 6. d; 7. a; 8. c; 9. c; 10. c; 11. c

CHAPTER 24: HEMOGLOBINOPATHIES (STRUCTURAL DEFECTS IN HEMOGLOBIN)

Case Study

1. The confirmatory test that should be performed is acid hemoglobin electrophoresis, which separates hemoglobin (Hb) C from Hb A_2, Hb O, and Hb E, and separates Hb S from Hb D and Hb G (Figure 24.7). High-performance liquid chromatography (HPLC) can also be performed.

2. The characteristic morphologic feature on the peripheral blood film is a Hb SC crystal. They appear as finger-like or quartz-like crystals of dense hemoglobin protruding from the red blood cell (RBC) membrane.

3. On the basis of the electrophoretic pattern and RBC morphology, Hb SC disease is likely.

4. With parents of the genotypes SC and AS, 25% of the offspring would have each of the following genotypes: AS, SS, AC, and SC.

Review Questions

1. d; 2. b; 3. c; 4. b; 5. d; 6. b; 7. a; 8. b; 9. c; 10. a; 11. b; 12. d; 13. d; 14. b; 15. c; 16. d

CHAPTER 25: THALASSEMIAS

Case Study

1. The family history revealed a Mediterranean ethnic background; both α- and β-thalassemia are common in the Mediterranean population. The student's mother had always been anemic, and her gallbladder attacks were probably caused by pigmented gallstones (calcium bilirubinate), which resulted from the mild hemolytic anemia of heterozygous β-thalassemia. A cousin on the mother's side had children with thalassemia major. Because of the family history, it is quite likely that the student has β-thalassemia minor. Note that his mother was periodically given iron therapy. It is a common mistake to treat a thalassemic individual for iron deficiency anemia, especially in areas in which thalassemia is not common in the general population, because both iron deficiency anemia and thalassemia are microcytic, hypochromic anemias.

2. The student had a mild hypochromic (decreased mean cell hemoglobin concentration) and microcytic (decreased mean cell volume) anemia with target cells and basophilic stippling on his peripheral blood film. He had an elevated level of hemoglobin A_2, which is a marker for β-thalassemia minor. His serum ferritin level was within the reference interval, which ruled out a diagnosis of iron deficiency anemia.

3. A microcytic, hypochromic anemia could be due to α- or β-thalassemia, Hb E disease or trait, iron deficiency anemia, or, more rarely, sideroblastic anemia (including lead poisoning) or anemia of chronic inflammation (Figure 16.2). Iron deficiency anemia is the most common of these. Iron studies can differentiate these conditions. An incorrect presumption that a patient has iron deficiency may lead to inappropriate iron therapy or to unnecessary diagnostic procedures.

4. The potential mother should be screened for β-thalassemia trait, and if she is heterozygous for a β-thalassemia gene mutation, the couple should be advised that there is a 25% chance of having a baby with β-thalassemia major (homozygous or compound heterozygous for a β-thalassemia mutation). In addition, there is a 25% chance of having a baby who is homozygous for normal β-globin genes and a 50% chance of having a baby heterozygous for a β-thalassemia mutation (β-thalassemia trait). Molecular genetic testing of the *HBB* gene is performed for carrier detection in couples seeking preconception counseling.

Review Questions

1. b; 2. c; 3. d; 4. d; 5. a; 6. a; 7. b; 8. c; 9. d; 10. a; 11. d; 12. d; 13. c; 14. d; 15. a

CHAPTER 26: NONMALIGNANT LEUKOCYTE DISORDERS

Case Study

1. No, the cell is not a myelocyte. The morphologic features are consistent with Pelger-Huët anomaly. The chromatin is clumped and the cytoplasmic color and granulation matches that of a mature neutrophil. Although the nuclear shape is round/oval, the nucleus-to-cytoplasm (N:C) ratio is lower than what would be expected in a myelocyte.

2. Pelger-Huët anomaly is the condition suspected. Other cells in the myelocytic series with morphology similar to the cell in the image are also likely to be Pelger-Huët neutrophils.

3. It is best to not identify Pelger-Huët cells as immature as this can be misleading to the clinician. One alternative would be to identify all cells with Pelger-Huët morphology as segmented neutrophils with a comment such as "few/moderate/many cells identified as segmented neutrophils exhibit Pelger-Huët morphology," or similar comment. Note: When changing previously reported test results, it is important to notify the clinician.

4. The clinical implications of erroneously reporting the patient's results as a substantial left shift may lead to an incorrect presumption of an infection. This could lead to unwarranted cultures and other diagnostic tests as well as inappropriate and potentially harmful treatments. In addition the patient could be subjected to unnecessary distress, lost time, and expense.

Review Questions

1. a; 2. d; 3. c; 4. b; 5. d; 6. c; 7. d; 8. c; 9. b; 10. c

CHAPTER 27: INTRODUCTION TO HEMATOLOGIC NEOPLASMS

Case Study

1. The nucleated cells in the figure are large, with round or slightly irregular nuclei with smooth chromatin and indistinct nucleoli, and an increased nucleus-to-cytoplasm (N:C) ratio. These cells should be reported as blasts. The inclusions are Auer rods and they are significant in that they are only found in leukemic myeloblasts, promyelocytes, or monoblasts. They are not found in lymphoblasts.

2. Given the presence of blasts with Auer rods, the most likely diagnosis is acute myeloid leukemia (AML). The World Health Organization criterion for acute leukemia is the finding of at least 20% blasts in the bone marrow.

3. A bone marrow aspirate is required and the following tests are performed: a differential count to determine the % blasts, immunophenotyping by flow cytometry to confirm the lineage and maturation stage of the blasts, cytogenetic analysis (karyotyping) to detect chromosome abnormalities, and molecular genetic testing to detect certain recurring mutations associated with AML.

4. In acute leukemia there is a rapid expansion of blasts in bone marrow, which replace the normal hematopoietic precursors and result in peripheral cytopenias. Anemia (low hemoglobin concentration) can cause weakness; the neutropenia increases the risk of infection and resulting fever; and the severe thrombocytopenia can cause generalized ecchymoses as well as other mucocutaneous bleeding symptoms. In acute leukemia the sudden onset of these symptoms are common at presentation.

5. A maturation arrest or a block in differentiation may occur as a result of mutation in genes coding for nuclear transcription factors or other genes needed for myeloid differentiation or as a result of aberrant changes in their epigenetic regulation, which prevent the expression of the genes needed for myeloid differentiation.

Review Questions

1. a; 2. b; 3. d; 4. c; 5. c; 6. c; 7. d; 8. d; 9. c; 10. a

CHAPTER 28: FLOW CYTOMETRIC ANALYSIS IN HEMATOLOGIC DISORDERS

Case Studies

Case 1

1. The lymphoid population is the most prominent. Forward scatter demonstrates small to medium-sized cells. These cells are characterized by low side scatter indicative of sparse agranular cytoplasm.

2. The majority of cells express CD19, CD10, and κ light chain. There is also a small population of T cells positive for CD5 and negative for CD19 antigen.

3. Prominent κ light chain expression indicates a monoclonal B cell population that is characteristic of lymphoma.

Case 2

1. The low density of CD45 antigen coupled with relatively low side scatter is characteristic of a blast population. Such a prominent blast population can only be seen in acute leukemias.

2. The expression of immature markers (CD34 and HLA-DR) coupled with positivity for myeloid and megakaryoblastic antigens (CD33, CD41, and CD61) is seen in acute megakaryoblastic leukemias.

Review Questions

1. c; 2. b; 3. a; 4. d; 5. b; 6. a; 7. a; 8. a; 9. c; 10. a; 11. b

CHAPTER 29: MOLECULAR DIAGNOSTICS IN HEMATOPATHOLOGY

Case Study

1. *JAK2* mutation testing is typically performed on blood specimens collected with an EDTA anticoagulant but can also be performed on bone marrow aspirates.

2. The patient specimen demonstrates amplification with both the VIC (WT) and FAM (MU) probes as seen by the amplification curves in panels A and B of Figure 29.1.

3. The patient specimen amplifies with both mutant and wild type probes indicating the presence of both wild-type and mutant DNA in the specimen. This indicates that the *JAK2* mutation is heterozygous.

4. Based on the laboratory results as well as the molecular testing results it is likely that the patient has polycythemia vera (PV). The 2016 World Health Organization guidelines describe PV as a myeloproliferative neoplasm with three major diagnostic criteria: elevated hemoglobin or hematocrit or red blood cell mass, hypercellular bone marrow, and the presence of a *JAK2* p.Val617Phe or exon 12 mutation (Chapter 32). The patient fulfills these diagnostic criteria.

Review Questions

1. a; 2. b; 3. d; 4. b; 5. b; 6. c; 7. a; 8. c; 9. b; 10. b

CHAPTER 30: CYTOGENETICS

Case Study

1. G banding uses Giemsa staining to differentiate chromosomes into bands for identification of specific chromosomes. The chromosomes must be pretreated with the proteolytic enzyme trypsin.

2. The mutation is an example of a structural rearrangement between chromosomes 9 and 22, called the *Philadelphia chromosome*. The Philadelphia chromosome represents a balanced translocation between the long arms of chromosomes 9 and 22. At the molecular level, the gene for *ABL1*, an oncogene, joins a gene on chromosome 22 named *BCR*. The result of the fusion of these two genes is a new fusion protein.

3. Fluorescence in situ hybridization (FISH) is a molecular technique that uses DNA or RNA probes labeled directly with a fluorescent nucleotide or with a hapten (e.g., dinitrophenyl, digoxigenin, or biotin). The DNA in the probe and either the metaphase or interphase cells are made single-stranded (denatured) and then hybridized together. Cells hybridized with a direct-label probe are viewed with a fluorescence microscope. If the probe was labeled with a hapten, antibodies to the hapten, carrying a fluorescent tag, are applied to the cells. Once the antibodies bind to the RNA or DNA probe, the cells can be viewed using a fluorescence microscope. FISH complements standard chromosome analysis by confirming the G-band analysis and by improving resolution, which allows for analysis at the molecular level.

Review Questions

1. c; 2. d; 3. a; 4. d; 5. a; 6. c; 7. d; 8. c; 9. c; 10. b

CHAPTER 31: ACUTE LEUKEMIAS

Case Study

1. Because of the presence of blasts on the peripheral blood film, the most likely diagnosis is acute leukemia. The thrombocytopenia and anemia support that diagnosis. According to the World Health Organization (WHO) classification, ≥20% blasts in the bone marrow is required for diagnosis of acute leukemia; an exception to this criterion are those cases that have specific genetic abnormalities (delineated in the WHO classification) that are diagnostic, regardless of blast count. Acute lymphoblastic leukemia (ALL) is more common in children. Immunophenotyping by flow cytometry determines the lineage and maturation stage of the blasts. Testing for genetic abnormalities is required for diagnosis and prognosis.

2. This child has clinical and laboratory features indicative of a favorable prognosis: young age, a white blood cell count less than 20×10^9 /L (i.e., low tumor burden), and hyperdiploidy. The strongest predictor of patient outcome is the presence of certain genetic abnormalities; the immunophenotype also contributes to the prognosis.

3. Hyperdiploidy carries a favorable prognosis in B cell ALL in children.

Review Questions

1. b; 2. b; 3. a; 4. d; 5. b; 6. d; 7. c; 8. c; 9. b; 10. b; 11. b; 12. b

CHAPTER 32: MYELOPROLIFERATIVE NEOPLASMS

Case Study

1. An elevated white blood cell (WBC) count with a left shift suggests a myeloproliferative neoplasm or a leukemoid reaction (reactive neutrophilia). However, in this patient the WBC count was extremely elevated, the left shift was rather deep (presence of promyelocytes and blasts), and basophilia was present, which suggests that a myeloproliferative neoplasm is likely present. Chronic myeloid (myelogenous) leukemia (CML) is the most likely cause of these laboratory findings.

2. The leukocyte alkaline phosphatase (LAP) score is low in CML as a result of inappropriate LAP synthesis in the secondary granules, whereas LAP is elevated in bacterial infections as a result of activation of enzyme synthesis.

3. The *BCR/ABL1* fusion gene must be identified to confirm the diagnosis of CML. *BCR/ABL1* can be demonstrated from a karyotype analysis showing the t(9;22) reciprocal translocation known as the *Philadelphia chromosome* (Chapter 30), by demonstration of the *BCR/ABL1* fusion gene using fluorescence in situ hybridization (Chapter 30), or by demonstration of the *BCR/ABL1* fusion mRNA by qualitative reverse transcriptase polymerase chain reaction (Chapter 29). Patients who have complete blood count and differential results that resemble those in CML but test negative for *BCR/ABL1* are considered to have atypical CML, and the disorder is classified as myelodysplastic syndrome/myeloproliferative neoplasm (Chapter 33).

4. Cytogenetic studies are likely to show the t(9;22) mutation.

5. The t(9;22) translocation produces the *BCR/ABL1* chimeric gene, which is observed in four primary molecular forms that produce three versions of the BCR/ABL chimeric protein: p190, p210, and p230.

6. First-line therapy for CML is the tyrosine kinase inhibitor imatinib mesylate. Allogeneic stem cell transplantation should be considered for all CML patients because it is the only potentially curative treatment for CML. However, few CML patients qualify for allogeneic stem cell transplantation because most do not meet the criteria for low risk: age younger than 40 years, disease in the chronic phase, transplantation within 1 year of diagnosis, and availability of an HLA-matched donor. For those patients who qualify for allogeneic stem cell transplantation, imatinib is used to induce remission before transplant, to treat minimum residual disease, and to provide rescue therapy if the transplant fails. Imatinib is continued as lifelong therapy until drug resistance is detected.

7. The majority of cases of imatinib resistance result from two primary causes: acquisition of additional *BCR/ABL1* mutations and expression of point mutations in the adenosine triphosphate (ATP) binding site. Additional *BCR/ABL1* mutations can occur through the usual translocation of the remaining unaffected chromosomes 9 and 22, which converts the hematopoietic stem cell from heterozygous to homozygous for the *BCR/ABL1* mutation. A double dose of *BCR/ABL1* can also be acquired from gene duplication during mitosis and accounts for 10% of secondary mutations. An additional *BCR/ABL1* mutation will double the tyrosine kinase activity, which makes the imatinib dosage inadequate. In these cases higher dosages of imatinib will restore remission in most patients. More than 60 mutations have been identified in the ATP binding site, and these account for the remaining 50% to 90% of secondary mutations. Mutations in the ATP binding site reduce the binding affinity of imatinib, producing some level of resistance.

Review Questions

1. b; 2. c; 3. d; 4. c; 5. c; 6. c; 7. b; 8. d; 9. a; 10. c

CHAPTER 33: MYELODYSPLASTIC SYNDROMES

Case Study

1. The differential diagnosis of patients with pancytopenia should include megaloblastic anemia (vitamin B_{12} or folate deficiency), aplastic anemia, liver disease, alcoholism, and myelodysplastic syndromes (MDS).

2. The probable diagnosis is MDS.

3. This patient's MDS should be classified as myelodysplastic syndrome with ring sideroblasts with multilineage dysplasia (MDS-RS-MLD).

Review Questions

1. d; 2. a; 3. b; 4. b; 5. c; 6. c; 7. a; 8. d; 9. c; 10. c

CHAPTER 34: MATURE LYMPHOID NEOPLASMS

Case Study

1. The CBC results indicate a lymphocytosis, with cells that appear mature along with large numbers of smudge cells. It suggests that this patient has chronic lymphocytic leukemia.
2. In cases of suspected chronic lymphocytic leukemia, a peripheral blood specimen should be sent for flow cytometry to determine the immunophenotype of the lymphocytes. A cytospin stained for cyclin D1 or florescence in situ hybridization (FISH) for t(11;14) can be performed to rule out mantle cell lymphoma when there are inconsistencies in the immunophenotype.
3. Tests and assessments that are used in staging and determining prognosis include Rai and Binet staging, age of the patient, serum B_2 microglobulin level, flow cytometry for ZAP70 and CD38 expression, and cytogenetic/molecular tests for immunoglobulin heavy chain variable region (IGHV) status and del17/TP59 and other genetic abnormalities.

Review Questions

1. d; 2. c; 3. d; 4. d; 5. b; 6. b; 7. b; 8. a; 9. c; 10. a

CHAPTER 35: NORMAL HEMOSTASIS

Case Study

1. Given the family history, this may be an inherited condition, although pregnancy is an independent risk factor for thrombosis.
2. Thrombosis is probably caused by the deficiency of a coagulation inhibitor such as protein C, protein S, or antithrombin. It may be caused by a procoagulant gain-of-function mutation such as the factor V Leiden mutation or the prothrombin G20210A mutation.

Review Questions

1. b; 2. c; 3. b; 4. d; 5. b; 6. d; 7. b; 8. c; 9. c; 10. a; 11. a; 12. d; 13. a

CHAPTER 36: HEMORRHAGIC DISORDERS AND LABORATORY ASSESSMENT

Case Study

1. The combination of thrombocytopenia and prolonged prothrombin time (PT) and partial thromboplastin time (PTT) indicate probable liver disease. In the absence of a full medical history, the patient's hemarthroses and description of himself as a "bleeder" lead to the presumption of hemophilia, possibly hemophilia A. It is possible that he contracted hepatitis C from an untreated blood product. Treatment of factor concentrates for viral disease began in 1984. Before 1984 most hemophilia patients eventually developed hepatitis B or C from factor concentrates. Hepatitis A is also a possibility. Liver disease may be confirmed using bilirubin and liver enzyme assays.

In advanced liver disease, poor liver circulation causes pressure in the portal circulation. This enlarges the spleen (splenomegaly). The enlarged spleen sequesters and clears platelets more rapidly than normal, a condition called hypersplenism, which causes thrombocytopenia. In most cases, platelet function is reduced. This reduced platelet function can be demonstrated in the laboratory using platelet aggregometry and is the reason for the patient's epistaxis.

Vitamin K deficiency is also a possibility. To differentiate vitamin K deficiency from liver disease, a factor V and VII activity assay is performed. In vitamin K deficiency, factor VII activity is reduced but factor V activity is normal. In liver disease, both are reduced.

2. In early liver disease the vitamin K-dependent factors II (prothrombin), VII, IX, and X are produced with diminished function. This can be corrected with a trial dose of oral or intravenous vitamin K. In people with true vitamin K deficiency secondary to an altered diet, the vitamin K therapy corrects bleeding and normalizes the PT and PTT, but in liver disease vitamin K may not have a lasting effect. This is because the liver cannot process the vitamin K normally.

In addition to vitamin K therapy, thawed frozen plasma (FP) transfusion at 1 to 2 units/day is effective in supplementing the liver's production of all the coagulation factors. Cryoprecipitate may also be used to raise the fibrinogen concentration, and platelet concentrate may be used if the platelet count drops to less than 50,000/μL and there is continued evidence of mucocutaneous bleeding. Administration of vitamin K, FP, cryoprecipitate, and platelets does not cure liver disease; these therapies only treat the bleeding symptoms.

Review Questions

1. a; 2. d; 3. b; 4. c; 5. b; 6. b; 7. d; 8. a; 9. a; 10. c; 11. c

CHAPTER 37: QUALITATIVE DISORDERS OF PLATELETS AND VASCULATURE

Case Study

1. Storage pool disease, aspirin-like defects, and use of antiplatelet agents such as aspirin are possibilities.
2. Storage pool disease or aspirin-like defects seem most likely.
3. Based on the results of the quantitative test for adenosine triphosphate release, the likely cause is dense granule storage pool disease.

These results were confirmed by the findings of electron microscopy of the patient's platelets, which revealed the absence of detectable dense granules. Because the patient's bleeding problems are due to an inherited abnormality that typically results in only mild bleeding problems, the patient was counseled to avoid antiplatelet agents, particularly aspirin, because they are known to exacerbate the bleeding problems encountered by patients with dense granule deficiency.

Review Questions

1. d; 2. a; 3. b; 4. c; 5. c; 6. d; 7. a; 8. d; 9. a; 10. a; 11. c; 12. b

CHAPTER 38: THROMBOCYTOPENIA AND THROMBOCYTOSIS

Case Study

1. Patients with end-stage liver disease completely remodel the blood circulating through the liver and all acquire portal venous hypertension and splenomegaly, sometimes severe. Enlarged spleens sequester circulating platelets. The disorder manifested in this patient represents an example of an abnormal distribution/hemodilution of platelets.

2. Consideration should be given to sorting out other differentials for thrombocytopenia:
   - Laboratory evidence could be sought to rule in or rule out infection including sources in the blood, sputum, urine, etc.
   - Laboratory tests to assess the likelihood of DIC (such as fibrin-split products, D-dimers, fibrinogen level) could be considered.
   - Because the history specifies multiple prior pregnancies, consideration could be given to assessing the degree, if any, of alloimmunization to class I HLA antigens.

3. Tissue-matched platelets can provide benefit in HLA-alloimmunized patients, however providing them in this clinical setting represents poor stewardship of expensive blood components. Any transfused platelets will suffer the same untimely, extravascular splenic sequestration as the patient's own platelets. They will not circulate long enough to provide any patient benefit.

Review Questions

1. c; 2. c; 3. b; 4. c; 5. c; 6. b; 7. b; 8. c; 9. d; 10. a; 11. d; 12. c

CHAPTER 39: THROMBOTIC DISORDERS AND LABORATORY ASSESSMENT

Case Study

1. The following tests for congenital and acquired risk factors are included in a thrombophilia profile. Results for the items with asterisks are valid only when the test is performed 10 to 14 days after termination of anticoagulant therapy or resolution of a thrombotic event.
   - Homocysteine
   - Lupus anticoagulant profile*
   - Prothrombin G20210A mutation
   - Activated protein C resistance*
   - Factor V Leiden mutation (confirmatory for activated protein C resistance)
   - Anticardiolipin antibodies by immunoassay
   - Protein C functional assay* and follow-up immunoassay
   - Protein S functional assay* and follow-up immunoassay
   - Antithrombin functional assay* and follow-up immunoassay

2. The most common acquired thrombotic risk factors are antiphospholipid antibodies and lupus anticoagulant, and these are most often implicated in a thrombotic event.

3. Patients with thrombotic risk factors may be instructed to avoid situations and practices that may trigger thrombosis, such as immobilization, smoking, and use of oral contraceptives or hormone replacement therapy. They may be provided with prophylactic anticoagulant therapy at times when circumstances increasing thrombotic risk cannot be avoided, such as when undergoing orthopedic surgery. Specific coagulation tests are available when monitoring of anticoagulation therapy is required.

Review Questions

1. b; 2. a; 3. d; 4. c; 5. a; 6. b; 7. a; 8. a; 9. c; 10. d; 11. d; 12. d; 13. d; 14. c; 15. a

CHAPTER 40: ANTITHROMBOTIC THERAPIES AND THEIR LABORATORY ASSESSMENT

Case Study

1. The increase in anticoagulation could be caused by a change in diet, dietary supplements, or drugs. Any new drug that interferes with the cytochrome oxidase P-450 enzyme 2C9 pathway could reduce Coumadin breakdown and excretion and increase its effectiveness.

2. Determine what has caused the change in Coumadin efficacy and eliminate it if possible, adjust the Coumadin dosage, or give vitamin K orally or intravenously to stop bleeding if necessary.

3. The chromogenic factor X assay.

Review Questions

1. c; 2. a; 3. c; 4. a; 5. d; 6. b; 7. d; 8. c; 9. b; 10. b; 11. a; 12. a; 13. a; 14. d

CHAPTER 41: LABORATORY EVALUATION OF HEMOSTASIS

Case Study

1. The laboratory director questioned the phlebotomist about the problem. The phlebotomist admitted that he had erroneously collected blood in a red- and gray-stoppered "tiger-top" tube and, responding to the patient's remark, had immediately poured the blood into a blue-stoppered tube for analysis. He thought the specimen would be okay because it had not clotted yet.

2. The red and gray marbleized stopper designates a serum separator tube. The phlebotomist poured the blood into the blue-stoppered tube before it had begun to clot; however, the activator from the tiger-top tube shortened the clotting time on the prothrombin time (PT) test, thus causing an erroneously short PT and low international normalized ratio (INR).

3. Unexpectedly short PTs during oral anticoagulant therapy are generally indicators of patient noncompliance to the drug regimen. The second most common circumstance that affects the PT is dietary changes, most often an increased intake of vitamin K-rich foods such as green leafy vegetables, liver, or avocado. In this instance the patient had been fully compliant, carefully following the prescribed dosage

and timing, and her diet had not changed. These facts led the laboratory director to consider a specimen collection error.

Specimens collected in 3.2% sodium citrate may be stored for up to 24 hours at room temperature without a change in the PT. However, specimens stored at higher than 24° C deteriorate rapidly, which causes prolongation of the PT and increase in the INR. Prolonged storage at 2° C to 4° C may activate factor VII, which slightly shortens the PT and slightly decreases the INR.

Many serum separator tubes contain particulate materials that hasten in vitro clotting. Core laboratory managers select these tubes to improve test result turnaround time when the required specimen is serum. When blood is collected into a series of tubes that includes a blue-stoppered tube for hemostasis testing, the blue-stoppered tube should be filled first or should be filled after a tube without additives. It should not be filled immediately after filling a serum separator tube with clot activators because the activators may carry over to the hemostasis specimen and affect test results.

In this case an observant patient provided clues that led to identification of the preanalytical error. The phlebotomist was carefully counseled about the effects of tube additives on hemostasis tests.

Review Questions

1. c; 2. b; 3. a; 4. b; 5. a; 6. d; 7. b; 8. b; 9. b; 10. a; 11. b; 12. d; 13. d; 14. d; 15. b

CHAPTER 42: HEMOSTASIS AND COAGULATION INSTRUMENTATION

Case Study

1. No. The flag on the result indicates a problem as the lower limit for the test was exceeded; further investigation of the quality set points within the instrument revealed a flag for a clotted specimen. The results of the prothrombin time/ international normalized ratio (PT/INR) for day 3 are consistent with Coumadin anticoagulation; however, the results for day 5 are not consistent with Coumadin anticoagulation and not similar to the result of day 3. Any PT/ INR lower than the lower limit of the reference value has no clinical meaning. The test results on day 5 are not valid and should not be reported.

2. The medical laboratory scientist must call the floor and explain that there was something wrong with the specimen, an invalid result was obtained, and a new specimen needs to be drawn. The scientist needs to explain the following to the nurse: the proper order of filling blood collection tubes, avoiding contaminating the blood specimen with substances being given intravenously, the proper amount of blood for the collection tube with proper mixing, and that the specimen should be immediately sent to the laboratory for testing.

3. Because the patient has a prolonged PT/INR and is taking Coumadin, she is at risk for bleeding if her dosage is not adjusted properly. Because her PT/INR on day 3 was in the therapeutic range she is likely safe from a bleeding episode, but a current test result is needed. Because the erroneous result on day 5 likely was due to an improper specimen, there is no information to infer that the patient is at risk of bleeding. If the repeat draw on the patient is higher than the therapeutic range for Coumadin (INR 2.0 to 3.0), then the patient is at risk for bleeding.

Review Questions

1. d; 2. a; 3. c; 4. b; 5. c; 6. b; 7. a; 8. d; 9. a; 10. d

CHAPTER 43: HEMATOLOGY AND HEMOSTASIS IN SELECTED POPULATIONS

Case Study

1. Yes, the newborn reference interval for hemoglobin is 16.5 to 21.5 g/dL and for the hematocrit it is 48% to 68%.

2. These values are normal for newborns. Erythrocytes of a newborn are markedly macrocytic. There may be 2 to 24 nucleated red blood cells on the first postnatal day, but they are not present by day 5. The polychromasia reflects the reticulocytosis that persists for about 4 days.

3. These values are within the reference intervals for newborns. The white blood cell count of a newborn fluctuates a great deal, with a reference interval of 9.0 to 37.0 $\times$ 10^9/L, and leukocytosis without evidence of infection is common. The differential may show an increase in neutrophils rather than the lymphocyte predominance seen after 2 weeks. In this case the neutrophils and lymphocytes were present in equal amounts, but no immature neutrophils were seen.

Review Questions

1. d; 2. b; 3. b; 4. c; 5. d; 6. b; 7. a; 8. d; 9. c; 10. a

abetalipoproteinemia (ABL): Autosomal recessive disorder of lipoprotein metabolism, caused by mutations in the *MTTP* (microsomal triglyceride transfer protein) gene, in which lipoproteins containing apolipoprotein B (chylomicrons, very-low-density lipoproteins, and low-density lipoproteins) are not synthesized. Characterized by fat malabsorption, ataxia, neuropathy, peripheral blood film acanthocytes, and low plasma cholesterol and triglyceride levels.

absolute neutrophil count (ANC): Neutrophils per liter of blood calculated by multiplying the total white blood cell count by the percentage of segmented neutrophils and bands, or may be counted directly using an automated blood cell analyzer.

absolute reticulocyte count (ARC): Reticulocytes per liter of blood calculated by multiplying the patient's visual reticulocyte count (reticulocyte percentage) by the red blood cell count or may be measured directly using an automated blood cell analyzer.

acanthocyte (spur cell): Small, dense, red blood cell with a few, irregularly spaced, spiny projections of varying lengths on a peripheral blood film. Contrast with the burr cell (echinocyte), which has short, evenly spaced projections.

acanthocytosis: Presence of acanthocytes in the blood. Associated with abnormalities of lipid metabolism, such as severe liver disease and neuroacanthocytosis (abetalipoproteinemia and McLeod syndrome).

accuracy: Extent to which an assay result matches its true value. Computed by comparing assay results with the results from an established reference assay or a primary standard.

achlorhydria: Pathologic absence of free hydrochloric acid from gastric secretions after stimulation.

acid elution slide test (Kleihauer-Betke stain): Test for detecting fetal red blood cells in the maternal circulation. Blood films are immersed in an acid buffer, which causes adult hemoglobin (Hb A) to be eluted from the cells. The film is stained, and red blood cells that have fetal hemoglobin (Hb F) take up the stain.

acquired immunodeficiency syndrome (AIDS): Late-stage immune system suppression characterized by depletion of CD4⁺ T lymphocytes and depression of cellular immunity causing susceptibility to opportunistic infections and neoplasms. Caused by infection with human immunodeficiency virus (HIV), a retrovirus.

acrocentric: Describes the appearance of a metaphase chromosome with the centromere near one end, which causes the q (long) arm to be much longer than the p (short) arm.

acrocyanosis: Persistent cyanosis (blotchy blue discoloration) in the skin of the fingers, toes, feet, nose, and ears on prolonged exposure to cold.

activated clotting time (ACT): Whole-blood clotting time test often used in cardiac surgical suites. A particulate activator is added to blood, the mixture is rocked, and the interval to clotting is recorded. Employed to monitor high-dose unfractionated heparin therapy during cardiac catheterization or cardiac surgeries using the cardiopulmonary bypass extracorporeal circuit.

activated partial thromboplastin time (APTT, partial thromboplastin time, PTT): Clot-based screening test to measure the activity of prekallikrein, high-molecular-weight kininogen, coagulation factors XII, XI, IX, VIII, X, V, and II (prothrombin), and fibrinogen. Calcium chloride, phospholipid, and negatively charged particulate activator are added to patient plasma and the time to form a clot is recorded. Used to monitor unfractionated heparin therapy and to screen for intrinsic and common pathway deficiencies, specific factor inhibitors, and lupus anticoagulant.

activated protein C (APC): Coagulation pathway regulatory protein activated by the thrombin-thrombomodulin complex that, when bound and stabilized by protein S, hydrolyzes and inactivates factor Va and factor VIIIa.

activated protein C resistance (APCR): Inherited condition in which activated coagulation factor V (Va) resists digestion by activated protein C, resulting in an increased risk of venous thrombosis. In 90% of cases, APCR is caused by the factor V Leiden mutation.

activated prothrombin complex concentrate (APCC): Therapeutic plasma preparation that bypasses factor VIII activation and is used to treat bleeding episodes in hemophilic patients who have developed factor VIII inhibitor; also used to treat other types of bleeding episodes. Contains *activated* factors II (prothrombin), VII, IX, and X. Contrast with prothrombin complex concentrate (PCC).

acute: Describes diseases whose symptoms begin abruptly with marked intensity and then may subside after a relatively short period.

acute leukemia: Malignant, unregulated proliferation of hematopoietic progenitors of the myeloid or lymphoid cell lines in the bone marrow with the appearance of blasts and other immature forms in the peripheral blood. Characterized by abrupt onset of symptoms and, if left untreated, death within months of the time of diagnosis.

acute myocardial infarction (AMI): Occlusion of a coronary artery by a clot, causing ischemia and necrosis (tissue death) of surrounding heart muscle. Commonly called a heart attack.

acute phase reactant: Protein produced by the liver, which undergoes a change in its serum concentration in response to inflammation. Positive acute phase reactants increase in concentration during inflammation (examples include C-reactive protein, hepcidin, ferritin, and fibrinogen). Negative acute phase reactants decrease in concentration during inflammation (examples include albumin and transferrin).

adenopathy: Enlargement of one or more lymph nodes.

adenosine diphosphate (ADP): Purine nucleotide that activates platelets by binding platelet receptor P2Y₁ and P2Y₁₂. Produced by hydrolysis of adenosine triphosphate.

adenosine triphosphate (ATP): Purine nucleotide that stores energy in the form of high-energy phosphate bonds, releasing energy on hydrolysis to drive metabolic reactions.

adhesion: Property of binding or remaining in proximity; for example, attachment of platelets to surfaces such as subendothelial collagen.

adipocyte: Fat cell; adipocytes make up adipose tissue and the yellow portion of the bone marrow.

afibrinogenemia: Complete absence of plasma fibrinogen.

agammaglobulinemia: Immunodeficiency characterized by an absence or extremely reduced level of plasma gamma globulin and reduced levels of immunoglobulins. Associated with increased risk of infection.

agglutination: Cross-linking of antigen-bearing cells or particles by a specific antibody to form visible clumps.

aggregation: Clustering or clumping of similar cell types or particles; for example, attachment of platelets to other platelets or red blood cells to other red blood cells.

agnogenic: Of idiopathic or unknown origin.

agonist: Reagent used in platelet aggregation tests that binds to specific platelet receptors and induces an activation signaling pathway that results in activation of the glycoprotein IIb/IIIa receptor, which allows platelet-platelet binding via fibrinogen.

agranulocytosis: Any condition involving decreased numbers of granulocytes (segmented neutrophils or band neutrophils).

albinism: Hereditary condition characterized by partial or total lack of melanin pigment in the body; skin, hair, and eyes may be affected. Individuals with total albinism have pale skin that does not tan, white hair, and pink eyes. Often associated with platelet storage pool deficiency.

Alder-Reilly anomaly: Autosomal dominant polysaccharide metabolism disorder in which white blood cells (WBCs) of the myelocytic series, and sometimes all WBCs, contain coarse azurophilic mucopolysaccharide granules.

allele: One of two or more alternative forms of a gene that occupy corresponding loci on homologous chromosomes. Each allele encodes a certain inherited characteristic. An individual normally has two alleles for each gene, one contributed by the mother and one by the father. If both alleles are the same, the individual is homozygous, but if the alleles are different, the individual is heterozygous. In heterozygous individuals, one of the alleles may be dominant and the other recessive.

alloantibody (isoantibody): Antibody that is produced in response to the presence of foreign antigens; for instance, an antibody to a therapeutic coagulation factor that may render factor therapy ineffective, or an antibody produced to a donor red blood cell antigen that can cause immune destruction of the donor's red blood cells after transfusion.

alloimmune: Producing antibodies to antigens derived from a genetically dissimilar individual of the same species.

alloimmune hemolytic anemia: Anemia caused by antibodies stimulated by exposure to foreign red blood cell antigens. Antibodies bind to and shorten the life span of circulating red blood cells, which is the pathologic basis for immune-mediated hemolytic transfusion reactions and hemolytic disease of the fetus and newborn.

α-granules: Platelet granules that store and release a variety of hemostasis proteins. There are 50 to 80 α-granules per platelet. In transmission electron microscopy, α-granules appear light gray, in contrast to dense granules, which appear black.

α-thalassemia: See thalassemia.

amyloidosis: Disease in which a waxy, starch-like glycoprotein (amyloid) accumulates in tissues and organs, impairing their function.

analogue drugs: Drugs that are chemically similar to one another but, because of minor structural differences, may have different physiologic actions.

anaplastic: Characterized by loss of differentiation and growth without structure or form. Anaplasia is a characteristic of cancer.

anatomic bleeding disorder: Chronic episodic bleeding into soft tissue such as muscles, joints, and body cavities. Indicates a coagulation factor deficiency such as hemophilia or an acquired coagulation factor inhibitor. Contrast with mucocutaneous bleeding disorder.

anemia: Diminished delivery of oxygen to tissues, as evidenced by pallor, muscle weakness, and dyspnea. May be caused by blood loss, decreased red blood cell production, or increased red blood cell destruction (shortened life span).

aneuploidy: An abnormal number of chromosomes that is not an exact multiple of the normal haploid number (23 in humans), such as trisomy (presence of an extra chromosome) or monosomy (absence of one chromosome from a pair).

anisocytosis: Abnormal red blood cell (RBC) morphology characterized by considerable variation in RBC volume or RBC diameter on a peripheral blood film.

anoxia: Inadequate tissue oxygenation caused by poor lung perfusion or a diminished blood supply.

antagonist: Drug that nullifies the action of another drug or that reduces a normal cellular response. Aspirin is a platelet antagonist because it reduces platelet activation.

antecubital fossa: Concavity opposite the elbow.

antibody (Ab): Specialized protein (immunoglobulin) that is produced by B lymphocytes and plasma cells when the immune system is exposed to foreign antigens from bacteria, viruses, or other biologic materials. An antibody molecule has a specific amino acid sequence in its variable region that enables it to bind to the antigen that originally stimulated its production.

anticardiolipin antibody (ACL, ACA): Member of the antiphospholipid antibody family that includes anti-β2-glycoprotein I and lupus anticoagulant. An ACL antibody is an autoantibody detected in a solid-phase immunoassay system using cardiolipin as the target antigen. The chronic presence of ACL antibodies is associated with venous and arterial thrombotic disease.

anticoagulant: Therapeutic agent that delays blood coagulation, such as heparin or Coumadin, used to treat thrombosis and to prevent thrombotic events in patients who are at risk. Also an additive to blood specimen collection tubes that prevents in vitro blood clotting, such as sodium citrate or ethylenediaminetetraacetate (EDTA).

antigen: Molecule that the immune system recognizes as foreign and that subsequently evokes an immune response.

antihemophilic factor (AHF): Therapeutic concentration of coagulation factor VIII produced through chemical fractionation, immunoaffinity column, or recombinant synthesis. Prescribed in the treatment of hemophilia A, a hereditary deficiency of factor VIII.

antineoplastic: Chemotherapeutic agent that controls or kills cancer cells.

antiphospholipid antibody (APL, APA): Member of the antibody family that includes anticardiolipin, anti-β2-glycoprotein I, and lupus anticoagulant. Binds phospholipid-binding proteins, such as β2-glycoprotein. Associated with venous and arterial thrombotic disease.

antiphospholipid syndrome (APS): Group of thrombotic disorders related to the chronic presence of an antiphospholipid antibody, such as anticardiolipin, anti-β2-glycoprotein I, or lupus anticoagulant. Manifestations include migraine, transient ischemic attacks, strokes, acute myocardial infarction, peripheral artery disease, venous thromboembolism, and spontaneous abortion.

antithrombin (AT, antithrombin III, AT III): Plasma serine protease inhibitor produced in the liver and activated by therapeutic heparin or vascular heparan sulfate. When activated, antithrombin controls the coagulation pathway because it neutralizes all the serine proteases except factor VIIa, most importantly factors IIa (thrombin) and Xa.

antithrombotic: A property of a cell or a therapeutic agent that prevents or reduces the formation of blood clots.

aperture: Optical device in a microscope substage light path that controls the diameter of the light column that reaches the specimen. Also in electrical impedance instruments for blood cell analysis, an opening in a tube immersed in a conducting solution with a flowing electrical current through which cells traverse to be sized and counted by changes they cause in electrical resistance.

aplasia: Failure of the normal process of cell generation and development. Bone marrow aplasia is the loss of all bone marrow cellular elements.

aplastic anemia: Deficiency of all of the formed elements of blood, representing a failure of the blood cell-generating capacity of bone marrow.

apoferritin: Cage-like protein that stores ferric iron to form ferritin. Apoferritin can bind more than 4000 ferric ions.

apoptosis: Self-inflicted, programmed cell death characterized by nuclear condensation and cellular fragmentation into membrane-bound apoptotic bodies, which are phagocytized by macrophages without an inflammatory response. Physiologic process to eliminate unwanted or aging cells, as well as cells that are damaged, virally infected, or mutated.

aspirin (acetylsalicylic acid, ASA): Acetylsalicylic acid irreversibly acetylates platelet cyclooxygenase and reduces platelet activation. Most commonly used antiplatelet therapy.

asynchrony: Disturbance of coordination that causes processes to occur at abnormal times. In hematopoietic cell development, a difference in rate between cytoplasmic and nuclear maturation.

atrial fibrillation (AFIB): Uncontrolled and ineffective atrial heartbeat that raises the risk for stroke. The risk is controlled using long-term anticoagulation therapy, such as Coumadin.

atypical lymphocyte: See reactive lymphocyte.

Auer rod: Abnormal needle-shaped dark pink or purple inclusion in the cytoplasm of leukemic myeloblasts, promyelocytes, or monoblasts; composed of condensed primary granules. Found in certain types of acute myeloid leukemia and myelodysplastic syndromes.

autoantibody: Antibody produced by an individual that recognizes and binds an antigen on the individual's own tissues.

autoimmune: Describes a pathologic condition in which an antibody-mediated or cell-mediated immune response is mounted to self-antigens; for instance, in autoimmune hemolytic anemia (to red blood cell antigens), pernicious anemia (to intrinsic factor or gastric parietal cell antigens), or acquired aplastic anemia (to hematopoietic stem cell antigens).

autoimmune hemolytic anemia: Anemia characterized by premature red blood cell destruction. Autoantibodies bind to red blood cell antigens, causing their destruction either by macrophages in the spleen (extravascular or macrophage-mediated hemolysis) or by direct lysis usually within the blood vessels (intravascular or fragmentation hemolysis).

autologous: Related to self or belonging to the same organism; for example, used to describe blood that is donated by patients before surgery for the purpose of transfusion to themselves during or after surgery.

autosomal dominant inheritance: Pattern of inheritance in which the transmission of a dominant allele on an autosome causes a trait to be expressed in heterozygotes.

autosomal inheritance: Inheritance of traits located on non-sex chromosomes.

autosomal recessive inheritance: Pattern of inheritance on non-sex chromosomes, resulting from the transmission of a recessive allele that is not expressed in heterozygotes.

autosome: Any of the 22 pairs of chromosomes in humans other than the sex chromosomes, X and Y.

autosplenectomy: Progressive damage, shrinkage, and loss of function of the spleen as a result of infarction secondary to a hemolytic anemia, such as sickle cell anemia.

azurophilic: Having cellular structures that stain blue with Giemsa stain and red-purple with Wright stain.

azurophilic granules: Primary cytoplasmic granules in myelocytic cells that, when stained with Wright stain, appear reddish purple. Azurophilic granules of different composition may also appear in a minority of lymphocytes.

Babesia: Protozoal parasite transmitted by ticks that infects human red blood cells and causes babesiosis, a malaria-like illness.

band neutrophil (band): Immediate precursor of the mature segmented neutrophil with a nonsegmented, usually curved, nucleus. Present in the bone marrow and in low numbers in the peripheral blood.

Bartonellosis: Acute febrile infection caused by the bacterium *Bartonella bacilliformis*, which is transmitted by the bite of a sandfly. The first stage of the disease is associated with severe hemolytic anemia.

base pair: Pair of nucleotides in complementary strands of a DNA molecule that interact through hydrogen bonding across the axis of the DNA helix. One of the nucleotides in each pair is a purine (either adenine or guanine), and the other is a pyrimidine (either thymine or cytosine). Adenine always pairs with thymine, and guanine always pairs with cytosine.

basophil (baso): Mature, granulocytic white blood cell characterized by cytoplasmic granules that stain bluish black with Wright stain. Cytoplasmic granules of basophils are of variable size and may obscure the nucleus.

basophilia: Increase in the number of basophils in the peripheral blood to more than the reference interval; also a description of cytoplasm that stains dark blue with Wright stain, such as radial basophilia or diffuse basophilia.

basophilic normoblast (prorubricyte): Second identifiable stage in bone marrow erythroid maturation, derived from the pronormoblast (rubriblast). Typically 10 to 15 μm in diameter, it has cytoplasm that stains dark blue with Wright stain.

basophilic stippling: Dark blue-purple, fine or coarse granules evenly distributed within a red blood cell stained with Wright stain. Composed of precipitated ribosomal proteins and ribonucleic acid (RNA) and found in various anemias and in toxic states such as lead poisoning.

B cell (B lymphocyte): Lymphocyte that participates in humoral immunity and the production of antibodies; develops into a plasma cell.

Bence Jones protein: Protein found almost exclusively in the urine of patients with plasma cell myeloma (multiple myeloma), consisting of the light chains of the abnormal immunoglobulins produced.

benign: Noncancerous or nonmalignant.

Bernard-Soulier syndrome (BSS): Mild to moderate mucocutaneous bleeding disorder caused by a mutation in platelet glycoprotein Ib (GPIb) or GPIX, part of the GPIb/IX/V von Willebrand factor receptor complex. The disorder is a defect of platelet adhesion.

β2-glycoprotein I (β2-GPI): Plasma globulin that is a target of the antiphospholipid antibody anti-β2-glycoprotein I.

β-thalassemia: See thalassemia.

bilirubin: Gold-red-brown pigment, the main component of bile and a major metabolic product of the heme portion of hemoglobin, released from senescent red blood cells. Elevated bilirubin imparts a gold color to plasma and urine and may indicate hemolytic anemia, liver disease, or bile duct occlusion.

bilirubinemia (icterus, hyperbilirubinemia): Excess bilirubin in plasma. Imparts a gold color to plasma and may indicate hemolytic anemia, liver disease, or bile duct occlusion.

2,3-bisphosphoglycerate (2,3-BPG, 2,3-diphosphoglycerate, 2,3-DPG): Product of red blood cell glycolysis that is generated in the Rapoport-Luebering shunt. One of the main regulators of oxygen uptake and delivery by hemoglobin, it decreases hemoglobin's affinity for oxygen, which enables it to more readily release oxygen to the tissues.

blast: Earliest, least differentiated stage of hematopoietic maturation that can be identified by its morphology in a Wright-stained bone marrow smear; for example, myeloblast, pronormoblast (rubriblast), lymphoblast.

bleeding time (BT): Time interval required for blood to stop flowing from a puncture wound 2 mm long and 1 mm deep on the volar surface of the forearm. The test is performed to evaluate vascular and platelet function.

Bohr effect: Effect of carbon dioxide and hydrogen ions on the affinity of hemoglobin for oxygen. Increasing carbon dioxide and hydrogen ion concentration (lower pH) decreases the affinity of hemoglobin for oxygen, allows hemoglobin to more readily release oxygen to tissues, and decreases oxygen saturation; decreasing concentration of carbon dioxide and hydrogen ion (higher pH) increases the affinity and oxygen saturation.

bone marrow: Gelatinous red and yellow tissue filling the medullary cavities of bones. In infants and young children, red marrow (active hematopoietic tissue) occupies the cavities of all bones. With age, yellow marrow (mostly adipocytes or fat cells) replaces much of the red marrow so that in adults the flat bones contain approximately half red and half yellow marrow, and the shaft of long bones contain yellow marrow with some red marrow at the extreme proximal ends. Diagnostic marrow specimens are usually collected from the posterior iliac crest in adults.

bone marrow aspirate specimen: A 1- to 1.5-mL aliquot of semiliquid marrow obtained by passing a needle into the marrow cavity and applying negative pressure. Spread as a smear on a microscope slide, stained, and examined for hematologic or systemic disease. Provides for analysis of individual cell morphology.

bone marrow biopsy specimen: A 1- to 1.5-cm cylinder of marrow tissue obtained by passing a biopsy cannula into the marrow cavity, rotating, and withdrawing. The tissue cylinder is fixed in formalin, sectioned, stained, and examined for hematologic or systemic disease. Provides for analysis of bone marrow architecture.

buffy coat: Gray-white layer of white blood cells and platelets that accumulates at the red blood cell-plasma interface when a tube of anticoagulated blood is allowed to stand or is centrifuged. May be used to harvest white blood cells for microscopic analysis when the count is low. An enlarged buffy coat may indicate leukemia.

Burkitt lymphoma: Lymphatic solid malignant tumor composed of mature B lymphocytes with a characteristic morphology, called Burkitt cells. Burkitt cells appear in lymph node biopsies, bone marrow, and occasionally in peripheral blood and have dark blue cytoplasm with multiple vacuoles creating a "starry sky" pattern.

burr cell (echinocyte): Red blood cell with short, equally spaced, blunt or pointed projections. Found in uremia and pyruvate kinase deficiency, and observed in all fields of a peripheral blood film. Differentiate from crenated red blood cells that are formed by cellular dehydration (drying artifact), and are not observed in all fields.

burst-forming unit (BFU): Early hematopoietic progenitor cell stage of the erythroid and megakaryocytic cell lines characterized by their tissue culture growth pattern in which large colonies are produced. Contrast with the more differentiated colony-forming unit (CFU) that produces smaller colonies.

C banding: In cytogenetic analysis, a specialized Giemsa stain technique employing first an acid and then a basic buffer, which highlights the centromeres of chromosomes. The stained centromere is the C band, which helps to identify the chromosome.

Cabot rings: Thread-like structures that appear as purple-blue loops or rings in Wright-stained red blood cell cytoplasm. Remnants of mitotic spindle fibers that indicate hematologic disease such as megaloblastic or refractory anemia.

calibrator (secondary standard): Preserved material in which the analyte concentration has been assigned by reference to a primary standard or by controlled reference assays in expert laboratories. Used for assays in which there are no primary standards, such as blood cell counts or coagulation assays.

carboxyhemoglobin: Hemoglobin that has bound carbon monoxide, which prevents normal oxygen exchange. Imparts a cherry-red color to venous blood, and its reduced oxygen capacity is the basis for carbon monoxide poisoning.

carcinoma: Malignant neoplasm of epithelial cell origin that invades surrounding tissue and may metastasize to distant regions of the body.

cardiopulmonary bypass (CPB): An extracorporeal device used in cardiac surgery to serve the functions of the heart and lungs of the patient. High levels of heparin, monitored by the ACT, are required.

cell membrane: Cell surface composed of two layers of phospholipids intermixed with cholesterol and a variety of specialized proteins that support cell structure, signaling, and ion transport.

cellular immunity (cell-mediated immunity, CMI): Immune response initiated and mediated by T lymphocytes (helper, cytotoxic, and regulatory), as well as natural killer cells and macrophages. Involved in graft rejection, delayed hypersensitivity, and responses to viral infections and tumors.

centriole: Cylindrical organelle composed of microtubules. Two centrioles typically orient perpendicular to each other forming the centrosome, located near the nucleus. During mitosis they replicate and move to opposite ends of the cell where they bind to spindle fibers that attach to the centromeres of chromosomes and effect their movement during metaphase.

centromere: Constricted portion of a chromosome that attaches to a spindle fiber to effect movement during metaphase. Categorized by their location as acrocentric (near one end), metacentric (near the center), or submetacentric (off center).

cerebrospinal fluid (CSF): Fluid that flows through and protects the four ventricles of the brain, the subarachnoid spaces, and the spinal canal. Derived from plasma and is the site of bacterial and viral infections called meningitis or encephalitis. Collected by lumbar puncture.

cerebrovascular accident (CVA): Stroke; occlusion of an artery of the brain or brain hemorrhage resulting in necrosis of brain tissue and loss of function.

Charcot-Leyden crystals: Crystalline structures that are shaped like narrow double pyramids and are found in the sputum of asthma patients and the feces of dysentery patients. Formed from the granules of disintegrating eosinophils.

Chédiak-Higashi anomaly: Autosomal recessive disorder characterized by partial albinism, photophobia, susceptibility to infection, and the presence of large blue granules in the cytoplasm of Wright-stained white blood cells and platelets.

chelation: Chemical formation of a ring-shaped molecular complex in which a metal ion is covalently bound. Chelating agents such as ethylenediaminetetraacetic acid (EDTA) or sodium citrate trap calcium ions and are used as blood specimen anticoagulants. Also used to treat lead poisoning or iron overload.

chemotaxis: Cellular movement toward or away from a chemical stimulus. Characteristic of neutrophils and monocytes, whose phagocytic activity is influenced by chemical factors released by invading microorganisms, damaged cells, or other white blood cells.

chemotherapy: Treatment of neoplastic disease (cancer) by chemical agents.

chromogen: Chemical that produces color in a reaction; used in spectrophotometric or microscopic analytical methods.

chromogenic substrate: A synthetic peptide that mimics the active site of an enzyme substrate with an attached chromophore; color is produced when the specified enzyme cleaves off the chromophore. Chromogenic substrate assays are used to quantify specific hemostatic enzymes.

chromophore: The portion of a molecule that absorbs incident light and emits colored light. Colored portions of chromogens that are synthesized in molecules to provide measurable color in laboratory assays.

chromosome: Thread-like nuclear structure composed of condensed DNA that transmits genetic information. In humans there are 46 chromosomes, including 22 homologous pairs of autosomes and 1 pair of sex chromosomes, XX in females and XY in males.

chronic: Persisting over a long period, often for the remainder of a person's life.

chronic leukemia: Malignant, unregulated proliferation of myelocytic or lymphocytic cells in the bone marrow in which increased numbers of their more differentiated and mature stages appear in peripheral blood. Characterized by slow onset and progression of symptoms.

Clinical and Laboratory Standards Institute (CLSI): Global nonprofit agency that uses consensus to develop and publish health care guidelines and standards.

Clinical Laboratory Improvement Amendments (CLIA) of 1988: Law establishing the Clinical Laboratory Improvement Amendments Committee (CLIAC), which sets and enforces standards for quality testing in the clinical laboratory.

clone: Group of genetically identical cells derived from a single common cell through mitosis.

Clostridium perfringens: Anaerobic gram-positive bacteria that cause gangrene, intravascular hemolysis, and thrombosis.

cluster of differentiation (CD): Cell surface membrane receptor or marker used to identify the lineage and maturation stage of hematopoietic cells. CD profiling (immunophenotyping) is used in flow cytometry to identify cell types and cell clones associated with lymphoid and myeloid neoplasms.

coagulation: Process in which soluble fibrinogen is converted into an insoluble fibrin clot.

coagulation cascade: Series of enzymatic reactions beginning with activation of factor VII by tissue factor (extrinsic pathway) or factor XII by a negatively charged surface (intrinsic pathway) and proceeding through the common pathway to the formation of an insoluble fibrin clot.

coagulation factors: Plasma proteins, also called procoagulants, that circulate as inactive forms. When activated in the process of coagulation, they participate in the coagulation cascade to form a fibrin clot. The units for the level of a coagulation factor is given as % or units/dL, where the number value is the same for both. Fibrinogen is always represented in units of mg/dL.

codocyte: See target cell.

coefficient of variation (CV, percent CV, CV%): Statistical measure of the deviation of a variable from its mean divided by the mean, usually expressed as a percentage.

colchicine: Alkaloid that blocks microtubule formation and prevents cell division. Colcemid, a colchicine derivative, is used in cytogenetic studies to arrest mitosis in metaphase so that chromosomes may be karyotyped.

cold agglutinin: Immunoglobulin M autoantibody specific for a red blood cell membrane antigen usually of the Ii system that typically reacts optimally at 4° C.

cold agglutinin disease (CAD): Acquired autoimmune hemolytic anemia resulting from red blood cell (RBC) agglutination by pathologic immunoglobulin M autoantibodies that react with RBCs at temperatures greater than 30° C. Symptoms include pallor, fatigue, dyspnea, and acrocyanosis or bluish discoloration of the extremities after exposure to cold. Acute CAD occurs secondary to *Mycoplasma pneumonia* or viral infections, whereas chronic CAD may occur secondary to lymphoproliferative neoplasms.

colony-forming unit (CFU): Hematopoietic progenitor cell derived from the pluripotent hematopoietic stem cell and gives rise to different hematopoietic cell lineages. Named because of its ability to form colonies in tissue culture.

colony-forming unit-granulocyte, erythrocyte, monocyte, and megakaryocyte (CFU-GEMM): Hematopoietic progenitor cell capable of differentiating into the granulocytic (myelocytic), erythrocytic (normoblastic), monocytic, or megakaryocytic cell lines.

colony-stimulating factor (CSF): Cytokine that promotes the division and differentiation of hematopoietic cells.

common coagulation pathway: The steps in the coagulation cascade from the activation of factor X through the conversion of fibrinogen to fibrin. The common pathway begins at the junction of the intrinsic and extrinsic pathways and involves factors X, V, II (prothrombin), and fibrinogen, in order of reaction.

complement (C): System of at least 20 serum proteins that responds to an antigen-antibody reaction to stimulate white blood cell chemotaxis, generate inflammation, or cause red blood cell lysis.

compound heterozygous: Having two different mutant alleles at the same locus on homologous chromosomes. An example is hemoglobin SC disease, with an S mutation at the β-globin chain locus on one chromosome, and a C mutation at the same locus on the other paired chromosome.

condenser: Substage microscope device that focuses light on the slide-mounted specimen to promote visual clarity.

confidence interval (CI): Range of values expected to contain the measured value (parameter) with a predetermined degree of statistical confidence. For instance, the 95% confidence interval is expected to include 95% of all values of a parameter measured in a normal population, which corresponds closely to ±2 standard deviations.

congenital: Describes a condition that exists at, and presumably before, birth. Often refers to a hereditary condition.

Coombs test: See direct antiglobulin test.

coronary artery bypass grafting (CABG): Cardiac surgery in which occluded sections of coronary arteries are replaced with grafts taken from nearby arteries, such as the internal mammary artery; requires cardiopulmonary bypass extracorporeal circulation with heparin anticoagulation.

corrected reticulocyte count: Calculation performed to correct the visual reticulocyte count for specimens with a hematocrit below 45% to the equivalent reticulocyte count at a hematocrit of 45%. In anemia, the visual reticulocyte percentage is misleadingly elevated because whole blood contains fewer red blood cells relative to reticulocytes.

Coumadin: Vitamin K antagonist used as an oral anticoagulant to prevent thrombosis in people at risk of developing a blood clot such as with atrial fibrillation, cardiac insufficiency, or after orthopedic surgery. Also used to treat people with a thromboembolic event. Suppresses vitamin K and reduces the activity of the vitamin K-dependent coagulation factors II (prothrombin), VII, IX, and X.

crenated cell: Red blood cell formed by cellular dehydration (drying artifact) and not observed in all fields on a peripheral blood film.

cryoglobulin: Any of numerous serum globulins, typically immunoglobulins, that precipitate at around 4° C and become resuspended at 37° C.

cryoprecipitate (CRYO): Therapeutic agent rich in fibrinogen, factor VIII, and factor XIII, used to treat bleeding disorders in fibrinogen deficiency, factor XIII deficiency, and hemorrhagic trauma. Collected from human plasma that has been frozen and slowly thawed.

cyanosis: Bluish discoloration of the skin, sclera, and mucous membranes caused by poor tissue oxygenation. Usually a sign of anemia.

cyclooxygenase: An enzyme responsible for the formation of prostaglandins from arachidonic acid; in the platelet the end product is thromboxane A2; in endothelial cells the end product is prostacyclin.

cytochemical analysis: Use of specialized stains to detect cellular enzymes and other substances in peripheral blood films and bone marrow aspirate smears.

cytogenetics: Branch of genetics devoted to the laboratory study of visible chromosome abnormalities, such as deletions, translocations, and aneuploidy.

cytokine: Cellular product that influences the function or activity of other cells. Includes colony-stimulating factors, interferons, interleukins, and lymphokines.

cytomegalovirus (CMV): Group of DNA viruses of the family *Herpesviridae*. CMV infection is asymptomatic in healthy adults but can be transmitted to a fetus, causing serious health and developmental problems, congenital abnormalities, or pregnancy loss. Can be transmitted by blood transfusion and is detected using serologic and molecular diagnostic techniques.

cytopenia: Reduced cell count in one or more of any blood cell line—red blood cells, white blood cells, or platelets.

cytosol: Fluid portion of the cytoplasm, less granules and organelles, as separated by ultracentrifugation.

cytotoxic: Describes a compound or agent that destroys or damages cells.

dacryocyte: See teardrop cell.

D-dimer (D:D, D-D): One of the fibrin degradation products composed of two fibrin D fragments covalently joined by the enzymatic action of factor XIII. The D-dimer assay is used to rule out venous thromboembolic disease and disseminated intravascular coagulation and may be used to monitor the efficacy and length of Coumadin therapy.

deep vein thrombosis (DVT, deep venous thrombosis): Pathologic formation of a clot in a deep leg vein such as the femoral vein. A manifestation of venous thromboembolic disease that is associated with a number of acquired or congenital thrombotic risk factors and raises the risk of a pulmonary embolus.

dehydrated hereditary stomatocytosis (DHS, hereditary xerocytosis, HX): Hereditary, autosomal dominant, red blood cell membrane disorder caused by a mutation in a membrane protein that disrupts membrane cation permeability, resulting in a mild to moderate hemolytic anemia. Characterized by the presence of dehydrated (desiccated) red blood cells, stomatocytes, target cells, and burr cells on the peripheral blood film.

11-dehydrothromboxane B2 (11-DHT): Measurable urine product of the platelet cyclooxygenase (eicosanoid) activation pathway. Employed clinically to measure in vivo platelet activation and aspirin resistance.

delayed hemolytic transfusion reaction: Hemolysis that occurs days or weeks after a blood transfusion, caused by an anamnestic response to an antigen in transfused donor red blood cells in a patient alloimmunized from a previous pregnancy or transfusion.

δ check (delta check): Quality control process in which a current analyte result is compared with the result for the same analyte from the previous specimen from the same patient.

dense granule (dense body, δ-granule): Platelet organelle that contains and secretes the small molecules adenosine diphosphate, adenosine triphosphate, serotonin, calcium (Ca^{2+}), and magnesium (Mg^{2+}). There are two to seven dense granules per platelet, and they are named by their opaque appearance in transmission electron microscopy.

deoxyhemoglobin: Hemoglobin that is not combined with oxygen, formed when oxyhemoglobin releases its oxygen to the tissues.

deoxyribonucleic acid (DNA): Double-stranded, helical nucleic acid that carries genetic information. Composed of nucleotide sequences with four repeating bases: adenine, cytosine, guanine, and thymine. During mitosis, condenses to form chromosomes.

des-γ-carboxyl coagulation factors and coagulation control proteins: See PIVKA factors.

desquamation: Shedding of epithelial elements, chiefly of the skin, in scales or sheets; endothelial cells that line the internal lumen of blood vessels can also shed.

Diamond-Blackfan anemia (DBA, congenital pure red cell aplasia): Rare congenital anemia with mostly an autosomal dominant inheritance as a result of mutations in structural ribosomal protein genes and evident within the first year of life. Anemia is severe as a result of erythroid hypoplasia in the bone marrow, but platelet and white blood cell counts are normal. Physical malformations may be present.

diapedesis: Outward passage of white blood cells through intact vessel walls.

differential white blood cell count: Review, classification, and tabulation of usually 100 white blood cells (WBCs) in a stained peripheral blood film. The different types of WBCs are counted and reported as absolute counts or percentages of total WBCs. In automated blood cell analyzers, the differential WBC count is accomplished by counting thousands of WBCs using various technologies.

dilute Russell viper venom time (DRVVT): Coagulation test in which Russell viper venom activates the common coagulation pathway at the level of factor X. Prolonged by lupus anticoagulant, and the test is used in screening for this antibody.

diploid: Having two sets of chromosomes, as normally found in nuclei of somatic cells. In humans the normal diploid number is 46.

direct antiglobulin test (DAT, formerly Coombs test): Screening procedure in which antihuman globulin is used to detect antibodies and complement bound to red blood cells in vivo.

direct thrombin inhibitors (DTIs): Class of anticoagulants including the intravenous use argatroban and bivalirudin, and the oral dabigatran that suppress coagulation (fibrin formation) by directly neutralizing thrombin.

disseminated intravascular coagulation (DIC): Uncontrolled generation of thrombin and consumption of coagulation factors, platelets, and fibrinolytic proteins secondary to many initiating events, including infection, inflammation, shock, and trauma. Most commonly evidenced by diffuse mucocutaneous bleeding.

DOAC (direct acting oral anticoagulant; new, novel, non-VKA oral anticoagulant, NOAC): Drugs that directly bind coagulation serine proteases and do not require a co-factor such as antithrombin to produce anticoagulant activity. Current examples are dabigatran, rivaroxaban, apixaban, edoxaban, and betrixaban.

Döhle bodies: In Wright-stained peripheral blood films, gray to light blue round or oval inclusions composed of ribosomal RNA found singly or in multiples near the inner membrane surface of granulocyte cytoplasm.

dominant: Denoting an inherited allele whose trait is expressed whenever the gene is present, even in heterozygotes.

Donath-Landsteiner (D-L) autoantibody: IgG autoantibody with anti-P specificity that binds red blood cells and partially activates complement at temperatures below 20° C and fully activates complement causing hemolysis at 37° C. Causes paroxysmal cold hemoglobinuria, an autoimmune hemolytic anemia.

double heterozygous: Having two different heterozygous mutant alleles at different loci. An example is hemoglobin SG-Philadelphia in which an individual is heterozygous for a β-globin chain mutation (hemoglobin S) and heterozygous for an α-globin chain mutation (hemoglobin G-Philadelphia).

Down syndrome: Congenital group of physical, mental, and functional abnormalities including distinctive facial features, congenital heart disease, muscular hypotonia, and mental retardation, associated with trisomy 21. Increases the risk of developing transient myeloproliferative disease and acute myeloid or acute lymphoblastic leukemia.

drepanocyte: See sickle cell.

drug-induced hemolytic anemia: Hemolytic anemia caused directly by a drug or secondary to an antibody-mediated response stimulated by the drug.

dry tap: Term used when an inadequate sample of bone marrow fluid is obtained during bone marrow aspiration. Occurs when the marrow is packed, such as in chronic myeloid (myelogenous) leukemia, or when it is fibrotic, as in primary myelofibrosis.

duodenum: Proximal and first part of the small intestine adjacent to the stomach.

dyscrasia: Disorder of a hematologic cell line or lines.

dyserythropoiesis: Deranged erythropoiesis producing cells with abnormal morphology; usually applied to congenital dyserythropoietic anemia and myelodysplastic syndromes.

dysfibrinogenemia: Presence in the plasma of structurally abnormal fibrinogen; often a result of liver disease, occasionally congenital.

dysmegakaryopoiesis: Defective megakaryocytic production and maturation characterized by cells with abnormal morphology and increased or decreased megakaryocyte counts.

dysmyelopoiesis: Defective myelocytic production and maturation characterized by cells with abnormal morphology; often applied to myelodysplastic syndromes.

dysplasia: Abnormal development or growth pattern of cells or tissues; may indicate a precancerous condition.

dyspnea: Difficult or painful breathing.

ecchymosis: Hemorrhagic spot, 1 cm or larger in diameter, in the skin or mucous membranes, typically forming an irregular blue or purplish patch. Also known as a bruise.

echinocyte: See burr cell.

eclampsia: Potentially life-threatening disorder during pregnancy characterized by hypertension, edema, proteinuria, and seizures.

edema: Accumulation of excess serous fluid in a fluid compartment or tissue.

effusion: Seepage and accumulation of plasma-derived fluid into a body cavity from blood vessels as a result of blood vessel damage or hydrostatic pressure.

electronic impedance: Opposition to the flow of electrical current. The impedance principle of cell counting is based on the detection and measurement of changes in electrical resistance produced by cells as they transverse a small aperture in a conducting solution.

electrophoresis: Separation and identification of proteins, nucleic acids, and hemoglobin types based on their relative rates of migration through agarose or polyacrylamide gel in an applied electrical field. Depending on the component, the rate of migration may be based on molecular mass and/or net charge.

elliptocyte (ovalocyte): Elliptical or oval red blood cell found on a peripheral blood film in hereditary elliptocytosis, which is caused by a mutation in a cytoskeletal protein that disrupts horizontal protein interactions. May also be found in low numbers in healthy states and in other anemias such as iron deficiency and thalassemia.

elliptocytosis: See hereditary elliptocytosis.

Embden-Meyerhof pathway (EMP, glycolysis): A series of enzymatically catalyzed reactions by which glucose and other sugars are metabolized to yield lactic acid (anaerobic glycolysis) or pyruvic acid (aerobic glycolysis). Metabolism releases energy in the form of adenosine triphosphate (ATP).

embolism: Pathologic event in which an object travels through the bloodstream, becomes lodged in an artery, and obstructs blood flow, causing tissue ischemia, necrosis, and loss of function. The embolus is often a blood clot, but it may be a fat globule, air bubble, piece of tissue, or clump of bacteria. A pulmonary embolism is a blood clot in a lung artery and is often fatal.

endoplasmic reticulum (ER): Extensive network of membrane-bound, branching, flattened sacs and tubules in the cytoplasm of cells. Its membrane is continuous with the nuclear membrane and provides for the flow of molecules between the nucleus and the cytoplasm. Rough endoplasmic reticulum (RER) is rich in ribosomes that synthesize most membrane-bound proteins and proteins destined for secretion from the cell. Smooth endoplasmic reticulum is continuous with the RER and synthesizes phospholipids and steroids, detoxifies drugs, and stores calcium.

endothelial cells: Cell layer that lines the inner surface of all blood vessels. Intact endothelial cells prevent thrombosis because they present a smooth, nonactivating surface and secrete antiplatelet and anticoagulant substances. Injured endothelial cells promote clotting through expression of tissue factor and secretion of coagulation-promoting factors, such as von Willebrand factor.

enterocytes: Epithelial cells that form the inner lining of the intestine. Absorbs nutrients from the intestinal lumen and transports them to the portal circulation.

eosinophil: Granulocyte with large uniform cytoplasmic granules that stain orange to pink with Wright stain. Granules usually do not obscure the segmented nucleus.

eosinophilia: Increase in the number of eosinophils in the peripheral blood to more than the reference interval. Associated with allergies, parasitic infections, or some hematologic neoplasms.

epigenetic: Describes heritable mutations in a cell that change the expression of a gene without changing the DNA sequence of the gene itself. Examples include hyper- and hypomethylation of CpG islands in gene promoters, mutations in histone acetyltransferases or excessive recruitment of histone deacetylases to transcription sites that keep chromatin in a closed inactive state, and microRNAs that inhibit gene expression by specifically binding to targeted mRNA transcripts.

epiphyses: Ends of long bones that normally contain active hematopoietic tissue.

epistaxis: Hemorrhage from the nose; a nosebleed that requires intervention.

Epstein-Barr virus (EBV): Herpesvirus that causes infectious mononucleosis and leads to the appearance of reactive lymphocytes on the peripheral blood film.

erythroblastosis fetalis: See hemolytic disease of the fetus and newborn.

erythrocyte (red blood cell, RBC): Nonnucleated biconcave disk-shaped peripheral blood cell containing hemoglobin. Its primary function is oxygen transport and delivery to tissues.

erythrocyte sedimentation rate (ESR): Distance that red blood cells fall in a column of anticoagulated blood in a specified period. Elevated sedimentation rates are not specific for any disorder but indicate the presence of inflammation.

erythrocytosis: Increase in the number of red blood cells in the peripheral blood to more than the reference interval.

erythroferrone (ERFE): Hormone secreted by erythroblasts that suppresses hepcidin production in the liver, thus allowing increased iron absorption in the intestines.

erythropoiesis-stimulating agent (ESA): Recombinant erythropoietin used to treat anemia caused by conditions such as chronic kidney disease and chemotherapy.

erythroleukemia (Di Guglielmo disease, FAB M6): Acute leukemia characterized by a proliferation of erythroid and myeloid precursors in bone marrow, with erythroblasts with bizarre lobulated nuclei and abnormal myeloblasts in peripheral blood.

erythron: The entirety of all erythroid cells in the body including red blood cells circulating in the peripheral blood and vascular spaces of organs, and their precursors in the bone marrow. Differentiate from red cell mass which represents only the red blood cells in circulation.

erythropoiesis: Bone marrow process of red blood cell production.

erythropoietin (EPO): Glycoprotein hormone synthesized primarily in the kidneys and released into the blood in response to hypoxia. Binds to the erythropoietin receptor on erythroid progenitors in the bone marrow to stimulate and regulate the production of red blood cells.

essential thrombocythemia: Myeloproliferative neoplasm characterized by marked thrombocytosis and dysfunctional platelets. Patients may experience bleeding or thrombosis.

etiology: Causes or origin of a disease, for instance, genetic factors, infection, toxins, or trauma. Contrast with pathogenesis, which is the physiologic and biochemical mechanisms by which a disease progresses.

euchromatin: Portion of DNA that is active in gene expression and stains lightly with Wright stain.

exogenous: Originating from outside the body or produced by external causes; used, for example, to describe a disease caused by a bacterial or viral agent foreign to the body, or administration of a therapeutic synthesized outside the body (such as recombinant erythropoietin).

exon: Portion of a DNA molecule that becomes translated to form a protein product. Exons and introns are transcribed from DNA to heteronuclear RNA, where the introns are excised to form messenger RNA.

extramedullary hematopoiesis: Production of blood cells outside the bone marrow, such as in the spleen, liver, or lymph nodes. Usually occurs in response to severe anemia or bone marrow fibrosis causing loss of hematopoiesis.

extranodal: Located outside a lymph node.

extravascular hemolysis (macrophage-mediated hemolysis): Destruction of red blood cells outside of a blood vessel, typically by splenic macrophage phagocytosis.

extrinsic coagulation pathway: Primary coagulation pathway. Exposure of tissue factor activates factor VII. Factor VIIa activates factors IX and X, which triggers the common pathway of coagulation and formation of fibrin.

exudate: Fluid (effusion) that leaks from blood vessels and accumulates in a body cavity as a result of inflammation caused by bacterial or viral infections, malignancy, or other abnormalities. It has a high concentration of white blood cells and protein and appears cloudy, yellow or amber, or grossly bloody.

factor assay: Clot-based or chromogenic assay to quantify specific coagulation factor activity. The units for the level of a coagulation factor is given as % or units/dL, where the number value is the same for both. Fibrinogen is always represented in units of mg/dL.

factor V Leiden mutation: Mutation in the coagulation factor V gene which substitutes arginine with glutamine at position 506 in the factor V protein. The resultant factor V resists digestion by activated protein C. Results in increased thrombin production and is a thrombosis risk factor.

Fanconi anemia: Congenital aplastic anemia with autosomal dominant or X-linked recessive inheritance caused by a mutation in a DNA repair gene and resulting in chromosome instability. Physical malformations may be present at birth such as skeletal malformations, skin pigmentation, abnormalities of eyes, kidneys, genitals, and developmental delay. Pancytopenia and related symptoms usually manifest at 5 to 10 years of age.

favism: Acute hemolytic anemia caused by ingestion of fava beans or inhalation of the pollen of the plant. Usually occurs in individuals with an inherited deficiency of glucose-6-phosphate dehydrogenase in red blood cells.

ferritin: Iron-apoferritin complex, a major form in which iron is stored in the liver.

ferrokinetics: Study of iron metabolism, including the movement of iron among the storage, transport, and functional iron compartments.

ferroportin: Transport protein in the membrane of enterocytes (serosal side), macrophages, and hepatocytes that facilitates iron transport one way out of the cell; transport inhibited by the binding of hepcidin.

fibrin: Fibrillar protein produced by the action of thrombin on fibrinogen in the clotting process. Responsible for the semisolid character of a blood clot.

fibrin degradation products (FDPs, fibrin split products, FSPs): Fragments X, Y, D, and E and D-dimer produced from fibrinogen and fibrin degradation by the action of plasmin during fibrinolysis.

fibrinogen: Plasma glycoprotein that is converted to fibrin by thrombin digestion.

fibrinolysis: Process of digestion of fibrinogen or fibrin by plasmin that has been activated by plasminogen activator. Fibrinolysis is the normal mechanism for the removal of fibrin clots.

fibroblast: Connective tissue cell that differentiates into numerous cells, which comprise the fibrous tissue of the body, for instance, tissue in the walls of arteries.

Fitzgerald factor: See high-molecular-weight kininogen.

Fletcher factor: See prekallikrein.

flow cytometer: Instrument in which cells suspended in fluid flow one at a time through a focused beam of light. The light is scattered in patterns characteristic of the cells and their components. A sensor detecting the scattered or emitted light measures the volume and other characteristics of individual cells.

fluorescence in situ hybridization (FISH): Laboratory technique in which fluorescence-labeled nucleic acid probes hybridize to selected DNA or RNA sequences in fixed tissue. Allows for the visual microscopic detection of aneuploidy (trisomy, monosomy) and mutations such as the *BCR-ABL1* fusion in cell or tissue specimens.

fluorophore: Portion of a molecule that absorbs incident light and emits fluorescent light at a different wavelength.

free erythrocyte protoporphyrin (FEP): Porphyrin precursor of heme that is present in low concentrations in normal red blood cells (RBCs). Elevated RBC concentrations indicate iron deficiency or impaired iron insertion into heme.

French-American-British (FAB) classification: International classification system for acute leukemias, myeloproliferative neoplasms, and myelodysplastic syndromes developed in the 1970s and 1980s. Still in use, although it has largely been replaced by the World Health Organization classification.

fresh frozen plasma (FFP): Plasma that is separated by centrifugation from donor whole blood and frozen within 8 hours of collection. Contains all plasma procoagulants and control proteins, including the labile factors V and VIII. Used for replacement therapy in acquired multiple-factor deficiencies or in single-factor deficiencies when factor concentrates are not available.

G banding (GTG banding): In cytogenetic analysis, a procedure in which metaphase chromosomes are treated with trypsin and then stained with Giemsa dye. The areas rich in adenine-thymine, called G+, stain intensely, whereas the areas rich in guanine-cytosine (G−) stain more lightly. The G+ bands correspond with Q bands in Q banding. Banding patterns are used for the identification of chromosomes.

gammopathy: Plasma protein imbalance caused by a markedly increased concentration of gamma globulin (immunoglobulin). A monoclonal gammopathy is characterized by one type of immunoglobulin produced by a single clone of plasma cells or B lymphocytes and is mainly found in malignant neoplasms such as plasma cell (multiple) myeloma, although it can be found in some benign conditions. It is seen as a single sharp spike or band on protein electrophoresis. A polyclonal gammopathy is an increase in several types of immunoglobulins and can be found in a variety of benign conditions, such as infections or inflammatory states.

Gaucher disease: Rare autosomal recessive lysosomal lipid storage disorder caused by β-glucocerebrosidase deficiency and characterized by histiocytic hyperplasia and damage in the liver, spleen, lymph nodes, and bone marrow. The characteristic Gaucher cells, which are lipid-filled macrophages whose cytoplasm resembles crumpled tissue paper, are found on the Wright-stained bone marrow aspirate smear.

Gaussian distribution: Frequency distribution that approximates the distribution of many random variables and is portrayed graphically as a symmetric bell-shaped curve. The peak represents the mean of the distribution and the width of the curve represents the dispersion or variability, which is generally expressed in terms of standard deviation from the mean. Also called a normal distribution.

gene: Segment of a DNA molecule that contains all the information required for synthesis of a protein, including both coding (exon) and noncoding (intron) sequences. Each gene occupies a specific position (locus) on a particular chromosome.

gene rearrangement: Reorganization of the DNA sequences of a gene. Rearrangement of B cell and T cell genes is a normal process that produces cells with an infinite variety of sequences in the variable region of their antigen receptors to respond to a vast array of antigens. A clonal gene rearrangement occurs mainly in malignant lymphoid neoplasms and is detected by flow cytometry and molecular diagnostic methods.

gestational age: Age of the fetus, usually expressed as the time elapsed from the first day of the mother's last menstrual period.

Glanzmann thrombasthenia (GT): Severe mucocutaneous bleeding disorder caused by a mutation in platelet glycoprotein (GP) IIb or IIIa. Normal GPIIb/IIIa recognizes and binds the arginine-glycine-aspartate peptide sequence receptor complex found in fibrinogen and von Willebrand factor. Causes a defect of fibrinogen-dependent platelet aggregation.

globin: Protein constituent of hemoglobin. Two pairs of globin chains bind four heme molecules to form the hemoglobin tetramer.

globulins: Class of proteins that are insoluble in water or highly concentrated salt solutions but are soluble in moderately concentrated salt solutions. All plasma proteins are globulins except albumin and prealbumin.

glossitis: Inflammation of the tongue that causes it to be red and smooth.

glucose-6-phosphate dehydrogenase (G6PD): First enzyme of the glucose monophosphate shunt from the Embden-Meyerhof pathway. Catalyzes the oxidation of glucose-6-phosphate to 6-phosphogluconate, converting the oxidized form of nicotinamide adenine dinucleotide phosphate (NADP) to the reduced form (NADPH).

glucose-6-phosphate dehydrogenase deficiency: X-linked deficiency of glucose-6-phosphate dehydrogenase usually characterized by episodes of acute intravascular hemolysis under conditions of oxidative stress, including infections and exposure to oxidizing drugs such as primaquine.

glycocalyx: Glycoprotein and polysaccharide covering that surrounds many cells. The platelet glycocalyx is thicker than that of other cells and provides a procoagulant environment.

glycolysis: See Embden-Meyerhof pathway.

glycophorin: Transmembrane red blood cell protein that carries several blood group antigens.

glycoprotein: Conjugated protein containing one or more covalently linked carbohydrate residues.

glycoprotein IIb/IIIa (GPIIb/IIIa): Pair of glycoproteins that function as a receptor for the arginine-glycine-aspartate sequence in fibrinogen and von Willebrand factor. The combination of fibrinogen and glycoprotein IIb/IIIa is essential to platelet aggregation.

Golgi apparatus: System of stacked, membrane-bound flattened sacs (cisternae) and associated vesicles. Contains numerous enzymes for the posttranslational modification and packaging of proteins and lipids destined for delivery to other organelles or secretion out of the cell.

gout: Painful inflammation caused by excessive plasma uric acid, which becomes deposited as monosodium urate monohydrate in joint capsules and adjacent tendons.

graft-versus-host disease (GVHD): Condition including tissue rejection that occurs when immunologically competent cells or their precursors are transplanted into an immunocompromised host who is not histocompatible with the donor. The donor cells engraft and mount an immune response against the host.

granulocytes: Class of white blood cells characterized by cytoplasmic granules; includes basophils, eosinophils, and neutrophils.

granuloma: Nodular, delimited aggregation of inflammatory cells, macrophages, and macrophage-derived multinucleate giant cells surrounded by a rim of lymphocytes and fibroblasts. Major sites of cell-mediated immune response to particulate antigens, and may occur in many organs in chronic granulomatous disease.

GTG banding: See G banding.

guaiac test: Test performed on stool emulsions to detect hemoglobin as evidence of gastrointestinal bleeding. Small amounts of blood may be invisible; therefore it is known as a test for occult (hidden) blood. The peroxidase activity of hemoglobin in blood reacts with guaiac to yield a blue color.

hairy cell: Malignant B lymphocyte seen in the peripheral blood and bone marrow in hairy cell leukemia. Characterized by delicate gray cytoplasm with projections resembling hairs.

haploid: Referring to the number of chromosomes found in sperm or ova, which is only one of each pair of chromosomes found in somatic (diploid) cells. In humans the haploid number is 23.

haptoglobin: Plasma protein that irreversibly binds free hemoglobin, forming a complex that is removed by macrophages while conserving iron. Serum level decreases due to consumption in intravascular hemolysis.

Heinz body: Round blue to purple inclusion of denatured hemoglobin attached to the inner red blood cell membrane and only visible with a supravital stain, such as new methylene blue. Found in unstable hemoglobin disorders, glucose-6-phosphate dehydrogenase deficiency, and after exposure to oxidant drugs or chemicals.

helmet cell: Helmet-shaped schistocyte (fragmented red blood cell) that may appear in microangiopathic hemolytic anemia.

hemacytometer (counting chamber): Device used to perform visual blood and body fluid cell counts, consisting of a microscopic slide with a depression whose polished glass base is marked with grids and into which a measured volume of a specimen of diluted blood or body fluid is placed and covered with a cover glass. The number of cells in selected squares of the grid is counted under a microscope and used as a representative sample for calculating the number of cells in a given volume (usually per µL or L).

hemarthroses: Chronic joint bleeds that cause inflammation and immobilization; a symptom of severe hemophilia.

hematemesis: Vomiting of bright red blood.

hematocrit (HCT, packed cell volume, PCV): Proportion of whole blood that consists of red blood cells, expressed as a percentage of the total blood volume.

hematoidin: Golden yellow, brown, or red crystals that are chemically similar to bilirubin. Indicates a hemorrhage site when present in a tissue preparation.

hematology: Clinical study of blood cells and blood-forming tissues.

hematoma: Localized collection of extravasated blood (blood that has escaped from vessel into tissue), usually clotted, in an organ space or tissue; in skin it gives the appearance of a bruise.

hematopathology: Study of the diseases of blood cells and hematopoietic tissue.

hematopoiesis: Formation and development of blood cells that normally occurs in the bone marrow and peripheral lymphatic tissues.

hematopoietic microenvironment: Matrix of bone marrow stromal cells and tissue that supports hematopoiesis both structurally and through the production of cytokines and colony-stimulating factors.

hematopoietic progenitor cell: Actively dividing cell that is committed to a specific blood cell lineage and is not capable of self-renewal. Therapeutic hematopoietic progenitor cell products intended for transplantation provide both hematopoietic stem cells and progenitor cells.

hematopoietic stem cell (HSC): Actively dividing cell that is capable of self-renewal and of differentiation into any blood cell lineage (pluripotent); identified by expression of membrane CD34.

hematuria: Abnormal presence of intact red blood cells in the urine; indicative of kidney or urinary tract disease.

heme: Pigmented iron-containing nonprotein part of the hemoglobin molecule. There are four heme groups in a hemoglobin molecule, each containing one ferrous ion in the center. Oxygen binds the ferrous ion and is transported from an area of high to low oxygen concentration.

hemochromatosis: Hereditary disease of iron metabolism that is characterized by excess deposition of iron in the tissues; caused most commonly by mutations in the *HFE* gene. Differentiate from transfusion-related hemosiderosis in which excess iron accumulates in tissues as a complication of a transfusion-dependent hemolytic anemia, such as β-thalassemia major.

hemoconcentration: Elevation of the red blood cell, white blood cell, and platelet counts resulting from a decrease in plasma volume, for example, in dehydration.

hemodialysis: Extracorporeal circulation process that substitutes for the kidneys and removes wastes from the blood; used to treat patients with renal failure. The patient's blood is shunted from the body through a dialysis machine for diffusion and ultrafiltration and is then returned to the patient's circulation.

hemoglobin (Hb, HGB): Tetramer composed of two different pairs of globin polypeptide chains, each of which binds a heme group containing a central ferrous iron. Normal Hb A contains 2 α-globin and 2 β-globin chains. Primary constituent of red blood cell cytoplasm and transports molecular oxygen from the lungs to the tissues.

hemoglobin C crystal: Hexagonal, dense cytoplasmic red blood cell crystal described as a "gold bar," or "Washington monument." Characteristic of homozygous hemoglobin C disease, crystals form as hemoglobin C polymerizes.

hemoglobin electrophoresis: Separation, identification, and quantification of normal and abnormal hemoglobin types based on their relative rates of migration through agarose or polyacrylamide gel in an applied electric field. The rate of migration depends mainly on net charge. Examples of hemoglobin types include Hb A, Hb C, Hb F, and Hb S.

hemoglobin SC crystal: Finger-like or quartz-like crystal of dense hemoglobin protruding from the red blood cell membrane. Characteristic of compound heterozygous hemoglobin SC disease, the crystals form as hemoglobin S and C polymerize.

hemoglobinemia: Presence of free hemoglobin in the plasma; indicative of intravascular hemolysis.

hemoglobinopathy: Condition characterized by structural variations in globin genes that result in the formation of abnormal globin chains. Examples are sickle cell anemia and hemoglobin C disease.

hemoglobinuria: Free hemoglobin in the urine; indicative of intravascular hemolysis.

hemolysis: Disruption of red blood cell membrane integrity that destroys the cell and releases hemoglobin and the other cell contents.

hemolytic anemia: Anemia characterized by premature hemolysis and shortened red blood cell life span with an inability of bone marrow erythropoiesis to adequately compensate. Caused by disorders extrinsic or intrinsic to the red blood cell.

hemolytic disease of the fetus and newborn (HDFN, erythroblastosis fetalis): Alloimmune anemia caused by maternal IgG antibody that crosses the placenta and binds fetal red blood cell antigens inherited from the father: for instance, maternal anti-D with fetal D antigen. Characterized by hemolytic anemia, hyperbilirubinemia, and extramedullary erythropoiesis.

hemolytic uremic syndrome (HUS): Severe microangiopathic hemolytic anemia that often follows infection of the gastrointestinal tract by *Escherichia coli* serotype O157:H7, which produces an exotoxin. Characterized by renal failure, thrombocytopenia, the appearance of schistocytes on the peripheral blood film, and severe mucocutaneous hemorrhage.

hemopexin: Plasma glycoprotein produced in the liver; binds free plasma heme or metheme to prevent iron loss in the urine.

hemophilia: Group of hereditary anatomic bleeding disorders caused by a deficiency of a single coagulation factor. The two most common forms are hemophilia A and hemophilia B.

hemophilia A (classic hemophilia): X-linked recessive anatomic bleeding disorder caused by a deficiency of coagulation factor VIII.

hemophilia B (Christmas disease): X-linked recessive anatomic bleeding disorder caused by a deficiency of coagulation factor IX.

hemophilia C (Rosenthal syndrome): Autosomal anatomic bleeding disorder caused by a deficiency of coagulation factor XI.

hemorrhage: Blood loss either outside the body or within a body cavity as a result of ruptured blood vessels. May be acute or a sudden loss of blood requiring immediate intervention and transfusions, or chronic with small volume blood loss over a long period of time. Chronic hemorrhage results in iron loss and can lead to iron deficiency anemia and microcytic red blood cells.

hemorrhagic disease of the newborn: Neonatal anatomic bleeding caused by vitamin K deficiency.

hemosiderin: Intracellular storage form of iron found predominantly in liver, spleen, and bone marrow cells as a breakdown product of ferritin. Appears in iron overload conditions and is detected microscopically using the Prussian blue iron stain.

hemosiderinuria: Presence in the urine of hemosiderin, which can be visualized using Prussian blue iron stain; most often an indicator of chronic intravascular hemolysis.

hemosiderosis: See transfusion-related hemosiderosis.

hemostasis: Process by which a series of platelet, endothelial cell, and plasma enzyme systems prevent blood loss through clot formation and maintain blood vessel patency.

heparin: See unfractionated heparin.

heparin-induced thrombocytopenia (HIT): Effect of unfractionated heparin therapy in which antibodies to heparin-platelet factor 4 complex develop. The antibody and target antigen complex bind platelet Fc receptors and activate platelets causing thrombocytopenia. Associated venous and arterial thrombosis can lead to amputation and death.

hepatitis: Inflammation of the liver that damages hepatocytes and releases bilirubin into the plasma.

hepatitis B virus (HBV): Causative agent of hepatitis B; transmitted by contaminated blood or blood products, by sexual contact with an infected person, or by the use of contaminated needles and instruments. Severe infection may cause prolonged illness, liver cell destruction, cirrhosis, increased risk of liver cancer, or death.

hepatocyte: Parenchymal liver cell.

hepatomegaly: Abnormal enlargement of the liver; usually a sign of disease.

hepatosplenomegaly: Abnormal enlargement of the spleen and liver.

hepcidin: Major regulator of iron homeostasis; binds to ferroportin in membranes of enterocytes (serosal side), macrophages, and hepatocytes and prevents iron transport out of the cell, thus reducing intestinal absorption of iron and iron transport out of storage sites. The liver increases hepcidin synthesis in iron excess states, and decreases synthesis in iron-depleted states. Inflammation increases hepcidin production as a protective mechanism to sequester iron from invading microorganisms and malignant cells that need iron for growth.

hereditary elliptocytosis (HE): Hereditary, autosomal dominant, red blood cell membrane disorder caused by a mutation in a cytoskeletal membrane protein (usually α- or β-spectrin) that disrupts horizontal membrane protein interactions. Often asymptomatic but may cause a mild hemolytic anemia and is characterized by the presence of elliptocytes or ovalocytes on the peripheral blood film.

hereditary pyropoikilocytosis (HPP): Rare hereditary, autosomal recessive, red blood cell membrane disorder caused by homozygous or compound heterozygous mutations in spectrin, which severely disrupt horizontal membrane protein interactions. Causes severe hemolytic anemia presenting in childhood and is characterized by the presence of extreme poikilocytosis on the peripheral blood film.

hereditary spherocytosis (HS): Hereditary, usually autosomal dominant, red blood cell membrane disorder caused by a mutation in a cytoskeletal or transmembrane protein that disrupts vertical membrane protein interactions resulting in loss of red blood cell membrane and a decreased surface area-to-volume ratio. Causes asymptomatic to severe hemolytic anemia characterized by numerous spherocytes on the peripheral blood film.

hereditary stomatocytosis: See dehydrated hereditary stomatocytosis and overhydrated hereditary stomatocytosis.

hereditary xerocytosis: See dehydrated hereditary stomatocytosis.

heterochromatin: Portion of DNA that is inactive during transcription to messenger RNA and stains deeply with Wright stain.

heterophile antibody: Antibody that reacts with an antigen from a species other than that of the antigen that stimulated its production. For example, patients with infectious mononucleosis caused by the Epstein-Barr virus produce an antibody to the virus but also produce heterophile antibodies that react with sheep or horse red blood cells.

heterozygous: Having two different alleles at corresponding loci on homologous chromosomes. An individual who is heterozygous for a trait has inherited an allele for that trait from one parent and an alternative allele from the other parent. A person who is heterozygous for a genetic disease will manifest the disorder if it is caused by a dominant allele but will remain asymptomatic if the disease is caused by a recessive allele.

high-molecular-weight kininogen (HMWK, Fitzgerald factor): Member of the kinin inflammatory system that is digested and activated by kallikrein to form bradykinin. One of the contact activators of the coagulation system, which also include prekallikrein and factor XII.

histiocyte: See macrophage.

histochemical analysis: Use of specialized stains to detect enzymes and other chemicals in tissues, usually by microscopy.

histocompatibility: Quality or state of immunologic similarity that allows cells or tissues from one individual to be successfully transplanted into another individual. The degree of compatibility is controlled by surface markers of the human leukocyte antigen (HLA) system of the major histocompatibility complex. Grafts from sibling donors have a greater chance of being fully HLA compatible with the recipient than those from unrelated donors.

histogram: Graph of a frequency distribution. In hematology a line graph generated by an automated blood cell analyzer that depicts the frequencies of platelet, white blood cell, or red blood cell volumes in a cell population.

histology: Science concerned with the microscopic identification of cells and tissues used to identify cellular and tissue disease.

histone: Nuclear protein that complexes with DNA to form chromatin. Provides for DNA folding and condensation and helps regulate replication and transcription.

Hodgkin lymphoma: Solid, malignant tumor, usually initiating in peripheral lymph nodes, with a biopsy characterized by Reed-Sternberg cells in a reactive background of benign small lymphocytes and other reactive white blood cells.

homocysteine: Naturally occurring sulfur-containing amino acid formed in the metabolism of dietary methionine to cysteine.

homocysteinemia: See hyperhomocysteinemia.

homocystinuria: Rare, autosomal recessive disorder involving a deficiency in an enzyme of the methionine-homocysteine metabolic pathway; characterized by markedly increased concentrations of homocysteine in the blood and urine as well as physical deformities, developmental delay, and cardiovascular and thromboembolic disease.

homozygous: Having two identical alleles at corresponding loci on homologous chromosomes. An individual who is homozygous for a trait has inherited one identical allele for that trait from each parent. A person who is homozygous for a genetic disease caused by a pair of recessive alleles manifests the disorder.

Howell-Jolly (HJ) body: Round, dark blue to purple inclusion in red blood cells, usually one per cell, visible on a Wright-stained peripheral blood film; composed of DNA and found in severe anemia or postsplenectomy.

human leukocyte antigen (HLA, major histocompatibility complex, MHC): Cell membrane glycoprotein system that forms the basis for antigen presentation in cellular and humoral immunity and enables the immune system to distinguish between self and nonself. HLA class I molecules (HLA-A, -B, -C) are found on most nucleated cells and on platelets. Class II antigens (HLA-DP, -DQ, -DR) are expressed on B lymphocytes, monocytes, macrophages, and dendritic cells.

humoral immunity: Immune response mediated by B lymphocytes, which produce circulating antibodies (immunoglobulins) in reaction to infectious organisms and other foreign antigens.

hybridization: In molecular biology, formation of a partially or wholly complementary nucleic acid duplex by association of single strands; used to detect and identify specific nucleic acid sequences.

hydrops fetalis: Gross edema of the entire body of a fetus or newborn infant, associated with severe anemia and occurring in conditions such as hemolytic disease of the fetus and newborn.

hyperbilirubinemia: See bilirubinemia.

hypercellular bone marrow: Bone marrow showing an abnormal increase in the concentration of nucleated hematopoietic cells; potentially associated with leukemia or hemolytic anemia.

hypercoagulability (thrombophilia): Abnormally increased tendency to develop pathologic thromboses (blood clots) caused by a number of acquired and congenital factors.

hyperhomocysteinemia: Elevated plasma homocysteine caused by a deficiency in vitamin B_6, vitamin B_{12}, or folate, and associated with an increased risk of arterial thrombosis. Also caused by an inherited deficiency of methylene tetrahydrofolate reductase (MTHFR).

hyperplasia: Abnormally increased number of cells per unit volume of tissue caused by increased cellular division or abnormal retention. In bone marrow, evident in hypercellularity. May cause bone deformities in children such as an enlarged forehead, called frontal bossing.

hypersegmented neutrophil: Neutrophil with six or more nuclear lobes or segments; associated with megaloblastic anemia.

hypersplenism: Increased hemolytic activity of the spleen caused by splenomegaly, resulting in deficiency of peripheral blood cells and compensatory hypercellularity of the bone marrow.

hypertension: Persistently elevated blood pressure.

hyperuricemia: Excess of plasma uric acid or urates; sometimes associated with gout.

hypocellular bone marrow: Abnormal decrease in the number of nucleated hematopoietic cells present in the bone marrow; may be associated with aplastic anemia or fibrosis.

hypochromia: Decrease in the hemoglobin content of red blood cells so that they appear pale with a larger central pallor on a peripheral blood film; called hypochromic and have a reduced mean cell hemoglobin concentration (MCHC).

hypodiploid: Having fewer than the normal number of somatic cell chromosomes; for example, fewer than 46 chromosomes in humans.

hypoplasia: Underdevelopment of an organ or tissue, usually resulting from a fewer-than-normal number of cells. A hypoplastic bone marrow is one in which the number of hematopoietic cells is reduced, as in aplastic anemia or fibrosis.

hypoxia: Diminished availability of oxygen to body tissues, usually secondary to decreased lung capacity or decreased oxygen-carrying capacity of the blood.

icterus: Dark yellow-amber color of plasma due to an elevated bilirubin level; also yellow-orange color of skin or sclera called jaundice.

idiopathic: Without a known cause.

immediate transfusion reaction: Hemolysis that begins within minutes or hours of a blood transfusion and is most commonly caused by an incompatibility of the ABO system.

immersion oil: Optically clear oil placed in the space between a microscopic specimen and the microscope objective lens. Raises the refractive index, improving resolution.

immune hemolytic anemia: Anemia resulting from premature hemolysis and shortened red blood cell (RBC) life span caused by antibodies to RBC membrane antigens with or without complement activation. The immunoglobulin- or complement-coated RBCs are cleared by macrophages in spleen or liver (extravascular or macrophage-mediated hemolysis) or the RBCs are directly lysed in circulation (intravascular or fragmentation hemolysis). Anemia results when the bone marrow fails to compensate for the RBC destruction.

immune thrombocytopenic purpura (ITP): Mucocutaneous bleeding secondary to thrombocytopenia caused by a platelet-specific autoantibody that shortens platelet life span. Acute ITP occurs more often in children, whereas chronic ITP occurs more often in middle-aged adults, more commonly in women than in men.

immunoblast: Large mitotically active T or B lymphocyte formed as a result of antigenic stimulation.

immunocompromised: Unable to mount an adequate immune response because of disease or treatment with an immunosuppressive agent. An immunocompromised patient is highly susceptible to infections.

immunocytochemical assay: Laboratory test in which antibodies labeled with chromophores or fluorophores bind to specific cellular proteins to produce a measurable color or fluorescent reaction.

immunoglobulin (antibody): Protein of the γ-globulin fraction produced by B lymphocytes and plasma cells that recognizes and binds a specific antigen; basis of humoral immunity.

immunophenotyping: Classification of blood cells by their membrane antigens. Synthetic antibodies, often monoclonal antibodies produced by hybridoma technology, are used to identify the antigens, called CD antigens, by flow cytometry. Important technique in the classification, diagnosis, and monitoring of hematologic malignancies.

immunosuppression: Abnormal state of the immune system characterized by its inability to respond to antigenic stimuli. Immunosuppressive drugs are used to reduce immune responses, particularly in tissue transplant therapy.

infectious mononucleosis: Acute infection caused by the Epstein-Barr virus, a herpesvirus. Characterized by fever, sore throat, lymphadenopathy, reactive lymphocytes, splenomegaly, hepatomegaly, abnormal liver function, and bruising. Laboratory tests used to identify the disease include blood film review for reactive lymphocytes, serologic mononucleosis testing, and molecular identification of Epstein-Barr virus.

integrin: Any of a family of cell-adhesion receptors that mediate interactions between cells and between cells and the extracellular matrix.

interferon: Natural glycoprotein produced by lymphocytes exposed to a virus or another foreign particle. Inhibits viral replication and provides other cells protection against the original as well as other viruses. Recombinant interferon-α is used to treat various viral infections and cancers.

interleukin (IL): A group of compounds that are synthesized by lymphocytes, macrophages, and matrix cells in the bone marrow and interact with cells to initiate, stimulate, or influence the development of blood cells.

international normalized ratio (INR): Index computed to normalize prothrombin time (PT) results worldwide. The activity of a PT reagent (thromboplastin) is characterized by manufacturers using the international sensitivity index (ISI), which compares the reagent to the international reference thromboplastin preparation provided by the World Health Organization. Local PT results are adjusted using the following formula: $INR = (PT_{patient}/PT_{normal})^{ISI}$, where $PT_{patient}$ is the individual patient's PT and PT_{normal} is the geometric mean of the PT reference interval.

international reference preparation (IRP) of thromboplastin: Human brain-derived thromboplastin maintained by the World Health Organization. Thromboplastin manufacturers worldwide compare their reagents' sensitivity with that of this reference preparation using orthogonal regression to generate an international sensitivity index (ISI) for their products.

international sensitivity index (ISI): Index comparing the sensitivity of a given thromboplastin preparation with the sensitivity of the international reference preparation as determined using orthogonal regression. The international sensitivity index is used as an exponent in the equation for calculating the international normalized ratio.

intracranial hemorrhage (ICH, hemorrhagic stroke): Bleeding into the brain causing tissue death. Fifteen percent of strokes are caused by intracranial hemorrhage; the remainder are caused by vascular occlusion (ischemia).

intramedullary hematopoiesis: Formation and development of blood cells within the marrow cavity of a bone.

intramuscular (IM): Injected into muscle tissue.

intravascular hemolysis (fragmentation hemolysis): Red blood cell destruction that occurs within the blood vessels at a rate exceeding splenic macrophage clearance capacity, releasing hemoglobin into the plasma. Seen in acute hemolytic episodes such as those associated with transfusion reaction, glucose-6-phosphate dehydrogenase deficiency, and sickle cell anemia crisis.

intrinsic coagulation pathway: Sequence of serine protease reactions leading to fibrin formation, beginning with the contact activation of coagulation factor XII, followed by the sequential activation of factors XI and IX, and with factor VIII as a cofactor, resulting in the activation of factor X, which initiates the common pathway of coagulation.

intrinsic factor (IF): Glycoprotein secreted by parietal cells of the gastric mucosa that is essential for the intestinal absorption of vitamin B_{12}. An autoantibody to intrinsic factor results in vitamin B_{12} deficiency and pernicious anemia.

intron: Nontranslated sequence in a gene. Introns are transcribed to heteronuclear RNA and are excised during the subsequent formation of messenger RNA.

inversion: Structural chromosome alteration caused by breaks at two locations, reversal of direction of the detached sequence, and reattachment.

iron deficiency anemia (IDA): Microcytic, hypochromic anemia caused by inadequate supply of the iron needed to synthesize hemoglobin and characterized by pallor, fatigue, and weakness. Caused by insufficient dietary iron intake, chronic blood loss, or impaired iron absorption.

isoantibody: See alloantibody.

jaundice: Orange-yellow discoloration of the skin, mucous membranes, and sclera. Caused by elevated plasma bilirubin, which signals hepatitis, hemolytic anemia, or common bile duct obstruction.

karyogram: An image of all the chromosome pairs aligned from 1 to 22 plus the sex chromosomes after analysis in a cytogenetic laboratory.

karyorrhexis: Nuclear necrosis in which the nucleus ruptures and chromatin disintegrates into formless granules.

karyotype: Number, form, size, and arrangement of the chromosomes within the nucleus. In cytogenetic laboratory assays mitosis is halted in metaphase and the chromosomes are visually examined and counted to generate the karyotype. Digital images or photomicrographs are used to confirm and record the microscopic examination.

kinin: Any of a group of polypeptides that trigger inflammatory activity such as contraction of smooth muscle, vascular permeability, and vasodilation; an example of a kinin is bradykinin.

Kleihauer-Betke stain (acid elution slide test): Test for detecting fetal red blood cells (RBCs) in the maternal circulation. Blood films are immersed in an acid buffer, which causes adult hemoglobin (Hb A) to be eluted from RBCs. The film is stained, and RBCs that have fetal hemoglobin (Hb F) take up the stain.

koilonychia: Dystrophy of the fingernails in which they become thin, ridged, and concave. Associated with iron deficiency anemia.

Kupffer cells: Fixed, highly phagocytic macrophages that line the liver sinusoids. Function like splenic macrophages to clear senescent red blood cells, immune complexes, and foreign materials.

lactate dehydrogenase (LD, LDH): Enzyme that catalyzes the reversible conversion of pyruvate to lactate; widespread in tissues and is particularly abundant in the kidneys, skeletal muscle, liver, red blood cells, and myocardium. The LD assay may be used to detect and monitor cell necrosis in these organs, for instance, acute myocardial infarction or as an indicator of intravascular hemolysis.

leptocyte: Abnormal mature red blood cell that is thin and flat with hemoglobin at the periphery and increased central pallor.

leukemia: Group of malignant neoplasms of hematopoietic tissues characterized by diffuse replacement of bone marrow or lymph nodes with abnormal proliferating blood cells and the presence of leukemic cells in the peripheral blood. May be chronic or acute and myeloid or lymphoid.

leukemogenesis: The initiation and maintenance of leukemia; usually a multistep process in which a hematopoietic cell accumulates multiple, independent mutations that affect various cellular processes, which eventually transforms it into a malignant clone.

leukemoid reaction: See reactive neutrophilia.

leukocyte (white blood cell, WBC): One of the formed elements of the blood. The five families of WBCs are lymphocytes, monocytes, neutrophils, basophils, and eosinophils. WBCs function as phagocytes of bacteria, fungi, and viruses; detoxifiers of toxic proteins that may be produced by allergic reactions and cellular injury; and immune system cells.

leukocytosis: Increase in the number of white blood cells in the peripheral blood to more than the reference interval.

leukoerythroblastic: Characterized by the presence of immature red blood cells and granulocytes in the peripheral blood and bone marrow.

leukopenia: Decrease in the number of white blood cells in the peripheral blood below the reference interval.

leukopoiesis: Process by which white blood cells form and develop in the bone marrow and lymph nodes.

Levey-Jennings chart: Quality control chart used to plot periodic test results for control specimens. Indicates the mean and the 1, 2, and 3 standard deviation intervals on both sides of the mean. Deviation from this standard distribution indicates the occurrence of a systematic analytical error.

ligand: Molecule, ion, or group bound to the central atom of a chemical compound—for example, the oxygen molecule in hemoglobin, which is bound to the central iron atom. Also, a molecule that binds to another molecule; used especially to refer to a small molecule that specifically binds to a larger molecule, such as a cell membrane receptor.

low-molecular-weight heparin (LMWH): Heparin with an average molecular weight of 5000 to 8000 Daltons produced by enzymatic or chemical digestion of unfractionated heparin. Most often used for prophylaxis against venous thrombosis in at risk patients. Monitoring, by the chromogenic antifactor Xa heparin assay, is required only in conditions of fluid imbalance, such as obesity, renal disease, and pregnancy.

lupus anticoagulant (LA, LAC): Acquired autoantibodies to phospholipid-protein complexes; the phospholipid binding proteins include β2-glycoprotein I, annexin V, and prothrombin. May be present as a primary condition or secondary to a collagen disorder such as systemic lupus erythematosus, Sjögren syndrome, or rheumatoid arthritis. Chronic lupus anticoagulant is associated with venous and arterial thrombosis and spontaneous abortion.

lymphadenopathy: Any disorder characterized by a localized or generalized enlargement of the lymph nodes.

lymphoblast: Immature cell found in the bone marrow and lymph nodes but not normally in the peripheral blood; the most primitive, morphologically recognizable precursor in the lymphocytic series, which develops into the prolymphocyte.

lymphocyte: Mononuclear, nonphagocytic white blood cell found in the blood, lymph, and lymphoid tissues, categorized as B and T lymphocytes and natural killer cells. Responsible for humoral and cellular immunity and tumor surveillance.

lymphocytopenia (lymphopenia): Decrease in the number of lymphocytes in the peripheral blood to less than the reference interval.

lymphocytosis: Increase in the number of lymphocytes in the peripheral blood to more than the reference interval.

lymphoid: Resembling or pertaining to lymph or tissue and cells of the lymphoid system.

lymphokines: Biologic response mediators released by both B and T lymphocytes.

lymphoma: Solid tumor neoplasm of lymphoid tissue categorized as Hodgkin or non-Hodgkin lymphoma and defined by lymphocyte morphology and the histologic features of the lymph nodes.

lymphopoiesis: Formation and production of lymphocytes, predominantly in the lymph nodes.

lymphoproliferative: Pertaining to the proliferation of lymphoid cells resulting in abnormally increased lymphocyte counts in peripheral blood, indicating a reactive or neoplastic condition.

lysosome: Membrane-bound sac of varying size distributed randomly in the cytoplasm of white blood cells and platelets; contains hydrolytic enzymes that digest bacteria and other foreign materials.

macrocyte: Large red blood cell with an increased mean cell volume (>100 fL) and an increased diameter on a peripheral blood film (>8 μm). Associated with folate and vitamin B_{12} deficiency (megaloblastic anemia), bone marrow failure, myelodysplastic syndromes, and chronic liver disease.

macroglobulin: High-molecular-weight plasma globulin, such as α_2-macroglobulin or an immunoglobulin of the M isotype. Abnormal monoclonal immunoglobulin M proteins are seen in Waldenström macroglobulinemia.

macrophage (histiocyte): Mononuclear phagocyte found in all tissues; part of the immune system.

major histocompatibility complex: See human leukocyte antigen.

malaise: Vague feeling of discomfort and fatigue, often associated with cancer or anemia.

malaria: Infectious disease caused by one or more of five species of the protozoan genus *Plasmodium*. Transmitted from human to human by a bite from an infected *Anopheles* mosquito.

malignant: Describes a cancerous disease that threatens life through its ability to metastasize.

marker chromosome: In cytogenetic analysis, a chromosome of abnormal size or shape that is an early indicator of neoplastic disease, for instance, the Philadelphia chromosome in chronic myeloid (myelogenous) leukemia.

mast cell: Connective tissue cell that has large basophilic granules containing heparin, serotonin, bradykinin, and histamine, which are released from the cell in response to immunoglobulin E stimulation.

May-Hegglin anomaly: Rare autosomal dominant disorder characterized by thrombocytopenia, giant platelets, and granulocytes that contain cytoplasmic inclusions similar to Döhle bodies.

mean: Value that is derived by dividing the total of a set of values by the number of items in the set; the arithmetic average.

mean cell hemoglobin (MCH): Average red blood cell (RBC) hemoglobin mass in picograms computed from the RBC count and hemoglobin level.

mean cell hemoglobin concentration (MCHC): Average relative hemoglobin concentration per red blood cell (RBC), expressed in grams per deciliter (g/dL), computed from the hemoglobin and hematocrit. Relates to RBC color intensity on a peripheral blood film.

mean cell volume (MCV): Average red blood cell (RBC) volume in femtoliters computed from the RBC count and hematocrit or directly measured by an automated blood cell analyzer. Relates to RBC diameter on a peripheral blood film.

megakaryoblast: Least differentiated visually identifiable megakaryocyte precursor in a bone marrow aspirate smear; cannot be distinguished visually from the myeloblast but is identified using specific surface antigens.

megakaryocyte: Largest cell in the bone marrow, measuring 30 to 50 μm and having a multilobed nucleus. Its cytoplasm is composed of platelets, which are released to the blood through the extension of proplatelet processes into the vascular sinuses of the bone marrow. Identified and enumerated microscopically at low (10×) power on a bone marrow aspirate smear.

megakaryopoiesis (megakaryocytopoiesis): Production and development of megakaryocytes, the precursors to platelets, in the bone marrow.

megaloblast: Abnormally large, nucleated, immature precursor of the erythrocytic series in which the nucleus appears more immature than the cytoplasm; an abnormal counterpart to the pronormoblast. Develops into a macrocytic red blood cell and is associated with megaloblastic anemia, usually caused by folate or vitamin B_{12} deficiency.

menorrhagia: Abnormally heavy or prolonged menstrual periods.

metacentric: Describes a mitotic chromosome having the centromere at the center, with one arm equal in length to the other.

metamyelocyte: Stage in the development of the granulocyte series, located between the myelocyte and the band stage. Characterized by mature, granulated cytoplasm and a bean-shaped nucleus.

metaphase: Phase of mitosis in which the chromosomes are aligned at the equatorial plate. Chromosomes at metaphase are maximally contracted and are most easily identified in cytogenetic analysis.

metarubricyte: See orthochromic normoblast.

metastasis: Extension or spread of tumor cells to distant parts of the body, usually through the lymphatics or blood vessels.

methemoglobin: Abnormal form of hemoglobin in which the ferrous ion is oxidized to the ferric state; cannot carry oxygen.

microangiopathic hemolytic anemia (MAHA): Condition in which narrowing or obstruction of small blood vessels by fibrin or platelet aggregates results in distortion and fragmentation of red blood cells, hemolysis, and anemia. The platelet count is decreased and schistocytes are found on the peripheral blood film.

microcyte: Small red blood cell with a reduced mean cell volume (<80 fL) and reduced diameter on a peripheral blood film (<6 μm). Associated with iron deficiency anemia, thalassemia, Hb E disease and trait, and some sideroblastic anemias and anemia of inflammation.

microfilament: Intracellular double-stranded intertwined structure of actin, 5 to 7 nm in diameter, that supports the cytoskeleton and assists with cell motility, contraction, and intracellular transport.

microtubule: Hollow cylinder of α- and β-tubulin, 25 nm in diameter, that maintains cell shape, contributes to motility, and makes up mitotic spindle fibers and centrioles.

mitochondrion: Round or oval structure distributed randomly in the cytoplasm of a cell. Contains mitochondrial DNA, ribosomes, and various enzymes and proteins, and produces most of the adenosine triphosphate (ATP) for the cell by oxidative phosphorylation (aerobic respiration).

mitosis: Ordinary process of somatic cell division resulting in the production of two daughter cells that have identical diploid complements of chromosomes.

mixing study: A clot-based test in which 1 part normal plasma and 1 part patient plasma is combined then tested by the partial thromboplastin time (PTT), immediately or after an incubation period. A factor deficiency of the patient will show a correction to a normal PPT for the mix. An inhibitor in the patient plasma will not correct to a normal PTT with the mix.

monoblast: Most undifferentiated morphologically identifiable precursor of the bone marrow monocytic series; develops into the promonocyte.

monoclonal: Pertaining to or designating a group of identical cells derived from a single cell. Also used to describe products from a clone of cells, such as monoclonal antibodies.

monocyte: Mononuclear phagocytic white blood cell having a round to horseshoe-shaped nucleus with abundant gray-blue cytoplasm filled with fine reddish granules. Circulating precursor to the macrophage, the primary phagocytic cell of most tissues.

monocytopenia: Decrease in the number of monocytes in the peripheral blood to less than the reference interval.

monocytosis: Increase in the number of monocytes in the peripheral blood to more than the reference interval; may indicate infection or a neoplasm.

mononuclear: Cell having only one nucleus. Used to describe cells such as monocytes or lymphocytes as distinct from neutrophils, which have nuclei with 2 to 5 connected lobes and hence are called segmented or polymorphonuclear.

monosomy: Absence of one chromosome from a pair.

Mott cell: Plasma cell containing colorless cytoplasmic inclusions of immunoglobulin called Russell bodies, which appear similar to vacuoles.

mucocutaneous bleeding disorder: Chronic episodic bleeding evidenced by bilateral petechiae and purpura, epistaxis, hematemesis, and menorrhagia. Systemic bleeding indicates a coagulopathy of the primary hemostasis system such as thrombocytopenia, von Willebrand disease, or a qualitative platelet disorder.

multiple myeloma: See plasma cell myeloma.

mutation: Acquired or inherited permanent transmissible change in the DNA sequence in a cell. Includes chromosomal rearrangement (such as translocation or inversion), gain or loss of chromosomes (aneuploidy), total or partial gene deletion, point mutation, insertion, or gene duplication or amplification. Results in the production of abnormal proteins, excessive production of normal proteins, or loss of essential proteins.

myelo-: Prefix relating to the bone marrow and used to identify precursors of neutrophils.

myeloblast: Least differentiated morphologically identifiable bone marrow precursor of the granulocytic cells; develops into the promyelocyte.

myelocyte: Third stage of bone marrow granulocytic cell differentiation, intermediate in development between a promyelocyte and a metamyelocyte. A neutrophilic myelocyte has a round nucleus that may be flattened on one side, and primary and secondary (specific) granules in the cytoplasm.

myelodysplastic syndromes (MDS): Group of acquired clonal hematologic malignancies characterized by progressive peripheral blood cytopenias that reflect defects in erythroid, myeloid, or megakaryocytic maturation.

myelofibrosis: Replacement of bone marrow with fibrous connective tissue.

myeloid: General term used to denote granulocytic cells and their precursors, including basophils, eosinophils, and neutrophils. Lymphoid and erythroid cell lines are excluded, and most morphologists also exclude the monocytic and megakaryocytic cell lines.

myeloid-to-erythroid (M:E) ratio: Proportion of myeloid cells to nucleated erythroid precursors in bone marrow aspirate. Excluded from the myeloid cell count are monocytic and lymphoid precursors and plasma cells. Used to evaluate hematopoietic cell production, and in healthy adults the M:E ratio varies from approximately 1.5:1 to 3.3:1, reflecting the larger proportion of myeloid cells in the bone marrow.

myeloperoxidase (MPO): Enzyme that occurs in primary granules of promyelocytes, myelocytes, and neutrophils and exhibits bactericidal, fungicidal, and viricidal properties. Cytochemical staining and flow cytometry are used to detect MPO in myeloid precursors in acute leukemia.

myeloproliferative neoplasms (MPN): Group of malignant neoplasms characterized by proliferation of myeloid cells and elevations in one or more myeloid cell types in the peripheral blood. Includes chronic myeloid (myelogenous) leukemia, polycythemia vera, essential thrombocythemia, and primary myelofibrosis.

myoglobin: Monomeric heme-containing protein in muscle. Combines with oxygen released by red blood cells, stores it, and transports it to the mitochondria of muscle cells, where it generates energy.

necrosis: Localized tissue death that occurs in groups of cells in response to disease or injury.

neonatal: Pertaining to the first 28 days after birth.

neoplasm: Any abnormal growth of new tissue; can be malignant or benign. Usually applied to cancerous cells.

neuropathy: Any disorder affecting the nervous system.

neutropenia: Decrease in the number of neutrophils in the peripheral blood to less than the reference interval. Often associated with chemotherapy, it exposes the patient to the risk of infection.

neutrophil (NEUT, segmented neutrophil, seg, polymorphonuclear neutrophil, PMN): Mature white blood cell with a condensed nucleus consisting of 2 to 5 lobes connected by filaments, with fine lavender-staining cytoplasmic granules in a Wright-stained peripheral blood film. Ingests bacteria and cellular debris and are the first-line defense against invading organisms.

neutrophilia: Increase in the number of neutrophils in the peripheral blood to more than the reference interval. Often indicates bacterial infection and may be associated with chronic myeloid (myelogenous) leukemia.

nondisjunction: Faulty distribution of chromosomal elements during mitosis or meiosis.

non-Hodgkin lymphoma (NHL): Solid tumors of lymphoid tissue classified by histologic features and lymphocytic morphology. Should be distinguished from Hodgkin lymphoma, which is characterized by a proliferation of Reed-Sternberg cells and accumulation of reactive peripheral blood cells.

nonsteroidal antiinflammatory drug (NSAID): Antiinflammatory, analgesic, and antiplatelet drug, other than steroids. Includes aspirin, which acetylates cyclooxygenase and reduces platelet activation, as well as naproxen, acetaminophen, and ibuprofen.

normochromic: Describes a Wright-stained red blood cell with normal color and normal hemoglobin content with a mean cell hemoglobin concentration within the reference interval.

normocyte: Normal, mature red blood cell with a mean cell volume within the reference interval.

nucleated red blood cell (NRBC): Immature red blood cell in peripheral blood that possesses a nucleus. Their presence in the peripheral blood falsely increases the manual white blood cell count and requires a calculation to correct the count.

nucleolus: Round or irregular light-stained structure in the nucleus consisting of ribosomal RNA, the genes that code it, and accessory proteins. Synthesizes ribosomal RNA and assembles ribosome subunits, and found in cells engaged in active protein synthesis, such as blasts.

nucleoside: A pentose (5-carbon sugar) linked to a nitrogenous purine or pyrimidine base, but without a phosphate group. In RNA and DNA the pentose sugars are ribose and deoxyribose, respectively.

nucleotide: Building blocks of DNA and RNA composed of a pentose (5-carbon sugar), a nitrogenous base, and a phosphate group. The phosphate group allows for the formation of phosphodiester bonds between the 3′ carbon of one nucleotide with the 5′ phosphate group of the downstream nucleotide to form strands of DNA and RNA.

nucleus: Cellular organelle surrounded by an inner and outer phospholipid bilayer membrane and containing DNA, RNA, and nuclear proteins. Stores the genetic code and controls cell division and cell functions.

nucleus-to-cytoplasm (N:C) ratio: Estimated volume of a Wright-stained nucleus compared with the volume of the cytoplasm. Used to differentiate cell developmental stages.

objective: Microscope lens closest to the specimen. Most clinical grade microscopes provide 10× dry, 40× dry or 50× oil immersion, and 100× oil immersion objectives.

ocular: Microscope lens, usually 10×, nearest the eye.

oncogene: A mutated protooncogene that imparts the ability to convert normal cells into cancer cells. Protooncogenes code for essential cellular proteins involved in signaling pathways, cell proliferation, cell differentiation, and apoptosis.

opsonization: Process by which an antibody or complement attaches itself to foreign material (such as bacteria), triggering or enhancing phagocytosis.

optical scatter: Scattering of light caused by the interaction of absorption, diffraction, refraction, and reflection. Automated blood cell analyzers use both laser and nonlaser light to apply the principle of light scatter to perform cell counting and identification. The angle of light scatter correlates with various cell features such as volume, density, and cellular complexity.

orthochromic normoblast (metarubricyte): Fourth stage of bone marrow erythropoiesis and the last in which the cell retains a nucleus. The nucleus is fully condensed with no parachromatin; the cytoplasm is bluish-pink as a result of the presence of hemoglobin and residual RNA.

osmotic fragility test: Assay in which whole blood is pipetted to each of a series of saline solutions of graduated concentration. The series begins with water and increases in concentration to normal (0.85%) saline. The osmotic fragility test detects spherocytes because they rupture in saline concentrations slightly lower than 0.85%.

osteoblast: Bone-forming cell.

osteoclast: Large multinuclear cell associated with the absorption and removal of bone. May be confused with a megakaryocyte under microscopic evaluation.

oval macrocyte: Oval red blood cell with an increased diameter on a peripheral blood film. Characteristic of megaloblastic anemia.

ovalocyte: See elliptocyte.

overhydrated hereditary stomatocytosis (OHS): Very rare hereditary, autosomal dominant, red blood cell membrane disorder caused by a mutation in a membrane protein, which disrupts membrane cation permeability, increases cell volume, and decreases mean cell hemoglobin concentration (MCHC). Causes a moderate to severe hemolytic anemia characterized by the presence of stomatocytes and macrocytes on the peripheral blood film.

oxygen affinity: Ability of hemoglobin to bind oxygen molecules.

oxygen dissociation curve: A graphic expression of the affinity of hemoglobin for oxygen, which plots the percent oxygen saturation of hemoglobin versus the partial pressure of oxygen. The sigmoidal-shaped curve reflects low hemoglobin affinity for oxygen at low oxygen tension and high hemoglobin affinity for oxygen at high oxygen tension.

oxyhemoglobin: Hemoglobin that contains bound oxygen.

p arm: Smaller (petite) arm of a chromosome.

packed cell volume (PCV): See hematocrit.

pallor: Excessive paleness or absence of color from the skin.

pancytopenia: Marked reduction in the count of red blood cells, white blood cells, and platelets in peripheral blood.

Pappenheimer bodies (siderotic granules): Red blood cell inclusions composed of non-heme ferric iron. On Prussian blue iron stain preparations, they appear as multiple dark blue irregular granules. On Wright stain preparations they appear as unevenly stained pale blue clusters. Found in conditions such as thalassemia, hemoglobinopathies, sideroblastic anemia, and megaloblastic anemia.

parachromatin: Pale-staining portion of the nucleus, roughly equivalent to euchromatin.

parenteral: Pertaining to administration of drugs or other compounds by means other than oral administration; includes intramuscular and intravenous administration.

paroxysmal cold hemoglobinuria (PCH): Rare acquired autoimmune hemolytic anemia in which the Donath-Landsteiner autoantibody, an immunoglobulin G with anti-P specificity, binds red blood cells during exposure to cold, producing acute hemolysis and hematuria on warming.

paroxysmal nocturnal hemoglobinuria (PNH): Rare acquired hemolytic anemia as a result of a hematopoietic stem cell clonal mutation in the *PIGA* gene that causes cells to lack glycosylphosphatidylinositol (GPI)-anchored proteins, including CD55 and CD59, two proteins that normally protect the red blood cell (RBC) from complement activation and hemolysis. RBCs therefore have an increased susceptibility to complement, which results in intravascular hemolysis and hemoglobinuria that occur in irregular episodes.

partial thromboplastin time: See activated partial thromboplastin time.

pathogenesis: Chemical and biologic events in cells and tissue by which disease occurs and progresses.

pathognomonic: Specifically characteristic of a given disease; indicating a sign or symptom from which a diagnosis can be made.

Pelger-Huët anomaly: Autosomal dominant asymptomatic anomaly of neutrophil nuclei, which fail to segment and appear dumbbell shaped or peanut shaped ("pince-nez" nuclei). Pelgeroid nuclei are acquired and more common, resembling the nuclei of Pelger-Huët anomaly, but may indicate myelodysplasia or may appear during chemotherapy.

pentasaccharide: Sequence of five specific heparin carbohydrate units that produce a high-affinity binding to antithrombin, which inhibits factor Xa. This heparin pentasaccharide can be synthesized; the therapeutic agent is fondaparinux. Activity is measured by the chromogenic anti-factor Xa heparin assay.

percutaneous coronary intervention (PCI): Any catheter-based technique for the management of coronary artery occlusion, such as angiography, angioplasty, stent placement within a coronary artery, or cardiac catheterization.

peripheral artery occlusion (PAO): Blockage of a noncardiac, noncerebral artery by thrombus formation. Vessels in the lower limbs most commonly are affected.

pernicious anemia: Progressive autoimmune disorder that results in megaloblastic anemia as a result of a lack of, or antibodies to, parietal cells or intrinsic factor essential for the absorption of vitamin B_{12}.

personal protective equipment (PPE): Clothing that is used to prevent blood or other potentially infectious biologic substances from contacting clothing, eyes, mouth, or mucous membranes. Includes, for example, gloves, fluid-impermeable laboratory coats, and eye protection.

petechiae: Pinpoint purple or red spots on the skin or mucous membranes, approximately 1 mm in diameter, indicating small bleeds within the dermal or submucosal layers. May indicate a systemic bleeding disorder caused by a platelet defect.

phagocyte: Cell that is able to surround, engulf, and digest microorganisms and cellular debris. Examples are macrophages and neutrophils.

phagocytosis: Ingestion of large particles or live microorganisms into a cell.

phagosome: Membrane-bound cytoplasmic vesicle in a phagocyte containing the phagocytosed material.

Philadelphia chromosome (Ph chromosome): Abnormally short chromosome 22 as a result of a reciprocal translocation between chromosome 9 and chromosome 22 (t9;22); definitive for the diagnosis of chronic myeloid (myelogenous) leukemia. Results in the fusion of the *BCR* and *ABL1* genes and abnormal tyrosine kinase production.

phlebotomy: Use of a needle to puncture a vein and collect blood.

pitting: Removal by the spleen of material from within red blood cells (RBCs) without damage to the RBCs; for example, removal of nuclei or Howell-Jolly bodies.

PIVKA factors (proteins induced by vitamin K antagonists): Des-γ-carboxyl coagulation factors and coagulation control proteins. During synthesis of factors II, VII, IX, and X and proteins C, S, and Z, under conditions of vitamin K absence or antagonism (such as with Coumadin treatment) a second carboxyl group is not attached to the terminal glutamic acid of the protein. Because this structure is required for binding Ca^{2+} and phospholipid, PIVKA factors do not participate in the coagulation process.

plasma: Fluid portion of the blood in which the formed elements (white blood cells, red blood cells, and platelets) and all hemostasis proteins are suspended. The portion of an anticoagulated blood specimen that remains after centrifuging to remove the cellular elements.

plasma cell: Fully differentiated B lymphocyte, found in the bone marrow and lymphoid tissue and occasionally in peripheral blood, which secretes antibody in the humoral immune response. Contains an eccentric nucleus with deeply staining chromatin and abundant dark blue cytoplasm. The Golgi apparatus produces a perinuclear halo because of its high lipid content.

plasma cell myeloma (formerly multiple myeloma): Malignant neoplasm in which plasma cells proliferate in the bone marrow, destroying bone and resulting in pain, fractures, and excess production of a monoclonal plasma immunoglobulin.

plasma frozen within 24 hours (FP24): Plasma that is separated from whole-blood donations and frozen within 24 hours of collection and contains all the plasma procoagulants and control proteins, including adequate levels of the labile factors V and VIII. Used for replacement therapy in acquired multiple-factor deficiencies or in single-factor deficiencies when factor concentrates are not available.

plasmin: Active form of plasminogen after cleavage by a plasminogen activator. Digests fibrin to form fibrin degradation products in the fibrinolytic process. Also degrades fibrinogen.

plasminogen: Inactive (zymogen) precursor of plasmin found in plasma.

plasminogen activator: Substance that cleaves plasminogen and converts it to plasmin; includes urokinase secreted by renal endothelial cells, and tissue plasminogen activator secreted by all endothelial cells. Synthetic plasminogen activators are used therapeutically to lyse coronary artery clots after acute myocardial infarction.

plasminogen activator inhibitor-1 (PAI-1): Inhibitor of tissue plasminogen activator secreted from endothelial cells; controls fibrinolysis.

platelet (thrombocyte): Smallest of the formed elements in blood; disk-shaped, 2 to 4 μm in diameter, nonnucleated cell formed in the bone marrow from the cytoplasm of megakaryocytes. Triggers blood coagulation and controls bleeding.

platelet adhesion: Platelet attachment to subendothelial collagen, part of a sequential mechanism leading to the initiation and formation of a thrombus or hemostatic plug. Platelet adhesion requires von Willebrand factor and platelet receptor glycoprotein Ib/IX/V.

platelet aggregation: Platelet-to-platelet binding, part of a sequential mechanism leading to the initiation and formation of a thrombus or hemostatic plug. Requires fibrinogen and platelet membrane receptor glycoprotein IIb/IIIa.

platelet factor 4 (PF4): Protein released from platelet α-granules that binds and inhibits heparin. Antibodies that form to the heparin-PF4 complex are the cause of heparin-induced thrombocytopenia.

platelet free plasma (PFP): Plasma double-centrifuged to achieve a platelet count of less than 5,000/μL. Required for certain coagulation tests such as lupus anticoagulant testing; optimal for specimens to be frozen.

platelet-poor plasma (PPP): Plasma centrifuged to achieve a platelet count of less than 10,000/μL. Required for all coagulation testing; PPP may be frozen.

platelet-rich plasma (PRP): Plasma centrifuged at 50 xg to achieve a platelet count of 200,000/μL to 300,000/μL. Used for light-transmission platelet aggregometry.

platelet satellitosis (satellitism): Antibody-mediated in vitro adhesion of platelets to segmented neutrophils. Occurs primarily in specimens anticoagulated with ethylenediaminetetraacetic acid (EDTA) and causes pseudothrombocytopenia.

pleomorphic: Occurring in various distinct forms; having the ability to exist in various forms and to change from one form to another.

pluripotential hematopoietic stem cell: See hematopoietic stem cell.

pneumatic tube system: System of tubes for transporting blood specimens or other small materials throughout a hospital by forced air.

poikilocytosis: Presence of red blood cells with varying or bizarre shapes on a peripheral blood film.

point-of-care (POC) testing: Rapid-turnaround clinical tests performed outside the clinical laboratory at or near the patient; usually performed by nonlaboratory personnel but managed for quality by laboratory personnel.

polychromatic (polychromatophilic): Having a staining quality in which both acid and basic stains are incorporated. Usually used to denote a mixture of pink and blue in the cytoplasm of Wright-stained cells.

polychromatic normoblast (polychromatophilic normoblast, rubricyte): Precursor in the erythrocytic maturation series, intermediate between the basophilic normoblast (prorubricyte) and the orthochromic normoblast (metarubricyte). In this stage, differentiation is based on the decreasing cell diameter and the gray-blue cytoplasm as hemoglobin first becomes visible.

polychromatic or polychromatophilic red blood cell (reticulocyte): Immature but anucleate red blood cell (RBC) with bluish-pink cytoplasm on a Wright-stained peripheral blood film. An increase in polychromatic RBCs on a peripheral blood film is called polychromatophilia or polychromasia. When stained with a vital stain such as new methylene blue, the cell is called a reticulocyte and its cytoplasm has a mesh-like pattern of dark blue threads and particles of residual ribosomal RNA.

polychromatophilia (polychromasia, reticulocytosis): An increase in polychromatic RBCs on a peripheral blood film; corresponds to an elevated reticulocyte count. Polychromatophilia and reticulocytosis indicates bone marrow regeneration activity in hemolytic anemia or acute blood loss.

polyclonal: Describes a group of cells derived from multiple different cells. Each cell is identical to its parent cells (i.e., a clone), but because all cells of the group did not derive from the same cell, the group of cells is mixed. A polyclonal antibody is developed within a laboratory animal and not a hybridoma.

polycythemia (erythrocytosis): Elevated red blood cell count, hemoglobin concentration, and hematocrit in peripheral blood to more than the reference interval for age and sex. Relative polycythemia is due to a decrease in plasma volume without a change in red cell mass. Absolute polycythemia is an increase in red cell mass. Absolute polycythemia can be primary, such as polycythemia vera, or secondary, usually in response to chronic hypoxia.

polycythemia vera (PV): Myeloproliferative clonal neoplasm in which a somatic mutation in a hematopoietic stem cell leads to a marked increase in the red blood cell count, hematocrit, hemoglobin, white blood cell count, platelet count, and red blood cell mass. Approximately 95% of patients with PV have a mutation in the *JAK2* gene that substitutes valine with phenylalanine at position 617 in the JAK2 signaling protein.

polymerase chain reaction (PCR): Laboratory process in which a double-stranded segment of DNA is replicated to produce millions of copies.

polymorphonuclear neutrophil: See neutrophil.

polyploid: Having more than the characteristic diploid set of chromosomes; for example, triploid (3×) or tetraploid (4×).

porphyria: Hereditary anemia caused by impaired heme synthesis with the accumulation of porphyrin and its precursors. Acquired porphyria may be seen in acute lead poisoning.

porphyrin: Product of the metabolism of a group of iron-free pyrrole derivatives such as protoporphyrin and protoporphyrinogen that incorporates ferrous iron to form heme.

posttransfusion purpura: Antibody-induced thrombocytopenia in patients who have received multiple transfusions of red blood cells or platelet concentrate. Antibodies to donor platelets cross-react with patient platelets to cause potentially life-threatening thrombocytopenia.

postmenstrual age: Time elapsed between the first day of the mother's last menstrual period and birth (gestational age) plus the time elapsed after birth (chronologic age). For example, a preterm infant born at a gestational age of 32 weeks who is currently 10 weeks old (chronologic age) would have a postmenstrual age of 42 weeks.

precision: Degree to which the results of replicate analyses of a specimen parallel each other, often expressed as coefficient of variation or percent coefficient of variation; expression of reproducibility or dispersion about the mean.

precursor: Differentiating, immature hematopoietic cell stage that is morphologically identifiable as belonging to a given cell line; for example, pronormoblasts (rubriblasts) are precursors of basophilic normoblasts (prorubricytes) in erythropoiesis. May also refer to the inactive zymogen forms of coagulation factors; for example, prothrombin is a precursor of thrombin.

preeclampsia: Pathologic condition of late pregnancy characterized by hypertension, edema, and proteinuria; may lead to eclampsia, which presents with seizures and can be fatal.

prekallikrein (PK, pre-K, Fletcher factor): Member of the kinin inflammatory system that forms active kallikrein on digestion by kininogen. Helps to trigger coagulation via the contact activation system. Pre-K deficiency prolongs the activated partial thromboplastin time but has no clinical consequence.

primary hemostasis: First phase of hemostasis in which the blood vessels contract to seal the wound and platelets and von Willebrand factor fill the open space by forming a platelet plug.

primary standard: Reference material that is of fixed and known composition and is capable of being prepared in essentially pure form.

primer: Short piece of synthetic DNA complementary to a target DNA sequence. Acts as a point from which DNA replication can proceed, as in a polymerase chain reaction.

procoagulant: Coagulation (clotting) factor. During the coagulation process, inactive procoagulants become activated to form serine proteases or cofactors and function together to generate thrombin that converts soluble fibrinogen into insoluble fibrin.

progenitor: Undifferentiated (immature) hematopoietic cell that is committed to a cell line but cannot be identified morphologically.

prolymphocyte: Developmental form in the lymphocytic series that is intermediate between the lymphoblast and the lymphocyte.

promegakaryocyte: Morphologically identifiable bone marrow cell stage that is intermediate between the megakaryoblast and the megakaryocyte.

promonocyte: Precursor in the monocytic series; the cell stage intermediate in development between the monoblast and the monocyte.

promyelocyte: Precursor in the granulocytic (myelocytic) series that is intermediate in development between a myeloblast and a myelocyte; contains primary granules.

pronormoblast (rubriblast): Undifferentiated (immature) hematopoietic cell that is the most primitive morphologically identifiable precursor in the erythrocytic series; differentiates into the basophilic normoblast (prorubricyte).

prorubricyte: See basophilic normoblast.

prostaglandin (PG): Any of a family of unsaturated 20-carbon fatty acids that are generated from enzymatic reactions on the fatty acid arachidonic acid derived from phospholipids that are cleaved from cell membranes; serves as intracellular activators and inhibitors. Includes thromboxane A_2, a platelet activator produced by platelets, and prostacyclin, a platelet inhibitor produced by endothelial cells.

protein C (PC): Vitamin K-dependent coagulation control protein. A plasma serine protease activated by thrombin-thrombomodulin and stabilized by its cofactor, protein S; protein C inhibits coagulation by inactivating factors Va and VIIIa.

protein S (PS): Vitamin K-dependent coagulation control protein. Serves as a stabilizing cofactor for protein C, enabling activated protein C, a serine protease, to inactivate factors Va and VIIIa.

proteolytic: Pertaining to any substance that digests protein by hydrolyzing primary peptide bonds.

prothrombin (coagulation factor II): Plasma precursor of the coagulation factor thrombin; converted to thrombin by activated factor X complexed to activated factor V.

prothrombin complex concentrate (PCC): Therapeutic plasma preparation of coagulation factors II, IX and X (some contain factor VII) used to treat bleeding episodes. Contrast with activated prothrombin complex concentrate (APCC).

prothrombin G20210A: A guanine to adenine mutation at base 20210 of the 3′ untranslated region of the prothrombin (coagulation factor II) gene that causes mildly elevated prothrombin activity and is a thrombosis risk factor.

prothrombin time (protime, PT): Clot-based screening test to measure the activity of coagulation factors I (fibrinogen), II (prothrombin), V, VII, and X. Thromboplastin (tissue factor) and calcium chloride are added to plasma and the time to form a clot is recorded. Used to monitor Coumadin therapy and to screen for extrinsic and common pathway coagulation factor deficiencies.

protooncogene: Normal gene controlling essential cell functions such as signaling pathways, cell proliferation, differentiation, and apoptosis that, on mutation, may become an oncogene.

pseudo-Pelger- Huët cell (Pelgeroid cell): Hyposegmented, hypogranular neutrophil that resembles a Pelger-Huët cell. Helpful in the diagnosis of myeloproliferative neoplasms and myelodysplastic syndromes.

pseudoleukocytosis: Falsely increased white blood cell count as a result of transient mobilization of neutrophils from the marginated neutrophil pool (MNP) to the circulating neutrophil pool (CNP) and caused by conditions such as strenuous physical activity, cold, or epinephrine administration. Also a falsely elevated white blood cell count caused by interferences such as platelet clumping or lysis-resistant red blood cells.

pseudothrombocytopenia: Falsely decreased platelet count caused by platelet clumping, platelet satellitosis, or the presence of giant platelets.

pulmonary embolism (PE): Pathologic movement of a proximal fragment of clot from a deep vein thrombosis through the right side of the heart to the pulmonary circulation, where it lodges in an artery and causes infarction of the lung. Approximately one third of pulmonary emboli are fatal within 1 hour.

purpura: Purple skin discoloration, typically rounded with a diameter greater than 3 mm, seen in mucocutaneous bleeding. Usually seen in thrombocytopenia, platelet disorders, von Willebrand disease, or vascular disorders such as scurvy.

pyknosis: Degeneration of a cell in which the nucleus shrinks in size and the chromatin condenses to a solid, structureless mass or masses. Part of the process of apoptosis, or indicative of the effects of chemotherapy.

pyropoikilocytosis: See hereditary pyropoikilocytosis.

pyruvate kinase (PK): Enzyme that converts phosphoenolpyruvate to pyruvate generating two molecules of adenosine triphosphate; essential for aerobic and anaerobic glycolysis.

pyruvate kinase deficiency: Autosomal recessive disorder resulting in a deficiency of pyruvate kinase, the enzyme that converts phosphoenolpyruvate to pyruvate; causes hemolytic anemia by reducing red blood cell life span. Most common enzyme deficiency of the Embden-Meyerhof pathway.

q arm: Long arm of a chromosome.

Q banding (quinacrine banding): In cytogenetic analysis, a procedure in which metaphase chromosomes are stained with fluorescent quinacrine dye. The areas rich in adenine-thymine, called Q+, fluoresce intensely, whereas the areas rich in guanine-cytosine (Q–) fluoresce more lightly. The Q+ bands correspond with G bands in Giemsa stain-based G banding. Banding patterns are used to identify chromosomes.

qualitative analysis: Determination of the presence, but not the concentration, of an analyte or nucleic acid sequence in a specimen.

quality control: Term used to refer to the control and monitoring of the testing process to ensure that the results are valid and reproducible.

quantitative analysis: Determination of the concentration of an analyte or the copy number of a nucleic acid sequence in a specimen.

radiotherapy: Treatment of neoplastic disease using x-rays or gamma rays to deter the proliferation of malignant cells by disrupting mitosis or impairing DNA synthesis.

reactive lymphocyte (atypical, transformed, or variant lymphocyte): Lymphocyte whose altered morphology is heterogeneous and includes a variety of morphologic features such as increased basophilic cytoplasm, variable nuclear-to-cytoplasmic ratio, radial basophilia of the cytoplasm, lobular or irregular nuclei, clumped or smooth nuclear chromatin, or the presence of nucleoli. Indicates immune stimulation, usually by a virus, an example being Epstein-Barr virus, which causes infectious mononucleosis. The term *reactive* is preferred to *atypical* or *transformed* in that the latter may imply a premalignant or malignant condition.

reactive neutrophilia (leukemoid reaction): Clinical syndrome resembling leukemia in which the white blood cell count is elevated to greater than 50,000/μL in response to a nonmalignant condition such as an infection or inflammation. It involves neutrophils with some immature forms and is distinguished from chronic myeloid (myelogenous) leukemia (CML) by the absence of molecular and cytogenetic markers for CML and by an increased leukocyte alkaline phosphatase index.

recessive: Denoting an allele whose product or effect is masked by a dominant allele at the corresponding locus. When an individual has two recessive genes, he or she is homozygous recessive and the trait is expressed.

red blood cell (RBC) indices: Numerical representations of average RBC volume (mean cell volume), hemoglobin mass (mean cell hemoglobin), and relative hemoglobin concentration (mean cell hemoglobin concentration). Computed from the RBC count, hemoglobin, and hematocrit values. The mean cell volume is directly measured by some blood cell analyzers.

red cell distribution width (RDW): Coefficient of variation of red blood cell volume. An increased value indicates anisocytosis.

red cell mass: Represents all the red blood cells in the peripheral circulation. Differentiate from erythron, which includes the entirety of all immature and mature erythroid cells in the body including those in organs and bone marrow, as well as those in the peripheral circulation.

red marrow: Hematopoietic bone marrow, in contrast to yellow, fatty bone marrow.

Reed-Sternberg cell: Large cell typically with two nuclei or a bilobed nucleus with prominent nucleoli and abundant cytoplasm. Definitive histologic characteristic of Hodgkin lymphoma.

reference interval (RI): Range of test results for a given analyte that is seen in a healthy population of individuals, typically computed as the mean plus or minus two times the standard deviation. Each laboratory must define the reference interval for the instrument that is being used and for the population that is being served.

refractive index: Speed at which light travels in air, divided by the speed at which light travels through another medium, such as immersion oil. The refractive index of oil is similar to the refractive index of glass.

reliability: Extent to which a method is able to maintain both accuracy and precision over a defined period.

remission: Partial or complete disappearance of the clinical and laboratory characteristics of a chronic or malignant disease.

replication: DNA duplication or synthesis prior to mitosis; may also be used to refer to mitosis.

reptilase: Thrombin-like enzyme isolated from the venom of *Bothrops atrox* that catalyzes the conversion of fibrinogen to fibrin in a manner similar to thrombin.

resolution: In microscopy, the smallest distance between which two adjacent objects can be distinguished. A measure of image and lens quality that relates to the smallest feature that can be seen with a set of lenses.

restriction endonuclease: Enzyme that cleaves DNA at a specific nucleotide site.

reticulocyte (polychromatic or polychromatophilic red blood cell): Immature but anucleate red blood cell (RBC) that shows a mesh-like pattern of dark blue threads and particles of residual ribosomal RNA when stained with a supravital stain such as new methylene blue. In a Wright-stained blood film, no filaments are seen, but the cytoplasm stains bluish-pink and the cell is called a polychromatic or polychromatophilic RBC. Reticulocytes can be enumerated in an automated blood cell analyzer or visually counted on a supravital-stained blood film.

reticulocyte production index (RPI): Index calculated to correct for a low hematocrit and the presence of shift reticulocytes that otherwise may falsely elevate the visual reticulocyte count.

reticulocytosis (polychromasia, polychromatophilia): Elevated reticulocyte count more than the reference interval. On a Wright-stained peripheral blood film, reticulocytes stain as polychromatic cells, and their increase is called polychromasia or polychromatophilia. Reticulocytosis, polychromasia or polychromatophilia indicates bone marrow regeneration activity in hemolytic anemia or acute blood loss.

reticuloendothelial system (RES): System of fixed and motile phagocytic macrophages and their precursor monocytes engaged in the immune response. Macrophages are found in every organ and tissue.

retrovirus: Any of a family of RNA viruses containing the enzyme reverse transcriptase.

reverse transcription polymerase chain reaction (RT-PCR): Polymerase chain reaction amplification process that produces complementary DNA from the messenger RNA present in an RNA specimen extracted from patient cells.

Rh deficiency syndrome (Rh null disease): Rare mild to moderate hemolytic anemia in which Rh membrane proteins are absent (Rh null) or decreased (Rh mod). Stomatocytes and occasional spherocytes are observed on the peripheral blood film.

Rh immune globulin (RhIg): Solution containing antibodies specific for the Rh(D) antigen given intramuscularly to an Rh(D)-negative mother with an Rh(D)-positive fetus or infant to prevent sensitization of the mother to the infant's D antigen. Given antepartum at 28 weeks' gestation and again within 72 hours of delivery.

Rh-null disease: See Rh deficiency syndrome.

ribonucleic acid (RNA): Single strand of nucleotides connected by ribose molecules. Messenger RNA base sequences are transcribed from DNA and are the basis for translation to proteins. Major types include messenger RNA, ribosomal RNA, and transfer RNA.

ribosome: Macromolecular complex of ribosomal RNA and protein, consisting of small and large subunits, embedded in the outer membrane of rough endoplasmic reticulum or found free in the cytoplasm. Site for protein synthesis in which the genetic code on messenger RNA is translated to protein using transfer RNA.

ring sideroblast: Nucleated red blood cell precursor with at least five iron granules that circle at least one third of the nucleus. These cells, visible with Prussian blue stain, are the pathognomonic finding in refractory anemia with ring sideroblasts.

ristocetin: Antibiotic no longer in clinical use that facilitates the in vitro interaction of von Willebrand factor (VWF) with platelet membrane glycoprotein Ib/IX/V. Used as an agonist in the platelet aggregation test for von Willebrand disease and in the ristocetin cofactor assay to quantify VWF activity.

Romanowsky stain: Prototype of the many eosin-methylene blue stains for blood cells and malarial parasites, including Wright and Giemsa stain.

rouleaux: Aggregation of stacked red blood cells caused by elevated plasma proteins and abnormal monoclonal proteins.

rubriblast: See pronormoblast.

rubricyte: See polychromatic normoblast.

Russell bodies: Plasma cell cytoplasmic inclusions that appear similar to vacuoles containing aggregates of immunoglobulins. Plasma cells with Russell bodies are called Mott cells.

Russell viper venom time: Coagulation assay similar to the prothrombin time. Russell viper venom activates the coagulation factor common pathway at the level of factor X. The dilute Russell viper venom time assay is used in lupus anticoagulant screening.

scatterplot: Plot on rectangular coordinates of paired observations of two random variables, with each observation plotted as one point on the graph; the scatter or clustering of points provides an indication of the relationship between the two variables. In hematology a typical scatterplot graphs cell volume against cytoplasmic complexity.

schistocyte (schizocyte): Fragmented red blood cell characteristic of microangiopathic hemolytic anemia (such as in thrombotic thrombocytopenic purpura, hemolytic uremic syndrome, disseminated intravascular coagulation), severe burns, and prosthetic cardiac valve mechanical trauma.

scurvy: Deficiency of vitamin C (ascorbic acid) causing connective tissue breakdown. Marked by weakness, anemia, spongy gums, and a tendency to mucocutaneous bleeding.

secondary hemostasis: Second phase of hemostasis involving the activation of plasma coagulation proteins to produce a fibrin clot, which secures the platelet plug at the site of injury.

secondary standard (calibrator): Calibration material for which the analyte concentration has been ascertained by reference to a primary standard or by controlled reference assays.

segmented neutrophil: See neutrophil.

selectin: Any of a family of cell adhesion molecules that mediate the binding of white blood cells and platelets to the vascular endothelium.

senescent: Aging or growing old. A senescent red blood cell loses its deformability and is cleared mainly by macrophages in the spleen.

sensitivity: In laboratory testing, diagnostic sensitivity is the probability that a person with a given disease will be correctly identified as having it by a clinical test. Analytical sensitivity is the lowest level of a substance that can be detected by a laboratory test procedure.

sepsis (septicemia): Proliferation of pathologic organisms in the blood.

sequestration: Transfer of blood cells from the circulation into a limited vascular area, such as the spleen. Platelets may be sequestered in the spleen, which results in a decrease in their circulating numbers.

serine protease: Any of a group of proteolytic enzymes of the trypsin family that include activated procoagulants (thrombin and factors VIIa, IXa, Xa, XIa, and XIIa) and the inhibitor activated protein C. Synthesized as inactive zymogens, activation occurs when the zymogen is cleaved at one or more specific sites by the action of another protease during the coagulation process.

serine protease inhibitor (serpin): Plasma proteins, for instance, antithrombin and heparin cofactor II, which control the coagulation cascade by inhibiting the serine proteases, particularly factors IIa and Xa, such that thrombin generation is controlled.

serotonin: Potent vasoconstrictor released from the dense granules of activated platelets.

serum: Fluid portion of the blood that remains after the blood has clotted; blood cells, coagulation factors, and coagulation control proteins, consumed in clot formation, are essentially absent.

Sézary cell: Mononuclear cell with a cerebriform nucleus and a narrow rim of cytoplasm. Characteristic finding in cutaneous T cell lymphomas.

Sézary syndrome: Cutaneous T cell lymphoma characterized by exfoliative erythroderma, peripheral lymphadenopathy, and the presence of Sézary cells in the skin, lymph nodes, and peripheral blood.

shift reticulocyte: Immature, anucleate red blood cell with gray-blue cytoplasm and increased diameter released from the bone marrow prematurely to compensate for hemolytic anemia or acute blood loss. Requires more than 1 day in the peripheral blood to lose residual RNA and gain a mature-looking pink cytoplasm.

sickle cell (drepanocyte): Abnormal crescent-shaped red blood cell on a peripheral blood film containing hemoglobin S. Characteristic of sickle cell anemia (Hb SS) but also found in compound heterozygous sickle cell–β-thalassemia (Hb S-β-thal).

sickle cell anemia: Severe chronic hemoglobinopathy in individuals who are homozygous for hemoglobin S. The abnormal hemoglobin results in distortion of red blood cells into sickle cells and leads to crises characterized by joint pain, anemia, thrombosis, fever, and splenomegaly.

sickle cell disease: Group of symptomatic hemoglobinopathies characterized by sickle cell formation and the associated crises. Includes individuals who are homozygous for hemoglobin S (Hb SS) and compound heterozygous for Hb S and another β-globin chain mutation, most often Hb S-β-thalassemia and Hb SC.

sickle cell crisis: Any of several acute conditions occurring as part of sickle cell disease, such as aplastic crisis, which is temporary bone marrow aplasia; hemolytic crisis, which is acute red blood cell destruction; and vasoocclusive crisis, which is severe pain caused by blockage of blood vessels.

sickle cell trait: Asymptomatic heterozygous condition characterized by the presence of both hemoglobin S and hemoglobin A.

sideroblast: Bone marrow erythrocytic precursor that shows excessive iron granules (siderotic granules) with Prussian blue staining.

siderocyte: Nonnucleated red blood cell in which particles of iron (siderotic granules) are visible with Prussian blue staining.

siderotic granules: See Pappenheimer bodies.

Southeast Asian ovalocytosis (SAO): Hereditary, autosomal dominant, red blood cell membrane disorder caused by a mutation in transmembrane protein, band 3. Prevalent in some areas of Southeast Asia; usually asymptomatic but may be associated with mild hemolytic anemia. Characterized by the presence of oval red blood cells with 1 or 2 transverse ridges on the peripheral blood film.

Southern blotting: Technique in which DNA fragments separated by gel electrophoresis are transferred to a nitrocellulose filter on which specific fragments can then be detected by their hybridization to probes.

specificity: In laboratory testing, diagnostic specificity is the probability that a person who does not have a specific disease will be correctly identified as not having it by a clinical test. Analytic specificity is the ability of an assay to distinguish an analyte from interfering substances. Also used to describe the attribute of antibodies that are able to bind only with the antigen that stimulated their production.

spectrin: Major cytoskeletal protein, composed of α- and β-spectrin heterodimers, forming a lattice at the cytoplasmic surface of the cell membrane that provides lateral support to the membrane and thus maintains its shape.

spherocyte: Abnormal spherical red blood cell with a decreased surface area–to–volume ratio. Appears dense, without a central pallor, and has a reduced diameter on a peripheral blood film. Associated with hereditary spherocytosis and warm autoimmune hemolytic anemia.

spleen: Large organ in the upper left quadrant of the abdomen, just under the stomach. Has the body's largest collection of macrophages, which are responsible for phagocytosis and elimination of senescent red blood cells. Also houses many lymphoid cells.

splenectomy: Excision of the spleen.

splenomegaly: Enlargement of the spleen.

spur cell: See acanthocyte.

standard deviation: Mathematic expression of the dispersion of a set of values or scores about the mean.

standard precautions (formerly universal precautions): Practices to control bloodborne disease in which all human blood and body fluids are treated as if infectious. Infection is prevented by a series of protective methods including the use of sterile gloves, fluid-impermeable clothing, and eye protection.

steatorrhea: Fat in the stool, usually because of malabsorption. Stool may be oily, pale or colorless, and foul smelling.

stem cell: See hematopoietic stem cell.

stomatocyte: Abnormal cup-shaped mature red blood cell that has a slit-like area of central pallor. Found in hereditary stomatocytosis (dehydrated and overhydrated), Rh deficiency syndrome, and in acquired conditions such as liver disease. May also be found on the peripheral blood film as an artifact.

storage pool disorder: Inadequacy of platelet dense granule release function or dense granule contents that causes mucocutaneous bleeding. Usually hereditary and related to conditions with oculocutaneous albinism, such as Hermansky-Pudlak syndrome, Chédiak-Higashi syndrome, and Wiskott-Aldrich syndrome. Acquired storage pool disorder is sometimes associated with myelodysplastic syndrome.

stroma: Supporting tissue or matrix of an organ.

subcutaneous (SC): Injected within the subdermal or dermal layer.

sulfhemoglobin: Hemoglobin with a sulfur atom on one of its porphyrin rings, which makes it ineffective for transporting oxygen. Results from ingestion or exposure to drugs or chemicals containing sulfur.

supernatant: Clear upper liquid part of a suspension after it has been centrifuged.

supravital stain (vital stain): Stain such as new methylene blue that colors living tissues or cells.

surface-connected canalicular system (SCCS): System of channels distributed throughout platelets that extends the plasma membrane inward. Binds numerous coagulation factors and provides a route for secretion of the protein contents of α-granules.

syncope: Brief lapse in consciousness; fainting.

systemic lupus erythematosus (SLE): Chronic autoimmune inflammatory disease manifested by severe vasculitis, renal involvement, and lesions of the skin and nervous system.

T cell (T lymphocyte): Lymphocyte that participates in cellular immunity, including cell-to-cell communication. Major categories are helper cells and suppressor-cytotoxic cells.

target cell (codocyte): Poorly hemoglobinized red blood cell found in hemoglobinopathies, thalassemia, and liver disease. Appears as a "bull's eye" on a peripheral blood film because hemoglobin concentrates in the center of the cell and around the periphery

teardrop cell (dacryocyte): Red blood cell with a single pointed extension, resembling a teardrop, and often seen in primary myelofibrosis and myelophthisic anemia.

telangiectasia: Permanent dilation of capillaries, arterioles, and venules that creates focal red lesions, usually in the skin or mucous membranes.

telomere: Repeating DNA sequences at a chromosome terminus which protects the ends of the chromosomes from damage. Shortened telomeres are associated with cell aging.

tetraploid: Possessing a double diploid chromosome complement, or four of each chromosome (4N).

thalassemia: Inherited, mild to severe anemia characterized by microcytic, hypochromic red blood cells caused by deficient or absent synthesis of one of the globin chains of hemoglobin. For example, α-thalassemia is a deficiency or absence of α-globin chains, β-thalassemia, a deficiency or absence of β-globin chains.

thrombin: Principle serine protease of coagulation. Factors Xa and Va combine to cleave prothrombin to produce thrombin. Cleaves fibrinopeptides A and B from fibrinogen to initiate fibrin polymerization, potentiates coagulation by activating platelets and factors XI, VIII, V, and XIII, and also activates the coagulation control protein, protein C.

thrombin clotting time (TCT, thrombin time, TT): Coagulation test that measures the interval to clot formation after the addition of thrombin to plasma. Often used to test for the presence of heparin.

thrombocyte: See platelet.

thrombocythemia: Abnormally high platelet count with dysfunctional platelets; seen in the myeloproliferative neoplasm known as essential thrombocythemia.

thrombocytopenia: Decrease in the number of platelets in the peripheral blood to less than the reference interval; usually less than 150,000/μL.

thrombocytopoiesis (thrombopoiesis): Production of platelets from bone marrow megakaryocytes. Megakaryocyte cytoplasm is composed of platelets that are released into the blood by extension of proplatelet processes into the vascular sinuses of the bone marrow.

thrombocytosis: Increase in the number of platelets in the peripheral blood to more than the reference interval; usually more than 450,000/μL.

thrombophilia (hypercoagulability): Abnormally increased tendency to form blood clots caused by a number of acquired or congenital factors.

thrombopoietin (TPO): Hormone produced primarily by the liver that promotes hematopoietic stem cells to differentiate into the megakaryocyte lineage and stimulates megakaryocyte mitosis and maturation in response to thrombocytopenia.

thrombosis: Formation, development, or presence of a clot in a blood vessel (i.e., a thrombus).

thrombospondin: Adhesive glycoprotein secreted by endothelial cells and platelet α-granules.

thrombotic thrombocytopenic purpura (TTP): Congenital or acquired deficiency of ADAMTS13, an endothelial cell von Willebrand factor-cleaving protease. Ultralarge von Willebrand factor multimers bind platelets and form platelet-rich clots in the microvasculature, causing severe thrombocytopenia with mucocutaneous bleeding, microangiopathic hemolytic anemia, and neuropathy.

thromboxane A$_2$: Metabolically active product of the eicosanoid synthesis (cyclooxygenase, prostaglandin) pathway in platelets; binds platelet membrane receptor and activates platelets.

thromboxane B$_2$: Metabolically inactive measurable plasma metabolite of thromboxane A$_2$.

thrombus: In vivo blood clot causing vascular occlusion and tissue ischemia.

tissue factor (TF): Constitutive membrane protein of subendothelial cells. Exposure to tissue factor activates factor VII and the tissue factor (extrinsic) coagulation pathway. Expressed on monocytes and endothelial cells in chronic inflammation.

tissue plasminogen activator (TPA): See plasminogen activator.

toxic granulation: Presence of abnormally large, dark-staining, or dominant primary granules in neutrophils associated with bacterial infections.

transcription: Process by which messenger RNA is produced from a DNA template.

transferrin: Plasma iron-transport protein that moves iron from sites of absorption and storage to hematopoietic tissue for incorporation into developing normoblasts.

transformed lymphocyte: See reactive lymphocyte.

transfusion-related hemosiderosis: Excess iron accumulation in tissues as a complication of a transfusion-dependent hemolytic anemia, such as β-thalassemia major. Differentiate from hereditary hematochromatosis, which is iron accumulation in tissues as a result of a mutation in a gene involved in iron metabolism.

translation: Process by which the genetic information carried by nucleotides in messenger RNA directs the sequence of amino acids in the synthesis of a specific polypeptide.

translocation: Rearrangement of DNA within a chromosome or transfer of a segment of one chromosome to a nonhomologous one.

transudate: Fluid (effusion) that leaks from blood vessels and accumulates in a body cavity as a result of increased pressure, increased production, or decreased resorption. It has a low concentration of white blood cells and protein and appears clear or straw colored. May occur in conditions such as congestive heart failure or nephrotic syndrome.

triploid: Possessing a single addition chromosome complement, resulting in three of each chromosome (3N).

trisomy: Presence of an extra chromosome in addition to a homologous pair; for example, trisomy 21 in Down syndrome.

unfractionated heparin (UFH, standard heparin): Naturally occurring anticoagulant classified as a glycosaminoglycan; extracted from porcine mucosa. Mixture of linear chains of variably sulfated repeating disaccharide units with an average molecular weight of 15,000 Daltons (range 3000 to 30,000 Daltons). Binds antithrombin, which binds to and inhibits thrombin, activated factor Xa, and other serine proteases. Common intravenous anticoagulant used to treat and prevent blood clotting and to prevent blood clot formation during procedures such as cardiac surgery and interventional cardiology. Requires monitoring with the chromogenic anti-factor Xa heparin assay, partial thromboplastin time, or activated clotting time assay, depending on the dose.

urobilinogen: Colorless water-soluble compound formed in the intestine through the breakdown of bilirubin by bacteria; low levels appear in the urine in healthy states.

urokinase: Enzyme produced by kidney endothelial cells that acts as a plasminogen activator.

vacuole: Any clear space or cavity formed in the cytoplasm of a cell.

vacuolization: Formation of vacuoles.

variant lymphocyte: See reactive lymphocyte.

vasoconstriction: Reduction in blood vessel diameter as a result of smooth muscle constriction.

venipuncture: Use of a needle to puncture a vein and collect blood.

venous thromboembolism (VTE): A term that encompasses deep venous thrombosis (DVT) and pulmonary embolism (PE); these blood clots form in a vein, typically in a lower extremity (DVT), and small pieces of clot that break away travel through the blood only to lodge in the lungs (PE).

vertigo: Sensation of rotation or movement of oneself or one's surroundings; dizziness.

viscosity: Resistance of a liquid to flow.

vital stain: See supravital stain.

vitamin B$_{12}$ (cyanocobalamin): Complex vitamin involved in the metabolism of protein and fats, DNA synthesis, normal blood cell formation, and nerve function.

vitamin K: Natural phylloquinone occurring in green leafy vegetables and liver and produced by commensal intestinal organisms. Catalyzes the γ-carboxylation of glutamic acid in a number of calcium-binding proteins, including the vitamin K–dependent coagulation factors II (prothrombin), VII, IX, and X and control proteins C, S, and Z.

vitamin K antagonist (VKA): Substance that inhibits the action of vitamin K; for example, warfarin (Coumadin), which is used in oral anticoagulant therapy.

von Willebrand disease: Congenital autosomal dominant disorder with variable mucocutaneous bleeding characterized by a deficiency of von Willebrand factor activity and antigen, and subsequent impairment of platelet adhesion.

waived testing: Test classification defined by the Clinical Laboratory Improvement Amendments that includes tests that are simple and accurate and can be performed by noncertified personnel.

Waldenström macroglobulinemia: Form of monoclonal gammopathy in which immunoglobulin M is overproduced by the clone of a plasma cell. Increased viscosity of the blood may result in circulatory impairment, and normal immunoglobulin synthesis is decreased, which increases susceptibility to infections.

warfarin: Vitamin K antagonist that reduces the activity of the vitamin K-dependent coagulation factors II (prothrombin), VII, IX, and X, and the regulatory proteins protein C, protein S, and protein Z.

warm antibody: Immunoglobulin G antibody that reacts optimally at a temperature of 37° C.

warm autoimmune hemolytic anemia: Most common autoimmune hemolytic anemia, which results from the reaction of immunoglobulin G autoantibodies with red blood cells at an optimal temperature of 37° C.

Wiskott-Aldrich syndrome: Immunodeficiency disorder characterized by oculocutaneous albinism, thrombocytopenia, inadequate T and B cell function, and an increased susceptibility to viral, bacterial, and fungal infections.

xanthochromic: Having a yellowish color. Used to describe cerebrospinal fluid, in which xanthochromia indicates the presence of bilirubin and thus serves as evidence of a prior episode of bleeding into the brain.

X-linked: Pertaining to genes or to the characteristics or conditions they transmit that are carried on the X chromosome.

X-linked recessive inheritance: Pattern of inheritance in which a recessive allele is carried on the X chromosome; results in the carrier state in females and development of disease characteristics in males because they do not have a normal X chromosome to compensate.

zymogen: Inactive precursor that is converted to an active form by an enzyme; inactive coagulation factor, such as prothrombin.